ADVANCES IN NEURAL INFORMATION PROCESSING SYSTEMS 18

ADVANCES IN NEURAL INFORMATION PROCESSING SYSTEMS

ADVANCES IN NEURAL INFORMATION PROCESSING SYSTEMS 18

Proceedings of the 2005 Conference

edited by
Yair Weiss, Bernard Schölkopf, and John C. Platt

A Bradford Book
The MIT Press
Cambridge, Massachusetts
London, England

ISSN: 1049-5258

ISBN: 0-262-23253-7

Contents

xi

Preface

This volume, entitled *Advances in Neural Information Processing Systems 18*, contains the papers presented at the nineteenth [sic] annual conference on Neural Information Processing Systems (NIPS). The conference was held in British Columbia, Canada from December 5 through 10, 2005. NIPS started as an interdisciplinary conference for researchers from a wide variety of fields, brought together by an excitement about synthetic and natural neural networks. The field has since matured: this maturation is owed in large part to NIPS and the many people that have shaped NIPS. Today, the interdisciplinary nature of NIPS complements its stellar reputation as the premier meeting of scientists interested in inference from empirical data. Papers in the NIPS proceedings are widely held to be of journal quality. In 2005, they were reviewed by at least three referees (drawing from a pool of 435 reviewers), the authors read the reviews and wrote short rebuttals (a novelty for NIPS), and the reviewers got to discuss and revise their reviews. Many papers were additionally read by members of the 20-person program committee (representing 11 countries and five continents) during its meeting in Tübingen, Germany. Size constraints and the policy of having only a single track of oral presentations makes NIPS very selective; out of 752 submissions, only 206 were accepted. The fact that the number of registrants has nevertheless grown to a record number of 949 speaks loudly. The volume you are holding in your hands contains revised versions of the accepted papers, submitted after the conference. Authors were given the chance to take into account both the reviewers' reports and the many comments made during late night discussions at the conference poster boards.

The outstanding student paper prizes went to *The Forgetron: A Kernel-Based Perceptron on a Fixed Budget* by Ofer Dekel, Shai Shalev-Shwartz, and Yoram Singer; *Robust Design of Biological Experiments* by Patrick Flaherty, Michael Jordan, and Adam Arkin; *Unbiased Estimator of Shape Parameter for Spiking Irregularities under Changing Environments* by Keiji Miura, Masato Okada, and Shun-ichi Amari; and *How Fast to Work: Response Vigor, Motivation and Tonic Dopamine* by Yael Niv, Nathaniel Daw, and Peter Dayan. The keynote talks were given by Urs Hölzle (*Petabyte Processing Made Easy*), Alessandro Vespignani (*Evolution and Structure of the Internet*), György Buzsáki (*Oscillations Organize Cell Assemblies*), Jim Hudspeth (*Making an Effort to Listen: Mechanical Amplification by Myosin Molecules and Ion Channels in Hair Cells of the Inner Ear*), and Christos Papadimitriou (*Games, Algorithms and Networks*). As usual, the conference was followed by two days of lively workshops in a nearby ski resort (Whistler), and preceded by a day of tutorials. The latter were presented by Lawrence Saul (*Spectral Methods for Dimensionality Reduction*), Satinder Singh (*Reinforcement Learning in Artificial Intelligence: Learning, Planning and Knowledge Representation*), Stuart Russell & Brian Milch (*First-Order Probabilistic Languages: Into the Unknown*), Bruno Olshausen (*Natural Scene Statistics and Biological Vision: from Pixels to Percepts*), Michael Jordan (*Nonparametric Bayesian Methods: Dirichlet Processes, Chinese Restaurant Processes and All That*), and Nancy Kanwisher & Frank Tong (*Reading Brains: fMRI Studies of Human Vision*).

A conference of this scale relies on contributions of many people and organizations, some of whom are listed on the following pages. We thank all of them, in particular Rosemary Miller, who has been organizing the conference for years, and Wolf Kienzle, this year's workflow master. Finally, we wish to thank the real heroes of any conference — the scientists around the world who submit papers describing their latest work. Ultimately, the most rewarding part of organizing a conference like NIPS is the remarkably high quality of the papers. We thank each and every author for making our jobs so much more pleasant.

Yair Weiss, Hebrew University of Jerusalem
Bernhard Schölkopf, Max Planck Institute for Biological Cybernetics
John Platt, Microsoft Research

January 2006

Donors

NIPS gratefully acknowledges the generosity of those individuals and organizations who have provided financial support for the NIPS*2005 conference. The financial support enabled us to sponsor student travel and participation, the outstanding student paper awards, the demonstration track and the opening buffet.

NIPS Foundation Officers and Board Members

Organizing Committee

General Chair
      YAIR WEISS, Hebrew University of Jerusalem
Program Chair
      BERNHARD SCHÖLKOPF, Max Planck Institute for Biological Cybernetics
Tutorial Chair
      JOSH TENENBAUM, Massachusetts Institute of Technology
Demonstration Co-Chairs
      TIMOTHY HORIUCHI, University of Maryland
      ALAN STOCKER, New York University
Workshop Co-Chairs
      DANIEL LEE, University of Pennsylvania
      CHARLES ISBELL, Georgia Tech
Publications Chair
      JOHN PLATT, Microsoft Research
Publicity Chair
      MARINA MEILA, University of Washington
Online Proceedings Chair
      ANDREW MCCALLUM, University of Massachusetts Amherst
Volunteers Chair
      KEVIN MURPHY, University of British Columbia

Program Committee

Program Chair
      BERNHARD SCHÖLKOPF, Max Planck Institute for Biological Cybernetics
Program Co-Chairs
      JEFF BILMES, University of Washington
      NIELS BIRBAUMER, Eberhard Karls University Tübingen
      OLIVIER BOUSQUET, Pertinence
      CHRIS J. C. BURGES, Microsoft Research
      MICHAEL COLLINS, Massachusetts Institute of Technology
      NANDO DE FREITAS, University of British Columbia
      THORE GRAEPEL, Microsoft Research
      TOM GRIFFITHS, Brown University
      NEIL LAWRENCE, University of Sheffield
      SHIH-CHII LIU, Swiss Federal Institute of Technology Zurich
      ANDREW NG, Stanford University
      PARTHA NIYOGI, University of Chicago
      KLAUS PAWELZIK, Bremen University
      CORDELIA SCHMID, INRIA
      YORAM SINGER, Google and Hebrew University of Jerusalem
      FRITZ SOMMER, Redwood Neuroscience Institute and UC Berkeley
      KOJI TSUDA, AIST Tokyo
      CHRIS WATKINS, Royal Holloway, University of London
      DAPHNA WEINSHALL, Hebrew University of Jerusalem

Reviewers

Pieter Abbeel
Felix Agakov
Yasemin Altun
Charlie Anderson
David Andre
Christophe Andrieu
Chris Atkeson
Jean-Yves Audibert
Peter Auer
Jonas August
Francis Bach
Drew Bagnell
Chris Baker
Pierre Baldi
Aharon Bar Hillel
David Barber
Kobus Barnard
Andrew Barto
Matthew Beal
Mikhail Belkin
Tony Bell
Serge Belongie
Asa Ben Hur
Shai Ben-David
Samy Bengio
Yoshua Bengio
Kristin Bennett
Matthias Bethge
Jeff Bilmes
Niels Birbaumer
Rahul Biswas
Andrew Blake
Gilles Blanchard
David Blei
Leon Bottou
Olivier Bousquet
Christoph Braun
Seth Bridges
Mark Briers
Nicolas Brunel
Joachim Buhmann
Wray Buntine
Giedrius Buracas
Stephane Canu
Andrea Caponnetto
Peter Carbonetto
Miguel Carreira-Perpinan
Rich Caruana
Olivier Catoni
Gert Cauwenberghs
Nicolo Cesa-Bianchi
Ozgur Cetin
Shantanu Chakrabartty
Frances Chance
Yu-Han Chang
Olivier Chapelle

Nick Chater
Gal Chechik
Ciprian Chelba
Kumar Chellapilla
Zhiyi Chi
Max Chickering
Dmitri Chklovskii
Ken Church
Alex Clark
Michael Collins
Robert Collins
Dorin Comaniciu
Adrian Corduneanu
Corinna Cortes
Gary Cottrell
James Coughlan
Aaron Courville
Koby Crammer
Lehel Csato
Florence d'Alche-Buc
David Danks
Trevor Darrell
Sanjoy Dasgupta
Denver Dash
Tim Davison
Nathaniel Daw
Peter Dayan
Tijl De Bie
Nando de Freitas
Virginia de Sa
Dennis DeCoste
Ofer Dekel
Li Deng
Simon Dennis
James DiCarlo
James Diebel
Thomas Dietterich
Arnaud Doucet
Kenji Doya
Shimon Edelman
Jan Eichhorn
Michael Eisele
Andre Elisseeff
Ran El-Yaniv
Yaakov Engel
Michael Erb
Udo Ernst
Ralph Etienne-Cummings
Jacob Feldman
Mario Figueiredo
Miguel Figueroa
Andrew Fitzgibbon
David Forsyth
Eric Fosler-Lussier
Matthias Franz
William Freeman

Learning vehicular dynamics, with application to modeling helicopters

Pieter Abbeel
Computer Science Dept.
Stanford University
Stanford, CA 94305

Varun Ganapathi
Computer Science Dept.
Stanford University
Stanford, CA 94305

Andrew Y. Ng
Computer Science Dept.
Stanford University
Stanford, CA 94305

Abstract

We consider the problem of modeling a helicopter's dynamics based on state-action trajectories collected from it. The contribution of this paper is two-fold. First, we consider the linear models such as learned by CIFER (the industry standard in helicopter identification), and show that the linear parameterization makes certain properties of dynamical systems, such as inertia, fundamentally difficult to capture. We propose an alternative, acceleration based, parameterization that does not suffer from this deficiency, and that can be learned as efficiently from data. Second, a Markov decision process model of a helicopter's dynamics would explicitly model only the one-step transitions, but we are often interested in a model's predictive performance over longer timescales. In this paper, we present an efficient algorithm for (approximately) minimizing the prediction error over long time scales. We present empirical results on two different helicopters. Although this work was motivated by the problem of modeling helicopters, the ideas presented here are general, and can be applied to modeling large classes of vehicular dynamics.

1 Introduction

In the last few years, considerable progress has been made in finding good controllers for helicopters. [7, 9, 2, 4, 3, 8] In designing helicopter controllers, one typically begins by constructing a model for the helicopter's dynamics, and then uses that model to design a controller. In our experience, after constructing a simulator (model) of our helicopters, policy search [7] almost always learns to fly (hover) very well in simulation, but may perform less well on the real-life helicopter. These differences between simulation and real-life performance can therefore be directly attributed to errors in the simulator (model) of the helicopter, and building accurate helicopter models remains a key technical challenge in autonomous flight. Modeling dynamical systems (also referred to as system identification) is one of the most basic and important problems in control. With an emphasis on helicopter aerodynamics, in this paper we consider the problem of learning good dynamical models of vehicles.

Helicopter aerodynamics are, to date, somewhat poorly understood, and (unlike most fixed-wing aircraft) no textbook models will accurately predict the dynamics of a helicopter from only its dimensions and specifications. [5, 10] Thus, at least part of the dynamics must be learned from data. CIFER® (Comprehensive Identification from Frequency Responses) is the industry standard for learning helicopter (and other rotorcraft) models from data. [11, 6]

CIFER uses frequency response methods to identify a linear model.

The models obtained from CIFER fail to capture some important aspects of the helicopter dynamics, such as the effects of inertia. Consider a setting in which the helicopter is flying forward, and suddenly turns sideways. Due to inertia, the helicopter will continue to travel in the same direction as before, so that it has "sideslip," meaning that its orientation is not aligned with its direction of motion. This is a non-linear effect that depends both on velocity and angular rates. The linear CIFER model is unable to capture this. In fact, the models used in [2, 8, 6] all suffer from this problem. The core of the problem is that the naive body-coordinate representation used in all these settings makes it fundamentally difficult for the learning algorithm to capture certain properties of dynamical systems such as inertia and gravity. As such, one places a significantly heavier burden than is necessary on the learning algorithm.

In Section 4, we propose an alternative parameterization for modeling dynamical systems that does not suffer from this deficiency. Our approach can be viewed as a hybrid of physical knowledge and learning. Although helicopter dynamics are not fully understood, there are also many properties—such as the direction and magnitude of acceleration due to gravity; the effects of inertia; symmetry properties of the dynamical system; and so on—which apply to *all* dynamical systems, and which are well-understood. All of this can therefore be encoded as prior knowledge, and there is little need to demand that our learning algorithms learn them. It is not immediately obvious how such prior knowledge can be encoded into a complex learning algorithm, but we will describe an acceleration based parameterization in which this can be done.

Given any model class, we can choose the parameter learning criterion used to learn a model within the class. CIFER finds the parameters that minimize a frequency domain error criterion. Alternatively, we can minimize the squared one-step prediction error in the time domain. Forward simulation on a held-out test set is a standard way to assess model quality, and we use it to compare the linear models learned using CIFER to the same linear models learned by optimizing the one-step prediction error. As suggested in [1], one can also learn parameters so as to optimize a "lagged criterion" that directly measures simulation accuracy—i.e., predictive accuracy of the model over long time scales. However, the EM algorithm given in [1] is expensive when applied in a continuous state-space setting. In this paper, we present an efficient algorithm that approximately optimizes the lagged criterion. Our experiments show that the resulting model consistently outperforms the linear models trained using CIFER or using the one-step error criterion. Combining this with the acceleration based parameterization results in our best helicopter model.

2 Helicopter state, input and dynamics

The helicopter state s comprises its position (x, y, z), orientation (roll ϕ, pitch θ, yaw ω), velocity $(\dot{x}, \dot{y}, \dot{z})$ and angular velocity $(\dot{\phi}, \dot{\theta}, \dot{\omega})$. The helicopter is controlled via a 4-dimensional action space:

1. u_1 and u_2: The longitudinal (front-back) and latitudinal (left-right) cyclic pitch controls cause the helicopter to pitch forward/backward or sideways, and can thereby also affect acceleration in the longitudinal and latitudinal directions.

2. u_3: The tail rotor collective pitch control affects tail rotor thrust, and can be used to yaw (turn) the helicopter.

3. u_4: The main rotor collective pitch control affects the pitch angle of the main rotor's blades, by rotating the blades around an axis that runs along the length of the blade. As the main rotor blades sweep through the air, the resulting amount of upward thrust (generally) increases with this pitch angle; thus this control affects the main rotor's thrust.

2

Following standard practice in system identification ([8, 6]), the original 12-dimensional helicopter state is reduced to an 8-dimensional state represented in body (or robot-centric) coordinates $s^b = (\phi, \theta, \dot{x}, \dot{y}, \dot{z}, \dot{\phi}, \dot{\theta}, \dot{\omega})$. Where there is risk of confusion, we will use superscript s and b to distinguish between spatial (world) coordinates and body coordinates. The body coordinate representation specifies the helicopter state using a coordinate frame in which the x, y, and z axes are forwards, sideways, and down relative to the current orientation of the helicopter, instead of north, east and down. Thus, $\dot{x}^b$ is the forward velocity, whereas $\dot{x}^s$ is the velocity in the northern direction. (ϕ and θ are always expressed in world coordinates, because roll and pitch relative to the body coordinate frame is always zero.) By using a body coordinate representation, we encode into our model certain "symmetries" of helicopter flight, such as that the helicopter's dynamics are the same regardless of its absolute position (x, y, z) and heading ω (assuming the absence of obstacles). Even in the reduced coordinate representation, only a subset of the state variables needs to be modeled explicitly using learning. Given a model that predicts only the angular velocities $(\dot{\phi}, \dot{\theta}, \dot{\omega})$, we can numerically integrate to obtain the orientation (ϕ, θ, ω).

We can integrate the reduced body coordinate states to obtain the complete world coordinate states. Integrating body-coordinate angular velocities to obtain world-coordinate angles is nonlinear, thus the model resulting from this process is necessarily nonlinear.

3   Linear model

The linear model we learn with CIFER has the following form:

$$\dot{\phi}^b_{t+1} - \dot{\phi}^b_t = \left(C_\phi \dot{\phi}^b_t + C_1(u_1)_t + D_1\right)\Delta t, \qquad \dot{x}^b_{t+1} - \dot{x}^b_t = \left(C_x \dot{x}^b_t - g\theta_t\right)\Delta t,$$

$$\dot{\theta}^b_{t+1} - \dot{\theta}^b_t = \left(C_\theta \dot{\theta}^b_t + C_2(u_2)_t + D_2\right)\Delta t, \qquad \dot{y}^b_{t+1} - \dot{y}^b_t = \left(C_y \dot{y}^b_t + g\phi_t + D_0\right)\Delta t,$$

$$\dot{\omega}^b_{t+1} - \dot{\omega}^b_t = \left(C_\omega \dot{\omega}^b_t + C_3(u_3)_t + D_3\right)\Delta t, \qquad \dot{z}^b_{t+1} - \dot{z}^b_t = \left(C_z \dot{z}^b_t + g + C_4(u_4)_t + D_4\right)\Delta t,$$

$$\phi_{t+1} - \phi_t = \dot{\phi}^b_t \Delta t, \qquad\qquad\qquad\qquad \theta_{t+1} - \theta_t = \dot{\theta}^b_t \Delta t.$$

Here $g = 9.81 m/s^2$ is the acceleration due to gravity and Δt is the time discretization, which is 0.1 seconds in our experiments. The free parameters in the model are $C_x, C_y, C_z, C_\phi, C_\theta, C_\omega$, which model damping, and $D_0, C_1, D_1, C_2, D_2, C_3, D_3, C_4, D_4$, which model the influence of the inputs on the states.[1] This parameterization was chosen using the "coherence" feature selection algorithm of CIFER. CIFER takes as input the state-action sequence $\{(\dot{x}^b_t, \dot{y}^b_t, \dot{z}^b_t, \dot{\phi}^b_t, \dot{\theta}^b_t, \dot{\omega}^b_t, \phi_t, \theta_t, u_t)\}_t$ and learns the free parameters using a frequency domain cost function. See [11] for details.

Frequency response methods (as used in CIFER) are not the only way to estimate the free parameters. Instead, we can minimize the average squared prediction error of next state given current state and action. Doing so only requires linear regression. In our experiments (see Section 6) we compare the simulation accuracy over several time-steps of the differently learned linear models. We also compare to learning by directly optimizing the simulation accuracy over several time-steps. The latter approach is presented in Section 5.

4   Acceleration prediction model

Due to inertia, if a forward-flying helicopter turns, it will have sideslip (i.e., the helicopter will not be aligned with its direction of motion). The linear model is unable to capture the sideslip effect, since this effect depends non-linearly on velocity and angular rates. In fact, the models used in [2, 8, 6] all suffer from this problem. More generally, these models do not capture conservation of momentum well. Although careful engineering of (many) additional non-linear features might fix individual effects such as, e.g., sideslip, it is unclear how to capture inertia compactly in the naive body-coordinate representation.

---

[1] D_0 captures the sideways acceleration caused by the tail rotor's thrust.

From physics, we have the following update equation for velocity in body-coordinates:

$$(\dot{x}, \dot{y}, \dot{z})^b_{t+1} = R\left((\dot{\phi}, \dot{\theta}, \dot{\omega})^b_t\right) * \left((\dot{x}, \dot{y}, \dot{z})^b_t + (\ddot{x}, \ddot{y}, \ddot{z})^b_t \Delta t\right). \tag{1}$$

Here, $R\left((\dot{\phi}, \dot{\theta}, \dot{\omega})^b_t\right)$ is the rotation matrix that transforms from the body-coordinate frame at time t to the body-coordinate frame at time $t+1$ (and is determined by the angular velocity $(\dot{\phi}, \dot{\theta}, \dot{\omega})^b_t$ at time t); and $(\ddot{x}, \ddot{y}, \ddot{z})^b_t$ denotes the acceleration vector in body-coordinates at time t. Forces and torques (and thus accelerations) are often a fairly simple function of inputs and state. This suggests that a model which learns to predict the accelerations, and then uses Eqn. (1) to obtain velocity over time, may perform well. Such a model would naturally capture inertia, by using the velocity update of Eqn. (1). In contrast, the models of Section 3 try to predict changes in body-coordinate velocity. *But the change in body-coordinate velocity does not correspond directly to physical accelerations, because the body-coordinate velocity at times t and $t + 1$ are expressed in different coordinate frames.* Thus, $\dot{x}^b_{t+1} - \dot{x}^b_t$ is not the forward acceleration—because $\dot{x}^b_{t+1}$ and $\dot{x}^b_t$ are expressed in different coordinate frames. To capture inertia, these models therefore need to predict not only the physical accelerations, but also the non-linear influence of the angular rates through the rotation matrix. This makes for a difficult learning problem, and puts an unnecessary burden on the learning algorithm. Our discussion above has focused on linear velocity, but a similar argument also holds for angular velocity.

The previous discussion suggests that we learn to *predict physical accelerations* and then integrate the accelerations to obtain the state trajectories. To do this, we propose:

$$\ddot{\phi}^b_t = C_\phi \dot{\phi}_t + C_1(u_1)_t + D_1, \quad \ddot{x}^b_t = C_x \dot{x}^b_t + (g_x)^b_t,$$
$$\ddot{\theta}^b_t = C_\theta \dot{\theta}_t + C_2(u_2)_t + D_2, \quad \ddot{y}^b_t = C_y \dot{y}^b_t + (g_y)^b_t + D_0,$$
$$\ddot{\omega}^b_t = C_\omega \dot{\omega}_t + C_3(u_3)_t + D_3, \quad \ddot{z}^b_t = C_z \dot{z}^b_t + (g_z)^b_t + C_4(u_4)_t + D_4.$$

Here $(g_x)^b_t, (g_y)^b_t, (g_z)^b_t$ are the components of the gravity acceleration vector in each of the body-coordinate axes at time t; and $C., D.$ are the free parameters to be learned from data. The model predicts accelerations in the body-coordinate frame, and is therefore able to take advantage of the same invariants as discussed earlier, such as invariance of the dynamics to the helicopter's (x, y, z) position and heading (ω). Further, it additionally captures the fact that the dynamics are invariant to roll (ϕ) and pitch (θ) once the (known) effects of gravity are subtracted out.

Frequency domain techniques cannot be used to learn the acceleration model above, because it is non-linear. Nevertheless, the parameters can be learned as easily as for the linear model in the time domain: Linear regression can be used to find the parameters that minimize the squared error of the one-step prediction in acceleration.[2]

5   The lagged error criterion

To evaluate the performance of a dynamical model, it is standard practice to run a simulation using the model for a certain duration, and then compare the simulated trajectory with the real state trajectory. To do well on this evaluation criterion, it is therefore important for the dynamical model to give not only accurate one-step predictions, but also predictions that are accurate at longer time-scales. Motivated by this, [1] suggested learning the model parameters by optimizing the following "lagged criterion":

$$\sum_{t=1}^{T-H} \sum_{h=1}^{H} \|\hat{s}_{t+h|t} - s_{t+h}\|^2_2. \tag{2}$$

Here, H is the time horizon of the simulation, and $\hat{s}_{t+h|t}$ is the estimate (from simulation) of the state at time $t + h$ given the state at time t.

---

[2]Note that, as discussed previously, the one-step difference of body coordinate velocities is not the acceleration. To obtain actual accelerations, the velocity at time $t + 1$ must be rotated into the body-frame at t before taking the difference.

Unfortunately the EM-algorithm given in [1] is prohibitively expensive in our continuous state-action space setting. We therefore present a simple and fast algorithm for (approximately) minimizing the lagged criterion. We begin by considering a linear model with update equation:

$$s_{t+1} - s_t = As_t + Bu_t, \tag{3}$$

where A, B are the parameters of the model. Minimizing the one-step prediction error would correspond to finding the parameters that minimize the expected squared difference between the left and right sides of Eqn. (3).

By summing the update equations for two consecutive time steps, we get that, for simulation to be exact over two time steps, the following needs to hold:

$$s_{t+2} - s_t = As_t + Bu_t + A\hat{s}_{t+1|t} + Bu_{t+1}. \tag{4}$$

Minimizing the expected squared difference between the left and right sides of Eqn. (4) would correspond to minimizing the two-step prediction error. More generally, by summing up the update equations for h consecutive timesteps and then minimizing the left and right sides' expected squared difference, we can minimize the h-step prediction error. Thus, it may seem that we can directly solve for the parameters that minimize the lagged criterion of Eqn. (2) by running least squares on the appropriate set of linear combinations of state update equations.

The difficulty with this procedure is that the intermediate states in the simulation—for example, $\hat{s}_{t+1|t}$ in Eqn. (4)—are also an implicit function of the parameters A and B. This is because $\hat{s}_{t+1|t}$ represents the result of a one-step simulation from s_t using our model. Taking into account the dependence of the intermediate states on the parameters makes the right side of Eqn. (4) non-linear in the parameters, and thus the optimization is non-convex. If, however, we make an approximation and neglect this dependence, then optimizing the objective can be done simply by solving a linear least squares problem.

This gives us the following algorithm. We will alternate between a simulation step that finds the necessary predicted intermediate states, and a least squares step that solves for the new parameters.

LEARN-LAGGED-LINEAR:

1. Use least squares to minimize the one-step squared prediction error criterion to obtain an initial model $A^{(0)}, B^{(0)}$. Set $i = 1$.

2. For all $t = 1, \ldots, T, h = 1, \ldots, H$, simulate in the current model to compute $\hat{s}_{t+h|t}$.

3. Solve the following least squares problem:
   $$(\bar{A}, \bar{B}) = \arg\min_{A,B} \sum_{t=1}^{T-H} \sum_{h=1}^{H} \|(s_{t+h} - s_t) - (\sum_{\tau=0}^{h-1} A\hat{s}_{t+\tau|t} + Bu_{t+\tau})\|_2^2.$$

4. Set $A^{(i+1)} = (1 - \alpha)A^{(i)} + \alpha\bar{A}$, $B^{(i+1)} = (1 - \alpha)B^{(i)} + \alpha\bar{B}$.[3]

5. If $\|A^{(i+1)} - A^{(i)}\| + \|B^{(i+1)} - B^{(i)}\| \le \epsilon$ exit. Otherwise go back to step 2.

Our helicopter acceleration prediction model is not of the simple form $s_{t+1} - s_t = As_t + Bu_t$ described above. However, a similar derivation still applies: The change in velocity over several time-steps corresponds to the sum of changes in velocity over several single time-steps. Thus by adding the one-step acceleration prediction equations as given in Section 4, we might expect to obtain equations corresponding to the acceleration over several time-steps. However, the acceleration equations at different time-steps are in different coordinate frames. Thus we first need to rotate the equations and then add them. In the algorithm described below, we rotate all accelerations into the world coordinate frame. The acceleration equations from Section 4 give us $(\ddot{x}, \ddot{y}, \ddot{z})_t^b = A_{\text{pos}}s_t + B_{\text{pos}}u_t$, and

---

[3]This step of the algorithm uses a simple line search to choose the stepsize α.

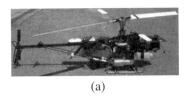 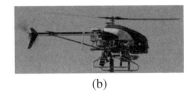

(a)   (b)

Figure 1: The XCell Tempest (a) and the Bergen Industrial Twin (b) used in our experiments.

$(\ddot{\phi}, \ddot{\theta}, \dot{\omega})^b_t = A_{\text{rot}} s_t + B_{\text{rot}} u_t$, where $A_{\text{pos}}, B_{\text{pos}}, A_{\text{rot}}, B_{\text{rot}}$ are (sparse) matrices that contain the parameters to be learned.[4] This gives us the LEARN-LAGGED-ACCELERATION algorithm, which is identical to LEARN-LAGGED-LINEAR except that step 3 now solves the following least squares problems:

$$(\bar{A}_{\text{pos}}, \bar{B}_{\text{pos}}) = \arg\min_{A,B} \sum_{t=1}^{T-H} \sum_{h=1}^{H} \| \sum_{\tau=0}^{h-1} \hat{R}^{b_{t+\tau} \to s} \left((\ddot{x}, \ddot{y}, \ddot{z})^b_{t+\tau} - (A\hat{s}_{t+\tau|t} + Bu_{t+\tau}) \right) \|_2^2$$

$$(\bar{A}_{\text{rot}}, \bar{B}_{\text{rot}}) = \arg\min_{A,B} \sum_{t=1}^{T-H} \sum_{h=1}^{H} \| \sum_{\tau=0}^{h-1} \hat{R}^{b_{t+\tau} \to s} \left((\ddot{\phi}, \ddot{\theta}, \dot{\omega})^b_{t+\tau} - (A\hat{s}_{t+\tau|t} + Bu_{t+\tau}) \right) \|_2^2$$

Here $\hat{R}^{b_t \to s}$ denotes the rotation matrix (estimated from simulation using the current model) from the body frame at time t to the world frame.

6 Experiments

We performed experiments on two RC helicopters: an XCell Tempest and a Bergen Industrial Twin helicopter. (See Figure 1.) The XCell Tempest is a competition-class aerobatic helicopter (length 54", height 19"), is powered by a 0.91-size, two-stroke engine, and has an unloaded weight of 13 pounds. It carries two sensor units: a Novatel RT2 GPS receiver and a Microstrain 3DM-GX1 orientation sensor. The Microstrain package contains triaxial accelerometers, rate gyros, and magnetometers, which are used for inertial sensing. The larger Bergen Industrial Twin helicopter is powered by a twin cylinder 46cc, two-stroke engine, and has an unloaded weight of 18 lbs. It carries three sensor units: a Novatel RT2 GPS receiver, MicroStrain 3DM-G magnetometers, and an Inertial Science ISIS-IMU (triaxial accelerometers and rate gyros).

For each helicopter, we collected data from two separate flights. The XCell Tempest train and test flights were 800 and 540 seconds long, the Bergen Industrial Twin train and test flights were each 110 seconds long. A highly optimized Kalman filter integrates the sensor information and reports (at 100Hz) 12 numbers corresponding to the helicopter's state $(x, y, z, \dot{x}, \dot{y}, \dot{z}, \phi, \theta, \omega, \dot{\phi}, \dot{\theta}, \dot{\omega})$. The data is then downsampled to 10Hz before learning. For each of the helicopters, we learned the following models:

1. Linear-One-Step: The linear model from Section 3 trained using linear regression to minimize the one-step prediction error.

2. Linear-CIFER: The linear model from Section 3 trained using CIFER.

3. Linear-Lagged: The linear model from Section 3 trained minimizing the lagged criterion.

4. Acceleration-One-Step: The acceleration prediction model from Section 4 trained using linear regression to minimize the one step prediction error.

5. Acceleration-Lagged: The acceleration prediction model from Section 4 trained minimizing the lagged criterion.

---

[4]For simplicity of notation we omit the intercept parameters here, but they are easily incorporated, e.g., by having one additional input which is always equal to one.

For Linear-Lagged and Acceleration-Lagged we used a horizon H of two seconds (20 simulation steps). The CPU times for training the different algorithms were: Less than one second for linear regression (algorithms 1 and 4 in the list above); one hour 20 minutes (XCell Tempest data) or 10 minutes (Bergen Industrial Twin data) for the lagged criteria (algorithms 3 and 5 above); about 5 minutes for CIFER. Our algorithm optimizing the lagged criterion appears to converge after at most 30 iterations. Since this algorithm is only approximate, we can then use coordinate descent search to further improve the lagged criterion.[5] This coordinate descent search took an additional four hours for the XCell Tempest data and an additional 30 minutes for the Bergen Industrial Twin data. We report results both with and without this coordinate descent search. Our results show that the algorithm presented in Section 5 works well for fast approximate optimization of the lagged criterion, but that locally greedy search (coordinate descent) may then improve it yet further.

For evaluation, the test data was split in consecutive non-overlapping two second windows. (This corresponds to 20 simulation steps, $s_0, \ldots, s_{20}$.) The models are used to predict the state sequence over the two second window, when started in the true state s_0. We report the average squared prediction error (difference between the simulated and true state) at each timestep $t = 1, \ldots, 20$ throughout the two second window. The orientation error is measured by the squared magnitude of the minimal rotation needed to align the simulated orientation with the true orientation. Velocity, position, angular rate and orientation errors are measured in m/s, m, rad/s and rad (squared) respectively. (See Figure 2.)

We see that Linear-Lagged consistently outperforms Linear-CIFER and Linear-One-Step. Similarly, for the acceleration prediction models, we have that Acceleration-Lagged consistently outperforms Acceleration-One-Step. These experiments support the case for training with the lagged criterion.

The best acceleration prediction model, Acceleration-Lagged, is significantly more accurate than any of the linear models presented in Section 3. This effect is mostly present in the XCell Tempest data, which contained data collected from many different parts of the state space (e.g., flying in a circle); in contrast, the Bergen Industrial Twin data was collected mostly near hovering (and thus the linearization assumptions were somewhat less poor there).

7 Summary

We presented an acceleration based parameterization for learning vehicular dynamics. The model predicts accelerations, and then integrates to obtain state trajectories. We also described an efficient algorithm for approximately minimizing the lagged criterion, which measures the predictive accuracy of the algorithm over both short and long time-scales. In our experiments, learning with the acceleration parameterization and using the lagged criterion gave significantly more accurate models than previous approaches. Using this approach, we have recently also succeeded in learning a model for, and then autonomously flying, a "funnel" aerobatic maneuver, in which the helicopter flies in a circle, keeping the tail pointed at the center of rotation, and the body of the helicopter pitched backwards at a steep angle (so that the body of the helicopter traces out the surface of a funnel). (Details will be presented in a forthcoming paper.)

Acknowledgments. We give warm thanks to Adam Coates and to helicopter pilot Ben Tse for their help on this work.

---

[5]We used coordinate descent on the criterion of Eqn. (2), but reweighted the errors on velocity, angular velocity, position and orientation to scale them to roughly the same order of magnitude.

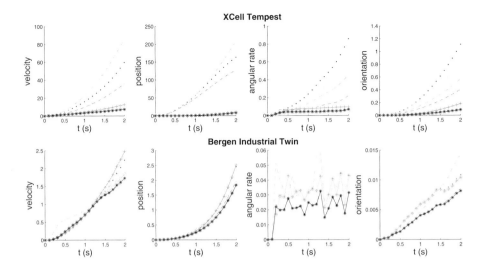

Figure 2: (Best viewed in color.) Average squared prediction errors throughout two-second simulations. Blue, dotted: Linear-One-Step. Green, dash-dotted: Linear-CIFER. Yellow, triangle: Linear-Lagged learned with fast, approximate algorithm from Section 5. Red, dashed: Linear-Lagged learned with fast, approximate algorithm from Section 5 followed by greedy coordinate descent search. Magenta, solid: Acceleration-One-Step. Cyan, circle: Acceleration-Lagged learned with fast, approximate algorithm from Section 5. Black,*: Acceleration-Lagged learned with fast, approximate algorithm from Section 5 followed by greedy coordinate descent search. The magenta, cyan and black lines (visually) coincide in the XCell position plots. The blue, yellow, magenta and cyan lines (visually) coincide in the Bergen angular rate and orientation plots. The red and black lines (visually) coincide in the Bergen angular rate plot. See text for details.

References

[1] P. Abbeel and A. Y. Ng. Learning first order Markov models for control. In *NIPS 18*, 2005.

[2] J. Bagnell and J. Schneider. Autonomous helicopter control using reinforcement learning policy search methods. In *International Conference on Robotics and Automation*. IEEE, 2001.

[3] V. Gavrilets, I. Martinos, B. Mettler, and E. Feron. Control logic for automated aerobatic flight of miniature helicopter. In *AIAA Guidance, Navigation and Control Conference*, 2002.

[4] V. Gavrilets, I. Martinos, B. Mettler, and E. Feron. Flight test and simulation results for an autonomous aerobatic helicopter. In *AIAA/IEEE Digital Avionics Systems Conference*, 2002.

[5] J. Leishman. *Principles of Helicopter Aerodynamics*. Cambridge University Press, 2000.

[6] B. Mettler, M. Tischler, and T. Kanade. System identification of small-size unmanned helicopter dynamics. In *American Helicopter Society, 55th Forum*, 1999.

[7] Andrew Y. Ng, Adam Coates, Mark Diel, Varun Ganapathi, Jamie Schulte, Ben Tse, Eric Berger, and Eric Liang. Autonomous inverted helicopter flight via reinforcement learning. In *International Symposium on Experimental Robotics*, 2004.

[8] Andrew Y. Ng, H. Jin Kim, Michael Jordan, and Shankar Sastry. Autnonomous helicopter flight via reinforcement learning. In *NIPS 16*, 2004.

[9] Jonathan M. Roberts, Peter I. Corke, and Gregg Buskey. Low-cost flight control system for a small autonomous helicopter. In *IEEE Int'l Conf. on Robotics and Automation*, 2003.

[10] J. Seddon. *Basic Helicopter Aerodynamics*. AIAA Education Series. America Institute of Aeronautics and Astronautics, 1990.

[11] M.B. Tischler and M.G. Cauffman. Frequency response method for rotorcraft system identification: Flight application to BO-105 couple rotor/fuselage dynamics. *Journal of the American Helicopter Society*, 1992.

Policy-Gradient Methods for Planning

Douglas Aberdeen
Statistical Machine Learning, National ICT Australia, Canberra
doug.aberdeen@anu.edu.au

Abstract

Probabilistic temporal planning attempts to find good policies for acting in domains with concurrent durative tasks, multiple uncertain outcomes, and limited resources. These domains are typically modelled as Markov decision problems and solved using dynamic programming methods. This paper demonstrates the application of reinforcement learning — in the form of a policy-gradient method — to these domains. Our emphasis is large domains that are infeasible for dynamic programming. Our approach is to construct simple policies, or agents, for each planning task. The result is a general probabilistic temporal planner, named the Factored Policy-Gradient Planner (FPG-Planner), which can handle hundreds of tasks, optimising for probability of success, duration, and resource use.

1 Introduction

To date, only a few planning tools have attempted to handle general probabilistic temporal planning problems. These tools have only been able to produce good policies for relatively trivial examples. We apply policy-gradient reinforcement learning (RL) to these domains with the goal of creating tools that produce good policies in real-world domains rather than perfect policies in toy domains. We achieve this by: (1) factoring the policy into simple independent policies for starting each task; (2) presenting each policy with critical observations instead of the entire state; (3) using function approximators for each policy; (4) using local optimisation methods instead of global optimisation; and (5) using algorithms with memory requirements that are independent of the state space size.

Policy gradient methods do not enumerate states and are applicable to multi-agent settings with function approximation [1, 2], thus they are a natural match for our approach to handling large planning problems. We use the GPOMDP algorithm [3] to estimate the gradient of a long-term average reward of the planner's performance, with respect to the parameters of each task policy. We show that maximising a simple reward function naturally minimises plan durations and maximises the probability of reaching the plan goal.

A frequent criticism of policy-gradient methods compared to traditional forward chaining planners — or even compared to value-based RL methods — is the lack of a clearly interpretable policy. A minor contribution of this paper is a description of how policy-gradient methods can be used to prune a decision tree over possible policies. After training, the decision tree can be translated into a list of policy rules.

Previous probabilistic temporal planners include CPTP [4], Prottle [5], Tempastic [6] and a military operations planner [7]. Most these algorithms use some form of dynamic programming (either RTDP [8] or AO*) to associate values with each state/action pair. However, this requires values to be stored for each encountered state. Even though these algorithms do not enumerate the entire state space their ability to scale is limited by memory size. Even problems with only tens of tasks can produce millions of relevant states. CPTP, Prottle, and Tempastic minimise either plan duration or failure probability, not both. The FPG-Planner minimises both of these metrics and can easily optimise over resources too.

2   Probabilistic temporal planning

Tasks are the basic planning unit corresponding to grounded[1] durative actions. Tasks have the effect of setting condition variables to true or false. Each task has a set of preconditions, effects, resource requirements, and a fixed probability of failure. Durations may be fixed or dependent on how long it takes for other conditions to be established. A task is *eligible* to begin when its preconditions are satisfied and sufficient resources are available. A starting task may have some immediate effects. As tasks end a set of effects appropriate to the outcome are applied. Typically, but not necessarily, succeeding tasks set some facts to true, while failing tasks do nothing or negate facts. Resources are occupied during task execution and consumed when the task ends. Different outcomes can consume varying levels of resources. The planning goal is to set a subset of the conditions to a desired value.

The closest work to that presented here is described by Peshkin et al. [1] which describes how a policy-gradient approach can be applied to multi-agent MDPs. This work lays the foundation for this application, but does not consider the planning domain specifically. It is also applied to relatively small domains, where the state space could be enumerated.

Actions in temporal planning consist of launching multiple tasks concurrently. The number of candidate actions available in a given state is the power set of the tasks that are eligible to start. That is, with N eligible tasks there are 2^N possible actions. Current planners explore this action space systematically, pruning actions that lead to low rewards. When combined with probabilistic outcomes the state space explosion cripples existing planners for tens of tasks and actions. A key reason treat each task as an individual policy agent is to deal with this explosion of the action space. We replace the single agent choosing from the power-set of eligible tasks with a single simple agent for each task. The policy learnt by each agent is whether to start its associated task given its observation, independent of the decisions made by the other agents. This idea alone does not simplify the problem. Indeed, if the agents received perfect state information they could learn to predict the decision of the other agents and still act optimally. The significant reduction in complexity arises from: (1) restricting the class of functions that represent agents, (2) providing only partial state information, (3) optimising locally, using gradient ascent.

3   POMDP formulation of planning

Our intention is to deliberately use simple agents that only consider partial state information. This requires us to explicitly consider partial observability. A finite partially observable Markov decision process consists of: a finite set of states $s \in \mathcal{S}$; a finite set of actions $\mathbf{a} \in \mathcal{A}$; probabilities $\Pr[s'|s, \mathbf{a}]$ of making state transition $s \rightarrow s'$ under action $\mathbf{a}$; a reward for each state $r(s) : \mathcal{S} \rightarrow \mathbb{R}$; and a finite set of observation vectors $\mathbf{o} \in \mathcal{O}$ seen by the agent in place of the complete state descriptions. For this application, observations are drawn deterministically given the state, but more generally may be stochastic. *Goal states* are states where all the goal state variables are satisfied. From *failure states* it is impossible to reach a goal state, usually because time or resources have run out. These two classes of state are combined to form the set of *reset* states that produce an immediate reset to the

---

[1]Grounded means that tasks do not have parameters that can be instantiated.

initial state s_0. A single trajectory through the state space consists of many individual trials that automatically reset to s_0 each time a goal state or failure state is reached.

Policies are stochastic, mapping observation vectors **o** to a probability over actions. Let N be the number of basic tasks available to the planner. In our setting an action **a** is a binary vector of length N. An entry of 1 at index n means 'Yes' begin task n, and a 0 entry means 'No' do not start task n. The probability of actions is $\Pr[\mathbf{a}|\mathbf{o}, \theta]$, where conditioning on θ reflects the fact that the policy is controlled by a set of real valued parameters $\theta \in \mathbb{R}^p$. This paper assumes that all stochastic policies (i.e., any values for θ) reach reset states in finite time when executed from s_0. This is enforced by limiting the maximum duration of a plan. This ensures that the underlying MDP is *ergodic*, a necessary condition for GPOMDP. The GPOMDP algorithm maximises the long-term average reward

$$\eta(\theta) = \lim_{T \to \infty} \frac{1}{T} \sum_{t=0}^{T-1} r(s_t).$$

In the context of planning, the instantaneous reward provides the agent with a measure of progress toward the goal. A simple reward scheme is to set $r(s) = 1$ for all states s that represent the goal state, and 0 for all other states. To maximise $\eta(\theta)$, successful planning outcomes must be reached as frequently as possible. This has the desired property of simultaneously minimising plan duration, as well as maximising the probability of reaching the goal (failure states achieve no reward). It is tempting to provide a negative reward for failure states, but this can introduce poor local maxima in the form of policies that avoid negative rewards by avoiding progress altogether. We provide a reward of 1000 each time the goal is achieved, plus an admissible heuristic reward for progress toward the goal. This additional *shaping* reward provides a reward of 1 for every goal state variable achieved, and -1 for every goal variable that becomes unset. Policies that are optimal with the additional shaping reward are still optimal under the basic goal state reward [9].

3.1 Planning state space

For probabilistic temporal planning our state description contains [7]: the state's absolute time, a queue of impending events, the status of each task, the truth value of each condition, and the available resources. In a particular state, only a subset of the eligible tasks will satisfy all preconditions for execution. We call these tasks *eligible*. When a decision to start a fixed duration task is made an end-task event is added to a time ordered event queue. The event queue holds a list of events that the planner is committed to, although the outcome of those events may be uncertain.

The generation of successor states is shown in Alg. 1. The algorithm begins by starting the tasks given by the current action, implementing any immediate effects. An end-task event is added at an appropriate time in the queue. The state update then proceeds to process events until there is at least one task that is eligible to begin. Events have probabilistic outcomes. Line 20 of Alg. 1 samples one possible outcome from the distribution imposed by probabilities in the problem definition. Future states are only generated at points where tasks can be started. Thus, if an event outcome is processed and no tasks are enabled, the search recurses to the next event in the queue.

4 Factored Policy-Gradient

We assume the presence of policy agents, parameterised with independent sets of parameters for each agent $\theta = \{\theta_1, \ldots, \theta_N\}$. We seek to adjust the parameters of the policy to maximise the long-term average reward $\eta(\theta)$. The GPOMDP algorithm [3] estimates the gradient $\nabla \eta(\theta)$ of the long-term average reward with respect to the current set of policy

Alg. 1: **findSuccessor(State** s, **Action** $\mathbf{a}$**)**
1: **for** each $a_n =$ 'Yes' in $\mathbf{a}$ **do**
2:     s.beginTask(n)
3:     s.addEvent(n, s.time+taskDuration(n))
4: **end for**
5: **repeat**
6:     **if** s.time > maximum makespan **then**
7:         s.failureLeaf=true
8:         return
9:     **end if**
10:     **if** s.operationGoalsMet() **then**
11:         s.goalLeaf=true
12:         return
13:     **end if**
14:     **if** $\neg s$.anyEligibleTasks() **then**
15:         s.failureLeaf=true
16:         return
17:     **end if**
18:     $event = s$.nextEvent()
19:     s.time = $event$.time
20:     sample $outcome$ from $event$
21:     s.implementEffects($outcome$)
22: **until** s.anyEligibleTasks()

Alg. 2: **Gradient Estimator**
1: Set s_0 to initial state, $t = 0$, $\mathbf{e}_t = [0]$
2: **while** $t < T$ **do**
3:     $\mathbf{e}_t = \beta \mathbf{e}_{t-1}$
4:     Generate observation $\mathbf{o}_t$ of s_t
5:     **for** Each eligible task n **do**
6:         Sample $a_{tn} =$ Yes or $a_{tn} =$ No
7:         $\mathbf{e}_t = \mathbf{e}_t + \nabla \log \Pr[a_{tn}|\mathbf{o}, \theta_n]$
8:     **end for**
9:     Try action $\mathbf{a}_t = \{a_{t1}, a_{t2}, \ldots, a_{tN}\}$
10:     **while** mutex prohibits $\mathbf{a}_t$ **do**
11:         randomly disable task in $\mathbf{a}_t$
12:     **end while**
13:     $s_{t+1} = $ findSuccessor(s_t, $\mathbf{a}_t$)
14:     $\hat{\nabla}_t \eta(\theta) = \hat{\nabla}_{t-1} \eta(\theta) - \frac{1}{t+1}(r(s_{t+1})\mathbf{e}_t - \hat{\nabla}_{t-1}\eta(\theta))$
15:     $t \leftarrow t + 1$
16: **end while**
17: Return $\hat{\nabla}_T \eta(\theta)$

parameters. Once an estimate $\hat{\nabla}\eta(\theta)$ is computed over T simulation steps, we maximise the long-term average reward with the gradient ascent $\theta \leftarrow \theta + \alpha \hat{\nabla}\eta(\theta)$, where α is a small step size. The experiments in this paper use a line search to determine good values of α. We do not guarantee that the best representable policy is found, but our experiments have produced policies comparable to global methods like real-time dynamic programming [8].

The algorithm works by sampling a single long trajectory through the state space (Fig. 4): (1) the first state represents time 0 in the plan; (2) the agents all receive the vector observation $\mathbf{o}_t$ of the current state s_t; (3) each agent representing an eligible task emits a probability of starting; (4) each agent samples start or do not start and issues it as a planning action; (5) the state transition is sampled with Alg. 1; (6) the agents receive the global reward for the new state action and update their gradient estimates. Steps 1 to 6 are repeated T times.

Each vector action $\mathbf{a}_t$ is a combination of independent 'Yes' or 'No' choices made by each eligible agent. Each agent is parameterised by an independent set of parameters that make up $\theta \in \mathbb{R}^p$: $\theta_1, \theta_2, \ldots, \theta_N$. If a_{tn} represents the binary decision made by agent n at time t about whether to start its corresponding task, then the policy factors into

$$\Pr[\mathbf{a}_t|\mathbf{o}_t, \theta] = \Pr[a_{t1}, \ldots, a_{tN}|\mathbf{o}_t, \theta_1, \ldots, \theta_N]$$
$$= \Pr[a_{t1}|\mathbf{o}_t, \theta_1] \times \cdots \times \Pr[a_{tN}|\mathbf{o}_t, \theta_N].$$

It is not necessary for all agents to receive the same observation, and it may be advantageous to show different agents different parts of the state, leading to a *decentralised* planning algorithm. Similar approaches are adopted by Peshkin et al. [1], Tao et al. [2], using policy-gradient methods to train multi-agent systems. The main requirement for each policy-agent is that $\log \Pr[a_{tn}|\mathbf{o}_t, \theta_n]$ be differentiable with respect to the parameters for each choice task start $a_{tn} =$ 'Yes' or 'No'. We now describe two such agents.

4.1 Linear approximator agents

One representation of agents is a linear network mapped into probabilities using a logistic regression function:

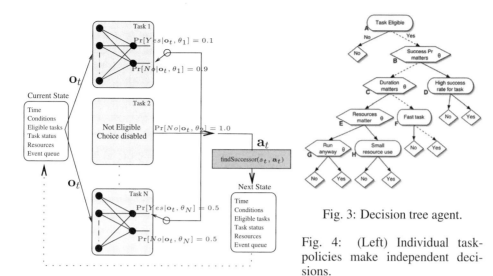

Fig. 3: Decision tree agent.

Fig. 4: (Left) Individual task-policies make independent decisions.

$$\Pr[a_{tn} = Yes | \mathbf{o}_t, \theta_n] = \frac{exp(\mathbf{o}_t^\top \theta_n)}{exp(\mathbf{o}_t^\top \theta_n) + 1} \tag{1}$$

If the dimension of the observation vector is $|\mathbf{o}|$ then each set of parameters θ_n can be thought of as an $|\mathbf{o}|$ vector that represents the approximator weights for task n. The log derivatives, necessary for Alg. 2, are given in [10]. Initially, the parameters are set to small random values: a near uniform random policy. This encourages exploration of the action space. Each gradient step typically moves the parameters closer to a deterministic policy. After some experimentation we chose an observation vector that is a binary description of the eligible tasks and the state variable truth values plus a constant 1 bit to provide bias to the agents' linear networks.

4.2 Decision tree agents

Often we have a selection of potential control rules. A decision tree can represent all such control rules at the leaves. The nodes are additional parameterised or hardwired rules that select between different branches, and therefore different control rules. An action a is selected by starting at the root node and following a path down the tree, visiting a set of decision nodes $\mathcal{D}$. At each node we either applying a hard coded branch selection rule, or sample a stochastic branch rule from the probability distribution invoked by the parameterisation. Assuming the independence of decisions at each node, the probability or reaching an action leaf l equals the product of branch probabilities at each decision node

$$\Pr[a = l | \mathbf{o}, \theta] = \prod_{d \in \mathcal{D}} \Pr[d' | \mathbf{o}, \theta_d], \tag{2}$$

where d represents the current decision node, and d' represents the next node visited in the tree. The final next node d' is the leaf l. The probability of a branch followed as a result of a hard-coded rule is 1. The individual $\Pr(d' | \mathbf{o}, \theta_d)$ functions can be any differentiable function of the observation vector $\mathbf{o}$.

For multi-agent domains, such as our formulation of planning, we have a decision tree for each task agent. We use the same initial tree (with different parameters), for each agent, shown in Fig. 3. Nodes A, D, F, H represent hard coded rules that switch with probability one between the Yes and No branches based on a boolean observation that gives the truth of the statement in the node for the current state. Nodes B, C, E, G are parameterised so

13

that they select branches stochastically. For this application, the probability of choosing the Yes or No branches is a single parameter logistic function that is independent of the observations. Parameter adjustments have the simple effect of pruning parts the tree that represent poor policies, leaving the hard coded rules to choose the best action given the observation. The policy encoded by the parameter is written in the node label. For example for task agent n, and decision node C "task duration matters?", we have the probability

$$\Pr(Yes|\mathbf{o}, \theta_{n,C}) = \Pr(Yes|\theta_{n,C}) = \frac{exp(\theta_{n,C})}{exp(\theta_{n,C}) + 1}$$

The log gradient of this function is given in [10]. If set parameters to always select the dashed branch in Fig. 3 we would be following the policy: *if the task IS eligible, and probability this task success does NOT matter, and the duration of this task DOES matter, and this task IS fast, then start, otherwise do not start.* Apart from being easy to interpret the optimised decision tree as a set of — possibly stochastic — if-then rules, we can also encode highly expressive policies with only a few parameters.

4.3   GPOMDP for planning

Alg. 4 describes the algorithm for computing $\hat{\nabla}\eta(\theta)$, based on GPOMDP [3]. The vector quantity $\mathbf{e}_t$ is an eligibility trace. It has dimension p (the total number of parameters), and can be thought of as storing the eligibility of each parameter for being reinforced after receiving a reward. The gradient estimate provably converges to a biased estimate of $\nabla\eta(\theta)$ as $T \to \infty$. The quantity $\beta \in [0, 1)$ controls the degree of bias in the estimate. As β approaches 1, the bias of the estimates drop to 0. However if $\beta = 1$, estimates exhibit infinite variance in the limit as $T \to \infty$. Thus the parameter β is used to achieve a bias/variance tradeoff in our stochastic gradient estimates. GPOMDP gradient estimates have been proven to converge, even under partial observability.

Line 8 computes the log gradient of the sampled action probability and adds the gradient for the n'th agent's parameters into the eligibility trace. The gradient for parameters not relating to agent n is 0. We do not compute $\Pr[a_{tn}|\mathbf{o}_t, \theta_n]$ or gradients for tasks with unsatisfied preconditions. If all eligible agents decide *not* to start their tasks, we issue a null-action. If the state event queue is not empty, we process the next event, otherwise time is incremented by 1 to ensure all possible policies will eventually reach a reset state.

5   Experiments

5.1   Comparison with previous work

We compare the FPG-Planner with that of our earlier RTDP based planner for military operations [7], which is based on real-time dynamic programming with [8]. The domains come from the Australian Defence Science and Technology Organisation, and represent military operations planning scenarios. There are two problems, the first with 18 tasks and 12 conditions, and the second with 41 tasks and 51 conditions. The goal is to set the "Objective island secured" variable to true. There are multiple interrelated tasks that can lead to the goal state. Tasks fail or succeed with a known probability and can only execute once, leading to relatively large probabilities of failure even for optimal plans. See [7] for details. Unless stated, FPG-Planner experiments used $T = 500,000$ gradient estimation steps and $\beta = 0.9$. Optimisation time was limited to 20 minutes wall clock time on a single user 3GHz Pentium IV with 1GB ram. All evaluations are based on 10,000 simulated executions of finalised policies. Results quote the average duration, resource consumption, and the percentage of plans that terminate in a failure state.

We repeat the comparison experiments 50 times with different random seeds and report

Table 1: Two domains compared with a dynamic programming based planner.

Problem	RTDP			Factored Linear			Factored Tree		
	Dur	**Res**	**Fail%**	**Dur**	**Res**	**Fail%**	**Dur**	**Res**	**Fail%**
Assault Ave	171	8.0	26.1	105	8.3	26.6	115	8.3	27.1
Assault Best	113	6.2	24.0	93.1	8.7	23.1	112	8.4	25.6
Webber Ave	245	4.4	58.1	193	4.1	57.9	186	4.1	58.0
Webber Best	217	4.2	57.7	190	4.1	57.0	181	4.1	57.3

Table 2: Effect of different observations.

Observation	**Dur**	**Res**	**Fail%**
Eligible & Conds	105	8.3	26.6
Conds only	112	8.1	28.1
Eligible only	112	8.1	29.6

Table 3: Results for the Art45/25 domain.

Policy	**Dur**	**Res**	**Fail%**
Random	394	206	83.4
Naive	332	231	78.6
Linear	121	67	7.4
Dumb Tree	157	92	19.1
Prob Tree	156	62	10.9
Dur Tree	167	72	17.4
Res Tree	136	53	8.50

mean and best results in Table 1. The "Best" plan minimises an arbitrarily chosen combined metric of $10 \times fail\% + dur$. FPG-Planning with a linear approximator significantly shortens the duration of plans, without increasing the failure rate. The very simple decision tree performs less well than than the linear approximator, but better than the dynamic programming algorithm. This is somewhat surprising given the simplicity of the tree for each task. The shorter duration for the Webber decision tree is probably due to the slightly higher failure rate. Plans failing early produces shorter durations.

Table 1 assumes that the observation vector **o** presented to linear agents is a binary description of the eligible tasks and the condition truth values plus a constant 1 bit to provide bias to the agents' linear networks. Table 2 shows that giving the agents less information in the observation harms performance.

5.2 Large artificial domains

Each scenario consists of N tasks and C state variables. The goal state of the synthetic scenarios is to assert 90% of the state variables, chosen during scenario synthesis, to be true. See [10] for details. All generated problems have scope for choosing tasks instead of merely scheduling them. All synthetic scenarios are guaranteed to have at least one policy which will reach the operation goal assuming all tasks succeed. Even a few tens of tasks and conditions can generate a state space too large for main memory.

We generated 37 problems, each with 40 tasks and 25 conditions (Art40/25). Although the number of tasks and conditions is similar to the Webber problem described above, these problems demonstrate significantly more choices to the planner, making planning non-trivial. Unlike the initial experiments, all tasks can be repeated as often as necessary so the overall probability of failure depends on how well the planner chooses and orders tasks to avoid running out of time and resources. Our RTDP based planner was not able to perform any significant optimisation in 20m due to memory problems. Thus, to demonstrate FPG-Planning is having some effect, we compared the optimised policies to two simple policies. The *random* policy starts each eligible task with probability 0.5. The *naive* policy starts all eligible tasks. Both of these policies suffer from excessive resource consumption and negative effects that can cause failure.

Table 3 shows that the linear approximator produces the best plans, but it requires $C + 1$ parameters per task. The results for the decision tree illustrated in Fig. 3 are given in the

"Prob Tree" row. This tree uses a constant 4 parameters per task, and subsequently requires fewer operations when computing gradients. The "Dumb" row is a decision stub, with one parameter per task that simply learns whether to start when eligible. The remaining "Dur" and "Res" Tree rows re-order the nodes in Fig. 3 to swap the nodes C and E respectively with node B. This tests the sensitivity of the tree to node ordering. There appears to be significant variation in the results. For example, when node E is swapped with B, the resultant policies use less resources.

We also performed optimisation of a 200 task, 100 condition problem generated using the same rules as the Art40/25 domain. The naive policy had a failure rate of 72.4%. No time limit was applied. Linear network agents (20,200 parameters) optimised for 14 hours, before terminating with small gradients, and resulted in a plan with 20.8% failure rate. The decision tree agent (800 parameters) optimised for 6 hours before terminating with a 1.7% failure rate. The smaller number of parameters and a priori policies embedded in the tree, allow the decision tree to perform well in very large domains. Inspection of the resulting parameters demonstrated that different tasks pruned different regions of the decision tree.

6 Conclusion

We have demonstrated an algorithm with great potential to produce good policies in real-world domains. Further work will refine our parameterised agents, and validate this approach on realistic larger domains. We also wish to characterise possible local minima.

Acknowledgements

Thank you to Olivier Buffet and Sylvie Thiébaux for many helpful comments. National ICT Australia is funded by the Australian Government's Backing Australia's Ability program and the Centre of Excellence program. This project was also funded by the Australian Defence Science and Technology Organisation.

References

[1] L. Peshkin, K.-E. Kim, N. Meuleau, and L. P. Kaelbling. Learning to cooperate via policy search. In *UAI*, 2000.

[2] Nigel Tao, Jonathan Baxter, and Lex Weaver. A multi-agent, policy-gradient approach to network routing. In *Proc. ICML'01*. Morgan Kaufmann, 2001.

[3] J. Baxter, P. Bartlett, and L. Weaver. Experiments with infinite-horizon, policy-gradient estimation. *JAIR*, 15:351–381, 2001.

[4] Mausam and Daniel S. Weld. Concurrent probabilistic temporal planning. In *Proc. International Conference on Automated Planning and Scheduling*, Moneteray, CA, June 2005. AAAI.

[5] I. Little, D. Aberdeen, and S. Thiébaux. Prottle: A probabilistic temporal planner. In *Proc. AAAI'05*, 2005.

[6] Hakan L. S. Younes and Reid G. Simmons. Policy generation for continuous-time stochastic domains with concurrency. In *Proc. of ICAPS'04*, volume 14, 2005.

[7] Douglas Aberdeen, Sylvie Thiébaux, and Lin Zhang. Decision-theoretic military operations planning. In *Proc. ICAPS*, volume 14, pages 402–411. AAAI, June 2004.

[8] A.G. Barto, S. Bradtke, and S. Singh. Learning to act using real-time dynamic programming. *Artificial Intelligence*, 72, 1995.

[9] A.Y. Ng, D. Harada, and S. Russell. Policy invariance under reward transformations: Theory and application to reward shaping. In *Proc. ICML'99*, 1999.

[10] Douglas Aberdeen. The factored policy-gradient planner. Technical report, NICTA, 2005.

Kernelized Infomax Clustering

Felix V. Agakov
Edinburgh University
Edinburgh EH1 2QL, U.K.
felixa@inf.ed.ac.uk

David Barber
IDIAP Research Institute
CH-1920 Martigny Switzerland
david.barber@idiap.ch

Abstract

We propose a simple information-theoretic approach to soft clustering based on maximizing the mutual information $I(\mathsf{x}, y)$ between the unknown cluster labels y and the training patterns x with respect to parameters of specifically constrained encoding distributions. The constraints are chosen such that patterns are likely to be clustered similarly if they lie close to specific unknown vectors in the feature space. The method may be conveniently applied to learning the optimal affinity matrix, which corresponds to learning parameters of the kernelized encoder. The procedure does not require computations of eigenvalues of the Gram matrices, which makes it potentially attractive for clustering large data sets.

1 Introduction

Let $\mathsf{x} \in \mathbb{R}^{|\mathsf{x}|}$ be a visible pattern, and $y \in \{y_1, \ldots, y_{|y|}\}$ its discrete unknown cluster label. Rather than learning a density model of the observations, our goal here will be to learn a mapping $\mathsf{x} \rightarrow y$ from the observations to the latent codes (cluster labels) by optimizing a formal measure of coding efficiency. Good codes y should be in some way informative about the underlying high-dimensional source vectors x, so that the useful information contained in the sources is not lost. The fundamental measure in this context is the mutual information

$$I(\mathsf{x}, y) \overset{\text{def}}{=} H(\mathsf{x}) - H(\mathsf{x}|y) \equiv H(y) - H(y|\mathsf{x}), \tag{1}$$

which indicates the decrease in uncertainty about the pattern x due to the knowledge of the underlying cluster label y (e.g. Cover and Thomas (1991)). Here $H(y) \equiv -\langle \log p(y) \rangle_{p(y)}$ and $H(y|\mathsf{x}) \equiv -\langle \log p(y|\mathsf{x}) \rangle_{p(\mathsf{x},y)}$ are marginal and conditional entropies respectively, and the brackets $\langle \ldots \rangle_p$ represent averages over p. In our case the *encoder* model is defined as

$$p(\mathsf{x}, y) \propto \sum_{m=1}^{M} \delta(\mathsf{x} - \mathsf{x}^{(m)}) p(y|\mathsf{x}), \tag{2}$$

where $\{\mathsf{x}^{(m)} | m = 1, \ldots, M\}$ is a set of training patterns.

Our goal is to maximize (1) with respect to parameters of a constrained encoding distribution $p(y|\mathsf{x})$. In contrast to most applications of the *infomax* principle

(Linsker (1988)) in stochastic channels (e.g. Brunel and Nadal (1998); Fisher and Principe (1998); Torkkola and Campbell (2000)), optimization of the objective (1) is computationally tractable since the cardinality of the code space $|y|$ (the number of clusters) will typically be low. Indeed, had the code space been high-dimensional, computation of $I(\mathsf{x}, y)$ would have required evaluation of the generally intractable entropy of the mixture $H(\mathsf{y})$, and approximations would have needed to be considered (e.g. Barber and Agakov (2003); Agakov and Barber (2006)).

Maximization of the mutual information with respect to parameters of the encoder model effectively defines a *discriminative unsupervised* optimization framework, where the model is parameterized similarly to a conditionally trained classifier, but where the cluster allocations are generally unknown. Training such models $p(y|\mathsf{x})$ by maximizing the likelihood $p(\mathsf{x})$ would be meaningless, as the cluster variables would marginalize out, which motivates also our information theoretic approach. In this way we may extract soft cluster allocations directly from the training set, with no additional information about class labels, relevance patterns, etc. required. This is an important difference from other clustering techniques making a recourse to information theory, which consider different channels and generally require additional information about relevance or irrelevance variables (*cf* Tishby et al. (1999); Chechik and Tishby (2002); Dhillon and Guan (2003)).

Our infomax approach is in contrast with probabilistic methods based on likelihood maximization. There the task of finding an optimal cluster allocation y for an observed pattern x may be viewed as an inference problem in *generative* models $y \rightarrow \mathsf{x}$, where the probability of the data $p(\mathsf{x}) = \sum_y p(y)p(\mathsf{x}|y)$ is defined as a mixture of $|y|$ processes. The key idea of fitting such models to data is to find a constrained probability distribution $p(\mathsf{x})$ which would be likely to generate the visible patterns $\{\mathsf{x}^{(1)}, \ldots, \mathsf{x}^{(M)}\}$ (this is commonly achieved by maximizing the marginal likelihood for deterministic parameters of the constrained distribution). The unknown clusters y corresponding to each pattern x may then be assigned according to the posterior $p(y|\mathsf{x}) \propto p(y)p(\mathsf{x}|y)$. Such generative approaches are well-known but suffer from the constraint that $p(\mathsf{x}|y)$ is a correctly normalised distribution in x. In high dimensions $|\mathsf{x}|$ this restricts the class of generative distributions usually to (mixtures of) Gaussians whose mean is dependent (in a linear or non-linear way) on the latent cluster y. Typically data will lie on low dimensional curved manifolds embedded in the high dimensional x-space. If we are restricted to using mixtures of Gaussians to model this curved manifold, typically a very large number of mixture components will be required. No such restrictions apply in the infomax case so that the mappings $p(y|\mathsf{x})$ may be very complex, subject only to sensible clustering constraints.

2   Clustering in Nonlinear Encoder Models

Arguably, there are at least two requirements which a meaningful cluster allocation procedure should satisfy. Firstly, clusters should be, in some sense, locally smooth. For example, each pair of source vectors should have a high probability of being assigned to the same cluster if the vectors satisfy specific geometric constraints. Secondly, we may wish to avoid assigning unique cluster labels to outliers (or other constrained regions in the data space), so that under-represented regions in the data space are not over-represented in the code space. Note that degenerate cluster allocations are generally suboptimal under the objective (1), as they would lead to a reduction in the marginal entropy $H(y)$. On the other hand, it is intuitive that maximization of the mutual information $I(\mathsf{x}, y)$ favors hard assignments of cluster labels to equiprobable data regions, as this would result in the growth in $H(y)$ and reduction in $H(y|\mathsf{x})$.

2.1 Learning Optimal Parameters

Local smoothness and "softness" of the clusters may be enforced by imposing appropriate constraints on $p(y|\mathsf{x})$. A simple choice of the encoder is

$$p(y_j|\mathsf{x}^{(i)}) \propto \exp\{-\|\mathsf{x}^{(i)} - \mathsf{w}_j\|^2/s_j + b_j\}, \tag{3}$$

where the cluster centers $\mathsf{w}_j \in \mathbb{R}^{|\mathsf{x}|}$, the dispersions s_j, and the biases b_j are the encoder parameters to be learned. Clearly, under the encoding distribution (3) patterns x lying close to specific centers w_j in the *data* space will tend to be clustered similarly. In principle, we could consider other choices of $p(y|\mathsf{x})$; however (3) will prove to be particularly convenient for the kernelized extensions.

Learning the optimal cluster allocations corresponds to maximizing (1) with respect to the encoder parameters (3). The gradients are given by

$$\frac{\partial I(\mathsf{x}, y)}{\partial \mathsf{w}_j} = \frac{1}{M} \sum_{m=1}^{M} p(y_j|\mathsf{x}^{(m)}) \frac{(\mathsf{x}^{(m)} - \mathsf{w}_j)}{s_j} \alpha_j^{(m)} \tag{4}$$

$$\frac{\partial I(\mathsf{x}, y)}{\partial s_j} = \frac{1}{M} \sum_{m=1}^{M} p(y_j|\mathsf{x}^{(m)}) \frac{\|\mathsf{x}^{(m)} - \mathsf{w}_j\|^2}{2s_j^2} \alpha_j^{(m)}. \tag{5}$$

Analogously, we get $\partial I(\mathsf{x}, y)/\partial b_j = \sum_{m=1}^{M} p(y_j|\mathsf{x}^{(m)})\alpha_j^{(m)}/M$.

Expressions (4) and (5) have the form of the weighted EM updates for isotropic Gaussian mixtures, with the weighting coefficients $\alpha_j^{(m)}$ defined as

$$\alpha_j^{(m)} \stackrel{\text{def}}{=} \alpha_j(\mathsf{x}^{(m)}) \stackrel{\text{def}}{=} \log \frac{p(y_j|\mathsf{x}^{(m)})}{p(y_j)} - KL\left(p(y|\mathsf{x}^{(m)})\|\langle p(y|\mathsf{x})\rangle_{\tilde{p}(\mathsf{x})}\right), \tag{6}$$

where KL defines the Kullback-Leibler divergence (e.g. Cover and Thomas (1991)), and $\tilde{p}(\mathsf{x}) \propto \sum_m \delta(\mathsf{x} - \mathsf{x}^{(m)})$ is the empirical distribution. Clearly, if $\alpha_j^{(m)}$ is kept fixed for all $m = 1, \ldots, M$ and $j = 1, \ldots, |y|$, the gradients (4) are identical to those obtained by maximizing the log-likelihood of a Gaussian mixture model (up to irrelevant constant pre-factors). Generally, however, the coefficients $\alpha_j^{(m)}$ will be functions of w_l, s_l, and b_l for all cluster labels $l = 1, \ldots, |y|$.

In practice, we may impose a simple construction ensuring that $s_j > 0$, for example by assuming that $s_j = \exp\{\tilde{s}_j\}$ where $\tilde{s}_j \in \mathbb{R}$. For this case, we may re-express the gradients for the variances as $\partial I(\mathsf{x}, y)/\partial \tilde{s}_j = s_j \partial I(\mathsf{x}, y)/\partial s_j$. Expressions (4) and (5) may then be used to perform gradient ascent on $I(\mathsf{x}, y)$ for $\mathsf{w}_j, \tilde{s}_j$, and b_j, where $j = 1, \ldots, |y|$. After training, the optimal cluster allocations may be assigned according to the encoding distribution $p(y|\mathsf{x})$.

2.2 Infomax Clustering with Kernelized Encoder Models

We now extend (3) by considering a kernelized parameterization of a nonlinear encoder. Let us assume that the source patterns $\mathsf{x}^{(i)}$, $\mathsf{x}^{(j)}$ have a high probability of being assigned to the same cluster if they lie close to a specific cluster center in some *feature* space. One choice of the encoder distribution for this case is

$$p(y_j|\mathsf{x}^{(i)}) \propto \exp\{-\|\phi(\mathsf{x}^{(i)}) - \mathsf{w}_j\|^2/s_j + b_j\}, \tag{7}$$

where $\phi(\mathsf{x}^{(i)}) \in \mathbb{R}^{|\phi|}$ is the feature vector corresponding to the source pattern $\mathsf{x}^{(i)}$, and $\mathsf{w}_j \in \mathbb{R}^{|\phi|}$ is the (unknown) cluster center in the feature space. The feature space may be very high- or even infinite-dimensional.

Since each cluster center $\mathsf{w}_i \in \mathbb{R}^{|\phi|}$ lives in the same space as the projected sources $\phi(\mathsf{x}^{(i)})$, it is representable in the basis of the projections as

$$\mathsf{w}_j = \sum_{m=1}^{M} \alpha_{mj} \phi(\mathsf{x}^{(m)}) + \mathsf{w}_j^{\perp}, \tag{8}$$

where $\tilde{\mathsf{w}}_i^{\perp} \in \mathbb{R}^{|\phi|}$ is orthogonal to the span of $\phi(\mathsf{x}_1), \ldots, \phi(\mathsf{x}_M)$, and $\{\alpha_{mj}\}$ is a set of coefficients (here j and m index $|y|$ codes and M patterns respectively). Then we may transform the encoder distribution (7) to

$$p(y_j|\mathsf{x}^{(m)}) \quad \propto \quad \exp\left\{ - \left(K_{mm} - 2\mathsf{k}^T(\mathsf{x}^{(m)})\mathsf{a}_j + \mathsf{a}_j^T \mathsf{K}\mathsf{a}_j + c_j \right) / s_j \right\}$$

$$\stackrel{\text{def}}{=} \quad \exp\{-f_j(\mathsf{x}^{(m)})\}, \tag{9}$$

where $\mathsf{k}(\mathsf{x}^{(m)})$ corresponds to the mth column (or row) of the Gram matrix $\mathsf{K} \stackrel{\text{def}}{=} \{K_{ij}\} \stackrel{\text{def}}{=} \{\phi(\mathsf{x}^{(i)})^T \phi(\mathsf{x}^{(j)})\} \in \mathbb{R}^{M \times M}$, $\mathsf{a}_j \in \mathbb{R}^M$ is the jth column of the matrix of the coefficients $\mathsf{A} \stackrel{\text{def}}{=} \{a_{mj}\} \in \mathbb{R}^{M \times |y|}$, and $c_j = (\mathsf{w}_j^{\perp})^T \mathsf{w}_j^{\perp} - s_j b_j$. Without loss of generality, we may assume that $\mathsf{c} = \{c_j\} \in \mathbb{R}^{|y|}$ is a free unconstrained parameter. Additionally, we will ensure positivity of the dispersions s_j by considering a construction constraint $s_j = \exp\{\tilde{s}_j\}$, where $\tilde{s}_j \in \mathbb{R}$.

Learning Optimal Parameters

First we will assume that the Gram matrix $\mathsf{K} \in \mathbb{R}^{M \times M}$ is *fixed* and *known* (which effectively corresponds to considering a fixed affinity matrix, see e.g. Dhillon et al. (2004)). Objective (1) should be optimized with respect to the log-dispersions $\tilde{s}_j \equiv \log(s_j)$, biases c_j, and coordinates $\mathsf{A} \in \mathbb{R}^{M \times |y|}$ in the space spanned by the feature vectors $\{\phi(\mathsf{x}^{(i)}) | i = 1, \ldots, M\}$. From (9) we get

$$\frac{\partial I(\mathsf{x}, y)}{\partial \mathsf{a}_j} \quad = \quad \frac{1}{s_j} \langle p(y_j|\mathsf{x})\,(\mathsf{k}(\mathsf{x}) - \mathsf{K}\mathsf{a}_j)\,\alpha_j(\mathsf{x}) \rangle_{\tilde{p}(\mathsf{x})} \in \mathbb{R}^M, \tag{10}$$

$$\frac{\partial I(\mathsf{x}, y)}{\partial \tilde{s}_j} \quad = \quad \frac{1}{2 s_j} \langle p(y_j|\mathsf{x}) f_j(\mathsf{x}) \alpha_j(\mathsf{x}) \rangle_{\tilde{p}(\mathsf{x})}, \tag{11}$$

where $\tilde{p}(\mathsf{x}) \propto \sum_{m-1}^{M} \delta(\mathsf{x} - \mathsf{x}^{(m)})$ is the empirical distribution. Analogously, we obtain

$$\partial I(\mathsf{x}, y)/\partial c_j = \langle \alpha_j(\mathsf{x}) \rangle_{\tilde{p}(\mathsf{x})}, \tag{12}$$

where the coefficients $\alpha_j(\mathsf{x})$ are given by (6). For a known Gram matrix $\mathsf{K} \in \mathbb{R}^{M \times M}$, the gradients $\partial I/\partial \mathsf{a}_j$, $\partial I/\partial \tilde{s}_j$, and $\partial I/\partial c_j$ given by expressions (10) – (12) may be used in numerical optimization for the model parameters. Note that the matrix multiplication in (10) is performed once for each a_j, so that the complexity of computing the gradient is $\sim O(M^2|y|)$ per iteration. We also note that one could potentially optimize (1) by applying the iterative Arimoto-Blahut algorithm for maximizing the channel capacity (see e.g. Cover and Thomas (1991)). However, for any given *constrained* encoder it is generally difficult to derive closed-form updates for the parameters of $p(y|\mathsf{x})$, which motivates a numerical optimization.

Learning Optimal Kernels

Since we presume that explicit computations in $\mathbb{R}^{|\phi|}$ are expensive, we cannot compute the Gram matrix by trivially applying its definition $\mathsf{K} = \{\phi(\mathsf{x}_i)^T \phi(\mathsf{x}_j)\}$. Instead, we may interpret scalar products in feature spaces as *kernel functions*

$$\phi(\mathsf{x}^{(i)})^T \phi(\mathsf{x}^{(j)}) = \mathcal{K}_{\Theta}(\mathsf{x}^{(i)}, \mathsf{x}^{(j)}; \Theta), \quad \forall \mathsf{x}^{(i)}, \mathsf{x}^{(j)} \in \mathcal{R}_{\mathsf{x}}, \tag{13}$$

where $\mathcal{K}_\Theta : \mathcal{R}_x \times \mathcal{R}_x \to \mathbb{R}$ satisfies Mercer's kernel properties (e.g. Scholkopf and Smola (2002)). We may now apply our *unsupervised* framework to implicitly learn the optimal nonlinear features by optimizing $I(x, y)$ with respect to the parameters Θ of the kernel function $\mathcal{K}_\Theta$. After some algebraic manipulations, we get

$$M \frac{\partial I(x, y)}{\partial \Theta} = \sum_{m=1}^{M} KL(p(y|x^{(m)}) \| p(y)) \sum_{k=1}^{|y|} \frac{\partial f_k(x^{(m)})}{\partial \Theta} p(y_k|x^{(m)})$$

$$- \sum_{m=1}^{M} \sum_{j=1}^{|y|} \frac{\partial f_j(x^{(m)})}{\partial \Theta} p(y_j|x^{(m)}) \log \frac{p(y_j|x^{(m)})}{p(y_j)} \quad (14)$$

where $f_k(x^{(m)})$ is given by (9). The computational complexity of computing the updates for Θ is $O(M|y|^2)$, where M is the number of training patterns and $|y|$ is the number of clusters (which is assumed to be small). Note that in contrast to spectral methods (see e.g. Shi and Malik (2000), Ng et al. (2001)) neither the objective (1) nor its gradients require inversion of the Gram matrix $\mathsf{K} \in \mathbb{R}^{M \times M}$ or computations of its eigenvalue decomposition.

In the special case of the radial basis function (RBF) kernels

$$\mathcal{K}_\beta(x^{(i)}, x^{(j)}) = \exp\{-\beta \| x^{(i)} - x^{(j)} \|^2\}, \quad (15)$$

the gradients of the encoder potentials are simply given by

$$\frac{\partial f_j(x^{(m)})}{\partial \beta} = \frac{1}{s_j} \left(\mathsf{a}_j^T \tilde{\mathsf{K}} \mathsf{a}_j - 2\tilde{\mathsf{k}}^T(x^{(m)}) \mathsf{a}_j \right), \quad (16)$$

where $\tilde{\mathsf{K}} \stackrel{\text{def}}{=} \{\tilde{K}_{ij}\} \stackrel{\text{def}}{=} K(x^{(i)}, x^{(j)})(1 - \delta(x^{(i)} - x^{(j)}))$, and δ is the Kronecker delta. By substituting (16) into the general expression (14), we obtain the gradient of the mutual information with respect to the RBF kernel parameters.

3 Demonstrations

We have empirically compared our kernelized information-theoretic clustering approach with Gaussian mixture, k-means, feature-space k-means, non-kernelized information-theoretic clustering (see Section 2.1), and a multi-class spectral clustering method optimizing the *normalized cuts*. We illustrate the methods on datasets that are particularly easy to visualize. Figure 1 shows a typical application of the methods to the spiral data, where $x_1(t) = t \cos(t)/4$, $x_2(t) = t \sin(t)/4$ correspond to different coordinates of $x \in \mathbb{R}^{|x|}$, $|x| = 2$, and $t \in [0, 3.(3)\pi]$. The kernel parameters β of the RBF-kernelized encoding distribution were initialized at $\beta_0 = 2.5$ and learned according to (16). The initial settings of the coefficients $\mathsf{A} \in \mathbb{R}^{M \times |y|}$ in the feature space were sampled from $\mathcal{N}_{A_{ij}}(0, 0.1)$. The log-variances $\tilde{s}_1, \dots, \tilde{s}_{|y|}$ were initialized at zeros. The encoder parameters A and $\{\tilde{s}_j | j = 1, \dots, |y|\}$ (along with the RBF kernel parameter β) were optimized by applying the scaled conjugate gradients. We found that Gaussian mixtures trained by maximizing the likelihood usually resulted in highly stochastic cluster allocations; additionally, they led to a large variation in cluster sizes. The Gaussian mixtures were initialized using k-means – other choices usually led to worse performance. We also see that the k-means effectively breaks, as the similarly clustered points lie close to each other in $\mathbb{R}^2$ (according to the L_2-norm), but the allocated clusters are *not* locally smooth in t. On the other hand, our method with the RBF-kernelized encoders typically led to locally smooth cluster allocations.

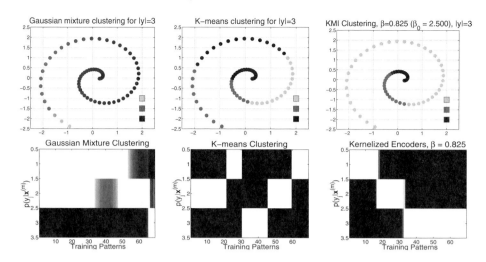

Figure 1: Cluster allocations (*top*) and the corresponding responsibilities (*bottom*) $p(y_j|\mathsf{x}^{(m)})$ for $|\mathsf{x}| = 2$, $|y| = 3$, $M = 70$ (the patterns are sorted to indicate local smoothness in the phase parameter). *Left:* Gaussian mixtures; *middle:* K-means; *right:* information-maximization for the (RBF-)kernelized encoder (the learned parameter $\beta \approx 0.825$). Light, medium, and dark-gray squares show the cluster colors corresponding to deterministic cluster allocations. The color intensity of each training point $\mathsf{x}^{(m)}$ is the average of the pure cluster intensities, weighted by the responsibilities $p(y_j|\mathsf{x}^{(m)})$. Nearly indistinguishable dark colors of the Gaussian mixture clustering indicate soft cluster assignments.

Figure 2 shows typical results for spatially translated letters with $|\mathsf{x}| = 2$, $M = 150$, and $|y| = 2$ (or $|y| = 3$), where we compare Gaussian mixture, feature-space k-means, the spectral method of Ng et al. (2001), and our information-theoretic clustering method. The initializations followed the same procedure as the previous experiment. The results produced by our kernelized infomax method were generally stable under different initializations, provided that β_0 was not too large or too small. In contrast to Gaussian mixture, spectral, and feature-space k-means clustering, the clusters produced by kernelized infomax for the cases considered are arguably more anthropomorphically appealing. Note that feature-space k-means, as well as the spectral method, presume that the kernel matrix $\mathsf{K} \in \mathbb{R}^{M \times M}$ is fixed and known (in the latter case, the Gram matrix defines the edge weights of the graph). For illustration purposes, we show the results for the fixed Gram matrices with kernel parameters β set to the initial values $\beta_0 = 1$ or the learned values $\beta \approx 0.604$ of the kernelized infomax method for $|y| = 2$. One may potentially improve the performance of these methods by running the algorithms several times (with different kernel parameters β), and choosing β which results in tightest clusters (Ng et al. (2001)). We were indeed able to apply the spectral method to obtain clusters for TA and T (for $\beta \approx 1.1$). While being useful in some situations, the procedure generally requires multiple runs. In contrast, the kernelized infomax method typically resulted in meaningful cluster allocations (TT and A) after a single run of the algorithm (see Figure 2 (*c*)), with the results qualitatively consistent under a variety of initializations.

Additionally, we note that in situations when we used simpler encoder models (see expression (3)) or did not adapt parameters of the kernel functions, the extracted clusters were often more intuitive than those produced by rival methods, but inferior

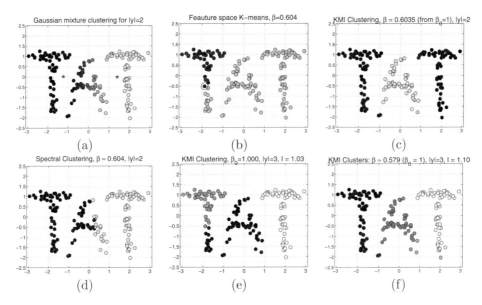

Figure 2: Learning cluster allocations for $|y| = 2$ and $|y| = 3$. Where appropriate, the stars show the cluster centers. *(a)* two-component Gaussian mixture trained by the EM algorithm; *(b)* feature-space k-means with $\beta = 1.0$ and $\beta \approx 0.604$ (the only pattern clustered differently (under identical initializations) is shown by ⊚); *(c)* kernelized infomax clustering for $|y| = 2$ (the inverse variance β of the RBF kernel varied from $\beta_0 = 1$ (at the initialization) to $\beta \approx 0.604$ after convergence); *(d)* spectral clustering for $|y| = 2$ and $\beta \approx 0.604$; *(e)* kernelized infomax clustering for $|y| = 3$ with a *fixed* Gram matrix; *(f)* kernelized infomax clustering for $|y| = 3$ started at $\beta_0 = 1$ and reaching $\beta \approx 0.579$ after convergence.

to the ones produced by (7) with the optimal learned β. Our results suggest that by learning kernel parameters we may often obtain higher values of the objective $I(\mathsf{x}, y)$, as well as more appealing cluster labeling (e.g. for the examples shown on Figure 2 *(e)*, *(f)* we get $I(\mathsf{x}, y) \approx 1.03$ and $I(\mathsf{x}, y) \approx 1.10$ respectively). Undoubtedly, a careful choice of the kernel function could potentially lead to an even better visualization of the locally smooth, non-degenerate structure.

4   Discussion

The proposed information-theoretic clustering framework is fundamentally different from the generative latent variable clustering approaches. Instead of explicitly parameterizing the data-generating process, we impose constraints on the *encoder* distributions, transforming the clustering problem to learning optimal discrete encodings of the unlabeled data. Many possible parameterizations of such distributions may potentially be considered. Here we discussed one such choice, which implicitly utilizes projections of the data to high-dimensional feature spaces.

Our method suggests a formal information-theoretic procedure for learning optimal cluster allocations. One potential disadvantage of the method is a potentially large number of local optima; however, our empirical results suggest that the method is stable under different initializations, provided that the initial variances are sufficiently large. Moreover, the results suggest that in the cases considered the method favorably compares with the common generative clustering techniques, k-means, feature-space k-means, and the variants of the method which do not use nonlinearities or do not learn parameters of kernel functions.

A number of interesting interpretations of clustering approaches in feature spaces are possible. Recently, it has been shown (Bach and Jordan (2003); Dhillon et al. (2004)) that spectral clustering methods optimizing normalized cuts (Shi and Malik (2000); Ng et al. (2001)) may be viewed as a form of weighted feature-space k-means, for a specific fixed similarity matrix. We are currently relating our method to the common spectral clustering approaches and a form of annealed weighted feature-space k-means. We stress, however, that our information-maximizing framework suggests a principled way of learning optimal similarity matrices by adapting parameters of the kernel functions. Additionally, our method does not require computations of eigenvalues of the similarity matrix, which may be particularly beneficial for large datasets. Finally, we expect that the proper information-theoretic interpretation of the encoder framework may facilitate extensions of the information-theoretic clustering method to richer families of encoder distributions.

References

Agakov, F. V. and Barber, D. (2006). Auxiliary Variational Information Maximization for Dimensionality Reduction. In *Proceedings of the PASCAL Workshop on Subspace, Latent Structure and Feature Selection Techniques*. Springer. To appear.

Bach, F. R. and Jordan, M. I. (2003). Learning spectral clustering. In *NIPS*. MIT Press.

Barber, D. and Agakov, F. V. (2003). The IM Algorithm: A Variational Approach to Information Maximization. In *NIPS*. MIT Press.

Brunel, N. and Nadal, J.-P. (1998). Mutual Information, Fisher Information and Population Coding. *Neural Computation*, 10:1731–1757.

Chechik, G. and Tishby, N. (2002). Extracting relevant structures with side information. In *NIPS*, volume 15. MIT Press.

Cover, T. M. and Thomas, J. A. (1991). *Elements of Information Theory*. Wiley, NY.

Dhillon, I. S. and Guan, Y. (2003). Information Theoretic Clustering of Sparse Co-Occurrence Data. In *Proceedings of the 3rd IEEE International Conf. on Data Mining*.

Dhillon, I. S., Guan, Y., and Kulis, B. (2004). Kernel k-means, Spectral Clustering and Normalized Cuts. In *KDD*. ACM.

Fisher, J. W. and Principe, J. C. (1998). A methodology for information theoretic feature extraction. In *Proc. of the IEEE International Joint Conference on Neural Networks*.

Linsker, R. (1988). Towards an Organizing Principle for a Layered Perceptual Network. In *Advances in Neural Information Processing Systems*. American Institute of Physics.

Ng, A. Y., Jordan, M., and Weiss, Y. (2001). On spectral clustering: Analysis and an algorithm. In *NIPS*, volume 14. MIT Press.

Scholkopf, B. and Smola, A. (2002). *Learning with Kernels*. MIT Press.

Shi, J. and Malik, J. (2000). Normalized Cuts and Image Segmentation. *IEEE Transactions on Pattern Analysis and Machine Intelligence*, 22(8):888–905.

Tishby, N., Pereira, F. C., and Bialek, W. (1999). The information bottleneck method. In *Proceedings of the 37-th Annual Allerton Conference on Communication, Control and Computing*. Kluwer Academic Publishers.

Torkkola, K. and Campbell, W. M. (2000). Mutual Information in Learning Feature Transformations. In *ICML*. Morgan Kaufmann.

Large-scale biophysical parameter estimation in single neurons via constrained linear regression

Misha B. Ahrens[*], **Quentin J.M. Huys**[*], **Liam Paninski**
Gatsby Computational Neuroscience Unit
University College London
{ahrens, qhuys, liam}@gatsby.ucl.ac.uk

Abstract

Our understanding of the input-output function of single cells has been substantially advanced by biophysically accurate multi-compartmental models. The large number of parameters needing hand tuning in these models has, however, somewhat hampered their applicability and interpretability. Here we propose a simple and well-founded method for automatic estimation of many of these key parameters: 1) the spatial distribution of channel densities on the cell's membrane; 2) the spatiotemporal pattern of synaptic input; 3) the channels' reversal potentials; 4) the intercompartmental conductances; and 5) the noise level in each compartment. We assume experimental access to: a) the spatiotemporal voltage signal in the dendrite (or some contiguous subpart thereof, e.g. via voltage sensitive imaging techniques), b) an approximate kinetic description of the channels and synapses present in each compartment, and c) the morphology of the part of the neuron under investigation. The key observation is that, given data a)-c), all of the parameters 1)-4) may be simultaneously inferred by a version of constrained linear regression; this regression, in turn, is efficiently solved using standard algorithms, without any "local minima" problems despite the large number of parameters and complex dynamics. The noise level 5) may also be estimated by standard techniques. We demonstrate the method's accuracy on several model datasets, and describe techniques for quantifying the uncertainty in our estimates.

1 Introduction

The usual tradeoff in parameter estimation for single neuron models is between realism and tractability. Typically, the more biophysical accuracy one tries to inject into the model, the harder the computational problem of fitting the model's parameters becomes, as the number of (nonlinearly interacting) parameters increases (sometimes even into the thousands, in the case of complex multicompartmental models).

---

[*]These authors contributed equally. Support contributed by the Gatsby Charitable Foundation (LP, MA), a Royal Society International Fellowship (LP), the BIBA consortium and the UCL School of Medicine (QH). We are indebted to P. Dayan, M. Häusser, M. London, A. Roth, and S. Roweis for helpful and interesting discussions, and to R. Wood for channel definitions.

Previous authors have noted the difficulties of this large-scale, simultaneous parameter estimation problem, which are due both to the highly nonlinear nature of the "cost functions" minimized (e.g., the percentage of correctly-predicted spike times [1]) and the abundance of local minima on the very large-dimensional allowed parameter space [2, 3].

Here we present a method that is both computationally tractable and biophysically detailed. Our goal is to simultaneously infer the following dendritic parameters: 1) the spatial distribution of channel densities on the cell's membrane; 2) the spatiotemporal pattern of synaptic input; 3) the channels' reversal potentials; 4) the intercompartmental conductances; and 5) the noise level in each compartment. Achieving this somewhat ambitious goal comes at a price: our method assumes that the experimenter a) knows the geometry of the cell, b) has a good understanding of the kinetics of the channels present in each compartment, and c) most importantly, is able to observe the spatiotemporal voltage signal on the dendritic tree, or at least a fraction thereof (e.g. by voltage-sensitive imaging methods; in electrotonically compact cells, single electrode recordings can be used).

The key to the proposed method is to recognise that, when we condition on data a)-c), the dynamics governing this observed spatiotemporal voltage signal become *linear* in the parameters we are seeking to estimate (even though the system itself may behave highly nonlinearly), so that the parameter estimation can be recast into a simple constrained linear regression problem (see also [4, 5]). This implies, somewhat counterintuitively, that optimizing the likelihood of the parameters in this setting is a *convex* problem, with no non-global local extrema. Moreover, linearly constrained quadratic optimization is an extremely well-studied problem, with many efficient algorithms available. We give examples of the resulting methods successfully applied to several types of model data below. In addition, we discuss methods for incorporating prior knowledge and analyzing uncertainty in our estimates, again basing our techniques on the well-founded probabilistic regression framework.

2 Methods

Biophysically accurate models of single cells are typically formulated compartmentally – a set of first-order coupled differential equations that form a spatially discrete approximation to the cable equations. Modeling the cell under investigation in this discretized manner, a typical equation describing the voltage in compartment x is

$$C_x dV_x(t) = \left(\sum_i a_{i,x} J_{i,x}(t) + I_x(t) \right) dt + \sigma_x dN_{x,t}. \tag{1}$$

Here $\sigma_x N_{x,t}$ is evolution (current) noise and $I_x(t)$ is externally injected current. Dropping the subscript x where possible, the terms $a_i \cdot J_i(t)$ represent currents due to:

1. voltage mismatch in neighbouring compartments, $f_{x,y}(V_y(t) - V_x(t))$,
2. synaptic input, $g_s(t)(E_s - V(t))$,
3. membrane channels, active (voltage-dependent) or passive, $\bar{g}_j g_j(t)(E_j - V(t))$.

Here a_i are parameters to be inferred:

1. the intercompartmental conductances $f_{x,y}$,
2. the spatiotemporal input from synapse s, $u_s(t)$, from which $g_s(t)$ is obtained by

$$dg_s(t)/dt = -g_s(t)/\tau_s + u_s(t), \tag{2}$$

a linear convolution operation (the synaptic kinetic parameter τ_s is assumed known) which may be written in matrix notation $\mathbf{g}_s = \mathbf{Ku}$.

3. the ion channel concentrations $\bar{g}_j$. The open probabilities of channel j, $g_j(t)$, are obtained from the *channel kinetics*, which are assumed to evolve deterministically, with a known dependence on V, as in the Hodgkin-Huxley model, $g_{Na} = m^3 h$,

$$\tau_m dm(t)/dt = m_\infty(V) - m, \tag{3}$$

and similarly for h. Again, we emphasize that the kinetic parameters τ_m and $m_\infty(V)$ are assumed known; only the inhomogeneous concentrations are unknown. (For passive channels g_j is taken constant and independent of voltage.)

The parameters 1-3 are relative to membrane capacitance C_x.[1]

When modeling the dynamics of a single neuron according to (1), the voltage $V(t)$ and channel kinetics $g_j(t)$ are typically evolved in parallel, according to the injected current $I(t)$ and synaptic inputs $u_s(t)$. Suppose, on the other hand, that we have observed the voltage $V_x(t)$ in each compartment. Since we have assumed we also know the channel kinetics (equation 3), the synaptic kinetics (equation 2) and the reversal potentials E_j of the channels present in each compartment, we may decouple the equations and determine the open probabilities $g_{j,x}(t)$ for $t \in [0, T]$. This, in turn, implies that the currents $J_{i,x}(t)$ and voltage differentials $\dot{V}_x(t)$ are all known, and we may interpret equation 1 as a *regression equation*, linear in the unknown parameters a_i, instead of an evolution equation. This is the key observation of this work.

Thus we can use linear regression methods to simultaneously infer optimal values of the parameters $\{\bar{g}_{j,x}, u_{s,x}(t), f_{x,y}\}$[2]. More precisely, rewrite equation (1) in matrix form, $\dot{\mathbf{V}} = \mathbf{Ma} + \sigma\eta$, where each column of the matrix $\mathbf{M}$ is composed of one of the known currents $\{J_i(t), t \in [0, T]\}$ (with T the length of the experiment) and the column vectors $\dot{\mathbf{V}}$, $\mathbf{a}$, and η are defined in the obvious way. Then

$$\hat{\mathbf{a}}_{opt} = \arg\min_{\mathbf{a}} \|\dot{\mathbf{V}} - \mathbf{Ma}\|_2^2. \tag{4}$$

In addition, since on physical grounds the channel concentrations, synaptic input, and conductances must be non-negative, we require our solution $a_i \geq 0$. The resulting linearly-constrained quadratic optimization problem has no local minima (due to the convexity of the objective function and of the domain $g_i \geq 0$), and allows quadratic programming (QP) tools (e.g., quadprog.m in Matlab) to be employed for highly efficient optimization.

Quadratic programming tactics: As emphasized above, the dimension d of the parameter space to be optimized over in this application is quite large ($d \sim N_{comp}(TN_{syn} + N_{chan})$, with N denoting the number of compartments, synapse types, and membrane channel types respectively). While our problem is convex, and therefore tractable in the sense of having no nonglobal local optima, the time-complexity of QP, implemented naively, is $\mathcal{O}(d^3)$, which is too slow for our purposes.

Fortunately, the correlational structure of the parameters allows us to perform this optimization more efficiently, by several natural decompositions: in particular, given the spatiotemporal voltage signal $V_x(t)$, parameters which are distant in space (e.g., the densities of channels in widely-separated compartments) and time (i.e., the synaptic input $u_{s,x}(t)$ for $t = t_i$ and t_j with $|t_i - t_j|$ large) may be optimized independently. This amounts to a kind of "coordinate descent" algorithm, in which we decompose our parameter set into a set of (not necessarily disjoint) subsets, and iteratively optimize the parameters in each subset

---

[1] Note that C_x is the proportionality constant between the externally injected electrode current and $\frac{dV}{dt}$. It is linear in the data and can be included with the other parameters a_i in the joint estimation.

[2] In the case that the reversal potentials E_j are unknown as well, we may estimate these terms by separating the term $\bar{g}_j g_j(t)(V(t) - E_j)$ into $\bar{g}_j g_j(t)V(t)$ and $(\bar{g}_j E_j)g_j(t)$, thereby increasing the number of parameters in the regression by one per channel; E_j is then set to $(\bar{g}_j E_j)/\bar{g}_j$.

while holding all the other parameters fixed. (The quadratic nature of the original problem guarantees that each of these subset problems will be quadratic, with no local minima.) Empirically, we found that this decomposition / sequential optimization approach reduced the computation time from $\mathcal{O}(d^3)$ to near $\mathcal{O}(d)$.

2.1 The probabilistic framework

If we assume the noise $N_{x,t}$ is Gaussian and white, then the mean-square regression solution for $\mathbf{a}$ described above coincides exactly with the (constrained) maximum likelihood estimate, $\hat{\mathbf{a}}_{ML} = \arg\min_{\mathbf{a}} \|\dot{\mathbf{V}} - \mathbf{Ma}\|_2^2 / 2\sigma^2$. (The noise scale σ may also be estimated via maximum likelihood.) This suggests several straightforward likelihood-based techniques for representing the uncertainty in our estimates.

Posterior confidence intervals: The assumption of Gaussian noise implies that the posterior distribution of the parameters $\mathbf{a}$ is of the form $p(\mathbf{a}|\mathbf{V}) = \frac{1}{Z} p(\mathbf{a}) G_{\mu,\Sigma}(\mathbf{a})$, with Z a normalizing constant, the prior $p(\mathbf{a})$ supported on $a_i \geq 0$, and the mean and covariance of the likelihood Gaussian $G(\mathbf{a})$ given by $\mu = (\mathbf{M}^T\mathbf{M})^{-1}\mathbf{M}^T\dot{\mathbf{V}}$ and $\Sigma^{-1} = \mathbf{M}^T\mathbf{M}/\sigma^2$. We will assume a flat prior distribution $p(\mathbf{a})$ (that is, no prior knowledge) on the non-synaptic parameters $\{\bar{g}_{j,x}, f_{x,y}\}$ (although clearly non-flat priors can be easily incorporated here [6]); for the synaptic parameters $u_{s,x}(t)$ it will be convenient to use a product-of-exponentials prior, $p(\mathbf{u}) = \prod_i \lambda_i \exp(-\lambda_i u_i)$. In each case, computing confidence intervals for a_i reduces to computing moments of multidimensional Gaussian distributions, truncated to $a_i \geq 0$.

We use importance sampling methods [7] to compute these moments for the channel parameters. Sampling from high-dimensional truncated Gaussians via sample-reject is inefficient (since samples from the non-truncated Gaussian – call this distribution $p^*(\mathbf{a}|\mathbf{V})$ – may violate the constraint $a_i \geq 0$ with high probability). Therefore we sample instead from a proposal density $q(\mathbf{a})$ with support on $a_i \geq 0$ (specifically, a product of univariate truncated Gaussians with mean a_i and appropriate variance) and evaluate the second moments around $\mathbf{a}_{ML}$ by

$$\mathbb{E}[(a_i - a_{MLi})^2 | \mathbf{V}] \approx \frac{1}{Z} \sum_{n=1}^{N} \frac{p^*(\mathbf{a}^n|\mathbf{V})}{q(\mathbf{a}^n)}(a_i^n - a_{MLi})^2 \qquad \text{where} \qquad Z = \sum_{n=1}^{N} \frac{p^*(\mathbf{a}^n|\mathbf{V})}{q(\mathbf{a}^n)}. \tag{5}$$

Hessian Principal Components Analysis: The procedure described above allows us to quantify the uncertainty of individual estimated parameters a_i. We are also interested in the uncertainty of our estimates in a joint sense (e.g., in the posterior covariance instead of just the individual variances). The negative Hessian of the loglikelihood function, $\mathbf{A} \sim \mathbf{M}^T\mathbf{M}$, contains a great deal of this information, which may be extracted via a kind of principal components analysis: the eigenvectors of $\mathbf{A}$ corresponding to the greatest eigenvalues tell us in which directions the model is most strongly constrained by the data, while low eigenvalues correspond to directions in which the likelihood changes relatively slowly, e.g. channels whose corresponding currents are highly correlated (and therefore approximately interchangeable). These ideas will be illustrated in section 3.4.

3 Results

To test the validity, efficiency and accuracy of the proposed method we apply it to model data of varying complexity.

3.1 Inferring channel conductances in a multicompartmental model

We take a simple 14-compartment model neuron, described by

$$C_x \frac{dV_x}{dt} = \sum_{c=1}^{N_{chan}} \bar{g}_c g_c(V_x, t)(E_c - V_x(t)) + \sum_y f_{x,y} \cdot (V_y(t) - V_x(t)) + I_x(t) + \sigma_x dN_{x,t};$$

recall $f_{x,y}$ are the intercompartmental conductances, $g_c(V, t)$ is channel c's conductance state given the voltage history up to time t, and $\bar{g}_c$ is the channel concentration. We minimize a vectorized expression as above (equation 4). On biophysical grounds we require $f_{x,y} = f_{y,x}$; we enforce this (linear) constraint by only including one parameter for each connected pair of compartments (x, y). In this case the true channel kinetics were of standard Hodgkin-Huxley form (Na$^+$, K$^+$ and leak), with inhomogeneous densities (figure 1). To test the selectivity of the estimation procedure, we fitted $N_{chan} = 8$ candidate channels from [8, 9, 10] (five of which were absent in the true model cell). Figure 1 shows the performance of the inference; despite the fact that we used only 20 ms of model data, the last 7 ms of which were used for the actual fitting (the first 13 ms were used to evolve the random initial conditions to an approximately correct value), the fit is near perfect in the $\sigma = 0$ case, with vanishingly small errorbars. The concentrations of the five channels that were not present when generating the data were set to approximately zero, as desired (data not shown). The lower panels demonstrate the robustness of the methods on highly noisy (large σ) data, in which case the estimated errorbars become significant, but the performance degrades only slightly.

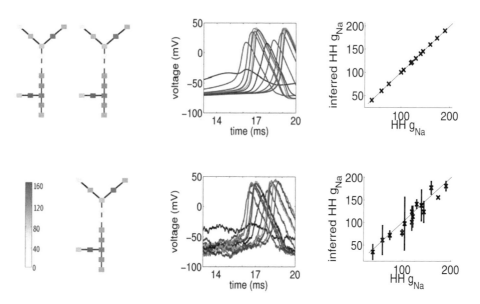

Figure 1: Top panels: $\sigma = 0$. 14 compartment model neuron, Na$^+$ channel concentration indicated by grey scale; estimated Na$^+$ channel concentrations in the noiseless case; observed voltage traces (one per compartment); estimated concentrations. Bottom panels: σ large. Na$^+$ channel concentration legend, values relative to C_m (e.g. in mS/cm^2 if $C_m = 1\mu F/cm^2$); estimated Na$^+$ concentrations in the noisy case; noisy voltage traces; estimated channel concentrations. K$^+$ channel concentrations and intercompartmental conductances $f_{x,y}$ not shown (similar performance).

3.2 Inferring synaptic input in a passive model

Next we simulated a single-compartment, leaky neuron (i.e., no voltage-sensitive membrane channels) with synaptic input from three synapses, two excitatory (glutamatertic;

$\tau = 3$ ms, $E = 0$ mV) and one inhibitory (GABA$_\text{A}$; $\tau = 5$ ms, $E = -75$ mV). When we attempted to estimate the synaptic input $u_s(t)$ via the ML estimator described above (figure 2, left), we observe an *overfitting* phenomenon: the current noise due to N_t is being "explained" by competing balanced excitatory and inhibitory synaptic inputs. This overfitting is unsurprising, given that we are modeling a T-dimensional observation, $\dot{\mathbf{V}}$, with $2T$ regressor variables, $u_-(t)$ and $u_+(t), 0 < t < T$ (indeed, overfitting is much less apparent in the case that only one synapse is modeled, where no balance of excitation and inhibition is possible; data not shown).

Once again, we may make use of well-known techniques from the regression literature to solve this problem: in this case, we need to regularize our estimated synaptic parameters. Instead of maximizing the likelihood, $\mathbf{u}_{ML}$, we maximize the *posterior* likelihood

$$\hat{\mathbf{u}}_{MAP} = \arg\min_{\mathbf{u}} \frac{1}{2\sigma^2} \|\dot{\mathbf{V}} - \mathbf{MKu}\|_2^2 + \lambda\mathbf{u} \cdot \mathbf{n} \qquad \text{with} \quad u_t \geq 0 \quad \forall t, \qquad (6)$$

where $\mathbf{n}$ is a vector of ones and λ is the Lagrange multiplier for the regularizer, or equivalently parametrizes the exponential prior distribution over $u(t)$. As mentioned above, this maximum *a posteriori* (MAP) estimate corresponds to a product exponential prior on the synaptic input u_t; the multiplier λ may be chosen as the expected synaptic input per unit time. It is well known that this type of prior has a sparsening effect, shrinking small values of $u_{ML}(t)$ to zero. This is visible in figure 2 (right); we see that the small, noise-matching synaptic activity is effectively suppressed, permitting much more accurate detection of the true input spike timing.

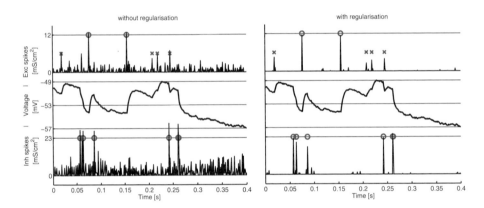

Figure 2: Inferring synaptic inputs to a passive membrane. Top traces: excitatory inputs; bottom: inhibitory inputs; middle: the resulting voltage trace. Left panels: synaptic inputs inferred by ML; right: MAP estimates under the exponential (shrinkage) prior. Note the overfitting by the ML estimate (left) and the higher accuracy under the MAP estimate (right); in particular note that the two excitatory synapses of differing magnitudes may easily be distinguished.

3.3 Inferring synaptic input and channel distribution in an active model

The optimization is, as mentioned earlier, jointly convex in both channel densities and synaptic input. We illustrate the simultaneous inference of channel densities and synaptic inputs in a single compartment, writing the model as:

$$\frac{dV}{dt} = \sum_{c=1}^{N_{chan}} \bar{g}_c g_c(V,t)(V_c - V(t)) + \sum_{s=1}^{S} g_s(t)(V_s - V(t)) + \sigma dN(t), \qquad (7)$$

with the same channels and synapse types as above. The combination of leak conductance and inhibitory synaptic input leads to very small eigenvalues in $\mathbf{A}$ and slow convergence when applying the above decomposition; thus, to speed convergence here we coarsened the time resolution of the synaptic input from 0.1 ms to 0.2 ms. Figure 3 demonstrates the accuracy of the results.

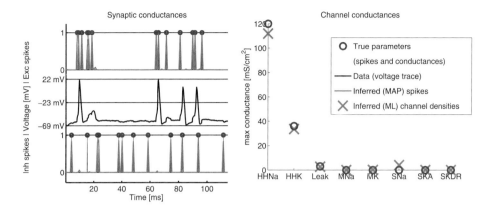

Figure 3: Joint inference of synaptic input and channel densities. The true parameters are in blue, the inferred parameters in red. The top left panel shows the excitatory synaptic input, the middle left panel the voltage trace (the only data) and the bottom left traces the inhibitory synaptic input. The right panel shows the true and inferred channel densities; channels are the same as in 3.1.

3.4 Eigenvector analysis for a single-compartment model

Finally, as discussed above, the eigenvectors ("principal components") of the loglikelihood Hessian $\mathbf{A}$ carry significant information about the dependence and redundancy of the parameters under study here. An example is given in figure 4; for simplicity, we restrict our attention again to the single-compartment case. In the leftmost panels, we see that the direction $\mathbf{a}_{most}$ most highly-constrained by the data – the eigenvector corresponding to the largest eigenvalue of $\mathbf{A}$ – turns out to have the intuitive form of the balance between Na^+ and K^+ channels. When we perturb this balance slightly (that is, when we shift the model parameters slightly along this direction in parameter space, $\mathbf{a}_{ML} \rightarrow \mathbf{a}_{ML} + \epsilon \mathbf{a}_{most}$), the cell's behavior changes dramatically. Conversely, the least-sensitive direction, $\mathbf{a}_{least}$, corresponds roughly to the balance between the concentrations of two Na^+ channels with similar kinetics, and moving in this direction in parameter space ($\mathbf{a}_{ML} \rightarrow \mathbf{a}_{ML} + \epsilon \mathbf{a}_{least}$) has a negligible effect on the model's dynamical behavior.

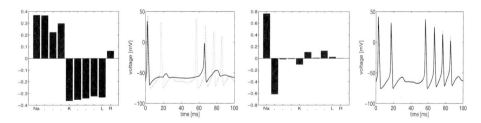

Figure 4: Eigenvectors of $\mathbf{A}$ corresponding to largest ($\mathbf{a}_{most}$, left) and smallest ($\mathbf{a}_{least}$, right) eigenvalues, and voltage traces of the model neuron after equal sized perturbations by both (solid line: perturbed model; dotted line: original model). The first four parameters are the concentrations of four Na^+ channels (the first two of which are in fact the same Hodgkin-Huxley channel, but with slightly different kinetic parameters); the next four of K^+ channels; the next of the leak channel; the last of $1/C$.

4   Discussion and future work

We have developed a probabilistic regression framework for estimation of biophysical single neuron properties and synaptic input. This framework leads directly to efficient, globally-convergent algorithms for determining these parameters, and also to well-founded methods for analyzing the uncertainty of the estimates. We believe this is a key first step towards applying these techniques in detailed, quantitative studies of dendritic input and processing *in vitro* and *in vivo*. However, some important caveats – and directions for necessary future work – should be emphasized.

Observation noise: While we have explicitly allowed current noise in our main evolution equation (1) (and experimented with a variety of other current- and conductance-noise terms; data not shown), we have assumed that the resulting voltage $V(t)$ is observed noiselessly, with sufficiently high sampling rates. This is a reasonable assumption when voltage is recorded directly, via patch-clamp methods. However, while voltage-sensitive imaging techniques have seen dramatic improvements over the last few years (and will continue to do so in the near future), currently these methods still suffer from relatively low signal-to-noise ratios and spatiotemporal sampling rates. While the procedure proved to be robust to low-level noise of various forms (data not shown), it will be important to relax the noiseless-observation assumption, most likely by adapting standard techniques from the hidden Markov model signal processing literature [11].

Hidden branches: Current imaging and dye technologies allow for the monitoring of only a fraction of a dendritic tree; therefore our focus will be on estimating the properties of these sub-structures. Furthermore, these dyes diffuse very slowly and may miss small branches of dendrites, thereby effectively creating unobserved current sources.

Misspecified channel kinetics and channels with chemical dependence: Channels dependent on unobserved variables (e.g., Ca^{++}-dependent K^{+} channels), have not been included in the model. The techniques described here may thus be applied unmodified to experimental data for which such channels have been blocked pharmacologically. However, we should note that our methods extend directly to the case where simultaneous access to voltage and calcium signals is possible; more generally, one could develop a semi-realistic model of calcium concentration, and optimize over the parameters of this model as well. We have discussed in some detail (e.g. figure 1) the effect of misspecifications of voltage-dependent channel kinetics and how the most relevant channels may be selected by supplying sufficiently rich "channel libraries". Such libraries can also contain several "copies" of the same channel, with one or more systematically varying parameters, thus allowing for a limited search in the nonlinear space of channel kinetics. Finally, in our discussion of "equivalence classes" of channels (figure 4), we illustrate how eigenvector analysis of our objective function allows for insights into the joint behaviour of channels.

References

[1] Jolivet, Lewis, and Gerstner, 2004. J. Neurophysiol., 92, 959-976.

[2] Vanier and Bower, 1999. J. Comput. Neurosci., 7(2), 149-171.

[3] Goldman, Golowasch, Marder and Abbott, 2001. J. Neurosci., 21(14), 5229-5238.

[4] Wood, Gurney and Wilson, 2004. Neurocomputing, 58-60, 1109-1116.

[5] Morse, Davison and Hines, 2001. Soc. Neurosci. Abs., 606.5.

[6] Baldi, Vanier and Bower, 1998. J. Comp. Neurosci., 5(3), 285-314.

[7] Press et al., 1992. Numerical Recipes in C, CUP.

[8] Hodgkin and Huxley, 1952. J. Physiol., 117.

[9] Poirazi, Brannon and Mel, 2003. Neuron, 37(6), 977-87.

[10] Mainen, Joerges, Huguenard, and Sejnowski, 1995. Neuron, 15(6), 1427-39.

[11] Rabiner, 1989. Proc. IEEE, 77(2), 257-286.

Maximum Margin Semi-Supervised Learning for Structured Variables

Y. Altun, D. McAllester
TTI at Chicago
Chicago, IL 60637
altun,mcallester@tti-c.org

M. Belkin
Department of Computer Science
University of Chicago
Chicago, IL 60637
misha@cs.uchicago.edu

Abstract

Many real-world classification problems involve the prediction of multiple inter-dependent variables forming some structural dependency. Recent progress in machine learning has mainly focused on supervised classification of such structured variables. In this paper, we investigate structured classification in a semi-supervised setting. We present a discriminative approach that utilizes the intrinsic geometry of input patterns revealed by unlabeled data points and we derive a maximum-margin formulation of semi-supervised learning for structured variables. Unlike transductive algorithms, our formulation naturally extends to new test points.

1 Introduction

Discriminative methods, such as Boosting and Support Vector Machines have significantly advanced the state of the art for classification. However, traditionally these methods do not exploit dependencies between class labels where more than one label is predicted. Many real-world classification problems, on the other hand, involve sequential or structural dependencies between multiple labels. For example labeling the words in a sentence with their part-of-speech tags involves sequential dependency between part-of-speech tags; finding the parse tree of a sentence involves a structural dependency among the labels in the parse tree. Recently, there has been a growing interest in generalizing kernel methods to predict structured and inter-dependent variables in a supervised learning setting, such as dual perceptron [7], SVMs [2, 15, 14] and kernel logistic regression [1, 11]. These techniques combine the efficiency of dynamic programming methods with the advantages of the state-of-the-art learning methods. In this paper, we investigate classification of structured objects in a semi-supervised setting.

The goal of semi-supervised learning is to leverage the learning process from a small sample of labeled inputs with a large sample of unlabeled data. This idea has recently attracted a considerable amount of interest due to ubiquity of unlabeled data. In many applications from data mining to speech recognition it is easy to produce large amounts of unlabeled data, while labeling is often manual and expensive. This is also the case for many structured classification problems. A variety of methods ranging from Naive Bayes [12], Cotraining [4], to Transductive SVM [9] to Cluster Kernels [6] and graph-based approaches [3] and references therein, have been proposed. The intuition behind many of these methods is that the classification/regression function should be smooth with respect to the geometry of the data, i. e. the labels of two inputs x and $\bar{x}$ are likely to be the same if x and $\bar{x}$ are similar. This idea is often represented as the *cluster assumption* or the *manifold assumption*. The unlabeled points reveal the intrinsic structure, which is then utilized by the classification algorithm. A discriminative approach to semi-supervised learning was developed by Belkin, Sindhwani and Niyogi [3, 13], where the Laplacian operator associated with unlabeled data is used as an additional penalty (regularizer) on the space of functions in a Reproducing Kernel Hilbert Space. The additional regularization from the unlabeled data can be represented as a new kernel — a "graph regularized" kernel.

In this paper, building on [3, 13], we present a discriminative semi-supervised learning formulation for problems that involve structured and inter-dependent outputs and give experimental results on max-margin semi-supervised structured classification using graph-regularized kernels. The solution of the optimization problem that utilizes both labeled and unlabeled data is a linear combination of the graph regularized kernel evaluated at the *parts* of the *labeled inputs only*, leading to a large reduction in the number of parameters. It is important to note that our classification function is defined on all input points whereas some previous work is only defined for the input points in the (labeled and unlabeled) training sample, as they use standard graph kernels, which are restricted to in-sample data points by definition.

There is an the extensive literature on semi-supervised learning and the growing number of studies on learning structured and inter-dependent variables. Delaleau et. al. [8] propose a semi-supervised learning method for standard classification that extends to out-of-sample points. Brefeld et. al. [5] is one of the first studies investigating semi-supervised structured learning problem in a discriminative framework. The most relevant previous work is the transductive structured learning proposed by Lafferty et. al. [11].

2 Supervised Learning for Structured Variables

In structured learning, the goal is to learn a mapping $h : \mathcal{X} \rightarrow \mathcal{Y}$ from *structured* inputs to *structured* response values, where the inputs and response values form a dependency structure. For each input x, there is a set of feasible outputs, $\mathcal{Y}(x) \subseteq \mathcal{Y}$. For simplicity, let us assume that $\mathcal{Y}(x)$ is finite for all $x \in \mathcal{X}$, which is the case in many real world problems and in all our examples. We denote the set of feasible input-output pairs by $\mathcal{Z} \subseteq \mathcal{X} \times \mathcal{Y}$.

It is common to construct a discriminant function $F : \mathcal{Z} \rightarrow \Re$ which maps the feasible input-output pairs to a compatibility score of the pair. To make a prediction for x, this score is maximized over the set of feasible outputs,

$$h(x) = \operatorname*{argmax}_{y \in \mathcal{Y}(x)} F(x, y). \tag{1}$$

The score of an $\langle x, y \rangle$ pair is computed from local fragments, or "parts", of $\langle x, y \rangle$. In Markov random fields, x is a graph, y is a labeling of the nodes of x and a local fragment (a part) of $\langle x, y \rangle$ is a clique in x and its labeling y. In parsing with probabilistic context free grammars, a local fragment (a part) of $\langle x, y \rangle$ consist of a branch of the tree y, where a branch is an internal node in y together with its children, plus all pairs of a leaf node in y with the word in x labeled by that node. Note that a given branch structure, such as NP → Det N, can occur more than once in a given parse tree.

In general, we let $\mathcal{P}$ be a set of (all possible) parts. We assume a "counting function", c, such that for $p \in \mathcal{P}$ and $\langle x, y \rangle \in Z$, $c(p, \langle x, y \rangle)$ gives the number of times that the part p occurs in the pair $\langle x, y \rangle$ (the count of p in $\langle x, y \rangle$). For a Mercer kernel $k : \mathcal{P} \times \mathcal{P} \to \Re$ on $\mathcal{P}$, there is an associated RHKS $\mathcal{H}_k$ of functions $f : \mathcal{P} \to \Re$, where f measures the *goodness* of a part p. For any $f \in \mathcal{H}_k$, we define a function F_f on $\mathcal{Z}$ as

$$F_f(x, y) = \sum_{p \in \mathcal{P}} c(p, \langle x, y \rangle) f(p). \tag{2}$$

Consider a simple chain example. Let Γ be a set of possible observations and Σ be a set of possible hidden states. We take the input x to be a sequence $x_1, \ldots, x_\ell$ with $x_i \in \Gamma$ and we take $\mathcal{Y}(x)$ to be the set of all sequences $y_1, \ldots, y_\ell$ with the same length as x and with $y_i \in \Sigma$. We can take $\mathcal{P}$ to be the set of all pairs $\langle s, \bar{s} \rangle$ plus all pairs $\langle s, u \rangle$ with $s, \bar{s} \in \Sigma$ and $u \in \Gamma$. Often Σ is taken to be a finite set of "states" and $\Gamma = \Re^d$ is a set of possible feature vectors. $k(p, p')$ is commonly defined as

$$k(\langle s, \bar{s} \rangle, \langle s', \bar{s}' \rangle) = \delta(s, s') \delta(\bar{s}, \bar{s}'), \tag{3}$$
$$k(\langle s, u \rangle, \langle s', u' \rangle) = \delta(s, s') k_o(u, u'), \tag{4}$$

where $\delta(w, w')$ denotes the Kronecker-δ. Note that in this example there are two types of parts — pairs of hidden states and pairs of a hidden state and an observation. Here we take $k(p, p')$ to be 0 if p and p' are of different types.

In the supervised learning scenario, we are given a sample S of ℓ pairs $(\langle x^1, y^1 \rangle, \ldots, \langle x^\ell, y^\ell \rangle)$ drawn i. i. d. from an unknown but fixed probability distribution P on $\mathcal{Z}$. The goal is to learn a function f on the local parts $\mathcal{P}$ with small expected loss $E_P[\mathcal{L}(x, y, f)]$ where $\mathcal{L}$ is a prescribed loss function. This is commonly realized by learning f that minimizes the regularized loss functional

$$f^* = \underset{f \in \mathcal{H}_k}{\text{argmin}} \sum_{i=1}^{\ell} \mathcal{L}(x^i, y^i, f) + \lambda \|f\|_k^2, \tag{5}$$

where $\|.\|_k$ is the norm corresponding to $\mathcal{H}_k$ measuring the complexity of f. A variety of loss functions $\mathcal{L}$ have been considered in the literature. In kernel conditional random fields (CRFs) [11], the loss function is given by

$$\mathcal{L}(x, y, f) = -F_f(x, y) + \log \sum_{\hat{y} \in \mathcal{Y}(x)} \exp(F_f(x, \hat{y}))$$

In structured Support Vector Machines (SVM), the loss function is given by

$$\mathcal{L}(x, y, f) = \max_{\hat{y} \in \mathcal{Y}(x)} \Delta(x, y, \hat{y}) + F_f(x, \hat{y}) - F_f(x, y), \tag{6}$$

where $\Delta(x, y, \hat{y})$ is some measure of distance between y and $\hat{y}$ for a given observation x. A natural choice for Δ is to take $\Delta(x, y, \hat{y})$ to be the indicator $1_{[y \neq \hat{y}]}$ [2]. Another choice is to take $\Delta(x, y, \hat{y})$ to be the size of the symmetric difference between the sets $\mathcal{P}(\langle x, y \rangle)$ and $\mathcal{P}(\langle x, \hat{y} \rangle)$ [14].

Let $\mathcal{P}(x) \subseteq \mathcal{P}$ be the set of parts having nonzero count in some pair $\langle x, y \rangle$ for $y \in \mathcal{Y}(x)$. Let $\mathcal{P}(S)$ be the union of all sets $\mathcal{P}(x^i)$ for x^i in the sample. Then, we have following straightforward variant of the Representer Theorem [10], which was also presented in [11].

Definition: A loss $\mathcal{L}$ is *local* if $\mathcal{L}(x, y, f)$ is determined by the value of f on the set $\mathcal{P}(x)$, i.e., for $f, g : \mathcal{P} \rightarrow \Re$ we have that if $f(p) = g(p)$ for all $p \in \mathcal{P}(x)$ then $\mathcal{L}(x, y, f) = \mathcal{L}(x, y, g)$.

Theorem 1. *For any local loss function $\mathcal{L}$ and sample S there exist weights α_p for $p \in \mathcal{P}(S)$ such that f^* as defined by (5) can be written as follows.*

$$f^*(p) = \sum_{p' \in \mathcal{P}(S)} \alpha_{p'} k(p', p) \tag{7}$$

Thus, even though the set of feasible outputs for x generally scales exponentially with the size of output, the solution can be represented in terms of the parts of the sample, which commonly scales polynomially. This is true for any loss function that partitions into parts, which is the case for loss functions discussed above.

3   A Semi-Supervised Learning Approach to Structured Variables

In semi-supervised learning, we are given a sample S consisting of l input-output pairs $\{(x^1, y^1), \dots, (x^\ell, y^\ell)\}$ drawn i. i. d. from the probability distribution P on $\mathcal{Z}$ and u unlabeled input patterns $\{x^{\ell+1}, \dots, x^{\ell+u}\}$ drawn i. i. d from the marginal distribution $P_\mathcal{X}$, where usually $l < u$. Let $\mathcal{X}(S)$ be the set $\{x^1, \dots, x^{\ell+u}\}$ and let $\mathcal{Z}(S)$ be the set of all pairs $\langle x, y \rangle$ with $x \in \mathcal{X}(S)$ and $y \in \mathcal{Y}(x)$.

If the true classification function is smooth wrt the underlying marginal distribution, one can utilize unlabeled data points to favor functions that are smooth in this sense. Belkin et. al. [3] implement this assumption by introducing a new regularizer to the standard RHKS optimization framework (as opposed to introducing a new kernel as discussed in Section 5)

$$f^* = \underset{f \in \mathcal{H}_k}{\operatorname{argmin}} \sum_{i=1}^{\ell} \mathcal{L}(x^i, y^i, f) + \lambda_1 ||f||_k^2 + \lambda_2 ||f||_{k_S}^2, \tag{8}$$

where k_S is a kernel representing the intrinsic measure of the marginal distribution. Sindhwani et. al.[13] prove that the minimizer of (8) is in the span of a new kernel function (details below) evaluated at labeled data only. Here, we generalize this framework to structured variables and give a simplified derivation of the new kernel.

The smoothness assumption in the structured setting states that f should be smooth on the underlying density on the parts $\mathcal{P}$, thus we enforce f to assign similar *goodness* scores to two parts p and p', if p and p' are *similar*, for all parts of $\mathcal{Z}(S)$. Let $\mathcal{P}(S)$ be the union of all sets $\mathcal{P}(z)$ for $z \in \mathcal{Z}(S)$ and let W be symmetric matrix where $W_{p,p'}$ represents the similarity of p and p' for $p, p' \in \mathcal{P}(S)$.

$$
\begin{aligned}
f^* &= \underset{f \in \mathcal{H}_k}{\operatorname{argmin}} \sum_{i=1}^{\ell} \mathcal{L}(x^i, y^i, f) + \lambda_1 ||f||_k^2 + \lambda_2 \sum_{p,p' \in \mathcal{P}(S)} W_{p,p'} (f(p) - f(p'))^2 \\
&= \underset{f \in \mathcal{H}_k}{\operatorname{argmin}} \sum_{i=1}^{\ell} \mathcal{L}(x^i, y^i, f) + \lambda_1 ||f||_k^2 + \lambda_2 \mathbf{f}^T L \mathbf{f}
\end{aligned}
\tag{9}
$$

Here W is a similarity matrix (like a nearest neighbor graph) and L is the Laplacian of W, $L = D - W$, where D is a diagonal matrix defined by $D_{p,p} = \sum_{p'} W_{p,p'}$. $\mathbf{f}$ denotes the vector of $f(p)$ for all $p \in \mathcal{P}(S)$. Note that the last term depends only on the value of f on the parts in the set $\mathcal{P}(S)$. Then, for any local loss $\mathcal{L}(x, y, f)$, we immediately have the following Representer Theorem for the semi-supervised structured case where S includes the labeled and the unlabeled data.

$$f_\alpha^*(p) = \sum_{p' \in \mathcal{P}(S)} \alpha_{p'} k(p', p) \tag{10}$$

Substituting (10) into (9) leads to the following optimization problem

$$\alpha^* = \underset{\alpha}{\operatorname{argmin}} \sum_{i=1}^\ell \mathcal{L}(x^i, y^i, f_\alpha) + \alpha^T Q \alpha, \tag{11}$$

where $Q = \lambda_1 K + \lambda_2 KLK$, K is the matrix of $k(p, p')$ for all $p, p' \in \mathcal{P}(S)$ and f_α, as a vector in the space $\mathcal{H}_k$, is a linear function of the vector α. Note that (11) applies to any local loss function and if $\mathcal{L}(x, y, f)$ is convex in f, as in the case for logistic or hinge loss, then (11) is convex in α.

We now have a loss function over labeled data regularized by the L_2 norm (wrt the inner product Q), for which we can re-evoke the Representer Theorem. Let S^ℓ be the set of labeled inputs $\{x^1, \ldots, x^\ell\}$, $\mathcal{Z}(S^\ell)$ be the set of all pairs $\langle x, y \rangle$ with $x \in \mathcal{X}(S^\ell)$ and $y \in \mathcal{Y}(x)$ and $\mathcal{P}(S^\ell)$ be the set of al parts having nonzero count for some pair in $\mathcal{Z}(S^\ell)$. Let δ_p be a vector whose pth component is 1 and 0 elsewhere. Using the standard orthogonality argument, let α^* decompose into two: the vector in the span of $\gamma_p = \delta_p K Q^{-1}$ for all $p \in \mathcal{P}(S^\ell)$, and the vector in the orthogonal component (under the inner product Q).

$$\alpha = \sum_{p \in \mathcal{P}(S^\ell)} \beta_p \gamma_p + \alpha_\perp$$

$\alpha_\perp$ can only increase the quadratic term in the optimization problem. Notice that the first term in (11) depends only on $f_\alpha(p)$ for $p \in \mathcal{P}(S^\ell)$,

$$f_\alpha(p) = \delta_p K \alpha = (\delta_p K Q^{-1}) Q \alpha = \gamma_p Q \alpha.$$

Since $\gamma_p Q \alpha_\perp = 0$, we conclude that the optimal solution to (11) is given by

$$\alpha^* = \sum_{p \in \mathcal{P}(S^\ell)} \beta_p \gamma_p = \beta K Q^{-1}, \tag{12}$$

where β is required to be sparse, such that only parts from the labeled data are nonzero. Plugging this into original equations we get

$$\tilde{k}(p, p') = k_p Q^{-1} k_{p'} \tag{13}$$

$$f_\beta(p') = \sum_{p \in \mathcal{P}(S^\ell)} \beta_p \tilde{k}(p, p') \tag{14}$$

$$\beta^* = \underset{\beta}{\operatorname{argmin}} \mathcal{L}(S^\ell, f_\beta) + \beta^T \tilde{K} \beta \tag{15}$$

where k_p is the vector of $k(p, p')$ for all $p' \in \mathcal{P}(S)$ and $\tilde{K}$ is the matrix of $\tilde{k}(p, p')$ for all p, p' in $\mathcal{P}(S^\ell)$. $\tilde{k}$ is the same as in [13].

We call $\tilde{k}$ the *graph-regularized* kernel, in which unlabeled data points are used to augment the base kernel k wrt the standard graph kernel to take the underlying density on parts into account. This kernel is defined over the complete part space, where as standard graph kernels are restricted to $\mathcal{P}(S)$ only.

Given the graph-regularized kernel, the semi-supervised structured learning problem is reduced to supervised structured learning. Since in semi-supervised learning problems, in general, labeled data points are far fewer than unlabeled data, the dimensionality of the optimization problems is greatly reduced by this reduction.

4 Structured Max-Margin Learning

We now investigate optimizing the hinge loss as defined by (6) using graph-regularized kernel $\tilde{k}$. Defining $\gamma^{x,y}$ to be the vector where $\gamma_p^{x,y} = c(p, \langle x, y \rangle)$ is the count of p in $\langle x, y \rangle$, the linear discriminant can be written in matrix notation for $x \in S^\ell$ as

$$F_{f_\beta}(x,y) = \beta^T \tilde{K} \gamma^{x,y}.$$

Then, the optimization problem for margin maximization is

$$\beta^* = \underset{\beta}{\text{argmin}} \min_\xi \sum_{i=1}^l \xi_i + \beta^T \tilde{K} \beta$$

$$\xi_i \geq \max_{\hat{y} \in \mathcal{Y}(x^i)} \triangle(\hat{y}, y^i) - \beta^T \tilde{K} \left(\gamma^{x^i, y^i} - \gamma^{x^i, \hat{y}} \right) \quad \forall i \leq l.$$

This gives a convex quadratic program over the vectors indexed by $\mathcal{P}(S)$, a polynomial size problem in terms of the size of the structures. Following [2], we replace the convex constraints by linear constraints for all $y \in \mathcal{Y}(x)$ and using Lagrangian duality techniques, we get the following dual Quadratic program:

$$\theta^* = \underset{\theta}{\text{argmin}} \, \theta^T dR\, \theta - \Delta^T \theta \tag{16}$$

$$\theta_{(x^i, y)} \geq 0, \quad \sum_{y \in \mathcal{Y}(x)} \theta_{(x^i, y)} = 1, \quad \forall y \in \mathcal{Y}(x^i), \quad \forall i \leq l,$$

where Δ is a vector of $\triangle(y, \hat{y})$ for all $y \in \mathcal{Y}(x)$ of all labeled observations x, $d\gamma$ is a matrix whose (x^i, y)th column $d\gamma., (x^i, y) = \gamma^{x^i, y^i} - \gamma^{x^i, y}$ and $dR = d\gamma^T \tilde{K} d\gamma$. Due to the sparse structure of the constraint matrix, even though this is an exponential sized QP, the algorithm proposed in [2] is proven to solve (16) to η proximity in polynomial time in $\mathcal{P}(S^l)$ and $\frac{1}{\eta}$[15].

5 Semi-Supervised vs Transductive Learning

Since one major contribution of this paper is learning a classifier for structured objects that is defined over the complete part space $\mathcal{P}$, we now examine the differences of semi-supervised and transductive learning in more detail. The most common approach to realize the smoothness assumption is to construct a data dependent kernel k_S derived from the graph Laplacian on a nearest neighbor graph on the labeled and unlabeled input patterns in the sample S. Thus, k_S is not defined on observations that are out of the sample. Given k_S, one can construct a function $\tilde{f}^*$ on S as

$$\tilde{f}^* = \underset{f \in \mathcal{H}_{k_S}}{\text{argmin}} \sum_{i=1}^\ell \mathcal{L}(x^i, y^i, f) + \lambda \|f\|_{k_S}^2. \tag{17}$$

It is well known that kernels can be combined linearly to yield new kernels. This observation in the transductive setting leads to the following optimization problem, when the kernel of the optimization problem is taken to be a linear combination of a graph kernel k_S and a standard kernel k restricted to $\mathcal{P}(S)$.

$$\bar{f}^* = \underset{f \in \mathcal{H}_{(\mu_1 k + \mu_2 k_S)}}{\text{argmin}} \sum_{i=1}^\ell \mathcal{L}(x^i, y^i, f) + \lambda \|f\|_{(\mu_1 k + \mu_2 k_S)}^2 \tag{18}$$

A structured semi-supervised algorithm based on (18) has been evaluated in [11]. The kernel is (18) is the weighted mean of k and k_S, whereas the graph-regularized kernel, resulting from weighted mean of two regularizers, is the harmonic mean of k and k_S [16]. An important distinction between $\bar{f}^*$ and f^* in (8), the optimization performed in this paper, is that $\bar{f}^*$ is only defined on $\mathcal{P}(S)$ (only on observations in the training data) while f^* is defined on all of $\mathcal{P}$ and can be used for novel (out of sample) inputs x. We note that in general $\mathcal{P}$ is infinite. Out-of-sample extension is already a serious limitation for transductive learning, but it is even more severe in the structured case where parts of $\mathcal{P}$ can be composed of multiple observation tokens.

6   Experiments

Similarity Graph: We build the similarity matrix W over $\mathcal{P}(S)$ using K-nearest neighborhood relationship. $W_{p,p'}$ is 0 if p and p' are not in the K-nearest neighborhood of each other or if p and p' are of different types. Otherwise, the similarity is given by a heat kernel. In our applications, the structure is a simple chain, therefore the cliques involved single observation label pairs,

$$W_{p,p'} = \delta(y(u_p), y(u'_{p'}))e^{\frac{\|u_p - u'_{p'}\|^2}{t}}, \tag{19}$$

where u_p denotes the observation part of p and $y(u)$ denotes the labeling of u [1]. In cases where $k(p, p') = W_{p,p'} = 0$ for p, p' of different types, as in our experiments, the Gram matrix K and the Laplacian L can be presented as block diagonal matrices, which significantly reduces the computational complexity, the computation of Q^{-1} in particular.

Applications: We performed experiments using a simple chain model for pitch accent (PA) prediction and OCR. In PA prediction, $\mathcal{Y}(x) = \{0, 1\}^T$ with $T = |x|$ and $x_t \in \Re^{31}, \forall t$. In OCR, $x_t \in \{0, 1\}^{128}$ and $|\Sigma| = 15$.

We ran experiments comparing semi-supervised structured (referred as STR) and unstructured (referred as SVM) max-margin optimization. For both SVM and STR, we used RBF kernel as the base kernel k_o in (4) and a 5-nearest neighbor graph to construct the Laplacian.

PA	U:0	U:80	U:0	U:80	U:200
SVM	65.92	68.83	70.34	71.27	73.68
	-	69.94	-	72.00	73.11
STR	65.81	70.28	72.15	74.92	76.37
	-	70.72	-	75.66	77.45

Table 1: Per-label accuracy for Pitch Accent.

We chose the width of the RBF kernel by cross-validation on SVM and used the same value for STR. Following [3], we fixed $\lambda_1 : \lambda_2$ ratio at $1 : 9$. We report the average results of experiments with 5 random selection of labeled sequences in Table 1 and 2, with number of labeled sequences 4 on the left side of Table 1, 40 on the right side, and 10 in Table 2. We varied the number of unlabeled sequences and reported the per-label accuracy of test sequences (on top of each cell) and of unlabeled sequences (bottom) (when $U > 0$). The results in pitch accent prediction shows the advantage of a sequence model over a non-structured

---

[1]For more complicated parts, different measures can apply. For example, in sequence classification, if the classifier is evaluated wrt the correctly classified individual labels in the sequence, W can be s. t. $W_{p,p'} = \sum_{u \in p, u' \in p'} \delta(y(u), y(u'))\tilde{s}(u, u')$ where $\tilde{s}$ denotes some similarity measure such as the heat kernel. If the evaluation is over segments of the sequence, the similarity can be $W_{p,p'} = \delta(y(p), y'(p')) \sum_{u \in p, u' \in p'} \tilde{s}(u, u')$ where $y(p)$ denotes all the label nodes in the part p.

model, where STR consistently performs better than SVM. We also observe the usefulness of unlabeled data both in the structured and unstructured models, where as U increases, so does the accuracy. The improvement from unlabeled data and from structured classification can be considered as additive. The small difference between the accuracy of in-sample unlabeled data and the test data indicates the natural extension of our framework to new data points.

In OCR, on the other hand, STR does not improve over SVM. Even though unlabeled data improves accuracy, performing sequence classification is not helpful due to the sparsity of structural information. Since $|\Sigma| = 15$ and there are only 10 labeled sequences with average length 8.3, the statistics of label-label dependency is quite noisy.

OCR	U:0	U:412
SVM	43.62	49.96
	-	47.56
STR	49.25	49.91
	-	49.65

Table 2: OCR

7 Conclusions

We presented a discriminative approach to semi-supervised learning of structured and inter-dependent response variables. In this framework, we derived a maximum margin formulation and presented experiments for a simple chain model. Our approach naturally extends to the classification of unobserved structured inputs and this is supported by our empirical results which showed similar accuracy on in-sample unlabeled data and out-of-sample test data.

References

[1] Y. Altun, T. Hofmann, and A. Smola. Gaussian process classification for segmenting and annotating sequences. In *ICML*, 2004.

[2] Y. Altun, I. Tsochantaridis, and T. Hofmann. Hidden markov support vector machines. In *ICML*, 2003.

[3] M. Belkin, P. Niyogi, and V. Sindhwani. Manifold regularization: a geometric framework for learning from examples. Technical Report 06, UChicago CS, 2004.

[4] Avrim Blum and Tom Mitchell. Combining labeled and unlabeled data with co-training. In *COLT*, 1998.

[5] U. Brefeld, C. Büscher, and T. Scheffer. Multi-view discriminative sequential learning. In *(ECML)*, 2005.

[6] O. Chappelle, J. Weston, and B. Scholkopf. Cluster kernels for semi-supervised learning. In *(NIPS)*, 2002.

[7] M. Collins and N.l Duffy. Convolution kernels for natural language. In *(NIPS)*, 2001.

[8] Olivier Delalleau, Yoshua Bengio, and Nicolas Le Roux. Efficient non-parametric function induction in semi-supervised learning. In *Proceedings of AISTAT*, 2005.

[9] Thorsten Joachims. Transductive inference for text classification using support vector machines. In *(ICML)*, pages 200–209, 1999.

[10] G. Kimeldorf and G. Wahba. Some results on tchebychean spline functions. *Journal of Mathematics Analysis and Applications*, 33:82–95, 1971.

[11] John Lafferty, Yan Liu, and Xiaojin Zhu. Kernel conditional random fields: Representation, clique selection, and semi-supervised learning. In *(ICML)*, 2004.

[12] K. Nigam, A. K. McCallum, S. Thrun, and T. M. Mitchell. Learning to classify text from labeled and unlabeled documents. In *Proceedings of AAAI-98*, pages 792–799, Madison, US, 1998.

[13] V. Sindhwani, P. Niyogi, and M. Belkin. Beyond the point cloud: from transductive to semi-supervised learning. In *(ICML)*, 2005.

[14] B. Taskar, C. Guestrin, and D. Koller. Max-margin markov networks. In *NIPS*, 2004.

[15] I. Tsochantaridis, T. Hofmann, T. Joachims, and Y. Altun. Support vector machine learning for interdependent and structured output spaces. In *(ICML)*, 2004.

[16] T. Zhang. personal communication.

Large scale networks fingerprinting and visualization using the k-core decomposition

J. Ignacio Alvarez-Hamelin[*]
LPT (UMR du CNRS 8627),
Université de Paris-Sud,
91405 ORSAY Cedex France
Ignacio.Alvarez-Hamelin@lri.fr

Luca Dall'Asta
LPT (UMR du CNRS 8627),
Université de Paris-Sud,
91405 ORSAY Cedex France
Luca.Dallasta@th.u-psud.fr

Alain Barrat
LPT (UMR du CNRS 8627),
Université de Paris-Sud,
91405 ORSAY Cedex France
Alain.Barrat@th.u-psud.fr

Alessandro Vespignani
School of Informatics,
Indiana University,
Bloomington, IN 47408, USA
alexv@indiana.edu

Abstract

We use the k-core decomposition to develop algorithms for the analysis of large scale complex networks. This decomposition, based on a recursive pruning of the least connected vertices, allows to disentangle the hierarchical structure of networks by progressively focusing on their central cores. By using this strategy we develop a general visualization algorithm that can be used to compare the structural properties of various networks and highlight their hierarchical structure. The low computational complexity of the algorithm, $\mathcal{O}(n + e)$, where n is the size of the network, and e is the number of edges, makes it suitable for the visualization of very large sparse networks. We show how the proposed visualization tool allows to find specific structural fingerprints of networks.

1 Introduction

In recent times, the possibility of accessing, handling and mining large-scale networks datasets has revamped the interest in their investigation and theoretical characterization along with the definition of new modeling frameworks. In particular, mapping projects of the World Wide Web and the physical Internet offered the first chance to study topology and traffic of large-scale networks. Other studies followed describing population networks of practical interest in social science, critical infrastructures and epidemiology [1, 2, 3]. The study of large scale networks, however, faces us with an array of new challenges. The definitions of centrality, hierarchies and structural organizations are hindered by the large size of these networks and the complex interplay of connectivity patterns, traffic flows and geographical, social and economical attributes characterizing their basic elements. In this

---

[*]Further author information: J.I.A-H. is also with Facultad de Ingeniería, Universidad de Buenos Aires, Paseo Colón 850, C 1063 ACV Buenos Aires, Argentina.

41

context, a large research effort is devoted to provide effective visualization and analysis tools able to cope with graphs whose size may easily reach millions of vertices.

In this paper, we propose a visualization algorithm based on the k-core decomposition able to uncover in a two-dimensional layout several topological and hierarchical properties of large scale networks. The k-core decomposition [4] consists in identifying particular subsets of the graph, called k-cores, each one obtained by recursively removing all the vertices of degree smaller than k, until the degree of all remaining vertices is larger than or equal to k. Larger values of the index k clearly correspond to vertices with larger degree and more central position in the network's structure.

This visualization tool allows the identification of real or computer-generated networks' fingerprints, according to properties such as hierarchical arrangement, degree correlations and centrality. The distinction between networks with seemingly similar properties is achieved by inspecting the different layouts generated by the visualization algorithm. In addition, the running time of the algorithm grows only linearly with the size of the network, granting the scalability needed for the visualization of very large sparse networks. The proposed (publicly available [5]) algorithm appears therefore as a convenient method for the general analysis of large scale complex networks and the study of their architecture.

The paper is organized as follows: after a brief survey on k-core studies (section 2), we present the basic definitions and the graphical algorithms in section 3 along with the basic features of the visualization layout. Section 4 shows how the visualizations obtained with the present algorithm may be used for network fingerprinting, and presents two examples of visualization of real networks.

2 Related work

While a large number of algorithms aimed at the visualization of large scale networks have been developed (e.g., see [6]), only a few consider explicitly the k-core decomposition. Vladimir Batagelj *et al.* [7] studied the k-core decomposition applied to visualization problems, introducing some graphical tools to analyse the cores, mainly based on the visualization of the adjacency matrix of certain k-cores. To the best of our knowledge, the algorithm presented by Baur *et al.* in [8] is the only one completely based on a k-core analysis and directly targeted at the study of large information networks. This algorithm uses a spectral layout to place vertices having the largest shell index. A combination of barycentric and iteratively directed-forces allows to place the vertices of each k-shell, in decreasing order. Finally, the network is drawn in three dimensions, using the z axis to place each shell in a distinct horizontal layer. Note that the spectral layout is not able to distinguish two or more disconnected components. The algorithm by Baur *et al.* is also tuned for representing AS graphs and its total complexity depends on the size of the highest k-core (see [9] for more details on spectral layout), making the computation time of this proposal largely variable. In this respect, the algorithm presented here is different in that it can represent networks in which k-cores are composed by several connected components. Another difference is that representations in 2D are more suited for information visualization than other representations (see [10] and references therein). Finally, the algorithm parameters can be universally defined, yielding a fast and general tool for analyzing all types of networks.

It is interesting to note that the notion of k-cores has been recently used in biologically related contexts, where it was applied to the analysis of protein interaction networks [11] or in the prediction of protein functions [12, 13]. Further applications in Internet-related areas can be found in [14], where the k-core decomposition is used for filtering out peripheral Autonomous Systems (ASes), and in [15] where the scale invariant structure of degree correlations and mapping biases in AS maps is shown. Finally in [16, 17], an interesting approach based on the k-core decomposition has been used to provide a conceptual and structural model of the Internet; the so-called medusa model for the Internet.

3 Graphical representation

Let us consider a graph $G = (V, E)$ of $|V| = n$ vertices and $|E| = e$ edges; a k-core is defined as follows [4]:

-A subgraph $H = (C, E|C)$ induced by the set $C \subseteq V$ is a *k-core* or a core of order k iff $\forall v \in C : \text{degree}_H(v) \geq k$, and H is the maximum subgraph with this property.

A k-core of G can therefore be obtained by recursively removing all the vertices of degree less than k, until all vertices in the remaining graph have at least degree k. Furthermore, we will use the following definitions:

-A vertex i has *shell index* c if it belongs to the c-core but not to $(c + 1)$-core. We denote by c_i the shell index of vertex i.

-A shell C_c is composed by all the vertices whose shell index is c. The maximum value c such that C_c is not empty is denoted $c_{\max}$. The k-core is thus the union of all shells C_c with $c \geq k$.

-Each connected set of vertices having the same shell index c is a *cluster* Q^c. Each shell C_c is thus composed by clusters Q_m^c, such that $C_c = \cup_{1 \leq m \leq q_{\max}^c} Q_m^c$, where $q_{\max}^c$ is the number of clusters in C_c.

The visualization algorithm we propose places vertices in 2 dimensions, the position of each vertex depending on its shell index and on the index of its neighbors. A color code allows for the identification of shell indices, while the vertex's original degree is provided by its size that depends logarithmically on the degree. For the sake of clarity, our algorithm represents a small percentage of the edges, chosen uniformly at random. As mentioned, a central role in our visualization method is played by multi-components representation of k-cores. In the most general situation, indeed, the recursive removal of vertices having degree less than a given k can break the original network into various connected components, each of which might even be once again broken by the subsequent decomposition. Our method takes into account this possibility, however we will first present the algorithm in the simplified case, in which none of the k-cores is fragmented. Then, this algorithm will be used as a subroutine for treating the general case (Table 1).

3.1 Drawing algorithm for k-cores with single connected component

k-core decomposition. The shell index of each vertex is computed and stored in a vector $\mathcal{C}$, along with the shells C_c and the maximum index c_{max}. Each shell is then decomposed into clusters Q_m^c of connected vertices, and each vertex i is labeled by its shell index c_i and by a number q_i representing the cluster it belongs to.

The two dimensional graphical layout. The visualization is obtained assigning to each vertex i a couple of polar coordinates (ρ_i, α_i): the radius ρ_i is a function of the shell index of the vertex i and of its neighbors; the angle α_i depends on the cluster number q_i. In this way, k-shells are displayed as layers with the form of circular shells, the innermost one corresponding to the set of vertices with highest shell index. A vertex i belongs to the $c_{\max} - c_i$ layer from the center.

More precisely, ρ_i is computed according to the following formula:

$$\rho_i = (1 - \epsilon)(c_{\max} - c_i) + \frac{\epsilon}{|V_{c_j \geq c_i}(i)|} \sum_{j \in V_{c_j \geq c_i}(i)} (c_{\max} - c_j) \;, \tag{1}$$

$V_{c_j \geq c_i}(i)$ is the set of neighbors of i having shell index c_j larger or equal to c_i. The parameter ϵ controls the possibility of rings overlapping, and is one of the only three external parameters required to tune image's rendering.

Inside a given shell, the angle α_i of a vertex i is computed as follow:

$$\alpha_i = 2\pi \sum_{1 \leq m < q_i} \frac{|Q_m|}{|C_{c_i}|} + \mathbf{N}\left(\frac{|Q_{q_i}|}{2|C_{c_i}|} \ , \ \pi \cdot \frac{|Q_{q_i}|}{|C_{c_i}|}\right) \ , \tag{2}$$

where Q_{q_i} and C_{c_i} are respectively the cluster q_i and c_i-shell the vertex belongs to, $\mathbf{N}$ is a normal distribution of mean $|Q_{q_i}|/(2|C_{c_i}|)$ and width $2\pi|Q_{q_i}|/|C_{c_i}|$. Since we are interested in distinguishing different clusters in the same shell, the first term on the right side of Eq. 2, referring to clusters with $m < q_i$, allows to allocate a correct partition of the angular sector to each cluster. The second term on the right side of Eq. 2, on the other hand, specifies a random position for the vertex i in the sector assigned to the cluster Q_{q_i}.

Colors and size of vertices. Colors depend on the shell index: vertices with shell index 1 are violet, and the maximum shell index vertices are red, following the rainbow color scale. The diameter of each vertex corresponds to the logarithm of its degree, giving a further information on vertex's properties. The vertices with largest shell index are placed uniformly in a disk of radius u, which is the unit length ($u = 1$ for this reduced algorithm).

3.2 Extended algorithm for networks with many k-cores components

The algorithm presented in the previous section can be used as the basic routine to define an extended algorithm aimed at the visualization of networks for which some k-cores are fragmented; i.e. made by more than one connected component. This issue is solved by assigning to each connected component of a k-core a center and a size, which depends on the relative sizes of the various components. Larger components are put closer to the global center of the representation (which has Cartesian coordinates $(0,0)$), and have larger sizes.

The algorithm begins with the center at the origin $(0,0)$. Whenever a connected component of a k-core, whose center p had coordinates (X_p, Y_p), is broken into several components by removing all vertices of degree k, i.e. by applying the next decomposition step, a new center is computed for each new component. The center of the component h has coordinates (X_h, Y_h), defined by

$$X_h = X_p + \delta(c_{\max} - c_h) \cdot u_p \cdot \varrho_h \cdot \cos(\phi_h) \ ; \ Y_h = Y_p + \delta(c_{\max} - c_h) \cdot u_p \cdot \varrho_h \cdot \sin(\phi_h) \ , \tag{3}$$

where δ scales the distance between components, $c_{\max}$ is the maximum shell index and c_h is the core number of component h (the components are numbered by $h = 1, \cdots, h_{max}$ in an arbitrary order), u_p is the unit length of its parent component, ϱ_h and ϕ_h are the radial and angular coordinates of the new center with respect to the parent center (X_p, Y_p). We define ϱ_h and ϕ_h as follows:

$$\varrho_h = 1 - \frac{|S_h|}{\sum_{1 \leq j \leq h_{max}} |S_j|} \ ; \ \phi_h = \phi_{ini} + \frac{2\pi}{\sum_{1 \leq j \leq h_{max}} |S_j|} \sum_{1 \leq j \leq h} |S_j| \ , \tag{4}$$

where S_h is the set of vertices in the component h, $\sum_j |S_j|$ is the sum of the sizes of all components having the same parent component. In this way, larger components will be closer to the original parent component's center p. The angle ϕ_h has two contributions. The initial angle ϕ_{ini} is chosen uniformly at random[1], while the angle sector is the sum of component angles whose number is less than or equal to the actual component number h.

---

[1]Note that if ϕ_{ini} is fixed, all the centers of the various components are aligned in the final representation.

Algorithm 1

1	$k := 1$ and $end := \texttt{false}$
2	while not end do
3	$\quad (end, C) \leftarrow \texttt{make\_core } k$
4	$\quad (Q, T) \leftarrow \texttt{compute\_clusters } k - 1$, if $k > 1$
5	$\quad S \leftarrow \texttt{compute\_components } k$
6	$\quad (X, Y) \leftarrow \texttt{compute\_origin\_coordinates\_cmp } k$ (Eqs. from 3 to 4)
7	$\quad U \leftarrow \texttt{compute\_unit\_size\_cmp } k$ (Eq. 5)
8	$\quad k := k + 1$
9	for each node i do
10	$\quad$ if $c_i == c_{\max}$ then
11	$\quad\quad$ set ρ_i and α_i according to a uniform distribution in the disk of radius u (u is the core representation unit size)
12	$\quad$ else
13	$\quad\quad$ set ρ_i and α_i according to Eqs. 1 and 2
14	$(\mathcal{X}, \mathcal{Y}) \leftarrow \texttt{compute\_final\_coordinates } \rho\, \alpha\, U\, X\, Y$ (Eq. 6)

Table 1: Algorithm for the representation of networks using k-cores decomposition

Finally, the unit length u_h of a component h is computed as

$$u_h = \frac{|S_h|}{\sum_{1 \leq j \leq h_{max}} |S_j|} \cdot u_p \ , \tag{5}$$

where u_p is the unit length of its parent component. Larger unit length and size are therefore attributed to larger components.

For each vertex i, radial and angular coordinates are computed by equations 1 and 2 as in the previous algorithm. These coordinates are then considered as relative to the center (X_h, Y_h) of the component to which i belongs. The position of i is thus given by

$$x_i = X_h + \gamma \cdot u_h \cdot \rho_i \cdot \cos(\alpha_i); \quad y_i = Y_h + \gamma \cdot u_h \cdot \rho_i \cdot \sin(\alpha_i) \tag{6}$$

where γ is a parameter controlling the component's diameter.

The global algorithm is formally presented in Table 1. The main loop is composed by the following functions. First, the function $\{(end, C) \leftarrow \texttt{make\_core } k\}$ recursively removes all vertices of degree $k - 1$, obtaining the k-core, and stores into C the shell index $k - 1$ of the removed vertices. The boolean variable end is set to $true$ if the k-core is empty, otherwise it is set to $false$. The function $\{(Q, T) \leftarrow \texttt{compute\_clusters } k - 1\}$ operates the decomposition of the $(k - 1)$-shell into clusters, storing for each vertex the cluster label into the vector Q, and filling table T, which is indexed by the shell index c and cluster label q: $T(c, q) = (\sum_{1 \leq m < q} |Q_m|/|C_c|, |Q_q|/|C_c|)$. The possible decomposition of the k-core into connected components is determined by function $\{S \leftarrow \texttt{compute\_components } k\}$, that also collects into a vector S the number of vertices contained in each component. At the following step, functions $\{(X, Y) \leftarrow \texttt{compute\_origin\_coordinates\_cmp } k\}$ and $\{U \leftarrow \texttt{compute\_unit\_size\_cmp } k\}$ get, respectively, the center and size of each component of the k-core, gathering them in vectors X, Y and U. Finally, the coordinates of each vertex are computed and stored in the vectors $\mathcal{X}$ and $\mathcal{Y}$.

Algorithm complexity. Batagelj and Zversnik [18] present an algorithm to perform the k-core decomposition, and show that its time complexity is $\mathcal{O}(e)$ (where e is the number of edges) for a connected graph. For a general graph it is $\mathcal{O}(n + e)$, where n is the number of nodes, which makes the algorithm very efficient for sparse graphs where e is of order n.

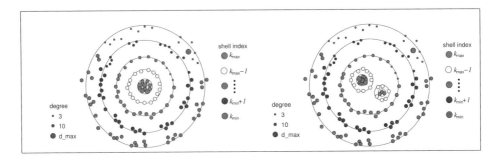

Figure 1: Structure of a typical layout in two important cases: on the left, all k-cores are connected; on the right, some k-cores are composed by more than one connected component. The vertices are arranged in a series of concentric shells corresponding to the various k-shells. The diameter of each shell depends on both the shell index and, in case of multiple components (right) also on the relative fraction of vertices belonging to the different components.

3.3 Basic features of the visualization's layout

The main features of the layout's structure obtained with the above algorithms are visible in Fig.1 where, for the sake of simplicity, we do not show any edge.

The two-dimensional layout is composed of a series of concentric *circular shells*. Each shell corresponds to a single *shell index* and all vertices in it are therefore drawn with the *same color*. A color scale allows to distinguish different *shell indices*: the violet is used for the minimum shell index k_{min}, then we use a graduated rainbow scale for higher and higher shell indices up to the maximum value k_{max} that is colored in red. The diameter of each k-shell depends on the *shell index* k, and is proportional to $k_{max} - k$ (In Fig.1, the position of each shell is identified by a circle having the corresponding diameter). The presence of a trivial order relation in the shell indices ensures that all shells are placed in a concentric arrangement. On the other hand, when a k-core is fragmented in two or more components, the diameters of the different components depend also on the relative number of vertices belonging to each of them, i.e. the fraction between the number of vertices belonging to that component and the total number of vertices in that core. This is a very important information, providing a way to distinguish between multiple components at a given shell index. Finally, the size of each node is proportional to the *original degree* of that vertex; we use a logarithmic scale for the size of the drawn bullets.

4 Network fingerprinting

The k-core decomposition peels the network layer by layer, revealing the structure of the different shells from the outmost one to the more internal ones. The algorithm provides a direct way to distinguish the network's different hierarchies and structural organization by means of some simple quantities: the radial width of the shells, the presence and size of clusters of vertices in the shells, the correlations between degree and shell index, the distribution of the edges interconnecting vertices of different shells, etc.

1) *Shells Width:* The thickness of a shell depends on the shell index properties of the neighbors of the vertices in the corresponding shell. For a given shell-diameter (black circle in the median position of shells in Fig.2), each vertex can be placed more internal or more external with respect to this reference. Nodes with more neighbors in higher shells are closer to the center and viceversa: in Fig.2, node y is more internal than node x because it

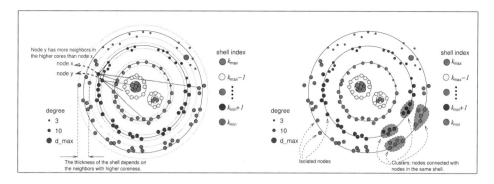

Figure 2: Left: each shell has a certain radial width. This width depends on the correlation's properties of the vertices in the shell. In the second shell, we have pinpointed two nodes x and y. Node y is more internal than x because a larger part of its neighbors belongs to higher k-shells compared to x's neighbors. The figure on the right shows the clustering properties of nodes in the same k-shell. In each k-shell, nodes that are directly connected between them (in the original graph) are drawn close one to the other, as in a cluster. Some of these sets of nodes are circled and highlighted in gray. Three examples of isolated nodes are also indicated; these nodes have no connections with the others of the same shell.

has three edges towards higher index nodes, while x has only one. The maximum thickness of the shells is controlled by the ϵ parameter (Eq. 1).

2) *Shell Clusters:* The angular distribution of vertices in the shells is not completely homogeneous. Fig.2 shows that clusters of vertices can be observed. The idea is to group together all nodes of the same shell that are directly linked in the original graph and to represent them close one to another. Thus, a shell is divided in many angular sectors, each containing a cluster of vertices. This feature allows to figure out at a glance if the shells are composed of a single large connected component rather than divided into many small clusters, or even if there are isolated vertices (i.e. disconnected from all other nodes in the shell, not from the rest of the k-core!).

3) *Degree-Shell index Correlation:* Another property that can be studied from the obtained layouts is the correlation between the degree of the nodes and the shell index. Both quantities are centrality measures and the nature of their correlations is a very important feature characterizing a network's topology. The nodes displayed in the most internal shells are those forming the central core of the network; the presence of degree-index correlations then corresponds to the fact that the central nodes are most likely high-degree hubs of the network. This effect is observed in many real communication networks with a clear hierarchical structure, such as the Internet at the Autonomous System level or the World Wide Air-transportation network [5]. On the contrary, the presence of hubs in external shells is typical of less hierarchically structured networks such as the World-Wide Web or the Internet Router Level. In this case, star-like configurations appear with high degree vertices connected only to very low degree vertices. These vertices are rapidly pruned out in the k-core decomposition even if they have a very high degree, leading to the presence of local hubs in external shells, as in Fig. 3.

4) *Edges:* The visualization shows only a homogeneously randomly sampled fraction of the edges, which can be tuned in order to get the better trade-off between the clarity of visualization and the necessity of giving information on the way the nodes are mainly connected. Edge-reduction techniques can be implemented to improve the algorithm's capacity in representing edges; however, a homogeneous sampling does not alter the extraction of topological information, ensuring a low computational cost. Finally, the two halves of each

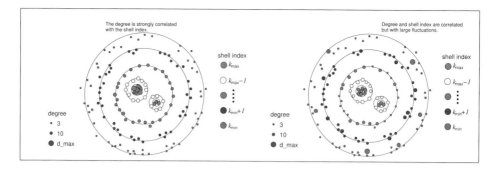

Figure 3: Correlations between shell index and degree. On the left, we report a graph with strong correlation: the size of the nodes grows from the periphery to the center, in correspondence with the shell index. In the right-hand case, the degree-index correlations are blurred by large fluctuations, as stressed by the presence of hubs in the external shells.

edge are colored with the color of the corresponding extremities to emphasize the connection among vertices in different shells.

5) *Disconnected components:* The fragmentation of any given k-core in two or more disconnected components is represented by the presence of a corresponding number of circular shells with different centers (Fig. 1). The diameter of these circles is related with the number of nodes of each component and modulated by the γ parameter (Eq. 6). The distance between components is controlled by the δ parameter (Eq. 3).

In summary, the proposed algorithm makes possible a direct, visual investigation of a series of properties: hierarchical structures of networks, connectivity and clustering properties inside a given shell; relations and interconnectivity between different levels of the hierarchy, correlations between degree and shell index, i.e. between different measures of centrality.

Numerous examples of the application of this tool to the visualization of real and computer generated networks can be found on the web page of the publicly available tool [5]. For example, the lack of hierarchy and structure of the Erdös-Rényi random graph is clearly identified. Similarly the time correlations present in the Barabási-Albert network find a clear fingerprint in our visualization layout. Here we display another interesting illustration of the use and capabilities of the proposed algorithm in the analysis of large sparse graphs: the identification of the different hierarchical arrangement of the Internet network when visualized at the Autonomous system (AS) and the Router (IR) levels [2]. The AS level is represented by collected routes of *Oregon route-views* [19] project, from May 2001. For the IR level, we use the graph obtained by an exploration of Govindan and Tangmunarunkit [20] in 2000. These networks are composed respectively by about 11500 and 200000 nodes.

Figures 4 and 5 display the representations of these two different maps of Internet. At the AS level, all shells are populated, and, for any given shell, the vertices are distributed on a relatively large range of the radial coordinate, which means that their neighborhoods are variously composed. The shell index and the degree are very correlated, with a clear hierarchical structure, and links go principally from one shell to another. The hierarchical structure exhibited by our analysis of the AS level is a striking property; for instance, one might exploit it for showing that in the Internet high-degree vertices are naturally (as an implicit result of the self-organizing growth) placed in the innermost structure. At higher resolution, i.e. at the IR level, Internet's properties are less structured: external layers, of

---

[2]The parameters are here set to the values $\epsilon = 0.18$, $\delta = 1.3$ and $\gamma = 1.5$.

lowest shell index, contain vertices with large degree. For instance, we find 20 vertices with degree larger than 100 but index smaller than 6. The correlation between shell index and degree is thus clearly of a very different nature in the maps of Internet obtained at different granularities.

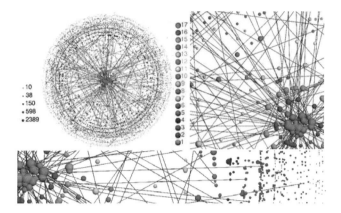

Figure 4: Graphical representation of the AS network. The three snapshots correspond to the full network (top left), with the color scale of the shell index and the size scale for the nodes' degrees, and to two magnifications showing respectively a more central part (top right) and a radial slice of the layout (bottom).

5 Conclusions

Exploiting k-core decomposition, and the corresponding natural hierarchical structures, we develop a visualization algorithm that yields a layout encoding a considerable amount of the information needed for network fingerprinting in the simplicity of a 2D representation. One can easily read basic features of the graph (degree, hierarchical structure, etc.) as well as more entangled features, e.g. the relation between a vertex and the hierarchical position of its neighbors. The present visualization strategy is a useful tool to discriminate between networks with different topological properties and structural arrangement, and may be also used for comparison of models with real data, providing a further interesting tool for model

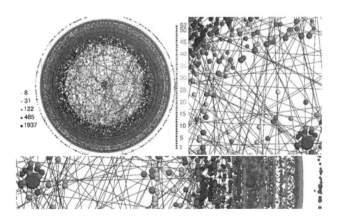

Figure 5: Same as Fig. 4, for the graphical representation of the IR network.

validation. Finally, we also provide a publicly available tool for visualizing networks [5].

Acknowledgments: This work has been partially funded by the European Commission - Fet Open project COSIN IST-2001-33555 and contract 001907 (DELIS).

References

[1] R. Albert and A.-L. Barabási, "Statistical mechanics of complex networks," *Rev. Mod. Phys.* **74**, pp. 47–97, 2000.

[2] S. N. Dorogovtsev and J. F. F. Mendes, *Evolution of networks: From biological nets to the Internet and WWW*, Oxford University Press, 2003.

[3] R. Pastor-Satorras and A. Vespignani, *Evolution and structure of the Internet: A statistical physics approach*, Cambridge University Press, 2004.

[4] V. Batagelj and M. Zaversnik, "Generalized Cores," *cs.DS/0202039* , 2002.

[5] LArge NETwork VIsualization tool.
http://xavier.informatics.indiana.edu/lanet-vi/.

[6] http://http://i11www.ira.uka.de/cosin/tools/index.php.

[7] V. Batagelj, A. Mrvar, and M. Zaversnik, "Partitioning Approach to Visualization of Large Networks," in *Graph Drawing '99, Castle Stirin, Czech Republic, LNCS 1731*, pp. 90–98, 1999.

[8] M. Baur, U. Brandes, M. Gaertler, and D. Wagner, "Drawing the AS Graph in 2.5 Dimensions," in *"12th International Symposium on Graph Drawing, Springer-Verlag editor"*, pp. 43–48, 2004.

[9] U. Brandes and S. Cornelsen, "Visual Ranking of Link Structures," *Journal of Graph Algorithms and Applications* **7**(2), pp. 181–201, 2003.

[10] B. Shneiderman, "Why not make interfaces better than 3d reality?," *IEEE Computer Graphics and Applications* **23**, pp. 12–15, November/December 2003.

[11] G. D. Bader and C. W. V. Hogue, "An automated method for finding molecular complexes in large protein interaction networks," *BMC Bioinformatics* **4**(2), 2003.

[12] M. Altaf-Ul-Amin, K. Nishikata, T. Koma, T. Miyasato, Y. Shinbo, M. Arifuzzaman, C. Wada, M. Maeda, T. Oshima, H. Mori, and S. Kanaya, "Prediction of Protein Functions Based on K-Cores of Protein-Protein Interaction Networks and Amino Acid Sequences," *Genome Informatics* **14**, pp. 498–499, 2003.

[13] S. Wuchty and E. Almaas, "Peeling the Yeast protein network," *Proteomics. 2005 Feb;5(2):444-9.* **5**(2), pp. 444–449, 2005.

[14] M. Gaertler and M. Patrignani, "Dynamic Analysis of the Autonomous System Graph," in *IPS 2004, International Workshop on Inter-domain Performance and Simulation, Budapest, Hungary*, pp. 13–24, 2004.

[15] I. Alvarez-Hamelin, L. Dall'Asta, A. Barrat, and A. Vespignani, "k-core decomposition: a tool for the analysis of large scale internet graphs," *cs.NI/0511007* .

[16] S. Carmi, S. Havlin, S. Kirkpatrick, Y. Shavitt, and E. Shir, 2005. http://www.cs.huji.ac.il/~kirk/Jellyfish_Dimes.ppt.

[17] S. Carmi, S. Havlin, S. Kirkpatrick, Y. Shavitt, and E. Shir, "Medusa - new model of internet topology using k-shell decomposition," *cond-mat/0601240* .

[18] V. Batagelj and M. Zaversnik, "An O(m) Algorithm for Cores Decomposition of Networks," *cs.DS/0310049* , 2003.

[19] University of Oregon Route Views Project. http://www.routeviews.org/.

[20] R. Govindan and H. Tangmunarunkit, "Heuristics for Internet Map Discovery," in *IEEE INFOCOM 2000*, pp. 1371–1380, IEEE, (Tel Aviv, Israel), March 2000.

Fast Information Value
for Graphical Models

Brigham S. Anderson
School of Computer Science
Carnegie Mellon University
Pittsburgh, PA 15213
brigham@cmu.edu

Andrew W. Moore
School of Computer Science
Carnegie Mellon University
Pittsburgh, PA 15213
awm@cs.cmu.edu

Abstract

Calculations that quantify the dependencies between variables are vital to many operations with graphical models, e.g., active learning and sensitivity analysis. Previously, pairwise information gain calculation has involved a cost quadratic in network size. In this work, we show how to perform a similar computation with cost linear in network size. The loss function that allows this is of a form amenable to computation by dynamic programming. The message-passing algorithm that results is described and empirical results demonstrate large speedups without decrease in accuracy. In the cost-sensitive domains examined, superior accuracy is achieved.

1 Introduction

In a diagnosis problem, one wishes to select the best test (or observation) to make in order to learn the most about a system of interest. Medical settings and disease diagnosis immediately come to mind, but sensor management (Krishnamurthy, 2002), sensitivity analysis (Kjrulff & van der Gaag, 2000), and active learning (Anderson & Moore, 2005) all make use of similar computations. These generally boil down to an all-pairs analysis between observable variables (queries) and the variables of interest (targets.)

A common technique in the field of diagnosis is to compute the mutual information between each query and target, then select the query that is expected to provide the most information (Agostak & Weiss, 1999). Likewise, a sensitivity analysis between the query variable and the target variables can be performed (Laskey, 1995; Kjrulff & van der Gaag, 2000). However, both suffer from a quadratic blowup with respect to the number of queries and targets.

In the current paper we present a loss function which can be used in a message-passing framework to perform the all-pairs computation with cost linear in network size. We describe the loss function in Section 2, we describe a polynomial expression for network-wide expected loss in Section 3, and in Section 4 we present a message-passing scheme to perform this computation efficiently for each node in the network. Section 5 shows the empirical speedups and accuracy gains achieved by the algorithm.

1.1 Graphical Models

To simplify presentation, we will consider only Bayesian networks, but the results generalize to any graphical model. We also restrict the class of networks to those without undirected loops, or polytrees, of which Junction trees are a member. We have a Bayesian Network $\mathcal{B}$, which is composed of an independence graph, $\mathcal{G}$ and parameters for CPT tables. The independence graph $\mathcal{G} = (\mathcal{X}, \mathcal{E})$ is a directed acyclic graph (DAG) in which $\mathcal{X}$ is a set of N discrete random variables $\{x_1, x_2, ..., x_N\} \in \mathcal{X}$, and the edges define the independence relations. We will denote the marginal distribution of a single node $P(x|\mathcal{B})$ by π_x, where $(\pi_x)_i$ is $P(x = i)$. We will omit conditioning on $\mathcal{B}$ for the remainder of the paper. We indicate the number states a node x can assume as $|x|$.

Additionally, each node x is assigned a *cost matrix* C_x, in which $(C_x)_{ij}$ is the cost of believing $x = j$ when in fact the true value $x^* = i$. A cost matrix of all zeros indicates that one is not interested in the node's value. The cost matrix C is useful because inhomogeneous costs are a common feature in most realistic domains. This ubiquity results from the fact that information almost always has a *purpose*, so that some variables are more relevant than others, some states of a variable are more relevant than others, and confusion between some pairs of states are more relevant than between other pairs.

For our task, we are given $\mathcal{B}$, and wish to estimate $P(\mathcal{X})$ accurately by iteratively selecting the next node to observe. Although typically only a subset of the nodes are queryable, we will for the purposes of this paper assume that any node can be queried. How do we select the most informative node to query? We must first define our objective function, which is determined by our definition of error.

2 Risk Due to Uncertainty

The underlying error function for the information gain computation will be denoted $Error(P(\mathcal{X})||\mathcal{X}^*)$, which quantifies the loss associated with the current belief state, $P(\mathcal{X})$ given the true values $\mathcal{X}^*$. There are several common candidates for this role, a log-loss function, a log-loss function over marginals, and an expected 0-1 misclassification rate (Kohavi & Wolpert, 1996). Constant factors have been omitted.

$$Error_{log}(P(\mathcal{X})||\mathcal{X}^*) = -\log P(\mathcal{X}^*) \tag{1}$$

$$Error_{mlog}(P(\mathcal{X})||\mathcal{X}^*) = -\sum_{u \in \mathcal{X}} \log P(u^*) \tag{2}$$

$$Error_{01}(P(\mathcal{X})||\mathcal{X}^*) = -\sum_{u \in \mathcal{X}} P(u^*) \tag{3}$$

Where $\mathcal{X}$ is the set of nodes, and u^* is the true value of node u. The error function of Equation 1 will prove insufficient for our needs as it cannot target individual node errors, while the error function of Equation 2 results in an objective function that is quadratic in cost to compute.

We will be exploring a more general form of Equation 3 which allows arbitrary weights to be placed on different *types* of misclassifications. For instance, we would like to specify that misclassifying a node's state as 0 when it is actually 1 is different from misclassifying it as 0 when it is actually in state 2. Different costs for each node can be specified with cost matrices C_u for $u \in \mathcal{X}$. The final error function is

$$Error(P(\mathcal{X})||\mathcal{X}^*) = \sum_{u \in \mathcal{X}} \sum_{i}^{|u|} P(u = i) C_u[u^*, i] \tag{4}$$

Where $C[i, j]$ is the ijth element of the matrix C, and $|u|$ is the number of states that the node u can assume. The presence of the cost matrix C_u in Equation 4 constitutes a significant advantage in real applications, as they often need to specify inhomogeneous costs.

There is a separate consideration, that of *query cost*, or $cost(x)$, which is the cost incurred by the action of observing x (e.g., the cost of a medical test.) If both the query cost and the misclassification cost C are formulated in the same units, e.g., dollars, then they form a coherent decision framework. The query costs will be omitted from this presentation for clarity.

In general, one does not actually know the true values $\mathcal{X}^*$ of the nodes, so one cannot directly minimize the error function as described. Instead, the expected error, or risk, is used.

$$Risk(P(\mathcal{X})) = \sum_{\mathbf{x}} P(\mathbf{x}) Error P(\mathcal{X}||\mathbf{x}) \tag{5}$$

which for the error function of Equation 4 reduces to

$$Risk(P(\mathcal{X})) = \sum_{u \in \mathcal{X}} \sum_{j} \sum_{k} P(u = j) P(u = k) C_u[j, k] \tag{6}$$

$$= \sum_{u \in \mathcal{X}} \pi_u^T C_u \pi_u \tag{7}$$

where $(\pi_u)_i = P(u = i)$. This is the objective we will minimize. It quantifies "On average, how much is our current ignorance going cost us?" For comparison, note that the log-loss function, $Error_{log}$, results in an entropy risk function $Risk_{log}(P(\mathcal{X})) = H(\mathcal{X})$, and the log-loss function over the marginals, $Error_{mlog}$, results in the risk function $Risk_{mlog}(P(\mathcal{X})) = \sum_{u \in \mathcal{X}} H(u)$.

Ultimately, we want to find the nodes that have the greatest effect on $Risk(P(\mathcal{X}))$, so we must condition $Risk(P(\mathcal{X}))$ on the beliefs at each node. In other words, if we learned that the true marginal probabilities of node x were π_x, what effect would that have on our current risk, or rather, what is $Risk(P(\mathcal{X})|P(x) = \pi_x)$? Discouragingly, however, any change in π_x propagates to all the other beliefs in the network. It seems as if we must perform several network evaluations for each node, a prohibitive cost for networks of any appreciable size. However, we will show that in fact dynamic programming can perform this computation for all nodes in only two passes through the network.

3 Risk Calculation

To clarify our objective, we wish to construct a function $R_a(\pi)$ for each node a, where $R_a(\pi) = Risk(P(\mathcal{X})|P(a) = \pi)$. Suppose, for instance, that we learn that the value of node a is equal to 3. Our $P(\mathcal{X})$ is now constrained to have the marginal $P(a) = \pi_a'$, where $(\pi_a')_3 = 1$ and equals zero elsewhere. If we had the function R_a in hand, we could simply evaluate $R_a(\pi_a')$ to immediately compute our new network-wide risk, which would account for all the changes in beliefs to all the other nodes due to learning that $a = 3$. This is exactly our objective; we would like to precompute R_a for all $a \in \mathcal{X}$. Define

$$R_a(\pi) = Risk(P(\mathcal{X})|P(a) = \pi) \tag{8}$$

$$= \left. \sum_{u \in \mathcal{X}} \pi_u^T C_u \pi_u \right|_{P(a)=\pi} \tag{9}$$

This simply restates the risk definition of Equation 7 under the condition that $P(a) = \pi$. As shown in the next theorem, the function R_a has a surprisingly simple form.

Theorem 3.1. *For any node x, the function $R_x(\pi)$ is a second-degree polynomial function of the elements of π*

Proof. Define the matrix $\mathbf{P}_{u|v}$ for every pair of nodes (u, v), such that $(\mathbf{P}_{u|v})_{ij} = P(u = j|v = i)$. Recall that the the beliefs at node x have a strictly linear relationship to the beliefs of node u, since

$$(\pi_u)_i = \sum_k P(u = i|x = k)P(x = k) \tag{10}$$

is equivalent to $\pi_u = \mathbf{P}_{u|x}\pi_x$. Substituting $\mathbf{P}_{u|x}\pi_x$ for π_u in Equation 9 obtains

$$R_x(\pi) = \sum_{u \in \mathcal{X}} \pi_x^T \mathbf{P}_{u|x}^T C_u \mathbf{P}_{u|x}\pi_x \Bigg|_{\pi_x = \pi} \tag{11}$$

$$= \pi^T \left(\sum_{u \in \mathcal{X}} \mathbf{P}_{u|x}^T C_u \mathbf{P}_{u|x} \right) \pi \tag{12}$$

$$= \pi^T \Theta_x \pi \tag{13}$$

Where Θ_x is an $|x| \times |x|$ matrix.

$\square$

Note that the matrix Θ_x is sufficient to completely describe R_x, so we only need to consider the computation of Θ_x for $x \in \mathcal{X}$. From Equation 12, we see a simple equation for computing these Θ_x directly (though expensively):

$$\Theta_x = \sum_{u \in \mathcal{X}} \mathbf{P}_{u|x}^T C_u \mathbf{P}_{u|x} \tag{14}$$

Example #1
Given the 2-node network $a \to b$, how do we calculate $R_a(\pi)$, the total risk associated with our beliefs about the value of node a? Our objective is thus to determine

$$R_a(\pi) = Risk(P(a, b)|P(a) = \pi) \tag{15}$$

$$= \pi^T \Theta_a \pi \tag{16}$$

Equation 14 will give Θ_a as

$$\Theta_a = \mathbf{P}_{a|a}^T C_a \mathbf{P}_{a|a} + \mathbf{P}_{b|a}^T C_b \mathbf{P}_{b|a} \tag{17}$$

$$= C_a + \mathbf{P}_{b|a}^T C_b \mathbf{P}_{b|a} \tag{18}$$

with $\mathbf{P}_{a|a} = \mathbf{I}$ by definition. The individual coefficients of Θ_a are thus

$$\theta_{aij} = C_{aij} + \sum_k \sum_l P(b = k|a = i)P(b = l|a = j)C_{bkl} \tag{19}$$

Now we can compute the relation between any marginal π at node a and our total network-wide risk via $R_a(\pi)$. However, using Equation 14 to compute all the Θ would require evaluating the entire network once per node. The function can, however, be decomposed further, which will enable much more efficient computation of Θ_x for $x \in \mathcal{X}$.

3.1 Recursion

To create an efficient message-passing algorithm for computing Θ_x for all $x \in \mathcal{X}$, we will introduce $\Theta_x^{\mathcal{W}}$, where $\mathcal{W}$ is a *subset* of the network over which $Risk(P(\mathcal{X}))$ is summed.

$$\Theta_x^{\mathcal{W}} = \sum_{u \in \mathcal{W}} \mathbf{P}_{u|x}^T C_u \mathbf{P}_{u|x} \qquad (20)$$

This is otherwise identical to Equation 14. It implies, for instance, that $\Theta_x^x = C_x$. More importantly, these matrices can be usefully decomposed as follows.

Theorem 3.2. $\Theta_x^{\mathcal{W}} = \mathbf{P}_{y|x}^T \Theta_y^{\mathcal{W}} \mathbf{P}_{y|x}$ *if x and $\mathcal{W}$ are conditionally independent given y.*

Proof. Note that $\mathbf{P}_{u|x} = \mathbf{P}_{u|y} \mathbf{P}_{y|x}$ for $u \in \mathcal{X}$, since

$$(\mathbf{P}_{u|y} \mathbf{P}_{y|x})_{ij} = \sum_k^{|y|} P(u = i|y = k) P(y = k|x = j) \qquad (21)$$

$$= P(u = i|x = j) \qquad (22)$$

$$= (\mathbf{P}_{u|x})_{ij} \qquad (23)$$

Step (21) is only true if x and u are conditionally independent given y. Substituting this result into Equation 20, we conclude

$$\Theta_x^{\mathcal{W}} = \sum_{u \in \mathcal{W}} \mathbf{P}_{u|x}^T C_u \mathbf{P}_{u|x} \qquad (24)$$

$$= \sum_{u \in \mathcal{W}} \mathbf{P}_{y|x}^T \mathbf{P}_{u|y}^T \Theta_u^u \mathbf{P}_{u|y} \mathbf{P}_{y|x} \qquad (25)$$

$$= \mathbf{P}_{y|x}^T \left(\sum_{u \in \mathcal{W}} \mathbf{P}_{u|y}^T \Theta_u^u \mathbf{P}_{u|y} \right) \mathbf{P}_{y|x} \qquad (26)$$

$$= \mathbf{P}_{y|x}^T \Theta_y^{\mathcal{W}} \mathbf{P}_{y|x} \qquad (27)$$

$$\square$$

Example #2

Suppose we now have a 3-node network, $a \to b \to c$, and we are only interested in the effect that node a has on the network-wide $Risk$. Our objective is to compute

$$R_a(\pi) = Risk(P(a, b, c)|P(a) = \pi) \qquad (28)$$

$$= \pi^T \Theta_a \pi \qquad (29)$$

where Θ_a is by definition

$$\Theta_a = \Theta_a^{abc} \qquad (30)$$

$$= C_a + \mathbf{P}_{b|a}^T C_b \mathbf{P}_{b|a} + \mathbf{P}_{c|a}^T C_c \mathbf{P}_{c|a} \qquad (31)$$

Using Theorem 3.2 and the fact that a is conditionally independent of c given b, we know

$$\Theta_a^{abc} = \Theta_a^a + \mathbf{P}_{b|a}^T \Theta_b^{bc} \mathbf{P}_{b|a} \qquad (32)$$

$$\Theta_b^{bc} = \Theta_b^b + \mathbf{P}_{c|b}^T \Theta_c^c \mathbf{P}_{c|b} \qquad (33)$$

Substituting 33 into 32

$$\Theta_a = \Theta_a^a + \mathbf{P}_{b|a}^T \left(\Theta_b^b + \mathbf{P}_{c|b}^T \Theta_c^c \mathbf{P}_{c|b} \right) \mathbf{P}_{b|a} \qquad (34)$$

$$= C_a + \mathbf{P}_{b|a}^T \left(C_b + \mathbf{P}_{c|b}^T C_c \mathbf{P}_{c|b} \right) \mathbf{P}_{b|a} \qquad (35)$$

Note that the coefficient Θ_a is obtained from probabilities between neighboring nodes only, without having to explicitly compute $\mathbf{P}_{c|a}$.

4 Message Passing

We are now ready to define message passing. Messages are of two types; *in*-messages and *out*-messages. They are denoted by λ and μ, respectively. Out-messages μ are passed from parent to child, and in-messages λ are passed from child to parent. The messages from x to y will be denoted as μ_{xy} and λ_{xy}. In the discrete case, μ_{xy} and λ_{xy} will both be matrices of size $|y| \times |y|$. The messages summarize the effect that y has on the part of the network that y is d-separated from by x. Messages relate to the Θ coefficients by the following definition

$$\lambda_{yx} = \Theta_x^{\backslash y} \tag{36}$$

$$\mu_{yx} = \Theta_x^{\backslash y} \tag{37}$$

where the (nonstandard) notation $\Theta_x^{\backslash y}$ indicates the matrix $\Theta_x^{\mathcal{V}}$ for which $\mathcal{V}$ is the set of all the nodes in $\mathcal{X}$ that are reachable by x if y were removed from the graph. In other words, $\Theta_x^{\backslash y}$ is summarizing the effect that x has on the entire network *except* for the part of the network that x can only reach through y.

Propagation: The message-passing scheme is organized to recursively compute the Θ matrices using Theorem 3.2. As can be seen from Equations 36 and 37, the two types of messages are very similar in meaning. They differ only in that passing a message from a parent to child automatically separates the child from the rest of the network the parent is connected to, while a child-to-parent message does not necessarily separate the parent from the rest of the network that the child is connected to (due to the "explaining away" effect.)

The contruction of the μ-message involves a short sequence of basic linear algebra. The μ-message from x to child c is created from all other messages entering x except those from c. The definition is

$$\mu_{xc} = \mathbf{P}_{x|c}^T \left(C_x + \sum_{u \in pa(x)} \mu_{ux} + \sum_{v \in ch(x)\backslash c} \lambda_{vx} \right) \mathbf{P}_{x|c} \tag{38}$$

The λ-messages from x to parent u are only slightly more involved. To account for the "explaining away" effect, we must construct λ_{xu} directly from the parents of x.

$$\lambda_{xu} = \mathbf{P}_{x|u}^T \left(C_x + \sum_{c \in ch(x)} \lambda_{cx} \right) \mathbf{P}_{x|u} +$$

$$\sum_{w \in pa(x)\backslash u} \mathbf{P}_{w|u}^T \left(C_w + \sum_{v \in pa(w)} \mu_{vw} + \sum_{c \in ch(w)\backslash x} \lambda_{cw} \right) \mathbf{P}_{w|u} \tag{39}$$

Messages are constructed (or "sent") whenever all of the required incoming messages are present *and* that particular message has not already been sent. For example, the out-message μ_{xc} can be sent only when messages from all the parents of x and all the children of x (save c) are present. The overall effect of this constraint is a single leaves-inward propagation followed by a single root-outward propagation.

Initialization and Termination: Initialization occurs naturally at any singly-connected (leaf) node x, where the message is by definition C_x. Termination occurs when no more messages meet the criteria for sending. Once all message propagation is finished, for each node x the coefficients Θ_x can be computed by a simple summation:

$$\Theta_x = \sum_{c \in ch(x)} \lambda_{cx} + \sum_{u \in par(x)} \mu_{ux} + C_x \tag{40}$$

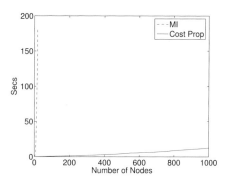

Figure 1: Comparison of execution times with synthetic polytrees.

Propagation runs in time linear in the number of nodes once the initial local probabilities are calculated. The local probabilities required are the matrices $\mathbf{P}$ for each parent-child probability, e.g., $P(child = j|parent = i)$, and for each *pair* (not set) of parents that share a child, $P(parent = j|coparent = i)$. These are all immediately available from a junction tree, or they can be obtained with a run of belief propagation.

It is worth noting that the apparent complexity of the λ, μ message propagation equations is due to the Bayes Net representation. The equivalent factor graph equations (not shown) are markedly more succinct.

5 Experiments

The performance of the message-passing algorithm (hereafter CostProp) was compared with a standard information gain algorithm which uses mutual information (hereafter MI). The error function used by MI is from Equation 2, where $Error_{mlog}(P(\mathcal{X})||\mathcal{X}^*) = \sum_{x \in \mathcal{X}} \log P(x^*)$, with a corresponding risk function $Risk(P(\mathcal{X})) = \sum_{x \in \mathcal{X}} H(x)$. This corresponds to selecting the node x that has the highest summed mutual information with each of the target nodes (in this case, the set of target nodes is $\mathcal{X}$ and the set of query nodes is also $\mathcal{X}$.) The computational cost of MI grows quadratically as the product of the number of queries and of targets.

In order to test the speed and relative accuracy of CostProp, we generated random polytrees with varying numbers of trinary nodes. The CPT tables were randomly generated with a slight bias towards lower-entropy probabilities. The code was written in Matlab using the Bayes Net Toolbox (Murphy, 2005).

Speed: We generated polytrees of sizes ranging from 2 to 1000 nodes and ran the MI algorithm, the CostProp algorithm, and a random-query algorithm on each. The two non-random algorithms were run using a junction tree, the build time of which was not included in the reported run times of either algorithm. Even with the relatively slow Matlab code, the speedup shown in Figure 1 is obvious. As expected, CostProp is many orders of magnitude faster than the MI algorithm, and shows a qualitative difference in scaling properties.

Accuracy: Due to the slow running time of MI, the accuracy comparison was performed on polytrees of size 20. For each run, a true assignment $\mathcal{X}^*$ was generated from the tree, but were initially hidden from the algorithms. Each algorithm would then determine for itself the best node to observe, receive the true value of that node, then select the next node to observe, et cetera. The true error at each step was computed as the 0-1 error of Equation 3. The reduction in error plotted against number of queries is shown in Figure 2. With uniform

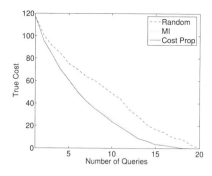

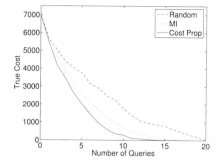

Figure 2: Performance on synthetic poly-trees with symmetric costs.

Figure 3: Performance on synthetic poly-trees with asymmetric costs.

cost matrices, performance of MI and CostProp are approximately equal on this task, but both are better than random. We next made the cost matrices asymmetric by initializing them such that confusing one pair of states was 100 times more costly than confusing the other two pairs. The results of Figure 3 show that CostProp reduces error faster than MI, presumably because it can accomodate the cost matrix information.

6 Discussion

We have described an all-pairs information gain calculation that scales linearly with network size. The objective function used has a polynomial form that allows for an efficient message-passing algorithm. Empirical results demonstrate large speedups and even improved accuracy in cost-sensitive domains. Future work will explore other applications of this method, including sensitivity analysis and active learning. Further research into other uses for the belief polynomials will also be explored.

References

Agostak, J. M., & Weiss, J. (1999). Active Fusion for Diagnosis Guided by Mutual Information. *Proceedings of the 2nd International Conference on Information Fusion*.

Anderson, B. S., & Moore, A. W. (2005). Active learning for hidden markov models: Objective functions and algorithms. *Proceedings of the 22nd International Conference on Machine Learning*.

Kjrulff, U., & van der Gaag, L. (2000). Making sensitivity analysis computationally efficient.

Kohavi, R., & Wolpert, D. H. (1996). Bias Plus Variance Decomposition for Zero-One Loss Functions. *Machine Learning : Proceedings of the Thirteenth International Conference*. Morgan Kaufmann.

Krishnamurthy, V. (2002). Algorithms for optimal scheduling and management of hidden markov model sensors. *IEEE Transactions on Signal Processing, 50*, 1382–1397.

Laskey, K. B. (1995). Sensitivity Analysis for Probability Assessments in Bayesian Networks. *IEEE Transactions on Systems, Man, and Cybernetics*.

Murphy, K. (2005). *Bayes net toolbox for matlab*. U. C. Berkeley. http://www.ai.mit.edu/~murphyk/Software/BNT/bnt.html.

A Cortically-Plausible Inverse Problem Solving Method Applied to Recognizing Static and Kinematic 3D Objects

David W. Arathorn

Center for Computational Biology,

Montana State University

Bozeman, MT 59717

`dwa@cns.montana.edu`

General Intelligence Corporation
`dwa@giclab.com`

Abstract

Recent neurophysiological evidence suggests the ability to interpret biological motion is facilitated by a neuronal "mirror system" which maps visual inputs to the pre-motor cortex. If the common architecture and circuitry of the cortices is taken to imply a common computation across multiple perceptual and cognitive modalities, this visual-motor interaction might be expected to have a unified computational basis. Two essential tasks underlying such visual-motor cooperation are shown here to be simply expressed and directly solved as transformation-discovery inverse problems: (a) discriminating and determining the pose of a primed 3D object in a real-world scene, and (b) interpreting the 3D configuration of an articulated kinematic object in an image. The recently developed map-seeking method provides a mathematically tractable, cortically-plausible solution to these and a variety of other inverse problems which can be posed as the discovery of a composition of transformations between two patterns. The method relies on an ordering property of superpositions and on decomposition of the transformation spaces inherent in the generating processes of the problem.

1 Introduction

A variety of "brain tasks" can be tersely posed as transformation-discovery problems. Vision is replete with such problems, as is limb control. The problem of recognizing the 2D projection of a known 3D object is an inverse problem of finding both the visual and pose transformations relating the image and the 3D model of the object. When the object in the image may be one of many known objects another step is added to the inverse problem, because there are multiple candidates each of which must be mapped to the input image with possibly different transformations. When the known object is not rigid, the determination of articulations and/or morphings is added to the inverse problem. This includes the general problem of recognition of biological articulation and motion, a task recently attributed to a neuronal mirror-system linking visual and motor cortical areas [1].

Though the aggregate transformation space implicit in such problems is vast, a recently developed method for exploring vast transformation spaces has allowed some significant progress with a simple unified approach. The map-seeking method [2,4] is a general purpose mathematical procedure for finding the decomposition of the aggregate transformation between two patterns, even when that aggregate transformation space is vast and there is no prior information is available to restrict the search space. The problem of concurrently searching a large collection of memories can be treated as a subset of the transformation problem and consequently the same method can be applied to find the best transformation between an input image and a collection of memories (numbering at least thousands in practice to date) during a single convergence. In the last several years the map-seeking method has been applied to a variety of practical problems, most of them related to vision, a few related to kinematics, and some which do not correspond to usual categories of "brain functions." The generality of the method is due to the fact that only the mappings are specialized to the task. The mathematics of the search, whether expressed in an algorithm or in a neuronal or electronic circuit, do not change. From an evolutionary biological point of view this is a satisfying characteristic for a model of cortical function because only the connectivity which implements the mappings must be varied to specialize a cortex to a task. All the rest – organization and dynamics – would remain the same across cortical areas.

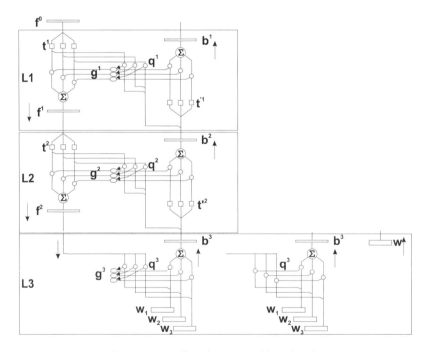

Figure 1. Data flow in map-seeking circuit

Cortical neuroanatomy offers emphatic hints about the characteristics of its solution in the vast neuronal resources allocated to creating reciprocal top-down and bottom-up pathways. More specifically, recent evidence suggests this reciprocal pathway architecture appears to be organized with reciprocal, co-centered fan outs in the opposing directions [3], quite possibly implementing inverse mappings. The data flow of map-seeking computations, seen in Figure 1, is architecturally compatibility with these features of cortical organization. Though not within the scope of this discussion, it has been demonstrated [4] that the mathematical expression of the map-seeking method, seen in equations 6-9 below, has an isomorphic implementation in neuronal circuitry with reasonably realistic dendritic architecture and dynamics (e.g. compatible with [5]) and oscillatory dynamics.

2 The basis for tractable transformation-discovery

The related problems of recognition/interpretation of 2D images of static and articulated kinematic 3D objects illustrate how cleanly significant vision problems may be posed and solved as transformation-discovery inverse problems. The visual and pose (in the sense of orientation) transformations, t^{visual} and t^{pose}, between a given 3D model m_1 and the extent of an input image containing a 2D projection $P(o_1)$ of an object o_1 mappable to m_1 can be expressed

$$P(o_1) = t_j^{visual} \circ t_k^{pose}(m_1) \qquad t_j^{visual} \in T^{visual}, t_k^{pose} \in T^{pose} \qquad \text{eq. 1}$$

If we now consider that the model m_1 may be constructed by the one-to-many mapping of a base vector or feature $\mathbf{e}$, and that arbitrarily other models m_i may be similarly constructed by different mappings, then the transformation $t^{formation}$ corresponding to the correct "memory" converts the memory database search problem into another transformation-discovery problem with one more composed transformation[1]

$$P(o_1) = t_j^{visual} \circ t_k^{pose} \circ t_{m_1}^{formation}(\mathbf{e}) \qquad t_{m_1}^{formation} \in T^{formation}$$

$$t_{m_1}^{formation}(\mathbf{e}) = m_l \quad m_l \in M \qquad \text{eq. 2}$$

Finally, if we allow a morphable object to be "constructed" by a generative model, whose various configurations or articulations may be generated by a composition of transformations $t^{generative}$ of some root or seed feature $\mathbf{e}$, the problem of explicitly recognizing the particular configuration of morph becomes a transformation-discovery problem of the form

$$P(C_l(o)) = t_j^{visual} \circ t_k^{pose} \circ t_l^{generative}(\mathbf{e}) \qquad t_l^{generative} \in T^{generative} \qquad \text{eq. 3}$$

These unifying formulations are only useful, however, if there is a tractable method of solving for the various transformations. That is what the map-seeking method provides. Abstractly the problem is the discovery of a composition of transformations between two patterns. In general the transformations express the generating process of the problem. Define correspondence c between vectors $\mathbf{r}$ and $\mathbf{w}$ through a composition of L transformations $t_{j_1}^1, t_{j_2}^2, \cdots, t_{j_L}^L$ where $t_{jl}^l \in t_1^l, t_2^l, \cdots, t_{nl}^l$

---

[1] This illustrates that forming a superposition of memories is equivalent to forming superpositions of transformations. The first is a more practical realization, as seen in Figure 1. Though not demonstrated in this paper, the multi-memory architecture has proved robust with 1000 or more memory patterns from real-world datasets.

$$c(\mathbf{j}) = \left\langle \overset{L}{\underset{i=1}{\circ}} t^i_{j_i}(\mathbf{r}), \mathbf{w} \right\rangle \qquad\qquad \text{eq. 4}$$

where the composition operator is defined

$$\overset{L}{\underset{i=\varnothing,1}{\circ}} t^l_{j_i}(\mathbf{r}) = \begin{cases} l=1\cdots L & t^L_{j_L} \circ t^{L-1}_{j_{L-1}} \cdots \circ t^1_{j_1}(\mathbf{r}) \\ l=\varnothing & \mathbf{r} \end{cases}$$

Let $\mathbf{C}$ be an L dimensional matrix of values of $c(\mathbf{j})$ whose dimensions are $n_1 \ldots n_L$. The problem, then is to find

$$\mathbf{x} = \arg\max \; c(\mathbf{j}) \qquad\qquad \text{eq. 5}$$

The indices $\mathbf{x}$ specify the sequence of transformations that best correspondence between vectors $\mathbf{r}$ and $\mathbf{w}$. The problem is that $\mathbf{C}$ is too large a space to search for $\mathbf{x}$ by conventional means. Instead, a continuous embedding of $\mathbf{C}$ permits a search with resources proportional to the sum of sizes of the dimensions of $\mathbf{C}$ instead of their product.

C is embedded in a superposition dot product space Q defined

$$Q : \mathbb{R}^{\sum_{l=1}^{L} n_l} \to \mathbb{R}^1$$

$$Q(\mathbf{G}) = \left\langle \overset{m-1}{\underset{l=1}{\circ}} \left(\sum_i g^l_i \cdot t^l_i \right)(\mathbf{r}), \overset{m+1}{\underset{l=\varnothing,L}{\circ}} \left(\sum_i g^l_i \cdot t^{\prime l}_i \right)(\mathbf{w}) \right\rangle \qquad \text{eq. 6}$$

where $\mathbf{G} = \left[g^m_{x_m} \right]$ $m = 1 \cdots L, x_m = 1 \cdots n_m$ n_m is number of t in layer m, $g^m_{x_m} \in [0,1]$, $t^{\prime l}_i$ is adjoint of t^l_i.

In Q space, the solution to eq. 5 lies along a single axis in the set of axes represented each row of $\mathbf{G}$. That is, $\mathbf{g}^m = <0,\cdots,u_{x_m},\cdots,0>$ $u_{x_m} > 0$ which corresponds to the best fitting transformation t_{x_m}, where $\mathbf{x}_m$ is the mth index in $\mathbf{x}$ in eq. 5. This state is reached from an initial state $\mathbf{G} = [1]$ by a process termed *superposition culling* in which the components of grad Q are used to compute a path in steps Δg,

$$\frac{\partial Q(\mathbf{G})}{g^m_j} = \left\langle t^m_j \overset{m-1}{\underset{l=\varnothing,1}{\circ}} \left(\sum_i g^l_i \cdot t^l_i \right)(\mathbf{r}), \overset{m+1}{\underset{l=\varnothing,L}{\circ}} \left(\sum_i g^l_i \cdot t^{\prime l}_i \right)(\mathbf{w}) \right\rangle \qquad \text{eq. 7}$$

$$\Delta \mathbf{g}^m = f\left(\frac{\partial Q(\mathbf{G})}{\partial g^m_1}, \cdots, \frac{\partial Q(\mathbf{G})}{\partial g^m_{n_m}} \right) \qquad\qquad \text{eq. 8}$$

The function f preserves the maximal component and reduces the others: in neuronal terms, *lateral inhibition*. The resulting path along the surface Q can be thought of as a "high traverse" in contrast to the gradient ascent or descent usual in optimization methods. The price for moving the problem into superposition dot product space is that *collusions* of components of the superpositions can result in better matches for incorrect mappings than for the mappings of the correct solution. If this occurs it is almost always a temporary state early in the convergence. This is a consequence of the *ordering property of superpositions* (OPS) [2,4], which, as applied here, describes the characteristics of the surface Q. For example, let three superpositions $\mathbf{r} = \sum_{i=1}^{n} \mathbf{u}_i$, $\mathbf{s} = \sum_{j=1}^{m} \mathbf{v}_j$ and $\mathbf{s}' = \sum_{k=1}^{m} \mathbf{v}_k$ be formed from three sets of sparse vectors $\mathbf{u}_i \in \mathbf{R}$, $\mathbf{v}_j \in \mathbf{S}$ and $\mathbf{v}_k \in \mathbf{S}'$ where $\mathbf{R} \cap \mathbf{S} = \emptyset$ and $\mathbf{R} \cap \mathbf{S}' = \mathbf{v}_q$. Then the following relationship expresses the OPS:

define $P_{correct} = P(\mathbf{r} \bullet \mathbf{s}' > \mathbf{r} \bullet \mathbf{s})$, $P_{incorrect} = P(\mathbf{r} \bullet \mathbf{s}' \leq \mathbf{r} \bullet \mathbf{s})$

then $P_{correct} > P_{incorrect}$ or $P_{correct} > 0.5$

and as $n, m \to 1$ $P_{correct} \to 1.0$

Applied to eq. 8, this means that for superpositions composed of vectors which satisfy the distribution properties of sparse, decorrelating encodings[2] (a biologically plausible assumption [6]), the probability of the maximum components of grad Q moving the solution in the correct direction is always greater than 0.5 and increases toward 1.0 as the $\mathbf{G}$ becomes sparser. In other words, the probability of the occurrence of collusion decreases with the decrease in numbers of contributing components in the superposition(s), and/or the decrease in their gating coefficients.

3 The map-seeking method and application

A map-seeking circuit (MSC) is composed of several transformation or mapping layers between the input at one end and a memory layer at the other, as seen in Figure 1. The compositional structure is evident in the simplicity of the equations (eqs. 9-12 below) which define a circuit of any dimension. In a multi-layer circuit of L layers plus memory with n_l mappings in layer l the forward path signal for layer m is computed

$$\mathbf{f}^m = \sum_{j=1}^{n_m} g_j^m \cdot t_j^m (\mathbf{f}^{m-1}) \qquad \text{for } m = 1 \dots L \qquad\qquad \text{eq. 9}$$

The backward path signal for layer m is computed

$$\mathbf{b}^m = \begin{cases} \sum_{j=1}^{n_l} g_j^m \cdot t_j'^m (\mathbf{b}^{m+1}) & \text{for } m = 1 \dots L \\ \sum_{k} z(\mathbf{w}_k \bullet \mathbf{f}^L) \cdot \mathbf{w}_k \quad or \quad \sum_{k=1}^{n_w} g_k^m \cdot \mathbf{w}_k \quad or \quad \mathbf{w} & \text{for } m = L+1 \end{cases} \qquad \text{eq. 10}$$

The mapping coefficients g are updated by the recurrence

$$g_i^m := \kappa\left(g_i^m, t_i^m(\mathbf{f}^{m-1}) \bullet \mathbf{b}^{m+1}\right) \text{ for } m = 1 \dots L, i = 1 \dots n_l$$
$$g_i^{L+1} := \kappa\left(g_i^{L+1}, \mathbf{f}^L \bullet \mathbf{w}_k\right) \text{ for } k = 1 \dots n_w \text{ (optional)} \qquad \text{eq. 11}$$

where match operator $\mathbf{u} \bullet \mathbf{v} = q$, q is a scalar measure of goodness-of-match between $\mathbf{u}$ and $\mathbf{v}$, and may be non-linear. When $\bullet$ is a dot product, the second argument of κ is the same as $\partial Q / g$ in eq. 7. The competition function κ is a realization of lateral inhibition function f in eq. 8. It may optionally be applied to the memory layer, as seen in eq. 11.

---

[2] A restricted case of the superposition ordering property using non-sparse representation is exploited by HRR distributed memory. See [7] for an analysis which is also applicable here.

$$\kappa(g_i, q_i) = \max\left(0,\ g_i - k_1 \cdot \left(1 - \frac{q_i}{\max \mathbf{q}}\right)^{k_2}\right)$$ eq. 12

Thresholds are normally applied to $\mathbf{q}$ and $\mathbf{g}$, below which they are set to zero to speed convergence. In above, $\mathbf{f}^0$ is the input signal, $t_j^m, t_j'^m$ are the jth forward and backward mappings for the mth layer, $\mathbf{w}_k$ is the kth memory pattern, $z(\ )$ is a non-linearity applied to the response of each memory. $\mathbf{g}^m$ is the set of mapping coefficients g_j^m for the mth layer, each of which is associated with mapping t_j^m and is modified over time by the competition function $\kappa(\ )$.

Recognizing 2D projections of 3D objects under real operating conditions

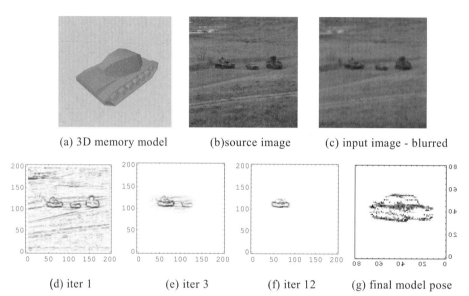

(a) 3D memory model (b)source image (c) input image - blurred

(d) iter 1 (e) iter 3 (f) iter 12 (g) final model pose

Figure 2. Recognizing target among distractor vehicles. (a) M60 3D memory model; (b) source image, Fort Carson Data Set; (c) Gaussian blurred input image; (d-f) isolation of target in layer 0, iterations 1, 3, 12; (g) pose determination in final iteration, layer 4 backward - presented left-right mirrored to reflect mirroring determined in layer 3. M-60 model courtesy Colorado State University.

Real world problems of the form expressed in eq. 1 often present objects at distances or in conditions which so limit the resolution that there are no alignable features other than the shape of the object itself, which is sufficiently blurred as to prevent generating reliable edges in a feed-forward manner (e.g. Fig. 2c). In the map-seeking approach, however, the top-down (in biological parlance) inverse-mappings of the 3D model are used to create a set of edge hypotheses on the backward path out of layer 1 into layer 0. In layer 0 these hypotheses are used to gate the input image. As convergence proceeds, the edge hypotheses are reduced to a single edge hypothesis that best fits the grayscale input image. Figure 2 shows this process applied to one of a set of deliberately blurred images from the Fort Carson Imagery Data Set. The MSC used four layers of visual transformations: 14,400 translational, 31 rotational, 41 scaling, 481 3D projection. The MSC had no difficulty distinguishing the location and orientation of the tank, despite distractors and background clutter: in all tests in the dataset target was correctly located. In effect, once primed with a top-down expectation, attentional behavior is an emergent property of application of the map-seeking method to vision [8].

Adapting generative models by transformation

"The direct-matching hypothesis of the interpretation of biological motion] holds that we understand actions when we map the visual representation of the observed action onto our motor representation of the same action." [1] This mapping, attributed to a neuronal mirror-system for which there is gathering neurobiological evidence (as reviewed in [1]), requires a mechanism for projecting between the visual space and the constrained skeletal joint parameter (kinematic) space to disambiguate the 2D projection of body structure.[4] Though this problem has been solved to various degrees by other computational methods, a review of which is beyond the scope of this discussion, to the author's knowledge none of these have biological plausibility. The present purpose is to show how simply the problem can be expressed by the generative model interpretation problem introduced in eq. 3 and solve by map-seeking circuits. An idealized example is the problem of interpreting the shape of a featureless "snake" articulated into any configuration, as appears in Fig. 3.

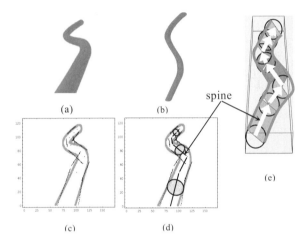

Figure 3. Projection between visual and kinematic spaces with two map-seeking circuits. (a) input view, (b) top view, (c) projection of 3D occluding contours, (d,e) projections of relationship of occluding contours to generating spine.

The solution to this problem involves two coupled map-seeking circuits. The kinematic circuit layers model the multiple degrees of freedom (here two angles, variable length and optionally variable radius from spine to surface) of each of the connected spine segments. The other circuit determines the visual transformations, as seen in the earlier example. The surface of the articulated cylinder is mapped from an axial spine. The points where that surface is tangent to the viewpoint vectors define the occluding contours which, projected in 2D, become the object silhouette. The problem is to find the articulations, segment lengths (and optionally segment diameter) which account for the occluding contour matching the silhouette in the input image. In the MSC solution, the initial state all possible articulations of the snake spine are superposed, and all the occluding contours from a range of viewing angles are projected into 2D. The latter superposition serves as the backward input to the visual space map-seeking circuit. Since the snake surfaceis determined by all of the layers of the kinematic circuit, these are projected in parallel to form the backward (biologically top-down) 2D input to the visual transformation-discovery circuit. A matching operation between the contributors to the 2D occluding contour superposition and the forward transformations of the input image modulates the gain of each mapping in the kinematic circuit via a_i^m in eqs. 13, 14 (modified from eq. 11). In eqs. 13, 14 K indicates kinematic circuit, V indicates visual circuit.

$$\overset{K}{g_i^m} := comp\left(\overset{K}{g_i^m}, \overset{VK}{a_i^m} \cdot \overset{K}{t_i^m}\left(\overset{K}{\mathbf{f}_{m-1}} \right) \bullet \overset{K}{\mathbf{b}^{m+1}} \right) \text{ for } m = 1\ldots\overset{K}{L}, i = 1\ldots\overset{K}{n_i} \qquad \text{eq. 13}$$

$$\overset{VK}{a_i^m} = \left(\overset{V}{\mathbf{f}^L} \right) \bullet t^{3D \to 2D} \circ t^{surface} \circ \overset{K}{t_i'^m}\left(\overset{K}{\mathbf{b}^{m+1}} \right) \qquad \text{eq. 14}$$

The process converges concurrently in both circuits to a solution, as seen in Figure 3. The match of the occluding contours and the input image, Figure 3a, is seen in Figure 3b,c, with its three dimensional structure is clarified in Figure 3d. Figure 3e shows a view of the 3D structure as determined directly from the mapping parameters defining the snake "spine" after convergence.

4 Conclusion

The investigations reported here expand the envelope of vision-related problems amenable to a pure transformation-discovery approach implemented by the map-seeking method. The recognition of static 3D models, as seen in Figure 2, and other problems [9] solved by MSC have been well tested with real-world input. Numerous variants of Figure 3 have demonstrated the applicability of MSC to recognizing generative models of high dimensionality, and the principle has recently been applied successfully to real-world domains. Consequently, the research to date does suggest that a single cortical computational mechanism could span a significant range of the brain's visual and kinematic computing.

References

[1] G. Rizzolati, L. Fogassi, V. Gallese, Neurophysiological mechanisms underlying the understanding and imitation of action, *Nature Reviews Neuroscience*, 2, 2001, 661-670

[2] D. Arathorn, Map-Seeking: Recognition Under Transformation Using A Superposition Ordering Property. *Electronics Letters* 37(3), 2001 pp164-165

[3] A. Angelucci, B. Levitt, E. Walton, J.M. Hupé, J. Bullier, J. Lund, Circuits for Local and Global Signal Integration in Primary Visual Cortex, *Journal of Neuroscience*, 22(19) , 2002 pp 8633-8646

[4] D. Arathorn, *Map-Seeking Circuits in Visual Cognition*, Palo Alto, Stanford Univ Press, 2002

[5] A. Polsky, B. Mel, J. Schiller, Computational Subunits in Thin Dendrites of Pyramidal Cells, *Nature Neuroscience* 7(6), 2004 pp 621-627

[6] B.A. Olshausen, D.J. Field, Emergence of Simple-Cell Receptive Field Properties by Learning a Sparse Code for Natural Images, *Nature,* 381, 1996 pp607-609

[7] T. Plate, *Holographic Reduced Representation*, CSLI publications, Stanford, California, 2003

[8] D. Arathorn, Memory-driven visual attention: an emergent behavior of map-seeking circuits, in *Neurobiology of Attention*, Eds Itti L, Rees G, Tsotsos J, Academic/Elsevier, 2005

[9] C. Vogel, D. Arathorn, A. Parker, and A. Roorda, "Retinal motion tracking in adaptive optics scanning laser ophthalmoscopy", *Proceedings of OSA Conference on Signal Recovery and Synthesis*, Charlotte NC, June 2005.

Combining Graph Laplacians for Semi–Supervised Learning

Andreas Argyriou,   Mark Herbster,   Massimiliano Pontil

Department of Computer Science
University College London
Gower Street, London WC1E 6BT, England, UK
{*a.argyriou, m.herbster, m.pontil*}@*cs.ucl.ac.uk*

Abstract

A foundational problem in semi-supervised learning is the construction
of a graph underlying the data. We propose to use a method which optimally combines a number of differently constructed graphs. For each
of these graphs we associate a basic graph kernel. We then compute
an optimal *combined* kernel. This kernel solves an extended regularization problem which requires a joint minimization over both the data and
the set of graph kernels. We present encouraging results on different
OCR tasks where the optimal combined kernel is computed from graphs
constructed with a variety of distances functions and the 'k' in nearest
neighbors.

1   Introduction

Semi-supervised learning has received significant attention in machine learning in recent
years, see, for example, [2, 3, 4, 8, 9, 16, 17, 18] and references therein. The defining insight
of semi-supervised methods is that unlabeled data may be used to improve the performance
of learners in a supervised task. One of the key semi-supervised learning methods builds
on the assumption that the data is situated on a low dimensional manifold within the ambient space of the data and that this manifold can be approximated by a weighted discrete
graph whose vertices are identified with the empirical (labeled and unlabeled) data, [3, 17].
Graph construction consists of two stages, first selection of a distance function and then
application of it to determine the graph's edges (or weights thereof). For example, in this
paper we consider distances between images based on the Euclidean distance, Euclidean
distance combined with image transformations, and the related tangent distance [6]; we
determine the edge set of the graph with k-nearest neighbors. Another common choice is
to weight edges by a decreasing function of the distance d such as $e^{-\beta d^2}$.

Although a surplus of unlabeled data may improve the quality of the empirical approximation of the manifold (via the graph) leading to improved performances, practical experience
with these methods indicates that their performance significantly depends on how the graph
is constructed. Hence, the model selection problem must consider both the selection of the
distance function and the parameters k or β used in the graph building process described
above. A diversity of methods have been proposed for graph construction; in this paper

we do not advocate *selecting* a single graph but, rather we propose *combining* a number of graphs. Our solution implements a method based on regularization which builds upon the work in [1]. For a given dataset each combination of distance functions and edge set specifications from the distance will lead to a specific graph. Each of these graphs may then be associated with a kernel. We then apply regularization to select the best convex combination of these kernels; the minimizing function will trade off its fit to the data against its norm. What is unique about this regularization is that the minimization is not over a single kernel space but rather over a space corresponding to all convex combinations of kernels. Thus all data (labeled vertices) may be conserved for training rather than reduced by cross-validation which is not an appealing option when the number of labeled vertices per class is very small.

Figure 3 in Section 4 illustrates our algorithm on a simple example. There, three different distances for 400 images of the digits 'six' and 'nine' are depicted, namely, the Euclidean distance, a distance invariant under small centered image rotations from $[-10°, 10°]$ and a distance invariant under rotations from $[-180°, 180°]$. Clearly, the last distance is problematic as sixes become similar to nines. The performance of our graph regularization learning algorithm discussed in Section 2.2 with these distances is reported below each plot; as expected, this performance is much lower in the case that the third distance is used. The paper is constructed as follows. In Section 2 we discuss how regularization may be applied to single graphs. First, we review regularization in the context of reproducing kernel Hilbert spaces (Section 2.1); then in Section 2.2 we specialize our discussion to Hilbert spaces of functions defined over a graph. Here we review the (normalized) Laplacian of the graph and a kernel which is the pseudoinverse of the graph Laplacian. In Section 3 we detail our algorithm for learning an optimal convex combination of Laplacian kernels. Finally, in Section 4 we present experiments on the USPS dataset with our algorithm trained over different classes of Laplacian kernels.

2 Background on graph regularization

In this section we review graph regularization [2, 9, 14] from the perspective of reproducing kernel Hilbert spaces, see e.g. [12].

2.1 Reproducing kernel Hilbert spaces

Let X be a set and $K : X \times X \to \mathbb{R}$ a kernel function. We say that $\mathcal{H}_K$ is a reproducing kernel Hilbert space (RKHS) of functions $f : X \to \mathbb{R}$ if (i): for every $x \in X$, $K(x, \cdot) \in \mathcal{H}_K$ and (ii): the *reproducing kernel property* $f(x) = \langle f, K(x, \cdot) \rangle_K$ holds for every $f \in \mathcal{H}_K$ and $x \in X$, where $\langle \cdot, \cdot \rangle_K$ is the inner product on $\mathcal{H}_K$. In particular, (ii) tells us that for $x, t \in X$, $K(x, t) = \langle K(x, \cdot), K(t, \cdot) \rangle_K$, implying that the $n \times n$ matrix $(K(t_i, t_j) : i, j \in \mathbb{N}_p)$ is symmetric and positive semi-definite for *any* set of inputs $\{t_i : i \in \mathbb{N}_p\} \subseteq X$, $p \in \mathbb{N}$, where we use the notation $\mathbb{N}_p := \{1, \ldots, p\}$.

Regularization in an RKHS learns a function $f \in \mathcal{H}_K$ on the basis of available input/output examples $\{(x_i, y_i) : i \in \mathbb{N}_\ell\}$ by solving the variational problem

$$E_\gamma(K) := \min \left\{ \sum_{i=1}^{\ell} V(y_i, f(x_i)) + \gamma \|f\|_K^2 : f \in \mathcal{H}_K \right\} \tag{2.1}$$

where $V : \mathbb{R} \times \mathbb{R} \to [0, \infty)$ is a loss function and γ a positive parameter. Moreover, if f is a solution to problem (2.1) then it has the form

$$f(x) = \sum_{i=1}^{\ell} c_i K(x_i, x), \ \ x \in X \tag{2.2}$$

68

for some real vector of coefficients $\mathbf{c} = (c_i : i \in \mathbb{N}_\ell)^\top$, see, for example, [12], where "$\top$" denotes transposition. This vector can be found by replacing f by the right hand side of equation (2.2) in equation (2.1) and then optimizing with respect to $\mathbf{c}$. However, in many practical situations it is more convenient to compute $\mathbf{c}$ by solving the dual problem to (2.1), namely

$$-E_\gamma(K) := \min \left\{ \frac{1}{4\gamma} \mathbf{c}^\top \widetilde{\mathbf{K}} \mathbf{c} + \sum_{i=1}^\ell V^*(y_i, c_i) : \mathbf{c} \in \mathbb{R}^\ell \right\} \qquad (2.3)$$

where $\widetilde{\mathbf{K}} = (K(x_i, x_j))_{i,j=1}^\ell$ and the function $V^* : \mathbb{R} \times \mathbb{R} \to \mathbb{R} \cup \{+\infty\}$ is the conjugate of the loss function V which is defined, for every $z, \alpha \in \mathbb{R}$, as $V^*(z, \alpha) := \sup\{\lambda\alpha - V(z, \lambda) : \lambda \in \mathbb{R}\}$, see, for example, [1] for a discussion. The choice of the loss function V leads to different learning methods among which the most prominent are square loss regularization and support vector machines, see, for example [15].

2.2 Graph regularization

Let G be an undirected graph with m vertices and an $m \times m$ adjacency matrix $\mathbf{A}$ such that $A_{ij} = 1$ if there is an edge connecting vertices i and j and zero otherwise[1]. The graph Laplacian $\mathbf{L}$ is the $m \times m$ matrix defined as $\mathbf{L} := \mathbf{D} - \mathbf{A}$, where $\mathbf{D} = \mathrm{diag}(d_i : i \in \mathbb{N}_m)$ and d_i is the degree of vertex i, that is $d_i = \sum_{j=1}^m A_{ij}$.

We identify the linear space of real-valued functions defined on the graph with $\mathbb{R}^m$ and introduce on it the semi-inner product

$$\langle \mathbf{u}, \mathbf{v} \rangle := \mathbf{u}^\top \mathbf{L} \mathbf{v}, \quad \mathbf{u}, \mathbf{v} \in \mathbb{R}^m.$$

The induced semi-norm is $\|\mathbf{v}\| := \sqrt{\langle \mathbf{v}, \mathbf{v} \rangle}$, $\mathbf{v} \in \mathbb{R}^m$. It is a semi-norm since $\|\mathbf{v}\| = 0$ if $\mathbf{v}$ is a constant vector, as can be verified by noting that $\|\mathbf{v}\|^2 = \frac{1}{2} \sum_{i,j=1}^m (v_i - v_j)^2 A_{ij}$.

We recall that G has r connected components if and only if $\mathbf{L}$ has r eigenvectors with zero eigenvalues. Those eigenvectors are piece-wise constant on the connected components of the graph. In particular, G is connected if and only if the constant vector is the only eigenvector of $\mathbf{L}$ with zero eigenvalue [5]. We let $\{\sigma_i, \mathbf{u}_i\}_{i=1}^m$ be a system of eigenvalues/vectors of $\mathbf{L}$ where the eigenvalues are non-decreasing in order, $\sigma_i = 0$, $i \in \mathbb{N}_r$, and define the linear subspace $\mathcal{H}(G)$ of $\mathbb{R}^m$ which is orthogonal to the eigenvectors with zero eigenvalue, that is,

$$\mathcal{H}(G) := \{\mathbf{v} : \mathbf{v}^\top \mathbf{u}_i = 0, \ i \in \mathbb{N}_r\}.$$

Within this framework, we wish to learn a function $\mathbf{v} \in \mathcal{H}(G)$ on the basis of a set of labeled vertices. Without loss of generality we assume that the first $\ell \leq m$ vertices are labeled and let $y_1, ..., y_\ell \in \{-1, 1\}$ be the corresponding labels. Following [2] we prescribe a loss function V and compute the function $\mathbf{v}$ by solving the optimization problem

$$\min \left\{ \sum_{i=1}^\ell V(y_i, v_i) + \gamma \|\mathbf{v}\|^2 : \mathbf{v} \in \mathcal{H}(G) \right\}. \qquad (2.4)$$

We note that a similar approach is presented in [17] where $\mathbf{v}$ is (essentially) obtained as the minimal norm interpolant in $\mathcal{H}(G)$ to the labeled vertices. The functional (2.4) balances the error on the labeled points with a smoothness term measuring the complexity of $\mathbf{v}$ on the graph. Note that this last term contains the information of both the labeled and unlabeled vertices via the graph Laplacian.

---

[1]The ideas we discuss below naturally extend to weighted graphs.

Method (2.4) is a special case of problem (2.1). Indeed, the restriction of the semi-norm $\|\cdot\|$ on $\mathcal{H}(G)$ is a norm. Moreover, the pseudoinverse of the Laplacian, $\mathbf{L}^+$, is the reproducing kernel of $\mathcal{H}(G)$, see, for example, [7] for a proof. This means that for every $\mathbf{v} \in \mathcal{H}(G)$ and $i \in \mathbb{N}_m$ there holds the reproducing kernel property $v_i = \langle \mathbf{L}_i^+, \mathbf{v} \rangle$, where $\mathbf{L}_i^+$ is the i-th column of $\mathbf{L}^+$. Hence, by setting $X \equiv \mathbb{N}_m$, $f(i) = v_i$ and $K(i,j) = L_{ij}^+$, $i,j \in \mathbb{N}_m$, we see that $\mathcal{H}_K \equiv \mathcal{H}(G)$. We note that the above analysis naturally extends to the case that $\mathbf{L}$ is replaced by any positive semidefinite matrix. In particular, in our experiments below we will use the normalized Laplacian matrix given by $\mathbf{D}^{-\frac{1}{2}} \mathbf{L} \mathbf{D}^{-\frac{1}{2}}$.

Typically, problem (2.4) is solved by optimizing over $\mathbf{v} = (v_i : i \in \mathbb{N}_m)$. In particular, for square loss regularization [2] and minimal norm interpolation [17] this requires solving a squared linear system of m and $m - \ell$ equations respectively. On the contrary, in this paper we use the representer theorem to express $\mathbf{v}$ as

$$\mathbf{v} = \Big(\sum_{j=1}^{\ell} L_{ij}^+ c_j : i \in \mathbb{N}_m \Big).$$

This approach is advantageous if $\mathbf{L}^+$ can be computed off-line because, typically, $\ell \ll m$. A further advantage of this approach is that multiple problems may be solved with the same Laplacian kernel. The coefficients c_i are obtained by solving problem (2.3) with $\widetilde{\mathbf{K}} = (L_{ij}^+)_{i,j=1}^{\ell}$. For example, for square loss regularization the computation of the parameter vector $\mathbf{c} = (c_i : i \in \mathbb{N}_\ell)$ involves solving a linear system of ℓ equations, namely

$$(\widetilde{\mathbf{K}} + \gamma \mathbf{I})\mathbf{c} = \mathbf{y}. \tag{2.5}$$

3   Learning a convex combination of Laplacian kernels

We now describe our framework for learning with multiple graph Laplacians. We assume that we are given n graphs $G^{(q)}$, $q \in \mathbb{N}_n$, all having m vertices, with corresponding Laplacians $\mathbf{L}^{(q)}$, kernels $K^{(q)} = (\mathbf{L}^{(q)})^+$, Hilbert spaces $\mathcal{H}^{(q)} := \mathcal{H}(G^{(q)})$ and norms $\|\mathbf{v}\|_q^2 := \mathbf{v}^\top \mathbf{L}^{(q)} \mathbf{v}$, $\mathbf{v} \in \mathcal{H}^{(q)}$. We propose to learn an optimal convex combination of graph kernels, that is, we solve the optimization problem

$$\rho = \min \Big\{ \sum_{i=1}^{\ell} V(y_i, v_i) + \gamma \|\mathbf{v}\|_{K(\boldsymbol{\lambda})}^2 : \boldsymbol{\lambda} \in \Lambda, \ \mathbf{v} \in \mathcal{H}_{K(\boldsymbol{\lambda})} \Big\} \tag{3.1}$$

where we have defined the set $\Lambda := \{ \boldsymbol{\lambda} \in \mathbb{R}^n : \lambda_q \geq 0, \sum_{q=1}^n \lambda_q = 1 \}$ and, for each $\boldsymbol{\lambda} \in \Lambda$, the kernel $K(\boldsymbol{\lambda}) := \sum_{q=1}^n \lambda_q K^{(q)}$. The above problem is motivated by observing that

$$\rho \leq \min \big\{ E_\gamma(K^{(q)}) : q \in \mathbb{N}_n \big\}.$$

Hence an optimal convex combination of kernels has a smaller right hand side than that of any individual kernel, motivating the expectation of improved performance. Furthermore, large values of the components of the minimizing $\boldsymbol{\lambda}$ identify the most relevant kernels.

Problem (3.1) is a special case of the problem of *jointly* minimizing functional (2.1) over $\mathbf{v} \in \mathcal{H}_K$ and $K \in co(\mathcal{K})$, the convex hull of kernels in a prescribed set $\mathcal{K}$. This problem is discussed in detail in [1, 12], see also [10, 11] where the case that $\mathcal{K}$ is finite is considered. Practical experience with this method [1, 10, 11] indicates that it can enhance the performance of the learning algorithm and, moreover, it is computationally efficient to solve. When solving problem (3.1) it is important to require that the kernels $K^{(q)}$ satisfy a normalization condition such as that they all have the same trace or the same Frobenius norm, see [10] for a discussion.

Initialization: Choose $K^{(1)} \in co\{K^{(q)} : q \in \mathbb{N}_n\}$
For t = 1 to T:

1. compute $c^{(t)}$ to be the solution of problem (2.3) with $K = K^{(t)}$;
2. find $q \in \mathbb{N}_n : (c^{(t)}, K^{(q)}c^{(t)}) > (c^{(t)}, K^{(t)}c^{(t)})$. If such q does not exist terminate;
3. compute $\hat{p} = \operatorname{argmin}\left\{E_\gamma(pK^{(q)} + (1-p)K^{(t)}) : p \in (0,1]\right\}$;
4. set $K^{(t+1)} = \hat{p}K^{(q)} + (1-\hat{p})K^{(t)}$.

Figure 1: Algorithm to compute an optimal convex combination of kernels in the set $co\{K^{(q)} : q \in \mathbb{N}_n\}$.

Using the dual problem formulation discussed above (see equation (2.3)) in the inner minimum in (3.1) we can rewrite this problem as

$$-\rho = \max\left\{\min\left\{\frac{1}{4\gamma}\mathbf{c}^\top\widetilde{\mathbf{K}}(\boldsymbol{\lambda})\mathbf{c} + \sum_{i=1}^{\ell} V^*(y_i, c_i) : \mathbf{c} \in \mathbb{R}^\ell\right\} : \boldsymbol{\lambda} \in \Lambda\right\}. \tag{3.2}$$

The variational problem (3.2) expresses the optimal convex combination of the kernels as the solution to a saddle point problem. This problem is simpler to solve than the original problem (3.1) since its objective function is linear in $\boldsymbol{\lambda}$, see [1] for a discussion. Several algorithms can be used for computing a saddle point $(\hat{\mathbf{c}}, \hat{\boldsymbol{\lambda}}) \in \mathbb{R}^\ell \times \Lambda$. Here we adapt an algorithm from [1] which alternately optimizes over $\mathbf{c}$ and $\boldsymbol{\lambda}$. For reproducibility of the algorithm, it is reported in Figure 1. Note that once $\hat{\boldsymbol{\lambda}}$ is computed $\hat{\mathbf{c}}$ is given by a minimizer of problem (2.3) for $K = K(\hat{\boldsymbol{\lambda}})$. In particular, for square loss regularization this requires solving the equation (2.5) with $\widetilde{\mathbf{K}} = (K_{ij}(\hat{\boldsymbol{\lambda}}) : i, j \in \mathbb{N}_\ell)$.

4 Experiments

In this section we present our experiments on optical character recognition. We observed the following. First, the optimal convex combination of kernels computed by our algorithm is competitive with the best base kernels. Second, by observing the 'weights' of the convex combination we can distinguish the strong from the weak candidate kernels. We proceed by discussing the details of the experimental design interleaved with our results.

We used the USPS dataset[2] of 16×16 images of handwritten digits with pixel values ranging between -1 and 1. We present the results for 5 pairwise classification tasks of varying difficulty and for odd vs. even digit classification. For pairwise classification, the training set consisted of the first 200 images for each digit in the USPS training set and the number of labeled points was chosen to be 4, 8 or 12 (with equal numbers for each digit). For odd vs. even digit classification, the training set consisted of the first 80 images per digit in the USPS training set and the number of labeled points was 10, 20 or 30, with equal numbers for each digit. Performance was averaged over 30 random selections, each with the same number of labeled points.

In each experiment, we constructed $n = 30$ graphs $G^{(q)}$ ($q \in \mathbb{N}_n$) by combining k-nearest neighbors ($k \in \mathbb{N}_{10}$) with three different distances. Then, n corresponding Laplacians were computed together with their associated kernels. We chose as the loss function V the square loss. Since kernels obtained from different types of graphs can vary widely, it was necessary to renormalize them. Hence, we chose to normalize each kernel during the

[2]Available at: *http://www-stat-class.stanford.edu/~tibs/ElemStatLearn/data.html*

Task \ Labels %	Euclidean (10 kernels)			Transf. (10 kernels)			Tangent dist. (10 kernels)			All (30 kernels)		
	1%	2%	3%	1%	2%	3%	1%	2%	3%	1%	2%	3%
1 vs. 7	1.55	1.53	1.50	1.45	1.45	1.38	1.01	1.00	1.00	1.28	1.24	1.20
	0.08	0.05	0.15	0.10	0.11	0.12	0.00	0.09	0.11	0.28	0.27	0.22
2 vs. 3	3.08	3.34	3.38	0.80	0.85	0.82	0.73	0.19	0.03	0.79	0.25	0.10
	0.85	1.21	1.29	0.40	0.38	0.32	0.93	0.51	0.09	0.93	0.61	0.21
2 vs. 7	4.46	4.04	3.56	3.27	2.92	2.96	2.95	2.30	2.14	3.51	2.54	2.41
	1.17	1.21	0.82	1.16	1.26	1.08	1.79	0.76	0.53	1.92	0.97	0.89
3 vs. 8	7.33	7.30	7.03	6.98	6.87	6.50	4.43	4.22	3.96	4.80	4.32	4.20
	1.67	1.49	1.43	1.57	1.77	1.78	1.21	1.36	1.25	1.57	1.46	1.53
4 vs. 7	2.90	2.64	2.25	1.81	1.82	1.69	0.88	0.90	0.90	1.04	1.14	1.13
	0.77	0.78	0.77	0.26	0.42	0.45	0.17	0.20	0.20	0.37	0.42	0.39
Labels	10	20	30	10	20	30	10	20	30	10	20	30
Odd vs. Even	18.6	15.5	13.4	15.7	11.7	8.52	14.66	10.50	8.38	17.07	10.98	8.74
	3.98	2.40	2.67	4.40	3.14	1.32	4.37	2.30	1.90	4.38	2.61	2.39

Table 1: Misclassification error percentage (*top*) and standard deviation (*bottom*) for the best convex combination of kernels on different handwritten digit recognition tasks, using different distances. See text for description.

training process by the Frobenius norm of its submatrix corresponding to the labeled data. We also observed that similar results were obtained when normalizing with the trace of this submatrix. The regularization parameter was set to 10^{-5} in all algorithms. For convex minimization, as the starting kernel in the algorithm in Figure 1 we always used the average of the n kernels and as the maximum number of iterations $T = 100$.

Table 1 shows the results obtained using three distances as combined with k-NN ($k \in \mathbb{N}_{10}$). The first distance is the *Euclidean* distance between images. The second method is *transformation*, where the distance between two images is given by the smallest Euclidean distance between any pair of transformed images as determined by applying a number of affine transformations and a thickness transformation[3], see [6] for more information. The third distance is *tangent distance*, as described in [6], which is a first-order approximation to the above transformations. For the first three columns in the table the Euclidean distance was used, for columns 4–6 the image transformation distance was used, for columns 7–9 the tangent distance was used. Finally, in the last three columns all three methods were jointly compared. As the results indicate, when combining different types of kernels, the algorithm tends to select the most effective ones (in this case the tangent distance kernels and to a lesser degree the transformation distance kernels which did not work very well because of the Matlab optimization routine we used). We also noted that within each of the methods the performance of the convex combination is comparable to that of the best kernels. Figure 2 reports the weight of each individual kernel learned by our algorithm when 2% labels are used in the pairwise tasks and 20 labels are used for odd vs. even. With the exception of the easy 1 vs. 7 task, the large weights are associated with the graphs/kernels built with the tangent distance.

The effectiveness of our algorithm in selecting the good graphs/kernels is better demonstrated in Figure 3, where the Euclidean and the transformation kernels are combined with a "low-quality" kernel. This "low-quality" kernel is induced by considering distances invariant over rotation in the range $[-180°, 180°]$, so that the image of a 6 can easily have a small distance from an image of a 9, that is, if $\mathbf{x}$ and $\mathbf{t}$ are two images and $T_\theta(\mathbf{x})$ is the image obtained by rotating $\mathbf{x}$ by θ degrees, we set

$$d(\mathbf{x}, \mathbf{t}) = \min\{\|T_\theta(\mathbf{x}) - T_{\theta'}(\mathbf{t})\| : \theta, \theta' \in [-180°, 180°]\}.$$

---

[3]This distance was approximated using Matlab's constrained minimization function.

The figure shows the distance matrix on the set of labeled and unlabeled data for the Euclidean, transformation and "low-quality distance" respectively. The best error among 15 different values of k within each method, the error of the learned convex combination and the total learned weights for each method are shown below each plot. It is clear that the solution of the algorithm is dominated by the good kernels and is not influenced by the ones with low performance. As a result, the error of the convex combination is comparable to that of the Euclidean and transformation methods. The final experiment (see Figure 4) demonstrates that unlabeled data improves the performance of our method.

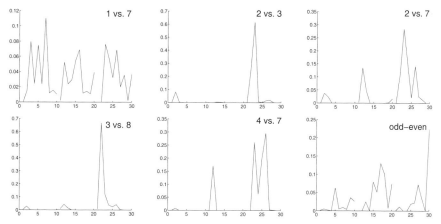

Figure 2: Kernel weights for Euclidean (first 10), Transformation (middle 10) and Tangent (last 10). See text for more information.

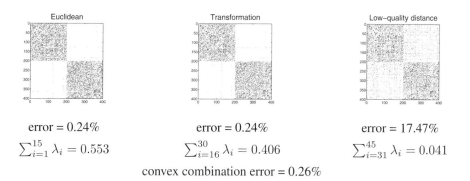

error = 0.24%   error = 0.24%   error = 17.47%

$\sum_{i=1}^{15} \lambda_i = 0.553$ $\sum_{i=16}^{30} \lambda_i = 0.406$ $\sum_{i=31}^{45} \lambda_i = 0.041$

convex combination error = 0.26%

Figure 3: Similarity matrices and corresponding learned coefficients of the convex combination for the 6 vs. 9 task. See text for description.

5 Conclusion

We have presented a method for computing an optimal kernel within the framework of regularization over graphs. The method consists of a minimax problem which can be efficiently solved by using an algorithm from [1]. When tested on optical character recognition tasks, the method exhibits competitive performance and is able to select good graph structures. Future work will focus on out-of-sample extensions of this algorithm and on continuous optimization versions of it. In particular, we may consider a continuous family of graphs each corresponding to a different weight matrix and study graph kernel combinations over this class.

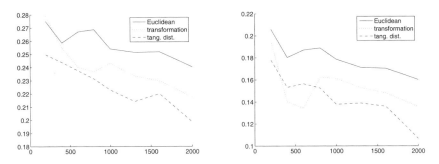

Figure 4: Misclassification error vs. number of training points for odd vs. even classification. The number of labeled points is 10 on the left and 20 on the right.

References

[1] A. Argyriou, C.A. Micchelli and M. Pontil. Learning convex combinations of continuously parameterized basic kernels. Proc. 18-th Conf. on Learning Theory, 2005.

[2] M. Belkin, I. Matveeva and P. Niyogi. Regularization and semi-supervised learning on large graphs. Proc. of 17–th Conf. Learning Theory (COLT), 2004.

[3] M. Belkin and P. Niyogi. Semi-supervised learning on Riemannian manifolds. *Mach. Learn.*, 56: 209–239, 2004.

[4] A. Blum and S. Chawla. Learning from Labeled and Unlabeled Data using Graph Mincuts, Proc. of 18–th International Conf. on Learning Theory, 2001.

[5] F.R. Chung. *Spectral Graph Theory*. Regional Conference Series in Mathematics, Vol. 92, 1997.

[6] T. Hastie and P. Simard. Models and Metrics for Handwritten Character Recognition. *Statistical Science*, 13(1): 54–65, 1998.

[7] M. Herbster, M. Pontil, L. Wainer. Online learning over graphs. Proc. 22-nd Int. Conf. Machine Learning, 2005.

[8] T. Joachims. Transductive Learning via Spectral Graph Partitioning. Proc. of the Int. Conf. Machine Learning (ICML), 2003.

[9] R.I. Kondor and J. Lafferty. Diffusion kernels on graphs and other discrete input spaces. Proc. 19-th Int. Conf. Machine Learning, 2002.

[10] G. R. G. Lanckriet, N. Cristianini, P. Bartlett, L. El Ghaoui, M. I. Jordan. Learning the kernel matrix with semidefinite programming. *J. Machine Learning Research,* 5: 27–72, 2004.

[11] Y. Lin and H.H. Zhang. Component selection and smoothing in smoothing spline analysis of variance models – COSSO. Institute of Statistics Mimeo Series 2556, NCSU, January 2003.

[12] C. A. Micchelli and M. Pontil. Learning the kernel function via regularization, *J. Machine Learning Research*, 6: 1099–1125, 2005.

[13] C.S. Ong, A.J. Smola, and R.C. Williamson. Hyperkernels. *Advances in Neural Information Processing Systems*, 15, S. Becker et al. (Eds.), MIT Press, Cambridge, MA, 2003.

[14] A.J. Smola and R.I Kondor. Kernels and regularization on graphs. Proc. of 16–th Conf. Learning Theory (COLT), 2003.

[15] V.N. Vapnik. *Statistical Learning Theory*. Wiley, New York, 1998.

[16] D. Zhou, O. Bousquet, T.N. Lal, J. Weston and B. Scholkopf. Learning with local and global consistency. *Advances in Neural Information Processing Systems*, 16, S. Thrun et al. (Eds.), MIT Press, Cambridge, MA, 2004.

[17] X. Zhu, Z. Ghahramani and J. Lafferty. Semi-supervised learning using Gaussian fields and harmonic functions. Proc. 20–th Int. Conf. Machine Learning, 2003.

[18] X. Zhu, J. Kandola, Z, Ghahramani, J. Lafferty. Nonparametric transforms of graph kernels for semi-supervised learning. *Advances in Neural Information Processing Systems*, 17, L.K. Saul et al. (Eds.), MIT Press, Cambridge, MA, 2005.

Learning in Silicon: Timing is Everything

John V. Arthur and Kwabena Boahen
Department of Bioengineering
University of Pennsylvania
Philadelphia, PA 19104
{jarthur, boahen}@seas.upenn.edu

Abstract

We describe a neuromorphic chip that uses binary synapses with spike timing-dependent plasticity (STDP) to learn stimulated patterns of activity and to compensate for variability in excitability. Specifically, STDP preferentially potentiates (turns on) synapses that project from excitable neurons, which spike early, to lethargic neurons, which spike late. The additional excitatory synaptic current makes lethargic neurons spike earlier, thereby causing neurons that belong to the same pattern to spike in synchrony. Once learned, an entire pattern can be recalled by stimulating a subset.

1 Variability in Neural Systems

Evidence suggests precise spike timing is important in neural coding, specifically, in the hippocampus. The hippocampus uses timing in the spike activity of place cells (in addition to rate) to encode location in space [1]. Place cells employ a *phase code*: the timing at which a neuron spikes relative to the phase of the inhibitory theta rhythm (5-12Hz) conveys information. As an animal approaches a place cell's preferred location, the place cell not only increases its spike rate, but also spikes at earlier phases in the theta cycle.

To implement a phase code, the theta rhythm is thought to prevent spiking until the input synaptic current exceeds the sum of the neuron threshold and the decreasing inhibition on the downward phase of the cycle [2]. However, even with identical inputs and common theta inhibition, neurons do not spike in synchrony. Variability in excitability spreads the activity in phase. Lethargic neurons (such as those with high thresholds) spike late in the theta cycle, since their input exceeds the sum of the neuron threshold and theta inhibition only after the theta inhibition has had time to decrease. Conversely, excitable neurons (such as those with low thresholds) spike early in the theta cycle. Consequently, variability in excitability translates into variability in timing.

We hypothesize that the hippocampus achieves its precise spike timing (about 10ms) through *plasticity enhanced phase-coding* (PEP). The source of hippocampal timing precision in the presence of variability (and noise) remains unexplained. Synaptic plasticity can compensate for variability in excitability if it increases excitatory synaptic input to neurons in inverse proportion to their excitabilities. Recasting this in a phase-coding framework, we desire a learning rule that increases excitatory synaptic input to neurons directly related to their phases. Neurons that lag require additional synaptic input, whereas neurons that lead

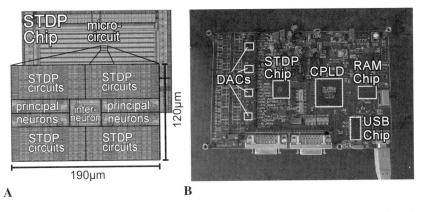

Figure 1: STDP Chip. **A** The chip has a 16-by-16 array of microcircuits; one microcircuit includes four principal neurons, each with 21 STDP circuits. **B** The STDP Chip is embedded in a circuit board including DACs, a CPLD, a RAM chip, and a USB chip, which communicates with a PC.

require none. The spike timing-dependent plasticity (STDP) observed in the hippocampus satisfies this requirement [3]. It requires repeated pre-before-post spike pairings (within a time window) to potentiate and repeated post-before-pre pairings to depress a synapse.

Here we validate our hypothesis with a model implemented in silicon, where variability is as ubiquitous as it is in biology [4]. Section 2 presents our silicon system, including the STDP Chip. Section 3 describes and characterizes the STDP circuit. Section 4 demonstrates that PEP compensates for variability and provides evidence that STDP is the compensation mechanism. Section 5 explores a desirable consequence of PEP: unconventional associative pattern recall. Section 6 discusses the implications of the PEP model, including its benefits and applications in the engineering of neuromorphic systems and in the study of neurobiology.

2   Silicon System

We have designed, submitted, and tested a silicon implementation of PEP. The STDP Chip was fabricated through MOSIS in a 1P5M 0.25μm CMOS process, with just under 750,000 transistors in just over 10mm^2 of area. It has a 32 by 32 array of excitatory principal neurons commingled with a 16 by 16 array of inhibitory interneurons that are not used here (Figure 1A). Each principal neuron has 21 STDP synapses. The address-event representation (AER) [5] is used to transmit spikes off chip and to receive afferent and recurrent spike input.

To configure the STDP Chip as a recurrent network, we embedded it in a circuit board (Figure 1B). The board has five primary components: a CPLD (complex programmable logic device), the STDP Chip, a RAM chip, a USB interface chip, and DACs (digital-to-analog converters). The central component in the system is the CPLD. The CPLD handles AER traffic, mediates communication between devices, and implements recurrent connections by accessing a lookup table, stored in the RAM chip. The USB interface chip provides a bidirectional link with a PC. The DACs control the analog biases in the system, including the leak current, which the PC varies in real-time to create the global inhibitory theta rhythm.

The principal neuron consists of a refractory period and calcium-dependent potassium circuit (RCK), a synapse circuit, and a soma circuit (Figure 2A). RCK and the synapse are

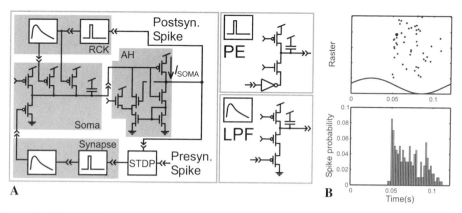

Figure 2: Principal neuron. **A** A simplified schematic is shown, including: the synapse, refractory and calcium-dependent potassium channel (RCK), soma, and axon-hillock (AH) circuits, plus their constituent elements, the pulse extender (PE) and the low-pass filter (LPF). **B** Spikes (dots) from 81 principal neurons are temporally dispersed, when excited by poisson-like inputs (58Hz) and inhibited by the common 8.3Hz theta rhythm (solid line). The histogram includes spikes from five theta cycles.

composed of two reusable blocks: the low-pass filter (LPF) and the pulse extender (PE). The soma is a modified version of the LPF, which receives additional input from an axon-hillock circuit (AH).

RCK is inhibitory to the neuron. It consists of a PE, which models calcium influx during a spike, and a LPF, which models calcium buffering. When AH fires a spike, a packet of charge is dumped onto a capacitor in the PE. The PE's output activates until the charge decays away, which takes a few milliseconds. Also, while the PE is active, charge accumulates on the LPF's capacitor, lowering the LPF's output voltage. Once the PE deactivates, this charge leaks away as well, but this takes tens of milliseconds because the leak is smaller. The PE's and the LPF's inhibitory effects on the soma are both described below in terms of the sum (I_{SHUNT}) of the currents their output voltages produce in pMOS transistors whose sources are at Vdd (see Figure 2A). Note that, in the absence of spikes, these currents decay exponentially, with a time-constant determined by their respective leaks.

The synapse circuit is excitatory to the neuron. It is composed of a PE, which represents the neurotransmitter released into the synaptic cleft, and a LPF, which represents the bound neurotransmitter. The synapse circuit is similar to RCK in structure but differs in function: It is activated not by the principal neuron itself but by the STDP circuits (or directly by afferent spikes that bypass these circuits, i.e., fixed synapses). The synapse's effect on the soma is also described below in terms of the current (I_{SYN}) its output voltage produces in a pMOS transistor whose source is at Vdd.

The soma circuit is a leaky integrator. It receives excitation from the synapse circuit and shunting inhibition from RCK and has a leak current as well. Its temporal behavior is described by:

$$\tau \frac{dI_{\mathrm{SOMA}}}{dt} + I_{\mathrm{SOMA}} = \frac{I_{\mathrm{SYN}} \, \mathrm{I}_0}{I_{\mathrm{SHUNT}}}$$

where I_{SOMA} is the current the capacitor's voltage produces in a pMOS transistor whose source is at Vdd (see Figure 2A). I_{SHUNT} is the sum of the leak, refractory, and calcium-dependent potassium currents. These currents also determine the time constant: $\tau = \frac{C \, U_t}{\kappa I_{\mathrm{SHUNT}}}$, where I_0 and κ are transistor parameters and U_t is the thermal voltage.

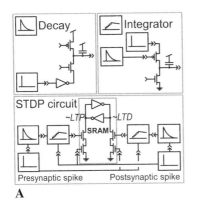
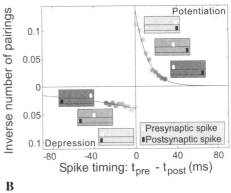

Figure 3: STDP circuit design and characterization. **A** The circuit is composed of three subcircuits: decay, integrator, and SRAM. **B** The circuit potentiates when the presynaptic spike precedes the postsynaptic spike and depresses when the postsynaptic spike precedes the presynaptic spike.

The soma circuit is connected to an AH, the locus of spike generation. The AH consists of model voltage-dependent sodium and potassium channel populations (modified from [6] by Kai Hynna). It initiates the AER signaling process required to send a spike off chip.

To characterize principal neuron variability, we excited 81 neurons with poisson-like 58Hz spike trains (Figure 2B). We made these spike trains poisson-like by starting with a regular 200Hz spike train and dropping spikes randomly, with probability of 0.71. Thus spikes were delivered to neurons that won the coin toss in synchrony every 5ms. However, neurons did not lock onto the input synchrony due to filtering by the synaptic time constant (see Figure 2B). They also received a common inhibitory input at the theta frequency (8.3Hz), via their leak current. Each neuron was prevented from firing more than one spike in a theta cycle by its model calcium-dependent potassium channel population.

The principal neurons' spike times were variable. To quantify the spike variability, we used timing precision, which we define as twice the standard deviation of spike times accumulated from five theta cycles. With an input rate of 58Hz the timing precision was 34ms.

3 STDP Circuit

The STDP circuit (related to [7]-[8]), for which the STDP Chip is named, is the most abundant, with 21,504 copies on the chip. This circuit is built from three subcircuits: decay, integrator, and SRAM (Figure 3A). The decay and integrator are used to implement potentiation, and depression, in a symmetric fashion. The SRAM holds the current binary state of the synapse, either potentiated or depressed.

For potentiation, the decay remembers the last presynaptic spike. Its capacitor is charged when that spike occurs and discharges linearly thereafter. A postsynaptic spike samples the charge remaining on the capacitor, passes it through an exponential function, and dumps the resultant charge into the integrator. This charge decays linearly thereafter. At the time of the postsynaptic spike, the SRAM, a cross-coupled inverter pair, reads the voltage on the integrator's capacitor. If it exceeds a threshold, the SRAM switches state from depressed to potentiated ($\sim LTD$ goes high and $\sim LTP$ goes low). The depression side of the STDP circuit is exactly symmetric, except that it responds to postsynaptic activation followed by presynaptic activation and switches the SRAM's state from potentiated to depressed ($\sim LTP$ goes high and $\sim LTD$ goes low). When the SRAM is in the potentiated state, the presynaptic

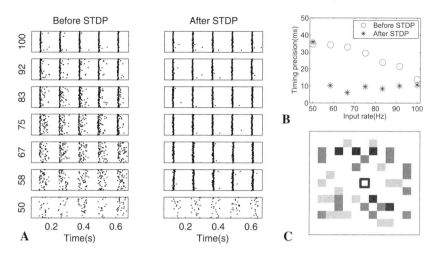

Figure 4: Plasticity enhanced phase-coding. **A** Spike rasters of 81 neurons (9 by 9 cluster) display synchrony over a two-fold range of input rates after STDP. **B** The degree of enhancement is quantified by timing precision. **C** Each neuron (center box) sends synapses to (dark gray) and receives synapses from (light gray) twenty-one randomly chosen neighbors up to five nodes away (black indicates both connections).

spike activates the principal neuron's synapse; otherwise the spike has no effect.

We characterized the STDP circuit by activating a plastic synapse and a fixed synapse– which elicits a spike at different relative times. We repeated this pairing at 16Hz. We counted the number of pairings required to potentiate (or depress) the synapse. Based on this count, we calculated the efficacy of each pairing as the inverse number of pairings required (Figure 3B). For example, if twenty pairings were required to potentiate the synapse, the efficacy of that pre-before-post time-interval was one twentieth. The efficacy of both potentiation and depression are fit by exponentials with time constants of 11.4ms and 94.9ms, respectively. This behavior is similar to that observed in the hippocampus: potentiation has a shorter time constant and higher maximum efficacy than depression [3].

4 Recurrent Network

We carried out an experiment designed to test the STDP circuit's ability to compensate for variability in spike timing through PEP. Each neuron received recurrent connections from 21 randomly selected neurons within an 11 by 11 neighborhood centered on itself (see Figure 4C). Conversely, it made recurrent connections to randomly chosen neurons within the same neighborhood. These connections were mediated by STDP circuits, initialized to the depressed state. We chose a 9 by 9 cluster of neurons and delivered spikes at a mean rate of 50 to 100Hz to each one (dropping spikes with a probability of 0.75 to 0.5 from a regular 200Hz train) and provided common theta inhibition as before.

We compared the variability in spike timing after five seconds of learning with the initial distribution. Phase coding was enhanced after STDP (Figure 4A). Before STDP, spike timing among neurons was highly variable (except for the very highest input rate). After STDP, variability was virtually eliminated (except for the very lowest input rate). Initially, the variability, characterized by timing precision, was inversely related to the input rate, decreasing from 34 to 13ms. After five seconds of STDP, variability decreased and was largely independent of input rate, remaining below 11ms.

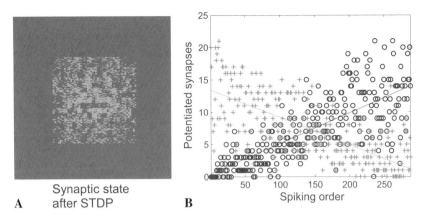

	Synaptic state	
A	after STDP	**B**

Figure 5: Compensating for variability. **A** Some synapses (dots) become potentiated (light) while others remain depressed (dark) after STDP. **B** The number of potentiated synapses neurons make (pluses) and receive (circles) is negatively (r = -0.71) and positively (r = 0.76) correlated to their rank in the spiking order, respectively.

Comparing the number of potentiated synapses each neuron made or received with its excitability confirmed the PEP hypothesis (i.e., leading neurons provide additional synaptic current to lagging neurons via potentiated recurrent synapses). In this experiment, to eliminate variability due to noise (as opposed to excitability), we provided a 17 by 17 cluster of neurons with a regular 200Hz excitatory input. Theta inhibition was present as before and all synapses were initialized to the depressed state. After 10 seconds of STDP, a large fraction of the synapses were potentiated (Figure 5A). When the number of potentiated synapses each neuron made or received was plotted versus its rank in spiking order (Figure 5B), a clear correlation emerged (r = -0.71 or 0.76, respectively). As expected, neurons that spiked early made more and received fewer potentiated synapses. In contrast, neurons that spiked late made fewer and received more potentiated synapses.

5 Pattern Completion

After STDP, we found that the network could recall an entire pattern given a subset, thus the same mechanisms that compensated for variability and noise could also compensate for lack of information. We chose a 9 by 9 cluster of neurons as our pattern and delivered a poisson-like spike train with mean rate of 67Hz to each one as in the first experiment. Theta inhibition was present as before and all synapses were initialized to the depressed state. Before STDP, we stimulated a subset of the pattern and only neurons in that subset spiked (Figure 6A). After five seconds of STDP, we stimulated the same subset again. This time they recruited spikes from other neurons in the pattern, completing it (Figure 6B).

Upon varying the fraction of the pattern presented, we found that the fraction recalled increased faster than the fraction presented. We selected subsets of the original pattern randomly, varying the fraction of neurons chosen from 0.1 to 1.0 (ten trials for each). We classified neurons as active if they spiked in the two second period over which we recorded. Thus, we characterized PEP's pattern-recall performance as a function of the probability that the pattern in question's neurons are activated (Figure 6C). At a fraction of 0.50 presented, nearly all of the neurons in the pattern are consistently activated (0.91±0.06), showing robust pattern completion. We fitted the recall performance with a sigmoid that reached 0.50 recall fraction with an input fraction of 0.30. No spurious neurons were activated during any trials.

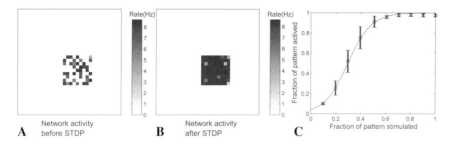

A Network activity before STDP

B Network activity after STDP

C

Figure 6: Associative recall. **A** Before STDP, half of the neurons in a pattern are stimulated; only they are activated. **B** After STDP, half of the neurons in a pattern are stimulated, and all are activated. **C** The fraction of the pattern activated grows faster than the fraction stimulated.

6 Discussion

Our results demonstrate that PEP successfully compensates for graded variations in our silicon recurrent network using binary (on–off) synapses (in contrast with [8], where weights are graded). While our chip results are encouraging, variability was not eliminated in every case. In the case of the lowest input (50Hz), we see virtually no change (Figure 4A). We suspect the timing remains imprecise because, with such low input, neurons do not spike every theta cycle and, consequently, provide fewer opportunities for the STDP synapses to potentiate. This shortfall illustrates the system's limits; it can only compensate for variability within certain bounds, and only for activity appropriate to the PEP model.

As expected, STDP is the mechanism responsible for PEP. STDP potentiated recurrent synapses from leading neurons to lagging neurons, reducing the disparity among the diverse population of neurons. Even though the STDP circuits are themselves variable, with different efficacies and time constants, when using timing the sign of the weight-change is always correct (data not shown). For this reason, we chose STDP over other more physiological implementations of plasticity, such as membrane-voltage-dependent plasticity (MVDP), which has the capability to learn with graded voltage signals [9], such as those found in active dendrites, providing more computational power [10].

Previously, we investigated a MVDP circuit, which modeled a voltage-dependent NMDA-receptor-gated synapse [11]. It potentiated when the calcium current analog exceeded a threshold, which was designed to occur only during a dendritic action potential. This circuit produced behavior similar to STDP, implying it could be used in PEP. However, it was sensitive to variability in the NMDA and potentiation thresholds, causing a fraction of the population to potentiate anytime the synapse received an input and another fraction to never potentiate, rendering both subpopulations useless. Therefore, the simpler, less biophysical STDP circuit won out over the MVDP circuit: In our system *timing is everything*.

Associative storage and recall naturally emerge in the PEP network when synapses between neurons coactivated by a pattern are potentiated. These synapses allow neurons to recruit their peers when a subset of the pattern is presented, thereby completing the pattern. However, this form of pattern storage and completion differs from Hopfield's attractor model [12] . Rather than forming symmetric, recurrent neuronal circuits, our recurrent network forms asymmetric circuits in which neurons make connections exclusively to less excitable neurons in the pattern. In both the poisson-like and regular cases (Figures 4 & 5), only about six percent of potentiated connections were reciprocated, as expected by chance. We plan to investigate the storage capacity of this asymmetric form of associative memory.

Our system lends itself to modeling brain regions that use precise spike timing, such as the hippocampus. We plan to extend the work presented to store and recall sequences of patterns, as the hippocampus is hypothesized to do. Place cells that represent different locations spike at different phases of the theta cycle, in relation to the distance to their preferred locations. This sequential spiking will allow us to link patterns representing different locations in the order those locations are visited, thereby realizing episodic memory.

We propose PEP as a candidate neural mechanism for information coding and storage in the hippocampal system. Observations from the CA1 region of the hippocampus suggest that basal dendrites (which primarily receive excitation from recurrent connections) support submillisecond timing precision, consistent with PEP [13]. We have shown, in a silicon model, PEP's ability to exploit such fast recurrent connections to sharpen timing precision as well as to associatively store and recall patterns.

Acknowledgments

We thank Joe Lin for assistance with chip generation. The Office of Naval Research funded this work (Award No. N000140210468).

References

[1] O'Keefe J. & Recce M.L. (1993). Phase relationship between hippocampal place units and the EEG theta rhythm. *Hippocampus* **3**(3):317-330.

[2] Mehta M.R., Lee A.K. & Wilson M.A. (2002) Role of experience and oscillations in transforming a rate code into a temporal code. *Nature* **417**(6890):741-746.

[3] Bi G.Q. & Wang H.X. (2002) Temporal asymmetry in spike timing-dependent synaptic plasticity. *Physiology & Behavior* **77**:551-555.

[4] Rodriguez-Vazquez, A., Linan, G., Espejo S. & Dominguez-Castro R. (2003) Mismatch-induced trade-offs and scalability of analog preprocessing visual microprocessor chips. *Analog Integrated Circuits and Signal Processing* **37**:73-83.

[5] Boahen K.A. (2000) Point-to-point connectivity between neuromorphic chips using address events. *IEEE Transactions on Circuits and Systems II* **47**:416-434.

[6] Culurciello E.R., Etienne-Cummings R. & Boahen K.A. (2003) A biomorphic digital image sensor. *IEEE Journal of Solid State Circuits* **38**:281-294.

[7] Bofill A., Murray A.F & Thompson D.P. (2005) Citcuits for VLSI Implementation of Temporally Asymmetric Hebbian Learning. In: *Advances in Neural Information Processing Systems 14*, MIT Press, 2002.

[8] Cameron K., Boonsobhak V., Murray A. & Renshaw D. (2005) Spike timing dependent plasticity (STDP) can ameliorate process variations in neuromorphic VLSI. *IEEE Transactions on Neural Networks* **16**(6):1626-1627.

[9] Chicca E., Badoni D., Dante V., D'Andreagiovanni M., Salina G., Carota L., Fusi S. & Del Giudice P. (2003) A VLSI recurrent network of integrate-and-fire neurons connected by plastic synapses with long-term memory. *IEEE Transaction on Neural Networks* **14**(5):1297-1307.

[10] Poirazi P., & Mel B.W. (2001) Impact of active dendrites and structural plasticity on the memory capacity of neural tissue. *Neuron* **29**(3)779-796.

[11] Arthur J.V. & Boahen K. (2004) Recurrently connected silicon neurons with active dendrites for one-shot learning. In: *IEEE International Joint Conference on Neural Networks* **3**, pp.1699-1704.

[12] Hopfield J.J. (1984) Neurons with graded response have collective computational properties like those of two-state neurons. *Proceedings of the National Academy of Science* **81**(10):3088-3092.

[13] Ariav G., Polsky A. & Schiller J. (2003) Submillisecond precision of the input-output transformation function mediated by fast sodium dendritic spikes in basal dendrites of CA1 pyramidal neurons. *Journal of Neuroscience* **23**(21):7750-7758.

Learning Topology with the Generative Gaussian Graph and the EM Algorithm

Michaël Aupetit
CEA - DASE
BP 12 - 91680
Bruyères-le-Châtel, France
`aupetit@dase.bruyeres.cea.fr`

Abstract

Given a set of points and a set of prototypes representing them, how to create a graph of the prototypes whose topology accounts for that of the points? This problem had not yet been explored in the framework of statistical learning theory. In this work, we propose a generative model based on the Delaunay graph of the prototypes and the Expectation-Maximization algorithm to learn the parameters. This work is a first step towards the construction of a topological model of a set of points grounded on statistics.

1 Introduction

1.1 Topology what for?

Given a set of points in a high-dimensional euclidean space, we intend to extract the topology of the manifolds from which they are drawn. There are several reasons for this among which: increasing our knowledge about this set of points by measuring its topological features (connectedness, intrinsic dimension, Betti numbers (number of voids, holes, tunnels...)) in the context of exploratory data analysis [1], allowing to compare two sets of points *wrt* their topological characteristics or to find clusters as connected components in the context of pattern recognition [2], or finding shortest path along manifolds in the context of robotics [3].

There are two families of approaches which deal with "topology" : on one hand, the "topology preserving" approaches based on nonlinear projection of the data in lower dimensional spaces with a constrained topology to allow visualization [4, 5, 6, 7, 8]; on the other hand, the "topology modelling" approaches based on the construction of a structure whose topology is not constrained *a priori*, so it is expected to better account for that of the data [9, 10, 11] at the expense of the visualisability. Much work has been done about the former problem also called "manifold learning", from Generative Topographic Mapping [4] to Multi-Dimensional Scaling and its variants [5, 6], Principal Curves [7] and so on. In all these approaches, the intrinsic dimension of the model is fixed *a priori* which eases the visualization but arbitrarily forces the topology of the model. And when the dimension is not fixed as in the mixture of Principal Component Analyzers [8], the connectedness is lost. The latter problem we deal with had never been explored in the statistical learning perspective. Its aim is not to project and visualize a high-dimensional set of points, but to extract the topological information from it directly in the high-dimensional space, so that the model must be freed as much as possible from any *a priori* topological constraint.

1.2 Learning topology: a state of the art

As we may learn a complicated function combining simple basis functions, we shall learn a complicated manifold[1] combining simple basis manifolds. A simplicial complex[2] is such a model based on the combination of simplices, each with its own dimension (a 1-simplex is a line segment, a 2-simplex is a triangle...a k-simplex is the convex hull of a set of $k+1$ points). In a simplicial complex, the simplices are exclusively connected by their vertices or their faces. Such a structure is appealing because it is possible to extract from it topological information like Betti numbers, connectedness and intrinsic dimension [10]. A particular simplicial complex is the Delaunay complex defined as the set of simplices whose Voronoï cells[3] of the vertices are adjacent assuming general position for the vertices. The Delaunay graph is made of vertices and edges of the Delaunay complex [12].

All the previous work about topology modelling is grounded on the result of Edelsbrunner and Shah [13] which prove that given a manifold $\mathcal{M} \subset \mathbb{R}^D$ and a set of N_0 vector prototypes $\underline{w} \in (\mathbb{R}^D)^{N_0}$ nearby $\mathcal{M}$, it exists a simplicial subcomplex of the Delaunay complex of $\underline{w}$ which has the same topology as $\mathcal{M}$ under what we call the "ES-conditions".

In the present work, the manifold $\mathcal{M}$ is not known but through a finite set of M data points $\underline{v} \in \mathcal{M}^M$. Martinetz and Schulten proposed to build a graph of the prototypes with an algorithm called "Competitive Hebbian Learning" (CHL)[11] to tackle this problem. Their approach has been extended to simplicial complexes by De Silva and Carlsson with the definition of "weak witnesses" [10]. In both cases, the ES-conditions about $\mathcal{M}$ are weakened so they can be verified by a finite sample $\underline{v}$ of $\mathcal{M}$, so that the graph or the simplicial complex built over $\underline{w}$ is proved to have the same topology as $\mathcal{M}$ if $\underline{v}$ is a sufficiently dense sampling of $\mathcal{M}$.

The CHL consists in connecting two prototypes in $\underline{w}$ if they are the first and the second closest neighbors to a point of $\underline{v}$ (closeness *wrt* the Euclidean norm). Each point of $\underline{v}$ leads to an edge, and is called a "weak witness" of the connected prototypes [10]. The topology representing graph obtained is a subgraph of the Delaunay graph. The region of $\mathbb{R}^D$ in which any data point would connect the same prototypes, is the "region of influence" (ROI) of this edge (see Figure 2 d-f). This principle is extended to create k-simplices connecting $k+1$ prototypes, which are part of the Delaunay simplicial-complex of $\underline{w}$ [10].

Therefore, the model obtained is based on regions of influence: a simplex exists in the model if there is at least one datum in its ROI. Hence, the capacity of this model to correctly represent the topology of a set of points, strongly depends on the shape and location of the ROI *wrt* the points, and on the presence of noise in the data. Moreover, as far as $N_0 > 2$, it cannot exist an isolated prototype allowing to represent an isolated bump in the data distribution, because any datum of this bump will have two closest prototypes to connect to each other. An aging process has been proposed by Martinetz and Schulten to filter out the noise, which works roughly such that edges with fewer data than a threshold in there ROI are pruned from the graph. This looks like a filter based on the probability density of the data distribution, but no statistical criterion is proposed to tune the parameters. Moreover the area of the ROI may be intractable in high dimension and is not trivially related to the

---

[1]For simplicity, we call "manifold" what can be actually a set of manifolds connected or not to each other with possibly various intrinsic dimensions.

[2]The terms "simplex" or "graph" denote both the abstract object and its geometrical realization.

[3]Given a set of points $\underline{w}$ in $\mathbb{R}^D$, $V_i = \{v \in \mathbb{R}^D | (v - w_i)^2 \leq (v - w_j)^2, \forall j\}$ defines the Voronoï cell associated to $w_i \in \underline{w}$.

corresponding line segment, so measuring the frequency over such a region is not relevant to define a useful probability density. At last, the line segment associated to an edge of the graph is not part of the model: data are not projected on it, data drawn from such a line segment may not give rise to the corresponding edge, and the line segment may not intersect at all its associated ROI. In other words, the model is not self-consistent, that is the geometrical realization of the graph is not always a good model of its own topology whatever the density of the sampling.

We proposed to define Voronoï cells of line segments as ROI for the edges and defined a criterion to cut edges with a lower density of data projecting on their middle than on their borders [9]. This solves some of the CHL limits but it still remains one important problem common to both approaches: they rely on the visual control of their quality, *i.e.* no criterion allows to assess the quality of the model especially in dimension greater than 3.

1.3 Emerging topology from a statistical generative model

For all the above reasons, we propose another way for modelling topology. The idea is to construct a "good" statistical generative model of the data taking the noise into account, and to assume that its topology is therefore a "good" model of the topology of the manifold which generated the data. The only constraint we impose on this generative model is that its topology must be as "flexible" as possible and must be "extractible". "Flexible" to avoid at best any *a priori* constraint on the topology so as to allow the modelling of any one. "Extractible" to get a "white box" model from which the topological characteristics are tractable in terms of computation. So we propose to define a "generative simplicial complex". However, this work being preliminary, we expose here the simpler case of defining a "generative graph" (a simplicial complex made only of vertices and edges) and tuning its parameters. This allows to demonstrate the feasibility of this approach and to foresee future difficulties when it is extended to simplicial complexes.

It works as follows. Given a set of prototypes located over the data distribution using *e.g.* Vector Quantization [14], the Delaunay graph (DG) of the prototypes is constructed [15]. Then, each edge and each vertex of the graph is the basis of a generative model so that the graph generates a mixture of gaussian density functions. The maximization of the likelihood of the data *wrt* the model, using Expectation-Maximization, allows to tune the weights of this mixture and leads to the emergence of the expected topology representing graph through the edges with non-negligible weights that remain after the optimization process.

We first present the framework and the algorithm we use in section 2. Then we test it on artificial data in section 3 before the discussion and conclusion in section 4.

2 A Generative Gaussian Graph to learn topology

2.1 The Generative Gaussian Graph

In this work, $\mathcal{M}$ is the support of the probability density function (pdf) p from which are drawn the data $\underline{v}$. In fact, this is not the topology of $\mathcal{M}$ which is of interest, but the topology of manifolds $\mathcal{M}^{prin}$ called "principal manifolds" of the distribution p (in reference to the definition of Tibshirani [7]) which can be viewed as the manifold $\mathcal{M}$ without the noise. We assume the data have been generated by some set of points and segments constituting the set of manifolds $\mathcal{M}^{prin}$ which have been corrupted with additive spherical gaussian noise with mean 0 and unknown variance σ_{noise}^2. Then, we define a gaussian mixture model to account for the observed data, which is based on both gaussian kernels that we call "gaussian-points", and what we call "gaussian-segments", forming a "Generative Gaussian Graph" (GGG).

The value at point $v_j \in \underline{v}$ of a normalized gaussian-point centered on a prototype $w_i \in \underline{w}$ with variance σ^2 is defined as: $g^0(v_j, w_i, \sigma) = (2\pi\sigma^2)^{-D/2} \exp(-\frac{(v_j - w_i)^2}{2\sigma^2})$

A normalized gaussian-segment is defined as the sum of an infinite number of gaussian-points evenly spread on a line segment. Thus, this is the integral of a gaussian-point along a line segment. The value at point v_j of the gaussian-segment $[w_{a_i} w_{b_i}]$ associated to the ith edge $\{a_i, b_i\}$ in DG with variance σ^2 is:

$$
\begin{aligned}
g^1(v_j, \{w_{a_i}, w_{b_i}\}, \sigma) &= \frac{\int_{w_{a_i}}^{w_{b_i}} \exp\left(-\frac{(v_j - w)^2}{2\sigma^2}\right) dw}{(2\pi\sigma^2)^{\frac{D}{2}} L_{a_i b_i}} \\
&= \frac{\exp\left(-\frac{(v_j - q_i^j)^2}{2\sigma^2}\right)}{(2\pi\sigma^2)^{\frac{D-1}{2}}} \cdot \frac{\mathrm{erf}\left(\frac{Q_{a_i b_i}^j}{\sigma\sqrt{2}}\right) - \mathrm{erf}\left(\frac{Q_{a_i b_i}^j - L_{a_i b_i}}{\sigma\sqrt{2}}\right)}{2 L_{a_i b_i}}
\end{aligned}
\tag{1}
$$

where $L_{a_i b_i} = \|w_{b_i} - w_{a_i}\|$, $Q_{a_i b_i}^j = \frac{\langle v_j - w_{a_i} | w_{b_i} - w_{a_i} \rangle}{L_{a_i b_i}}$ and $q_i^j = w_{a_i} + (w_{b_i} - w_{a_i}) \frac{Q_{a_i b_i}^j}{L_{a_i b_i}}$ is the orthogonal projection of v_j on the straight line passing through w_{a_i} and w_{b_i}. In the case where $w_{a_i} = w_{b_i}$, we set $g^1(v_j, \{w_{a_i}, w_{b_i}\}, \sigma) = g^0(v_j, w_{a_i}, \sigma)$.

The left part of the dot product accounts for the gaussian noise orthogonal to the line segment, and the right part for the gaussian noise integrated along the line segment. The functions g^0 and g^1 are positive and we can prove that: $\int_{\mathbb{R}^D} g^0(v, w_i, \sigma) dv = 1$ and $\int_{\mathbb{R}^D} g^1(v, \{w_a, w_b\}, \sigma) dv = 1$, so they are both probability density functions. A gaussian-point is associated to each prototype in $\underline{w}$ and a gaussian-segment to each edge in DG.

The gaussian mixture is obtained by a weighting sum of the N_0 gaussian-points and N_1 gaussian-segments, such that the weights π sum to 1 and are non-negative:

$$
p(v_j | \underline{\pi}, \underline{w}, \sigma, DG) = \sum_{k=0}^{1} \sum_{i=1}^{N_k} \pi_i^k g^k(v_j, s_i^k, \sigma)
\tag{2}
$$

with $\sum_{k=0}^{1} \sum_{i=1}^{N_k} \pi_i^k = 1$ and $\forall i, k, \ \pi_i^k \geq 0$, where $s_i^0 = w_i$ and $s_i^1 = \{w_{a_i}, w_{b_i}\}$ such that $\{a_i, b_i\}$ is the ith edge in DG. The weight π_i^0 (resp. π_i^1) is the probability that a datum v was drawn from the gaussian-point associated to w_i (resp. the gaussian-segment associated to the ith edge of DG).

2.2 Measure of quality

The function $p(v_j | \underline{\pi}, \underline{w}, \sigma, DG)$ is the probability density at v_j given the parameters of the model. We measure the likelihood P of the data $\underline{v}$ wrt the parameters of the GGG model:

$$
P = P(\underline{\pi}, \underline{w}, \sigma, DG) = \prod_{j=1}^{M} p(v_j | \underline{\pi}, \underline{w}, \sigma, DG)
\tag{3}
$$

2.3 The Expectation-Maximization algorithm

In order to maximize the likelihood P or equivalently to minimize the negative log-likelihood $L = -\log(P)$ wrt $\underline{\pi}$ and σ, we use the Expectation-Maximization algorithm.

We refer to [2] (pages $59 - 73$) and [16] for further details. The minimization of the negative log-likelihood consists in t_{max} iterative steps updating π and σ which ensure the decrease of L. The updating rules take into account the constraints about positivity or sum to unity of the parameters:

$$
\begin{aligned}
\pi_i^{k[\text{new}]} &= \frac{1}{M} \sum_{j=1}^M P(k,i|v_j) \\
\sigma^{2[\text{new}]} &= \frac{1}{DM} \sum_{j=1}^M \left[\sum_{i=1}^{N_0} P(0,i|v_j)(v_j - w_i)^2 \right. \\
&\left. + \sum_{i=1}^{N_1} P(1,i|v_j) \frac{(2\pi\sigma^2)^{-D/2} \exp(-\frac{(v_j - q_i^j)^2}{2\sigma^2})(I_1[(v_j-q_i^j)^2 + \sigma^2] + I_2)}{L_{a_i b_i} \cdot g^1(v_j, \{w_{a_i}, w_{b_i}\}, \sigma)} \right]
\end{aligned} \tag{4}
$$

where

$$
\begin{aligned}
I_1 &= \sigma \sqrt{\frac{\pi}{2}} \left(\text{erf}\left(\frac{Q_{a_i b_i}^j}{\sigma \sqrt{2}}\right) - \text{erf}\left(\frac{Q_{a_i b_i}^j - L_{a_i b_i}}{\sigma \sqrt{2}}\right) \right) \\
I_2 &= \sigma^2 \left((Q_{a_i b_i}^j - L_{a_i b_i}) \exp\left(-\frac{(Q_{a_i b_i}^j - L_{a_i b_i})^2}{2\sigma^2}\right) - Q_{a_i b_i}^j \exp\left(-\frac{(Q_{a_i b_i}^j)^2}{2\sigma^2}\right) \right)
\end{aligned} \tag{5}
$$

and $P(k,i|v_j) = \frac{\pi_i^k g^k(v_j, s_i^k, \sigma)}{p(v_j|\pi, w, \sigma, DG)}$ is the posterior probability that the datum v_j was generated by the component associated to (k, i).

2.4 Emerging topology by maximizing the likelihood

Finally, to get the topology representing graph from the generative model, the core idea is to prune from the initial DG the edges for which there is probability ϵ they generated the data. The complete algorithm is the following:

1. Initialize the location of the prototypes w using vector quantization [14].
2. Construct the Delaunay graph DG of the prototypes.
3. Initialize the weights π to $1/(N_0 + N_1)$ to give equiprobability to each vertices and edges.
4. Given w and DG, use updating rules (4) to find σ^{2*} and π^* maximizing the likelihood P.
5. Prune the edges $\{a_i b_i\}$ of DG associated to the gaussian segments with probability $\pi_i^1 \leq \epsilon$ where $\pi_i^1 \in \pi^*$.

The topology representing graph emerges from the edges with probabilities $\pi^* > \epsilon$. It is the graph which best models the topology of the data in the sense of the maximum likelihood *wrt* π, σ, ϵ and the set of prototypes w and their Delaunay graph.

3 Experiments

In these experiments, given a set of points and a set of prototypes located thanks to vector quantization [14], we want to verify the relevance of the GGG to learn the topology in various noise conditions. The principle of the GGG is shown in the Figure 1. In the Figure 2, we show the comparison of the GGG to a CHL for which we filter out edges which have a number of hits lower than a threshold T. The data and prototypes are the same for both algorithms. We set T^* such that the graph obtained matches visually as close as possible the expected solution. We optimize σ and π using (4) for $t_{max} = 100$ steps and $\epsilon = 0.001$. Conditions and conclusions of the experiments are given in the captions.

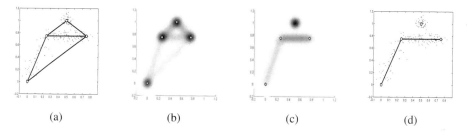

(a)   (b)   (c)   (d)

Figure 1: **Principle of the Generative Gaussian Graph**: (a) Data drawn from an oblique segment, an horizontal one and an isolated point with respective density $\{0.25; 0.5; 0.25\}$. The prototypes are located at the extreme points of the segments, and at the isolated point. They are connected with edges from the Delaunay graph. (b) The corresponding initial Generative Gaussian Graph. (c) The optimal GGG obtained after optimization of the likelihood according to σ and π. (d) The edges of the optimal GGG associated to non-negligible probabilities model the topology of the data.

4 Discussion

We propose that the problem of learning the topology of a set of points can be posed as a statistical learning problem: we assume that the topology of a statistical generative model of a set of points is an estimator of the topology of the principal manifold of this set. From this assumption, we define a topologically flexible statistical generative mixture model that we call Generative Gaussian Graph from which we can extract the topology. The final topology representing graph emerges from the edges with non-negligible probability. We propose to use the Delaunay graph as an initial graph assuming it is rich enough to contain as a subgraph a good topological model of the data. The use of the likelihood criterion makes possible cross-validation to select the best generative model hence the best topological model in terms of generalization capacities.

The GGG allows to avoid the limits of the CHL for modelling topology. In particular, it allows to take into account the noise and to model isolated bumps. Moreover, the likelihood of the data *wrt* the GGG is maximized during the learning, allowing to measure the quality of the model even when no visualization is possible. For some particular data distributions where all the data lie on the Delaunay line segments, no maximum of the likelihood exists. This case is not a problem because $\sigma = 0$ effectively defines a good solution (no noise in a data set drawn from a graph). If only some of the data lie exactly on the line segments, a maximum of the likelihood still exists because σ^2 defines the variance for all the generative gaussian points and segments at the same time so it cannot vanish to 0. The computing time complexity of the GGG is $o(D(N_0 + N_1)Mt_{max})$ plus the time $O(DN_0^3)$ [15] needed to build the Delaunay graph which dominates the overall worst time complexity. The Competitive Hebbian Learning is in time $o(DN_0M)$. As in general, the CHL builds too much edges than needed to model the topology, it would be interesting to use the Delaunay subgraph obtained with the CHL as a starting point for the GGG model.

The Generative Gaussian Graph can be viewed as a generalization of gaussian mixtures to points and segments: a gaussian mixture is a GGG with no edge. GGG provides at the same time an estimation of the data distribution density more accurate than the gaussian mixture based on the same set of prototypes and the same noise isovariance hypothesis (because it adds gaussian-segments to the pool of gaussian-points), and intrinsically an explicit model of the topology of the data set which provides most of the topological information at once. In contrast, other generative models do not provide any insight about the topology of the data, except the Generative Topographic Map (GTM) [4], the revisited Principal Manifolds [7] or the mixture of Probabilistics Principal Component Analysers (PPCA) [8]. However, in the two former cases, the intrinsic dimension of the model is fixed *a priori* and

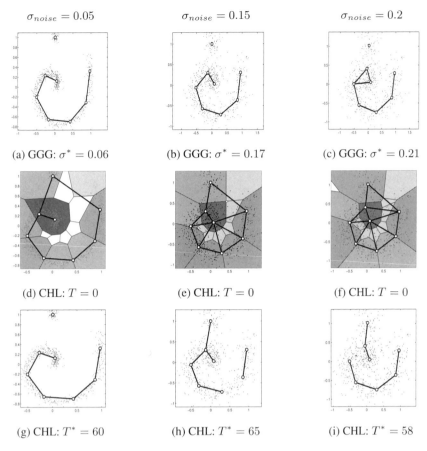

$\sigma_{noise} = 0.05$ $\sigma_{noise} = 0.15$ $\sigma_{noise} = 0.2$

(a) GGG: $\sigma^* = 0.06$ (b) GGG: $\sigma^* = 0.17$ (c) GGG: $\sigma^* = 0.21$

(d) CHL: $T = 0$ (e) CHL: $T = 0$ (f) CHL: $T = 0$

(g) CHL: $T^* = 60$ (h) CHL: $T^* = 65$ (i) CHL: $T^* = 58$

Figure 2: **Learning the topology of a data set**: 600 data drawn from a spirale and an isolated point corrupted with additive gaussian noise with mean 0 and variance σ_{noise}^2. Prototypes are located by vector quantization [14]. (a-c) The edges of the GGG with weights greater than ϵ allow to recover the topology of the principal manifolds except for large noise variance (c) where a triangle was created at the center of the spirale. σ^* over-estimates σ_{noise} because the model is piecewise linear while the true manifolds are non-linear. (d-f) The CHL without threshold (T=0) is not able to recover the true topology of the data for even small σ_{noise}. In particular, the isolated bump cannot be recovered. The grey cells correspond to ROI of the edges (darker cells contain more data). It shows these cells are not intuitively related to the edges they are associated to (*e.g.* they may have very tiny areas (e), and may partly (d) or never (f) contain the corresponding line segment). (g-h) The CHL with a threshold T allows to recover the topology of the data only for small noise variance (g) (Notice $T_1 < T_2 \Rightarrow DG_{CHL}(T_2) \subseteq DG_{CHL}(T_1)$). Moreover, setting T requires visual control and is not associated to the optimum of any energy function which prevents its use in higher dimensional space.

not learned from the data, while in the latter the local intrinsic dimension is learned but the connectedness between the local models is not.

One obvious way to follow to extend this work is considering a simplicial complex in place of the graph to get the full topological information extractible. Some other interesting questions arise about the curse of the dimension, the selection of the number of prototypes and the threshold ϵ, the theoretical grounding of the connection between the likelihood and some topological measure of accuracy, the possibility to devise a "universal topology estimator", the way to deal with data sets with multi-scale structures or background noise...

This preliminary work is an attempt to bridge the gap between Statistical Learning Theory [17] and Computational Topology [18][19]. We wish it to cross-fertilize and to open new perspectives in both fields.

References

[1] M. Aupetit and T. Catz. High-dimensional labeled data analysis with topology representing graphs. *Neurocomputing, Elsevier*, 63:139–169, 2005.

[2] C. M. Bishop. *Neural Networks for Pattern Recognition*. Oxford Univ. Press, New York, 1995.

[3] M. Zeller, R. Sharma, and K. Schulten. Topology representing network for sensor-based robot motion planning. *World Congress on Neural Networks, INNS Press*, pages 100–103, 1996.

[4] C. M. Bishop, M. Svensén, and C. K. I. Williams. Gtm: the generative topographic mapping. *Neural Computation, MIT Press*, 10(1):215–234, 1998.

[5] V. de Silva and J. B. Tenenbaum. Global versus local methods for nonlinear dimensionality reduction. *In S. Becker, S. Thrun, K. Obermayer (Eds) Advances in Neural Information Processing Systems, MIT Press,Cambridge, MA*, 15:705–712, 2003.

[6] J. A. Lee, A. Lendasse, and M. Verleysen. Curvilinear distance analysis versus isomap. *Europ. Symp. on Art. Neural Networks, Bruges (Belgium), d-side eds.*, pages 185–192, 2002.

[7] R. Tibshirani. Principal curves revisited. *Statistics and Computing*, (2):183–190, 1992.

[8] M. E. Tipping and C. M. Bishop. Mixtures of probabilistic principal component analysers. *Neural Computation*, 11(2):443–482, 1999.

[9] M. Aupetit. Robust topology representing networks. *European Symp. on Artificial Neural Networks, Bruges (Belgium), d-side eds.*, pages 45–50, 2003.

[10] V. de Silva and G. Carlsson. Topological estimation using witness complexes. *In M. Alexa and S. Rusinkiewicz (Eds) Eurographics Symposium on Point-Based Graphics, ETH, Zürich,Switzerland, June 2-4*, 2004.

[11] T. M. Martinetz and K. J. Schulten. Topology representing networks. *Neural Networks, Elsevier London*, 7:507–522, 1994.

[12] A. Okabe, B. Boots, and K. Sugihara. *Spatial tessellations: concepts and applications of Voronoï diagrams*. John Wiley, Chichester, 1992.

[13] H. Edelsbrunner and N. R. Shah. Triangulating topological spaces. *International Journal on Computational Geometry and Applications*, 7:365–378, 1997.

[14] T. M. Martinetz, S. G. Berkovitch, and K. J. Schulten. "neural-gas" network for vector quantization and its application to time-series prediction. *IEEE Trans. on NN*, 4(4):558–569, 1993.

[15] E. Agrell. A method for examining vector quantizer structures. *Proceedings of IEEE International Symposium on Information Theory, San Antonio, TX*, page 394, 1993.

[16] A. Dempster, N. Laird, and D. Rubin. Maximum likelihood from incomplete data via the em algorithm. *Journal of the Royal Statistical Society, Series B*, 39(1):1–38, 1977.

[17] V.N. Vapnik. *Statistical Learning Theory*. John Wiley, 1998.

[18] T. Dey, H. Edelsbrunner, and S. Guha. Computational topology. *In B. Chazelle, J. Goodman and R. Pollack, editors, Advances in Discrete and Computational Geometry. American Math. Society, Princeton, NJ*, 1999.

[19] V. Robins, J. Abernethy, N. Rooney, and E. Bradley. Topology and intelligent data analysis. *IDA-03 (International Symposium on Intelligent Data Analysis), Berlin*, 2003.

On Local Rewards and Scaling Distributed Reinforcement Learning

J. Andrew Bagnell
Robotics Institute
Carnegie Mellon University
Pittsburgh, PA 15213
dbagnell@ri.cmu.edu

Andrew Y. Ng
Computer Science Department
Stanford University
Stanford, CA 94305
ang@cs.stanford.edu

Abstract

We consider the scaling of the number of examples necessary to achieve good performance in distributed, cooperative, multi-agent reinforcement learning, as a function of the the number of agents n. We prove a worst-case lower bound showing that algorithms that rely solely on a *global* reward signal to learn policies confront a fundamental limit: They require a number of real-world examples that scales roughly linearly in the number of agents. For settings of interest with a very large number of agents, this is impractical. We demonstrate, however, that there is a class of algorithms that, by taking advantage of *local* reward signals in large distributed Markov Decision Processes, are able to ensure good performance with a number of samples that scales as $O(\log n)$. This makes them applicable even in settings with a very large number of agents n.

1 Introduction

Recently there has been great interest in distributed reinforcement learning problems where a collection of agents with independent action choices attempts to optimize a joint performance metric. Imagine, for instance, a traffic engineering application where each traffic signal may independently decide when to switch colors, and performance is measured by aggregating the throughput at all traffic stops. Problems with such factorizations where the *global* reward decomposes in to a sum of *local* rewards are common and have been studied in the RL literature. [10]

The most straightforward and common approach to solving these problems is to apply one of the many well-studied single agent algorithms to the global reward signal. Effectively, this treats the multi-agent problem as a single agent problem with a very large action space. Peshkin et al. [9] establish that policy gradient learning factorizes into independent policy gradient learning problems for each agent using the global reward signal. Chang et al. [3] use global reward signals to estimate effective local rewards for each agent. Guestrin et al. [5] consider coordinating agent actions using the global reward. We argue from an information theoretic perspective that such algorithms are fundamentally limited in their scalability. In particular, we show in Section 3 that as a function of the number of agents n, such algorithms will need to see[1] $\tilde{\Omega}(n)$ trajectories in the worst case to achieve good performance.

We suggest an alternate line of inquiry, pursued as well by other researchers (including

---

[1] Big-$\tilde{\Omega}$ notation omits logarithmic terms, similar to how big-Ω notation drops constant values.

notably [10]), of developing algorithms that capitalize on the availability of local reward signals to improve performance. Our results show that such local information can dramatically reduce the number of examples necessary for learning to $O(\log n)$. One approach that the results suggest to solving such distributed problems is to estimate model parameters from all local information available, and then to solve the resulting model offline. Although this clearly still carries a high *computational* burden, it is much preferable to requiring a large amount of real-world experience. Further, useful approximate multiple agent Markov Decision Process (MDP) solvers that take advantage of local reward structure have been developed. [4]

2 Preliminaries

We consider distributed reinforcement learning problems, modeled as MDPs, in which there are n (cooperative) agents, each of which can directly influence only a small number of its neighbors. More formally, let there be n agents, each with a finite state space S of size $|S|$ states and a finite action space A of size $|A|$. The joint state space of all the agents is therefore S^n, and the joint action space A^n. If $s_t \in S^n$ is the joint state of the agents at time t, we will use $s_t^{(i)}$ to denote the state of agent i. Similarly, let $a_t^{(i)}$ denote the action of agent i.

For each agent $i \in \{1, \ldots, n\}$, we let $\text{neigh}(i) \subseteq \{1, \ldots, n\}$ denote the subset of agents that i's state directly influences. For notational convenience, we assume that if $i \in \text{neigh}(j)$, then $j \in \text{neigh}(i)$, and that $i \in \text{neigh}(i)$. Thus, the agents can be viewed as living on the vertices of a graph, where agents have a direct influence on each other's state only if they are connected by an edge. This is similar to the graphical games formalism of [7], and is also similar to the Dynamic Bayes Net (DBN)-MDP formalisms of [6] and [2]. (Figure 1 depicts a DBN and an agent influence graph.) DBN formalisms allow the more refined notion of directionality in the influence between neighbors.

More formally, each agent i is associated with a CPT (conditional probability table) $P_i(s_{t+1}^{(i)}|s_t^{(\text{neigh}(i))}, a_t^{(i)})$, where $s_t^{(\text{neigh}(i))}$ denotes the state of agent i's neighbors at time t. Given the joint action a of the agents, the joint state evolves according to

$$p(s_{t+1}|s_t, a_t) = \prod_{i=1}^{n} p(s_{t+1}^{(i)}|s_t^{(\text{neigh}(i))}, a_t^{(i)}). \tag{1}$$

For simplicity, we have assumed that agent i's state is directly influenced by the states of $\text{neigh}(i)$ but not their actions; the generalization offers no difficulties. The initial state s_1 is distributed according to some initial-state distribution $\mathcal{D}$.

A policy is a map $\pi : S^n \mapsto A^n$. Writing π out explicitly as a vector-valued function, we have $\pi(s) = (\pi_1(s), \ldots, \pi_n(s))$, where $\pi_i(s) : S^n \mapsto A$ is the local policy of agent i. For some applications, we may wish to consider only policies in which agent i chooses its local action as a function of only its local state $s^{(i)}$ (and possibly its neighbors); in this case, π_i can be restricted to depend only on $s^{(i)}$.

Each agent has a **local reward function** $R_i(s^{(i)}, a^{(i)})$, which takes values in the unit interval $[0, 1]$. The total payoff in the MDP at each step is $R(s, a) = (1/n) \sum_{i=1}^{n} R(s^{(i)}, a^{(i)})$. We call this $R(s, a)$ the **global reward function**, since it reflects the total reward received by the joint set of agents. We will consider the finite-horizon setting, in which the MDP terminates after T steps. Thus, the utility of a policy π in an MDP M is

$$U(\pi) = U_M(\pi) = \mathrm{E}_{s_1 \sim \mathcal{D}}[V^\pi(s_1)] = \mathrm{E}\left[\frac{1}{n}\sum_{t=1}^{T}\sum_{i=1}^{n} R_i(s_t^{(i)}, a_t^{(i)})|\pi\right].$$

In the reinforcement learning setting, the dynamics (CPTs) and rewards of the problem are unknown, and a learning algorithm has to take actions in the MDP and use the resulting observations of state transitions and rewards to learn a good policy. Each "trial" taken by a reinforcement learning algorithm shall consist of a T-step sequence in the MDP.

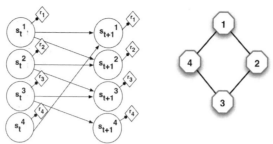

Figure 1: (Left) A DBN description of a multi-agent MDP. Each row of (round) nodes in the DBN corresponds to one agent. (Right) A graphical depiction of the influence effects in a multi-agent MDP. A connection between nodes in the graph implies arrows connecting the nodes in the DBN.

Our goal is to characterize the scaling of the sample complexity for various reinforcement learning approaches (i.e., how many trials they require in order to learn a near-optimal policy) for large numbers of agents n. Thus, in our bounds below, no serious attempt has been made to make our bounds tight in variables other than n.

3   Global rewards hardness result

Below we show that if an RL algorithm uses only the global reward signal, then there exists a very simple MDP—one with horizon, $T = 1$, only one state/trivial dynamics, and two actions per agent—on which the learning algorithm will require $\tilde{\Omega}(n)$ trials to learn a good policy. Thus, such algorithms do not scale well to large numbers of agents. For example, consider learning in the traffic signal problem described in the introduction with $n = 100,000$ traffic lights. Such an algorithm may then require on the order of $100,000$ days of experience (trials) to learn. In contrast, in Section 4, we show that if a reinforcement learning algorithm is given access to the local rewards, it can be possible to learn in such problems with an exponentially smaller $O(\log n)$ sample complexity.

Theorem 3.1: *Let any* $0 < \epsilon < 0.05$ *be fixed. Let any reinforcement learning algorithm* $\mathcal{L}$ *be given that only uses the* global *reward signal* $R(s)$, *and does not use the local rewards* $R_i(s^{(i)})$ *to learn (other than through their sum). Then there exists an MDP with time horizon* $T = 1$, *so that:*

1. *The MDP is very "simple" in that it has only one state ($|S| = 1$, $|S^n| = 1$); trivial state transition probabilities (since $T = 1$); two actions per agent ($|A| = 2$); and deterministic binary (0/1)-valued local reward functions.*

2. *In order for* $\mathcal{L}$ *to output a policy* $\hat{\pi}$ *that is near-optimal satisfying[2]* $U(\hat{\pi}) \geq \max_\pi U(\pi) - \epsilon$, *it is necessary that the number of trials* m *be at least*

$$m \geq \frac{0.32n + \log(1/4)}{\log(n+1)} = \tilde{\Omega}(n).$$

Proof. For simplicity, we first assume that $\mathcal{L}$ is a deterministic learning algorithm, so that in each of the m trials, its choice of action is some deterministic function of the outcomes of the earlier trials. Thus, in each of the m trials, $\mathcal{L}$ chooses a vector of actions $a \in A^N$, and receives the global reward signal $R(s,a) = \frac{1}{n}\sum_{i=1}^n R(s^{(i)}, a^{(i)})$. In our MDP, each local reward $R(s^{(i)}, a^{(i)})$ will take values only 0 and 1. Thus, $R(s,a)$ can take only $n+1$ different values (namely, $\frac{0}{n}, \frac{1}{n}, \ldots, \frac{n}{n}$). Since $T = 1$, the algorithm receives only one such reward value in each trial.

Let $r_1, \ldots, r_m$ be the m global reward signals received by $\mathcal{L}$ in the m trials. Since $\mathcal{L}$ is deterministic, its output policy $\hat{\pi}$ will be chosen as some deterministic function of these

---

[2] For randomized algorithms we consider instead the expectation of $U(\hat{\pi})$ under the algorithm's randomization.

rewards $r_1, \ldots, r_m$. But the vector $(r_1, \ldots, r_m)$ can take on only $(n+1)^m$ different values (since each r_t can take only $n+1$ different values), and thus $\hat{\pi}$ itself can also take only at most $(n+1)^m$ different values. Let Π_m denote this set of possible values for $\hat{\pi}$. ($|\Pi_m| \leq (n+1)^m$).

Call each local agent's two actions a_1, a_2. We will generate an MDP with randomly chosen parameters. Specifically, each local reward $R_i(s^{(i)}, a^{(i)})$ function is randomly chosen with equal probability to either give reward 1 for action a_1 and reward 0 for action a_2; or vice versa. Thus, each local agent has one "right" action that gives reward 1, but the algorithm has to learn which of the two actions this is. Further, by choosing the right actions, the optimal policy π^* attains $U(\pi^*) = 1$.

Fix any policy π. Then $U_M(\pi) = \frac{1}{n} \sum_{i=1}^{n} R(s^{(i)}, \pi(s^{(i)}))$ is the mean of n independent Bernoulli(0.5) random variables (since the rewards are chosen randomly), and has expected value 0.5. Thus, by the Hoeffding inequality, $P(U_M(\pi) \geq 1 - 2\epsilon) \leq \exp(-2(0.5 - 2\epsilon)^2 n)$. Thus, taking a union bound over all policies $\pi \in \Pi_M$, we have

$$P(\exists \pi \in \Pi_M \text{ s.t. } U_M(\pi) \geq 1 - 2\epsilon) \leq |\Pi_M| \exp(-2(0.5 - 2\epsilon)^2 n) \qquad (2)$$
$$\leq (n+1)^m \exp(-2(0.5 - 2\epsilon)^2 n) \qquad (3)$$

Here, the probability is over the random MDP M. But since $\mathcal{L}$ outputs a policy in Π_M, the chance of $\mathcal{L}$ outputting a policy $\hat{\pi}$ with $U_M(\hat{\pi}) \geq 1 - 2\epsilon$ is bounded by the chance that there exists such a policy in Π_M. Thus,

$$P(U_M(\hat{\pi}) \geq 1 - 2\epsilon) \leq (n+1)^m \exp(-2(0.5 - 2\epsilon)^2 n). \qquad (4)$$

By setting the right hand side to $1/4$ and solving for m, we see that so long as

$$m < \frac{2(0.5 - 2\epsilon)^2 n + \log(1/4)}{\log(n+1)} \leq \frac{0.32n + \log(1/4)}{\log(n+1)}, \qquad (5)$$

we have that $P(U_M(\hat{\pi}) \geq 1 - 2\epsilon) < 1/4$. (The second equality above follows by taking $\epsilon < 0.05$, ensuring that no policy will be within 0.1 of optimal.) Thus, under this condition, by the standard probabilistic method argument [1], there must be at least one such MDP under which $\mathcal{L}$ fails to find an ϵ-optimal policy.

For randomized algorithms $\mathcal{L}$, we can define for each string of input random numbers to the algorithm ω a deterministic algorithm $\mathcal{L}^\omega$. Given m samples above, the expected performance of algorithm $\mathcal{L}^\omega$ over the distribution of MDPs

$$E_{p(M)}[\mathcal{L}^\omega] \leq Pr(U_M(\mathcal{L}^\omega) \geq 1 - 2\epsilon)1 + (1 - Pr(U_M(\mathcal{L}^\omega) \geq 1 - 2\epsilon))(1 - 2\epsilon)$$
$$< \frac{1}{4} + \frac{3}{4}(1 - 2\epsilon) < 1 - \epsilon$$

Since

$$E_{p(M)}E_{p(\omega)}[U_M(\mathcal{L}^\omega)] = E_{p(\omega)}E_{p(M)}[U_M(\mathcal{L}^\omega)] < E_{p(\omega)}[1 - \epsilon]$$

it follows again from the probabilistic method there must be at least one MDP for which the $\mathcal{L}$ has expected performance less than $1 - \epsilon$. $\qquad \square$

4 Learning with local rewards

Assuming the existence of a good exploration policy, we now show a positive result that if our learning algorithm has access to the local rewards, then it is possible to learn a near-optimal policy after a number of trials that grows only *logarithmically* in the number of agents n. In this section, we will assume that the neighborhood structure (encoded by $\text{neigh}(i)$) is known, but that the CPT parameters of the dynamics and the reward functions are unknown. We also assume that the size of the largest neighborhood is bounded by $\max_i |\text{neigh}(i)| = B$.

Definition. A policy π_{explore} is a (ρ, ν)-exploration policy if, given any i, any configuration of states $s^{(\text{neigh}(i))} \in S^{|\text{neigh}(i)|}$, and any action $a^{(i)} \in A$, on a trial of length T the policy π_{explore} has at least a probability $\nu \cdot \rho^B$ of executing action $a^{(i)}$ while i and its neighbors are in state $s^{(\text{neigh}(i))}$.

Proposition 4.1: *Suppose the MDP's initial state distribution is random, so that the state $s_i^{(i)}$ of each agent i is chosen independently from some distribution D_i. Further, assume that D_i assigns probability at least $\rho > 0$ to each possible state value $s \in S$. Then the "random" policy π (that on each time-step chooses each agent's action uniformly at random over A) is a $(\rho, \frac{1}{|A|})$-exploration policy.*

Proof. For agent i, the initial state of $s^{(\text{neigh}(i))}$ has has at least a ρ^B chance of being any particular vector of values, and the random action policy has a $1/|A|$ chance of taking any particular action from this state. □

In general, it is a fairly strong assumption to assume that we have an exploration policy. However, this assumption serves to decouple the problem of exploration from the "sample complexity" question of how much data we need from the MDP. Specifically, it guarantees that we visit each local configuration sufficiently often to have a reasonable amount of data to estimate each CPT. [3]

In the envisioned procedure, we will execute an exploration policy for m trials, and then use the resulting data we collect to obtain the maximum-likelihood estimates for the CPT entries and the rewards. We call the resulting estimates $\hat{p}(s_{t+1}^{(i)}|s_t^{(\text{neigh}(i))}, a_t^{(i)})$ and $\hat{R}(s^{(i)}, a^{(i)})$.[4] The following simple lemma shows that, with a number of trials that grows only logarithmically in n, this procedure will give us good estimates for all CPTs and local rewards.

Lemma 4.2: *Let any $\epsilon_0 > 0, \delta > 0$ be fixed. Suppose $|\text{neigh}(i)| \leq B$ for all i, and let a (ρ, ν)-exploration policy be executed for m trials. Then in order to guarantee that, with probability at least $1 - \delta$, the CPT and reward estimates are ϵ_0-accurate:*

$$|\hat{p}(s_{t+1}^{(i)}|s_t^{(\text{neigh}(i))}, a_t^{(i)}) - p(s_{t+1}^{(i)}|s_t^{(\text{neigh}(i))}, a_t^{(i)})| \leq \epsilon_0 \qquad \text{for all } i, s_{t+1}^{(i)}, s_t^{(\text{neigh}(i))}, a_t^{(i)}$$

$$|\hat{R}(s^{(i)}, a^{(i)})| - R(s^{(i)}, a^{(i)})| \leq \epsilon_0 \qquad \text{for all } i, s^{(i)}, a^{(i)}, \qquad (6)$$

it suffices that the number of trials be

$$m = O((\log n) \cdot \text{poly}(\frac{1}{\epsilon_0}, \frac{1}{\delta}, |S|, |A|, 1/(\nu\rho^B), B, T)).$$

Proof (Sketch). Given c examples to estimate a particular CPT entry (or a reward table entry), the probability that this estimate differs from the true value by more than ϵ_0 can be controlled by the Hoeffding bound:

$$P(|\hat{p}(s_{t+1}^{(i)}|s_t^{(\text{neigh}(i))}, a_t^{(i)}) - p(s_{t+1}^{(i)}|s_t^{(\text{neigh}(i))}, a_t^{(i)})| \geq \epsilon_0) \leq 2\exp(-2\epsilon_0^2 c).$$

Each CPT has at most $|A||S|^{B+1}$ entries and there are n such tables. There are also $n|S||A|$ possible local reward values. Taking a union bound over them, setting our probability of incorrectly estimating any CPTs or rewards to $\delta/2$, and solving for c gives $c \geq \frac{2}{\epsilon_0^2}\log(\frac{4\,n\,|A||S|^{B+1}}{\delta})$. For each agent i we see each local configurations of states and actions $(s^{(\text{neigh}(i))}, a^{(i)})$ with probability $\geq \rho^B\nu$. For m trajectories the expected number

---

[3]Further, it is possible to show a stronger version of our result than that stated below, showing that a random action policy can always be used as our exploration policy, to obtain a sample complexity bound with the same logarithmic dependence on n (but significantly worse dependencies on T and B). This result uses ideas from the random trajectory method of [8], with the key observation that local configurations that are not visited reasonably frequently by the random exploration policy will not be visited frequently by *any* policy, and thus inaccuracies in our estimates of their CPT entries will not significantly affect the result.

[4]We let $\hat{p}(s_{t+1}^{(i)}|s_t^{(\text{neigh}(i))}, a_t^{(i)})$ be the uniform distribution if $(s_t^{(\text{neigh}(i))}, a_t^{(i)})$ was never observed in the training data, and similarly let $\hat{R}(s^{(i)}, a^{(i)}) = 0$ if $\hat{R}(s^{(i)}, a^{(i)})$ was never observed.

of samples we see for each CPT entry is at least $m\rho^B\nu$. Call $S_m^{(s^{(\text{neigh}(i))},a^{(i)})}$ the number of samples we've seen of a configuration $(s^{(\text{neigh}(i))},a^{(i)})$ in m trajectories. Note then that:

$$P(S_m^{(s^{(\text{neigh}(i))},a^{(i)})} \leq c) \leq P(S_m^{(s^{(\text{neigh}(i))},a^{(i)})} - E[S_m^{(s^{(\text{neigh}(i))},a^{(i)})}] \leq c - m\rho^B\nu).$$

and another application of Hoeffding's bound ensures that:

$$P(S_m^{(s^{(\text{neigh}(i))},a^{(i)})} - E[S_m^{(s^{(\text{neigh}(i))},a^{(i)})}] \leq c - m\rho^B\nu) \leq \exp(\frac{-2}{mT^2}(c - m\rho^B\nu)^2).$$

Applying again the union bound to ensure that the probability of failure here is $\leq \delta/2$ and solving for m gives the result. $\qquad\square$

Definition. Define the **radius of influence** $r(t)$ after t steps to be the maximum number of nodes that are within t steps in the neighborhood graph of any single node.

Viewed differently, $r(t)$ upper bounds the number of nodes in the t-th timeslice of the DBN (as in Figure 1) which are decendants of any single node in the 1-st timeslice. In a DBN as shown in Figure 1, we have $r(t) = O(t)$. If the neighborhood graph is a 2-d lattice in which each node has at most 4 neighbors, then $r(t) = O(t^2)$. More generally, we might expect to have $r(t) = O(t^2)$ for "most" planar neigborhood graphs. Note that, even in the worst case, by our assumption of each node having B neighbors, we still have the bound $r(t) \leq B^t$, which is a bound independent of the number of agents n.

Theorem 4.3: *Let any $\epsilon > 0, \delta > 0$ be fixed. Suppose $|\text{neigh}(i)| \leq B$ for all i, and let a (ρ, ν)-exploration policy be executed for m trials in the MDP M. Let $\hat{M}$ be the maximum likelihood MDP, estimated from data from these m trials. Let Π be a policy class, and let*

$$\hat{\pi} = \arg\max_{\pi \in \Pi} U_{\hat{M}}(\pi)$$

be the best policy in the class, as evaluated on $\hat{M}$. Then to ensure that, with probability $1 - \delta$, we have that $\hat{\pi}$ is near-optimal within Π, i.e., that

$$U_M(\hat{\pi}) \geq \max_{\pi \in \Pi} U_M(\pi) - \epsilon,$$

it suffices that the number of trials be:

$$m = O((\log n) \cdot \text{poly}(1/\epsilon, 1/\delta, |S|, |A|, 1/(\nu\rho^B)), B, T, r(T)).$$

Proof. Our approach is essentially constructive: we show that for any policy, finite-horizon value-iteration using approximate CPTs and rewards in its backups will correctly estimate the true value function for that policy within $\epsilon/2$. For simplicity, we assume that the initial state distribution is known (and thus the same in $\hat{M}$ and M); the generalization offers no difficulties. By lemma (4.2) with m samples we can know both CPTs and rewards with the probability required within any required ϵ_0.

Note also that for any MDP with the given DBN or neighborhood graph structure (including both M and $\hat{M}$) the value function for every policy π and at each time-step has a property of *bounded variation*:

$$|\hat{V}_t(s^{(1)}, \ldots s^{(n)}) - \hat{V}_t(s^{(1)}, \ldots s^{(i-1)}, s^{(i)}_{\text{changed}}, s^{(i+1)}, \ldots, s^{(n)})| \leq \frac{r(T)T}{n}$$

This follows since a change in state can effect at most $r(T)$ agents' states, so the resulting change in utility must be bounded by $r(T)T/n$.

To compute a bound on the error in our estimate of overall utility we compute a bound on the error induced by a one-step Bellman backup $||B\hat{V} - \hat{B}\hat{V}||_\infty$. This quantity can be bounded in turn by considering the sequence of partially correct backup operators $\hat{B}_0, \ldots, \hat{B}_n$ where $\hat{B}_i$ is defined as the Bellman operator for policy π using the exact transitions and rewards for agents $1, 2, \ldots, i$, and the estimated transitions rewards/transitions

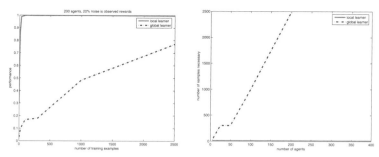

Figure 2: (Left) Scaling of performance as a function of the number of trajectories seen for a global reward and local reward algorithms. (Right) Scaling of the number of samples necessary to achieve near optimal reward as a function of the number of agents.

for agents $i + 1, \ldots, n$. From this definition it is immediate that the total error is equivalent to the telescoping sum:

$$||B\hat{V} - \hat{B}\hat{V}||_\infty = ||\hat{B}_0\hat{V} - \hat{B}_1\hat{V} + \hat{B}_1\hat{V} - \ldots + \hat{B}_{n-1}\hat{V} - \hat{B}_n\hat{V}||_\infty \qquad (7)$$

That sum is upper-bounded by the sum of term-by-term errors $\sum_{i=0}^{n-1} ||\hat{B}_i\hat{V} - \hat{B}_{i+1}\hat{V}||_\infty$. We can show that each of the terms in the sum is less than $\epsilon_0 r(T)(T+1)/n$ since the Bellman operators $\hat{B}_i\hat{V} - \hat{B}_{i+1}\hat{V}$ differ in the immediate reward contribution of agent $i+1$ by $\leq \epsilon_0$ and differ in computing the expected value of the future value by

$$E_{\prod_{j=1}^{i+1} p(s_{t+1}^j|s_t,\pi) \prod_{j=i+2}^{n} p(s_{t+1}^j|s_t,\pi)}[\sum_{s^{i+1}} \Delta p(s_{t+1}^{i+1}|s_t, \pi)\hat{V}_{t+1}(s)],$$

with $\Delta p(s_{t+1}^{i+1}|s_t, \pi) \leq \epsilon_0$ the difference in the CPTs between $\hat{B}_i$ and $\hat{B}_{i+1}$. By the bounded variation argument this total is then less than $\epsilon_0 r(T)T|S|/n$. It follows then $\sum_i ||\hat{B}_i\hat{V} - \hat{B}_{i+1}\hat{V}||_\infty \leq \epsilon_0 \, r(T) \, (T+1)|S|$. We now appeal to finite-horizon bounds on the error induced by Bellman backups [11] to show that the $||\hat{V} - V||_\infty \leq T||B\hat{V} - \hat{B}\hat{V}||_\infty \leq T(T+1) \, \epsilon_0 \, r(T)|S|$. Taking the expectation of $\hat{V}$ with respect to the initial state distribution D and setting m according to Lemma (4.2) with $\epsilon_0 = \frac{\epsilon}{2\lceil S \rceil r(T) T(T+1)}$ completes the proof. $\qquad \square$

5 Demonstration

We first present an experimental domain that hews closely to the theory in Section (3) above to demonstrate the importance of local rewards. In our simple problem there are $n = 400$ independent agents who each choose an action in $\{0, 1\}$. Each agent has a "correct" action that earns it reward $R_i = 1$ with probability 0.8, and reward 0 with probability 0.2. Equally, if the agents chooses the wrong action, it earns reward $R_i = 1$ with probability 0.2.

We compare two methods on this problem. Our first *global* algorithm uses only the global rewards R and uses this to build a model of the local rewards, and finally solves the resulting estimated MDP exactly. The local reward functions are learnt by a least-squares procedure with basis functions for each agent. The second algorithm also learns a local reward function, but does so taking advantage of the local rewards it observes as opposed to only the global signal. Figure (2) demonstrates the advantages of learning using a global reward signal.[5] On the right in Figure (2), we compute the time required to achieve $\frac{1}{4}$ of optimal reward for each algorithm, as a function of the number of agents.

In our next example, we consider a simple variant of the multi-agent SYSADMIN[6] prob-

----

[5]A gradient-based model-free approach using the global reward signal was also tried, but its performance was significantly poorer than that of the two algorithms depicted in Figure (2, left).

[6]In SYSADMIN there is a network of computers that fail randomly. A computer is more likely to fail if a neighboring computer (arranged in a ring topology) fails. The goal is to reboot machines in such a fashion so a maximize the number of running computers.

lem [4]. Again, we consider two algorithms: a global REINFORCE [9] learner, and a RE-INFORCE algorithm run using only local rewards, even through the local REINFORCE algorithm run in this way is not guaranteed to converge to the globally optimal (cooperative) solution. We note that the local algorithm learns much more quickly than using the global reward. (Figure 3) The learning speed we observed for the global algorithm correlates well with the observations in [5] that the number of samples needed scales roughly linearly in the number of agents. The local algorithm continued to require essentially the same number of examples for all sizes used (up to over 100 agents) in our experiments.

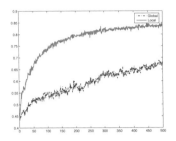 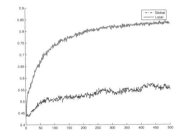

Figure 3: REINFORCE applied to the multi-agent SYSADMIN problem. *Local* refers to REINFORCE applied using only neighborhood (local) rewards while *global* refers to standard REINFORCE (applied to the global reward signal). (Left) shows averaged reward performance as a function of number of iterations for 10 agents. (Right) depicts the performance for 20 agents.

References

[1]   N. Alon and J. Spencer. *The Probabilistic Method*. Wiley, 2000.

[2]   C. Boutilier, T. Dean, and S. Hanks. Decision theoretic planning: Structural assumptions and computational leverage. *Journal of Artificial Intelligence Research*, 1999.

[3]   Y. Chang, T. Ho, and L. Kaelbling. All learning is local: Multi-agent learning in global reward games. In *Advances in NIPS 14*, 2004.

[4]   C. Guestrin, D. Koller, and R. Parr. Multi-agent planning with factored MDPs. In *NIPS-14*, 2002.

[5]   C. Guestrin, M. Lagoudakis, and R. Parr. Coordinated reinforcement learning. In *ICML*, 2002.

[6]   M. Kearns and D. Koller. Efficient reinforcement learning in factored mdps. In *IJCAI 16*, 1999.

[7]   M. Kearns, M. Littman, and S. Singh. Graphical models for game theory. In *UAI*, 2001.

[8]   M. Kearns, Y. Mansour, and A. Ng. Approximate planning in large POMDPs via reusable trajectories. *(extended version of paper in NIPS 12)*, 1999.

[9]   L. Peshkin, K-E. Kim, N. Meleau, and L. Kaelbling. Learning to cooperate via policy search. In *UAI 16*, 2000.

[10] J. Schneider, W. Wong, A. Moore, and M. Riedmiller. Distributed value functions. In *ICML*, 1999.

[11] R. Williams and L. Baird. Tight performance bounds on greedy policies based on imperfect value functions. Technical report, Northeastern University, 1993.

Bayesian models of human action understanding

Chris L. Baker, Joshua B. Tenenbaum & Rebecca R. Saxe
{clbaker,jbt,saxe}@mit.edu
Department of Brain and Cognitive Sciences
Massachusetts Institute of Technology

Abstract

We present a Bayesian framework for explaining how people reason about and predict the actions of an intentional agent, based on observing its behavior. Action-understanding is cast as a problem of inverting a probabilistic generative model, which assumes that agents tend to act rationally in order to achieve their goals given the constraints of their environment. Working in a simple sprite-world domain, we show how this model can be used to infer the goal of an agent and predict how the agent will act in novel situations or when environmental constraints change. The model provides a qualitative account of several kinds of inferences that preverbal infants have been shown to perform, and also fits quantitative predictions that adult observers make in a new experiment.

1 Introduction

A woman is walking down the street. Suddenly, she turns 180 degrees and begins running in the opposite direction. Why? Did she suddenly realize she was going the wrong way, or change her mind about where she should be headed? Did she remember something important left behind? Did she see someone she is trying to avoid? These explanations for the woman's behavior derive from taking the *intentional stance*: treating her as a rational agent whose behavior is governed by beliefs, desires or other mental states that refer to objects, events, or states of the world [5].

Both adults and infants have been shown to make robust and rapid intentional inferences about agents' behavior, even from highly impoverished stimuli. In "sprite-world" displays, simple shapes (e.g., circles) move in ways that convey a strong sense of agency to adults, and that lead to the formation of expectations consistent with goal-directed reasoning in infants [9, 8, 14]. The importance of the intentional stance in interpreting everyday situations, together with its robust engagement even in preverbal infants and with highly simplified perceptual stimuli, suggest that it is a core capacity of human cognition.

In this paper we describe a computational framework for modeling intentional reasoning in adults and infants. Interpreting an agent's behavior via the intentional stance poses a highly underconstrained inference problem: there are typically many configurations of beliefs and desires consistent with any sequence of behavior. We define a probabilistic generative model of an agent's behavior, in which behavior is dependent on hidden variables representing beliefs and desires. We then model intentional reasoning as a Bayesian inference about these hidden variables given observed behavior sequences.

It is often said that "vision is inverse graphics" – the inversion of a causal physical process of scene formation. By analogy, our analysis of intentional reasoning might be called "inverse planning", where the observer infers an agent's intentions, given observations of the agent's behavior, by inverting a model of how intentions cause behavior. The intentional stance assumes that an agent's actions depend causally on mental states via the *principle of rationality*: rational agents tend to act to achieve their desires as optimally as possible, given their beliefs. To achieve their desired goals, agents must typically not only select single actions but must construct *plans*, or sequences of intended actions. The standards of "optimal plan" may vary with agent or circumstance: possibilities include achieving goals "as quickly as possible", "as cheaply ...", "as reliably ...", and so on. We assume a soft, probabilistic version of the rationality principle, allowing that agents can often only approximate the optimal sequence of actions, and occasionally act in unexpected ways.

The paper is organized as follows. We first review several theoretical accounts of intentional reasoning from the cognitive science and artificial intelligence literatures, along with some motivating empirical findings. We then present our computational framework, grounding the discussion in a specific sprite-world domain. Lastly, we present results of our model on two sprite-world examples inspired by previous experiments in developmental psychology, and results of the model on our own experiments.

2 Empirical studies of intentional reasoning in infants and adults

2.1 Inferring an invariant goal

The ability to predict how an agent's behavior will adapt when environmental circumstances change, such as when an obstacle is inserted or removed, is a critical aspect of intentional reasoning. Gergely, Csibra and colleagues [8, 4] showed that preverbal infants can infer an agent's goal that appears to be invariant across different circumstances, and can predict the agent's future behavior by effectively assuming that it will act to achieve its goal in an efficient way, subject to the constraints of its environment. Their experiments used a looking-time (violation-of-expectation) paradigm with sprite-world stimuli. Infant participants were assigned to one of two groups. In the "obstacle" condition, infants were habituated to a sprite (a colored circle) moving ("jumping") in a curved path over an obstacle to reach another object. The size of the obstacle varied across trials, but the sprite always followed a near-shortest path over the obstacle to reach the other object. In the "no obstacle" group, infants were habituated to the sprite following the same curved "jumping" trajectory to the other object, but without an obstacle blocking its path. Both groups were then presented with the same test conditions, in which the obstacle was placed out of the sprite's way, and the sprite followed either the old, curved path or a new direct path to the other object. Infants from the "obstacle" group looked longer at the sprite following the unobstructed curved path, which (in the test condition) was now far from the most efficient route to the other object. Infants in the "no obstacle" group looked equally at both test stimuli. That is, infants in the "obstacle" condition appeared to interpret the sprite as moving in a rational goal-directed fashion, with the other object as its goal. They expected the sprite to plan a path to the goal that was maximally efficient, subject to environmental constraints when present. Infants in the "no obstacle" group appeared more uncertain about whether the sprite's movement was actually goal-directed or about what its goal was: was it simply to reach the other object, or something more complex, such as reaching the object via a particular curved path?

2.2 Inferring goals of varying complexity: rational means-ends analysis

Gergely et al. [6], expanding on work by Meltzoff [11], showed that infants can infer goals of varying complexity, again by interpreting agents' behaviors as rational responses to environmental constraints. In two conditions, infants saw an adult demonstrate an unfamiliar complex action: illuminating a light-box by pressing its top with her forehead. In the "hands occupied" condition, the demonstrator pretended to be cold and wrapped a blanket around herself, so that she was incapable of using a more typical means (i.e., her hands) to achieve the same goal. In the "hands free" condition the demonstrator had no such constraint. Most infants in the "hands free" condition spontaneously performed the head-press action when shown the light-box one week later, but only a few infants in the "hands occupied" condition did so; the others illuminated the light-box simply by pressing it with their hands. Thus infants appear to assume that rational agents will take the most efficient path to their goal, and that if an agent appears to systematically employ an inefficient means, it is likely because the agent has adopted a more complex goal that includes not only the end state but also the means by which that end should be achieved.

2.3 Inductive inference in intentional reasoning

Gergely and colleagues interpret their findings as if infants are reasoning about intentional action in an almost logical fashion, deducing the goal of an agent from its observed behavior, the rationality principle, and other implicit premises. However, from a computational point of view, it is surely oversimplified to think that the intentional stance could be implemented in a deductive system. There are too many sources of uncertainty and the inference problem is far too underconstrained for a logical approach to be successful. In contrast, our model posits that intentional reasoning is probabilistic. People's inferences about an agent's goal should be graded, reflecting a tradeoff between the prior probability of a candidate goal and its likelihood in light of the agent's observed behavior. Inferences should become more confident as more of the agent's behavior is observed.

To test whether human intentional reasoning is consistent with a probabilistic account, it is necessary to collect data in greater quantities and with greater precision than infant studies allow. Hence we designed our own sprite-world experimental paradigm, to collect richer quantitative judgments from adult observers. Many experiments are possible in this paradigm, but here we describe just one study of statistical effects on goal inference.

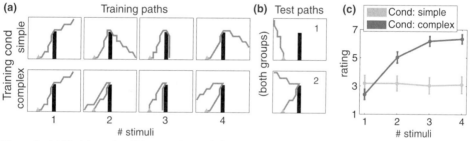

Figure 1: (a) Training stimuli in complex and simple goal conditions. (b) Test stimuli 1 and 2. Test stimuli was the same for each group. (c) Mean of subjects' ratings with standard error bars (n=16).

Sixteen observers were told that they would be watching a series of animations of a mouse running in a simple maze (a box with a single internal wall). The displays were shown from an overhead perspective, with an animated schematic trace of the mouse's path as it ran through the box. In each display, the mouse was placed in a different starting location and ran to recover a piece of cheese at a fixed, previously learned location. Observers were told that the mouse had learned to follow a more-or-less direct path to the cheese, regardless of its starting location. Subjects saw two conditions in counterbalanced order. In one condition ("simple goal"), observers saw four displays consistent with this prior knowledge. In another condition ("complex goal"), observers saw movements suggestive of a more complex, path-dependent goal for the mouse: it first ran directly to a particular location in the middle of the box (the "via-point"), and only then ran to the cheese. Fig. 1(a) shows the mouse's four trajectories in each of these conditions. Note that the first trajectory was the same in both conditions, while the next three were different. Also, all four trajectories in both conditions passed through the same hypothetical via-point in the middle of the box, which was not marked in any conspicuous way. Hence both the simple goal ("get to the cheese") and complex goal ("get to the cheese via point X") were logically possible interpretations in both conditions.

Observers' interpretations were assessed after viewing each of the four trajectories, by showing them diagrams of two test paths (Fig. 1(b)) running from a novel starting location to the cheese. They were asked to rate the probability of the mouse taking one or the other test path using a 1-7 scale: 1 = definitely path 1, 7 = definitely path 2, with intermediate values expressing intermediate degrees of confidence. Observers in the simple-goal condition always leaned towards path 1, the direct route that was consistent with the given prior knowledge. Observers in the complex-goal condition initially leaned just as much towards path 1, but after seeing additional trajectories they became increasingly confident that the mouse would follow path 2 (Fig. 1(c)). Importantly, the latter group increased its average confidence in path 2 with each subsequent trajectory viewed, consistent with the notion that goal inference results from something like a Bayesian integration process: prior probability favors the simple goal, but successive observations are more likely under the complex goal.

3 Previous models of intentional reasoning

The above phenomena highlight two capacities than any model of intentional reasoning should capture. First, representations of agents' mental states should include at least primitive planning capacities, with a constrained space of candidate goals and subgoals (or intended paths) that can refer to objects or locations in space, and the tendency to choose action sequences that achieve goals as efficiently as possible. Second, inferences about agents' goals should be probabilistic, and be sensitive to both prior knowledge about likely goals as well as statistical evidence for more complex or less likely goals that better account for observed actions.

These two components are clearly not sufficient for a complete account of human intentional reasoning, but most previous accounts do not include even these capacities. Gergely, Csibra and colleagues [7] have proposed an informal (noncomputational) model in which agents are essentially treated as rational planners, but inferences about agents' goals are purely deductive, without a role for probabilistic expectations or gradations of confidence.

A more statistically sophisticated computational framework for inferring goals from behavior has been proposed by [13], but this approach does not incorporate planning capacities. In this framework, the observer learns to represent an agent's policies, conditional on the agent's goals. Within a static environment, this knowledge allows an observer to infer the goal of an agent's actions, predict subsequent actions, and perform imitation, but it does not support generalization to new environments where the agent's policy must adapt in response. Further, because generalization is not based on strong prior knowledge such as the principle of rationality, many observations are needed for good performance. Likewise, probabilistic approaches to plan recognition in AI (e.g., [3, 10]) typically represent plans in terms of policies (state-action pairs) that do not generalize when the structure of the environment changes in some unexpected way, and that require much data to learn from observations of behavior.

Perhaps closest to how people reason with the intentional stance are methods for *inverse reinforcement learning* (IRL) [12], or methods for learning an agent's utility function [2]. Both approaches assume a rational agent who maximizes expected utility, and attempt to infer the agent's utility function from observations of its behavior. However, the utility functions that people attribute to intentional agents are typically much more structured and constrained than in conventional IRL. Goals are typically defined as relations towards objects or other agents, and may include subgoals, preferred paths, or other elements. In the next section we describe a Bayesian framework for modeling intentional reasoning that is similar in spirit to IRL, but more focused on the kinds of goal structures that are cognitively natural to human adults and infants.

4 The Bayesian framework

We propose to model intentional reasoning by combining the inferential power of statistical approaches to action understanding [12, 2, 13] with simple versions of the representational structures that psychologists and philosophers [5, 7] have argued are essential in theory of mind. This section first presents our general approach, and then presents a specific mathematical model for the "mouse" sprite-world introduced above.

Most generally, we assume a world that can be represented in terms of entities, attributes, and relations. Some attributes and relations are *dynamic*, indexed by a time dimension. Some entities are *agents*, who can perform actions at any time t with the potential to change the world state at time $t+1$. We distinguish between environmental state, denoted W, and agent states, denoted S. For simplicity, we will assume that there is exactly one intentional agent in the world, and that the agent's actions can only affect its own state $s \in S$. Let $s_{0:T}$ be a sequence of $T+1$ agent states. Typically, observations of multiple state sequences of the agent are available, and in general each may occur in a separate environment. Let $s_{0:T}^{1:N}$ be a set of N state sequences, and let $w^{1:N}$ be a set of N corresponding environments. Let A_s be the set of actions available to the agent from state s, and let $C(a)$ be the cost to the agent of action $a \in A_s$. Let $P(s_{t+1}|a_t, s_t, w)$ be the distribution over the agent's next state s_{t+1}, given the current state s_t, an action $a_t \in A_{s_t}$, and the environmental state w.

The agent's actions are assumed to depend on mental states such as *beliefs* and *desires*. In our context, beliefs correspond to knowledge about the environmental state. Desires may be simple or complex. A simple desire is an *end goal*: a world state or class of states that the agent will act to bring about. There are many possibilities for more complex goals, such as achieving a certain end by means of a certain route, achieving a certain sequence of states in some order, and so on. We specify a particular goal space G of simple and complex goals for sprite-worlds in the next subsection. The agent draws goals $g \in G$ from a prior distribution $P(g|w^{1:N})$, which constrains goals to be feasible in the environments $w^{1:N}$ from which observations of the agent's behavior are available.

Given the agent's goal g and an environment w, we can define a value $V_{g,w}(s)$ for each state s. The value function can be defined in various ways depending on the domain, task, and agent type. We specify a particular value function in the next subsection that reflects the goal structure of our sprite-world agent. The agent is assumed to choose actions according to a probabilistic policy, with a preference for actions with greater expected increases in value. Let $Q_{g,w}(s,a) = \sum_{s'} P(s'|a,s,w)V_{g,w}(s') - C(a)$ be the expected value of the state resulting from action a, minus the cost of the action. The agent's policy is

$$P(a_t|s_t, g, w) \propto \exp(\beta Q_{g,w}(s_t, a_t)). \qquad (1)$$

The parameter β controls how likely the agent is to select the most valuable action. This policy embodies a "soft" principle of rationality, which allows for inevitable sources of suboptimal planning, or unexplained deviations from the direct path. A graphical model illustrating the relationship between the environmental state, and the agent's goals, actions, and states is shown in Fig. 2.

The observer's task is to infer g from the agent's behavior. We assume that state sequences are independent given the environment and the goal. The observer infers g from $s_{0:T}^{1:N}$ via Bayes' rule, conditional on $w^{1:N}$:

$$P(g|s_{0:T}^{1:N}, w^{1:N}) \propto P(g|w^{1:N}) \prod_{i=1}^{N} P(s_{0:T}^i|g, w^i). \qquad (2)$$

We assume that state transition probabilities and action probabilities are conditionally independent given the agent's goal g, the agent's current state s_t, and the environment w. The likelihood of a state sequence $s_{0:T}$ given a goal g and an environment w is computed by marginalizing over possible actions generating state transitions:

$$P(s_{0:T}|g, w) = \prod_{t=0}^{T-1} \sum_{a_t \in A_{s_t}} P(s_{t+1}|a_t, s_t, w)P(a_t|s_t, g, w). \qquad (3)$$

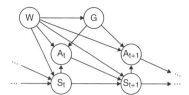

Figure 2: Two time-slice dynamic Bayes net representation of our model, where W is the environmental state, G is the agent's goal, S_t is the agent's state at time t, and A_t is the agent's action at time t. Beliefs, desires, and actions intuitively map onto W, G and A, respectively.

4.1 Modeling sprite-world inferences

Several additional assumptions are necessary to apply the above framework to any specific domain, such as the sprite-worlds discussed in §2. The size of the grid, the location of obstacles, and likely goal points (such as the location of the cheese in our experimental stimuli) are represented by W, and assumed to be known to both the agent and the observer. The agent's state space S consists of valid locations in the grid. All state sequences are assumed to be of the same length. The action space A_s consists of moves in all compass directions $\{N, S, E, W, NE, NW, SE, SW\}$, except where blocked by an obstacle, and action costs are Euclidean. The agent can also choose to remain still with cost 1. We assume $P(s_{t+1}|a_t, s_t, w)$ takes the agent to the desired adjacent grid point deterministically.

The set of possible goals G includes both simple and complex goals. Simple goals will just be specific end states in S. While many kinds of complex goals are possible, we assume here that a complex goal is just the combination of a desired end state with a desired means to achieving that end. In our sprite-worlds, we identify "desired means" with a constraint that the agent must pass through an additional specified location enroute, such as the via-point in the experiment from §2.3. Because the number of complex goals defined in this way is much larger than the number of simple goals, the likelihood of each complex goal is small relative to the likelihood of individual simple goals. In addition, although path-dependent goals are possible, they should not be likely a priori. We thus set the prior $P(g|w^{1:N})$ to favor simple goals by a factor of γ. For simplicity, we assume that the agent draws just a single invariant goal $g \in G$ from $P(g|w^{1:N})$, and we assume that this prior distribution is known to the observer. More generally, an agent's goals may vary across different environments, and the prior $P(g|w^{1:N})$ may have to be learned.

We define the value of a state $V_{g,w}(s)$ as the expected total cost to the agent of achieving g while following the policy given in Eq. 1. We assume the desired end-state is absorbing and cost-free, which implies that the agent attempts the *stochastic shortest path* (with respect to its probabilistic policy) [1]. If g is a complex goal, $V_{g,w}(s)$ is based on the stochastic shortest path through the specified via-point. The agent's value function is computed using the value iteration algorithm [1] with respect to the policy given in Eq. 1.

Finally, to compare our model's predictions with behavioral data from human observers, we must specify how to compute the probability of novel trajectories $s'_{0:T}$ in a new environment w', such as the test stimuli in Fig. 1, conditioned on an observed sequence $s_{0:T}$ in environment w. This is just an average over the predictions for each possible goal g:

$$P(s'_{0:T}|s_{0:T}, w, w') = \sum_{g \in G} P(s'_{0:T}|g, w')P(g|s_{0:T}, w, w'). \qquad (4)$$

5 Sprite-world simulations

5.1 Inferring an invariant goal

As a starting point for testing our model, we return to the experiments of Gergely et al. [8, 4, 7], reviewed in §2.1. Our input to the model, shown in Fig. 3(a,b), differs slightly from the original stimuli used in [8], but the relevant details of interest are spared: goal-directed action in the presence of constraints. Our model predictions, shown in Fig. 3(c), capture the qualitative results of these experiments, showing a large contrast between the straight path and the curved path in the condition with an obstacle, and a relatively small contrast in the condition with no obstacle. In the "no obstacle" condition, our model infers that the agent has a more complex goal, constrained by a via-point. This significantly increases the probability of the curved test path, to the point where the difference between the probability of observing curved and straight paths is negligible.

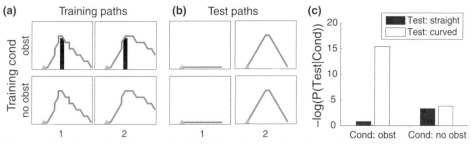

Figure 3: Inferring an invariant goal. (a) Training input in obstacle and no obstacle conditions. (b) Test input is the same in each condition. (c) Model predictions: negative log likelihoods of test paths 1 and 2 given data from training condition. In the obstacle condition, a large dissociation is seen between path 1 and path 2, with path 1 being much more likely. In the no obstacle condition, there is not a large preference for either path 1 or path 2, qualitatively matching Gergely et al.'s results [8].

5.2 Inferring goals of varying complexity: rational means-ends analysis

Our next example is inspired by the studies of Gergely et al. [6] described in §2.2. In our sprite-world version of the experiment, we varied the amount of evidence for a simple versus a complex goal, by inputting the same three trajectories with and without an obstacle present (Fig. 4(a)). In the "obstacle" condition, the trajectories were all approximately shortest paths to the goal, because the agent was forced to take indirect paths around the obstacle. In the "no obstacle" condition, no such constraint was present to explain the curved paths. Thus a more complex goal is inferred, with a path constrained to pass through a via-point. Given a choice of test paths, shown in Fig. 4(b), the model shows a double-dissociation between the probability of the direct path and the curved path through the putative via-point, given each training condition (Fig. 4(c)), similar to the results in [6].

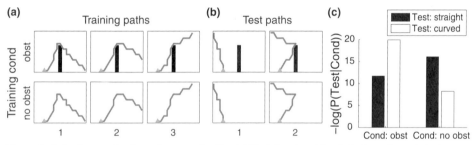

Figure 4: Inferring goals of varying complexity. (a) Training input in obstacle and no obstacle conditions. (b) Test input in each condition. (c) Model predictions: a double dissociation between probability of test paths 1 and 2 in the two conditions. This reflects a preference for the straight path in the first condition, where there is an obstacle to explain the agent's deflections in the training input, and a preference for the curved path in the second condition, where a complex goal is inferred.

5.3 Inductive inference in intentional reasoning

Lastly, we present the results of our model on our own behavioral experiment, first described in §2.3 and shown in Fig. 1. These data demonstrated the statistical nature of people's intentional inferences. Fig. 5 compares people's judgments of the probability that the agent takes a particular test path with our model's predictions. To place model predictions and human judgments on a comparable scale, we fit a sigmoidal psychometric transformation to the computed log posterior odds for the curved test path versus the straight path. The Bayesian model captures the graded shift in people's expectations in the "complex goal" condition, as evidence accumulates that the agent always seeks to pass through an arbitrary via-point enroute to the end state.

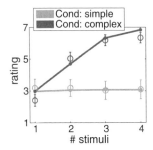

Figure 5: Experimental results: model fit for behavioral data. Mean ratings are plotted as hollow circles. Error bars give standard error. The log posterior odds from the model were fit to subjects' ratings using a scaled sigmoid function with range $(1, 7)$. The sigmoid function includes bias and gain parameters, which were fit to the human data by minimizing the sum-squared error between the model predictions and mean subject ratings.

6 Conclusion

We presented a Bayesian framework to explain several core aspects of intentional reasoning: inferring the goal of an agent based on observations of its behavior, and predicting how the agent will act when constraints or initial conditions for action change. Our model captured basic qualitative inferences that even preverbal infants have been shown to perform, as well as more subtle quantitative inferences that adult observers made in a novel experiment. Two future challenges for our computational framework are: representing and learning multiple agent types (e.g. rational, irrational, random, etc.), and representing and learning hierarchically structured goal spaces that vary across environments, situations and even domains. These extensions will allow us to further test the power of our computational framework, and will support its application to the wide range of intentional inferences that people constantly make in their everyday lives.

Acknowledgments: We thank Whitman Richards, Konrad Körding, Kobi Gal, Vikash Mansinghka, Charles Kemp, and Pat Shafto for helpful comments and discussions.

References

[1] D. P. Bertsekas. *Dynamic Programming and Optimal Control*. Athena Scientific, Belmont, MA, 2nd edition, 2001.

[2] U. Chajewska, D. Koller, and D. Ormoneit. Learning an agent's utility function by observing behavior. In *Proc. of the 18th Intl. Conf. on Machine Learning (ICML)*, pages 35–42, 2001.

[3] E. Charniak and R. Goldman. A probabilistic model of plan recognition. In *Proc. AAAI*, 1991.

[4] G. Csibra, G. Gergely, S. Biró, O. Koós, and M. Brockbank. Goal attribution without agency cues: the perception of 'pure reason' in infancy. *Cognition*, 72:237–267, 1999.

[5] D. C. Dennett. *The Intentional Stance*. Cambridge, MA: MIT Press, 1987.

[6] G. Gergely, H. Bekkering, and I. Király. Rational imitation in preverbal infants. *Nature*, 415:755, 2002.

[7] G. Gergely and G. Csibra. Teleological reasoning in infancy: the naïve theory of rational action. *Trends in Cognitive Sciences*, 7(7):287–292, 2003.

[8] G. Gergely, Z. Nádasdy, G. Csibra, and S. Biró. Taking the intentional stance at 12 months of age. *Cognition*, 56:165–193, 1995.

[9] F. Heider and M. A. Simmel. An experimental study of apparent behavior. *American Journal of Psychology*, 57:243–249, 1944.

[10] L. Liao, D. Fox, and H. Kautz. Learning and inferring transportation routines. In *Proc. AAAI*, pages 348–353, 2004.

[11] A. N. Meltzoff. Infant imitation after a 1-week delay: Long-term memory for novel acts and multiple stimuli. *Developmental Psychology*, 24:470–476, 1988.

[12] A. Y. Ng and S. Russell. Algorithms for inverse reinforcement learning. In *Proc. of the 17th Intl. Conf. on Machine Learning (ICML)*, pages 663–670, 2000.

[13] R. P. N. Rao, A. P. Shon, and A. N. Meltzoff. A Bayesian model of imitation in infants and robots. In *Imitation and Social Learning in Robots, Humans, and Animals*. (in press).

[14] B. J. Scholl and P. D. Tremoulet. Perceptual causality and animacy. *Trends in Cognitive Sciences*, 4(8):299–309, 2000.

The Curse of Highly Variable Functions for Local Kernel Machines

Yoshua Bengio, Olivier Delalleau, Nicolas Le Roux
Dept. IRO, Université de Montréal
P.O. Box 6128, Downtown Branch, Montreal, H3C 3J7, Qc, Canada
{bengioy,delallea,lerouxni}@iro.umontreal.ca

Abstract

We present a series of theoretical arguments supporting the claim that a large class of modern learning algorithms that rely solely on the smoothness prior – with similarity between examples expressed with a local kernel – are sensitive to the curse of dimensionality, or more precisely to the variability of the target. Our discussion covers supervised, semi-supervised and unsupervised learning algorithms. These algorithms are found to be local in the sense that crucial properties of the learned function at x depend mostly on the neighbors of x in the training set. This makes them sensitive to the curse of dimensionality, well studied for classical non-parametric statistical learning. We show in the case of the Gaussian kernel that when the function to be learned has many variations, these algorithms require a number of training examples proportional to the number of variations, which could be large even though there may exist short descriptions of the target function, i.e. their Kolmogorov complexity may be low. This suggests that there exist non-local learning algorithms that at least have the potential to learn about such structured but apparently complex functions (because locally they have many variations), while not using very specific prior domain knowledge.

1 Introduction

A very large fraction of the recent work in statistical machine learning has been focused on non-parametric learning algorithms which rely solely, explicitly or implicitely, on the **smoothness prior**, which says that we prefer as solution functions f such that when $x \approx y$, $f(x) \approx f(y)$. Additional prior knowledge is expressed by choosing the space of the data and the particular notion of similarity between examples (typically expressed as a kernel function). This class of learning algorithms therefore includes most of the kernel machine algorithms (Schölkopf, Burges and Smola, 1999), such as Support Vector Machines (SVMs) (Boser, Guyon and Vapnik, 1992; Cortes and Vapnik, 1995) or Gaussian processes (Williams and Rasmussen, 1996), but also unsupervised learning algorithms that attempt to capture the manifold structure of the data, such as Locally Linear Embedding (Roweis and Saul, 2000), Isomap (Tenenbaum, de Silva and Langford, 2000), kernel PCA (Schölkopf, Smola and Müller, 1998), Laplacian Eigenmaps (Belkin and Niyogi, 2003), Manifold Charting (Brand, 2003), and *spectral clustering* algorithms (see (Weiss, 1999) for a review). More recently, there has also been much interest in non-parametric *semi-supervised learning algorithms*, such as (Zhu, Ghahramani and Lafferty, 2003; Zhou et al., 2004; Belkin, Matveeva and Niyogi, 2004; Delalleau, Bengio and Le Roux, 2005), which also fall in this category, and share many ideas with manifold learning algorithms.

Since this is a very large class of algorithms and it is attracting so much attention, it is worthwhile to investigate its limitations, and this is the main goal of this paper. Since these methods share many characteristics with classical non-parametric statistical learning algorithms (such as the k-nearest neighbors and the Parzen windows regression and density estimation algorithms (Duda and Hart, 1973)), which have been shown to suffer from the so-called *curse of dimensionality*, it is logical to investigate the following question: to what extent do these modern kernel methods suffer from a similar problem?

In this paper, we focus on algorithms in which the learned function is expressed in terms of a linear combination of kernel functions applied on the training examples:

$$f(x) = b + \sum_{i=1}^{n} \alpha_i K_D(x, x_i) \qquad (1)$$

where optionally a bias term b is added, $D = \{z_1, \ldots, z_n\}$ are training examples ($z_i = x_i$ for unsupervised learning, $z_i = (x_i, y_i)$ for supervised learning, and y_i can take a special "missing" value for semi-supervised learning). The α_i's are scalars chosen by the learning algorithm using D, and $K_D(\cdot, \cdot)$ is the kernel function, a symmetric function (sometimes expected to be positive definite), which may be chosen by taking into account all the x_i's. A typical kernel function is the Gaussian kernel,

$$K_\sigma(u, v) = e^{-\frac{1}{\sigma^2}||u-v||^2}, \qquad (2)$$

with the width σ controlling how local the kernel is. See (Bengio et al., 2004) to see that LLE, Isomap, Laplacian eigenmaps and other spectral manifold learning algorithms such as spectral clustering can be generalized to be written as in eq. 1 for a test point x.

One obtains consistency of classical non-parametric estimators by appropriately varying the hyper-parameter that controls the locality of the estimator as n increases. Basically, the kernel should be allowed to become more and more local, so that statistical bias goes to zero, but the "effective number of examples" involved in the estimator at x (equal to k for the k-nearest neighbor estimator) should increase as n increases, so that statistical variance is also driven to 0. For a wide class of kernel regression estimators, the unconditional variance and squared bias can be shown to be written as follows (Härdle et al., 2004):

$$\text{expected error} = \frac{C_1}{n\sigma^d} + C_2\sigma^4,$$

with C_1 and C_2 not depending on n nor on the dimension d. Hence an optimal bandwidth is chosen proportional to $n^{\frac{-1}{4+d}}$, and the resulting generalization error (not counting the noise) converges in $n^{-4/(4+d)}$, which becomes very slow for large d. Consider for example the increase in number of examples required to get the same level of error, in 1 dimension versus d dimensions. If n_1 is the number of examples required to get a level of error e, to get the same level of error in d dimensions requires on the order of $n_1^{(4+d)/5}$ examples, i.e. the **required number of examples is exponential in** d. For the k-nearest neighbor classifier, a similar result is obtained (Snapp and Venkatesh, 1998):

$$\text{expected error} = E_\infty + \sum_{j=2}^{\infty} c_j n^{-j/d}$$

where E_∞ is the asymptotic error, d is the dimension and n the number of examples.

Note however that, if the data distribution is concentrated on a lower dimensional manifold, it is the **manifold dimension** that matters. Indeed, for data on a smooth lower-dimensional manifold, the only dimension that say a k-nearest neighbor classifier sees is the dimension of the manifold, since it only uses the Euclidean distances between the near neighbors, and if they lie on such a manifold then the local Euclidean distances approach the local geodesic distances on the manifold (Tenenbaum, de Silva and Langford, 2000).

2 Minimum Number of Bases Required

In this section we present results showing the number of required bases (hence of training examples) of a kernel machine with Gaussian kernel may grow linearly with the "variations" of the target function that must be captured in order to achieve a given error level.

2.1 Result for Supervised Learning

The following theorem informs us about the number of sign changes that a Gaussian kernel machine can achieve, when it has k bases (i.e. k support vectors, or at least k training examples).

Theorem 2.1 (Theorem 2 of (Schmitt, 2002)). *Let $f : \mathbb{R} \to \mathbb{R}$ computed by a Gaussian kernel machine (eq. 1) with k bases (non-zero α_i's). Then f has at most $2k$ zeros.*

We would like to say something about kernel machines in $\mathbb{R}^d$, and we can do this simply by considering a straight line in $\mathbb{R}^d$ and the number of sign changes that the solution function f can achieve along that line.

Corollary 2.2. *Suppose that the learning problem is such that in order to achieve a given error level for samples from a distribution P with a Gaussian kernel machine (eq. 1), then f must change sign at least $2k$ times along some straight line (i.e., in the case of a classifier, the decision surface must be crossed at least $2k$ times by that straight line). Then the kernel machine must have at least k bases (non-zero α_i's).*

Proof. Let the straight line be parameterized by $x(t) = u + tw$, with $t \in \mathbb{R}$ and $\|w\| = 1$ without loss of generality. Define $g : \mathbb{R} \to \mathbb{R}$ by

$$g(t) = f(u + tw).$$

If f is a Gaussian kernel classifier with k' bases, then g can be written

$$g(t) = b + \sum_{i=1}^{k'} \beta_i \exp\left(-\frac{(t - t_i)^2}{2\sigma^2}\right)$$

where $u + t_i w$ is the projection of x_i on the line $D_{u,w} = \{u + tw, t \in \mathbb{R}\}$, and $\beta_i \neq 0$. The number of bases of g is $k'' \leq k'$, as there may exist $x_i \neq x_j$ such that $t_i = t_j$. Since g must change sign at least $2k$ times, thanks to theorem 2.1, we can conclude that g has at least k bases, i.e. $k \leq k'' \leq k'$. $\qquad\square$

The above theorem tells us that if we are trying to represent a function that locally varies a lot (in the sense that its sign along a straight line changes many times), then we need many training examples to do so with a Gaussian kernel machine. Note that it says nothing about the dimensionality of the space, but we might expect to have to learn functions that vary more when the data is high-dimensional. The next theorem confirms this suspicion in the special case of the d-bits parity function:

$$\text{parity} : (b_1, \ldots, b_d) \in \{0, 1\}^d \mapsto \begin{cases} 1 \text{ if } \sum_{i=1}^{d} b_i \text{ is even} \\ -1 \text{ otherwise} \end{cases}$$

We will show that learning this apparently simple function with Gaussians centered on points in $\{0, 1\}^d$ is difficult, in the sense that it requires a number of Gaussians exponential in d (for a fixed Gaussian width). Note that our corollary 2.2 does not apply to the d-bits parity function, so it represents another type of local variation (not along a line). However, we are also able to prove a strong result about that case. We will use the following notations:

$$
\begin{aligned}
X_d &= \{0,1\}^d = \{x_1, x_2, \ldots, x_{2^d}\} \\
H_d^0 &= \{(b_1, \ldots, b_d) \in X_d \mid b_d = 0\} \\
H_d^1 &= \{(b_1, \ldots, b_d) \in X_d \mid b_d = 1\}
\end{aligned}
\tag{3}
$$

$$
\tag{4}
$$

We say that a decision function $f : \mathbb{R}^d \to \mathbb{R}$ solves the parity problem if $\mathrm{sign}(f(x_i)) = \mathrm{parity}(x_i)$ for all i in $\{1, \ldots, 2^d\}$.

Lemma 2.3. *Let* $f(x) = \sum_{i=1}^{2^d} \alpha_i K_\sigma(x_i, x)$ *be a linear combination of Gaussians with same width* σ *centered on points* $x_i \in X_d$. *If* f *solves the parity problem, then* $\alpha_i \mathrm{parity}(x_i) > 0$ *for all* i.

Proof. We prove this lemma by induction on d. If $d = 1$ there are only 2 points. Obviously one Gaussian is not enough to classify correctly x_1 and x_2, so both α_1 and α_2 are non-zero, and $\alpha_1 \alpha_2 < 0$ (otherwise f is of constant sign). Without loss of generality, assume $\mathrm{parity}(x_1) = 1$ and $\mathrm{parity}(x_2) = -1$. Then $f(x_1) > 0 > f(x_2)$, which implies $\alpha_1(1 - K_\sigma(x_1, x_2)) > \alpha_2(1 - K_\sigma(x_1, x_2))$ and $\alpha_1 > \alpha_2$ since $K_\sigma(x_1, x_2) < 1$. Thus $\alpha_1 > 0$ and $\alpha_2 < 0$, i.e. $\alpha_i \mathrm{parity}(x_i) > 0$ for $i \in \{1, 2\}$.
Suppose now lemma 2.3 is true for $d = d' - 1$, and consider the case $d = d'$. We denote by x_i^0 the points in H_d^0 and by α_i^0 their coefficient in the expansion of f (see eq. 3 for the definition of H_d^0). For $x_i^0 \in H_d^0$, we denote by $x_i^1 \in H_d^1$ its projection on H_d^1 (obtained by setting its last bit to 1), whose coefficient in f is α_i^1. For any $x \in H_d^0$ and $x_j^1 \in H_d^1$ we have:

$$
\begin{aligned}
K_\sigma(x_j^1, x) &= \exp\left(-\frac{\|x_j^1 - x\|^2}{2\sigma^2}\right) = \exp\left(-\frac{1}{2\sigma^2}\right)\exp\left(-\frac{\|x_j^0 - x\|^2}{2\sigma^2}\right) \\
&= \gamma K_\sigma(x_j^0, x)
\end{aligned}
$$

where $\gamma = \exp\left(-\frac{1}{2\sigma^2}\right) \in (0, 1)$. Thus $f(x)$ for $x \in H_d^0$ can be written

$$
\begin{aligned}
f(x) &= \sum_{x_i^0 \in H_d^0} \alpha_i^0 K_\sigma(x_i^0, x) + \sum_{x_j^1 \in H_d^1} \alpha_j^1 \gamma K_\sigma(x_j^0, x) \\
&= \sum_{x_i^0 \in H_d^0} \left(\alpha_i^0 + \gamma \alpha_i^1\right) K_\sigma(x_i^0, x).
\end{aligned}
$$

Since H_d^0 is isomorphic to X_{d-1}, the restriction of f to H_d^0 implicitly defines a function over X_{d-1} that solves the parity problem (because the last bit in H_d^0 is 0, the parity is not modified). Using our induction hypothesis, we have that for all $x_i^0 \in H_d^0$:

$$
\left(\alpha_i^0 + \gamma \alpha_i^1\right) \mathrm{parity}(x_i^0) > 0.
\tag{5}
$$

A similar reasoning can be made if we switch the roles of H_d^0 and H_d^1. One has to be careful that the parity is modified between H_d^1 and its mapping to X_{d-1} (because the last bit in H_d^1 is 1). Thus we obtain that the restriction of $(-f)$ to H_d^1 defines a function over X_{d-1} that solves the parity problem, and the induction hypothesis tells us that for all $x_j^1 \in H_d^1$:

$$
\left(-\left(\alpha_j^1 + \gamma \alpha_j^0\right)\right)\left(-\mathrm{parity}(x_j^1)\right) > 0.
\tag{6}
$$

and the two negative signs cancel out. Now consider any $x_i^0 \in H_d^0$ and its projection $x_i^1 \in H_d^1$. Without loss of generality, assume $\mathrm{parity}(x_i^0) = 1$ (and thus $\mathrm{parity}(x_i^1) = -1$). Using eq. 5 and 6 we obtain:

$$
\begin{aligned}
\alpha_i^0 + \gamma \alpha_i^1 &> 0 \\
\alpha_i^1 + \gamma \alpha_i^0 &< 0
\end{aligned}
$$

It is obvious that for these two equations to be simultaneously verified, we need α_i^0 and α_i^1 to be non-zero and of opposite sign. Moreover, because $\gamma \in (0,1)$, $\alpha_i^0 + \gamma\alpha_i^1 > 0 > \alpha_i^1 + \gamma\alpha_i^0 \Rightarrow \alpha_i^0 > \alpha_i^1$, which implies $\alpha_i^0 > 0$ and $\alpha_i^1 < 0$, i.e. $\alpha_i^0 \text{parity}(x_i^0) > 0$ and $\alpha_i^1 \text{parity}(x_i^1) > 0$. Since this is true for all x_i^0 in H_d^0, we have proved lemma 2.3. $\qquad\square$

Theorem 2.4. *Let* $f(x) = b + \sum_{i=1}^{2^d} \alpha_i K_\sigma(x_i, x)$ *be an affine combination of Gaussians with same width* σ *centered on points* $x_i \in X_d$. *If* f *solves the parity problem, then there are at least* 2^{d-1} *non-zero coefficients* α_i.

Proof. We begin with two preliminary results. First, given any $x_i \in X_d$, the number of points in X_d that differ from x_i by exactly k bits is $\binom{d}{k}$. Thus,

$$\sum_{x_j \in X_d} K_\sigma(x_i, x_j) = \sum_{k=0}^{d} \binom{d}{k} \exp\left(-\frac{k^2}{2\sigma^2}\right) = c_\sigma. \tag{7}$$

Second, it is possible to find a linear combination (i.e. without bias) of Gaussians g such that $g(x_i) = f(x_i)$ for all $x_i \in X_d$. Indeed, let

$$g(x) = f(x) - b + \sum_{x_j \in X_d} \beta_j K_\sigma(x_j, x). \tag{8}$$

g verifies $g(x_i) = f(x_i)$ iff $\sum_{x_j \in X_d} \beta_j K_\sigma(x_j, x_i) = b$, i.e. the vector β satisfies the linear system $M_\sigma \beta = b\mathbf{1}$, where M_σ is the kernel matrix whose element (i,j) is $K_\sigma(x_i, x_j)$ and $\mathbf{1}$ is a vector of ones. It is well known that M_σ is invertible as long as the x_i are all different, which is the case here (Micchelli, 1986). Thus $\beta = bM_\sigma^{-1}\mathbf{1}$ is the only solution to the system.

We now proceed to the proof of the theorem. By contradiction, suppose f solves the parity problem with less than 2^{d-1} non-zero coefficients α_i. Then there exist two points x_s and x_t in X_d such that $\alpha_s = \alpha_t = 0$ and $\text{parity}(x_s) = 1 = -\text{parity}(x_t)$. Consider the function g defined as in eq. 8 with $\beta = bM_\sigma^{-1}\mathbf{1}$. Since $g(x_i) = f(x_i)$ for all $x_i \in X_d$, g solves the parity problem with a linear combination of Gaussians centered points in X_d. Thus, applying lemma 2.3, we have in particular that $\beta_s \text{parity}(x_s) > 0$ and $\beta_t \text{parity}(x_t) > 0$ (because $\alpha_s = \alpha_t = 0$), so that $\beta_s \beta_t < 0$. But, because of eq. 7, $M_\sigma \mathbf{1} = c_\sigma \mathbf{1}$, which means $\mathbf{1}$ is an eigenvector of M_σ with eigenvalue $c_\sigma > 0$. Consequently, $\mathbf{1}$ is also an eigenvector of M_σ^{-1} with eigenvalue $c_\sigma^{-1} > 0$, and $\beta = bM_\sigma^{-1}\mathbf{1} = bc_\sigma^{-1}\mathbf{1}$, which is in contradiction with $\beta_s \beta_t < 0$: f must therefore have at least 2^{d-1} non-zero coefficients. $\qquad\square$

The bound in theorem 2.4 is tight, since it is possible to solve the parity problem with exactly 2^{d-1} Gaussians and a bias, for instance by using a negative bias and putting a positive weight on each example satisfying $\text{parity}(x_i) = 1$. When trained to learn the parity function, a SVM may learn a function that looks like the opposite of the parity on test points (while still performing optimally on training points), but it is an artefact of the specific geometry of the problem, and only occurs when the training set size is appropriate compared to $|X_d| = 2^d$ (see (Bengio, Delalleau and Le Roux, 2005) for details). Note that if the centers of the Gaussians are not restricted anymore to be points in X_d, it is possible to solve the parity problem with only $d + 1$ Gaussians and no bias (Bengio, Delalleau and Le Roux, 2005).

One may argue that parity is a simple discrete toy problem of little interest. But even if we have to restrict the analysis to discrete samples in $\{0, 1\}^d$ for mathematical reasons, the parity function can be extended to a smooth function on the $[0, 1]^d$ hypercube depending only on the continuous sum $b_1 + \ldots + b_d$. Theorem 2.4 is thus a basis to argue that the number of Gaussians needed to learn a function with many variations in a continuous space may scale linearly with these variations, and thus possibly exponentially in the dimension.

2.2 Results for Semi-Supervised Learning

In this section we focus on algorithms of the type described in recent papers (Zhu, Ghahramani and Lafferty, 2003; Zhou et al., 2004; Belkin, Matveeva and Niyogi, 2004; Delalleau, Bengio and Le Roux, 2005), which are graph-based non-parametric semi-supervised learning algorithms. Note that transductive SVMs, which are another class of semi-supervised algorithms, are already subject to the limitations of corollary 2.2. The graph-based algorithms we consider here can be seen as minimizing the following cost function, as shown in (Delalleau, Bengio and Le Roux, 2005):

$$C(\hat{Y}) = \|\hat{Y}_l - Y_l\|^2 + \mu \hat{Y}^\top L \hat{Y} + \mu\epsilon \|\hat{Y}\|^2 \tag{9}$$

with $\hat{Y} = (\hat{y}_1, \ldots, \hat{y}_n)$ the estimated labels on both labeled and unlabeled data, and L the (un-normalized) graph Laplacian derived from a similarity function W between points such that $W_{ij} = W(x_i, x_j)$ corresponds to the weights of the edges in the graph. Here, $\hat{Y}_l = (\hat{y}_1, \ldots, \hat{y}_l)$ is the vector of estimated labels on the l labeled examples, whose known labels are given by $Y_l = (y_1, \ldots, y_l)$, and one may constrain $\hat{Y}_l = Y_l$ as in (Zhu, Ghahramani and Lafferty, 2003) by letting $\mu \to 0$. We define a region with constant label as a connected subset of the graph where all nodes x_i have the same estimated label (sign of $\hat{y}_i$), and such that no other node can be added while keeping these properties.

Proposition 2.5. *After running a label propagation algorithm minimizing the cost of eq. 9, the number of regions with constant estimated label is less than (or equal to) the number of labeled examples.*

Proof. By contradiction, if this proposition is false, then there exists a region with constant estimated label that does not contain any labeled example. Without loss of generality, consider the case of a positive constant label, with $x_{l+1}, \ldots, x_{l+q}$ the q samples in this region. The part of the cost of eq. 9 depending on their labels is

$$C(\hat{y}_{l+1}, \ldots, \hat{y}_{l+q}) = \frac{\mu}{2} \sum_{i,j=l+1}^{l+q} W_{ij}(\hat{y}_i - \hat{y}_j)^2$$

$$+ \mu \sum_{i=l+1}^{l+q} \left(\sum_{j \notin \{l+1, \ldots, l+q\}} W_{ij}(\hat{y}_i - \hat{y}_j)^2 \right) + \mu\epsilon \sum_{i=l+1}^{l+q} \hat{y}_i^2.$$

The second term is stricly positive, and because the region we consider is maximal (by definition) all samples x_j outside of the region such that $W_{ij} > 0$ verify $\hat{y}_j < 0$ (for x_i a sample in the region). Since all $\hat{y}_i$ are strictly positive for $i \in \{l+1, \ldots, l+q\}$, this means this second term can be strictly decreased by setting all $\hat{y}_i$ to 0 for $i \in \{l+1, \ldots, l+q\}$. This also sets the first and third terms to zero (i.e. their minimum), showing that the set of labels $\hat{y}_i$ are not optimal, which conflicts with their definition as labels minimizing C. $\square$

This means that if the class distributions are such that there are many distinct regions with constant labels (either separated by low-density regions or regions with samples from the other class), we will need at least the same number of labeled samples as there are such regions (assuming we are using a sparse local kernel such as the k-nearest neighbor kernel, or a thresholded Gaussian kernel). But this number could *grow exponentially with the dimension of the manifold(s) on which the data lie*, for instance in the case of a labeling function varying highly along each dimension, *even if the label variations are "simple" in a non-local sense*, e.g. if they alternate in a regular fashion. When the kernel is not sparse (e.g. Gaussian kernel), obtaining such a result is less obvious. However, there often exists a sparse approximation of the kernel. Thus we conjecture the same kind of result holds for dense weight matrices, if the weighting function is local in the sense that it is close to zero when applied to a pair of examples far from each other.

3   Extensions and Conclusions

In (Bengio, Delalleau and Le Roux, 2005) we present additional results that apply to unsupervised learning algorithms such as non-parametric manifold learning algorithms (Roweis
and Saul, 2000; Tenenbaum, de Silva and Langford, 2000; Schölkopf, Smola and Müller,
1998; Belkin and Niyogi, 2003). We find that when the underlying manifold varies a lot
in the sense of having high curvature in many places, then a large number of examples is
required. Note that the tangent plane is defined by the derivatives of the kernel machine
function f, for such algorithms. The core result is that the manifold tangent plane at x
is mostly defined by the near neighbors of x in the training set (more precisely it is constrained to be in the span of the vectors $x - x_i$, with x_i a neighbor of x). Hence one needs
to cover the manifold with small enough linear patches with at least $d + 1$ examples per
patch (where d is the dimension of the manifold).

In the same paper, we present a conjecture that generalizes the results presented here for
Gaussian kernel classifiers to a larger class of local kernels, using the same notion of locality of the derivative summarized above for manifold learning algorithms. In that case the
derivative of f represents the normal of the decision surface, and we find that at x it mostly
depends on the neighbors of x in the training set.

It could be argued that if a function has many local variations (hence is not very smooth),
then it is not learnable unless having strong prior knowledge at hand. However, this is not
true. For example consider functions that have low Kolmogorov complexity, i.e. can be
described by a short string in some language. The only prior we need in order to quickly
learn such functions (in terms of number of examples needed) is that functions that are
simple to express in that language (e.g. a programming language) are preferred. For example, the functions $g(x) = sin(x)$ or $g(x) = parity(x)$ would be easy to learn using
the C programming language to define the prior, even though the number of variations of
$g(x)$ can be chosen to be arbitrarily large (hence also the number of required training examples when using only the smoothness prior), while keeping the Kolmogorov complexity
constant. We do not propose to necessarily focus on the Kolmogorov complexity to design
new learning algorithms, but we use this example to illustrate that it is possible to learn
apparently complex functions (because they vary a lot), as long as one uses a "non-local"
learning algorithm, corresponding to a broad prior, not solely relying on the smoothness
prior. Of course, if additional domain knowledge about the task is available, it should be
used, but without abandoning research on learning algorithms that can address a wider
scope of problems. We hope that this paper will stimulate more research into such learning
algorithms, since we expect local learning algorithms (that only rely on the smoothness
prior) will be insufficient to make significant progress on complex problems such as those
raised by research on Artificial Intelligence.

Acknowledgments

The authors would like to thank the following funding organizations for support: NSERC,
MITACS, and the Canada Research Chairs. The authors are also grateful for the feedback
and stimulating exchanges that helped shape this paper, with Yann Le Cun and Léon Bottou,
as well as for the anonymous reviewers' helpful comments.

References

Belkin, M., Matveeva, I., and Niyogi, P. (2004). Regularization and semi-supervised learn-
     ing on large graphs. In Shawe-Taylor, J. and Singer, Y., editors, *COLT'2004*. Springer.

Belkin, M. and Niyogi, P. (2003). Using manifold structure for partially labeled classi-
     fication. In Becker, S., Thrun, S., and Obermayer, K., editors, *Advances in Neural*

Information Processing Systems 15, Cambridge, MA. MIT Press.

Bengio, Y., Delalleau, O., and Le Roux, N. (2005). The curse of dimensionality for local kernel machines. Technical Report 1258, Département d'informatique et recherche opérationnelle, Université de Montréal.

Bengio, Y., Delalleau, O., Le Roux, N., Paiement, J.-F., Vincent, P., and Ouimet, M. (2004). Learning eigenfunctions links spectral embedding and kernel PCA. *Neural Computation*, 16(10):2197–2219.

Boser, B., Guyon, I., and Vapnik, V. (1992). A training algorithm for optimal margin classifiers. In *Fifth Annual Workshop on Computational Learning Theory*, pages 144–152, Pittsburgh.

Brand, M. (2003). Charting a manifold. In Becker, S., Thrun, S., and Obermayer, K., editors, *Advances in Neural Information Processing Systems 15*. MIT Press.

Cortes, C. and Vapnik, V. (1995). Support vector networks. *Machine Learning*, 20:273–297.

Delalleau, O., Bengio, Y., and Le Roux, N. (2005). Efficient non-parametric function induction in semi-supervised learning. In Cowell, R. and Ghahramani, Z., editors, *Proceedings of the Tenth International Workshop on Artificial Intelligence and Statistics, Jan 6-8, 2005, Savannah Hotel, Barbados*, pages 96–103. Society for Artificial Intelligence and Statistics.

Duda, R. and Hart, P. (1973). *Pattern Classification and Scene Analysis*. Wiley, New York.

Härdle, W., Müller, M., Sperlich, S., and Werwatz, A. (2004). *Nonparametric and Semiparametric Models*. Springer, http://www.xplore-stat.de/ebooks/ebooks.html.

Micchelli, C. A. (1986). Interpolation of scattered data: distance matrices and conditionally positive definite functions. *Constructive Approximation*, 2:11–22.

Roweis, S. and Saul, L. (2000). Nonlinear dimensionality reduction by locally linear embedding. *Science*, 290(5500):2323–2326.

Schmitt, M. (2002). Descartes' rule of signs for radial basis function neural networks. *Neural Computation*, 14(12):2997–3011.

Schölkopf, B., Burges, C. J. C., and Smola, A. J. (1999). *Advances in Kernel Methods — Support Vector Learning*. MIT Press, Cambridge, MA.

Schölkopf, B., Smola, A., and Müller, K.-R. (1998). Nonlinear component analysis as a kernel eigenvalue problem. *Neural Computation*, 10:1299–1319.

Snapp, R. R. and Venkatesh, S. S. (1998). Asymptotic derivation of the finite-sample risk of the k nearest neighbor classifier. Technical Report UVM-CS-1998-0101, Department of Computer Science, University of Vermont.

Tenenbaum, J., de Silva, V., and Langford, J. (2000). A global geometric framework for nonlinear dimensionality reduction. *Science*, 290(5500):2319–2323.

Weiss, Y. (1999). Segmentation using eigenvectors: a unifying view. In *Proceedings IEEE International Conference on Computer Vision*, pages 975–982.

Williams, C. and Rasmussen, C. (1996). Gaussian processes for regression. In Touretzky, D., Mozer, M., and Hasselmo, M., editors, *Advances in Neural Information Processing Systems 8*, pages 514–520. MIT Press, Cambridge, MA.

Zhou, D., Bousquet, O., Navin Lal, T., Weston, J., and Schölkopf, B. (2004). Learning with local and global consistency. In Thrun, S., Saul, L., and Schölkopf, B., editors, *Advances in Neural Information Processing Systems 16*, Cambridge, MA. MIT Press.

Zhu, X., Ghahramani, Z., and Lafferty, J. (2003). Semi-supervised learning using Gaussian fields and harmonic functions. In *ICML'2003*.

Non-Local Manifold Parzen Windows

Yoshua Bengio, Hugo Larochelle and Pascal Vincent
Dept. IRO, Université de Montréal
P.O. Box 6128, Downtown Branch, Montreal, H3C 3J7, Qc, Canada
{*bengioy,larocheh,vincentp*}@*iro.umontreal.ca*

Abstract

To escape from the curse of dimensionality, we claim that one can learn non-local functions, in the sense that the value and shape of the learned function at x must be inferred using examples that may be far from x. With this objective, we present a non-local non-parametric density estimator. It builds upon previously proposed Gaussian mixture models with regularized covariance matrices to take into account the local shape of the manifold. It also builds upon recent work on non-local estimators of the tangent plane of a manifold, which are able to generalize in places with little training data, unlike traditional, local, non-parametric models.

1 Introduction

A central objective of statistical machine learning is to discover structure in the joint distribution between random variables, so as to be able to make predictions about new combinations of values of these variables. A central issue in obtaining generalization is how information from the training examples can be used to make predictions about new examples and, without strong prior assumptions (i.e. in non-parametric models), this may be fundamentally difficult, as illustrated by the curse of dimensionality.

(Bengio, Delalleau and Le Roux, 2005) and (Bengio and Monperrus, 2005) present several arguments illustrating some fundamental limitations of modern kernel methods due to the curse of dimensionality, when the kernel is local (like the Gaussian kernel). These arguments are all based on the locality of the estimators, i.e., that very important information about the predicted function at x is derived mostly from the near neighbors of x in the training set. This analysis has been applied to supervised learning algorithms such as SVMs as well as to unsupervised manifold learning algorithms and graph-based semi-supervised learning. The analysis in (Bengio, Delalleau and Le Roux, 2005) highlights intrinsic limitations of such local learning algorithms, that can make them fail when applied on problems where one has to look beyond what happens locally in order to overcome the curse of dimensionality, or more precisely when the function to be learned has many variations while there exist more compact representations of these variations than a simple enumeration.

This strongly suggests to investigate **non-local learning methods**, which can in principle generalize at x using information gathered at training points x_i that are far from x. We present here such a non-local learning algorithm, in the realm of density estimation.

The proposed non-local non-parametric density estimator builds upon the Manifold Parzen density estimator (Vincent and Bengio, 2003) that associates a regularized Gaussian with each training point, and upon recent work on non-local estimators of the tangent plane of a manifold (Bengio and Monperrus, 2005). The *local* covariance matrix characterizing the density in the immediate neighborhood of a data point is learned as a **function** of that data point, with *global* parameters. This allows to potentially generalize in places with little or no training data, unlike traditional, local, non-parametric models. Here, the implicit assumption is that there is some kind of regularity in the shape of the density, such that learning about its shape in one region could be informative of the shape in another region that is not adjacent. Note that the smoothness assumption typically underlying non-parametric models relies on a simple form of such transfer, but only for neighboring regions, which is not very helpful when the intrinsic dimension of the data (the dimension of the manifold on which or near which it lives) is high or when the underlying density function has many variations (Bengio, Delalleau and Le Roux, 2005). The proposed model is also related to the Neighborhood Component Analysis algorithm (Goldberger et al., 2005), which learns a global covariance matrix for use in the Mahalanobis distance within a non-parametric classifier. Here we generalize this global matrix to one that is a function of the datum x.

2 Manifold Parzen Windows

In the Parzen Windows estimator, one puts a spherical (*isotropic*) Gaussian around each training point x_i, with a single shared variance hyper-parameter. One approach to improve on this estimator, introduced in (Vincent and Bengio, 2003), is to use not just the presence of x_i and its neighbors but also their geometry, trying to infer the principal characteristics of the local shape of the manifold (where the density concentrates), which can be summarized in the covariance matrix of the Gaussian, as illustrated in Figure 1. If the data concentrates in certain directions around x_i, we want that covariance matrix to be "flat" (near zero variance) in the orthogonal directions.

One way to achieve this is to parametrize each of these covariance matrices in terms of "principal directions" (which correspond to the tangent vectors of the manifold, if the data concentrates on a manifold). In this way we do not need to specify individually all the entries of the covariance matrix. The only required assumption is that the "noise directions" orthogonal to the "principal directions" all have the same variance.

$$\hat{p}(y) = \frac{1}{n} \sum_{i=1}^{n} N(y; x_i + \mu(x_i), S(x_i)) \tag{1}$$

where $N(y; x_i + \mu(x_i), S(x_i))$ is a Gaussian density at y, with mean vector $x_i + \mu(x_i)$ and covariance matrix $S(x_i)$ represented compactly by

$$S(x_i) = \sigma_{noise}^2(x_i)I + \sum_{j=1}^{d} s_j^2(x_i)v_j(x_i)v_j(x_i)' \tag{2}$$

where $s_j^2(x_i)$ and $\sigma_{noise}^2(x_i)$ are scalars, and $v_j(x_i)$ denotes a "principal" direction with variance $s_j^2(x_i) + \sigma_{noise}^2(x_i)$, while $\sigma_{noise}^2(x_i)$ is the noise variance (the variance in all the other directions). $v_j(x_i)'$ denotes the transpose of $v_j(x_i)$.

In (Vincent and Bengio, 2003), $\mu(x_i) = 0$, and $\sigma_{noise}^2(x_i) = \sigma_0^2$ is a global hyper-parameter, while $(\lambda_j(x_i), v_j) = (s_j^2(x_i) + \sigma_{noise}^2(x_i), v_j(x_i))$ are the leading (eigenvalue,eigenvector) pairs from the eigen-decomposition of a locally weighted covariance matrix (e.g. the empirical covariance of the vectors $x_l - x_i$, with x_l a near neighbor of x_i). The "noise level" hyper-parameter σ_0^2 must be chosen such that the principal eigenvalues are all greater than σ_0^2. Another hyper-parameter is the number d of principal components to keep. Alternatively, one can choose $\sigma_{noise}^2(x_i)$ to be the $(d+1)^{th}$ eigenvalue, which guarantees that $\lambda_j(x_i) > \sigma_{noise}^2(x_i)$, and gets rid of a hyper-parameter. This very simple model was found to be consistently better than the ordinary Parzen density estimator in numerical experiments in which all hyper-parameters are chosen by cross-validation.

3 Non-Local Manifold Tangent Learning

In (Bengio and Monperrus, 2005) a manifold learning algorithm was introduced in which the tangent plane of a d-dimensional manifold at x is learned as a function of $x \in \mathbb{R}^D$, using globally estimated parameters. The output of the predictor function $F(x)$ is a $d \times D$ matrix whose d rows are the d (possibly non-orthogonal) vectors that span the tangent plane. The training information about the tangent plane is obtained by considering pairs of near neighbors x_i and x_j in the training set. Consider the predicted tangent plane of the manifold at x_i, characterized by the rows of $F(x_i)$. For a good predictor we expect the vector $(x_i - x_j)$ to be close to its projection on the tangent plane, with local coordinates $w \in \mathbb{R}^d$. w can be obtained analytically by solving a linear system of dimension d.

The training criterion chosen in (Bengio and Monperrus, 2005) then minimizes the sum over such (x_i, x_j) of the sinus of the projection angle, i.e. $||F'(x_i)w - (x_j - x_i)||^2 / ||x_j - x_i||^2$. It is a heuristic criterion, which will be replaced in our new algorithm by one derived from the maximum likelihood criterion, considering that $F(x_i)$ indirectly provides the principal eigenvectors of the local covariance matrix at x_i. Both criteria gave similar results experimentally, but the model proposed here yields a complete density estimator. In both cases $F(x_i)$ can be interpreted as specifying the directions in which one expects to see the most variations when going from x_i to one of its near neighbors in a finite sample.

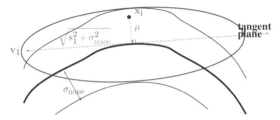

Figure 1: *Illustration of the local parametrization of local or Non-Local Manifold Parzen. The examples around training point x_i are modeled by a Gaussian. $\mu(x_i)$ specifies the center of that Gaussian, which should be non-zero when x_i is off the manifold. v_k's are principal directions of the Gaussian and are tangent vectors of the manifold. σ_{noise} represents the thickness of the manifold.*

4 Proposed Algorithm: Non-Local Manifold Parzen Windows

In equations (1) and (2) we wrote $\mu(x_i)$ and $S(x_i)$ as if they were **functions** of x_i rather than simply using indices μ_i and S_i. This is because we introduce here a non-local version of Manifold Parzen Windows inspired from the non-local manifold tangent learning algorithm, i.e., in which we can **share information about the density across different regions of space**. In our experiments we use a neural network of $nhid$ hidden neurons, with x_i in input to predict $\mu(x_i)$, $\sigma^2_{noise}(x_i)$, and the $s_j^2(x_i)$ and $v_j(x_i)$. The vectors computed by the neural network do not need to be orthonormal: we only need to consider the subspace that they span. Also, the vectors' squared norm is used to infer $s_j^2(x_i)$, instead of having a separate output for them. We will note $F(x_i)$ the matrix whose rows are the vectors output of the neural network. From it we obtain the $s_j^2(x_i)$ and $v_j(x_i)$ by performing a singular value decomposition, i.e. $F'F = \sum_{j=1}^d s_j^2 v_j v_j'$. Moreover, to make sure σ^2_{noise} does not get too small, which could make the optimization unstable, we impose $\sigma^2_{noise}(x_i) = s^2_{noise}(x_i) + \sigma_0^2$, where $s_{noise}(\cdot)$ is an output of the neural network and σ_0^2 is a fixed constant.

Imagine that the data were lying near a lower dimensional manifold. Consider a training example x_i near the manifold. The Gaussian centered near x_i tells us how neighbors of

x_i are expected to differ from x_i. Its "principal" vectors $v_j(x_i)$ span the tangent of the manifold near x_i. The Gaussian center variation $\mu(x_i)$ tells us how x_i is located with respect to its projection on the manifold. The noise variance $\sigma^2_{noise}(x_i)$ tells us how far from the manifold to expect neighbors, and the directional variances $s^2_j(x_i) + \sigma^2_{noise}(x_i)$ tell us how far to expect neighbors on the different local axes of the manifold, near x_i's projection on the manifold. Figure 1 illustrates this in 2 dimensions.

The important element of this model is that the parameters of the predictive neural network can potentially represent non-local structure in the density, i.e., they allow to potentially discover shared structure among the different covariance matrices in the mixture. Here is the pseudo code algorithm for training Non-Local Manifold Parzen (NLMP):

Algorithm NLMP::Train$(X, d, k, k_\mu, \mu(\cdot), S(\cdot), \sigma^2_0)$

Input: training set X, chosen number of principal directions d, chosen number of neighbors k and k_μ, initial functions $\mu(\cdot)$ and $S(\cdot)$, and regularization hyper-parameter σ^2_0.

(1) For $x_i \in X$

(2)   Collect max(k,k_μ) nearest neighbors of x_j.
Below, call y_j one of the k nearest neighbors, y^μ_j one of the k_μ nearest neighbors.

(3)   Perform a stochastic gradient step on parameters of $S(\cdot)$ and $\mu(\cdot)$,
using the negative log-likelihood error signal on the y_j, with a Gaussian
of mean $x_i + \mu(x_i)$ and of covariance matrix $S(x_i)$.

The approximate gradients are:

$$\frac{\partial C(y^\mu_j, x_i)}{\partial \mu(x_i)} = -\frac{1}{n_{k_\mu}(y^\mu_j)} S(x_i)^{-1}(y^\mu_j - x_i - \mu(x_i))$$

$$\frac{\partial C(y_j, x_i)}{\partial \sigma^2_{noise}(x_i)} = 0.5 \frac{1}{n_k(y_j)} \left(Tr(S(x_i)^{-1}) - ||(y_j - x_i - \mu(x_i))'S(x_i)^{-1}||^2 \right)$$

$$\frac{\partial C(y_j, x_i)}{\partial F(x_i)} = \frac{1}{n_k(y_j)} F(x_i) S(x_i)^{-1} \left(I - (y_j - x_i - \mu(x_i))(y_j - x_i - \mu(x_i))'S(x_i)^{-1} \right)$$

where $n_k(y) = |\mathcal{N}_k(y)|$ is the number of points in the training set that
have y among their k nearest neighbors.

(4) Go to **(1)** until a given criterion is satisfied (e.g. average NLL of NLMP density estimation on a validation set stops decreasing)

Result: trained $\mu(\cdot)$ and $S(\cdot)$ functions, with corresponding σ^2_0.

Deriving the gradient formula (the derivative of the log-likelihood with respect to the neural network outputs) is lengthy but straightforward. The main trick is to do a Singular Value Decomposition of the basis vectors computed by the neural network, and to use known simplifying formulas for the derivative of the inverse of a matrix and of the determinant of a matrix. Details on the gradient derivation and on the optimization of the neural network are given in the technical report (Bengio and Larochelle, 2005).

5 Computationally Efficient Extension: Test-Centric NLMP

While the NLMP algorithm appears to perform very well, one of its main practical limitation for density estimation, that it shares with Manifold Parzen, is the large amount of computation required upon testing: for *each* test point x, the complexity of the computation is $O(n.d.D)$ (where D is the dimensionality of input space $\mathbb{R}^D$).

However there may be a different and cheaper way to compute an estimate of the density at x. We build here on an idea suggested in (Vincent, 2003), which yields an estimator that does not exactly integrate to one, but this is not an issue if the estimator is to be used for applications such as classification. Note that in our presentation of NLMP, we are using "hard" neighborhoods (i.e. a local weighting kernel that assigns a weight of 1 to the k nearest neighbors and 0 to the rest) but it could easily be generalized to "soft" weighting, as in (Vincent, 2003).

Let us decompose the true density at x as: $p(x) = p(x|x \in B_k(x))P(B_k(x))$, where $B_k(x)$ represents the spherical ball centered on x and containing the k nearest neighbors of x (i.e., the ball with radius $\|x - N_k(x)\|$ where $N_k(x)$ is the k-th neighbor of x in the training set).

It can be shown that the above NLMP learning procedure looks for functions $\mu(\cdot)$ and $S(\cdot)$ that best characterize the distribution of the k training-set nearest neighbors of x as the normal $N(\cdot; x + \mu(x), S(x))$. If we trust this locally normal (unimodal) approximation of the neighborhood distribution to be appropriate then we can approximate $p(x|x \in B_k(x))$ by $N(x; x + \mu(x), S(x))$. The approximation should be good when $B_k(x)$ is small and $p(x)$ is continuous. Moreover as $B_k(x)$ contains k points among n we can approximate $P(B_k(x))$ by $\frac{k}{n}$.

This yields the estimator $\hat{p}(x) = N(x; x + \mu(x), S(x))\frac{k}{n}$, which requires only $O(d.D)$ time to evaluate at a test point. We call this estimator *Test-centric NLMP*, since it considers only the Gaussian predicted at the test point, rather than a mixture of all the Gaussians obtained at the training points.

6   Experimental Results

We have performed comparative experiments on both toy and real-world data, on density estimation and classification tasks. All hyper-parameters are selected by cross-validation, and the costs on a large test set is used to compare final performance of all algorithms.

Experiments on toy 2D data. To understand and validate the non-local algorithm we tested it on toy 2D data where it is easy to understand what is being learned. The **sinus** data set includes examples sampled around a sinus curve. In the **spiral** data set examples are sampled near a spiral. Respectively, 57 and 113 examples are used for training, 23 and 48 for validation (hyper-parameter selection), and 920 and 3839 for testing. The following algorithms were compared:
• Non-Local Manifold Parzen Windows. The hyper-parameters are the number of principal directions (i.e., the dimension of the manifold), the number of nearest neighbors k and k_μ, the minimum constant noise variance σ_0^2 and the number of hidden units of the neural network.
• Gaussian mixture with full but regularized covariance matrices. Regularization is done by setting a minimum constant value σ_0^2 to the eigenvalues of the Gaussians. It is trained by EM and initialized using the k-means algorithm. The hyper-parameter is σ_0^2, and early stopping of EM iterations is done with the validation set.
• Parzen Windows density estimator, with a spherical Gaussian kernel. The hyper-parameter is the spread of the Gaussian kernel.
• Manifold Parzen density estimator. The hyper-parameters are the number of principal components, k of the nearest neighbor kernel and the minimum eigenvalue σ_0^2.

Note that, for these experiments, the number of principal directions (or components) was fixed to 1 for both NLMP and Manifold Parzen.

Density estimation results are shown in table 1. To help understand why Non-Local Manifold Parzen works well on these data, figure 2 illustrates the learned densities for the sinus and spiral data. Basically, it works better here because it yields an estimator that is less sensitive to the specific samples around each test point, thanks to its ability to share structure

Algorithm	sinus	spiral
Non-Local MP	**1.144**	**-1.346**
Manifold Parzen	1.345	-0.914
Gauss Mix Full	1.567	-0.857
Parzen Windows	1.841	-0.487

Table 1: *Average out-of-sample negative log-likelihood on two toy problems, for Non-Local Manifold Parzen, a Gaussian mixture with full covariance, Manifold Parzen, and Parzen Windows. The non-local algorithm dominates all the others.*

Algorithm	Valid.	Test
Non-Local MP	**-73.10**	**-76.03**
Manifold Parzen	65.21	58.33
Parzen Windows	77.87	65.94

Table 2: *Average Negative Log-Likelihood on the digit rotation experiment, when testing on a digit class (1's) not used during training, for Non-Local Manifold Parzen, Manifold Parzen, and Parzen Windows. The non-local algorithm is clearly superior.*

across the whole training set.

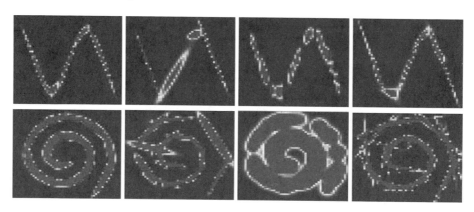

Figure 2: *Illustration of the learned densities (sinus on top, spiral on bottom) for four compared models. From left to right: Non-Local Manifold Parzen, Gaussian mixture, Parzen Windows, Manifold Parzen. Parzen Windows wastes probability mass in the spheres around each point, while leaving many holes. Gaussian mixtures tend to choose too few components to avoid overfitting. The Non-Local Manifold Parzen exploits global structure to yield the best estimator.*

Experiments on rotated digits. The next experiment is meant to show both qualitatively and quantitatively the power of non-local learning, by using 9 classes of rotated digit images (from 729 first examples of the USPS training set) to learn about the rotation manifold and testing on the left-out class (digit 1), not used for training. Each training digit was rotated by 0.1 and 0.2 radians and all these images were used as training data. We used NLMP for training, and for testing we formed an augmented mixture with Gaussians centered not only on the training examples, but also on the original unrotated 1 digits. We tested our estimator on the rotated versions of each of the 1 digits. We compared this to Manifold Parzen trained on the training data containing both the original and rotated images of the training class digits and the unrotated 1 digits. The objective of the experiment was to see if the model was able to infer the density correctly around the original unrotated images, i.e., to predict a high probability for the rotated versions of these images. In table 2 we see quantitatively that the non-local estimator predicts the rotated images much better.

As qualitative evidence, we used small steps in the principal direction predicted by *Test-centric NLMP* to rotate an image of the digit 1. To make this task even more illustrative of the generalization potential of non-local learning, we followed the tangent in the direction opposite to the rotations of the training set. It can be seen in figure 3 that the rotated

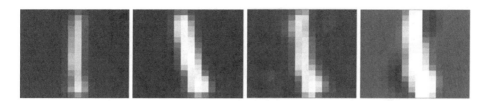

Figure 3: *From left to right: original image of a digit 1; rotated analytically by -0.2 radians; Rotation predicted using Non-Local MP; rotation predicted using MP. Rotations are obtained by following the tangent vector in small steps.*

digit obtained is quite similar to the same digit analytically rotated. For comparison, we tried to apply the same rotation technique to that digit, but by using the principal direction, computed by Manifold Parzen, of its nearest neighbor's Gaussian component in the training set. This clearly did not work, and hence shows how crucial non-local learning is for this task.

In this experiment, to make sure that NLMP focusses on the tangent plane of the rotation manifold, we fixed the number of principal directions $d = 1$ and the number of nearest neighbors $k = 1$, and also imposed $\mu(\cdot) = 0$. The same was done for Manifold Parzen.

Experiments on Classification by Density Estimation. The USPS data set was used to perform a classification experiment. The original training set (7291) was split into a training (first 6291) and validation set (last 1000), used to tune hyper-parameters. One density estimator for each of the 10 digit classes is estimated. For comparison we also show the results obtained with a Gaussian kernel Support Vector Machine (already used in (Vincent and Bengio, 2003)). **Non-local MP*** refers to the variation described in (Bengio and Larochelle, 2005), which attemps to train faster the components with larger variance. The t-test statistic for the null hypothesis of no difference in the average classification error on the test set of 2007 examples between Non-local MP and the strongest competitor (Manifold Parzen) is shown in parenthesis. Figure 4 also shows some of the invariant transformations learned by **Non-local MP** for this task.

Note that better SVM results (about 3% error) can be obtained using prior knowledge about image invariances, e.g. with virtual support vectors (Decoste and Scholkopf, 2002). However, as far as we know the NLMP performance is the best on the original USPS dataset among algorithms that do not use prior knowledge about images.

Algorithm	Valid.	Test	Hyper-Parameters
SVM	1.2%	4.68%	$C = 100, \sigma = 8$
Parzen Windows	1.8%	5.08%	$\sigma = 0.8$
Manifold Parzen	0.9%	4.08%	$d = 11, k = 11, \sigma_0^2 = 0.1$
Non-local MP	**0.6%**	**3.64% (-1.5218)**	$d = 7, k = 10, k_\mu = 10,$ $\sigma_0^2 = 0.05, n_{hid} = 70$
Non-local MP*	**0.6%**	**3.54% (-1.9771)**	$d = 7, k = 10, k_\mu = 4,$ $\sigma_0^2 = 0.05, n_{hid} = 30$

Table 3: *Classification error obtained on USPS with SVM, Parzen Windows and Local and Non-Local Manifold Parzen Windows classifiers. The hyper-parameters shown are those selected with the validation set.*

7 Conclusion

We have proposed a non-parametric density estimator that, unlike its predecessors, is able to generalize far from the training examples by capturing global structural features of the

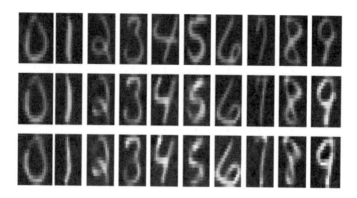

Figure 4: *Tranformations learned by* **Non-local MP**. *The top row shows digits taken from the USPS training set, and the two following rows display the results of steps taken by one of the 7 principal directions learned by* **Non-local MP**, *the third one corresponding to more steps than the second one.*

density. It does so by learning a function with global parameters that successfully predicts the local shape of the density, i.e., the tangent plane of the manifold along which the density concentrates. Three types of experiments showed that this idea works, yields improved density estimation and reduced classification error compared to its local predecessors.

Acknowledgments

The authors would like to thank the following funding organizations for support: NSERC, MITACS, and the Canada Research Chairs. The authors are also grateful for the feedback and stimulating exchanges that helped to shape this paper, with Sam Roweis and Olivier Delalleau.

References

Bengio, Y., Delalleau, O., and Le Roux, N. (2005). The curse of dimensionality for local kernel machines. Technical Report 1258, Département d'informatique et recherche opérationnelle, Université de Montréal.

Bengio, Y. and Larochelle, H. (2005). Non-local manifold parzen windows. Technical report, Département d'informatique et recherche opérationnelle, Université de Montréal.

Bengio, Y. and Monperrus, M. (2005). Non-local manifold tangent learning. In Saul, L., Weiss, Y., and Bottou, L., editors, *Advances in Neural Information Processing Systems 17*. MIT Press.

Decoste, D. and Scholkopf, B. (2002). Training invariant support vector machines. *Machine Learning*, 46:161–190.

Goldberger, J., Roweis, S., Hinton, G., and Salakhutdinov, R. (2005). Neighbourhood component analysis. In Saul, L., Weiss, Y., and Bottou, L., editors, *Advances in Neural Information Processing Systems 17*. MIT Press.

Vincent, P. (2003). *Modèles à Noyaux à Structure Locale*. PhD thesis, Université de Montréal, Département d'informatique et recherche opérationnelle, Montreal, Qc., Canada.

Vincent, P. and Bengio, Y. (2003). Manifold parzen windows. In Becker, S., Thrun, S., and Obermayer, K., editors, *Advances in Neural Information Processing Systems 15*, Cambridge, MA. MIT Press.

Convex Neural Networks

Yoshua Bengio, Nicolas Le Roux, Pascal Vincent, Olivier Delalleau, Patrice Marcotte
Dept. IRO, Université de Montréal
P.O. Box 6128, Downtown Branch, Montreal, H3C 3J7, Qc, Canada
{bengioy,lerouxni,vincentp,delallea,marcotte}@iro.umontreal.ca

Abstract

Convexity has recently received a lot of attention in the machine learning community, and the lack of convexity has been seen as a major disadvantage of many learning algorithms, such as multi-layer artificial neural networks. We show that training multi-layer neural networks in which the number of hidden units is learned can be viewed as a convex optimization problem. This problem involves an infinite number of variables, but can be solved by incrementally inserting a hidden unit at a time, each time finding a linear classifier that minimizes a weighted sum of errors.

1 Introduction

The objective of this paper is not to present yet another learning algorithm, but rather to point to a previously unnoticed relation between multi-layer neural networks (NNs),Boosting (Freund and Schapire, 1997) and convex optimization. Its main contributions concern the mathematical analysis of an algorithm that is similar to previously proposed incremental NNs, with L^1 regularization on the output weights. This analysis helps to understand the underlying convex optimization problem that one is trying to solve.

This paper was motivated by the unproven conjecture (based on anecdotal experience) that when the number of hidden units is "large", the resulting average error is rather insensitive to the random initialization of the NN parameters. One way to justify this assertion is that to really stay stuck in a local minimum, one must have second derivatives positive simultaneously in all directions. When the number of hidden units is large, it seems implausible for none of them to offer a descent direction. Although this paper does not prove or disprove the above conjecture, in trying to do so we found an interesting **characterization of the optimization problem for NNs as a convex program** if the output loss function is convex in the NN output and if the output layer weights are regularized by a convex penalty. More specifically, if the regularization is the L^1 norm of the output layer weights, then we show that a "reasonable" solution exists, involving a finite number of hidden units (no more than the number of examples, and in practice typically much less). We present a theoretical algorithm that is reminiscent of Column Generation (Chvátal, 1983), in which hidden neurons are inserted one at a time. Each insertion requires solving a weighted classification problem, very much like in Boosting (Freund and Schapire, 1997) and in particular Gradient Boosting (Mason et al., 2000; Friedman, 2001).

Neural Networks, Gradient Boosting, and Column Generation

Denote $\tilde{x} \in \mathbb{R}^{d+1}$ the extension of vector $x \in \mathbb{R}^d$ with one element with value 1. What we call "Neural Network" (NN) here is a predictor for supervised learning of the form $\hat{y}(x) = \sum_{i=1}^{m} w_i h_i(x)$ where x is an input vector, $h_i(x)$ is obtained from a linear discriminant function $h_i(x) = s(v_i \cdot \tilde{x})$ with e.g. $s(a) = \mathrm{sign}(a)$, or $s(a) = \tanh(a)$ or $s(a) = \frac{1}{1+e^{-a}}$. A learning algorithm must specify how to select m, the w_i's and the v_i's.

The classical solution (Rumelhart, Hinton and Williams, 1986) involves (a) selecting a loss function $Q(\hat{y}, y)$ that specifies how to penalize for mismatches between $\hat{y}(x)$ and the observed y's (target output or target class), (b) optionally selecting a regularization penalty that favors "small" parameters, and (c) choosing a method to approximately minimize the sum of the losses on the training data $D = \{(x_1, y_1), \dots, (x_n, y_n)\}$ plus the regularization penalty. Note that in this formulation, an output non-linearity can still be used, by inserting it in the loss function Q. Examples of such loss functions are the quadratic loss $||\hat{y} - y||^2$, the hinge loss $\max(0, 1 - y\hat{y})$ (used in SVMs), the cross-entropy loss $-y \log \hat{y} - (1 - y) \log(1 - \hat{y})$ (used in logistic regression), and the exponential loss $e^{-y\hat{y}}$ (used in Boosting).

Gradient Boosting has been introduced in (Friedman, 2001) and (Mason et al., 2000) as a non-parametric greedy-stagewise supervised learning algorithm in which one adds a function at a time to the current solution $\hat{y}(x)$, in a steepest-descent fashion, to form an additive model as above but with the functions h_i typically taken in other kinds of sets of functions, such as those obtained with decision trees. In a stagewise approach, when the $(m+1)$-th basis h_{m+1} is added, only w_{m+1} is optimized (by a line search), like in *matching pursuit* algorithms. Such a greedy-stagewise approach is also at the basis of Boosting algorithms (Freund and Schapire, 1997), which is usually applied using decision trees as bases and Q the exponential loss. It may be difficult to minimize exactly for w_{m+1} and h_{m+1} when the previous bases and weights are fixed, so (Friedman, 2001) proposes to "follow the gradient" in function space, i.e., look for a base learner h_{m+1} that is best correlated with the gradient of the average loss on the $\hat{y}(x_i)$ (that would be the residue $\hat{y}(x_i) - y_i$ in the case of the square loss). The algorithm analyzed here also involves maximizing the correlation between Q' (the derivative of Q with respect to its first argument, evaluated on the training predictions) and the next basis h_{m+1}. However, we follow a "stepwise", less greedy, approach, in which all the output weights are optimized at each step, in order to obtain convergence guarantees.

Our approach adapts the Column Generation principle (Chvátal, 1983), a decomposition technique initially proposed for solving linear programs with many variables and few constraints. In this framework, active variables, or "columns", are only generated as they are required to decrease the objective. In several implementations, the column-generation subproblem is frequently a combinatorial problem for which efficient algorithms are available. In our case, the subproblem corresponds to determining an "optimal" linear classifier.

2   Core Ideas

Informally, consider the set $\mathcal{H}$ of all possible hidden unit functions (i.e., of all possible hidden unit weight vectors v_i). Imagine a NN that has all the elements in this set as hidden units. We might want to impose precision limitations on those weights to obtain either a countable or even a finite set. For such a NN, we only need to learn the output weights. If we end up with a finite number of non-zero output weights, we will have at the end an ordinary feedforward NN. This can be achieved by using a regularization penalty on the output weights that yields sparse solutions, such as the L^1 penalty. If in addition the loss function is convex in the output layer weights (which is the case of squared error, hinge loss, ϵ-tube regression loss, and logistic or softmax cross-entropy), then it is easy to show that the overall training criterion is convex in the parameters (which are now only the output weights). The only problem is that there are as many variables in this convex program as there are elements in the set $\mathcal{H}$, which may be very large (possibly infinite). However, we find that with L^1 regularization, a finite solution is obtained, and that such a solution can be obtained by greedily inserting one hidden unit at a time. Furthermore, it is theoretically possible to check that the global optimum has been reached.

Definition 2.1. *Let $\mathcal{H}$ be a set of functions from an input space $\mathcal{X}$ to $\mathbb{R}$. Elements of $\mathcal{H}$ can be understood as "hidden units" in a NN. Let $\mathcal{W}$ be the Hilbert space of functions from $\mathcal{H}$ to $\mathbb{R}$, with an inner product denoted by $a \cdot b$ for $a, b \in \mathcal{W}$. An element of $\mathcal{W}$ can be understood as the output weights vector in a neural network. Let $h(x) : \mathcal{H} \to \mathbb{R}$ the function that maps any element h_i of $\mathcal{H}$ to $h_i(x)$. $h(x)$ can be understood as the vector of activations* *of hidden units when input x is observed. Let $w \in \mathcal{W}$ represent a* parameter *(the output weights). The NN prediction is denoted $\hat{y}(x) = w \cdot h(x)$. Let $Q : \mathbb{R} \times \mathbb{R} \to \mathbb{R}$ be a cost function convex in its first argument that takes a scalar prediction $\hat{y}(x)$ and a scalar target value y and returns a scalar cost. This is the cost to be minimized on example pair (x, y). Let $D = \{(x_i, y_i) : 1 \le i \le n\}$ a training set. Let $\Omega : \mathcal{W} \to \mathbb{R}$ be a convex regularization functional that penalizes for the choice of more "complex" parameters (e.g., $\Omega(w) = \lambda ||w||_1$ according to a 1-norm in $\mathcal{W}$, if $\mathcal{H}$ is countable). We define the* convex NN *criterion $C(\mathcal{H}, Q, \Omega, D, w)$ with parameter w as follows:*

$$C(\mathcal{H}, Q, \Omega, D, w) = \Omega(w) + \sum_{t=1}^{n} Q(w \cdot h(x_t), y_t). \tag{1}$$

The following is a trivial lemma, but it is conceptually very important as it is the basis for the rest of the analysis in this paper.

Lemma 2.2. *The convex NN cost $C(\mathcal{H}, Q, \Omega, D, w)$ is a convex function of w.*

Proof. $Q(w \cdot h(x_t), y_t)$ is convex in w and Ω is convex in w, by the above construction. C is additive in $Q(w \cdot h(x_t), y_t)$ and additive in Ω. Hence C is convex in w. $\square$

Note that there are no constraints in this convex optimization program, so that at the global minimum all the partial derivatives of C with respect to elements of w cancel.

Let $|\mathcal{H}|$ be the cardinality of the set $\mathcal{H}$. If it is not finite, it is not obvious that an optimal solution can be achieved in finitely many iterations.

Lemma 2.2 says that training NNs from a very large class (with one or more hidden layer) can be seen as convex optimization problems, usually in a very high dimensional space, **as long as we allow the number of hidden units to be selected by the learning algorithm**. By choosing a regularizer that promotes **sparse** solutions, we obtain a solution that has a **finite** number of "active" hidden units (non-zero entries in the output weights vector w). This assertion is proven below, in theorem 3.1, for the case of the hinge loss.

However, even if the solution involves a finite number of active hidden units, the convex optimization problem could still be computationally intractable because of the large number of variables involved. One approach to this problem is to apply the principles already successfully embedded in Gradient Boosting, but more specifically in Column Generation (an optimization technique for very large scale linear programs), i.e., add one hidden unit at a time in an incremental fashion. The **important ingredient here is a way to know that we have reached the global optimum, thus not requiring to actually visit all the possible hidden units.** We show that this can be achieved as long as we can solve the sub-problem of finding a linear classifier that minimizes the weighted sum of classification errors. This can be done exactly only on low dimensional data sets but can be well approached using weighted linear SVMs, weighted logistic regression, or Perceptron-type algorithms.

Another idea (not followed up here) would be to consider first a smaller set $\mathcal{H}_1$, for which the convex problem can be solved in polynomial time, and whose solution can theoretically be selected as initialization for minimizing the criterion $C(\mathcal{H}_2, Q, \Omega, D, w)$, with $\mathcal{H}_1 \subset \mathcal{H}_2$, and where $\mathcal{H}_2$ may have infinite cardinality (countable or not). In this way we could show that we can find a solution whose cost satisfies $C(\mathcal{H}_2, Q, \Omega, D, w) \le C(\mathcal{H}_1, Q, \Omega, D, w)$, i.e., is at least as good as the solution of a more restricted convex optimization problem. The second minimization can be performed with a local descent algorithm, without the necessity to guarantee that the global optimum will be found.

3 Finite Number of Hidden Neurons

In this section we consider the special case with $Q(\hat{y}, y) = max(0, 1 - y\hat{y})$ the hinge loss, and L^1 regularization, and we show that the global optimum of the convex cost involves at most $n + 1$ hidden neurons, using an approach already exploited in (Rätsch, Demiriz and Bennett, 2002) for L^1-loss regression Boosting with L^1 regularization of output weights.

The training criterion is $C(w) = K\|w\|_1 + \sum_{t=1}^{n} \max(0, 1 - y_t w \cdot h(x_t))$. Let us rewrite this cost function as the constrained optimization problem:

$$\min_{w,\xi} \ L(w, \xi) = K\|w\|_1 + \sum_{t=1}^{n} \xi_t \quad \text{s.t.} \quad \left\{ \begin{array}{ll} y_t \left[w \cdot h(x_t)\right] \geq 1 - \xi_t & (C_1) \\ \text{and} \ \ \xi_t \geq 0, t = 1, \ldots, n & (C_2) \end{array} \right.$$

Using a standard technique, the above program can be recast as a linear program. Defining $\lambda = (\lambda_1, \ldots, \lambda_n)$ the vector of Lagrangian multipliers for the constraints C_1, its dual problem (P) takes the form (in the case of a finite number J of base learners):

$$(P): \quad \max_{\lambda} \sum_{t=1}^{n} \lambda_t \quad \text{s.t.} \quad \left\{ \begin{array}{ll} \lambda \cdot Z_i - K \leq 0, i \in I \\ \text{and} \ \ \lambda_t \leq 1, t = 1, \ldots, n \end{array} \right.$$

with $(Z_i)_t = y_t h_i(x_t)$. In the case of a finite number J of base learners, $I = \{1, \ldots, J\}$. If the number of hidden units is uncountable, then I is a closed bounded interval of $\mathbb{R}$.

Such an optimization problem satisfies all the conditions needed for using Theorem 4.2 from (Hettich and Kortanek, 1993). Indeed:

- I is compact (as a closed bounded interval of $\mathbb{R}$);
- $F : \lambda \mapsto \sum_{t=1}^{n} \lambda_t$ is a concave function (it is even a linear function);
- $g : (\lambda, i) \mapsto \lambda \cdot Z_i - K$ is convex in λ (it is actually linear in λ);
- $\nu(P) \leq n$ (therefore finite) ($\nu(P)$ is the largest value of F satisfying the constraints);
- for every set of $n + 1$ points $i_0, \ldots, i_n \in I$, there exists $\tilde{\lambda}$ such that $g(\tilde{\lambda}, i_j) < 0$ for $j = 0, \ldots, n$ (one can take $\tilde{\lambda} = 0$ since $K > 0$).

Then, from Theorem 4.2 from (Hettich and Kortanek, 1993), the following theorem holds:

Theorem 3.1. *The solution of (P) can be attained with constraints C_2' and only $n + 1$ constraints C_1' (i.e., there exists a subset of $n+1$ constraints C_1' giving rise to the same maximum as when using the whole set of constraints). Therefore, the primal problem associated is the minimization of the cost function of a NN with $n + 1$ hidden neurons.*

4 Incremental Convex NN Algorithm

In this section we present a stepwise algorithm to optimize a NN, and show that there is a criterion that allows to verify whether the global optimum has been reached. This is a specialization of minimizing $C(\mathcal{H}, Q, \Omega, D, w)$, with $\Omega(w) = \lambda\|w\|_1$ and $\mathcal{H} = \{h : h(x) = s(v \cdot \tilde{x})\}$ is the set of soft or hard linear classifiers (depending on choice of $s(\cdot)$).

Algorithm ConvexNN(D,Q,λ,s)

Input: training set $D = \{(x_1, y_1), \ldots, (x_n, y_n)\}$, convex loss function Q, and scalar regularization penalty λ. s is either the *sign* function or the *tanh* function.

(1) Set $v_1 = (0, 0, \ldots, 1)$ and select $w_1 = \mathrm{argmin}_{w_1} \sum_t Q(w_1 s(1), y_t) + \lambda|w_1|$.

(2) Set $i = 2$.

(3) Repeat

(4)   Let $q_t = Q'(\sum_{j=1}^{i-1} w_j h_j(x_t), y_t)$

(5)   If $s = \mathrm{sign}$

(5a)   train linear classifier $h_i(x) = \mathrm{sign}(v_i \cdot \tilde{x})$ with examples $\{(x_t, \mathrm{sign}(q_t))\}$ and errors weighted by $|q_t|, t = 1 \ldots n$ (i.e., *maximize* $\sum_t q_t h_i(x_t)$)

(5b)   else ($s = \tanh$)

(5c)   train linear classifier $h_i(x) = \tanh(v_i \cdot \tilde{x})$ to *maximize* $\sum_t q_t h_i(x_t)$.

(6)   If $\sum_t q_t h_i(x_t) < \lambda$, **stop**.

(7)   Select $w_1, \ldots, w_i$ (and optionally $v_2, \ldots, v_i$) minimizing (exactly or approximately) $C = \sum_t Q(\sum_{j=1}^{i} w_j h_j(x_t), y_t) + \lambda \sum_{j=1}^{i} |w_j|$ such that $\frac{\partial C}{\partial w_j} = 0$ for $j = 1 \ldots i$.

(8) Return the predictor $\hat{y}(x) = \sum_{j=1}^{i} w_j h_j(x)$.

A key property of the above algorithm is that, at termination, the global optimum is reached, i.e., no hidden unit (linear classifier) can improve the objective. In the case where $s = \text{sign}$, we obtain a Boosting-like algorithm, i.e., it involves finding a classifier which minimizes the weighted cost $\sum_t q_t \text{sign}(v \cdot \tilde{x}_t)$.

Theorem 4.1. *Algorithm* **ConvexNN** *stops when it reaches the global optimum of*
$$C(w) = \sum_t Q(w \cdot h(x_t), y_t) + \lambda ||w||_1.$$

Proof. Let w be the output weights vector when the algorithm stops. Because the set of hidden units $\mathcal{H}$ we consider is such that when h is in $\mathcal{H}$, $-h$ is also in $\mathcal{H}$, we can assume all weights to be non-negative. By contradiction, if $w' \neq w$ is the global optimum, with $C(w') < C(w)$, then, since C is convex in the output weights, for any $\epsilon \in (0, 1)$, we have $C(\epsilon w' + (1 - \epsilon)w) \leq \epsilon C(w') + (1 - \epsilon)C(w) < C(w)$. Let $w_\epsilon = \epsilon w' + (1 - \epsilon)w$. For ϵ small enough, we can assume all weights in w that are strictly positive to be also strictly positive in w_ϵ. Let us denote by I_p the set of strictly positive weights in w (and w_ϵ), by I_z the set of weights set to zero in w but to a non-zero value in w_ϵ, and by $\delta_{\epsilon k}$ the difference $w_{\epsilon,k} - w_k$ in the weight of hidden unit h_k between w and w_ϵ. We can assume $\delta_{\epsilon j} < 0$ for $j \in I_z$, because instead of setting a small positive weight to h_j, one can decrease the weight of $-h_j$ by the same amount, which will give either the same cost, or possibly a lower one when the weight of $-h_j$ is positive. With $o(\epsilon)$ denoting a quantity such that $\epsilon^{-1}o(\epsilon) \to 0$ when $\epsilon \to 0$, the difference $\Delta_\epsilon(w) = C(w_\epsilon) - C(w)$ can now be written:

$$\Delta_\epsilon(w) = \lambda (||w_\epsilon||_1 - ||w||_1) + \sum_t (Q(w_\epsilon \cdot h(x_t), y_t) - Q(w \cdot h(x_t), y_t))$$

$$= \lambda \left(\sum_{i \in I_p} \delta_{\epsilon i} + \sum_{j \in I_z} -\delta_{\epsilon j} \right) + \sum_t \sum_k (Q'(w \cdot h(x_t), y_t)\delta_{\epsilon k} h_k(x_t)) + o(\epsilon)$$

$$= \sum_{i \in I_p} \left(\lambda \delta_{\epsilon i} + \sum_t q_t \delta_{\epsilon i} h_i(x_t) \right) + \sum_{j \in I_z} \left(-\lambda \delta_{\epsilon j} + \sum_t q_t \delta_{\epsilon j} h_j(x_t) \right) + o(\epsilon)$$

$$= \sum_{i \in I_p} \delta_{\epsilon i} \frac{\partial C}{\partial w_i}(w) + \sum_{j \in I_z} \left(-\lambda \delta_{\epsilon j} + \sum_t q_t \delta_{\epsilon j} h_j(x_t) \right) + o(\epsilon)$$

$$= 0 + \sum_{j \in I_z} \left(-\lambda \delta_{\epsilon j} + \sum_t q_t \delta_{\epsilon j} h_j(x_t) \right) + o(\epsilon)$$

since for $i \in I_p$, thanks to step (7) of the algorithm, we have $\frac{\partial C}{\partial w_i}(w) = 0$. Thus the inequality $\epsilon^{-1}\Delta_\epsilon(w) < 0$ rewrites into

$$\sum_{j \in I_z} \epsilon^{-1}\delta_{\epsilon j} \left(-\lambda + \sum_t q_t h_j(x_t) \right) + \epsilon^{-1}o(\epsilon) < 0$$

which, when $\epsilon \to 0$, yields (note that $\epsilon^{-1}\delta_{\epsilon j}$ does not depend on ϵ since $\delta_{\epsilon j}$ is linear in ϵ):

$$\sum_{j \in I_z} \epsilon^{-1}\delta_{\epsilon j} \left(-\lambda + \sum_t q_t h_j(x_t) \right) \leq 0 \tag{2}$$

But, h_i being the optimal classifier chosen in step (5a) or (5c), all hidden units h_j verify $\sum_t q_t h_j(x_t) \leq \sum_t q_t h_i(x_t) < \lambda$ and $\forall j \in I_z$, $\epsilon^{-1}\delta_{\epsilon j}(-\lambda + \sum_t q_t h_j(x_t)) > 0$ (since $\delta_{\epsilon j} < 0$), contradicting eq. 2. □

(Mason et al., 2000) prove a related global convergence result for the AnyBoost algorithm, a non-parametric Boosting algorithm that is also similar to Gradient Boosting (Friedman, 2001). Again, this requires solving as a sub-problem an exact minimization to find a function $h_i \in \mathcal{H}$ that is maximally correlated with the gradient Q' on the output. We now show a simple procedure to select a hyperplane with the best weighted classification error.

Exact Minimization

In step (5a) we are required to find a linear classifier that minimizes the weighted sum of classification errors. Unfortunately, this is an NP-hard problem (w.r.t. d, see theorem 4 in (Marcotte and Savard, 1992)). However, an exact solution can be easily found in $O(n^3)$ computations for $d = 2$ inputs.

Proposition 4.2. *Finding a linear classifier that minimizes the weighted sum of classification error can be achieved in $O(n^3)$ steps when the input dimension is $d = 2$.*

Proof. We want to maximize $\sum_i c_i \text{sign}(u \cdot x_i + b)$ with respect to u and b, the c_i's being in $\mathbb{R}$. Consider u **fixed** and sort the x_i's according to their dot product with u and denote r the function which maps i to $r(i)$ such that $x_{r(i)}$ is in i-th position in the sort. Depending on the value of b, we will have $n + 1$ possible sums, respectively $-\sum_{i=1}^{k} c_{r(i)} + \sum_{i=k+1}^{n} c_{r(i)}$, $k = 0, \ldots, n$. It is obvious that those sums only depend on the order of the products $u \cdot x_i$, $i = 1, \ldots, n$. When u varies smoothly on the unit circle, as the dot product is a continuous function of its arguments, the changes in the order of the dot products will occur only when there is a pair (i, j) such that $u \cdot x_i = u \cdot x_j$. Therefore, there are at most as many order changes as there are pairs of different points, i.e., $n(n-1)/2$. In the case of $d = 2$, we can enumerate all the different angles for which there is a change, namely $a_1, \ldots, a_z$ with $z \leq \frac{n(n-1)}{2}$. We then need to test at least one $u = [\cos(\theta), \sin(\theta)]$ for each interval $a_i < \theta < a_{i+1}$, and also one u for $\theta < a_1$, which makes a total of $\frac{n(n-1)}{2}$ possibilities. $\square$

It is possible to generalize this result in higher dimensions, and as shown in (Marcotte and Savard, 1992), one can achieve $O(\log(n)n^d)$ time.

Algorithm 1 Optimal linear classifier search

> **Maximizing** $\sum_{i=1}^{n} c_i \delta(\text{sign}(w \cdot x_i), y_i)$ **in dimension 2**
> **(1)** for $i = 1, \ldots, n$ for $j = i + 1, \ldots, n$
> **(3)** $\quad \Theta_{i,j} = \theta(x_i, x_j) + \frac{\pi}{2}$ where $\theta(x_i, x_j)$ is the angle between x_i and x_j
> **(6)** sort the $\Theta_{i,j}$ in increasing order
> **(7)** $w_0 = (1, 0)$
> **(8)** for $k = 1, \ldots, \frac{n(n-1)}{2}$
> **(9)** $\quad w_k = (\cos \Theta_{i,j}, \sin \Theta_{i,j})$, $u_k = \frac{w_k + w_{k-1}}{2}$
> **(10)** $\quad$ sort the x_i according to the value of $u_k \cdot x_i$
> **(11)** $\quad$ compute $S(u_k) = \sum_{i=1}^{n} c_i \delta(u_k \cdot x_i), y_i)$
> **(12)** output: $\text{argmax}_{u_k} S$

Approximate Minimization

For data in higher dimensions, the exact minimization scheme to find the optimal linear classifier is not practical. Therefore it is interesting to consider approximate schemes for obtaining a linear classifier with weighted costs. Popular schemes for doing so are the linear SVM (i.e., linear classifier with hinge loss), the logistic regression classifier, and variants of the Perceptron algorithm. In that case, step (5c) of the algorithm is not an exact minimization, and one cannot guarantee that the global optimum will be reached. However, it might be reasonable to believe that finding a linear classifier by minimizing a weighted hinge loss should yield solutions close to the exact minimization. Unfortunately, this is not generally true, as we have found out on a simple toy data set described below. On the other hand, if in step (7) one performs an optimization not only of the output weights w_j ($j \leq i$) but also of the corresponding weight vectors v_j, then the algorithm finds a solution close to the global optimum (we could only verify this on 2D data sets, where the exact solution can be computed easily). It means that at the end of each stage, one first performs a few training iterations of the whole NN (for the hidden units $j \leq i$) with an ordinary gradient descent mechanism (we used conjugate gradients but stochastic gradient descent would work too), optimizing the w_j's and the v_j's, and then one fixes the v_j's and obtains the optimal w_j's for these v_j's (using a convex optimization procedure). In our experiments we used a quadratic Q, for which the optimization of the output weights can be done with a neural network, using the outputs of the hidden layer as inputs.

Let us consider now a bit more carefully what it means to tune the v_j's in step (7). Indeed, changing the weight vector v_j of a selected hidden neuron to decrease the cost is **equivalent to a change in the output weights w's**. More precisely, consider the step in which the value of v_j becomes v'_j. This is equivalent to the following operation on the w's, when w_j is the corresponding output weight value: the output weight associated with the value v_j of a hidden neuron is set to 0, and the output weight associated with the value v'_j of a hidden neuron is set to w_j. This corresponds to an exchange between two variables in the convex program. We are justified to take any such step as long as it allows us to decrease the cost $C(w)$. The fact that we are simultaneously making such exchanges on all the hidden units when we tune the v_j's allows us to move faster towards the global optimum.

Extension to multiple outputs

The multiple outputs case is more involved than the single-output case because it is not enough to check the condition $\sum_t h_t q_t > \lambda$. Consider a new hidden neuron whose output is h_i when the input is x_i. Let us also denote $\alpha = [\alpha_1, \ldots, \alpha_{n_o}]'$ the vector of output weights between the new hidden neuron and the n_o output neurons. The gradient with respect to α_j is $g_j = \frac{\partial C}{\partial \alpha_j} = \sum_t h_t q_{tj} - \lambda \text{sign}(\alpha_j)$ with q_{tj} the value of the j-th output neuron with input x_t. This means that if, for a given j, we have $|\sum_t h_t q_{tj}| < \lambda$, moving α_j away from 0 can only increase the cost. Therefore, the right quantity to consider is $(|\sum_t h_t q_{tj}| - \lambda)_+$.

We must therefore find $\text{argmax}_v \sum_j (|\sum_t h_t q_{tj}| - \lambda)_+^2$. As before, this sub-problem is not convex, but it is not as obvious how to approximate it by a convex problem. The stopping criterion becomes: if there is no j such that $|\sum_t h_t q_{tj}| > \lambda$, then all weights must remain equal to 0 and a global minimum is reached.

Experimental Results

We performed experiments on the 2D double moon toy dataset (as used in (Delalleau, Bengio and Le Roux, 2005)), to be able to compare with the exact version of the algorithm. In these experiments, $Q(w \cdot h(x_t), y_t) = [w \cdot h(x_t) - y_t]^2$. The set-up is the following:
• Select a new linear classifier, either (a) the optimal one or (b) an approximate using logistic regression.
• Optimize the output weights using a convex optimizer.
• In case (b), tune both input and output weights by conjugate gradient descent on C and finally re-optimize the output weights using LASSO regression.
• Optionally, remove neurons whose output weight has been set to 0.

Using the approximate algorithm yielded for 100 training examples an average penalized ($\lambda = 1$) squared error of 17.11 (over 10 runs), an average test classification error of 3.68% and an average number of neurons of 5.5 . The exact algorithm yielded a penalized squared error of 8.09, an average test classification error of 5.3%, and required 3 hidden neurons. A penalty of $\lambda = 1$ was nearly optimal for the exact algorithm whereas a smaller penalty further improved the test classification error of the approximate algorithm. Besides, when running the approximate algorithm for a long time, it converges to a solution whose quadratic error is extremely close to the one of the exact algorithm.

5   Conclusion

We have shown that training a NN can be seen as a convex optimization problem, and have analyzed an algorithm that can exactly or approximately solve this problem. We have shown that the solution with the hinge loss involved a number of non-zero weights bounded by the number of examples, and much smaller in practice. We have shown that there exists a stopping criterion to verify if the global optimum has been reached, but it involves solving a sub-learning problem involving a linear classifier with weighted errors, which can be computationally hard if the exact solution is sought, but can be easily implemented for toy data sets (in low dimension), for comparing exact and approximate solutions.

The above experimental results are in agreement with our initial conjecture: when there are many hidden units we are much less likely to stall in the optimization procedure, because there are many more ways to descend on the convex cost $C(w)$. They also suggest, based on experiments in which we can compare with the exact sub-problem minimization, that applying Algorithm **ConvexNN** with an approximate minimization for adding each hidden unit **while continuing to tune the previous hidden units** tends to lead to fast convergence to the global minimum. What can get us stuck in a "local minimum" (in the traditional sense, i.e., of optimizing w's and v's together) is simply the **inability to find a new hidden unit weight vector that can improve the total cost (fit and regularization term) even if there exists one**.

Note that as a side-effect of the results presented here, we have a simple way to train **neural networks with hard-threshold hidden units**, since increasing $\sum_t Q'(\hat{y}(x_t), y_t) \mathrm{sign}(v_i x_t)$ can be either achieved exactly (at great price) or approximately (e.g. by using a cross-entropy or hinge loss on the corresponding linear classifier).

Acknowledgments

The authors thank the following for support: NSERC, MITACS, and the Canada Research Chairs. They are also grateful for the feedback and stimulating exchanges with Sam Roweis, Nathan Srebro, and Aaron Courville.

References

Chvátal, V. (1983). *Linear Programming*. W.H. Freeman.

Delalleau, O., Bengio, Y., and Le Roux, N. (2005). Efficient non-parametric function induction in semi-supervised learning. In Cowell, R. and Ghahramani, Z., editors, *Proceedings of AISTATS'2005*, pages 96–103.

Freund, Y. and Schapire, R. E. (1997). A decision theoretic generalization of on-line learning and an application to boosting. *Journal of Computer and System Science*, 55(1):119–139.

Friedman, J. (2001). Greedy function approximation: a gradient boosting machine. *Annals of Statistics*, 29:1180.

Hettich, R. and Kortanek, K. (1993). Semi-infinite programming: theory, methods, and applications. *SIAM Review*, 35(3):380–429.

Marcotte, P. and Savard, G. (1992). Novel approaches to the discrimination problem. *Zeitschrift fr Operations Research (Theory)*, 36:517–545.

Mason, L., Baxter, J., Bartlett, P. L., and Frean, M. (2000). Boosting algorithms as gradient descent. In *Advances in Neural Information Processing Systems 12*, pages 512–518.

Rätsch, G., Demiriz, A., and Bennett, K. P. (2002). Sparse regression ensembles in infinite and finite hypothesis spaces. *Machine Learning*.

Rumelhart, D., Hinton, G., and Williams, R. (1986). Learning representations by back-propagating errors. *Nature*, 323:533–536.

Non-Gaussian Component Analysis: a Semi-parametric Framework for Linear Dimension Reduction

G. Blanchard[1], M. Sugiyama[1,2], M. Kawanabe[1], V. Spokoiny[3], K.-R. Müller[1,4]

[1] Fraunhofer FIRST.IDA, Kekuléstr. 7, 12489 Berlin, Germany

[2] Dept. of CS, Tokyo Inst. of Tech., 2-12-1, O-okayama, Meguro-ku, Tokyo, 152-8552, Japan

[3]Weierstrass Institute and Humboldt University, Mohrenstr. 39, 10117 Berlin, Germany

[4] Dept. of CS, University of Potsdam, August-Bebel-Strasse 89, 14482 Potsdam, Germany

spokoiny@wias-berlin.de   {blanchar,sugi,nabe,klaus}@first.fhg.de

Abstract

We propose a new *linear* method for dimension reduction to identify non-Gaussian components in high dimensional data. Our method, NGCA (non-Gaussian component analysis), uses a very general semi-parametric framework. In contrast to existing projection methods we define what is *un*interesting (Gaussian): by projecting out uninterestingness, we can estimate the relevant non-Gaussian subspace. We show that the estimation error of finding the non-Gaussian components tends to zero at a parametric rate. Once NGCA components are identified and extracted, various tasks can be applied in the data analysis process, like data visualization, clustering, denoising or classification. A numerical study demonstrates the usefulness of our method.

1 Introduction

Suppose $\{X_i\}_{i=1}^n$ are i.i.d. samples in a high dimensional space $\mathbb{R}^d$ drawn from an unknown distribution with density $p(x)$. A general multivariate distribution is typically too complex to analyze from the data, thus dimensionality reduction is necessary to decrease the complexity of the model (see, e.g., [4, 11, 10, 12, 1]). We will follow the rationale that in most real-world applications the 'signal' or 'information' contained in the high-dimensional data is essentially non-Gaussian while the 'rest' can be interpreted as high dimensional Gaussian noise. Thus we implicitly fix what is *not* interesting (Gaussian part) and learn its orthogonal complement, i.e. what is interesting. We call this approach non-Gaussian components analysis (NGCA).

We want to emphasize that we do *not* assume the Gaussian components to be of *smaller* order of magnitude than the signal components. This setting therefore excludes the use of common (nonlinear) dimensionality reduction methods such as Isomap [12], LLE [10], that are based on the assumption that the data lies, say, on a lower dimensional manifold, up to some small noise distortion. In the restricted setting where the number of Gaussian components is *at most one* and all the non-Gaussian components are mutually independent, *Independent Component Analysis (ICA)* techniques (e.g., [9]) are applicable to identify the non-Gaussian subspace.

A framework closer in spirit to NGCA is that of *projection pursuit (PP)* algorithms [5, 7, 9], where the goal is to extract non-Gaussian components in a general setting, i.e., the number of Gaussian components can be more than one and the non-Gaussian components can be dependent. Projection pursuit methods typically proceed by fixing a *single* index which measures the non-Gaussianity (or 'interestingness') of a projection direction. This index is then optimized to find a good direction of projection, and the procedure is iterated to find further directions. Note that some projection indices are suitable for finding super-Gaussian components (heavy-tailed distribution) while others are suited for identifying sub-Gaussian components (light-tailed distribution) [9]. Therefore, traditional PP algorithms may not work effectively if the data contains, say, both super- and sub-Gaussian components.

Technically, the NGCA approach to identify the non-Gaussian subspace uses a very general semi-parametric framework based on a central property: there exists a linear mapping $h \mapsto \beta(h) \in \mathbb{R}^d$ which, to any *arbitrary* (smooth) nonlinear function $h : \mathbb{R}^d \rightarrow \mathbb{R}$, associates a vector β lying in the non-Gaussian subspace. Using a whole family of different nonlinear functions h then yields a family of different vectors $\widehat{\beta}(h)$ which all approximately lie in, and span, the non-Gaussian subspace. We finally perform PCA on this family of vectors to extract the principal directions and estimate the target space. Our main theoretical contribution in this paper is to prove consistency of the NGCA procedure, i.e. that the above estimation error vanishes at a rate $\sqrt{\log(n)/n}$ with the sample size n. In practice, we consider functions of the particular form $h_{\omega,a}(x) = f_a(\langle \omega, x \rangle)$ where f is a function class parameterized, say, by a parameter a, and $\|\omega\| = 1$.

Apart from the conceptual point, defining uninterestingness as the point of departure instead of interestingness, another way to look at our method is to say that it allows the combination of information coming from different indices h: here the above function f_a (for fixed a) plays a role similar to that of a non-Gaussianity index in PP, but we do combine a rich family of such functions (by varying a and even by considering several function classes at the same time). The important point here is while traditional projection pursuit does not provide a well-founded justification for combining directions obtained from different indices, our framework allows to do precisely this – thus implicitly selecting, in a given family of indices, the ones which are the most informative for the data at hand (while always maintaining consistency).

In the following section we will outline our main theoretical contribution, a novel semi-parametric theory for *linear* dimension reduction. Section 3 discusses the algorithmic procedures and simulation results underline the usefulness of NGCA; finally a brief conclusion is given.

2 Theoretical framework

The model. We assume the unknown probability density function $p(x)$ of the observations in $\mathbb{R}^d$ is of the form

$$p(x) = g(Tx)\phi_\Gamma(x), \tag{1}$$

where T is an unknown linear mapping from $\mathbb{R}^d$ to another space $\mathbb{R}^m$ with $m \leq d$, g is an unknown function on $\mathbb{R}^m$, and ϕ_Γ is a centered Gaussian density with unknown covariance matrix Γ. The above decomposition may be possible for any density p since g can be any function. Therefore, this decomposition is not restrictive in general.

Note that the model (1) includes as particular cases both the pure parametric ($m = 0$) and pure non-parametric ($m = d$) models. We effectively consider an intermediate case where d is large and m is rather small. In what follows we denote by $\mathcal{I}$ the m-dimensional *linear* subspace in $\mathbb{R}^d$ generated by the dual operator $T^\top$:

$$\mathcal{I} = Ker(T)^\perp = Range(T^\top).$$

We call $\mathcal{I}$ the *non-Gaussian subspace*. Note how this definition implements the general point of view outlined in the introduction: by this model we define rather what is considered *uninteresting*, i.e. the null space of T; the target space is defined indirectly as the orthogonal of the uninteresting component. More precisely, using the orthogonal decomposition $X = X_0 + X_{\mathcal{I}}$, where $X_0 \in Ker(T)$ and $X_{\mathcal{I}} \in \mathcal{I}$, equation (1) implies that conditionally to $X_{\mathcal{I}}$, X_0 has a Gaussian distribution. X_0 is therefore 'not interesting' and we wish to project it out.

Our goal is therefore to estimate $\mathcal{I}$ by some subspace $\widehat{\mathcal{I}}$ computed from i.i.d. samples $\{X_i\}_{i=1}^n$ which follows the distribution with density $p(x)$. In this paper we assume the effective dimension m to be known or fixed *a priori* by the user. Note that we do *not* estimate Γ, g, and T when estimating $\mathcal{I}$.

Population analysis. The main idea underlying our approach is summed up in the following Proposition (proof in Appendix). Whenever variable X has covariance matrix identity, this result allows, from an *arbitrary* smooth real function h on $\mathbb{R}^d$, to find a vector $\beta(h) \in \mathcal{I}$.

Proposition 1 *Let X be a random variable whose density function $p(x)$ satisfies (1) and suppose that $h(x)$ is a smooth real function on $\mathbb{R}^d$. Assume furthermore that $\Sigma = \mathbb{E}\left[XX^\top\right] = I_d$. Then under mild regularity conditions the following vector belongs to the target space $\mathcal{I}$:*

$$\beta(h) = \mathbb{E}\left[\nabla h - X h(X)\right] . \tag{2}$$

Estimation using empirical data. Since the unknown density $p(x)$ is used to define β by Eq.(2), one can not directly use this formula in practice, and it must be approximated using the empirical data. We therefore have to estimate the population expectations using empirical ones. A bound on the corresponding approximation error is then given by the following theorem:

Theorem 1 *Let h be a smooth function. Assume that $\sup_y \max\left(\|\nabla h(y)\|, \|h(y)\|\right) < B$ and that X has covariance matrix $\mathbb{E}\left[XX^\top\right] = I_d$ and is such that for some $\lambda_0 > 0$:*

$$\mathbb{E}\left[\exp\left(\lambda_0 \|X\|\right)\right] \le a_0 < \infty. \tag{3}$$

Denote $\widetilde{h}(x) = \nabla h(x) - x h(x)$. Suppose $X_1, \ldots, X_n$ are i.i.d. copies of X and define

$$\widehat{\beta}(h) = \frac{1}{n}\sum_{i=1}^n \widetilde{h}(X_i), \text{ and } \widehat{\sigma}(h) = \frac{1}{n}\sum_{i=1}^n \left\|\widetilde{h}(X_i) - \widehat{\beta}(h)\right\|^2 ; \tag{4}$$

then with probability $1 - 4\delta$ the following holds:

$$dist\left(\widehat{\beta}(h), \mathcal{I}\right) \le 2\sqrt{\widehat{\sigma}(h)\frac{\log \delta^{-1} + \log d}{n}} + C(\lambda_0, a_0, B, d)\left(\frac{\log(n\delta^{-1})\log \delta^{-1}}{n^{\frac{3}{4}}}\right) .$$

Comments. 1. The proof of the theorem relies on standard tools using Chernoff's bounding method and is omitted for space. In this theorem, the covariance matrix of X is assumed to be *known* and equal to identity which is not a realistic assumption; in practice, we use a standard "whitening" procedure (see next section) using the empirical covariance matrix. Of course there is an additional error coming from this step, since the covariance matrix is also estimated empirically. In the extended version of the paper [3], we prove (under somewhat stronger assumptions) a bound for the entirely empirical procedure including whitening, resulting in an approximation error of the same order in n (up to a logarithmic factor). This result was omitted here due to space constraints.

2. Fixing δ, Theorem 1 implies that the vector $\widehat{\beta}(h)$ obtained from any $h(x)$ converges to the unknown non-Gaussian subspace $\mathcal{I}$ at a "parametric" rate of order $1/\sqrt{n}$. Furthermore, the theorem gives us an estimation of the relative size of the estimation error for different functions h through the (computable from the data) factor $\sqrt{\widehat{\sigma}(h)}$ in the main term of the bound. This suggests using this quantity as a renormalizing factor so that the typical approximation error is (roughly) independent of the function h used. This normalization principle will be used in the main procedure.

3. Note the theorem results in an *exponential deviation inequality* (the dependence in the confidence level δ is logarithmic). As a consequence, using the union bound over a finite net, we can obtain as a corollary of the above theorem a uniform deviation bound of the same form over a (discretized) set of functions (where the log-cardinality of the set appears as an additional factor). For instance, if we consider a $1/n$-discretization net of functions with d parameters, hence of size $\mathcal{O}(n^d)$, then the above bounds holds uniformly when replacing the $\log \delta^{-1}$ term by $d \log n + \log \delta^{-1}$. This does not change fundamentally the bound (up to an additional complexity factor $\sqrt{d \log(n)}$), and justifies that we consider simultaneously such a family of functions in the main algorithm.

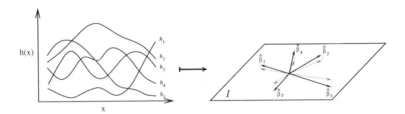

Figure 1: The NGCA main idea: from a varied family of real functions h, compute a family of vectors $\widehat{\beta}$ belonging to the target space up to small estimation error.

3 The NGCA algorithm

In the last section, we have established that given an arbitrary smooth real function h on $\mathbb{R}^d$, we are able to construct a vector $\widehat{\beta}(h)$ which belongs to the target space $\mathcal{I}$ up to a small estimation error. The main idea is now to consider a large family of such functions (h_k), giving rise to a family of vectors $\widehat{\beta}_k$ (see Fig. 1). Theorem 1 ensures that the estimation error remains controlled uniformly, and we can also normalize the vectors such that the estimation error is of the same order for all vectors (see Comments 2 and 3 above). Under this condition, it can be shown that vectors with a longer norm are more informative about the target subspace, and that vectors with too small a norm are uninformative. We therefore throw out the smaller vectors, then estimate the target space $\mathcal{I}$ by applying a principal components analysis to the remaining vector family.

In the proposed algorithm we will restrict our attention to functions of the form $h_{f,\omega}(x) = f(\langle \omega, x \rangle)$, where $\omega \in \mathbb{R}^d, \|\omega\| = 1$, and f belongs to a finite family $\mathcal{F}$ of smooth real functions of real variable. Our theoretical setting allows to ensure that the approximation error remains small uniformly over $\mathcal{F}$ and ω (rigorously, ω should be restricted to a finite ε-net of the unit sphere in order to consider a finite family of functions: in practice we will overlook this weak restriction). However, it is not feasible in practice to sample the whole parameter space for ω as soon as it has more than a few dimensions. To overcome this difficulty, we advocate using a well-known PP algorithm, FastICA [8], as a proxy to find good candidates for ω_f for a fixed f. Note that this does not make NGCA equivalent to FastICA: the important point is that FastICA, as a stand-alone procedure, requires to fix the "index function" f beforehand. The crucial novelty of our method is that we provide a theoretical setting and a methodology which allows to *combine* the results of this projection pursuit method when used over a possibly large spectrum of arbitrary index functions f.

<u>NGCA ALGORITHM.</u>

Input: Data points $(X_i) \in \mathbb{R}^d$, dimension m of target subspace.

Parameters: Number $T_{\max}$ of FastICA iterations; threshold ϵ;
           family of real functions (f_k).

Whitening.

    The data X_i is recentered by subtracting the empirical mean.

    Let $\widehat{\Sigma}$ denote the empirical covariance matrix of the data sample (X_i);

    put $\widehat{Y}_i = \widehat{\Sigma}^{-\frac{1}{2}} X_i$ the empirically whitened data.

Main Procedure.

    Loop on $k = 1, \ldots, L$:

       Draw ω_0 at random on the unit sphere of $\mathbb{R}^d$.

        Loop on $t = 1, \ldots, T_{\max}$: *[FastICA loop]*

$$\text{Put } \widehat{\beta}_t \leftarrow \frac{1}{n} \sum_{i=1}^{n} \left(\widehat{Y}_i f_k(\langle \omega_{t-1}, \widehat{Y}_i \rangle) - f'_k(\langle \omega_{t-1}, \widehat{Y}_i \rangle) \omega_{t-1} \right).$$

           Put $\omega_t \leftarrow \widehat{\beta}_t / \|\widehat{\beta}_t\|$.

        End Loop on t

      Let N_i be the trace of the empirical covariance matrix of $\widehat{\beta}_{T_{\max}}$:

$$N_i = \frac{1}{n} \sum_{i=1}^{n} \left\| \widehat{Y}_i f_k(\langle \omega_{T_{\max}-1}, \widehat{Y}_i \rangle) - f'_k(\langle \omega_{T_{\max}-1}, \widehat{Y}_i \rangle) \omega_{T_{\max}-1} \right\|^2 - \left\| \widehat{\beta}_{T_{\max}} \right\|^2.$$

      Store $v^{(k)} \leftarrow \widehat{\beta}_{T_{\max}} * \sqrt{n/N_i}$. *[Normalization]*

    End Loop on k

Thresholding.

    From the family $v^{(k)}$, throw away vectors having norm smaller than threshold ϵ.

PCA step.

    Perform PCA on the set of remaining $v^{(k)}$.

    Let V_m be the space spanned by the first m principal directions.

Pull back in original space.

    Output: $W_m = \widehat{\Sigma}^{-\frac{1}{2}} V_m$.

Summing up, the NGCA algorithm finally consists of the following steps (see above pseudocode): (1) Data whitening (see Comment 1 in the previous section), (2) Apply FastICA to each function $f \in \mathcal{F}$ to find a promising candidate value for ω_f, (3) Compute the corresponding family of vectors $(\widehat{\beta}(h_{f,\omega_f}))_{f \in \mathcal{F}}$ (using Eq. (4)), (4) Normalize the vectors appropriately; threshold and throw out uninformative ones, (5) Apply PCA, (6) Pull back in original space (de-whitening). In the implementation tested, we have used the following forms of the functions f_k: $f_\sigma^{(1)}(z) = z^3 \exp(-z^2/2\sigma^2)$ (Gauss-Pow3), $f_b^{(2)}(z) = \tanh(bz)$ (Hyperbolic Tangent), $f_a^{(3)}(z) = \{\sin, \cos\}(az)$ (Fourier). More precisely, we consider discretized ranges for $a \in [0, A], b \in [0, B], \sigma \in [\sigma_{\min}, \sigma_{\max}]$; this gives rise to a finite family (f_k) (which includes *simultaneously* functions of the three different above families).

4   Numerical results

Parameters used. All the experiments presented where obtained with exactly the same set of parameters: $a \in [0, 4]$ for the Fourier functions; $b \in [0, 5]$ for the Hyperbolic Tangent functions; $\sigma^2 \in [0.5, 5]$ for the Gauss-pow3 functions. Each of these ranges was divided

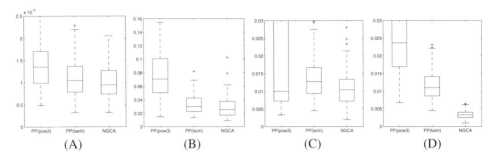

(A)   (B)   (C)   (D)

Figure 2: Boxplots of the error criterion $\mathcal{E}(\widehat{\mathcal{I}}, \mathcal{I})$ over 100 training samples of size 1000.

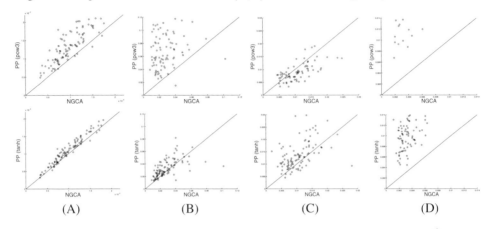

(A)   (B)   (C)   (D)

Figure 3: Sample-wise performance comparison plots (for error criterion $\mathcal{E}(\widehat{\mathcal{I}}, \mathcal{I})$) of NGCA versus FastICA; top: versus pow3 index; bottom: versus tanh index. Each point represents a different sample of size 1000. In (C)-top, about 25% of the points corresponding to a failure of FastICA fall outside of the range and were not represented.

into 1000 equispaced values, thus yielding a family (f_k) of size 4000 (Fourier functions count twice because of the sine and cosine parts). Some preliminary calibration suggested to take $\varepsilon = 1.5$ as the threshold under which vectors are not informative. Finally we fixed the number of FastICA iterations $T_{\max} = 10$. With this choice of parameters, with 1000 points of data the computation time is typically of the order of 10 seconds on a modern PC under a Matlab implementation.

Tests in a controlled setting. We performed numerical experiments using various synthetic data. We report exemplary results using 4 data sets. Each data set includes 1000 samples in 10 dimensions, and consists of 8-dimensional independent standard Gaussian and 2 non-Gaussian components as follows:

(A) Simple Gaussian Mixture: 2-dimensional independent bimodal Gaussian mixtures;
(B) Dependent super-Gaussian: 2-dimensional density is proportional to $\exp(-\|x\|)$;
(C) Dependent sub-Gaussian: 2-dimensional uniform on the unit circle;
(D) Dependent super- and sub-Gaussian: 1-dimensional Laplacian with density proportional to $\exp(-|x_{Lap}|)$ and 1-dimensional dependent uniform $U(c, c+1)$, where $c = 0$ for $|x_{Lap}| \leq \log 2$ and $c = -1$ otherwise.

We compare the NGCA method against stand-alone FastICA with two different index functions. Figure 2 shows boxplots and Figure 3 sample-wise comparison plots, over 100 samples, of the error criterion $\mathcal{E}(\widehat{\mathcal{I}}, \mathcal{I}) = m^{-1} \sum_{i=1}^{m} \|(I_d - P_{\mathcal{I}})\widehat{v}_i\|^2$, where $\{\widehat{v}_i\}_{i=1}^{m}$ is an

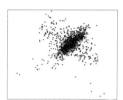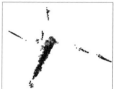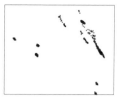

Figure 4: 2D projection of the "oil flow" (12-dimensional) data obtained by different algorithms, from left two right: PCA, Isomap, FastICA (tanh index), NGCA. In each case, the data was first projected in 3D using the respective methods, from which a 2D projection was chosen visually so as to yield the clearest cluster structure. Available label information was not used to determine the projections.

orthonormal basis of $\widehat{\mathcal{I}}$, I_d is the identity matrix, and $P_{\mathcal{I}}$ denotes the orthogonal projection on $\mathcal{I}$. In datasets (A),(B),(C), NGCA appears to be on par with the best FastICA method. As expected, the best index for FastICA is data-dependent: the 'tanh' index is more suited to the super-Gaussian data (B), while the 'pow3' index works best with the sub-Gaussian data (C) (although, in this case, FastICA with this index has a tendency to get caught in local minima, leading to a disastrous result for about 25% of the samples. Note that NGCA does *not* suffer from this problem). Finally, the advantage of the implicit index adaptation feature of NGCA can be clearly observed in the data set (D), which includes both sub- and super-Gaussian components. In this case, neither of the two FastICA index functions taken alone does well, and NGCA gives significantly lower error than either FastICA flavor.

Example of application for realistic data: visualization and clustering   We now give an example of application of NGCA to visualization and clustering of realistic data. We consider here "oil flow" data, which has been obtained by numerical simulation of a complex physical model. This data was already used before for testing techniques of dimension reduction [2]. The data is 12-dimensional and our goal is to visualize the data, and possibly exhibit a clustered structure. We compared results obtained with the NGCA methodology, regular PCA, FastICA with tanh index and Isomap. The results are shown on Figure 4. A 3D projection of the data was first computed using these methods, which was in turn projected in 2D to draw the figure; this last projection was chosen manually so as to make the cluster structure as visible as possible in each case. The NGCA result appears better with a clearer clustered structure appearing. This structure is only partly visible in the Isomap result; the NGCA method additionally has the advantage of a clear geometrical interpretation (linear orthogonal projection). Finally, datapoints in this dataset are distributed in 3 classes. This information was not used in the different procedures, but we can see *a posteriori* that only NGCA clearly separates the classes in distinct clusters. Clustering applications on other benchmark datasets is presented in the extended paper [3].

5   Conclusion

We proposed a new semi-parametric framework for constructing a linear projection to separate an uninteresting, possibly of large amplitude multivariate Gaussian 'noise' subspace from the 'signal-of-interest' subspace. We provide generic consistency results on how well the non-Gaussian directions can be identified (Theorem 1). Once the low-dimensional 'signal' part is extracted, we can use it for a variety of applications such as data visualization, clustering, denoising or classification.

Numerically we found comparable or superior performance to, e.g., FastICA in deflation mode as a generic representative of the family of PP algorithms. Note that in general, PP methods need to pre-specify a projection index with which they search non-Gaussian components. By contrast, an important advantage of our method is that we are able to simultaneously use several families of nonlinear functions; moreover, also inside a same function family we are able to use an entire range of parameters (such as frequency for Fourier functions). Thus, NGCA provides higher flexibility, and less restricting assumptions *a priori* on the data. In a sense, the functional indices that are the most relevant for the data at hand are automatically selected.

Future research will adapt the theory to simultaneously estimate the dimension of the non-Gaussian subspace. Extending the proposed framework to non-linear projection scenarios [4, 11, 10, 12, 1, 6] and to finding the most discriminative directions using labels are examples for which the current theory could be taken as a basis.

Acknowledgements: This work was supported in part by the PASCAL Network of Excellence (EU # 506778).

Proof of Proposition 1 Put $\alpha = \mathbb{E}\left[Xh(X)\right]$ and $\psi(x) = h(x) - \alpha^\top x$. Note that $\nabla\psi = \nabla h - \alpha$, hence $\beta(h) = \mathbb{E}\left[\nabla\psi(X)\right]$. Furthermore, it holds by change of variable that

$$\int \psi(x+u)p(x)dx = \int \psi(x)p(x-u)dx.$$

Under mild regularity conditions on $p(x)$ and $h(x)$, differentiating this with respect to u gives

$$\mathbb{E}\left[\nabla\psi(X)\right] = \int \nabla\psi(x)p(x)dx = -\int \psi(x)\nabla p(x)dx = -\mathbb{E}\left[\psi(X)\nabla\log p(X)\right],$$

where we have used $\nabla p(x) = \nabla\log p(x)\,p(x)$. Eq.(1) now implies $\nabla\log p(x) = \nabla\log g(Tx) - \Gamma^{-1}x$, hence

$$\beta(\psi) = -\mathbb{E}\left[\psi(X)\nabla\log g(TX)\right] + \mathbb{E}\left[\psi(X)\Gamma^{-1}X\right]$$

$$= -T^\top\mathbb{E}\left[\psi(X)\nabla g(TX)/g(TX)\right] + \Gamma^{-1}\mathbb{E}\left[Xh(X) - XX^\top\mathbb{E}\left[Xh(X)\right]\right].$$

The last term above vanishes because we assumed $\mathbb{E}\left[XX^\top\right] = I_d$. The first term belongs to $\mathcal{I}$ by definition. This concludes the proof. $\square$

References

[1] M. Belkin and P. Niyogi. Laplacian eigenmaps for dimensionality reduction and data representation. *Neural Computation*, 15(6):1373–1396, 2003.

[2] C.M. Bishop, M. Svensen and C.K.I. Wiliams. GTM: The generative topographic mapping. *Neural Computation*, 10(1):215–234, 1998.

[3] G. Blanchard, M. Sugiyama, M. Kawanabe, V. Spokoiny, K.-R. Müller. *In search of non-Gaussian components of a high-dimensional distribution.* Technical report of the Weierstrass Institute for Applied Analysis and Stochastics, 2006.

[4] T.F. Cox and M.A.A. Cox. *Multidimensional Scaling.* Chapman & Hall, London, 2001.

[5] J.H. Friedman and J.W. Tukey. A projection pursuit algorithm for exploratory data analysis. *IEEE Transactions on Computers*, 23(9):881–890, 1975.

[6] S. Harmeling, A. Ziehe, M. Kawanabe and K.-R. Müller. Kernel-based nonlinear blind source separation. *Neural Computation*, 15(5):1089–1124, 2003.

[7] P.J. Huber. Projection pursuit. *The Annals of Statistics*, 13:435–475, 1985.

[8] A. Hyvärinen. Fast and robust fixed-point algorithms for independent component analysis. *IEEE Transactions on Neural Networks*, 10(3):626–634, 1999.

[9] A. Hyvärinen, J. Karhunen and E. Oja. *Independent component analysis.* Wiley, 2001.

[10] S. Roweis and L. Saul. Nonlinear dimensionality reduction by locally linear embedding. *Science*, 290(5500):2323–2326, 2000.

[11] B. Schölkopf, A.J. Smola and K.–R. Müller. Nonlinear component analysis as a kernel Eigenvalue problem. *Neural Computation*, 10(5):1299–1319, 1998.

[12] J.B. Tenenbaum, V. de Silva and J.C. Langford. A global geometric framework for nonlinear dimensionality reduction. *Science*, 290(5500):2319–2323, 2000.

From Weighted Classification to Policy Search

D. Blatt
Department of Electrical Engineering
and Computer Science
University of Michigan
Ann Arbor, MI 48109-2122
dblatt@eecs.umich.edu

A. O. Hero
Department of Electrical Engineering
and Computer Science
University of Michigan
Ann Arbor, MI 48109-2122
hero@eecs.umich.edu

Abstract

This paper proposes an algorithm to convert a T-stage stochastic decision problem with a continuous state space to a sequence of supervised learning problems. The optimization problem associated with the trajectory tree and random trajectory methods of Kearns, Mansour, and Ng, 2000, is solved using the Gauss-Seidel method. The algorithm breaks a multi-stage reinforcement learning problem into a sequence of single-stage reinforcement learning subproblems, each of which is solved via an exact reduction to a weighted-classification problem that can be solved using off-the-self methods. Thus the algorithm converts a reinforcement learning problem into simpler supervised learning subproblems. It is shown that the method converges in a finite number of steps to a solution that cannot be further improved by componentwise optimization. The implication of the proposed algorithm is that a plethora of classification methods can be applied to find policies in the reinforcement learning problem.

1 Introduction

There has been increased interest in applying tools from supervised learning to problems in reinforcement learning. The goal is to leverage techniques and theoretical results from supervised learning for solving the more complex problem of reinforcement learning [3]. In [6] and [4], classification was incorporated into approximate policy iterations. In [2], regression and classification are used to perform dynamic programming. Bounds on the performance of a policy which is built from a sequence of classifiers were derived in [8] and [9].

Similar to [8], we adopt the generative model assumption of [5] and tackle the problem of finding good policies within an infinite class of policies, where performance is evaluated in terms of empirical averages over a set of trajectory trees. In [8] the T-step reinforcement learning problem was converted to a set of weighted classification problems by trying to fit the classifiers to the maximal path on the trajectory tree of the decision process.

In this paper we take a different approach. We show that while the task of finding the global optimum within a class of non-stationary policies may be overwhelming, the componen-twise search leads to single step reinforcement learning problems which can be reduced to a sequence of weighted classification problems. Our reduction is exact and is different from the one proposed in [8]; it gives more weight to regions of the state space in which the difference between the possible actions in terms of future reward is large, rather than giving more weight to regions in which the maximal future reward is large. The weighted classification problems can be solved by applying weights-sensitive classifiers or by further reducing the weighted classification problem to a standard classification problem using re-sampling methods (see [7], [1], and references therein for a description of both approaches). Based on this observation, an algorithm that converts the policy search problem into a sequence of weighted classification problems is given. It is shown that the algorithm converges in a finite number of steps to a solution, which cannot be further improved by changing the control of a single stage while holding the rest of the policy fixed.

2 Problem Formulation

The results are presented in the context of MDPs but can be applied to POMDPs and non-Markovian decision processes as well. Consider a T-step MDP $\mathcal{M} = \{\mathcal{S}, \mathcal{A}, D, P_{s,a}\}$, where $\mathcal{S}$ is a (possibly continuous) state space, $\mathcal{A} = \{0, \ldots, L-1\}$ is a finite set of possible actions, D is the distribution of the initial state, and $P_{s,a}$ is the distribution of the next state given that the current state is s and the action taken is a. The reward granted when taking action a at state s and making a transition to state s' is assumed to be a known deterministic and bounded function of s' denoted by $r : \mathcal{S} \rightarrow [-M, M]$. No generality is lost in specifying a known deterministic reward since it is possible to augment the state variable by an additional random component whose distribution depends on the previous state and action, and specify the function r to extract this random component. Denote by $S_0, S_1, \ldots, S_T$ the random state variables.

A non-stationary deterministic policy $\pi = (\pi_0, \pi_1, \ldots, \pi_{T-1})$ is a sequence of mappings $\pi_t : \mathcal{S} \rightarrow \mathcal{A}$, which are called controls. The control π_t specifies the action taken at time t as a function of the state at time t. The expected sum of rewards of a non-stationary deterministic policy π is given by

$$V(\pi) = \mathrm{E}_\pi \left\{ \sum_{t=1}^T r(S_t) \right\}, \tag{1}$$

where the expectation is taken with respect to the distribution over the random state variables induced by the policy π. We call $V(\pi)$ the value of policy π. Non-stationary deterministic policies are considered since the optimal policy for a finite horizon MDP is non-stationary and deterministic [10]. Usually the optimal policy is defined as the policy that maximizes the value conditioned on the initial state, i.e.,

$$V_\pi(s) = \mathrm{E}_\pi \left\{ \sum_{t=1}^T R(S_t) \,|\, S_0 = s \right\}, \tag{2}$$

for any realization s of S_0 [10]. The policy that maximizes the conditional value given each realization of the initial state also maximizes the value averaged over the initial state, and it is the unique maximizer if the distribution of the initial state D is positive over $\mathcal{S}$. Therefore, when optimizing over all possible policies, the maximization of (1) and (2) are equivalent. When optimizing (1) over a restricted class of policies, which does not contain the optimal policy, the distribution over the initial state specifies the importance of different regions of the state space in terms of the approximation error. For example, assigning high probability to a certain region of $\mathcal{S}$ will favor policies that well approximate the optimal policy over that region. Alternatively, maximizing (1) when D is a point mass at state s is equivalent to maximizing (2).

Following the generative model assumption of [5], the initial distribution D and the conditional distribution $P_{s,a}$ are unknown but it is possible to generate realization of the initial state according to D and the next state according to $P_{s,a}$ for arbitrary state-action pairs (s, a). Given the generative model, n trajectory trees are constructed in the following manner. The root of each tree is a realization of S_0 generated according to the distribution D. Given the realization of the initial state, realizations of the next state S_1 given the L possible actions, denoted by $S_1|a$, $a \in \mathcal{A}$, are generated. Note that this notation omits the dependence on the value of the initial state. Each of the L realizations of S_1 is now the root of the subtree. These iterations continue to generate a depth T tree. Denote by $S_t|i_0, i_1, \ldots, i_{t-1}$ the random variable generated at the node that follows the sequence of actions $i_0, i_1, \ldots, i_{t-1}$. Hence, each tree is constructed using a single call to the initial state generator and $L^T - 2$ calls to the next state generator.

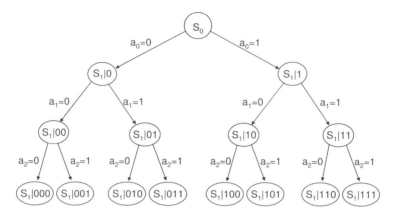

Figure 1: A binary trajectory tree.

Consider a class of policies Π, i.e., each element of Π is a sequence of T mappings from $\mathcal{S}$ to $\mathcal{A}$. It is possible to estimate the value of any policy in the class from the set of trajectory trees by simply averaging the sum of rewards on each tree along the path that agrees with the policy [5]. Denote by $\widehat{V}^i(\pi)$ the observed value on the i'th tree along the path that corresponds to the policy π. Then the value of the policy π is estimated by

$$\widehat{V}_n(\pi) = n^{-1} \sum_{i=1}^{n} \widehat{V}^i(\pi). \qquad (3)$$

In [5], the authors show that with high probability (over the data set) $\widehat{V}_n(\pi)$ converges uniformly to $V(\pi)$ (1) with rates that depend on the VC-dimension of the policy class. This result motivates the use of policies π with high $\widehat{V}_n(\pi)$, since with high probability these policies have high values of $V(\pi)$. In this paper, we consider the problem of finding policies that obtain high values of $\widehat{V}_n(\pi)$.

3 A Reduction From a Single Step Reinforcement Learning Problem to Weighted Classification

The building block of the proposed algorithm is an exact reduction from a single step reinforcement learning to a weighted classification problem. Consider the single step decision process. An initial state S_0 generated according to the distribution D is followed by one of L possible actions $A \in \{0, 1, \ldots, L-1\}$, which leads to a transition to state S_1 whose conditional distribution given the initial state is s and the action is a is given by $P_{s,a}$. Given a class of policies Π, where policy in Π is a map from $\mathcal{S}$ to $\mathcal{A}$, the goal is to find

$$\widehat{\pi} \in \arg \max_{\pi \in \Pi} \widehat{V}_n(\pi). \qquad (4)$$

In this single step problem the data are n realization of the random element $\{S_0, S_1|0, S_1|1, \ldots, S_1|L-1\}$. Denote the i'th realization by $\{s_0^i, s_1^i|0, s_1^i|1, \ldots, s_1^i|L-1\}$. In this case, $\widehat{V}_n(\pi)$ can be written explicitly by

$$\widehat{V}_n(\pi) = \mathrm{E}_n\left\{\sum_{l=0}^{L-1} r(S_1|l)I(\pi(S_0) = l)\right\}, \tag{5}$$

where for a function f, $\mathrm{E}_n\{f(S_0, S_1|0, S_1|1, \ldots, S_1|L-1)\}$ is its empirical expectation $n^{-1}\sum_{i=1}^n f(s_0^i, s_1^i|0, s_1^i|1, \ldots, s_1^i|L-1)$, and $I(\cdot)$ is the indicator function taking a value of one when its argument is true and zero otherwise.

The following proposition shows that the problem of maximizing the empirical reward (5) is equivalent to a weighted classification problem.

Proposition 1 *Given a class of policies Π and a set of n trajectory trees,*

$$\arg\max_{\pi\in\Pi} \mathrm{E}_n\left\{\sum_{l=0}^{L-1} r(S_1|l)I(\pi(S_0) = l)\right\}$$

$$= \arg\min_{\pi\in\Pi} \mathrm{E}_n\left\{\sum_{l=0}^{L-1}\left[\max_k r(S_1|k) - r(S_1|l)\right]I(\pi(S_0) = l)\right\}. \tag{6}$$

The proposition implies that the maximizer of the empirical reward over a class of policies is the output of an optimal weights dependent classifier for the data set:

$$\left\{\left(s_0^i, \arg\max_k r(s_1^i|k), w^i\right)\right\}_{i=1}^n,$$

where for each sample, the first argument is the example, the second is the label, and

$$w^i = \left[\max_k r(s_1^i|k) - r(s_1^i|0), \max_k r(s_1^i|k) - r(s_1^i|1), \ldots, \max_k r(s_1^i|k) - r(s_1^i|L-1)\right]$$

is the realization of the L costs of classifying example i to each of the possible labels. Note that the realizations of the costs are always non-negative and the cost of the correct classification ($\arg\max_k r(s_1^i|k)$) is always zero. The solution to the weighted classification problem is a map from $\mathcal{S}$ to $\mathcal{A}$ which minimizes the empirical weighted misclassification error (6). The proposition asserts that this mapping is also the control which maximizes the empirical reward (5).

Proof 1 *For all $j \in \{0, 1, \ldots, L-1\}$,*

$$\sum_{l=0}^{L-1} r(S_1|l)I(\pi(S_0) = l) = r(S_1|j) + (r(S_1|0) - r(S_1|j))I(\pi(s) = 0) + \tag{7}$$

$$(r(S_1|1) - r(S_1|j))I(\pi(s) = 1) + \ldots + (r(S_1|L-1) - r(S_1|j))I(\pi(s) = L-1).$$

In addition,

$$\mathrm{E}_n\left\{\sum_{l=0}^{L-1} r(S_1|l)I(\pi(S_0) = l)\right\} =$$

$$\mathrm{E}_n\left\{I(\arg\max_k r(S_1|k) = 0)\sum_{l=0}^{L-1} r(S_1|l)I(\pi(S_0) = l)\right\} +$$

$$\mathrm{E}_n \left\{ I(\arg\max_k r(S_1|k) = 1) \sum_{l=0}^{L-1} r(S_1|l) I(\pi(S_0) = l) \right\} + \ldots +$$

$$\mathrm{E}_n \left\{ I(\arg\max_k r(S_1|k) = L-1) \sum_{l=0}^{L-1} r(S_1|l) I(\pi(S_0) = l) \right\}.$$

Substituting (7) we obtain

$$\mathrm{E}_n \left\{ \sum_{l=0}^{L-1} r(S_1|l) I(\pi(S_0) = l) \right\} =$$

$$\sum_{j=0}^{L-1} \mathrm{E}_n \{ I(\arg\max_k r(S_1|k) = j)[r(S_1|j) -$$

$$(\max_k r(S_1|k) - r(S_1|0)) I(\pi(S_0) = 0) -$$

$$(\max_k r(S_1|k) - r(S_1|1)) I(\pi(S_0) = 1) - \ldots -$$

$$(\max_k r(S_1|k) - r(S_1|L-1)) I(\pi(S_0) = L-1)]\} =$$

$$\sum_{j=0}^{L-1} \mathrm{E}_n \left\{ I(\arg\max_k r(S_1|k) = j) r(S_1|j) \right\} -$$

$$\mathrm{E}_n \left\{ \sum_{l=0}^{L-1} \left[\max_k R(S_1|k) - R(S_1|l) \right] I(\pi(S_0) = l) \right\}$$

The term in the second to last line is independent of $\pi(s)$ and the result follows.

In the binary case, the optimization problem is

$$\arg\min_{\pi \in \Pi} \mathrm{E}_n \left\{ |r(S_1|0) - r(S_1|1)| I(\pi(S_0) \neq \arg\max_k r(S_1|k)) \right\},$$

i.e., the single step reinforcement learning problem reduces to the weighted classification problem with samples

$$\left\{ \left(s_0^i, \arg\max_{k \in \{0,1\}} r(s_1^i|k), |r(s_1^i|0) - r(s_1^i|1)| \right) \right\}_{i=1}^n,$$

where for each sample, the first argument is the example, the second is the label, and the third is a realization of the cost incurred when misclassifying the example. Note that this is different from the reduction in [8]. When applying the reduction in [8] to our single step problem the costs are taken to be $\max_{k \in \{0,1\}} r(s_1^i|k)$ rather than $|r(s_1^i|0) - r(s_1^i|1)|$. Setting the costs to $\max_{k \in \{0,1\}} r(s_1^i|k)$ instead of $|r(s_1^i|0) - r(s_1^i|1)|$ favors classifiers which perform well in regions where the maximal reward is large (regardless of the difference between the two actions) instead of regions where the difference between the rewards that result from the two actions is large. It is easy to set an example of a simple MDP and a restricted class of policies, which do not include the optimal policy, in which the classifier that minimizes the weighted misclassification problem with costs $\max_{k \in \{0,1\}} r(s_1^i|k)$ is not equivalent to the optimal policy. When using our reduction, they are always equivalent. On the other hand, in [8] the choice $\max_{k \in \{0,1\}} r(s_1^i|k)$ led to a bound on the performance of the policy in terms of the performance of the classifier. We do not pursue this type of bounds here since given the classifier, the performance of the resulting policy can be directly estimated from (5). Given a sequence of classifiers, the value of the induced sequence of controls (or policy) can be estimated directly by (3) with generalization guarantees provided by the bounds in [5]. In [2], a certain single step binary reinforcement learning problem is converted to weighted classification by averaging multiple realizations of the rewards under the two possible actions for each state. As seen here, this Monte Carlo approach is not necessary; it is sufficient to sample the rewards once for each state.

4 Finding Good Policies for a T-Step Markov Decision Processes By Solving a Sequence of Weighted Classification Problems

Given the class of policies Π, the algorithm updates the controls $\pi_0, \ldots, \pi_{T-1}$ one at a time in a cyclic manner while holding the rest constant. Each update is formulated as a single step reinforcement learning problem which is then converted to a weighted classification problem. In practice, if the weighted classification problem is only approximately solved, then the new control is accepted only if it leads to higher value of $\widehat{V}$. When updating π_t, the trees are pruned from the root to stage t by keeping only the branch which agrees with the controls $\pi_0, \pi_1, \ldots, \pi_{t-1}$. Then a single step reinforcement learning is formulated at time step t, where the realization of the reward which follows action $a \in \mathcal{A}$ at stage t is the immediate reward obtained at the state which follows action a plus the sum of rewards which are accumulated along the branch which agrees with the controls $\pi_{t+1}, \pi_{t+2}, \ldots, \pi_{T-1}$. The iterations end after the first complete cycle with no parameter modifications.

Note that when updating π_t, each tree contributes one realization of the state at time t. A result of the pruning process is that the ensemble of state realization are drawn from the distribution induced by the policy up to time $t - 1$. In other words, the algorithm relaxes the requirement in [2] to have access to a baseline distribution - a distribution over the states that is induced by a good policy. Our algorithm automatically generates samples from distributions that are induced by a sequence of monotonically improving policies.

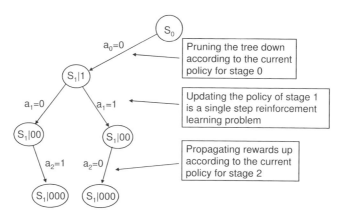

Figure 2: Updating π_1. In the example: pruning down according to $\pi_0(S_0) = 0$, propagating rewards up according to $\pi_2(S_2|00) = 1$, and $\pi_2(S_2|01) = 0$.

Proposition 2 *The algorithm converges after a finite number of iterations to a policy that cannot be further improved by changing one of the controls and holding the rest fixed.*

Proof 2 *Writing the empirical average sum of rewards $\widehat{V}_n(\pi)$ explicitly as*

$$\widehat{V}_n(\pi) = \mathrm{E}_n \left\{ \sum_{i_0,\ldots,i_{T-1} \in \mathcal{A}^T} I(\pi_0(S^0) = i_0) I(\pi_1(S^1|i^0) = i^1) \ldots \right.$$

144

$$I(\pi_{T-1}(S^{T-1}|i^0, i^1, \dots, i^{T-2}) = i^{T-1}) \sum_{t=1}^{T} r(S^t|i^0, i^1, \dots, i^{t-1})\Bigg\},$$

it can be seen that the algorithm is a Gauss-Seidel algorithm for maximizing $\widehat{V}_n(\pi)$, where, at each iteration, optimization of π_t is carried out at one of the stages t while keeping $\pi_{t'}$, $t' \neq t$ fixed. At each iteration the previous control is a valid solution and hence the objective function is non decreasing. Since $\widehat{V}_n(\pi)$ is evaluated using a finite number of trees, it can take only a finite set of values. Therefore, we must reach a cycle with no updates after a finite number of iterations. A cycle with no improvements implies that we cannot increase the empirical average sum of rewards by updating one of the π_t's.

5   Initialization

There are two possible initial policies that can be extracted from the set of trajectory trees. One possible initial policy is the myopic policy which is computed from the root of the tree downwards. Staring from the root, π_0 is found by solving the single stage reinforcement learning resulting from taking into account only the immediate reward at the next state. Once the weighted classification problem is solved the trees are pruned by following the action which agrees with π_0. The remaining realizations of state S_1 follow the distribution induced by the myopic control of the first stage. The process is continued to stage $T - 1$. The second possible initial policy is computed from the leaves backward to the root. Note that the distribution of the state at a leaf that is chosen at random is the distribution of the state when a randomized policy is used. Therefore, to find the best control at stage $T - 1$, given that the previous $T - 2$ controls choose random actions, we solve the weighted classification problem induced by considering all the realization of the state S_{T-1} from all the trees (these are not independent observations) or choose randomly one realization from each tree (these are independent realizations). Given the classifier, we use the equivalent control π_{T-1} to propagated the rewards up to the previous stage and solve the resulting weighted classification problem. This is carried out recursively up to the root of the tree.

6   Extensions

The results presented in this paper generalize to the non-Markovian setting as well. In particular, when the state space, action space, and the reward function depend on time, and the distribution over the next state depends on all past states and actions, we will be dealing with non-stationary deterministic policies $\pi = (\pi_0, \pi_1, \dots, \pi_{T-1})$; $\pi_t : S_0 \times A_0 \times \dots \times S_{t-1} \times A_{t-1} \times S_t \rightarrow A_t$, $t = 0, 1, \dots, T - 1$. POMDPs can be dealt with in terms of the belief states as a continuous state space MDP or as a non-Markovian process in which policies depend directly on all past observations.

While we focused on the trajectory tree method, the algorithm can be easily modified to solve the optimization problem associated with the random trajectory method [5] by adjusting the single step reinforcement learning reduction and the pruning method presented here.

7   Illustrative Example

The following example illustrates the aspects of the problem and the components of our solution. The simulated system is a two-step MDP, with continuous state space $S = [0, 1]$ and a binary action space $A = \{0, 1\}$. The distribution over the initial state is uniform. Given state s and action a the next state s' is generated by $s' = \mathrm{mod}(s + 0.33a + 0.1\mathrm{randn}, 1)$, where $\mathrm{mod}(x, 1)$ is the fraction part of x, and randn is a Gaussian random variable independent of the other variables in the problem. The reward function is $r(s) = s \sin(\pi s)$. We consider a class of policies parameterized by a continuous parameter: $\Pi = \{\pi(\cdot; \theta) | \theta = (\theta_0, \theta_1) \in [0, 2]^2\}$, where $\pi_i(s; \theta_i) = 1$ when $\theta_i \leq 1$ and $s > \theta_i$ or when $\theta_i > 1$ and $s < \theta_i - 1$ and zero otherwise, $i = 0, 1$.

In Figure 3 the objective function $\widehat{V}_n(\pi(\theta))$, estimated from $n = 20$ trees, is presented as a function of θ_0 and θ_1. The path taken by the algorithm supperimposed on the contour plot of $\widehat{V}_n(\pi(\theta))$ is also presented. Starting from the arbitrary point 0, the algorithm performs optimization with respect to one of the coordinates at a time and converges after 3 iterations.

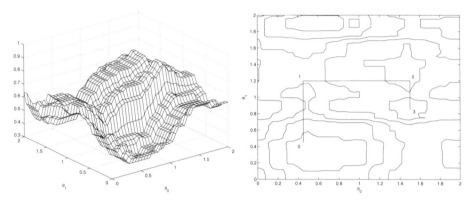

Figure 3: The objective function $\widehat{V}_n(\pi(\theta))$ and the path taken by the algorithm.

References

[1] N. Abe, B. Zadrozny, and J. Langford. An iterative method for multi-class cost-sensitive learning. In *Proceedings of the Tenth ACM SIGKDD International Conference on Knowledge Discovery and Data Mining*, pages 3–11, 2004.

[2] J. Bagnell, S. Kakade, A. Ng, and J. Schneider. Policy search by dynamic programming. In *Advances in Neural Information Processing Systems*, volume 16. MIT Press, 2003.

[3] A. G. Barto and T. G. Dietterich. Reinforcement learning and its relationship to supervised learning. In J. Si, A. Barto, W. Powell, and D. Wunsch, editors, *Handbook of learning and approximate dynamic programming*. John Wiley and Sons, Inc, 2004.

[4] A. Fern, S. Yoon, and R. Givan. Approximate policy iteration with a policy language bias. In *Advances in Neural Information Processing Systems*, volume 16, 2003.

[5] M. Kearns, Y. Mansour, and A. Ng. Approximate planning in large POMDPs via reusable trajectories. In *Advances in Neural Information Processing Systems*, volume 12. MIT Press, 2000.

[6] M. Lagoudakis and R. Parr. Reinforcement learning as classification: Leveraging modern classifiers. In *Proceedings of the Twentieth International Conference on Machine Learning*, 2003.

[7] J. Langford and A. Beygelzimer. Sensitive error correcting output codes. In *Proceedings of the 18th Annual Conference on Learning Theory*, pages 158–172, 2005.

[8] J. Langford and B. Zadrozny. Reducing T-step reinforcement learning to classification. http://hunch.net/~jl/projects/reductions/reductions.html, 2003.

[9] J. Langford and B. Zadrozny. Relating reinforcement learning performance to classification performance. In *Proceedings of the Twenty Second International Conference on Machine Learning*, pages 473–480, 2005.

[10] M. L. Puterman. *Markov decision processes: discrete stochastic dynamic programming*. John Wiley & Sons, Inc, 1994.

Correlated Topic Models

David M. Blei
Department of Computer Science
Princeton University

John D. Lafferty
School of Computer Science
Carnegie Mellon University

Abstract

Topic models, such as latent Dirichlet allocation (LDA), can be useful tools for the statistical analysis of document collections and other discrete data. The LDA model assumes that the words of each document arise from a mixture of *topics*, each of which is a distribution over the vocabulary. A limitation of LDA is the inability to model topic correlation even though, for example, a document about genetics is more likely to also be about disease than x-ray astronomy. This limitation stems from the use of the Dirichlet distribution to model the variability among the topic proportions. In this paper we develop the correlated topic model (CTM), where the topic proportions exhibit correlation via the logistic normal distribution [1]. We derive a mean-field variational inference algorithm for approximate posterior inference in this model, which is complicated by the fact that the logistic normal is not conjugate to the multinomial. The CTM gives a better fit than LDA on a collection of OCRed articles from the journal *Science*. Furthermore, the CTM provides a natural way of visualizing and exploring this and other unstructured data sets.

1 Introduction

The availability and use of unstructured historical collections of documents is rapidly growing. As one example, JSTOR (`www.jstor.org`) is a not-for-profit organization that maintains a large online scholarly journal archive obtained by running an optical character recognition engine over the original printed journals. JSTOR indexes the resulting text and provides online access to the scanned images of the original content through keyword search. This provides an extremely useful service to the scholarly community, with the collection comprising nearly three million published articles in a variety of fields.

The sheer size of this unstructured and noisy archive naturally suggests opportunities for the use of statistical modeling. For instance, a scholar in a narrow subdiscipline, searching for a particular research article, would certainly be interested to learn that the topic of that article is highly correlated with another topic that the researcher may not have known about, and that is not explicitly contained in the article. Alerted to the existence of this new related topic, the researcher could browse the collection in a topic-guided manner to begin to investigate connections to a previously unrecognized body of work. Since the archive comprises millions of articles spanning centuries of scholarly work, automated analysis is essential.

147

Several statistical models have recently been developed for automatically extracting the topical structure of large document collections. In technical terms, a topic model is a generative probabilistic model that uses a small number of distributions over a vocabulary to describe a document collection. When fit from data, these distributions often correspond to intuitive notions of topicality. In this work, we build upon the latent Dirichlet allocation (LDA) [4] model. LDA assumes that the words of each document arise from a mixture of topics. The topics are shared by all documents in the collection; the topic proportions are document-specific and randomly drawn from a Dirichlet distribution. LDA allows each document to exhibit multiple topics with different proportions, and it can thus capture the heterogeneity in grouped data that exhibit multiple latent patterns. Recent work has used LDA in more complicated document models [9, 11, 7], and in a variety of settings such as image processing [12], collaborative filtering [8], and the modeling of sequential data and user profiles [6]. Similar models were independently developed for disability survey data [5] and population genetics [10].

Our goal in this paper is to address a limitation of the topic models proposed to date: they fail to directly model correlation between topics. In many—indeed most—text corpora, it is natural to expect that subsets of the underlying latent topics will be highly correlated. In a corpus of scientific articles, for instance, an article about genetics may be likely to also be about health and disease, but unlikely to also be about x-ray astronomy. For the LDA model, this limitation stems from the independence assumptions implicit in the Dirichlet distribution on the topic proportions. Under a Dirichlet, the components of the proportions vector are nearly independent; this leads to the strong and unrealistic modeling assumption that the presence of one topic is not correlated with the presence of another.

In this paper we present the *correlated topic model* (CTM). The CTM uses an alternative, more flexible distribution for the topic proportions that allows for covariance structure among the components. This gives a more realistic model of latent topic structure where the presence of one latent topic may be correlated with the presence of another. In the following sections we develop the technical aspects of this model, and then demonstrate its potential for the applications envisioned above. We fit the model to a portion of the JSTOR archive of the journal *Science*. We demonstrate that the model gives a better fit than LDA, as measured by the accuracy of the predictive distributions over held out documents. Furthermore, we demonstrate qualitatively that the correlated topic model provides a natural way of visualizing and exploring such an unstructured collection of textual data.

2   The Correlated Topic Model

The key to the correlated topic model we propose is the logistic normal distribution [1]. The logistic normal is a distribution on the simplex that allows for a general pattern of variability between the components by transforming a multivariate normal random variable. Consider the *natural parameterization* of a K-dimensional multinomial distribution:

$$p(z \mid \eta) = \exp\{\eta^T z - a(\eta)\}. \tag{1}$$

The random variable Z can take on K values; it can be represented by a K-vector with exactly one component equal to one, denoting a value in $\{1, \ldots, K\}$. The cumulant generating function of the distribution is

$$a(\eta) = \log \left(\sum_{i=1}^{K} \exp\{\eta_i\} \right). \tag{2}$$

The mapping between the mean parameterization (i.e., the simplex) and the natural parameterization is given by

$$\eta_i = \log \theta_i / \theta_K. \tag{3}$$

Notice that this is not the minimal exponential family representation of the multinomial because multiple values of η can yield the same mean parameter.

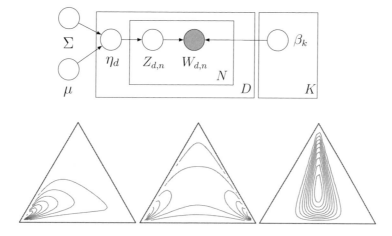

Figure 1: Top: Graphical model representation of the correlated topic model. The logistic normal distribution, used to model the latent topic proportions of a document, can represent correlations between topics that are impossible to capture using a single Dirichlet. Bottom: Example densities of the logistic normal on the 2-simplex. From left: diagonal covariance and nonzero-mean, negative correlation between components 1 and 2, positive correlation between components 1 and 2.

The logistic normal distribution assumes that η is normally distributed and then mapped to the simplex with the inverse of the mapping given in equation (3); that is, $f(\eta_i) = \exp \eta_i / \sum_j \exp \eta_j$. The logistic normal models correlations between components of the simplicial random variable through the covariance matrix of the normal distribution. The logistic normal was originally studied in the context of analyzing observed compositional data such as the proportions of minerals in geological samples. In this work, we extend its use to a hierarchical model where it describes the *latent* composition of topics associated with each document.

Let $\{\mu, \Sigma\}$ be a K-dimensional mean and covariance matrix, and let topics $\beta_{1:K}$ be K multinomials over a fixed word vocabulary. The correlated topic model assumes that an N-word document arises from the following generative process:

1. Draw $\eta \mid \{\mu, \Sigma\} \sim \mathcal{N}(\mu, \Sigma)$.
2. For $n \in \{1, \ldots, N\}$:
    (a) Draw topic assignment $Z_n \mid \eta$ from $\mathrm{Mult}(f(\eta))$.
    (b) Draw word $W_n \mid \{z_n, \beta_{1:K}\}$ from $\mathrm{Mult}(\beta_{z_n})$.

This process is identical to the generative process of LDA except that the topic proportions are drawn from a logistic normal rather than a Dirichlet. The model is shown as a directed graphical model in Figure 1.

The CTM is more expressive than LDA. The strong independence assumption imposed by the Dirichlet in LDA is not realistic when analyzing document collections, where one may find strong correlations between topics. The covariance matrix of the logistic normal in the CTM is introduced to model such correlations. In Section 3, we illustrate how the higher order structure given by the covariance can be used as an exploratory tool for better understanding and navigating a large corpus of documents. Moreover, modeling correlation can lead to better predictive distributions. In some settings, such as collaborative filtering, the goal is to predict unseen items conditional on a set of observations. An LDA model will predict words based on the latent topics that the observations suggest, but the CTM has the ability to predict items associated with *additional* topics that are correlated with the conditionally probable topics.

2.1 Posterior inference and parameter estimation

Posterior inference is the central challenge to using the CTM. The posterior distribution of the latent variables conditional on a document, $p(\eta, z_{1:N} \mid w_{1:N})$, is intractable to compute; once conditioned on some observations, the topic assignments $z_{1:N}$ and log proportions η are dependent. We make use of mean-field variational methods to efficiently obtain an approximation of this posterior distribution.

In brief, the strategy employed by mean-field variational methods is to form a factorized distribution of the latent variables, parameterized by free variables which are called the variational parameters. These parameters are fit so that the Kullback-Leibler (KL) divergence between the approximate and true posterior is small. For many problems this optimization problem is computationally manageable, while standard methods, such as Markov Chain Monte Carlo, are impractical. The tradeoff is that variational methods do not come with the same theoretical guarantees as simulation methods. See [13] for a modern review of variational methods for statistical inference.

In graphical models composed of conjugate-exponential family pairs and mixtures, the variational inference algorithm can be automatically derived from general principles [2, 14]. In the CTM, however, the logistic normal is *not* conjugate to the multinomial. We will therefore derive a variational inference algorithm by taking into account the special structure and distributions used by our model.

We begin by using Jensen's inequality to bound the log probability of a document:

$$\log p(w_{1:N} \mid \mu, \Sigma, \beta) \geq \tag{4}$$
$$\mathrm{E}_q\left[\log p(\eta \mid \mu, \Sigma)\right] + \sum_{n=1}^N (\mathrm{E}_q\left[\log p(z_n \mid \eta)\right] + \mathrm{E}_q\left[\log p(w_n \mid z_n, \beta)\right]) + \mathrm{H}\left(q\right),$$

where the expectation is taken with respect to a variational distribution of the latent variables, and $\mathrm{H}\left(q\right)$ denotes the entropy of that distribution. We use a factorized distribution:

$$q(\eta_{1:K}, z_{1:N} \mid \lambda_{1:K}, \nu_{1:K}^2, \phi_{1:N}) = \prod_{i=1}^K q(\eta_i \mid \lambda_i, \nu_i^2) \prod_{n=1}^N q(z_n \mid \phi_n). \tag{5}$$

The variational distributions of the discrete variables $z_{1:N}$ are specified by the K-dimensional multinomial parameters $\phi_{1:N}$. The variational distribution of the continuous variables $\eta_{1:K}$ are K independent univariate Gaussians $\{\lambda_i, \nu_i\}$. Since the variational parameters are fit using a *single* observed document $w_{1:N}$, there is no advantage in introducing a non-diagonal variational covariance matrix.

The nonconjugacy of the logistic normal leads to difficulty in computing the expected log probability of a topic assignment:

$$\mathrm{E}_q\left[\log p(z_n \mid \eta)\right] = \mathrm{E}_q\left[\eta^T z_n\right] - \mathrm{E}_q\left[\log(\sum_{i=1}^K \exp\{\eta_i\})\right]. \tag{6}$$

To preserve the lower bound on the log probability, we upper bound the log normalizer with a Taylor expansion,

$$\mathrm{E}_q\left[\log\left(\sum_{i=1}^K \exp\{\eta_i\}\right)\right] \leq \zeta^{-1}(\sum_{i=1}^K \mathrm{E}_q\left[\exp\{\eta_i\}\right]) - 1 + \log(\zeta), \tag{7}$$

where we have introduced a new variational parameter ζ. The expectation $\mathrm{E}_q\left[\exp\{\eta_i\}\right]$ is the mean of a log normal distribution with mean and variance obtained from the variational parameters $\{\lambda_i, \nu_i^2\}$; thus, $\mathrm{E}_q\left[\exp\{\eta_i\}\right] = \exp\{\lambda_i + \nu_i^2/2\}$ for $i \in \{1, \dots, K\}$.

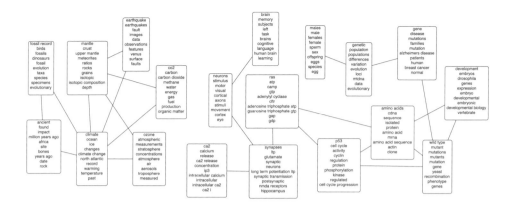

Figure 2: A portion of the topic graph learned from 16,351 OCR articles from *Science*. Each node represents a topic, and is labeled with the five most probable phrases from its distribution (phrases are found by the "turbo topics" method [3]). The interested reader can browse the full model at http://www.cs.cmu.edu/~lemur/science/.

Given a model $\{\beta_{1:K}, \mu, \Sigma\}$ and a document $w_{1:N}$, the variational inference algorithm optimizes equation (4) with respect to the variational parameters $\{\lambda_{1:K}, \nu_{1:K}, \phi_{1:N}, \zeta\}$. We use coordinate ascent, repeatedly optimizing with respect to each parameter while holding the others fixed. In variational inference for LDA, each coordinate can be optimized analytically. However, iterative methods are required for the CTM when optimizing for λ_i and ν_i^2. The details are given in Appendix A.

Given a collection of documents, we carry out parameter estimation in the correlated topic model by attempting to maximize the likelihood of a corpus of documents as a function of the topics $\beta_{1:K}$ and the multivariate Gaussian parameters $\{\mu, \Sigma\}$. We use variational expectation-maximization (EM), where we maximize the bound on the log probability of a collection given by summing equation (4) over the documents.

In the E-step, we maximize the bound with respect to the variational parameters by performing variational inference for each document. In the M-step, we maximize the bound with respect to the model parameters. This is maximum likelihood estimation of the topics and multivariate Gaussian using expected sufficient statistics, where the expectation is taken with respect to the variational distributions computed in the E-step. The E-step and M-step are repeated until the bound on the likelihood converges. In the experiments reported below, we run variational inference until the relative change in the probability bound of equation (4) is less than 10^{-6}, and run variational EM until the relative change in the likelihood bound is less than 10^{-5}.

3   Examples and Empirical Results: Modeling *Science*

In order to test and illustrate the correlated topic model, we estimated a 100-topic CTM on 16,351 *Science* articles spanning 1990 to 1999. We constructed a graph of the latent topics and the connections among them by examining the most probable words from each topic and the between-topic correlations. Part of this graph is illustrated in Figure 2. In this subgraph, there are three densely connected collections of topics: material science, geology, and cell biology. Furthermore, an estimated CTM can be used to explore otherwise unstructured observed documents. In Figure 4, we list articles that are assigned to the cognitive science topic and articles that are assigned to both the cog-

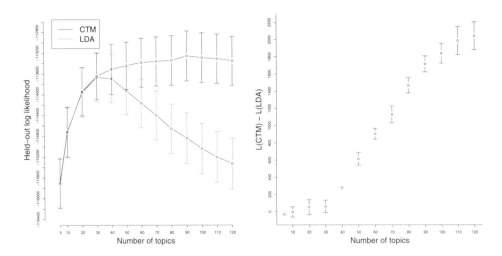

Figure 3: (L) The average held-out probability; CTM supports more topics than LDA. See figure at right for the standard error of the difference. (R) The log odds ratio of the held-out probability. Positive numbers indicate a better fit by the correlated topic model.

nitive science and visual neuroscience topics. The interested reader is invited to visit http://www.cs.cmu.edu/~lemur/science/ to interactively explore this model, including the topics, their connections, and the articles that exhibit them.

We compared the CTM to LDA by fitting a smaller collection of articles to models of varying numbers of topics. This collection contains the 1,452 documents from 1960; we used a vocabulary of 5,612 words after pruning common function words and terms that occur once in the collection. Using ten-fold cross validation, we computed the log probability of the held-out data given a model estimated from the remaining data. A better model of the document collection will assign higher probability to the held out data. To avoid comparing bounds, we used importance sampling to compute the log probability of a document where the fitted variational distribution is the proposal.

Figure 3 illustrates the average held out log probability for each model and the average difference between them. The CTM provides a better fit than LDA and supports more topics; the likelihood for LDA peaks near 30 topics while the likelihood for the CTM peaks close to 90 topics. The means and standard errors of the *difference* in log-likelihood of the models is shown at right; this indicates that the CTM always gives a better fit.

Another quantitative evaluation of the relative strengths of LDA and the CTM is how well the models predict the remaining words after observing a portion of the document. Suppose we observe words $w_{1:P}$ from a document and are interested in which model provides a better predictive distribution $p(w \mid w_{1:P})$ of the remaining words. To compare these distributions, we use *perplexity*, which can be thought of as the effective number of equally likely words according to the model. Mathematically, the perplexity of a word distribution is defined as the inverse of the per-word geometric average of the probability of the observations,

$$\text{Perp}(\Phi) \;=\; \left(\prod_{d=1}^{D} \prod_{i=P+1}^{N_d} p(w_i \mid \Phi, w_{1:P}) \right)^{\frac{-1}{\sum_{d=1}^{D}(N_d - P)}},$$

where Φ denotes the model parameters of an LDA or CTM model. Note that lower numbers denote more predictive power.

The plot in Figure 4 compares the predictive perplexity under LDA and the CTM. When a

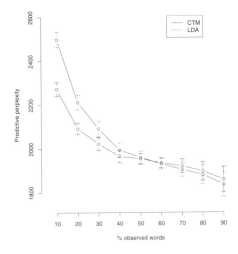

Top Articles with
{brain, memory, human, visual, cognitive}

(1) Separate Neural Bases of Two Fundamental Memory
    Processes in the Human Medial Temporal Lobe
(2) Inattentional Blindness Versus Inattentional Amnesia for
    Fixated but Ignored Words
(3) Making Memories: Brain Activity that Predicts How Well
    Visual Experience Will be Remembered
(4) The Learning of Categories: Parallel Brain Systems for
    Item Memory and Category Knowledge
(5) Brain Activation Modulated by Sentence Comprehension

Top Articles with
{brain, memory, human, visual, cognitive} and
{computer, data, information, problem, systems}

(1) A Head for Figures
(2) Sources of Mathematical Thinking: Behavioral and Brain
    Imaging Evidence
(3) Natural Language Processing
(4) A Romance Blossoms Between Gray Matter and Silicon
(5) Computer Vision

Figure 4: (Left) Exploring a collection through its topics. (Right) Predictive perplexity for partially observed held-out documents from the 1960 *Science* corpus.

small number of words have been observed, there is less uncertainty about the remaining words under the CTM than under LDA—the perplexity is reduced by nearly 200 words, or roughly 10%. The reason is that after seeing a few words in one topic, the CTM uses topic correlation to infer that words in a related topic may also be probable. In contrast, LDA cannot predict the remaining words as well until a large portion of the document as been observed so that all of its topics are represented.

Acknowledgments Research supported in part by NSF grants IIS-0312814 and IIS-0427206 and by the DARPA CALO project.

References

[1] J. Aitchison. The statistical analysis of compositional data. *Journal of the Royal Statistical Society, Series B*, 44(2):139–177, 1982.

[2] C. Bishop, D. Spiegelhalter, and J. Winn. VIBES: A variational inference engine for Bayesian networks. In *NIPS 15*, pages 777–784. Cambridge, MA, 2003.

[3] D. Blei, J. Lafferty, C. Genovese, and L. Wasserman. Turbo topics. In progress, 2006.

[4] D. Blei, A. Ng, and M. Jordan. Latent Dirichlet allocation. *Journal of Machine Learning Research*, 3:993–1022, January 2003.

[5] E. Erosheva. *Grade of membership and latent structure models with application to disability survey data*. PhD thesis, Carnegie Mellon University, Department of Statistics, 2002.

[6] M. Girolami and A. Kaban. Simplicial mixtures of Markov chains: Distributed modelling of dynamic user profiles. In *NIPS 16*, pages 9–16, 2004.

[7] T. Griffiths, M. Steyvers, D. Blei, and J. Tenenbaum. Integrating topics and syntax. In *Advances in Neural Information Processing Systems 17*, 2005.

[8] B. Marlin. Collaborative filtering: A machine learning perspective. Master's thesis, University of Toronto, 2004.

[9] A. McCallum, A. Corrada-Emmanuel, and X. Wang. The author-recipient-topic model for topic and role discovery in social networks. 2004.

[10] J. Pritchard, M. Stephens, and P. Donnelly. Inference of population structure using multilocus genotype data. *Genetics*, 155:945–959, June 2000.

[11] M. Rosen-Zvi, T. Griffiths, M. Steyvers, and P. Smith. In *UAI '04: Proceedings of the 20th Conference on Uncertainty in Artificial Intelligence*, pages 487–494.

[12] J. Sivic, B. Rusell, A. Efros, A. Zisserman, and W. Freeman. Discovering object categories in image collections. Technical report, CSAIL, MIT, 2005.

[13] M. Wainwright and M. Jordan. A variational principle for graphical models. In *New Directions in Statistical Signal Processing*, chapter 11. MIT Press, 2005.

[14] E. Xing, M. Jordan, and S. Russell. A generalized mean field algorithm for variational inference in exponential families. In *Proceedings of UAI*, 2003.

A Variational Inference

We describe a coordinate ascent optimization algorithm for the likelihood bound in equation (4) with respect to the variational parameters.

The first term of equation (4) is

$$E_q \left[\log p(\eta \mid \mu, \Sigma) \right] = (1/2) \log |\Sigma^{-1}| - (K/2) \log 2\pi - (1/2) E_q \left[(\eta - \mu)^T \Sigma^{-1} (\eta - \mu) \right], \tag{8}$$

where

$$E_q \left[(\eta - \mu)^T \Sigma^{-1} (\eta - \mu) \right] = \mathrm{Tr}(\mathrm{diag}(\nu^2) \Sigma^{-1}) + (\lambda - \mu)^T \Sigma^{-1} (\lambda - \mu). \tag{9}$$

The second term of equation (4), using the additional bound in equation (7), is

$$E_q \left[\log p(z_n \mid \eta) \right] = \sum_{i=1}^{K} \lambda_i \phi_{n,i} - \zeta^{-1} \left(\sum_{i=1}^{K} \exp\{\lambda_i + \nu_i^2/2\} \right) + 1 - \log \zeta. \tag{10}$$

The third term of equation (4) is

$$E_q \left[\log p(w_n \mid z_n, \beta) \right] = \sum_{i=1}^{K} \phi_{n,i} \log \beta_{i,w_n}. \tag{11}$$

Finally, the fourth term is the entropy of the variational distribution:

$$\sum_{i=1}^{K} \tfrac{1}{2} (\log \nu_i^2 + \log 2\pi + 1) - \sum_{n=1}^{N} \sum_{i=1}^{k} \phi_{n,i} \log \phi_{n,i}. \tag{12}$$

We maximize the bound in equation (4) with respect to the variational parameters $\lambda_{1:K}$, $\nu_{1:K}$, $\phi_{1:N}$, and ζ. We use a coordinate ascent algorithm, iteratively maximizing the bound with respect to each parameter.

First, we maximize equation (4) with respect to ζ, using the second bound in equation (7). The derivative with respect to ζ is

$$f'(\zeta) = N \left(\zeta^{-2} \left(\sum_{i=1}^{K} \exp\{\lambda_i + \nu_i^2/2\} \right) - \zeta^{-1} \right), \tag{13}$$

which has a maximum at

$$\hat{\zeta} = \sum_{i=1}^{K} \exp\{\lambda_i + \nu_i^2/2\}. \tag{14}$$

Second, we maximize with respect to ϕ_n. This yields a maximum at

$$\hat{\phi}_{n,i} \propto \exp\{\lambda_i\} \beta_{i,w_n}, \quad i \in \{1, \dots, K\}. \tag{15}$$

Third, we maximize with respect to λ_i. Since equation (4) is not amenable to analytic maximization, we use a conjugate gradient algorithm with derivative

$$dL/d\lambda = -\Sigma^{-1}(\lambda - \mu) + \sum_{n=1}^{N} \phi_{n,1:K} - (N/\zeta) \exp\{\lambda + \nu^2/2\}. \tag{16}$$

Finally, we maximize with respect to ν_i^2. Again, there is no analytic solution. We use Newton's method for each coordinate, constrained such that $\nu_i > 0$:

$$dL/d\nu_i^2 = -\Sigma_{ii}^{-1}/2 - N/2\zeta \exp\{\lambda + \nu_i^2/2\} + 1/(2\nu_i^2). \tag{17}$$

Iterating between these optimizations defines a coordinate ascent algorithm on equation (4).

Saliency Based on Information Maximization

Neil D.B. Bruce and John K. Tsotsos
Department of Computer Science and Centre for Vision Research
York University, Toronto, ON, M2N 5X8
{neil,tsotsos}@cs.yorku.ca

Abstract

A model of bottom-up overt attention is proposed based on the principle of maximizing information sampled from a scene. The proposed operation is based on Shannon's self-information measure and is achieved in a neural circuit, which is demonstrated as having close ties with the circuitry existent in the primate visual cortex. It is further shown that the proposed saliency measure may be extended to address issues that currently elude explanation in the domain of saliency based models. Results on natural images are compared with experimental eye tracking data revealing the efficacy of the model in predicting the deployment of overt attention as compared with existing efforts.

1 Introduction

There has long been interest in the nature of eye movements and fixation behavior following early studies by Buswell [1] and Yarbus [2]. However, a complete description of the mechanisms underlying these peculiar fixation patterns remains elusive. This is further complicated by the fact that task demands and contextual knowledge factor heavily in how sampling of visual content proceeds.

Current bottom-up models of attention posit that *saliency* is the impetus for selection of fixation points. Each model differs in its definition of saliency. In perhaps the most popular model of bottom-up attention, saliency is based on centre-surround contrast of units modeled on known properties of primary visual cortical cells [3]. In other efforts, saliency is defined by more *ad hoc* quantities having less connection to biology [4]. In this paper, we explore the notion that *information* is the driving force behind attentive sampling.

The application of information theory in this context is not in itself novel. There exist several previous efforts that define saliency based on Shannon entropy of image content defined on a local neighborhood [5, 6, 7, 8]. The model presented in this work is based on the closely related quantity of self-information [9]. In section 2.2 we discuss differences between entropy and self-information in this context, including why self-information may present a more appropriate metric than entropy in this domain. That said, contributions of this paper are as follows:

1. A bottom-up model of overt attention with selection based on the self-information of local image content.

2. A qualitative and quantitative comparison of predictions of the model with human

eye tracking data, contrasted against the model of Itti and Koch [3].

3. Demonstration that the model is neurally plausible via implementation based on a neural circuit resembling circuitry involved in early visual processing in primates.

4. Discussion of how the proposal generalizes to address issues that deny explanation by existing saliency based attention models.

2 The Proposed Saliency Measure

There exists much evidence indicating that the primate visual system is built on the principle of establishing a sparse representation of image statistics. In the most prominent of such studies, it was demonstrated that learning a sparse code for natural image statistics results in the emergence of simple-cell receptive fields similar to those appearing in the primary visual cortex of primates [10, 11]. The apparent benefit of such a representation comes from the fact that a sparse representation allows certain independence assumptions with regard to neural firing. This issue becomes important in evaluating the likelihood of a set of local image statistics and is elaborated on later in this section.

In this paper, saliency is determined by quantifying the self-information of each local image patch. Even for a very small image patch, the probability distribution resides in a very high dimensional space. There is insufficient data in a single image to produce a reasonable estimate of the probability distribution. For this reason, a representation based on independent components is employed for the independence assumption it affords. ICA is performed on a large sample of 7x7 RGB patches drawn from natural images to determine a suitable basis. For a given image, an estimate of the distribution of each basis coefficient is learned across the entire image through non-parametric density estimation. The probability of observing the RGB values corresponding to a patch centred at any image location may then be evaluated by independently considering the likelihood of each corresponding basis coefficient. The product of such likelihoods yields the joint likelihood of the entire set of basis coefficients. Given the basis determined by ICA, the preceding computation may be realized entirely in the context of a biologically plausible neural circuit. The overall architecture is depicted in figure 1. Details of each of the aforesaid model components including the details of the neural circuit are as follows:

Projection into independent component space provides, for each local neighborhood of the image, a vector w consisting of N variables w_i with values v_i. Each w_i specifies the contribution of a particular basis function to the representation of the local neighborhood. As mentioned, these basis functions, learned from statistical regularities observed in a large set of natural images show remarkable similarity to V1 cells [10, 11]. The ICA projection then allows a representation w, in which the components w_i are as independent as possible. For further details on the ICA projection of local image statistics see [12]. In this paper, we propose that salience may be defined based on a strategy for maximum information sampling. In particular, Shannon's self-information measure [9], $-log(p(x))$, applied to the joint likelihood of statistics in a local neighborhood decribed by w, provides an appropriate transformation between probability and the degree of information inherent in the local statistics. It is in computing the observation likelihood that a sparse representation is instrumental: Consider the probability density function $p(w_1 = v_1, w_2 = v_2, ..., w_n = v_n)$ which quantifies the likelihood of observing the local statistics with values $v_1, ..., v_n$ within a particular context. An appropriate context may include a larger area encompassing the local neigbourhood described by w, or the entire scene in question. The presumed independence of the ICA decomposition means that $p(w_1 = v_1, w_2 = v_2, ..., w_n = v_n) = \prod_{i=1}^{n} p(w_i = v_i)$. Thus, a sparse representation allows the estimation of the n-dimensional space described by w to be derived from n one dimensional probability density functions. Evaluating $p(w_1 = v_1, w_2 = v_2, ..., w_n = v_n)$ requires considering the distribution of values taken on by each w_i in a more global context. In practice, this might be derived on the basis of a nonparametric or histogram density estimate. In the section that follows, we demonstrate that an operation equivalent to a non-parametric density estimate may be achieved using a suitable neural circuit.

2.1 Likelihood Estimation in A Neural Circuit

In the following formulation, we assume an estimate of the likelihood of the components of w based on a Gaussian kernel density estimate. Any other choice of kernel may be substituted, with a Gaussian window chosen only for its common use in density estimation and without loss of generality.

Let $w_{i,j,k}$ denote the set of independent coefficients based on the neighborhood centered at j, k. An estimate of $p(w_{i,j,k} = v_{i,j,k})$ based on a Gaussian window is given by:

$$\frac{1}{\sigma\sqrt{2\pi}} \sum_{\forall s,t \in \Psi} \omega(s,t) e^{-(v_{i,j,k} - v_{i,s,t})^2 / 2\sigma^2} \tag{1}$$

with $\sum_{s,t} \omega(s,t) = 1$ where Ψ is the context on which the probability estimate of the coefficients of ω is based. $\omega(s,t)$ describes the degree to which the coefficient ω at coordinates s, t contributes to the probability estimate. On the basis of the form given in equation 1 it is evident that this operation may equivalently be implemented by the neural circuit depicted in figure 2. Figure 2 demonstrates only coefficients derived from a horizontal cross-section. The two dimensional case is analogous with parameters varying in i, j, and k dimensions. K consists of the Kernel function employed for density estimation. In our case this is a Gaussian of the form $\frac{1}{\sigma\sqrt{2\pi}} e^{-x^2/2\sigma^2}$. $\omega(s,t)$ is encoded based on the weight of connections to K. As $x = v_{i,j,k} - v_{i,s,t}$ the output of this operation encodes the impact of the Kernel function with mean $v_{i,s,t}$ on the value of $p(w_{i,j,k} = v_{i,j,k})$. Coefficients at the input layer correspond to coefficients of v. The logarithmic operator at the final stage might also be placed before the product on each incoming connection, with the product then becoming a summation. It is interesting to note that the structure of this circuit at the level of within feature spatial competition is remarkably similar to the standard feedforward model of lateral inhibition, a ubiquitous operation along the visual pathways thought to play a chief role in attentional processing [14]. The similarity between independent components and V1 cells, in conjunction with the aforementioned consideration lends credibility to the proposal that *information* may contribute to driving overt attentional selection.

One aspect lacking from the preceding description is that the saliency map fails to take into account the dropoff in visual acuity moving peripherally from the fovea. In some instances the maximum information accommodating for visual acuity may correspond to the center of a cluster of salient items, rather than centered on one such item. For this reason, the resulting saliency map is convolved with a Gaussian with parameters chosen to correspond approximately to the dropoff in visual acuity observed in the human visual system.

2.2 Self-Information versus Entropy

It is important to distinguish between self-information and entropy since these terms are often confused. The difference is subtle but important on two fronts. The first consideration lies in the expected behavior in *popout* paradigms and the second in the neural circuitry involved.

Let $X = [x_1, x_2, ..., x_n]$ denote a vector of RGB values corresponding to image patch X, and D a probability density function describing the distribution of some feature set over X. For example, D might correspond to a histogram estimate of intensity values within X or the relative contribution of different orientations within a local neighborhood situated on the boundary of an object silhouette [6]. Assuming an estimate of D based on N

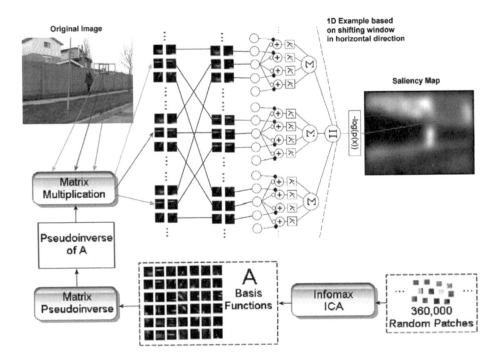

Figure 1: The framework that achieves the desired information measure. Shown is the computation corresponding to three horizontally adjacent neighbourhoods with flow through the network indicated by the orange, purple, and cyan windows and connections. The connections shown facilitate computation of the information measure corresponding to the pixel centered in the purple window. The network architecture produces this measure on the basis of evaluating the probability of these coefficients with consideration to the values of such coefficients in neighbouring regions.

bins, the entropy of D is given by: $-\sum_{i=1}^{N} D_i log(D_i)$. In this example, entropy characterizes the extent to which the feature(s) characterized by D are *uniformly* distributed on X. Self-information in the proposed saliency measure is given by $-log(p(X))$. That is, Self-information characterizes the raw likelihood of the specific n-dimensional vector of RGB values given by X. $p(X)$ in this case is based on observing a number of n-dimensional feature vectors based on patches drawn from the area surrounding X. Thus, $p(X)$ characterizes the raw likelihood of observing X based on its surround and $-log(p(X))$ becomes closer to a measure of local contrast whereas entropy as defined in the usual manner is closer to a measure of local activity. The importance of this distinction is evident in considering figure 3. Figure 3 depicts a variety of candles of varying orientation, and color. There is a tendency to fixate the empty region on the left, which is the location of lowest entropy in the image. In contrast, this region receives the highest confidence from the algorithm proposed in this paper as it is highly informative in the context of this image. In classic popout experiments, a vertical line among horizontal lines presents a highly salient target. The same vertical line among many lines of random orientations is not, although the entropy associated with the second scenario is much greater.

With regard to the neural circuitry involved, we have demonstrated that self-information may be computed using a neural circuit in the absence of a representation of the entire probability distribution. Whether an equivalent operation may be achieved in a biologically plausible manner for the computation of entropy remains to be established.

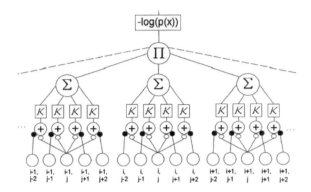

Figure 2: A 1D depiction of the neural architecture that computes the self-information of a set of local statistics. The operation is equivalent to a Kernel density estimate. Coefficients correspond to subscripts of $v_{i,j,k}$. The small black circles indicate an inhibitory relationship and the small white circles an excitatory relationship

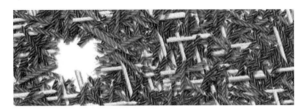

Figure 3: An image that highlights the difference between entropy and self-information. Fixation invariably falls on the empty patch, the locus of minimum entropy in orientation and color but maximum in self-information when the surrounding context is considered.

3 Experimental Validation

The following section evaluates the output of the proposed algorithm as compared with the bottom-up model of Itti and Koch [3]. The model of Itti and Koch is perhaps the most popular model of saliency based attention and currently appears to be the yardstick against which other models are measured.

3.1 Experimental eye tracking data

The data that forms the basis for performance evaluation is derived from eye tracking experiments performed while subjects observed 120 different color images. Images were presented in random order for 4 seconds each with a mask between each pair of images. Subjects were positioned 0.75m from a 21 inch CRT monitor and given no particular instructions except to observe the images. Images consist of a variety of indoor and outdoor scenes, some with very salient items, others with no particular regions of interest. The eye tracking apparatus consisted of a standard non head-mounted device. The parameters of the setup are intended to quantify salience in a general sense based on stimuli that one might expect to encounter in a typical urban environment. Data was collected from 20 different subjects for the full set of 120 images.

The issue of comparing between the output of a particular algorithm, and the eye tracking data is non-trivial. Previous efforts have selected a number of fixation points based on the saliency map, and compared these with the experimental fixation points derived from a small number of subjects and images (7 subjects and 15 images in a recent effort [4]). There are a variety of methodological issues associated with such a representation. The most important such consideration is that the representation of perceptual importance is typically based on a saliency map. Observing the output of an algorithm that selects fixation points based on the underlying saliency map obscures observation of the degree to which the saliency maps predict important and unimportant content and in particular, ignores confidence away from highly salient regions. Secondly, it is not clear how many fixation points should be selected. Choosing this value based on the experimental data will bias output based on information pertaining to the content of the image and may produce artificially good results.

The preceding discussion is intended to motivate the fact that selecting discrete fixation co-ordinates based on the saliency map for comparison may not present the most appropriate representation to use for performance evaluation. In this effort, we consider two different measures of performance. Qualitative comparison is based on the representation proposed in [16]. In this representation, a fixation density map is produced for each image based on all fixation points, and subjects. Given a fixation point, one might consider how the image under consideration is sampled by the human visual system as photoreceptor density drops steeply moving peripherally from the centre of the fovea. This dropoff may be modeled based on a 2D Gaussian distribution with appropriately chosen parameters, and centred on the measured fixation point. A continuous fixation density map may be derived for a particular image based on the sum of all 2D Gaussians corresponding to each fixation point, from each subject. The density map then comprises a measure of the extent to which each pixel of the image is sampled on average by a human observer based on observed fixations. This affords a representation for which similarity to a saliency map may be considered at a glance. Quantitative performance evaluation is achieved based on the measure proposed in [15]. The saliency maps produced by each algorithm are treated as binary classifiers for fixation versus non-fixation points. The choice of several different thresholds and assessment of performance in predicting fixated versus not fixated pixel locations allows an ROC curve to be produced for each algorithm.

3.2 Experimental Results

Figure 4 affords a qualitative comparison of the output of the proposed model with the experimental eye tracking data for a variety of images. Also depicted is the output of the Itti and Koch algorithm for comparison.

In the implementation results shown, the ICA basis set was learned from a set of 360,000 7x7x3 image patches from 3600 natural images using the Lee et al. extended infomax algorithm [17]. Processed images are 340 by 255 pixels. Ψ consists of the entire extent of the image and $\omega(s,t) = \frac{1}{p} \forall s,t$ with p the number of pixels in the image. One might make a variety of selections for these variables based on arguments related to the human visual system, or based on performance. In our case, the values have been chosen on the basis of simplicity and do not appear to dramatically affect the predictive capacity of the model in the simulation results. In particular, we wished to avoid tuning these parameters to the available data set. Future work may include a closer look at some of the parameters involved in order to determine the most appropriate choices. The ROC curves appearing in figure 5 give some sense of the efficacy of the model in predicting which regions of a scene human observers tend to fixate. As may be observed, the predictive capacity of the model is on par with the approach of Itti and Koch. Encouraging is the fact that similar performance is achieved using a method derived from first principles, and with no parameter tuning or *ad hoc* design choices.

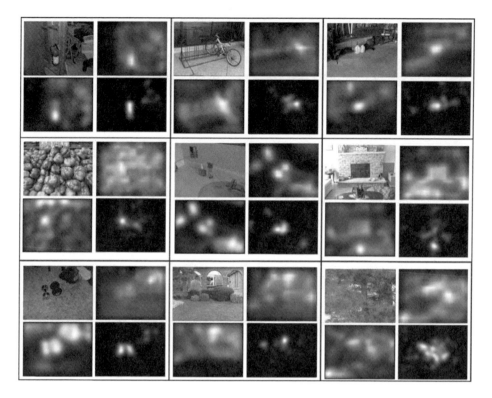

Figure 4: Results for qualitative comparison. Within each boxed region defined by solid lines: (Top Left) Original Image (Top Right) Saliency map produced by Itti + Koch algorithm. (Bottom Left) Saliency map based on information maximization. (Bottom Right) Fixation density map based on experimental human eye tracking data.

4 On Biological Plausibility

Although the proposed approach, along with the model of Itti and Koch describe saliency on the basis of a single topographical saliency map, there is mounting evidence that saliency in the primate brain is represented at several levels based on a hierarchical representation [18] of visual content. The proposed approach may accommodate such a configuration with the single necessary condition being a sparse representation at each layer.

As we have described in section 2, there is evidence that suggests the possibility that the primate visual system may consist of a multi-layer sparse coding architecture [10, 11]. The proposed algorithm quantifies information on the basis of a neural circuit, on units with response properties corresponding to neurons appearing in the primary visual cortex. However, given an analogous representation corresponding to higher visual areas that encode form, depth, convexity etc. the proposed method may be employed without any modification. Since the *popout* of features can occur on the basis of more complex properties such as a convex surface among concave surfaces [19], this is perhaps the next stage in a system that encodes saliency in the same manner as primates. Given a multi-layer architecture, the mechanism for selecting the locus of attention becomes less clear. In the model of Itti and Koch, a multi-layer winner-take-all network acts directly on the saliency map and there is no hierarchical representation of image content. There are however attention models that subscribe to a distributed representation of saliency (e.g. [20]), that may implement attentional selection with the proposed neural circuit encoding saliency at each layer.

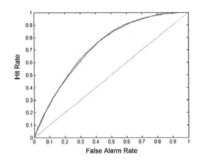

Figure 5: ROC curves for Self-information (blue) and Itti and Koch (red) saliency maps. Area under curves is 0.7288 and 0.7277 respectively.

5   Conclusion

We have described a strategy that predicts human attentional deployment on the principle of maximizing information sampled from a scene. Although no computational machinery is included strictly on the basis of biological plausibility, nevertheless the formulation results in an implementation based on a neurally plausible circuit acting on units that resemble those that facilitate early visual processing in primates. Comparison with an existing attention model reveals the efficacy of the proposed model in predicting salient image content. Finally, we demonstrate that the proposal might be generalized to facilitate selection based on high-level features provided an appropriate sparse representation is available.

References

[1]   G.T. Buswell, How people look at pictures. Chicago: The University of Chicago Press.

[2]   A. Yarbus, Eye movements and vision. New York: Plenum Press.

[3]   L. Itti, C. Koch, E. Niebur, IEEE T PAMI, 11:1254-1259, 1998.

[4]   C. M. Privitera and L.W. Stark, IEEE T PAMI 22:970-981, 2000.

[5]   F. Fritz, C. Seifert, L. Paletta, H. Bischof, Proc. WAPCV, Graz, Austria, 2004.

[6]   L.W. Renninger, J. Coughlan, P. Verghese, J. Malik, Proceedings NIPS 17, Vancouver, 2004.

[7]   T. Kadir, M. Brady, IJCV 45(2):83-105, 2001.

[8]   T.S. Lee, S. Yu, Advances in NIPS 12:834-840 , Ed. S.A. Solla, T.K. Leen, K. Muller, MIT Press.

[9]   C. E. Shannon, The Bell Systems Technical Journal, 27:93-154, 1948.

[10]   D.J. Field, and B. A. Olshausen, Nature 381:607-609, 1996.

[11]   A.J. Bell, T.J. Sejnowski, Vision Research 37:3327-3338, 1997.

[12]   N. Bruce, Neurocomputing, 65-66:125-133, 2005.

[13]   P. Comon, Signal Processing 36(3):287-314, 1994.

[14]   M.W. Cannon and S.C. Fullenkamp, Vision Research 36(8):1115-1125, 1996.

[15]   B.W. Tatler, R.J. Baddeley, I.D. Gilchrist, Vision Research 45(5):643-659, 2005.

[16]   H. Koesling, E. Carbone, H. Ritter, University of Bielefeld, Technical Report, 2002.

[17]   T.W. Lee, M. Girolami, T.J. Sejnowski, Neural Computation 11:417-441, 1999.

[18]   J. Braun, C. Koch, D. K. Lee, L. Itti, In: Visual Attention and Cortical Circuits, (J. Braun, C. Koch, J. Davis Ed.), 215-242, Cambridge, MA:MIT Press, 2001.

[19]   J. Hullman, W. Te Winkel, F. Boselie, Perception and Psychophysics 62:162-174, 2000.

[20]   J.K. Tsotsos, S. Culhane, W. Wai, Y. Lai, N. Davis, F. Nuflo, Art. Intell. 78(1-2):507-547, 1995.

Active Learning For Identifying Function Threshold Boundaries

Brent Bryan
Center for Automated Learning and Discovery
Carnegie Mellon University
Pittsburgh, PA 15213
bryanba@cs.cmu.edu

Jeff Schneider
Robotics Institute
Carnegie Mellon University
Pittsburgh, PA 15213
schneide@cs.cmu.edu

Robert C. Nichol
Institute of Cosmology and Gravitation
University of Portsmouth
Portsmouth, PO1 2EG, UK
bob.nichol@port.ac.uk

Christopher J. Miller
Observatorio Cerro Tololo
Observatorio de AURA en Chile
La Serena, Chile
cmiller@noao.edu

Christopher R. Genovese
Department of Statistics
Carnegie Mellon University
Pittsburgh, PA 15213
genovese@stat.cmu.edu

Larry Wasserman
Department of Statistics
Carnegie Mellon University
Pittsburgh, PA 15213
larry@stat.cmu.edu

Abstract

We present an efficient algorithm to actively select queries for learning the boundaries separating a function domain into regions where the function is above and below a given threshold. We develop experiment selection methods based on entropy, misclassification rate, variance, and their combinations, and show how they perform on a number of data sets. We then show how these algorithms are used to determine simultaneously valid $1 - \alpha$ confidence intervals for seven cosmological parameters. Experimentation shows that the algorithm reduces the computation necessary for the parameter estimation problem by an order of magnitude.

1 Introduction

In many scientific and engineering problems where one is modeling some function over an experimental space, one is not necessarily interested in the precise value of the function over an entire region. Rather, one is curious about determining the set of points for which the function exceeds some particular value. Applications include determining the functional range of wireless networks [1], factory optimization analysis, and gaging the extent of environmental regions in geostatistics. In this paper, we use this idea to compute confidence intervals for a set of cosmological parameters that affect the shape of the temperature power spectrum of the Cosmic Microwave Background (CMB).

In one dimension, the threshold discovery problem is a root-finding problem where no

163

hints as to the location or number of solutions are given; several methods exist which can be used to solve this problem (e.g. bisection, Newton-Raphson). However, one dimensional algorithms cannot be easily extended to the multivariate case. In particular, the ideas of root bracketing and function transversal are not well defined [2]; given a particular bracket of a continuous surface, there will be an infinite number of solutions to the equation $f(\vec{x}) - t = 0$, since the solution in multiple dimensions is a set of surfaces, rather than a set of points.

Numerous active learning papers deal with similar problems in multiple dimensions. For instance, [1] presents a method for picking experiments to determine the localities of local extrema when the input space is discrete. Others have used a variety of techniques to reduce the uncertainty over the problem's entire domain to map out the function (e.g. [3], and [4]), or locate the optimal value (e.g. [5]).

We are interested in locating the subset of the input space wherein the function is above a given threshold. Algorithms that merely find a local optimum and search around it will not work in general, as there may be multiple disjoint regions above the threshold. While techniques that map out the entire surface of the underlying function will correctly identify those regions which are above a given threshold, we assert that methods can be developed that are more efficient at localizing a particular contour of the function. Intuitively, points on the function that are located far from the boundary are less interesting, regardless of their variance. In this paper, we make the following contributions to the literature:

- We present a method for choosing experiments that is more efficient than global variance minimization, as well as other heuristics, when one is solely interested in localizing a function contour.
- We show that this heuristic can be used in continuous valued input spaces, without defining *a priori* a set of possible experiments (e.g. imposing a grid).
- We use our function threshold detection method to determine $1 - \alpha$ simultaneously valid confidence intervals of CMB parameters, making no assumptions about the model being fit and few assumptions about the data in general.

2 Algorithm

We begin by formalizing the problem. Assume that we are given a bounded sample space $S \subset \mathbb{R}^n$ and a scoring function: $f : S \rightarrow \mathbb{R}$, but possibly no data points ($\{s, f(s)\}, s \in S$). Given a threshold t, we want to find the set of points S' where f is equal to or above the threshold: $\{s \in S' | s \in S, f(s) \geq t\}$. If f is invertible, then the solution is trivial. However, it is often the case that f is not trivially invertible, such as the CMB model mentioned in §1. In these cases, we can discover S' by modeling S given some experiments. Thus, we wish to know how to choose experiments that help us determine S' efficiently.

We assume that the cost to compute $f(s)$ given s is significant. Thus, care should be taken when choosing the next experiment, as picking optimum points may reduce the runtime of the algorithm by orders of magnitude. Therefore, it is preferable to analyze current knowledge about the underlying function and select experiments which quickly refine the estimate of the function around the threshold of interest. There are several methods one could use to create a model of the data, notably some form of parametric regression. However, we chose to approximate the unknown boundary as a Gaussian Process (GP), as many forms of regression (e.g. linear) necessarily smooths the data, ignoring subtle features of the function that may become pronounced with more data. In particular, we use ordinary kriging, a form of GPs, which assumes that the semivariogram ($\mathcal{K}(\cdot, \cdot)$ is a linear function of the distance between samples [6]; this estimation procedure assumes the the sampled data are normal with mean equal to the true function and variance given by the sampling noise . The expected value of $\mathcal{K}(s_i, s_j)$ for $s_i, s_j \in S$, is can be written as

$$E[\mathcal{K}(s_i, s_j)] = \frac{k}{2} \left[\sum_{l=1}^{n} \alpha_l (s_{il} - s_{jl})^2 \right]^{1/2} + c$$

where k is a constant — known as the kriging parameter — which is an estimated limit on the first derivate of the function, α_l is a scaling factor for each dimension, and c is the variance (e.g. experimental noise) of the sampled points. Since, the joint distribution of a finite set of sampled points for GPs is Gaussian, the predicted distribution of a query point s_q given a known set A is normal with mean and variance given by

$$\mu_{s_q} = \mu_A + \Sigma'_{Aq}\Sigma^{-1}_{AA}(y_A - \mu_A) \tag{1}$$

$$\sigma^2_{s_q} = \Sigma'_{Aq}\Sigma^{-1}_{AA}\Sigma_{Aq} \tag{2}$$

where Σ_{Aq} denotes the column vector with the ith entry equal to $\mathcal{K}(s_i, s_q)$, Σ_{AA} denotes the semivariance matrix between the elements of A (the ij element of Σ_{AA} is $\mathcal{K}(s_i, s_j)$), y_A denotes the column vector with the ith entry equal to $f(s_i)$, the true value of the function for each point in A, and μ_A is the mean of the y_A's.

As given, prediction with GP requires $O(n^3)$ time, as an $n \times n$ linear system of equations must be solved. However, for many GPs — and ordinary kriging in particular — the correlation between two points decreases as a function of distance. Thus, the full GP model can be approximated well by a local GP, where only the k nearest neighbors of the query point are used to compute the prediction value; this reduces the computation time to $O(k^3 \log(n))$ per prediction, since $O(\log(n))$ time is required to find the k-nearest neighbors using spatial indexing structures such as balanced kd-trees.

Since we have assumed that experimentation is expensive, it would be ideal to iteratively analyze the entire input space and pick the next experiment in such a manner that minimized the total number of experiments necessary. If the size of the parameter space ($|S|$) is finite, such an approach may be feasible. However, if $|S|$ is large or infinite, testing all points may be impractical. Instead of imposing some arbitrary structure on the possible experimental points (such as using a grid), our algorithm chooses candidate points uniformly at random from the input space, and then selects the candidate point with the highest score according to the metrics given in §2.1. This allows the input space to be fully explored (in expectation), and ensures that interesting regions of space that would have fallen between successive grid points are not missed; in §4 we show how imposing a grid upon the input space results in just such a situation. While the algorithm is unable to consider the entire space for each sampling iteration, over multiple iterations it does consider most of the space, resulting in the function boundaries being quickly localized, as can be seen in §3.

2.1 Choosing experiments from among candidates

Given a set of random input points, the algorithm evaluates each one and chooses the point with the highest score as the location for the next experiment. Below is the list of evaluation methods we considered.

Random: One of the candidate points is chosen uniformly at random. This method serves as a baseline for comparison,

Probability of incorrect classification: Since we are trying to map the boundary between points above and below a threshold, we consider choosing the point from our random sample which has the largest probability of being misclassified by our model. Using the distribution defined by Equations 1 and 2, the probability, p, that the point is above the given threshold can be computed. The point is predicted to be above the threshold if $p > 0.5$ and thus the expected misclassification probability is $\min(p, 1 - p)$.

Entropy: Instead of misclassification probability we can consider entropy: $-p \log_2(p) - (1 - p) \log_2(1 - p)$. Entropy is a monotonic function of the misclassification rate so these two will not choose different experiments. They are listed separately because they have different effects when mixed with other evaluations. Both entropy and misclassification will choose points near the boundary. Unfortunately, they have the drawback that once they find a point near the boundary they continue to choose points near that location and will not explore the rest of the parameter space.

Variance: Both entropy and probability of incorrect classification suffer from a lack of incentive to explore the space. To rectify this problem, we consider the variance of each query point (given by Equation 2) as an evaluation metric. This metric is common in active learning methods whose goal is to map out an entire function. Since variance is related to the distance to nearest neighbors, this strategy chooses points that are far from areas currently searched, and hence will not get stuck at one boundary point. However, it is well known that such approaches tend to spend a large portion of their time on the edges of the parameter space and ultimately cover the space exhaustively [7].

Information gain: Information gain is a common myopic metric used in active learning. Information gain at the query point is the same as entropy in our case because all run experiments are assumed to have the same variance. Computing a full measure of information gain over the whole state space would provide an optimal 1-step experiment choice. In some discrete or linear problems this can be done, but it is intractable for continuous non-linear spaces. We believe the good performance of the evaluation metrics proposed below stems from their being heuristic proxies for global information gain or reduction in misclassification error.

Products of metrics: One way to rectify the problems of point policies that focus solely on points near the boundary or points with large variance regardless of their relevance to refining the predictive model, is to combine the two measures. Intuitively, doing this can mimic the idea of information gain; the entropy of a query point measures the classification uncertainty, while the variance is a good estimator of how much impact a new observation would have in this region, and thus what fraction the uncertainty would be reduced. [1] proposed scoring points based upon the product of their entropy and variance to identify the presence of local maxima and minima, a problem closely related to boundary detection. We shall also consider scoring points based upon the product of their probability of incorrect classification and variance. Note that while entropy and probability of incorrect classification are monotonically related, entropy times variance and probability of incorrect classification times variance are not.

Straddle: Using the same intuition as for products of heuristics, we define straddle heuristic, as $\text{straddle}(s_q) = 1.96\hat{\sigma}_q - |\hat{f}(s_q) - t|$, The straddle algorithm scores points highest that are both unknown and near the boundary. As such, the straddle algorithm prefers points near the threshold, but far from previous examples. The straddle score for a point may be negative, which indicates that the model currently estimates the probability that the point is on a boundary is less than five percent. Since the straddle heuristic relies on the variance estimate, it is also subject to oversampling edge positions.

3 Experiments

We now assess the accuracy with which our model reproduces a known function for the point policies just described. This is done by computing the fraction of test points in which the predictive model agrees with the true function about which side of the threshold the test points are on after some fixed number of experiments. This process is repeated several times to account for variations due to the random sampling of the input space.

The first model we consider is a 2D sinusoidal function given by

$$f(x, y) = \sin(10x) + \cos(4y) - \cos(3xy) \qquad x \in [0, 1], \quad y \in [0, 2],$$

with a boundary threshold of $t = 0$. This function and threshold were examined for the following reasons: 1) the target threshold winds through the plot giving ample length to

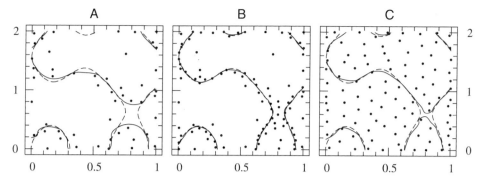

Figure 1: Predicted function boundary (solid), true function boundary (dashed), and experiments (dots) for the 2D sinusoid function after A) 50 experiments and B) 100 experiments using the straddle heuristic and C) 100 experiments using the variance heuristic.

Table 1: Number of experiments required to obtain 99% classification accuracy for the 2D models and 95% classification accuracy for the 4D model for various heuristics. Heuristics requiring more than 10,000 experiments to converge are labeled "did not converge".

	2D Sin.(1K Cand.)	2D Sin.(31 Cand.)	2D DeBoor	4D Sinusoid
Random	617 ± 158	617 ± 158	7727 ± 987	6254 ± 364
Entropy	did not converge	did not converge	did not converge	6121 ± 1740
Variance	207 ± 7	229 ± 9	4306 ± 573	2320 ± 57
Entropy $\times$ Var	117 ± 5	138 ± 6	1621 ± 201	1210 ± 43
Prob. Incor. $\times$ Std	113 ± 11	129 ± 14	740 ± 117	1362 ± 89
Straddle	106 ± 5	123 ± 6	963 ± 136	1265 ± 94

test the accuracy of the approximating model, 2) the boundary is discontinuous with several small pieces, 3) there is an ambiguous region (around $(0.9, 1)$, where the true function is approximately equal to the threshold, and the gradient is small and 4) there are areas in the domain where the function is far from the threshold and hence we can ensure that the algorithm is not oversampling in these regions.

Table 1 shows the number of experiments necessary to reach a 99% and 95% accuracy for the 2D and 4D models, respectively. Note that picking points solely on entropy does not converge in many cases, while both the straddle algorithm and probability incorrect times standard deviation heuristic result in approximations that are significantly better than random and variance heuristics. Figures 1A-C confirm that the straddle heuristic is aiding in boundary prediction. Note that most of the 50 experiments sampled between Figures 1A and 1B are chosen near the boundary. The 100 experiments chosen to minimize the variance result in an even distribution over the input space and a worse boundary approximation, as seen in Figure 1C. These results indicate that the algorithm is correctly modeling the test function and choosing experiments that pinpoint the location of the boundary.

From the Equations 1 and 2, it is clear that the algorithm does not depend on data dimensionality directly. To ensure that heuristics are not exploiting some feature of the 2D input space, we consider the 4D sinusoidal function

$$f(\vec{x}) = \sin(10x_1) + \cos(4x_2) - \cos(3x_1x_2) + \cos(2x_3) + \cos(3x_4) - \sin(5x_3x_4)$$

where $\vec{x} \in [(0, 0, 1, 0), (1, 2, 2, 2)]$ and $t = 0$. Comparison of the 2D and 4D results in Table 1 reveals that the relative performance of the heuristics remains unchanged, indicating that the best heuristic for picking experiments is independent of the problem dimension.

To show that the decrease in the number candidate points relative to the input parameter space that occurs with higher dimensional problems is not an issue, we reconsider the 2D sinusoidal problem. Now, we use only 31 candidate points instead of 1000 to simulate the point density difference between 4D and 2D. Results shown in Table 1, indicate that reducing the number of candidate points does not drastically alter the realized performance. Additional experiments were performed on a discontinuous 2D function (the DeBoor function given in [1]) with similar results, as can be seen in Table 1.

4 Statistical analysis of cosmological parameters

Let us now look at a concrete application of this work: a statistical analysis of cosmological parameters that affect formation and evolution of our universe. One key prediction of the Big Bang model for the origin of our universe is the presence of a $2.73K$ cosmic microwave background radiation (CMB). Recently, the Wilkinson Microwave Anisotropy Project (WMAP) has completed a detailed survey of the this radiation exhibiting small CMB temperature fluctuations over the sky [8]. It is believed that the size and spatial proximity of these temperature fluctuations depict the types and rates of particle interactions in the early universe and consequently characterize the formation of large scale structure (galaxies, clusters, walls and voids) in the current observable universe. It is conjectured that this radiation permeated through the universe unchanged since its formation 15 billion years ago. Therefore, the sizes and angular separations of these CMB fluctuations give an unique picture of the universe immediately after the Big Bang and have a large implication on our understanding of primordial cosmology.

An important summary of the temperature fluctuations is the CMB power spectrum shown in Figure 2, which gives the temperature variance of the CMB as a function of spatial frequency (or multi-pole moment). It is well known that the shape of this curve is affected by at least seven cosmological parameters: optical depth (τ), dark energy mass fraction (Ω_Λ), total mass fraction (Ω_m), baryon density (ω_b), dark matter density (ω_{dm}), neutrino fraction (f_n), and spectral index (n_s). For instance, the height of first peak is determined by the total energy density of the universe, while the third peak is related to the amount of dark matter. Thus, by fitting models of the CMB power spectrum for given values of the seven parameters, we can determine how the parameters influence the shape of the model spectrum. By examining those models that fit the data, we can then establish the ranges of the parameters that result in models which fit the data.

Previous work characterizing confidence intervals for cosmological parameters either used marginalization over the other parameters, or made assumptions about the values of the parameters and/or the shape of the CMB power spectrum. However, [9] notes that "CMB data have now become so sensitive that the key issue in cosmological parameter determination is not always the accuracy with which the CMB power spectrum features can be measured, but often what prior information is used or assumed." In this analysis, we make no assumptions about the ranges or values of the parameters, and assume only that the data are normally distributed around the unknown CMB spectrum with covariance known up to a constant multiple. Using the method of [10], we create a non-parametric confidence ball (under a weighted squared-error loss) for the unknown spectrum that is centered on a nonparametric estimate with a radius for each specified confidence level derived from the asymptotic distribution of a pivot statistic[1]. For any candidate spectrum, membership in the confidence ball can be determined by comparing the ball's radius to the variance weighted sum of squares deviation between the candidate function and the center of the ball.

One advantage of this method is that it gives us simultaneously valid confidence intervals on all seven of our input parameters; this is not true for $1 - \alpha$ confidence intervals derived from a collection of χ^2 distributions where the confidence intervals often have substantially lower coverage [11]. However, there is no way to invert the modeling process to determine parameter ranges given a fixed sum of squared error. Thus, we use the algorithm detailed

---

[1]See Appendix 3 in [10] for the derivation of this radius

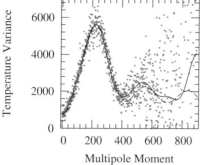

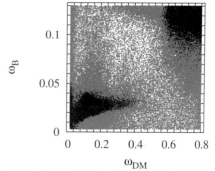

Figure 2: WMAP data, overlaid with regressed model (solid) and an example of a model CMB spectrum that barely fits at the 95% confidence level (dashed; parameter values are $\omega_{DM} = 0.1$ and $\omega_B = 0.028$).

Figure 3: 95% confidence bounds for ω_B as a function of ω_{DM}. Gray dots denote models which are rejected at a 95% confidence level, while the black dots denote those that are not.

in §2 to map out the confidence surface as a function of the input parameters; that is, we use the algorithm to pick a location in the seven dimensional parameter space to perform an experiment, and then run CMBFast [12] to create simulated power spectrum given this set of input parameters. We can then compute the sum of squares of error for this spectrum (relative to the regressed model) and easily tell if the 7D input point is inside the confidence ball. In practice, we model the sum of squared error, not the confidence level of the model. This creates a more linear output space, as the confidence level for most of the models is zero, and thus it is impossible to distinguish between poor and terrible model fits.

Due to previous efforts on this project, we were able to estimate the semivariogram of the GP from several hundred thousand random points already run through CMBFast. For this work, we chose the α_l's such that the partials in each dimension where approximately unity, resulting in $k \simeq 1$; c was set to a small constant to account for instabilities in the simulator. These points also gave a starting point for our algorithm[2]. Subsequently, we have run several hundred thousand more CMBFast models. We find that it takes 20 seconds to pick an experiment from among a set of 2,000 random candidates. CMBFast then takes roughly 3 minutes to compute the CMB spectrum given our chosen point in parameter space.

In Figure 3, we show a plot of baryon density (ω_B) versus the dark matter density (ω_{DM}) of the universe over all values of the other five parameters ($\tau, \Omega_{DE}, \Omega_M, f_n, n_s$). Experiments that are within a 95% confidence ball given the CMB data are plotted in black, while those that are rejected at the 95% level are gray. Note how there are areas that remain unsampled, while the boundary regions (transitions between gray and black points) are heavily sampled, indicating that our algorithm is choosing reasonable points. Moreover, the results of Figure 3 agree well with results in the literature (derived using parametric models and Bayesian analysis), as well as with predictions favored by nucleosynthesis [9].

While hard to distinguish in Figure 3, the bottom left group of points above the 95% confidence boundary splits into two separate peaks in parameter space. The one to the left is the concordance model, while the second peak (the one to the right) is not believed to represent the correct values of the parameters (due to constraints from other data). The existence of high probability points in this region of the parameter space has been suggested before, but computational limitations have prevented much characterization of it. Moreover, the third peak, near the top right corner of Figure 3 was basically ignored by previous grid based approaches. Comparison of the number of experiments performed by our straddle

---

[2]While initial values are not required (as we have seen in §3), it is possible to incorporate this background knowledge into the model to help the algorithm converge more quickly.

Table 2: Number of points found in the three peaks for the grid based approach of [9] and our straddle algorithm.

| | Peak Center | | # Points in Effective Radius | |
	ω_{DM}	ω_B	Grid	Straddle
Concordance Model	0.116	0.024	2118	16055
Peak 2	0.165	0.023	2825	9634
Peak 3	0.665	0.122	0	5488
Total Points			5613300	603384

algorithm with the grid based approach used by [9] is shown in Table 2. Even with only 10% of the experiments used in the grid approach, we sampled the concordance peak 8 times more frequently, and the second peak 3.4 times more frequently than the grid based approach. Moreover, it appears that the grid completely missed the third peak, while our method sampled it over 5000 times. These results dramatically illustrate the power of our adaptive method, and show how it does not suffer from assumptions made by a grid-based approaches. We are following up on the scientific ramifications of these results in a separate astrophysics paper.

5 Conclusions

We have developed an algorithm for locating a specified contour of a function while minimizing the number queries necessary. We described and showed how several different methods for picking the next experimental point from a group of candidates perform on synthetic test functions. Our experiments indicate that the straddle algorithm outperforms previously published methods, and even handles functions with large discontinuities. Moreover, the algorithm is shown to work on multi-dimensional data, correctly classifying the boundary at a 99% level with half the points required for variance minimizing methods. We have then applied this algorithm to a seven dimensional statistical analysis of cosmological parameters affecting the Cosmic Microwave Background. With only a few hundred thousand simulations we are able to accurately describe the interdependence of the cosmological parameters, leading to a better understanding of fundamental physical properties.

References

[1] N. Ramakrishnan, C. Bailey-Kellogg, S. Tadepalli, and V. N. Pandey. Gaussian processes for active data mining of spatial aggregates. In *Proceedings of the SIAM International Conference on Data Mining*, 2005.

[2] W. H. Press, S. A. Teukolsky, W. T. Vetterling, and B. P. Flannery. *Numerical Recipes in C*. Cambridge University Press, 2nd edition, 1992.

[3] D. A. Cohn, Z. Ghahramani, and M. I. Jordan. Active learning with statistical models. In G. Tesauro, D. Touretzky, and T. Leen, editors, *Advances in Neural Information Processing Systems*, volume 7, pages 705–712. The MIT Press, 1995.

[4] Simon Tong and Daphne Koller. Active learning for parameter estimation in bayesian networks. In *NIPS*, pages 647–653, 2000.

[5] A. Moore and J. Schneider. Memory-based stochastic optimization. In D. Touretzky, M. Mozer, and M. Hasselm, editors, *Neural Information Processing Systems 8*, volume 8, pages 1066–1072. MIT Press, 1996.

[6] Noel A. C. Cressie. *Statistics for Spatial Data*. Wiley, New York, 1991.

[7] D. MacKay. Information-based objective functions for active data selection. *Neural Computation*, 4(4):590–604, 1992.

[8] C. L. Bennett et al. First-Year Wilkinson Microwave Anisotropy Probe (WMAP) Observations: Preliminary Maps and Basic Results. *Astrophysical Journal Supplement Series*, 148:1–27, September 2003.

[9] M. Tegmark, M. Zaldarriaga, and A. J. Hamilton. Towards a refined cosmic concordance model: Joint 11-parameter constraints from the cosmic microwave background and large-scale structure. *Physical Review D*, 63(4), February 2001.

[10] C. Genovese, C. J. Miller, R. C. Nichol, M. Arjunwadkar, and L. Wasserman. Nonparametric inference for the cosmic microwave background. *Statistic Science*, 19(2):308–321, 2004.

[11] C. J. Miller, R. C. Nichol, C. Genovese, and L. Wasserman. A non-parametric analysis of the cmb power spectrum. *Bulletin of the American Astronomical Society*, 33:1358, December 2001.

[12] U. Seljak and M. Zaldarriaga. A Line-of-Sight Integration Approach to Cosmic Microwave Background Anisotropies. *Astrophyical Journal*, 469:437–+, October 1996.

Subsequence Kernels for Relation Extraction

Razvan C. Bunescu
Department of Computer Sciences
University of Texas at Austin
1 University Station C0500
Austin, TX 78712
razvan@cs.utexas.edu

Raymond J. Mooney
Department of Computer Sciences
University of Texas at Austin
1 University Station C0500
Austin, TX 78712
mooney@cs.utexas.edu

Abstract

We present a new kernel method for extracting semantic relations between entities in natural language text, based on a generalization of subsequence kernels. This kernel uses three types of subsequence patterns that are typically employed in natural language to assert relationships between two entities. Experiments on extracting protein interactions from biomedical corpora and top-level relations from newspaper corpora demonstrate the advantages of this approach.

1 Introduction

Information Extraction (IE) is an important task in natural language processing, with many practical applications. It involves the analysis of text documents, with the aim of identifying particular types of entities and relations among them. Reliably extracting relations between entities in natural-language documents is still a difficult, unsolved problem. Its inherent difficulty is compounded by the emergence of new application domains, with new types of narrative that challenge systems developed for other, well-studied domains. Traditionally, IE systems have been trained to recognize names of people, organizations, locations and relations between them (MUC [1], ACE [2]). For example, in the sentence "*protesters seized several pumping stations*", the task is to identify a LOCATED AT relationship between *protesters* (a PERSON entity) and *stations* (a LOCATION entity). Recently, substantial resources have been allocated for automatically extracting information from biomedical corpora, and consequently much effort is currently spent on automatically identifying biologically relevant entities, as well as on extracting useful biological relationships such as protein interactions or subcellular localizations. For example, the sentence "*TR6 specifically binds Fas ligand*", asserts an interaction relationship between the two proteins *TR6* and *Fas ligand*. As in the case of the more traditional applications of IE, systems based on manually developed extraction rules [3, 4] were soon superseded by information extractors learned through training on supervised corpora [5, 6]. One challenge posed by the biological domain is that current systems for doing part-of-speech (POS) tagging or parsing do not perform as well on the biomedical narrative as on the newspaper corpora on which they were originally trained. Consequently, IE systems developed for biological corpora need to be robust to POS or parsing errors, or to give reasonable performance using shallower but more reliable information, such as chunking instead of parsing.

Motivated by the task of extracting protein-protein interactions from biomedical corpora, we present a generalization of the subsequence kernel from [7] that works with sequences containing combinations of words and word classes. This generalized kernel is further tailored for the task of relation extraction. Experimental results show that the new relation kernel outperforms two previous rule-based methods for interaction extraction. With a small modification, the same kernel is used for extracting top-level relations from ACE corpora, providing better results than a recent approach based on dependency tree kernels.

2 Background

One of the first approaches to extracting protein interactions is that of Blaschke *et al.*, described in [3, 4]. Their system is based on a set of manually developed rules, where each rule (or frame) is a sequence of words (or POS tags) and two protein-name tokens. Between every two adjacent words is a number indicating the maximum number of intervening words allowed when matching the rule to a sentence. An example rule is "*interaction of (3) <P> (3) with (3) <P>*", where '*<P>*' is used to denote a protein name. A sentence matches the rule if and only if it satisfies the word constraints in the given order and respects the respective word gaps.

In [6] the authors described a new method ELCS (Extraction using Longest Common Subsequences) that automatically learns such rules. ELCS' rule representation is similar to that in [3, 4], except that it currently does not use POS tags, but allows disjunctions of words. An example rule learned by this system is "- *(7) interaction (0) [between | of] (5) <P> (9) <P> (17)* .". Words in square brackets separated by '|' indicate disjunctive lexical constraints, i.e. one of the given words must match the sentence at that position. The numbers in parentheses between adjacent constraints indicate the maximum number of unconstrained words allowed between the two.

3 Extraction using a Relation Kernel

Both Blaschke and ELCS do interaction extraction based on a limited set of matching rules, where a rule is simply a sparse (gappy) subsequence of words or POS tags anchored on the two protein-name tokens. Therefore, the two methods share a common limitation: either through manual selection (Blaschke), or as a result of the greedy learning procedure (ELCS), they end up using only a subset of all possible anchored sparse subsequences. Ideally, we would want to use all such anchored sparse subsequences as features, with weights reflecting their relative accuracy. However explicitly creating for each sentence a vector with a position for each such feature is infeasible, due to the high dimensionality of the feature space. Here we can exploit dual learning algorithms that process examples only via computing their dot-products, such as the Support Vector Machines (SVMs) [8]. Computing the dot-product between two such vectors amounts to calculating the number of common anchored subsequences between the two sentences. This can be done very efficiently by modifying the dynamic programming algorithm used in the string kernel from [7] to account only for common sparse subsequences constrained to contain the two protein-name tokens. We further prune down the feature space by utilizing the following property of natural language statements: when a sentence asserts a relationship between two entity mentions, it generally does this using one of the following three patterns:

- **[FB]** Fore–Between: words before and between the two entity mentions are simultaneously used to express the relationship. Examples: 'interaction of $\langle P_1 \rangle$ with $\langle P_2 \rangle$', 'activation of $\langle P_1 \rangle$ by $\langle P_2 \rangle$'.

- **[B]** Between: only words between the two entities are essential for asserting the relationship. Examples: '$\langle P_1 \rangle$ interacts with $\langle P_2 \rangle$', '$\langle P_1 \rangle$ is activated by $\langle P_2 \rangle$'.

- **[BA]** Between–After: words between and after the two entity mentions are simultaneously used to express the relationship. Examples: '$\langle P_1 \rangle - \langle P_2 \rangle$ complex', '$\langle P_1 \rangle$ and $\langle P_2 \rangle$ interact'.

Another observation is that all these patterns use at most 4 words to express the relationship (not counting the two entity names). Consequently, when computing the relation kernel, we restrict the counting of common anchored subsequences only to those having one of the three types described above, with a maximum word-length of 4. This type of feature selection leads not only to a faster kernel computation, but also to less overfitting, which results in increased accuracy (see Section 5 for comparative experiments).

The patterns enumerated above are completely lexicalized and consequently their performance is limited by data sparsity. This can be alleviated by categorizing words into classes with varying degrees of generality, and then allowing patterns to use both words and their classes. Examples of word classes are POS tags and generalizations over POS tags such as Noun, Active Verb or Passive Verb. The entity type can also be used, if the word is part of a known named entity, as well as the type of the chunk containing the word, when chunking information is available. Content words such as nouns and verbs can also be related to their synsets via WordNet. Patterns then will consist of sparse subsequences of words, POS tags, general POS (GPOS) tags, entity and chunk types, or WordNet synsets. For example, 'Noun of $\langle P_1 \rangle$ by $\langle P_2 \rangle$' is an FB pattern based on words and general POS tags.

4 Subsequence Kernels for Relation Extraction

We are going to show how to compute the relation kernel described in the previous section in two steps. First, in Section 4.1 we present a generalization of the subsequence kernel from [7]. This new kernel works with patterns construed as mixtures of words and word classes. Based on this generalized subsequence kernel, in Section 4.2 we formally define and show the efficient computation of the relation kernel used in our experiments.

4.1 A Generalized Subsequence Kernel

Let $\Sigma_1, \Sigma_2, ..., \Sigma_k$ be some disjoint feature spaces. Following the example in Section 3, Σ_1 could be the set of words, Σ_2 the set of POS tags, etc. Let $\Sigma_\times = \Sigma_1 \times \Sigma_2 \times ... \times \Sigma_k$ be the set of all possible feature vectors, where a feature vector would be associated with each position in a sentence. Given two feature vectors $x, y \in \Sigma_\times$, let $c(x, y)$ denote the number of common features between x and y. The next notation follows that introduced in [7]. Thus, let s, t be two sequences over the finite set $\Sigma_\times$, and let $|s|$ denote the length of $s = s_1...s_{|s|}$. The sequence $s[i:j]$ is the contiguous subsequence $s_i...s_j$ of s. Let $\mathbf{i} = (i_1, ..., i_{|\mathbf{i}|})$ be a sequence of $|\mathbf{i}|$ indices in s, in ascending order. We define the length $l(\mathbf{i})$ of the index sequence $\mathbf{i}$ in s as $i_{|\mathbf{i}|} - i_1 + 1$. Similarly, $\mathbf{j}$ is a sequence of $|\mathbf{j}|$ indices in t.

Let $\Sigma_\cup = \Sigma_1 \cup \Sigma_2 \cup ... \cup \Sigma_k$ be the set of all possible features. We say that the sequence $u \in \Sigma_\cup^*$ is a (sparse) subsequence of s if there is a sequence of $|u|$ indices $\mathbf{i}$ such that $u_k \in s_{i_k}$, for all $k = 1, ..., |u|$. Equivalently, we write $u \prec s[\mathbf{i}]$ as a shorthand for the component-wise '$\in$' relationship between u and $s[\mathbf{i}]$.

Finally, let $K_n(s, t, \lambda)$ (Equation 1) be the number of weighted sparse subsequences u of length n common to s and t (i.e. $u \prec s[\mathbf{i}]$, $u \prec t[\mathbf{j}]$), where the weight of u is $\lambda^{l(\mathbf{i})+l(\mathbf{j})}$, for some $\lambda \leq 1$.

$$K_n(s, t, \lambda) = \sum_{u \in \Sigma_\cup^n} \sum_{\mathbf{i}:u \prec s[\mathbf{i}]} \sum_{\mathbf{j}:u \prec t[\mathbf{j}]} \lambda^{l(\mathbf{i})+l(\mathbf{j})} \qquad (1)$$

Because for two fixed index sequences $\mathbf{i}$ and $\mathbf{j}$, both of length n, the size of the set $\{u \in \Sigma_\cup^n | u \prec s[\mathbf{i}], u \prec t[\mathbf{j}]\}$ is $\prod_{k=1}^n c(s_{i_k}, t_{j_k})$, then we can rewrite $K_n(s, t, \lambda)$ as in Equation 2:

$$K_n(s, t, \lambda) = \sum_{\mathbf{i}:|\mathbf{i}|=n} \sum_{\mathbf{j}:|\mathbf{j}|=n} \prod_{k=1}^n c(s_{i_k}, t_{j_k}) \lambda^{l(\mathbf{i})+l(\mathbf{j})} \qquad (2)$$

We use λ as a decaying factor that penalizes longer subsequences. For sparse subsequences, this means that wider gaps will be penalized more, which is exactly the desired behavior for our patterns. Through them, we try to capture head-modifier dependencies that are important for relation extraction; for lack of reliable dependency information, the larger the word gap is between two words, the less confident we are in the existence of a head-modifier relationship between them.

To enable an efficient computation of K_n, we use the auxiliary function K'_n with a similar definition as K_n, the only difference being that it counts the length from the beginning of the particular subsequence u to the end of the strings s and t, as illustrated in Equation 3:

$$K'_n(s,t,\lambda) = \sum_{u \in \Sigma^n_U} \sum_{i:u \prec s[i]} \sum_{j:u \prec t[j]} \lambda^{|s|+|t|-i_1-j_1+2} \tag{3}$$

An equivalent formula for $K'_n(s,t,\lambda)$ is obtained by changing the exponent of λ from Equation 2 to $|s| + |t| - i_1 - j_1 + 2$.

Based on all definitions above, K_n can be computed in $O(kn|s||t|)$ time, by modifying the recursive computation from [7] with the new factor $c(x, y)$, as shown in Figure 1. In this figure, the sequence sx is the result of appending x to s (with ty defined in a similar way). To avoid clutter, the parameter λ is not shown in the argument list of K and K', unless it is instantiated to a specific constant.

$$
\begin{aligned}
K'_0(s,t) &= 1, \text{ for all } s,t \\
K''_i(sx, ty) &= \lambda K''_i(sx,t) + \lambda^2 K'_{i-1}(s,t) \cdot c(x,y) \\
K'_i(sx,t) &= \lambda K'_i(s,t) + K''_i(sx,t) \\
K_n(sx,t) &= K_n(s,t) + \sum_j \lambda^2 K'_{n-1}(s, t[1:j-1]) \cdot c(x, t[j])
\end{aligned}
$$

Figure 1: Computation of subsequence kernel.

4.2 Computing the Relation Kernel

As described in Section 2, the input consists of a set of sentences, where each sentence contains exactly two entities (protein names in the case of interaction extraction). In Figure 2 we show the segments that will be used for computing the relation kernel between two example sentences s and t. In sentence s for instance, x_1 and x_2 are the two entities, s_f is the sentence segment before x_1, s_b is the segment between x_1 and x_2, and s_a is the sentence segment after x_2. For convenience, we also include the auxiliary segment $s'_b = x_1 s_b x_2$, whose span is computed as $l(s'_b) = l(s_b) + 2$ (in all length computations, we consider x_1 and x_2 as contributing one unit only).

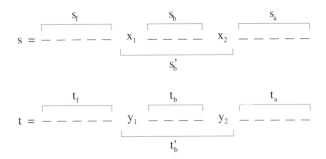

Figure 2: Sentence segments.

The relation kernel computes the number of common patterns between two sentences s and t, where the set of patterns is restricted to the three types introduced in Section 3. Therefore, the kernel $rK(s,t)$ is expressed as the sum of three sub-kernels: $fbK(s,t)$ counting the

$$rK(s,t) = fbK(s,t) + bK(s,t) + baK(s,t)$$

$$bK_i(s,t) = K_i(s_b, t_b, 1) \cdot c(x_1, y_1) \cdot c(x_2, y_2) \cdot \lambda^{l(s_b') + l(t_b')}$$

$$fbK(s,t) = \sum_{i,j} bK_i(s,t) \cdot K_j'(s_f, t_f), \quad 1 \leq i,\ 1 \leq j,\ i+j < \text{fb}_{\max}$$

$$bK(s,t) = \sum_i bK_i(s,t), \quad 1 \leq i \leq \text{b}_{\max}$$

$$baK(s,t) = \sum_{i,j} bK_i(s,t) \cdot K_j'(s_a^-, t_a^-), \quad 1 \leq i,\ 1 \leq j,\ i+j < \text{ba}_{\max}$$

Figure 3: Computation of relation kernel.

number of common fore–between patterns, $bK(s,t)$ for between patterns, and $baK(s,t)$ for between–after patterns, as in Figure 3.

All three sub-kernels include in their computation the counting of common subsequences between s_b' and t_b'. In order to speed up the computation, all these common counts can be calculated separately in bK_i, which is defined as the number of common subsequences of length i between s_b' and t_b', anchored at x_1/x_2 and y_1/y_2 respectively (i.e. constrained to start at x_1/y_1 and to end at x_2/y_2). Then fbK simply counts the number of subsequences that match j positions before the first entity and i positions between the entities, constrained to have length less than a constant fb_{max}. To obtain a similar formula for baK we simply use the reversed (mirror) version of segments s_a and t_a (e.g. s_a^- and t_a^-). In Section 3 we observed that all three subsequence patterns use at most 4 words to express a relation, therefore we set constants fb_{max}, b_{max} and ba_{max} to 4. Kernels K and K' are computed using the procedure described in Section 4.1.

5 Experimental Results

The relation kernel (ERK) is evaluated on the task of extracting relations from two corpora with different types of narrative, which are described in more detail in the following sections. In both cases, we assume that the entities and their labels are known. All pre-processing steps – sentence segmentation, tokenization, POS tagging and chunking – were performed using the OpenNLP[1] package. If a sentence contains n entities ($n \geq 2$), it is replicated into $\binom{n}{2}$ sentences, each containing only two entities. If the two entities are known to be in a relationship, then the replicated sentence is added to the set of corresponding positive sentences, otherwise it is added to the set of negative sentences. During testing, a sentence having n entities ($n \geq 2$) is again replicated into $\binom{n}{2}$ sentences in a similar way.

The relation kernel is used in conjunction with SVM learning in order to find a decision hyperplane that best separates the positive examples from negative examples. We modified the LibSVM[2] package by plugging in the kernel described above. In all experiments, the decay factor λ is set to 0.75. The performance is measured using *precision* (percentage of correctly extracted relations out of total extracted) and *recall* (percentage of correctly extracted relations out of total number of relations annotated in the corpus). When PR curves are reported, the precision and recall are computed using output from 10-fold cross-validation. The graph points are obtained by varying a threshold on the minimum acceptable extraction confidence, based on the probability estimates from LibSVM.

---

[1]URL: http://opennlp.sourceforge.net
[2]URL:http://www.csie.ntu.edu.tw/~cjlin/libsvm/

5.1 Interaction Extraction from AImed

We did comparative experiments on the AImed corpus, which has been previously used for training the protein interaction extraction systems in [6]. It consists of 225 Medline abstracts, of which 200 are known to describe interactions between human proteins, while the other 25 do not refer to any interaction. There are 4084 protein references and around 1000 tagged interactions in this dataset.

We compare the following three systems on the task of retrieving protein interactions from AImed (assuming gold standard proteins):

• [**Manual**]: We report the performance of the rule-based system of [3, 4].

• [**ELCS**]: We report the 10-fold cross-validated results from [6] as a PR graph.

• [**ERK**]: Based on the same splits as ELCS, we compute the corresponding precision-recall graph. In order to have a fair comparison with the other two systems, which use only lexical information, we do not use any word classes here.

The results, summarized in Figure 4(a), show that the relation kernel outperforms both ELCS and the manually written rules.

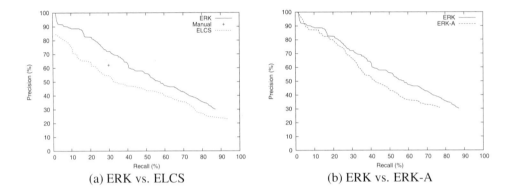

(a) ERK vs. ELCS   (b) ERK vs. ERK-A

Figure 4: PR curves for interaction extractors.

To evaluate the impact that the three types of patterns have on performance, we compare ERK with an ablated system (ERK-A) that uses all possible patterns, constrained only to be anchored on the two entity names. As can be seen in Figure 4(b), the three patterns (FB, B, BA) do lead to a significant increase in performance, especially for higher recall levels.

5.2 Relation Extraction from ACE

To evaluate how well this relation kernel ports to other types of narrative, we applied it to the problem of extracting top-level relations from the ACE corpus [2], the version used for the September 2002 evaluation. The training part of this dataset consists of 422 documents, with a separate set of 97 documents allocated for testing. This version of the ACE corpus contains three types of annotations: coreference, named entities and relations. There are five types of entities – PERSON, ORGANIZATION, FACILITY, LOCATION, and GEO-POLITICAL ENTITY – which can participate in five general, top-level relations: ROLE, PART, LOCATED, NEAR, and SOCIAL. A recent approach to extracting relations is described in [9]. The authors use a generalized version of the tree kernel from [10] to compute a kernel over relation examples, where a relation example consists of the smallest dependency tree containing the two entities of the relation. Precision and recall values are reported for the task of extracting the 5 top-level relations in the ACE corpus under two different scenarios:

– [**S1**] This is the classic setting: one multi-class SVM is learned to discriminate among the 5 top-level classes, plus one more class for the no-relation cases.

– **[S2]** One binary SVM is trained for *relation detection*, meaning that all positive relation instances are combined into one class. The thresholded output of this binary classifier is used as training data for a second multi-class SVM, trained for *relation classification*.

We trained our relation kernel, under the first scenario, to recognize the same 5 top-level relation types. While for interaction extraction we used only the lexicalized version of the kernel, here we utilize more features, corresponding to the following feature spaces: Σ_1 is the word vocabulary, Σ_2 is the set of POS tags, Σ_3 is the set of generic POS tags, and Σ_4 contains the 5 entity types. We also used chunking information as follows: all (sparse) subsequences were created exclusively from the chunk heads, where a head is defined as the last word in a chunk. The same criterion was used for computing the length of a subsequence – all words other than head words were ignored. This is based on the observation that in general words other than the chunk head do not contribute to establishing a relationship between two entities outside of that chunk. One exception is when both entities in the example sentence are contained in the same chunk. This happens very often due to noun-noun ('U.S. troops') or adjective-noun ('Serbian general') compounds. In these cases, we let one chunk contribute both entity heads. Also, an important difference from the interaction extraction case is that often the two entities in a relation do not have any words separating them, as for example in noun-noun compounds. None of the three patterns from Section 3 capture this type of dependency, therefore we introduced a fourth type of pattern, the modifier pattern **M**. This pattern consists of a sequence of length two formed from the head words (or their word classes) of the two entities. Correspondingly, we updated the relation kernel from Figure 3 with a new kernel term mK, as illustrated in Equation 4.

$$rK(s,t) = fbK(s,t) + bK(s,t) + baK(s,t) + mK(s,t) \tag{4}$$

The sub-kernel mK corresponds to a product of counts, as shown in Equation 5.

$$mK(s,t) = c(x_1, y_1) \cdot c(x_2, y_2) \cdot \lambda^{2+2} \tag{5}$$

We present in Table 1 the results of using our updated relation kernel to extract relations from ACE, under the first scenario. We also show the results presented in [9] for their best performing kernel K4 (a sum between a bag-of-words kernel and the dependency kernel) under both scenarios.

Table 1: Extraction Performance on ACE.

Method	Precision	Recall	F-measure
(S1) ERK	**73.9**	**35.2**	**47.7**
(S1) K4	70.3	26.3	38.0
(S2) K4	67.1	35.0	45.8

Even though it uses less sophisticated syntactic and semantic information, ERK in S1 significantly outperforms the dependency kernel. Also, ERK already performs a few percentage points better than K4 in S2. Therefore we expect to get an even more significant increase in performance by training our relation kernel in the same cascaded fashion.

6   Related Work

In [10], a tree kernel is defined over shallow parse representations of text, together with an efficient algorithm for computing it. Experiments on extracting PERSON-AFFILIATION and ORGANIZATION-LOCATION relations from 200 news articles show the advantage of using this new type of tree kernels over three feature-based algorithms. The same kernel was slightly generalized in [9] and applied on dependency tree representations of sentences, with dependency trees being created from head-modifier relationships extracted from syntactic parse trees. Experimental results show a clear win of the dependency tree kernel over a bag-of-words kernel. However, in a bag-of-words approach the word order is completely lost. For relation extraction, word order is important, and our experimental results support this claim – all subsequence patterns used in our approach retain the order between words.

177

The tree kernels used in the two methods above are *opaque* in the sense that the semantics of the dimensions in the corresponding Hilbert space is not obvious. For subsequence kernels, the semantics is known by definition: each subsequence pattern corresponds to a dimension in the Hilbert space. This enabled us to easily restrict the types of patterns counted by the kernel to the three types that we deemed relevant for relation extraction.

7   Conclusion and Future Work

We have presented a new relation extraction method based on a generalization of subsequence kernels. When evaluated on a protein interaction dataset, the new method showed better performance than two previous rule-based systems. After a small modification, the same kernel was evaluated on the task of extracting top-level relations from the ACE corpus, showing better performance when compared with a recent dependency tree kernel.

An experiment that we expect to lead to better performance was already suggested in Section 5.2 – using the relation kernel in a cascaded fashion, in order to improve the low recall caused by the highly unbalanced data distribution. Another performance gain may come from setting the factor λ to a more appropriate value based on a development dataset.

Currently, the method assumes the named entities are known. A natural extension is to integrate named entity recognition with relation extraction. Recent research [11] indicates that a global model that captures the mutual influences between the two tasks can lead to significant improvements in accuracy.

8   Acknowledgements

This work was supported by grants IIS-0117308 and IIS-0325116 from the NSF. We would like to thank Rohit J. Kate and the anonymous reviewers for helpful observations.

References

[1] R. Grishman, Message Understanding Conference 6, http://cs.nyu.edu/cs/faculty/grishman/muc6.html (1995).

[2] NIST, ACE – Automatic Content Extraction, http://www.nist.gov/speech/tests/ace (2000).

[3] C. Blaschke, A. Valencia, Can bibliographic pointers for known biological data be found automatically? protein interactions as a case study, Comparative and Functional Genomics 2 (2001) 196–206.

[4] C. Blaschke, A. Valencia, The frame-based module of the Suiseki information extraction system, IEEE Intelligent Systems 17 (2002) 14–20.

[5] S. Ray, M. Craven, Representing sentence structure in hidden Markov models for information extraction, in: Proceedings of the Seventeenth International Joint Conference on Artificial Intelligence (IJCAI-2001), Seattle, WA, 2001, pp. 1273–1279.

[6] R. Bunescu, R. Ge, R. J. Kate, E. M. Marcotte, R. J. Mooney, A. K. Ramani, Y. W. Wong, Comparative experiments on learning information extractors for proteins and their interactions, Artificial Intelligence in Medicine (special issue on Summarization and Information Extraction from Medical Documents) 33 (2) (2005) 139–155.

[7] H. Lodhi, C. Saunders, J. Shawe-Taylor, N. Cristianini, C. Watkins, Text classification using string kernels, Journal of Machine Learning Research 2 (2002) 419–444.

[8] V. N. Vapnik, Statistical Learning Theory, John Wiley & Sons, 1998.

[9] A. Culotta, J. Sorensen, Dependency tree kernels for relation extraction, in: Proceedings of the 42nd Annual Meeting of the Association for Computational Linguistics (ACL-04), Barcelona, Spain, 2004, pp. 423–429.

[10] D. Zelenko, C. Aone, A. Richardella, Kernel methods for relation extraction, Journal of Machine Learning Research 3 (2003) 1083–1106.

[11] D. Roth, W. Yih, A linear programming formulation for global inference in natural language tasks, in: Proceedings of the Annual Conference on Computational Natural Language Learning (CoNLL), Boston, MA, 2004, pp. 1–8.

Faster Rates in Regression via Active Learning

Rui Castro
Rice University
Houston, TX 77005
rcastro@rice.edu

Rebecca Willett
University of Wisconsin
Madison, WI 53706
willett@cae.wisc.edu

Robert Nowak
University of Wisconsin
Madison, WI 53706
nowak@engr.wisc.edu

Abstract

This paper presents a rigorous statistical analysis characterizing regimes in which active learning significantly outperforms classical passive learning. Active learning algorithms are able to make queries or select sample locations in an online fashion, depending on the results of the previous queries. In some regimes, this extra flexibility leads to significantly faster rates of error decay than those possible in classical passive learning settings. The nature of these regimes is explored by studying fundamental performance limits of active and passive learning in two illustrative nonparametric function classes. In addition to examining the theoretical potential of active learning, this paper describes a practical algorithm capable of exploiting the extra flexibility of the active setting and provably improving upon the classical passive techniques. Our active learning theory and methods show promise in a number of applications, including field estimation using wireless sensor networks and fault line detection.

1 Introduction

In this paper we address the theoretical capabilities of active learning for estimating functions in noise. Several empirical and theoretical studies have shown that selecting samples or making strategic queries in order to learn a target function/classifier can outperform commonly used passive methods based on random or deterministic sampling [1–5]. There are essentially two different scenarios in active learning: (i) *selective sampling*, where we are presented a pool of examples (possibly very large), and for each of these we can decide whether to collect a label associated with it, the goal being learning with the least amount of carefully selected labels [3]; (ii) *adaptive sampling*, where one chooses an experiment/sample location based on previous observations [4,6]. We consider adaptive sampling in this paper. Most previous analytical work in active learning regimes deals with very stringent conditions, like the ability to make perfect or nearly perfect decisions at every stage in the sampling procedure. Our working scenario is significantly less restrictive, and based on assumptions that are more reasonable for a broad range of practical applications.

We investigate the problem of nonparametric function regression, where the goal is to estimate a function from noisy point-wise samples. In the classical (passive) setting the sampling locations are chosen *a priori*, meaning that the selection of the sample locations precedes the gathering of the function observations. In the active sampling setting, however, the sample locations are chosen in an online fashion: the decision of where to sample next depends on all the observations made previously, in the spirit of the "Twenty Questions" game (in passive sampling all the questions need to be asked before any answers are given). The extra degree of flexibility garnered through active learning can lead to significantly better function estimates than those possible using classical (passive) methods. However, there are very few analytical methodologies for these Twenty Questions problems when the answers are not entirely reliable (see for example [6–8]); this precludes performance guarantees and limits the applicability of many such methods. To address this critical issue, in this paper we answer several pertinent questions regarding the fundamental performance limits of active learning in the context of regression under noisy conditions.

Significantly faster rates of convergence are generally achievable in cases involving functions whose complexity (in a the Kolmogorov sense) is highly concentrated in small regions of space (e.g., functions that are smoothly varying apart from highly localized abrupt changes such as jumps or edges). We illustrate this by characterizing the fundamental limits of active learning for two broad nonparametric function classes which map $[0, 1]^d$ onto the real line: (i) Hölder smooth functions (spatially homogeneous complexity) and (ii) piecewise constant functions that are constant except on a $d − 1$ dimensional *boundary set* or discontinuity embedded in the d dimensional function domain (spatially concentrated complexity). The main result of this paper is two-fold. First, when the complexity of the function is spatially homogeneous, passive learning algorithms are near-minimax optimal over all estimation methods and all (active or passive) learning schemes, indicating that active learning methods cannot provide faster rates of convergence in this regime. Second, for piecewise constant functions, active learning methods can capitalize on the highly localized nature of the boundary by focusing the sampling process in the estimated vicinity of the boundary. We present an algorithm that provably improves on the best possible passive learning algorithm and achieves faster rates of error convergence. Furthermore, we show that this performance cannot be significantly improved on by any other active learning method (in a minimax sense). Earlier existing work had focused on one dimensional problems [6, 7], and very specialized multidimensional problems that can be reduced to a series of one dimensional problems [8]. Unfortunately these techniques cannot be extended to more general piecewise constant/smooth models, and to the best of our knowledge our work is the first addressing active learning in this class of models.

Our active learning theory and methods show promise for a number of problems. In particular, in imaging techniques such as laser scanning it is possible to adaptively vary the scanning process. Using active learning in this context can significantly reduce image acquisition times. Wireless sensor network constitute another key application area. Because of necessarily small batteries, it is desirable to limit the number of measurements collected as much as possible. Incorporating active learning strategies into such systems can dramatically lengthen the lifetime of the system. In fact, active learning problems like the one we pose in Section 4 have already found application in fault line detection [7] and boundary estimation in wireless sensor networking [9].

2   Problem Statement

Our goal is to estimate $f : [0, 1]^d \to \mathbb{R}$ from a finite number of noise-corrupted samples. We consider two different scenarios: (a) *passive learning*, where the location of the sample points is chosen statistically independently of the measurement outcomes; and (b) *active learning*, where the location of the ith sample point can be chosen as a function of the samples points and samples collected up to that instant. The statistical model we consider builds on the following assumptions:

(A1) The observations $\{Y_i\}_{i=1}^n$ are given by
$$Y_i = f(\boldsymbol{X_i}) + W_i, \ i \in \{1, \dots, n\}.$$

(A2) The random variables W_i are Gaussian zero mean and variance σ^2. These are independent and identically distributed (i.i.d.) and independent of $\{X_i\}_{i=1}^n$.

(A3.1) Passive Learning: The sample locations $X_i \in [0,1]^d$ are either deterministic or random, but independent of $\{Y_j\}_{j \neq i}$. They do not depend in any way on f.

(A3.2) Active Learning: The sample locations X_i are random, and depend only on $\{X_j, Y_j\}_{j=1}^{i-1}$. In other words the sample locations X_i have only a causal dependency on the system variables $\{X_i, Y_i\}$. Finally, given $\{X_j, Y_j\}_{j=1}^{i-1}$ the random variable X_i does not depend in any way on f.

Let $\hat{f}_n : [0,1]^d \to \mathbb{R}$ denote an estimator based on the training samples $\{X_i, Y_i\}_{i=1}^n$. When constructing an estimator under the active learning paradigm there is another degree of freedom: we are allowed to choose our *sampling strategy*, that is, we can specify $X_i | X_1 \ldots X_{i-1}, Y_1 \ldots Y_{i-1}$. We will denote the sampling strategy by S_n. The pair $(\hat{f}_n, S_n)$ is called the *estimation strategy*. Our goal is to construct estimation strategies which minimize the expected squared error,

$$\mathbb{E}_{f,S_n}[\|\hat{f}_n - f\|^2],$$

where $\mathbb{E}_{f,S_n}$ is the expectation with respect to the probability measure of $\{X_i, Y_i\}_{i=1}^n$ induced by model f and sampling strategy S_n, and $\|\cdot\|$ is the usual L_2 norm.

3 Learning in Classical Smoothness Spaces

In this section we consider classes of functions whose complexity is homogeneous over the entire domain, so that there are no localized features, as in Figure 1(a). In this case we do not expect the extra flexibility of the active learning strategies to provide any substantial benefit over passive sampling strategies, since a simple uniform sampling scheme is naturally matched to the homogeneous "distribution" of the target function's complexity. To exemplify this consider the Hölder smooth function class: a function $f : [0,1]^d \to \mathbb{R}$ is *Hölder smooth* if it has continuous partial derivatives up to order $k = \lfloor \alpha \rfloor$ [1] and

$$\forall\, z, x \in [0,1]^d : \quad |f(z) - P_x(z)| \leq L\|z - x\|^\alpha,$$

where $L, \alpha > 0$, and $P_x(\cdot)$ denotes the order k Taylor polynomial approximation of f expanded around x. Denote this class of functions by $\Sigma(L, \alpha)$. Functions in $\Sigma(L, \alpha)$ are essentially C^α functions when $\alpha \in \mathbb{N}$. The first of our two main results is a minimax lower bound on the performance of all active estimation strategies for this class of functions.

Theorem 1. *Under the requirements of the active learning model we have the minimax bound*

$$\inf_{(\hat{f}_n, S_n) \in \Theta_{active}} \sup_{f \in \Sigma(L, \alpha)} \mathbb{E}_{f,S_n}[\|\hat{f}_n - f\|^2] \geq cn^{-\frac{2\alpha}{2\alpha+d}}, \tag{1}$$

where $c \equiv c(L, \alpha, \sigma^2) > 0$ and Θ_{active} is the set of all active estimation strategies (which includes also passive strategies).

Note that the rate in Theorem 1 is the same as the classical passive learning rate [10, 11] but the class of estimation strategies allowed is now much bigger. The proof of Theorem 1 is presented in our technical report [12] and uses standard tools of minimax analysis, such as Assouad's Lemma. The key idea of the proof is to reduce the problem of estimating a function in $\Sigma(L, \alpha)$ to the problem of deciding among a finite number of hypotheses. The key aspects of the proof for the passive setting [13] apply to the active scenario due to the fact that we can choose an adequate set of hypotheses without knowledge of the sampling strategy, although some modifications are required due to the extra flexibility of the sampling strategy. There are various practical estimators achieving the performance predicted by Theorem 1, including some based on kernels, splines or wavelets [13].

---

[1] $k = \lfloor \alpha \rfloor$ is the maximal integer such that $k < \alpha$.

4 The Active Advantage

In this section we address two key questions: (i) when does active learning provably yield better results, and (ii) what are the fundamental limitations of active learning? These are difficult questions to answer in general. We expect that, for functions whose complexity is spatially non-uniform and highly concentrated in small subsets of the domain, the extra spatial adaptivity of the active learning paradigm can lead into significant performance gains. We study a class of functions which highlights this notion of "spatially concentrated complexity". Although this is a canonical example and a relatively simple function class, it is general enough to provide insights into methodologies for broader classes.

A function $f : [0,1]^d \to \mathbb{R}$ is called *piecewise constant* if it is locally constant[2] in any point $\boldsymbol{x} \in [0,1]^d \setminus B(f)$, where $B(f) \subset [0,1]^d$, the *boundary set*, has upper box-counting dimension at most $d-1$. Furthermore let f be uniformly bounded on $[0,1]^d$ (that is, $|f(\boldsymbol{x})| \le M$, $\forall \boldsymbol{x} \in [0,1]^d$) and let $B(f)$ satisfy $N(r) \le \beta r^{-(d-1)}$ for all $r > 0$, where $\beta > 0$ is a constant and $N(r)$ is the minimal number of closed balls of diameter r that covers $B(f)$. The set of all piecewise constant functions f satisfying the above conditions is denoted by $\mathrm{PC}(\beta, M)$.

The conditions above mean that (a) the functions are constant except along $d-1$-dimensional "boundaries" where they are discontinuous and (b) the boundaries between the various constant regions are $(d-1)$-dimensional non-fractal sets. If the boundaries $B(f)$ are smooth then β is an approximate bound on their total $d-1$ dimensional volume (*e.g.*, the length if $d = 2$). An example of such a function is depicted in Figure 1(b). The class $\mathrm{PC}(\beta, M)$ has the main ingredients that make active learning appealing: a function f is "well-behaved" everywhere on the unit square, except on a small subset $B(f)$. We will see that the critical task for any good estimator is to accurately find the location of the boundary $B(f)$.

4.1 Passive Learning Framework

To obtain minimax lower bounds for $\mathrm{PC}(\beta, M)$ we consider a smaller class of functions, namely the boundary fragment class studied in [11]. Let $g : [0,1]^{d-1} \to [0,1]$ be a Lipshitz function with graph in $[0,1]^d$, that is

$$|g(\boldsymbol{x}) - g(\boldsymbol{z})| \le \|\boldsymbol{x} - \boldsymbol{z}\|,\ 0 \le g(\boldsymbol{x}) \le 1,\ \forall\, \boldsymbol{x}, \boldsymbol{z} \in [0,1]^{d-1}.$$

Define $G = \{(\boldsymbol{x}, y) : 0 \le y \le g(\boldsymbol{x}),\ \boldsymbol{x} \in [0,1]^{d-1}\}$. Finally define $f : [0,1]^d \to \mathbb{R}$ by $f(\boldsymbol{x}) = 2M\mathbf{1}_G(\boldsymbol{x}) - M$. The class of all the functions of this form is called the *boundary fragment* class (usually $M = 1$), denoted by $\mathrm{BF}(M)$. Note that there are only two regions, and the boundary separating those is a function of the first $d-1$ variables.

It is straightforward to show that $\mathrm{BF}(M) \subseteq \mathrm{PC}(\beta, M)$ for a suitable constant β; therefore a minimax lower bound for the boundary fragment class is trivially a lower bound for the piecewise constant class. From the results in [11] we have

$$\inf_{(\hat{f}_n, S_n) \in \Theta_{\text{passive}}} \sup_{f \in \mathrm{PC}(\beta, M)} \mathbb{E}_{f, S_n}[d^2(\hat{f}_n, f)] \ge cn^{-\frac{1}{d}}, \tag{2}$$

where $c \equiv c(\beta, M, \sigma^2) > 0$.

There exist practical passive learning strategies that are near-minimax optimal. For example, tree-structured estimators based on *Recursive Dyadic Partitions* (RDPs) are capable of

---

[2] A function $f : [0,1]^d \to \mathbb{R}$ is locally constant at a point $\boldsymbol{x} \in [0,1]^d$ if

$$\exists \epsilon > 0 \ : \forall \boldsymbol{y} \in [0,1]^d : \quad \|\boldsymbol{x} - \boldsymbol{y}\| < \epsilon \Rightarrow f(\boldsymbol{y}) = f(\boldsymbol{x}).$$

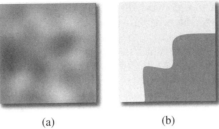

(a)   (b)

Figure 1: Examples of functions in the classes considered: (a) Hölder smooth function. (b) Piecewise constant function.

nearly attaining the minimax rate above [14]. These estimators are constructed as follows: (i) Divide $[0,1]^d$ into 2^d equal sized hypercubes. (ii) Repeat this process again on each hypercube. Repeating this process $\log_2 m$ times gives rise to a partition of the unit hypercube into m^d hypercubes of identical size. This process can be represented as a 2^d-ary tree structure (where a leaf of the tree corresponds to a partition cell). Pruning this tree gives rise to an RDP with non-uniform resolution. Let Π denote the class of all possible pruned RDPs. The estimators we consider are constructed by decorating the elements of a partition with constants. Let π be an RDP; the estimators built over this RDP have the form $\tilde{f}^{(\pi)}(\boldsymbol{x}) \equiv \sum_{A \in \pi} c_A \mathbf{1}\{x \in A\}$.

Since the location of the boundary is *a priori* unknown it is natural to distribute the sample points uniformly over the unit cube. There are various ways of doing this; for example, the points can be placed deterministically over a lattice, or randomly sampled from a uniform distribution. We will use the latter strategy. Assume that $\{\boldsymbol{X}_i\}_{i=1}^n$ are i.i.d. uniform over $[0,1]^d$. Define the *complexity regularized estimator* as

$$\hat{f}_n \equiv \arg \min_{\tilde{f}^{(\pi)}:\pi \in \Pi} \left\{ \frac{1}{n} \sum_{i=1}^n \left(\tilde{f}^{(\pi)}(\boldsymbol{X}_i) - Y_i \right)^2 + \lambda \frac{\log n}{n} |\pi| \right\}, \tag{3}$$

where $|\pi|$ denotes the number of elements of π and $\lambda > 0$. The above optimization can be solved efficiently in $O(n)$ operations using a bottom-up tree pruning algorithm [14].

The performance of the estimator in (3) can be assessed using bounding techniques in the spirit of [14, 15]. From that analysis we conclude that

$$\sup_{f \in \mathrm{PC}(\beta,M)} \mathbb{E}_f[\|\hat{f}_n - f\|^2] \leq C(n/\log n)^{-\frac{1}{d}}, \tag{4}$$

where $C \equiv C(\beta, M, \sigma^2) > 0$. This shows that, up to a logarithmic factor, the rate in (2) is the optimal rate of convergence for passive strategies. A complete derivation of the above result is available in [12].

4.2   Active Learning Framework

We now turn our attention to the active learning scenario. In [8] this was studied for the boundary fragment class. From that work and noting again that $\mathrm{BF}(M) \subseteq \mathrm{PC}(\beta,M)$ we have, for $d \geq 2$,

$$\inf_{(\hat{f}_n, S_n) \in \Theta_{\mathrm{active}}} \sup_{f \in \mathrm{PC}(\beta,M)} \mathbb{E}_{f,S_n}[\|\hat{f}_n - f\|^2] \geq cn^{-\frac{1}{d-1}}, \tag{5}$$

where $c \equiv c(M, \sigma^2) > 0$.

In contrast with (2), we observe that with active learning we have a potential performance gain over passive strategies, effectively equivalent to a dimensionality reduction. Essentially the exponent in (5) depends now on the dimension of the boundary set, $d-1$, instead of the dimension of the entire domain, d. In [11] an algorithm capable of achieving the above rate for the boundary fragment class is presented, but this algorithm takes advantage of the very special functional form of the boundary fragment functions. The algorithm begins by dividing the unit hypercube into "strips" and performing a one-dimensional change-point estimation in each of the strips. This change-point detection can be performed extremely accurately using active learning, as shown in the pioneering work of Burnashev and Zigangirov [6]. Unfortunately, the boundary fragment class is very restrictive and impractical for most applications. Recall that boundary fragments consist of only two regions, separated by a boundary that is a function of the first $d - 1$ coordinates. The class PC(β, M) is much larger and more general and the algorithmic ideas that work for boundary fragments can no longer be used. A completely different approach is required, using radically different tools.

We now propose an active learning scheme for the piecewise constant class. The proposed scheme is a two-step approach based in part on the tree-structured estimators described above for passive learning. In the first step, called the *preview step*, a rough estimator of f is constructed using $n/2$ samples (assume for simplicity that n is even), distributed uniformly over $[0, 1]^d$. In the second step, called the *refinement step*, we select $n/2$ samples near the perceived locations of the boundaries (estimated in the preview step) separating constant regions. At the end of this process we will have half the samples concentrated in the vicinity of the boundary set $B(f)$. Since accurately estimating f near $B(f)$ is key to obtaining faster rates, the strategy described seems quite sensible. However, it is *critical* that the preview step is able to detect the boundary with very high probability. If part of the boundary is missed, then the error incurred is going to propagate into the final estimate, ultimately degrading the performance. Therefore extreme care must be taken to detect the boundary in the preview step, as described below.

Preview: The goal of this stage is to provide a coarse estimate of the location of $B(f)$. Specifically, collect $n' \equiv n/2$ samples at points distributed uniformly over $[0, 1]^d$. Next proceed by using the passive learning algorithm described before, but restrict the estimator to RDPs with leafs at a maximum depth of $J = \frac{d-1}{(d-1)^2+d} \log(n'/\log(n'))$. This ensures that, on average, every element of the RDP contains many sample points; therefore we obtain a low variance estimate, although the estimator bias is going to be large. In other words, we obtain a very "stable" coarse estimate of f, where stable means that the estimator does not change much for different realizations of the data.

The above strategy ensures that most of the time, leafs that intersect the boundary are at the maximum allowed depth (because otherwise the estimator would incur too much empirical error) and leafs away from the boundary are at shallower depths. Therefore we can "detect" the rough location of the boundary just by looking at the deepest leafs. Unfortunately, if the set $B(f)$ is somewhat aligned with the dyadic splits of the RDP, leafs intersecting the boundary can be pruned without incurring a large error. This is illustrated in Figure 2(b); the cell with the arrow was pruned and contains a piece of the boundary, but the error incurred by pruning is small since that region is mostly a constant region. However, worst-case analysis reveals that the squared bias induced by these small volumes can add up, precluding the desired rates. A way of mitigating this issue is to consider multiple RDP-based estimators, each one using RDPs appropriately shifted. We use $d + 1$ estimators in the preview step: one on the initial uniform partition, and d over partitions whose dyadic splits have been translated by 2^{-J} in each one of the d coordinates. Any leaf that is at the maximum depth of any of the $d + 1$ RDPs pruned in the preview step indicates the highly probable presence of a boundary, and will be refined in the next stage.

Refinement: With high probability, the boundary is contained in the leafs at the maximum depth. In the refinement step we collect additional $n/2$ samples in the corresponding partition cells, using these to obtain a refined estimate of the function f by again applying

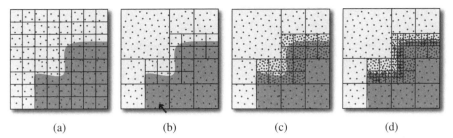

| (a) | (b) | (c) | (d) |

Figure 2: The two step procedure for $d = 2$: (a) Initial unpruned RDP and $n/2$ samples. (b) Preview step RDP. Note that the cell with the arrow was pruned, but it contains a part of the boundary. (c) Additional sampling for the refinement step. (d) Refinement step.

an RDP-based estimator. This produces a higher resolution estimate in the vicinity of the boundary set $B(f)$, yielding better performance than the passive learning technique.

To formally show that this algorithm attains the faster rates we desire we have to consider a further technical assumption, namely that the boundary set is "cusp-free"[3]. This condition is rather technical, but it is not very restrictive, and encompasses many interesting situations, including of course boundary fragments. For a more detailed explanation see [12]. Under this condition we have the following:

Theorem 2. *Under the active learning scenario we have, for $d \geq 2$ and functions f whose boundary is cusp-free,*

$$\mathbb{E}\left[\|\hat{f}_n - f\|^2\right] \leq C\left(\frac{n}{\log n}\right)^{-\frac{1}{d-1+1/d}}, \tag{6}$$

where $C > 0$.

This bound improves on (4), demonstrating that this technique performs better than the best possible passive learning estimator. The proof of Theorem 2 is quite involved and is presented in detail in [12]. The main idea behind the proof is to decompose the error of the estimator for three different cases: (i) the error incurred during the preview stage in regions "away" from the boundary; (ii) the error incurred by not detecting a piece of the boundary (and therefore not performing the refinement step in that area); (iii) the error remaining in the refinement region at the end of the process. By restricting the maximum depth of the trees in the preview stage we can control the type-(i) error, ensuring that it does not exceed the error rate in (6). Type-(ii) error corresponds to the situations when a part of the boundary was not detected in the preview step. This can happen because of the inherent randomness of the noise and sampling distribution, or because the boundary is somewhat aligned with the dyadic splits. The latter can be a problem and this is why one needs to perform $d + 1$ preview estimates over shifted partitions. If the boundary is cusp-free then it is guaranteed that one of those preview estimators is going to "feel" the boundary since it is not aligned with the corresponding partition. Finally, the type-(iii) error is very easy to analyze, using the same techniques we used for the passive estimator.

A couple of remarks are important at this point. Instead of a two-step procedure one can reiterate this idea, performing multiple steps (*e.g.*, for a three-step approach replace the refinement step with the two-step approach described above). Doing so can further improve the performance. One can show that the expected error will decay like $n^{-1/(d-1+\epsilon)}$, with $\epsilon > 0$, given a sufficiently large number of steps. Therefore we can get rates arbitrarily close to the lower bound rates in (5).

---

[3]A cusp-free boundary cannot have the behavior you observe in the graph of $|x|^{1/2}$ at the origin. Less "aggressive" kinks are allowed, such as in the graph of $|x|$.

185

5 Final Remarks

The results presented in this paper show that in certain scenarios active learning attains provable gains over the classical passive approaches. Active learning is an intuitively appealing idea and may find application in many practical problems. Despite these draws, the analysis of such active methods is quite challenging due to the loss of statistical independence in the observations (recall that now the sample locations are coupled with all the observations made in the past). The two function classes presented are non-trivial canonical examples illustrating under what conditions one might expect active learning to improve rates of convergence. The algorithm presented here for actively learning members of the piecewise constant class demonstrates the possibilities of active learning. In fact, this algorithm has already been applied in the context of field estimation using wireless sensor networks [9]. Future work includes the further development of the ideas presented here to the context of binary classification and active learning of the Bayes decision boundary.

References

[1] D. Cohn, Z. Ghahramani, and M. Jordan, "Active learning with statistical models," *Journal of Artificial Intelligence Research*, pp. 129–145, 1996.

[2] D. J. C. Mackay, "Information-based objective functions for active data selection," *Neural Computation*, vol. 4, pp. 698–714, 1991.

[3] Y. Freund, H. S. Seung, E. Shamir, and N. Tishby, "Information, prediction, and query by committee," *Proc. Advances in Neural Information Processing Systems*, 1993.

[4] K. Sung and P. Niyogi, "Active learning for function approximation," *Proc. Advances in Neural Information Processing Systems*, vol. 7, 1995.

[5] G. Blanchard and D. Geman, "Hierarchical testing designs for pattern recognition," to appear in Annals of Statistics, 2005.

[6] M. V. Burnashev and K. Sh. Zigangirov, "An interval estimation problem for controlled observations," *Problems in Information Transmission*, vol. 10, pp. 223–231, 1974.

[7] P. Hall and I. Molchanov, "Sequential methods for design-adaptive estimation of discontinuities in regression curves and surfaces," *The Annals of Statistics*, vol. 31, no. 3, pp. 921–941, 2003.

[8] Alexander Korostelev, "On minimax rates of convergence in image models under sequential design," *Statistics & Probability Letters*, vol. 43, pp. 369–375, 1999.

[9] R. Willett, A. Martin, and R. Nowak, "Backcasting: Adaptive sampling for sensor networks," in *Proc. Information Processing in Sensor Networks*, 26-27 April, Berkeley, CA, USA, 2004.

[10] Charles J. Stone, "Optimal rates of convergence for nonparametric estimators," *The Annals of Statistics*, vol. 8, no. 6, pp. 1348–1360, 1980.

[11] A.P. Korostelev and A.B. Tsybakov, *Minimax Theory of Image Reconstruction*, Springer Lecture Notes in Statistics, 1993.

[12] R. Castro, R. Willett, and R. Nowak, "Fast rates in regression via active learning," Tech. Rep., University of Wisconsin, Madison, June 2005, ECE-05-3 Technical Report (available at http://homepages.cae.wisc.edu/ rcastro/ECE-05-3.pdf).

[13] Alexandre B. Tsybakov, *Introduction à l'estimation non-paramétrique*, Mathématiques et Applications, 41. Springer, 2004.

[14] R. Nowak, U. Mitra, and R. Willett, "Estimating inhomogeneous fields using wireless sensor networks," *IEEE Journal on Selected Areas in Communication*, vol. 22, no. 6, pp. 999–1006, 2004.

[15] Andrew R. Barron, "Complexity regularization with application to artificial neural networks," in *Nonparametric Functional Estimation and Related Topics*. 1991, pp. 561–576, Kluwer Academic Publishers.

Gradient Flow Independent Component Analysis in Micropower VLSI

Abdullah Celik, Milutin Stanacevic and Gert Cauwenberghs
Johns Hopkins University, Baltimore, MD 21218
{acelik,miki,gert}@jhu.edu

Abstract

We present micropower mixed-signal VLSI hardware for real-time blind separation and localization of acoustic sources. Gradient flow representation of the traveling wave signals acquired over a miniature (1cm diameter) array of four microphones yields linearly mixed instantaneous observations of the time-differentiated sources, separated and localized by independent component analysis (ICA). The gradient flow and ICA processors each measure 3mm × 3mm in 0.5 μm CMOS, and consume 54 μW and 180 μW power, respectively, from a 3 V supply at 16 ks/s sampling rate. Experiments demonstrate perceptually clear (12dB) separation and precise localization of two speech sources presented through speakers positioned at 1.5m from the array on a conference room table. Analysis of the multipath residuals shows that they are spectrally diffuse, and void of the direct path.

1 Introduction

Time lags in acoustic wave propagation provide cues to localize an acoustic source from observations across an array. The time lags also complicate the task of separating multiple co-existing sources using independent component analysis (ICA), which conventionally assumes instantaneous mixture observations.

Inspiration from biology suggests that for very small aperture (spacing between acoustic sensors *i.e.,* tympanal membranes), small differences (gradients) in sound pressure *level* are more effective in resolving source direction than actual (microsecond scale) time differences. The remarkable auditory localization capability of certain insects at a small (1%) fraction of the wavelength of the source owes to highly sensitive differential processing of sound pressure through inter-tympanal mechanical coupling [1] or inter-aural coupled neural circuits [2].

We present a mixed-signal VLSI system that operates on spatial and temporal differences (gradients) of the acoustic field at very small aperture to separate and localize mixtures of traveling wave sources. The real-time performance of the system is characterized through experiments with speech sources presented through speakers in a conference room setting.

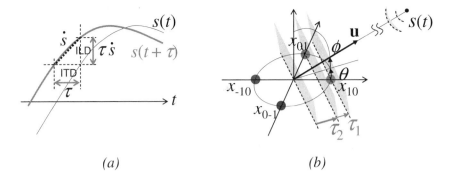

(a)   *(b)*

Figure 1: *(a)* Gradient flow principle. At low aperture, interaural level differences (ILD) and interaural time differences (ITD) are directly related, scaled by the temporal derivative of the signal. *(b)* 3-D localization (azimuth θ and elevation ϕ) of an acoustic source using a planar geometry of four microphones.

2   Gradient Flow Independent Component Analysis

Gradient flow [3, 4] is a signal conditioning technique for source separation and localization suited for arrays of very small aperture, *i.e.,* of dimensions significantly smaller than the shortest wavelength in the sources. The principle is illustrated in Figure 1 (a). Consider a traveling acoustic wave impinging on an array of four microphones, in the configuration of Figure 1 (b). The 3-D direction cosines of the traveling wave **u** are implied by propagation delays τ_1 and τ_2 in the source along directions p and q in the sensor plane. Direct measurement of these delays is problematic as they require sampling in excess of the bandwidth of the signal, increasing noise floor and power requirements. However, indirect estimates of the delays are obtained, to first order, by relating spatial and temporal derivatives of the acoustic field:

$$
\begin{aligned}
\xi_{10}(t) &\approx \tau_1 \dot{\xi}_{00}(t) \\
\xi_{01}(t) &\approx \tau_2 \dot{\xi}_{00}(t)
\end{aligned}
\tag{1}
$$

where ξ_{10} and ξ_{01} represent spatial gradients in p and q directions around the origin ($p = q = 0$), ξ_{00} the spatial common mode, and $\dot{\xi}_{00}$ its time derivative. Estimates of ξ_{00}, ξ_{10} and ξ_{01} for the sensor geometry of Figure 1 can be obtained as:

$$
\begin{aligned}
\xi_{00} &\approx \tfrac{1}{4}\left(x_{-1,0} + x_{1,0} + x_{0,-1} + x_{0,1}\right) \\
\xi_{10} &\approx \tfrac{1}{2}\left(x_{1,0} - x_{-1,0}\right) \\
\xi_{01} &\approx \tfrac{1}{2}\left(x_{0,1} - x_{0,-1}\right)
\end{aligned}
\tag{2}
$$

A single source can be localized by estimating direction cosines τ_1 and τ_2 from (1), a principle known for years in monopulse radar, exploited by parasite insects [1], and implemented in mixed-signal VLSI hardware [6]. As shown in Figure 1 (b), the planar geometry of four microphones allows to localize a source in 3-D, with both azimuth and elevation [1]. More significantly, multiple coexisting sources $s^\ell(t)$ can be jointly separated and localized

---

[1]An alternative using two microphones, exploiting shape of the pinna, is presented in [5]

188

using essentially the same principle [3, 4]:

$$\xi_{00}(t) = \sum_{\ell} s^{\ell}(t) + \nu_{00}(t)$$

$$\xi_{10}(t) = \sum_{\ell} \tau_1^{\ell} \dot{s}^{\ell}(t) + \nu_{10}(t) \qquad (3)$$

$$\xi_{01}(t) = \sum_{\ell} \tau_2^{\ell} \dot{s}^{\ell}(t) + \nu_{01}(t)$$

where ν_{00}, ν_{10} and ν_{01} represent common mode and spatial derivative components of additive noise in the sensor observations. Taking the time derivative of ξ_{00}, we thus obtain from the sensors a linear instantaneous mixture of the time-differentiated source signals,

$$\begin{bmatrix} \dot{\xi}_{00} \\ \dot{\xi}_{10} \\ \dot{\xi}_{01} \end{bmatrix} \approx \begin{bmatrix} 1 & \cdots & 1 \\ \tau_1^1 & \cdots & \tau_1^L \\ \tau_2^1 & \cdots & \tau_2^L \end{bmatrix} \begin{bmatrix} \dot{s}^1 \\ \vdots \\ \dot{s}^L \end{bmatrix} + \begin{bmatrix} \dot{\nu}_{00} \\ \dot{\nu}_{10} \\ \dot{\nu}_{01} \end{bmatrix}, \qquad (4)$$

an equation in the standard form $\mathbf{x} = \mathbf{A}\mathbf{s} + \mathbf{n}$, where $\mathbf{x}$ is given and the mixing matrix $\mathbf{A}$ and sources $\mathbf{s}$ are unknown. Ignoring the noise term $\mathbf{n}$, the problem setting is standard in Independent Component Analysis (ICA), and three independent sources can be identified from the three gradient observations.

Various formulations of ICA exist to arrive at estimates of the unknown $\mathbf{s}$ and $\mathbf{A}$ from observations $\mathbf{x}$. ICA algorithms typically specify some sort of statistical independence assumption on the sources $\mathbf{s}$ either in distribution over amplitude [7] or over time [8]. Most forms specify ICA to be *static*, in assuming that the observations contain static (instantaneous) linear mixtures of the sources. Note that this definition of *static* ICA includes methods for blind source separation that make use of temporal structure in the dynamics within the sources themselves [8], as long as the observed mixture of the sources is static. In contrast, 'convolutive' ICA techniques explicitly assume convolutive or delayed mixtures in the source observations. Convolutive ICA techniques (*e.g.,* [10]) are usually much more involved and require a large number of parameters and long adaptation time horizons for proper convergence.

The instantaneous static formulation of gradient flow (4) is convenient,[2] and avoids the need for non-static (convolutive) ICA to separate delayed mixtures of traveling wave sources (in free space) $x_{pq}(t) = \sum_{\ell} s^{\ell}(t + p\tau_1 + q\tau_2)$. Reverberation in multipath wave propagation contributes delayed mixture components in the observations which limit the effectiveness of a static ICA formulation. As shown in the experiments below, static ICA still produces reasonable results (12 dB of perceptually clear separation) in typical enclosed acoustic environments (conference room).

3 Micropower VLSI Implementation

Various analog VLSI implementations of ICA exist in the literature, *e.g.,* [11, 12], and digital implementations using DSP are common practice in the field. By adopting a mixed-signal architecture in the implementation, we combine advantages of both approaches: an analog datapath directly interfaces with inputs and outputs without the need for data conversion; and digital adaptation offers the flexibility of reconfigurable ICA learning rules.

---

[2] The time-derivative in the source signals (4) is immaterial, and can be removed by time-integrating the separated signals obtained by applying ICA directly to the gradient flow signals.

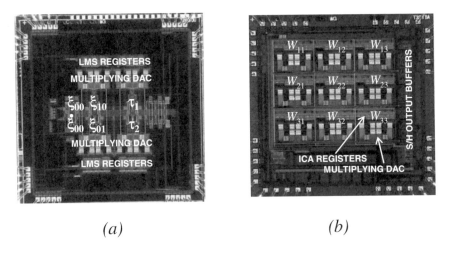

(a)   (b)

Figure 2: *(a)* Gradient flow processor. *(b)* Reconfigurable ICA processor. Dimensions of both processors are 3mm × 3mm in 0.5 μm CMOS technology.

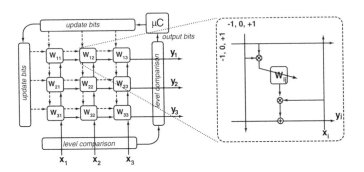

Figure 3: Reconfigurable mixed-signal ICA architecture implementing general outer-product forms of ICA update rules.

3.1 Gradient Flow Processor

The mixed-signal VLSI processor implementing gradient flow is presented in [6]. A micrograph of the chip is shown in Figure 2 (a). Precise analog gradients $\dot{\xi}_{00}$, ξ_{10} and ξ_{01} are acquired from the microphone signals by correlated double sampling (CDS) in fully differential switched-capacitor circuits. Least-mean-squares (LMS) cancellation of common-mode leakage in the gradient signals further increases differential sensitivity. The adaptation is performed in the digital domain using counting registers, and couples to the switched-capacitor circuits using capacitive multiplying DAC arrays. An additional stage of LMS adaptation produces digital estimates of direction cosines τ_1 and τ_2 for a single source. In the present setup this stage is bypassed, and the common-mode corrected gradient signals are presented as inputs to the ICA chip for localization and separation of up to three independent sources.

3.2 Reconfigurable ICA Processor

A general mixed-signal parallel architecture, that can be configured for implementation of various ICA update rules in conjunction with gradient flow, is shown in Figure 3 [9]. Here

190

we briefly illustrate the architecture with a simple configuration designed to separate two sources, and present CMOS circuits that implement the architecture. The micrograph of the reconfigurable ICA chip is shown in Figure 2 (a).

3.2.1 ICA update rule

Efficient implementation in parallel architecture requires a simple form of the update rule, that avoids excessive matrix multiplications and inversions. A variety of ICA update algorithms can be cast in a common, unifying framework of outer-product rules [9].

To obtain estimates $y = \hat{s}$ of the sources s, a linear transformation with matrix $\mathbf{W}$ is applied to the gradient signals x, $y = \mathbf{W}x$. Diagonal terms are fixed $w_{ii} \equiv 1$, and off-diagonal terms adapt according to

$$\Delta w_{ij} = -\mu\, f(y_i) g(y_j), \qquad i \neq j \tag{5}$$

The implemented update rule can be seen as the gradient of *InfoMax* [7] multiplied by $\mathbf{W}^T$, rather than the natural gradient multiplication factor $\mathbf{W}^T\mathbf{W}$. To obtain the full natural gradient in outer-product form, it is necessary to include a back-propagation path in the network architecture, and thus additional silicon resources, to implement the vector contribution y^T. Other equivalences with standard ICA algorithms are outlined in [9].

3.2.2 Architecture

Level comparison provides implementation of discrete approximations of any scalar function $f(y)$ and $g(y)$ appearing in different learning rules. Since speech signals are approximately Laplacian distributed, the nonlinear scalar function $f(y)$ is approximated by $\text{sign}(y)$ and implemented using single bit quantization. Conversely, a linear function $g(y) \equiv y$ in the learning rule is approximated by a 3-level staircase function $(-1, 0, +1)$ using 2-bit quantization. The quantization of the f and g terms in the update rule (5) simplifies the implementation to that of discrete counting operations.

The functional block diagram of a 3×3 outer-product incremental ICA architecture, supporting a quantized form of the general update rule (5), is shown in Figure 3 [9]. Un-mixing coefficients are stored digitally in each cell of the architecture. The update is performed locally by once or repeatedly incrementing, decrementing or holding the current value of counter based on the learning rule served by the micro-controller. The 8 most significant bits of the 14-bit counter holding and updating the coefficients are presented to a multiplying D/A capacitor array [6] to linearly unmix the separated signal. The remaining 6 bits in the coefficient registers provide flexibility in programming the update rate to tailor convergence.

3.2.3 Circuit implementation

As in the implementation of the gradient flow processor [6], the mixed-signal ICA architecture is implemented using fully differential switched-capacitor sampled-data circuits. Correlated double sampling performs common mode offset rejection and 1/f noise reduction. An external micro-controller provides flexibility in the implementation of different learning rules. The ICA architecture is integrated on a single $3mm \times 3mm$ chip fabricated in 0.5 μm 3M2P CMOS technology.

The block diagram of ICA prototype in Figure 3 indicates its main functionality is a vector(3x1)-matrix(3x3) multiplication with adaptive matrix elements.

Each cell in the implemented architecture contains a 14-bit counter, decoder and D/A capacitor arrays. Adaptation is performed in outer-product fashion by incrementing, decrementing or holding the current value of the counters. The most significant 8 bits of the

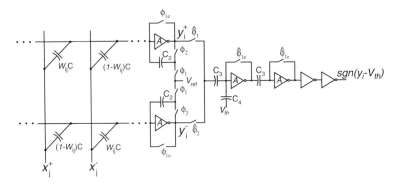

Figure 4: Correlated double sampling (CDS) switched-capacitor fully differential circuits implementing linearly weighted summing in the mixed-signal ICA architecture.

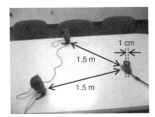

Figure 5: Experimental setup for separation of two acoustic sources in a conference room enviroment.

counter are presented to the multiplying D/A capacitor arrays to construct the source estimation. Figure 4 shows the circuits one output component in the architecture, linearly summing the input contributions. The implementation of the multiplying capacitor arrays are identical to those discussed in [6]. Each output signal y_i is is computed by accumulating outputs from the all the cells in the ith row. The accumulation is performed on C_2 by switch-cap amplifier yielding the estimated signals during Φ_2 phase. While the estimation signals are valid, $y_i{}^+$ is sampled at $\hat{\Phi}_1$ by the comparator circuit. The sign of the comparison of y_i with variable level threshold V_{th} is computed in the evaluate phase, through capacitive coupling into the amplifier input node.

4   Experimental Results

To demonstrate source separation and localization in a real environment, the mixed-signal VLSI ASICs were interfaced with four omnidirectional miniature microphones (Knowles FG-3629), arranged in a circular array with radius 0.5 cm. At the front-end, the microphone signals were passed through second-order bandpass filters with low-frequency cutoff at 130 Hz and high-frequency cutoff at 4.3 kHz. The signals were also amplified by a factor of 20.

The experimental setup is shown in Figure 5. The speech signals were presented through loudspeakers positioned at 1.5 m distance from the array. The system sampling frequency of both chips was set to 16 kHz. A male and female speakers from TIMIT database were chosen as sound sources. To provide the ground truth data and full characterization of the systems, speech segments were presented individually through either loudspeaker at different time instances. The data was recorded for both speakers, archived, and presented to the

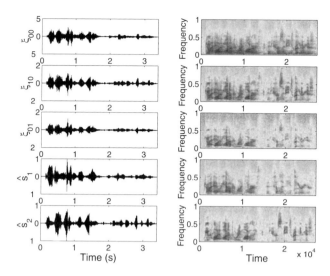

Figure 6: Time waveforms and spectrograms of the presented sources s_1 and s_2, observed common-mode and gradient signals ξ_{00}, ξ_{10} and ξ_{01} by the gradient flow chip, and recovered sources $\hat{s}_1$ and $\hat{s}_2$ by the ICA chip.

Table 1: Localization Performance

	Male speaker	Female speaker
Single-source LMS localization	-31.11	40.95
Dual-source ICA localization	-30.35	43.55

gradient flow chip. Localization results obtained by gradient flow chip through LMS adaptation are reported in Table 1. The two recorded datasets were then added, and presented to the gradient flow ASIC. The gradient signals obtained from the chip were then presented to the ICA processor, configured to implement the outerproduct update algorithm in (5). The observed convergence time was around 2 seconds. From the recorded 14-bit digital weights, the angles of incidence of the sources relative to the array were derived. These estimated angles are reported in Table 1. As seen, the angles obtained through LMS bearing estimation under individual source presentation are very close to the angles produced by ICA under joint presentation of both sources. The original sources and the recorded source signal estimates, along with recorded common-mode signal and first-order spatial gradients, are shown in Figure 6.

5 Conclusions

We presented a mixed-signal VLSI system that operates on spatial and temporal differences (gradients) of the acoustic field at very small aperture to separate and localize mixtures of traveling wave sources. The real-time performance of the system was characterized through experiments with speech sources presented through speakers in a conference room setting. Although application of static ICA is limited by reverberation, the perceptual quality of the separated outputs owes to the elimination of the direct path in the residuals. Miniature size of the microphone array enclosure (1 cm diameter) and micropower consumption of the VLSI hardware (250 μW) are key advantages of the approach, with applications to hearing aids, conferencing, multimedia, and surveillance.

Acknowledgments

This work was supported by grants of the Catalyst Foundation (New York), the National Science Foundation, and the Defense Intelligence Agency.

References

[1] D. Robert, R.N. Miles, and R.R. Hoy, "Tympanal Hearing in the Sarcophagid Parasitoid Fly Emblemasoma sp.: the Biomechanics of Directional Hearing," *J. Experimental Biology*, vol. 202, pp 1865-1876, 1999.

[2] R. Reeve and B. Webb, "New neural circuits for robot phonotaxis", *Philosophical Transactions of the Royal Society A*, vol. **361**, pp. 2245-2266, 2002.

[3] G. Cauwenberghs, M. Stanacevic, and G. Zweig, "Blind Broadband Source Localization and Separation in Miniature Sensor Arrays," *Proc. IEEE Int. Symp. Circuits and Systems (ISCAS'2001)*, Sydney, Australia, May 6-9, 2001.

[4] J. Barrère and G. Chabriel, "A Compact Sensor Array for Blind Separation of Sources", *IEEE Transactions Circuits and Systems, Part I*, vol. **49** (5), pp. 565-574, 2002.

[5] J.G. Harris, C.-J. Pu, J.C. Principe, "A Neuromorphic Monaural Sound Localizer," *Proc. Neural Inf. Proc. Sys. (NIPS*1998)*, Cambridge MA: MIT Press, vol. 10, pp. 692-698, 1999.

[6] G. Cauwenberghs and M. Stanacevic, "Micropower Mixed-Signal Acoustic Localizer," *Proc. IEEE Eur. Solid State Circuits Conf. (ESSCIRC'2003)*, Estoril Portugal, Sept. 16-18, 2003.

[7] A.J. Bell and T.J. Sejnowski, "An Information Maximization Approach to Blind Separation and Blind Deconvolution," *Neural Comp*, vol. **7** (6), pp 1129-1159, Nov 1995.

[8] L. Molgedey and G. Schuster, "Separation of a mixture of independent signals using time delayed correlations," *Physical Review Letters*, vol. 72, no. 23, pp. 3634–3637, 1994.

[9] A. Celik, M. Stanacevic and G. Cauwenberghs, "Mixed-Signal Real-Time Adaptive Blind Source Separation," *Proc. IEEE Int. Symp. Circuits and Systems (ISCAS'2004)*, Vancouver Canada, May 23-26, 2004.

[10] R. Lambert and A. Bell, "Blind separation of multiple speakers in a multipath environment," *Proc. ICASSP'97*, München, 1997.

[11] Cohen, M.H., Andreou, A.G. "Analog CMOS Integration and Experimentation with an Autoadaptive Independent Component Analyzer," *IEEE Trans. Circuits and Systems II*, vol 42 (2), pp 65-77, Feb. 1995.

[12] Gharbi, A.B.A., Salam, F.M.A. "Implementation and Test Results of a Chip for the Separation of Mixed Signals," *Proc. Int. Symp. Circuits and Systems (ISCAS'95)*, May 1995.

[13] M. Cohen and G. Cauwenberghs, "Blind Separation of Linear Convolutive Mixtures through Parallel Stochastic Optimization," *Proc. IEEE Int. Symp. Circuits and Systems (ISCAS'98)*, Monterey CA, vol. 3, pp. 17-20, 1998.

Improved Risk Tail Bounds
for On-Line Algorithms [*]

Nicolò Cesa-Bianchi
DSI, Università di Milano
via Comelico 39
20135 Milano, Italy
cesa-bianchi@dsi.unimi.it

Claudio Gentile
DICOM, Università dell'Insubria
via Mazzini 5
21100 Varese, Italy
gentile@dsi.unimi.it

Abstract

We prove the strongest known bound for the risk of hypotheses selected from the ensemble generated by running a learning algorithm incrementally on the training data. Our result is based on proof techniques that are remarkably different from the standard risk analysis based on uniform convergence arguments.

1 Introduction

In this paper, we analyze the risk of hypotheses selected from the ensemble obtained by running an arbitrary on-line learning algorithm on an i.i.d. sequence of training data. We describe a procedure that selects from the ensemble a hypothesis whose risk is, with high probability, at most

$$M_n + O\left(\frac{(\ln n)^2}{n} + \sqrt{\frac{M_n}{n}\ln n}\right),$$

where M_n is the average cumulative loss incurred by the on-line algorithm on a training sequence of length n. Note that this bound exhibits the "fast" rate $(\ln n)^2/n$ whenever the cumulative loss nM_n is $O(1)$.

This result is proven through a refinement of techniques that we used in [2] to prove the substantially weaker bound $M_n + O\left(\sqrt{(\ln n)/n}\right)$. As in the proof of the older result, we analyze the empirical process associated with a run of the on-line learner using exponential inequalities for martingales. However, this time we control the large deviations of the on-line process using Bernstein's maximal inequality rather than the Azuma-Hoeffding inequality. This provides a much tighter bound on the average risk of the ensemble. Finally, we relate the risk of a specific hypothesis within the ensemble to the average risk. As in [2], we select this hypothesis using a deterministic sequential testing procedure, but the use of Bernstein's inequality makes the analysis of this procedure far more complicated.

The study of the statistical risk of hypotheses generated by on-line algorithms, initiated by Littlestone [5], uses tools that are sharply different from those used for uniform convergence analysis, a popular approach based on the manipulation of suprema of empirical

---

[*] Part of the results contained in this paper have been presented in a talk given at the NIPS 2004 workshop on "(Ab)Use of Bounds".

processes (see, e.g., [3]). Unlike uniform convergence, which is tailored to empirical risk minimization, our bounds hold for *any* learning algorithm. Indeed, disregarding efficiency issues, any learner can be run incrementally on a data sequence to generate an ensemble of hypotheses.

The consequences of this line of research to kernel and margin-based algorithms have been presented in our previous work [2].

Notation. An *example* is a pair (x, y), where $x \in \mathcal{X}$ (which we call *instance*) is a data element and $y \in \mathcal{Y}$ is the *label* associated with it. Instances x are tuples of numerical and/or symbolic attributes. Labels y belong to a finite set of symbols (the class elements) or to an interval of the real line, depending on whether the task is classification or regression. We allow a learning algorithm to output hypotheses of the form $h : \mathcal{X} \to \mathcal{D}$, where $\mathcal{D}$ is a decision space not necessarily equal to $\mathcal{Y}$. The goodness of hypothesis h on example (x, y) is measured by the quantity $\ell(h(x), y)$, where $\ell : \mathcal{D} \times \mathcal{Y} \to \mathbb{R}$ is a nonnegative and bounded *loss function*.

2 A bound on the average risk

An on-line algorithm A works in a sequence of trials. In each trial $t = 1, 2, \ldots$ the algorithm takes in input a hypothesis H_{t-1} and an example $Z_t = (X_t, Y_t)$, and returns a new hypothesis H_t to be used in the next trial. We follow the standard assumptions in statistical learning: the sequence of examples $Z^n = ((X_1, Y_1), \ldots, (X_n, Y_n))$ is drawn i.i.d. according to an unknown distribution over $\mathcal{X} \times \mathcal{Y}$. We also assume that the loss function ℓ satisfies $0 \le \ell \le 1$. The success of a hypothesis h is measured by the *risk* of h, denoted by $\mathrm{risk}(h)$. This is the expected loss of h on an example (X, Y) drawn from the underlying distribution, $\mathrm{risk}(h) = \mathbb{E}\,\ell(h(X), Y)$. Define also $\mathrm{risk_{emp}}(h)$ to be the empirical risk of h on a sample Z^n,

$$\mathrm{risk_{emp}}(h) = \frac{1}{n} \sum_{t=1}^{n} \ell(h(X_t), Y_t) \,.$$

Given a sample Z^n and an on-line algorithm A, we use $H_0, H_1, \ldots, H_{n-1}$ to denote the *ensemble of hypotheses generated by* A. Note that the ensemble is a function of the random training sample Z^n. Our bounds hinge on the sample statistic

$$M_n = M_n(Z^n) = \frac{1}{n} \sum_{t=1}^{n} \ell(H_{t-1}(X_t), Y_t)$$

which can be easily computed as the on-line algorithm is run on Z^n.

The following bound, a consequence of Bernstein's maximal inequality for martingales due to Freedman [4], is of primary importance for proving our results.

Lemma 1 *Let $L_1, L_2, \ldots$ be a sequence of random variables, $0 \le L_t \le 1$. Define the bounded martingale difference sequence $V_t = \mathbb{E}[L_t \mid L_1, \ldots, L_{t-1}] - L_t$ and the associated martingale $S_n = V_1 + \ldots + V_n$ with conditional variance $K_n = \sum_{t=1}^{n} \mathrm{Var}[L_t \mid L_1, \ldots, L_{t-1}]$. Then, for all $s, k \ge 0$,*

$$\mathbb{P}\left(S_n \ge s, K_n \le k\right) \le \exp\left(-\frac{s^2}{2k + 2s/3}\right) \,.$$

The next proposition, derived from Lemma 1, establishes a bound on the average risk of the ensemble of hypotheses.

Proposition 2 *Let $H_0, \ldots, H_{n-1}$ be the ensemble of hypotheses generated by an arbitrary on-line algorithm $\mathbb{A}$. Then, for any $0 < \delta \leq 1$,*

$$\mathbb{P}\left(\frac{1}{n}\sum_{t=1}^{n}\mathrm{risk}(H_{t-1}) \geq M_n + \frac{36}{n}\ln\left(\frac{n\,M_n + 3}{\delta}\right) + 2\sqrt{\frac{M_n}{n}\ln\left(\frac{n\,M_n + 3}{\delta}\right)}\right) \leq \delta.$$

The bound shown in Proposition 2 has the same rate as a bound recently proven by Zhang [6, Theorem 5]. However, rather than deriving the bound from Bernstein inequality as we do, Zhang uses an ad hoc argument.

Proof. Let

$$\mu_n = \frac{1}{n}\sum_{t=1}^{n}\mathrm{risk}(H_{t-1}) \quad \text{and} \quad V_{t-1} = \mathrm{risk}(H_{t-1}) - \ell(H_{t-1}(X_t), Y_t) \quad \text{for } t \geq 1.$$

Let κ_t be the conditional variance $\mathrm{Var}\big(\ell(H_{t-1}(X_t), Y_t) \mid Z_1, \ldots, Z_{t-1}\big)$. Also, set for brevity $K_n = \sum_{t=1}^{n}\kappa_t$, $K'_n = \lfloor\sum_{t=1}^{n}\kappa_t\rfloor$, and introduce the function $A(x) = 2\ln\frac{(x+1)(x+3)}{\delta}$ for $x \geq 0$. We find upper and lower bounds on the probability

$$\mathbb{P}\left(\sum_{t=1}^{n}V_{t-1} \geq A(K_n) + \sqrt{A(K_n)\,K_n}\right). \tag{1}$$

The upper bound is determined through a simple stratification argument over Lemma 1. We can write

$$\mathbb{P}\left(\sum_{t=1}^{n}V_{t-1} \geq A(K_n) + \sqrt{A(K_n)\,K_n}\right)$$

$$\leq \mathbb{P}\left(\sum_{t=1}^{n}V_{t-1} \geq A(K'_n) + \sqrt{A(K'_n)\,K'_n}\right)$$

$$\leq \sum_{s=0}^{n}\mathbb{P}\left(\sum_{t=1}^{n}V_{t-1} \geq A(s) + \sqrt{A(s)\,s},\ K'_n = s\right)$$

$$\leq \sum_{s=0}^{n}\mathbb{P}\left(\sum_{t=1}^{n}V_{t-1} \geq A(s) + \sqrt{A(s)\,s},\ K_n \leq s+1\right)$$

$$\leq \sum_{s=0}^{n}\exp\left(-\frac{(A(s) + \sqrt{A(s)\,s})^2}{\frac{2}{3}(A(s) + \sqrt{A(s)\,s}) + 2(s+1)}\right) \quad \text{(using Lemma 1).}$$

Since $\dfrac{(A(s)+\sqrt{A(s)\,s})^2}{\frac{2}{3}\left(A(s)+\sqrt{A(s)\,s}\right)+2(s+1)} \geq A(s)/2$ for all $s \geq 0$, we obtain

$$(1) \leq \sum_{s=0}^{n}e^{-A(s)/2} = \sum_{s=0}^{n}\frac{\delta}{(s+1)(s+3)} < \delta. \tag{2}$$

As far as the lower bound on (1) is concerned, we note that our assumption $0 \leq \ell \leq 1$ implies $\kappa_t \leq \mathrm{risk}(H_{t-1})$ for all t which, in turn, gives $K_n \leq n\mu_n$. Thus

$$(1) = \mathbb{P}\left(n\mu_n - nM_n \geq A(K_n) + \sqrt{A(K_n)\,K_n}\right)$$

$$\geq \mathbb{P}\left(n\mu_n - nM_n \geq A(n\mu_n) + \sqrt{A(n\mu_n)\,n\mu_n}\right)$$

$$= \mathbb{P}\left(2n\mu_n \geq 2nM_n + 3A(n\mu_n) + \sqrt{4n\,M_n\,A(n\mu_n) + 5A(n\mu_n)^2}\right)$$

$$= \mathbb{P}\left(x \geq B + \tfrac{3}{2}A(x) + \sqrt{B\,A(x) + \tfrac{5}{4}A^2(x)}\right),$$

where we set for brevity $x = n\mu_n$ and $B = n M_n$. We would like to solve the inequality

$$x \geq B + \tfrac{3}{2}A(x) + \sqrt{B\,A(x) + \tfrac{5}{4}A^2(x)} \qquad (3)$$

w.r.t. x. More precisely, we would like to find a suitable upper bound on the (unique) x^* such that the above is satisfied as an equality.

A (tedious) derivative argument along with the upper bound $A(x) \leq 4 \ln\left(\frac{x+3}{\delta}\right)$ show that

$$x' = B + 2\sqrt{B \ln\left(\tfrac{B+3}{\delta}\right)} + 36 \ln\left(\tfrac{B+3}{\delta}\right)$$

makes the left-hand side of (3) larger than its right-hand side. Thus x' is an upper bound on x^*, and we conclude that

$$(1) \geq \mathbb{P}\left(x \geq B + 2\sqrt{B \ln\left(\tfrac{B+3}{\delta}\right)} + 36 \ln\left(\tfrac{B+3}{\delta}\right)\right)$$

which, recalling the definitions of x and B, and combining with (2), proves the bound. $\square$

3 Selecting a good hypothesis from the ensemble

If the decision space $\mathcal{D}$ of A is a convex set and the loss function ℓ is convex in its first argument, then via Jensen's inequality we can directly apply the bound of Proposition 2 to the risk of the *average hypothesis* $\overline{H} = \frac{1}{n}\sum_{t=1}^{n} H_{t-1}$. This yields

$$\mathbb{P}\left(\mathrm{risk}(\overline{H}) \geq M_n + \frac{36}{n} \ln\left(\frac{n M_n + 3}{\delta}\right) + 2\sqrt{\frac{M_n}{n} \ln\left(\frac{n M_n + 3}{\delta}\right)}\right) \leq \delta. \qquad (4)$$

Observe that this is a $O(1/n)$ bound whenever the cumulative loss $n M_n$ is $O(1)$.

If the convexity hypotheses do not hold (as in the case of classification problems), then the bound in (4) applies to a hypothesis randomly drawn from the ensemble (this was investigated in [1] though with different goals).

In this section we show how to deterministically pick from the ensemble a hypothesis whose risk is close to the average ensemble risk.

To see how this could be done, let us first introduce the functions

$$\mathcal{E}_\delta(r, t) = \frac{8B}{3(n-t)} + \sqrt{\frac{2Br}{n-t}} \quad \text{and} \quad c_\delta(r, t) = \mathcal{E}_\delta\left(r + \sqrt{\frac{2Br}{n-t}}, t\right),$$

with $B = \ln\frac{n(n+2)}{\delta}$.

Let $\mathrm{risk_{emp}}(H_t, t+1) + \mathcal{E}_\delta(\mathrm{risk_{emp}}(H_t, t+1), t)$ be the *penalized empirical risk* of hypothesis H_t, where

$$\mathrm{risk_{emp}}(H_t, t+1) = \frac{1}{n-t} \sum_{i=t+1}^{n} \ell(H_t(X_i), Y_i)$$

is the empirical risk of H_t on the remaining sample $Z_{t+1}, \ldots, Z_n$. We now analyze the performance of the learning algorithm that returns the hypothesis $\widehat{H}$ minimizing the penalized risk estimate over all hypotheses in the ensemble, i.e., [1]

$$\widehat{H} = \underset{0 \leq t < n}{\mathrm{argmin}}\left(\mathrm{risk_{emp}}(H_t, t+1) + \mathcal{E}_\delta(\mathrm{risk_{emp}}(H_t, t+1), t)\right). \qquad (5)$$

---

[1] Note that, from an algorithmic point of view, this hypothesis is fairly easy to compute. In particular, if the underlying on-line algorithm is a standard kernel-based algorithm, $\widehat{H}$ can be calculated via a single sweep through the example sequence.

Lemma 3 *Let $H_0, \ldots, H_{n-1}$ be the ensemble of hypotheses generated by an arbitrary on-line algorithm $\mathtt{A}$ working with a loss ℓ satisfying $0 \leq \ell \leq 1$. Then, for any $0 < \delta \leq 1$, the hypothesis $\widehat{H}$ satisfies*

$$\mathbb{P}\left(\mathtt{risk}(\widehat{H}) > \min_{0 \leq t < n}\left(\mathtt{risk}(H_t) + 2\,c_\delta(\mathtt{risk}(H_t), t)\right)\right) \leq \delta.$$

Proof. We introduce the following short-hand notation

$$R_t \;=\; \mathtt{risk_{emp}}(H_t, t+1), \qquad \widehat{T} = \operatorname*{argmin}_{0 \leq t < n}\left(R_t + \mathcal{E}_\delta(R_t, t)\right)$$

$$T^* \;=\; \operatorname*{argmin}_{0 \leq t < n}\left(\mathtt{risk}(H_t) + 2c_\delta(\mathtt{risk}(H_t), t)\right).$$

Also, let $H^* = H_{T^*}$ and $R^* = \mathtt{risk_{emp}}(H_{T^*}, T^* + 1) = R_{T^*}$. Note that $\widehat{H}$ defined in (5) coincides with $H_{\widehat{T}}$. Finally, let

$$Q(r, t) = \frac{\sqrt{2B(2B + 9r(n-t))} - 2B}{3(n-t)}.$$

With this notation we can write

$$\mathbb{P}\left(\mathtt{risk}(\widehat{H}) > \mathtt{risk}(H^*) + 2c_\delta(\mathtt{risk}(H^*), T^*)\right)$$

$$\leq \quad \mathbb{P}\left(\mathtt{risk}(\widehat{H}) > \mathtt{risk}(H^*) + 2c_\delta\left(R^* - Q(R^*, T^*), T^*\right)\right)$$

$$+ \quad \mathbb{P}\left(\mathtt{risk}(H^*) < R^* - Q(R^*, T^*)\right)$$

$$\leq \quad \mathbb{P}\left(\mathtt{risk}(\widehat{H}) > \mathtt{risk}(H^*) + 2c_\delta\left(R^* - Q(R^*, T^*), T^*\right)\right)$$

$$+ \quad \sum_{t=0}^{n-1} \mathbb{P}\left(\mathtt{risk}(H_t) < R_t - Q(R_t, t)\right).$$

Applying the standard Bernstein's inequality (see, e.g., [3, Ch. 8]) to the random variables R_t with $|R_t| \leq 1$ and expected value $\mathtt{risk}(H_t)$, and upper bounding the variance of R_t with $\mathtt{risk}(H_t)$, yields

$$\mathbb{P}\left(\mathtt{risk}(H_t) < R_t - \frac{B + \sqrt{B(B + 18(n-t)\mathtt{risk}(H_t))}}{3(n-t)}\right) \leq e^{-B}.$$

With a little algebra, it is easy to show that

$$\mathtt{risk}(H_t) < R_t - \frac{B + \sqrt{B(B + 18(n-t)\mathtt{risk}(H_t))}}{3(n-t)}$$

is equivalent to $\mathtt{risk}(H_t) < R_t - Q(R_t, t)$. Hence, we get

$$\mathbb{P}\left(\mathtt{risk}(\widehat{H}) > \mathtt{risk}(H^*) + 2c_\delta(\mathtt{risk}(H^*), T^*)\right)$$

$$\leq \quad \mathbb{P}\left(\mathtt{risk}(\widehat{H}) > \mathtt{risk}(H^*) + 2c_\delta\left(R^* - Q(R^*, T^*), T^*\right)\right) + n\,e^{-B}$$

$$\leq \quad \mathbb{P}\left(\mathtt{risk}(\widehat{H}) > \mathtt{risk}(H^*) + 2\mathcal{E}_\delta(R^*, T^*)\right) + n\,e^{-B}$$

where in the last step we used

$$Q(r,t) \leq \sqrt{\frac{2Br}{n-t}} \quad \text{and} \quad c_\delta\left(r - \sqrt{\frac{2Br}{n-t}}, t\right) = \mathcal{E}_\delta(r,t).$$

Set for brevity $\mathcal{E} = \mathcal{E}_\delta(R^*, T^*)$. We have

$$\mathbb{P}\left(\text{risk}(\widehat{H}) > \text{risk}(H^*) + 2\mathcal{E}\right)$$

$$= \mathbb{P}\left(\text{risk}(\widehat{H}) > \text{risk}(H^*) + 2\mathcal{E}, \; R_{\widehat{T}} + \mathcal{E}_\delta(R_{\widehat{T}}, \widehat{T}) \leq R^* + \mathcal{E}\right)$$

(since $R_{\widehat{T}} + \mathcal{E}_\delta(R_{\widehat{T}}, \widehat{T}) \leq R^* + \mathcal{E}$ holds with certainty)

$$\leq \sum_{t=0}^{n-1} \mathbb{P}\left(R_t + \mathcal{E}_\delta(R_t, t) \leq R^* + \mathcal{E}, \; \text{risk}(H_t) > \text{risk}(H^*) + 2\mathcal{E}\right). \qquad (6)$$

Now, if $R_t + \mathcal{E}_\delta(R_t, t) \leq R^* + \mathcal{E}$ holds, then at least one of the following three conditions
$R_t \leq \text{risk}(H_t) - \mathcal{E}_\delta(R_t, t), \quad R^* > \text{risk}(H^*) + \mathcal{E}, \quad \text{risk}(H_t) - \text{risk}(H^*) < 2\mathcal{E}$
must hold. Hence, for any fixed t we can write

$$\mathbb{P}\left(R_t + \mathcal{E}_\delta(R_t, t) \leq R^* + \mathcal{E}, \; \text{risk}(H_t) > \text{risk}(H^*) + 2\mathcal{E}\right)$$

$$\leq \mathbb{P}\left(R_t \leq \text{risk}(H_t) - \mathcal{E}_\delta(R_t, t), \; \text{risk}(H_t) > \text{risk}(H^*) + 2\mathcal{E}\right)$$

$$+ \mathbb{P}\left(R^* > \text{risk}(H^*) + \mathcal{E}, \; \text{risk}(H_t) > \text{risk}(H^*) + 2\mathcal{E}\right)$$

$$+ \mathbb{P}\left(\text{risk}(H_t) - \text{risk}(H^*) < 2\mathcal{E}, \; \text{risk}(H_t) > \text{risk}(H^*) + 2\mathcal{E}\right)$$

$$\leq \mathbb{P}\left(R_t \leq \text{risk}(H_t) - \mathcal{E}_\delta(R_t, t)\right) + \mathbb{P}\left(R^* > \text{risk}(H^*) + \mathcal{E}\right). \qquad (7)$$

Plugging (7) into (6) we have

$$\mathbb{P}\left(\text{risk}(\widehat{H}) > \text{risk}(H^*) + 2\mathcal{E}\right)$$

$$\leq \sum_{t=0}^{n-1} \mathbb{P}\left(R_t \leq \text{risk}(H_t) - \mathcal{E}_\delta(R_t, t)\right) + n\,\mathbb{P}\left(R^* > \text{risk}(H^*) + \mathcal{E}\right)$$

$$\leq n e^{-B} + n \sum_{t=0}^{n-1} \mathbb{P}\left(R_t \geq \text{risk}(H_t) + \mathcal{E}_\delta(R_t, t)\right) \leq n e^{-B} + n^2 e^{-B},$$

where in the last two inequalities we applied again Bernstein's inequality to the random variables R_t with mean $\text{risk}(H_t)$. Putting together we obtain

$$\mathbb{P}\left(\text{risk}(\widehat{H}) > \text{risk}(H^*) + 2c_\delta(\text{risk}(H^*), T^*)\right) \leq (2n + n^2)e^{-B}$$

which, recalling that $B = \ln \frac{n(n+2)}{\delta}$, implies the thesis. $\qquad \square$

Fix $n \geq 1$ and $\delta \in (0, 1)$. For each $t = 0, \ldots, n-1$, introduce the function

$$f_t(x) = x + \frac{11C}{3} \frac{\ln(n-t) + 1}{n-t} + 2\sqrt{\frac{2Cx}{n-t}}, \quad x \geq 0,$$

where $C = \ln \frac{2n(n+2)}{\delta}$. Note that each f_t is monotonically increasing. We are now ready to state and prove the main result of this paper.

Theorem 4 *Fix any loss function ℓ satisfying $0 \le \ell \le 1$. Let $H_0, \ldots, H_{n-1}$ be the ensemble of hypotheses generated by an arbitrary on-line algorithm $\mathbb{A}$ and let $\widehat{H}$ be the hypothesis minimizing the penalized empirical risk expression obtained by replacing c_δ with $c_{\delta/2}$ in (5). Then, for any $0 < \delta \le 1$, $\widehat{H}$ satisfies*

$$\mathbb{P}\left(\mathrm{risk}(\widehat{H}) \ge \min_{0 \le t < n} f_t\left(M_{t,n} + \frac{36}{n-t} \ln \frac{2n(n+3)}{\delta} + 2\sqrt{\frac{M_{t,n} \ln \frac{2n(n+3)}{\delta}}{n-t}} \right) \right) \le \delta,$$

where $M_{t,n} = \frac{1}{n-t} \sum_{i=t+1}^{n} \ell(H_{i-1}(X_i), Y_i)$. *In particular, upper bounding the minimum over t with $t = 0$ yields*

$$\mathbb{P}\left(\mathrm{risk}(\widehat{H}) \ge f_0\left(M_n + \frac{36}{n} \ln \frac{2n(n+3)}{\delta} + 2\sqrt{\frac{M_n \ln \frac{2n(n+3)}{\delta}}{n}} \right) \right) \le \delta. \quad (8)$$

For $n \to \infty$, bound (8) shows that $\mathrm{risk}(\widehat{H})$ is bounded with high probability by

$$M_n + O\left(\frac{\ln^2 n}{n} + \sqrt{\frac{M_n \ln n}{n}} \right).$$

If the empirical cumulative loss $n M_n$ is small (say, $M_n \le c/n$, where c is constant with n), then our penalized empirical risk minimizer $\widehat{H}$ achieves a $O((\ln^2 n)/n)$ risk bound. Also, recall that, in this case, under convexity assumptions the average hypothesis $\overline{H}$ achieves the sharper bound $O(1/n)$.

Proof. Let $\mu_{t,n} = \frac{1}{n-t} \sum_{i=t}^{n-1} \mathrm{risk}(H_i)$. Applying Lemma 3 with $c_{\delta/2}$ we obtain

$$\mathbb{P}\left(\mathrm{risk}(\widehat{H}) > \min_{0 \le t < n} \left(\mathrm{risk}(H_t) + c_{\delta/2}(\mathrm{risk}(H_t), t) \right) \right) \le \frac{\delta}{2}. \quad (9)$$

We then observe that

$$\min_{0 \le t < n} \left(\mathrm{risk}(H_t) + c_{\delta/2}(\mathrm{risk}(H_t), t) \right)$$

$$= \min_{0 \le t < n} \min_{t \le i < n} \left(\mathrm{risk}(H_i) + c_{\delta/2}(\mathrm{risk}(H_i), i) \right)$$

$$\le \min_{0 \le t < n} \frac{1}{n-t} \sum_{i=t}^{n-1} \left(\mathrm{risk}(H_i) + c_{\delta/2}(\mathrm{risk}(H_i), i) \right)$$

$$\le \min_{0 \le t < n} \left(\mu_{t,n} + \frac{1}{n-t} \sum_{i=t}^{n-1} \frac{8}{3} \frac{C}{n-i} + \frac{1}{n-t} \sum_{i=t}^{n-1} \left(\sqrt{\frac{2C \, \mathrm{risk}(H_i)}{n-i}} + \frac{C}{n-i} \right) \right)$$

$$\quad \text{(using the inequality } \sqrt{x+y} \le \sqrt{x} + \frac{y}{2\sqrt{x}} \text{)}$$

$$= \min_{0 \le t < n} \left(\mu_{t,n} + \frac{1}{n-t} \sum_{i=t}^{n-1} \frac{11}{3} \frac{C}{n-i} + \frac{1}{n-t} \sum_{i=t}^{n-1} \sqrt{\frac{2C \, \mathrm{risk}(H_i)}{n-i}} \right)$$

$$\le \min_{0 \le t < n} \left(\mu_{t,n} + \frac{11C}{3} \frac{\ln(n-t)+1}{n-t} + 2\sqrt{\frac{2C\mu_{t,n}}{n-t}} \right)$$

$$\quad \text{(using } \sum_{i=1}^{k} 1/i \le 1 + \ln k \text{ and the concavity of the square root)}$$

$$= \min_{0 \le t < n} f_t(\mu_{t,n}).$$

201

Now, it is clear that Proposition 2 can be immediately generalized to imply the following set of inequalities, one for each $t = 0, \ldots, n-1$,

$$\mathbb{P}\left(\mu_{t,n} \geq M_{t,n} + \frac{36\,A}{n-t} + 2\sqrt{\frac{M_{t,n}\,A}{n-t}}\right) \leq \frac{\delta}{2n} \qquad (10)$$

where $A = \ln \frac{2n(n+3)}{\delta}$. Introduce the random variables $K_0, \ldots, K_{n-1}$ to be defined later. We can write

$$\mathbb{P}\left(\min_{0 \leq t < n}\left(\texttt{risk}(H_t) + c_{\delta/2}(\texttt{risk}(H_t), t)\right) \geq \min_{0 \leq t < n} K_t\right)$$

$$\leq \mathbb{P}\left(\min_{0 \leq t < n} f_t(\mu_{t,n}) \geq \min_{0 \leq t < n} K_t\right) \leq \sum_{t=0}^{n-1}\mathbb{P}\left(f_t(\mu_{t,n}) \geq K_t\right).$$

Now, for each $t = 0, \ldots, n-1$, define $K_t = f_t\left(M_{t,n} + \frac{36\,A}{n-t} + 2\sqrt{\frac{M_{t,n}\,A}{n-t}}\right)$. Then (10) and the monotonicity of $f_0, \ldots, f_{n-1}$ allow us to obtain

$$\mathbb{P}\left(\min_{0 \leq t < n}\left(\texttt{risk}(H_t) + c_{\delta/2}(\texttt{risk}(H_t), t)\right) \geq \min_{0 \leq t < n} K_t\right)$$

$$\leq \sum_{t=0}^{n-1}\mathbb{P}\left(f_t(\mu_{t,n}) \geq f_t\left(M_{t,n} + \frac{36\,A}{n-t} + 2\sqrt{\frac{M_{t,n}\,A}{n-t}}\right)\right)$$

$$= \sum_{t=0}^{n-1}\mathbb{P}\left(\mu_{t,n} \geq M_{t,n} + \frac{36\,A}{n-t} + 2\sqrt{\frac{M_{t,n}\,A}{n-t}}\right) \leq \delta/2.$$

Combining with (9) concludes the proof. $\qquad\qquad\square$

4   Conclusions and current research issues

We have shown tail risk bounds for specific hypotheses selected from the ensemble generated by the run of an arbitrary on-line algorithm. Proposition 2, our simplest bound, is proven via an easy application of Bernstein's maximal inequality for martingales, a quite basic result in probability theory. The analysis of Theorem 4 is also centered on the same martingale inequality. An open problem is to simplify this analysis, possibly obtaining a more readable bound. Also, the bound shown in Theorem 4 contains $\ln n$ terms. We do not know whether these logarithmic terms can be improved to $\ln(M_n n)$, similarly to Proposition 2. A further open problem is to prove lower bounds, even in the special case when $n M_n$ is bounded by a constant.

References

[1] A. Blum, A. Kalai, and J. Langford. Beating the hold-out. In *Proc. 12th COLT*, 1999.

[2] N. Cesa-Bianchi, A. Conconi, and C. Gentile. On the generalization ability of on-line learning algorithms. *IEEE Trans. on Information Theory*, 50(9):2050–2057, 2004.

[3] L. Devroye, L. Győrfi, and G. Lugosi. *A Probabilistic Theory of Pattern Recognition*. Springer Verlag, 1996.

[4] D. A. Freedman. On tail probabilities for martingales. *The Annals of Probability*, 3:100–118, 1975.

[5] N. Littlestone. From on-line to batch learning. In *Proc. 2nd COLT*, 1989.

[6] T. Zhang. Data dependent concentration bounds for sequential prediction algorithms. In *Proc. 18th COLT*, 2005.

Layered Dynamic Textures

Antoni B. Chan   **Nuno Vasconcelos**
Department of Electrical and Computer Engineering
University of California, San Diego
abchan@ucsd.edu, nuno@ece.ucsd.edu

Abstract

A dynamic texture is a video model that treats a video as a sample from a spatio-temporal stochastic process, specifically a linear dynamical system. One problem associated with the dynamic texture is that it cannot model video where there are multiple regions of distinct motion. In this work, we introduce the layered dynamic texture model, which addresses this problem. We also introduce a variant of the model, and present the EM algorithm for learning each of the models. Finally, we demonstrate the efficacy of the proposed model for the tasks of segmentation and synthesis of video.

1 Introduction

Traditional motion representations, based on optical flow, are inherently local and have significant difficulties when faced with aperture problems and noise. The classical solution to this problem is to regularize the optical flow field [1, 2, 3, 4], but this introduces undesirable smoothing across motion edges or regions where the motion is, by definition, not smooth (e.g. vegetation in outdoors scenes). More recently, there have been various attempts to model video as a superposition of layers subject to homogeneous motion. While layered representations exhibited significant promise in terms of combining the advantages of regularization (use of global cues to determine local motion) with the flexibility of local representations (little undue smoothing), this potential has so far not fully materialized. One of the main limitations is their dependence on parametric motion models, such as affine transforms, which assume a piece-wise planar world that rarely holds in practice [5, 6]. In fact, layers are usually formulated as "cardboard" models of the world that are warped by such transformations and then stitched to form the frames in a video stream [5]. This severely limits the types of video that can be synthesized: while layers showed most promise as models for scenes composed of ensembles of objects subject to homogeneous motion (e.g. leaves blowing in the wind, a flock of birds, a picket fence, or highway traffic), very little progress has so far been demonstrated in actually modeling such scenes.

Recently, there has been more success in modeling complex scenes as *dynamic textures* or, more precisely, samples from stochastic processes defined over space and time [7, 8, 9, 10]. This work has demonstrated that modeling both the dynamics and appearance of video as stochastic quantities leads to a much more powerful generative model for video than that of a "cardboard" figure subject to parametric motion. In fact, the dynamic texture model has shown a surprising ability to abstract a wide variety of complex patterns of motion and appearance into a *simple* spatio-temporal model. One major current limitation of the dynamic texture framework, however, is its inability to account for visual processes consisting of *multiple, co-occurring, dynamic textures*. For example, a flock of birds flying in front of a water fountain, highway traffic moving at different speeds, video containing both trees in the background and people in the foreground, and so forth. In such cases, the existing dynamic texture model is inherently incorrect, since it must represent multiple motion fields with a single dynamic process.

In this work, we address this limitation by introducing a new generative model for video, which we denote by the *layered dynamic texture* (LDT). This consists of augmenting the dynamic texture with a discrete *hidden* variable, that enables the assignment of different dynamics to different regions of the video. Conditioned on the state of this hidden variable, the video is then modeled as a simple dynamic texture. By introducing a shared dynamic representation for all the pixels in the same region, the new model is a layered representation. When compared with traditional layered models, it replaces the process of layer formation based on "warping of cardboard figures" with one based on sampling from the generative model (for both dynamics and appearance) provided by the dynamic texture. This enables a much richer video representation. Since each layer is a dynamic texture, the model can also be seen as a multi-state dynamic texture, which is capable of assigning different dynamics and appearance to different image regions.

We consider two models for the LDT, that differ in the way they enforce consistency of layer dynamics. One model enforces stronger consistency but has no closed-form solution for parameter estimates (which require sampling), while the second enforces weaker consistency but is simpler to learn. The models are applied to the segmentation and synthesis of sequences that are challenging for traditional vision representations. It is shown that stronger consistency leads to superior performance, demonstrating the benefits of sophisticated layered representations. The paper is organized as follows. In Section 2, we introduce the two layered dynamic texture models. In Section 3 we present the EM algorithm for learning both models from training data. Finally, in Section 4 we present an experimental evaluation in the context of segmentation and synthesis.

2   Layered dynamic textures

We start with a brief review of dynamic textures, and then introduce the layered dynamic texture model.

2.1   Dynamic texture

A dynamic texture [7] is a generative model for video, based on a linear dynamical system. The basic idea is to separate the visual component and the underlying dynamics into two processes. While the dynamics are represented as a time-evolving state process $x_t \in \mathbb{R}^n$, the appearance of frame $y_t \in \mathbb{R}^N$ is a linear function of the current state vector, plus some observation noise. Formally, the system is described by

$$\begin{cases} x_t = Ax_{t-1} + Bv_t \\ y_t = Cx_t + \sqrt{r}w_t \end{cases} \tag{1}$$

where $A \in \mathbb{R}^{n \times n}$ is a transition matrix, $C \in \mathbb{R}^{N \times n}$ a transformation matrix, $Bv_t \sim_{iid} \mathcal{N}(0, Q,)$ and $\sqrt{r}w_t \sim_{iid} \mathcal{N}(0, rI_N)$ the state and observation noise processes parameterized by $B \in \mathbb{R}^{n \times n}$ and $r \in \mathbb{R}$, and the initial state $x_0 \in \mathbb{R}^n$ is a constant. One interpretation of the dynamic texture model is that the columns of C are the principal components of the video frames, and the state vectors the PCA coefficients for each video frame. This is the case when the model is learned with the method of [7].

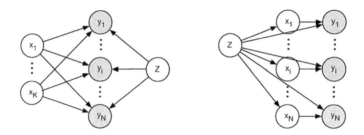

Figure 1: The layered dynamic texture (left), and the approximate layered dynamic texture (right). y_i is an observed pixel over time, x_j is a hidden state process, and Z is the collection of layer assignment variables z_i that assigns each pixels to one of the state processes.

An alternative interpretation considers a single pixel as it evolves over time. Each coordinate of the state vector x_t defines a one-dimensional random trajectory in time. A pixel is then represented as a weighted sum of random trajectories, where the weighting coefficients are contained in the corresponding row of C. This is analogous to the discrete Fourier transform in signal processing, where a signal is represented as a weighted sum of complex exponentials although, for the dynamic texture, the trajectories are not necessarily orthogonal. This interpretation illustrates the ability of the dynamic texture to model the same motion under different intensity levels (e.g. cars moving from the shade into sunlight) by simply scaling the rows of C. Regardless of interpretation, the simple dynamic texture model has only one state process, which restricts the efficacy of the model to video where the motion is homogeneous.

2.2 Layered dynamic textures

We now introduce the *layered dynamic texture* (LDT), which is shown in Figure 1 (left). The model addresses the limitations of the dynamic texture by relying on a set of state processes $X = \{x^{(j)}\}_{j=1}^{K}$ to model different video dynamics. The layer assignment variable z_i assigns pixel y_i to one of the state processes (layers), and conditioned on the layer assignments, the pixels in the same layer are modeled as a dynamic texture. In addition, the collection of layer assignments $Z = \{z_i\}_{i=1}^{N}$ is modeled as a Markov random field (MRF) to ensure spatial layer consistency. The linear system equations for the layered dynamic texture are

$$
\begin{cases}
x_t^{(j)} = A^{(j)} x_{t-1}^{(j)} + B^{(j)} v_t^{(j)} & j \in \{1, \cdots, K\} \\
y_{i,t} = C_i^{(z_i)} x_t^{(z_i)} + \sqrt{r^{(z_i)}} w_{i,t} & i \in \{1, \cdots, N\}
\end{cases}
\tag{2}
$$

where $C_i^{(j)} \in \mathbb{R}^{1 \times n}$ is the transformation from the hidden state to the observed pixel domain for each pixel y_i and each layer j, the noise parameters are $B^{(j)} \in \mathbb{R}^{n \times n}$ and $r^{(j)} \in \mathbb{R}$, the iid noise processes are $w_{i,t} \sim_{iid} \mathcal{N}(0,1)$ and $v_t^{(j)} \sim_{iid} \mathcal{N}(0, I_n)$, and the initial states are drawn from $x_1^{(j)} \sim \mathcal{N}(\mu^{(j)}, S^{(j)})$. As a generative model, the layered dynamic texture assumes that the state processes X and the layer assignments Z are independent, i.e. layer motion is independent of layer location, and vice versa. As will be seen in Section 3, this makes the expectation-step of the EM algorithm intractable to compute in closed-form. To address this issue, we also consider a slightly different model.

2.3 Approximate layered dynamic texture

We now consider a different model, the approximate layered dynamic texture (ALDT), shown in Figure 1 (right). Each pixel y_i is associated with its own state process x_i, and a different dynamic texture is defined for each pixel. However, dynamic textures associated with the same layer share the same set of dynamic parameters, which are assigned by the layer assignment variable z_i. Again, the collection of layer assignments Z is modeled as an MRF but, unlike the first model, conditioning on the layer assignments makes all the pixels independent. The model is described by the following linear system equations

$$\begin{cases} x_{i,t} = A^{(z_i)}x_{i,t-1} + B^{(z_i)}v_{i,t} & i \in \{1, \cdots, N\} \\ y_{i,t} = C_i^{(z_i)}x_{i,t} + \sqrt{r^{(z_i)}}w_{i,t} \end{cases} \tag{3}$$

where the noise processes are $w_{i,t} \sim_{iid} \mathcal{N}(0, 1)$ and $v_{i,t} \sim_{iid} \mathcal{N}(0, I_n)$, and the initial states are given by $x_{i,1} \sim \mathcal{N}(\mu^{(z_i)}, S^{(z_i)})$. This model can also be seen as a video extension of the popular image MRF models [11], where class variables for each pixel form an MRF grid and each class (e.g. pixels in the same segment) has some class-conditional distribution (in our case a linear dynamical system).

The main difference between the two proposed models is in the enforcement of consistency of dynamics within a layer. With the LDT, consistency of dynamics is strongly enforced by requiring each pixel in the layer to be associated with the *same* state process. On the other hand, for the ALDT, consistency within a layer is weakly enforced by allowing the pixels to be associated with *many* instantiations of the state process (instantiations associated with the same layer sharing the same dynamic parameters). This weaker dependency structure enables a more efficient learning algorithm.

2.4 Modeling layer assignments

The MRF which determines layer assignments has the following distribution

$$p(Z) = \frac{1}{\mathcal{Z}} \prod_i \psi_i(z_i) \prod_{(i,j) \in \mathcal{E}} \psi_{i,j}(z_i, z_j) \tag{4}$$

where $\mathcal{E}$ is the set of edges in the MRF grid, $\mathcal{Z}$ a normalization constant (partition function), and ψ_i and $\psi_{i,j}$ potential functions of the form

$$\psi_i(z_i) = \begin{cases} \alpha_1 & , z_i = 1 \\ \vdots & \vdots \\ \alpha_K & , z_i = K \end{cases} \qquad \psi_{i,j}(z_i, z_j) = \begin{cases} \gamma_1 & , z_i = z_j \\ \gamma_2 & , z_i \neq z_j \end{cases} \tag{5}$$

The potential function ψ_i defines a prior likelihood for each layer, while $\psi_{i,j}$ attributes higher probability to configurations where neighboring pixels are in the same layer. While the parameters for the potential functions could be learned for each model, we instead treat them as constants that can be estimated from a database of manually segmented training video.

3   Parameter estimation

The parameters of the model are learned using the Expectation-Maximization (EM) algorithm [12], which iterates between estimating hidden state variables X and hidden layer assignments Z from the current parameters, and updating the parameters given the current hidden variable estimates. One iteration of the EM algorithm contains the following two steps

- E-Step: $\mathcal{Q}(\Theta; \hat{\Theta}) = \mathrm{E}_{X,Z|Y;\hat{\Theta}}(\log p(X, Y, Z; \Theta))$
- M-Step: $\hat{\Theta}^* = \mathrm{argmax}_\Theta \mathcal{Q}(\Theta; \hat{\Theta})$

In the remainder of this section, we briefly describe the EM algorithm for the two proposed models. Due to the limited space available, we refer the reader to the companion technical report [13] for further details.

3.1 EM for the layered dynamic texture

The E-step for the layered dynamic texture computes the conditional mean and covariance of $x_t^{(j)}$ given the observed video Y. These expectations are intractable to compute in closed-form since it is not known to which state process each of the pixels y_i is assigned, and it is therefore necessary to marginalize over all configurations of Z. This problem also appears for the computation of the posterior layer assignment probability $p(z_i = j|Y)$. The method of approximating these expectations which we currently adopt is to simply average over draws from the posterior $p(X, Z|Y)$ using a Gibbs sampler. Other approximations, e.g. variational methods or belief propagation, could be used as well. We plan to consider them in the future. Once the expectations are known, the M-step parameter updates are analogous to those required to learn a regular linear dynamical system [15, 16], with a minor modification in the updates if the transformation matrices $C_i^{(j)}$. See [13] for details.

3.2 EM for the approximate layered dynamic texture

The ALDT model is similar to the mixture of dynamic textures [14], a video clustering model that treats a collection of videos as a sample from a collection of dynamic textures. Since, for the ALDT model, each pixel is sampled from a set of one-dimensional dynamic textures, the EM algorithm is similar to that of the mixture of dynamic textures. There are only two differences. First, the E-step computes the posterior assignment probability $p(z_i|Y)$ given all the observed data, rather than conditioned on a single data point $p(z_i|y_i)$. The posterior $p(z_i|Y)$ can be approximated by sampling from the full posterior $p(Z|Y)$ using Markov-Chain Monte Carlo [11], or with other methods, such as loopy belief propagation. Second, the transformation matrix $C_i^{(j)}$ is different for each pixel, and the E and M steps must be modified accordingly. Once again, the details are available in [13].

4 Experiments

In this section, we show the efficacy of the proposed model for segmentation and synthesis of several videos with multiple regions of distinct motion. Figure 2 shows the three video sequences used in testing. The first (top) is a composite of three distinct video textures of water, smoke, and fire. The second (middle) is of laundry spinning in a dryer. The laundry in the bottom left of the video is spinning in place in a circular motion, and the laundry around the outside is spinning faster. The final video (bottom) is of a highway [17] where the traffic in each lane is traveling at a different speed. The first, second and fourth lanes (from left to right) move faster than the third and fifth. All three videos have multiple regions of motion and are therefore properly modeled by the models proposed in this paper, but not by a regular dynamic texture.

Four variations of the video models were fit to each of the three videos. The four models were the layered dynamic texture and the approximate layered dynamic texture models (LDT and ALDT), and those two models without the MRF layer assignment (LDT-iid and ALDT-iid). In the latter two cases, the layers assignments z_i are distributed as iid multinomials. In all the experiments, the dimension of the state space was $n = 10$. The MRF grid was based on the eight-neighbor system (with cliques of size 2), and the parameters of the potential functions were $\gamma_1 = 0.99$, $\gamma_2 = 0.01$, and $\alpha_j = 1/K$. The expectations required by the EM algorithm were approximated using Gibbs sampling for the LDT and LDT-iid models and MCMC for the ALDT model. We first present segmentation results, to show that the models can effectively separate layers with different dynamics, and then discuss results relative to video synthesis from the learned models.

4.1 Segmentation

The videos were segmented by assigning each of the pixels to the most probable layer conditioned on the observed video, i.e.

$$z_i^* = \operatorname*{argmax}_j p(z_i = j|Y) \tag{6}$$

Another possibility would be to assign the pixels by maximizing the posterior of all the pixels $p(Z|Y)$. While this maximizes the true posterior, in practice we obtained similar results with the two methods. The former method was chosen because the individual posterior distributions are already computed during the E-step of EM.

The columns of Figure 3 show the segmentation results obtained with for the four models: LDT and LDT-iid in columns (a) and (b), and ALDT and ALDT-iid in columns (c) and (d). The segmented video is also available at [18]. From the segmentations produced by the iid models, it can be concluded that the composite and laundry videos can be reasonably well segmented without the MRF prior. This confirms the intuition that the various video regions contain very distinct dynamics, which can only be modeled with separate state processes. Otherwise, the pixels should be either randomly assigned among the various layers, or uniformly assigned to one of them. The segmentations of the traffic video using the iid models are poor. While the dynamics are different, the differences are significantly more subtle, and segmentation requires stronger enforcement of layer consistency. In general, the segmentations using LDT-iid are better than to those of the ALDT-iid, due to the weaker form of layer consistency imposed by the ALDT model. While this deficiency is offset by the introduction of the MRF prior, the stronger consistency enforced by the LDT model always results in better segmentations. This illustrates the need for the design of sophisticated layered representations when the goal is to model video with subtle inter-layer variations. As expected, the introduction of the MRF prior improves the segmentations produced by both models. For example, in the composite sequence all erroneous segments in the water region are removed, and in the traffic sequence, most of the speckled segmentation also disappears.

In terms of the overall segmentation quality, both LDT and ALDT are able to segment the composite video perfectly. The segmentation of the laundry video by both models is plausible, as the laundry tumbling around the edge of the dryer moves faster than that spinning in place. The two models also produce reasonable segmentations of the traffic video, with the segments roughly corresponding to the different lanes of traffic. Much of the errors correspond to regions that either contain intermittent motion (e.g. the region between the lanes) or almost no motion (e.g. truck in the upper-right corner and flat-bed truck in the third lane). Some of these errors could be eliminated by filtering the video before segmentation, but we have attempted no pre or post-processing. Finally, we note that the laundry and traffic videos are not trivial to segment with standard computer vision techniques, namely methods based on optical flow. This is particularly true in the case of the traffic video where the abundance of straight lines and flat regions makes computing the correct optical flow difficult due to the aperture problem.

4.2 Synthesis

The layered dynamic texture is a generative model, and hence a video can be synthesized by drawing a sample from the learned model. A synthesized composite video using the LDT, ALDT, and the normal dynamic texture can be found at [18]. When modeling a video with multiple motions, the regular dynamic texture will average different dynamics.

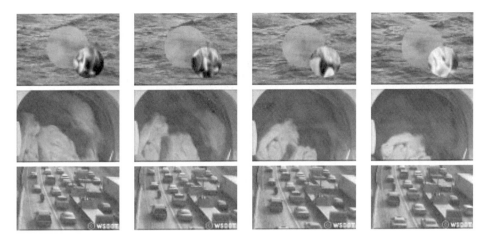

Figure 2: Frames from the test video sequences: (top) composite of water, smoke, and fire video textures; (middle) spinning laundry in a dryer; and (bottom) highway traffic with lanes traveling at different speeds.

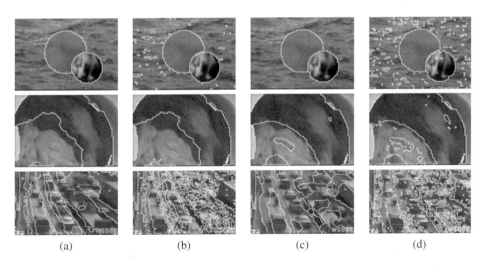

(a)   (b)   (c)   (d)

Figure 3: Segmentation results for each of the test videos using: (a) the layered dynamic texture, and (b) the layered dynamic texture without MRF; (c) the approximate layered dynamic texture, and (d) the approximate LDT without MRF.

This is noticeable in the synthesized video, where the fire region does not flicker at the same speed as in the original video. Furthermore, the motions in different regions are coupled, e.g. when the fire begins to flicker faster, the water region ceases to move smoothly. In contrast, the video synthesized from the layered dynamic texture is more realistic, as the fire region flickers at the correct speed, and the different regions follow their own motion patterns. The video synthesized from the ALDT appears noisy because the pixels evolve from different instantiations of the state process. Once again this illustrates the need for sophisticated layered models.

References

[1] B. K. P. Horn. *Robot Vision*. McGraw-Hill Book Company, New York, 1986.

[2] B. Horn and B. Schunk. Determining optical fbw. *Artificial Intelligence*, vol. 17, 1981.

[3] B. Lucas and T. Kanade. An iterative image registration technique with an application to stereo vision. *Proc. DARPA Image Understanding Workshop*, 1981.

[4] J. Barron, D. Fleet, and S. Beauchemin. Performance of optical fbw techniques. *International Journal of Computer Vision*, vol. 12, 1994.

[5] J. Wang and E. Adelson. Representing moving images with layers. *IEEE Trans. on Image Processing*, vol. 3, September 1994.

[6] B. Frey and N. Jojic. Estimating mixture models of images and inferring spatial transformations using the EM algorithm. In *IEEE Conference on Computer Vision and Pattern Recognition*, 1999.

[7] G. Doretto, A. Chiuso, Y. N. Wu, and S. Soatto. Dynamic textures. *International Journal of Computer Vision*, vol. 2, pp. 91-109, 2003.

[8] G. Doretto, D. Cremers, P. Favaro, and S. Soatto. Dynamic texture segmentation. In *IEEE International Conference on Computer Vision*, vol. 2, pp. 1236-42, 2003.

[9] P. Saisan, G. Doretto, Y. Wu, and S. Soatto. Dynamic texture recognition. In *IEEE Conference on Computer Vision and Pattern Recognition, Proceedings*, vol. 2, pp. 58-63, 2001.

[10] A. B. Chan and N. Vasconcelos. Probabilistic kernels for the classifi cation of auto-regressive visual processes. In *IEEE Conference on Computer Vision and Pattern Recognition*, vol. 1, pp. 846-51, 2005.

[11] S. Geman and D. Geman. Stochastic relaxation, Gibbs distribution, and the Bayesian restoration of images. *IEEE Transactions on Pattern Analysis and Machine Intelligence*, vol. 6(6), pp. 721-41, 1984.

[12] A. P. Dempster, N. M. Laird, and D. B. Rubin. Maximum likelihood from incomplete data via the EM algorithm. *Journal of the Royal Statistical Society B*, vol. 39, pp. 1-38, 1977.

[13] A. B. Chan and N. Vasconcelos. The EM algorithm for layered dynamic textures. *Technical Report SVCL-TR-2005-03*, June 2005. http://www.svcl.ucsd.edu/.

[14] A. B. Chan and N. Vasconcelos. Mixtures of dynamic textures. In *IEEE International Conference on Computer Vision*, vol. 1, pp. 641-47, 2005.

[15] R. H. Shumway and D. S. Stoffer. An approach to time series smoothing and forecasting using the EM algorithm. *Journal of Time Series Analysis*, vol. 3(4), pp. 253-64, 1982.

[16] S. Roweis and Z. Ghahramani. A unifying review of linear Gaussian models. *Neural Computation*, vol. 11, pp. 305-45, 1999.

[17] http://www.wsdot.wa.gov

[18] http://www.svcl.ucsd.edu/~abc/nips05/

Size Regularized Cut for Data Clustering

Yixin Chen
Department of CS
Univ. of New Orleans
yixin@cs.uno.edu

Ya Zhang
Department of EECS
Uinv. of Kansas
yazhang@ittc.ku.edu

Xiang Ji
NEC-Labs America, Inc.
xji@sv.nec-labs.com

Abstract

We present a novel spectral clustering method that enables users to incorporate prior knowledge of the size of clusters into the clustering process. The cost function, which is named size regularized cut (SRcut), is defined as the sum of the inter-cluster similarity and a regularization term measuring the relative size of two clusters. Finding a partition of the data set to minimize SRcut is proved to be NP-complete. An approximation algorithm is proposed to solve a relaxed version of the optimization problem as an eigenvalue problem. Evaluations over different data sets demonstrate that the method is not sensitive to outliers and performs better than normalized cut.

1 Introduction

In recent years, spectral clustering based on graph partitioning theories has emerged as one of the most effective data clustering tools. These methods model the given data set as a weighted undirected graph. Each data instance is represented as a node. Each edge is assigned a weight describing the similarity between the two nodes connected by the edge. Clustering is then accomplished by finding the best cuts of the graph that optimize certain predefined cost functions. The optimization usually leads to the computation of the top eigenvectors of certain graph affinity matrices, and the clustering result can be derived from the obtained eigen-space [12, 6]. Many cost functions, such as the ratio cut [3], average association [15], spectral k-means [19], normalized cut [15], min-max cut [7], and a measure using conductance and cut [9] have been proposed along with the corresponding eigen-systems for the data clustering purpose.

The above data clustering methods, as well as most other methods in the literature, bear a common characteristic that manages to generate results maximizing the intra-cluster similarity, and/or minimizing the inter-cluster similarity. These approaches perform well in some cases, but fail drastically when target data sets possess complex, extreme data distributions, and when the user has special needs for the data clustering task. For example, it has been pointed out by several researchers that normalized cut sometimes displays sensitivity to outliers [7, 14]. Normalized cut tends to find a cluster consisting of a very small number of points if those points are far away from the center of the data set [14].

There has been an abundance of prior work on embedding user's prior knowledge of the data set in the clustering process. Kernighan and Lin [11] applied a local search procedure that maintained two equally sized clusters while trying to minimize the association between the clusters. Wagstaff et al. [16] modified k-means method to deal with *a priori* knowledge about must-link and cannot link constraints. Banerjee and Ghosh [2] proposed a method to balance the size of the clusters by considering an explicit soft constraint. Xing et al. [17] presented a method to learn a clustering metric over user specified samples. Yu and Shi [18] introduced a method to include must-link grouping cues in normalized cut. Other related works include leaving ϵ fraction of the points unclustered to avoid the effect of outliers [4] and enforcing minimum cluster size constraint [10].

In this paper, we present a novel clustering method based on graph partitioning. The new method enables users to incorporate prior knowledge of the expected size of clusters into the clustering process. Specifically, the cost function of the new method is defined as the sum of the inter-cluster similarity and a regularization term that measures the relative size of two clusters. An "optimal" partition corresponds to a tradeoff between the inter-cluster similarity and the relative size of two clusters. We show that the size of the clusters generated by the optimal partition can be controlled by adjusting the weight on the regularization term. We also prove that the optimization problem is NP-complete. So we present an approximation algorithm and demonstrate its performance using two document data sets.

2 Size regularized cut

We model a given data set using a weighted undirected graph $\mathbb{G} = \mathbb{G}(\mathcal{V}, \mathcal{E}, \mathbf{W})$ where $\mathcal{V}$, $\mathcal{E}$, and $\mathbf{W}$ denote the vertex set, edge set, and graph affinity matrix, respectively. Each vertex $i \in \mathcal{V}$ represents a data point, and each edge $(i, j) \in \mathbb{E}$ is assigned a nonnegative weight $\mathbf{W}_{ij}$ to reflect the similarity between the data points i and j. A graph partitioning method attempts to organize vertices into groups so that the intra-cluster similarity is high, and/or the inter-cluster similarity is low. A simple way to quantify the cost for partitioning vertices into two disjoint sets $\mathcal{V}_1$ and $\mathcal{V}_2$ is the cut size

$$\text{cut}(\mathcal{V}_1, \mathcal{V}_2) = \sum_{i \in \mathcal{V}_1, j \in \mathcal{V}_2} \mathbf{W}_{ij} \, ,$$

which can be viewed as the similarity or association between $\mathcal{V}_1$ and $\mathcal{V}_2$. Finding a binary partition of the graph that minimizes the cut size is known as the minimum cut problem. There exist efficient algorithms for solving this problem. However, the minimum cut criterion favors grouping small sets of isolated nodes in the graph [15].

To capture the need for more balanced clusters, it has been proposed to include the cluster size information as a multiplicative penalty factor in the cost function, such as average cut [3] and normalized cut [15]. Both cost functions can be uniformly written as [5]

$$\text{cost}(\mathcal{V}_1, \mathcal{V}_2) = \text{cut}(\mathcal{V}_1, \mathcal{V}_2) \left(\frac{1}{|\mathcal{V}_1|_{\boldsymbol{\beta}}} + \frac{1}{|\mathcal{V}_1|_{\boldsymbol{\beta}}} \right) . \tag{1}$$

Here, $\boldsymbol{\beta} = [\beta_1, \cdots, \beta_N]^T$ is a weight vector where β_i is a nonnegative weight associated with vertex i, and N is the total number of vertices in $\mathcal{V}$. The penalty factor for "unbalanced partition" is determined by $|\mathcal{V}_j|_{\boldsymbol{\beta}}$ ($j = 1, 2$), which is a weighted cardinality (or weighted size) of $\mathcal{V}_j$, i.e.,

$$|\mathcal{V}_j|_{\boldsymbol{\beta}} = \sum_{i \in \mathcal{V}_j} \beta_i \, . \tag{2}$$

Dhillon [5] showed that if $\beta_i = 1$ (for all i), the cost function (1) becomes average cut. If $\beta_i = \sum_j \mathbf{W}_{ij}$, then (1) turns out to be normalized cut.

In contrast with minimum cut, average cut and normalized cut tend to generate more balanced clusters. However, due to the multiplicative nature of their cost functions, average cut and normalized cut are still sensitive to outliers. This is because the cut value for separating outliers from the rest of the data points is usually close to zero, and thus makes the multiplicative penalty factor void. To avoid the drawback of the above multiplicative cost functions, we introduce an additive cost function for graph bi-partitioning. The cost function is named *size regularized cut* (SRcut), and is defined as

$$\text{SRcut}(\mathcal{V}_1, \mathcal{V}_2) = \text{cut}(\mathcal{V}_1, \mathcal{V}_2) - \alpha |\mathcal{V}_1|_\beta |\mathcal{V}_2|_\beta \tag{3}$$

where $|\mathcal{V}_j|_\beta$ ($j = 1, 2$) is described in (2), β and $\alpha > 0$ are given a priori. The last term in (3), $\alpha |\mathcal{V}_1|_\beta |\mathcal{V}_2|_\beta$, is the size regularization term, which can be interpreted as below.

Since $|\mathcal{V}_1|_\beta + |\mathcal{V}_2|_\beta = |\mathcal{V}|_\beta = \beta^T \mathbf{e}$ where $\mathbf{e}$ is a vector of 1's, it is straightforward to show that the following inequality $|\mathcal{V}_1|_\beta |\mathcal{V}_2|_\beta \le \left(\frac{\beta^T \mathbf{e}}{2}\right)^2$ holds for arbitrary $\mathcal{V}_1, \mathcal{V}_2 \in \mathcal{V}$ satisfying $\mathcal{V}_1 \cup \mathcal{V}_2 = \mathcal{V}$ and $\mathcal{V}_1 \cap \mathcal{V}_2 = \emptyset$. In addition, the equality holds if and only if

$$|\mathcal{V}_1|_\beta = |\mathcal{V}_2|_\beta = \frac{\beta^T \mathbf{e}}{2}.$$

Therefore, $|\mathcal{V}_1|_\beta |\mathcal{V}_2|_\beta$ achieves the maximum value when two clusters are of equal weighted size. Consequently, *minimizing SRcut is equivalent to minimizing the similarity between two clusters and, at the same time, searching for a balanced partition*. The tradeoff between the inter-cluster similarity and the balance of the cut depends on the α parameter, which needs to be determined by the prior information on the size of clusters. If $\alpha = 0$, minimum SRcut will assign all vertices to one cluster. On the other end, if $\alpha \gg 0$, minimum SRcut will generate two clusters of equal size (if N is an even number). We defer the discussion on the choice of α to Section 5.

In a spirit similar to that of (3), we can define *size regularized association* (SRassoc) as

$$\text{SRassoc}(\mathcal{V}_1, \mathcal{V}_2) = \sum_{i=1,2} \text{cut}(\mathcal{V}_i, \mathcal{V}_i) + 2\alpha |\mathcal{V}_1|_\beta |\mathcal{V}_2|_\beta$$

where $\text{cut}(\mathcal{V}_i, \mathcal{V}_i)$ measures the intra-cluster similarity. An important property of SRassoc and SRcut is that they are naturally related:

$$\text{SRcut}(\mathcal{V}_1, \mathcal{V}_2) = \frac{\text{cut}(\mathcal{V}, \mathcal{V}) - \text{SRassoc}(\mathcal{V}_1, \mathcal{V}_2)}{2}.$$

Hence, minimizing size regularized cut is in fact identical to maximizing size regularized association. In other words, *minimizing the size regularized inter-cluster similarity is equivalent to maximizing the size regularized intra-cluster similarity*. In this paper, we will use SRcut as the clustering criterion.

3   Size ratio monotonicity

Let $\mathcal{V}_1$ and $\mathcal{V}_2$ be a partition of $\mathcal{V}$. The size ratio $r = \frac{\min(|\mathcal{V}_1|_\beta, |\mathcal{V}_2|_\beta)}{\max(|\mathcal{V}_1|_\beta, |\mathcal{V}_2|_\beta)}$ defines the relative size of two clusters. It is always within the interval $[0, 1]$, and a larger value indicates a more balanced partition. The following theorem shows that by controlling the parameter α in the SRcut cost function, one can control the balance of the optimal partition. In addition, the size ratio increases monotonically as the increase of α.

Theorem 3.1 (Size Ratio Monotonicity) *Let $\mathcal{V}_1^i$ and $\mathcal{V}_2^i$ be the clusters generated by the minimum SRcut with $\alpha = \alpha_i$, and the corresponding size ratio, r_i, be defined as*

$$r_i = \frac{\min(|\mathcal{V}_1^i|_\beta, |\mathcal{V}_2^i|_\beta)}{\max(|\mathcal{V}_1^i|_\beta, |\mathcal{V}_2^i|_\beta)}.$$

If $\alpha_1 > \alpha_2 \ge 0$, then $r_1 \ge r_2$.

Proof: Given vertex weight vector β, let $\mathcal{S}$ be the collection of all distinct values that the size regularization term in (3) can have, i.e.,

$$\mathcal{S} = \{S \mid \mathcal{V}_1 \cup \mathcal{V}_2 = \mathcal{V},\ \mathcal{V}_1 \cap \mathcal{V}_2 = \emptyset,\ S = |\mathcal{V}_1|_\beta |\mathcal{V}_2|_\beta\}\ .$$

Clearly, $|\mathcal{S}|$, the number of elements in $\mathcal{S}$, is less than or equal to 2^{N-1} where N is the size of $\mathcal{V}$. Hence we can write the elements in $\mathcal{S}$ in ascending order as

$$0 = S_1 < S_2 < \cdots\cdots < S_{|\mathcal{S}|} \le \left(\frac{\beta^T \mathbf{e}}{2}\right)^2\ .$$

Next, we define cut_i be the minimal cut satisfying $|\mathcal{V}_1|_\beta |\mathcal{V}_2|_\beta = S_i$, i.e.,

$$\mathrm{cut}_i = \min_{\substack{|\mathcal{V}_1|_\beta |\mathcal{V}_2|_\beta = S_i \\ \mathcal{V}_1 \cup \mathcal{V}_2 = \mathcal{V} \\ \mathcal{V}_1 \cap \mathcal{V}_2 = \emptyset}} \mathrm{cut}(\mathcal{V}_1, \mathcal{V}_2)\ ,$$

then

$$\min_{\substack{\mathcal{V}_1 \cup \mathcal{V}_2 = \mathcal{V} \\ \mathcal{V}_1 \cap \mathcal{V}_2 = \emptyset}} \mathrm{SRcut}(\mathcal{V}_1, \mathcal{V}_2) = \min_{i=1,\cdots,|\mathcal{S}|} (\mathrm{cut}_i - \alpha S_i)\ .$$

If $\mathcal{V}_1^2$ and $\mathcal{V}_2^2$ are the clusters generated by the minimum SRcut with $\alpha = \alpha_2$, then $|\mathcal{V}_1^2|_\beta |\mathcal{V}_2^2|_\beta = S_{k^*}$ where $k^* = \mathrm{argmin}_{i=1,\cdots,|\mathcal{S}|} (\mathrm{cut}_i - \alpha_2 S_i)$. Therefore, for any $1 \le t < k^*$,

$$\mathrm{cut}_{k^*} - \alpha_2 S_{k^*} \le \mathrm{cut}_t - \alpha_2 S_t\ . \tag{4}$$

If $\alpha_1 > \alpha_2$, we have

$$(\alpha_2 - \alpha_1) S_{k^*} < (\alpha_2 - \alpha_1) S_t\ . \tag{5}$$

Adding (4) and (5) gives $\mathrm{cut}_{k^*} - \alpha_1 S_{k^*} < \mathrm{cut}_t - \alpha_1 S_t$, which implies

$$k^* \le \mathrm{argmin}_{i=1,\cdots,|\mathcal{S}|} (\mathrm{cut}_i - \alpha_1 S_i)\ . \tag{6}$$

Now, let $\mathcal{V}_1^1$ and $\mathcal{V}_2^1$ be the clusters generated by the minimum SRcut with $\alpha = \alpha_1$, and $|\mathcal{V}_1^1|_\beta |\mathcal{V}_2^1|_\beta = S_{j^*}$ where $j^* = \mathrm{argmin}_{i=1,\cdots,|\mathcal{S}|} (\mathrm{cut}_i - \alpha_1 S_i)$. From (6) we have $j^* \ge k^*$, therefore $S_{j^*} \ge S_{k^*}$, or equivalently $|\mathcal{V}_1^1|_\beta |\mathcal{V}_2^1|_\beta \ge |\mathcal{V}_1^2|_\beta |\mathcal{V}_2^2|_\beta$. Without loss of generality, we can assume that $|\mathcal{V}_1^1|_\beta \le |\mathcal{V}_2^1|_\beta$ and $|\mathcal{V}_1^2|_\beta \le |\mathcal{V}_2^2|_\beta$, therefore $|\mathcal{V}_1^1|_\beta \le \frac{|\mathcal{V}|_\beta}{2}$ and $|\mathcal{V}_1^2|_\beta \le \frac{|\mathcal{V}|_\beta}{2}$. Considering the fact that $f(x) = x(|\mathcal{V}|_\beta - x)$ is strictly monotonically increasing as $x \le \frac{|\mathcal{V}|_\beta}{2}$ and $f(|\mathcal{V}_1^1|_\beta) \ge f(|\mathcal{V}_1^2|_\beta)$, we have $|\mathcal{V}_1^1|_\beta \ge |\mathcal{V}_1^2|_\beta$. This leads to $r_1 = \frac{|\mathcal{V}_1^1|_\beta}{|\mathcal{V}_2^1|_\beta} \ge r_2 = \frac{|\mathcal{V}_1^2|_\beta}{|\mathcal{V}_2^2|_\beta}$. $\qquad\square$

Unfortunately, minimizing size regularized cut for an arbitrary α is an NP-complete problem. This is proved in the following section.

4 Size regularized cut and graph bisection

The decision problem for minimum SRcut can be formulated as: whether, given an undirected graph $\mathbb{G}(\mathcal{V}, \mathcal{E}, \mathbf{W})$ with weight vector β and regularization parameter α, a partition exists such that SRcut is less than a given cost. This decision problem is clearly NP because we can verify in polynomial time the SRcut value for a given partition. Next we show that graph bisection can be reduced, in polynomial time, to minimum SRcut. Since graph bisection is a classified NP-complete problem [1], so is minimum SRcut.

Definition 4.1 (Graph Bisection) *Given an undirected graph $\mathbb{G} = \mathbb{G}(\mathcal{V}, \mathcal{E}, \mathbf{W})$ with even number of vertices where $\mathbf{W}$ is the adjacency matrix, find a pair of disjoint subsets $\mathcal{V}_1, \mathcal{V}_2 \subset \mathcal{V}$ of equal size and $\mathcal{V}_1 \cup \mathcal{V}_2 = \mathcal{V}$, such that the number of edges between vertices in $\mathcal{V}_1$ and vertices in $\mathcal{V}_2$, i.e., $\mathrm{cut}(\mathcal{V}_1, \mathcal{V}_2)$, is minimal.*

Theorem 4.2 (Reduction of Graph Bisection to SRcut) *For any given undirected graph* $\mathbb{G} = \mathbb{G}(\mathcal{V}, \mathcal{E}, \mathbf{W})$ *where* $\mathbf{W}$ *is the adjacency matrix, finding the minimum bisection of* $\mathbb{G}$ *is equivalent to finding a partition of* $\mathbb{G}$ *that minimizes the SRcut cost function with weights* $\beta = \mathbf{e}$ *and the regularization parameter* $\alpha > d^*$ *where*

$$d^* = \max_{i=1,\cdots,N} \sum_{j=1,\cdots,N} \mathbf{W}_{ij} .$$

Proof: Without loss of generality, we assume that N is even (if not, we can always add an isolated vertex). Let cut_i be the minimal cut with the size of the smaller subset is i, i.e.,

$$\text{cut}_i = \min_{\substack{\min(|\mathcal{V}_1|,|\mathcal{V}_2|) = i \\ \mathcal{V}_1 \cup \mathcal{V}_2 = \mathcal{V} \\ \mathcal{V}_1 \cap \mathcal{V}_2 = \emptyset}} \text{cut}(\mathcal{V}_1, \mathcal{V}_2) .$$

Clearly, we have $d^* \geq \text{cut}_{i+1} - \text{cut}_i$ for $0 \leq i \leq \frac{N}{2} - 1$. If $0 \leq i \leq \frac{N}{2} - 1$, then $N - 2i - 1 \geq 1$. Therefore, for any $\alpha > d^*$, we have

$$\alpha(N - 2i - 1) > d^* \geq \text{cut}_{i+1} - \text{cut}_i .$$

This implies that $\text{cut}_i - \alpha i(N - i) > \text{cut}_{i+1} - \alpha(i+1)(N - i - 1)$, or, equivalently,

$$\min_{\substack{\min(|\mathcal{V}_1|,|\mathcal{V}_2|) = i \\ \mathcal{V}_1 \cup \mathcal{V}_2 = \mathcal{V} \\ \mathcal{V}_1 \cap \mathcal{V}_2 = \emptyset}} \text{cut}(\mathcal{V}_1, \mathcal{V}_2) - \alpha|\mathcal{V}_1||\mathcal{V}_2| > \min_{\substack{\min(|\mathcal{V}_1|,|\mathcal{V}_2|) = i + 1 \\ \mathcal{V}_1 \cup \mathcal{V}_2 = \mathcal{V} \\ \mathcal{V}_1 \cap \mathcal{V}_2 = \emptyset}} \text{cut}(\mathcal{V}_1, \mathcal{V}_2) - \alpha|\mathcal{V}_1||\mathcal{V}_2|$$

for $0 \leq i \leq \frac{N}{2} - 1$. Hence, for any $\alpha > d^*$, minimizing SRcut is identical to minimizing

$$\text{cut}(\mathcal{V}_1, \mathcal{V}_2) - \alpha|\mathcal{V}_1||\mathcal{V}_2|$$

with the constraint that $|\mathcal{V}_1| = |\mathcal{V}_2| = \frac{N}{2}$, $\mathcal{V}_1 \cup \mathcal{V}_2 = \mathcal{V}$, and $\mathcal{V}_1 \cap \mathcal{V}_2 = \emptyset$, which is exactly the graph bisection problem since $\alpha|\mathcal{V}_1||\mathcal{V}_2| = \alpha\frac{N^2}{4}$ is a constant. $\qquad\square$

5 An approximation algorithm for SRcut

Given a partition of vertex set $\mathcal{V}$ into two sets $\mathcal{V}_1$ and $\mathcal{V}_2$, let $\mathbf{x} \in \{-1, 1\}^N$ be an indicator vector such that $x_i = 1$ if $i \in \mathcal{V}_1$ and $x_i = -1$ if $i \in \mathcal{V}_2$. It is not difficult to show that

$$\text{cut}(\mathcal{V}_1, \mathcal{V}_2) = \frac{(\mathbf{e} + \mathbf{x})^T}{2} \mathbf{W} \frac{(\mathbf{e} - \mathbf{x})}{2} \quad \text{and} \quad |\mathcal{V}_1|_\beta |\mathcal{V}_2|_\beta = \frac{(\mathbf{e} + \mathbf{x})^T}{2} \beta\beta^T \frac{(\mathbf{e} - \mathbf{x})}{2} .$$

We can therefore rewrite SRcut in (3) as a function of the indicator vector $\mathbf{x}$:

$$\begin{aligned} \text{SRcut}(\mathcal{V}_1, \mathcal{V}_2) &= \frac{(\mathbf{e} + \mathbf{x})^T}{2} (\mathbf{W} - \alpha\beta\beta^T) \frac{(\mathbf{e} - \mathbf{x})}{2} \\ &= -\frac{1}{4}\mathbf{x}^T(\mathbf{W} - \alpha\beta\beta^T)\mathbf{x} + \frac{1}{4}\mathbf{e}^T(\mathbf{W} - \alpha\beta\beta^T)\mathbf{e} . \end{aligned} \tag{7}$$

Given $\mathbf{W}$, α, and β, we have

$$\text{argmin}_{\mathbf{x} \in \{-1,1\}^N} \text{SRcut}(\mathbf{x}) = \text{argmax}_{\mathbf{x} \in \{-1,1\}^N} \mathbf{x}^T(\mathbf{W} - \alpha\beta\beta^T)\mathbf{x}$$

If we define a normalized indicator vector, $\mathbf{y} = \frac{1}{\sqrt{N}}\mathbf{x}$ (i.e., $\|\mathbf{y}\| = 1$), then minimum SRcut can be found by solving the following discrete optimization problem

$$\mathbf{y} = \text{argmax}_{\mathbf{y} \in \{-\frac{1}{\sqrt{N}}, \frac{1}{\sqrt{N}}\}^N} \mathbf{y}^T(\mathbf{W} - \alpha\beta\beta^T)\mathbf{y} , \tag{8}$$

which is NP-complete. However, if we relax all the elements in the indicator vector $\mathbf{y}$ from discrete values to real values and keep the unit length constraint on $\mathbf{y}$, the above optimization problem can be easily solved. And the solution is the eigenvector corresponding to the largest eigenvalue of $\mathbf{W} - \alpha\beta\beta^T$ (or named the largest eigenvector).

Similar to other spectral graph partitioning techniques that use top eigenvectors to approximate "optimal" partitions, the largest eigenvector of $\mathbf{W} - \alpha\boldsymbol{\beta}\boldsymbol{\beta}^T$ provides a linear search direction, along which a splitting point can be found. We use a simple approach by checking each element in the largest eigenvector as a possible splitting point. The vertices, whose continuous indicators are greater than or equal to the splitting point, are assigned to one cluster. The remaining vertices are assigned to the other cluster. The corresponding SRcut value is then computed. The final partition is determined by the splitting point with the minimum SRcut value. The relaxed optimization problem provides a lower bound on the optimal SRcut value, SRcut*. Let λ_1 be the largest eigenvalue of $\mathbf{W} - \alpha\boldsymbol{\beta}\boldsymbol{\beta}^T$. From (7) and (8), it is straightforward to show that

$$\text{SRcut}^* \geq \frac{\mathbf{e}^T(\mathbf{W} - \alpha\boldsymbol{\beta}\boldsymbol{\beta}^T)\mathbf{e} - N\lambda_1}{4}.$$

The SRcut value of the partition generated by the largest eigenvector provides an upper bound for SRcut*.

As implied by SRcut cost function in (3), the partition of the dataset depends on the value of α, which determines the tradeoff between inter-cluster similarity and the balance of the partition. Moreover, Theorem 3.1 indicates that with the increase of α, the size ratio of the clusters generated by the optimal partition increase monotonically, i.e., the partition becomes more balanced. Even though, we do not have a counterpart of Theorem 3.1 for the approximated partition derived above, our empirical study shows that, in general, the size ratio of the approximated partition increases along with α. Therefore, we use the prior information on the size of the clusters to select α. Specifically, we define expected size ratio, R, as $R = \frac{\min(s_1, s_2)}{\max(s_1, s_2)}$ where s_1 and s_2 are the expected size of the two clusters (known a priori). We then search for a value of α such that the resulting size ratio is close to R. A simple one-dimensional search method based on bracketing and bisection is implemented [13]. The pseudo code of the searching algorithm is given in Algorithm 1 along with the rest of the clustering procedure. The input of the algorithm is the graph affinity matrix $\mathbf{W}$, the weight vector $\boldsymbol{\beta}$, the expected size ratio R, and $\alpha_0 > 0$ (the initial value of α). The output is a partition of $\mathcal{V}$. In our experiments, α_0 is chosen to be $10\frac{\mathbf{e}^T\mathbf{W}\mathbf{e}}{N^2}$.

If the expected size ratio R is unknown, one can estimate R assuming that the data are i.i.d. samples and a sample belongs to the smaller cluster with probability $p \leq 0.5$ (i.e., $R = \frac{p}{1-p}$). It is not difficult to prove that $\hat{p}$ of n randomly selected samples from the data set is an unbiased estimator of p. Moreover, the distribution of $\hat{p}$ can be well approximated by a normal distribution with mean p and variance $\frac{p(1-p)}{n}$ when n is sufficiently large (say $n > 30$). Hence $\hat{p}$ converges to p as the increase of n. This suggests a simple strategy for SRcut with unknown R. One can manually examine $n \ll N$ randomly selected data instances to get $\hat{p}$ and the 95% confidence interval $[p_{low}, p_{high}]$, from which one can evaluate the invertal $[R_{low}, R_{high}]$ for R. Algorithm 1 is then applied to a number of evenly distributed R's within the interval to find the corresponding partitions. The final partition is chosen to be the one with the minimum cut value by assuming that a "good" partition should have a small cut.

6 Time complexity

The time complexity of each iteration is determined by that of computing the largest eigenvector. Using power method or Lanczos method [8], the running time is $O(MN^2)$ where M is the number of matrix-vector computations required and N is the number of vertices. Hence the overall time complexity is $O(KMN^2)$ where K is the number of iterations in searching α. Similar to other spectral graph clustering methods, the time complexity of SRcut can be significantly reduced if the affinity matrix $\mathbf{W}$ is sparse, i.e., the graph is only

Algorithm 1: Size Regularized Cut

```
1 initialize α_l to 2α_0 and α_h to α_0/2
2 REPEAT
3    α_l ← α_l/2, y ← largest eigenvector of W − α_l ββ^T
4    partition V using y and compute size ratio r
5 UNTIL (r < R)
6 REPEAT
7    α_h ← 2α_h, y ← largest eigenvector of W − α_h ββ^T
8    partition V using y and compute size ratio r
9 UNTIL (r ≥ R)
10 REPEAT
11    α ← (α_l+α_h)/2, y ← largest eigenvector of W − α ββ^T
12    partition V using y and compute size ratio r
13    IF (r < R)
14       α_l ← α
15    ELSE
16       α_h ← α
17    END IF
18 UNTIL (|r − R| < 0.01R or α_h − α_l < 0.01α_0)
```

locally connected. Although $\mathbf{W} - \alpha\boldsymbol{\beta}\boldsymbol{\beta}^T$ is in general not sparse, the time complexity of power method is still $O(MN)$. This is because $(\mathbf{W} - \alpha\boldsymbol{\beta}\boldsymbol{\beta}^T)\mathbf{y}$ can be evaluated as the sum of $\mathbf{W}\mathbf{y}$ and $\alpha\boldsymbol{\beta}(\boldsymbol{\beta}^T\mathbf{y})$, each requiring $O(N)$ operations. Therefore, by enforcing the sparsity, the overall time complexity of SRcut is $O(KMN)$.

7 Experiments

We test the SRcut algorithm using two data sets, Reuters-21578 document corpus and 20-Newsgroups. Reuters-21578 data set contains 21578 documents that have been manually assigned to 135 topics. In our experiments, we discarded documents with multiple category labels, and removed the topic classes containing less than 5 documents. This leads to a data set of 50 clusters with a total of 9102 documents. The 20-Newsgroups data set contains about 20000 documents collected from 20 newsgroups, each corresponding to a distinct topic. The number of news articles in each cluster is roughly the same. We pair each cluster with another cluster to form a data set, so that 190 test data sets are generated. Each document is represented by a term-frequency vector using TF-IDF weights.

We use the normalized mutual information as our evaluation metric. Normalized mutual information is always within the interval $[0, 1]$, with a larger value indicating a better performance. A simple sampling scheme described in Section 5 is used to estimate the expected size ratio. For the Reuters-21578 data set, 50 test runs were conducted, each on a test set created by mixing 2 topics randomly selected from the data set. The performance score in Table 1 was obtained by averaging the scores from 50 test runs. The results for 20-Newsgroups data set were obtained by averaging the scores from 190 test data sets. Clearly, SRcut outperforms the normalized cut on both data sets. SRcut performs significantly better than normalized cut on the 20-Newsgroups data set. In comparison with Reuters-21578, many topic classes in the 20-Newsgroups data set contain outliers. The results suggest that SRcut is less sensitive to outliers than normalized cut.

8 Conclusions

We proposed size regularized cut, a novel method that enables users to specify prior knowledge of the size of two clusters in spectral clustering. The SRcut cost function takes into

Table 1: Performance comparison for SRcut and Normalized Cut. The numbers shown are the normalized mutual information. A larger value indicates a better performance.

Algorithms	Reuters-21578	20-Newsgroups
SRcut	**0.7330**	**0.7315**
Normalized Cut	0.7102	0.2531

account inter-cluster similarity and the relative size of two clusters. The "optimal" partition of the data set corresponds to a tradeoff between the inter-cluster similarity and the balance of the partition. We proved that finding a partition with minimum SRcut is an NP-complete problem. We presented an approximation algorithm to solve a relaxed version of the optimization problem. Evaluations over different data sets indicate that the method is not sensitive to outliers and performs better than normalized cut. The SRcut model can be easily adapted to solve multiple-clusters problem by applying the clustering method recursively/iteratively on data sets. Since graph bisection can be reduced to SRcut, the proposed approximation algorithm provides a new spectral technique for graph bisection. Comparing SRcut with other graph bisection algorithms is therefore an interesting future work.

References

[1] S. Arora, D. Karger, and M. Karpinski, "Polynomial Time Approximation Schemes for Dense Instances of NP-hard Problems," *Proc. ACM Symp. on Theory of Computing*, pp. 284-293, 1995.

[2] A. Banerjee and J. Ghosh, "On Scaling up Balanced Clustering Algorithms," *Proc. SIAM Int'l Conf. on Data Mining*, pp. 333-349, 2002.

[3] P. K. Chan, D. F. Schlag, and J. Y. Zien, "Spectral k-Way Ratio-Cut Partitioning and Clustering," *IEEE Trans. on Computer-Aided Design of Integrated Circuits and Systems*, 13:1088-1096, 1994.

[4] M. Charikar, S. Khuller, D. M. Mount, and G. Narasimhan, "Algorithms for Facility Location Problems with Outliers," *Proc. ACM-SIAM Symp. on Discrete Algorithms*, pp. 642-651, 2001.

[5] I. S. Dhillon, "Co-clustering Documents and Words using Bipartite Spectral Graph Partitioning," *Proc. ACM SIGKDD Conf. Knowledge Discovery and Data Mining*, pp. 269-274, 2001.

[6] C. Ding, "Data Clustering: Principal Components, Hopfield and Self-Aggregation Networks," *Proc. Int'l Joint Conf. on Artificial Intelligence*, pp. 479-484, 2003.

[7] C. Ding, X. He, H. Zha, M. Gu, and H. Simon, "Spectral Min-Max Cut for Graph Partitioning and Data Clustering," *Proc. IEEE Int'l Conf. Data Mining*, pp. 107-114, 2001.

[8] G. H. Golub and C. F. Van Loan, *Matrix Computations*, John Hopkins Press, 1999.

[9] R. Kannan, S. Vempala, and A. Vetta, "On Clusterings - Good, Bad and Spectral," *Proc. IEEE Symp. on Foundations of Computer Science*, pp. 367-377, 2000.

[10] D. R. Karget and M. Minkoff, "Building Steiner Trees with Incomplete Global Knowledge," *Proc. IEEE Symp. on Foundations of Computer Science*, pp. 613-623, 2000

[11] B. Kernighan and S. Lin, "An Efficient Heuristic Procedure for Partitioning Graphs," *The Bell System Technical Journal*, 49:291-307, 1970.

[12] A. Y. Ng, M. I. Jordan, and Y. Weiss, "On Spectral Clustering: Analysis and an Algorithm," *Advances in Neural Information Processing Systems 14*, pp. 849-856, 2001.

[13] W. H. Press, S. A. Teukolsky, W. T. Vetterling, and B. P. Flannery, *Numerical Recipes in C*, second edition, Cambridge University Press, 1992.

[14] A. Rahimi and B. Recht, "Clustering with Normalized Cuts is Clustering with a Hyperplane," *Statistical Learning in Computer Vision*, 2004.

[15] J. Shi and J. Malik, "Normalized Cuts and Image Segmentation," *IEEE Trans. on Pattern Analysis and Machine Intelligence*, 22:888-905, 2000.

[16] K. Wagstaff, C. Cardie, S. Rogers, and S. Schrodl, "Constrained K-means Clustering with Background Knowledge," *Proc. Int'l Conf. on Machine Learning*, pp. 577-584, 2001.

[17] E. P. Xing, A. Y. Ng, M. I. Jordan, and S. Russell, "Distance Metric Learning, with Applications to Clustering with Side Information," *Advances in Neural Information Processing Systems 15*, pp. 505-512, 2003.

[18] X. Yu and J. Shi, "Segmentation Given Partial Grouping Constraints," *IEEE Trans. on Pattern Analysis and Machine Intelligence*, 26:173-183, 2004.

[19] H. Zha, X. He, C. Ding, H. Simon, and M. Gu, "Spectral Relaxation for K-means Clustering," *Advances in Neural Information Processing Systems 14*, pp. 1057-1064, 2001.

Learning from Data of Variable Quality

Koby Crammer, Michael Kearns, Jennifer Wortman
Computer and Information Science
University of Pennsylvania
Philadelphia, PA 19103
{crammer,mkearns,wortmanj}@cis.upenn.edu

Abstract

We initiate the study of learning from multiple sources of limited data, each of which may be corrupted at a different rate. We develop a complete theory of which data sources should be used for two fundamental problems: estimating the bias of a coin, and learning a classifier in the presence of label noise. In both cases, efficient algorithms are provided for computing the optimal subset of data.

1   Introduction

In many natural machine learning settings, one is not only faced with data that may be corrupted or deficient in some way (classification noise or other label errors, missing attributes, and so on), but with data that is not *uniformly* corrupted. In other words, we might be presented with data of *variable quality* — perhaps some small amount of entirely "clean" data, another amount of slightly corrupted data, yet more that is significantly corrupted, and so on. Furthermore, in such circumstances we may often know at least an upper bound on the rate and type of corruption in each pile of data. An extreme example is the recent interest in settings where one has a very limited set of correctly labeled examples, and an effectively unlimited set of entirely unlabeled examples, as naturally arises in problems such as classifying web pages [1]. Another general category of problems that falls within our interest is when multiple piles of data are drawn from processes that differ perhaps slightly and in varying amounts from the process we wish to estimate. For example, we might wish to estimate a conditional distribution $P(X|Y = y)$ but have only a small number of observations in which $Y = y$, but a larger number of observations in which $Y = y'$ for values of y' "near" to y. In such circumstances it might make sense to base our model on a larger number of observations, at least for those y' closest to y.

While there is a large body of learning theory both for uncorrupted data and for data that is uniformly corrupted in some way [2, 3], there is no general framework and theory for learning from data of variable quality. In this paper we introduce such a framework, and develop its theory, for two basic problems: estimating a bias from corrupted coins, and learning a classifier in the presence of varying amounts of label noise. For the corrupted coins case we provide an upper bound on the error that is expressed as a trade-off between weighted approximation errors and larger amounts of data. This bound provides a building block for the classification noise setting, in which we are able to give a bound on the generalization error of empirical risk minimization that specifies the optimal subset of the data to use. Both bounds can computed by simple and efficient algorithms. We illustrate both problems and our algorithms with numerical simulations.

2 Estimating the Bias from Corrupted Coins

We begin by considering perhaps the simplest possible instance of the general class of problems in which we are interested — namely, the problem of estimating the unknown bias of a coin. In this version of the variable quality model, we will have access to different amounts of data from "corrupted" coins whose bias differs from the one we wish to estimate. We use our solution for this simple problem as a building block for the classification noise setting in Section 3.

2.1 Problem Description

Suppose we wish to estimate the bias β of a coin given K piles of training observations $N_1, ..., N_K$. Each pile N_i contains n_i outcomes of flips of a coin with bias β_i, where the only information we are provided is that $\beta_i \in [\beta - \epsilon_i, \beta + \epsilon_i]$, and $0 \le \epsilon_1 \le \epsilon_2 \le ... \le \epsilon_K$. We refer to the ϵ_i as bounds on the *approximation errors* of the corrupted coins. We denote by h_i the number of heads observed in the ith pile. Our immediate goal is to determine which piles should be considered in order to obtain the best estimate of the true bias β.

We consider estimates for β obtained by merging some subset of the data into a single unified pile, and computing the maximum likelihood estimate for β, which is simply the fraction of times heads appears as an outcome in the unified pile. Although one can consider using *any* subset of the data, it can be proved (and is intuitively obvious) that an optimal estimate (in the sense that will be defined shortly) always uses a *prefix* of the data, i.e. all data from the piles indexed 1 to k for some $k \le K$, and possibly a subset of the data from pile $k + 1$. In fact, it will be shown that only complete piles need to be considered. Therefore, from this point on we restrict ourselves to estimates of this form, and identify them by the maximal index k of the piles used. The associated estimate is then simply

$$\hat{\beta}_k = \frac{h_1 + \ldots + h_k}{n_1 + \ldots + n_k} .$$

We denote the expectation of this estimate by

$$\bar{\beta}_k = \mathrm{E}\left[\hat{\beta}_k\right] = \frac{n_1 \beta_1 + \ldots + n_k \beta_k}{n_1 + \ldots + n_k} .$$

To simplify the presentation we denote by $n_{i,j}$ the number of outcomes in piles $N_i, \ldots, N_j$, that is, $n_{i,j} = \sum_{m=i}^{j} n_m$.

We now bound the deviation of the estimate $\hat{\beta}_k$ from the true bias of the coin β using the expectation $\bar{\beta}_k$:

$$
\begin{aligned}
|\beta - \hat{\beta}_k| &= |\beta - \bar{\beta}_k + \bar{\beta}_k - \hat{\beta}_k| \\
&\le |\beta - \bar{\beta}_k| + |\bar{\beta}_k - \hat{\beta}_k| \\
&\le \sum_{i=1}^{k} \frac{n_i}{n_{1,k}} \epsilon_i + |\bar{\beta}_k - \hat{\beta}_k|
\end{aligned}
$$

The first inequality follows from the triangle inequality and the second from our assumptions. Using the Hoeffding inequality we can bound the second term and find that with high probability for an appropriate choice of δ we have

$$|\beta - \hat{\beta}_k| \le \sum_{i=1}^{k} \frac{n_i}{n_{1,k}} \epsilon_i + \sqrt{\frac{\log(2K/\delta)}{2n_{1,k}}} . \tag{1}$$

To summarize, we have proved the following theorem.

Theorem 1 *Let $\hat{\beta}_k$ be the estimate obtained by using only the data from the first k piles. Then for any $\delta > 0$, with probability $\geq 1 - \delta$ we have*

$$\left| \beta - \hat{\beta}_k \right| \leq \sum_{i=1}^{k} \frac{n_i}{n_{1,k}} \epsilon_i + \sqrt{\frac{\log(2K/\delta)}{2n_{1,k}}}$$

simultaneously for all $k = 1, \ldots, K$.

Two remarks are in place here. First, the theorem is data-independent since it does not take into account the actual outcomes of the experiments $h_1, \ldots, h_K$. Second, the two terms in the bound reflect the well-known trade-off between bias (approximation error) and variance (estimation error). The first term bounds the approximation error of replacing the true coin β with the average $\bar{\beta}_k$. The second term corresponds to the estimation error which arises as a result of our finite sample size.

This theorem implies a natural algorithm to choose the number of piles k^* as is the minimizer of the bound over the number of piles used:

$$k^* = \operatorname*{argmin}_{k \in \{1, \ldots, K\}} \left\{ \sum_{i=1}^{k} \frac{n_i}{n_{1,k}} \epsilon_i + \sqrt{\frac{\log(2K/\delta)}{2n_{1,k}}} \right\}.$$

To conclude this section we argue that our choice of using a prefix of piles is optimal. First, note that by adding a new pile with a corruption level ϵ smaller then the current corruption level, we can always reduce the bounds. Thus it is optimal to use prefix of the piles and not to ignore piles with low corruption levels. Second, we need to show that if we decide to use a pile, it will be optimal to use all of it. Note that we can choose to view each coin toss as a separate pile with a single observation, thus yielding $n_{1,K}$ piles of size 1. The following technical lemma states that under this view of singleton piles, once we decide to add a pile with some corruption level, it will be optimal to use all singleton piles with the same corruption level. The proof of this lemma is omitted due to lack of space.

Lemma 1 *Assume that all the piles are of size $n_i = 1$ and that $\epsilon_k \leq \epsilon_{p+k} = \epsilon_{p+k+1}$. Then the following two inequalities cannot hold simultaneously:*

$$\sum_{i=1}^{k} \frac{n_i}{n_{1,k}} \epsilon_i + \sqrt{\frac{\log(2n_{1,K}/\delta)}{2n_{1,k}}} > \sum_{i=1}^{k+p} \frac{n_i}{n_{1,k+p}} \epsilon_i + \sqrt{\frac{\log(2n_{1,K}/\delta)}{2n_{1,k+p}}}$$

$$\sum_{i=1}^{k+p+1} \frac{n_i}{n_{1,k+p+1}} \epsilon_i + \sqrt{\frac{\log(2n_{1,K}/\delta)}{2n_{1,k+p+1}}} \geq \sum_{i=1}^{k+p} \frac{n_i}{n_{1,k+p}} \epsilon_i + \sqrt{\frac{\log(2n_{1,K}/\delta)}{2n_{1,k+p}}}.$$

In other words, if the bound on $|\beta - \hat{\beta}_{k+p}|$ is smaller than the bound on $|\beta - \hat{\beta}_k|$, then the bound on $|\beta - \hat{\beta}_{k+p+1}|$ must be smaller than both unless $\epsilon_{k+p+1} > \epsilon_{k+p}$. Thus if the pth and $p+1$th samples are from the same original pile (and $\epsilon_{k+p+1} = \epsilon_{k+p}$), then once we decide to use samples through p, we will always want to include sample $p + 1$. It follows that we must only consider using complete piles of data.

2.2 Corrupted Coins Simulations

The theory developed so far can be nicely illustrated via some simple simulations. We briefly describe just one such experiment in which there were $K = 8$ piles. The target coin was fair: $\beta = 0.5$. The approximation errors of the corrupted coins were

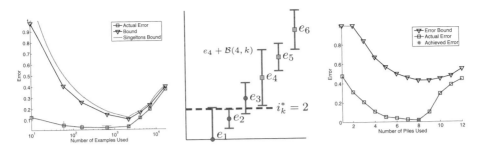

Figure 1: **Left:** Illustration of the actual error and our error bounds for estimating the bias of a coin. The error bars show one standard deviation. **Center:** Illustration of the interval construction. **Right:** Illustration of actual error of a 20 dimensional classification problem and the error bounds found using our methods.

$\vec{\epsilon} = (0.001, 0.01, 0.02, 0.03, 0.04, 0.2, 0.3, 0.5)$, and number of outcomes in the corresponding piles were $\vec{n} = (10, 50, 100, 500, 1500, 2000, 3000, 10000)$. The following process was repeated $1,000$ times. We set the probability of the ith coin to be $\beta_i = \beta + \epsilon_i$ and sampled n_i times from it. We then used all possible prefixes $1, \ldots, k$ of piles to estimate β. For each k, we computed the bound for the estimate using piles $1, \ldots, k$ using the theory developed in the previous section. To illustrate Lemma 1 we also computed the bound using partial piles. This bound is slightly higher than the suggested bound since we use effectively more piles ($n_{1,K}$ instead of K). As the lemma predicts, it is not valuable to use subsets of piles. Simulations with other values of K, $\vec{\epsilon}$ and $\vec{n}$ yield similar qualitative behavior. We note that a strength of the theory developed is its generality, as it provides bounds for any model parameters.

The leftmost panel of Figure 1 summarizes the simulation results. Empirically, the best estimate of the target coin is using the first four piles, while our algorithm suggests using the first five piles. However, the empirical difference in quality between the two estimates is negligible, so the theory has given near-optimal guidance in this case. We note that while our bounds have essentially the right shape (which is what matters for the computation of k^*), numerically they are quite loose compared to the true behavior. There are various limits to the numerical precision we should expect without increasing the complexity of the theory — for example, the precision is limited by accuracy of constants in the Hoeffding inequality and the use of the union bound.

3   Classification with Label Noise

We next explore the problem of classification in the presence of multiple data sets with varying amounts of *label noise*. The setting is as follows. We assume there is a fixed and unknown binary function $f : X \to \{0, 1\}$ and a fixed and unknown distribution P on the inputs X to f. We are presented again with K piles of data, $N_1, ..., N_K$. Now each pile N_i contains n_i labeled examples (x, y) that are generated from the target function f with label noise at rate η_i, where $0 \le \eta_1 < \eta_2 < \ldots < \eta_K$. In other words, for each example (x, y) in pile N_i, $y = f(x)$ with probability $1 - \eta_i$ and $y = \neg f(x)$ with probability η_i. The goal is to decide which piles of data to use in order to choose a function h from a set of hypothesis functions $\mathcal{H}$ with minimal *generalization (true) error* $e(h)$ with respect to f and P. As before, for any prefix of piles $N_1, \ldots, N_k$, we examine the most basic estimator based on this data, namely the hypothesis minimizing the observed or training error:

$$\hat{h}_k = \underset{h \in \mathcal{H}}{\operatorname{argmin}} \{\hat{e}_k(h)\}$$

where $\hat{e}_k(h)$ is the fraction of times $h(x) \neq y$ over all $(x, y) \in N_1 \cup \cdots \cup N_k$. Thus we examine the standard empirical risk minimization framework [2]. Generalizing from the biased coin setting, we are interested in three primary questions: what can we say about the deviation $|e(\hat{h}_k) - \hat{e}(\hat{h}_k)|$, which is the gap between the true and observed error of the estimator $\hat{h}_k$; what is the optimal value of k; and how can we compute the corresponding bounds?

We note that the classification noise setting can naturally be viewed as a special case of a more general and challenging "agnostic" classification setting that we discuss briefly in Section 4. Here we provide a more specialized solution that exploits particular properties of class label noise.

We begin by observing that for any *fixed* function h, the question of how $\hat{e}_k(h)$ is related to $e(h)$ bears great similarity to the biased coin setting. More precisely, the expected classification error of h on pile N_i only is

$$(1 - \eta_i)e(h) + \eta_i(1 - e(h)) = e(h) + \eta_i(1 - 2e(h)) .$$

Thus if we set

$$\beta = e(h), \quad \epsilon_i = \eta_i |1 - 2e(h)| \tag{2}$$

and if we were only concerned with making the best use of the data in estimating $e(h)$, we could attempt to apply the theory developed in Section 2 using the reduction above. There are two distinct and obvious difficulties. The first difficulty is that even restricting attention to estimating $e(h)$ for a fixed h, the values for ϵ_i above (and thus the bounds computed by the methods of Section 2) depend on $e(h)$, which is exactly the unknown quantity we would like to estimate. The second difficulty is that in order to bound the performance of empirical error minimization within $\mathcal{H}$, we must say something about the probability of *any* $h \in \mathcal{H}$ being selected. We address each of these difficulties in turn.

3.1 Computing the Error Bound Matrix

For now we assume that $\{e(h) : h \in \mathcal{H}\}$ is a finite set containing M values $e_1 < \ldots < e_M$. This assumption clearly holds if $|\mathcal{H}|$ is finite, and can be removed entirely by discretizing the values in $\{e(h) : h \in \mathcal{H}\}$. For convenience we assume that for all levels e_i there exists a function $h \in \mathcal{H}$ such that $e(h) = e_i$. This assumption can also be removed (details of both omitted due to space considerations). We define a matrix $\mathcal{B}$ of estimation errors as follows. Each row i of $\mathcal{B}$ represents one possible value of $e(h) = e_i$, while each column k represents the use of only piles $N_1, \ldots, N_k$ of noisy labeled examples of the target f. The entry $\mathcal{B}(i, k)$ will contain a bound on $|e(h) - \hat{e}_k(h)|$ that is valid simultaneously for all $h \in \mathcal{H}$ with $e(h) = e_i$. In other words, for any such h, with high probability $\hat{e}_k(h)$ falls in the range $[e_i - \mathcal{B}(i, k), e_i + \mathcal{B}(i, k)]$. It is crucial to note that we do not need to know *which* functions $h \in \mathcal{H}$ satisfy $e(h) = e_i$ in order to either compute or use the bound $\mathcal{B}(i, k)$, as we shall see shortly. Rather, it is enough to know that for each $h \in \mathcal{H}$, some row of $\mathcal{B}$ will provide estimation error bounds for each k.

The values in $\mathcal{B}$ can be now be calculated using the settings provided by Eq. (2) and the bound in Eq. (1). However, since Eq. (1) applies to the case of a single biased coin and here we have many (essentially one for each function at a given generalization error e_i), we must modify it slightly. We can (pessimistically) bound the VC dimension of all functions with error rate $e(h) = e_i$ by the VC dimension d of the entire class $\mathcal{H}$. Formally, we replace the square root term in Eq. (1) with the following expression, which is a simple application of VC theory [2, 3]:

$$\mathcal{O}\left(\sqrt{\frac{1}{n_{1,k}}\left(d\log\left(\frac{n_{1,k}}{d}\right) + \log\left(\frac{KM}{\delta}\right)\right)}\right) . \tag{3}$$

We note that in cases where we have more information on the structure of the generalization errors in $\mathcal{H}$, an accordingly modified equation can be used, which may yield considerably improved bounds. For example, in the statistical physics theory of learning curves[4] it is common to posit knowledge of the density or number of functions in $\mathcal{H}$ at a given generalization error e_i. In such a case we could clearly substitute the VC dimension d by the (potentially much smaller) VC dimension d_i of just this subclass.

In a moment we describe how the matrix $\mathcal{B}$ can be used to choose the number k of piles to use, and to compute a bound on the generalization error of $\hat{h}_k$. We first formalize the development above as an intermediate result.

Lemma 2 *Suppose $\mathcal{H}$ is a set of binary functions with VC dimension d. Let M be the number of noise levels and K be the number of piles. Then for all $\delta > 0$, with probability at least $1 - \delta$, for all $i \in \{1, \ldots, M\}$, for all $h \in \mathcal{H}$ with $e(h) = e_i$, and for all $k \in \{1, \ldots, K\}$ we have*

$$|e(h) - \hat{e}_k(h)| \leq \mathcal{B}(i, k).$$

The matrix $\mathcal{B}$ can be computed in time linear in its size $\mathcal{O}(KM)$.

3.2 Putting It All Together

By Lemma 2, the matrix $\mathcal{B}$ gives, for each possible generalization error e_i and each k, an upper bound on the deviation between observed and true errors for functions of true error e_i when using piles $N_1, \ldots, N_k$. It is thus natural to try to use column k of $\mathcal{B}$ to bound the error of $\hat{h}_k$, the function minimizing the observed error on these piles.

Suppose we fix the number of piles used to be k. The observed error of any function with true generalization error e_i must, with high probability, lie in the interval $I_{i,k} = [e_i - \mathcal{B}(i, k), e_i + \mathcal{B}(i, k)]$. By simultaneously considering these intervals for all values of e_i, we can put a bound on the generalization error of the best function in the hypothesis class. This process is best illustrated by an example.

Consider a hypothesis space in which the generalization error of the available functions can take on the discrete values 0, 0.1, 0.2, 0.3, 0.4, and 0.5. Suppose the matrix $\mathcal{B}$ has been calculated as above and the kth column is (0.16, 0.05, 0.08, 0.14, 0.07, 0.1). We know, for example, that all functions with true generalization error $e_2 = 0.1$ will show an error in the range $I_{2,k} = [0.05, 0.15]$, and that all functions with true generalization error $e_4 = 0.3$ will show an error in the range $I_{4,k} = [0.16, 0.44]$. The center panel of Figure 1 illustrates the span of each interval.

Examining this diagram, it becomes clear that the function $\hat{h}_k$ minimizing the error on $N_1 \cup \cdots \cup N_k$ could not possibly be a function with true error e_4 or higher as long as $\mathcal{H}$ contains at least one function with true error e_2 since the observed error of the latter would necessarily be lower (with high probability). Likewise, it would not be possible for a function with true error e_5 or e_6 to be chosen. However, a function with true error e_3 could produce a lower observed error than one with true error e_1 or e_2 (since $e_3 - \mathcal{B}(3, k) < e_2 + \mathcal{B}(2, k)$ and $e_3 - \mathcal{B}(3, k) < e_1 + \mathcal{B}(1, k)$), and thus could be chosen as $\hat{h}_k$. Therefore, the smallest bound we can place on the true error of $\hat{h}_k$ in this example is $e_3 = 0.2$.

In general, we know that $\hat{h}_k$ will have true error corresponding to the midpoint of an a interval which overlaps with the interval with the least upper bound ($I_{2,k}$ in this example). This leads to an intuitive procedure for calculating a bound on the true error of $\hat{h}_k$. First, we determine the interval with the smallest upper bound, $i_k^* = \operatorname{argmin}_i \{e_i + \mathcal{B}(i, k)\}$. Consider the set of intervals which overlap with i_k^*, namely $J_k = \{i : e_i - \mathcal{B}(i, k) \leq e_{i_k^*} + \mathcal{B}(i_k^*, k)\}$. It is possible for the smallest observed error to come from a function corresponding to any of the intervals in J_k. Thus, a bound on the true error of $\hat{h}_k$ can be obtained by taking the maximum $e(h)$ value for any function in J_k, i.e. $\mathcal{C}(k) \stackrel{\text{def}}{=} \max_{i \in J_k} \{e_i\}$.

Our overall algorithm for bounding $e(\hat{h}_k)$ and choosing k^* can thus be summarized:

1. Compute the matrix $\mathcal{B}$ as described in Section 3.1 .
2. Compute the vector $\mathcal{C}$ described above.
3. Output $k^* = \operatorname{argmin}_k \{\mathcal{C}(k)\}$.

We have established the following theorem.

Theorem 2 *Suppose $\mathcal{H}$ is a set of binary functions with VC dimension d. Let M be the number of noise levels and K be the number of piles. For all $k = 1, ..., K$, let $\hat{h}_k = \operatorname{argmin}_h \{\hat{e}_k(h)\}$ be the function in $\mathcal{H}$ with the lowest empirical error evaluated using the first k piles of data. Then for all $\delta > 0$, with probability at least $1 - \delta$,*

$$e(\hat{h}_k) \leq \mathcal{C}(k)$$

The suggested choice of k is thus $k^* = \operatorname{argmin}_k \{\mathcal{C}(k)\}$.

3.3 Classification Noise Simulations

In order to illustrate the methodology described in this section, simulations were run on a classification problem in which samples $\vec{x} \in \{0, 1\}^{20}$ were chosen uniformly at random, and the target function $f(\vec{x})$ was 1 if and only if $\sum_{i=1}^{20} x_i > 10$.

Classification models were created for $k = 1, ..., K$ by training using the first k piles of data using logistic regression with a learning rate of 0.0005 for a maximum of $5,000$ iterations. The generalization error for each model was determined by testing on a noise-free sample of 500 examples drawn from the same uniform distribution. Bounds were calculated using the algorithm described above with functions binned into 101 evenly spaced error values $\vec{e} = (0, 0.01, 0.02, ..., 1)$ with $\delta = 0.001$.

The right panel of Figure 1 shows an example of the bounds found with $K = 12$ piles, noise levels $\vec{\eta} = (0.001, 0.002, 0.01, 0.02, 0.03, 0.04, 0.05, 0.1, 0.2, 0.3, 0.4, 0.5)$, and sample sizes $\vec{n} = (20, 150, 300, 400, 500, 600, 700, 1000, 1500, 2000, 3000, 5000)$. The algorithm described above correctly predicts that the eighth pile should be chosen as the cutoff, yielding an optimal error value of 0.018. It is interesting to note that although the error bounds shown are significantly higher than the actual error, the shapes of the curves are similar. This phenomena is common to many uniform convergence bounds.

Further experimentation has shown that the algorithm described here works well in general when there are small piles of low noise data and large piles of high noise data. Its predictions are more useful in higher dimensional space, since it is relatively easy to get good predictions without much available data in lower dimensions.

4   Further Research

In research subsequent to the results presented here [5], we examine a considerably more general "agnostic" classification setting [6]. As before, we assume there is a fixed and unknown binary function $f : X \rightarrow \{0, 1\}$ and a fixed and unknown distribution P on the inputs X to f. We are presented again with K piles of data, $N_1, ..., N_K$. Now each pile N_i contains n_i labeled examples (x, y) that are generated from an unknown function h_i such that $e(h_i) = e(h_i, f) = \Pr_P[h_i(x) \neq f(x)] \leq \epsilon_i$ for given values $\epsilon_1 \leq \ldots \leq \epsilon_K$. Thus

225

we are provided piles of labeled examples of unknown functions "nearby" the unknown target f, where "nearby" is quantified by the sequence of ϵ_i.

In forthcoming work [5] we show that with high probability, for any $k \leq K$

$$e(\hat{h}_k, f) \leq \min_{h \in \mathcal{H}} \{e(f, h)\} + 2 \sum_{i=1}^{k} \left(\frac{n_i}{n_{1,k}} \right) \epsilon_i + \mathcal{O} \left(\sqrt{\frac{1}{n_{1,k}} \left(d \log \left(\frac{n_{1,k}}{d} \right) + \log \left(\frac{K}{\delta} \right) \right)} \right)$$

This result again allows us to express the optimal number of piles as a trade-off between weighted approximation errors and increasing sample size. We suspect the result can be extended to a wider class of loss functions that just classification.

References

[1] A. Blum and T. Mitchell. Combining labeled and unlabeled data with co-training. In *Proceedings of the Eleventh Annual Conference on Computational Learning Theory*, pages 92–100, 1998.

[2] V. N. Vapnik. *Statistical Learning Theory*. Wiley, 1998.

[3] M. J. Kearns and U. V. Vazirani. *An Introduction to Computational Learning Theory*. MIT Press, 1994.

[4] D. Haussler, M. Kearns, H.S. Seung, and N. Tishby. Rigorous learning curve bounds from statistical mechanics. In *Proceedings of the Seventh Annual ACM Conference on Computational Learning Theory*, pages 76–87, 1994.

[5] K. Crammer, M. Kearns, and J. Wortman. Forthcoming. 2006.

[6] M. Kearns, R. Schapire, and L. Sellie. Towards efficient agnostic learning. *Machine Learning*, 17:115–141, 1994.

Efficient estimation of hidden state dynamics from spike trains

Márton G. Danóczy
Inst. for Theoretical Biology
Humboldt University, Berlin
Invalidenstr. 43
10115 Berlin, Germany
m.danoczy@biologie.hu-berlin.de

Richard H. R. Hahnloser
Inst. for Neuroinformatics
UNIZH / ETHZ
Winterthurerstrasse 190
8057 Zurich, Switzerland
rich@ini.phys.ethz.ch

Abstract

Neurons can have rapidly changing spike train statistics dictated by the underlying network excitability or behavioural state of an animal. To estimate the time course of such state dynamics from single- or multiple neuron recordings, we have developed an algorithm that maximizes the likelihood of observed spike trains by optimizing the state lifetimes and the state-conditional *interspike-interval* (ISI) distributions. Our non-parametric algorithm is free of time-binning and spike-counting problems and has the computational complexity of a Mixed-state Markov Model operating on a state sequence of length equal to the total number of recorded spikes. As an example, we fit a two-state model to paired recordings of premotor neurons in the sleeping songbird. We find that the two state-conditional ISI functions are highly similar to the ones measured during waking and singing, respectively.

1 Introduction

It is well known that neurons can suddenly change firing statistics to reflect a macroscopic change of a nervous system. Often, firing changes are not accompanied by an immediate behavioural change, as is the case, for example, in paralysed patients, during sleep [1], during covert discriminative processing [2], and for all in-vitro studies [3]. In all of these cases, changes in some hidden macroscopic state can only be detected by close inspection of single or multiple spike trains. Our goal is to develop a powerful, but computationally simple tool for point processes such as spike trains. From spike train data, we want to the extract continuously evolving hidden variables, assuming a discrete set of possible states.

Our model for classifying spikes into discrete hidden states is based on three assumptions:

1. Hidden states form a continuous-time Markov process and thus have exponentially distributed lifetimes

2. State switching can occur only at the time of a spike (where there is observable evidence for a new state).

3. In each of the hidden states, spike trains are generated by mutually independent renewal processes.

1. For a continuous-time Markov process, the probability of staying in state $S = i$ for a time interval $T > t$ is given by $P_i(t) = \exp(-r_i t)$, where r_i is the escape rate (or hazard rate) of state i. The mean lifetime τ_i is defined as the inverse of the escape rate, $\tau_i = 1/r_i$.

As a corollary, it follows that the probability of staying in state i for a particular duration equals the probability of surviving for a fraction of that duration times the probability of surviving for the remaining time, i.e., the state survival probability $P_i(t)$ satisfies the product identity

$$P_i(t_1 + t_2) = P_i(t_1)P_i(t_2).$$

2. According to the second assumption, state switching can occur at any spike, irrespective of which neuron fired the spike. In the following, we shall refer to a spike fired by any of the neurons as an *event* (where state switching might occur). Note that if two (or more) neurons happen to fire a spike at exactly the same time, the respective spikes are regarded as two (or more) distinct events. The collection of event times is denoted by t_e.

Combining the first two assumptions, we formulate the hidden state sequence at the events (i.e. observation points) as a non-homogeneous discrete Markov chain. Accordingly, the probability of remaining in state i for the duration of the *interevent-interval* (IEI) $\Delta t_e = t_e - t_{e-1}$ is given by the state survival probability $P_i(\Delta t_e)$. The probability to change state is then $1 - P_i(\Delta t_e)$.

3. In each state i, the spike trains are assumed to be generated by a renewal process that randomly draws *interspike-intervals* (ISIs) t from a *probability density function* (pdf) $h_i(t)$. Because every IEI is only a fraction of an ISI, instead of working with ISI distributions, we use an equivalent formulation based on the *conditional intensity function* (CIF) $\lambda_i(\varphi)$ [4]. The CIF, also called hazard function in reliability theory, is a generalization of the Poisson firing rate. It is defined as the probability density of spiking in the time interval $[\varphi, \varphi + d\varphi]$, given that no spike has occurred in the interval $[0, \varphi)$ since the last spike. In the following, the variable φ, i.e. the time that has elapsed since the last spike, shall be referred to as *phase* [5]. Using the CIF, the ISI pdf can be expressed by the fundamental equation of renewal theory,

$$h_i(t) = \exp\left(-\int_0^t \lambda_i(\varphi)\, d\varphi \right) \lambda_i(t). \tag{1}$$

At each event e, we observe the phase trajectory of every neuron traced out since the last event. It is clear that in multiple electrode recordings the phase trajectories between events are not independent, since they have to start where the previous trajectory ended. Therefore, our model violates the observation independence assumption of standard *Hidden Markov Models* (HMMs). Our model is, in formal terms, a mixed-state Markov model [6], with the architecture of a double-chain [7]. Such models are generalizations of HMMs in that the observable outputs may not only be dependent on the current hidden state, but also on past observations (formally, the mixed state is formed by combining the hidden and observable states).

In our model, hidden state transition probabilities are characterized by the escape rates r_i and observable state transition probabilities by the CIFs λ_i^n for neuron n in hidden state i. Our goal is to find a set Ψ of model parameters, such that the likelihood

$$\Pr\{\mathbf{O}|\Psi\} = \sum_{S \in \mathfrak{S}} \Pr\{\mathbf{S}, \mathbf{O}|\Psi\}$$

of the observation sequence $\mathbf{O}$ is maximized.

As a first step, we will derive an expression for the combined likelihood $\Pr\{\mathbf{S}, \mathbf{O}|\Psi\}$. Then, we will apply the *expectation maximization* (EM) algorithm to find the optimal parameter set.

2 Transition probabilities

The mixed state at event e shall be composed of the hidden state S_e and the observable outputs O_e^n (for neurons $n \in \{1, \dots, N\}$).

Hidden state transitions   In classical mixed-state Markov models, the hidden state transition probabilities are constant. In our model, however, we describe time as a continuous quantity and observe the system whenever a spike occurs, thus in non-equidistant intervals. Consequently, hidden state transitions depend explicitly on the elapsed time since the last observation, i.e., on the IEIs Δt_e. The transition probability $a_{ij}(\Delta t_e)$ from hidden state i to hidden state j is then given by

$$a_{ij}(\Delta t_e) = \begin{cases} \exp(-r_j \Delta t_e) & \text{if } i = j, \\ [1 - \exp(-r_j \Delta t_e)] g_{ij} & \text{otherwise,} \end{cases} \tag{2}$$

where g_{ij} is the conditional probability of making a transition from state i into a new state j, given that $j \neq i$. Thus, g_{ij} has to satisfy the constraint $\sum_j g_{ij} = 1$, with $g_{ii} = 0$.

Observable state transitions   The observation at event e is defined as $O_e = \{\Phi_e^n, v_e\}$, where v_e contains the index of the neuron that has triggered event e by emitting a spike, and $\Phi_e^n = (\inf \Phi_e^n, \sup \Phi_e^n]$ is the phase interval traced out by neuron n since its last spike. Observations form a cascade. After a spike, the phase of the respective neuron is immediately reset to zero. The interval's bounds are thus defined by

$$\sup \Phi_e^n = \inf \Phi_e^n + \Delta t_e \quad \text{and} \quad \inf \Phi_e^n = \begin{cases} 0 & \text{if } v_{e-1} = n, \\ \sup \Phi_{e-1}^n & \text{otherwise.} \end{cases}$$

The observable transition probability $p_i(O_e) = \Pr\{O_e \mid O_{e-1}, S_e = i\}$ is the probability of observing output O_e, given the previous output O_{e-1} and the current hidden state S_e. With our independence assumption (3.), we can give its density as the product of every neuron's probability of having survived the respective phase interval Φ_e^n that it has traced out since its last spike, multiplied by the spiking neuron's firing rate (compare equation 1):

$$p_i(O_e) = \left[\prod_n \exp \left(-\int_{\Phi_e^n} \lambda_i^n(\varphi) \, d\varphi \right) \right] \lambda_i^{v_e}(\sup \Phi_e^{v_e}). \tag{3}$$

Note that in case of a single neuron recording, this reduces to the ISI pdf.

To give a closed form of the observable transition pdf, several approaches are thinkable. Here, for the sake of flexibility and computational simplicity, we approximate the CIF λ_i^n for neuron n in state i by a step function, assuming that its value is constant inside small, arbitrarily spaced bins $B^n(b), b \in \{1, \dots, N_{\text{bins}}^n\}$. That is, $\lambda_i^n(\varphi) \approx \ell_i^n(b), \forall \varphi \in B^n(b)$.

In order to use the discretized CIFs $\ell_i^n(b)$, we also discretize Φ_e^n: the fractions $f_e^n(b) \in [0, 1]$ represent how much of neuron n's phase bin $B^n(b)$ has been traced out since the last event. For example, if event $e - 1$ happened in the middle of neuron n's phase bin 2 and event e happened ten percent into its phase bin 4, then $f_e^n(2) = 0.5$, $f_e^n(3) = 1$, and $f_e^n(4) = 0.1$, whereas $f_e^n(i) = 0$ for other i, Figure 1.

Making use of these discretizations, the integral in equation 3 is approximated by a sum:

$$p_i(O_e) \approx \left[\prod_n \exp \left(-\sum_{b=1}^{N_{\text{bins}}^n} f_e^n(b) \, \ell_i^n(b) \, \|B^n(b)\| \right) \right] \lambda_i^{v_e}(\sup \Phi_e^{v_e}), \tag{4}$$

with $\|B^n(b)\|$ denoting the width of neuron n's phase bin b.

Equations 2 and 4 fully describe transitions in our mixed-state Markov model. Next, we apply the EM algorithm to find optimal values of the escape rates r_i, the conditional hidden state transition probabilities g_{ij} and the discretized CIFs $\ell_i^n(b)$, given a set of spike trains.

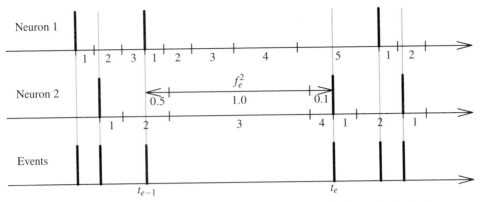

Figure 1: Two spike trains are combined to form the event train shown in the bottom row. The phase bins are shown below the spike trains, they are labelled with the corresponding bin number. As an example, for the second neuron, the fractions $f_e^2(b)$ of its phase bins that have been traced out since event $e-1$ are indicated by the horizontal arrow. They are nonzero for $b = 2, 3$, and 4.

3 Parameter estimation

Our goal is to find model parameters $\Psi = \{r_i, g_{ij}, \ell_i^n(b)\}$, such that the likelihood $\Pr\{\mathbf{O} \mid \Psi\}$ of observation sequence $\mathbf{O}$ is maximized. According to the EM algorithm, we can find such values by iterating over models

$$\Psi^{\text{new}} = \arg\max_{\Psi} \sum_{S \in \mathfrak{S}} \Pr\{\mathbf{S} \mid \mathbf{O}, \Psi^{\text{old}}\} \ln(\Pr\{\mathbf{S}, \mathbf{O} \mid \psi\}), \tag{5}$$

where $\mathfrak{S}$ is the set of all possible hidden state sequences. The product of equations 2 and 4 over all events is proportional to the combined likelihood $\Pr\{\mathbf{S}, \mathbf{O} \mid \psi\}$:

$$\Pr\{\mathbf{S}, \mathbf{O} \mid \psi\} \sim \prod_e a_{S_{e-1} S_e}(\Delta t_e) \, p_{S_e}(O_e).$$

Because of the logarithm in equation 5, the maximization over escape rates can be separated from the maximization over conditional intensity functions. We define the abbreviations $\xi_{ij}(e) = \Pr\{S_{e-1} = i, S_e = j \mid \mathbf{O}, \Psi^{\text{old}}\}$ and $\gamma_i(e) = \Pr\{S_e = i \mid \mathbf{O}, \Psi^{\text{old}}\}$ for the posterior probabilities appearing in equation 5. In practice, both expressions are computed in the expectation step by the classic forward-backward algorithm [8], using equations 2 and 4 as the transition probabilities. With the abbreviations defined above, equation 5 is split to

$$r_j^{\text{new}} = \arg\max_r \left(\sum_e \xi_{jj}(e)(-r\Delta t_e) + \sum_{e, i \neq j} \xi_{ij}(e) \ln[1 - \exp(-r\Delta t_e)] \right) \tag{6}$$

$$\ell_i^n(b)^{\text{new}} = \arg\max_{\ell} \left(-\ell \sum_e \gamma_i(e) f_e^n(b) \|B^n(b)\| + \ln \ell \sum_{\substack{e: \, v_e = n \, \wedge \\ \sup \Phi_e^n \in B^n(b)}} \gamma_i(e) \right) \tag{7}$$

$$g_{ij}^{\text{new}} = \arg\max_g \left(\ln g \sum_e \xi_{ij}(e) \right) \text{ with } g_{ii}^{\text{new}} = 0 \text{ and } \sum_j g_{ij}^{\text{new}} = 1. \tag{8}$$

In order to perform the maximization in equation 6, we compute its derivative with respect to r and set it to zero:

$$0 = \sum_e \xi_{jj}(e) \Delta t_e + \left(\Delta t_e - \frac{\Delta t_e}{1 - \exp\left(-r_j^{\text{new}} \Delta t_e\right)} \right) \sum_{i \neq j} \xi_{ij}(e)$$

This equation cannot be solved analytically, but being just a one dimensional optimization problem, a solution can be found using numerical methods, such as the Levenberg-Marquardt algorithm. The singularity in case of $\Delta t_e = 0$, which arises when two or more spikes occur at the same time, needs the special treatment of replacing the respective fraction by its limit: $1/r_i^{new}$.

To obtain the reestimation formula for the discretized CIFs, equation 7's derivative with respect to ℓ is set to zero. The result can be solved directly and yields

$$\ell_i^n(b)^{new} = \sum_{\substack{e: v_e = n \wedge \\ \sup \Phi_e^n \in B^n(b)}} \gamma_i(e) \Big/ \sum_e \gamma_i(e) f_e^n(b) \|B^n(b)\|.$$

Finally, to obtain the reestimation formula for the conditional hidden state transition probabilities g_{ij}, we solve equation 8 using Lagrange multipliers, resulting in

$$g_{i \neq j}^{new} = \sum_e \xi_{ij}(e) \Big/ \sum_{e, k \neq i} \xi_{ik}(e).$$

4 Application to spike trains from the sleeping songbird

We have applied our model to spike train data from sleeping songbirds [9]. It has been found that during sleep, neurons in vocal premotor area RA exhibit spontaneous activity that at times resembles premotor activity during singing [10, 9].

We train our model on the spike train of a single RA neuron in the sleeping bird with $N_{bins} = 100$, where the first bin extends from the sample time to 1ms and the consecutive 99 steps are logarithmically spaced up to the largest ISI. After convergence, we find that the ISI pdfs associated with the two hidden states qualitatively agree with the pdfs recorded in the awake non-singing bird and the awake singing bird, respectively, Figure 2. ISI pdfs were derived from the CIFs by using equation 1. For the state-conditional ISI histograms we first ran the Viterbi algorithm to find the most likely hidden-state sequence and then sorted spikes into two groups, for which the ISIs histograms were computed.

We find that sleep-related activity in the RA neuron of Figure 2 is best described by random switching between a singing-like state of lifetime $\tau_1 = 1.18s \pm 0.38s$ and an awake, non-singing-like state of lifetime $\tau_2 = 2.26s \pm 0.42s$. Standard deviations of lifetime estimates were computed by dividing the spike train into 30 data windows of 10s duration each and computing the Jackknife variance [11] on the truncated spike trains. The difference between the singing-like state in our model and the true singing ISI pdf shown in Figure 2 is more likely due to generally reduced burst rates during sleep, rather than to a particularity of the examined neuron.

Next we applied our model to simultaneous recordings from pairs of RA neurons. By fitting two separate models (with identical phase binning) to the two spike trains, and after running the Viterbi algorithm to find the most likely hidden state sequences, we find good agreement between the two sequences, Figure 3 (top row) and 4c. The correspondence of hidden state sequences suggests a common network mechanism for the generation of the singing-like states in both neurons. We thus applied a single model to both spike trains and found again good agreement with hidden-state sequences determined for the separate models, Figure 3 (bottom row) and 4f. The lifetime histograms for both states look approximatively exponential, justifying our assumption for the state dynamics, Figure 4g and h.

For the model trained on neuron one we find lifetimes $\tau_1 = 0.63s \pm 0.37s$ and $\tau_2 = 1.71s \pm 0.45s$, and for the model trained on neuron two we find $\tau_1 = 0.42s \pm 0.11s$ and $\tau_2 = 1.23s \pm 0.17s$. For the combined model, lifetimes are $\tau_1 = 0.58s \pm 0.25s$ and

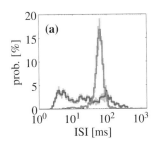 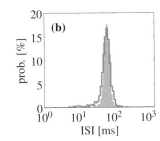 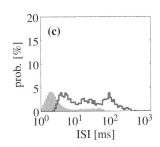

Figure 2: **(a)**: The two state-conditional ISI histograms of an RA neuron during sleep are shown by the red and green curves, respectively. Gray patches represent Jackknife standard deviations. **(b)**: After waking up the bird by pinching his tail, the new ISI histogram shown by the gray area becomes almost indistinguishable from the ISI histogram of state 1 (green line). **(c)**: In comparison to the average ISI histogram of many RA neurons during singing (shown by the gray area, reproduced from [12]), the ISI histogram corresponding to state 2 (red line) is shifted to the right, but looks otherwise qualitatively similar.

$\tau_2 = 1.13s \pm 0.15s$. Thus, hidden-state switching seems to occur more frequently in the combined model. The reason for this increase might be that evidence for the song-like state appears more frequently with two neurons, as a single neuron might not be able to indicate song-like firing statistics with high temporal fidelity.

We have also analysed the correlations between state dynamics in the different models. The hidden state function $S(t)$ is a binary function that equals one when in hidden state 1 and zero when in state 2. For the case where we modelled the two spike trains separately, we have two such hidden state functions, $S^1(t)$ for neuron one and $S^2(t)$ for neuron two. We find that all correlation functions $C_{SS^1}(t)$, $C_{SS^2}(t)$, and $C_{S^1S^2}(t)$, have a peak at zero time lag, with a high peak correlation of about 0.7, Figure 4c and f (the correlation function is defined as the cross-covariance function divided by the autocovariance functions).

We tested whether our model is a good generative model for the observed spike trains by applying the time rescaling theorem, after which the ISIs of a good generative model with known CIFs should reduce to a Poisson process with unit rate, which, after another transformation, should lead to a uniform probability density in the interval $(0, 1)$ [4]. Performing this test, we found that the transformed ISI densities of the combined model are uniform, thus validating our model (95% Kolmogorov-Smirnov test, Figure 4i).

5 Discussion

We have presented a mixed-state Markov model for point processes, assuming generation by random switching between renewal processes. Our algorithm is suited for systems in which neurons make discrete state transitions simultaneously. Previous attempts of fitting spike train data with Markov models exhibited weaknesses due to time binning. With large time bins and the number of spikes per bin treated as observables [13, 14], state transitions can only be detected when they are accompanied by firing rate changes. In our case, RA neurons have a roughly constant firing rate throughout the entire recording, and so such approaches fail.

We were able to model the hidden states in continuous time, but had to bin the ISIs in order to deal with limited data. In principle, the algorithm can operate on any binning scheme for the ISIs. Our choice of logarithmic bins keeps the number of parameters small (proportional to N_{bins}), but preserves a constant temporal resolution.

The hidden-state dynamics form Poisson processes characterized by a lifetime. By esti-

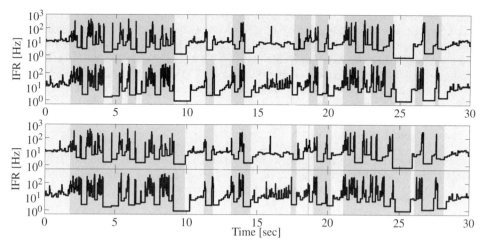

Figure 3: Shown are the instantaneous firing rate (IFR) functions of two simultaneously recorded RA neurons (at any time, the IFR corresponds to the inverse of the current ISI). The green areas show the times when in the first (awake-like) hidden state, and the red areas when in the song-like hidden state. The top two rows show the result of computing two independent models on the two neurons, whereas the bottom rows show the result of a single model.

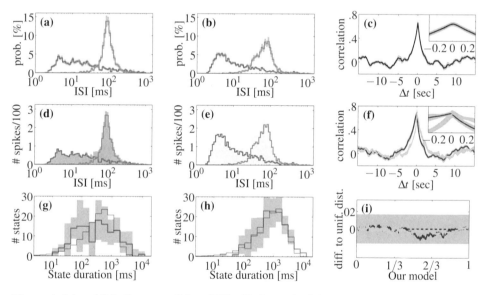

Figure 4: **(a)** and **(b)**: State-conditional ISI pdfs for each of the two neurons. **(d)** and **(e)**: ISI histograms (blue and yellow) for neurons 1 and 2, respectively, as well as state-conditional ISI histograms (red and green), computed as in Figure 2a. **(g)** and **(h)**: State lifetime histograms for the song-like state (red) and for the awake-like state (green). Theoretical (exponential) histograms with escape rates r_1 and r_2 (fine black lines) show good agreement with the measured histograms, especially in F. **(c)**: Correlation between state functions of the two separate models. **(f)**: Correlation between the state functions of the combined model with separate model 1 (blue) and separate model 2 (yellow). **(i)**: Kolmogorov-Smirnov plot after time rescaling. After transforming the ISIs, the resulting densities for both neurons remain within the 95% confidence bounds of the uniform density (gray area). In **(a)**–**(c)** and **(f)**–**(h)**, Jackknife standard deviations are shown by the gray areas.

mating this lifetime, we hope it might be possible to form a link between the hidden states and the underlying physical process that governs the dynamics of switching. Despite the apparent limitation of Poisson statistics, it is a simple matter to generalize our model to hidden state distributions with long tails (e.g., power-law lifetime distributions): By cascading many hidden states into a chain (with fixed CIFs), a power-law distribution can be approximated by the combination of multiple exponentials with different lifetimes. Our code is available at http://www.ini.unizh.ch/~rich/software/.

Acknowledgements

We would like to thank Sam Roweis for advice on Hidden Markov models and Maria Minkoff for help with the manuscript. R. H. is supported by the Swiss National Science Foundation. M. D. is supported by Stiftung der Deutschen Wirtschaft.

References

[1] Z. Nádasdy, H. Hirase, A. Czurkó, J. Csicsvári, and G. Buzsáki. Replay and time compression of recurring spike sequences in the hippocampus. *J Neurosci*, 19(21):9497–9507, Nov 1999.

[2] K. G. Thompson, D. P. Hanes, N. P. Bichot, and J. D. Schall. Perceptual and motor processing stages identified in the activity of macaque frontal eye field neurons during visual search. *J Neurophysiol*, 76(6):4040–4055, Dec 1996.

[3] R. Cossart, D. Aronov, and R. Yuste. Attractor dynamics of network UP states in the neocortex. *Nature*, 423(6937):283–288, May 2003.

[4] E. N. Brown, R. Barbieri, V. Ventura, R. E. Kass, and L. M. Frank. The time-rescaling theorem and its application to neural spike train data analysis. *Neur Comp*, 14(2):325–346, Feb 2002.

[5] J. Deppisch, K. Pawelzik, and T. Geisel. Uncovering the synchronization dynamics from correlated neuronal activity quantifies assembly formation. *Biol Cybern*, 71(5):387–399, 1994.

[6] A. M. Fraser and A. Dimitriadis. Forecasting probability densities by using hidden Markov models with mixed states. In Weigend and Gershenfeld, editors, *Time Series Prediction: Forecasting the Future and Understanding the Past*, pages 265–82. Addison-Wesley, 1994.

[7] A. Berchtold. The double chain Markov model. *Comm Stat Theor Meths*, 28:2569–2589, 1999.

[8] L. R. Rabiner. A tutorial on hidden Markov models and selected applications in speech recognition. *Proc IEEE*, 77(2):257–286, Feb 1989.

[9] R. H. R. Hahnloser, A. A. Kozhevnikov, and M. S. Fee. An ultra-sparse code underlies the generation of neural sequences in a songbird. *Nature*, 419(6902):65–70, Sep 2002.

[10] A. S. Dave and D. Margoliash. Song replay during sleep and computational rules for sensorimotor vocal learning. *Science*, 290(5492):812–816, Oct 2000.

[11] D. J. Thomson and A. D. Chave. Jackknifed error estimates for spectra, coherences, and transfer functions. In Simon Haykin, editor, *Advances in Spectrum Analysis and Array Processing*, volume 1, chapter 2, pages 58–113. Prentice Hall, 1991.

[12] A. Leonardo and M. S. Fee. Ensemble coding of vocal control in birdsong. *J Neurosci*, 25(3):652–661, Jan 2005.

[13] G. Radons, J. D. Becker, B. Dülfer, and J. Krüger. Analysis, classification, and coding of multielectrode spike trains with hidden Markov models. *Biol Cybern*, 71(4):359–373, 1994.

[14] I. Gat, N. Tishby, and M. Abeles. Hidden Markov modelling of simultaneously recorded cells in the associative cortex of behaving monkeys. *Network: Computation in Neural Systems*, 8(3):297–322, 1997.

Coarse sample complexity bounds for active learning

Sanjoy Dasgupta
UC San Diego
dasgupta@cs.ucsd.edu

Abstract

We characterize the sample complexity of active learning problems in terms of a parameter which takes into account the distribution over the input space, the specific target hypothesis, and the desired accuracy.

1   Introduction

The goal of active learning is to learn a classifier in a setting where data comes unlabeled, and any labels must be explicitly requested and paid for. The hope is that an accurate classifier can be found by buying just a few labels.

So far the most encouraging theoretical results in this field are [7, 6], which show that if the hypothesis class is that of homogeneous (i.e. through the origin) linear separators, and the data is distributed uniformly over the unit sphere in $\mathbb{R}^d$, and the labels correspond perfectly to one of the hypotheses (i.e. the separable case) then at most $O(d \log d/\epsilon)$ labels are needed to learn a classifier with error less than ϵ. This is exponentially smaller than the usual $\Omega(d/\epsilon)$ sample complexity of learning linear classifiers in a supervised setting.

However, generalizing this result is non-trivial. For instance, if the hypothesis class is expanded to include non-homogeneous linear separators, then even in just two dimensions, under the same benign input distribution, we will see that there are some target hypotheses for which active learning does not help much, for which $\Omega(1/\epsilon)$ labels are needed. In fact, in this example the label complexity of active learning depends heavily on the specific target hypothesis, and ranges from $O(\log 1/\epsilon)$ to $\Omega(1/\epsilon)$.

In this paper, we consider arbitrary hypothesis classes $\mathcal{H}$ of VC dimension $d < \infty$, and learning problems which are separable. We characterize the sample complexity of active learning in terms of a parameter which takes into account: (1) the distribution $\mathbb{P}$ over the input space $\mathcal{X}$; (2) the specific target hypothesis $h^* \in \mathcal{H}$; and (3) the desired accuracy ϵ.

Specifically, we notice that distribution $\mathbb{P}$ induces a natural topology on $\mathcal{H}$, and we define a *splitting index* ρ which captures the relevant local geometry of $\mathcal{H}$ in the vicinity of h^*, at scale ϵ. We show that this quantity fairly tightly describes the sample complexity of active learning: any active learning scheme requires $\Omega(1/\rho)$ labels and there is a generic active learner which always uses at most $\tilde{O}(d/\rho)$ labels[1].

This ρ is always at least ϵ; if it is ϵ we just get the usual sample complexity of supervised

---

[1] The $\tilde{O}(\cdot)$ notation hides factors polylogarithmic in $d, 1/\epsilon, 1/\delta$, and $1/\tau$.

learning. But sometimes ρ is a constant, and in such instances active learning gives an exponential improvement in the number of labels needed.

We look at various hypothesis classes and derive splitting indices for target hypotheses at different levels of accuracy. For homogeneous linear separators and the uniform input distribution, we easily find ρ to be a constant – perhaps the most direct proof yet of the efficacy of active learning in this case. Most proofs have been omitted for want of space; the full details, along with more examples, can be found at [5].

2 Sample complexity bounds

2.1 Motivating examples

Linear separators in $\mathbb{R}^1$

Our first example is taken from [3, 4]. Suppose the data lie on the real line, and the classifiers are simple thresholding functions, $\mathcal{H} = \{h_w : w \in \mathbb{R}\}$:

$$h_w(x) = \begin{cases} 1 & \text{if } x \geq w \\ 0 & \text{if } x < w \end{cases}$$

VC theory tells us that if the underlying distribution $\mathbb{P}$ is separable (can be classified perfectly by some hypothesis in $\mathcal{H}$), then in order to achieve an error rate less than ϵ, it is enough to draw $m = O(1/\epsilon)$ random labeled examples from $\mathbb{P}$, and to return any classifier consistent with them. But suppose we instead draw m *unlabeled* samples from $\mathbb{P}$. If we lay these points down on the line, their hidden labels are a sequence of 0's followed by a sequence of 1's, and the goal is to discover the point w at which the transition occurs. This can be done with a binary search which asks for just $\log m = O(\log 1/\epsilon)$ labels. Thus, in this case active learning gives an *exponential* improvement in the number of labels needed.

Can we always achieve a label complexity proportional to $\log 1/\epsilon$ rather than $1/\epsilon$? A natural next step is to consider linear separators in *two* dimensions.

Linear separators in $\mathbb{R}^2$

Let $\mathcal{H}$ be the hypothesis class of linear separators in $\mathbb{R}^2$, and suppose the input distribution $\mathbb{P}$ is some density supported on the perimeter of the unit circle. It turns out that the positive results of the one-dimensional case do not generalize: there are some target hypotheses in $\mathcal{H}$ for which $\Omega(1/\epsilon)$ labels are needed to find a classifier with error rate less than ϵ, no matter what active learning scheme is used.

To see this, consider the following possible target hypotheses (Figure 1, left): h_0, for which all points are positive; and h_i ($1 \leq i \leq 1/\epsilon$), for which all points are positive except for a small slice B_i of probability mass ϵ.

The slices B_i are explicitly chosen to be disjoint, with the result that $\Omega(1/\epsilon)$ labels are needed to distinguish between these hypotheses. For instance, suppose nature chooses a target hypothesis at random from among the $h_i, 1 \leq i \leq 1/\epsilon$. Then, to identify this target with probability at least $1/2$, it is necessary to query points in at least (about) half the B_i's.

Thus for these particular target hypotheses, active learning offers no improvement in sample complexity. What about other target hypotheses in $\mathcal{H}$, for instance those in which the positive and negative regions are most evenly balanced? Consider the following active learning scheme:

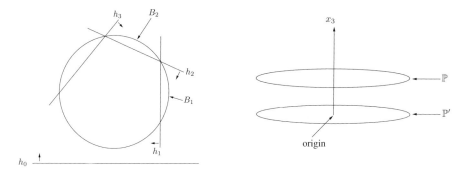

Figure 1: *Left:* The data lie on the circumference of a circle. Each B_i is an arc of probability mass ϵ. *Right:* The same distribution $\mathbb{P}$, lifted to 3-d, and with trace amounts of another distribution $\mathbb{P}'$ mixed in.

1. Draw a pool of $O(1/\epsilon)$ unlabeled points.

2. From this pool, choose query points at random until at least one positive and one negative point have been found. (If all points have been queried, then halt.)

3. Apply binary search to find the two boundaries between positive and negative on the perimeter of the circle.

For any $h \in \mathcal{H}$, define $i(h) = \min\{$positive mass of h, negative mass of $h\}$. It is not hard to see that when the target hypothesis is h, step (2) asks for $O(1/i(h))$ labels (with probability at least $9/10$, say) and step (3) asks for $O(\log 1/\epsilon)$ labels.

Thus even within this simple hypothesis class, the label complexity of active learning can run anywhere from $O(\log 1/\epsilon)$ to $\Omega(1/\epsilon)$, depending on the specific target hypothesis.

Linear separators in $\mathbb{R}^3$

In our two previous examples, the amount of unlabeled data needed was $O(1/\epsilon)$, exactly the usual sample complexity of supervised learning. We next turn to a case in which it is helpful to have significantly more unlabeled data than this.

Consider the distribution of the previous 2-d example: for concreteness, fix $\mathbb{P}$ to be uniform over the unit circle in $\mathbb{R}^2$. Now lift it into three dimensions by adding to each point $x = (x_1, x_2)$ a third coordinate $x_3 = 1$. Let $\mathcal{H}$ consist of *homogeneous* linear separators in $\mathbb{R}^3$. Clearly the bad cases of the previous example persist.

Suppose, now, that a trace amount τ of a second distribution $\mathbb{P}'$ is mixed in with $\mathbb{P}$ (Figure 1, right), where $\mathbb{P}'$ is uniform on the circle $\{x_1^2 + x_2^2 = 1, x_3 = 0\}$. The "bad" linear separators in $\mathcal{H}$ cut off just a small portion of $\mathbb{P}$ but nonetheless divide $\mathbb{P}'$ perfectly in half. This permits a three-stage algorithm: (1) using binary search on points from $\mathbb{P}'$, approximately identify the two places at which the target hypothesis h^* cuts $\mathbb{P}'$; (2) use this to identify a positive and negative point of $\mathbb{P}$ (look at the midpoints of the positive and negative intervals in $\mathbb{P}'$); (3) do binary search on points from $\mathbb{P}$. Steps (1) and (3) each use just $O(\log 1/\epsilon)$ labels.

This $O(\log 1/\epsilon)$ label complexity is made possible by the presence of $\mathbb{P}'$ and is only achievable if the amount of unlabeled data is $\Omega(1/\tau)$, which could potentially be enormous. With less unlabeled data, the usual $\Omega(1/\epsilon)$ label complexity applies.

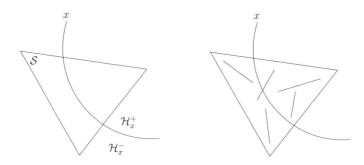

Figure 2: (a) x is a cut through $\mathcal{H}$; (b) splitting edges.

2.2 Basic definitions

The sample complexity of supervised learning is commonly expressed as a function of the error rate ϵ and the underlying distribution $\mathbb{P}$. For active learning, the previous three examples demonstrate that it is also important to take into account the target hypothesis and the amount of unlabeled data. The main goal of this paper is to present one particular formalism by which this can be accomplished.

Let $\mathcal{X}$ be an instance space with underlying distribution $\mathbb{P}$. Let $\mathcal{H}$ be the hypothesis class, a set of functions from $\mathcal{X}$ to $\{0, 1\}$ whose VC dimension is $d < \infty$.

We are operating in a non-Bayesian setting, so we are not given a measure (prior) on the space $\mathcal{H}$. In the absence of a measure, there is no natural notion of the "volume" of the current version space. However, the distribution $\mathbb{P}$ does induce a natural distance function on $\mathcal{H}$, a pseudometric:

$$d(h, h') = \mathbb{P}\{x : h(x) \neq h'(x)\}.$$

We can likewise define the notion of neighborhood: $B(h, r) = \{h' \in \mathcal{H} : d(h, h') \leq r\}$.

We will be dealing with a *separable* learning scenario, in which all labels correspond perfectly to some concept $h^* \in \mathcal{H}$, and the goal is to find $h \in \mathcal{H}$ such that $d(h^*, h) \leq \epsilon$. To do this, it is sufficient to whittle down the version space to the point where it has diameter at most ϵ, and to then return any of the remaining hypotheses. Likewise, if the diameter of the current version space is more than ϵ then any hypothesis chosen from it will have error more than $\epsilon/2$ with respect to the worst-case target. Thus, in a non-Bayesian setting, active learning is about *reducing the diameter* of the version space.

If our current version space is $\mathcal{S} \subset \mathcal{H}$, how can we quantify the amount by which a point $x \in \mathcal{X}$ reduces its diameter? Let $\mathcal{H}_x^+$ denote the classifiers that assign x a value of 1, $\mathcal{H}_x^+ = \{h \in \mathcal{H} : h(x) = 1\}$, and let $\mathcal{H}_x^-$ be the remainder, which assign it a value of 0. We can think of x as a cut through hypothesis space; see Figure 2(a). In this example, x is clearly helpful, but it doesn't reduce the diameter of $\mathcal{S}$. And we cannot say that it reduces the *average* distance between hypotheses, since again there is no measure on $\mathcal{H}$. What x seems to be doing is to reduce the diameter in a certain "direction". Is there some notion in arbitrary metric spaces which captures this intuition?

Consider any finite $Q \subset \mathcal{H} \times \mathcal{H}$. We will think of an element $(h, h') \in Q$ as an *edge* between *vertices* h and h'. For us, each such edge will represent a pair of hypotheses which need to be distinguished from one another: that is, they are relatively far apart, so there is no way to achieve our target accuracy if both of them remain in the version space. We would hope that for any finite set of edges Q, there are queries that will remove a substantial fraction of them.

To this end, a point $x \in \mathcal{X}$ is said to *ρ-split* Q if its label is guaranteed to reduce the number

of edges by a fraction $\rho > 0$, that is, if:
$$\max\{|Q \cap (\mathcal{H}_x^+ \times \mathcal{H}_x^+)|, \ |Q \cap (\mathcal{H}_x^- \times \mathcal{H}_x^-)|\} \ \le \ (1 - \rho)|Q|.$$
For instance, in Figure 2(b), the edges are $3/5$-split by x.

If our target accuracy is ϵ, we only really care about edges of length more than ϵ. So define
$$Q_\epsilon = \{(h, h') \in Q : d(h, h') > \epsilon\}.$$
Finally, we say that a subset of hypotheses $S \subset \mathcal{H}$ is (ρ, ϵ, τ)-*splittable* if for all finite edge-sets $Q \subset S \times S$,
$$\mathbb{P}\{x : x \ \rho\text{-splits} \ Q_\epsilon\} \ge \tau.$$
Paraphrasing, at least a τ fraction of the distribution $\mathbb{P}$ is useful for splitting S.[2] This τ gives a sense of how many unlabeled samples are needed. If τ is miniscule, then there are good points to query, but these will emerge only in an enormous pool of unlabeled data. It will soon transpire that the parameters ρ, τ play roughly the following roles:

$$\text{\# labels needed} \propto 1/\rho, \quad \text{\# of unlabeled points needed} \propto 1/\tau$$

A first step towards understanding them is to establish a trivial lower bound on ρ.

Lemma 1 *Pick any $0 < \alpha, \epsilon < 1$, and any set S. Then S is $((1 - \alpha)\epsilon, \epsilon, \alpha\epsilon)$-splittable.*

Proof. Pick any finite edge-set $Q \subset S \times S$. Let Z denote the number of edges of Q_ϵ cut by a point x chosen at random from $\mathbb{P}$. Since the edges have length at least ϵ, this x has at least an ϵ chance of cutting any of them, whereby $\mathbb{E}Z \ge \epsilon|Q_\epsilon|$. Now,
$$\epsilon|Q_\epsilon| \ \le \ \mathbb{E}Z \ \le \ \mathbb{P}(Z \ge (1 - \alpha)\epsilon|Q_\epsilon|) \cdot |Q_\epsilon| \ + \ (1 - \alpha)\epsilon|Q_\epsilon|,$$
which after rearrangement becomes $\mathbb{P}(Z \ge (1 - \alpha)\epsilon|Q_\epsilon|) \ge \alpha\epsilon$, as claimed. $\blacksquare$

Thus, ρ is always $\Omega(\epsilon)$; but of course, we hope for a much larger value. We will now see that the splitting index roughly characterizes the sample complexity of active learning.

2.3 Lower bound

We start by showing that if some region of the hypothesis space has a low splitting index, then it must contain hypotheses which are not conducive to active learning.

Theorem 2 *Fix a hypothesis space $\mathcal{H}$ and distribution $\mathbb{P}$. Suppose that for some $\rho, \epsilon < 1$ and $\tau < 1/2$, $S \subset \mathcal{H}$ is not (ρ, ϵ, τ)-splittable. Then any active learner which achieves an accuracy of ϵ on all target hypotheses in S, with confidence $> 3/4$ (over the random sampling of data), either needs $\ge 1/\tau$ unlabeled samples or $\ge 1/\rho$ labels.*

Proof. Let Q_ϵ be the set of edges of length $> \epsilon$ which defies splittability, with vertices $V = \{h : (h, h') \in Q_\epsilon$ for some $h' \in \mathcal{H}\}$. We'll show that in order to distinguish between hypotheses in V, either $1/\tau$ unlabeled samples or $1/\rho$ queries are needed.

So pick less than $1/\tau$ unlabeled samples. With probability at least $(1 - \tau)^{1/\tau} \ge 1/4$, none of these points ρ-splits Q_ϵ; put differently, each of these potential queries has a bad outcome ($+$ or $-$) in which at most $\rho|Q_\epsilon|$ edges are eliminated. In this case there must be a target hypothesis in V for which at least $1/\rho$ labels are required. $\blacksquare$

In our examples, we will apply this lower bound through the following simple corollary.

---

[2]Whenever an edge of length $l \ge \epsilon$ can be constructed in S, then by taking Q to consist solely of this edge, we see that $\tau \le l$. Thus we typically expect τ to be at most about ϵ, although of course it might be a good deal smaller than this.

Let S_0 be an ϵ_0-cover of $\mathcal{H}$
for $t = 1, 2, \ldots, T = \lg 2/\epsilon$:
$\quad S_t = \text{split}(S_{t-1}, 1/2^t)$
return any $h \in S_T$

function split(S, Δ)
Let $Q_0 = \{(h, h') \in S \times S : d(h, h') > \Delta\}$
Repeat for $t = 0, 1, 2, \ldots$:
$\quad$ Draw m unlabeled points $x_{t1}, \ldots, x_{tm}$
$\quad$ Query the x_{ti} which maximally splits Q_t
$\quad$ Let Q_{t+1} be the remaining edges
until $Q_{t+1} = \emptyset$
return remaining hypotheses in S

Figure 3: A generic active learner.

Corollary 3 *Suppose that in some neighborhood* $B(h_0, \Delta)$*, there are hypotheses* $h_1, \ldots, h_N$ *such that: (1)* $d(h_0, h_i) > \epsilon$ *for all* i*; and (2) the "disagree sets"* $\{x : h_0(x) \neq h_i(x)\}$ *are disjoint for different* i*.*

Then for any τ *and any* $\rho > 1/N$*, the set* $B(h_0, \Delta)$ *is not* (ρ, ϵ, τ)*-splittable . Any active learning scheme which achieves an accuracy of* ϵ *on all of* $B(h_0, \Delta)$ *must use at least* N *labels for some of the target hypotheses, no matter how much unlabeled data is available.*

In this case, the distance metric on $h_0, h_1, \ldots, h_N$ can accurately be depicted as a *star* with h_0 at the center and with spokes leading to each h_i. Each query only cuts off one spoke, so N queries are needed.

2.4 Upper bound

We now show a loosely matching upper bound on sample complexity, via an algorithm (Figure 3) which repeatedly halves the diameter of the remaining version space. For some ϵ_0 less than half the target error rate ϵ, it starts with an ϵ_0-cover of $\mathcal{H}$: a set of hypotheses $S_0 \subset \mathcal{H}$ such that any $h \in \mathcal{H}$ is within distance ϵ_0 of S_0. It is well-known that it is possible to find such an S_0 of size $\leq 2(2e/\epsilon_0 \ln 2e/\epsilon_0)^d$ [9](Theorem 5). The ϵ_0-cover serves as a surrogate for the hypothesis class – for instance, the final hypothesis is chosen from it.

The algorithm is hopelessly intractable and is meant only to demonstrate the following upper bound.

Theorem 4 *Let the target hypothesis be some* $h^* \in \mathcal{H}$*. Pick any target accuracy* $\epsilon > 0$ *and confidence level* $\delta > 0$*. Suppose* $B(h^*, 4\Delta)$ *is* (ρ, Δ, τ)*-splittable for all* $\Delta \geq \epsilon/2$*. Then there is an appropriate choice of* ϵ_0 *and* m *for which, with probability at least* $1 - \delta$*, the algorithm will draw* $\tilde{O}((1/\epsilon) + (d/\rho\tau))$ *unlabeled points, make* $\tilde{O}(d/\rho)$ *queries, and return a hypothesis with error at most* ϵ*.*

This theorem makes it possible to derive label complexity bounds which are fine-tuned to the specific target hypothesis. At the same time, it is extremely loose in that no attempt has been made to optimize logarithmic factors.

3 Examples

3.1 Simple boundaries on the line

Returning to our first example, let $\mathcal{X} = \mathbb{R}$ and $\mathcal{H} = \{h_w : w \in \mathbb{R}\}$, where each h_w is a threshold function $h_w(x) = \mathbf{1}(x \geq w)$. Suppose $\mathbb{P}$ is the underlying distribution on $\mathcal{X}$; for simplicity we'll assume it's a density, although the discussion can easily be generalized.

The distance measure $\mathbb{P}$ induces on $\mathcal{H}$ is

$$d(h_w, h_{w'}) = \mathbb{P}\{x : h_w(x) \neq h_{w'}(x)\} = \mathbb{P}\{x : w \leq x < w'\} = \mathbb{P}[w, w']$$

(assuming $w' \geq w$). Pick any accuracy $\epsilon > 0$ and consider any finite set of edges $Q = \{(h_{w_i}, h_{w'_i}) : i = 1, \ldots, n\}$, where without loss of generality the w_i are in nondecreasing order, and where each edge has length greater than ϵ: $\mathbb{P}[w_i, w'_i) > \epsilon$. Pick w so that $\mathbb{P}[w_{n/2}, w) = \epsilon$. It is easy to see that any $x \in [w_{n/2}, w)$ must eliminate at least half the edges in Q. Therefore, $\mathcal{H}$ is $(\rho = 1/2, \epsilon, \epsilon)$-splittable for any $\epsilon > 0$.

This echoes the simple fact that active-learning $\mathcal{H}$ is just a binary search.

3.2   Intervals on the line

The next case we consider is almost identical to our earlier example of 2-d linear separators (and the results carry over to that example, within constant factors). The hypotheses correspond to intervals on the real line: $\mathcal{X} = \mathbb{R}$ and $\mathcal{H} = \{h_{a,b} : a, b \in \mathbb{R}\}$, where $h_{a,b}(x) = 1(a \leq x \leq b)$. Once again assume $\mathbb{P}$ is a density. The distance measure it induces is $d(h_{a,b}, h_{a',b'}) = \mathbb{P}\{x : x \in [a, b] \cup [a', b'], x \notin [a, b] \cap [a', b']\} = \mathbb{P}([a, b]\Delta[a', b'])$, where $S\Delta T$ denotes symmetric difference $(S \cup T) \setminus (S \cap T)$.

Even in this very simple class, some hypotheses are much easier to active-learn than others.

Hypotheses not amenable to active-learning. Divide the real line into $1/\epsilon$ disjoint intervals, each with probability mass ϵ, and let $\{h_i : i = 1, \ldots, 1/\epsilon\}$ denote the hypotheses taking value 1 on the corresponding intervals. Let h_0 be the everywhere-zero concept. Then these h_i satisfy the conditions of Corollary 3; their star-shaped configuration forces a ρ-value of ϵ, and active learning doesn't help at all in choosing amongst them.

Hypotheses amenable to active learning. The bad hypotheses are the ones whose intervals have small probability mass. We'll now see that larger concepts are not so bad; in particular, for any h whose interval has mass $> 4\epsilon$, $B(h, 4\epsilon)$ is $(\rho = \Omega(1), \epsilon, \Omega(\epsilon))$-splittable.

Pick any $\epsilon > 0$ and any $h_{a,b}$ such that $\mathbb{P}[a, b] = r > 4\epsilon$. Consider a set of edges Q whose endpoints are in $B(h_{a,b}, 4\epsilon)$ and which all have length $> \epsilon$. In the figure below, all lengths denote probability masses. Any concept in $B(h_{a,b}, 4\epsilon)$ (more precisely, its interval) must lie within the outer box and must contain the inner box (this inner box might be empty).

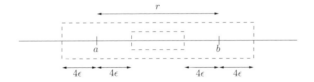

Any edge $(h_{a',b'}, h_{a'',b''}) \in Q$ has length $> \epsilon$, so $[a', b']\Delta[a'', b'']$ (either a single interval or a union of two intervals) has total length $> \epsilon$ and lies between the inner and outer boxes.

Now pick x at random from the distribution $\mathbb{P}$ restricted to the space between the two boxes. This space has mass at most 16ϵ and at least 4ϵ, of which at least ϵ is occupied by $[a', b']\Delta[a'', b'']$. Therefore x separates $h_{a',b'}$ from $h_{a'',b''}$ with probability $\geq 1/16$.

Now let's look at all of Q. The expected number of edges split by our x is at least $|Q|/16$, and therefore the probability that more than $|Q|/32$ edges are split is at least $1/32$. So $\mathbb{P}\{x : x \ (1/32)\text{-splits } Q\} \geq 4\epsilon/32 = \epsilon/8$.

To summarize, for any hypothesis $h_{a,b}$, let $i(h_{a,b}) = \mathbb{P}[a, b]$ denote the probability mass of its interval. Then for any $h \in \mathcal{H}$ and any $\epsilon < i(h)/4$, the set $B(h, 4\epsilon)$ is $(1/32, \epsilon, \epsilon/8)$-splittable. In short, once the version space is whittled down to $B(h, i(h)/4)$, efficient active learning is possible. And the initial phase of getting to $B(h, i(h)/4)$ can be managed by random sampling, using $\tilde{O}(1/i(h))$ labels: not too bad when $i(h)$ is large.

3.3 Linear separators under the uniform distribution

The most encouraging positive result for active learning to date has been for learning homogeneous (through the origin) linear separators with data drawn uniformly from the surface of the unit sphere in $\mathbb{R}^d$. The splitting indices for this case [5] bring this out immediately:

Theorem 5 *For any $h \in \mathcal{H}$, any $\epsilon \leq 1/(32\pi^2\sqrt{d})$, $B(h, 4\epsilon)$ is $(\frac{1}{8}, \epsilon, \Omega(\epsilon/\sqrt{d}))$-splittable.*

4 Related work and open problems

There has been a lot of work on a related model in which the points to be queried are synthetically constructed, rather than chosen from unlabeled data [1]. The expanded role of $\mathbb{P}$ in our model makes it substantially different, although a few intuitions do carry over – for instance, Corollary 3 generalizes the notion of *teaching dimension*[8].

We have already discussed [7, 4, 6]. One other technique which seems useful for active learning is to look at the unlabeled data and then place bets on certain target hypotheses, for instance the ones with large margin. This insight – nicely formulated in [2, 10] – is not specific to active learning and is orthogonal to the search issues considered in this paper.

In all the positive examples in this paper, a random data point which intersects the version space has a good chance of $\Omega(1)$-splitting it. This permits a naive active learning strategy, also suggested in [3]: just pick a random point whose label you are not yet sure of. On what kinds of problems will this work, and what are prototypical cases where more intelligent querying is needed?

Acknowledgements. I'm grateful to Yoav Freund for introducing me to this field; to Peter Bartlett, John Langford, Adam Kalai and Claire Monteleoni for helpful discussions; and to the anonymous NIPS reviewers for their detailed and perceptive comments.

References

[1] D. Angluin. Queries revisited. *ALT*, 2001.

[2] M.-F. Balcan and A. Blum. A PAC-style model for learning from labeled and unlabeled data. *Eighteenth Annual Conference on Learning Theory*, 2005.

[3] D. Cohn, L. Atlas, and R. Ladner. Improving generalization with active learning. *Machine Learning*, 15(2):201–221, 1994.

[4] S. Dasgupta. Analysis of a greedy active learning strategy. *NIPS*, 2004.

[5] S. Dasgupta. Full version of this paper at www.cs.ucsd.edu/˜dasgupta/papers/sample.ps.

[6] S. Dasgupta, A. Kalai, and C. Monteleoni. Analysis of perceptron-based active learning. *Eighteenth Annual Conference on Learning Theory*, 2005.

[7] Y. Freund, S. Seung, E. Shamir, and N. Tishby. Selective sampling using the query by committee algorithm. *Machine Learning Journal*, 28:133–168, 1997.

[8] S. Goldman and M. Kearns. On the complexity of teaching. *Journal of Computer and System Sciences*, 50(1):20–31, 1995.

[9] D. Haussler. Decision-theoretic generalizations of the PAC model for neural net and other learning applications. *Information and Computation*, 100(1):78–150, 1992.

[10] J. Shawe-Taylor, P. Bartlett, R. Williamson, and M. Anthony. Structural risk minimization over data-dependent hierarchies. *IEEE Transactions on Information Theory*, 44(5):1926–1940, 1998.

Norepinephrine and Neural Interrupts

Peter Dayan
Gatsby Computational Neuroscience Unit
University College London
17 Queen Square, London WC1N 3AR, UK
dayan@gatsby.ucl.ac.uk

Angela J. Yu
Center for Brain, Mind & Behavior
Green Hall, Princeton University
Princeton, NJ 08540, USA
ajyu@princeton.edu

Abstract

Experimental data indicate that norepinephrine is critically involved in aspects of vigilance and attention. Previously, we considered the function of this neuromodulatory system on a time scale of minutes and longer, and suggested that it signals global uncertainty arising from gross changes in environmental contingencies. However, norepinephrine is also known to be activated phasically by familiar stimuli in well-learned tasks. Here, we extend our uncertainty-based treatment of norepinephrine to this phasic mode, proposing that it is involved in the detection and reaction to state uncertainty *within* a task. This role of norepinephrine can be understood through the metaphor of neural interrupts.

1 Introduction

Theoretical approaches to understanding neuromodulatory systems are plagued by the latter's neural ubiquity, evolutionary longevity, and temporal promiscuity. Neuromodulators act in potentially different ways over many different time-scales [14]. There are various general notions about their roles, such as regulating sleeping and waking [13] and changing the signal to noise ratios of cortical neurons [11]. However, these are slowly giving way to more specific computational ideas [20, 7, 10, 24, 25, 5], based on such notions as optimal gain scheduling, prediction error and uncertainty.

In this paper, we focus on the short term activity of norepinephrine (NE) neurons in the locus coeruleus [18, 1, 2, 3, 16, 4]. These neurons project NE to subcortical structures and throughout the entire cortex, with individual neurons having massive axonal arborizations [12]. Over medium and short time-scales, norepinephrine is implicated in various ways in attention, vigilance, and learning. Given the widespread distribution and effects of NE in key cognitive tasks, it is very important to understand what it is in a task that drives the activity of NE neurons, and thus what computational effects it may be exerting.

Figure 1 illustrates some of the key data that has motivated theoretical treatments of NE. Figure 1A;B;C show more tonic responses operating around a time-scale of minutes. Figures 1D;E;F show the short-term effects that are our main focus here.

Briefly, Figures 1A;B show that when the rules of a task are reversed, NE influences the speed of adaptation to the changed contingency (Figure 1A) and the activity of noradrenergic cells is tonically elevated (Figure 1B). Based on these data, we suggested [24, 25] that medium-term NE reports *unexpected uncertainty* arising from unpredicted changes in an environment or task. This signal is a key part of a strategy for inference in potentially labile contexts. It operates in collaboration with a putatively cholinergic signal which reports on *expected uncertainty* that arises, for instance, from known variability or noise.

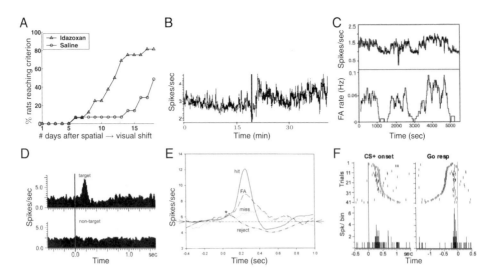

Figure 1: NE activity and effects. (A) Rats solve a sequential decision problem in a linear maze. When the relevant cues are switched after a few days of learning (from spatial to visual), rats with pharmacologically boosted NE ("idazoxan") learn to use the new set of cues *faster* than the controls. Adapted from [9]. (B) In a vigilance task, monkeys respond to rare targets and ignore common distractor stimuli. The trace shows the activity of a single NE neuron in the locus coeruleus (LC) around the time of a target-distractor reversal (vertical line). Tonic activity is elevated for a considerable period. Adapted from [2]. (C) Correlation between the gross fluctuations in the tonic activity of a single NE neuron (upper) and performance in the task (lower, measured by false alarm rate). Adapted from [20]. (D) Single NE cells are activated on a phasic time-scale stimulus locked (vertical line) to the target (upper plot) and not the distractor (lower plot). Adapted from [16]. (E) The average responses of a large number of norepinephrine cells (over a total of 41,454 trials) stimulus locked (vertical line) to targets or distractors, sorted by the nature and rectitude of the response. The asterisk marks (similar) early activation of the neurons by the stimulus. Adapted from [16]. (F) In a GO/NO-GO olfactory discrimination task for rats, single units are activated by the target odor (and not by the distractor odor), but are temporally much more tightly locked to the response (right) than the stimulus (left). Trials are ordered according to the time between stimulus (blue) and response (red). Adapted from [4].

However, Figures 1D;E;F, along with other substantial neurophysiological data on the activity of NE neurons [18, 4], show NE neurons have phasic response properties that lie outside this model. The data in Figure 1D;E come from a vigilance task [1], in which subjects can gain reward by reacting to a rare target (a rectangle oriented one way), while ignoring distractors (a rectangle oriented in the orthogonal direction). Under these circumstances, NE is consistently activated by the target and *not* the distractor (Figure 1D). There are also clear correlations in the magnitude of the NE activity and the nature of a trial: hit, miss, false alarm, correct reject (Figure 1E). It is known that the activity is weaker if the targets are more common [17] (though the lack of response to rare distractors shows that NE is not driven by mere rarity), and disappears if no action need be taken in response to the target [18]. In fact, the signal is more tightly related in time to the subsequent action than the preceding stimulus (Figure 1F). The signal has been qualitatively described in terms of influencing or controlling the allocation of behavioral or cognitive resources [20, 4].

Since it arises on every trial in an extremely well-learned task with stable stimulus contingencies, this NE signal clearly cannot be indicating unpredicted task changes. Brown *et al* [5] have recently made the seminal suggestion that it reports changes in the statistical structure of the input (stimulus-present versus stimulus-absent) to decision-making circuits that are involved in initiating differential responding to distinct target stimuli. A statistically necessary consequence of the change in the input structure is that afferent information should be integrated differently: sensory responses should be ignored if no target is present, but taken seriously otherwise. Their suggestion is that NE, by changing the gain of neurons in the decision-making circuit, has exactly this optimizing effect.

In this paper, we argue for a related, but distinct, notion of phasic NE, suggesting that it reports on unexpected *state* changes within a task. This is a significant, though natural, extension of its role in reporting unexpected *task* changes [25]. We demonstrate that it accounts well for the neurophysiological data. In agreement with the various accounts of the effects of phasic NE, we consider its role as a form of internal *interrupt* signal [6]. Computers use interrupts to organize the correct handling of internal and external events such as timers or peripheral input. Higher-level programs specify what interrupts are allowed to gain control, and the consequences thereof. We argue that phasic NE is the medium for a somewhat similar neural interrupt, allowing the correct handling of statistically *atypical* events. This notion relates comfortably to many existing views of phasic NE, and provides a computational correlate for quantitative models.

2 The Model

Figure 2A illustrates a simple hidden Markov generative model (HMM) of the vigilance task in Figure 1B-E. The (start) state models the condition established when the monkey fixates the light and initiates a trial. Following a somewhat variable delay, either the target (target) or the distractor (distractor) is presented, and the monkey must respond appropriately (release a continuously depressed bar for target and continue pressing for distractor) The transition out of start is uniformly distributed between timesteps 6 and 10, implemented by a time-varying transition function for this node:

$$P(s_t|s_{t-1} = \text{start}) = \begin{cases} 1 - q_t & s_t = \text{start} \\ 0.8q_t & s_t = \text{distractor} \\ 0.2q_t & s_t = \text{target} \end{cases} \quad (1)$$

where $q_t = 1/(11-t)$ for ($6 \leq t \leq 10$) and $q_t = 0$ otherwise. The start and target states are assumed to be absorbing states (self-transition probability $= 1$). This transition function ensures that the stimulus onset has a uniform distribution between 6 and 10 timesteps (and 0 otherwise). Given that a transition out of start (into either target or distractor) takes place, the probability is .2 for entering target and .8 for start, as in the actual task.

In addition, it is assumed that the node start does not emit observations, while target emits $x_t = $ t with probability $\eta > 0.5$ and d with probability $1 - \eta$, and distractor emits $x_t = $ d with probability η and t with probability $1 - \eta$. The transition out of start is evident as soon as the first d or t is observed, while the magnitude of η controls the "confusability" of the target and distractor states. Figure 2B shows a typical run from this generative model. The transition into target happens on step 10 (top), and the outputs generated are a mixture of t and d(middle), with an overall prevalence of t (bottom).

Exact inference on this model can be performed in a manner similar to the forward pass in a standard HMM:

$$P(s_t|x_1, \ldots, x_t) \propto p(x_t|s_t) \sum_{s_{t-1}} P(s_t|s_{t-1})P(s_{t-1}|x_1, \ldots, x_{t-1}) . \quad (2)$$

Because start does not produce outputs, as soon as the first t is observed, the probability of start plummets to 0. There then ensues an inferential battle between target and distractor, with the latter having the initial advantage, since its prior probability is 80%.

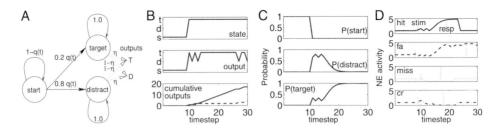

Figure 2: The model. (A) Task is modeled as a hidden Markov model (HMM), with transitions from start to either distractor (probability .8) or target (probability .2). The transitions happen between timesteps 6 and 10 with uniform probability; distractor and target are absorbing states. The only outputs are from the absorbing states, and the two have overlapping output distributions over t and d with probabilities $\eta > .5$ for their "own" output (t for target, and d for distractor), and $1 - \eta$ for the other output. (B) Sample run with a transition from start to target at timestep 10 (upper). The outputs favor target once the state has changed (middle), more clearly shown in the cumulative plot (bottom). (C) Correct probabilistic inference in the task leads to the probabilities for the three states as shown. The distractor's initial advantage arises from a base rate effect, as it is the more likely default transition. (D) Model NE signal for four trials including one for hit (top; same trials as in B;C), a false alarm (fa), a miss (miss) and a correct rejection (cr). The second vertical line represents the point at which the decision was taken (target vs. distractor).

Because of the preponderance of transitions to distractor over target, the distractor state can be thought of as the *reference* or *default* state. Evidence against that default state is a form of unexpected uncertainty within a task, and we propose that phasic NE reports this uncertainty. More specifically, NE signals $P(\text{target}|x_1, \ldots, x_t)/P(\text{target})$, where $P(\text{target}) = .2$ is the prior probability of observing a target trial. We assume that a target-response is initiated when $P(s_t|x_1, \ldots, x_t)$ exceeds 0.95, or equivalently, when the NE signal exceeds $0.95/P(\text{target})$. This implies the following intuitive relationship: the smaller the probability of the non-default state target the greater the NE-mediated "surprise" signal has to be in order to convince the inferential system that an anomalous stimulus has been observed. We also assume that if the posterior probability of target reaches 0.01, then the trial ends with no action (either a cr or a miss). The asymmetry in the thresholds arises from the asymmetry in the response contingencies of the task. Further, to model non-inferential errors, we assume that there is probability of 0.0005 per timestep of releasing the bar after the transition out of start. Once a decision is reached, the NE signal is set back to baseline (1, for equal prior and posterior) after a delay of 5 timesteps.

Note that the precise form of the mapping from unexpected uncertainty to NE spikes is rather arbitrary. In particular, there may be a strong non-linearity, such as a thresholded response profile. For simplicity, we assume a linear mapping between the two.

The NE activity during the start state is also rather arbitrary. Activity is at baseline before the stimulus comes on, since prior and posterior match when there is no explicit information from the world. When the stimulus comes on, the divisive normalization makes the activity go above baseline because although the transition was expected, its occurrence was not predicted with perfect precision. The magnitude of this activity depends on the precision of the model of the time of the transition; and the uncertainty in the interval timer. We set it to a small super-baseline level to match the data.

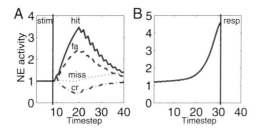

Figure 3: NE activity. (A) NE activity locked to the stimulus onset (*ie* the transition out of start). (B) NE activity response-locked to the decision to act, just for hit and fa trials. Note the difference in scale between the two figures.

3 Results

Figure 2C illustrates the inferential performance of the model for the sample run in Figure 2B;C. When the first t is observed on timestep 10, the probability of start drops to 0 and the probability of distractor, which has an initial advantage over target due to its higher probability, eventually loses out to target as the evidence overwhelms the prior. Figure 2D shows the model's NE signal for one example each of hit, fa, miss, and cr trials.

Figure 3 presents our main results. Figure 3A shows the average NE signal for the four classes of responses (hit, false alarm, miss, and correct rejection), time-locked to the start of the stimulus. These traces should be compared with those in Figure 1E. The basic form of the *rise* of the signal in the model is broadly similar to that in the data; as we have argued, the fall is rather arbitrary. Figure 3B shows the average signal locked to the time of reaction (for hit and false alarm trials) rather than stimulus onset. As in the data (Figure 1F), response-locked activities are much more tightly clustered, although this flatters the model somewhat, since we do not allow for any variability in the response time as a function of when the probability of state target reaches the threshold. Since the decay of the signal following a response is unconstrained, the trace terminates when the response is determined, usually when the probability of target reaches threshold, but also sometimes when there is an accidental erroneous response.

Figure 4 shows some additional features of the NE signal in this case. Figure 4A compares the effect of making the discrimination between target and distractor more or less difficult in the model (upper) and in the data (lower; [16]). As in the data, the stimulus-locked NE signal is somewhat broader for the more difficult case, since information has to build up over a longer period. Also as in the data, correct rejections are much less affected than hits. Figure 4B shows response locked NE. Although it is correctly slightly broader for the more difficult discrimination, the timing is not quite the same. This is largely due to the lack of a realistic model tying the defeat of the default state assumption to a behavioral response. For the easy task ($\eta = 0.675$), there were 19% hits, 1.5% false alarms, 1% misses and 77% correct rejections. For the difficult task ($\eta = 0.65$) the main difference was an increase in the number of misses to 1.5%, largely at the expense of hits. Note that since the NE signal is calculated relative to the prior likelihood, making target *more* likely would *reduce* the NE signal exactly proportionally. The data certainly hint at such a reduction [17] although the precise proportionality is not clear.

4 Discussion

The present model of the phasic activity of NE cells is a direct and major extension of our previous model of tonic aspects of this neuromodulator. The key difference is that

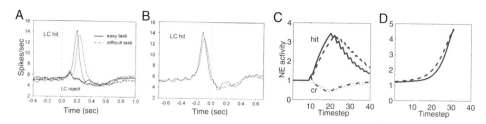

Figure 4: NE activities and task difficulty. (A) Stimulus-locked LC responses are slower and broader for a more difficult discrimination; where difficulty is controlled by the similarity of target and distractor stimuli. (B) When aligned to response, LC activities for easy and difficult discriminations are more similar, although their response in the more difficult condition is still somewhat attenuated compared to the easy one. Data in A;B adapted from [16]. (C) Discrimination difficulty in the model is controlled by the parameter η. When η is reduced from 0.675 (easy; solid) to 0.65 (hard; dashed), simulated NE activity also becomes slower and broader when aligned to stimulus. (D) Same traces aligned to response indicate NE activity in the difficult condition is attenuated in the model.

unexpected uncertainty is now about the state *within* a current characterization of the task rather than about the characterization as a whole. These aspects of NE functionality are likely quite widespread, and allow us to account for a much wider range of data on this neuromodulator.

In the model, NE activity is explicitly normalized by prior probabilities arising from the default state transitions in tasks. This is necessary to measure specifically *unexpected* uncertainty, and explains the decrement in NE phasic response as a function of the **target** probability [17]. It is also associated with the small activation to the stimulus onset, although the precise form of this deserves closer scrutiny. For instance, if subjects were to build a richer model of the statistics of the time of the transition out of the **start** state, then we should see this reflected directly in the NE signal even before the stimulus comes on, for instance related to the inverse of the survival function for the transition. We would also expect this transition to effect a different NE signature if stimuli were expected during **start** that could also be confused with those expected during **target** and **distractor**.

If NE indeed reports on the failure of the current state within the model of the task to account successfully for the observations, then what effect should it have? One useful way to think about the signal is in terms of an *interrupt* signal in computers. In these, a control program establishes a set of conditions (*eg* keyboard input) under which normal processing should be interrupted, in order that the consequence of the interrupt (*eg* a keystroke) can be appropriately handled. Computers have highly centralized processing architecture, and therefore the interrupt signal only needs a very limited spatial extent to exert a widespread effect on the course of computation. By contrast, processing in the brain is highly distributed, and therefore it is necessary for the interrupt signal to have a widespread distribution, so that the full ramifications of the failure of the current state can be felt. Neuromodulatory systems are ideal vehicles for the signal.

The interrupt signal should engage mechanisms for establishing the new state, which then allows a new set of conditions to be established as to which interrupts will be allowed to occur, and also to take any appropriate action (as in the task we modeled). The interrupt signal can be expected to be beneficial, for instance, when there is competition between tasks for the use of neural resources such as receptive fields [8].

Apart from interrupts such as these under sophisticated top-down control, there are also more basic contingencies from things such as critical potential threats and stressors that should exert a rapid and dramatic effect on neural processing (these also have computational analogues in signals such as that power is about to fail). The NE system is duly subject to what might be considered as bottom-up as well as top-down influences [21].

The interrupt-based account is a close relative of existing notions of phasic NE. For instance, NE has been implicated in the process of alerting [23]. The difference from our account is perhaps the stronger tie in the latter to actual behavioral output. A task with second-order contingencies may help to differentiate the two accounts. There are also close relations with theories [20, 5] that suggest how NE may be an integral part of an optimal decisional strategy. These propose that NE controls the gain in competitive decision-making networks that implement sequential decision-making [22], essentially by reporting on the changes in the statistical structure of the inputs induced by stimulus onset. It is also suggested that a more extreme change in the gain, destabilizing the competitive networks through explosive symmetry breaking, can be used to freeze or lock-in any small difference in the competing activities.

The idea that NE can signal the change in the input statistics occasioned by the (temporally-unpredictable) occurrence of the target is highly appealing. However, the statistics of the input change when either the target *or* the distractor appears, and so the preference for responding to the target at the expense of the distractor is strange. The effect of forcing the decision making network to become unstable, and therefore enforcing a speeded decision is much closer to an interrupt; but then it is not clear why this signal should decrease as the target becomes more common. Further, since in the unstable regime, the statistical optimality of integration is effectively abandoned, the computational appeal of the signal is somewhat weakened. However, this alternative theory does make an important link to sequential statistical analysis [22], raising issues about things like thresholds for deciding target and distractor that should be important foci of future work here too.

Figure 1C shows an additional phenomenon that has arisen in a task when subjects were not even occasionally taxed with difficult discrimination problems. The overall performance fluctuates dramatically (shown by the changing false alarm rate), in a manner that is tightly correlated with fluctuations in tonic NE activity. Periods of high tonic activity are correlated with low phasic activation to the targets (data not shown). Aston-Jones, Cohen and their colleagues [20, 3] have suggested that NE regulates the balance between exploration and exploitation. The high tonic phase is associated with the former, with subjects failing to concentrate on the contingencies that lead to their current rewards in order to search for stimuli or actions that might be associated with better rewards. Increasing the ease of interruptability to either external cues or internal state changes, could certainly lead to apparently exploratory behavior. However, there is little evidence as to how this sort of exploration is being actively determined, since, for instance, the macroscopic fluctuations evident in Figure 1C do not arise in response to any experimental contingency. Given the relationship between phasic and tonic firing, further investigation of these periodic fluctuations and their implications would be desirable.

Finally, in our previous model [24, 25], tonic NE was closely coupled with tonic acetylcholine (ACh), with the latter reporting expected rather than unexpected uncertainty. The account of ACh should transfer somewhat directly into the short-term contingencies within a task – we might expect it to be involved in reporting on aspects of the known variability associated with each state, including each distinct stimulus state as well as the no-stimulus state. As such, this ACh signal might be expected to be relatively more tonic than NE (an effect that is also apparent in our previous work on more tonic interactions between ACh and NE (*eg* Figure 2 of [24]). One attractive target for an account along these lines is the sustained attention task studied by Sarter and colleagues, which involves temporal uncertainty. Performance in this task is exquisitely sensitive to cholinergic manipulation [19], but unaffected by gross noradrenergic manipulation [15]. We may again expect there to be interesting part-opponent and part-synergistic interactions between the neuromodulators.

Acknowledgements

We are grateful to Gary Aston-Jones, Sebastien Bouret, Jonathan Cohen, Peter Latham, Susan Sara, and Eric Shea-Brown for helpful discussions. Funding was from the Gatsby Charitable Foundation, the EU BIBA project and the ACI Neurosciences Intégratives et Computationnelles of the French Ministry of Research.

References

[1] Aston-Jones, G, Rajkowski, J, Kubiak, P & Alexinsky, T (1994). Locus coeruleus neurons in monkey are selectively activated by attended cues in a vigilance task. *J. Neurosci.* **14**:4467-4480.

[2] Aston-Jones, G, Rajkowski, J & Kubiak, P (1997). Conditioned responses of monkey locus coeruleus neurons anticipate Acquisition of discriminative behavior in a vigilance task. *Neuroscience* **80**:697-715.

[3] Aston-Jones, G, Rajkowski, J & Cohen, J (2000). Locus coeruleus and regulation of behavioral flexibility and attention. *Prog. Brain Res.* **126**:165-182.

[4] Bouret, S & Sara, SJ (2004). Reward expectation, orientation of attention and locus coeruleus-medial frontal cortex interplay during learning. *Eur. J. Neurosci.* **20**:791-802.

[5] Brown, E, Gao, J, Holmes, P, Bogacz, R, Gilzenrat, M & Cohen, JD (2005). Simple neural networks that optimize decisions. *Int. J. Bif. & Chaos*, in press.

[6] David Johnson, J (2003). Noradrenergic control of cognition: global attenuation and an interrupt function. *Med. Hypoth.* **60**:689-692.

[7] Dayan, P & Yu, AJ (2001). ACh, uncertainty, and cortical inference. *NIPS 2001.*

[8] Desimone, R & Duncan, J (1995). Neural mechanisms of selective visual attention. *Annual Reviews in Neuroscience* **18**:193-222.

[9] Devauges, V & Sara, SJ (1990). Activation of the noradrenergic system facilitates an attentional shift in the rat. *Beh. Brain Res.* **39**:19-28.

[10] Doya, K (2002). Metalearning and neuromodulation. *Neur. Netw.* **15**:495-506.

[11] Foote, SL, Freedman, R & Oliver, AP (1975). Effects of putative neurotransmitters on neuronal activity in monkey auditory cortex. *Brain Res.* **86**:229-242.

[12] Freedman, R, Foote, SL & Bloom, FE (1975) Histochemical characterization of a neocortical projection of the nucleus locus coeruleus in the squirrel monkey. *J. Comp. Neurol.* **164**:209-231.

[13] Jouvet, M (1969). Biogenic amines and the states of sleep. *Science* **163**:32-41.

[14] Marder, E & Thirumalai, V (2002). Cellular, synaptic and network effects of neuromodulation. *Neur. Netw.* **15**:479-493.

[15] McGaughy, J, Sandstrom, M, Ruland, S, Bruno JP & Sarter, M (1997). Lack of effects of lesions of the dorsal noradrenergic bundle on behavioral vigilance. *Beh. Neurosci.* **111**:646-652.

[16] Rajkowski, J, Majczynski, H, Clayton, E & Aston-Jones, G (2004). Activation of monkey locus coeruleus neurons varies with difficulty and performance in a target detection task. *J. Neurophysiol.* **92**:361-371.

[17] Rajkowski, J, Majczynski, H, Clayton, E, Cohen, JD & Aston-Jones, G (2002). Phasic activation of monkey locus coeruleus (LC) neurons with recognition of motivationally relevant stimuli. *Society for Neuroscience, Abstracts* 86.10.

[18] Sara, SJ & Segal, M (1991). Plasticity of sensory responses of locus coeruleus neurons in the behaving rat: implications for cognition. *Prog. Brain Res.* **88**:571-585.

[19] Turchi, J & Sarter, M (2001). Bidirectional modulation of basal forebrain NMDA receptor function differentially affects visual attention but not visual discrimination performance. *Neuroscience* **104**:407-417.

[20] Usher, M, Cohen, JD, Servan-Schreiber, D, Rajkowski, J & Aston-Jones, G (1999). The role of locus coeruleus in the regulation of cognitive performance. *Science* **283**:549-554.

[21] Van Bockstaele, EJ, Chan, J & Pickel, VM (1996). Input from central nucleus of the amygdala efferents to pericoerulear dendrites, some of which contain tyrosine hydroxylase immunoreactivity. *Journal of Neuroscience Research* **45**:289-302.

[22] Wald, A (1947). *Sequential Analysis.* New York, NY: John Wiley & Sons.

[23] Witte, EA & Marrocco, RT (1997). Alteration of brain noradrenergic activity in rhesus monkeys affects the alerting component of covert orienting. *Psychopharmacology* **132**:315-323.

[24] Yu, AJ & Dayan, P (2003). Expected and unexpected uncertainty. ACh and NE in the neocortex. *NIPS 2002.*

[25] Yu, AJ & Dayan, P (2005). Uncertainty, neuromodulation, and attention. *Neuron* **46**, 681-692.

Fast Krylov Methods for N-Body Learning

Nando de Freitas
Department of Computer Science
University of British Columbia
nando@cs.ubc.ca

Yang Wang
School of Computing Science
Simon Fraser University
ywang12@cs.sfu.ca

Maryam Mahdaviani
Department of Computer Science
University of British Columbia
maryam@cs.ubc.ca

Dustin Lang
Department of Computer Science
University of Toronto
dalang@cs.ubc.ca

Abstract

This paper addresses the issue of numerical computation in machine learning domains based on similarity metrics, such as kernel methods, spectral techniques and Gaussian processes. It presents a general solution strategy based on Krylov subspace iteration and fast N-body learning methods. The experiments show significant gains in computation and storage on datasets arising in image segmentation, object detection and dimensionality reduction. The paper also presents theoretical bounds on the stability of these methods.

1 Introduction

Machine learning techniques based on similarity metrics have gained wide acceptance over the last few years. Spectral clustering [1] is a typical example. Here one forms a Laplacian matrix $\mathbf{L} = \mathbf{D}^{-1/2}\mathbf{W}\mathbf{D}^{-1/2}$, where the entries of $\mathbf{W}$ measure the similarity between data points $\mathbf{x}_i \in \mathcal{X}, i = 1, \ldots, N$. For example, a popular choice is to set the entries of $\mathbf{W}$ to

$$w_{ij} = e^{-\frac{1}{\sigma}\|\mathbf{x}_i - \mathbf{x}_j\|^2}$$

where σ is a user-specified parameter. $\mathbf{D}$ is a normalizing diagonal matrix with entries $d_i = \sum_j w_{ij}$. The clusters can be found by running, say, K-means on the eigenvectors of $\mathbf{L}$. K-means generates better clusters on this nonlinear embedding of the data provided one adopts a suitable similarity metric.

The list of machine learning domains where one forms a covariance or similarity matrix (be it $\mathbf{W}$, $\mathbf{D}^{-1}\mathbf{W}$ or $\mathbf{D} - \mathbf{W}$) is vast and includes ranking on nonlinear manifolds [2], semi-supervised and active learning [3], Gaussian processes [4], Laplacian eigen-maps [5], stochastic neighbor embedding [6], multi-dimensional scaling, kernels on graphs [7] and many other kernel methods for dimensionality reduction, feature extraction, regression and classification. In these settings, one is interested in either inverting the similarity matrix or finding some of its eigenvectors. The computational cost of both of these operations is $O(N^3)$ while the storage requirement is $O(N^2)$. These costs are prohibitively large in applications where one encounters massive quantities of data points or where one is interested in real-time solutions such as spectral image segmentation for mobile robots [8]. In this paper, we present general numerical techniques for reducing the computational cost to $O(N \log N)$, or even $O(N)$ in specific cases, and the storage cost to $O(N)$. These reductions are achieved by combining Krylov subspace iterative solvers (such as Arnoldi, Lanczos, GMRES and conjugate gradients) with fast kernel density estimation (KDE) techniques (such as fast multipole expansions, the fast Gauss transform and dual tree recursions [9, 10, 11]).

Specific Krylov methods have been applied to kernel problems. For example, [12] uses Lanczos for spectral clustering and [4] uses conjugate gradients for Gaussian processes. However, the use of fast KDE methods, in particular fast multipole methods, to further accelerate these techniques has only appeared in the context of interpolation [13] and our paper on semi-supervised learning [8]. Here, we go for a more general exposition and present several new examples, such as fast nonlinear embeddings and fast Gaussian processes. More importantly, we attack the issue of stability of these methods. Fast KDE techniques have guaranteed error bounds. However, if these techiques are used inside iterative schemes based on orthogonalization of the Krylov subspace, there is a danger that the errors might grow over iterations. In practice, good behaviour has been observed. In Section 4, we present theoretical results that explain these observations and shed light on the behaviour of these algorithms. Before doing so, we begin with a very brief review of Krylov solvers and fast KDE methods.

2   Krylov subspace iteration

This section is a compressed overview of Krylov subspace iteration. The main message is that Krylov methods are very efficient algorithms for solving linear systems and eigenvalue problems, but they require a matrix vector multiplication at each iteration. In the next section, we replace this expensive matrix-vector multiplication with a call to fast KDE routines. Readers happy with this message and familiar with Krylov methods, such as conjugate gradients and Lanczos, can skip the rest of this section.

For ease of presentation, let the similarity matrix be simply $\mathbf{A} = \mathbf{W} \in \mathbb{R}^{N \times N}$, with entries $a_{ij} = a(\mathbf{x}_i, \mathbf{x}_j)$. (One can easily handle other cases, such as $\mathbf{A} = \mathbf{D}^{-1}\mathbf{W}$ and $\mathbf{A} = \mathbf{D} - \mathbf{W}$.) Typical measures of similarity include polynomial $a(\mathbf{x}_i, \mathbf{x}_j) = (\mathbf{x}_i \mathbf{x}_j^T + b)^p$, Gaussian $a(\mathbf{x}_i, \mathbf{x}_j) = e^{-\frac{1}{\sigma}(\mathbf{x}_i - \mathbf{x}_j)(\mathbf{x}_i - \mathbf{x}_j)^T}$ and sigmoid $a(x_i, x_j) = tanh(\alpha \mathbf{x}_i \mathbf{x}_j^T - \beta)$ kernels, where $\mathbf{x}_i \mathbf{x}_j^T$ denotes a scalar inner product. Our goal is to solve linear systems $\mathbf{A}\mathbf{x} = \mathbf{b}$ and (possibly generalized) eigenvalue problems $\mathbf{A}\mathbf{x} = \lambda\mathbf{x}$. The former arise, for example, in semi-supervised learning and Gaussian processes, while the latter arise in spectral clustering and dimensionality reduction. One could attack these problems with naive iterative methods such as the power method, Jacobi and Gauss-Seidel [14]. The problem with these strategies is that the estimate $\mathbf{x}^{(t)}$, at iteration t, only depends on the previous estimate $\mathbf{x}^{(t-1)}$. Hence, these methods do typically take too many iterations to converge. It is well accepted in the numerical computation field that Krylov methods [14, 15], which make use of the entire history of solutions $\{\mathbf{x}^{(1)}, \ldots, \mathbf{x}^{(t-1)}\}$, converge at a faster rate.

The intuition behind Krylov subspace methods is to use the history of the solutions we have already computed. We formulate this intuition in terms of projecting an N-dimensional problem onto a lower dimensional subspace. Given a matrix $\mathbf{A}$ and a vector $\mathbf{b}$, the associated Krylov matrix is:

$$\mathbf{K} = [\mathbf{b} \quad \mathbf{A}\mathbf{b} \quad \mathbf{A}^2\mathbf{b} \quad \ldots].$$

The *Krylov subspaces* are the spaces spanned by the column vectors of this matrix. In order to find a new estimate of $\mathbf{x}^{(t)}$ we could project onto the Krylov subspace. However, $\mathbf{K}$ is a poorly conditioned matrix. (As in the power method, $\mathbf{A}^t\mathbf{b}$ is converging to the eigenvector corresponding to the largest eigenvalue of $\mathbf{A}$.) We therefore need to construct a well-conditioned orthogonal matrix $\mathbf{Q}^{(t)} = [\mathbf{q}^{(1)} \cdots \mathbf{q}^{(t)}]$, with $\mathbf{q}^{(i)} \in \mathbb{R}^N$, that spans the Krylov space. That is, the leading t columns of $\mathbf{K}$ and $\mathbf{Q}$ span the same space. This is easily done using the QR-decomposition of $\mathbf{K}$ [14], yielding the following *Arnoldi relation* (augmented Schuur factorization):

$$\mathbf{A}\mathbf{Q}^{(t)} = \mathbf{Q}^{(t+1)}\widetilde{\mathbf{H}}^{(t)},$$

where $\widetilde{\mathbf{H}}^{(t)}$ is the augmented Hessenberg matrix:

$$\widetilde{\mathbf{H}}^{(t)} = \begin{pmatrix} h_{1,1} & h_{1,2} & h_{1,3} & \cdots & & h1,t \\ h_{2,1} & h_{2,2} & h_{2,3} & \cdots & & h_{2,t} \\ \vdots & \vdots & \vdots & \vdots & & \vdots \\ 0 & \cdots & 0 & h_{t,t-1} & h_{t,t} \\ 0 & \cdots & 0 & 0 & h_{t+1,t} \end{pmatrix}.$$

The eigenvalues of the smaller $(t + 1) \times t$ Hessenberg matrix approximate the eigenvalues of $\mathbf{A}$ as t increases. These eigenvalues can be computed efficiently by applying the Arnoldi relation recursively as shown in Figure 1. (If $\mathbf{A}$ is symmetric, then $\widetilde{\mathbf{H}}$ is tridiagonal and we obtain the Lanczos algorithm.) *Notice that the matrix vector multiplication $\mathbf{v} = \mathbf{A}\mathbf{q}$ is the expensive step in the Arnoldi algorithm.* Most Krylov algorithms resemble the Arnoldi algorithm in this. To solve systems of equations, we can minimize either the residual

Initialization: $\mathbf{b} = arbitrary$, $\quad \mathbf{q}^{(1)} = \mathbf{b}/\|\mathbf{b}\|$
FOR $t = 1, 2, 3, \ldots$

- $\mathbf{v} = \mathbf{A}\mathbf{q}^{(t)}$
- FOR $j = 1, \ldots, N$
  - $h_{j,t} = \mathbf{q}^{(t)T}\mathbf{v}$
  - $\mathbf{v} = \mathbf{v} - h_{j,t}\mathbf{q}^{(j)}$
- $h_{t+1,t} = \|\mathbf{v}\|$
- $\mathbf{q}^{(t+1)} = \mathbf{v}/h_{t+1,t}$

Initialization: $\mathbf{q}^{(1)} = \mathbf{b}/\|\mathbf{b}\|$
FOR $t = 1, 2, 3, \ldots$

- Perform step t of the Arnoldi algorithm
- $\min_{\mathbf{y}} \left\|\widetilde{\mathbf{H}}^{(t)}\mathbf{y} - \|\mathbf{b}\|\mathbf{i}\right\|$
- Set $\mathbf{x}^{(t)} = \mathbf{Q}^{(t)}\mathbf{y}^{(t)}$

Figure 1: The Arnoldi (left) and GMRES (right) algorithms.

$\mathbf{r}^{(t)} \triangleq \mathbf{b} - \mathbf{A}\mathbf{x}^{(t)}$, leading to the GMRES and MINRES algorithms, or the A-norm, leading to conjugate gradients (CG) [14]. GMRES, MINRES and CG apply to general, symmetric, and spd matrices respectively. For ease of presentation, we focus on the GMRES algorithm.

At step t of GMRES, we approximate the solution by the vector in the Krylov subspace $\mathbf{x}^{(t)} \in \mathcal{K}^{(t)}$ that minimizes the norm of the residual. Since $\mathbf{x}^{(t)}$ is in the Krylov subspace, it can be written as a linear combination of the columns of the Krylov matrix $\mathbf{K}^{(t)}$. Our problem therefore reduces to finding the vector $\mathbf{y} \in \mathbb{R}^t$ that minimizes $\|\mathbf{A}\mathbf{K}^{(t)}\mathbf{y} - \mathbf{b}\|$. As before, stability considerations force us to use the QR decomposition of $\mathbf{K}^{(t)}$. That is, instead of using a linear combination of the columns of $\mathbf{K}^{(t)}$, we use a linear combination of the columns of $\mathbf{Q}^{(t)}$. So our least squares problem becomes $\mathbf{y}^{(t)} = \min_{\mathbf{y}} \|\mathbf{A}\mathbf{Q}^{(t)}\mathbf{y} - \mathbf{b}\|$. Since $\mathbf{A}\mathbf{Q}^{(t)} = \mathbf{Q}^{(t+1)}\widetilde{\mathbf{H}}^{(t)}$, we only need to solve a problem of dimension $(t + 1) \times t$: $\mathbf{y}^{(t)} = \min_{\mathbf{y}} \|\mathbf{Q}^{(t+1)}\widetilde{\mathbf{H}}^{(t)}\mathbf{y} - \mathbf{b}\|$. Keeping in mind that the columns of the projection matrix $\mathbf{Q}$ are orthonormal, we can rewrite this least squares problem as $\min_{\mathbf{y}} \|\widetilde{\mathbf{H}}^{(t)}\mathbf{y} - \mathbf{Q}^{(t+1)T}\mathbf{b}\|$. We start the iterations with $\mathbf{q}^{(1)} = \mathbf{b}/\|\mathbf{b}\|$ and hence $\mathbf{Q}^{(t+1)T}\mathbf{b} = \|\mathbf{b}\|\mathbf{i}$, where $\mathbf{i}$ is the unit vector with a 1 in the first entry. The final form of our least squares problem at iteration t is:

$$\mathbf{y}^{(t)} = \min_{\mathbf{y}} \left\| \widetilde{\mathbf{H}}^{(t)} \mathbf{y} - \|\mathbf{b}\| \mathbf{i} \right\|,$$

with solution $\mathbf{x}^{(t)} = \mathbf{Q}^{(t)} \mathbf{y}^{(t)}$. The algorithm is shown in Figure 1. The least squares problem of size $(t + 1) \times t$ to compute $\mathbf{y}^{(t)}$ can be solved in $O(t)$ steps using Givens rotations [14]. *Notice again that the expensive step in each iteration is the matrix-vector product* $\mathbf{v} = \mathbf{A}\mathbf{q}$. *This is true also of CG and other Krylov methods.*

One important property of the Arnoldi relation is that the residuals are orthogonal to the space spanned by the columns of $\mathbf{V} = \mathbf{Q}^{(t+1)} \widetilde{\mathbf{H}}^{(t)}$. That is,

$$\mathbf{V}^T \mathbf{r}^{(t)} = \widetilde{\mathbf{H}}^{(t)T} \mathbf{Q}^{(t+1)T} (\mathbf{b} - \mathbf{Q}^{(t+1)} \widetilde{\mathbf{H}}^{(t)} \mathbf{y}^{(t)}) = \widetilde{\mathbf{H}}^{(t)T} \|\mathbf{b}\| \mathbf{i} - \widetilde{\mathbf{H}}^{(t)T} \widetilde{\mathbf{H}}^{(t)} \mathbf{y}^{(t)} = 0$$

In the following section, we introduce methods to speed up the matrix-vector product $\mathbf{v} = \mathbf{A}\mathbf{q}$. These methods will incur, at most, a pre-specified (tolerance) error $\mathbf{e}^{(t)}$ at iteration t. Later, we present theoretical bounds on how these errors affect the residuals and the orthogonality of the Krylov subspace.

3   Fast KDE

The expensive step in Krylov methods is the operation $\mathbf{v} = \mathbf{A}\mathbf{q}^{(t)}$. This step requires that we solve two $O(N^2)$ kernel estimates:

$$v_i = \sum_{j=1}^{N} q_j^{(t)} a(\mathbf{x}_i, \mathbf{x}_j) \qquad i = 1, 2, \ldots, M.$$

It is possible to reduce the storage and computational cost to $O(N)$ at the expense of a small specified error tolerance ϵ, say 10^{-6}, using the *fast Gauss transform* (FGT) algorithm [16, 17]. This algorithm is an instance of more general fast multipole methods for solving N-body interactions [9]. The FGT applies when the problem is low dimensional, say $\mathbf{x}_k \in \mathbb{R}^3$. However, to attack larger dimensions one can adopt clustering-based partitions as in the improved fast Gauss transform (IFGT) [10].

Fast multipole methods tend to work only in low dimensions and are specific to the choice of similarity metric. Dual tree recursions based on KD-trees and ball trees [11, 18] overcome these difficulties, but on average cost $O(N \log N)$. Due to space constraints, we can only mention these techniques here, but refer the reader to [18] for a thorough comparison.

4   Stability results

The problem with replacing the matrix-vector multiplication at each iteration of the Krylov methods is that we do not know how the errors accumulate over successive iterations. In this section, we will derive bounds that describe what factors influence these errors. In particular, the bounds will state what properties of the similarity metric and measurable quantities affect the residuals and the orthogonality of the Krylov subspaces.

Several papers have addressed the issue of Krylov subspace stability [19, 20, 21]. Our approach follows from [21]. For presentation purposes, we focus on the GMRES algorithm.

Let $\mathbf{e}^{(t)}$ denote the errors introduced in the approximate matrix-vector multiplication at each iteration of Arnoldi. For the purposes of upper-bounding, this is the tolerance of the fast KDE methods. Then, the fast KDE methods change the *Arnoldi relation* to:

$$\mathbf{A}\mathbf{Q}^{(t)} + \mathbf{E}^{(t)} = \left[\mathbf{A}\mathbf{q}^{(1)} + \mathbf{e}^{(1)}, \ldots, \mathbf{A}\mathbf{q}^{(t)} + \mathbf{e}^{(t)} \right] = \mathbf{Q}^{(t+1)} \widetilde{\mathbf{H}}^{(t)},$$

where $\mathbf{E}^{(t)} = \left[\mathbf{e}^{(1)}, \ldots, \mathbf{e}^{(t)} \right]$. The new true residuals are therefore:

$$\mathbf{r}^{(t)} = \mathbf{b} - \mathbf{A}\mathbf{x}^{(t)} = \mathbf{b} - \mathbf{A}\mathbf{Q}^{(t)}\mathbf{y}^{(t)} = \mathbf{b} - \mathbf{Q}^{(t+1)}\widetilde{\mathbf{H}}^{(t)}\mathbf{y}^{(t)} + \mathbf{E}^{(t)}\mathbf{y}^{(t)}$$

and $\widetilde{\mathbf{r}}^{(t)} = \mathbf{b} - \mathbf{Q}^{(t+1)}\widetilde{\mathbf{H}}^{(t)}\mathbf{y}^{(t)}$ are the *measured residuals*.

We need to ensure two bounds when using fast KDE methods in Krylov iterations. First, the measured residuals $\widetilde{\mathbf{r}}^{(t)}$ should not deviate too far from the true residuals $\mathbf{r}^{(t)}$. Second, deviations from orthogonality should be upper-bounded. Let us address the first question. The deviation in residuals is given by

$$\|\widetilde{\mathbf{r}}^{(t)} - \mathbf{r}^{(t)}\| = \|\mathbf{E}^{(t)}\mathbf{y}^{(t)}\|.$$

Let $\mathbf{y}^{(t)} = [y_1, \ldots, y_t]^T$. Then, this deviation satisfies:

$$\|\widetilde{\mathbf{r}}^{(t)} - \mathbf{r}^{(t)}\| = \left\| \sum_{k=1}^{t} y_k \mathbf{e}^{(k)} \right\| \leq \sum_{k=1}^{t} |y_k| \|\mathbf{e}^{(k)}\|. \tag{1}$$

The deviation from orthogonality can be upper-bounded in a similar fashion:

$$\|\mathbf{V}^T\mathbf{r}^{(t)}\| = \|\widetilde{\mathbf{H}}^{(t)T}\mathbf{Q}^{(t+1)T}(\widetilde{\mathbf{r}}^{(t)} + \mathbf{E}^{(t)}\mathbf{y}^{(t)})\| = \left\| \widetilde{\mathbf{H}}^{(t)T}\mathbf{E}^{(t)}\mathbf{y}^{(t)} \right\| \leq \|\widetilde{\mathbf{H}}^{(t)}\| \sum_{k=1}^{t} |y_k| \|\mathbf{e}^{(k)}\|$$

$$\tag{2}$$

The following lemma provides a relation between the y_k and the measured residuals $\widetilde{\mathbf{r}}^{(k-1)}$.

Lemma 1. *[21, Lemma 5.1] Assume that t iterations of the inexact Arnoldi method have been carried out. Then, for any $k = 1, \ldots, t$,*

$$|y_k| \leq \frac{1}{\sigma_t(\widetilde{\mathbf{H}}^{(t)})} \|\widetilde{\mathbf{r}}^{(k-1)}\| \tag{3}$$

where $\sigma_t(\widetilde{\mathbf{H}}^{(t)})$ denotes the t-th singular value of $\widetilde{\mathbf{H}}^{(t)}$.

The proof of the lemma follows from the QR decomposition of $\widetilde{\mathbf{H}}^{(t)}$, see [15, 21]. This lemma, in conjunction with equations (1) and (2), allows us to establish the main theoretical result of this section:

Proposition 1. *Let $\epsilon > 0$. If for every $k \leq t$ we have*

$$\|\mathbf{e}^{(k)}\| < \frac{\sigma_t(\widetilde{\mathbf{H}}^{(t)})}{t} \frac{1}{\|\widetilde{\mathbf{r}}^{(k-1)}\|} \epsilon,$$

then $\|\widetilde{\mathbf{r}}^{(t)} - \mathbf{r}^{(t)}\| < \epsilon$. Moreover, if

$$\|\mathbf{e}^{(k)}\| < \frac{\sigma_t(\widetilde{\mathbf{H}}^{(t)})}{t\|\widetilde{\mathbf{H}}^{(t)}\|} \frac{1}{\|\widetilde{\mathbf{r}}^{(k-1)}\|} \epsilon,$$

then $\|\mathbf{V}^T\mathbf{r}^{(t)}\| < \epsilon$.

Proof: First, we have

$$\|\widetilde{\mathbf{r}}^{(t)} - \mathbf{r}^{(t)}\| \leq \sum_{k=1}^{t} |y_k| \|\mathbf{e}^{(k)}\| < \sum_{k=1}^{t} \frac{\sigma_t(\widetilde{\mathbf{H}}^{(t)})}{t} \frac{1}{\|\widetilde{\mathbf{r}}^{(k-1)}\|} \epsilon \frac{1}{\sigma_t(\widetilde{\mathbf{H}}^{(t)})} \|\widetilde{\mathbf{r}}^{(k-1)}\| = \epsilon.$$

and similarly, $\|\mathbf{V}^T\mathbf{r}^{(t)}\| \leq \|\widetilde{\mathbf{H}}^{(t)}\| \sum_{k=1}^{t} |y_k| \|\mathbf{e}^{(k)}\| < \epsilon$ □

Proposition 1 tells us that in order to keep the residuals bounded while ensuring bounded deviations from orthogonality at iteration k, we need to monitor the eigenvalues of $\widetilde{\mathbf{H}}^{(t)}$ and the measured residuals $\widetilde{\mathbf{r}}^{(k-1)}$. Of course, we have no access to $\widetilde{\mathbf{H}}^{(t)}$. However, monitoring the residuals is of practical value. If the residuals decrease, we can increase the tolerance of the fast KDE algorithms and viceversa. The bounds do lead to a natural way of constructing adaptive algorithms for setting the tolerance of the fast KDE algorithms.

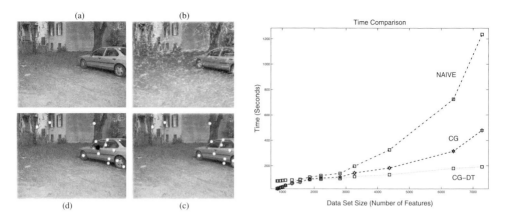

Figure 2: Figure (a) shows a test image from the PASCAL database. Figure (b) shows the SIFT features extracted from the image. Figure (c) shows the positive feature predictions for the label "car". Figure (d) shows the centroid of the positive features as a black dot. The plot on the right shows the computational gains obtained by using fast Krylov methods.

5 Experimental results

The results of this section demonstrate that significant computational gains may be obtained by combining fast KDE methods with Krylov iterations. We present results in three domains: spectral clustering and image segmentation [1, 12], Gaussian process regression [4] and stochastic neighbor embedding [6].

5.1 Gaussian processes with large dimensional features

In this experiment we use Gaussian processes to predict the labels of 128-dimensional SIFT features [22] for the purposes of object detection and localization as shown in Figure 2. There are typically thousands of features per image, so it is of paramount importance to generate fast predictions. The hard computational task here involves inverting the covariance matrix of the Gaussian process. The figure shows that it is possible to do this efficiently, under the same ROC error, by combining conjugate gradients [4] with dual trees.

5.2 Spectral clustering and image segmentation

We applied spectral clustering to color image segmentation; a generalized eigenvalue problem. The types of segmentations obtained are shown in Figure 3. There are no perceptible differences between them. We observed that fast Krylov methods run approximately twice as fast as the Nystrom method. One should note that the result of Nystrom depends on the quality of sampling, while fast N-body methods enable us to work directly with the full matrix, so the solution is less sensitive. Once again, fast KDE methods lead to significant computational improvements over Krylov algorithms (Lanczos in this case).

5.3 Stochastic neighbor embedding

Our final example is again a generalized eigenvalue problem arising in dimensionality reduction. We use the stochastic neighbor embedding algorithm of [6] to project two 3-D structures to 2-D, as shown in Figure 4. Again, we observe significant computational improvements.

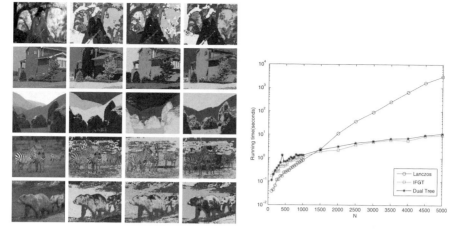

Figure 3: (left) Segmentation results (order: original image, IFGT, dual trees and Nystrom) and (right) computational improvements obtained in spectral clustering.

6 Conclusions

We presented a general approach for combining Krylov solvers and fast KDE methods to accelerate machine learning techniques based on similarity metrics. We demonstrated some of the methods on several datasets and presented results that shed light on the stability and convergence properties of these methods. One important point to make is that these methods work better when there is structure in the data. There is no computational gain if there is not statistical information in the data. This is a fascinating relation between computation and statistical information, which we believe deserves further research and understanding. One question is how can we design pre-conditioners in order to improve the convergence behavior of these algorithms. Another important avenue for further research is the application of the bounds presented in this paper in the design of adaptive algorithms.

Acknowledgments

We would like to thank Arnaud Doucet, Firas Hamze, Greg Mori and Changjiang Yang.

References

[1] A Y Ng, M I Jordan, and Y Weiss. On spectral clustering: Analysis and algorithm. In *Advances in Neural Information Processing Systems*, pages 849–856, 2001.

[2] D Zhou, J Weston, A Gretton, O Bousquet, and B Scholkopf. Ranking on data manifolds. In *Advances on Neural Information Processing Systems*, 2004.

[3] X Zhu, J Lafferty, and Z Ghahramani. Semi-supervised learning using Gaussian fields and harmonic functions. In *International Conference on Machine Learning*, pages 912–919, 2003.

[4] M N Gibbs. Bayesian Gaussian processes for regression and classification. In *PhD Thesis, University of Cambridge*, 1997.

[5] M Belkin and P Niyogi. Laplacian eigenmaps for dimensionality reduction and data representation. *Neural Computation*, 15(6):1373–1396, 2003.

[6] G Hinton and S Roweis. Stochastic neighbor embedding. In *Advances in Neural Information Processing Systems*, pages 833–840, 2002.

[7] A Smola and R Kondor. Kernels and regularization of graphs. In *Computational Learning Theory*, pages 144–158, 2003.

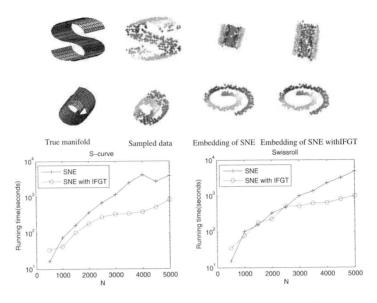

Figure 4: Examples of embedding on S-curve and Swiss-roll datasets.

[8] M Mahdaviani, N de Freitas, B Fraser, and F Hamze. Fast computational methods for visually guided robots. In *IEEE International Conference on Robotics and Automation*, 2004.

[9] L Greengard and V Rokhlin. A fast algorithm for particle simulations. *Journal of Computational Physics*, 73:325–348, 1987.

[10] C Yang, R Duraiswami, N A Gumerov, and L S Davis. Improved fast Gauss transform and efficient kernel density estimation. In *International Conference on Computer Vision*, Nice, 2003.

[11] A Gray and A Moore. Rapid evaluation of multiple density models. In *Artificial Iintelligence and Statistics*, 2003.

[12] J Shi and J Malik. Normalized cuts and image segmentation. In *IEEE Conference on Computer Vision and Pattern Recognition*, pages 731–737, 1997.

[13] R K Beatson, J B Cherrie, and C T Mouat. Fast fitting of radial basis functions: Methods based on preconditioned GMRES iteration. *Advances in Computational Mathematics*, 11:253–270, 1999.

[14] J W Demmel. *Applied Numerical Linear Algebra*. SIAM, 1997.

[15] Y Saad. *Iterative Methods for Sparse Linear Systems*. The PWS Publishing Company, 1996.

[16] L Greengard and J Strain. The fast Gauss transform. *SIAM Journal of Scientific Statistical Computing*, 12(1):79–94, 1991.

[17] B J C Baxter and G Roussos. A new error estimate of the fast Gauss transform. *SIAM Journal of Scientific Computing*, 24(1):257–259, 2002.

[18] D Lang, M Klaas, and N de Freitas. Empirical testing of fast kernel density estimation algorithms. Technical Report TR-2005-03, Department of Computer Science, UBC, 2005.

[19] G H Golub and Q Ye. Inexact preconditioned conjugate gradient method with inner-outer iteration. *SIAM Journal of Scientific Computing*, 21:1305–1320, 1999.

[20] G W Stewart. Backward error bounds for approximate Krylov subspaces. *Linear Algebra and Applications*, 340:81–86, 2002.

[21] V Simoncini and D B Szyld. Theory of inexact Krylov subspace methods and applications to scientific computing. *SIAM Journal on Scientific Computing*, 25:454–477, 2003.

[22] D G Lowe. Object recognition from local scale-invariant features. In *ICCV*, 1999.

The Forgetron:
A Kernel-Based Perceptron on a Fixed Budget

Ofer Dekel   Shai Shalev-Shwartz   Yoram Singer
School of Computer Science & Engineering
The Hebrew University, Jerusalem 91904, Israel
{oferd,shais,singer}@cs.huji.ac.il

Abstract

The Perceptron algorithm, despite its simplicity, often performs well on online classification tasks. The Perceptron becomes especially effective when it is used in conjunction with kernels. However, a common difficulty encountered when implementing kernel-based online algorithms is the amount of memory required to store the online hypothesis, which may grow unboundedly. In this paper we present and analyze the Forgetron algorithm for kernel-based online learning on a fixed memory budget. To our knowledge, this is the first online learning algorithm which, on one hand, maintains a *strict* limit on the number of examples it stores while, on the other hand, entertains a relative mistake bound. In addition to the formal results, we also present experiments with real datasets which underscore the merits of our approach.

1   Introduction

The introduction of the Support Vector Machine (SVM) [8] sparked a widespread interest in kernel methods as a means of solving (binary) classification problems. Although SVM was initially stated as a batch-learning technique, it significantly influenced the development of kernel methods in the online-learning setting. Online classification algorithms that can incorporate kernels include the Perceptron [6], ROMMA [5], ALMA [3], NORMA [4], Ballseptron [7], and the Passive-Aggressive family of algorithms [1]. Each of these algorithms observes examples in a sequence of rounds, and constructs its classification function incrementally, by storing a subset of the observed examples in its internal memory. The classification function is then defined by a kernel-dependent combination of the stored examples. This set of stored examples is the online equivalent of the *support set* of SVMs, however in contrast to the support, it continually changes as learning progresses. In this paper, we call this set the *active set*, as it includes those examples that actively define the current classifier. Typically, an example is added to the active set every time the online algorithm makes a prediction mistake, or when its confidence in a prediction is inadequately low. A rapid growth of the active set can lead to significant computational difficulties. Naturally, since computing devices have bounded memory resources, there is the danger that an online algorithm would require more memory than is physically available. This problem becomes especially eminent in cases where the online algorithm is implemented as part of a specialized hardware system with a small memory, such as a mobile telephone or an autonomous robot. Moreover, an excessively large active set can lead to unacceptably long running times, as the time-complexity of each online round scales linearly with the size of the active set.

Crammer, Kandola, and Singer [2] first addressed this problem by describing an online kernel-based modification of the Perceptron algorithm in which the active set does not exceed a predefined *budget*. Their algorithm removes redundant examples from the active set so as to make the best use of the limited memory resource. Weston, Bordes and Bottou [9] followed with their own online kernel machine on a budget. Both techniques work relatively well in practice, however they both lack a theoretical guarantee on their prediction accuracy. In this paper we present the Forgetron algorithm for online kernel-based classification. To the best of our knowledge, the Forgetron is the first online algorithm with a fixed memory budget which also entertains a formal worst-case mistake bound. We name our algorithm the Forgetron since its update builds on that of the Perceptron and since it gradually forgets active examples as learning progresses.

This paper is organized as follows. In Sec. 2 we begin with a more formal presentation of our problem and discuss some difficulties in proving mistake bounds for kernel-methods on a budget. In Sec. 3 we present an algorithmic framework for online prediction with a predefined budget of active examples. Then in Sec. 4 we derive a concrete algorithm within this framework and analyze its performance. Formal proofs of our claims are omitted due to the lack of space. Finally, we present an empirical evaluation of our algorithm in Sec. 5.

2 Problem Setting

Online learning is performed in a sequence of consecutive rounds. On round t the online algorithm observes an instance $\mathbf{x}_t$, which is drawn from some predefined instance domain $\mathcal{X}$. The algorithm predicts the binary label associated with that instance and is then provided with the correct label $y_t \in \{-1, +1\}$. At this point, the algorithm may use the instance-label pair $(\mathbf{x}_t, y_t)$ to improve its prediction mechanism. The goal of the algorithm is to correctly predict as many labels as possible.

The predictions of the online algorithm are determined by a *hypothesis* which is stored in its internal memory and is updated from round to round. We denote the hypothesis used on round t by f_t. Our focus in this paper is on margin based hypotheses, namely, f_t is a function from $\mathcal{X}$ to $\mathbb{R}$ where $\text{sign}(f_t(\mathbf{x}_t))$ constitutes the actual binary prediction and $|f_t(\mathbf{x}_t)|$ is the confidence in this prediction. The term $yf(\mathbf{x})$ is called the *margin* of the prediction and is positive whenever y and $\text{sign}(f(\mathbf{x}))$ agree. We can evaluate the performance of a hypothesis on a given example $(\mathbf{x}, y)$ in one of two ways. First, we can check whether the hypothesis makes a prediction mistake, namely determine whether $y = \text{sign}(f(\mathbf{x}))$ or not. Throughout this paper, we use M to denote the number of prediction mistakes made by an online algorithm on a sequence of examples $(\mathbf{x}_1, y_1), \ldots, (\mathbf{x}_T, y_T)$. The second way we evaluate the predictions of a hypothesis is by using the *hinge-loss* function, defined as,

$$\ell(f; (\mathbf{x}, y)) = \begin{cases} 0 & \text{if } yf(\mathbf{x}) \geq 1 \\ 1 - yf(\mathbf{x}) & \text{otherwise} \end{cases} . \tag{1}$$

The hinge-loss penalizes a hypothesis for any margin less than 1. Additionally, if $y \neq \text{sign}(f(\mathbf{x}))$ then $\ell(f, (\mathbf{x}, y)) \geq 1$ and therefore the *cumulative hinge-loss* suffered over a sequence of examples upper bounds M. The algorithms discussed in this paper use kernel-based hypotheses that are defined with respect to a kernel operator $K : \mathcal{X} \times \mathcal{X} \to \mathbb{R}$ which adheres to Mercer's positivity conditions [8]. A kernel-based hypothesis takes the form,

$$f(\mathbf{x}) = \sum_{i=1}^{k} \alpha_i K(\mathbf{x}_i, \mathbf{x}) , \tag{2}$$

where $\mathbf{x}_1, \ldots, \mathbf{x}_k$ are members of $\mathcal{X}$ and $\alpha_1, \ldots, \alpha_k$ are real weights. To facilitate the derivation of our algorithms and their analysis, we associate a reproducing kernel Hilbert space (RKHS) with K in the standard way common to all kernel methods. Formally, let $\mathcal{H}_K$ be the closure of the set of all hypotheses of the form given in Eq. (2). For any two functions, $f(\mathbf{x}) = \sum_{i=1}^{k} \alpha_i K(\mathbf{x}_i, \mathbf{x})$ and $g(\mathbf{x}) = \sum_{j=1}^{l} \beta_j K(\mathbf{z}_j, \mathbf{x})$, define the inner product between them to be, $\langle f, g \rangle = \sum_{i=1}^{k} \sum_{j=1}^{l} \alpha_i \beta_j K(\mathbf{x}_i, \mathbf{z}_j)$. This inner-product naturally induces a norm defined by $\|f\| = \langle f, f \rangle^{1/2}$ and a metric $\|f - g\| = (\langle f, f \rangle - 2\langle f, g \rangle + \langle g, g \rangle)^{1/2}$. These definitions play an important role in the analysis of our algorithms. Online kernel methods typically restrict themselves to hypotheses that are defined by some subset of the examples observed on previous rounds. That is, the hypothesis used on round t takes the form, $f_t(\mathbf{x}) = \sum_{i \in I_t} \alpha_i K(\mathbf{x}_i, \mathbf{x})$, where I_t is a subset of $\{1, \ldots, (t\text{-}1)\}$ and $\mathbf{x}_i$ is the example observed by the algorithm on round i. As stated above, I_t is called the active set, and we say that example $\mathbf{x}_i$ is *active* on round t if $i \in I_t$.

Perhaps the most well known online algorithm for binary classification is the Perceptron [6]. Stated in the form of a kernel method, the hypotheses generated by the Perceptron take the form $f_t(\mathbf{x}) = \sum_{i \in I_t} y_i K(\mathbf{x}_i, \mathbf{x})$. Namely, the weight assigned to each active example is either $+1$ or -1, depending on the label of that example. The Perceptron initializes I_1 to be the empty set, which implicitly sets f_1 to be the zero function. It then updates its hypothesis only on rounds where a prediction mistake is made. Concretely, on round t, if $f_t(\mathbf{x}_t) \neq y_t$ then the index t is inserted into the active set. As a consequence, the size of the active set on round t equals the number of prediction mistakes made on previous rounds. A relative mistake bound can be proven for the Perceptron algorithm. The bound holds for any sequence of instance-label pairs, and compares the number of mistakes made by the Perceptron with the cumulative hinge-loss of any fixed hypothesis $g \in \mathcal{H}_K$, even one defined with prior knowledge of the sequence.

Theorem 1. *Let K be a Mercer kernel and let $(\mathbf{x}_1, y_1), \ldots, (\mathbf{x}_T, y_T)$ be a sequence of examples such that $K(\mathbf{x}_t, \mathbf{x}_t) \leq 1$ for all t. Let g be an arbitrary function in $\mathcal{H}_K$ and define $\hat{\ell}_t = \ell(g; (\mathbf{x}_t, y_t))$. Then the number of prediction mistakes made by the Perceptron on this sequence is bounded by, $M \leq \|g\|^2 + 2 \sum_{t=1}^{T} \hat{\ell}_t$.*

Although the Perceptron is guaranteed to be competitive with any fixed hypothesis $g \in \mathcal{H}_K$, the fact that its active set can grow without a bound poses a serious computational problem. In fact, this problem is common to most kernel-based online methods that do not explicitly monitor the size of I_t.

As discussed above, our goal is to derive and analyze an online prediction algorithm which resolves these problems by enforcing a *fixed* bound on the size of the active set. Formally, let B be a positive integer, which we refer to as the *budget parameter*. We would like to devise an algorithm which enforces the constraint $|I_t| \leq B$ on every round t. Furthermore, we would like to prove a relative mistake bound for this algorithm, analogous to the bound stated in Thm. 1. Regretfully, this goal turns out to be impossible without making additional assumptions. We show this inherent limitation by presenting a simple counterexample which applies to any online algorithm which uses a prediction function of the form given in Eq. (2), and for which $|I_t| \leq B$ for all t. In this example, we show a hypothesis $g \in \mathcal{H}_K$ and an arbitrarily long sequence of examples such that the algorithm makes a prediction mistake on every single round whereas g suffers no loss at all. We choose the instance space $\mathcal{X}$ to be the set of $B+1$ standard unit vectors in $\mathbb{R}^{B+1}$, that is $\mathcal{X} = \{e_i\}_{i=1}^{B+1}$ where e_i is the vector with 1 in its i'th coordinate and zeros elsewhere. K is set to be the standard inner-product in $\mathbb{R}^{B+1}$, that is $K(\mathbf{x}, \mathbf{x}') = \langle \mathbf{x}, \mathbf{x}' \rangle$. Now for every t, f_t is a linear combination of at most B vectors from $\mathcal{X}$. Since $|\mathcal{X}| = B + 1$, there exists a vector $\mathbf{x}_t \in \mathcal{X}$ which is currently not in the active set. Furthermore, $\mathbf{x}_t$ is orthogonal to all of the active vectors and therefore $f_t(\mathbf{x}_t) = 0$. Assume without loss of generality that the online algorithm we are using predicts y_t to be -1 when $f_t(\mathbf{x}) = 0$. If on every round we were to present the online algorithm with the example $(\mathbf{x}_t, +1)$ then the online algorithm would make a prediction mistake on every round. On the other hand, the hypothesis $\bar{g} = \sum_{i=1}^{B+1} e_i$ is a member of $\mathcal{H}_K$ and attains a zero hinge-loss on every round. We have found a sequence of examples and a fixed hypothesis (which is indeed defined by more than B vectors from $\mathcal{X}$) that attains a cumulative loss of zero on this sequence, while the number of mistakes made by the online algorithm equals the number of rounds. Clearly, a theorem along the lines of Thm. 1 cannot be proven.

One way to resolve this problem is to limit the set of hypotheses we compete with to a subset of $\mathcal{H}_K$, which would naturally exclude $\bar{g}$. In this paper, we limit the set of competitors to hypotheses with small norms. Formally, we wish to devise an online algorithm which is competitive with every hypothesis $g \in \mathcal{H}_K$ for which $\|g\| \leq U$, for some constant U. Our counterexample indicates that we cannot prove a relative mistake bound with U set to at least $\sqrt{B+1}$, since that was the norm of $\bar{g}$ in our counterexample. In this paper we come close to this upper bound by proving that our algorithms can compete with any hypothesis with a norm bounded by $\frac{1}{4}\sqrt{(B+1)/\log(B+1)}$.

3   A Perceptron with "Shrinking" and "Removal" Steps

The Perceptron algorithm will serve as our starting point. Recall that whenever the Perceptron makes a prediction mistake, it updates its hypothesis by adding the element t to I_t. Thus, on any given round, the size of its active set equals the number of prediction mistakes it has made so far. This implies that the Perceptron may violate the budget constraint $|I_t| \leq B$. We can solve this problem by removing an example from the active set whenever its size exceeds B. One simple strategy is to remove the oldest example in the active set whenever $|I_t| > B$. Let t be a round on which the Perceptron makes a prediction mistake. We apply the following two step update. First, we perform the Perceptron's update by adding t to I_t. Let $I_t' = I_t \cup \{t\}$ denote the resulting active set. If $|I_t'| \leq B$ we are done and we set $I_{t+1} = I_t'$. Otherwise, we apply a *removal* step by finding the oldest example in the active set, $r_t = \min I_t'$, and setting $I_{t+1} = I_t' \setminus \{r_t\}$. The resulting algorithm is a simple modification of the kernel Perceptron, which conforms with a fixed budget constraint. While we are unable to prove a mistake bound for this algorithm, it is nonetheless an important milestone on the path to an algorithm with a fixed budget and a formal mistake bound.

The removal of the oldest active example from I_t may significantly change the hypothesis and effect its accuracy. One way to overcome this obstacle is to reduce the weight of old examples in the definition of the current hypothesis. By controlling the weight of the oldest active example, we can guarantee that the removal step will not significantly effect the accuracy of our predictions. More formally, we redefine our hypothesis to be,

$$f_t = \sum_{i \in I_t} \sigma_{i,t} y_i K(\mathbf{x}_i, \cdot) \ ,$$

where each $\sigma_{i,t}$ is a weight in $(0, 1]$. Clearly, the effect of removing r_t from I_t depends on the magnitude of $\sigma_{r_t, t}$.

Using the ideas discussed above, we are now ready to outline the Forgetron algorithm. The Forgetron initializes I_1 to be the empty set, which implicitly sets f_1 to be the zero function. On round t, if a prediction mistake occurs, a three step update is performed. The first step is the standard Perceptron update, namely, the index t is inserted into the active set and the weight $\sigma_{t,t}$ is set to be 1. Let I_t' denote the active set which results from this update, and let f_t' denote the resulting hypothesis, $f_t'(\mathbf{x}) = f_t(\mathbf{x}) + y_t K(\mathbf{x}_t, \mathbf{x})$. The second step of the update is a *shrinking* step in which we scale f' by a coefficient $\phi_t \in (0, 1]$. The value of

ϕ_t is intentionally left unspecified for now. Let f_t'' denote the resulting hypothesis, that is, $f_t'' = \phi_t f_t'$. Setting $\sigma_{i,t+1} = \phi_t \sigma_{i,t}$ for all $i \in I_t'$, we can write,

$$f_t''(\mathbf{x}) = \sum_{i \in I_t'} \sigma_{i,t+1} y_i K(\mathbf{x}_i, \mathbf{x}) \ .$$

The third and last step of the update is the removal step discussed above. That is, if the budget constraint is violated and $|I_t'| > B$ then I_{t+1} is set to be $I_t' \setminus \{r_t\}$ where $r_t = \min I_t'$. Otherwise, I_{t+1} simply equals I_t'. The recursive definition of the weight $\sigma_{i,t}$ can be unraveled to give the following explicit form, $\sigma_{i,t} = \prod_{j \in I_{t-1} \wedge j \geq i} \phi_j$. If the shrinking coefficients ϕ_t are sufficiently small, then the example weights $\sigma_{i,t}$ decrease rapidly with t, and particularly the weight of the oldest active example can be made arbitrarily small. Thus, if ϕ_t is small enough, then the removal step is guaranteed not to cause any significant damage. Alas, aggressively shrinking the online hypothesis with every update might itself degrade the performance of the online hypothesis and therefore ϕ_t should not be set too small. The delicate balance between safe removal of the oldest example and over-aggressive scaling is our main challenge. To formalize this tradeoff, we begin with the mistake bound in Thm. 1 and investigate how it is effected by the shrinking and removal steps.

We focus first on the removal step. Let J denote the set of rounds on which the Forgetron makes a prediction mistake and define the function,

$$\Psi(\sigma, \phi, \mu) = (\sigma \phi)^2 + 2\sigma \phi(1 - \phi\mu) \ .$$

Let $t \in J$ be a round on which $|I_t| = B$. On this round, example r_t is removed from the active set. Let $\mu_t = y_{r_t} f_t'(\mathbf{x}_{r_t})$ be the signed margin attained by f_t' on the active example being removed. Finally, we abbreviate,

$$\Psi_t = \begin{cases} \Psi(\sigma_{r_t,t}, \phi_t, \mu_t) & \text{if } t \in J \wedge |I_t| = B \\ 0 & \text{otherwise} \end{cases} \ .$$

Lemma 1 below states that removing example r_t from the active set on round t increases the mistake bound by Ψ_t. As expected, Ψ_t decreases with the weight of the removed example, $\sigma_{r_t,t+1}$. In addition, it is clear from the definition of Ψ_t that μ_t also plays a key role in determining whether $\mathbf{x}_{r_t}$ can be safely removed from the active set. We note in passing that [2] used a heuristic criterion similar to μ_t to dynamically choose which active example to remove on each online round.

Turning to the shrinking step, for every $t \in J$ we define,

$$\Phi_t = \begin{cases} 1 & \text{if } \|f_{t+1}\| \geq U \\ \phi_t & \text{if } \|f_t'\| \leq U \wedge \|f_{t+1}\| < U \\ \frac{\phi_t \|f_t'\|}{U} & \text{if } \|f_t'\| > U \wedge \|f_{t+1}\| < U \end{cases} \ .$$

Lemma 1 below also states that applying the shrinking step on round t increases the mistake bound by $U^2 \log(1/\Phi_t)$. Note that if $\|f_{t+1}\| \geq U$ then $\Phi_t = 1$ and the shrinking step on round t has no effect on our mistake bound. Intuitively, this is due to the fact that, in this case, the shrinking step does not make the norm of f_{t+1} smaller than the norm of our competitor, g.

Lemma 1. *Let* $(\mathbf{x}_1, y_1), \ldots, (\mathbf{x}_T, y_T)$ *be a sequence of examples such that* $K(\mathbf{x}_t, \mathbf{x}_t) \leq 1$ *for all t and assume that this sequence is presented to the Forgetron with a budget constraint* B. *Let g be a function in $\mathcal{H}_K$ for which* $\|g\| \leq U$, *and define* $\hat{\ell}_t = \ell(g; (\mathbf{x}_t, y_t))$. *Then,*

$$M \leq \left(\|g\|^2 + 2 \sum_{t=1}^T \hat{\ell}_t \right) + \left(\sum_{t \in J} \Psi_t + U^2 \sum_{t \in J} \log(1/\Phi_t) \right) \ .$$

The first term in the bound of Lemma 1 is identical to the mistake bound of the standard Perceptron, given in Thm. 1. The second term is the consequence of the removal and shrinking steps. If we set the shrinking coefficients in such a way that the second term is at most $\frac{M}{2}$, then the bound in Lemma 1 reduces to $M \leq \|g\|^2 + 2\sum_t \hat{\ell}_t + \frac{M}{2}$. This can be restated as $M \leq 2\|g\|^2 + 4\sum_t \hat{\ell}_t$, which is twice the bound of the Perceptron algorithm. The next lemma states sufficient conditions on ϕ_t under which the second term in Lemma 1 is indeed upper bounded by $\frac{M}{2}$.

Lemma 2. *Assume that the conditions of Lemma 1 hold and that $B \geq 83$. If the shrinking coefficients ϕ_t are chosen such that,*

$$\sum_{t \in J} \Psi_t \leq \frac{15}{32} M \quad and \quad \sum_{t \in J} \log\left(1/\Phi_t\right) \leq \frac{\log(B+1)}{2(B+1)} M ,$$

then the following holds, $\sum_{t \in J} \Psi_t + U^2 \sum_{t \in J} \log\left(1/\Phi_t\right) \leq \frac{M}{2}$.

In the next section, we define the specific mechanism used by the Forgetron algorithm to choose the shrinking coefficients ϕ_t. Then, we conclude our analysis by arguing that this choice satisfies the sufficient conditions stated in Lemma 2, and obtain a mistake bound as described above.

4   The Forgetron Algorithm

We are now ready to define the specific choice of ϕ_t used by the Forgetron algorithm. On each round, the Forgetron chooses ϕ_t to be the maximal value in $(0, 1]$ for which the damage caused by the removal step is still manageable. To clarify our construction, define $J_t = \{i \in J : i \leq t\}$ and $M_t = |J_t|$. In words, J_t is the set of rounds on which the algorithm made a mistake up until round t, and M_t is the size of this set. We can now rewrite the first condition in Lemma 2 as,

$$\sum_{t \in J_T} \Psi_t \leq \frac{15}{32} M_T . \tag{3}$$

Instead of the above condition, the Forgetron enforces the following stronger condition,

$$\forall i \in \{1, \dots, T\}, \quad \sum_{t \in J_i} \Psi_t \leq \frac{15}{32} M_i . \tag{4}$$

This is done as follows. Define, $Q_i = \sum_{t \in J_{i-1}} \Psi_t$. Let i denote a round on which the algorithm makes a prediction mistake and on which an example must be removed from the active set. The i'th constraint in Eq. (4) can be rewritten as $\Psi_i + Q_i \leq \frac{15}{32} M_i$. The Forgetron sets ϕ_i to be the maximal value in $(0, 1]$ for which this constraint holds, namely, $\phi_i = \max\{\phi \in (0, 1] : \Psi(\sigma_{r_i,i}, \phi, \mu_i) + Q_i \leq \frac{15}{32} M_i\}$. Note that Q_i does not depend on ϕ and that $\Psi(\sigma_{r_i,i}, \phi, \mu_i)$ is a quadratic expression in ϕ. Therefore, the value of ϕ_i can be found analytically. The pseudo-code of the Forgetron algorithm is given in Fig. 1.

Having described our algorithm, we now turn to its analysis. To prove a mistake bound it suffices to show that the two conditions stated in Lemma 2 hold. The first condition of the lemma follows immediately from the definition of ϕ_t. Using strong induction on the size of J, we can show that the second condition holds as well. Using these two facts, the following theorem follows as a direct corollary of Lemma 1 and Lemma 2.

INPUT: Mercer kernel $K(\cdot,\cdot)$; budget parameter $B > 0$

INITIALIZE: $I_1 = \emptyset$; $f_1 \equiv 0$; $Q_1 = 0$; $M_0 = 0$

For $t = 1, 2, \ldots$

    receive instance $\mathbf{x}_t$; predict label: $\text{sign}(f_t(\mathbf{x}_t))$

    receive correct label y_t

    If $y_t f_t(\mathbf{x}_t) > 0$

        set $I_{t+1} = I_t$, $Q_{t+1} = Q_t$, $M_t = M_{t-1}$, and $\forall i \in I_t$ set $\sigma_{i,t+1} = \sigma_{i,t}$

    Else

        set $M_t = M_{t-1} + 1$

        (1) set $I_t' = I_t \cup \{t\}$

        If $|I_t'| \leq B$

            set $I_{t+1} = I_t'$, $Q_{t+1} = Q_t$, $\sigma_{t,t} = 1$, and $\forall i \in I_{t+1}$ set $\sigma_{i,t+1} = \sigma_{i,t}$

        Else

            (2) define $r_t = \min I_t$

            choose $\phi_t = \max\{\phi \in (0,1] : \Psi(\sigma_{r_t,t}, \phi, \mu_t) + Q_t \leq \frac{15}{32} M_t\}$

            set $\sigma_{t,t} = 1$ and $\forall i \in I_t'$ set $\sigma_{i,t+1} = \phi_t \sigma_{i,t}$

            set $Q_{t+1} = Q_t + \Psi_t$

            (3) set $I_{t+1} = I_t' \setminus \{r_t\}$

    define $f_{t+1} = \sum_{i \in I_{t+1}} \sigma_{i,t+1} y_i K(\mathbf{x}_i, \cdot)$

Figure 1: The Forgetron algorithm.

Theorem 2. *Let* $(\mathbf{x}_1, y_1), \ldots, (\mathbf{x}_T, y_T)$ *be a sequence of examples such that* $K(\mathbf{x}_t, \mathbf{x}_t) \leq 1$ *for all* t. *Assume that this sequence is presented to the Forgetron algorithm from Fig. 1 with a budget parameter* $B \geq 83$. *Let* g *be a function in* $\mathcal{H}_K$ *for which* $\|g\| \leq U$, *where* $U = \frac{1}{4}\sqrt{(B+1)/\log(B+1)}$, *and define* $\hat{\ell}_t = \ell(g; (\mathbf{x}_t, y_t))$. *Then, the number of prediction mistakes made by the Forgetron on this sequence is at most,*

$$M \leq 2\|g\|^2 + 4\sum_{t=1}^{T} \hat{\ell}_t$$

5 Experiments and Discussion

In this section we present preliminary experimental results which demonstrate the merits of the Forgetron algorithm. We compared the performance of the Forgetron with the method described in [2], which we abbreviate by CKS. When the CKS algorithm exceeds its budget, it removes the active example whose margin would be the largest after the removal. Our experiment was performed with two standard datasets: the MNIST dataset, which consists of 60,000 training examples, and the census-income (adult) dataset, with 200,000 examples. The labels of the MNIST dataset are the 10 digit classes, while the setting we consider in this paper is that of binary classification. We therefore generated binary problems by splitting the 10 labels into two sets of equal size in all possible ways, totaling $\binom{10}{5}/2 = 126$ classification problems. For each budget value, we ran the two algorithms on all 126 binary problems and averaged the results. The labels in the census-income dataset are already binary, so we ran the two algorithms on 10 different permutations of the examples and averaged the results. Both algorithms used a fifth degree non-homogeneous polynomial kernel. The results of these experiments are summarized in Fig. 2. The accuracy of the standard Perceptron (which does not depend on B) is marked in each plot

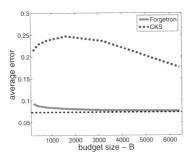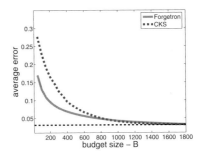

Figure 2: The error of different budget algorithms as a function of the budget size B on the census-income (adult) dataset (left) and on the MNIST dataset (right). The Perceptron's active set reaches a size of 14,626 for census-income and 1,886 for MNIST. The Perceptron's error is marked with a horizontal dashed black line.

using a horizontal dashed black line. Note that the Forgetron outperforms CKS on both datasets, especially when the value of B is small. In fact, on the census-income dataset, the Forgetron achieves almost the same performance as the Perceptron with only a fifth of the active examples. In contrast to the Forgetron, which performs well on both datasets, the CKS algorithm performs rather poorly on the census-income dataset. This can be partly attributed to the different level of difficulty of the two classification tasks. It turns out that the performance of CKS deteriorates as the classification task becomes more difficult. In contrast, the Forgetron seems to perform well on both easy and difficult classification tasks.

In this paper we described the Forgetron algorithm which is a kernel-based online learning algorithm with a fixed memory budget. We proved that the Forgetron is competitive with any hypothesis whose norm is upper bounded by $U = \frac{1}{4}\sqrt{(B+1)/\log(B+1)}$. We further argued that no algorithm with a budget of B active examples can be competitive with every hypothesis whose norm is $\sqrt{B+1}$, on every input sequence. Bridging the small gap between U and $\sqrt{B+1}$ remains an open problem. The analysis presented in this paper can be used to derive a family of online algorithms of which the Forgetron is only one special case. This family of algorithms, as well as complete proofs of our formal claims and extensive experiments, will be presented in a long version of this paper.

References

[1] K. Crammer, O. Dekel, J. Keshet, S. Shalev-Shwartz, and Y. Singer. Online passive aggressive algorithms. Technical report, The Hebrew University, 2005.

[2] K. Crammer, J. Kandola, and Y. Singer. Online classification on a budget. *NIPS*, 2003.

[3] C. Gentile. A new approximate maximal margin classification algorithm. *JMLR*, 2001.

[4] J. Kivinen, A. J. Smola, and R. C. Williamson. Online learning with kernels. *IEEE Transactions on Signal Processing*, 52(8):2165–2176, 2002.

[5] Y. Li and P. M. Long. The relaxed online maximum margin algorithm. *NIPS*, 1999.

[6] F. Rosenblatt. The Perceptron: A probabilistic model for information storage and organization in the brain. *Psychological Review*, 65:386–407, 1958.

[7] S. Shalev-Shwartz and Y. Singer. A new perspective on an old perceptron algorithm. *COLT*, 2005.

[8] V. N. Vapnik. *Statistical Learning Theory*. Wiley, 1998.

[9] J. Weston, A. Bordes, and L. Bottou. Online (and offline) on an even tighter budget. *AISTATS*, 2005.

Data-Driven Online to Batch Conversions

Ofer Dekel and Yoram Singer
School of Computer Science and Engineering
The Hebrew University, Jerusalem 91904, Israel
{oferd,singer}@cs.huji.ac.il

Abstract

Online learning algorithms are typically fast, memory efficient, and simple to implement. However, many common learning problems fit more naturally in the batch learning setting. The power of online learning algorithms can be exploited in batch settings by using *online-to-batch* conversions techniques which build a new batch algorithm from an existing online algorithm. We first give a unified overview of three existing online-to-batch conversion techniques which do not use training data in the conversion process. We then build upon these *data-independent* conversions to derive and analyze *data-driven* conversions. Our conversions find hypotheses with a small risk by explicitly minimizing data-dependent generalization bounds. We experimentally demonstrate the usefulness of our approach and in particular show that the data-driven conversions consistently outperform the data-independent conversions.

1 Introduction

Batch learning is probably the most common supervised machine-learning setting. In the batch setting, instances are drawn from a domain $\mathcal{X}$ and are associated with target values from a target set $\mathcal{Y}$. The learning algorithm is given a training set of examples, where each example is an instance-target pair, and attempts to identify an underlying rule that can be used to predict the target values of new unseen examples. In other words, we would like the algorithm to *generalize* from the training set to the entire domain of examples. The target space $\mathcal{Y}$ can be either discrete, as in the case of classification, or continuous, as in the case of regression. Concretely, the learning algorithm is confined to a predetermined set of candidate *hypotheses* $\mathcal{H}$, where each hypothesis $h \in H$ is a mapping from $\mathcal{X}$ to $\mathcal{Y}$, and the algorithm must select a "good" hypothesis from $\mathcal{H}$. The quality of different hypotheses in $\mathcal{H}$ is evaluated with respect to a loss function ℓ, where $\ell(y, y')$ is interpreted as the penalty for predicting the target value y' when the correct target is y. Therefore, $\ell(y, h(\mathbf{x}))$ indicates how well hypothesis h performs with respect to the example $(\mathbf{x}, y)$. When $\mathcal{Y}$ is a discrete set, we often use the 0-1 loss, defined by $\ell(y, y') = 1_{y \neq y'}$. We also assume that there exists a probability distribution $\mathcal{D}$ over the product space $\mathcal{X} \times \mathcal{Y}$, and that the training set was sampled i.i.d. from this distribution. Moreover, the existence of $\mathcal{D}$ enables us to reason about the average performance of an hypothesis over its entire domain. Formally, the *risk* of an hypothesis h is defined to be,

$$\text{Risk}_{\mathcal{D}}(h) = \mathbb{E}_{(\mathbf{x},y)\sim\mathcal{D}} [\ell(y, h(\mathbf{x}))] \ . \tag{1}$$

The goal of a batch learning algorithm is to use the training set to find a hypothesis that does well on average, or more formally, to find $h \in \mathcal{H}$ with a small risk.

In contrast to the batch learning setting, *online learning* takes place in a sequence of rounds. On any given round, t, the learning algorithm receives a single instance $\mathbf{x}_t \in \mathcal{X}$ and predicts its target value using an hypothesis h_{t-1}, which was generated on the previous round. On the first round, the algorithm uses a default hypothesis h_0. Immediately after the prediction is made, the correct target value y_t is revealed and the algorithm suffers an instantaneous loss of $\ell(y_t, h_{t-1}(\mathbf{x}_t))$. Finally, the online algorithm may use the newly obtained example $(\mathbf{x}_t, y_t)$ to improve its prediction strategy, namely to replace h_{t-1} with a new hypothesis h_t. Alternatively, the algorithm may choose to stick with its current hypothesis and sets $h_t = h_{t-1}$. An online algorithm is therefore defined by its default hypothesis h_0 and the update rule it uses to define new hypotheses. The *cumulative loss* suffered on a sequence of rounds is the sum of instantaneous losses suffered on each one of the rounds in the sequence. In the online setting there is typically no need for any statistical assumptions since there is no notion of generalization. The goal of the online algorithm is simply to suffer a small cumulative loss on the sequence of examples it is given, and examples that are not in this sequence are entirely irrelevant.

Throughout this paper, we assume that we have access to a good online learning algorithm $\mathcal{A}$ for the task on hand. Moreover, $\mathcal{A}$ is computationally efficient and easy to implement. However, the learning problem we face fits much more naturally within the batch learning setting. We would like to develop a batch algorithm $\mathcal{B}$ that exhibits the desirable characteristics of $\mathcal{A}$ but also has good generalization properties. A simple and powerful way to achieve this is to use an *online-to-batch conversion* technique. This is a general name for any technique which uses $\mathcal{A}$ as a building block in the construction of $\mathcal{B}$. Several different online-to-batch conversion techniques have been developed over the years. Littlestone and Warmuth [11] introduced an explicit relation between compression and learnability, which immediately lent itself to a conversion technique for classification algorithms. Gallant [7] presented the *Pocket algorithm*, a conversion of Rosenblatt's online *Perceptron* to the batch setting. Littlestone [10] presented the *Cross-Validation* conversion which was further developed by Cesa-Bianchi, Conconi and Gentile [2]. All of these techniques begin by presenting the training set $(\mathbf{x}_1, y_1), \ldots, (\mathbf{x}_m, y_m)$ to $\mathcal{A}$ in some arbitrary order. As $\mathcal{A}$ performs the m online rounds, it generates a sequence of online hypotheses which it uses to make predictions on each round. This sequence includes the default hypothesis h_0 and the m hypotheses $h_1, \ldots, h_m$ generated by the update rule. The aforementioned techniques all share a common property: they all choose h, the output of the batch algorithm $\mathcal{B}$, to be one of the online hypotheses $h_0, \ldots, h_m$.

In this paper, we focus on a second family of conversions, which evolved somewhat later and is due to the work of Helmbold and Warmuth [8], Freund and Schapire [6] and Cesa-Bianchi, Conconi and Gentile [2]. The conversion strategies in this family also begin by using $\mathcal{A}$ to generate the sequence of online hypotheses. However, instead of relying on a single hypothesis from the sequence, they set h to be some combination of the entire sequence. Another characteristic shared by these three conversions is that the training data does not play a part in determining how the online hypotheses are combined. That is, the training data is not used in any way other than to generate the sequence $h_0, \ldots, h_m$. In this sense, these conversion techniques are *data-independent*. In this paper, we build on the foundations of these data-independent conversions, and define conversion techniques that explicitly use the training data to derive the batch algorithm from the online algorithm. By doing so, we effectively define the *data-driven* counterparts of the algorithms in [8, 6, 2].

This paper is organized as follows. In Sec. 2 we review the data-independent conversion techniques from [8, 6, 2] and give a simple unified analysis for all three conversions. At the same time, we present a general framework which serves as a building-block for our data-driven conversions. Then, in Sec. 3, we derive three special cases of the general framework and demonstrate some useful properties of the data-driven conversions. Finally, in Sec. 4, we compare the different conversion techniques on several benchmark datasets and show that our data-driven approach outperforms the existing data-independent approach.

2 Voting, Averaging, and Sampling

The first conversion we discuss is the *voting* conversion [6], which applies to problems where the target space $\mathcal{Y}$ is discrete (and relatively small), such as classification problems. The conversion presents the training set $(\mathbf{x}_1, y_1), \ldots, (\mathbf{x}_m, y_m)$ to the online algorithm $\mathcal{A}$, which generates the sequence of online hypotheses, $h_0, \ldots, h_m$. The conversion then outputs the hypothesis h^{V}, which is defined as follows: given an input $\mathbf{x} \in \mathcal{X}$, each online hypothesis casts a vote of $h_i(\mathbf{x})$ and then h^{V} outputs the target value that receives the highest number of votes. For simplicity, assume that ties are broken arbitrarily. The second conversion is the *averaging* conversion [2] which applies to problems where $\mathcal{Y}$ is a convex set. For example, this conversion is applicable to margin-based online classifiers or to regression problems where, in both cases, $\mathcal{Y} = \mathbb{R}$. This conversion also begins by using $\mathcal{A}$ to generate $h_0, \ldots, h_m$. Then the batch hypothesis h^{A} is defined to be $\frac{1}{m+1} \sum_{i=0}^{m} h_i(\mathbf{x})$. The third and last conversion discussed here is the *sampling* conversion [8]. This conversion is the most general and applicable to any learning problem, however this generality comes at a price. The resulting hypothesis, h^{S}, is a stochastic function and not a deterministic one. In other words, if applied twice to the same instance, h^{S} may output different target values. Again, this conversion begins by applying $\mathcal{A}$ to the training set and obtaining the sequence of online hypotheses. Every time h^{S} is evaluated, it randomly selects one of $h_0, \ldots, h_m$ and uses it to make the prediction. Since h^{S} is a stochastic function, the definition of $\mathrm{Risk}_{\mathcal{D}}(h^{\mathrm{S}})$ changes slightly and expectation in Eq. (1) is taken also over the random function h^{S}.

Simple data-dependent bounds on the risk of h^{V}, h^{A} and h^{S} can be derived, and these bounds are special cases of the more general analysis given below. We now describe a simple generalization of these three conversion techniques. It is reasonable to assume that some of the online hypotheses generated by $\mathcal{A}$ are better than others. For instance, the default hypothesis h_0 is determined without observing even a single training example. This surfaces the question whether it is possible to isolate the "best" online hypotheses and only use them to define the batch hypothesis. Formally, let $[m]$ denote the set $\{0, \ldots, m\}$ and let I be some non-empty subset of $[m]$. Now define $h_I^{\mathrm{V}}(\mathbf{x})$ to be the hypothesis which performs voting as described above, with the single difference that only the members of $\{h_i : i \in I\}$ participate in the vote. Similarly, define $h_I^{\mathrm{A}}(\mathbf{x}) = (1/|I|) \sum_{i \in I} h_i(\mathbf{x})$, and let h_I^{S} be the stochastic function that randomly chooses a function from the set $\{h_i : i \in I\}$ every time it is evaluated, and predicts according to it. The data-independent conversions presented in the beginning of this section are obtained by setting $I = [m]$. Our idea is to use the training data to find a set I which induces the batch hypotheses h_I^{V}, h_I^{A}, and h_I^{S} with the smallest risk.

Since there is an exponential number of potential subsets of $[m]$, we need to restrict ourselves to a smaller set of candidate sets. Formally, let $\mathcal{I}$ be a family of subsets of $[m]$, and we restrict our search for I to the family $\mathcal{I}$. Following in the footsteps of [2], we make the simplifying assumption that none of the sets in $\mathcal{I}$ include the largest index m. This is a technical assumption which can be relaxed at the price of a slightly less elegant analysis. We use two intuitive concepts to guide our search for I. First, for any set $J \subseteq [m-1]$, define $L(J) = (1/|J|) \sum_{j \in J} \ell(y_{j+1}, h_j(\mathbf{x}_{j+1}))$. $L(J)$ is the empirical evaluation of the loss of the hypotheses indexed by J. We would like to find a set J for which $L(J)$ is small since we expect that good empirical loss of the online hypotheses indicates a low risk of the batch hypothesis. Second, we would like $|J|$ to be large so that the presence of a few bad online hypotheses in J will not have a devastating effect on the performance of the batch hypothesis. The trade-off between these two competing concepts can be formalized as follows. Let C be a non-negative constant and define,

$$\beta(J) \;=\; L(J) + C\,|J|^{-\frac{1}{2}} \;. \tag{2}$$

The function β decreases as the average empirical loss $L(J)$ decreases, and also as $|J|$ increases. It therefore captures the intuition described above. The function β serves as our yardstick when evaluating the candidates in $\mathcal{I}$. Specifically, we set $I \;=\; \arg\min_{J \in \mathcal{I}} \beta(J)$. Below we formally justify our choice of β, and specifically show that $\beta(J)$ is a rather tight upper bound on the risk of h_J^A, h_J^V and h_J^S. The first lemma relates the risk of these functions with the average risk of the hypotheses indexed by J.

Lemma 1. *Let* $(\mathbf{x}_1, y_1), \ldots, (\mathbf{x}_m, y_m)$ *be a sequence of examples which is presented to the online algorithm* $\mathcal{A}$ *and let* $h_0, \ldots, h_m$ *be the resulting sequence of online hypotheses. Let* J *be a non-empty subset of* $[m-1]$ *and let* $\ell : \mathcal{Y} \times \mathcal{Y} \to \mathbb{R}_+$ *be a loss function.* **(1)** *If* ℓ *is the 0-1 loss then* $\mathrm{Risk}_{\mathcal{D}}(h_J^V) \leq (2/|J|) \sum_{i \in J} \mathrm{Risk}_{\mathcal{D}}(h_i(\mathbf{x}))$. **(2)** *If* ℓ *is convex in its second argument then* $\mathrm{Risk}_{\mathcal{D}}(h_J^A) \leq (1/|J|) \sum_{i \in J} \mathrm{Risk}_{\mathcal{D}}(h_i(\mathbf{x}))$. **(3)** *For any loss function* ℓ *it holds that* $\mathrm{Risk}_{\mathcal{D}}(h_J^S) = (1/|J|) \sum_{i \in J} \mathrm{Risk}_{\mathcal{D}}(h_i(\mathbf{x}))$.

Proof. Beginning with the voting conversion, recall that the loss function being used is the 0-1 loss, namely there is a single correct prediction which incurs a loss of 0 and every other prediction incurs a loss of 1. For any example $(\mathbf{x}, y)$, if more than half of the hypotheses in $\{h_i\}_{i \in J}$ predict the correct outcome then clearly h_J^V also predicts this outcome and $\ell(y, h_J^V(\mathbf{x})) = 0$. Therefore, if $\ell(y, h_J^V(\mathbf{x})) = 1$ then at least half of the hypotheses in $\{h_i\}_{i \in J}$ make incorrect predictions and $(|J|/2) \leq \sum_{i \in J} \ell(y, h_i(\mathbf{x}))$. We therefore get,

$$\ell(y, h_J^V(\mathbf{x})) \;\leq\; \frac{2}{|J|} \sum_{i \in J} \ell(y, h_i(\mathbf{x})) \;.$$

The above holds for any example $(\mathbf{x}, y)$ and therefore also holds after taking expectations on both sides of the inequality. The bound now follows from the linearity of expectation and the definition of the risk function in Eq. (1).

Moving on to the second claim of the lemma, we assume that ℓ is convex in its second argument. The claim now follows from a direct application of Jensen's inequality.

Finally, h_J^S chooses its outcome by randomly choosing an hypothesis in $\{h_i : i \in J\}$, where the probability of choosing each hypothesis in this set equals $(1/|J|)$. Therefore, the expected loss suffered by h_J^S on an example $(\mathbf{x}, y)$ is $(1/|J|) \sum_{i \in J} \ell(y, h_i(\mathbf{x}))$. The risk of h_J^S is simply the expected value of this term with respect to the random selection of $(\mathbf{x}, y)$. Again using the linearity of expectation, we obtain the third claim of the lemma. $\quad\square$

The next lemma relates the average risk of the hypotheses indexed by J with the empirical performance of these hypotheses, $L(J)$. In the following lemma, we use capital letters to emphasize that we are dealing with random variables.

Lemma 2. *Let* $(X_1, Y_1), \ldots, (X_m, Y_m)$ *be a sequence of examples independently sampled according to* $\mathcal{D}$. *Let,* $H_0, \ldots, H_m$ *be the sequence of online hypotheses generated by* $\mathcal{A}$ *while observing this sequence of examples. Assume that the loss function* ℓ *is upper-bounded by* R. *Then for any* $J \subseteq [m-1]$,

$$\Pr\left[\frac{1}{|J|} \sum_{i \in J} \mathrm{Risk}_{\mathcal{D}}(H_i) > \beta(J)\right] < \exp\left(-\frac{C^2}{2R^2}\right) \;,$$

where C *is the constant used in the definition of* β *(Eq. (2)).*

The proof of this lemma is a direct application of Azuma's bound on the concentration of Lipschitz martingales [1], and is identical to that of Proposition 1 in [2]. For concreteness,

270

we now focus on the averaging conversion and note that the analyses of the other two conversion strategies are virtually identical. By combining the first claim of Lemma 1 with Lemma 2, we get that for any $J \in \mathcal{I}$ it holds that $\mathrm{Risk}_{\mathcal{D}}(h_J^A) \leq \beta(J)$ with probability at least $1 - \exp\left(-C^2/(2R^2)\right)$. Using the union bound, $\mathrm{Risk}_{\mathcal{D}}(h_J^A) \leq \beta(J)$ for all $J \in \mathcal{I}$ simultaneously with probability at least,

$$1 - |\mathcal{I}| \exp\left(-\frac{C^2}{2R^2}\right) \ .$$

The greater the value of C, the more β is influenced by the term $|J|$. On the other hand, a large value of C increases the probability that β indeed upper bounds $\mathrm{Risk}_{\mathcal{D}}(h_J^A)$ for all $J \in \mathcal{I}$. In conclusion, we have theoretically justified our choice of β in Eq. (2).

3 Concrete Data-Driven Conversions

In this section we build on the ideas of the previous section and derive three concrete data-driven conversion techniques.

Suffix Conversion: An intuitive argument against selecting $I = [m]$, as done by the data-independent conversions, is that many online algorithms tend to generate bad hypotheses during the first few rounds of learning. As previously noted, the default hypothesis h_0 is determined without observing any training data, and we should expect the first few online hypotheses to be inferior to those that are generated further along. This argument motivates us to consider subsets J of the form $\{a, a+1, \ldots, m-1\}$, where a is a positive integer less than or equal to $m-1$. Li [9] proposed this idea in the context of the voting conversion and gave a heuristic criterion for choosing a. Our formal setting gives a different criterion for choosing a. In this conversion we define $\mathcal{I}$ to be the set of all suffixes of $[m-1]$. After the algorithm generates $h_0, \ldots, h_m$, we set I to be $I = \arg\min_{J \in \mathcal{I}} \beta(J)$.

Interval Conversion: Kernel-based hypotheses are functions that take the form, $h(\mathbf{x}) = \sum_{j=1}^{n} \alpha_j K(\mathbf{z}_j, \mathbf{x})$, where K is a Mercer kernel, $\mathbf{z}_1, \ldots, \mathbf{z}_n$ are instances, often referred to as *support patterns* and $\alpha_1, \ldots, \alpha_n$ are real weights. A variety of different batch algorithms produce kernel-based hypotheses, including the Support Vector Machine [12]. An important learning problem, which is currently addressed by only a handful of algorithms, is to learn a kernel-based hypothesis h which is defined by at most B support patterns. The parameter B is a predefined constant often referred to as the *budget* of support patterns. Naturally, kernel-based hypotheses which are represented by a few support patterns are memory efficient and faster to calculate. A similar problem arises in the online learning setting where the goal is to construct online algorithms where each online hypothesis h_i is a kernel-based function defined by at most B vectors. Several online algorithms have been proposed for this problem [4, 13, 5]. First note that the data-independent conversions, with $I = [m]$, are inadequate for this setting. Although each individual online hypothesis is defined by at most B vectors, h^A is defined by the union of these sets, which can be much larger than B.

To convert a budget-constrained online algorithm $\mathcal{A}$ into a budget-constrained batch algorithm, we make an additional assumption on the update strategy employed by $\mathcal{A}$. We assume that whenever $\mathcal{A}$ updates its online hypothesis, it adds a single new support pattern into the set used to represent the kernel hypothesis, and possibly removes some other pattern from this set. The algorithms in [4, 13, 5] all fall into this category. Therefore, if we choose I to be the set $\{a, a+1, \ldots, b\}$ for some integers $0 \leq a < b < m$, and $\mathcal{A}$ updates its hypothesis k times during rounds $a+1$ through b, then h_I^A is defined by at most $B+k$ support patterns. Concretely, define $\mathcal{I}$ to be the set of all non-empty intervals in $[m-1]$. With C set properly, $\beta(J)$ bounds $\mathrm{Risk}_{\mathcal{D}}(h_J^A)$ for every $J \in \mathcal{I}$ with high probability. Next,

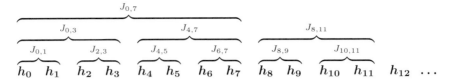

Figure 1: An illustration of the tree-based conversion.

generate $h_0, \ldots, h_m$ by running $\mathcal{A}$ with a budget parameter of $B/2$. Finally, choose I to be the set in $\mathcal{I}$ which contains at most $B/2$ updates and also minimizes the β function. By construction, the resulting hypothesis, h_I^A, is defined using at most B support patterns.

Tree-Based Conversion: A drawback of the suffix conversions is that it must be performed in two consecutive stages. First $h_0, \ldots, h_m$ are generated and stored in memory. Only then can we calculate $\beta(J)$ for every $J \in \mathcal{I}$ and perform the conversion. Therefore, the memory requirements of this conversions grow linearly with m. We now present a conversion that can sidestep this problem by interleaving the conversion with the online hypothesis generation. This conversion slightly deviates from the general framework described in the previous section: instead of predefining a set of candidates $\mathcal{I}$, we construct the optimal subset I in a recursive manner. As a consequence, the analysis in the previous section does not directly provide a generalization bound for this conversion. Assume for a moment that m is a power of 2. For all $0 \le a \le m - 1$ define $J_{a,a} = \{a\}$. Now, assume that we have already constructed the sets $J_{a,b}$ and $J_{c,d}$, where a, b, c, d are integers such that $a < d$, $b = (a + d - 1)/2$, and $c = b + 1$. Given these sets, define $J_{a,d}$ as follows:

$$J_{a,d} = \begin{cases} J_{a,b} & \text{if } \beta(J_{a,b}) \le \beta(J_{c,d}) \ \wedge \ \beta(J_{a,b}) \le \beta(J_{a,b} \cup J_{c,d}) \\ J_{c,d} & \text{if } \beta(J_{c,d}) \le \beta(J_{a,b}) \ \wedge \ \beta(J_{c,d}) \le \beta(J_{a,b} \cup J_{c,d}) \\ J_{a,b} \cup J_{c,d} & \text{otherwise} \end{cases} \quad . \tag{3}$$

Finally, define $I = J_{0,m-1}$ and output the batch hypothesis h_I^A. An illustration of this process is given in Fig. 1. Note that the definition of I requires only $m - 1$ recursive evaluations of Eq. (3). When m is not a power of 2, we can pad the sequence of online hypotheses with virtual hypotheses, each of which attains an infinite loss. This conversion can be performed in parallel with the online rounds since on round t we already have all of the information required to calculate $J_{a,b}$ for all $b < t$.

In the special case where the instances are vectors in $\mathbb{R}^n$, $h_0, \ldots, h_m$ are linear hypotheses and we use the averaging technique, the implementation of the tree-based conversion becomes memory efficient. Specifically, assume that each h_i takes the form $h_i(\mathbf{x}) = \mathbf{w}_i \cdot \mathbf{x}$ where $\mathbf{w}_i$ is a vector of weights in $\mathbb{R}^n$. In this case, storing an online hypothesis h_i is equivalent to storing its weight vector $\mathbf{w}_i$. For any $J \subseteq [m - 1]$, storing $\sum_{j \in J} h_j$ requires storing the single n-dimensional vector $\sum_{j \in J} \mathbf{w}_j$. Hence, once we calculate $J_{a,b}$ we can discard the original online hypotheses $h_a, \ldots, h_b$ and instead merely keep $h_{J_{a,b}}^\mathsf{A}$. Moreover, in order to calculate β we do not need to keep the set $J_{a,b}$ itself but rather the values $L(J_{a,b})$ and $|J_{a,b}|$. Overall, storing $h_{J_{a,b}}^\mathsf{A}$, $L(J_{a,b})$, and $|J_{a,b}|$ requires only a constant amount of memory. It can be verified using an inductive argument that the overall memory utilization of this conversion is $O(\log(m))$, which is significantly less than the $O(m)$ space required by the suffix conversion.

4 Experiments

We now turn to an empirical evaluation of the averaging and voting conversions. We chose multiclass classification as the underlying task and used the multiclass version of

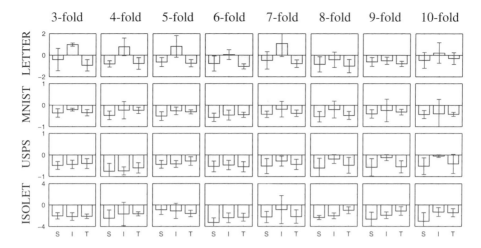

Figure 2: Comparison of the three data-driven averaging conversions with the data-independent averaging conversion, for different datasets (Y-axis) and different training-set sizes (X-axis). Each bar shows the difference between the error percentages of a data-driven conversion (*suffix* (S), *interval* (I) or *tree-based* (T)) and of the data-independent conversion. Error bars show standard deviation over the k folds.

the *Passive-Aggressive* (PA) algorithm [3] as the online algorithm. The PA algorithm is a kernel-based large-margin online classifier. To apply the voting conversion, $\mathcal{Y}$ should be a finite set. Indeed, in multiclass categorization problems the set $\mathcal{Y}$ consists of all possible labels. To apply the averaging conversion $\mathcal{Y}$ must be a convex set. To achieve this, we use the fact that PA associates a margin value with each class, and define $\mathcal{Y} = \mathbb{R}^s$ (where s is the number of classes).

In our experiments, we used the datasets LETTER, MNIST, USPS (training set only), and ISOLET. These datasets are of size 20000, 70000, 7291 and 7797 respectively. MNIST and USPS both contain images of handwritten digits and thus induce 10-class problems. The other datasets contain images (LETTER) and utterances (ISOLET) of the English alphabet. We did not use the standard splits into training set and test set and instead performed cross-validation in all of our experiments. For various values of k, we split each dataset into k parts, trained each algorithm using each of these parts and tested on the $k - 1$ remaining parts. Specifically, we ran this experiment for $k = 3, \ldots, 10$. The reason for doing this is that the experiment is most interesting when the training sets are small and the learning task becomes difficult.

We applied the data-independent averaging and voting conversions, as well as the three data-driven variants of these conversions (6 data-driven conversions in all). The interval conversion was set to choose an interval containing 500 updates. The parameter C was arbitrarily set to 3. Additionally, we evaluated the test error of the last hypothesis generated by the online algorithm, h_m. It is common malpractice amongst practitioners to use h_m as if it were a batch hypothesis, instead of using an online-to-batch conversion. As a byproduct of our experiments, we show that h_m performs significantly worse than any of the conversion techniques discussed in this paper. The kernel used in all of the experiments is the Gaussian kernel with default kernel parameters. We would like to emphasize that our goal was not to achieve state-of-the-art results on these datasets but rather to compare the different conversion strategies on the same sequence of hypotheses. To achieve the best results, one would have to tune C and the various kernel parameters.

The results for the different variants of the averaging conversion are depicted in Fig. 2.

	last	average	average-sfx	voting	voting-sfx
LETTER 5-fold	29.9 ± 1.8	21.2 ± 0.5	$\mathbf{20.5 \pm 0.6}$	23.4 ± 0.8	21.5 ± 0.8
LETTER 10-fold	37.3 ± 2.1	26.9 ± 0.7	$\mathbf{26.5 \pm 0.6}$	30.2 ± 1.0	27.9 ± 0.6
MNIST 5-fold	7.2 ± 0.5	5.9 ± 0.4	$\mathbf{5.3 \pm 0.6}$	7.0 ± 0.5	6.5 ± 0.5
MNIST 10-fold	13.8 ± 2.3	9.5 ± 0.8	9.1 ± 0.8	8.7 ± 0.5	$\mathbf{8.0 \pm 0.5}$
USPS 5-fold	9.7 ± 1.0	7.5 ± 0.4	$\mathbf{7.1 \pm 0.4}$	9.4 ± 0.4	8.8 ± 0.3
USPS 10-fold	12.7 ± 4.7	10.1 ± 0.7	$\mathbf{9.5 \pm 0.8}$	12.5 ± 1.0	11.3 ± 0.6
ISOLET 5-fold	20.1 ± 3.8	17.6 ± 4.1	$\mathbf{16.7 \pm 3.3}$	20.6 ± 3.4	18.3 ± 3.9
ISOLET 10-fold	28.6 ± 3.6	25.8 ± 2.8	$\mathbf{22.7 \pm 3.3}$	29.3 ± 3.1	26.7 ± 4.0

Table 1: Percent of errors averaged over the k folds with standard deviation. Results are given for the last online hypothesis (h_m), the data-independent averaging and voting conversions, and their suffix variants. The lowest error on each row is shown in bold.

For each dataset and each training-set size, we present a bar-plot which represents by how much each of the data-driven averaging conversions improves over the data-independent averaging conversion. For instance, the left bar in each plot shows the difference between the test errors of the suffix conversion and the data-independent conversion. A negative value means that the data-driven technique outperforms the data-independent one. The results clearly indicate that the suffix and tree-based conversions consistently improve over the data-independent conversion. The interval conversion does not improve as much and occasionally even looses to the data-independent conversion. However, this is a small price to pay in situations where it is important to generate a compact kernel-based hypothesis. Due to the lack of space, we omit a similar figure for the voting conversion and merely note that the plots are very similar to the ones in Fig. 2.

In Table 1 we give some concrete values of test error, and compare data-independent and data-driven versions of averaging and voting, using the suffix conversion. As a reference, we also give the results obtained by the last hypothesis generated by the online algorithm. In all of the experiments, the data-driven conversion outperforms the data-independent conversion. In general, averaging exhibits better results than voting, while the last online hypothesis is almost always inferior to all of the online-to-batch conversions.

References

[1] K. Azuma. Weighted sums of certain dependent random variables. *Tohoku Mathematical Journal*, 68:357–367, 1967.

[2] N. Cesa-Bianchi, A. Conconi, and C.Gentile. On the generalization ability of on-line learning algorithms. *IEEE Transactions on Information Theory*, 2004.

[3] K. Crammer, O. Dekel, J. Keshet, S. Shalev-Shwartz, and Y. Singer. Online passive aggressive algorithms. *Journal of Machine Learning Research*, 2006.

[4] K. Crammer, J. Kandola, and Y. Singer. Online classification on a budget. *NIPS 16*, 2003.

[5] O. Dekel, S. Shalev-Shwartz, and Y. Singer. The Forgetron: A kernel-based perceptron on a fixed budget. *NIPS 18*, 2005.

[6] Y. Freund and R. E. Schapire. Large margin classification using the perceptron algorithm. *Machine Learning*, 37(3):277–296, 1999.

[7] S. I. Gallant. Optimal linear discriminants. *ICPR 8*, pages 849–852. IEEE, 1986.

[8] D. P. Helmbold and M. K. Warmuth. On weak learning. *Journal of Computer and System Sciences*, 50:551–573, 1995.

[9] Y. Li. Selective voting for perceptron-like on-line learning. In *ICML 17*, 2000.

[10] N. Littlestone. From on-line to batch learning. *COLT 2*, pages 269–284, July 1989.

[11] N. Littlestone and M. Warmuth. Relating data compression and learnability. Unpublished manuscript, November 1986.

[12] V. N. Vapnik. *Statistical Learning Theory*. Wiley, 1998.

[13] J. Weston, A. Bordes, and L. Bottou. Online (and offline) on a tighter budget. *AISTAT 10*, 2005.

Beyond Gaussian Processes: On the Distributions of Infinite Networks

Ricky Der
Department of Mathematics
University of Pennsylvania
Philadelphia, PA 19104
rickyder@math.upenn.edu

Daniel Lee
Department of Electrical Engineering
University of Pennsylvania
Philadelphia, PA 19104
ddlee@seas.upenn.edu

Abstract

A general analysis of the limiting distribution of neural network functions is performed, with emphasis on non-Gaussian limits. We show that with i.i.d. symmetric stable output weights, and more generally with weights distributed from the normal domain of attraction of a stable variable, that the neural functions converge in distribution to stable processes. Conditions are also investigated under which Gaussian limits do occur when the weights are independent but not identically distributed. Some particularly tractable classes of stable distributions are examined, and the possibility of learning with such processes.

1 Introduction

Consider the model

$$f_n(x) = \frac{1}{s_n} \sum_{j=1}^{n} v_j h(x; u_j) \equiv \frac{1}{s_n} \sum_{j=1}^{n} v_j h_j(x) \tag{1}$$

which can be viewed as a multi-layer perceptron with input x, hidden functions h, weights u_j, output weights v_j, and s_n a sequence of normalizing constants. The work of Radford Neal [1] showed that, under certain assumptions on the parameter priors $\{v_j, h_j\}$, the distribution over the implied network functions f_n converged to that of a Gaussian process, in the large network limit $n \to \infty$. The main feature of this derivation consisted of an invocation of the classical Central Limit Theorem (CLT).

While one cavalierly speaks of "the" central limit theorem, there are in actuality many different CLTs, of varying generality and effect. All are concerned with the limits of suitably normalised sums of independent random variables (or where some condition is imposed so that no one variable dominates the sum[1]), but the limits themselves differ greatly: Gaussian, stable, infinitely divisible, or, discarding the infinitesimal assumption, none of these. It follows that in general, the asymptotic process for (1) may not be Gaussian. The following questions then arise: what is the relationship between choices of distributions on the model priors, and the asymptotic distribution over the induced neural functions? Under what conditions does the Gaussian approximation hold? If there do exist non-Gaussian limit points, is it possible to construct analogous generalizations of Gaussian process regression?

---

[1] Typically called an *infinitesimal* condition — see [4].

Previous work on these problems consists mainly in Neal's publication [1], which established that when the output weights v_j are *finite variance* and *i.i.d.*, the limiting distribution is a Gaussian process. Additionally, it was shown that when the weights are i.i.d. symmetric stable (SS), the first-order marginal distributions of the functions are also SS. Unfortunately, no mathematical analysis was presented to show that the higher-order distributions converged, though empirical evidence was suggestive of that hypothesis. Moreover, the exact form of the higher-dimensional distributions remained elusive.

This paper conducts a further investigation of these questions, with concentration on the cases where the weight priors can be 1) of infinite variance, and 2) non-i.i.d. Such assumptions fall outside the ambit of the classical CLT, but are amenable to more general limit methods. In Section 1, we give a general classification of the possible limiting processes that may arise under an i.i.d. assumption on output weights distributed from a certain class — roughly speaking, those weights with tails asymptotic to a power-law — and provide explicit formulae for all the joint distribution functions. As a byproduct, Neal's preliminary analysis is completed, a full multivariate prescription attained and the convergence of the finite-dimensional distributions proved. The subsequent section considers non-i.i.d. priors, specifically independent priors where the "identically distributed" assumption is discarded. An example where a finite-variance non-Gaussian process acts as a limit point for a nontrivial infinite network is presented, followed by an investigation of conditions under which the Gaussian approximation is valid, via the Lindeberg-Feller theorem. Finally, we raise the possibility of replacing network models with the processes themselves for learning applications: here, motivated by the foregoing limit theorems, the set of stable processes form a natural generalization to the Gaussian case. Classes of stable stochastic processes are examined where the parameterizations are particularly simple, as well as preliminary applications to the nonlinear regression problem.

2 Neural Network Limits

Referring to (1), we make the following assumptions: $h_j(x) \equiv h(x; u_j)$ are uniformly bounded in x (as for instance occurs if h is associated with some fixed nonlinearity), and $\{u_j\}$ is an i.i.d. sequence, so that $h_j(x)$ are i.i.d. for fixed x, and independent of $\{v_j\}$. With these assumptions, the choice of output priors v_j will tend to dictate large-network behavior, independently of u_j. In the sequel, we restrict ourselves to functions $f_n(x) : \mathbb{R} \to \mathbb{R}$, as the respective proofs for the generalizations of x and f_n to higher-dimensional spaces are routine. Finally, all random variables are assumed to be of zero mean whenever first moments exist. For brevity, we only present sketches of proofs.

2.1 Limits with i.i.d. priors

The Gaussian distribution has the feature that if X_1 and X_2 are statistically independent copies of the Gaussian variable X, then their linear combination is also Gaussian, i.e. $aX_1 + bX_2$ has the same distribution as $cX + d$ for some c and d. More generally, the *stable* distributions [5], [6, Chap. 17] are defined to be the set of all distributions satisfying the above "closure" property. If one further demands symmetry of the distribution, then they must have characteristic function $\Phi(t) = e^{-\sigma^\alpha |t|^\alpha}$, for parameters $\sigma > 0$ (called the spread), and $0 < \alpha \leq 2$, termed the index. Since the characteristic functions are not generally twice differentiable at $t = 0$, their variances are infinite, the Gaussian distribution being the only finite variance stable distribution, associated to index $\alpha = 2$.

The attractive feature of stable variables, by definition, is closure under the formation of linear combinations: the linear combination of any two independent stable variables is another stable variable of the same index. Moreover, the stable distributions are attraction points of distributions under a linear combiner operator, and indeed, the only such distributions in the following sense: if $\{Y_j\}$ are i.i.d., and $a_n + \frac{1}{s_n}\sum_{j=1}^{n} Y_j$ converges in distribution to X, then X must be stable [5]. This fact already has consequences for our network model (1), and implies that — under i.i.d. priors v_j, and assuming (1) converges at all — convergence can occur only to stable variables, for each x.

Multivariate analogues are defined similarly: we say a random vector $\mathbf{X}$ is (strictly) stable if, for every $a, b \in \mathbb{R}$, there exists a constant c such that $a\mathbf{X}_1 + b\mathbf{X}_2 = c\mathbf{X}$ where $\mathbf{X}_i$ are independent copies of $\mathbf{X}$ and the equality is in distribution. A *symmetric* stable random vector is one which is stable and for which the distribution of $\mathbf{X}$ is the same as $-\mathbf{X}$. The following important classification theorem gives an explicit Fourier domain description of all multivariate symmetric stable distributions:

Theorem 1. Kuelbs [5]. $\mathbf{X}$ *is a symmetric α-stable vector if and only if it has characteristic function*

$$\Phi(\mathbf{t}) = \exp\left\{-\int_{S^{d-1}} |\langle \mathbf{t}, \mathbf{s}\rangle|^\alpha \, d\Gamma(\mathbf{s})\right\} \tag{2}$$

where Γ is a finite measure on the unit $(d-1)$-sphere S^{d-1}, and $0 < \alpha \le 2$.

Remark: (2) remains unchanged replacing Γ by the symmetrized measure $\tilde{\Gamma} = \frac{1}{2}(\Gamma(A) + \Gamma(-A))$, for all Borel sets A. In this case, the (unique) symmetrized measure $\tilde{\Gamma}$ is called the *spectral* measure of the stable random vector $\mathbf{X}$.

Finally, stable *processes* are defined as indexed sets of random variables whose finite-dimensional distributions are (multivariate) stable.

First we establish the following preliminary result.

Lemma 1. *Let v be a symmetric stable random variable of index $0 < \alpha \le 2$, and spread $\sigma > 0$. Let h be independent of v and $E|h|^\alpha < \infty$. If $y = hv$, and $\{y_i\}$ are i.i.d. copies of y, then $S_n = \frac{1}{n^{1/\alpha}}\sum_{i=1}^{n} y_i$ converges in distribution to an α-stable variable with characteristic function $\Phi(t) = \exp\{-|\sigma t|^\alpha E|h|^\alpha\}$.*

Proof. This follows by computing the characteristic function Φ_{S_n}, then using standard theorems in measure theory (e.g. [4]), to obtain $\lim_{n\to\infty} \log \Phi_{S_n}(t) = -|\sigma t|^\alpha E|h|^\alpha$. ∎

Now we can state the first network convergence theorem.

Proposition 1. *Let the network (1) have symmetric stable i.i.d. weights v_j of index $0 < \alpha \le 2$ and spread σ. Then $f_n(x) = \frac{1}{n^{1/\alpha}}\sum_{j=1}^{n} v_j h_j(x)$ converges in distribution to a symmetric α-stable process $f(x)$ as $n \to \infty$. The finite-dimensional stable distribution of $(f(x_1), \ldots, f(x_d))$, where $x_i \in \mathbb{R}$, has characteristic function:*

$$\Psi(\mathbf{t}) = \exp\left(-\sigma^\alpha E_{\mathbf{h}} |\langle \mathbf{t}, \mathbf{h}\rangle|^\alpha\right) \tag{3}$$

where $\mathbf{h} = (h(x_1), \ldots, h(x_d))$, and $h(x)$ is a random variable with the common distribution (across j) of $h_j(x)$. Moreover, if $\mathbf{h} = (h(x_1), \ldots, h(x_d))$ has joint probability density $p(\mathbf{h}) = p(r\mathbf{s})$, with $\mathbf{s}$ on the S^{d-1} sphere and r the radial component of h, then the finite measure Γ corresponding to the multivariate stable distribution of $(f(x_1), \ldots, f(x_d))$ is given by

$$d\Gamma(\mathbf{s}) = \left(\int_0^\infty r^{\alpha+d-1} p(r\mathbf{s}) \, dr\right) d\mathbf{s} \tag{4}$$

where $d\mathbf{s}$ is Lebesgue measure on S^{d-1}.

Proof. It suffices to show that every finite-dimensional distribution of $f(x)$ converges to a symmetric multivariate stable characteristic function. We have $\sum_{i=1}^{d} t_i f_n(x_i) =$

$\frac{1}{n^{1/\alpha}} \sum_{j=1}^{n} v_j \sum_{i=1}^{d} t_i h_j(x_i)$ for constants $\{x_1, \ldots, x_d\}$ and $(t_1, \ldots, t_d) \in \mathbb{R}^d$. An application of Lemma 1 proves the statement. The relation between the expectation in (3) and the stable spectral measure (4) is derived from a change of variable to spherical coordinates in the d-dimensional space of $\mathbf{h}$. $\blacksquare$

Remark: When $\alpha = 2$, the exponent in the characteristic function (3) is a quadratic form in $\mathbf{t}$, and becomes the usual Gaussian multivariate distribution.

The above proposition is the rigorous completion of Neal's analysis, and gives the explicit form of the asymptotic process under i.i.d. SS weights. More generally, we can consider output weights from the *normal domain of attraction of index* α, which, roughly, consists of those densities whose tails are asymptotic to $|x|^{-(\alpha+1)}$, $0 < \alpha < 2$ [6, pg. 547]. With a similar proof to the previous theorem, one establishes

Proposition 2. *Let network (1) have i.i.d. weights v_j from the normal domain of attraction of an SS variable with index α, spread σ. Then $f_n(x) = \frac{1}{n^{1/\alpha}} \sum_{j=1}^{n} v_j h_j(x)$ converges in distribution to a symmetric α-stable process $f(x)$, with the joint characteristic functions given as in Proposition 1.*

2.1.1 Example: Distributions with step-function priors

Let $h(x) = \text{sgn}(a + ux)$, where a and u are independent Gaussians with zero mean. From (3) it is clear that the limiting network function $f(x)$ is a constant (in law, hence almost surely), as $|x| \to \infty$, so that the interesting behavior occurs in some "central region" $|x| < k$. Neal in [1] has shown that when the output weights v_j are Gaussian, then the choice of the signum nonlinearity for h gives rise to local Brownian motion in the central regime.

There is a natural generalization of the Brownian process within the context of symmetric stable processes, called the *symmetric α-stable Lévy motion*. It is characterised by an indexed sequence $\{w_t : t \in \mathbb{R}\}$ satisfying i) $w_0 = 0$ almost surely, ii) independent increments, and iii) $w_t - w_s$ is distributed symmetric α-stable with spread $\sigma = |t - s|^{1/\alpha}$. As we shall now show, the choice of step-function nonlinearity for h and symmetric α-stable priors for v_j lead to locally Lévy stable motion, which provide a theoretical exposition for the empirical observations in [1].

Fix two nearby positions x and y, and select $\sigma = 1$ for notational simplicity. From (3) the random variable $f(x) - f(y)$ is symmetric stable with spread parameter $[E_\mathbf{h}|h(x) - h(y)|^\alpha]^{1/\alpha}$. For step inputs, $|h(x) - h(y)|$ is non-zero only when the step located at $-a/u$ falls between x and y. For small $|x - y|$ approximate the density of this event to be uniform, so that $[E_\mathbf{h}|h(x) - h(y)|^\alpha] \sim |x - y|$. Hence locally, the increment $f(x) - f(y)$ is a symmetric stable variable with spread proportional to $|x - y|^{1/\alpha}$, which is condition (iii) of Lévy motion. Next let us demonstrate that the increments are independent. Consider the vector $(f(x_1) - f(x_2), f(x_2) - f(x_3), \ldots, f(x_{n-1}) - f(x_n))$, where $x_1 < x_2 < \ldots < x_n$. Its joint characteristic function in the variables $t_1, \ldots, t_{n-1}$ can be calculated to be

$$\Phi(t_1, \ldots, t_{n-1}) = \exp\left(-E_\mathbf{h}|t_1(h(x_1) - h(x_2)) + \cdots + t_{n-1}(h(x_{n-1}) - h(x_n))|^\alpha\right) \tag{5}$$

The disjointness of the intervals (x_{i-1}, x_i) implies that the only events which have non-zero probability within the range $[x_1, x_n]$ are the events $|h(x_i) - h(x_{i-1})| = 2$ for some i, and zero for all other indices. Letting p_i denote the probabilities of those events, (5) reads

$$\Phi(t_1, \ldots, t_{n-1}) = \exp\left(-2^\alpha(p_1|t_1|^\alpha + \cdots + p_{n-1}|t_{n-1}|^\alpha)\right) \tag{6}$$

which describes a vector of independent α-stable random variables, as the characteristic function splits. Thus the limiting process has independent increments.

The differences between sample functions arising from Cauchy priors as opposed to Gaussian priors is evident from Fig. 1, which displays sample paths from Gaussian and

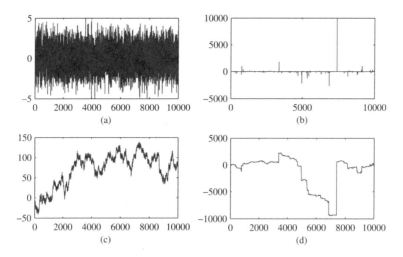

Figure 1: Sample functions: (a) i.i.d. Gaussian, (b) i.i.d. Cauchy, (c) Brownian motion, (d) Lévy Cauchy-Stable motion.

Cauchy i.i.d. processes w_n and their "integrated" versions $\sum_{i=1}^{n} w_i$, simulating the Lévy motions. The sudden jumps in the Cauchy motion arise from the presence of strong outliers in the respective Cauchy i.i.d. process, which would correspond, in the network, to hidden units with heavy weighting factors v_j.

2.2 Limits with non-i.i.d. priors

We begin with an interesting example, which shows that if the "identically distributed" assumption for the output weights is dispensed with, the limiting distribution of (1) can attain a non-stable (and non-Gaussian) form. Take v_j to be independent random variables with $P(v_j = 2^{-j}) = P(v_j = -2^{-j}) = 1/2$. The characteristic functions can easily be computed as $E[e^{itv_j}] = \cos(t/2^j)$. Now recall the Vieté formula:

$$\prod_{j=1}^{n} \cos(t/2^j) = \frac{\sin t}{2^n \sin(t/2^n)} \tag{7}$$

Taking $n \to \infty$ shows that the limiting characteristic function is a sinc function, which corresponds with the uniform density. Selecting the signum nonlinearity for h, it is not difficult to show with estimates on the tail of the product (7) that all finite-dimensional distributions of the neural process $f_n(x) = \sum_{j=1}^{n} v_j h_j(x)$ converge, so that f_n converges in distribution to a random process whose first-order distributions are uniform[2].

What conditions are required on independent, but not necessarily identically distributed priors v_j for convergence to the Gaussian? This question is answered by the classical Lindeberg-Feller theorem.

Theorem 2. Central Limit Theorem (Lindeberg-Feller) [4]. *Let v_j be a sequence of independent random variables each with zero mean and finite variance, define $s_n^2 = var[\sum_{j=1}^{n} v_j]$, and assume $s_1 \neq 0$. Then the sequence $\frac{1}{s_n}\sum_{j=1}^{n} v_j$ converges in distri-*

---

[2] An intuitive proof is as follows: one thinks of $\sum_j v_j$ as a binary expansion of real numbers in [-1,1]; the prescription of the probability laws for v_j imply all such expansions are equiprobable, manifesting in the uniform distribution.

bution to an $N(0, 1)$ variable, if

$$\lim_{n \to \infty} \frac{1}{s_n^2} \sum_{i=1}^{n} \int_{|v| \geq \epsilon s_n} v^2 \, dF_{v_j}(v) = 0 \tag{8}$$

for each $\epsilon > 0$, and where F_{v_j} is the distribution function for v_j.

Condition (8) is called the Lindeberg condition, and imposes an "infinitesimal" requirement on the sequence $\{v_j\}$ in the sense that no one variable is allowed to dominate the sum. This theorem can be used to establish the following non-i.i.d. network convergence result.

Proposition 3. *Let the network (1) have independent finite-variance weights v_j. Defining $s_n^2 = var[\sum_{j=1}^{n} v_j]$, if the sequence $\{v_j\}$ is Lindeberg then $f_n(x) = \frac{1}{s_n} \sum_{j=1}^{n} v_j h_j(x)$ converges in distribution to a Gaussian process $f(x)$ of mean zero and covariance function $C(f(x), f(y)) = E[h(x)h(y)]$ as $n \to \infty$, where $h(x)$ is a variable with the common distribution of the $h_j(x)$.*

Proof. Fix a finite set of points $\{x_1, \ldots, x_k\}$ in the input space, and look at the joint distribution $(f_n(x_1), \ldots, f_n(x_n))$. We want to show these variables are jointly Gaussian in the limit as $n \to \infty$, by showing that every linear combination of the components converges in distribution to a Gaussian distribution. Fixing k constants μ_i, we have $\sum_{i=1}^{k} \mu_i f(x_i) = \frac{1}{s_n} \sum_{j=1}^{n} v_j \sum_{i=1}^{k} \mu_i h_j(x_i)$. Define $\xi_j = \sum_{i=1}^{k} \mu_i h_j(x_i)$, and $\tilde{s}_n^2 = var(\sum_{j=1}^{n} v_j \xi_j) = (E\xi^2)s_n^2$, where ξ is a random variable with the common distribution of ξ_j. Then for some $c > 0$:

$$\frac{1}{\tilde{s}_n^2} \sum_{j=1}^{n} \int_{|v_j \xi_j| \geq \epsilon \tilde{s}_n} |v_j(\omega)\xi_j(\omega)|^2 \, dP(\omega) \leq \frac{c^2}{E\xi^2} \frac{1}{s_n^2} \sum_{j=1}^{n} \int_{|v_j| \geq \frac{(E\xi^2)^{1/2} s_n}{c}} |v_j(\omega)|^2 \, dP(\omega)$$

The right-hand side can be made arbitrarily small, from the Lindeberg assumption on $\{v_j\}$, hence $\{v_j \xi_j\}$ is Lindeberg, from which the theorem follows. The covariance function is easy to calculate. ∎

Corollary 1. *If the output weights $\{v_j\}$ are a uniformly bounded sequence of independent random variables, and $\lim_{n \to \infty} s_n = \infty$, then $f_n(x)$ in (1) converges in distribution to a Gaussian process.*

The preceding corollary, besides giving an easily verifiable condition for Gaussian limits, demonstrates that the non-Gaussian convergence in the example initialising Section 2.2 was made possible precisely because the weights v_j decayed sufficiently quickly with j, with the result that $\lim_n s_n < \infty$.

3   Learning with Stable Processes

One of the original reasons for focusing machine learning interest on Gaussian processes consisted in the fact that they act as limit points of suitably constructed parametric models [2], [3]. The problem of learning a regression function, which was previously tackled by Bayesian inference on a modelling neural network, could be reconsidered by directly placing a Gaussian process prior on the fitting functions themselves. Yet already in early papers introducing the technique, reservations had been expressed concerning such wholesale replacement [2]. Gaussian processes did not seem to capture the richness of finite neural networks — for one, the dependencies between multiple outputs of a network vanished in the Gaussian limit.

Consider the simplest regression problem, that of the estimation of a state process $u(x)$ from observations $y(x_i)$, under the model

$$y(x) = u(x) + \epsilon(x) \tag{9}$$

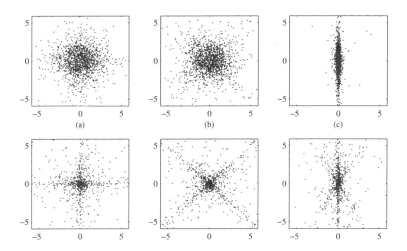

Figure 2: Scatter plots of bivariate symmetric α-stable distributions with discrete spectral measures. Top row: $\alpha = 1.5$; Bottom row: $\alpha = 0.5$. Left to right: (a) $\mathbf{H} = $ identity, (b) $\mathbf{H}$ a rotation, (c) $\mathbf{H}$ a 2×3 matrix with columns $(-1/16, \sqrt{3}/16)^T$, $(0,1)^T$, $(1/16, \sqrt{3}/16)^T$.

where $\epsilon(x)$ is noise independent of u. The obvious generalization of Gaussian process regression involves the placement of a stable process prior of index α on u, and setting ϵ as i.i.d. stable noise of the same index. Then the observations y also form a stable process of index α. Two advantages come with such generalization. First, the use of a heavy-tailed distribution for ϵ will tend to produce more robust regression estimates, relative to the Gaussian case; this robustness can be additionally controlled by the stability parameter α. Secondly, a glance at the classification of Theorem 1 indicates that the correlation structure of stable vectors (hence processes), is significantly richer than that of the Gaussian; the space of n-dimensional stable vectors is already characterised by a whole space of measures, rather than an $n \times n$ covariance matrix. The use of such priors on the data u afford a significant broadening in the number of interesting dependency relationships that may be assumed.

An understanding of the dependency structure of multivariate stable vectors can be first broached by considering the following basic class. Let $\mathbf{v}$ be a vector of i.i.d. symmetric stable variables of the same index, and let $\mathbf{H}$ be a matrix of appropriate dimension so that $\mathbf{x} = \mathbf{H}\mathbf{v}$ is well-defined. Then $\mathbf{x}$ has a symmetric stable characteristic function, where the spectral measure $\tilde{\Gamma}$ in Theorem 1 is *discrete*, i.e. concentrated on a finite number of points. Divergences in the correlation structure are readily apparent even within this class. In the Gaussian case, there is no advantage in the selection of non-square matrices $\mathbf{H}$, since the distribution of $\mathbf{x}$ can always be obtained by a square mixing matrix $\tilde{\mathbf{H}}$ with the same number of rows as $\mathbf{H}$. Not so when $\alpha < 2$, for then the characteristic function for $\mathbf{x}$ in general possesses n fundamental discontinuities in higher-order derivatives, where n is the number of columns of $\mathbf{H}$. Furthermore, in the square case, replacement of $\mathbf{H}$ with $\mathbf{HR}$, where $\mathbf{R}$ is any rotation matrix, leaves the distribution invariant when $\alpha = 2$; for non-Gaussian stable vectors, the mixing matrices $\mathbf{H}$ and $\mathbf{H}'$ give rise to the same distribution only when $|\mathbf{H}^{-1}\mathbf{H}'|$ is a permutation matrix, where $|\cdot|$ is defined component-wise. Figure 2 illustrates the variety of dependency structures which can be attained as $\mathbf{H}$ is changed. A number of techniques already exist in the statistical literature for the estimation of the spectral measure (and hence the mixing $\mathbf{H}$) of multivariate stable vectors from empirical data. The infinite-dimensional generalization of the above situation gives rise to the set of stable processes produced as time-varying filtered versions of i.i.d. stable noise, and similar to the Gaussian process, are parameterized by a centering (mean) function $\mu(x)$ and a bivariate filter function $h(x, \nu)$ encoding dependency information. Another simple family of stable processes consist of the so-called *sub-Gaussian processes*. These are processes defined by $u(x) = A^{1/2}G(x)$ where A is a totally right-skew $\alpha/2$ stable variable [5], and G a Gaussian process of mean zero and covariance K. The result is a symmetric α-stable random process with finite-dimensional characteristic functions of form

$$\Phi(\mathbf{t}) = \exp(-\frac{1}{2}|\langle \mathbf{t}, \mathbf{Kt} \rangle|^{\alpha/2}) \tag{10}$$

The sub-Gaussian processes are then completely parameterized by the statistics of the subordinating Gaussian process G. Even more, they have the following *linear* regression property [5]: if $Y_1, \ldots, Y_n$ are jointly sub-Gaussian, then

$$E[Y_n|Y_1, \ldots, Y_{n-1}] = a_1 Y_1 + \cdots a_{n-1} Y_{n-1}. \tag{11}$$

Unfortunately, the regression is somewhat trivial, because a calculation shows that the coefficients of regression $\{a_i\}$ are the *same* as the case where Y_i are assumed jointly Gaussian! Indeed, this curious property appears anytime the variables take the form $\mathbf{Y} = B\mathbf{G}$, for *any* fixed scalar random variable B and Gaussian vector $\mathbf{G}$. It follows that the predictive mean estimates for (10) employing sub-Gaussian priors are identical to the estimates under a Gaussian hypothesis. On the other hand, the conditional *distribution* of $Y_n|Y_1, \ldots, Y_{n-1}$ differs greatly from the Gaussian, and is neither stable nor symmetric about its conditional mean in general. From Fig. 2 one even sees that the conditional distribution may be multimodal, in which case the predictive mean estimates are not particularly valuable. More useful are MAP estimates, which in the Gaussian scenario coincide with the conditional mean. In any case, regression on stable processes suggest the need to compute and investigate the entire *a posteriori* probability law.

The main thrust of our foregoing results indicate that the class of possible limit points of network functions is significantly richer than the family of Gaussian processes, even under relatively restricted (e.g. i.i.d.) hypotheses. Gaussian processes are the appropriate models of large networks with finite variance priors in which no one component dominates another, but when the finite variance assumption is discarded, stable processes become the natural limit points. Non-stable processes can be obtained with the appropriate choice of non-i.i.d. parameters priors, even in an infinite network. Our discussion of the stable process regression problem has principally been confined to an exposition of the basic theoretical issues and principles involved, rather than to algorithmic procedures. Nevertheless, since simple closed-form expressions exist for the characteristic functions, the predictive probability laws can all in principle be computed with multi-dimensional Fourier transform techniques. Stable variables form mathematically natural generalisations of the Gaussian, with some fundamental, but compelling, differences which suggest additional variety and flexibility in learning applications.

References

[1] R. Neal, *Bayesian Learning for Neural Networks*. New York: Springer-Verlag, 1996.

[2] D. MacKay. *Introduction to Gaussian Processes*. Extended lecture notes, NIPS 1997.

[3] M. Seeger, *Gaussian Processes for Machine Learning*. International Journal of Neural Systems 14(2), 2004, 69–106.

[4] C. Burrill, *Measure, Integration and Probability*. New York: McGraw-Hill, 1972.

[5] G. Samorodnitsky & M. Taqqu, *Stable Non-Gaussian Random Processes*. New York: Chapman & Hall, 1994.

[6] W. Feller, *An Introduction to Probability Theory and Its Applications, Vol. 2*. New York: John Wiley & Sons, 1966.

Generalized Nonnegative Matrix Approximations with Bregman Divergences

Inderjit S. Dhillon   **Suvrit Sra**
Dept. of Computer Sciences
The Univ. of Texas at Austin
Austin, TX 78712.
{inderjit,suvrit}@cs.utexas.edu

Abstract

Nonnegative matrix approximation (NNMA) is a recent technique for dimensionality reduction and data analysis that yields a parts based, sparse nonnegative representation for nonnegative input data. NNMA has found a wide variety of applications, including text analysis, document clustering, face/image recognition, language modeling, speech processing and many others. Despite these numerous applications, the algorithmic development for computing the NNMA factors has been relatively deficient. This paper makes algorithmic progress by modeling and *solving* (using multiplicative updates) new generalized NNMA problems that minimize Bregman divergences between the input matrix and its low-rank approximation. The multiplicative update formulae in the pioneering work by Lee and Seung [11] arise as a special case of our algorithms. In addition, the paper shows how to use penalty functions for incorporating constraints other than nonnegativity into the problem. Further, some interesting extensions to the use of "link" functions for modeling nonlinear relationships are also discussed.

1 Introduction

Nonnegative matrix approximation (NNMA) is a method for dimensionality reduction and data analysis that has gained favor over the past few years. NNMA has previously been called *positive matrix factorization* [13] and *nonnegative matrix factorization*[1] [12]. Assume that $a_1, \ldots, a_N$ are N nonnegative input (M-dimensional) vectors. We organize these vectors as the columns of a nonnegative data matrix

$$A \triangleq \begin{bmatrix} a_1 & a_2 & \ldots & a_N \end{bmatrix}.$$

NNMA seeks a small set of K nonnegative representative vectors $b_1, \ldots, b_K$ that can be nonnegatively (or conically) combined to approximate the input vectors a_i. That is,

$$a_n \approx \sum_{k=1}^{K} c_{kn} b_k, \quad 1 \le n \le N,$$

---

[1] We use the word *approximation* instead of *factorization* to emphasize the inexactness of the process since, the input A is approximated by BC.

where the combining coefficients c_{kn} are restricted to be nonnegative. If c_{kn} and b_k are unrestricted, and we minimize $\sum_n \|a_n - Bc_n\|^2$, the Truncated Singular Value Decomposition (TSVD) of A yields the optimal b_k and c_{kn} values. If the b_k are unrestricted, but the coefficient vectors c_n are restricted to be indicator vectors, then we obtain the problem of hard-clustering (See [16, Chapter 8] for related discussion regarding different constraints on c_n and b_k).

In this paper we consider problems where all involved matrices are nonnegative. For many practical problems nonnegativity is a natural requirement. For example, color intensities, chemical concentrations, frequency counts etc., are all nonnegative entities, and approximating their measurements by nonnegative representations leads to greater interpretability. NNMA has found a significant number of applications, not only due to increased interpretability, but also because admitting only nonnegative combinations of the b_k leads to sparse representations.

This paper contributes to the algorithmic advancement of NNMA by generalizing the problem significantly, and by deriving efficient algorithms based on multiplicative updates for the generalized problems. The scope of this paper is primarily on generic methods for NNMA, rather than on specific applications. The multiplicative update formulae in the pioneering work by Lee and Seung [11] arise as a special case of our algorithms, which seek to minimize Bregman divergences between the nonnegative input A and its approximation. In addition, we discuss the use penalty functions for incorporating constraints other than nonnegativity into the problem. Further, we illustrate an interesting extension of our algorithms for handling non-linear relationships through the use of "link" functions.

2   Problems

Given a nonnegative matrix A as input, the classical NNMA problem is to approximate it by a lower rank nonnegative matrix of the form BC, where $B = [b_1, ..., b_K]$ and $C = [c_1, ..., c_N]$ are themselves nonnegative. That is, we seek the approximation,

$$A \approx BC, \qquad \text{where } B, C \geq 0. \tag{2.1}$$

We judge the goodness of the approximation in (2.1) by using a general class of distortion measures called *Bregman divergences*. For any strictly convex function $\varphi : S \subseteq \mathbb{R} \to \mathbb{R}$ that has a continuous first derivative, the corresponding **Bregman divergence** $D_\varphi : S \times \text{int}(S) \to \mathbb{R}_+$ is defined as $D_\varphi(x, y) \triangleq \varphi(x) - \varphi(y) - \nabla\varphi(y)(x - y)$, where $\text{int}(S)$ is the interior of set S [1, 2]. Bregman divergences are nonnegative, convex in the first argument and zero if and only if $x = y$. These divergences play an important role in convex optimization [2]. For the sequel we consider only separable Bregman divergences, i.e., $D_\varphi(X, Y) = \sum_{ij} D_\varphi(x_{ij}, y_{ij})$. We further require $x_{ij}, y_{ij} \in \text{dom}\varphi \cap \mathbb{R}_+$.

Formally, the resulting generalized nonnegative matrix approximation problems are:

$$\min_{B, C \geq 0} \quad D_\varphi(BC, A) + \alpha(B) + \beta(C), \tag{2.2}$$

$$\min_{B, C \geq 0} \quad D_\varphi(A, BC) + \alpha(B) + \beta(C). \tag{2.3}$$

The functions α and β serve as *penalty* functions, and they allow us to enforce regularization (or other constraints) on B and C. We consider both (2.2) and (2.3) since Bregman divergences are generally asymmetric. Table 1 gives a small sample of NNMA problems to illustrate the breadth of our formulation.

3   Algorithms

In this section we present algorithms that seek to optimize (2.2) and (2.3). Our algorithms are iterative in nature, and are directly inspired by the efficient algorithms of Lee and Seung [11]. Appealing properties include ease of implementation and computational efficiency.

Divergence D_φ	φ	α	β	Remarks
$\|A - BC\|_F^2$	$\frac{1}{2}x^2$	0	0	Lee and Seung [11, 12]
$\|A - BC\|_F^2$	$\frac{1}{2}x^2$	0	$\lambda 1^T C 1$	Hoyer [10]
$\|W \odot (A - BC)\|_F^2$	$\frac{1}{2}x^2$	0	0	Paatero and Tapper [13]
$\mathrm{KL}(A, BC)$	$x \log x$	0	0	Lee and Seung [11]
$\mathrm{KL}(A, WBC)$	$x \log x$	0	0	Guillamet et al. [9]
$\mathrm{KL}(A, BC)$	$x \log x$	$c 1 B^T B 1$	$-c' \|C\|_F^2$	Feng et al. [8]
$D_\varphi(A, W_1 B C W_2)$	$\varphi(x)$	$\alpha(B)$	$\beta(C)$	Weighted NNMA (new)

Table 1: Some example NNMA problems that may be obtained from (2.3). The corresponding asymmetric problem (2.2) has not been previously treated in the literature. $\mathrm{KL}(x, y)$
denotes the generalized KL-Divergence = $\sum_i x_i \log \frac{x_i}{y_i} - x_i + y_i$ (also called I-divergence).

Note that the problems (2.2) and (2.3) are not jointly convex in B and C, so it is not easy
to obtain globally optimal solutions in polynomial time. Our iterative procedures start by
initializing B and C randomly or otherwise. Then, B and C are alternately updated until
there is no further appreciable change in the objective function value.

3.1 Algorithms for (2.2)

We utilize the concept of auxiliary functions [11] for our derivations. It is sufficient to
illustrate our methods using a single column of C (or row of B), since our divergences are
separable.

Definition 3.1 (Auxiliary function). A function $G(c, c')$ is called an auxiliary function
for $F(c)$ if:

1. $G(c, c) = F(c)$, and

2. $G(c, c') \geq F(c)$ for all c'.

Auxiliary functions turn out to be useful due to the following lemma.

Lemma 3.2 (Iterative minimization). *If $G(c, c')$ is an auxiliary function for $F(c)$, then
F is non-increasing under the update*

$$c^{t+1} = \mathrm{argmin}_c \, G(c, c^t).$$

Proof. $F(c^{t+1}) \leq G(c^{t+1}, c^t) \leq G(c^t, c^t) = F(c^t).$ □

As can be observed, the sequence formed by the iterative application of Lemma 3.2 leads to
a monotonic decrease in the objective function value $F(c)$. For an algorithm that iteratively
updates c in its quest to minimize $F(c)$, the method for proving convergence boils down to
the construction of an appropriate auxiliary function. Auxiliary functions have been used
in many places before, see for example [5, 11].

We now construct simple auxiliary functions for (2.2) that yield multiplicative updates. To
avoid clutter we drop the functions α and β from (2.2), noting that our methods can easily
be extended to incorporate these functions.

Suppose B is fixed and we wish to compute an updated column of C. We wish to minimize

$$F(c) = D_\varphi(Bc, a), \qquad (3.1)$$

where a is the column of A corresponding to the column c of C. The lemma below shows
how to construct an auxiliary function for (3.1). For convenience of notation we use ψ to
denote $\nabla \varphi$ for the rest of this section.

Lemma 3.3 (Auxiliary function). *The function*

$$G(\boldsymbol{c}, \boldsymbol{c}') = \sum_{ij} \lambda_{ij} \varphi\left(\frac{b_{ij} c_j}{\lambda_{ij}}\right) - \left(\sum_i \varphi(a_i) + \psi(a_i)\big((\boldsymbol{Bc})_i - a_i\big)\right), \qquad (3.2)$$

with $\lambda_{ij} = (b_{ij} c'_j)/(\sum_l b_{il} c'_l)$, is an auxiliary function for (3.1). Note that by definition $\sum_j \lambda_{ij} = 1$, and as both b_{ij} and c'_j are nonnegative, $\lambda_{ij} \geq 0$.

Proof. It is easy to verify that $G(\boldsymbol{c}, \boldsymbol{c}) = F(\boldsymbol{c})$, since $\sum_j \lambda_{ij} = 1$. Using the convexity of φ, we conclude that if $\sum_j \lambda_{ij} = 1$ and $\lambda_{ij} \geq 0$, then

$$F(\boldsymbol{c}) = \sum_i \varphi\left(\sum_j b_{ij} c_j\right) - \varphi(a_i) - \psi(a_i)\big((\boldsymbol{Bc})_i - a_i\big)$$

$$\leq \sum_{ij} \lambda_{ij} \varphi\left(\frac{b_{ij} c_j}{\lambda_{ij}}\right) - \left(\sum_i \varphi(a_i) + \psi(a_i)\big((\boldsymbol{Bc})_i - a_i\big)\right)$$

$$= G(\boldsymbol{c}, \boldsymbol{c}'). \qquad \square$$

To obtain the update, we minimize $G(\boldsymbol{c}, \boldsymbol{c}')$ w.r.t. $\boldsymbol{c}$. Let $\psi(\boldsymbol{x})$ denote the vector $[\psi(x_1), \ldots, \psi(x_n)]^T$. We compute the partial derivative

$$\frac{\partial G}{\partial c_p} = \sum_i \lambda_{ip} \psi\left(\frac{b_{ip} c_p}{\lambda_{ip}}\right) \frac{b_{ip}}{\lambda_{ip}} - \sum_i b_{ip} \psi(a_i)$$

$$= \sum_i b_{ip} \psi\left(\frac{c_p}{c'_p}(\boldsymbol{Bc}')_i\right) - (\boldsymbol{B}^T \psi(\boldsymbol{a}))_p. \qquad (3.3)$$

We need to solve (3.3) for c_p by setting $\partial G/\partial c_p = 0$. Solving this equation analytically is not always possible. However, for a broad class of functions, we can obtain an analytic solution. For example, if ψ is multiplicative (i.e., $\psi(xy) = \psi(x)\psi(y)$) we obtain the following iterative update relations for $\boldsymbol{b}$ and $\boldsymbol{c}$ (see [7])

$$b_p \leftarrow b_p \cdot \psi^{-1}\left(\frac{[\psi(\boldsymbol{a}^T)\boldsymbol{C}^T]_p}{[\psi(\boldsymbol{b}^T \boldsymbol{C})\boldsymbol{C}^T]_p}\right), \qquad (3.4)$$

$$c_p \leftarrow c_p \cdot \psi^{-1}\left(\frac{[\boldsymbol{B}^T \psi(\boldsymbol{a})]_p}{[\boldsymbol{B}^T \psi(\boldsymbol{Bc})]_p}\right). \qquad (3.5)$$

It turns out that when φ is a convex function of Legendre type, then ψ^{-1} can be obtained by the derivative of the conjugate function φ^* of φ, i.e., $\psi^{-1} = \nabla\varphi^*$ [14].

Note. (3.4) & (3.5) coincide with updates derived by Lee and Seung [11], if $\varphi(x) = \frac{1}{2}x^2$.

3.1.1 Examples of New NNMA Problems

We illustrate the power of our generic auxiliary functions given above for deriving algorithms with multiplicative updates for some specific interesting problems.

First we consider the problem that seeks to minimize the divergence,

$$\mathrm{KL}(\boldsymbol{Bc}, \boldsymbol{a}) = \sum_i (\boldsymbol{Bc})_i \log \frac{(\boldsymbol{Bc})_i}{a_i} - (\boldsymbol{Bc})_i + a_i, \qquad \boldsymbol{B}, \boldsymbol{c} \geq 0. \qquad (3.6)$$

Let $\varphi(x) = x \log x - x$. Then, $\psi(x) = \log x$, and as $\psi(xy) = \psi(x) + \psi(y)$, upon substituting in (3.3), and setting the resultant to zero we obtain

$$\frac{\partial G}{\partial c_p} = \sum_i b_{ip} \log(c_p(\boldsymbol{Bc'})_i/c_p') - \sum_i b_{ip} \log a_i = 0,$$

$$\implies (\boldsymbol{B}^T \boldsymbol{1})_p \log \frac{c_p}{c_p'} = [\boldsymbol{B}^T \log \boldsymbol{a} - \boldsymbol{B}^T \log(\boldsymbol{Bc'})]_p$$

$$\implies c_p = c_p' \cdot \exp\left(\frac{[\boldsymbol{B}^T \log(\boldsymbol{a}/(\boldsymbol{Bc'}))]_p}{[\boldsymbol{B}^T \boldsymbol{1}]_p}\right).$$

The update for $\boldsymbol{b}$ can be derived similarly.

Constrained NNMA. Next we consider NNMA problems that have additional constraints. We illustrate our ideas on a problem with linear constraints.

$$\min_{\boldsymbol{x}} \quad D_\varphi(\boldsymbol{Bc}, \boldsymbol{a})$$
$$\text{s.t.} \quad \boldsymbol{Pc} \le \boldsymbol{0}, \quad \boldsymbol{c} \ge \boldsymbol{0}. \tag{3.7}$$

We can solve (3.7) problem using our method by making use of an appropriate (differentiable) penalty function that enforces $\boldsymbol{Pc} \le \boldsymbol{0}$. We consider,

$$F(\boldsymbol{c}) = D_\varphi(\boldsymbol{Bc}, \boldsymbol{a}) + \rho \|\max(0, \boldsymbol{Pc})\|^2, \tag{3.8}$$

where $\rho > 0$ is some penalty constant. Assuming multiplicative ψ and following the auxiliary function technique described above, we obtain the following updates for $\boldsymbol{c}$,

$$c_k \leftarrow c_k \cdot \psi^{-1}\left(\frac{[\boldsymbol{B}^T \psi(\boldsymbol{a})]_k - \rho[\boldsymbol{P}^T(\boldsymbol{Pc})^+]_k}{[\boldsymbol{B}^T \psi(\boldsymbol{Bc})]_k}\right),$$

where $(\boldsymbol{Pc})^+ = \max(0, \boldsymbol{Pc})$. Note that care must be taken to ensure that the addition of this penalty term does not violate the nonnegativity of $\boldsymbol{c}$, and to ensure that the argument of ψ^{-1} lies in its domain.

Remarks. Incorporating additional constraints into (3.6) is however easier, since the exponential updates ensure nonnegativity. Given $\boldsymbol{a} = \boldsymbol{1}$, with appropriate penalty functions, our solution to (3.6) can be utilized for maximizing entropy of $\boldsymbol{Bc}$ subject to linear or non-linear constraints on $\boldsymbol{c}$.

Nonlinear models with "link" functions. If $\boldsymbol{A} \approx h(\boldsymbol{BC})$, where h is a "link" function that models a nonlinear relationship between $\boldsymbol{A}$ and the approximant $\boldsymbol{BC}$, we may wish to minimize $D_\varphi(h(\boldsymbol{BC}), \boldsymbol{A})$. We can easily extend our methods to handle this case for appropriate h. Recall that the auxiliary function that we used, depended upon the convexity of φ. Thus, if $(\varphi \circ h)$ is a convex function, whose derivative $\nabla(\varphi \circ h)$ is "factorizable," then we can easily derive algorithms for this problem with link functions. We exclude explicit examples for lack of space and refer the reader to [7] for further details.

3.2 Algorithms using KKT conditions

We now derive efficient multiplicative update relations for (2.3), and these updates turn out to be simpler than those for (2.2). To avoid clutter, we describe our methods with $\alpha \equiv 0$, and $\beta \equiv 0$, noting that if α and β are differentiable, then it is easy to incorporate them in our derivations. For convenience we use $\zeta(x)$ to denote $\nabla^2(x)$ for the rest of this section.

Using matrix algebra, one can show that the gradients of $D_\varphi(\boldsymbol{A}, \boldsymbol{BC})$ w.r.t. $\boldsymbol{B}$ and $\boldsymbol{C}$ are,

$$\nabla_B D_\varphi(\boldsymbol{A}, \boldsymbol{BC}) = (\zeta(\boldsymbol{BC}) \odot (\boldsymbol{BC} - \boldsymbol{A}))\boldsymbol{C}^T$$
$$\nabla_C D_\varphi(\boldsymbol{A}, \boldsymbol{BC}) = \boldsymbol{B}^T(\zeta(\boldsymbol{BC}) \odot (\boldsymbol{BC} - \boldsymbol{A})),$$

where $\odot$ denotes the elementwise or Hadamard product, and ζ is applied elementwise to BC. According to the KKT conditions, there exist Lagrange multiplier matrices $\Lambda \geq 0$ and $\Omega \geq 0$ such that

$$\nabla_B D_\varphi(A, BC) = \Lambda, \qquad \nabla_C D_\varphi(A, BC) = \Omega, \qquad (3.9a)$$
$$\lambda_{mk} b_{mk} = \omega_{kn} c_{kn} = 0. \qquad (3.9b)$$

Writing out the gradient $\nabla_B D_\varphi(A, BC)$ elementwise, multiplying by b_{mk}, and making use of (3.9a,b), we obtain

$$\left[(\zeta(BC) \odot (BC - A))C^T\right]_{mk} b_{mk} = \lambda_{mk} b_{mk} = 0,$$

which suggests the iterative scheme

$$b_{mk} \leftarrow b_{mk} \frac{\left[(\zeta(BC) \odot A)C^T\right]_{mk}}{\left[(\zeta(BC) \odot BC)C^T\right]_{mk}}. \qquad (3.10)$$

Proceeding in a similar fashion we obtain a similar iterative formula for c_{kn}, which is

$$c_{kn} \leftarrow c_{kn} \frac{[B^T(\zeta(BC) \odot A)]_{kn}}{[B^T(\zeta(BC) \odot BC)]_{kn}}. \qquad (3.11)$$

3.2.1 Examples of New and Old NNMA Problems as Special Cases

We now illustrate the power of our approach by showing how one can easily obtain iterative update relations for many NNMA problems, including known and new problems. For more examples and further generalizations we refer the reader to [7].

Lee and Seung's Algorithms. Let $\alpha \equiv 0$, $\beta \equiv 0$. Now if we set $\varphi(x) = \frac{1}{2}x^2$ or $\varphi(x) = x \log x$, then (3.10) and (3.11) reduce to the Frobenius norm and KL-Divergence update rules originally derived by Lee and Seung [11].

Elementwise weighted distortion. Here we wish to minimize $\|W \odot (A - BC)\|_F^2$. Using $X \leftarrow \sqrt{W} \odot X$, and $A \leftarrow \sqrt{W} \odot A$ in (3.10) and (3.11) one obtains

$$B \leftarrow B \odot \frac{(W \odot A)C^T}{(W \odot (BC))C^T}, \qquad C \leftarrow C \odot \frac{B^T(W \odot A)}{B^T(W \odot (BC))}.$$

These iterative updates are significantly simpler than the PMF algorithms of [13].

The Multifactor NNMA Problem (new). The above ideas can be extended to the multi-factor NNMA problem that seeks to minimize the following divergence (see [7])

$$D_\varphi(A, B_1 B_2 \ldots B_R),$$

where all matrices involved are nonnegative. A typical usage of multifactor NNMA problem would be to obtain a three-factor NNMA, namely $A \approx RBC$. Such an approximation is closely tied to the problem of co-clustering [3], and can be used to produce relaxed co-clustering solutions [7].

Weighted NNMA Problem (new). We can follow the same derivation method as above (based on KKT conditions) for obtaining multiplicative updates for the weighted NNMA problem:

$$\min D_\varphi(A, W_1 B C W_2),$$

where W_1 and W_2 are nonnegative (and nonsingular) weight matrices. The work of [9] is a special case as mentioned in Table 1. Please refer to [7] for more details.

4   Experiments and Discussion

We have looked at generic algorithms for minimizing Bregman divergences between the input and its approximation. One important question arises: Which Bregman divergence should one use for a given problem? Consider the following factor analytic model

$$A = BC + N,$$

where N represents some additive noise present in the measurements A, and the aim is to recover B and C. If we assume that the noise is distributed according to some member of the exponential family, then minimizing the corresponding Bregman divergence [1] is appropriate. For e.g., if the noise is modeled as i.i.d. Gaussian noise, then the Frobenius norm based problem is natural.

Another question is: Which version of the problem we should use, (2.2) or (2.3)? For $\varphi(x) = \frac{1}{2}x^2$, both problems coincide. For other φ, the choice between (2.2) and (2.3) can be guided by computation issues or sparsity patterns of A. Clearly, further work is needed for answering this question in more detail.

Some other open problems involve looking at the class of minimization problems to which the iterative methods of Section 3.2 may be applied. For example, determining the class of functions h, for which these methods may be used to minimize $D_\varphi(A, h(BC))$. Other possible methods for solving both (2.2) and (2.3), such as the use of alternating projections (AP) for NNMA, also merit a study.

Our methods for (2.2) decreased the objective function monotonically (by construction). However, we did not demonstrate such a guarantee for the updates (3.10) & (3.11). Figure 1 offers encouraging empirical evidence in favor of a monotonic behavior of these updates. It is still an open problem to formally prove this monotonic decrease. Preliminary results that yield *new* monotonicity proofs for the Frobenius norm and KL-divergence NNMA problems may be found in [7].

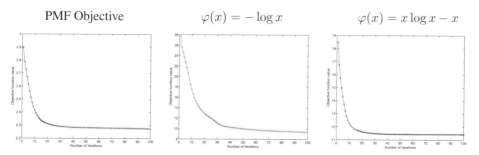

Figure 1: Objective function values over 100 iterations for different NNMA problems. The input matrix A was random 20×8 nonnegative matrix. Matrices B and C were 20×4, 4×8, respectively.

NNMA has been used in a large number of applications, a fact that attests to its importance and appeal. We believe that special cases of our generalized problems will prove to be useful for applications in data mining and machine learning.

5   Related Work

Paatero and Tapper [13] introduced NNMA as positive matrix factorization, and they aimed to minimize $\|W \odot (A - BC)\|_F$, where W was a fixed nonnegative matrix of weights. NNMA remained confined to applications in Environmetrics and Chemometrics before pioneering papers of Lee and Seung [11, 12] popularized the problem. Lee and Seung [11] provided simple and efficient algorithms for the NNMA problems that sought to minimize

$\|A - BC\|_F$ and $KL(A, BC)$. Lee & Seung called these problems *nonnegative matrix factorization* (NNMF), and their algorithms have inspired our generalizations.

NNMA was applied to a host of applications including text analysis, face/image recognition, language modeling, and speech processing amongst others. We refer the reader to [7] for pointers to the literature on various applications of NNMA.

Srebro and Jaakola [15] discuss elementwise weighted low-rank approximations without any nonnegativity constraints. Collins et al. [6] discuss algorithms for obtaining a low rank approximation of the form $A \approx BC$, where the loss functions are Bregman divergences, however, there is no restriction on B and C. More recently, Cichocki et al. [4] presented schemes for NNMA with Csiszár's φ-divergeneces, though rigorous convergence proofs seem to be unavailable. Our approach of Section 3.2 also yields heuristic methods for minimizing Csiszár's divergences.

Acknowledgments

This research was supported by NSF grant CCF-0431257, NSF Career Award ACI-0093404, and NSF-ITR award IIS-0325116.

References

[1] A. Banerjee, S. Merugu, I. S. Dhillon, and J. Ghosh. Clustering with Bregman Divergences. In *SIAM International Conf. on Data Mining*, Lake Buena Vista, Florida, April 2004. SIAM.

[2] Y. Censor and S. A. Zenios. *Parallel Optimization: Theory, Algorithms, and Applications*. Numerical Mathematics and Scientific Computation. Oxford University Press, 1997.

[3] H. Cho, I. S. Dhillon, Y. Guan, and S. Sra. Minimum Sum Squared Residue based Co-clustering of Gene Expression data. In *Proc. 4th SIAM International Conference on Data Mining (SDM)*, pages 114–125, Florida, 2004. SIAM.

[4] A. Cichocki, R. Zdunek, and S. Amari. Csiszár's Divergences for Non-Negative Matrix Factorization: Family of New Algorithms. In *6th Int. Conf. ICA & BSS*, USA, March 2006.

[5] M. Collins, R. Schapire, and Y. Singer. Logistic regression, adaBoost, and Bregman distances. In *Thirteenth annual conference on COLT*, 2000.

[6] M. Collins, S. Dasgupta, and R. E. Schapire. A Generalization of Principal Components Analysis to the Exponential Family. In *NIPS 2001*, 2001.

[7] I. S. Dhillon and S. Sra. Generalized nonnegative matrix approximations. Technical report, Computer Sciences, University of Texas at Austin, 2005.

[8] T. Feng, S. Z. Li, H-Y. Shum, and H. Zhang. Local nonnegative matrix factorization as a visual representation. In *Proceedings of the 2nd International Conference on Development and Learning*, pages 178–193, Cambridge, MA, June 2002.

[9] D. Guillamet, M. Bressan, and J. Vitrià. A weighted nonnegative matrix factorization for local representations. In *CVPR*. IEEE, 2001.

[10] P. O. Hoyer. Non-negative sparse coding. In *Proc. IEEE Workshop on Neural Networks for Signal Processing*, pages 557–565, 2002.

[11] D. D. Lee and H. S. Seung. Algorithms for nonnegative matrix factorization. In *NIPS*, pages 556–562, 2000.

[12] D. D. Lee and H. S. Seung. Learning the parts of objects by nonnegative matrix factorization. *Nature*, 401:788–791, October 1999.

[13] P. Paatero and U. Tapper. Positive matrix factorization: A nonnegative factor model with optimal utilization of error estimates of data values. *Environmetrics*, 5(111–126), 1994.

[14] R. T. Rockafellar. *Convex Analysis*. Princeton Univ. Press, 1970.

[15] N. Srebro and T. Jaakola. Weighted low-rank approximations. In *Proc. of 20th ICML*, 2003.

[16] J. A. Tropp. *Topics in Sparse Approximation*. PhD thesis, The Univ. of Texas at Austin, 2004.

An Application of Markov Random Fields to Range Sensing

James Diebel and Sebastian Thrun

Stanford AI Lab
Stanford University, Stanford, CA 94305

Abstract

This paper describes a highly successful application of MRFs to the problem of generating high-resolution range images. A new generation of range sensors combines the capture of low-resolution range images with the acquisition of registered high-resolution camera images. The MRF in this paper exploits the fact that discontinuities in range and coloring tend to co-align. This enables it to generate high-resolution, low-noise range images by integrating regular camera images into the range data. We show that by using such an MRF, we can substantially improve over existing range imaging technology.

1 Introduction

In recent years, there has been an enormous interest in developing technologies for measuring range. The set of commercially available technologies include passive stereo with two or more cameras, active stereo, triangulating light stripers, millimeter wavelength radar, and scanning and flash lidar. In the low-cost arena, systems such as the *Swiss Ranger* and the *CanestaVision* sensors provide means to acquire low-res range data along with passive camera images. Both of these devices capture high-res visual images along with lower-res depth information. This is the case for a number of devices at all price ranges, including the highly-praised range camera by *3DV Systems*.

This paper addresses a single shortcoming that (with the exception of stereo) is shared by most active range acquisition devices: Namely that range is captured at much lower resolution than images. This raises the question as to whether we *can turn a low-resolution depth imager into a high-resolution one, by exploiting conventional camera images?* A positive answer to this question would significantly advance the field of depth perception. Yet we lack techniques to fuse high-res conventional images with low-res depth images.

This paper applies graphical models to the problem of fusing low-res depth images with high-res camera images. Specifically, we propose a Markov Random Field (MRF) method for integrating both data sources. The intuition behind the MRF is that depth discontinuities in a scene often co-occur with color or brightness changes within the associated camera image. Since the camera image is commonly available at much higher resolution, this insight can be used to enhance the resolution and accuracy of the depth image.

Our approach performs this data integration using a multi-resolution MRF, which ties together image and range data. The mode of the probability distribution defined by the MRF provides us with a high-res depth map. Because we are only interested in finding the mode, we can apply fast optimization technique to the MRF inference problem, such as a

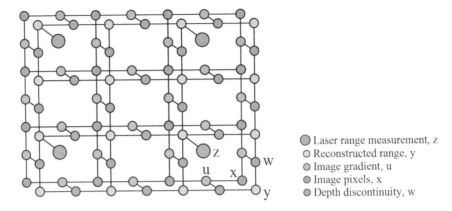

Laser range measurement, z
Reconstructed range, y
Image gradient, u
Image pixels, x
Depth discontinuity, w

Figure 1: The MRF is composed of 5 node types: The measurements mapped to two types of variables, the range measurement variables labeled z, image pixel variables labeled x. The density of image pixels is larger than those of the range measurements. The reconstructed range nodes, labeled y, are unobservable, but their density matches that of the image pixels. Auxiliary nodes labeled w and u mediate the information from the image and the depth map, as described in the text.

conjugate gradient algorithm. This approach leads to a high-res depth map within seconds, increasing the resolution of our depth sensor by an order of magnitude while improving local accuracy. To back up this claim, we provide several example results obtained using a low-res laser range finder paired with a conventional point-and-shot camera.

While none of the modeling or inference techniques in this paper are new, we believe that this paper provides a significant application of graphical modeling techniques to a problem that can dramatically alter an entire growing industry.

2 The Image-Range MRF

Figure 1 shows the MRF designed for our task. The input to the MRF occurs at two layers, through the variables labeled x_i and the variables labeled z_i. The variables x_i correspond to the image pixels, and their values are the three-dimensional RGB value of each pixel. The variables z_i are the range measurements. The range measurements are sampled much less densely than the image pixels, as indicated in this figure.

The key variables in this MRF are the ones labeled y, which model the reconstructed range at the same resolution as the image pixels. These variables are unobservable. Additional nodes labeled u and w leverage the image information into the estimated depth map y.

Specifically, the MRF is defined through the following potentials:

1. The *depth measurement potential* is of the form

$$\Psi = \sum_{i \in L} k \, (y_i - z_i)^2 \tag{1}$$

Here L is the set of indexes for which a depth measurement is available, and k is a constant weight placed on the depth measurements. This potential measures the quadratic distance between the estimated range in the high-res grid y and the measured range in the variables z, where available.

2. A *depth smoothness prior* is expressed by a potential of the form

$$\Phi = \sum_{i} \sum_{j \in N(i)} w_{ij} \, (y_i - y_j)^2 \tag{2}$$

Here $N(i)$ is the set of nodes adjacent to i. Φ is a weighted quadratic distance between neighboring nodes.

3. The *weighting factors* w_{ij} are a key element, in that they provide the link to the image layer in the MRF. Each w_{ij} is a deterministic function of the corresponding two adjacent image pixels, which is calculated as follows:

$$w_{ij} \;=\; \exp(-c\, u_{ij}) \tag{3}$$

$$u_{ij} \;=\; ||x_i - x_j||_2^2 \tag{4}$$

Here c is a constant that quantifies how unwilling we are to have smoothing occur across edges in the image.

The resulting MRF is now defined through the constraints Ψ and Φ. The conditional distribution over the target variables y is given by an expression of the form

$$p(y \mid x, z) \;=\; \frac{1}{Z}\exp(-\frac{1}{2}(\Psi + \Phi)) \tag{5}$$

where Z is a normalizer (partition function).

3 Optimization

Unfortunately, computing the full posterior is impossible for such an MRF, not least because the MRF may possesses many millions of nodes; even loopy belief propagation [19] requires enormous time for convergence. Instead, for the depth reconstruction problem we shall be content with computing the *mode* of the posterior.

Finding the mode of the log-posterior is, of course, a least square optimization problem, which we solve with the well-known conjugate gradient (CG) algorithm [12]. A typical single-image optimization with $2 \cdot 10^5$ nodes takes about a second to optimize on a modern computer.

The details of the CG algorithm are omitted for brevity, but can be found in contemporary texts. The resulting algorithm for probable depth image reconstruction is now remarkably simple: Simply set $y^{[0]}$ by the bilinear interpolation of z, and then iterate the CG update rule. The result is a probable reconstruction of the depth map at the same resolution as the camera image.

4 Results

Our experiments were performed with a SICK sweeping laser range finder and a Canon consumer digital camera with 5 mega pixels per image. Both were mounted on a rotating platform controlled by a servo actuator. This configuration allows us to survey an entire room from a consistent vantage point and with known camera and laser positions at all times. The output of this system is a set of pre-aligned laser range measurements and camera images.

Figure 2 shows a scan of a bookshelf in our lab. The top row contains several views of the raw measurements and the bottom row is the output of the MRF. The latter is clearly much sharper and less noisy; many features that are smaller than the resolution of the laser scanner are pulled out by the camera image. Figure 5 shows the same scene from much further back.

A more detailed look is taken in Figure 3. Here we examine the painted metal door frame to an office. The detailed structure is completely invisible in the raw laser scan but is easily drawn out when the image data is incorporated. It is notable that traditional mesh fairing algorithms would not be able to recover this fine structure, as there is simply insufficient evidence of it in the range data alone. Specifically, when running our MRF using a *fixed* value for w_{ij}, which effectively decouples the range image and the depth image, the depth reconstruction leads to a model that is either overly noise (for $w_{ij} = 1$ or

(a) Raw low-res depth map   **(b)** Raw low-res 3D model   **(c)** Image mapped onto 3D model

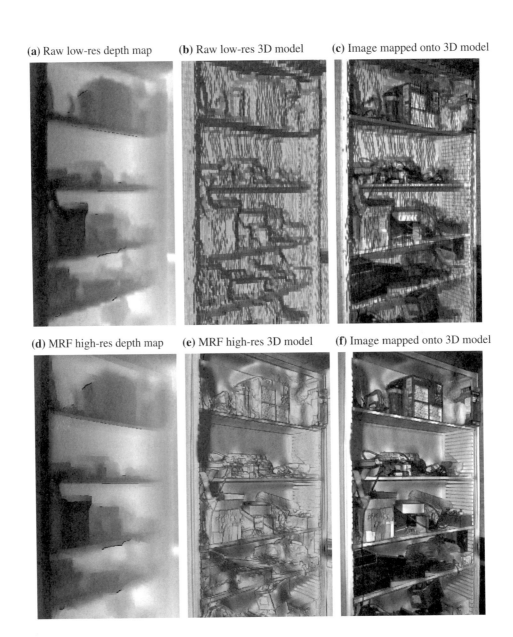

(d) MRF high-res depth map   **(e)** MRF high-res 3D model   **(f)** Image mapped onto 3D model

Figure 2: Example result of our MRF approach. Panels (a-c) show the raw data, the low-res depth map, a 3D model constructed from this depth map, and the same model with image texture superimposed. Panels (d-f) show the results of our algorithm. The depth map is now high-resolution, as is the 3D model. The 3D rendering is a substantial improvement over the raw sensor data; in fact, many small details are now visible.

smooths out the edge features for $w_{ij} = 5$. Our approach clearly recovers those corners, thanks to the use of the camera image.

Finally, in Fig. 4 we give one more example of a shipping crate next to a white wall. The coarse texture of the wooden surface is correctly inferred in contrast to the smooth white wall. This brings up the obvious problem that sharp color gradients do frequently occur on smooth surfaces; take, for example, posters. While this fact can sometimes lead to falsely-textured surfaces, it has been our experience that these flaws are often unnoticeable

(a) Raw 3D model, with and without color from the image

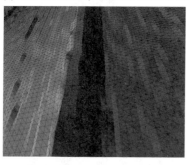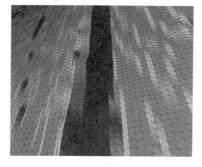

(b) Two results ignoring the image color information, for two different smoothers

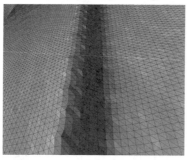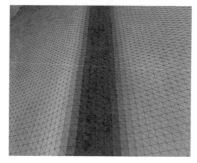

(c) Reconstruction with our MRF, integrating both depth and image color

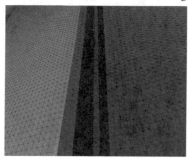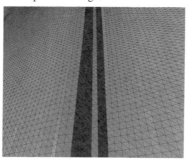

Figure 3: The important of the image information in depth recovery is illustrated in this figure. It shows a part of a door frame, for which a course depth map and a fine-grained image is available. The rendering labeled (b) show the result of our MRF when color is entirely ignored, for different fixed value of the weights w_{ij}. The images in (c) are the results of our approach, which clearly retains the sharp corner of the door frame.

and certainly no worse than the original scan. Clearly, the reconstruction of such depth maps is an ill-posed problem, and our approach generates a high-res model that is still significantly better than the original data. Notice, however, that the background wall is recovered accurately, and the corner of the room is visually enhanced.

5   Related Work

One of the primary acquisition techniques for depth is stereo. A good survey and comparison of stereo algorithms can is due to [14]. Our algorithm does not apply to stereo vision, since by definition the resolution of the image and the inferred depth map are equivalent.

(a) 3D model based on the raw range data, with and without texture

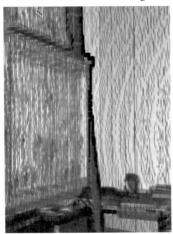 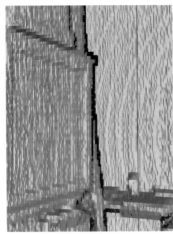

(b) Refined and super-resolved model, generated by our MRF

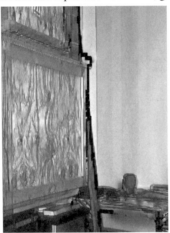 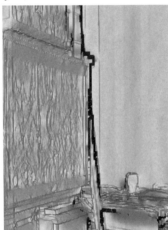

Figure 4: This example illustrate that the amount of smoothing in the range data is dependent on the image texture. On the left is a wooden box with an unsmooth surface that causes significant color variations. The 3D model generated from the MRF provides relatively little smoothing. In the background is a while wall with almost no color variation. Here our approach smooths the mesh significantly; in fact, it enhances the visibility of the room corner.

Passive stereo, in which the sensor does not carry its own light source, is unable to estimate ranges in the absence of texture (e.g., when imaging a featureless wall). Active stereo techniques supply their own light [4]. However, those techniques differ in characteristics from laser-based system to an extent that renders them practically inapplicable for many applications (most notably: long-range acquisition, where time-of-flight techniques are an order of magnitude more accurate then triangulation techniques, and bright-light outdoor environments). We remark that Markov Random fields have become a defining methodology in stereo reconstruction [15], along with layered EM-style methods [2, 16]; see the comparison in [14].

Similar work due to [20] relies on a different set of image cues to improve stereo shape estimates. In particular, learned regression coefficients are used to predict the band-passed shape of a scene from a band-passed image of that scene. The regression coefficients are

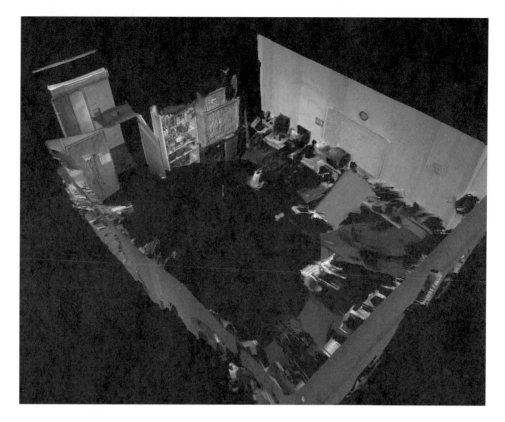

Figure 5: 3D model of a larger indoor environment, after applying our MRF.

learned from laser-stripe-scanned reference models with registered images.

For range images, surfaces, and point clouds, there exists a large literature on smoothing while preserving features such as edges. This includes work on diffusion processes [6], frequency-domain filtering [17], and anisotropic diffusion [5]; see also [3] and [1]. Most recently [10] proposed an efficient non-iterative technique for feature-preserving mesh smoothing, [9] adapted bilateral filtering for application to mesh denoising. and [7] developed anisotropic MRF techniques. None of these techniques, however, integrates high-resolution images to guide the smoothing process. Instead, they all operate on monochromatic 3D surfaces.

Our work can be viewed as generating super-resolution. Super-resolution techniques have long been popular in the computer vision field [8] and in aerial photogrammetry [11]. Here Bayesian techniques are often brought to bear for integrating multiple images into a single image of higher resolution. None of these techniques deal with range data. Finally, multiple range scans are often integrated into a single model [13, 18], yet none of these techniques involve image data.

6   Conclusion

We have presented a Markov Random Field that integrated high-res image data into low-res range data, to recover range data at the same resolution as the image data. This approach is specifically aimed at a new wave of commercially available sensors, which provide range at lower resolution than image data.

The significance of this work lies in the results. We have shown that our approach can truly fill the resolution gap between range and images, and use image data to effectively boost the resolution of a range finder. While none of the techniques used here are new (even though CG is usually not applied for inference in MRFs), we believe this is the first application of MRF to multimodal data integration. A large number of scientific fields would benefit from better range sensing; the present approach provides a solution that endows low-cost range finders with unprecedented resolution and accuracy.

References

[1] C.L. Bajaj and G. Xu. Anisotropic diffusion of surfaces and functions on surfaces. In *Proceedings of SIGGRAPH*, pages 4–32, 2003.

[2] S. Baker, R Szeliski, and P. Anandan. A layered approach to stereo reconstruction. In *Proceedings of the Conference on Computer Vision and Pattern Recognition (CVPR)*, pages 434–438, Santa Barbara, CA, 1998.

[3] U. Clarenz, U. Diewald, and M. Rumpf. Anisotropic geometric diffusion in surface processing. In *Proceedings of the IEEE Conference on Visualization*, pages 397–405, 2000.

[4] J. Davis, R. Ramamoothi, and S. Rusinkiewicz. Spacetime stereo: A unifying framework for depth from triangulation. In *Proceedings of the Conference on Computer Vision and Pattern Recognition (CVPR)*, 2003.

[5] M. Desbrun, M. Meyer, P. Schröder, and A. Barr. Anisotropic feature-preserving denoising of height fi elds and bivariate data. In *Proceedings Graphics Interface*, Montreal, Quebec, 2000.

[6] M. Desbrun, M. Meyer, P. Schröder, and A. H. Barr. Implicit fairing of irregular meshes using diffusion and curvature fbw. In *Proceedings of SIGGRAPH*, 1999.

[7] J. Diebel, S. Thrun, and M. Brüning. A bayesian method for probable surface reconstruction and decimation. *IEEE Transactions on Graphics*, 2005. To appear.

[8] M. Elad and A. Feuer. Restoration of single super-resolution image from several blurred. *IEEE Transcation on Image Processing*, 6(12):1646–1658, 1997.

[9] S. Fleishman, I. Drori, and D. Cohen-Or. Bilateral mesh denoising. In *Proceedings of SIGGRAPH*, pages 950–953, 2003.

[10] T.R. Jones, F. Durand, and M. Desbrun. Non-iterative, feature-preserving mesh smoothing. In *Proceedings of SIGGRAPH*, pages 943–949, 2003.

[11] I. K. Jung and S. Lacroix. High resolution terrain mapping using low altitude aerial stereo imagery. In *Proceedings of the International Conference on Computer Vision (ICCV)*, Nice, France, 2003.

[12] W. H. Press. *Numerical recipes in C: the art of scientific computing*. Cambridge University Press, Cambridge; New York, 1988.

[13] S. Rusinkiewicz and M. Levoy. Effi cient variants of the ICP algorithm. In *Proc. Third International Conference on 3D Digital Imaging and Modeling (3DIM)*, Quebec City, Canada, 2001. IEEEComputer Society.

[14] D. Scharstein and R. Szeliski. A taxonomy and evaluation of dense two-frame stereo correspondence algorithms. *International Journal of Computer Vision*, 47(1-3):7–42, 2002.

[15] J. Sun, H.-Y. Shum, and N.-N. Zheng. Stereo matching using belief propagation. *IEEE Transcation on PAMI*, 25(7), 2003.

[16] R. Szeliski. Stereo algorithms and representations for image-based rendering. In *Proceedings of the British Machine Vision Conference, Vol 2*, pages 314–328, 1999.

[17] G. Taubin. A signal processing approach to fair surface design. In *Proceedings of SIGGRAPH*, pages 351–358, 1995.

[18] S. Thrun, W. Burgard, and D. Fox. *Probabilistic Robotics*. MIT Press, Cambridge, MA, 2005.

[19] Y. Weiss and W.T. Freeman. Correctness of belief propagation in gaussian graphical models of arbitrary topology. *Neural Computation*, 13(10):2173–2200, 2001.

[20] W. T. Freeman and A. Torralba. Shape recipes: Scene representations that refer to the image. In *Advances in Neural Information Processing Systems (NIPS) 15*, Cambridge, MA, 2003. MIT Press.

Transfer learning for text classification

Chuong B. Do
Computer Science Department
Stanford University
Stanford, CA 94305

Andrew Y. Ng
Computer Science Department
Stanford University
Stanford, CA 94305

Abstract

Linear text classification algorithms work by computing an inner product between a test document vector and a parameter vector. In many such algorithms, including naive Bayes and most TFIDF variants, the parameters are determined by some simple, closed-form, function of training set statistics; we call this mapping mapping from statistics to parameters, the *parameter function*. Much research in text classification over the last few decades has consisted of manual efforts to identify better parameter functions. In this paper, we propose an algorithm for automatically *learning* this function from related classification problems. The parameter function found by our algorithm then defines a *new learning algorithm* for text classification, which we can apply to novel classification tasks. We find that our learned classifier outperforms existing methods on a variety of multiclass text classification tasks.

1 Introduction

In the multiclass text classification task, we are given a training set of documents, each labeled as belonging to one of K disjoint classes, and a new unlabeled test document. Using the training set as a guide, we must predict the most likely class for the test document. "Bag-of-words" linear text classifiers represent a document as a vector $\mathbf{x}$ of word counts, and predict the class whose score (a linear function of $\mathbf{x}$) is highest, i.e., $\arg\max_{k \in \{1,...,K\}} \sum_{i=1}^{n} \theta_{ki} x_i$. Choosing parameters $\{\theta_{ki}\}$ which give high classification accuracy on test data, thus, is the main challenge for linear text classification algorithms.

In this paper, we focus on linear text classification algorithms in which the parameters are pre-specified functions of training set statistics; that is, each θ_{ki} is a function $\theta_{ki} := g(\mathbf{u}_{ki})$ of some *fixed statistics* $\mathbf{u}_{ki}$ of the training set. Unlike discriminative learning methods, such as logistic regression [1] or support vector machines (SVMs) [2], which use numerical optimization to pick parameters, the learners we consider perform no optimization. Rather, in our technique, parameter learning involves tabulating statistics vectors $\{\mathbf{u}_{ki}\}$ and applying the closed-form function g to obtain parameters. We refer to g, this mapping from statistics to parameters, as the *parameter function*.

Many common text classification methods—including the multinomial and multivariate Bernoulli event models for naive Bayes [3], the vector space-based TFIDF classifier [4], and its probabilistic variant, PrTFIDF [5]—belong to this class of algorithms. Here, picking a good text classifier from this class is equivalent to finding the right parameter function for the available statistics.

In practice, researchers often develop text classification algorithms by trial-and-error, guided by empirical testing on real-world classification tasks (cf. [6, 7]). Indeed, one could argue that much of the 30-year history of information retrieval has consisted of manually trying TFIDF formula variants (i.e. adjusting the parameter function g) to optimize performance [8]. Even though this heuristic process can often lead to good parameter functions, such a laborious task requires much human ingenuity, and risks failing to find algorithm variations not considered by the designer.

In this paper, we consider the task of *automatically* learning a parameter function g for text classification. Given a set of example text classification problems, we wish to "meta-learn" a new *learning algorithm* (as specified by the parameter function g), which may then be applied new classification problems. The meta-learning technique we propose, which leverages data from a variety of related classification tasks to obtain a good classifier for new tasks, is thus an instance of *transfer learning*; specifically, our framework automates the process of finding a good parameter function for text classifiers, replacing hours of hand-tweaking with a straightforward, globally-convergent, convex optimization problem.

Our experiments demonstrate the effectiveness of learning classifier forms. In low training data classification tasks, the learning algorithm given by our automatically learned parameter function consistently outperforms human-designed parameter functions based on naive Bayes and TFIDF, as well as existing discriminative learning approaches.

2 Preliminaries

Let $\mathcal{V} = \{w_1, \ldots, w_n\}$ be a fixed vocabulary of words, and let $\mathcal{X} = \mathbb{Z}^n$ and $\mathcal{Y} = \{1, \ldots, K\}$ be the input and output spaces for our classification problem. A *labeled document* is a pair $(\mathbf{x}, y) \in \mathcal{X} \times \mathcal{Y}$, where $\mathbf{x}$ is an n-dimensional vector with x_i indicating the number of occurrences of word w_i in the document, and y is the document's class label. A *classification problem* is a tuple $\langle \mathcal{D}, S, (\mathbf{x}_{\text{test}}, y_{\text{test}}) \rangle$, where $\mathcal{D}$ is a distribution over $\mathcal{X} \times \mathcal{Y}$, $S = \{(\mathbf{x}_i, y_i)\}_{i=1}^M$ is a set of M training examples, $(\mathbf{x}_{\text{test}}, y_{\text{test}})$ is a single test example, and all $M + 1$ examples are drawn iid from $\mathcal{D}$. Given a training set S and a test input vector $\mathbf{x}_{\text{test}}$, we must predict the value of the test class label y_{test}.

In linear classification algorithms, we evaluate the score $f_k(\mathbf{x}_{\text{test}}) := \sum_i \theta_{ki} \mathbf{x}_{\text{test}\,i}$ for assigning $\mathbf{x}_{\text{test}}$ to each class $k \in \{1, \ldots, K\}$ and pick the class $y = \arg\max_k f_k(\mathbf{x}_{\text{test}})$ with the highest score. In our meta-learning setting, we define each θ_{ki} as the component-wise evaluation of the parameter function g on some vector of training set statistics $\mathbf{u}_{ki}$:

$$
\begin{bmatrix} \theta_{k1} \\ \theta_{k2} \\ \vdots \\ \theta_{kn} \end{bmatrix} := \begin{bmatrix} g(\mathbf{u}_{k1}) \\ g(\mathbf{u}_{k2}) \\ \vdots \\ g(\mathbf{u}_{kn}) \end{bmatrix}.
\tag{1}
$$

Here, each $\mathbf{u}_{ki} \in \mathbb{R}^q$ ($k = 1, \ldots, K$, $i = 1, \ldots, n$) is a vector whose components are computed from the training set S (we will provide specific examples later). Furthermore, $g : \mathbb{R}^q \to \mathbb{R}$ is the *parameter function* mapping from $\mathbf{u}_{ki}$ to its corresponding parameter θ_{ki}. To illustrate these definitions, we show that two specific cases of the naive Bayes and TFIDF classification methods belong to the class of algorithms described above.

Naive Bayes: In the multinomial variant of the naive Bayes classification algorithm,[1] the score for assigning a document $\mathbf{x}$ to class k is

$$
f_k^{\text{NB}}(\mathbf{x}) := \log \hat{p}(y = k) + \sum_{i=1}^n x_i \log \hat{p}(w_i \mid y = k).
\tag{2}
$$

The first term, $\hat{p}(y = k)$, corresponds to a "prior" over document classes, and the second term, $\hat{p}(w_i \mid y = k)$, is the (smoothed) relative frequency of word

---

[1]Despite naive Bayes' overly strong independence assumptions and thus its shortcomings as a probabilistic *model* for text documents, we can nonetheless view naive Bayes as simply an *algorithm* which makes predictions by computing certain functions of the training set. This view has proved useful for analysis of naive Bayes even when none of its probabilistic assumptions hold [9]; here, we adopt this view, without attaching any particular probabilistic meaning to the empirical frequencies $\hat{p}(\cdot)$ that happen to be computed by the algorithm.

w_i in training documents of class k. For balanced training sets, the first term is irrelevant. Therefore, we have $f_k^{NB}(\mathbf{x}) = \sum_i \theta_{ki} x_i$ where $\theta_{ki} = g_{NB}(\mathbf{u}_{ki})$,

$$
\mathbf{u}_{ki} := \begin{bmatrix} u_{ki1} \\ u_{ki2} \\ u_{ki3} \\ u_{ki4} \\ u_{ki5} \end{bmatrix} = \begin{bmatrix} \text{number of times } w_i \text{ appears in documents of class } k \\ \text{number of documents of class } k \text{ containing } w_i \\ \text{total number of words in documents of class } k \\ \text{total number of documents of class } k \\ \text{total number of documents} \end{bmatrix}, \quad (3)
$$

and

$$
g_{NB}(\mathbf{u}_{ki}) := \log \frac{u_{ki1} + \varepsilon}{u_{ki3} + n\varepsilon} \quad (4)
$$

where ε is a smoothing parameter. ($\varepsilon = 1$ gives Laplace smoothing.)

TFIDF: In the unnormalized TFIDF classifier, the score for assigning $\mathbf{x}$ to class k is

$$
f_k^{TFIDF}(\mathbf{x}) := \sum_{i=1}^n \left(\bar{x}_i|_{y=k} \cdot \log \frac{1}{\hat{p}(x_i > 0)} \right) \left(x_i \cdot \log \frac{1}{\hat{p}(x_i > 0)} \right), \quad (5)
$$

where $\bar{x}_i|_{y=k}$ (sometimes called the average term frequency of w_i) is the average ith component of all document vectors of class k, and $\hat{p}(x_i > 0)$ (sometimes called the document frequency of w_i) is the proportion of all documents containing w_i.[2] As before, we write $f_k^{TFIDF}(\mathbf{x}) = \sum_i \theta_{ki} x_i$ with $\theta_{ki} = g_{TFIDF}(\mathbf{u}_{ki})$. The statistics vector is again defined as in (3), but this time,

$$
g_{TFIDF}(\mathbf{u}_{ki}) := \frac{u_{ki1}}{u_{ki4}} \left(\log \frac{u_{ki5}}{u_{ki2}} \right)^2. \quad (6)
$$

Space constraints preclude a detailed discussion, but many other classification algorithms can similarly be expressed in this framework, using other definitions of the statistics vectors $\{\mathbf{u}_{ki}\}$. These include most other variants of TFIDF based on different TF and IDF terms [7], PrTFIDF [5], and various heuristically modified versions of naive Bayes [6].

3 Learning the parameter function

In the last section, we gave two examples of algorithms that obtain their parameters θ_{ki} by applying a function g to a statistics vector $\mathbf{u}_{ki}$. In each case, the parameter function was hand-designed, either from probabilistic (in the case of naive Bayes [3]) or geometric (in the case of TFIDF [4]) considerations. We now consider the problem of automatically learning a parameter function from example classification tasks. In the sequel, we assume fixed statistics vectors $\{\mathbf{u}_{ki}\}$ and focus on finding an optimal parameter function g.

In the standard supervised learning setting, we are given a training set of examples sampled from some unknown distribution $\mathcal{D}$, and our goal is to use the training set to make a prediction on a new test example also sampled from $\mathcal{D}$. By using the training examples to understand the statistical regularities in $\mathcal{D}$, we hope to predict y_{test} from $\mathbf{x}_{test}$ with low error.

Analogously, the problem of meta-learning g is again a supervised learning task; here, however, the training "examples" are now classification problems sampled from a distribution $\mathcal{D}$ over classification problems.[3] By seeing many instances of text classification problems

---

[2] Note that (5) implicitly defines $f_k^{TFIDF}(\mathbf{x})$ as a dot product of two vectors, each of whose components consist of a product of two terms. In the normalized TFIDF classifier, both vectors are normalized to unit length before computing the dot product, a modification that makes the algorithm more stable for documents of varying length. This too can be represented within our framework by considering appropriately normalized statistics vectors.

[3] Note that in our meta-learning problem, the output of our algorithm is a parameter function g mapping statistics to parameters. Our training data, however, do not explicitly indicate the best parameter function g^* for each example classification problem. Effectively then, in the meta-learning task, the central problem is to fit g to some *unseen* g^*, based on test examples in each training classification problem.

drawn from $\mathscr{D}$, we hope to learn a parameter function g that exploits the statistical regularities in problems from $\mathscr{D}$. Formally, let $\mathscr{S} = \{\langle \mathcal{D}^{(j)}, S^{(j)}, (\mathbf{x}^{(j)}, y^{(j)}) \rangle\}_{j=1}^{m}$ be a collection of m classification problems sampled iid from $\mathscr{D}$. For a new, test classification problem $\langle \mathcal{D}_{\text{test}}, S_{\text{test}}, (\mathbf{x}_{\text{test}}, y_{\text{test}}) \rangle$ sampled independently from $\mathscr{D}$, we desire that our learned g correctly classify $\mathbf{x}_{\text{test}}$ with high probability.

To achieve our goal, we first restrict our attention to parameter functions g that are *linear* in their inputs. Using the linearity assumption, we pose a convex optimization problem for finding a parameter function g that achieves small loss on test examples in the training collection. Finally, we generalize our method to the non-parametric setting via the "kernel trick," thus allowing us to learn complex, highly non-linear functions of the input statistics.

3.1 Softmax learning

Recall that in *softmax regression*, the class probabilities $p(y \mid \mathbf{x})$ are modeled as

$$p(y = k \mid \mathbf{x}; \{\theta_{ki}\}) := \frac{\exp(\sum_i \theta_{ki} x_i)}{\sum_{k'} \exp(\sum_i \theta_{k'i} x_i)}, \qquad k = 1, \ldots, K, \tag{7}$$

where the parameters $\{\theta_{ki}\}$ are learned from the training data S by maximizing the conditional log likelihood of the data. In this approach, a total of Kn parameters are trained jointly using numerical optimization. Here, we consider an alternative approach in which each of the Kn parameters is some function of the prespecified statistics vectors; in particular, $\theta_{ki} := g(\mathbf{u}_{ki})$. Our goal is to learn an appropriate g.

To pose our optimization problem, we start by learning the *linear form* $g(\mathbf{u}_{ki}) = \boldsymbol{\beta}^T \mathbf{u}_{ki}$. Under this parameterization, the conditional likelihood of an example $(\mathbf{x}, y)$ is

$$p(y = k \mid \mathbf{x}; \boldsymbol{\beta}) = \frac{\exp(\sum_i \boldsymbol{\beta}^T \mathbf{u}_{ki} x_i)}{\sum_{k'} \exp(\sum_i \boldsymbol{\beta}^T \mathbf{u}_{k'i} x_i)}, \qquad k = 1, \ldots, K. \tag{8}$$

In this setup, one natural approach for learning a linear function g is to maximize the (regularized) conditional log likelihood $\ell(\boldsymbol{\beta} : \mathscr{S})$ for the entire collection $\mathscr{S}$:

$$\ell(\boldsymbol{\beta} : \mathscr{S}) := \sum_{j=1}^{m} \log p(y^{(j)} \mid \mathbf{x}^{(j)}; \boldsymbol{\beta}) - C\|\boldsymbol{\beta}\|^2$$

$$= \sum_{j=1}^{m} \log \left(\frac{\exp\left(\boldsymbol{\beta}^T \sum_i \mathbf{u}_{y^{(j)}i}^{(j)} x_i^{(j)}\right)}{\sum_k \exp\left(\boldsymbol{\beta}^T \sum_i \mathbf{u}_{ki}^{(j)} x_i^{(j)}\right)} \right) - C\|\boldsymbol{\beta}\|^2. \tag{9}$$

In (9), the latter term corresponds to a Gaussian prior on the parameters $\boldsymbol{\beta}$, which provides a means for controlling the complexity of the learned parameter function g. The maximization of (9) is similar to softmax regression training except that here, instead of optimizing over the parameters $\{\theta_{ki}\}$ directly, we optimize over the choice of $\boldsymbol{\beta}$.

3.2 Nonparametric function learning

In this section, we generalize the technique of the previous section to nonlinear g. By the Representer Theorem [10], there exists a maximizing solution to (9) for which the optimal parameter vector $\boldsymbol{\beta}^*$ is a linear combination of training set statistics:

$$\boldsymbol{\beta}^* = \sum_{j=1}^{m} \sum_k \alpha_{jk}^* \sum_i \mathbf{u}_{ki}^{(j)} x_i^{(j)}. \tag{10}$$

From this, we reparameterize the original optimization over $\boldsymbol{\beta}$ in (9) as an equivalent optimization over training example weights $\{\alpha_{jk}\}$. For notational convenience, let

$$\mathcal{K}(j, j', k, k') := \sum_i \sum_{i'} x_i^{(j)} x_{i'}^{(j')} (\mathbf{u}_{ki}^{(j)})^T \mathbf{u}_{k'i'}^{(j')}. \tag{11}$$

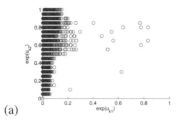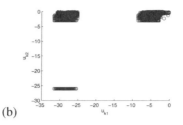

(a)   (b)

Figure 1: Distribution of unnormalized $\mathbf{u}_{ki}$ vectors in dmoz data (a) with and (b) without applying the log transformation in (15). In principle, one could alternatively use a feature vector representation using these frequencies directly, as in (a). However, applying the log transformation yields a feature space with fewer isolated points in $\mathbb{R}^2$, as in (b). When using the Gaussian kernel, a feature space with few isolated points is important as the topology of the feature space establishes locality of influence for support vectors.

Substituting (10) and (11) into (9), we obtain

$$\ell(\{\alpha_{jk}\} : \mathscr{S}) := \sum_{j'=1}^{m} \log \left(\frac{\exp\left(\sum_{j=1}^{m} \sum_{k} \alpha_{jk} \mathcal{K}(j, j', k, y^{(j')})\right)}{\sum_{k'} \exp\left(\sum_{j=1}^{m} \sum_{k} \alpha_{jk} \mathcal{K}(j, j', k, k')\right)} \right)$$

$$- C \sum_{j=1}^{m} \sum_{j'=1}^{m} \sum_{k} \sum_{k'} \alpha_{jk} \alpha_{j'k'} \mathcal{K}(j, j', k, k'). \tag{12}$$

Note that (12) is concave and differentiable, so we can train the model using any standard numerical gradient optimization procedure, such as conjugate gradient or L-BFGS [11].

The assumption that g is a linear function of $\mathbf{u}_{ki}$, however, places a severe restriction on the class of learnable parameter functions. Noting that the statistics vectors appear only as an inner product in (11), we apply the "kernel trick" to obtain

$$\mathcal{K}(j, j', k, k') := \sum_{i} \sum_{i'} x_i^{(j)} x_{i'}^{(j')} K(\mathbf{u}_{ki}^{(j)}, \mathbf{u}_{k'i'}^{(j')}), \tag{13}$$

where the kernel function $K(\mathbf{u}, \mathbf{v}) = \langle \Phi(\mathbf{u}), \Phi(\mathbf{v}) \rangle$ defines the inner product of some high-dimensional mapping $\Phi(\cdot)$ of its inputs.[4] In particular, choosing a Gaussian (RBF) kernel, $K(\mathbf{u}, \mathbf{v}) := \exp(-\gamma\|\mathbf{u} - \mathbf{v}\|^2)$, gives a *non-parametric* representation for g:

$$g(\mathbf{u}_{ki}) = \boldsymbol{\beta}^T \Phi(\mathbf{u}_{ki}) = \sum_{j=1}^{m} \sum_{k} \sum_{i} \alpha_{jk} x_i^{(j)} \exp(-\gamma\|\mathbf{u}_{ki}^{(j)} - \mathbf{u}_{ki}\|^2). \tag{14}$$

Thus, $g(\mathbf{u}_{ki})$ is a weighted combination of the values $\{\alpha_{jk} x_i^{(j)}\}$, where the weights depend exponentially on the squared ℓ_2-distance of $\mathbf{u}_{ki}$ to each of the statistics vectors $\{\mathbf{u}_{ki}^{(j)}\}$. As a result, we can approximate any sufficiently smooth bounded function of $\mathbf{u}$ arbitrarily well, given sufficiently many training classification problems.

4   Experiments

To validate our method, we evaluated its ability to learn parameter functions on a variety of email and webpage classification tasks in which the number of classes, K, was large ($K = 10$), and the number of number of training examples per class, m/K, was small ($m/K = 2$). We used the dmoz Open Directory Project hierarchy,[5] the 20 Newsgroups dataset,[6] the Reuters-21578 dataset,[7] and the Industry Sector dataset[8].

---

[4]Note also that as a consequence of our kernelization, $\mathcal{K}$ itself can be considered a 'kernel' between all statistics vectors from two entire documents.

[5]http://www.dmoz.org

[6]http://kdd.ics.uci.edu/databases/20newsgroups/20newsgroups.tar.gz

[7]http://www.daviddlewis.com/resources/testcollections/reuters21578/reuters21578.tar.gz

[8]http://www.cs.umass.edu/~mccallum/data/sector.tar.gz

Table 1: Test set accuracy on dmoz categories. Columns 2-4 give the proportion of correct classifications using non-discriminative methods: the learned g, Naive Bayes, and TFIDF, respectively. Columns 5-7 give the corresponding values for the discriminative methods: softmax regression, 1-vs-all SVMs, and multiclass SVMs. The best accuracy in each row is shown in bold.

Category	g	g_{NB}	g_{TFIDF}	softmax	1VA-SVM	MC-SVM
Arts	**0.421**	0.296	0.286	0.352	0.203	0.367
Business	**0.456**	0.283	0.286	0.336	0.233	0.340
Computers	**0.467**	0.304	0.327	0.344	0.217	0.387
Games	**0.411**	0.288	0.240	0.279	0.240	0.330
Health	**0.479**	0.282	0.337	0.382	0.213	0.337
Home	**0.640**	0.470	0.454	0.501	0.333	0.440
Kids and Teens	**0.252**	0.205	0.142	0.202	0.173	0.167
News	0.349	0.222	0.212	0.382	0.270	**0.397**
Recreation	**0.663**	0.487	0.529	0.477	0.353	0.590
Reference	**0.635**	0.415	0.458	0.602	0.383	0.543
Regional	**0.438**	0.268	0.258	0.329	0.260	0.357
Science	**0.363**	0.256	0.246	0.353	0.223	0.340
Shopping	**0.612**	0.456	0.556	0.483	0.373	0.550
Society	**0.435**	0.308	0.285	0.379	0.213	0.377
Sports	**0.619**	0.432	0.285	0.507	0.267	0.527
World	**0.531**	0.491	0.352	0.329	0.277	0.303
Average	**0.486**	0.341	0.328	0.390	0.264	0.397

The dmoz project is a hierarchical collection of webpage links organized by subject matter. The top level of the hierarchy consists of 16 major categories, each of which contains several subcategories. To perform cross-validated testing, we obtained classification problems from each of the top-level categories by retrieving webpages from each of their respective subcategories. For the 20 Newsgroups, Reuters-21578, and Industry Sector datasets, we performed similar preprocessing.[9] Given a dataset of documents, we sampled 10-class 2-training-examples-per-class classification problems by randomly selecting 10 different classes within the dataset, picking 2 training examples within each class, and choosing one test example from a randomly chosen class.

4.1 Choice of features

Theoretically, for the method described in this paper, any sufficiently rich set of features could be used to learn a parameter function for classification. For simplicity, we reduced the feature vector in (3) to the following two-dimensional representation,[10]

$$\mathbf{u}_{ki} = \begin{bmatrix} \log(\text{proportion of } w_i \text{ among words from documents of class } k) \\ \log(\text{proportion of documents containing } w_i) \end{bmatrix}. \quad (15)$$

Note that up to the log transformation, the components of $\mathbf{u}_{ki}$ correspond to the relative term frequency and document frequency of a word relative to class k (see Figure 1).

4.2 Generalization performance

We tested our meta-learning algorithm on classification problems taken from each of the 16 top-level dmoz categories. For each top-level category, we built a collection of 300 classification problems from that category; results reported here are averages over these

---

[9]For the Reuters data, we associated each article with its hand-annotated 'topic' label and discarded any articles with more than one topic annotation. For each dataset, we discarded all categories with fewer than 50 examples, and selected a 500-word vocabulary based on information gain.

[10]Features were rescaled to have zero mean and unit variance over the training set.

Table 2: Cross corpora classification accuracy, using classifiers trained on each of the four corpora. The best accuracy in each row is shown in bold.

Dataset	g_{dmoz}	g_{news}	g_{reut}	g_{indu}	g_{NB}	g_{TFIDF}	softmax	1VA-SVM	MC-SVM
dmoz	n/a	0.471	**0.475**	0.473	0.365	0.352	0.381	0.283	0.412
20 Newsgroups	0.369	n/a	**0.371**	0.369	0.223	0.184	0.217	0.206	0.248
Reuters-21578	0.567	0.567	n/a	**0.619**	0.463	0.475	0.463	0.308	0.481
Industry Sector	0.438	**0.459**	0.446	n/a	0.374	0.274	0.376	0.271	0.375

problems. To assess the accuracy of our meta-learning algorithm for a particular test category, we used the g learned from a set of 450 classification problems drawn from the *other* 15 top-level categories.[11] This ensured no overlap of training and testing data. In 15 out of 16 categories, the learned parameter function g outperforms naive Bayes and TFIDF in addition to the discriminative methods we tested (softmax regression, 1-vs-all SVMs [12], and multiclass SVMs [13][12]; see Table 1).[13]

Next, we assessed the ability of g to transfer across even more dissimilar corpora. Here, for each of the four corpora (dmoz, 20 Newsgroups, Reuters-21578, Industry Sector), we constructed independent training and testing datasets of 480 random classification problems. After training separate classifiers (g_{dmoz}, g_{news}, g_{reut}, and g_{indu}) using data from each of the four corpora, we tested the performance of each learned classifier on the remaining three corpora (see Table 2). Again, the learned parameter functions compare favorably to the other methods. Moreover, these tests show that a single parameter function may give an accurate classification algorithm for many different corpora, demonstrating the effectiveness of our approach for achieving transfer across related learning tasks.

5 Discussion and Related Work

In this paper, we presented an algorithm based on softmax regression for learning a parameter function g from example classification problems. Once learned, g defines a new learning algorithm that can be applied to novel classification tasks.

Another approach for learning g is to modify the multiclass support vector machine formulation of Crammer and Singer [13] in a manner analagous to the modification of softmax regression in Section 3.1, giving the following quadratic program:

$$\begin{aligned} &\underset{\boldsymbol{\beta}\in\mathbb{R}^n,\boldsymbol{\xi}\in\mathbb{R}^m}{\text{minimize}} \quad \tfrac{1}{2}||\boldsymbol{\beta}||^2 + C\sum_j \xi_j \\ &\text{subject to} \quad \boldsymbol{\beta}^T \sum_i x_i^{(j)}(\mathbf{u}_{y^{(j)}i}^{(j)} - \mathbf{u}_{ki}^{(j)}) \geq \mathbf{I}_{\{k\neq y^{(j)}\}} - \xi_j, \quad \forall k, \forall j. \end{aligned}$$

As usual, taking the dual leads naturally to an SMO-like procedure for optimization. We implemented this method and found that the learned g, like in the softmax formulation, outperforms naive Bayes, TFIDF, and the other discriminative methods.

The techniques described in this paper give one approach for achieving *inductive transfer* in classifier design—using labeled data from related example classification problems to solve a particular classification problem [16, 17]. Bennett et al. [18] also consider the issue of knowledge transfer in text classification in the context of ensemble classifiers, and propose a system for using related classification problems to learn the reliability of individual classifiers within the ensemble. Unlike their approach, which attempts to meta-learn *properties*

---

[11] For each execution of the learning algorithm, (C, γ) parameters were determined via grid search using a small holdout set of 160 classification problems. The same holdout set was used to select regularization parameters for the discriminative learning algorithms.

[12] We used LIBSVM [14] to assess 1VA-SVMs and SVM-Light [15] for multiclass SVMs.

[13] For larger values of m/K (e.g. $m/K = 10$), softmax and multiclass SVMs consistently outperform naive Bayes and TFIDF; nevertheless, the learned g achieves a performance on par with discriminative methods, despite being constrained to parameters which are explicit functions of training data statistics. This result is consistent with a previous study in which a heuristically hand-tuned version of Naive Bayes attained near-SVM text classification performance for large datasets [6].

of algorithms, our method uses meta-learning to *construct* a new classification algorithm. Though not directly applied to text classification, Teevan and Karger [19] consider the problem of automatically learning term distributions for use in information retrieval.

Finally, Thrun and O'Sullivan [20] consider the task of classification in a mobile robot domain. In this work, the authors describe a task-clustering (TC) algorithm in which learning tasks are grouped via a nearest neighbors algorithm, as a means of facilitating knowledge transfer. A similar concept is implicit in the kernelized parameter function learned by our algorithm, where the Gaussian kernel facilitates transfer between similar statistics vectors.

Acknowledgments

We thank David Vickrey and Pieter Abbeel for useful discussions, and the anonymous referees for helpful comments. CBD was supported by an NDSEG fellowship. This work was supported by DARPA under contract number FA8750-05-2-0249.

References

[1] K. Nigam, J. Lafferty, and A. McCallum. Using maximum entropy for text classification. In *IJCAI-99 Workshop on Machine Learning for Information Filtering*, pages 61–67, 1999.

[2] T. Joachims. Text categorization with support vector machines: Learning with many relevant features. In *Machine Learning: ECML-98*, pages 137–142, 1998.

[3] A. McCallum and K. Nigam. A comparison of event models for Naive Bayes text classification. In *AAAI-98 Workshop on Learning for Text Categorization*, 1998.

[4] G. Salton and C. Buckley. Term weighting approaches in automatic text retrieval. *Information Processing and Management*, 29(5):513–523, 1988.

[5] T. Joachims. A probabilistic analysis of the Rocchio algorithm with TFIDF for text categorization. In *Proceedings of ICML-97*, pages 143–151, 1997.

[6] J. D. Rennie, L. Shih, J. Teevan, and D. R. Karger. Tackling the poor assumptions of naive Bayes text classifiers. In *ICML*, pages 616–623, 2003.

[7] A. Moffat and J. Zobel. Exploring the similarity space. In *ACM SIGIR Forum 32*, 1998.

[8] C. Manning and H. Schutze. Foundations of statistical natural language processing, 1999.

[9] A. Ng and M. Jordan. On discriminative vs. generative classifiers: a comparison of logistic regression and naive Bayes. In *NIPS 14*, 2002.

[10] G. Kimeldorf and G. Wahba. Some results on Tchebycheffian spline functions. *J. Math. Anal. Appl.*, 33:82–95, 1971.

[11] J. Nocedal and S. J. Wright. *Numerical Optimization*. Springer, 1999.

[12] R. Rifkin and A. Klautau. In defense of one-vs-all classification. *J. Mach. Learn. Res.*, 5:101–141, 2004.

[13] K. Crammer and Y. Singer. On the algorithmic implementation of multiclass kernel-based vector machines. *J. Mach. Learn. Res.*, 2:265–292, 2001.

[14] C-C. Chang and C-J. Lin. *LIBSVM: a library for support vector machines*, 2001. Software available at http://www.csie.ntu.edu.tw/~cjlin/libsvm.

[15] T. Joachims. Making large-scale support vector machine learning practical. In *Advances in Kernel Methods: Support Vector Machines*. MIT Press, Cambridge, MA, 1998.

[16] S. Thrun. Lifelong learning: A case study. CMU tech report CS-95-208, 1995.

[17] R. Caruana. Multitask learning. *Machine Learning*, 28(1):41–75, 1997.

[18] P. N. Bennett, S. T. Dumais, and E. Horvitz. Inductive transfer for text classification using generalized reliability indicators. In *Proceedings of ICML Workshop on The Continuum from Labeled to Unlabeled Data in Machine Learning and Data Mining*, 2003.

[19] J. Teevan and D. R. Karger. Empirical development of an exponential probabilistic model for text retrieval: Using textual analysis to build a better model. In *SIGIR '03*, 2003.

[20] S. Thrun and J. O'Sullivan. Discovering structure in multiple learning tasks: The TC algorithm. In *International Conference on Machine Learning*, pages 489–497, 1996.

A Theoretical Analysis of Robust Coding over Noisy Overcomplete Channels

Eizaburo Doi[1], Doru C. Balcan[2], & Michael S. Lewicki[1,2]
[1]Center for the Neural Basis of Cognition,
[2]Computer Science Department,
Carnegie Mellon University, Pittsburgh, PA 15213
{edoi,dbalcan,lewicki}@cnbc.cmu.edu

Abstract

Biological sensory systems are faced with the problem of encoding a high-fidelity sensory signal with a population of noisy, low-fidelity neurons. This problem can be expressed in information theoretic terms as coding and transmitting a multi-dimensional, analog signal over a set of noisy channels. Previously, we have shown that robust, overcomplete codes can be learned by minimizing the reconstruction error with a constraint on the channel capacity. Here, we present a theoretical analysis that characterizes the optimal linear coder and decoder for one- and two-dimensional data. The analysis allows for an arbitrary number of coding units, thus including both under- and over-complete representations, and provides a number of important insights into optimal coding strategies. In particular, we show how the form of the code adapts to the number of coding units and to different data and noise conditions to achieve robustness. We also report numerical solutions for robust coding of high-dimensional image data and show that these codes are substantially more robust compared against other image codes such as ICA and wavelets.

1 Introduction

In neural systems, the representational capacity of a single neuron is estimated to be as low as 1 bit/spike [1, 2]. The characteristics of the optimal coding strategy under such conditions, however, remains an open question. Recent efficient coding models for sensory coding such as sparse coding and ICA have provided many insights into visual sensory coding (for a review, see [3]), but those models made the implicit assumption that the representational capacity of individual neurons was infinite. Intuitively, such a limit on representational precision should strongly influence the form of the optimal code. In particular, it should be possible to increase the number of limited capacity units in a population to form a more precise representation of the sensory signal. However, to the best of our knowledge, such a code has not been characterized analytically, even in the simplest case.

Here we present a theoretical analysis of this problem for one- and two-dimensional data for arbitrary numbers of units. For simplicity, we assume that the encoder and decoder are both linear, and that the goal is to minimize the mean squared error (MSE) of the reconstruction. In contrast to our previous report, which examined noisy overcomplete representations [4], the cost function does not contain a sparsity prior. This simplification makes the cost depend up to second order statistics, making it analytically tractable while preserving the robustness to noise.

2 The model

To define our model, we assume that the data is N-dimensional, has zero mean and covariance matrix $\Sigma_{\mathbf{x}}$, and define two matrices $\mathbf{W} \in \mathbb{R}^{M \times N}$ and $\mathbf{A} \in \mathbb{R}^{N \times M}$. For each data point $\mathbf{x}$, its representation $\mathbf{r}$ in the model is the linear transform of $\mathbf{x}$ through matrix $\mathbf{W}$, perturbed by the additive noise (i.e., channel noise) $\mathbf{n} \sim \mathcal{N}(\mathbf{0}, \sigma_n^2 \mathbf{I}_M)$:

$$\mathbf{r} = \mathbf{W}\mathbf{x} + \mathbf{n} = \mathbf{u} + \mathbf{n}. \tag{1}$$

We refer to $\mathbf{W}$ as the *encoding matrix* and its row vectors as *encoding vectors*. The reconstruction of a data point from its representation is simply the linear transform of the latter, using matrix $\mathbf{A}$:

$$\hat{\mathbf{x}} = \mathbf{A}\mathbf{r} = \mathbf{A}\mathbf{W}\mathbf{x} + \mathbf{A}\mathbf{n}. \tag{2}$$

We refer to $\mathbf{A}$ as the *decoding matrix* and its column vectors as *decoding vectors*. The term $\mathbf{A}\mathbf{W}\mathbf{x}$ in eq. 2 determines how the reconstruction depends on the data, while $\mathbf{A}\mathbf{n}$ reflects the channel noise in the reconstruction. When there is no channel noise ($\mathbf{n} = \mathbf{0}$), $\mathbf{A}\mathbf{W} = \mathbf{I}$ is equivalent to perfect reconstruction. A graphical description of this system is shown in Fig. 1.

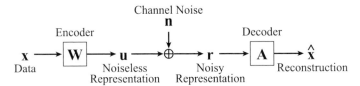

Figure 1: Diagram of the model.

The goal of the system is to form an accurate representation of the data that is robust to the presence of channel noise. We quantify the accuracy of the reconstruction by the mean squared error (MSE) over a set of data. The error of each sample is $\epsilon = \mathbf{x} - \hat{\mathbf{x}} = (\mathbf{I}_N - \mathbf{A}\mathbf{W})\mathbf{x} - \mathbf{A}\mathbf{n}$, and the MSE is expressed in matrix form:

$$\mathcal{E}(\mathbf{A}, \mathbf{W}) = \text{tr}\{(\mathbf{I}_N - \mathbf{A}\mathbf{W})\Sigma_{\mathbf{x}}(\mathbf{I}_N - \mathbf{A}\mathbf{W})^T\} + \sigma_n^2 \text{tr}\{\mathbf{A}\mathbf{A}^T\}, \tag{3}$$

where we used $\mathcal{E} = \langle \epsilon^T \epsilon \rangle = \text{tr}(\langle \epsilon \epsilon^T \rangle)$. Note that, due to the MSE objective along with the zero-mean assumptions, the optimal solution depends solely on second-order statistics of the data and the noise.

Since the SNR is limited in the neural representation [1, 2], we assume that each coding unit has a limited variance $\langle u_i^2 \rangle = \sigma_u^2$ so that the SNR is limited to the same constant value $\gamma^2 = \sigma_u^2/\sigma_n^2$. As the channel capacity of information is defined by $C = \frac{1}{2}\ln(\gamma^2 + 1)$, this is equivalent to limiting the capacity of each unit to the same level. We will call this constraint as *channel capacity constraint*.

Now our problem is to minimize eq. 3 under the channel capacity constraint. To solve it, we will include this constraint in the parametrization of $\mathbf{W}$. Let $\Sigma_{\mathbf{x}} = \mathbf{E}\mathbf{D}\mathbf{E}^T$ be the eigenvalue decomposition of the data covariance matrix, and denote $\mathbf{S} = \mathbf{D}^{\frac{1}{2}} = \text{diag}(\sqrt{\lambda_1}, \cdots, \sqrt{\lambda_M})$, where $\lambda_i \equiv \mathbf{D}_{ii}$ are the $\Sigma_{\mathbf{x}}$'s eigenvalues. As we will see shortly, it is convenient to define $\mathbf{V} \equiv \mathbf{W}\mathbf{E}\mathbf{S}/\sigma_u$, then the condition $\langle u_i^2 \rangle = \sigma_u^2$ implies that

$$\mathbf{V}\mathbf{V}^T = \mathbf{C}_{\mathbf{u}} = \langle \mathbf{u}\mathbf{u}^T \rangle / \sigma_u^2, \tag{4}$$

where $\mathbf{C}_{\mathbf{u}}$ is the correlation matrix of the representation $\mathbf{u}$. Now the problem is formulated as a constrained optimization: finding the parameters that satisfy eq. 4 and minimize $\mathcal{E}$.

3 The optimal solutions and their characteristics

In this section we analyze the optimal solutions in some simple cases, namely for 1-dimensional (1-D) and 2-dimensional (2-D) data.

3.1 1-D data

In the 1-D case the MSE (eq. 3) is expressed as

$$\mathcal{E} = \sigma_x^2(1 - \mathbf{aw})^2 + \sigma_n^2\|\mathbf{a}\|_2^2, \tag{5}$$

where $\sigma_x^2 = \Sigma_{\mathbf{x}} \in \mathbb{R}$, $\mathbf{a} = \mathbf{A} \in \mathbb{R}^{1 \times M}$ and $\mathbf{w} = \mathbf{W} \in \mathbb{R}^{M \times 1}$. By solving the necessary condition for the minimum, $\partial\mathcal{E}/\partial\mathbf{a} = \mathbf{0}$, with the channel capacity constraint (eq. 4), the entries of the optimal solutions are

$$w_i = \pm\frac{\sigma_u}{\sigma_x}, \quad a_i = \frac{1}{w_i} \cdot \frac{\gamma^2}{M \cdot \gamma^2 + 1}, \tag{6}$$

and the smallest value of the MSE is

$$\mathcal{E} = \frac{\sigma_x^2}{M \cdot \gamma^2 + 1}. \tag{7}$$

This minimum depends on the SNR (γ^2) and on the number of units (M), and it is monotonically decreasing with respect to both. Furthermore, we can compensate for a decrease in SNR by an increase of the number of units. Note that a_i are responsible for this adaptive behavior as w_i do not vary with either γ^2 or M, in the 1-D case. The second term in eq. 5 leads the optimal $\mathbf{a}$ into having as small norm as possible, while the first term prevents it from being arbitrarily small. The optimum is given by the best trade-off between them.

3.2 2-D data

In the 2-D case, the channel capacity constraint (eq. 4) restricts $\mathbf{V}$ such that the row vectors of $\mathbf{V}$ should be on the unit circle. Therefore $\mathbf{V}$ can be parameterized as

$$\mathbf{V} = \begin{pmatrix} \cos\theta_1 & \sin\theta_1 \\ \vdots & \vdots \\ \cos\theta_M & \sin\theta_M \end{pmatrix}, \tag{8}$$

where $\theta_i \in [0, 2\pi)$ is the angle between i-th row of $\mathbf{V}$ and the principal eigenvector of the data $\mathbf{e}_1$ ($\mathbf{E} = [\mathbf{e}_1, \mathbf{e}_2]$, $\lambda_1 \geq \lambda_2 > 0$). The necessary condition for the minimum $\partial\mathcal{E}/\partial\mathbf{A} = \mathbf{O}$ implies

$$\mathbf{A} = \sigma_u\mathbf{E}\mathbf{S}\mathbf{V}^T(\sigma_u^2\mathbf{V}\mathbf{V}^T + \sigma_n^2\mathbf{I}_M)^{-1}. \tag{9}$$

Using eqs. 8 and 9, the MSE can be expressed as

$$\mathcal{E} = \frac{(\lambda_1 + \lambda_2)\left(\frac{2}{M}\gamma^2 + 1\right) - \frac{\gamma^2}{2}(\lambda_1 - \lambda_2)\,\mathrm{Re}(Z)}{\left(\frac{M}{2}\gamma^2 + 1\right)^2 - \frac{1}{4}\gamma^4|Z|^2}, \tag{10}$$

where by definition

$$Z = \sum_{k=1}^{M} z_k = \sum_{k=1}^{M}[\cos(2\theta_k) + i\sin(2\theta_k)]. \tag{11}$$

Now the problem has been reduced to finding simply a complex number Z that minimizes $\mathcal{E}$. Note that Z defines θ_k in $\mathbf{V}$, which in turn defines $\mathbf{W}$ (by definition; see eq. 4) and $\mathbf{A}$ (eq. 9). In the following we analyze the problem in two complementary cases: when the data variance is isotropic (i.e., $\lambda_1 = \lambda_2$), and when it is anisotropic ($\lambda_1 > \lambda_2$). As we will see, the solutions are qualitatively different in these two cases.

3.2.1 Isotropic case

Isotropy of the data variance implies $\lambda_1 = \lambda_2 \equiv \sigma_x^2$, and (without loss of generality) $\mathbf{E} = \mathbf{I}$, which simplifies the MSE (eq. 10) as

$$\mathcal{E} = \frac{2\sigma_x^2 \left(1 + \frac{M}{2}\gamma^2\right)}{\left(\frac{2}{M}\gamma^2 + 1\right)^2 - \frac{1}{4}\gamma^4 |Z|^2}. \tag{12}$$

Therefore, $\mathcal{E}$ is minimized whenever $|Z|^2$ is minimized.

If $M = 1$, $|Z|^2 = |z_1|^2$ is always 1 by definition (eq. 11), yielding the optimal solutions

$$\mathbf{W} = \frac{\sigma_u}{\sigma_x}\mathbf{V}, \quad \mathbf{A} = \frac{\sigma_x}{\sigma_u} \cdot \frac{\gamma^2}{\gamma^2 + 1}\mathbf{V}^T, \tag{13}$$

where $\mathbf{V} = \mathbf{V}(\theta_1)$, $\forall\,\theta_1 \in [0, 2\pi)$. Eq. 13 means that the orientation of the encoding and decoding vectors is arbitrary, and that the length of those vectors is adjusted exactly as in the 1-D case (eq. 6 with $M = 1$; Fig. 2). The minimum MSE is given by

$$\mathcal{E} = \frac{\sigma_x^2}{\gamma^2 + 1} + \sigma_x^2. \tag{14}$$

The first term is the same as in the 1-D case (eq. 7 with $M = 1$), corresponding to the error component along the axis that the encoding/decoding vectors represent, while the second term is the whole data variance along the axis orthogonal to the encoding/decoding vectors, along which no reconstruction is made.

If $M \geq 2$, there exists a set of angles θ_k for which $|Z|^2$ is 0. This can be verified by representing Z in the complex plane (Z-diagram in Fig. 2) and observing that there is always a configuration of connected, unit-length bars that starts from, and ends up at the origin, thus indicating that $Z = |Z|^2 = 0$. Accordingly, the optimal solution is

$$\mathbf{W} = \frac{\sigma_u}{\sigma_x}\mathbf{V}, \quad \mathbf{A} = \frac{\sigma_x}{\sigma_u} \cdot \frac{\gamma^2}{\frac{M}{2}\gamma^2 + 1}\mathbf{V}^T, \tag{15}$$

where the optimal $\mathbf{V} = \mathbf{V}(\theta_1, \cdots, \theta_M)$ is given by such $\theta_1, \ldots, \theta_M$ for which $Z = 0$. Specifically, if $M = 2$, then z_1 and z_2 must be antiparallel but are not otherwise constrained, making the pair of decoding vectors (and that of encoding vectors) orthogonal, yet free to rotate. Note that both the encoding and the decoding vectors are parallel to the rows of $\mathbf{V}$ (eq. 15), and the angle of z_k from the real axis is twice as large as that of $\mathbf{a}_k$ (or $\mathbf{w}_k$). Likewise, if $M = 3$, the decoding vectors should be evenly distributed yet still free to rotate; if $M = 4$, the four vectors should just be two pairs of orthogonal vectors (not necessarily evenly distributed); if $M \geq 5$, there is no obvious regularity. With $Z = 0$, the MSE is minimized as

$$\mathcal{E} = \frac{2\sigma_x^2}{\frac{M}{2}\gamma^2 + 1}. \tag{16}$$

The minimum MSE (eq. 16) depends on the SNR (γ^2) and overcompleteness ratio (M/N) exactly in the same manner as explained in the 1-D case (eq. 7), considering that in both cases the numerator is the data variance, $\mathrm{tr}(\Sigma_x)$. We present examples in Fig 2: given $M = 2$, the reconstruction gets worse by lowering the SNR from 10 to 1; however, the reconstruction can be improved by increasing the number of units for a fixed SNR ($\gamma^2 = 1$). Just as in the 1-D case, the norm of the decoding vectors gets smaller by increasing M or decreasing γ^2, which is explicitly described by eq. 15.

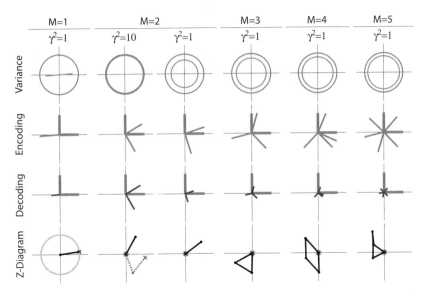

Figure 2: The optimal solutions for isotropic data. M is the number of units and γ^2 is the SNR in the representation. "Variance" shows the variance ellipses for the data (gray) and the reconstruction (magenta). For perfect reconstruction, the two ellipses should overlap. "Encoding" and "Decoding" show encoding vectors (red) and decoding vectors (blue), respectively. The gray vectors show the principal axes of the data, $\mathbf{e}_1$ and $\mathbf{e}_2$. "Z-Diagram" represents $Z = \Sigma_k z_k$ (eq. 11) in the complex plane, where each unit length bar corresponds to a z_k, and the end point indicated by "×" represents the coordinates of Z. The set of green dots in a plot corresponds to optimal values of Z; when this set reduces to a single dot, the optimal Z is unique. In general there could be multiple configurations of bars for a single Z, implying multiple equivalent solutions of $\mathbf{A}$ and $\mathbf{W}$ for a given Z. For $M = 2$ and $\gamma^2 = 10$, we drew with gray dotted bars an example of Z that is not optimal (corresponding encoding and decoding vectors not shown).

3.2.2 Anisotropic case

In the anisotropic condition $\lambda_1 > \lambda_2$, the MSE (eq. 10) is minimized when $Z = \mathrm{Re}(Z) \geq 0$ for a fixed value of $|Z|^2$. Therefore, the problem is reduced to seeking a real value $Z = y \in [0, M]$ that minimizes

$$\mathcal{E} = \frac{(\lambda_1 + \lambda_2)\left(\frac{M}{2}\gamma^2 + 1\right) - \frac{\gamma^2}{2}(\lambda_1 - \lambda_2)\,y}{\left(\frac{M}{2}\gamma^2 + 1\right)^2 - \frac{1}{4}\gamma^4 y^2}. \tag{17}$$

If $M = 1$, then $y = \cos 2\theta_1$ from eq. 11, and therefore, $\mathcal{E}$ in eq. 17 is minimized iff $\theta_1 = 0$, yielding the optimal solutions

$$\mathbf{W} = \frac{\sigma_u}{\sqrt{\lambda_1}}\mathbf{e}_1^T, \quad \mathbf{A} = \frac{\sqrt{\lambda_1}}{\sigma_u} \cdot \frac{\gamma^2}{\gamma^2 + 1}\mathbf{e}_1. \tag{18}$$

In contrast to the isotropic case with $M = 1$, the encoding and decoding vectors are specified along the principal axis ($\mathbf{e}_1$) as illustrated in Fig. 3. The minimum MSE is

$$\mathcal{E} = \frac{\lambda_1}{\gamma^2 + 1} + \lambda_2. \tag{19}$$

This is the same form as in the isotropic case (eq. 14) except that the first term is now related to the variance along the principal axis, λ_1, by which the encoding/decoding vectors can most effectively be utilized for representing the data, while the second term is specified as the data variance along the minor axis, λ_2, by which the loss of reconstruction is mostly minimized. Note that it is a similar mechanism of dimensionality reduction as using PCA.

If $M \geq 2$, then we can derive the optimal y from the necessary condition for the minimum, $d\mathcal{E}/dy = 0$, which yields

$$\left[\frac{\sqrt{\lambda_1} - \sqrt{\lambda_2}}{\sqrt{\lambda_1} + \sqrt{\lambda_2}} \left(M + \frac{2}{\gamma^2} \right) - y \right] \left[\frac{\sqrt{\lambda_1} + \sqrt{\lambda_2}}{\sqrt{\lambda_1} - \sqrt{\lambda_2}} \left(M + \frac{2}{\gamma^2} \right) - y \right] = 0. \tag{20}$$

Let γ_c^2 denote the SNR critical point, where

$$\gamma_c^2 = (\sqrt{\lambda_1/\lambda_2} - 1)/M. \tag{21}$$

If $\gamma^2 \geq \gamma_c^2$, then eq. 20 has a root within its domain $[0, M]$,

$$y = \frac{\sqrt{\lambda_1} - \sqrt{\lambda_2}}{\sqrt{\lambda_1} + \sqrt{\lambda_2}} \left(\frac{2}{\gamma^2} + M \right), \tag{22}$$

with $y = M$ if $\gamma^2 = \gamma_c^2$. Accordingly the optimal solutions are given by

$$\mathbf{W} = \mathbf{V} \begin{pmatrix} \sigma_u/\sqrt{\lambda_1} & 0 \\ 0 & \sigma_u/\sqrt{\lambda_2} \end{pmatrix} \mathbf{E}^T, \quad \mathbf{A} = \frac{\sqrt{\lambda_1} + \sqrt{\lambda_2}}{2\sigma_u} \cdot \frac{\gamma^2}{\frac{M}{2}\gamma^2 + 1} \mathbf{E}\mathbf{V}^T, \tag{23}$$

where the optimal $\mathbf{V} = \mathbf{V}(\theta_1, \cdots, \theta_M)$ is given by the Z-diagram as illustrated in Fig. 3, which we will describe shortly. The minimum MSE is given by

$$\mathcal{E} = \frac{1}{\frac{M}{2}\gamma^2 + 1} \frac{(\sqrt{\lambda_1} + \sqrt{\lambda_2})^2}{2}. \tag{24}$$

Note that eqs. 23–24 are reduced to eqs. 15–16 if $\lambda_1 = \lambda_2$.

If the SNR is smaller than γ_c^2, then $d\mathcal{E}/dy = 0$ does not have a root within the domain. However, $d\mathcal{E}/dy$ is always negative, and hence, $\mathcal{E}$ decreases monotonically on $[0, M]$. The minimum is therefore obtained when $y = M$, yielding the optimal solutions

$$\mathbf{W} = \frac{\sigma_u}{\sqrt{\lambda_1}} \mathbf{1}_M \mathbf{e}_1^T, \quad \mathbf{A} = \frac{\sqrt{\lambda_1}}{\sigma_u} \cdot \frac{\gamma^2}{M\gamma^2 + 1} \mathbf{e}_1 \mathbf{1}_M^T, \tag{25}$$

where $\mathbf{1}_M = (1, \cdots, 1)^T \in \mathbb{R}^M$, and the minimum is given by

$$\mathcal{E} = \frac{\lambda_1}{M\gamma^2 + 1} + \lambda_2. \tag{26}$$

Note that $\mathcal{E}$ takes the same form as in $M = 1$ (eq. 19) except that we can now decrease the error by increasing the number of units. To summarize, if the representational resource is too limited either by M or γ^2, the best strategy is to represent only the principal axis.

Now we describe the optimal solutions using the Z-diagram (Fig. 3). First, the optimal solutions differ depending on the SNR. If $\gamma^2 > \gamma_c^2$, the optimal Z is a certain point between 0 and M on the real axis. Specifically, for $M = 2$ the optimal configuration of the unit-length connected bars is unique (up to flipping about x-axis), meaning that the encoding/decoding vectors are symmetric about the principal axis; for $M \geq 3$, there are infinitely many configurations of the bars starting from the origin and ending at the optimal Z, and nothing can be added about their regularity. If $\gamma^2 \leq \gamma_c^2$, the optimal Z is M, and the optimal configuration is obtained only when all the bars align on the real axis. In this case, encoding/decoding vectors are all parallel to the principal axis ($\mathbf{e}_1$), as described by eq. 25. Such a degenerate representation is unique for the anisotropic case and is determined by γ_c^2 (eq. 21). We can

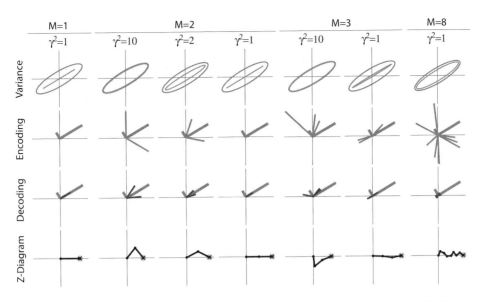

Figure 3: The optimal solutions for anisotropic data. Notations are as in Fig. 2. We set $\lambda_1 = 1.87$ and $\lambda_2 = 0.13$. $\gamma^2 > \gamma_c^2$ holds for all $M \geq 2$ but the one with $M = 2$ and $\gamma^2 = 1$.

avoid the degeneration either by increasing the SNR (e.g., Fig. 3, $M = 2$ with different γ^2) or by increasing the number of units ($\gamma^2 = 1$ with different M).

Also, the optimal solutions for the overcomplete representation are, in general, not obtained by simple replication (except in the degenerate case). For example, for $\gamma^2 = 1$ in Fig. 3, the optimal solution for $M = 8$ is not identical to the replication of the optimal solution for $M = 2$, and we can formally prove it by using eq. 22.

For $M = 1$ and for the degenerate case, where only one axis in two dimensional space is represented, the optimal strategy is to preserve information along the principal axis at the cost of losing all information along the minor axis. Such a biased representation is also found for the non-degenerate case. We can see in Fig. 3 that the data along the principal axis is more accurately reconstructed than that along the minor axis; if there is no bias, the ellipse for the reconstruction should be similar to that of the data. More precisely, we can prove that the error ratio along e_1 is smaller than that along e_2 at the ratio of $\sqrt{\lambda_2} : \sqrt{\lambda_1}$ (note the switch of the subscripts), which describes the representation bias toward the main axis.

4   Application to image coding

In the case of high-dimensional data we can employ an algorithm similar to the one in [4], to numerically compute optimal solutions that minimizes the MSE subject to the channel capacity constraint. Fig. 4 presents the performance of our model when applied to image coding in the presence of channel noise. The data were 8×8 pixel blocks taken from a large image, and for comparison we considered representations with $M = 64$ ("1×") and respectively, 512 ("8×") units. As for the channel capacity, each unit has 1.0 bit precision as in the neural representation [1]. The robust coding model shows a dramatic reduction in the reconstruction error, when compared to alternatives such as ICA and wavelet codes. This underscores the importance of taking into account the channel capacity constraint for better understanding the neural representation.

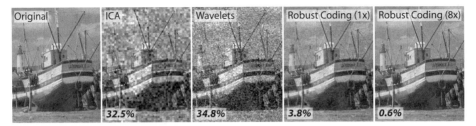

Figure 4: Reconstruction using one bit channel capacity representations. To ensure that all models had the same precision of 1.0 bit for each coefficient, we added Gaussian noise to the coefficients of the ICA and "Daubechies 9/7" wavelet codes as in the robust coding. For each representation, we displayed percentage error of the reconstruction. The results are consistent using other images, block size, or wavelet filters.

5 Discussion

In this study we measured the accuracy of the reconstruction by the MSE. An alternative measure could be, as in [5, 3], mutual information $I(\mathbf{x}, \hat{\mathbf{x}})$ between the data and the reconstruction. However, we can prove that this measure does not yield optimal solutions for the robust coding problem. Assuming the data is Gaussian and the representation is complete, we can prove that the mutual information is upper-bounded,

$$I(\mathbf{x}, \hat{\mathbf{x}}) = \frac{1}{2} \ln \det(\gamma^2 \mathbf{V}\mathbf{V}^T + \mathbf{I}_N) \leq \frac{N}{2} \ln(\gamma^2 + 1), \qquad (27)$$

with equality iff $\mathbf{V}\mathbf{V}^T = \mathbf{I}$, i.e., when the representation $\mathbf{u}$ is whitened (see eq. 4). This result holds even for anisotropic data, which is different from the optimal MSE code that can employ correlated, or even degenerate, representation. As ICA is one form of whitening, the results in Fig. 4 demonstrate the suboptimality of whitening in the MSE sense.

The optimal MSE code over noisy channels was examined previously in [6] for N-dimensional data. However, the capacity constraint was defined for a population and only examined the case of undercomplete codes. In the model studied here, motivated by the neural representation, the capacity constraint is imposed for individual units. Furthermore, the model allows for arbitrary number of units, which provides a way to arbitrarily improve the robustness of the code using a population code. The theoretical analysis for one- and two-dimensional cases quantifies the amount of error reduction as a function of the SNR and the number of units along with the data covariance matrix. Finally, our numerical results for higher-dimensional image data demonstrate a dramatic improvement in the robustness of the code over both conventional transforms such as wavelets and also representations optimized for statistical efficiency such as ICA.

References

[1] A. Borst and F. E. Theunissen. Information theory and neural coding. *Nature Neuroscience*, 2:947–957, 1999.

[2] N. K. Dhingra and R. G. Smith. Spike generator limits efficiency of information transfer in a retinal ganglion cell. *Journal of Neuroscience*, 24:2914–2922, 2004.

[3] A. Hyvarinen, J. Karhunen, and E. Oja. *Independent Component Analysis*. Wiley, 2001.

[4] E. Doi and M. S. Lewicki. Sparse coding of natural images using an overcomplete set of limited capacity units. In *Advances in NIPS*, volume 17, pages 377–384. MIT Press, 2005.

[5] J. J. Atick and A. N. Redlich. What does the retina know about natural scenes? *Neural Computation*, 4:196–210, 1992.

[6] K. I. Diamantaras, K. Hornik, and M. G. Strintzis. Optimal linear compression under unreliable representation and robust PCA neural models. *IEEE Trans. Neur. Netw.*, 10(5):1186–1195, 1999.

Optimizing spatio-temporal filters for improving Brain-Computer Interfacing

Guido Dornhege[1], Benjamin Blankertz[1], Matthias Krauledat[1,3],
Florian Losch[2], Gabriel Curio[2] and Klaus-Robert Müller[1,3]

[1]Fraunhofer FIRST.IDA, Kekuléstr. 7, 12 489 Berlin, Germany
[2]Campus Benjamin Franklin, Charité University Medicine Berlin,
Hindenburgdamm 30, 12 203 Berlin, Germany.
[3]University of Potsdam, August-Bebel-Str. 89, 14 482 Germany
{dornhege,blanker,kraulem,klaus}@first.fhg.de,
{florian-philip.losch,gabriel.curio}@charite.de

Abstract

Brain-Computer Interface (BCI) systems create a novel communication channel from the brain to an output device by bypassing conventional motor output pathways of nerves and muscles. Therefore they could provide a new communication and control option for paralyzed patients. Modern BCI technology is essentially based on techniques for the classification of single-trial brain signals. Here we present a novel technique that allows the simultaneous optimization of a spatial and a spectral filter enhancing discriminability of multi-channel EEG single-trials. The evaluation of 60 experiments involving 22 different subjects demonstrates the superiority of the proposed algorithm. Apart from the enhanced classification, the spatial and/or the spectral filter that are determined by the algorithm can also be used for further analysis of the data, e.g., for source localization of the respective brain rhythms.

1 Introduction

Brain-Computer Interface (BCI) research aims at the development of a system that allows direct control of, e.g., a computer application or a neuroprosthesis, solely by human intentions as reflected in suitable brain signals, cf. [1, 2, 3, 4, 5, 6, 7, 8, 9]. We will be focussing on noninvasive, electroencephalogram (EEG) based BCI systems. Such devices can be used as tools of communication for the disabled or for healthy subjects that might be interested in exploring a new path of man-machine interfacing, say when playing BCI operated computer games.

The classical approach to establish EEG-based control is to set up a system that is controlled by a specific EEG feature which is known to be susceptible to conditioning and to let the subjects learn the voluntary control of that feature. In contrast, the Berlin Brain-Computer Interface (BBCI) uses well established motor competences in control paradigms and a machine learning approach to extract subject-specific discriminability patterns from high-dimensional features. This approach has the advantage that the long subject training needed in the operant conditioning approach is replaced by a short calibration measurement

315

(20 minutes) and machine training (1 minute). The machine adapts to the specific characteristics of the brain signals of each subject, accounting for the high inter-subject variability. With respect to the topographic patterns of brain rhythm modulations the Common Spatial Patterns (CSP) (see [10]) algorithm has proven to be very useful to extract subject-specific, discriminative spatial filters. On the other hand the frequency band on which the CSP algorithm operates is either selected manually or unspecifically set to a broad band filter, cf. [10, 5]. Obviously, a simultaneous optimization of a frequency filter with the spatial filter is highly desirable. Recently, in [11] the CSSP algorithm was presented, in which very simple frequency filters (with one delay tap) for each channel are optimized together with the spatial filters. Although the results showed an improvement of the CSSP algorithm over CSP, the flexibility of the frequency filters is very limited. Here we present a method that allows to simultaneously optimize an arbitrary FIR filter within the CSP analysis. The proposed algorithm outperforms CSP and CSSP on average, and in cases where a separation of the discriminative rhythm from dominating non-discriminative rhythms is of importance, a considerable increase of classification accuracy can be achieved.

2 Experimental Setup

In this paper we investigate data from 60 EEG experiments with 22 different subjects. All experiments included so called training sessions which are used to train subject-specific classifiers. Many experiments also included feedback sessions in which the subject could steer a cursor or play a computer game like *brain-pong* by BCI control. Data from feedback sessions are not used in this a-posteriori study since they depend on an intricate interaction of the subject with the original classification algorithm.

In the experimental sessions used for the present study, labeled trials of brain signals were recorded in the following way: The subjects were sitting in a comfortable chair with arms lying relaxed on the armrests. All 4.5–6 seconds one of 3 different visual stimuli indicated for 3–3.5 seconds which mental task the subject should accomplish during that period. The investigated mental tasks were imagined movements of the left hand (*l*), the right hand (*r*), and one foot (*f*). Brain activity was recorded from the scalp with multi-channel EEG amplifiers using 32, 64 resp. 128 channels. Besides EEG channels, we recorded the electromyogram (EMG) from both forearms and the leg as well as horizontal and vertical electrooculogram (EOG) from the eyes. The EMG and EOG channels were used exclusively to make sure that the subjects performed no real limb or eye movements correlated with the mental tasks that could directly (artifacts) or indirectly (afferent signals from muscles and joint receptors) be reflected in the EEG channels and thus be detected by the classifier, which operates on the EEG signals only. Between 120 and 200 trials for each class were recorded. In this study we investigate only binary classifications, but the results can be expected to safely transfer to the multi-class case.

3 Neurophysiological Background

According to the well established model called homunculus, first described by [12], for each part of the human body there exists a corresponding region in the motor and somatosensory area of the neocortex. The 'mapping' from the body to the respective brain areas preserves in big parts topography, i.e., neighboring parts of the body are almost represented in neighboring parts of the cortex. While the region of the feet is located at the center of the vertex, the left hand is represented lateralized on the right hemisphere and the right hand on the left hemisphere. Brain activity during rest and wakefulness is describable by different rhythms located over different brain areas. These rhythms reflect functional states of different neuronal cortical networks and can be used for brain-computer interfacing. These rhythms are blocked by movements, independent of their active, passive or reflexive origin. Blocking effects are visible bilaterally but pronounced contralaterally in the cortical area that corresponds to the moved limb. This attenuation of brain rhythms is

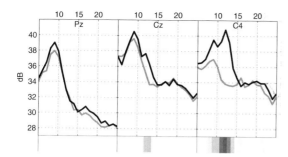

Figure 1: The plot shows the spectra for one subject during left hand (light line) and foot (dark line) motor imagery between 5 and 25 Hz at scalp positions Pz, Cz and C4. In both central channels two peaks, one at 8 Hz and one at 12 Hz are visible. Below each channel the r^2-value which measures discriminability is added. It indicates that the second peak contains more discriminative information.

termed event-related desynchronization (ERD), see [13]. Over sensorimotor cortex a so called idle- or μ-rhythm can be measured in the scalp EEG. The most common frequency band of μ-rhythm is about 10 Hz (precentral α- or μ-rhythm, [14]). Jasper and Penfield ([12]) described a strictly local so called beta-rhythm about 20 Hz over human motor cortex in electrocorticographic recordings. In Scalp EEG recording one can find μ-rhythm over motor areas mixed and superimposed by 20 Hz-activity. In this context μ-rhythm is sometimes interpreted as a subharmonic of cortical faster activity. These brain rhythms described above are of cortical origin but the role of a thalomo-cortical pacemaker has been discussed since the first description of EEG by Berger ([15]) and is still a point of discussion. Lopes da Silva ([16]) showed that cortico-cortical coherence is much larger than thalamo-cortical. However, since the focal ERD in the motor and/or sensory cortex can be observed even when a subject is only imagining a movement or sensation in the specific limb, this feature can well be used for BCI control. The discrimination of the imagination of movements of left hand vs. right hand vs. foot is based on the topography of the attenuation of the μ and/or β rhythm.

There are two problems when using ERD features for BCI control:

(1) The strength of the sensorimotor idle rhythms as measured by scalp EEG is known to vary strongly between subjects. This introduces a high intersubject variability on the accuracy with which an ERD-based BCI system works. There is another feature independent from the ERD reflecting imagined or intended movements, the movement related potentials (MRP), denoting a negative DC shift of the EEG signals in the respective cortical regions. See [17, 18] for an investigation of how this feature can be exploited for BCI use and combined with the ERD feature. This combination strategy was able to greatly enhance classification performance in offline studies. In this paper we focus only on improving the ERD-based classification, but all the improvements presented here can also be used in the combined algorithm.

(2) The precentral μ-rhythm is often superimposed by the much stronger posterior α-rhythm, which is the idle rhythm of the visual system. It is best articulated with eyes closed, but also present in awake and attentive subjects, see Fig. 1 at channel Pz. Due to volume conduction the posterior α-rhythm interferes with the precentral μ-rhythm in the EEG channels over motor cortex. Hence a μ-power based classifier is susceptible to modulations of the posterior α-rhythm that occur due to fatigue, change in attentional focus while performing tasks, or changing demands of visual processing. When the two rhythms have different spectral peaks as in Fig. 1, channels Cz and C4, a suitable frequency filter can help to weaken the interference. The optimization of such a filter integrated in the CSP algorithm is addressed in this paper.

4   Spatial Filter - the CSP Algorithm

The common spatial pattern (CSP) algorithm ([19]) is very useful in calculating spatial filters for detecting ERD effects ([20]) and for ERD-based BCIs, see [10], and has been extended to multi-class problems in [21]. Given two distributions in a high-dimensional space, the (supervised) CSP algorithm finds directions (i.e., spatial filters) that maximize variance for one class and at the same time minimize variance for the other class. After having band-pass filtered the EEG signals to the rhythms of interest, high variance reflects a strong rhythm and low variance a weak (or attenuated) rhythm. Let us take the example of discriminating left hand vs. right hand imagery. According to Sec. 3, the spatial filter that focusses on the area of the left hand is characterized by a strong motor rhythm during imagination of right hand movements (left hand is in idle state), and by an attenuated motor rhythm during left hand imagination.

This criterion is exactly what the CSP algorithm optimizes: maximizing variance for the class of right hand trials and at the same time minimizing variance for left hand trials. Furthermore the CSP algorithm calculates the dual filter that will focus on the area of the right hand (and it will even calculate several filters for both optimizations by considering orthogonal subspaces).

The CSP algorithm is trained on labeled data, i.e., we have a set of trials s_i, $i = 1, 2, ...$, where each trial consists of several channels (as rows) and time points (as columns). A spatial filter $w \in \mathbb{R}^{\#channels}$ projects these trials to the signal $\hat{s}_i(w) = w^\top s_i$ with only one channel. The idea of CSP is to find a spatial filter w such that the projected signal has high variance for one class and low variance for the other. In other words we maximize the variance for one class whereas the sum of the variances of both classes remains constant, which is expressed by the following optimization problem:

$$\max_w \sum_{i:\text{Trial in Class 1}} var(\hat{s}_i(w)), \quad \text{s.t.} \quad \sum_i var(\hat{s}_i(w)) = 1, \tag{1}$$

where $var(\cdot)$ is the variance of the vector. An analoguous formulation can be formed for the second class.

Using the definition of the variance we simplify the problem to

$$\max_w w^\top \Sigma_1 w, \quad s.t. \quad w^\top (\Sigma_1 + \Sigma_2) w = 1, \tag{2}$$

where Σ_y is the covariance matrix of the trial-concatenated matrix of dimension [channels $\times$ concatenated time-points] belonging to the respective class $y \in \{1, 2\}$.

Formulating the dual problem we can find that the problem can be solved by calculating a matrix Q and diagonal matrix D with elements in $[0, 1]$ such that

$$Q\Sigma_1 Q^\top = D \quad \text{and} \quad Q\Sigma_2 Q^\top = I - D \tag{3}$$

and by choosing the highest and lowest eigenvalue.

Equation (3) can be accomplished in the following way. First we *whiten* the matrix $\Sigma_1 + \Sigma_2$, i.e., determine a matrix P such that $P(\Sigma_1 + \Sigma_2)P^\top = I$ which is possible due to positive definiteness of $\Sigma_1 + \Sigma_2$. Then define $\hat{\Sigma}_y = P\Sigma_y P^\top$ and calculate an orthogonal matrix R and a diagonal maxtrix D by spectral theory such that $\hat{\Sigma}_1 = RDR^\top$. Therefore $\hat{\Sigma}_2 = R(I - D)R^\top$ since $\hat{\Sigma}_1 + \hat{\Sigma}_2 = I$ and $Q := R^\top P$ satisfies (3). The projection that is given by the j-th row of matrix R has a relative variance of d_j (j-th element of D) for trials of class 1 and relative variance $1 - d_j$ for trials of class 2. If d_j is near 1 the filter given by the j-th row of R maximizes variance for class 1, and since $1 - d_j$ is near 0, minimizes variance for class 2. Typically one would retain some projections corresponding to the highest eigenvalues d_j, i.e., CSPs for class 1, and some corresponding to the lowest eigenvalues, i.e., CSPs for class 2.

5 Spectral Filter

As discussed in Sec. 3 the content of discriminative information in different frequency bands is highly subject-dependent. For example the subject whose spectra are visualized in Fig. 1 shows a highly discriminative peak at 12 Hz whereas the peak at 8 Hz does not show good discrimination. Since the lower frequency peak is stronger a better performance in classification can be expected, if we reduce the influence of the lower frequency peak for this subject. However, for other subjects the situation looks differently, i.e., the classification might fail if we exclude this information. Thus it is desirable to optimize a spectral filter for better discriminability. Here are two approaches to this task.

CSSP. In [11] the following was suggested: Given s_i the signal s_i^τ is defined to be the signal s_i delayed by τ timepoints. In CSSP the usual CSP approach is applied to the concatenation of s_i and s_i^τ in the channel dimension, i.e., the delayed signals are treated as new channels. By this concatenation step the ability to neglect or emphasize specific frequency bands can be achieved and strongly depends on the choice of τ which can be accomplished by some validation approach on the training set. More complex frequency filters can be found by concatenating more delayed EEG-signals with several delays. In [11] it was concluded that in typical BCI situations where only small training sets are available, the choice of only one delay tap is most effective. The increased flexibility of a frequency filter with more delay taps does not trade off the increased complexity of the optimization problem.

CSSSP. The idea of our new CSSSP algorithm is to learn a complete global spatial-temporal filter in the spirit of CSP and CSSP.

A digital frequency filter consists of two sequences a and b with length n_a and n_b such that the signal x is filtered to y by

$$
\begin{aligned}
a(1)y(t) = \quad & b(1)x(t) + b(2)x(t-1) + \ldots + b(n_b)x(t-n_b-1) \\
- \quad & a(2)y(t-1) - \ldots - a(n_a)y(t-n_a-1)
\end{aligned}
$$

Here we restrict ourselves to FIR (finite impulse response) filters by defining $n_a = 1$ and $a = 1$. Furthermore we define $b(1) = 1$ and fix the length of b to some T with $T > 1$. By this restriction we resign some flexibility of the frequency filter but it allows us to find a suitable solution in the following way: We are looking for a real-valued sequence $b_{1,\ldots,T}$ with $b(1) = 1$ such that the trials

$$
s_{i,b} = s_i + \sum_{\tau=2,\ldots,T} b_\tau s_i^\tau \tag{4}
$$

can be classified better in some way. Using equation (1) we have to solve the problem

$$
\max_{w,b,b(1)=1} \sum_{i:\text{Trial in Class 1}} var(\hat{s}_{i,b}(w)), \quad \text{s.t.} \quad \sum_i var(\hat{s}_{i,b}(w)) = 1, \tag{5}
$$

which can be simplified to

$$
\max_{b,b(1)=1} \max_w \ w^\top \left(\sum_{\tau=0,\ldots,T-1} \left(\sum_{j=1,\ldots,T-\tau} b(j)b(j+\tau) \right) \Sigma_1^\tau \right) w,
$$

$$
\text{s.t.} \quad w^\top \left(\sum_{\tau=0,\ldots,T-1} \left(\sum_{j=1,\ldots,T-\tau} b(j)b(j+\tau) \right) (\Sigma_1^\tau + \Sigma_2^\tau) \right) w = 1. \tag{6}
$$

where $\Sigma_y^\tau = E(\langle s_i(s_i^\tau)^\top + s_i^\tau s_i^\top \mid i : \text{Trial in Class } y\rangle)$, namely the correlation between the signal and the by τ timepoints delayed signal.

Since we can calculate for each b the optimal w by the usual CSP techniques (see equation (2) and (3)) a $(T-1)$-dimensional ($b(1)=1$) problem remains which we can solve with usual line-search optimization techniques if T is not too large.

Consequently we get for each class a frequency band filter and a pattern (or similar to CSP more than one pattern by choosing the next eigenvectors).

However, with increasing T the complexity of the frequency filter has to be controlled in order to avoid overfitting. This control is achieved by introducing a regularization term in

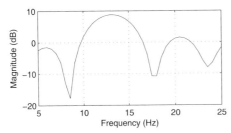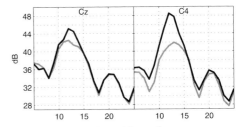

Figure 2: The plot on the left shows one learned frequency filter for the subject whose spectra was shown Fig. 1. In the plot on the right the resulting spectra are visualized after applying the frequency filter on the left. By this technique the classification error could be reduced from 12.9 % to 4.3 %.

the following way:

$$
\max_{b,b(1)=1} \max_{w} \quad w^\top \left(\sum_{\tau=0,\dots,T-1} \left(\sum_{j=1,\dots,T-\tau} b(j)b(j+\tau) \right) \Sigma_1^\tau \right) w - C/T \|b\|_1,
$$

$$
s.t. \quad w^\top \left(\sum_{\tau=0,\dots,T-1} \left(\sum_{j=1,\dots,T-\tau} b(j)b(j+\tau) \right) (\Sigma_1^\tau + \Sigma_2^\tau) \right) w = 1.
$$

(7)

Here C is a non-negative regularization constant, which has to be chosen, e.g., by cross-validation. Since a sparse solution for b is desired, we use the 1-norm in this formulation. With higher C we get sparser solutions for b until at one point the usual CSP approach remains, i.e., $b(1) = 1, b(m) = 0$ for $m > 1$. We call this approach *Common Sparse Spectral Spatial Pattern* (CSSSP) algorithm.

6 Feature Extraction, Classification and Validation

6.1 Feature Extraction

After choosing all channels except the EOG and EMG and a few of the outermost channels of the cap we apply a causal band-pass filter from 7–30 Hz to the data, which encompasses both the μ- and the β-rhythm. For classification we extract the interval 500–3500 ms after the presented visual stimulus. To these trials we apply the original CSP ([10]) algorithm (see Sec. 4), the extended CSSP ([11]), and the proposed CSSSP algorithm (see Sec. 5). For CSSP we choose the best τ by leave-one-out cross validation on the training set. For CSSSP we present the results for different regularization constants C with fixed $T = 16$. Here we use 3 patterns per class which leads to a 6-dimensional output signal. As a measure of the amplitude in the specified frequency band we calculate the logarithm of the variances of the spatio-temporally filtered output signals as feature vectors.

6.2 Classification and Validation

The presented preprocessing reduces the dimensionality of the feature vectors to six. Since we have 120 up to 200 samples per class for each data set, there is no need for regularization when using linear classifiers. When testing non-linear classification methods on these features, we could not observe any statistically significant gain for the given experimental setup when compared to Linear Discriminant Analysis (LDA) (see also [22, 6, 23]). Therefore we choose LDA for classification.

For validation purposes the (chronologically) first half of the data are used as training and the second half as test data.

7 Results

Fig. 2 shows one chosen frequency filter for the subject whose spectra are shown in Fig. 1 and the remaining spectrum after using this filter. As expected the filter detects that there

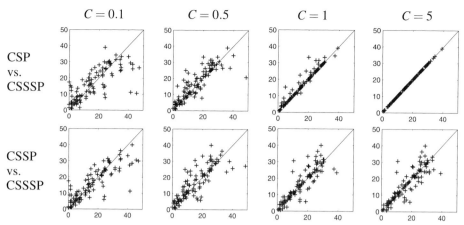

Figure 3: Each plots shows validation error of one algorithm against another, in row 1 that is CSP (*y*-axis) vs. CSSSP (*x*-axis), in row 2 that is CSSP (*y*-axis) vs. CSSSP (*x*-axis). In columns the regularization parameter of CSSSP is varied between 0.1, 0.5, 1 and 5. In each plot a cross above the diagonal marks a dataset where CSSSP outperforms the other algorithm.

is a high discrimination in frequencies at 12 Hz, but only a low discrimination in the frequency band at 8 Hz. Since the lower frequency peak is very predominant for this subject without having a high discrimination power, a filter is learned which drastically decreases the amplitude in this band, whereas full power at 12 Hz is retained.

Applied to all datasets and all pairwise class combinations of the datasets we get the results shown in Fig. 3. Only the results of those datasets are displayed whose classification accuracy exceeds 70 % for at least one classifier. First of all, it is obvious that a small choice of the regularization constant is problematic, since the algorithm tends to overfit. For high values CSSSP tends towards the CSP performance since using frequency filters is punished too hard. In between there is a range where CSSSP is better than CSP. Furthermore there are some datasets where the gain by CSSSP is huge.

Compared to CSSP the situation is similar, namely that CSSSP outperforms the CSSP in many cases and on average, but there are also a few cases, where CSSP is better.

An open issue is the choice of the parameter C. If we choose it constant at 1 for all datasets the figure shows that CSSSP will typically outperform CSP. Compared to CSSP both cases appear, namely that CSSP is better than CSSSP and vice versa.

A more refined way is to choose C individually for each dataset. One way to accomplish this choice is to perform cross-validations for a set of possible values of C and to select the C with minimum cross-validation error. We have done this, for example, for the dataset whose spectra are shown in Fig. 1. Here on the training set for C the value 0.3 is chosen. The classification error of CSSSP with this C is 4.3 %, whereas CSP has 12.9 % and CSSP 8.6 % classification error.

8   Concluding discussion

In past BCI research the CSP algorithm has proven to be very sucessful in determining spatial filters which extract discriminative brain rhythms. However the performance can suffer when a non-discriminative brain rhythm with an overlapping frequency range interferes. The presented CSSSP algorithm successful solves such problematic situations by optimizing simultaneously with the spatial filters a spectral filter. The trade-off between flexibility of the estimated frequency filter and the danger of overfitting is accounted for by a sparsity constraint which is weighted by a regularization constant. The successfulness of the proposed algorithm when compared to the original CSP and to the CSSP algorithm was demonstrated on a corpus of 60 EEG data sets recorded from 22 different subjects.

Acknowledgments   We thank S. Lemm for helpful discussions.   The studies were supported by BMBF-grants FKZ 01IBB02A and FKZ 01IBB02B, by the *Deutsche Forschungsgemeinschaft* (DFG), FOR 375/B1 and by the PASCAL Network of Excellence (EU # 506778).

References

[1] J. R. Wolpaw, N. Birbaumer, D. J. McFarland, G. Pfurtscheller, and T. M. Vaughan, "Brain-computer interfaces for communication and control", *Clin. Neurophysiol.*, 113: 767–791, 2002.

[2] E. A. Curran and M. J. Stokes, "Learning to control brain activity: A review of the production and control of EEG components for driving brain-computer interface (BCI) systems", *Brain Cogn.*, 51: 326–336, 2003.

[3] A. Kübler, B. Kotchoubey, J. Kaiser, J. Wolpaw, and N. Birbaumer, "Brain-Computer Communication: Unlocking the Locked In", *Psychol. Bull.*, 127(3): 358–375, 2001.

[4] N. Birbaumer, N. Ghanayim, T. Hinterberger, I. Iversen, B. Kotchoubey, A. Kübler, J. Perelmouter, E. Taub, and H. Flor, "A spelling device for the paralysed", *Nature*, 398: 297–298, 1999.

[5] G. Pfurtscheller, C. Neuper, C. Guger, W. Harkam, R. Ramoser, A. Schlögl, B. Obermaier, and M. Pregenzer, "Current Trends in Graz Brain-computer Interface (BCI)", *IEEE Trans. Rehab. Eng.*, 8(2): 216–219, 2000.

[6] B. Blankertz, G. Curio, and K.-R. Müller, "Classifying Single Trial EEG: Towards Brain Computer Interfacing", in: T. G. Diettrich, S. Becker, and Z. Ghahramani, eds., *Advances in Neural Inf. Proc. Systems (NIPS 01)*, vol. 14, 157–164, 2002.

[7] L. Trejo, K. Wheeler, C. Jorgensen, R. Rosipal, S. Clanton, B. Matthews, A. Hibbs, R. Matthews, and M. Krupka, "Multimodal Neuroelectric Interface Development", *IEEE Trans. Neural Sys. Rehab. Eng.*, (11): 199–204, 2003.

[8] L. Parra, C. Alvino, A. C. Tang, B. A. Pearlmutter, N. Yeung, A. Osman, and P. Sajda, "Linear spatial integration for single trial detection in encephalography", *NeuroImage*, 7(1): 223–230, 2002.

[9] W. D. Penny, S. J. Roberts, E. A. Curran, and M. J. Stokes, "EEG-Based Communication: A Pattern Recognition Approach", *IEEE Trans. Rehab. Eng.*, 8(2): 214–215, 2000.

[10] H. Ramoser, J. Müller-Gerking, and G. Pfurtscheller, "Optimal spatial filtering of single trial EEG during imagined hand movement", *IEEE Trans. Rehab. Eng.*, 8(4): 441–446, 2000.

[11] S. Lemm, B. Blankertz, G. Curio, and K.-R. Müller, "Spatio-Spectral Filters for Improved Classification of Single Trial EEG", *IEEE Trans. Biomed. Eng.*, 52(9): 1541–1548, 2005.

[12] H. Jasper and W. Penfield, "Electrocorticograms in man: Effects of voluntary movement upon the electrical activity of the precentral gyrus", *Arch. Psychiat. Nervenkr.*, 183: 163–174, 1949.

[13] G. Pfurtscheller and F. H. L. da Silva, "Event-related EEG/MEG synchronization and desynchronization: basic principles", *Clin. Neurophysiol.*, 110(11): 1842–1857, 1999.

[14] H. Jasper and H. Andrews, "Normal differentiation of occipital and precentral regions in man", *Arch. Neurol. Psychiat. (Chicago)*, 39: 96–115, 1938.

[15] H. Berger, "Über das Elektroenkephalogramm des Menschen", *Arch. Psychiat. Nervenkr.*, 99(6): 555–574, 1933.

[16] F. H. da Silva, T. H. van Lierop, C. F. Schrijer, and W. S. van Leeuwen, "Organization of thalamic and cortical alpha rhythm: Spectra and coherences", *Electroencephalogr. Clin. Neurophysiol.*, 35: 627–640, 1973.

[17] G. Dornhege, B. Blankertz, G. Curio, and K.-R. Müller, "Combining Features for BCI", in: S. Becker, S. Thrun, and K. Obermayer, eds., *Advances in Neural Inf. Proc. Systems (NIPS 02)*, vol. 15, 1115–1122, 2003.

[18] G. Dornhege, B. Blankertz, G. Curio, and K.-R. Müller, "Increase Information Transfer Rates in BCI by CSP Extension to Multi-class", in: S. Thrun, L. Saul, and B. Schölkopf, eds., *Advances in Neural Information Processing Systems*, vol. 16, 733–740, MIT Press, Cambridge, MA, 2004.

[19] K. Fukunaga, *Introduction to Statistical Pattern Recognition*, Academic Press, San Diego, 2nd edn., 1990.

[20] Z. J. Koles and A. C. K. Soong, "EEG source localization: implementing the spatio-temporal decomposition approach", *Electroencephalogr. Clin. Neurophysiol.*, 107: 343–352, 1998.

[21] G. Dornhege, B. Blankertz, G. Curio, and K.-R. Müller, "Boosting bit rates in non-invasive EEG single-trial classifications by feature combination and multi-class paradigms", *IEEE Trans. Biomed. Eng.*, 51(6): 993–1002, 2004.

[22] K.-R. Müller, C. W. Anderson, and G. E. Birch, "Linear and Non-Linear Methods for Brain-Computer Interfaces", *IEEE Trans. Neural Sys. Rehab. Eng.*, 11(2): 165–169, 2003.

[23] B. Blankertz, G. Dornhege, C. Schäfer, R. Krepki, J. Kohlmorgen, K.-R. Müller, V. Kunzmann, F. Losch, and G. Curio, "Boosting Bit Rates and Error Detection for the Classification of Fast-Paced Motor Commands Based on Single-Trial EEG Analysis", *IEEE Trans. Neural Sys. Rehab. Eng.*, 11(2): 127–131, 2003.

Correcting sample selection bias in maximum entropy density estimation

Miroslav Dudík, Robert E. Schapire
Princeton University
Department of Computer Science
35 Olden St, Princeton, NJ 08544
{mdudik,schapire}@princeton.edu

Steven J. Phillips
AT&T Labs − Research
180 Park Ave, Florham Park, NJ 07932
phillips@research.att.com

Abstract

We study the problem of maximum entropy density estimation in the presence of known sample selection bias. We propose three bias correction approaches. The first one takes advantage of unbiased sufficient statistics which can be obtained from biased samples. The second one estimates the biased distribution and then factors the bias out. The third one approximates the second by only using samples from the sampling distribution. We provide guarantees for the first two approaches and evaluate the performance of all three approaches in synthetic experiments and on real data from species habitat modeling, where maxent has been successfully applied and where sample selection bias is a significant problem.

1 Introduction

We study the problem of estimating a probability distribution, particularly in the context of species habitat modeling. It is very common in distribution modeling to assume access to independent samples from the distribution being estimated. In practice, this assumption is violated for various reasons. For example, habitat modeling is typically based on known occurrence locations derived from collections in natural history museums and herbariums as well as biological surveys [1, 2, 3]. Here, the goal is to predict the species' distribution as a function of climatic and other environmental variables. To achieve this in a statistically sound manner using current methods, it is necessary to assume that the sampling distribution and species distributions are not correlated. In fact, however, most sampling is done in locations that are easier to access, such as areas close to towns, roads, airports or waterways [4]. Furthermore, the independence assumption may not hold since roads and waterways are often correlated with topography and vegetation which influence species distributions. New unbiased sampling may be expensive, so much can be gained by using the extensive existing biased data, especially since it is becoming freely available online [5].

Although the available data may have been collected in a biased manner, we usually have some information available about the nature of the bias. For instance, in the case of habitat modeling, some factors influencing the sampling distribution are well known, such as distance from roads, towns, etc. In addition, a list of visited sites may be available and viewed as a sample of the sampling distribution itself. If such a list is not available, the set of sites where any species from a large group has been observed may be a reasonable approximation of all visited locations.

In this paper, we study probability density estimation under sample selection bias. We assume that the sampling distribution (or an approximation) is known during *training*, but we require that unbiased models not use any knowledge of sample selection bias during *testing*. This requirement is vital for habitat modeling where models are often applied to a different region or under different climatic conditions. To our knowledge this is the first work addressing sample selection bias in a statistically sound manner and in a setup suitable for species habitat modeling from presence-only data.

We propose three approaches that incorporate sample selection bias in a common density estimation technique based on the principle of maximum entropy (maxent). Maxent with ℓ_1-regularization has been successfully used to model geographic distributions of species under the assumption that samples are unbiased [3]. We review ℓ_1-regularized maxent with unbiased data in Section 2, and give details of the new approaches in Section 3.

Our three approaches make simple modifications to unbiased maxent and achieve analogous provable performance guarantees. The first approach uses a bias correction technique similar to that of Zadrozny et al. [6, 7] to obtain unbiased confidence intervals from biased samples as required by our version of maxent. We prove that, as in the unbiased case, this produces models whose log loss approaches that of the best possible Gibbs distribution (with increasing sample size).

In contrast, the second approach we propose first estimates the biased distribution and then factors the bias out. When the target distribution is a Gibbs distribution, the solution again approaches the log loss of the target distribution. When the target distribution is not Gibbs, we demonstrate that the second approach need not produce the optimal Gibbs distribution (with respect to log loss) even in the limit of infinitely many samples. However, we prove that it produces models that are almost as good as the best Gibbs distribution according to a certain Bregman divergence that depends on the selection bias. In addition, we observe good empirical performance for moderate sample sizes. The third approach is an approximation of the second approach which uses samples from the sampling distribution instead of the distribution itself.

One of the challenges in studying methods for correcting sample selection bias is that unbiased data sets, though not required during training, are needed as test sets to evaluate performance. Unbiased data sets are difficult to obtain — this is the very reason why we study this problem! Thus, it is almost inevitable that synthetic data must be used. In Section 4, we describe experiments evaluating performance of the three methods. We use both fully synthetic data, as well as a biological dataset consisting of a biased training set and an independently collected reasonably unbiased test set.

Related work. Sample selection bias also arises in econometrics where it stems from factors such as attrition, nonresponse and self selection [8, 9, 10]. It has been extensively studied in the context of linear regression after Heckman's seminal paper [8] in which the bias is first estimated and then a transform of the estimate is used as an additional regressor.

In the machine learning community, sample selection bias has been recently considered for classification problems by Zadrozny [6]. Here the goal is to learn a decision rule from a biased sample. The problem is closely related to cost-sensitive learning [11, 7] and the same techniques such as resampling or differential weighting of samples apply.

However, the methods of the previous two approaches do not apply directly to density estimation where the setup is "unconditional", i.e. there is no dependent variable, or, in the classification terminology, we only have access to positive examples, and the cost function (log loss) is unbounded. In addition, in the case of modeling species habitats, we face the challenge of sample sizes that are very small (2–100) by machine learning standards.

2 Maxent setup

In this section, we describe the setup for unbiased maximum entropy density estimation and review performance guarantees. We use a relaxed formulation which will yield an ℓ_1-regularization term in our objective function.

The goal is to estimate an unknown *target distribution* π over a known *sample space* $\mathcal{X}$ based on *samples* $x_1, \ldots, x_m \in \mathcal{X}$. We assume that samples are independently distributed according to π and denote the *empirical distribution* by $\tilde{\pi}(x) = |\{1 \leq i \leq m : x_i = x\}|/m$. The structure of the problem is specified by real valued functions $f_j : \mathcal{X} \to \mathbb{R}$, $j = 1, \ldots, n$, called *features* and by a distribution q_0 representing a *default estimate*. We assume that features capture all the relevant information available for the problem at hand and q_0 is the distribution we would choose if we were given no samples. The distribution q_0 is most often assumed uniform.

For a limited number of samples, we expect that $\tilde{\pi}$ will be a poor estimate of π under any reasonable distance measure. However, empirical averages of features will not be too different from their expectations with respect to π. Let $p[f]$ denote the expectation of a function $f(x)$ when x is chosen randomly according to distribution p. We would like to find a distribution p which satisfies

$$|p[f_j] - \tilde{\pi}[f_j]| \leq \beta_j \text{ for all } 1 \leq j \leq n, \tag{1}$$

for some estimates β_j of deviations of empirical averages from their expectations. Usually there will be infinitely many distributions satisfying these constraints. For the case when the default distribution q_0 is uniform, the maximum entropy principle tells us to choose the distribution of maximum entropy satisfying these constraints. In general, we should minimize the relative entropy from q_0. This corresponds to choosing the distribution that satisfies the constraints (1) but imposes as little additional information as possible when compared with q_0. Allowing for asymmetric constraints, we obtain the formulation

$$\min_{p \in \Delta} \text{RE}(p \parallel q_0) \text{ subject to } \forall 1 \leq j \leq n : a_j \leq p[f_j] \leq b_j. \tag{2}$$

Here, $\Delta \subseteq \mathbb{R}^{\mathcal{X}}$ is the simplex of probability distributions and $\text{RE}(p \parallel q)$ is the relative entropy (or Kullback-Leibler divergence) from q to p, an information theoretic measure of difference between the two distributions. It is non-negative, equal to zero only when the two distributions are identical, and convex in its arguments.

Problem (2) is a convex program. Using Lagrange multipliers, we obtain that the solution takes the form

$$q_\lambda(x) = q_0(x)e^{\lambda \cdot f(x)}/Z_\lambda \tag{3}$$

where $Z_\lambda = \sum_x q_0(x)e^{\lambda \cdot f(x)}$ is the normalization constant. Distributions q_λ of the form (3) will be referred to as q_0-Gibbs or just Gibbs when no ambiguity arises.

Instead of solving (2) directly, we solve its dual:

$$\min_{\lambda \in \mathbb{R}^n} \left(\log Z_\lambda - \tfrac{1}{2} \sum_j (b_j + a_j)\lambda_j + \tfrac{1}{2} \sum_j (b_j - a_j)|\lambda_j| \right). \tag{4}$$

We can choose from a range of general convex optimization techniques or use some of the algorithms in [12]. For the symmetric case when

$$[a_j, b_j] = [\tilde{\pi}[f_j] - \beta_j, \tilde{\pi}[f_j] + \beta_j], \tag{5}$$

the dual becomes

$$\min_{\lambda \in \mathbb{R}^n} \left(-\tilde{\pi}[\log q_\lambda] + \sum_j \beta_j |\lambda_j| \right). \tag{6}$$

The first term is the *empirical log loss* (negative log likelihood), the second term is an ℓ_1-*regularization*. Small values of log loss mean a good fit to the data. This is balanced by regularization forcing simpler models and hence preventing overfitting.

When all the primal constraints are satisfied by the target distribution π then the solution $\hat{q}$ of the dual is guaranteed to be not much worse an approximation of π than the best Gibbs distribution q^*. More precisely:

Theorem 1 (Performance guarantees, Theorem 1 of [12]). *Assume that the distribution π satisfies the primal constraints (2). Let $\hat{q}$ be the solution of the dual (4). Then for an arbitrary Gibbs distribution $q^* = q_{\lambda^*}$*

$$\text{RE}(\pi \parallel \hat{q}) \leq \text{RE}(\pi \parallel q^*) + \sum_j (b_j - a_j)|\lambda_j^*|.$$

Algorithm 1: DEBIASAVERAGES.

Table 1: *Example 1.* Comparison of distributions q^* and q^{**} minimizing $\mathrm{RE}(\pi \parallel q_\lambda)$ and $\mathrm{RE}(\pi s \parallel q_\lambda s)$.

x	$f(x)$	$\pi(x)$	$s(x)$	$\pi s(x)$	$q^*(x)$	$q^{**}s(x)$	$q^{**}(x)$
1	$(0,0)$	0.4	0.4	0.64	0.25	0.544	0.34
2	$(0,1)$	0.1	0.4	0.16	0.25	0.256	0.16
3	$(1,0)$	0.1	0.1	0.04	0.25	0.136	0.34
4	$(1,1)$	0.4	0.1	0.16	0.25	0.064	0.16

When features are bounded between 0 and 1, the symmetric box constraints (5) with $\beta_j = O(\sqrt{(\log n)/m})$ are satisfied with high probability by Hoeffding's inequality and the union bound. Then the relative entropy from $\hat{q}$ to π will not be worse than the relative entropy from any Gibbs distribution q^* to π by more than $O(\|\boldsymbol{\lambda}^*\|_1 \sqrt{(\log n)/m})$.

In practice, we set

$$\beta_j = (\beta/\sqrt{m}) \cdot \min \{\tilde{\sigma}[f_j], \sigma_{\max}[f_j]\} \tag{7}$$

where β is a tuned constant, $\tilde{\sigma}[f_j]$ is the sample deviation of f_j, and $\sigma_{\max}[f_j]$ is an upper bound on the standard deviation, such as $(\max_x f_j(x) - \min_x f_j(x))/2$. We refer to this algorithm for unbiased data as UNBIASEDMAXENT.

3 Maxent with sample selection bias

In the biased case, the goal is to estimate the target distribution π, but samples do not come directly from π. For nonnegative functions p_1, p_2 defined on $\mathcal{X}$, let $p_1 p_2$ denote the distribution obtained by multiplying weights $p_1(x)$ and $p_2(x)$ at every point and renormalizing:

$$p_1 p_2(x) = \frac{p_1(x) p_2(x)}{\sum_{x'} p_1(x') p_2(x')}.$$

Samples $x_1, \ldots, x_m$ come from the *biased distribution* πs where s is the *sampling distribution*. This setup corresponds to the situation when an event being observed occurs at the point x with probability $\pi(x)$ while we perform an independent observation with probability $s(x)$. The probability of observing an event at x given that we observe an event is then equal to $\pi s(x)$. The empirical distribution of m samples drawn from πs will be denoted by $\widetilde{\pi s}$. We assume that s is known (principal assumption, see introduction) and strictly positive (technical assumption).

Approach I: Debiasing Averages. In our first approach, we use the same algorithm as for the unbiased case but employ a different method to obtain confidence intervals $[a_j, b_j]$. Since we do not have direct access to samples from π, we use a version of the Bias Correction Theorem of Zadrozny [6] to convert expectations with respect to πs to expectations with respect to π.

Theorem 2 (Bias Correction Theorem [6], Translation Theorem [7]).

$$\pi s[\boldsymbol{f}/s]/\pi s[1/s] = \pi[\boldsymbol{f}].$$

Hence, it suffices to give confidence intervals for $\pi s[\boldsymbol{f}/s]$ and $\pi s[1/s]$ to obtain confidence intervals for $\pi[\boldsymbol{f}]$.

Corollary 3. *Assume that for some sample-derived bounds $c_j, d_j, 0 \le j \le n$, with high probability $0 < c_0 \le \pi s[1/s] \le d_0$ and $0 \le c_j \le \pi s[f_j/s] \le d_j$ for all $1 \le j \le n$. Then with at least the same probability $c_j/d_0 \le \pi[f_j] \le d_j/c_0$ for all $1 \le j \le n$.*

If s is bounded away from 0 then Chernoff bounds may be used to determine c_j, d_j. Corollary 3 and Theorem 1 then yield guarantees that this method's performance converges, with increasing sample sizes, to that of the "best" Gibbs distribution.

In practice, confidence intervals $[c_j, d_j]$ may be determined using expressions analogous to (5) and (7) for random variables f_j/s, $1/s$ and the empirical distribution $\widetilde{\pi s}$. After first restricting the confidence intervals in a natural fashion, this yields Algorithm 1. Alternatively, we could use bootstrap or other types of estimates for the confidence intervals.

Approach II: Factoring Bias Out. The second algorithm does not approximate π directly, but uses maxent to estimate the distribution πs and then converts this estimate into an approximation of π. If the default estimate of π is q_0, then the default estimate of πs is $q_0 s$. Applying unbiased maxent to the empirical distribution $\widetilde{\pi s}$ with the default $q_0 s$, we obtain a $q_0 s$-Gibbs distribution $q_0 s e^{\hat{\lambda} \cdot \boldsymbol{f}}$ approximating πs. We factor out s to obtain $q_0 e^{\hat{\lambda} \cdot \boldsymbol{f}}$ as an estimate of π. This yields the algorithm FACTORBIASOUT.

This approach corresponds to ℓ_1-regularized maximum likelihood estimation of π by q_0-Gibbs distributions. When π itself is q_0-Gibbs then the distribution πs is $q_0 s$-Gibbs. Performance guarantees for unbiased maxent imply that estimates of πs converge to πs as the number of samples increases. Now, if $\inf_x s(x) > 0$ (which is the case for finite $\mathcal{X}$) then estimates of π obtained by factoring out s converge to π as well.

When π is not q_0-Gibbs then πs is not $q_0 s$-Gibbs either. We approximate π by a q_0-Gibbs distribution $\hat{q} = q_{\hat{\lambda}}$ which, with an increasing number of samples, minimizes $\mathrm{RE}(\pi s \parallel q_\lambda s)$ rather than $\mathrm{RE}(\pi \parallel q_\lambda)$. Our next example shows that these two minimizers may be different.

Example 1. Consider the space $\mathcal{X} = \{1, 2, 3, 4\}$ with two features f_1, f_2. Features f_1, f_2, target distribution π, sampling distribution s and the biased distribution πs are given in Table 1. We use the uniform distribution as a default estimate. The minimizer of $\mathrm{RE}(\pi \parallel q_\lambda)$ is the unique uniform-Gibbs distribution q^* such that $q^*[\boldsymbol{f}] = \pi[\boldsymbol{f}]$. Similarly, the minimizer $q^{**} s$ of $\mathrm{RE}(\pi s \parallel q_\lambda s)$ is the unique s-Gibbs distribution for which $q^{**} s[\boldsymbol{f}] = \pi s[\boldsymbol{f}]$. Solving for these exactly, we find that q^* and q^{**} are as given in Table 1, and that these two distributions differ. $\square$

Even though FACTORBIASOUT does not minimize $\mathrm{RE}(\pi \parallel q_\lambda)$, we can show that it minimizes a different Bregman divergence. More precisely, it minimizes a Bregman divergence between certain projections of the two distributions. Bregman divergences generalize some common distance measures such as relative entropy or the squared Euclidean distance, and enjoy many of the same favorable properties. The Bregman divergence associated with a convex function F is defined as $D_F(u \parallel v) = F(u) - F(v) - \nabla F(v) \cdot (u - v)$.

Proposition 4. *Define $F : \mathbb{R}_+^{\mathcal{X}} \to \mathbb{R}$ as $F(u) = \sum_x s(x) u(x) \log u(x)$. Then F is a convex function and for all $p_1, p_2 \in \Delta$, $\mathrm{RE}(p_1 s \parallel p_2 s) = D_F(p_1' \parallel p_2')$, where $p_1'(x) = p_1(x)/\sum_{x'} s(x') p_1(x')$ and $p_2'(x) = p_2(x)/\sum_{x'} s(x') p_2(x')$ are projections of p_1, p_2 along lines $tp, t \in \mathbb{R}$ onto the hyperplane $\sum_x s(x) p(x) = 1$.*

Approach III: Approximating FACTORBIASOUT. As mentioned in the introduction, knowing the sampling distribution s exactly is unrealistic. However, we often have access to samples from s. In this approach we assume that s is unknown but that, in addition to samples $x_1, \ldots, x_m$ from πs, we are also given a separate set of samples $x_{(1)}, x_{(2)}, \ldots, x_{(N)}$ from s. We use the algorithm FACTORBIASOUT with the sampling distribution s replaced by the corresponding empirical distribution $\tilde{s}$.

To simplify the algorithm, we note that instead of using $q_0 \tilde{s}$ as a default estimate for πs, it suffices to replace the sample space $\mathcal{X}$ by $\mathcal{X}' = \{x_{(1)}, x_{(2)}, \ldots, x_{(N)}\}$ and use q_0

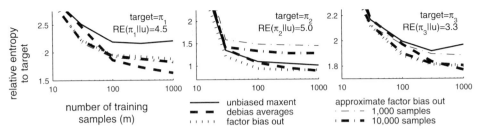

Figure 1: *Learning curves for synthetic experiments.* We use u to denote the uniform distribution. For the sampling distribution s, $\mathrm{RE}(s \parallel u) = 0.8$. Performance is measured in terms of relative entropy to the target distribution as a function of an increasing number of training samples. The number of samples is plotted on a log scale.

restricted to $\mathcal{X}'$ as a default. The last step of factoring out $\tilde{s}$ is equivalent to using $\hat{\lambda}$ returned for space $\mathcal{X}'$ on the entire space $\mathcal{X}$.

When the sampling distribution s is correlated with feature values, $\mathcal{X}'$ might not cover all feature ranges. In that case, reprojecting on $\mathcal{X}$ may yield poor estimates outside of these ranges. We therefore do "clamping", restricting values $f_j(x)$ to their ranges over $\mathcal{X}'$ and capping values of the exponent $\hat{\lambda} \cdot f(x)$ at its maximum over $\mathcal{X}'$. The resulting algorithm is called APPROXFACTORBIASOUT.

4 Experiments

Conducting real data experiments to evaluate bias correction techniques is difficult, because bias is typically unknown and samples from unbiased distributions are not available. Therefore, synthetic experiments are often a necessity for precise evaluation. Nevertheless, in addition to synthetic experiments, we were also able to conduct experiments with real-world data for habitat modeling.

Synthetic experiments. In synthetic experiments, we generated three target uniform-Gibbs distributions π_1, π_2, π_3 over a domain $\mathcal{X}$ of size 10,000. These distributions were derived from 65 features indexed as $f_i, 0 \leq i \leq 9$ and $f_{ij}, 0 \leq i \leq j \leq 9$. Values $f_i(x)$ were chosen independently and uniformly in $[0, 1]$, and we set $f_{ij}(x) = f_i(x)f_j(x)$. Fixing these features, we generated weights for each distribution. Weights λ_i and λ_{ii} were generated jointly to capture a range of different behaviors for values of f_i in the range $[0, 1]$.

Let U_S denote a random variable uniform over the set S. Each instance of U_S corresponds to a new independent variable. We set $\lambda_{ii} = U_{\{-1,0,1\}}U_{[1,5]}$ and λ_i to be $\lambda_{ii}U_{[-3,1]}$ if $\lambda_{ii} \neq 0$, and $U_{\{-1,1\}}U_{[2,10]}$ otherwise. Weights $\lambda_{ij}, i < j$ were chosen to create correlations between f_i's that would be observable, but not strong enough to dominate λ_i's and λ_{ii}'s. We set $\lambda_{ij} = -0.5$ or 0 or 0.5 with respective probabilities 0.05, 0.9 and 0.05. In maxent, we used a subset of features specifying target distributions and some irrelevant features. We used features $f_i', 0 \leq i \leq 9$ and their squares f_{ii}', where $f_i'(x) = f_i(x)$ for $0 \leq i \leq 5$ (relevant features) and $f_i'(x) = U_{[0,1]}$ for $6 \leq i \leq 9$ (irrelevant features). Once generated, we used the same set of features in all experiments. We generated a sampling distribution s correlated with target distributions. More specifically, s was a Gibbs distribution generated from features $f_i^{(s)}, 0 \leq i \leq 5$ and their squares $f_{ii}^{(s)}$, where $f_i^{(s)}(x) = U_{[0,1]}$ for $0 \leq i \leq 1$ and $f_i^{(s)} = f_{i+2}$ for $2 \leq i \leq 5$. We used weights $\lambda_i^{(s)} = 0$ and $\lambda_{ii}^{(s)} = -1$.

For every target distribution, we evaluated the performance of UNBIASEDMAXENT, DEBIASAVERAGES, FACTORBIASOUT and APPROXFACTORBIASOUT with 1,000 and 10,000 samples from the sampling distribution. The performance was evaluated in terms of relative entropy to the target distribution. We used training sets of sizes 10 to 1000. We considered five randomly generated training sets and took the average performance over these five sets for settings of β from the range $[0.05, 4.64]$. We report results for the best β, chosen separately for each average. The rationale behind this approach is that we want to

Table 2: *Results of real data experiments.* Average performance of unbiased maxent and three bias correction approaches over all species in six regions. The uniform distribution would receive the log loss of 14.2 and AUC of 0.5. Results of bias correction approaches are italicized if they are significantly worse and set in boldface if they are significantly better than those of the unbiased maxent according to a paired t-test at the level of significance 5%.

	average log loss						average AUC					
	awt	can	nsw	nz	sa	swi	awt	can	nsw	nz	sa	swi
unbiased maxent	13.78	12.89	13.40	13.77	13.14	12.81	0.69	0.58	0.71	0.72	0.78	0.81
debias averages	*13.92*	13.10	*13.88*	*14.31*	*14.10*	*13.59*	0.67	0.64	*0.65*	*0.67*	*0.68*	*0.78*
factor bias out	13.90	*13.13*	*14.06*	*14.20*	*13.66*	*13.46*	0.71	**0.69**	0.72	0.72	0.78	**0.83**
apx. factor bias out	13.89	*13.40*	*14.19*	*14.07*	*13.62*	*13.41*	**0.72**	**0.72**	0.73	0.73	0.78	**0.84**

explore the potential performance of each method.

Figure 1 shows the results at the optimal β as a function of an increasing number of samples. FACTORBIASOUT is always better than UNBIASEDMAXENT. DEBIASAVERAGES is worse than UNBIASEDMAXENT for small sample sizes, but as the number of training samples increases, it soon outperforms UNBIASEDMAXENT and eventually also outperforms FACTORBIASOUT. APPROXFACTORBIASOUT improves as the number of samples from the sampling distribution increases from 1,000 to 10,000, but both versions of APPROX-FACTORBIASOUT perform worse than UNBIASEDMAXENT for the distribution π_2.

Real data experiments. In this set of experiments, we evaluated maxent in the task of estimating species habitats. The sample space is a geographic region divided into a grid of cells and samples are known occurrence localities — cells where a given species was observed. Every cell is described by a set of *environmental variables*, which may be categorical, such as vegetation type, or continuous, such as altitude or annual precipitation. Features are real-valued functions derived from environmental variables. We used *binary indicator features* for different values of categorical variables and *binary threshold features* for continuous variables. The latter are equal to one when the value of a variable is greater than a fixed threshold and zero otherwise.

Species sample locations and environmental variables were all produced and used as part of the "Testing alternative methodologies for modeling species' ecological niches and predicting geographic distributions" Working Group at the National Center for Ecological Analysis and Synthesis (NCEAS). The working group compared modeling methods across a variety of species and regions. The training set contained presence-only data from unplanned surveys or incidental records, including those from museums and herbariums. The test set contained presence-absence data from rigorously planned independent surveys.

We compared performance of our bias correction approaches with that of the unbiased maxent which was among the top methods in the NCEAS comparison [13]. We used the full dataset consisting of 226 species in 6 regions with 2–5822 training presences per species (233 on average) and 102–19120 test presences/absences. For more details see [13].

We treated training occurrence locations for all species in each region as sampling distribution samples and used them directly in APPROXFACTORBIASOUT. In order to apply DEBIASAVERAGES and FACTORBIASOUT, we estimated the sampling distribution using unbiased maxent. Sampling distribution estimation is also the first step of [6]. In contrast with that work, however, our experiments do not use the sampling distribution estimate during evaluation and hence do not depend on its quality.

The resulting distributions were evaluated on test presences according to the log loss and on test presences and absences according to the *area under an ROC curve* (AUC) [14]. AUC quantifies how well the predicted distribution ranks test presences above test absences. Its value is equal to the probability that a randomly chosen presence will be ranked above a randomly chosen absence. The uniformly random prediction receives AUC of 0.5 while a perfect prediction receives AUC of 1.0.

In Table 2 we show performance of our three approaches compared with the unbiased maxent. All three algorithms yield on average a worse log loss than the unbiased maxent. This can perhaps be attributed to the imperfect estimate of the sampling distribution or to the sampling distribution being zero over large portions of the sample space. In contrast, when the performance is measured in terms of AUC, FACTORBIASOUT and APPROX-FACTORBIASOUT yield on average the same or better AUC as UNBIASEDMAXENT in all six regions. Improvements in regions *awt*, *can* and *swi* are dramatic enough so that both of these methods perform better than any method evaluated in [13].

5 Conclusions

We have proposed three approaches that incorporate information about sample selection bias in maxent and demonstrated their utility in synthetic and real data experiments. Experiments also raise several questions that merit further research: DEBIASAVERAGES has the strongest performance guarantees, but it performs the worst in real data experiments and catches up with other methods only for large sample sizes in synthetic experiments. This may be due to poor estimates of unbiased confidence intervals and could be possibly improved using a different estimation method. FACTORBIASOUT and APPROXFACTOR-BIASOUT improve over UNBIASEDMAXENT in terms of AUC over real data, but are worse in terms of log loss. This disagreement suggests that methods which aim to optimize AUC directly could be more successful in species modeling, possibly incorporating some concepts from FACTORBIASOUT and APPROXFACTORBIASOUT. APPROXFACTORBIAS-OUT performs the best on real world data, possibly due to the direct use of samples from the sampling distribution rather than a sampling distribution estimate. However, this method comes without performance guarantees and does not exploit the knowledge of the full sample space. Proving performance guarantees for APPROXFACTORBIASOUT remains open for future research.

Acknowledgments

This material is based upon work supported by NSF under grant 0325463. Any opinions, findings, and conclusions or recommendations expressed in this material are those of the authors and do not necessarily reflect the views of NSF. The NCEAS data was kindly shared with us by the members of the "Testing alternative methodologies for modeling species' ecological niches and predicting geographic distributions" Working Group, which was supported by the National Center for Ecological Analysis and Synthesis, a Center funded by NSF (grant DEB-0072909), the University of California and the Santa Barbara campus.

References

[1] Jane Elith. Quantitative methods for modeling species habitat: Comparative performance and an application to Australian plants. In Scott Ferson and Mark Burgman, editors, *Quantitative Methods for Conservation Biology*, pages 39–58. Springer-Verlag, 2002.

[2] A. Guisan and N. E. Zimmerman. Predictive habitat distribution models in ecology. *Ecological Modelling*, 135:147–186, 2000.

[3] Steven J. Phillips, Miroslav Dudík, and Robert E. Schapire. A maximum entropy approach to species distribution modeling. In *Proceedings of the Twenty-First International Conference on Machine Learning*, 2004.

[4] S. Reddy and L. M. Dávalos. Geographical sampling bias and its implications for conservation priorities in Africa. *Journal of Biogeography*, 30:1719–1727, 2003.

[5] Barbara R. Stein and John Wieczorek. Mammals of the world: MaNIS as an example of data integration in a distributed network environment. *Biodiversity Informatics*, 1(1):14–22, 2004.

[6] Bianca Zadrozny. Learning and evaluating classifiers under sample selection bias. In *Proceedings of the Twenty-First International Conference on Machine Learning*, 2004.

[7] Bianca Zadrozny, John Langford, and Naoki Abe. Cost-sensitive learning by cost-proportionate example weighting. In *Proceedings of the Third IEEE International Conference on Data Mining*, 2003.

[8] James J. Heckman. Sample selection bias as a specification error. *Econometrica*, 47(1):153–161, 1979.

[9] Robert M. Groves. *Survey Errors and Survey Costs*. Wiley, 1989.

[10] Roderick J. Little and Donald B. Rubin. *Statistical Analysis with Missing Data*. Wiley, second edition, 2002.

[11] Charles Elkan. The foundations of cost-sensitive learning. In *Proceedings of the Seventeenth International Joint Conference on Artificial Intelligence*, 2001.

[12] Miroslav Dudík, Steven J. Phillips, and Robert E. Schapire. Performance guarantees for regularized maximum entropy density estimation. In *17th Annual Conference on Learning Theory*, 2004.

[13] J. Elith, C. Graham, and NCEAS working group. Comparing methodologies for modeling species' distributions from presence-only data. In preparation.

[14] J. A. Hanley and B. S. McNeil. The meaning and use of the area under a receiver operating characteristic (ROC) curve. *Radiology*, 143:29–36, 1982.

Searching for Character Models

Jaety Edwards
Department of Computer Science
UC Berkeley
Berkeley, CA 94720
jaety@cs.berkeley.edu

David Forsyth
Department of Computer Science
UC Berkeley
Berkeley, CA 94720
daf@cs.berkeley.edu

Abstract

We introduce a method to automatically improve character models for a handwritten script without the use of transcriptions and using a minimum of document specific training data. We show that we can use searches for the words in a dictionary to identify portions of the document whose transcriptions are unambiguous. Using templates extracted from those regions, we retrain our character prediction model to drastically improve our search retrieval performance for words in the document.

1 Introduction

An active area of research in machine transcription of handwritten documents is reducing the amount and expense of supervised data required to train prediction models. Traditional OCR techniques require a large sample of hand segmented letter glyphs for training. This per character segmentation is expensive and often impractical to acquire, particularly if the corpora in question contain documents in many different scripts.

Numerous authors have presented methods for reducing the expense of training data by removing the need to segment individual characters. Both Kopec et al [3] and LeCun et al [5] have presented models that take as input images of lines of text with their ASCII transcriptions. Training with these datasets is made possible by explicitly modelling possible segmentations in addition to having a model for character templates.

In their research on "wordspotting", Lavrenko et al [4] demonstrate that images of entire words can be highly discriminative, even when the individual characters composing the word are locally ambiguous. This implies that images of many sufficiently long words should have unambiguous transcriptions, even when the character models are poorly tuned. In our previous work, [2], the discriminatory power of whole words allowed us to achieve strong search results with a model trained on a single example per character.

The above results have shown that A) one can learn new template models given images of text lines and their associated transcriptions, [3, 5] without needing an explicit segmentation and that B) entire words can often be identified unambiguously, even when the models for individual characters are poorly tuned. [2, 4]. The first of these two points implies that given a transcription, we can learn new character models. The second implies that for at least some parts of a document, we should be able to provide that transcription "for free", by matching against a dictionary of known words.

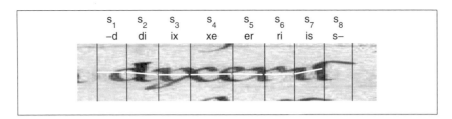

Figure 1: **A line, and the states that generate it.** *Each state s_t is defined by its left and right characters c_{tl} and c_{tr} (eg "x" and "e" for s_4). In the image, a state spans half of each of these two characters, starting just past the center of the left character and extending to the center of the right character, i.e. the right half of the "x" and the left half of the "e" in s_4. The relative positions of the two characters is given by a displacement vector d_t (superimposed on the image as white lines). Associating states with intracharacter spaces instead of with individual characters allows for the bounding boxes of characters to overlap while maintaining the independence properties of the Markov chain.*

In this work we combine these two observations in order to improve character models without the need for a document specific transcription. We provide a generic dictionary of words in the target language. We then identify "high confidence" regions of a document. These are image regions for which exactly one word from our dictionary scores highly under our model. Given a set of high confidence regions, we effectively have a training corpus of text images with associated transcriptions. In these regions, we infer a segmentation and extract new character examples. Finally, we use these new exemplars to learn an improved character prediction model. As in [2], our document in this work is a 12th century manuscript of Terence's Comedies obtained from Oxford's Bodleian library [1].

2   The Model

Hidden Markov Models are a natural and widely used method for modeling images of text. In their simplest incarnation, a hidden state represents a character and the evidence variable is some feature vector calculated at points along the line. If all characters were known to be of a single fixed width, this model would suffice. The probability of a line under this model is given as

$$p(line) = p(c_1|\alpha) \prod_{t>1} p(c_t|c_{t-1})p(im_{[w*(t-1):w*t]}|c_t) \tag{1}$$

where c_t represents the tth character on the line, α represents the start state, w is the width of a character, and $im_{[w(t-1)+1:wt]}$ represents the column of pixels beginning at column $w * (t - 1) + 1$ of the image and ending at column $w * t$, (i.e. the set of pixels spanned by c)

Unfortunately, character's widths do vary quite substantially and so we must extend the model to accommodate different possible segmentations. A generalized HMM allows us to do this. In this model a hidden state is allowed to emit a variable length series of evidence variables. We introduce an explicit distribution over the possible widths of a character. Letting d_t be the displacement vector associated with the tth character, and c_{tx} refer to the x location of the left edge of a character on the line, the probability of a line under this revised model is

$$p(line) = p(c_1|\alpha) \prod_{t>1} p(c_t|c_{t-1})p(d_t|c_t)p(im_{[c_{tx}+1:c_{tx}+d]}|d_t, c_t) \tag{2}$$

This is the model we used in [2]. It performs far better than using an assumption of fixed widths, but it still imposes unrealistic constraints on the relative positions of characters. In particular, the portion of the ink generated by the current character is assumed to be independent of the preceding character. In other words, the model assumes that the bounding boxes of characters do not overlap. This constraint is obviously unrealistic. Characters routinely overlap in our documents. "f"s, for instance, form ligatures with most following characters. In previous work, we treated this overlap as noise, hurting our ability to correctly localize templates. Under this model, local errors of alignment would also often propagate globally, adversely affecting the segmentation of the whole line. For search, this noisy segmentation still provides acceptable results. In this work, however, we need to extract new templates, and thus correct localization and segmentation of templates is crucial.

In our current work, we have relaxed this constraint, allowing characters to partially overlap. We achieve this by changing hidden states to represent character bigrams instead of single characters (Figure 1). In the image, a state now spans the pixels from just past the center of the left character to the pixel containing the center of the right character. We adjust our notation somewhat to reflect this change, letting s_t now represent the tth hidden state and c_{tl} and c_{tr} be the left and right characters associated with s. d_t is now the displacement vector between the centers of c_{tl} and c_{tr}.

The probability of a line under this, our actual, model is

$$p(line) = p(s_1|\alpha) \prod_{t>1} p(s_t|s_{t-1}) p(d_t|c_{tl}, c_{tr}) p(im_{[s_{tx}+1:s_{tx}+d_t]}|c_{tl}, c_{tr}, d_t) \qquad (3)$$

This model allows overlap of bounding boxes, but it does still make the assumption that the bounding box of the current character does not extend past the center of the previous character. This assumption does not fully reflect reality either. In Figure 1, for example, the left descender of the x extends back further than the center of the preceding character. It does, however, accurately reflect the constraints within the heart of the line (excluding ascenders and descenders). In practice, it has proven to generate very accurate segmentations. Moreover, the errors we do encounter no longer tend to affect the entire line, since the model has more flexibility with which to readjust back to the correct segmentation.

2.1 Model Parameters

Our transition distribution between states is simply a 3-gram character model. We train this model using a collection of ASCII Latin documents collected from the web. This set does not include the transcriptions of our documents.

Conditioned on displacement vector, the emission model for generating an image chunk given a state is a mixture of gaussians. We associate with each character a set of image windows extracted from various locations in the document. We initialize these sets with one example a piece from our hand cut set (Figure 2). We adjust the probability of an image given the state to include the distribution over blocks by expanding the last term of Equation 3 to reflect this mixture. Letting b_{ck} represent the kth exemplar in the set associated with character c, the conditional probability of an image region spanning the columns from x to x' is given as

$$p(im_{x:x'}|c_{tl}, c_{tr}, d_t) = \sum_{i,j} p(im_{x:x'}|b_{c_{tl}i}, b_{c_{tr}j}, d_t) \qquad (4)$$

In principle, the displacement vectors should now be associated with an individual block, not a character. This is especially true when we have both upper and lower case letters. However, our model does not seem particularly sensitive to this displacement distribution and so in practice, we have a single, fairly loose, displacement distribution per character.

Given a displacement vector, we can generate the maximum likelihood template image under our model by compositing the correct halves of the left and right blocks. Reshaping the image window into a vector, the likelihood of an image window is then modeled as a gaussian, using the corresponding pixels in the template as the means, and assuming a diagonal covariance matrix. The covariance matrix largely serves to mask out empty regions of a character's bounding box, so that we do not pay a penalty when the overlap of two characters' bounding boxes contains only whitespace.

2.2 Efficiency Considerations

The number of possible different templates for a state is $O(|B| \times |B| \times |D|)$, where $|B|$ is the number of different possible blocks and $|D|$ is the number of candidate displacement vectors. To make inference in this model computationally feasible, we first restrict the domain of d. For a given pair of blocks b_l and b_r, we consider only displacement vectors within some small x distance from a mean displacement m_{b_l,b_r}, and we have a uniform distribution within this region. m is initialized from the known size of our single hand cut template. In the current work, we do not relearn the m. These are held fixed and assumed to be the same for all blocks associated with the same letter.

Even when restricting the number of d's under consideration as discussed above, it is computationally infeasible to consider every possible location and pair of blocks. We therefore prune our candidate locations by looking at the likelihood of blocks in isolation and only considering locations where there is a local optimum in the response function and whose value is better than a given threshold. In this case our threshold for a given location is that $\mathcal{L}(block) < .7\mathcal{L}(background)$ (where $\mathcal{L}(x)$ represents the negative log likelihood of x). In other words, a location has to look at least marginally more like a given block than it looks like the background.

After pruning locations in this manner, we are left with a discrete set of "sites," where we define a site as the tuple (block type, x location, y location). We can enumerate the set of possible states by looking at every pair of sites whose displacement vector has a non-zero probability.

2.3 Inference In The Model

The statespace defined above is a directed acyclic graph, anchored at the left edge and right edges of a line of text. A path through this lattice defines both a transcription and a segmentation of the line into individual characters. Inference in this model is relatively straightforward because of our constraint that each character may overlap only one preceding and one following character, and our restriction of displacement vectors to a small discrete range. The first restriction means that we need only consider binary relations between templates. The second preserves the independence relationships of an HMM. A given state s_t is independent of the rest of the line given the values of all other states within d_{max} of either edge of s_t (where d_{max} is the legal displacement vector with the longest x component.) We can therefore easily calculate the best path or explicitly calculate the posterior of a node by traversing the state graph in topological order, sorted from left to right. The literature on Weighted Finite State Transducers ([6], [5]) is a good resource for efficient algorithms on these types of statespace graph.

3 Learning Better Character Templates

We initialize our algorithm with a set of handcut templates, exactly 1 per character, (Figure 2), and our goal is to construct more accurate character models automatically from unsupervised data. As noted above, we can easily calculate the posterior of a given site under our model. (Recall that a site is a particular character template at a given (x,y) location in the line.) The traditional EM approach to estimating new templates would be to use these

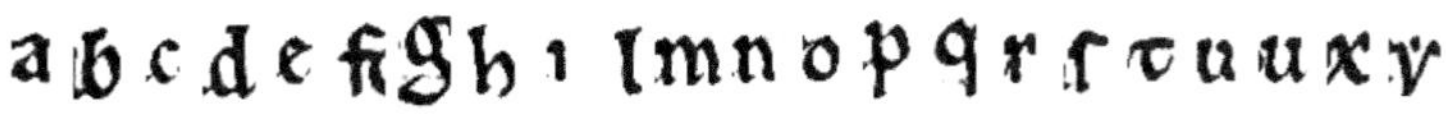

abcdefghi lmnopqrstuuxy

Figure 2: **Original Training Data** *These 22 glyphs are our only document specific training data. We use the model based on these characters to extract the new examples shown below*

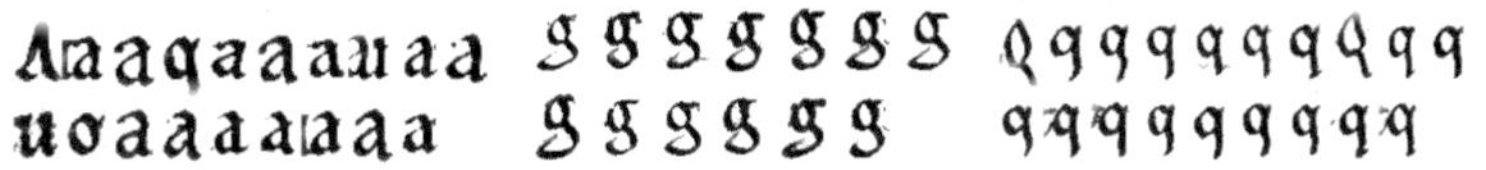

Aaaqaaauaa ſſ ſ ſ ſ ſ ſ ſ qqqqqqqqq
uoaaaaaaa ſ ſ ſ ſ ſ ſ qqqqqqqqq

Figure 3: **Examples of extracted templates** *We extract new templates from high confidence regions. From these, we choose a subset to incorporate into the model as new exemplars. Templates are chosen iteratively to best cover the space of training examples. Notice that for "q" and "a", we have extracted capital letters, of which there were no examples in our original set of glyphs. This happens when the combination of constraints from the dictionary the surrounding glyphs make a "q" or "a" the only possible explanation for this region, even though its local likelihood is poor.*

sites as training examples, weighted by their posteriors. Unfortunately, the constraints imposed by 3 and even 4-gram character models seem to be insufficient. The posteriors of sites are not discriminative enough to get learning off the ground.

The key to successfully learning new templates lies is the observation from our previous work [2], that even when the posteriors of individual characters are not discriminative, one can still achieve very good search results with the same model. The search word in effect serves as its own language model, only allowing paths through the state graph that actually contain it, and the longer the word the more it constrains the model. Whole words impose much tighter constraints than a 2 or 3-gram character model, and it is only with this added power that we can successfully learn new character templates.

We define the score for a search as the negative log likelihood of the best path containing that word. With sufficiently long words, it becomes increasingly unlikely that a spurious path will achieve a high score. Moreover, if we are given a large dictionary of words and no alternative word explains a region of ink nearly as well as the best scoring word, then we can be extremely confident that this is a true transcription of that piece of ink.

Starting with a weak character model, we do not expect to find many of these "high confidence" regions, but with a large enough document, we should expect to find some. From these regions, we can extract new, reliable templates with which to improve our character models. The most valuable of these new templates will be those that are significantly different from any in our current set. For example, in Figure 3, note that our system identifies capital Q's, even though our only input template was lower case. It identifies this ink as a Q in much the same way that a person solves a crossword puzzle. We can easily infer the missing character in the string "obv-ous" because the other letters constrain us to one possible solution. Similarly, if other character templates in a word match well, then we can unambiguously identify the other, more ambiguous ones. In our Latin case, "Quid" is the only likely explanation for "-uid".

3.1 Extracting New Templates and Updating The Model

Within a high confidence region we have both a transcription and a localization of template centers. It remains only to cut out new templates. We accomplish this by creating a template image for the column of pixels from the corresponding block templates and then assigning image pixels to the nearest template character (measured by Euclidean distance).

Given a set of templates extracted from high confidence regions, we choose a subset of

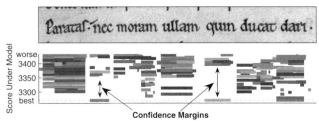

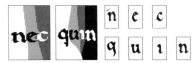

Figure 4: *Each line segment in the lower figure represents a proposed location for a word from our dictionary. It's vertical height is the score of that location under our model. A lower score represents a better fit. The dotted line is the score of our model's best possible path. Three correct words, "nec", "quin" and "dari", are actually on the best path. We define the* **confidence margin** *of a location as the difference in score between the best fitting word from our dictionary and the next best.*

Figure 5: **Extracting Templates** *For a region with sufficiently high confidence margin, we construct the maximum likelihood template from our current exemplars.* **left**, *and we assign pixels from the original image to a template based on its distance to the nearest pixel in the template image, extracting new glyph exemplars* **right**. *These new glyphs become the exemplars for our next round of training.*

templates that best explain the remaining examples. We do this in a greedy fashion by choosing the example whose likelihood is lowest under our current model and adding it to our set. Currently, we threshold the number of new templates for the sake of efficiency. Finally, given the new set of templates, we can add them to the model and rerun our searches, potentially identifying new high confidence regions.

4   Results

Our algorithm iteratively improves the character model by gathering new training data from high confidence regions. Figure 3 shows that this method finds new templates significantly different from the originals. In this document, our set of examples after one round appears to cover the space of character images well, at least those in lower case. Our templates are not perfect. The "a", for instance, has become associated with at least one block that is in fact an "o". These mistakes are uncommon, particularly if we restrict ourselves to longer words. Those that do occur introduce a tolerable level noise into our model. They make certain regions of the document more ambiguous locally, but that local ambiguity can be overcome with the context provided by surrounding characters and a language model.

Improved Character Models We evaluate the method more quantitatively by testing the impact of the new templates on the quality of searches performed against the document. To search for a given word, we rank lines by the ratio of the maximum likelihood transcription/segmentation that contains the search word to the likelihood of the best possible segmentation/transcription under our model. The lowest possible search score is 1, happening when the search word is actually a substring of the maximum likelihood transcription. Higher scores mean that the word is increasingly unlikely under our model. In Figure 7, the figure on the left shows the improvement in ranking of the lines that truly contain selected search words. The odd rows (in red) are search results using only the original 22 glyphs,

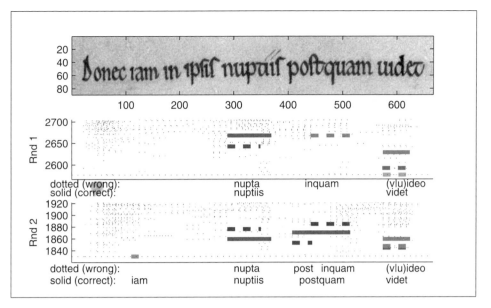

Figure 6: *Search Results with (Rnd 1) initial templates only and with (Rnd 2) templates extracted from high confidence regions. We show results that have a score within 5% of the best path.* **Solid Lines** *are the results for the correct word. Dotted lines represent other search results, where we have made a few larger in order to show those words that are the closest competitors to the true word. Many alternative searches, like the highlighted "post" are actually portions of the correct larger words. These restrict our selection of confidence regions, but do not impinge on search quality.*
Each correct word has significantly improved after one round of template reestimation. **"iam"** *has been correctly identified, and is a new high confidence region. Both* **"nuptiis"** *and* **"postquam"** *are now the highest likelihood words for their region barring smaller subsequences, and* **"videt"** *has narrowed the gap between its competitor "video".*

while the even rows (in green) use an additional 332 glyphs extracted from high confidence regions. Search results are markedly improved in the second model. The word "est", for instance, only had 15 of 24 of the correct lines in the top 100 under the original model, while under the learned model all 24 are not only present but also more highly ranked.

Improved Search *Figure 6* shows the improved performance of our refitted model for a single line. Most words have greatly improved relative to their next best alternative. "postquam" and "iam" were not even considered by the original model and now are nearly optimal. The *right of Figure 7* shows the average precision/recall curve under each model for 21 words with more than 4 occurrences in the dataset. Precision is the percentage of lines truly containing a word in the top n search results, and recall is the percentage of all lines containing the word returned in the top n results. The learned model clearly dominates. The new model also greatly improves performance for rare words. For 320 words ocurring just once in the dataset, 50% are correctly returned as the top ranked result under the original model. Under the learned model, this number jumps to 78%.

5   Conclusions and Future Work

In most fonts, characters are quite ambiguous locally. An "n" looks like a "u", looks like "ii", etc. This ambiguity is the major hurdle to the unsupervised learning of character templates. Language models help, but the standard n-gram models provide insufficient constraints, giving posteriors for character sites too uninformative to get EM off the ground.

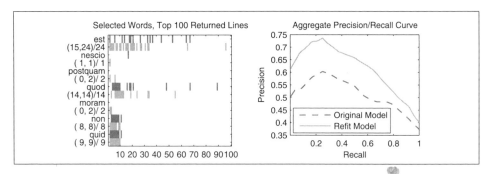

Figure 7: *The figure on the **left** shows the those lines with the top 100 scores that actually contain the specified word. The first of each set of two rows (in red) is the results from Round 1. The second (in green) is the results for Round 2. Almost all search words in our corpus show a significant improvement. The numbers to the right (x/y) mean that out of y lines that actually contained the search word in our document, x of them made it into the top ten. On the **right** are average precision/recall curves for 21 high frequency words under the model with our original templates (Rnd 1) and after refitting with new extracted templates (Rnd 2). Extracting new templates vastly improves our search quality*

An entire word is much different. Given a dictionary, we expect many word images to have a single likely transcription even if many characters are locally ambiguous. We show that we can identify these high confidence regions even with a poorly tuned character model. By extracting new templates only from these regions of the document, we overcome the noise problem and significantly improve our character models. We demonstrate this improvement for the task of search where the refitted models have drastically better search responses than with the original. Our method is indifferent to the form of the actual character emission model. There is a rich literature in character prediction from isolated image windows, and we expect that incorporating more powerful character models should provide even greater returns and help us in learning less regular scripts.

Finding high confidence regions to extract good training examples is a broadly applicable concept. We believe this work should extend to other problems, most notably speech recognition. Looked at more abstractly, our use of language model in this work is actually encoding spatial constraints. The probability of a character given an image window depends not only on the identify of surrounding characters but also on their spatial configuration. Integrating context into recognition problems is an area of intense research in the computer vision community, and we are investigating extending the idea of confidence regions to more general object recognition problems.

References

[1] Early Manuscripts at Oxford University. Bodleian library ms. auct. f. 2.13. *http://image.ox.ac.uk/*.

[2] J. Edwards, Y.W. Teh, D. Forsyth, R. Bock, M. Maire, and G. Vesom. Making latin manuscripts searchable using ghmm's. In *NIPS 17*, pages 385–392. 2005.

[3] G. Kopec and M. Lomelin. Document-specific character template estimation. In *Proceedings, Document Image Recognition III, SPIE*, 1996.

[4] V. Lavrenko, T. Rath, and R. Manmatha. Holistic word recognition for handwritten historical documents. In *dial*, pages 278–287, 2004.

[5] Y. LeCun, L. Bottou, Y. Bengio, and P. Haffner. Gradient-based learning applied to document recognition. *Proceedings of the IEEE*, 86(11):2278–2324, 1998.

[6] M. Mohri, F. Pereira, and M. Riley. Weighted finite state transducers in speech recognition. *ISCA ITRW Automatic Speech Recognition*, pages 97–106, 2000.

Hierarchical Linear/Constant Time SLAM Using Particle Filters for Dense Maps

Austin I. Eliazar   **Ronald Parr**
Department of Computer Science
Duke University
Durham, NC 27708
{*eliazar,parr*}*@cs.duke.edu*

Abstract

We present an improvement to the DP-SLAM algorithm for simultaneous localization and mapping (SLAM) that maintains multiple hypotheses about densely populated maps (one full map per particle in a particle filter) in time that is linear in all significant algorithm parameters and takes constant (amortized) time per iteration. This means that the asymptotic complexity of the algorithm is no greater than that of a pure localization algorithm using a single map and the same number of particles. We also present a hierarchical extension of DP-SLAM that uses a two level particle filter which models drift in the particle filtering process itself. The hierarchical approach enables recovery from the inevitable drift that results from using a finite number of particles in a particle filter and permits the use of DP-SLAM in more challenging domains, while maintaining linear time asymptotic complexity.

1   Introduction

The ability to construct and use a map of the environment is a critical enabling technology for many important applications, such as search and rescue or extraterrestrial exploration. Probabilistic approaches have proved successful at addressing the basic problem of localization using particle filters [6]. Expectation Maximization (EM) has been used successfully to address the problem of mapping [1] and Kalman filters [2, 10] have shown promise on the combined problem of simultaneous localization and mapping (SLAM).

SLAM algorithms ought to produce accurate maps with bounded resource consumption per sensor sweep. To the extent that it is possible, it is desirable to avoid explicit map correcting actions, which are computationally intensive and would be symptomatic of accumulating error in the map. One family of approaches to SLAM assumes relatively sparse, relatively unambiguous landmarks and builds a Kalman filter over landmark positions [2, 9, 10] . Other approaches assume dense sensor data which individually are not very distinctive, such as those available from a laser range finder [7, 8]. An advantage of the latter group is that they are capable of producing detailed maps that can be used for path planning.

In earlier work, we presented an algorithm called DP-SLAM [4], which produced extremely accurate, densely populated maps by maintaining a joint distribution over robot maps and poses using a particle filter. DP-SLAM uses novel data structures that exploit shared structure between maps, permitting efficient use of many joint map/pose particles.

This gives DP-SLAM the ability to resolve map ambiguities automatically, as a natural part of the particle filtering process, effectively obviating the explicit loop closing phase needed for other approaches [7, 12].

A known limitation of particle filters is that they can require a very large number of particles to track systems with diffuse posterior distributions. This limitation strongly affected earlier versions of DP-SLAM, which had a worst-case run time that scaled quadratically with the number of particles. In this paper, we present a significant improvement to DP-SLAM which reduces the run time to linear in the number of particles, giving multiple map hypothesis SLAM the same asymptotic complexity per particle as localization with a single map. The new algorithm also has a more straightforward analysis and implementation.

Unfortunately, even with linear time complexity, there exist domains which require infeasibly large numbers of particles for accurate mapping. The cumulative effect of very small errors (resulting from sampling or discretization) can cause drift. To address the issue of drift in a direct and principled manner, we propose a hierarchical particle filter method which can specifically model and recover from small amounts of drift, while maintaining particle diversity longer than in typical particle filters. The combined result is an algorithm that can produce extraordinarily detailed maps of large domains at close to real time speeds.

2   Linear Time Algorithm

A DP-SLAM *ancestry tree* contains all of the current particles as leaves. The parent of a given node represents the particle of the previous iteration from which that particle was resampled. An ancestry tree is *minimal* if the following two properties hold:

1. A node is a leaf node if and only if it corresponds to a current generation particle.
2. All interior nodes have at least two children.

The first property is ensured by simply removing particles that are not resampled from the ancestry tree. The second property is ensured by merging parents with only-child nodes. It is easy to see that for a particle filter with P particles, the corresponding minimal ancestry tree will have a branching factor of at least two and depth of no more than $O(P)$.

The complexity of maintaining a minimal ancestry tree will depend upon the manner in which observations, and thus maps, are associated with nodes in the tree. DP-SLAM distributes this information in the following manner: All map updates for all nodes in the ancestry tree are stored in a single global grid, while each node in the ancestry tree also maintains a list of all grid squares updated by that node. The information contained in these two data structures is integrated for efficient access at each cycle of the particle filter through a new data structure called an *map cache*.

2.1   Core Data Structures

The DP-SLAM map is a global occupancy grid-like array. Each grid cell contains an *observation vector* with one entry for each ancestry tree node that has made an observation of the grid cell. Each vector entry is an *observation node* containing the following fields:

opacity a data structure storing sufficient statistics for the current estimate of the opacity of the grid cell to the laser range finder. See Eliazar and Parr [4] for details.

parent a pointer to a parent observation node for which this node is an update. (If an ancestor of a current particle has seen this square already, then the opacity value for this square is considered an update to the previous value stored by the ancestor. However, both the update and the original observation are stored, since it may not be the case that all successors of the ancestor have made updates to this square.)

anode a pointer to the ancestry tree node associated with the current opacity estimate.

In previous versions of DP-SLAM, this information was stored using a balanced tree. This added significant overhead to the algorithm, both conceptual and computational, and is no longer required in the current version.

The DP-SLAM *ancestry tree* is a basic tree data structure with pointers to parents and children. Each node in the ancestry tree also contains an **onodes** vector, which contains pointers to observation nodes in the grid cells updated by the ancestry tree node.

2.2 Map cache

The main sacrifice that was made when originally designing DP-SLAM was that map accesses no longer took constant time, due to the need to search the observation vector at a given grid square. The map cache provides a way of returning to this constant time access, by reconstructing a separate local map which is consistent with the history of map updates for each particle. Each local map is only as large as the area currently observed, and therefore is of a manageable size.

For a localization procedure using P particles and observing an area of A grid squares, there is a total of $O(AP)$ map accesses. For the constant time accesses provided by the map cache to be useful, the time complexity to build the map cache needs to be $O(AP)$. This result can be achieved by constructing the cache in two passes.

The first pass is to iterate over all grid squares in the global map which could be within sensor range of the robot. For each of these grid squares, the observation vector stores all observations made of that grid square by any particle. This vector is traversed, and for each observation, we update the corresponding local map with a pointer back to the corresponding observation node. This creates a set of partial local maps that store pointers to map updates, but no inherited map information. Since the size of the observation vector can be no greater than the size of the ancestry tree, which has $O(P)$ nodes, the first pass takes $O(P)$ time per grid square.

In the second pass we fill holes in the local maps by propagating inherited map information. The entire ancestry tree is traced, depth first, and the local map is checked for each ancestor node encountered. If the local map for the current ancestor node was not filled during the first pass, then the hole is patched by inheritance from the ancestor node's parent. This will fill any gaps in the local maps for grid squares that have been seen by any current particle. As this pass is directly based on the size of the ancestry tree, it is also $O(P)$ per grid square. Therefore, the total complexity of building the map cache is $O(AP)$.

For each particle, the algorithm constructs a grid of pointers to observation nodes. This provides constant time access to the opacity values consistent with each particle's map. Localization now becomes trivial with this representation: Laser scans are traced through the corresponding local map, and the necessary opacity values are extracted via the pointers. With the constant time accesses afforded by the local maps, the total localization cost in DP-SLAM is now $O(AP)$.

2.3 Updates and Deletions

When the observations associated with a new particle's sensor sweep are integrated into the map, two basic steps are performed. First, a new observation is added to the observation vector of each grid square which was visited by the particle's laser casts. Next, a pointer to each new observation is added to this particle's **onodes** vector. The cost of this operation is obviously no more than that of localization.

There are two situations which require deleting nodes from the ancestry tree. The first is the simple case of removing a node from which the particle filter has not resampled. Each ancestor node maintains a vector of pointers to all observations attributed to it. Therefore, these entries can be removed from the observation vectors in the global grid in constant time. Since there can be no more deletions than there are updates, this process has an amortized cost of $O(AP)$.

The second case for deleting a node occurs when a node in the ancestry tree which has an only child is merged with that child. This involves replacing the opacity value for the parent with that of the child, and then removing that child's entry from the associated grid cell's observation vector. Therefore, this process is identical to the first case, except that each removal of an entry from the global map is preceded by a single update to the same grid square. Since the observation vector at each grid square is not ordered, additions to the vector can be done in constant time, and does not change the complexity from $O(AP)$.

3   Drift

A significant problem faced by current SLAM algorithms is that of drift. Small errors can accumulate over several iterations, and while the resulting map may seem locally consistent, there could be large total errors, which become apparent after the robot closes a large loop. In theory, drift can be avoided by some algorithms in situations where strong linear Gaussian assumptions hold [10]. In practice, it is hard to avoid drift, either as a consequence of violated assumptions or as a consequence of particle filtering. The best algorithms can only extend the distance that the robot travels before experiencing drift. Errors come from (at least) three sources: insufficient particle coverage, coarse precision, and resampling itself (particle depletion).

The first problem is a well known issue with particle filters. Given a finite number of particles, there will be unsampled gaps in the particle coverage of the state space and the proximity to the true state can be as coarse as the size of these gaps. This is exacerbated by the fact that particle filters are often applied to high dimensional state spaces with Gaussian noise, making it impossible to cover unlikely (but still possible) events in the tails of distribution with high particle density. The second issue is coarse precision. This can occur as a result of explicit discretization through an occupancy grid, or implicit discretization through the use of a sensor with finite precision. Coarse precision can make minor perturbations in the state appear identical from the perspective of the sensors and the particle weights. Finally, resampling itself can lead to drift by shifting a finite population of particles away from low probability regions of the state space. While this behavior of a particle filter is typically viewed as a desirable reallocation of computational resources, it can shift particles away from the true state in some cases.

The net effect of these errors can be the gradual accumulation of small errors resulting from failure to sample, differentiate, or remember a state vector that is sufficiently close to the true state. In practice, we have found that there exist large domains where high precision mapping is essentially impossible with any reasonable number of particles.

4   Hierarchical SLAM

In the first part of the paper, we presented an approach to SLAM that reduced the asymptotic complexity per particle to that of pure localization. This is likely as low as can reasonably be expected and should allow the use of large numbers of particles for mapping. However, the discussion of drift in the previous section underscores that the ability to use large numbers of particles may not be sufficient, and we would like techniques that delay the onset of drift as long as possible. We therefore propose a hierarchical approach to SLAM that is capable of recognizing, representing, and recovering from drift.

The basic idea is that the main sources of drift can be modeled as the cumulative effect of a sequence of random events. Through experimentation, we can quantify the expected amount of drift over a certain distance for a given algorithm, much in the same way that we create a probabilistic motion model for the noise in the robot's odometry. Since the total drift over a trajectory is assumed to be a summation of many small, largely independent sources of error, it will be close to a Gaussian distribution.

If we view the act of completing a small map *segment* as a random process with noise, we can then apply a higher level filter to the output of the map segment process in an attempt to track the underlying state more accurately. There are two benefits to this approach. First, it explicitly models and permits the correction of drift. Second, the coarser time granularity of the high level process implies fewer resampling steps and fewer opportunities for particle depletion. Thus, if we can model how much drift is expected to occur over a small section of the robot's trajectory, we can maintain this extra uncertainty longer, and resolve inaccuracies or ambiguities in the map in a natural fashion.

There are some special properties of the SLAM problem that make it particularly well suited to this approach. In the full generality of an arbitrary tracking problem, one should view drift as a problem that affects entire trajectories through state space and the complete belief state at any time. Sampling the space of drifts would then require sampling perturbations to the entire state vector. In this fully general case, the benefit of the hierarchical view would be unclear, as the end result would be quite similar to adding additional noise to the low level process. In SLAM, we can make two assumptions that simplify things. The first is that the robot state vector is highly correlated with the remaining state variables, and the second is that we have access to a low level mapping procedure with moderate accuracy and local consistency. Under these assumptions, the the effects of drift on low level maps can be accurately approximated by perturbations to the endpoints of the robot trajectory used to construct a low level map. By sampling drift only at endpoints, we will fail to sample some of the internal structure that is possible in drifts, e.g., we will fail to distinguish between a linear drift and a spiral pattern with the same endpoints. However, the existence of significant, complicated drift patterns within a map segment would violate our assumption of moderate accuracy and local consistency within our low level mapper.

To achieve a hierarchical approach to SLAM, we use a standard SLAM algorithm using a small portion of the robot's trajectory as input for the low level mapping process. The output is not only a distribution over maps, but also a distribution over robot trajectories. We can treat the distribution over trajectories as a distribution over motions in the higher level SLAM process, to which additional noise from drift is added. This allows us to use the output from each of our small mapping efforts as the input for a new SLAM process, working at a much higher level of time granularity.

For the high level SLAM process, we need to be careful to avoid double counting evidence. Each low level mapping process runs as an independent process intialized with an empty map. The distribution over trajectories returned by the low level mapping process incorporates the effects of the observations used by the low level mapper. To avoid double counting, the high level SLAM process can only weigh the match between the new observations and the existing high level maps. In other words, *all* of the observations for a single high level motion step (single low level trajectory) must be evaluated against the high level map, before any of those observations are used to update the map. We summarize the high level SLAM loop for each high level particle as follows:

1. Sample a high level SLAM state (high level map and robot state).

2. Perturb the sampled robot state by adding random drift.

3. Sample a low level trajectory from the distribution over trajectories returned by the low level SLAM process.

4. Compute a high level weight by evaluating the trajectory and robot observations against the

343

sampled high level map, starting from the perturbed robot state.

5. Update the high level map based upon the new observations.

In practice this can give a much greater improvement in accuracy over simply doubling the resources allocated to a single level SLAM algorithm because the high level is able to model and recover from errors much longer than would be otherwise possible with only a single particle filter. In our implementation we used DP-SLAM at both levels of the hierarchy to ensure a total computational complexity of $O(AP)$. However, there is reason to believe that this approach could be applied to any other sampling-based SLAM method just as effectively. We also implemented this idea with only one level of hierarchy, but multiple levels could provide additional robustness. We felt that the size of the domains on which we tested did not warrant any further levels.

5 Implementation and Empirical Results

Our description of the algorithm and complexity analysis assumes constant time updates to the vectors storing information in the core DP-SLAM data structures. This can be achieved in a straightforward manner using doubly linked lists, but a somewhat more complicated implementation using adjustable arrays is dramatically more efficient in practice. A careful implementation can also avoid caching maps for interior nodes of the ancestry tree.

As with previous versions of DP-SLAM, we generate many more particles than we keep at each iteration. Evaluating a particle requires line tracing 181 laser casts. However, many particles will have significantly lower probability than others and this can be discovered before they are fully evaluated. Using a technique we call *particle culling* we use partial scan information to identify and discard lower probability particles before they are evaluated fully. In practice, this leads to large reduction in the number of laser casts that are fully traced through the grid. Typically, less than one tenth of the particles generated are resampled.

For a complex algorithm like DP-SLAM, asymptotic analysis may not always give a complete picture of real world performance. Therefore, we provide a comparison of actual run times for each method on three different data logs. The particle counts provided are the minimum number of particles needed (at each level) to produce high-quality maps reliably. The improved run time for the linear algorithm also reflects the benefits of some improvements in our culling technique and a cleaner implementation permitted by the linear time algorithm. The quadratic code is simply too slow to run on the Wean Hall data. Log files for these runs are available from the DP-SLAM web page: http://www.cs.duke.edu/~parr/dpslam/. The results show a significant practical advantage for the linear code, and vast improvement, both in terms of time and number of particles, for the hierarchical implementation.

	Quadratic		Linear		Hierarchical	
Log	Particles	Minutes	Particles	Minutes	Particles (high/low)	Minutes
loop5	1500	55	1500	14	200/250	12
loop25	11000	1345	11000	690	2000/3000	289
Wean Hall	120000	N/A	120000	2535	2000/3000	293

Finally, in Figure 1 we include sample output from the hierarchical mapper on the Wean Hall data shown in our table. In this domain, the robot travels approximately 220m before returning to its starting position. Each low level SLAM process was run for 75 time steps, with an average motion of 12cm for each time step. The nonhierarchical approach can produce a very similar result, but requires at least 120,000 particles to do so reliably. (Smaller numbers of particles produced maps with noticeable drifts and errors.) This extreme difference in particle counts and computation time demonstrates the great improvement that can be realized with the hierarchical approach. (The Wean Hall dataset has been mapped

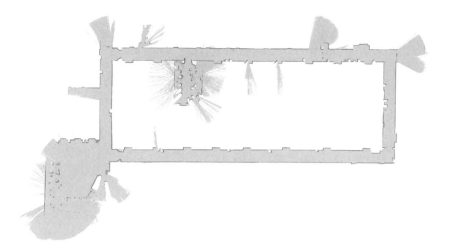

Figure 1: CMU's Wean Hall at 4cm resolution, using hierarchical SLAM. Please zoom in on the map using a software viewer to appreciate some of the fine detail.

successfully before at low resolution using a non-hierarchical approach with run time per iteration that grows with the number of iterations [8].)

6   Related Work

Other methods have attempted to preserve uncertainty for longer numbers of time steps. One approach seeks to delay the resampling step for several iterations, so as to address the total noise in a certain number of steps as one Gaussian with a larger variance [8]. In general, look-ahead methods can "peek" at future observations to use the information from later time steps to influence samples at a previous time step [3]. The HYMM approach[11] combines different types of maps. Another way to interpret hierarchical SLAM is in terms of a hierarchical hidden Markov model framework [5]. In a hierarchical HMM, each node in the HMM has the potential to invoke sub-HMMs to produce a series of observations. The main difference is that in hierarchical HMMs, there is assumed to be a single process that can be represented in different ways. In our hierarchical SLAM approach, only the lowest level models a physical process, while higher levels model the errors in lower levels.

7   Conclusions and Future Research

We have presented a SLAM algorithm which is the culmination of our efforts to make multiple hypothesis mapping practical for densely populated maps. Our first algorithmic accomplishment is to show that this requires no more effort, asymptotically, than pure localization using a particle filter. However, for mapping, the number of particles needed can be large and can still grow to be unmanageable for large domains due to drift. We therefore developed a method to improve the accuracy achieveable with a reasonable number of particles. This is accomplished through the use of a hierarchical particle filter. By allowing an additional level of sampling on top of a series of small particle filters, we can successfully maintain the necessary uncertainty to produce very accurate maps. This is due to the explicit modeling of the drift, a key process which differentiates this approach from previous attempts to preserve uncertainty in particle filters.

The hierarchical approach to SLAM has been shown to be very useful in improving DP-SLAM performance. This would lead us to believe that similar improvements could also be realized in applying this to other sampling based SLAM methods. SLAM is perhaps not the only viable application for hierarchical framework for particle filters. However, one of the key aspects of SLAM is that the drift can easily be represented by a very low dimensional descriptor. Other particle filter applications which have drift that must be modeled in many more dimensions could benefit much less from this hierarchical approach.

The work of Hahnel et al. [8] has made progress in increasing efficiency and reducing drift by using scan matching rather than pure sampling from a noisy proposal distribution. Since much of the computation time used by DP-SLAM is spent evaluating bad particles, a combination of DP-SLAM with scan matching could yield significant practical speedups.

Acknowledgments

This research was supported by SAIC, the Sloan foundation, and the NSF. The Wean Hall data were graciously provided by Dirk Hahnel and Dieter Fox.

References

[1] W. Burgard, D. Fox, H. Jans, C. Matenar, and S. Thrun. Sonar-based mapping with mobile robots using EM. In *Proc. of the International Conference on Machine Learning*, 1999.

[2] P. Cheeseman, P. Smith, and M. Self. Estimating uncertain spatial relationships in robotics. In *Autonomous Robot Vehicles*, pages 167–193. Springer-Verlag, 1990.

[3] N. de Freitas, R. Dearden, F. Hutter, R. Morales-Menendez, J. Mutch, and D. Poole. Diagnosis by a waiter and a Mars explorer. In *IEEE Special Issue on Sequential State Estimation*, pages 455–468, 2003.

[4] A. Eliazar and R. Parr. DP-SLAM 2.0. In *IEEE International Conference on Robotics and Automation (ICRA)*, 2004.

[5] Shai Fine, Yoram Singer, and Naftali Tishby. The hierarchical hidden markov model: Analysis and applications. *Machine Learning*, 32(1):41–62, 1998.

[6] Dieter Fox, Wolfram Burgard, Frank Dellaert, and Sebastian Thrun. Monte carlo localization: Efficient position estimation for mobile robots. In *AAAI-99*, 1999.

[7] J. Gutmann and K. Konolige. Incremental mapping of large cyclic environments. In *IEEE International Symposium on Computational Intelligence in Robotics and Automation (ICRA)*, pages 318–325, 2000.

[8] Dirk Hahnel, Wolfram Burgard, Dieter Fox, and Sebastian Thrun. An efficient fastslam algorithm for generating maps of large-scale cyclic environments from raw laser range measurements. In *Proceedings of the International Conference on Intelligent Robots and Systems*, 2003.

[9] John H. Leonard, , and Hugh F. Durrant-Whyte. Mobile robot localization by tracking geometric beacons. In *IEEE Transactions on Robotics and Automation*, pages 376–382. IEEE, June 1991.

[10] M. Montemerlo, S. Thrun, D. Koller, and B. Wegbreit. FastSLAM 2.0: An improved particle filtering algorithm for simultaneous localization and mapping that provably converges. In *IJCAI-03*, Morgan Kaufmann, 2003. 1151–1156.

[11] J. Nieto, J. Guivant, and E. Nebot. The HYbrid Metric Maps (HYMMS): A novel map representation for denseSLAM. In *IEEE International Conference on Robotics and Automation (ICRA)*, 2004.

[12] S. Thrun. A probabilistic online mapping algorithm for teams of mobile robots. *International Journal of Robotics Research*, 20(5):335–363, 2001.

Learning to Control an Octopus Arm with Gaussian Process Temporal Difference Methods

Yaakov Engel[*]
AICML, Dept. of Computing Science
University of Alberta
Edmonton, Canada
yaki@cs.ualberta.ca

Peter Szabo and Dmitry Volkinshtein
Dept. of Electrical Engineering
Technion Institute of Technology
Haifa, Israel
peter.z.szabo@gmail.com
dmitryvolk@gmail.com

Abstract

The Octopus arm is a highly versatile and complex limb. How the Octopus controls such a hyper-redundant arm (not to mention eight of them!) is as yet unknown. Robotic arms based on the same mechanical principles may render present day robotic arms obsolete. In this paper, we tackle this control problem using an online reinforcement learning algorithm, based on a Bayesian approach to policy evaluation known as Gaussian process temporal difference (GPTD) learning. Our substitute for the real arm is a computer simulation of a 2-dimensional model of an Octopus arm. Even with the simplifications inherent to this model, the state space we face is a high-dimensional one. We apply a GPTD-based algorithm to this domain, and demonstrate its operation on several learning tasks of varying degrees of difficulty.

1 Introduction

The Octopus arm is one of the most sophisticated and fascinating appendages found in nature. It is an exceptionally flexible organ, with a remarkable repertoire of motion. In contrast to skeleton-based vertebrate and present-day robotic limbs, the Octopus arm lacks a rigid skeleton and has virtually infinitely many degrees of freedom. As a result, this arm is highly hyper-redundant – it is capable of stretching, contracting, folding over itself several times, rotating along its axis at any point, and following the contours of almost any object. These properties allow the Octopus to exhibit feats requiring agility, precision and force. For instance, it is well documented that Octopuses are able to pry open a clam or remove the plug off a glass jar, to gain access to its contents [1].

The basic mechanism underlying the flexibility of the Octopus arm (as well as of other organs, such as the elephant trunk and vertebrate tongues) is the muscular hydrostat [2]. Muscular hydrostats are organs capable of exerting force and producing motion with the sole use of muscles. The muscles serve in the dual roles of generating the forces and maintaining the structural rigidity of the appendage. This is possible due to a constant volume constraint, which arises from the fact that muscle tissue is incompressible. Proper

---

[*]To whom correspondence should be addressed. Web site: www.cs.ualberta.ca/~yaki

use of this constraint allows muscle contractions in one direction to generate forces acting in perpendicular directions.

Due to their unique properties, understanding the principles governing the movement and control of the Octopus arm and other muscular hydrostats is of great interest to both physiologists and robotics engineers. Recent physiological and behavioral studies produced some interesting insights to the way the Octopus plans and controls its movements. Gutfreund et al. [3] investigated the reaching movement of an Octopus arm and showed that the motion is performed by a stereotypical forward propagation of a bend point along the arm. Yekutieli et al. [4] propose that the complex behavioral movements of the Octopus are composed from a limited number of "motion primitives", which are spatio-temporally combined to produce the arm's motion.

Although physical implementations of robotic arms based on the same principles are not yet available, recent progress in the technology of "artificial muscles" using electroactive polymers [5] may allow the construction of such arms in the near future. Needless to say, even a single such arm poses a formidable control challenge, which does not appear to be amenable to conventional control theoretic or robotics methodology. In this paper we propose a learning approach for tackling this problem. Specifically, we formulate the task of bringing some part of the arm into a goal region as a reinforcement learning (RL) problem. We then proceed to solve this problem using Gaussian process temporal difference learning (GPTD) algorithms [6, 7, 8].

2   The Domain

Our experimental test-bed is a finite-elements computer simulation of a planar variant of the Octopus arm, described in [9, 4]. This model is based on a decomposition of the arm into quadrilateral compartments, and the constant muscular volume constraint mentioned above is translated into a constant area constraint on each compartment. Muscles are modeled as dampened springs and the mass of each compartment is concentrated in point masses located at its corners[1]. Although this is a rather crude approximation of the real arm, even for a modest 10-segment model there are already 88 continuous state variables[2], making this a rather high dimensional learning problem. Figure 1 illustrates this model.

Since our model is 2–dimensional, all force vectors lie on the $x - y$ plane, and the arm's motion is planar. This limitation is due mainly to the high computational cost of the full 3–dimensional calculations for any arm of reasonable size. There are four types of forces acting on the arm: 1) The internal forces generated by the arm's muscles, 2) the vertical forces caused by the influence of gravity and the arm's buoyancy in the medium in which it is immersed (typically sea water), 3) drag forces produced by the arm's motion through this medium, and 4) internal pressure-induced forces responsible for maintaining the constant volume of each compartment. The use of simulation allows us to easily investigate different operating scenarios, such as zero or low gravity scenarios, different media, such as water, air or vacuum, and different muscle models. In this study, we used a simple linear model for the muscles. The force applied by a muscle at any given time t is

$$F(t) = \big(k_0 + (k_{max} - k_0)A(t)\big)\big(\ell(t) - \ell_{rest}\big) + c\frac{d\ell(t)}{dt}.$$

---

[1]For the purpose of computing volumes, masses, friction and muscle strength, the arm is effectively defined in three dimensions. However, no forces or motion are allowed in the third dimension. We also ignore the suckers located along the ventral side of the arm, and treat the arm as if it were symmetric with respect to reflection along its long axis. Finally, we comment that this model is restricted to modeling the mechanics of the arm and does not attempt to model its nervous system.

[2]10 segments result in 22 point masses, each being described by 4 state variables – the x and y coordinates and their respective first time-derivatives.

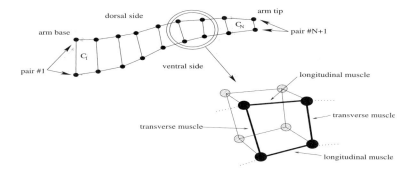

Figure 1: An N compartment simulated Octopus arm. Each constant area compartment C_i is defined by its surrounding 2 longitudinal muscles (ventral and dorsal) and 2 transverse muscles. Circles mark the $2N + 2$ point masses in which the arm's mass is distributed. In the bottom right one compartment is magnified with additional detail.

This equation describes a dampened spring with a controllable spring constant. The spring's length at time t is $\ell(t)$, its resting length, at which it does not apply any force is ℓ_{rest}.[3] The spring's stiffness is controlled by the activation variable $A(t) \in [0, 1]$. Thus, when the activation is zero, and the contraction is isometric (with zero velocity), the relaxed muscle exhibits a baseline passive stiffness k_0. In a fully activated isometric contraction the spring constant becomes k_{max}. The second term is a dampening, energy dissipating term, which is proportional to the rate of change in the spring's length, and (with $c > 0$) is directed to resist that change. This is a very simple muscle model, which has been chosen mainly due to its low computational cost, and the relative ease of computing the energy expended by the muscle (why this is useful will become apparent in the sequel). More complex muscle models can be easily incorporated into the simulator, but may result in higher computational overhead. For additional details on the modeling of the other forces and on the derivation of the equations of motion, refer to [4].

3 The Learning Algorithms

As mentioned above, we formulate the problem of controlling our Octopus arm as a RL problem. We are therefore required to define a Markov decision process (MDP), consisting of state and action spaces, a reward function and state transition dynamics. The states in our model are the Cartesian coordinates of the point masses and their first time-derivatives. A finite (and relatively small) number of actions are defined by specifying, for each action, a set of activations for the arm's muscles. The actions used in this study are depicted in Figure 2. Given the arm's current state and the chosen action, we use the simulator to compute the arm's state after a small fixed time interval. Throughout this interval the activations remain fixed, until a new action is chosen for the next interval. The reward is defined as -1 for non-goal states, and 10 for goal states. This encourages the controller to find policies that bring the arm to the goal as quickly as possible. In addition, in order to encourage smoothness and economy in the arm's movements, we subtract an energy penalty term from these rewards. This term is proportional to the total energy expended by all muscles during each action interval. Training is performed in an episodic manner: Upon reaching a goal, the current episode terminates and the arm is placed in a new initial position to begin a new episode. If a goal is not reached by some fixed amount of time, the

---

[3]It is assumed that at all times $\ell(t) \geq \ell_{rest}$. This is meant to ensure that our muscles can only apply force by contracting, as real muscles do. This can be assured by endowing the compartments with sufficiently high volumes, or equivalently, by setting ℓ_{rest} sufficiently low.

episode terminates regardless.

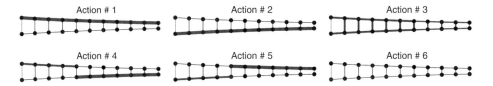

Figure 2: The actions used in the fixed-base experiments. Line thickness is proportional to activation intensity. For the rotating base experiment, these actions were augmented with versions of actions 1, 2, 4 and 5 that include clockwise and anti-clockwise torques applied to the arm's base.

The RL algorithms implemented in this study belong to the Policy Iteration family of algorithms [10]. Such algorithms require an algorithmic component for estimating the mean sum of (possibly discounted) future rewards collected along trajectories, as a function of the trajectory's initial state, also known as the *value function*. The best known RL algorithms for performing this task are *temporal difference* algorithms. Since the state space of our problem is very large, some form of function approximation must be used to represent the value estimator. Temporal difference methods, such as TD(λ) and LSTD(λ), are provably convergent when used with linearly parametrized function approximation architectures [10]. Used this way, they require the user to define a fixed set of basis functions, which are then linearly combined to approximate the value function. These basis functions must be defined over the entire state space, or at least over the subset of states that might be reached during learning. When local basis functions are used (e.g., RBFs or tile codes [11]), this inevitably means an exponential explosion of the number of basis functions with the dimensionality of the state space. Nonparametric GPTD learning algorithms[4] [8], offer an alternative to the conventional parametric approach. The idea is to define a nonparametric statistical generative model connecting the hidden values and the observed rewards, and a prior distribution over value functions. The GPTD modeling assumptions are that both the prior and the observation-noise distributions are Gaussian, and that the model equations relating values and rewards have a special linear form. During or following a learning session, in which a sequence of states and rewards are observed, Bayes' rule may be used to compute the posterior distribution over value functions, conditioned on the observed reward sequence. Due to the GPTD model assumptions, this distribution is also Gaussian, and is derivable in closed form. The benefits of using (nonparametric) GPTD methods are that 1) the resulting value estimates are generally not constrained to lie in the span of any predetermined set of basis functions, 2) no resources are wasted on unvisited state and action space regions, and 3) rather than the point estimates provided by other methods, GPTD methods provide complete probability distributions over value functions.

In [6, 7, 8] it was shown how the computation of the posterior value GP moments can be performed sequentially and online. This is done by a employing a forward selection mechanism, which is aimed at attaining a sparse approximation of the posterior moments, under a constraint on the resulting error. The input samples (states, or state-action pairs) used in this approximation are stored in a *dictionary*, the final size of which is often a good indicator of the problem's complexity. Since nonparametric GPTD algorithms belong to the family of kernel machines, they require the user to define a kernel function, which encodes her prior knowledge and beliefs concerning similarities and correlations in the domain at hand. More specifically, the kernel function $k(\cdot, \cdot)$ defines the *prior covariance* of the value process. Namely, for two arbitrary states $\mathbf{x}$ and $\mathbf{x}'$, $\mathbf{Cov}[V(\mathbf{x}), V(\mathbf{x}')] = k(\mathbf{x}, \mathbf{x}')$ (see [8] for details). In this study we experimented with several kernel functions, however, in this

---

[4]GPTD models can also be defined parametrically, see [8].

paper we will describe results obtained using a third degree polynomial kernel, defined by $k(\mathbf{x}, \mathbf{x}') = \left(\mathbf{x}^\top \mathbf{x}' + 1\right)^3$. It is well known that this kernel induces a feature space of monomials of degree 3 or less [12]. For our 88 dimensional input space, this feature space is spanned by a basis consisting of $\binom{91}{3} = 121{,}485$ linearly independent monomials.

We experimented with two types of policy-iteration based algorithms. The first was optimistic policy iteration (OPI), in which, in any given time-step, the current GPTD value estimator is used to evaluate the successor states resulting from each one of the actions available at the current state. Since, given an action, the dynamics are deterministic, we used the simulation to determine the identity of successor states. An action is then chosen according to a semi-greedy selection rule (more on this below). A more disciplined approach is provided by a *paired actor-critic* algorithm. Here, two independent GPTD estimators are maintained. The first is used to determine the policy, again, by some semi-greedy action selection rule, while its parameters remain fixed. In the meantime, the second GPTD estimator is used to evaluate the stationary policy determined by the first. After the second GPTD estimator is deemed sufficiently accurate, as indicated by the GPTD value variance estimate, the roles are reversed. This is repeated as many times as required, until no significant improvement in policies is observed.

Although the latter algorithm, being an instance of approximate policy iteration, has a better theoretical grounding [10], in practice it was observed that the GPTD-based OPI worked significantly faster in this domain. In the experiments reported in the next section we therefore used the latter. For additional details and experiments refer to [13]. One final wrinkle concerns the selection of the initial state in a new episode. Since plausible arm configurations cannot be attained by randomly drawing 88 state variable from some simple distribution, a more involved mechanism for setting the initial state in each episode has to be defined. The method we chose is tightly connected to the GPTD mode of operation: At the end of each episode, 10 random states were drawn from the GPTD dictionary. From these, the state with the highest posterior value variance estimate was selected as the initial state of the next episode. This is a form of *active learning*, which is made possible by employing GPTD, and that is applicable to general episodic RL problems.

4 Experiments

The experiments described in this section are aimed at demonstrating the applicability of GPTD-based algorithms to large-scale RL problems, such as our Octopus arm. In these experiments we used the simulated 10-compartment arm described in Section 2. The set of goal states consisted of a circular region located somewhere within the potential reach of the arm (recall that the arm has no fixed length). The action set depends on the task, as described in Figure 2. Training episode duration was set to 4 seconds, and the time interval between action decisions was 0.4 seconds. This allowed a maximum of 10 learning steps per trial. The discount factor was set to 1.

The exploration policy used was the ubiquitous ε-greedy policy: The greedy action (i.e. the one for which the sum of the reward and the successor state's estimated value is the highest) is chosen with probability $1 - \varepsilon$, and with probability ε a random action is drawn from a uniform distribution over all other actions. The value of ε is reduced during learning, until the policy converges to the greedy one. In our implementation, in each episode, ε was dependent on the number of successful episodes experienced up to that point. The general form of this relation is $\varepsilon = \varepsilon_0 N_{\frac{1}{2}}/(N_{\frac{1}{2}} + N_{goals})$, where N_{goals} is the number of successful episodes, ε_0 is the initial value of ε and $N_{\frac{1}{2}}$ is the number of successful episodes required to reduce ε to $\varepsilon_0/2$.

In order to evaluate the quality of learned solutions, 100 initial arm configurations were cre-

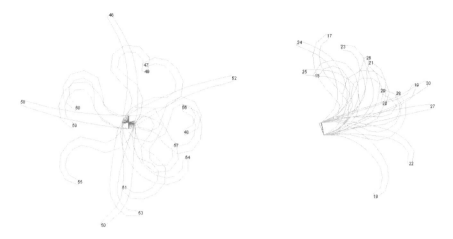

Figure 3: Examples of initial states for the rotating-base experiments (left) and the fixed-base experiments (right). Starting states also include velocities, which are not shown.

ated. This was done by starting a simulation from some fixed arm configuration, performing a long sequence of random actions, and sampling states randomly from the resulting trajectory. Some examples of such initial states are depicted in Figure 3. During learning, following each training episode, the GPTD-learned parameters were recorded on file. Each set of GPTD parameters defines a value estimator, and therefore also a greedy policy with respect to the posterior value mean. Each such policy was evaluated by using it, starting from each of the 100 initial test states. For each starting state, we recorded whether or not a goal state was reached within the episode's time limit (4 seconds), and the duration of the episode (successful episodes terminate when a goal state is reached). These two measures of performance were averaged over the 100 starting states and plotted against the episode index, resulting in two corresponding learning curves for each experiment[5].

We started with a simple task in which reaching the goal is quite easy. Any point of the arm entering the goal circle was considered as a success. The arm's base was fixed and the gravity constant was set to zero, corresponding to a scenario in which the arm moves on a horizontal frictionless plane. In the second experiment the task was made a little more difficult. The goal was moved further away from the base of the arm. Moreover, gravity was set to its natural level, of $9.8 \frac{m}{s^2}$, with the motion of the arm now restricted to a vertical plane. The learning curves corresponding to these two experiments are shown in Figure 4. A success rate of 100% was reached after 10 and 20 episodes, respectively. In both cases, even after a success rate of 100% is attained, the mean time-to-goal keeps improving. The final dictionaries contained about 200 and 350 states, respectively.

In our next two experiments, the arm had to reach a goal located so that it cannot be reached unless the base of the arm is allowed to rotate. We added base-rotating actions to the basic actions used in the previous experiments (see Figure 2 for an explanation). Allowing a rotating base significantly increases the size of the action set, as well the size of the reachable state space, making the learning task considerably more difficult. To make things even more difficult, we rewarded the arm only if it reached the goal with its tip, i.e. the two point-masses at the end of the arm. In the first experiment in this series, gravity was switched on. A 99% success rate was attained after 270 trials, with a final dictionary size of

---

[5]It is worth noting that this evaluation procedure requires by far more time than the actual learning, since each point in the graphs shown below requires us to perform 100 simulation runs. Whereas learning can be performed almost in real-time (depending on dictionary size), computing the statistics for a single learning run may take a day, or more.

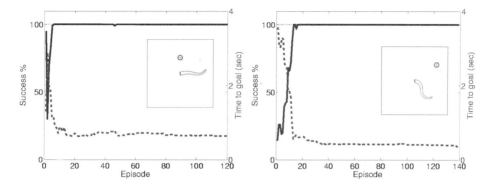

Figure 4: Success rate (solid) and mean time to goal (dashed) for a fixed-base arm in zero gravity (left), and with gravity (right). 100% success was reached after 10 and 20 trials, respectively. The insets illustrate one starting position and the location of the goal regions, in each case.

about 600 states. In the second experiment gravity was switched off, but a circular region of obstacle states was placed between the arm's base and the goal circle. If any part of the arm touched the obstacle, the episode immediately terminated with a negative reward of -2. Here, the success rate peaked at 40% after around 1000 episodes, and remained roughly constant thereafter. It should be taken into consideration that at least some of the 100 test starting states are so close to the obstacle that, regardless of the action taken, the arm cannot avoid hitting the obstacle. The learning curves are presented in Figure 5.

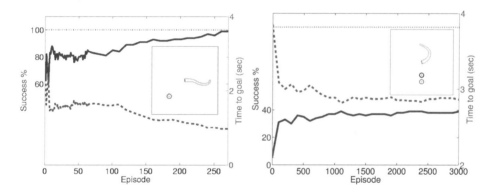

Figure 5: Success rate (solid) and mean time to goal (dashed) for a rotating-base arm with gravity switched on (left), and with gravity switched off but with an obstacle blocking the direct path to the goal (right). The arm has to rotate its base in order to reach the goal in either case (see insets). Positive reward was given only for arm-tip contact, any contact with the obstacle terminated the episode with a penalty. A 99% success rate was attained after 270 episodes for the first task, whereas for the second task success rate reached 40%.

Video movies showing the arm in various scenarios are available at www.cs.ualberta.ca/~yaki/movies/.

5 Discussion

Up to now, GPTD based RL algorithms have only been tested on low dimensional problem domains. Although kernel methods have handled high-dimensional data, such as handwritten digits, remarkably well in supervised learning domains, the applicability of the kernel-based GPTD approach to high dimensional RL problems has remained an open question. The results presented in this paper are, in our view, a clear indication that GPTD methods are indeed scalable, and should be considered seriously as a possible solution method by practitioners facing large-scale RL problems. Further work on the theory and practice of GPTD methods is called for. Standard techniques for model selection and tuning of hyper-parameters can be incorporated straightforwardly into GPTD algorithms. Value iteration-based variants, i.e. "GPQ-learning", would provide yet another useful set of tools.

The Octopus arm domain is of independent interest, both to physiologists and robotics engineers. The fact that reasonable controllers for such a complex arm can be learned from trial and error, in a relatively short time, should not be understated. Further work in this direction should be aimed at extending the Octopus arm simulation to a full 3-dimensional model, as well as applying our RL algorithms to real robotic arms based on the muscular hydrostat principle, when these become available.

Acknowledgments

Y. E. was partially supported by the AICML and the Alberta Ingenuity fund. We would also like to thank the Ollendorff Minerva Center, for supporting this project.

References

[1] G. Fiorito, C. V. Planta, and P. Scotto. Problem solving ability of Octopus Vulgaris Lamarck (Mollusca, Cephalopoda). *Behavioral and Neural Biology*, 53 (2):217–230, 1990.

[2] W.M. Kier and K.K. Smith. Tongues, tentacles and trunks: The biomechanics of movement in muscular-hydrostats. *Zoological Journal of the Linnean Society*, 83:307–324, 1985.

[3] Y. Gutfreund, T. Flash, Y. Yarom, G. Fiorito, I. Segev, and B. Hochner. Organization of Octopus arm movements: A model system for studying the control of flexible arms. *The journal of Neuroscience*, 16:7297–7307, 1996.

[4] Y. Yekutieli, R. Sagiv-Zohar, R. Aharonov, Y. Engel, B. Hochner, and T. Flash. A dynamic model of the Octopus arm. I. Biomechanics of the Octopus reaching movement. *Journal of Neurophysiology (in press)*, 2005.

[5] Y. Bar-Cohen, editor. *Electroactive Polymer (EAP) Actuators as Artificial Muscles - Reality, Potential and Challenges*. SPIE Press, 2nd edition, 2004.

[6] Y. Engel, S. Mannor, and R. Meir. Bayes meets Bellman: The Gaussian process approach to temporal difference learning. In *Proc. of the 20th International Conference on Machine Learning*, 2003.

[7] Y. Engel, S. Mannor, and R. Meir. Reinforcement learning with Gaussian processes. In *Proc. of the 22nd International Conference on Machine Learning*, 2005.

[8] Y. Engel. *Algorithms and Representations for Reinforcement Learning*. PhD thesis, The Hebrew University of Jerusalem, 2005. www.cs.ualberta.ca/~yaki/papers/thesis.ps.

[9] R. Aharonov, Y. Engel, B. Hochner, and T. Flash. A dynamical model of the octopus arm. In *Neuroscience letters. Supl. 48. Proceedings of the 6th annual meeting of the Israeli Neuroscience Society*, 1997.

[10] D.P. Bertsekas and J.N. Tsitsiklis. *Neuro-Dynamic Programming*. Athena Scientific, 1996.

[11] R.S. Sutton and Andrew G. Barto. *Reinforcement Learning: An Introduction*. MIT Press, 1998.

[12] J. Shawe-Taylor and N. Cristianini. *Kernel Methods for Pattern Analysis*. Cambridge University Press, Cambridge, England, 2004.

[13] Y. Engel, P. Szabo, and D. Volkinshtein. Learning to control an Octopus arm with Gaussian process temporal difference methods. Technical report, Technion Institute of Technology, 2005. www.cs.ualberta.ca/~yaki/reports/octopus.pdf.

Two view learning: SVM-2K, Theory and Practice

Jason D.R. Farquhar
jdrf99r@ecs.soton.ac.uk

David R. Hardoon
drh@ecs.soton.ac.uk

Hongying Meng
hongying@cs.york.ac.uk

John Shawe-Taylor
jst@ecs.soton.ac.uk

Sandor Szedmak
ss03v@ecs.soton.ac.uk

School of Electronics and Computer Science,
University of Southampton, Southampton, England

Abstract

Kernel methods make it relatively easy to define complex high-dimensional feature spaces. This raises the question of how we can identify the relevant subspaces for a particular learning task. When two views of the same phenomenon are available kernel Canonical Correlation Analysis (KCCA) has been shown to be an effective preprocessing step that can improve the performance of classification algorithms such as the Support Vector Machine (SVM). This paper takes this observation to its logical conclusion and proposes a method that combines this two stage learning (KCCA followed by SVM) into a single optimisation termed SVM-2K. We present both experimental and theoretical analysis of the approach showing encouraging results and insights.

1 Introduction

Kernel methods enable us to work with high dimensional feature spaces by defining weight vectors implicitly as linear combinations of the training examples. This even makes it practical to learn in infinite dimensional spaces as for example when using the Gaussian kernel. The Gaussian kernel is an extreme example, but techniques have been developed to define kernels for a range of different datatypes, in many cases characterised by very high dimensionality. Examples are the string kernels for text, graph kernels for graphs, marginal kernels, kernels for image data, etc.

With this plethora of high dimensional representations it is frequently helpful to assist learning algorithms by preprocessing the feature space in projecting the data into a low dimensional subspace that contains the relevant information for the learning task. Methods of performing this include principle components analysis (PCA) [7], partial least squares [8], kernel independent component analysis (KICA) [1] and kernel canonical correlation analysis (KCCA) [5].

The last method requires two views of the data both of which contain all of the relevant information for the learning task, but which individually contain representation specific details that are different and irrelevant. Perhaps the simplest example of this situation is a paired document corpus in which we have the same information in two languages. KCCA attempts to isolate feature space directions that correlate between the two views and hence might be expected to represent the common relevant information. Hence, one can view this preprocessing as a denoising of the individual representations through cross-correlating them.

Experiments have shown how using this as a preprocessing step can improve subsequent analysis in for example classification experiments using a support vector machine (SVM) [6]. This is explained by the fact that the signal to noise ratio has improved in the identified subspace.

Though the combination of KCCA and SVM seems effective, there appears no guarantee that the directions identified by KCCA will be best suited to the classification task. This paper therefore looks at the possibility of combining the two distinct stages of KCCA and SVM into a single optimisation that will be termed SVM-2K.

The next section introduces the new algorithm and discusses its structure. Experiments are then given showing the performance of the algorithm on an image classification task.

Though the performance is encouraging it is in many ways counter-intuitive, leading to speculation about why an improvement is seen. To investigate this question an analysis of its generalisation properties is given in the following two sections, before drawing conclusions.

2 SVM-2K Algorithm

We assume that we are given two views of the same data, one expressed through a feature projection ϕ_A with corresponding kernel κ_A and the other through a feature projection ϕ_B with kernel κ_B. A paired data set is then given by a set

$$S = \{(\phi_A(\mathbf{x}_1), \phi_B(\mathbf{x}_1)), \ldots, (\phi_A(\mathbf{x}_\ell), \phi_B(\mathbf{x}_\ell))\},$$

where for example ϕ_A could be the feature vector associated with one language and ϕ_B that associated with a second language. For a classification task each data item would also include a label.

The KCCA algorithm looks for directions in the two feature spaces such that when the training data is projected onto those directions the two vectors (one for each view) of values obtained are maximally correlated. One can also characterise these directions as those that minimise the two norm between the two vectors under the constraint that they both have norm 1 [5].

We can think of this as constraining the choice of weight vectors in the two spaces. KCCA would typically find a sequence of projection directions of dimension anywhere between 50 and 500 that can then be used as the feature space for training an SVM [6].

An SVM can be thought of as a 1-dimensional projection followed by thresholding, so SVM-2K combines the two steps by introducing the constraint of similarity between two 1-dimensional projections identifying two distinct SVMs one in each of the two feature spaces. The extra constraint is chosen slightly differently from the 2-norm that characterises KCCA. We rather take an ϵ-insensitive 1-norm using slack variables to measure the amount by which points fail to meet ϵ similarity:

$$|\langle \mathbf{w}_A, \phi_A(\mathbf{x}_i) \rangle + b_A - \langle \mathbf{w}_B, \phi_B(\mathbf{x}_i) \rangle - b_B| \leq \eta_i + \epsilon,$$

where $\mathbf{w}_A, b_A$ ($\mathbf{w}_B, b_B$) are the weight and threshold of the first (second) SVM.

Combining this constraint with the usual 1-norm SVM constraints and allowing different regularisation constants gives the following optimisation:

$$\min L = \frac{1}{2}\|\mathbf{w}_A\|^2 + \frac{1}{2}\|\mathbf{w}_B\|^2 + C^A\sum_{i=1}^{\ell}\xi_i^A + C^B\sum_{i=1}^{\ell}\xi_i^B + D\sum_{i=1}^{\ell}\eta_i$$

such that
$$|\langle\mathbf{w}_A,\phi_A(\mathbf{x}_i)\rangle + b_A - \langle\mathbf{w}_B,\phi_B(\mathbf{x}_i)\rangle - b_B| \leq \eta_i + \epsilon$$
$$y_i\left(\langle\mathbf{w}_A,\phi_A(\mathbf{x}_i)\rangle + b_A\right) \geq 1 - \xi_i^A$$
$$y_i\left(\langle\mathbf{w}_B,\phi_B(\mathbf{x}_i)\rangle + b_B\right) \geq 1 - \xi_i^B$$
$$\xi_i^A \geq 0,\quad \xi_i^B \geq 0,\quad \eta_i \geq 0\quad\text{all for}\quad 1 \leq i \leq \ell.$$

Let $\hat{\mathbf{w}}_A$, $\hat{\mathbf{w}}_B$, $\hat{b}_A$, $\hat{b}_B$ be the solution to this optimisation problem. The final SVM-2K decision function is then $h(x) = \mathrm{sign}(f(x))$, where

$$f(x) = 0.5\left(\langle\hat{\mathbf{w}}_A,\phi_A(x)\rangle + \hat{b}_A + \langle\hat{\mathbf{w}}_B,\phi_B(x)\rangle + \hat{b}_B\right) = 0.5\left(f_A(x) + f_B(x)\right).$$

Applying the usual Lagrange multiplier techniques we arrive at the following dual problem:

$$\max W = -\frac{1}{2}\sum_{i,j=1}^{\ell}\left(g_i^A g_j^A \kappa_A(\mathbf{x}_i,\mathbf{x}_j) + g_i^B g_j^B \kappa_B(\mathbf{x}_i,\mathbf{x}_j)\right) + \sum_{i=1}^{\ell}(\alpha_i^A + \alpha_i^B)$$

such that
$$g_i^A = \alpha_i^A y_i - \beta_i^+ + \beta_i^-,\quad g_i^B = \alpha_i^B y_i + \beta_i^+ - \beta_i^-,$$
$$\sum_{i=1}^{\ell}g_i^A = 0 = \sum_{i=1}^{\ell}g_i^B,$$
$$0 \leq \alpha_i^{A/B} \leq C^{A/B}$$
$$0 \leq \beta_i^{+/-},\quad \beta_i^+ + \beta_i^- \leq D$$

with the functions
$$f_{A/B}(x) = \sum_{i=1}^{\ell}g_i^{A/B}\kappa_{A/B}(\mathbf{x}_i,x) + b_{A/B}.$$

3 Experimental results

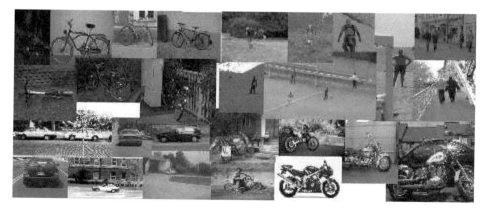

Figure 1: Typical example images from the PASCAL VOC challenge database. Classes are; Bikes (top-left), People (top-right), Cars (bottom-left) and Motorbikes (bottom-right).

The performance of the algorithms developed in this paper we evaluated on PASCAL Visual Object Classes (VOC) challenge dataset `test1`[1]. This is a new dataset consisting of four object classes in realistic scenes. The object classes are, motorbikes (M), bicycles (B), people (P) and cars (C) with the dataset containing 684 training set images consisting of (214, 114, 84, 272) images in each class and 689 test set images with (216, 114, 84, 275) for each class. As can be seen in Figure 1 this is a very challenging dataset with objects of widely varying type, pose, illumination, occlusion, background, etc.

The task is to classify the image according to whether it contains a given object type. We tested the images containing the object (i.e. categories M, B, C and P) against non-object images from the database (i.e. category N). The training set contained 100 positive and 100 negative images. The tests are carried out on 100 new images, half belonging to the learned class and half not.

Like many other successful methods [3, 4] we take a "set-of-patches" approach to this problem. These methods represent an image in terms of the features of a set of small image patches. By carefully choosing the patches and their features this representation can be made largely robust to the common types of image transformation, e.g. scale, rotation, perspective, occlusion.

Two views were provided of each image through the use of different patch types. One was from affine invariant interest point detectors with a moment invariant descriptor calculated for each interest point. The second were key point features from SIFT detectors. For one image, several hundred characteristic patches were detected according to the complexity of the images. These were then clustered around $K = 400$ centres for each feature space. Each image is then represented as a histogram over these centres. So finally, for one image there are two feature vectors of length 400 that provide the two views.

	Motorbike	Bicycle	People	Car
SVM 1	94.05	91.58	91.58	87.95
SVM 2	91.15	91.15	90.57	86.21
KCCA + SVM	94.19	90.28	90.57	88.68
SVM 2K	**94.34**	**93.47**	**92.74**	**90.13**

Table 1: Results for 4 datasets showing test accuracy of the individual SVMs and SVM-2K.

Figure 1 show the results of the test errors obtained for the different categories for the individual SVMs and the SVM-2K. There is a clear improvement in performance of the SVM-2K over the two individual SVMs in all four categories.

If we examine the structure of the optimisation, the restriction that the output of the two linear functions be similar seems to be an arbitrary restriction particularly for points that are far from the margin or are misclassified. Intuitively it would appear better to take advantage of the abilities of the different representations to better fit the data.

In order to understand this apparent contradiction we now consider a theoretical analysis of the generalisation of the SVM-2K using the framework provided by Rademacher complexity bounds.

4   Background theory

We begin with the definitions required for Rademacher complexity, see for example Bartlett and Mendelson [2] (see also [9] for an introductory exposition).

Definition 1. *For a sample $S = \{x_1, \cdots, x_\ell\}$ generated by a distribution D on a set*

---

[1] Available from `http://www.pascal-network.org/challenges/VOC/voc/160305_VOCdata.tar.gz`

X and a real-valued function class $\mathcal{F}$ with a domain X, the empirical Rademacher complexity of $\mathcal{F}$ is the random variable

$$\hat{R}_\ell(\mathcal{F}) = \mathbb{E}_\sigma \left[\sup_{f \in \mathcal{F}} \left| \frac{2}{\ell} \sum_{i=1}^\ell \sigma_i f(\mathbf{x}_i) \right| \Big| \mathbf{x}_1, \cdots, \mathbf{x}_\ell \right]$$

where $\sigma = \{\sigma_1, \cdots, \sigma_\ell\}$ are independent uniform $\{\pm 1\}$-valued Rademacher random variables. The Rademacher complexity of $\mathcal{F}$ is

$$R_\ell(\mathcal{F}) = \mathbb{E}_S \left[\hat{R}_\ell(\mathcal{F}) \right] = \mathbb{E}_{S\sigma} \left[\sup_{f \in \mathcal{F}} \left| \frac{2}{\ell} \sum_{i=1}^\ell \sigma_i f(\mathbf{x}_i) \right| \right]$$

We use $\mathbb{E}_\mathcal{D}$ to denote expectation with respect to a distribution $\mathcal{D}$ and $\mathbb{E}_S$ when the distribution is the uniform (empirical) distribution on a sample S.

Theorem 1. *Fix $\delta \in (0, 1)$ and let $\mathcal{F}$ be a class of functions mapping from S to $[0, 1]$. Let $(\mathbf{x}_i)_{i=1}^\ell$ be drawn independently according to a probability distribution $\mathcal{D}$. Then with probability at least $1 - \delta$ over random draws of samples of size ℓ, every $f \in \mathcal{F}$ satisfies*

$$\mathbb{E}_\mathcal{D}[f(x)] \leq \mathbb{E}_S[f(x)] + R_\ell(\mathcal{F}) + 3\sqrt{\frac{\ln(2/\delta)}{2\ell}}$$
$$\leq \mathbb{E}_S[f(x)] + \hat{R}_\ell(\mathcal{F}) + 3\sqrt{\frac{\ln(2/\delta)}{2\ell}}$$

Given a training set S the class of functions that we will primarily be considering are linear functions with bounded norm

$$\left\{ x \rightarrow \sum_{i=1}^\ell \alpha_i \kappa(\mathbf{x}_i, x) : \alpha' K \alpha \leq B^2 \right\}$$
$$\subseteq \{x \rightarrow \langle w, \phi(x) \rangle : \|w\| \leq B\} = \mathcal{F}_B$$

where ϕ is the feature mapping corresponding to the kernel κ and K is the corresponding kernel matrix for the sample S. The following result bounds the Rademacher complexity of linear function classes.

Theorem 2. *[2] If $\kappa : X \times X \rightarrow R$ is a kernel, and $S = \{\mathbf{x}_1, \cdots, \mathbf{x}_\ell\}$ is a sample of point from X, then the empirical Rademacher complexity of the class $\mathcal{F}_B$ satisfies*

$$\hat{R}_\ell(\mathcal{F}) \leq \frac{2B}{\ell} \sqrt{\sum_{i=1}^\ell \kappa(\mathbf{x}_i, \mathbf{x}_i)} = \frac{2B}{\ell} \sqrt{tr(K)}$$

4.1 Analysing SVM-2K

For SVM-2K, the two feature sets from the same objects are $(\phi_A(\mathbf{x}_i))_{i=1}^\ell$ and $(\phi_B(\mathbf{x}_i))_{i=1}^\ell$ respectively. We assume the notation and optimisation of SVM-2K given in section 2, equation (1).

First observe that an application of Theorem 1 shows that

$$\mathbb{E}_S[|f_A(x) - f_B(x)|] \leq \mathbb{E}_S[|\langle \hat{\mathbf{w}}_A, \phi_A(x) \rangle + \hat{b}_A - \langle \hat{\mathbf{w}}_B, \phi_B(x) \rangle - \hat{b}_B|]$$
$$\leq \epsilon + \frac{1}{\ell} \sum_{i=1}^\ell \eta_i + \frac{2C}{\ell} \sqrt{tr(K_A) + tr(K_B)} + 3\sqrt{\frac{\ln(2/\delta)}{2\ell}} =: D$$

with probability at least $1 - \delta$. We have assumed that $\|\mathbf{w}_A\|^2 + b_A^2 \leq C^2$ and $\|\mathbf{w}_B\|^2 + b_B^2 \leq C^2$ for some prefixed C. Hence, the class of functions we are considering when applying

SVM-2K to this problem can be restricted to

$$\mathcal{F}_{C,D} = \left\{ f \middle| f : x \rightarrow 0.5 \left(\sum_{i=1}^{\ell} [g_i^A \kappa_A(\mathbf{x}_i, x) + g_i^B \kappa_B(\mathbf{x}_i, x)] + b_A + b_B \right), \right.$$

$$\left. g^{A'} K_A g^A + b_A^2 \le C^2, g^{B'} K_B g^B + b_B^2 \le C^2, \mathbb{E}_S[|f_A(x) - f_B(x)|] \le D \right\}$$

The class $\mathcal{F}_{C,D}$ is clearly closed under negation.

Applying the usual Rademacher techniques for margin bounds on generalisation we obtain the following result.

Theorem 3. *Fix $\delta \in (0, 1)$ and let $\mathcal{F}_{C,D}$ be the class of functions described above. Let $(\mathbf{x}_i)_{i=1}^{\ell}$ be drawn independently according to a probability distribution $\mathcal{D}$. Then with probability at least $1 - \delta$ over random draws of samples of size ℓ, every $f \in \mathcal{F}_{C,D}$ satisfies*

$$P_{(x,y) \sim \mathcal{D}}(\operatorname{sign}(f(x)) \ne y) \le \frac{0.5}{\ell} \sum_{i=1}^{\ell} (\xi_i^A + \xi_i^B) + \hat{R}_{\ell}(\mathcal{F}_{C,D}) + 3\sqrt{\frac{\ln(2/\delta)}{2\ell}}.$$

It therefore remains to compute the empirical Rademacher complexity of $\mathcal{F}_{C,D}$, which is the critical discriminator between the bounds for the individual SVMs and that of the SVM-2K.

4.2 Empirical Rademacher complexity of $\mathcal{F}_{C,D}$

We now define an auxiliary function of two weight vectors $\mathbf{w}_A$ and $\mathbf{w}_B$,

$$D(\mathbf{w}_A, \mathbf{w}_B) := \mathbb{E}_{\mathcal{D}}[|\langle \mathbf{w}_A, \phi_A(x) \rangle + b_A - \langle \mathbf{w}_B, \phi_B(x) \rangle - b_B|]$$

With this notation we can consider computing the Rademacher complexity of the class $\mathcal{F}_{C,D}$.

$$\hat{R}_{\ell}(\mathcal{F}_{C,D}) = \mathbb{E}_{\sigma} \left[\sup_{f \in \mathcal{F}_{C,D}} \left| \frac{2}{\ell} \sum_{i=1}^{\ell} \sigma_i f(\mathbf{x}_i) \right| \right]$$

$$= \mathbb{E}_{\sigma} \left[\sup_{\substack{\|\mathbf{w}_A\| \le C, \|\mathbf{w}_B\| \le C \\ D(\mathbf{w}_A, \mathbf{w}_B) \le D}} \left| \frac{1}{\ell} \sum_{i=1}^{\ell} \sigma_i [\langle \mathbf{w}_A, \phi_A(\mathbf{x}_i) \rangle + b_A + \langle \mathbf{w}_B, \phi_B(\mathbf{x}_i) \rangle + b_B] \right| \right]$$

Our next observation follows from a reversed version of the basic Rademacher complexity theorem reworked to reverse the roles of the empirical and true expectations:

Theorem 4. *Fix $\delta \in (0, 1)$ and let $\mathcal{F}$ be a class of functions mapping from S to $[0, 1]$. Let $(\mathbf{x}_i)_{i=1}^{\ell}$ be drawn independently according to a probability distribution $\mathcal{D}$. Then with probability at least $1 - \delta$ over random draws of samples of size ℓ, every $f \in \mathcal{F}$ satisfies*

$$\mathbb{E}_S[f(x)] \le \mathbb{E}_{\mathcal{D}}[f(x)] + R_{\ell}(\mathcal{F}) + 3\sqrt{\frac{\ln(2/\delta)}{2\ell}}$$

$$\le \mathbb{E}_{\mathcal{D}}[f(x)] + \hat{R}_{\ell}(\mathcal{F}) + 3\sqrt{\frac{\ln(2/\delta)}{2\ell}}$$

The proof tracks that of Theorem 1 but is omitted through lack of space.

For weight vectors $\mathbf{w}_A$ and $\mathbf{w}_B$ satisfying $D(\mathbf{w}_A, \mathbf{w}_B) \le D$, an application of Theorem 4 shows that with probability at least $1 - \delta$ we have

$$
\begin{aligned}
\hat{D}(\mathbf{w}_A, \mathbf{w}_B) &:= \mathbb{E}_S[|\langle \mathbf{w}_A, \phi_A(x)\rangle + b_A - \langle \mathbf{w}_B, \phi_B(x)\rangle - b_B|] \\
&\leq D + \frac{2C}{\ell}\sqrt{\mathrm{tr}(K_A) + \mathrm{tr}(K_B)} + 3\sqrt{\frac{\ln(2/\delta)}{2\ell}} \\
&\leq \epsilon + \frac{1}{\ell}\sum_{i=1}^{\ell}\eta_i + \frac{4C}{\ell}\sqrt{\mathrm{tr}(K_A) + \mathrm{tr}(K_B)} + 6\sqrt{\frac{\ln(2/\delta)}{2\ell}} =: \hat{D}
\end{aligned}
$$

We now return to bounding the Rademacher complexity of $\mathcal{F}_{C,D}$. The above result shows that with probability greater than $1 - \delta$

$$
\begin{aligned}
&\hat{R}_\ell(\mathcal{F}_{C,D}) \\
&\leq \mathbb{E}_\sigma\left[\sup_{\substack{\|\mathbf{w}_A\|\leq C \\ \|\mathbf{w}_B\|\leq C \\ \hat{D}(\mathbf{w}_A,\mathbf{w}_B)\leq\hat{D}}} \left|\frac{1}{\ell}\sum_{i=1}^{\ell}\sigma_i\left[\langle \mathbf{w}_A, \phi_A(\mathbf{x}_i)\rangle + b_A + \langle \mathbf{w}_B, \phi_B(\mathbf{x}_i)\rangle + b_B\right]\right|\right]
\end{aligned}
$$

First note that the expression in square brackets is concentrated under the uniform distribution of Rademacher variables. Hence, we can estimate the complexity for a fixed instantiation $\hat{\sigma}$ of the the Rademacher variables σ. We now must find the value of $\mathbf{w}_A$ and $\mathbf{w}_B$ that maximises the expression

$$
\begin{aligned}
&\frac{1}{\ell}\left|\left[\left\langle \mathbf{w}_A, \sum_{i=1}^{\ell}\hat{\sigma}_i\phi_A(\mathbf{x}_i)\right\rangle + b_A\sum_{i=1}^{\ell}\hat{\sigma}_i + \left\langle \mathbf{w}_B, \sum_{i=1}^{\ell}\hat{\sigma}_i\phi_B(\mathbf{x}_i)\right\rangle + b_B\sum_{i=1}^{\ell}\hat{\sigma}_i\right]\right| \\
&= \frac{1}{\ell}\left|\hat{\sigma}'K_A g^A + \hat{\sigma}'K_B g^B + (b_A + b_B)\hat{\sigma}'\mathbf{j}\right|
\end{aligned}
$$

subject to the constraints $g^{A'}K_A g^A \leq C^2$, $g^{B'}K_B g^B \leq C^2$, and

$$
\frac{1}{\ell}\mathbf{1}'\mathrm{abs}(K_A g^A - K_B g^B + (b_A - b_B)\mathbf{1}) \leq \hat{D}
$$

where $\mathbf{1}$ is the all ones vector and $\mathrm{abs}(\mathbf{u})$ is the vector obtained by applying the abs function to $\mathbf{u}$ component-wise. The resulting value of the objective function is the estimate of the Rademacher complexity. This is the optimisation solved in the brief experiments described below.

4.3 Experiments with Rademacher complexity

We computed the Rademacher complexity for the problems considered in the experimental section above. We wished to verify that the Rademacher complexity of the space $\mathcal{F}_{C,D}$, where C and D are determined by applying the SVM-2K, are indeed significantly lower than that obtained for the SVMs in each space individually.

	Motorbike	Bicycle	People	Car
SVM 1	94.05	91.58	91.58	87.95
Rad 1	1.65	0.93	0.91	1.60
SVM 2	91.15	91.15	90.57	86.21
Rad 2	1.72	1.48	0.87	1.64
SVM 2K	94.34	93.47	92.74	90.13
Rad 2K	1.26	1.28	0.82	1.26

Table 2: Results for 4 datasets showing test accuracy and Rademacher complexity (Rad) of the individual SVMs and SVM-2K.

361

Table 2 shows the results for the motorbike, bicycle, people and car datasets. We show the Rademacher complexities for the individual SVMs and for the SVM-2K along with the generalisation results already given in Table 1. In the case of SVM-2K we sampled the Rademacher variables 10 times and give the corresponding standard deviation. As predicted the Rademacher complexity is significantly smaller for SVM-2K, hence confirming the intuition that led to the introduction of the approach, namely that the complexity of the class is reduced by restricting the weight vectors to align on the training data. Provided both representations contain the necessary data we can therefore expect an improvement in generalisation as observed in the reported experiments.

5 Conclusions

With the plethora of data now being collected in a wide range of fields there is frequently the luxury of having two views of the same phenomenon. The simplest example is paired corpora of documents in different languages, but equally we can think of examples from bioinformatics, machine vision, etc. Frequently it is also reasonable to assume that both views contain all of the relevant information required for a classification task.

We have demonstrated that in such cases it can be possible to leaver the correlation between the two views to improve classification accuracy. This has been demonstrated in experiments with a machine vision task. Furthermore, we have undertaken a theoretical analysis to illuminate the source and extent of the advantage that can be obtained, showing in the cases considered a significant reduction in the Rademacher complexity of the corresponding function classes.

References

[1] Francis R. Bach and Michael I. Jordan. Kernel independent component analysis. *Journal of Machine Learning Research*, 3:1–48, 2002.

[2] P. L. Bartlett and S. Mendelson. Rademacher and Gaussian complexities: risk bounds and structural results. *Journal of Machine Learning Research*, 3:463–482, 2002.

[3] G. Csurka, C. Bray, C. Dance, and L. Fan. Visual categorization with bags of keypoints. In *XRCE Research Reports, XEROX*. The 8th European Conference on Computer Vision - ECCV, Prague, 2004.

[4] R. Fergus, P. Perona, and A. Zisserman. Object class recognition by unsupervised scale-invariant learning. In *Proceedings of the IEEE Conference on Computer Vision and Pattern Recognition*, 2003.

[5] David Hardoon, Sandor Szedmak, and John Shawe-Taylor. Canonical correlation analysis: An overview with application to learning methods. *Neural Computation*, 16:2639–2664, 2004.

[6] Yaoyong Li and John Shawe-Taylor. Using kcca for japanese-english cross-language information retrieval and classification. *to appear in Journal of Intelligent Information Systems*, 2005.

[7] S. Mika, B. Schölkopf, A. Smola, K.-R. Müller, M. Scholz, and G. Rätsch. Kernel PCA and de-noising in feature spaces. In *Advances in Neural Information Processing Systems 11*, 1998.

[8] R. Rosipal and L. J. Trejo. Kernel partial least squares regression in reproducing kernel hilbert space. *Journal of Machine Learning Research*, 2:97–123, 2001.

[9] J. Shawe-Taylor and N. Cristianini. *Kernel Methods for Pattern Analysis*. Cambridge University Press, Cambridge, UK, 2004.

Robust design of biological experiments

Patrick Flaherty
EECS Department
University of California
Berkeley, CA 94720
flaherty@berkeley.edu

Michael I. Jordan
Computer Science and Statistics
University of California
Berkeley, CA 94720
jordan@cs.berkeley.edu

Adam P. Arkin
Bioengineering Department,
LBL, Howard Hughes Medical Institute
University of California
Berkeley, CA 94720
aparkin@lbl.gov

Abstract

We address the problem of robust, computationally-efficient design of biological experiments. Classical optimal experiment design methods have not been widely adopted in biological practice, in part because the resulting designs can be very brittle if the nominal parameter estimates for the model are poor, and in part because of computational constraints. We present a method for robust experiment design based on a semidefinite programming relaxation. We present an application of this method to the design of experiments for a complex calcium signal transduction pathway, where we have found that the parameter estimates obtained from the robust design are better than those obtained from an "optimal" design.

1 Introduction

Statistical machine learning methods are making increasing inroads in the area of biological data analysis, particularly in the context of genome-scale data, where computational efficiency is paramount. Learning methods are particularly valuable for their ability to fuse multiple sources of information, aiding the biologist to interpret a phenomenon in its appropriate cellular, genetic and evolutionary context. At least as important to the biologist, however, is to use the results of data analysis to aid in the design of further experiments. In this paper we take up this challenge—we show how recent developments in computationally-efficient optimization can be brought to bear on the problem of the design of experiments for complex biological data. We present results for a specific model of calcium signal transduction in which choices must be made among 17 kinds of RNAi knockdown experiments.

There are three main objectives for experiment design: parameter estimation, hypothesis testing and prediction. Our focus in this paper is parameter estimation, specifically in the setting of nonlinear kinetic models [1]. Suppose in particular that we have a nonlinear model $y = f(x, \theta) + \varepsilon, \varepsilon \sim \mathcal{N}(0, \sigma^2)$, where $x \in \mathcal{X}$ represents the controllable conditions of the experiment (such as dose or temperature), y is the experimental measurement and $\theta \in \mathbb{R}^p$ is the set of parameters to be estimated. We consider a finite menu of available experiments $\mathcal{X} = \{x_1, \ldots, x_m\}$. Our objective is to select the best set of N experiments (with repeats) from the menu. Relaxing the problem to a continuous representation, we solve for a distribution over the design points and then multiply the weights by N at the end [2]. The experiment design is thus

$$\xi = \left\{ \begin{array}{c} x_1, \ldots, x_m \\ w_1, \ldots, w_m \end{array} \right\}, \quad \sum_{i=1}^{m} w_i = 1, \quad w_i \geq 0, \forall i, \tag{1}$$

and it is our goal to select values of w_i that satisfy an experimental design criterion.

2 Background

We adopt a standard least-squares framework for parameter estimation. In the nonlinear setting this is done by making a Taylor series expansion of the model about an estimate θ_0 [3]

$$f(x, \theta) \approx f(x, \theta_0) + V(\theta - \theta_0), \tag{2}$$

where V is the Jacobian matrix of the model; the ith row of V is $v_i^T = \left. \frac{\partial f(x_i, \theta)}{\partial \theta} \right|_{\theta_0}$.

The least-squares estimate of θ is $\hat{\theta} = \theta_0 + \left(V^T W V \right)^{-1} V^T W \left(y - f(x, \theta_0) \right)$, where $W = \mathrm{diag}(w)$. The covariance matrix for the parameter estimate is $\mathrm{cov}(\hat{\theta}|\xi) = \sigma^2 \left(V^T W V \right)^{-1}$, which is the inverse of the observed Fisher information matrix.

The aim of optimal experiment design methods is to minimize the covariance matrix of the parameter estimate [4, 5, 6]. There are two well-known difficulties that must be surmounted in the case of nonlinear models [6]:

- The optimal design depends on an evaluation of the derivative of the model with respect to the parameters at a particular parameter estimate. Given that our goal is parameter estimation, this involves a certain circularity.

- Simple optimal design procedures tend to concentrate experimental weight on only a few design points [7]. Such designs are overly optimistic about the appropriateness of the model, and provide little information about possible lack of fit over a wider experimental range.

There have been three main responses to these problems: sequential experiment design [7], Bayesian methods [8], and maximin approaches [9].

In the sequential approach, a working parameter estimate is first used to construct a tentative experiment design. Data are collected under that design and the parameter estimate is updated. The procedure is iterated in stages. While heuristically reasonable, this approach is often inapplicable in practice because of costs associated with experiment set-up time.

In the Bayesian approach exemplified by [8], a proper prior distribution is constructed for the parameters to be estimated. The objective function is the KL divergence between the prior distribution and the expected posterior distribution; this KL divergence is *maximized* (thereby maximizing the amount of expected information in the experiment design). Sensitivity to priors is a serious concern, however, particularly in the biological setting in which it can be quite difficult to choose priors for quantities such as bulk rates for a complex process.

The maximin approach considers a bounded range for each parameter and finds the optimal design for the worst case parameters in that range. The major difficulties with this approach are computational, and its main applications have been to specialized problems [7].

The approach that we present here is closest in spirit to the maximin approach. We view both of the problems discussed above as arguments for a *robust* design, one which is insensitive to the linearization point and to model error. We work within the framework of E-optimal design (see below) and consider perturbations to the rank-one Fisher information matrix for each design point. An optimization with respect to such perturbations yields a robust semidefinite program [10, 11, 12].

3 Optimal Experiment Design

The three most common scalar measures of the size of the parameter covariance matrix in optimal experiment design are:

- *D-optimal design*: determinant of the covariance matrix.
- *A-optimal design*: trace of the covariance matrix.
- *E-optimal design*: maximum eigenvalue of the covariance matrix.

We adopt the E-optimal design criterion, and formulate the design problem as follows:

$$\mathcal{P}_0 : p_0^* = \min_w \lambda_{\max}\left[\left(\sum_{i=1}^m w_i v_i v_i^T\right)^{-1}\right] \quad s.t. \ \sum_{i=1}^m w_i = 1 \tag{3}$$

$$w_i \geq 0, \forall i,$$

where $\lambda_{\max}[M]$ is the maximum eigenvalue of a matrix M. This problem can be recast as the following semidefinite program [5]:

$$\mathcal{P}_0 : p_0^* = \max_{w,s} s \quad s.t. \ \sum_{i=1}^m w_i v_i v_i^T \geq s I_p \tag{4}$$

$$\sum_{i=1}^m w_i = 1, \quad w_i \geq 0, \forall i,$$

which forms the basis of the robust extension that we develop in the following section.

4 Robust Experiment Design

The uncertain parameters appear in the experiment design optimization problem through the Jacobian matrix, V. We consider additive unstructured perturbations on the Jacobian or "data" in this problem. The uncertain observed Fisher information matrix is $F(w, \Delta) = \sum_{i=1}^m w_i(v_i v_i^T - \Delta_i)$, where Δ_i is a $p \times p$ matrix for $i = 1, \ldots, m$. We consider a spectral norm bound on the magnitude of the perturbations such that $\|\mathbf{blkdiag}(\Delta_1, \ldots, \Delta_m)\| \leq \rho$.

Incorporating the perturbations, the E-optimal experiment design problem with uncertainty based on (4) can be cast as the following minimax problem:

$$\mathcal{P}_\rho : p_\rho^* = \min_{w,s} \max_{\|\Delta\| \leq \rho} -s$$

$$\text{subject to} \quad \sum_{i=1}^m w_i(v_i v_i^T - \Delta_i) \geq s I_p$$

$$\Delta = \mathbf{blkdiag}(\Delta_1, \ldots, \Delta_m) \tag{5}$$

$$\sum_{i=1}^m w_i = 1, \quad w_i \geq 0, \forall i.$$

We will call equation (5) an *E-robust experiment design*.

To implement the program efficiently, we can recast the linear matrix inequality in (5) in a linear fractional representation:

$$F(w, s, \Delta) = F(w, s) + L\Delta R(w) + R(w)^T \Delta^T L^T \geq 0,$$

where

$$F(w, s) = \sum_{i=1}^{m} w_i v_i v_i^T - sI_p, \qquad R(w) = \frac{1}{\sqrt{2}} (w \otimes I_p)$$

$$L = \frac{-1}{\sqrt{2}} \left(\mathbf{1}_m^T \otimes I_p \right), \quad \Delta = \mathbf{blkdiag}(\Delta_1, \ldots, \Delta_m).$$

Taking $\Delta_1 = \cdots = \Delta_m$, a special case of the S-procedure [11] yields the following semidefinite program:

$$\mathcal{P}_\rho : p_\rho^* = \min_{w, s, \tau} -s$$

subject to
$$\begin{bmatrix} \sum_{i=1}^{m} w_i v_i v_i^T - sI_p - \frac{m}{2}\tau I_p & w^T \otimes \frac{\rho}{\sqrt{2}} I_p \\ w \otimes \frac{\rho}{\sqrt{2}} I_p & \tau I_{mp} \end{bmatrix} \geq 0 \qquad (7)$$

$$\sum_{i=1}^{m} w_i = 1, \quad w_i \geq 0, \forall i.$$

If $\rho = 0$ we recover (4). Using the Schur complement the first constraint in (7) can be further simplified to

$$\sum_{i=1}^{m} w_i v_i v_i^T - \rho\sqrt{m}\|w\|_2 \geq sI_p, \qquad (8)$$

which makes the regularization of the optimization problem (4) explicit. The uncertainty bound, ρ, serves as a weighting parameter for a Tikhonov regularization term.

5   Results

We demonstrate the robust experiment design on two models of biological systems. The first model is the Michaelis-Menten model of a simple enzyme reaction system. This model, derived from mass-action kinetics, is a fundamental building block of many mechanistic models of biological systems. The second example is a model of a complex calcium signal transduction pathway in macrophage immune cells. In this example we consider RNAi knockdowns at a variety of ligand doses for the estimation of receptor level parameters.

5.1   Michaelis-Menten Reaction Model

The Michaelis-Menten model is a common approximation to an enzyme-substrate reaction [13]. The basic chemical reaction that leads to this model is $E + S \underset{k_{-1}}{\overset{k_{+1}}{\rightleftharpoons}} C \overset{k_2}{\longrightarrow} E + P$, where E is the enzyme concentration, S is the substrate concentration and P is the product concentration. We employ mass action kinetics to develop a differential equation model for this reaction system [13]. The velocity of the reaction is defined to be the rate of product formation, $V_0 = \frac{\partial P}{\partial t}\big|_{t_0}$. The initial velocity of the reaction is

$$V_0 \approx \frac{\theta_1 x}{\theta_2 + x}, \qquad (9)$$

where

$$\theta_1 = k_{+2} E_0, \quad \theta_2 = \frac{k_{-1} + k_{+2}}{k_{+1}}. \qquad (10)$$

We have taken the controllable factor, x, in this system to be the initial substrate concentration S_0. The parameter θ_1 is the saturating velocity and θ_2 is the initial substrate concentration at which product is formed at one-half the maximal velocity. In this example $\theta_1 = 2$ and $\theta_2 = 2$ are the total enzyme and initial substrate concentrations. We consider six initial substrate concentrations as the menu of experiments, $\mathcal{X} = \left\{\frac{1}{8}, 1, 2, 4, 8, 16\right\}$.

Figure 1 shows the robust experiment design weights as a function of the uncertainty parameter with the Jacobian computed at the true parameter values. When ρ is small, the experimental weight is concentrated on only two design points. As $\rho \to \rho_{\max}$ the design converges to a uniform distribution over the entire menu of design points. In a sense, this uniform allocation of experimental energy is most robust to parameter uncertainty. Intermediate values of ρ yield an allocation of design points that reflects a tradeoff between robustness and nominal optimality.

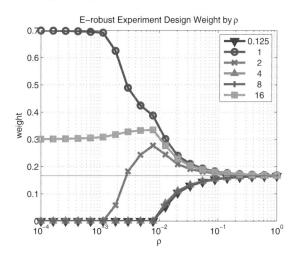

Figure 1: Michaelis-Menten model experiment design weights as a function of ρ.

For moderate values of ρ we gain significantly in terms of robustness to errors in $v_i v_i^T$, at a moderate cost to maximal value of the minimum eigenvalues of the parameter estimate covariance matrix. Figure 2 shows the efficiency of the experiment design as a function of ρ and the prior estimate θ_{02} used to compute the Jacobian matrix. The E-efficiency of a design is defined to be

$$\text{efficiency} \triangleq \frac{\lambda_{\max}\left[\text{cov}\left(\hat{\theta}|\theta, \xi_0\right)\right]}{\lambda_{\max}\left[\text{cov}\left(\hat{\theta}|\theta_0, \xi_\rho\right)\right]}. \tag{11}$$

If the Jacobian is computed at the correct point in parameter space the optimal design achieves maximal efficiency. As the distance between θ_0 and θ grows the efficiency of the optimal design decreases rapidly. If the estimate, θ_{02}, is eight instead of the true value, two, the efficiency of the optimal design at θ_0 is 36% of the optimal design at θ. However, at the cost of a decrease in efficiency for parameter estimates close to the true parameter value we guarantee the efficiency is better for points further from the true parameters with a robust design. For example, for $\rho = 0.001$ the robust design is less efficient for the range $0 < \theta_{02} < 7$, but is more efficient for $7 < \theta_{02} < 16$.

5.2 Calcium Signal Transduction Model

When certain small molecule ligands such as the anaphylatoxin C5a are introduced into the environment of an immune cell a complex chain of chemical reactions leads to the

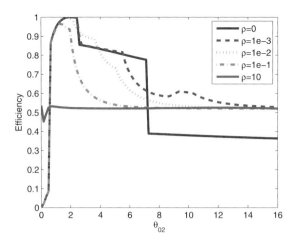

Figure 2: Efficiency of robust designs as a function of ρ and perturbations in the prior parameter estimate θ_{02}.

transduction of the extracellular ligand concentration information and a transient increase in the intracellular calcium concentration. This chain of reactions can be mathematically modeled using the principles of mass-action kinetics and nonlinear ordinary differential equations. We consider specifically the model presented in [14] which was developed for the P2Y2 receptor, modifying the model for our data on the C5a receptor.

The menu of available experiments is indexed by one of two different cell lines in combination with different ligand doses. The cell lines are: wild-type and a *GRK2* knockdown line. *GRK2* is a protein that represses signaling in the G-protein receptor complex. When its concentration is decreased with interfering RNA the repression of the signal due to *GRK2* is reduced. There are 17 experiments on the menu and we choose to do 100 experiments allocated according the experiment design. For each experiment we are able measure the transient calcium spike peak height using a fluorescent calcium dye. We are concerned with estimating three C5A receptor parameters: K_1, k_p, k_{deg} which are detailed in [14]. We have selected the initial parameter estimates based on a least-squares fit to a separate data set of 67 experiments on a wild-type cell line with a ligand concentration of 250nM. We have estimated, from experimental data, the mean and variance for all of the experiments in our menu. Observations are simulated from these data to obtain the least-squares parameter estimate for the optimal, robust ($\rho = 1.5 \times 10^{-6}$) and uniform experiment designs.

Figure 3 shows the model fits with associated 95% confidence bands for the wild-type and knockdown cell lines for the parameter estimates from the three experiment designs. A separate validation data set is generated uniformly across the design menu. Compared to the optimal design, the parameter estimates based on the robust design provide a better fit across the whole dose range for both cell types as measured by mean-squared residual error.

Note also that the measured response at high ligand concentration is better fit with parameters estimated from the robust design. Near $1\mu M$ of C5a concentration the peak height is predicted to decrease slightly in the wild-type cell line, but plateaus for the *GRK2* knockdown cell line. This matches the biochemical understanding that *GRK2* acts as a repressor of signaling.

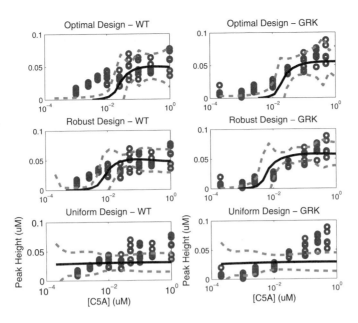

Figure 3: Model predictions based on the least squares parameter estimate using data observed from the optimal, robust and uniform design. The predicted peak height curve (black line) based on the robust design data is shifted to the left compared to the peak height curve based on the optimal design data and matches the validation sample (shown as blue dots) more accurately.

6 Discussion

The methodology of optimal experiment design leads to efficient algorithms for the construction of designs in general nonlinear situations [15]. However, these variance-minimizing designs fail to account for uncertainty in the nominal parameter estimate and the model. We present a methodology, based on recent advances in semidefinite programming, that retains the advantages of the general purpose algorithm while explicitly incorporating uncertainty.

We demonstrated this robust experiment design method on two example systems. In the Michaelis-Menten model, we showed that the E-optimal design is recovered for $\rho = 0$ and the uniform design is recovered as $\rho \rightarrow \rho_{\max}$. It was also shown that the robust design is more efficient than the optimal for large perturbations of the nominal parameter estimate away from the true parameter.

The second example, of a calcium signal transduction model, is a more realistic case of the need for experiment design in high-throughput biological research. The model captures some of the important kinetics of the system, but is far from complete. We require a reasonably accurate model to make further predictions about the system and drive a set of experiments to estimate critical parameters of the model more accurately. The resulting robust design spreads some experiments across the menu, but also concentrates on experiments that will help minimize the variance of the parameter estimates.

These robust experiment designs were obtained using SeDuMi 1.05 [16]. The design for the calcium signal transduction model takes approximately one second on a 2GHz processor, which is less time than required to compute the Jacobian matrix for the model.

Research in machine learning has led to significant advances in computationally-efficient data analysis methods, allowing increasingly complex models to be fit to biological data. Challenges in experimental design are the flip side of this coin—for complex models to be useful in closing the loop in biological research it is essential to begin to focus on the development of computationally-efficient experimental design methods.

Acknowledgments

We would like to thank Andy Packard for helpful discussions. We would also like to thank Robert Rebres and William Seaman for the data used in the second example. PF and APA would like to acknowledge support from the Howard Hughes Medical Institute and from the Alliance for Cellular Signaling through the NIH Grant Number 5U54 GM62114-05. MIJ would like to thank NIH R33 HG003070 for funding.

References

[1] I. Ford, D.M. Titterington, and C.P. Kitsos. Recent advances in nonlinear experiment design. *Technometrics*, 31(1):49–60, 1989.

[2] L. Vandenberghe, S. Boyd, and W. S.-P. Determinant maximization with linear matrix inequality constraints. *SIAM Journal on Matrix Analysis and Applications*, 19(2):499–533, 1998.

[3] G.A.F. Seber and C.J. Wild. *Nonlinear Regression*. Wiley-Interscience, Hoboken, NJ, 2003.

[4] A.C. Atkinson and A.N. Donev. *Optimum Experimental Designs*. Oxford University Press, 1992.

[5] S. Boyd and L. Vandenberghe. *Convex Optimization*. Cambridge University Press, 2003.

[6] G.E.P Box, W.G. Hunter, and J.S. Hunter. *Statistics for Experimenters: An Introduction to Design, Data Analysis, and Model Building*. John Wiley and Sons, New York, 1978.

[7] S.D. Silvey. *Optimal Design*. Chapman and Hall, London, 1980.

[8] D.V. Lindley. On the measure of information provided by an experiment. *The Annals of Mathematical Statistics*, 27(4):986–1005, 1956.

[9] L. Pronzato and E. Walter. Robust experiment design via maximin optimization. *Mathematical Biosciences*, 89:161–176, 1988.

[10] L. Vandenberghe and S. Boyd. Semidefinite programming. *SIAM Review*, 38(1):49–95, 1996.

[11] L. El Ghaoui, L. Oustry, and H. Lebret. Robust solutions to uncertain semidefinite programs. *SIAM J. Optimization*, 9(1):33–52, 1998.

[12] L. El Ghaoui and H. Lebret. Robust solutions to least squares problems with uncertain data. *SIAM J. Matrix Anal. Appl.*, 18(4):1035–1064, 1997.

[13] L.A. Segel and M. Slemrod. The quasi-steady state assumption: A case study in perturbation. *SIAM Review*, 31(3):446–477, 1989.

[14] G. Lemon, W.G. Gibson, and M.R. Bennett. Metabotropic receptor activation, desensitization and sequestrationi: modelling calcium and inositol 1,4,5-trisphosphate dynamics following receptor activation. *Journal of Theoretical Biology*, 223(1):93–111, 2003.

[15] A.C. Atkinson. The usefulness of optimum experiment designs. *JRSS B*, 58(1):59–76, 1996.

[16] J.F. Sturm. Using SeDuMi 1.02, a MATLAB toolbox for optimization over symmetric cones. *Optimization Methods and Software*, 11:625–653, 1999.

Pattern Recognition from One Example by Chopping

François Fleuret
CVLAB/LCN – EPFL
Lausanne, Switzerland
francois.fleuret@epfl.ch

Gilles Blanchard[*]
Fraunhofer FIRST
Berlin, Germany
blanchar@first.fhg.de

Abstract

We investigate the learning of the appearance of an object from a single image of it. Instead of using a large number of pictures of the object to recognize, we use a labeled reference database of pictures of other objects to learn invariance to noise and variations in pose and illumination. This acquired knowledge is then used to predict if two pictures of new objects, which do not appear on the training pictures, actually display the same object.

We propose a generic scheme called *chopping* to address this task. It relies on hundreds of random binary splits of the training set chosen to keep together the images of any given object. Those splits are extended to the complete image space with a simple learning algorithm. Given two images, the responses of the split predictors are combined with a Bayesian rule into a posterior probability of similarity.

Experiments with the COIL-100 database and with a database of 150 degraded LATEX symbols compare our method to a classical learning with several examples of the positive class and to a direct learning of the similarity.

1 Introduction

Pattern recognition has so far mainly focused on the following task: given many training examples labelled with their classes (the object they display), guess the class of a new sample which was not available during training. The various approaches all consist of going to some invariant feature space, and there using a classification method such as neural networks, decision trees, kernel techniques, Bayesian estimations based on parametric density models, etc. Providing a large number of examples results in good statistical estimates of the model parameters. Although such approaches have been successful in applications to many problems, their performance are still far from what biological visual systems can do, which is *one sample learning*. This can be defined as the ability, given one picture of an object, to spot instances of the same object, under the assumption that these new views can be induced by the single available example.

---

[*]Supported in part by the IST Programme of the European Community, under the PASCAL Network of Excellence, IST-2002-506778

Being able to perform that type of one-sample learning corresponds to the ability, given one example, to sort out which elements of a test set are of the same class (i.e. one class vs. the rest of the world). This can be done by comparing one by one all the elements of the test set with the reference example, and labelling as of the same class those which are *similar enough*. Learning techniques can be used to choose the similarity measure, which could be adaptive and learned from a large number of examples of classes not involved in the test.

Thus, given a large number of training images of a large number of objects labeled with their actual classes, and provided two pictures of unknown objects (objects which *do not appear in the training pictures*), we want to decide if these two objects are actually the same object. The first image of such a couple can be seen as a single training example, and the second image as a test example. Averaging the error rate by repeating that test several times provides with an estimate of a one-sample learning (OSL) error rate.

The idea of "learning how to learn" is not new and has been applied in various settings [12]. Taking into account and/or learning relevant geometric invariances for a given task has been studied under various forms [1, 8, 11], and in [7] with the goal to achieve learning from very few examples. Finally, the precise one-sample learning setting considered here has been the object of recent research [4, 3, 5] proposing different methods (hyperfeature learning, distance learning) for finding invariant features from a set of training reference objects distinct from the test objects. This principle has also been dubbed *interclass transfer*.

The present study proposes a generic approach, and avoids an explicit description of the space of deformations. We propose to build a large number of binary *splits* of the image space, designed to assign the same binary label to all the images common to a same object. The binary mapping associated to such a split is thus highly invariant across the images of a certain object while highly variant across images of different objects. We can define such a split on the training images, and train a predictor to extend it to the complete image space by induction. We expect the predictor to respond similarly on two images of a same object, and differently on two images of two different objects with probability $\frac{1}{2}$. The global criterion to compare two images consists roughly of counting how many such split-predictors responds similarly and compare the result to a fixed threshold.

The principle of transforming a multiclass learning problem into several binary ones by class grouping has a long history in Machine Learning [10]. From this point of view the collected output of several binary classifiers is used as a way for coding class membership. In [2] it was proposed to carefully choose the class groupings so as to yield optimal separation of codewords (ECOC methodology). While our method is related to this general principle, our goal is different since we are interested in recognizing yet-unseen objects. Hence, the goal is not to code multiclass membership; our focus is not on designing efficient codes – splits are chosen randomly and we take a large number of them – but rather on how to use the learned mappings for learning unknown objects.

2 Data and features

To make the rest of the paper clearer to the reader, we now introduce the data and feature sets we are using for our proof of concept experiments. However, note that while we have focused on image classification, our approach is generic and could be applied to any signals for which adaptive binary classifiers are available.

2.1 Data

We use two databases of pictures for our experiments. The first one is the standard COIL-100 database of pictures [9]. It contains 7200 images corresponding to 100 different objects

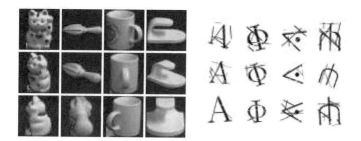

Figure 1: Four objects from the 100 objects of the COIL-100 database (downsampled to 38×38 grayscale pixels) and four symbols from the 150 symbols of our LaTeX symbol database (A, Φ, $<$ and ⋔, resolution 28×28). Each image of the later is generated by applying a rotation and a scaling, and by adding lines of random grayscales at random locations and orientations.

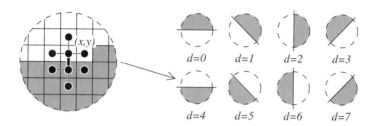

Figure 2: The figure on the left shows how an horizontal edge $\xi_{x,y,4}$ is detected: the six differences between pixels connected by a thin segment have to be all smaller in absolute value than the difference between the pixels connected by the thick segment. The relative values of the two pixels connected by the thick segment define the polarity of the edge (dark to light or light to dark). On the right are shown the eight different types of edges.

seen from 72 angles of view. We down-sample these images from their original resolution to 38×38 pixels, and convert them to grayscale. Examples are given in figure 1 (left). The second database contains images of 150 LaTeX symbols. We generated $1,000$ images of each symbol by applying a random rotation (angle is taken between -20 and $+20$ degrees) and a random scaling factor (up to 1.25). Noise is then added by adding random line segments of various gray scales, locations and orientations. The final resulting database contains $150,000$ images. Examples of these degraded images are given in figure 1 (right).

2.2 Features

All the classification processes in the rest of the paper are based on edge-based boolean features. Let $\xi_{x,y,d}$ denote a basic edge detector indexed by a location (x,y) in the image frame and an orientation d which can take eight different values, corresponding to four orientations and two polarities (see figure 2). Such an edge detector is equal to 1 if and only if an edge of the given location is detected at the specified location, and 0 otherwise. A feature $f_{x_0,y_0,x_1,y_1,d}$ is a disjunction of the ξ's in the rectangle defined by x_0, y_0, x_1, y_1. Thus, it is equal to one if and only if $\exists x, y, x_0 \leq x \leq x_1, y_0 \leq y \leq y_1, \xi_{x,y,d} = 1$. For pictures of size 32×32 there is a total of $N = \frac{1}{4}(32 \times 32)^2 \times 8 \simeq 2.10^6$ features.

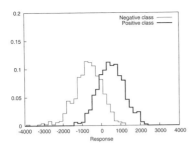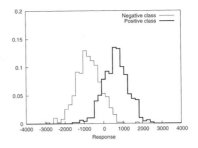

Figure 3: These two histograms are representative of the responses of two split predictors conditionally to the real arbitrary labelling $P(L \mid S)$.

3 Chopping

The main idea we propose in this paper consists of learning a large number of binary splits of the image space which would ideally assign the same binary label to all the images of any given object. In this section we define these splits and describe and justify how they are combined into a global rule.

3.1 Splits

A split is a binary labelling of the image space, with the property to give the same label to all images of a given object. We can trivially produce a labelling with that property on the training examples, but we need to be able to extend it to images not appearing in the training data, including images of other objects. We suppose that it is possible to infer a relevant split function on the complete image space, including images of other objects by looking at the problem as a binary classification problem. Inference is done by the mean of a simple learning scheme: a combination of a fast feature selection based on conditional mutual information (CMIM) [6] and a linear perceptron.

Thus, we create M arbitrary splits on the training sample by randomly assigning the label 1 to half of the N_T objects appearing in the training set, and 0 to the others. Since there are $\binom{N_T}{N_T/2}$ such balanced arbitrary labellings, with N_T of the order of a few tens, a very large number of splits is available and only a small subset of them will be actually used for learning. For each one of those splits, we train a predictor using the scheme described above. Let $(S_1, \ldots, S_M)$ denote the family of arbitrary splits and $(L_1, \ldots, L_M)$ the split-predictors. The continuous outputs of these predictors before thresholding will be combined in the final classification.

3.2 Combining splits

To combine the responses of the various split predictors, we rely on a set of simple conditional independence assumptions (comparable to the "naive Bayes" setting) on the distribution of the true class label C (each class corresponds to an object), the split labels (S_i) and the predictor outputs (L_i) for a single image. We do not assume that for test image pairs (I_1, I_2) the two images are independent, because we want to encompass the case where pairs of images of the same object are much more frequent than they would be if they were independent (typically in our test data we have arranged to have 50% of test pairs picturing the same object). We however still need some *conditional* independence assumption for the drawing of test image pairs. To simplify the notation we denote $L^1 = (L_i^1), L^2 = (L_i^2)$ the collection of predictor outputs for images 1 and 2, $S^1 = (S_i^1), S^2 = (S_i^2)$ the collection of their split labels and C_1, C_2 their true classes. The conditional indepence

374

assumptions we make are summed up in the following Markov dependency diagram:

$$
\begin{array}{ccccccccc}
L_1^2 & \!\!—\!\! & S_1^2 & & & & S_1^1 & \!\!—\!\! & L_1^1 \\
L_2^2 & \!\!—\!\! & S_2^2 & \!\!\!\searrow\!\!\! & & \nearrow & S_2^1 & \!\!—\!\! & L_2^1 \\
& & & C^2 & \!\!—\!\! & C^1 & & & \\
\cdots & & \cdots & \!\!\!\nearrow\!\!\! & & \searrow & \cdots & & \cdots \\
L_M^2 & \!\!—\!\! & S_M^2 & & & & S_M^1 & \!\!—\!\! & L_M^1
\end{array}
$$

In words, for each split i, the predictor output L_i is assumed to be independent of the true class C conditionally to the split label S_i; and conditionally to the split labels (S_1, S_2) of both images, the outputs of predictors on test pair images are assumed to be independent.

Finally, we make the additional symmetry hypothesis that conditionally to $C_1 = C_2$, for all $i : S_i^1 = S_i^2 = S_i$ and (S_i) are independent Bernoulli variables with parameter 0.5, while conditionally to $C_1 \neq C_2$ all split labels (S_i^1, S_i^2) are independent Bernoulli(0.5).

Under these assumptions we then want to compute the log-odds ratio

$$
\log \frac{P(C_1 = C_2 \mid L^1, L^2)}{P(C_1 \neq C_2 \mid L^1, L^2)} = \log \frac{P(L^1, L^2 \mid C_1 = C_2)}{P(L^1, L^2 \mid C_1 \neq C_2)} + \log \frac{P(C_1 = C_2)}{P(C_1 \neq C_2)}. \tag{1}
$$

In this formula and the next ones, when handling real-valued variables L_1, L_2 we are implicitly assuming that they have a density with respect to the Lebesgue measure and probabilities are to be interpreted as densities with some abuse of notation. We assume that the second term above is either known or can be reliably estimated. For the first term, under the aforementioned independence assumptions, the following holds (see appendix):

$$
\log \frac{P(L^1, L^2 \mid C_1 = C_2)}{P(L^1, L^2 \mid C_1 \neq C_2)} = N \log 2 + \sum_i \log \left(\alpha_i^1 \alpha_i^2 + (1 - \alpha_i^1)(1 - \alpha_i^2) \right), \tag{2}
$$

where $\alpha_i^j = P(S_i^j = 1 \mid L_i^j)$. As a quick check, note that if the predictor outputs (L_i) are uninformative (i.e. every probability α_i^j is 0.5), then the above formula gives a ratio of 1 which is what we expect. If they are perfectly informative (i.e. all α_i^j are 0 or 1), the odds ratio can take the values 0 (if for some j we can ensure $S_j^1 \neq S_j^2$, this excludes the case $C_1 = C_2$) or 2^N (if for all j we have $S_j^1 = S_j^2$ there is still a tiny chance that $C_1 \neq C_2$ if by chance C_1, C_2 are on the same side of each split).

To estimate the probabilities $P(S_j \mid L_j)$, we use a simple 1D Gaussian model for the output of the predictor given the true split label. Mean and variance are estimated from the training set for each predictor. Experimental findings show that this Gaussian modelling is realistic (see figure 3).

4 Experiments

We estimate the performance of the chopping approach by comparing it to classical learning with several examples of the positive class and to a direct learning of the similarity of two objects on different images. For every experiment, we use a family of $10,000$ features sampled uniformly in the complete set of features (see section 2.2)

4.1 Multiple example learning

In this procedure, we train a predictor with several pictures of a positive class and with a very large number of pictures of a negative class. The number of positive examples depends on the experiments (from 1 to 32) and the number of negative examples is $2,000$

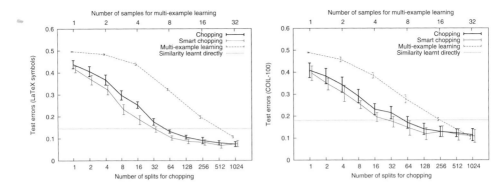

Figure 4: Error rates of the chopping, smart-chopping (see §4.2), multi-example learning and learnt similarity on the LATEX symbol (left) and the COIL-100 database (right). Each curve shows the average error and a two standard deviation interval, both estimated on ten experiments for each setting. The x-axis shows either the number of splits for chopping or the number of samples of the positive class for the multi-example learning.

for both the COIL-100 and the LATEX symbol databases. Note that to handle the unbalanced positive and negative populations, the perceptron bias is chosen to minimize a balanced error rate. In each case, and for each number of positive samples, we run 10 experiments. Each experiment consists of several cross-validation cycles so that the total number of test pictures is roughly the same as the number of pairs in one-sample techniques experiments below.

4.2 One-sample learning

For each experiment, whatever the predictor is, we first select 80 training objects from the COIL-100 database (respectively 100 symbols from the LATEX symbol database). The test error is computed with 500 pairs of images of the 20 unseen objects for the COIL-100, and 1,000 pairs of images of the 50 unseen objects for the LATEX symbols. These test sets are built to have as many pairs of images of the same object than pairs of images of different objects.

Learnt similarity: Note that one-sample learning can also be simply cast as a standard binary classification problem of pairs of images into the classes {*same, different*}. We therefore want to compare the Chopping method to a more standard learning method directly on pairs of images using a comparable set of features. For every single feature f on single images, we consider three features of a pair of images standing for the conjunction, disjunction and equality of the feature responses on the two images. From the 10,000 features on single images, we thus create a set of 30,000 features on pairs of images.

We generate a training set of 2,000 pairs of pictures for the experiments with the COIL-100 database and 5,000 for the LATEX symbols, half picturing the same object twice, half picturing two different objects. We then train a predictor similar to those used for the splits in the chopping scheme: feature selection with CMIM, and linear combination with a perceptron (see section 3.1), using the 30,000 features described above.

Chopping: The performance of the chopping approach is estimated for several numbers of splits (from 1 to 1024). For each split we select 50 objects from the training objects, and select at random 1,000 training images of these objects. We generate an arbitrary balanced binary labelling of these 50 objects and label the training images accordingly. We then build a predictor by selecting $2,000$ features with the CMIM algorithm, and combine them with a perceptron (see section 3.1).

To compensate for the limitation of our conditional independence assumptions we allow to add a fixed bias to the log-odds ratio (1). This type of correction is common when using naive-Bayes type assumptions. Using the remaining training objects as validation set, we compute this bias so as to minimize the validation error. We insist that no objects of the test classes be used for training.

To improve the performance of the splits, we also test a "smart" version of the chopping for which each split is built in two steps. The first step is similar to what is described above. From that first step, we remove the 10 objects for which the labelling prediction has the highest error rate, and re-build the split with the 40 remaining objects. This get rid of problematic objects or inconsistent labelling (for instance trying to force two similar objects to be in different halves of the split).

4.3   Results

The experiments demonstrate the good performance of chopping when only one example is available. Its optimal error rate, obtained for the largest number of splits, is 7.41% on the LaTeX symbol database and 11.42% on the COIL-100 database. By contrast, a direct learning of the similarity (see section 4.2), reaches respectively 15.54% and 18.1% respectively with $8,192$ features.

On both databases, the classical multi-sample learning scheme requires 32 samples to reach the same level of performances (10.51% on the COIL-100 and 10.7% on the LaTeX symbols).

The error curves (see figure 4) are all monotonic. There is no overfitting when the number of splits increases, which is consistent with the absence of global learning: splits are combined with an ad-hoc Bayesian rule, without optimizing a global functional, which generally also results in better robustness.

The smart splits (see section 4.2) achieve better performance initially but eventually reach the same error rates as the standard splits. There is no visible degradation of the asymptotic performance due to either a reduced independence between splits or a diminution of their separation power. However the computational cost is twice as high, since every predictor has to be built twice.

5   Conclusion

In this paper we have proposed an original approach to learning the appearance of an object from a single image. Our method relies on a large number of individual splits of the image space designed to keep together the images of any of the training objects. These splits are learned from a training set of examples and combined into a Bayesian framework to estimate the posterior probability for two images to show the same object.

This approach is very generic since it never makes the space of admissible perturbations explicit and relies on the generalization properties of the family of predictors. It can be applied to predict the similarity of two signals as soon as a family of binary predictors exists on the space of individual signals.

Since the learning is decomposed into the training of several splits independently, it can be easily parallelized. Also, because the combination rule is symmetric with respect to the splits, the learning can be incremental: splits can be added to the global rule progressively when they become available.

Appendix: Proof of formula (2). For the first factor, we have

$$P(L^1, L^2 \mid C_1 = C_2)$$

$$= \sum_{s^1, s^2} P(L^1, L^2 \mid C_1 = C_2, S^1 = s^1, S^2 = s^2) P(S^1 = s^1, S^2 = s^2 \mid C_1 = C_2)$$

$$= \sum_{s^1, s^2} P(L^1, L^2 \mid S^1 = s^1, S^2 = s^2) P(S^1 = s^1, S^2 = s^2 \mid C_1 = C_2)$$

$$= \sum_{s^1, s^2} \prod_i P(L_i^1 \mid S_i^1 = s_i^1) P(L_i^2 \mid S_i^2 = s_i^2) P((S_i^1, S_i^2) = (s_i^1, s_i^2) \mid C_1 = C_2)$$

$$= 2^{-N} \prod_i \left(P(L_i^1 \mid S_i^1 = 1) P(L_i^2 \mid S_i^2 = 1) + P(L_i^1 \mid S_i^1 = 0) P(L_i^2 \mid S_i^2 = 0) \right) .$$

In the second equality, we have used that L is independent of C given S. In the third equality, we have used that the (L_i^j) are independent given S. In the last equality, we have used the symmetry assumption on the distribution of (S_1, S_2) given $C_1 = C_2$. Similarly,

$$P(L^1, L^2 \mid C_1 \neq C_2) = 4^{-N} \prod_i \sum_{s_1, s_2} P(L_i^1 \mid S_i^1 = s_1) P(L_i^2 \mid S_i^2 = s_2)$$

$$= 4^{-N} \prod_i P(L_i^1) P(L_i^2) \sum_{s_1, s_2} \frac{P(S_i^1 = s_1 \mid L_i^1) P(S_i^2 = s_2 \mid L_i^2)}{P(S_i^1 = s_1) P(S_i^2 = s_2)}$$

$$= 4^{-2N} \prod_i P(L_i^1) P(L_i^2) ,$$

since $P(S_i^j = s) \equiv \frac{1}{2}$ by the symmetry hypothesis. Taking the ratio of the two factors and using the latter property again leads to the conclusion.

References

[1] Y. Bengio and M. Monperrus. Non-local manifold tangent learning. In *Advances in Neural Information Processing Systems 17*, pages 129–136. MIT press, 2005.

[2] T. Dietterich and G. Bakiri. Solving multiclass learning problems via error-correcting output codes. *Journal of Artificial Intelligence Research*, 2:263–286, 1995.

[3] A. Ferencz, E. Learned-Miller, and J. Malik. Learning hyper-features for visual identification. In *Advances in Neural Information Processing Systems 17*, pages 425–432. MIT Press, 2004.

[4] A. Ferencz, E. Learned-Miller, and J. Malik. Building a classification cascade for visual identification from one example. In *International Conference on Computer Vision (ICCV)*, 2005.

[5] M. Fink. Object classification from a single example utilizing class relevance metrics. In *Advances in Neural Information Processing Systems 17*, pages 449–456. MIT Press, 2005.

[6] F. Fleuret. Fast binary feature selection with conditional mutual information. *Journal of Machine Learning Research*, 5:1531–1555, November 2004.

[7] F. Li, R. Fergus, and P. Perona. A Bayesian approach to unsupervised one-shot learning of object categories. In *Proceedings of ICCV*, volume 2, page 1134, 2003.

[8] E. G. Miller, N. E. Matsakis, and P. A. Viola. Learning from one example through shared densities on transforms. In *Proceedings of the IEEE conference on Computer Vision and Pattern Recognition*, volume 1, pages 464–471, 2000.

[9] S. A. Nene, S. K. Nayar, and H. Murase. Columbia Object Image Library (COIL-100). Technical Report CUCS-006-96, Columbia University, 1996.

[10] T. Sejnowski and C. Rosenberg. Parallel networks that learn to pronounce english text. *Journal of Complex Systems*, 1:145–168, 1987.

[11] P. Simard, Y. Le Cun, and J. Denker. Efficient pattern recognition using a new transformation distance. In S. Hanson, J. Cowan, and C. Giles, editors, *Advances in Neural Information Processing Systems 5*, pages 50–68. Morgan Kaufmann, 1993.

[12] S. Thrun and L. Pratt, editors. *Learning to learn*. Kluwer, 1997.

Mixture Modeling by Affinity Propagation

Brendan J. Frey and Delbert Dueck
University of Toronto

Software and demonstrations available at www.psi.toronto.edu

Abstract

Clustering is a fundamental problem in machine learning and has been approached in many ways. Two general and quite different approaches include iteratively fitting a mixture model (*e.g.*, using EM) and linking together pairs of training cases that have high affinity (*e.g.*, using spectral methods). Pair-wise clustering algorithms need not compute sufficient statistics and avoid poor solutions by directly placing similar examples in the same cluster. However, many applications require that each cluster of data be accurately described by a prototype or model, so affinity-based clustering – and its benefits – cannot be directly realized. We describe a technique called "affinity propagation", which combines the advantages of both approaches. The method learns a mixture model of the data by recursively propagating affinity messages. We demonstrate affinity propagation on the problems of clustering image patches for image segmentation and learning mixtures of gene expression models from microarray data. We find that affinity propagation obtains better solutions than mixtures of Gaussians, the K-medoids algorithm, spectral clustering and hierarchical clustering, and is both able to find a pre-specified number of clusters and is able to automatically determine the number of clusters. Interestingly, affinity propagation can be viewed as belief propagation in a graphical model that accounts for pairwise training case likelihood functions and the identification of cluster centers.

1   Introduction

Many machine learning tasks involve clustering data using a mixture model, so that the data in each cluster is accurately described by a probability model from a pre-defined, possibly parameterized, set of models [1]. For example, words can be grouped according to common usage across a reference set of documents, and segments of speech spectrograms can be grouped according to similar speaker and phonetic unit. As researchers increasingly confront more challenging and realistic problems, the appropriate class-conditional models become more sophisticated and much more difficult to optimize.

By marginalizing over hidden variables, we can still view many hierarchical learning problems as mixture modeling, but the class-conditional models become complicated and non-linear. While such class-conditional models may more accurately describe the problem at hand, the optimization of the mixture model often becomes much more difficult. Exact computation of the data likelihoods may not be feasible and exact computation of the sufficient statistics needed to update parameterized models may not be feasible. Further, the complexity of the model and the approximations used for the likelihoods and the sufficient statistics often produce an optimization surface with a large number of poor local minima.

A different approach to clustering ignores the notion of a class-conditional model, and links together pairs of data points that have high affinity. The affinity or similarity (a real number in $[0, 1]$) between two training cases gives a direct indication of whether they should be in the same cluster. Hierarchical clustering and its Bayesian variants [2] is a popular affinity-based clustering technique, whereby a binary tree is constructed greedily from the leaves to the root, by recursively linking together pairs of training cases with high affinity. Another popular method uses a spectral decomposition of the *normalized* affinity matrix [4]. Viewing affinities as transition probabilities in a random walk on data points, modes of the affinity matrix correspond to clusters of points that are isolated in the walk [3,5].

We describe a new method that, for the first time to our knowledge, combines the advantages of model-based clustering and affinity-based clustering. Unlike previous techniques that construct and learn probability models of *transitions* between data points [6, 7], our technique learns a probability model of the data itself. Like affinity-based clustering, our algorithm directly examines pairs of nearby training cases to help ascertain whether or not they should be in the same cluster. However, like model-based clustering, our technique uses a probability model that describes the data as a mixture of class-conditional distributions. Our method, called "affinity propagation", can be viewed as the sum-product algorithm or the max-product algorithm in a graphical model describing the mixture model.

2 A greedy algorithm: K-medoids

The first step in obtaining the benefit of pair-wise training case comparisons is to replace the parameters of the mixture model with pointers into the training data. A similar representation is used in K-medians clustering or K-medoids clustering, where the goal is to identify K training cases, or *exemplars*, as cluster centers. Exact learning is known to be NP-hard (c.f. [8]), but a hard-decision algorithm can be used to find approximate solutions. While the algorithm makes greedy hard decisions for the cluster centers, it is a useful intermediate step in introducing affinity propagation.

For training cases $x_1, \ldots, x_N$, suppose the likelihood of training case x_i given that training case x_k is its cluster center is $P(x_i | x_i \text{ in } x_k)$ (e.g., a Gaussian likelihood would have the form $e^{-(x_i - x_k)^2 / 2\sigma^2} / \sqrt{2\pi\sigma^2}$). Given the training data, this likelihood depends only on i and k, so we denote it by L_{ik}. L_{ii} is set to the Bayesian prior probability that x_i is a cluster center. Initially, K training cases are chosen as exemplars, e.g., at random. Denote the current set of cluster center indices by $\mathcal{K}$ and the index of the current cluster center for x_i by s_i. K-medoids iterates between assigning training cases to exemplars (E step), and choosing a training case as the new exemplar for each cluster (M step). Assuming for simplicity that the mixing proportions are equal and denoting the responsibility likelihood ratio by $r_{ik} = P(x_i | x_i \text{ in } x_k) / P(x_i | x_i \text{ not in } x_k)^1$, the updates are

E step
For $i = 1, \ldots, N$:
    For $k \in \mathcal{K}$: $r_{ik} \leftarrow L_{ik} / (\sum_{j:j\neq k} L_{ij})$
    $s_i \leftarrow \text{argmax}_{k \in \mathcal{K}} r_{ik}$

Greedy M step
For $k \in \mathcal{K}$: Replace k in $\mathcal{K}$ with $\text{argmax}_{j:s_j=k} \left(\prod_{i:s_i=k} L_{ij} \right)$

This algorithm nicely replaces parameter-to-training case comparisons with pair-wise training case comparisons. However, in the greedy M step, specific training cases are chosen as exemplars. By not searching over all possible combinations of exemplars, the algorithm will frequently find poor local minima. We now introduce an algorithm that does approximately search over all possible combinations of exemplars.

---

[1] Note that using the traditional definition of responsibility, $r_{ik} \leftarrow L_{ik} / (\sum_j L_{ij})$, will give the same decisions as using the likelihood ratio.

3   Affinity propagation

The responsibilities in the greedy K-medoids algorithm can be viewed as messages that are sent from training cases to potential exemplars, providing soft evidence of the preference for each training case to be in each exemplar. To avoid making hard decisions for the cluster centers, we introduce messages called "availabilities". Availabilities are sent from exemplars to training cases and provide soft evidence of the preference for each exemplar to be available as a center for each training case.

Responsibilities are computed using likelihoods and availabilities, and availabilities are computed using responsibilities, recursively. We refer to both responsibilities and availabilities as affinities and we refer to the message-passing scheme as affinity propagation. Here, we explain the update rules; in the next section, we show that affinity propagation can be derived as the sum-product algorithm in a graphical model describing the mixture model. Denote the availability sent from candidate exemplar x_k to training case x_i by a_{ki}. Initially, these messages are set equal, *e.g.*, $a_{ki} = 1$ for all i and k. Then, the affinity propagation update rules are recursively applied:

Responsibility updates

$$r_{ik} \leftarrow L_{ik}/(\textstyle\sum_{j:j\neq k} a_{ij}L_{ij})$$

Availability updates

$$a_{kk} \leftarrow \textstyle\prod_{j:j\neq k}(1 + r_{jk}) - 1$$
$$a_{ki} \leftarrow 1/(\tfrac{1}{r_{kk}}\textstyle\prod_{j:j\neq k,j\neq i}(1 + r_{jk})^{-1} + 1 - \textstyle\prod_{j:j\neq k,j\neq i}(1 + r_{jk})^{-1})$$

The first update rule is quite similar to the update used in EM, except the likelihoods used to normalize the responsibilities are modulated by the availabilities of the competing exemplars. In this rule, the responsibility of a training case x_i as its own cluster center, r_{ii}, is high if no other exemplars are highly available to x_i and if x_i has high probability under the Bayesian prior, L_{ii}.

The second update rule also has an intuitive explanation. The availability of a training case x_k as its own exemplar, a_{kk}, is high if at least one other training case places high responsibility on x_k being an exemplar. The availability of x_k as a exemplar for x_i, a_{ki} is high if the self-responsibility r_{kk} is high ($1/r_{kk}-1$ approaches -1), but is decreased if other training cases compete in using x_k as an exemplar (the term $1/r_{kk}-1$ is scaled down if r_{jk} is large for some other training case x_j).

Messages may be propagated in parallel or sequentially. In our implementation, each candidate exemplar absorbs and emits affinities in parallel, and the centers are ordered according to the sum of their likelihoods, *i.e.* $\sum_i L_{ik}$. Direct implementation of the above propagation rules gives an N^2-time algorithm, but affinities need only be propagated between i and k if $L_{ik} > 0$. In practice, likelihoods below some threshold can be set to zero, leading to a sparse graph on which affinities are propagated.

Affinity propagation accounts for a Bayesian prior pdf on the exemplars and is able to automatically search over the appropriate number of exemplars. (Note that the number of exemplars is not pre-specified in the above updates.) In applications where a particular number of clusters is desired, the update rule for the responsibilities (in particular, the self-responsibilities r_{kk}, which determine the availabilities of the exemplars) can be modified, as described in the next section. Later, we describe applications where K is pre-specified and where K is automatically selected by affinity propagation.

The affinity propagation update rules can be derived as an instance of the sum-product

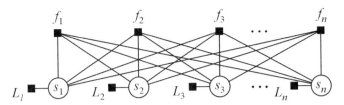

Figure 1: Affinity propagation can be viewed as belief propagation in this factor graph.

("loopy BP") algorithm in a graphical model. Using s_i to denote the index of the exemplar for x_i, the product of the likelihoods of the training cases and the priors on the exemplars is $\prod_{i=1}^{N} L_{is_i}$. (If $s_i = i$, x_i is an exemplar with *a priori* pdf L_{ii}.) The set of hidden variables $s_1, \ldots, s_N$ completely specifies the mixture model, but not all configurations of these variables are allowed: $s_i = k$ (x_i in cluster x_k) implies $s_k = k$ (x_k is an exemplar) and $s_k = k$ (x_k is an exemplar) implies $s_i = k$ for some $i \neq k$ (some other training case is in cluster x_k). The global indicator function for the satisfaction of these constraints can be written $\prod_{k=1}^{N} f_k(s_1, \ldots, s_N)$, where f_k is the constraint for candidate cluster x_k:

$$f_k(s_1, \ldots, s_N) = \begin{cases} 0 & \text{if } s_k = k \text{ and } s_i \neq k \text{ for all } i \neq k \\ 0 & \text{if } s_k \neq k \text{ and } s_i = k \text{ for some } i \neq k \\ 1 & \text{otherwise.} \end{cases}$$

Thus, the joint distribution of the mixture model and data factorizes as follows:

$$P = \prod_{i=1}^{N} L_{is_i} \prod_{k=1}^{N} f_k(s_1, \ldots, s_N).$$

The factor graph [10] in Fig. 1 describes this factorization. Each black box corresponds to a term in the factorization, and it is connected to the variables on which the term depends.

While exact inference in this factor graph is NP-hard, approximate inference algorithms can be used to infer the s variables. It is straightforward to show that the updates for affinity propagation correspond to the message updates for the sum-product algorithm or loopy belief propagation (see [10] for a tutorial). The responsibilities correspond to messages sent from the s's to the f's, while the availabilities correspond to messages sent from the f's to the s's. If the goal is to find K exemplars, an additional constraint $g(s_1, \ldots, s_N) = [K = \sum_{k=1}^{N}[s_k = k]]$ can be included, where $[\ ]$ indicates Iverson's notation ([true]=1 and [false] = 0). Messages can be propagated through this function in linear time, by implementing it as a Markov chain that accumulates exemplar counts.

Max-product affinity propagation. Max-product affinity propagation can be derived as an instance of the max-product algorithm, instead of the sum-product algorithm. The update equations for the affinities are modified and maximizations are used instead of summations. An advantage of max-product affinity propagation is that the algorithm is invariant to multiplicative constants in the *log-likelihoods*.

4 Image segmentation

A sensible model-based approach to image segmentation is to imagine that each patch in the image originates from one of a small number of prototype texture patches. The main difficulty is that in addition to standard additive or multiplicative pixel-level noise, another prevailing form of noise is due to transformations of the image features, and in particular translations.

Pair-wise affinity-based techniques and in particular spectral clustering has been employed with some success [4, 9], with the main disadvantage being that without an underlying

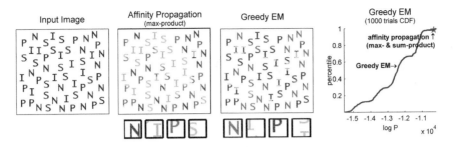

Figure 2: Segmentation of non-aligned gray-scale characters. Patches clustered by affinity propagation and K-medoids are colored according to classification (centers shown below solutions). Affinity propagation achieves a near-best score compared to 1000 runs of K-medoids.

model there is no sound basis for selecting good class representatives. Having a model with class representatives enables efficient synthesis (generation) of patches, and classification of test patches – requiring only K comparisons (to class centers) rather than N comparisons (to training cases).

We present results for segmenting two image types. First, as a toy example, we segment an image containing many noisy examples of the letters 'N' 'I' 'P' and 'S' (see Fig. 2). The original image is gray-scale with resolution 216×240 and intensities ranging from 0 (background color, white) to 1 (foreground color, black). Each training case x_i is a 24×24 image patch and x_i^m is the mth pixel in the patch. To account for translations, we include a hidden 2-D translation variable T. The match between patch x_i and patch x_k is measured by $\sum_m x_i^m \cdot f^m(x_k, T)$, where $f(x_k, T)$ is the patch obtained by applying a 2-D translation T plus cropping to patch x_k. f^m is the mth pixel in the translated, cropped patch. This metric is used in the likelihood function:

$$L_{ik} \propto \sum_T p(T) e^{\beta(\sum_m x_i^m \cdot f^m(x_k,T))/\bar{x}_i} \approx e^{\beta \max_T (\sum_m x_i^m \cdot f^m(x_k,T))/\bar{x}_i},$$

where $\bar{x}_i = \frac{1}{24^2} \sum_m x_i^m$ is used to normalize the match by the amount of ink in x_i. β controls how strictly x_i should match x_k to have high likelihood. Max-product affinity propagation is independent of the choice of β, and for sum-product affinity propagation we quite arbitrarily chose $\beta = 1$. The exemplar priors L_{kk} were set to $\text{median}_{i,k \neq i} L_{ik}$.

We cut the image in Fig. 2 into a 9×10 grid of non-overlapping 24×24 patches, computed the pair-wise likelihoods, and clustered them into $K = 4$ classes using the greedy EM algorithm (randomly chosen initial exemplars) and affinity propagation. (Max-product and sum-product affinity propagation yielded identical results.) We then took a much larger set of overlapping patches, classified them into the 4 categories, and then colored each pixel in the image according to the most frequent class for the pixel. The results are shown in Fig. 2. While affinity propagation is deterministic, the EM algorithm depends on initialization. So, we ran the EM algorithm 1000 times and in Fig. 2 we plot the cumulative distribution of the $\log P$ scores obtained by EM. The score for affinity propagation is also shown, and achieves near-best performance (98th percentile).

We next analyzed the more natural 192×192 image shown in Fig. 3. Since there is no natural background color, we use mean-squared pixel differences in HSV color space to measure similarity between the 24×24 patches:

$$L_{ik} \propto e^{-\beta \min_T \sum_{m \in W} (x_i^m - f^m(x_k,T))^2},$$

where W is the set of indices corresponding to a 16×16 window centered in the patch and $f^m(x_k, T)$ is the same as above. As before, we arbitrarily set $\beta = 1$ and L_{kk} to $\text{median}_{i,k \neq i} L_{ik}$.

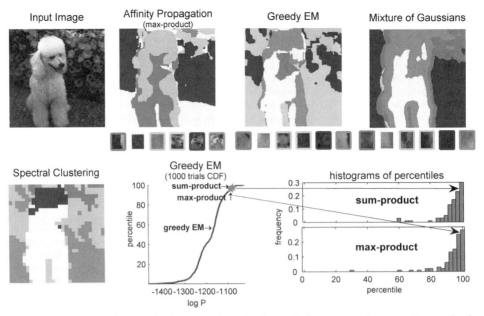

Figure 3: Segmentation results for several methods applied to a natural image. For methods other than affinity propagation, many parameter settings were tried and the best segmentation selected. The histograms show the percentile in score achieved by affinity propagation compared to 1000 runs of greedy EM, for different random training sets.

We cut the image in Fig. 3 into an 8×8 grid of non-overlapping 24×24 patches and clustered them into $K = 6$ classes using affinity propagation (both forms), greedy EM in our model, spectral clustering (using a normalized L-matrix based on a set of 29×29 overlapping patches), and mixtures of Gaussians[2]. For greedy EM, the affinity propagation algorithms, and mixtures of Gaussians, we then choose all possible 24×24 overlapping patches and calculated the likelihoods of them given each of the 6 cluster centers, classifying each patch according to its maximum likelihood.

Fig. 3 shows the segmentations for the various methods, where the central pixel of each patch is colored according to its class. Again, affinity propagation achieves a solution that is near-best compared to one thousand runs of greedy EM.

5 Learning mixtures of gene models

Currently, an important problem in genomics research is the discovery of genes and gene variants that are expressed as messenger RNAs (mRNAs) in normal tissues. In a recent study [11], we used DNA-based techniques to identify 837,251 possible exons ("putative exons") in the mouse genome. For each putative exon, we used an Agilent microarray probe to measure the amount of corresponding mRNA that was present in each of 12 mouse tissues. Each 12-D vector, called an "expression profile", can be viewed as a feature vector indicating the putative exon's function. By grouping together feature vectors for nearby probes, we can detect genes and variations of genes. Here, we compare affinity propagation with hierarchical clustering, which was previously used to find gene structures [12].

Fig. 4a shows a normalized subset of the data and gives three examples of groups of nearby

---

[2]For spectral clustering, we tried $\beta = 0.5$, 1 and 2, and for each of these tried clustering using 6, 8, 10, 12 and 14 eigenvectors. We then visually picked the best segmentation ($\beta = 1$, 10 eigenvectors). The eigenvector features were clustered using EM in a mixture of Gaussians and out of 10 trials, the solution with highest likelihood was selected. For mixtures of Gaussians applied directly to the image patches, we picked the model with highest likelihood in 10 trials.

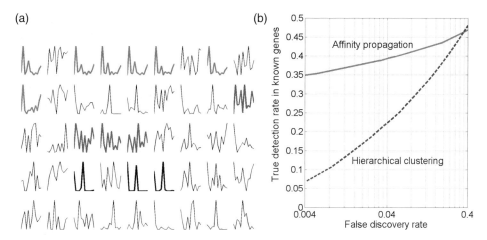

Figure 4: (a) A normalized subset of 837,251 tissue expression profiles – mRNA level versus tissue – for putative exons from the mouse genome (most profiles are much noisier than these). (b) The true exon detection rate (in known genes) versus the false discovery rate, for affinity propagation and hierarchical clustering.

feature vectors that are similar enough to provide evidence of gene units. The actual data is generally much noisier, and includes multiplicative noise (exon probe sensitivity can vary by two orders of magnitude), correlated additive noise (a probe can cross-hybridize in a tissue-independent manner to background mRNA sources), and spurious additive noise (due to a noisy measurement procedure and biological effects such as alternative splicing). To account for noise, false putative exons, and the distance between exons in the same gene, we used the following likelihood function:

$$L_{ij} = \lambda e^{-\lambda|i-j|}\left(q \cdot p_0(x_i) + (1-q)\int p(y,z,\sigma)\frac{e^{-\frac{1}{2\sigma^2}\Sigma_{m=1}^{12}(x_i^m - (y \cdot x_j^m + z))^2}}{\sqrt{2\pi\sigma^2}^{12}}dydzd\sigma\right)$$

$$\approx \lambda e^{-\lambda|i-j|}\left(q \cdot p_0(x_i) + (1-q)\max_{y,z,\sigma} p(y,z,\sigma)\frac{e^{-\frac{1}{2\sigma^2}\Sigma_{m=1}^{12}(x_i^m - (y \cdot x_j^m + z))^2}}{\sqrt{2\pi\sigma^2}^{12}}\right),$$

where x_i^m is the expression level for the mth tissue in the ith probe (in genomic order). We found that in this application, the maximum is a sufficiently good approximation to the integral. The distribution over the distance between probes in the same gene $|i - j|$ is assumed to be geometric with parameter λ. $p_0(x_i)$ is a background distribution that accounts for false putative exons and q is the probability of a false putative exon within a gene. We assumed y, z and σ are independent and uniformly distributed[3]. The Bayesian prior probability that x_k is an exemplar is set to $\theta \cdot p_0(x_k)$, where θ is a control knob used to vary the sensitivity of the system.

Because of the term $\lambda e^{-\lambda|i-j|}$ and the additional assumption that genes on the same strand do not overlap, it is not necessary to propagate affinities between all $837,251^2$ pairs of training cases. We assume $L_{ij} = 0$ for $|i - j| > 100$, in which case it is not necessary to propagate affinities between x_i and x_j. The assumption that genes do not overlap implies that if $s_i = k$, then $s_j = k$ for $j \in \{\min(i,k),\ldots,\max(i,k)\}$. It turns out that this constraint causes the dependence structure in the update equations for the affinities to reduce to a chain, so affinities need only be propagated forward and backward along the genome. After affinity propagation is used to automatically select the number of mixture

---

[3]Based on the experimental procedure and a set of previously-annotated genes (RefSeq), we estimated $\lambda = 0.05$, $q = 0.7$, $y \in [.025, 40]$, $z \in [-\mu, \mu]$ (where $\mu = \max_{i,m} x_i^m$), $\sigma \in (0, \mu]$. We used a mixture of Gaussians for $p_0(x_i)$, which was learned from the entire training set.

components and identify the mixture centers and the probes that belong to them (genes), each probe x_i is labeled as an exon or a non-exon depending on which of the two terms in the above likelihood function ($q \cdot p_0(x_i)$ or the large term to its right) is larger.

Fig. 4b shows the fraction of exons in known genes detected by affinity propagation versus the false detection rate. The curve is obtained by varying the sensitivity parameter, θ. The false detection rate was estimated by randomly permuting the order of the probes in the training set, and applying affinity propagation. Even for quite low false discovery rates, affinity propagation identifies over one third of the known exons. Using a variety of metrics, including the above metric, we also used hierarchical clustering to detect exons. The performance of hierarchical clustering using the metric with highest sensitivity is also shown. Affinity propagation has significantly higher sensitivity, *e.g.*, achieving a five-fold increase in true detection rate at a false detection rate of 0.4%.

6 Computational efficiency

The following table compares the MATLAB execution times of our implementations of the methods we compared on the problems we studied. For methods that first compute a likelihood or affinity matrix, we give the timing of this computation first. Techniques denoted by "*" were run many times to obtain the shown results, but the given time is for a single run.

	Affinity Prop	K-medoids*	Spec Clust*	MOG EM*	Hierarch Clust
NIPS	12.9 s + 2.0 s	12.9 s + .2 s	-	-	-
Dog	12.0 s + 1.5 s	12.0 s + 0.1 s	12.0 s + 29 s	3.3 s	-
Genes	16 m + 43 m	-	-	-	16 m + 28 m

7 Summary

An advantage of affinity propagation is that the update rules are deterministic, quite simple, and can be derived as an instance of the sum-product algorithm in a factor graph. Using challenging applications, we showed that affinity propagation obtains better solutions (in terms of percentile log-likelihood, visual quality of image segmentation and sensitivity-to-specificity) than other techniques, including K-medoids, spectral clustering, Gaussian mixture modeling and hierarchical clustering.

To our knowledge, affinity propagation is the first algorithm to combine advantages of pair-wise clustering methods that make use of bottom-up evidence and model-based methods that seek to fit top-down global models to the data.

References

[1] CM Bishop. *Neural Networks for Pattern Recognition*. Oxford University Press, NY, 1995.

[2] KA Heller, Z Ghahramani. Bayesian hierarchical clustering. *ICML*, 2005.

[3] M Meila, J Shi. Learning segmentation by random walks. *NIPS 14*, 2001.

[4] J Shi, J Malik. Normalized cuts and image segmentation. *Proc CVPR*, 731-737, 1997.

[5] A Ng, M Jordan, Y Weiss. On spectral clustering: Analysis and an algorithm. *NIPS 14*, 2001.

[6] N Shental A Zomet T Hertz Y Weiss. Pairwise clustering and graphical models *NIPS 16* 2003.

[7] R Rosales, BJ Frey. Learning generative models of affinity matrices. *Proc UAI*, 2003.

[8] M Charikar, S Guha, A Tardos, DB Shmoys. A constant-factor approximation algorithm for the k-median problem. *J Comp and Sys Sci*, **65:1**, 129-149, 2002.

[9] J Malik *et al.*. Contour and texture analysis for image segmentation. *IJCV* **43:1**, 2001.

[10] FR Kschischang, BJ Frey, H-A Loeliger. Factor graphs and the sum-product algorithm. *IEEE Trans Info Theory* **47:2**, 498-519, 2001.

[11] BJ Frey, QD Morris, M Robinson, TR Hughes. Finding novel transcripts in high-resolution genome-wide microarray data using the GenRate model. *Proc RECOMB 2005*, 2005.

[12] D. D. Shoemaker *et al.* Experimental annotation of the human genome using microarray technology. *Nature* **409**, 922-927, 2001.

Statistical Convergence of Kernel CCA

Kenji Fukumizu
Institute of Statistical Mathematics
Tokyo 106-8569 Japan
fukumizu@ism.ac.jp

Francis R. Bach
Centre de Morphologie Mathematique
Ecole des Mines de Paris, France
francis.bach@mines.org

Arthur Gretton
Max Planck Institute for Biological Cybernetics
72076 Tübingen, Germany
arthur.gretton@tuebingen.mpg.de

Abstract

While kernel canonical correlation analysis (kernel CCA) has been applied in many problems, the asymptotic convergence of the functions estimated from a finite sample to the true functions has not yet been established. This paper gives a rigorous proof of the statistical convergence of kernel CCA and a related method (NOCCO), which provides a theoretical justification for these methods. The result also gives a sufficient condition on the decay of the regularization coefficient in the methods to ensure convergence.

1 Introduction

Kernel canonical correlation analysis (kernel CCA) has been proposed as a nonlinear extension of CCA [1, 11, 3]. Given two random variables, kernel CCA aims at extracting the information which is shared by the two random variables, and has been successfully applied in various practical contexts. More precisely, given two random variables X and Y, the purpose of kernel CCA is to provide nonlinear mappings $f(X)$ and $g(Y)$ such that their correlation is maximized.

As in many statistical methods, the desired functions are in practice estimated from a finite sample. Thus, the convergence of the estimated functions to the population ones with increasing sample size is very important to justify the method. Since the goal of kernel CCA is to estimate a pair of functions, the convergence should be evaluated in an appropriate functional norm: thus, we need tools from functional analysis to characterize the type of convergence.

The purpose of this paper is to rigorously prove the statistical convergence of kernel CCA, and of a related method. The latter uses a NOrmalized Cross-Covariance Operator, and we call it NOCCO for short. Both kernel CCA and NOCCO require a regularization coefficient to enforce smoothness of the functions in the finite sample case (thus avoiding a trivial solution), but the decay of this regularisation with increased sample size has not yet been established. Our main theorems give a sufficient condition on the decay of the regularization coefficient for the finite sample

387

estimates to converge to the desired functions in the population limit. Another important issue in establishing the convergence is an appropriate distance measure for functions. For NOCCO, we obtain convergence in the norm of reproducing kernel Hilbert spaces (RKHS) [2]. This norm is very strong: if the positive definite (p.d.) kernels are continuous and bounded, it is stronger than the uniform norm in the space of continuous functions, and thus the estimated functions converge uniformly to the desired ones. For kernel CCA, we show convergence in the L_2 norm, which is a standard distance measure for functions. We also discuss the relation between our results and two relevant studies: COCO [9] and CCA on curves [10].

2 Kernel CCA and related methods

In this section, we review kernel CCA as presented by [3], and then formulate it with covariance operators on RKHS. In this paper, a Hilbert space always refers to a separable Hilbert space, and an operator to a linear operator. $\|T\|$ denotes the operator norm $\sup_{\|\varphi\|=1} \|T\varphi\|$, and $\mathcal{R}(T)$ denotes the range of an operator T.

Throughout this paper, $(\mathcal{H}_\mathcal{X}, k_\mathcal{X})$ and $(\mathcal{H}_\mathcal{Y}, k_\mathcal{Y})$ are RKHS of functions on measurable spaces $\mathcal{X}$ and $\mathcal{Y}$, respectively, with measurable p.d. kernels $k_\mathcal{X}$ and $k_\mathcal{Y}$. We consider a random vector $(X, Y) : \Omega \to \mathcal{X} \times \mathcal{Y}$ with distribution P_{XY}. The marginal distributions of X and Y are denoted P_X and P_Y. We always assume

$$E_X[k_\mathcal{X}(X, X)] < \infty \quad \text{and} \quad E_Y[k_\mathcal{Y}(Y, Y)] < \infty. \tag{1}$$

Note that under this assumption it is easy to see $\mathcal{H}_\mathcal{X}$ and $\mathcal{H}_\mathcal{Y}$ are continuously included in $L_2(P_X)$ and $L_2(P_Y)$, respectively, where $L_2(\mu)$ denotes the Hilbert space of square integrable functions with respect to the measure μ.

2.1 CCA in reproducing kernel Hilbert spaces

Classical CCA provides the linear mappings $a^T X$ and $b^T Y$ that achieve maximum correlation. Kernel CCA extends this by looking for functions f and g such that $f(X)$ and $g(Y)$ have maximal correlation. More precisely, kernel CCA solves

$$\max_{f \in \mathcal{H}_\mathcal{X}, g \in \mathcal{H}_\mathcal{Y}} \frac{\text{Cov}[f(X), g(Y)]}{\text{Var}[f(X)]^{1/2} \text{Var}[g(Y)]^{1/2}}. \tag{2}$$

In practice, we have to estimate the desired function from a finite sample. Given an i.i.d. sample $(X_1, Y_1), \ldots, (X_n, Y_n)$ from P_{XY}, an empirical solution of Eq. (2) is

$$\max_{f \in \mathcal{H}_\mathcal{X}, g \in \mathcal{H}_\mathcal{Y}} \frac{\widehat{\text{Cov}}[f(X), g(Y)]}{\left(\widehat{\text{Var}}[f(X)] + \varepsilon_n \|f\|_{\mathcal{H}_\mathcal{X}}^2\right)^{1/2} \left(\widehat{\text{Var}}[g(Y)] + \varepsilon_n \|g\|_{\mathcal{H}_\mathcal{Y}}^2\right)^{1/2}}, \tag{3}$$

where $\widehat{\text{Cov}}$ and $\widehat{\text{Var}}$ denote the empirical covariance and variance, such as

$$\widehat{\text{Cov}}[f(X), g(Y)] = \frac{1}{n}\sum_{i=1}^n \left(f(X_i) - \frac{1}{n}\sum_{j=1}^n f(X_j)\right)\left(g(Y_i) - \frac{1}{n}\sum_{j=1}^n g(Y_j)\right).$$

The positive constant ε_n is a regularization coefficient. As we shall see, the regularization terms $\varepsilon_n \|f\|_{\mathcal{H}_\mathcal{X}}^2$ and $\varepsilon_n \|g\|_{\mathcal{H}_\mathcal{Y}}^2$ make the problem well-formulated statistically, enforce smoothness, and enable operator inversion, as in Tikhonov regularization.

2.2 Representation with cross-covariance operators

Kernel CCA and related methods can be formulated using covariance operators [4, 7, 8], which make theoretical discussions easier. It is known that there exists a unique *cross-covariance operator* $\Sigma_{YX} : \mathcal{H}_\mathcal{X} \to \mathcal{H}_\mathcal{Y}$ for (X, Y) such that

$$\langle g, \Sigma_{YX} f \rangle_{\mathcal{H}_\mathcal{Y}} = E_{XY}\left[(f(X) - E_X[f(X)])(g(Y) - E_Y[g(Y)])\right] \quad (= \text{Cov}[f(X), g(Y)])$$

holds for all $f \in \mathcal{H}_{\mathcal{X}}$ and $g \in \mathcal{H}_{\mathcal{Y}}$. The cross covariance operator represents the covariance of $f(X)$ and $g(Y)$ as a bilinear form of f and g. In particular, if Y is equal to X, the self-adjoint operator Σ_{XX} is called the *covariance operator*.

Let $(X_1, Y_1), \ldots, (X_n, Y_n)$ be i.i.d. random vectors on $\mathcal{X} \times \mathcal{Y}$ with distribution P_{XY}. The *empirical cross-covariance operator* $\widehat{\Sigma}_{YX}^{(n)}$ is defined by the cross-covariance operator with the empirical distribution $\frac{1}{n} \sum_{i=1}^{n} \delta_{X_i} \delta_{Y_i}$. By definition, for any $f \in \mathcal{H}_{\mathcal{X}}$ and $g \in \mathcal{H}_{\mathcal{Y}}$, the operator $\widehat{\Sigma}_{YX}^{(n)}$ gives the empirical covariance as follows;

$$\langle g, \widehat{\Sigma}_{YX}^{(n)} f \rangle_{\mathcal{H}_{\mathcal{Y}}} = \widehat{\mathrm{Cov}}[f(X), g(Y)].$$

Let Q_X and Q_Y be the orthogonal projections which respectively map $\mathcal{H}_{\mathcal{X}}$ onto $\overline{\mathcal{R}(\Sigma_{XX})}$ and $\mathcal{H}_{\mathcal{Y}}$ onto $\overline{\mathcal{R}(\Sigma_{YY})}$. It is known [4] that Σ_{YX} can be represented as

$$\Sigma_{YX} = \Sigma_{YY}^{1/2} V_{YX} \Sigma_{XX}^{1/2}, \tag{4}$$

where $V_{YX} : \mathcal{H}_{\mathcal{X}} \to \mathcal{H}_{\mathcal{Y}}$ is a unique bounded operator such that $\|V_{YX}\| \leq 1$ and $V_{YX} = Q_Y V_{YX} Q_X$. We often write V_{YX} as $\Sigma_{YY}^{-1/2} \Sigma_{YX} \Sigma_{XX}^{-1/2}$ in an abuse of notation, even when $\Sigma_{XX}^{-1/2}$ or $\Sigma_{YY}^{-1/2}$ are not appropriately defined as operators.

With cross-covariance operators, the kernel CCA problem can be formulated as

$$\sup_{f \in \mathcal{H}_{\mathcal{X}}, g \in \mathcal{H}_{\mathcal{Y}}} \langle g, \Sigma_{YX} f \rangle_{\mathcal{H}_{\mathcal{Y}}} \quad \text{subject to} \quad \begin{cases} \langle f, \Sigma_{XX} f \rangle_{\mathcal{H}_{\mathcal{X}}} = 1, \\ \langle g, \Sigma_{YY} g \rangle_{\mathcal{H}_{\mathcal{Y}}} = 1. \end{cases} \tag{5}$$

As with classical CCA, the solution of Eq. (5) is given by the eigenfunctions corresponding to the largest eigenvalue of the following generalized eigenproblem:

$$\begin{pmatrix} O & \Sigma_{XY} \\ \Sigma_{YX} & O \end{pmatrix} \begin{pmatrix} f \\ g \end{pmatrix} = \rho_1 \begin{pmatrix} \Sigma_{XX} & O \\ O & \Sigma_{YY} \end{pmatrix} \begin{pmatrix} f \\ g \end{pmatrix}. \tag{6}$$

Similarly, the empirical estimator in Eq. (3) is obtained by solving

$$\sup_{f \in \mathcal{H}_{\mathcal{X}}, g \in \mathcal{H}_{\mathcal{Y}}} \langle g, \widehat{\Sigma}_{YX}^{(n)} f \rangle_{\mathcal{H}_{\mathcal{Y}}} \quad \text{subject to} \quad \begin{cases} \langle f, (\widehat{\Sigma}_{XX}^{(n)} + \varepsilon_n I) f \rangle_{\mathcal{H}_{\mathcal{X}}} = 1, \\ \langle g, (\widehat{\Sigma}_{YY}^{(n)} + \varepsilon_n I) g \rangle_{\mathcal{H}_{\mathcal{Y}}} = 1. \end{cases} \tag{7}$$

Let us assume that the operator V_{YX} is compact,[1] and let ϕ and ψ be the unit eigenfunctions of V_{YX} corresponding to the largest singular value; that is,

$$\langle \psi, V_{YX} \phi \rangle_{\mathcal{H}_{\mathcal{Y}}} = \max_{f \in \mathcal{H}_{\mathcal{X}}, g \in \mathcal{H}_{\mathcal{Y}}, \|f\|_{\mathcal{H}_{\mathcal{X}}} = \|g\|_{\mathcal{H}_{\mathcal{Y}}} = 1} \langle g, V_{YX} f \rangle_{\mathcal{H}_{\mathcal{Y}}}. \tag{8}$$

Given $\phi \in \overline{\mathcal{R}(\Sigma_{XX})}$ and $\psi \in \overline{\mathcal{R}(\Sigma_{YY})}$, the kernel CCA solution in Eq. (6) is

$$f = \Sigma_{XX}^{-1/2} \phi, \qquad g = \Sigma_{YY}^{-1/2} \psi. \tag{9}$$

In the empirical case, let $\widehat{\phi}_n \in \mathcal{H}_{\mathcal{X}}$ and $\widehat{\psi}_n \in \mathcal{H}_{\mathcal{Y}}$ be the unit eigenfunctions corresponding to the largest singular value of the finite rank operator

$$\widehat{V}_{YX}^{(n)} := (\widehat{\Sigma}_{YY}^{(n)} + \varepsilon_n I)^{-1/2} \widehat{\Sigma}_{YX}^{(n)} (\widehat{\Sigma}_{XX}^{(n)} + \varepsilon_n I)^{-1/2}. \tag{10}$$

As in Eq. (9), the empirical estimators $\widehat{f}_n$ and $\widehat{g}_n$ in Eq. (7) are equal to

$$\widehat{f}_n = (\widehat{\Sigma}_{XX}^{(n)} + \varepsilon_n I)^{-1/2} \widehat{\phi}_n, \qquad \widehat{g}_n = (\widehat{\Sigma}_{YY}^{(n)} + \varepsilon_n I)^{-1/2} \widehat{\psi}_n. \tag{11}$$

---

[1] A bounded operator $T : \mathcal{H}_1 \to \mathcal{H}_2$ is called *compact* if any bounded sequence $\{u_n\} \subset \mathcal{H}_1$ has a subsequence $\{u_{n'}\}$ such that $T u_{n'}$ converges in $\mathcal{H}_2$. One of the useful properties of a compact operator is that it admits a singular value decomposition (see [5, 6])

Note that all the above empirical operators and the estimators can be expressed in terms of *Gram matrices*. The solutions $\hat{f}_n$ and $\hat{g}_n$ are exactly the same as those given in [3], and are obtained by linear combinations of $k_{\mathcal{X}}(\cdot, X_i) - \frac{1}{n}\sum_{j=1}^{n} k_{\mathcal{X}}(\cdot, X_j)$ and $k_{\mathcal{Y}}(\cdot, Y_i) - \frac{1}{n}\sum_{j=1}^{n} k_{\mathcal{Y}}(\cdot, Y_j)$. The functions $\hat{\phi}_n$ and $\hat{\psi}_n$ are obtained similarly.

There exist additional, related methods to extract nonlinear dependence. The constrained covariance (COCO) [9] uses the unit eigenfunctions of Σ_{YX};

$$\max_{\substack{f \in \mathcal{H}_{\mathcal{X}}, g \in \mathcal{H}_{\mathcal{Y}} \\ \|f\|_{\mathcal{H}_{\mathcal{X}}} = \|g\|_{\mathcal{H}_{\mathcal{Y}}} = 1}} \langle g, \Sigma_{YX} f \rangle_{\mathcal{H}_{\mathcal{Y}}} = \max_{\substack{f \in \mathcal{H}_{\mathcal{X}}, g \in \mathcal{H}_{\mathcal{Y}} \\ \|f\|_{\mathcal{H}_{\mathcal{X}}} = \|g\|_{\mathcal{H}_{\mathcal{Y}}} = 1}} \mathrm{Cov}[f(X), g(Y)].$$

The statistical convergence of COCO has been proved in [8]. Instead of normalizing the covariance by the variances, COCO normalizes it by the RKHS norms of f and g. Kernel CCA is a more direct nonlinear extension of CCA than COCO. COCO tends to find functions with large variance for $f(X)$ and $g(Y)$, which may not be the most correlated features. On the other hand, kernel CCA may encounter situations where it finds functions with moderately large covariance but very small variance for $f(X)$ or $g(Y)$, since Σ_{XX} and Σ_{YY} can have arbitrarily small eigenvalues.

A possible compromise is to use ϕ and ψ for V_{YX}, the NOrmalized Cross-Covariance Operator (NOCCO). While the statistical meaning of NOCCO is not as direct as kernel CCA, it can incorporate the normalization by Σ_{XX} and Σ_{YY}. We will establish the convergence of kernel CCA and NOCCO in Section 3.

3 Main theorems: convergence of kernel CCA and NOCCO

We show the convergence of NOCCO in the RKHS norm, and the kernel CCA in L_2 sense. The results may easily be extended to the convergence of the eigenspace corresponding to the m-th largest eigenvalue.

Theorem 1. *Let $(\varepsilon_n)_{n=1}^{\infty}$ be a sequence of positive numbers such that*

$$\lim_{n \to \infty} \varepsilon_n = 0, \qquad \lim_{n \to \infty} n^{1/3} \varepsilon_n = \infty. \tag{12}$$

Assume V_{YX} is compact, and the eigenspaces given by Eq. (8) are one-dimensional. Let ϕ, ψ, $\hat{\phi}_n$, and $\hat{\psi}_n$ be the unit eigenfunctions of Eqs. (8) and (10). Then

$$|\langle \hat{\phi}_n, \phi \rangle_{\mathcal{H}_{\mathcal{X}}}| \to 1, \qquad |\langle \hat{\psi}_n, \psi \rangle_{\mathcal{H}_{\mathcal{Y}}}| \to 1$$

in probability, as n goes to infinity.

Theorem 2. *Let $(\varepsilon_n)_{n=1}^{\infty}$ be a sequence of positive numbers which satisfies Eq. (12). Assume that ϕ and ψ are included in $\mathcal{R}(\Sigma_{XX})$ and $\mathcal{R}(\Sigma_{YY})$, respectively, and that V_{YX} is compact. Then, for $f, g, \hat{f}_n$, and $\hat{g}_n$ in Eqs.(9), (11), we have*

$$\left\| (\hat{f}_n - E_X[\hat{f}_n(X)]) - (f - E_X[f(X)]) \right\|_{L_2(P_X)} \to 0,$$

$$\left\| (\hat{g}_n - E_Y[\hat{g}_n(Y)]) - (g - E_Y[g(Y)]) \right\|_{L_2(P_Y)} \to 0$$

in probability, as n goes to infinity.

The convergence of NOCCO in the RKHS norm is a very strong result. If $k_{\mathcal{X}}$ and $k_{\mathcal{Y}}$ are continuous and bounded, the RKHS norm is stronger than the uniform norm of the continuous functions. In such cases, Theorem 1 implies $\hat{\phi}_n$ and $\hat{\psi}_n$ converge uniformly to ϕ and ψ, respectively. This uniform convergence is useful in practice, because in many applications the function value at each point is important.

For any complete orthonormal systems (CONS) $\{\phi_i\}_{i=1}^\infty$ of $\mathcal{H}_\mathcal{X}$ and $\{\psi_i\}_{i=1}^\infty$ of $\mathcal{H}_\mathcal{Y}$, the compactness assumption on V_{YX} requires that the correlation of $\Sigma_{XX}^{-1/2}\phi_i(X)$ and $\Sigma_{YY}^{-1/2}\psi_i(Y)$ decay to zero as $i \to \infty$. This is not necessarily satisfied in general. A trivial example is the case of variables with $Y = X$, in which $V_{YX} = I$ is not compact. In this case, NOCCO is solved by an arbitrary function. Moreover, the kernel CCA does not have solutions, if Σ_{XX} has arbitrarily small eigenvalues.

Leurgans et al. ([10]) discuss CCA on curves, which are represented by stochastic processes on an interval, and use the Sobolev space of functions with square integrable second derivative. Since the Sobolev space is a RKHS, their method is an example of kernel CCA. They also show the convergence of estimators under the condition $n^{1/2}\varepsilon_n \to \infty$. Although the proof can be extended to a general RKHS, convergence is measured by the correlation,

$$\frac{|\langle \widehat{f}_n, \Sigma_{XX} f \rangle_{\mathcal{H}_\mathcal{X}}|}{(\langle \widehat{f}_n, \Sigma_{XX} \widehat{f}_n \rangle_{\mathcal{H}_\mathcal{X}})^{1/2}(\langle f, \Sigma_{XX} f \rangle_{\mathcal{H}_\mathcal{X}})^{1/2}} \;\to\; 1,$$

which is weaker than the L_2 convergence in Theorem 2. In fact, using $\langle f, \Sigma_{XX} f \rangle_{\mathcal{H}_\mathcal{X}} = 1$, it is easy to derive the above convergence from Theorem 2. On the other hand, convergence of the correlation does not necessarily imply $\langle (\widehat{f}_n - f), \Sigma_{XX}(\widehat{f}_n - f) \rangle_{\mathcal{H}_\mathcal{X}} \to 0$. From the equality

$$\langle (\widehat{f}_n - f), \Sigma_{XX}(\widehat{f}_n - f) \rangle_{\mathcal{H}_\mathcal{X}} = (\langle \widehat{f}_n, \Sigma_{XX} \widehat{f}_n \rangle_{\mathcal{H}_\mathcal{X}}^{1/2} - \langle f, \Sigma_{XX} f \rangle_{\mathcal{H}_\mathcal{X}}^{1/2})^2$$
$$+ 2\{1 - \langle \widehat{f}_n, \Sigma_{XX} f \rangle_{\mathcal{H}_\mathcal{X}}/(\|\Sigma_{XX}^{1/2} \widehat{f}_n\|_{\mathcal{H}_\mathcal{X}} \|\Sigma_{XX}^{1/2} f\|_{\mathcal{H}_\mathcal{X}})\} \|\Sigma_{XX}^{1/2} \widehat{f}_n\|_{\mathcal{H}_\mathcal{X}} \|\Sigma_{XX}^{1/2} f\|_{\mathcal{H}_\mathcal{X}},$$

we require $\langle \widehat{f}_n, \Sigma_{XX} \widehat{f}_n \rangle_{\mathcal{H}_\mathcal{X}} \to \langle f, \Sigma_{XX} f \rangle_{\mathcal{H}_\mathcal{X}} = 1$ in order to guarantee the left hand side converges to zero. However, with the normalization $\langle \widehat{f}_n, (\widehat{\Sigma}_{XX}^{(n)} + \varepsilon_n I)\widehat{f}_n \rangle_{\mathcal{H}_\mathcal{X}} = 1$, convergence of $\langle \widehat{f}_n, \Sigma_{XX} \widehat{f}_n \rangle_{\mathcal{H}_\mathcal{X}}$ is not clear. We use the stronger assumption $n^{1/3}\varepsilon_n \to \infty$ to prove $\langle (\widehat{f}_n - f), \Sigma_{XX}(\widehat{f}_n - f) \rangle_{\mathcal{H}_\mathcal{X}} \to 0$ in Theorem 2.

4 Outline of the proof of the main theorems

We show only the outline of the proof in this paper. See [6] for the detail.

4.1 Preliminary lemmas

We introduce some definitions for our proofs. Let $\mathcal{H}_1$ and $\mathcal{H}_2$ be Hilbert spaces. An operator $T : \mathcal{H}_1 \to \mathcal{H}_2$ is called *Hilbert-Schmidt* if $\sum_{i=1}^\infty \|T\varphi_i\|_{\mathcal{H}_2}^2 < \infty$ for a CONS $\{\varphi_i\}_{i=1}^\infty$ of $\mathcal{H}_1$. Obviously $\|T\| \leq \|T\|_{HS}$. For Hilbert-Schmidt operators, the Hilbert-Schmidt norm and inner product are defined as

$$\|T\|_{HS}^2 = \sum_{i=1}^\infty \|T\varphi_i\|_{\mathcal{H}_2}^2, \qquad \langle T_1, T_2 \rangle_{HS} = \sum_{i=1}^\infty \langle T_1\varphi_i, T_2\varphi_i \rangle_{\mathcal{H}_2}.$$

These definitions are independent of the CONS. For more details, see [5] and [8].

For a Hilbert space $\mathcal{F}$, a Borel measurable map $F : \Omega \to \mathcal{F}$ from a measurable space F is called a *random element* in $\mathcal{F}$. For a random element F in $\mathcal{F}$ with $E\|F\| < \infty$, there exists a unique element $E[F] \in \mathcal{F}$, called the *expectation* of F, such that

$$\langle E[F], g \rangle_{\mathcal{H}} = E[\langle F, g \rangle_{\mathcal{F}}] \qquad (\forall g \in \mathcal{F})$$

holds. If random elements F and G in $\mathcal{F}$ satisfy $E[\|F\|^2] < \infty$ and $E[\|G\|^2] < \infty$, then $\langle F, G \rangle_{\mathcal{F}}$ is integrable. Moreover, if F and G are independent, we have

$$E[\langle F, G \rangle_{\mathcal{F}}] = \langle E[F], E[G] \rangle_{\mathcal{F}}. \tag{13}$$

It is easy to see under the condition Eq. (1), the random element $k_{\mathcal{X}}(\cdot, X)k_{\mathcal{Y}}(\cdot, Y)$ in the direct product $\mathcal{H}_{\mathcal{X}} \otimes \mathcal{H}_{\mathcal{Y}}$ is integrable, i.e. $E[\|k_{\mathcal{X}}(\cdot, X)k_{\mathcal{Y}}(\cdot, Y)\|_{\mathcal{H}_{\mathcal{X}} \otimes \mathcal{H}_{\mathcal{Y}}}] < \infty$. Combining Lemma 1 in [8] and Eq. (13), we obtain the following lemma.

Lemma 3. *The cross-covariance operator Σ_{YX} is Hilbert-Schmidt, and*

$$\|\Sigma_{YX}\|_{HS}^2 = \left\|E_{YX}\left[\left(k_{\mathcal{X}}(\cdot, X) - E_X[k_{\mathcal{X}}(\cdot, X)]\right)\left(k_{\mathcal{Y}}(\cdot, Y) - E_Y[k_{\mathcal{Y}}(\cdot, Y)]\right)\right]\right\|_{\mathcal{H}_{\mathcal{X}} \otimes \mathcal{H}_{\mathcal{Y}}}^2.$$

The law of large numbers implies $\lim_{n \to \infty}\langle g, \widehat{\Sigma}_{YX}^{(n)} f\rangle_{\mathcal{H}_{\mathcal{Y}}} = \langle g, \Sigma_{YX} f\rangle_{\mathcal{H}_{\mathcal{Y}}}$ for each f and g in probability. The following lemma shows a much stronger uniform result.

Lemma 4.
$$\|\widehat{\Sigma}_{YX}^{(n)} - \Sigma_{YX}\|_{HS} = O_p(n^{-1/2}) \quad (n \to \infty).$$

Proof. Write for simplicity $F = k_{\mathcal{X}}(\cdot, X) - E_X[k_{\mathcal{X}}(\cdot, X)]$, $G = k_{\mathcal{Y}}(\cdot, Y) - E_Y[k_{\mathcal{Y}}(\cdot, Y)]$, $F_i = k_{\mathcal{X}}(\cdot, X_i) - E_X[k_{\mathcal{X}}(\cdot, X)]$, and $G_i = k_{\mathcal{Y}}(\cdot, Y_i) - E_Y[k_{\mathcal{Y}}(\cdot, Y)]$. Then, $F, F_1, \ldots, F_n$ are i.i.d. random elements in $\mathcal{H}_{\mathcal{X}}$, and a similar property also holds for $G, G_1, \ldots, G_n$. Lemma 3 and the same argument as its proof implies

$$\|\widehat{\Sigma}_{YX}^{(n)}\|_{HS}^2 = \left\|\tfrac{1}{n}\sum_{i=1}^{n}\left(F_i - \tfrac{1}{n}\sum_{j=1}^{n} F_j\right)\left(G_i - \tfrac{1}{n}\sum_{j=1}^{n} G_j\right)\right\|_{\mathcal{H}_{\mathcal{X}} \otimes \mathcal{H}_{\mathcal{Y}}},$$

$$\langle \Sigma_{YX}, \widehat{\Sigma}_{YX}^{(n)}\rangle_{HS} = \left\langle E[FG], \tfrac{1}{n}\sum_{i=1}^{n}\left(F_i - \tfrac{1}{n}\sum_{j=1}^{n} F_j\right)\left(G_i - \tfrac{1}{n}\sum_{j=1}^{n} G_j\right)\right\rangle_{\mathcal{H}_{\mathcal{X}} \otimes \mathcal{H}_{\mathcal{Y}}}.$$

From these equations, we have

$$\|\widehat{\Sigma}_{YX}^{(n)} - \Sigma_{YX}\|_{HS}^2 = \left\|\tfrac{1}{n}\sum_{i=1}^{n}\left(F_i - \tfrac{1}{n}\sum_{j=1}^{n} F_j\right)\left(G_i - \tfrac{1}{n}\sum_{j=1}^{n} G_j\right) - E[FG]\right\|_{\mathcal{H}_{\mathcal{X}} \otimes \mathcal{H}_{\mathcal{Y}}}^2$$

$$= \left\|\tfrac{1}{n}\left(1 - \tfrac{1}{n}\right)\sum_{i=1}^{n} F_i G_i - \tfrac{1}{n^2}\sum_{i=1}^{n}\sum_{j \neq i}(F_i G_j + F_j G_i) - E[FG]\right\|_{\mathcal{H}_{\mathcal{X}} \otimes \mathcal{H}_{\mathcal{Y}}}^2.$$

Using $E[F_i] = E[G_i] = 0$ and $E[F_i G_j F_k G_\ell] = 0$ for $i \neq j, \{k, \ell\} \neq \{i, j\}$, we have

$$E\|\widehat{\Sigma}_{YX}^{(n)} - \Sigma_{YX}\|_{HS}^2 = \tfrac{1}{n}E\left[\|FG\|_{\mathcal{H}_{\mathcal{X}} \otimes \mathcal{H}_{\mathcal{Y}}}^2\right] - \tfrac{1}{n}\|E[FG]\|_{\mathcal{H}_{\mathcal{X}} \otimes \mathcal{H}_{\mathcal{Y}}}^2 + O(1/n^2).$$

The proof is completed by Chebyshev's inequality. □

The following two lemmas are essential parts of the proof of the main theorems.

Lemma 5. *Let ε_n be a positive number such that $\varepsilon_n \to 0$ $(n \to \infty)$. Then*

$$\left\|\widehat{V}_{YX}^{(n)} - (\Sigma_{YY} + \varepsilon_n I)^{-1/2}\Sigma_{YX}(\Sigma_{XX} + \varepsilon_n I)^{-1/2}\right\| = O_p(\varepsilon_n^{-3/2} n^{-1/2}).$$

Proof. The operator on the left hand side is equal to

$$\left\{(\widehat{\Sigma}_{YY}^{(n)} + \varepsilon_n I)^{-1/2} - (\Sigma_{YY} + \varepsilon_n I)^{-1/2}\right\}\widehat{\Sigma}_{YX}^{(n)}(\widehat{\Sigma}_{XX}^{(n)} + \varepsilon_n I)^{-1/2}$$

$$+ (\Sigma_{YY} + \varepsilon_n I)^{-1/2}\left\{\widehat{\Sigma}_{YX}^{(n)} - \Sigma_{YX}\right\}(\widehat{\Sigma}_{XX}^{(n)} + \varepsilon_n I)^{-1/2}$$

$$+ (\Sigma_{YY} + \varepsilon_n I)^{-1/2}\Sigma_{YX}\left\{(\widehat{\Sigma}_{XX}^{(n)} + \varepsilon_n I)^{-1/2} - (\Sigma_{XX} + \varepsilon_n I)^{-1/2}\right\}. \quad (14)$$

From the equality $A^{-1/2} - B^{-1/2} = A^{-1/2}(B^{3/2} - A^{3/2})B^{-3/2} + (A - B)B^{-3/2}$, the first term in Eq. (14) is equal to

$$\left\{(\widehat{\Sigma}_{YY}^{(n)} + \varepsilon_n I)^{-\frac{1}{2}}(\Sigma_{YY}^{\frac{3}{2}} - \widehat{\Sigma}_{YY}^{(n)\frac{3}{2}}) + (\widehat{\Sigma}_{YY}^{(n)} - \Sigma_{YY})\right\}(\widehat{\Sigma}_{YY}^{(n)} + \varepsilon_n I)^{-\frac{3}{2}}\widehat{\Sigma}_{YX}^{(n)}(\widehat{\Sigma}_{XX}^{(n)} + \varepsilon_n I)^{-\frac{1}{2}}.$$

From $\|(\widehat{\Sigma}_{YY}^{(n)} + \varepsilon_n I)^{-1/2}\| \leq 1/\sqrt{\varepsilon_n}$, $\|(\widehat{\Sigma}_{YY}^{(n)} + \varepsilon_n I)^{-1/2}\widehat{\Sigma}_{YX}^{(n)}(\widehat{\Sigma}_{XX}^{(n)} + \varepsilon_n I)^{-1/2}\| \leq 1$ and Lemma 7, the norm of the above operator is upper-bounded by

$$\tfrac{1}{\varepsilon_n}\left\{\tfrac{3}{\sqrt{\varepsilon_n}}\max\{\|\Sigma_{YY}\|^{3/2}, \|\widehat{\Sigma}_{YY}^{(n)}\|^{3/2}\} + 1\right\}\|\widehat{\Sigma}_{YY}^{(n)} - \Sigma_{YY}\|.$$

A similar bound applies to the third term of Eq. (14), and the second term is upper-bounded by $\tfrac{1}{\varepsilon_n}\|\Sigma_{YX} - \widehat{\Sigma}_{YX}^{(n)}\|$. Thus, Lemma 4 completes the proof. □

Lemma 6. *Assume V_{YX} is compact. Then, for a sequence $\varepsilon_n \to 0$,*

$$\|(\Sigma_{YY} + \varepsilon_n I)^{-1/2}\Sigma_{YX}(\Sigma_{XX} + \varepsilon_n I)^{-1/2} - V_{YX}\| \to 0 \quad (n \to \infty).$$

Proof. It suffices to prove $\|\{(\Sigma_{YY} + \varepsilon_n I)^{-1/2} - \Sigma_{YY}^{-1/2}\}\Sigma_{YX}(\Sigma_{XX} + \varepsilon_n I)^{-1/2}\|$ and $\|\Sigma_{YY}^{-1/2}\Sigma_{YX}\{(\Sigma_{XX} + \varepsilon_n I)^{-1/2} - \Sigma_{XX}^{-1/2}\}\|$ converge to zero. The former is equal to

$$\|\{(\Sigma_{YY} + \varepsilon_n I)^{-1/2}\Sigma_{YY}^{1/2} - I\}V_{YX}\|. \tag{15}$$

Note that $\mathcal{R}(V_{YX}) \subset \overline{\mathcal{R}(\Sigma_{YY})}$, as remarked in Section 2.2. Let $v = \Sigma_{YY}u$ be an arbitrary element in $\mathcal{R}(V_{YX}) \cap \mathcal{R}(\Sigma_{YY})$. We have $\|\{(\Sigma_{YY} + \varepsilon_n I)^{-1/2}\Sigma_{YY}^{1/2} - I\}v\|_{\mathcal{H}_y} = \|(\Sigma_{YY} + \varepsilon_n I)^{-1/2}\Sigma_{YY}^{1/2}\{\Sigma_{YY}^{1/2} - (\Sigma_{YY} + \varepsilon_n I)^{1/2}\}\Sigma_{YY}^{1/2}u\|_{\mathcal{H}_y} \leq \|\Sigma_{YY}^{1/2} - (\Sigma_{YY} + \varepsilon_n I)^{1/2}\| \|\Sigma_{YY}^{1/2}u\|_{\mathcal{H}_y}$. Since $(\Sigma_{YY} + \varepsilon_n I)^{1/2} \to \Sigma_{YY}^{1/2}$ in norm, we obtain

$$\{(\Sigma_{YY} + \varepsilon_n I)^{-1/2}\Sigma_{YY}^{1/2} - I\}v \to 0 \quad (n \to \infty) \tag{16}$$

for all $v \in \mathcal{R}(V_{YX}) \cap \mathcal{R}(\Sigma_{YY})$. Because V_{YX} is compact, Lemma 8 in the Appendix shows Eq. (15) converges to zero. The convergence of the second norm is similar. $\square$

4.2 Proof of the main theorems

Proof of Thm. 1. This follows from Lemmas 5, 6, and Lemma 9 in Appendix. $\square$

Proof Thm. 2. We show only the convergence of $\widehat{f}_n$. W.l.o.g, we can assume $\widehat{\phi}_n \to \phi$ in $\mathcal{H}_x$. From $\|\Sigma_{XX}^{1/2}(\widehat{f}_n - f)\|_{\mathcal{H}_x}^2 = \|\Sigma_{XX}^{1/2}\widehat{f}_n\|_{\mathcal{H}_x}^2 - 2\langle\phi, \Sigma_{XX}^{1/2}\widehat{f}_n\rangle_{\mathcal{H}_x} + \|\phi\|_{\mathcal{H}_x}^2$, it suffices to show $\Sigma_{XX}^{1/2}\widehat{f}_n$ converges to ϕ in probability. We have

$$\|\Sigma_{XX}^{1/2}\widehat{f}_n - \phi\|_{\mathcal{H}_x} \leq \|\Sigma_{XX}^{1/2}\{(\widehat{\Sigma}_{XX}^{(n)} + \varepsilon_n I)^{-1/2} - (\Sigma_{XX} + \varepsilon_n I)^{-1/2}\}\widehat{\phi}_n\|_{\mathcal{H}_x}$$
$$+ \|\Sigma_{XX}^{1/2}(\Sigma_{XX} + \varepsilon_n I)^{-1/2}(\widehat{\phi}_n - \phi)\|_{\mathcal{H}_x} + \|\Sigma_{XX}^{1/2}(\Sigma_{XX} + \varepsilon_n I)^{-1/2}\phi - \phi\|_{\mathcal{H}_x}.$$

Using the same argument as the bound on the first term in Eq. (14), the first term on the R.H.S of the above inequality is shown to converge to zero. The convergence of the second term is obvious. Using the assumption $\phi \in \mathcal{R}(\Sigma_{XX})$, the same argument as the proof of Eq. (16) applies to the third term, which completes the proof. $\square$

5 Concluding remarks

We have established the statistical convergence of kernel CCA and NOCCO, showing that the finite sample estimators of the nonlinear mappings converge to the desired population functions. This convergence is proved in the RKHS norm for NOCCO, and in the L_2 norm for kernel CCA. These results give a theoretical justification for using the empirical estimates of NOCCO and kernel CCA in practice.

We have also derived a sufficient condition, $n^{1/3}\varepsilon_n \to \infty$, for the decay of the regularization coefficient ε_n, which ensures the convergence described above. As [10] suggests, the order of the sufficient condition seems to depend on the function norm used to determine convergence. An interesting consideration is whether the order $n^{1/3}\varepsilon_n \to \infty$ can be improved for convergence in the L_2 or RKHS norm.

Another question that remains to be addressed is when to use kernel CCA, COCO, or NOCCO in practice. The answer probably depends on the statistical properties of the data. It might consequently be helpful to determine the relation between the spectral properties of the data distribution and the solutions of these methods.

Acknowledgements

This work is partially supported by KAKENHI 15700241 and Inamori Foundation.

References

[1] S. Akaho. A kernel method for canonical correlation analysis. *Proc. Intern. Meeting on Psychometric Society (IMPS2001)*, 2001.

[2] N. Aronszajn. Theory of reproducing kernels. *Trans. American Mathematical Society*, 69(3):337–404, 1950.

[3] F. R. Bach and M. I. Jordan. Kernel independent component analysis. *J. Machine Learning Research*, 3:1–48, 2002.

[4] C. R. Baker. Joint measures and cross-covariance operators. *Trans. American Mathematical Society*, 186:273–289, 1973.

[5] N. Dunford and J. T. Schwartz. *Linear Operators, Part II*. Interscience, 1963.

[6] K. Fukumizu, F. R. Bach, and A. Gretton. Consistency of kernel canonical correlation. Research Memorandum 942, Institute of Statistical Mathematics, 2005.

[7] K. Fukumizu, F. R. Bach, and M. I. Jordan. Dimensionality reduction for supervised learning with reproducing kernel Hilbert spaces. *J. Machine Learning Research*, 5:73–99, 2004.

[8] A. Gretton, O. Bousquet, A. Smola, and B. Schölkopf. Measuring statistical dependence with Hilbert-Schmidt norms. Tech Report 140, Max-Planck-Institut für biologische Kybernetik, 2005.

[9] A. Gretton, A. Smola, O. Bousquet, R. Herbrich, B. Schölkopf, and N. Logothetis. Behaviour and convergence of the constrained covariance. Tech Report 128, Max-Planck-Institut für biologische Kybernetik, 2004.

[10] S. Leurgans, R. Moyeed, and B. Silverman. Canonical correlation analysis when the data are curves. *J. Royal Statistical Society, Series B*, 55(3):725–740, 1993.

[11] T. Melzer, M. Reiter, and H. Bischof. Nonlinear feature extraction using generalized canonical correlation analysis. *Proc. Intern. Conf. Artificial Neural Networks (ICANN2001)*, 353–360, 2001.

A   Lemmas used in the proofs

We list the lemmas used in Section 4. See [6] for the proofs.

Lemma 7. *Suppose A and B are positive self-adjoint operators on a Hilbert space such that $0 \leq A \leq \lambda I$ and $0 \leq B \leq \lambda I$ hold for a positive constant λ. Then*

$$\|A^{3/2} - B^{3/2}\| \leq 3\lambda^{3/2}\|A - B\|.$$

Lemma 8. *Let $\mathcal{H}_1$ and $\mathcal{H}_2$ be Hilbert spaces, and $\mathcal{H}_0$ be a dense linear subspace of $\mathcal{H}_2$. Suppose A_n and A are bounded operators on $\mathcal{H}_2$, and B is a compact operator from $\mathcal{H}_1$ to $\mathcal{H}_2$ such that $A_n u \to Au$ for all $u \in \mathcal{H}_0$, and $\sup_n \|A_n\| \leq M$ for some $M > 0$. Then $A_n B$ converges to AB in norm.*

Lemma 9. *Let A be a compact positive operator on a Hilbert space $\mathcal{H}$, and A_n ($n \in \mathbb{N}$) be bounded positive operators on $\mathcal{H}$ such that A_n converges to A in norm. Assume the eigenspace of A corresponding to the largest eigenvalue is one-dimensional and spanned by a unit eigenvector ϕ, and the maximum of the spectrum of A_n is attained by a unit eigenvector ϕ_n. Then we have $|\langle \phi_n, \phi \rangle_{\mathcal{H}}| \to 1$ as $n \to \infty$.*

Learning Rankings via Convex Hull Separation

Glenn Fung, Rómer Rosales, Balaji Krishnapuram
Computer Aided Diagnosis, Siemens Medical Solutions USA, Malvern, PA 19355
{glenn.fung, romer.rosales, balaji.krishnapuram}@siemens.com

Abstract

We propose efficient algorithms for learning ranking functions from order constraints between sets—*i.e.* classes—of training samples. Our algorithms may be used for maximizing the generalized Wilcoxon Mann Whitney statistic that accounts for the partial ordering of the classes: special cases include maximizing the area under the ROC curve for binary classification and its generalization for ordinal regression. Experiments on public benchmarks indicate that: (a) the proposed algorithm is at least as accurate as the current state-of-the-art; (b) computationally, it is several orders of magnitude faster and—unlike current methods—it is easily able to handle even large datasets with over 20,000 samples.

1 Introduction

Many machine learning applications depend on accurately ordering the elements of a set based on the known ordering of only some of its elements. In the literature, variants of this problem have been referred to as ordinal regression, ranking, and learning of preference relations. Formally, we want to find a function $f : \Re^n \to \Re$ such that, for a set of test samples $\{x_k \in \Re^n\}$, the output of the function $f(x_k)$ can be sorted to obtain a ranking. In order to learn such a function we are provided with training data, A, containing S sets (or classes) of training samples: $A = \bigcup_{j=1}^{S}(A^j = \{x_i^j\}_{i=1}^{m_j})$, where the j-th set A^j contains m_j samples, so that we have a total of $m = \sum_{j=1}^{S} m_j$ samples in A. Further, we are also provided with a directed *order graph* $G = (\mathcal{S}, \mathcal{E})$ each of whose vertices corresponds to a class A^j, and the existence of a directed edge $\mathcal{E}_{PQ}$—corresponding to $A^P \to A^Q$—means that all training samples $x_p \in A^P$ should be ranked higher than any sample $x_q \in A^Q$: *i.e.* $\forall\ (x_p \in A^P, x_q \in A^Q),\ f(x_p) \le f(x_q)$.

In general the number of constraints on the ranking function grows as $\mathcal{O}(m^2)$ so that naive solutions are computationally infeasible even for moderate sized training sets with a few thousand samples. Hence, we propose a *more stringent* problem with a larger (infinite) set of constraints, that is nevertheless much more tractably solved. In particular, we modify the constraints to: $\forall\ (x_p \in CH(A^P), x_q \in CH(A^Q)),\ f(x_p) \le f(x_q)$, where $CH(A^j)$ denotes the set of all points in the convex hull of A^j.

We show how this leads to: (a) a family of approximations to the original problem; and (b) considerably more efficient solutions that still enforce all of the original inter-group order constraints. Notice that, this formulation subsumes the standard ranking problem (*e.g.* [4]) as a special case when each set A^j is reduced to a singleton and the order graph is equal to

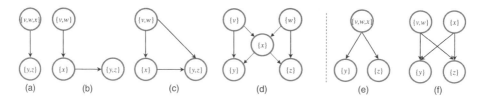

Figure 1: Various instances of the proposed ranking problem consistent with the training set $\{v, w, x, y, z\}$ satisfying $v > w > x > y > z$. Each problem instance is defined by an order graph. (a-d) A succession of order graphs with an increasing number of constraints (e-f) Two order graphs defining the same partial ordering but different problem instances.

a full graph. However, as illustrated in Figure 1, the formulation is more general and does not require a *total ordering* of the sets of training samples A^j, *i.e.* it allows any order graph G to be incorporated into the problem.

1.1 Generalized Wilcoxon-Mann-Whitney Statistics

A distinction is usually made between classification and ordinal regression methods on one hand, and ranking on the other. In particular, the loss functions used for classification and ordinal regression evaluate whether each test sample is correctly classified: in other words, the loss functions that are used to evaluate these algorithms—*e.g.* the 0–1 loss for binary classification—are computed for every sample individually, and then averaged over the training or test set.

By contrast, bipartite ranking solutions are evaluated using the *Wilcoxon-Mann-Whitney* (WMW) statistic which measures the (sample averaged) probability that any *pair of samples* is ordered correctly; intuitively, the WMW statistic may be interpreted as the *area under the ROC curve* (AUC). We define a slight generalization of the WMW statistic that accounts for our notion of class-ordering:

$$WMW(f, A) = \sum_{\mathcal{E}_{ij}} \frac{\sum_{k=1}^{m_i} \sum_{l=1}^{m_j} \delta\left(f(x_k^i) < f(x_l^j)\right)}{\sum_{k=1}^{m_i} \sum_{l=1}^{m_j} 1}.$$

Hence, if a sample is individually misclassified because it falls on the wrong side of the decision boundary between classes it incurs a penalty in ordinal regression, whereas, in ranking, it may be possible that it is still correctly ordered with respect to every other test sample, and thus it may incur no penalty in the WMW statistic.

1.2 Previous Work

Ordinal regression and methods for handling structured output classes: For a classic description of generalized linear models for ordinal regression, see [11]. A non-parametric Bayesian model for ordinal regression based on Gaussian processes (GP) was defined [1]. Several recent machine learning papers consider structured output classes: *e.g.* [13] presents SVM based algorithms for handling structured and interdependent output spaces, and [5] discusses automatic document categorization into pre-defined hierarchies or taxonomies of topics.

Learning Rankings: The problem of learning rankings was first treated as a classification problem on pairs of objects by Herbrich [4] and subsequently used on a web page ranking task by Joachims [6]; a variety of authors have investigated this approach recently. The major advantage of this approach is that it considers a more explicit notion of ordering— However, the naive optimization strategy proposed there suffers from the $\mathcal{O}(m^2)$ growth in the number of constraints mentioned in the previous section. This computational burden renders these methods impractical even for medium sized datasets with a few thousand samples. In other related work, boosting methods have been proposed for learning preferences [3], and a combinatorial structure called the ranking poset was used for conditional modeling of partially ranked data[8], in the context of combining ranked sets of web pages produced by various web-page search engines. Another, less related, approach is [2].

Relationship to the proposed work: Our algorithm penalizes wrong ordering of pairs of training instances in order to learn ranking functions (similar to [4]), but in addition, it can also utilize the notion of a structured class order graph. Nevertheless, using a formulation based on constraints over convex hulls of the training classes, our method avoids the prohibitive computational complexity of the previous algorithms for ranking.

1.3 Notation and Background

In the following, vectors will be assumed to be column vectors unless transposed to a row vector by a prime superscript $'$. For a vector x in the n-dimensional real space $\Re^n$, the cardinality of a set A will be denoted by #(A). The scalar (inner) product of two vectors x and y in the n-dimensional real space $\Re^n$ will be denoted by $x'y$ and the 2-norm of x will be denoted by $\|x\|$. For a matrix $A \in \Re^{m \times n}$, A_i is the ith row of A which is a row vector in $\Re^n$, while $A_{\cdot j}$ is the jth column of A. A column vector of ones of arbitrary dimension will be denoted by e. For $A \in \Re^{m \times n}$ and $B \in \Re^{n \times k}$, the kernel $K(A, B)$ maps $\Re^{m \times n} \times \Re^{n \times k}$ into $\Re^{m \times k}$. In particular, if x and y are column vectors in $\Re^n$ then, $K(x', y)$ is a real number, $K(x', A')$ is a row vector in $\Re^m$ and $K(A, A')$ is an $m \times m$ matrix. The identity matrix of arbitrary dimension will be denoted by I.

2 Convex Hull formulation

We are interested in learning a ranking function $f : \Re^n \to \Re$ given known ranking relationships between some *training instances* $A_i, A_j \subset A$. Let the ranking relationships be specified by a set $\mathcal{E} = \{(i, j)|A_i \prec A_j\}$

To begin with, let us consider the *linearly separable* binary ranking case which is equivalent to the problem of classifying m points in the n-dimensional real space $\Re^n$, represented by the $m \times n$ matrix A, according to membership of each point $x = A_i$ in the class A^+ or A^- as specified by a given vector of labels d. In others words, for binary classifiers, we want a linear ranking function $f_w(x) = w'x$ that satisfies the following constraints:

$$\forall \, (x^+ \in A^+, x^- \in A^-), \, f(x^-) \le f(x^+) \Rightarrow f(x^-) - f(x^+) = w'x^- - w'x^+ \le -1 \le 0. \tag{1}$$

Clearly, the number of constraints grows as $O(m^+ m^-)$, which is roughly quadratic in the number of training samples (unless we have severe class imbalance). While easily overcome–based on additional insights–in the separable problem, in the non-separable case, the quadratic growth in the number of constraints poses huge computational burdens on the optimization algorithm; indeed direct optimization with these constraints is infeasible even for moderate sized problems. We overcome this computational problem based on **three key insights** that are explained below.

First, notice that (by negation) the feasibility constraints in (1) can also be defined as:

$$\forall \, (x^+ \in A^+, x^- \in A^-), w'x^- - w'x^+ \le -1 \Leftrightarrow \nexists (x^+ \in A^+, x^- \in A^-), w'x^- - w'x^+ > -1.$$

In other words, a solution w is feasible iff there exist no pair of samples from the two classes such that $f_w(\cdot)$ orders them incorrectly.

Second, we will make the constraints in (1) *more stringent*: instead of requiring that equation (1) be satisfied for each possible pair $(x^+ \in A^+, x^- \in A^-)$ in the training set, we will

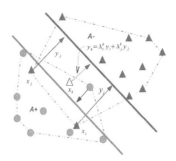

Figure 2: Example binary problem where points belonging to the A^+ and A^- sets are represented by blue circles and red triangles respectively. Note that two elements x_i and x_j of the set A^- are not correctly ordered and hence generate positive values of the corresponding slack variables y_i and y_j. Note that the point x_k (hollow triangle) is in the convex hull of the set A^- and hence the corresponding y_k error can be writen as a convex combination ($y_k = \lambda_i^k y_i + \lambda_j^k y_j$) of the two nonzero errors corresponding to points of A^-

require (1) to be satisfied for each pair $(x^+ \in CH(A^+), x^- \in CH(A^-))$, where $CH(A^i)$ denotes the convex hull of the set A^i [12]. Thus, our constraints become:

$$\forall(\lambda^+, \lambda^-) \quad \text{such that} \quad \left\{ \begin{array}{l} 0 \leq \lambda^+ \leq 1, \sum \lambda^+ = 1 \\ 0 \leq \lambda^- \leq 1, \sum \lambda^- = 1 \end{array} \right\}, \quad w'A^{-'}\lambda^- - w'A^{+'}\lambda^+ \leq -1 \quad (2)$$

Next, notice that all the linear inequality and equality constraints on (λ^+, λ^-) may be conveniently grouped together as $B\lambda \leq b$, where,

$$\lambda = \left[\begin{array}{c} \lambda^- \\ \lambda^+ \end{array} \right]_{m \times 1} \quad b^+ = \left[\begin{array}{c} \mathbf{0}^+_{m^+ \times 1} \\ 1 \\ -1 \end{array} \right]_{(m^+ +2) \times 1} \quad b^- = \left[\begin{array}{c} \mathbf{0}^-_{m^- \times 1} \\ 1 \\ -1 \end{array} \right]_{(m^- +2) \times 1} \quad b = \left[\begin{array}{c} b^+ \\ b^- \end{array} \right]$$

$$(3)$$

$$B^- = \left[\begin{array}{cc} -I_{m^-} & 0 \\ e' & 0 \\ -e' & 0 \end{array} \right]_{(m^- +2) \times m} \quad B^+ = \left[\begin{array}{cc} 0 & -I_{m^+} \\ 0 & e' \\ 0 & -e' \end{array} \right]_{(m^+ +2) \times m} \quad B = \left[\begin{array}{c} B^- \\ B^+ \end{array} \right]_{(m+4) \times m}$$

$$(4)$$

Thus, our constraints on w can be written as:

$$\forall \lambda \text{ s.t. } B\lambda \leq b, \ w'A^{-'}\lambda^- - w'A^{+'}\lambda^+ \leq -1 \quad (5)$$

$$\Leftrightarrow \nexists \lambda \text{ s.t. } B\lambda \leq b, \ w'A^{-'}\lambda^- - w'A^{+'}\lambda^+ > -1 \quad (6)$$

$$\Leftrightarrow \exists u \text{ s.t. } B'u - w'[A^{-'} - A^{+'}] = 0, \ b'u \leq -1, \ u \geq 0, \quad (7)$$

Where the second equivalent form of the constraints was obtained by negation (as before), and the third equivalent form results from our **third** key insight: the application of Farka's theorem of alternatives[9]. The resulting linear system of m equalities and $m + 5$ inequalities in $m + n + 4$ variables can be used while minimizing any regularizer (such as $\|w\|^2$) to obtain the linear ranking function that satisfies (1); notice, however, that we avoid the $O(m^2)$ scaling in constraints.

2.1 The binary non-separable case

In the non-separable case, $CH(A^+) \cap CH(A^-) \neq \emptyset$ so the requirements have to be relaxed by introducing slack variables. To this end, we allow one slack variable $y_i \geq 0$ for each training sample x_i, and consider the slack for any point *inside* the convex hull $CH(A^j)$ to also be a convex combination of y (see Fig. 2). For example, this implies that if only a subset of training samples have non-zero slacks $y_i > 0$ (*i.e.* they are possibly mis-classified), then the slacks of any points inside the convex hull also only depend on those y_i. Thus, our constraints now become:

$$\forall \lambda \text{ s.t. } B\lambda \leq b, \ w'A^{-'}\lambda^{-} - w'A^{+'}\lambda^{+} \leq -1 + (\lambda^{-}y^{-} + \lambda^{+}y^{+}), \ y^{+} \geq 0, \ y^{-} \geq 0. \quad (8)$$

Applying Farka's theorem of alternatives, we get:

$$(2) \Leftrightarrow \exists u \text{ s.t. } B'u - \begin{bmatrix} A^{-}w \\ -A^{+}w \end{bmatrix} + \begin{bmatrix} y^{-} \\ y^{+} \end{bmatrix} = 0, \ b'u \leq -1, \ u \geq 0 \quad (9)$$

Replacing B from equation (4) and defining $u' = [u^{-'} \quad u^{+'}] \geq 0$ we get the constraints:

$$B^{+'}u^{+} + A^{+}w + y^{+} = 0, \quad (10)$$
$$B^{-'}u^{-} - A^{-}w + y^{-} = 0, \quad (11)$$
$$b^{+}u^{+} + b^{-}u^{-} \leq -1, \ u \geq 0 \quad (12)$$

2.2 The general ranking problem

Now we can extend the idea presented in the previous section for any given arbitrary directed *order graph* $G = (\mathcal{S}, \mathcal{E})$, as stated in the introduction, each of whose vertices corresponds to a class A^j and the existence of a directed edge $\mathcal{E}_{ij}$ means that all training samples $x_i \in A^i$ should be ranked higher than any sample $x_j \in A^j$, that is:

$$f(x^j) \leq f(x^i) \Rightarrow f(x^j) - f(x^i) = w'x^j - w'x^i \leq -1 \leq 0 \quad (13)$$

Analogously we obtain the following set of equations that enforced the ordering between sets A^i and A^j:

$$B^{i'}u^{ij} + A^iw + y^i = 0 \quad (14)$$
$$B^{j'}\hat{u}^{ij} - A^jw + y^j = 0 \quad (15)$$
$$b^iu^{ij} + b^j\hat{u}^{ij} \leq -1 \quad (16)$$
$$u^{ij}, \hat{u}^{ij} \geq 0 \quad (17)$$

It can be shown that using the definitions of B^i, B^j, b^i, b^j and the fact that $u^{ij}, \hat{u}^{ij} \geq 0$, equations (14) can be rewritten in the following way:

$$\gamma^{ij} + A^iw + y^i \geq 0 \quad (18)$$
$$\hat{\gamma}^{ij} - A^jw + y^j \geq 0 \quad (19)$$
$$\gamma^{ij} + \hat{\gamma}^{ij} \leq -1 \quad (20)$$
$$y^i, y^j \geq 0 \quad (21)$$

where $\gamma^{ij} = b^iu^{ij}$ and $\hat{\gamma}^{ij} = b^j\hat{u}^{ij}$. Note that enforcing the constraints defined above indeed implies the desired ordering, since we have:

$$A^iw + y^i \geq -\gamma^{ij} \geq \hat{\gamma}^{ij} + 1 \geq \hat{\gamma}^{ij} \geq A^jw - y^j$$

It is also important to note the connection with Support Vector Machines (SVM) formulation [10, 14] for the binary case. If we impose the extra constraints $-\gamma^{ij} = \gamma + 1$ and $\hat{\gamma}^{ij} = \gamma - 1$, then equations (18) imply the constraints included in the standard primal SVM formulation. To obtain a more general formulation, we can "kernelize" equations (14) by making a transformation of the variable w as: $w = A'v$, where v can be interpreted as an arbitrary variable in R^m, This transformation can be motivated by duality theory [10], then equations (14) become:

$$\gamma^{ij} + A^iA'v + y^i \geq 0 \quad (22)$$
$$\hat{\gamma}^{ij} - A^jA'v + y^j \geq 0 \quad (23)$$
$$\gamma^{ij} + \hat{\gamma}^{ij} \leq -1 \quad (24)$$
$$y^i, y^j \geq 0 \quad (25)$$

If we now replace the linear kernels $A^i A'$ and $A^i A'$ by more general kernels $K(A^i, A')$ and $K(A^j, A')$ we obtain a "kernelized" version of equations (14)

$$E_{ij} \equiv \left\{ \begin{array}{rcl} \gamma^{ij} + K(A^i, A')v + y^i & \geq & 0 \\ \hat{\gamma}^{ij} - K(A^j, A')v + y^j & \geq & 0 \\ \gamma^{ij} + \hat{\gamma}^{ij} & \leq & -1 \\ y^i, y^j & \geq & 0 \end{array} \right\} \qquad (26)$$

Given a graph $\mathcal{G} = (\mathcal{V}, \mathcal{E})$ representing the ordering of the training data and using equations (26), we present next, a general mathematical programming formulation the ranking problem:

$$\min_{\{v, y^i, \gamma^{ij} \mid (i,j) \in \mathcal{E}\}} \quad \nu \epsilon(y) + R(v) \qquad (27)$$
$$\text{s.t.} \qquad E_{ij} \quad \forall (i,j) \in \mathcal{E}$$

Where ϵ is a given loss function for the slack variables y^i and $R(v)$ represents a regularizer on the normal to the hyperplane v. For an arbitrary kernel $K(x, x')$ the number of variables of formulation (27) is $2 * m + 2\#(\mathcal{E})$ and the number of linear equations(excluding the nonnegativity constraints) is $m\#(\mathcal{E}) + \#(\mathcal{E}) = \#(\mathcal{E})(m + 1)$. for a linear kernel i.e. $K(x, x') = xx'$ the number of variables of formulation (27) becomes $m + n + 2\#(\mathcal{E})$ and the number of linear equations remains the same. When using a linear kernel and using $\epsilon(x) = R(x) = \|x\|_2^2$, the optimization problem (27) becomes a linearly constrained quadratic optimization problem for which a unique solution exists due to the convexity of the objective function:

$$\min_{\{w, y^i, \gamma^{ij} \mid (i,j) \in \mathcal{E}\}} \quad \nu \|y\|_2^2 + \tfrac{1}{2} w'w \qquad (28)$$
$$\text{s.t.} \qquad E_{ij} \quad \forall (i,j) \in \mathcal{E}$$

Unlike other SVM-like methods for ranking that need a $O(m^2)$ number of slack variables y our formulation only require one slack variable for example, only m slack variables are used, giving our formulation computational advantage over ranking methods. Next, we demonstrate the effectiveness of our algorithm by comparing it to two state-of-the-art algorithms.

3 Experimental Evaluation

We test tested our approach in a set of nine publicly available datasets [1] shown in Tab. 1 (several large datasets are not reported since only the algorithm presented in this paper was able to run them). These datasets have been frequently used as a benchmark for ordinal regression methods (e.g. [1]). Here we use them for evaluating ranking performance. We compare our method against SVM for ranking (e.g. [4, 6]) using the SVM-light package [2] and an efficient Gaussian process method (the informative vector machine) [3] [7].

These datasets were originally designed for regression, thus the continuous *target* values for each dataset were discretized into five equal size bins. We use these bins to define our ranking constraints: all the datapoints with target value falling in the same bin were grouped together. Each dataset was divided into 10% for testing and 90% for training. Thus, the input to all of the algorithms tested was, for each point in the training set: (1) a vector in $\Re^n$ (where n is different for each set) and (2) a value from 1 to 5 denoting the rank of the group to which it belongs.

Performance is defined in terms of the Wilcoxon statistic. Since we do not employ information about the ranking of the elements within each group, order constraints within a group

---

[1] Available at http:\\www.liacc.up.pt\ĩtorgo\Regression\DataSets.html
[2] http:\\www.cs.cornell.edu\People\tj\svm_light\
[3] http:\\www.dcs.shef.ac.uk\ neil\ivm\

Table 1: Benchmark Datasets

Name	m	n	Name	m	n
1 Abalone	4177	9	6 Machine-CPU	209	7
2 Airplane Comp.	950	10	7 Pyrimidines	74	28
3 Auto-MPG	392	8	8 Triazines	186	61
4 CA Housing	20640	9	9 WI Breast Cancer	194	33
5 Housing-Boston	506	14			

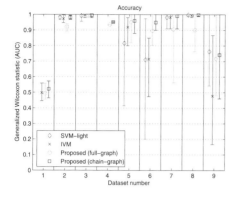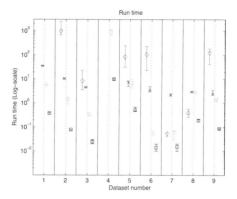

Figure 3: Experimental comparison of the ranking SVM, IVM and the proposed method on nine benchmark datasets. Along with the mean values in 10 fold cross-validation, the entire range of variation is indicated in the error-bars. (a) The overall accuracy for all the three methods is comparable. (b) The proposed method has a much lower run time than the other methods, even for the full graph case for medium to large size datasets. NOTE: Both SVM-light and IVM ran out of memory and crashed on dataset 4; on dataset 1, SVM-light failed to complete even one fold after more than 24 hours of run time, so its results could not be compiled in time for submission.

cannot be verified. Letting $b(m) = m(m-1)/2$, the total number of order constraints is equal to $b(m) - \sum_i b(m_i)$, where m_i is the number of instances in group i.

The results for all of the algorithms are shown in Fig.3. Our formulation was tested employing two order graphs, the full directed acyclic graph and the chain graph. The performance for all datasets is generally comparable or significantly better for our algorithm (when using a chain order graph). Note that the performance for the full graph is consistently lower than that for the chain graph. Thus, interestingly enforcing more order constraints does not necessarily imply better performance. We suspect that this is due to the role that the slack variables play in both formulations, since the number of slack variables remains the same while the number of constraints increases. Adding more slack variables may positively affect performance in the full graph, but this comes at a computational cost. An interesting problem is to find the right compromise. A different but potentially related problem is that of finding *good* order graph given a dataset. Note also that the chain graph is much more stable regarding performance overall. Regarding run-time, our algorithm runs an order of magnitude faster than current implementations of state-of-the-art methods, even approximate ones (like IVM).

4 Discussions and future work

We propose a general method for learning a ranking function from structured order constraints on sets of training samples. The proposed algorithm was illustrated on benchmark ranking problems with two different constraint graphs: (a) a chain graph; and (b) a full ordering graph. Although a chain graph was more accurate in the experiments shown in Figure 3, with either type of graph structure, the proposed method is at least as accurate (in terms of the WMW statistic for ordinal regression) as state-of-the-art algorithms such as the ranking-SVM and Gaussian Processes for ordinal regression.

Besides being accurate, the computational requirements of our algorithm scale much more favorably with the number of training samples as compared to other state-of-the-art methods. Indeed it was the only algorithm capable of handling several large datasets, while the other methods either crashed due to lack of memory or ran for so long that they were not practically feasible. While our experiments illustrate only specific order graphs, we stress that the method is general enough to handle arbitrary constraint relationships.

While the proposed formulation reduces the computational complexity of enforcing order constraints, it is entirely independent of the *regularizer* that is minimized (under these constraints) while learning the optimal ranking function. Though we have used a simple margin regularization (via $\|w\|^2$ in (28), and RKHS regularization in (27) in order to learn in a *supervised* setting, we can just as easily easily use a graph-Laplacian based regularizer that exploits unlabeled data, in order to learn in *semi-supervised* settings. We plan to explore this in future work.

References

[1] W. Chu and Z. Ghahramani, *Gaussian processes for ordinal regression*, Tech. report, University College London, 2004.

[2] K. Crammer and Y. Singer, *Pranking with ranking*, Neural Info. Proc. Systems, 2002.

[3] Y. Freund, R. Iyer, and R. Schapire, *An efficient boosting algorithm for combining preferences*, Journal of Machine Learning Research **4** (2003), 933–969.

[4] R. Herbrich, T. Graepel, and K. Obermayer, *Large margin rank boundaries for ordinal regression*, Advances in Large Margin Classifiers (2000), 115–132.

[5] T. Hofmann, L. Cai, and M. Ciaramita, *Learning with taxonomies: Classifying documents and words*, (NIPS) Workshop on Syntax, Semantics, and Statistics, 2003.

[6] T. Joachims, *Optimizing search engines using clickthrough data*, Proc. ACM Conference on Knowledge Discovery and Data Mining (KDD), 2002.

[7] N. Lawrence, M. Seeger, and R. Herbrich, *Fast sparse gaussian process methods: The informative vector machine*, Neural Info. Proc. Systems, 2002.

[8] G. Lebanon and J. Lafferty, *Conditional models on the ranking poset*, Neural Info. Proc. Systems, 2002.

[9] O. L. Mangasarian, *Nonlinear programming*, McGraw–Hill, New York, 1969, Reprint: SIAM Classic in Applied Mathematics 10, 1994, Philadelphia.

[10] ———, *Generalized support vector machines*, Advances in Large Margin Classifiers, 2000, pp. 135–146.

[11] P. McCullagh and J. Nelder, *Generalized linear models*, Chapman & Hall, 1983.

[12] R. T. Rockafellar, *Convex analysis*, Princeton University Press, Princeton, New Jersey, 1970.

[13] I. Tsochantaridis, T. Hofmann, T. Joachims, and Y. Altun, *Support vector machine learning for interdependent and structured output spaces*, Int.Conf. on Machine Learning, 2004.

[14] V. N. Vapnik, *The nature of statistical learning theory*, second ed., Springer, New York, 2000.

A Connectionist Model for Constructive Modal Reasoning

Artur S. d'Avila Garcez
Department of Computing, City University London
London EC1V 0HB, UK
aag@soi.city.ac.uk

Luís C. Lamb
Institute of Informatics, Federal University of Rio Grande do Sul
Porto Alegre RS, 91501-970, Brazil
LuisLamb@acm.org

Dov M. Gabbay
Department of Computer Science, King's College London
Strand, London, WC2R 2LS, UK
dg@dcs.kcl.ac.uk

Abstract

We present a new connectionist model for constructive, intuitionistic modal reasoning. We use ensembles of neural networks to represent intuitionistic modal theories, and show that for each intuitionistic modal program there exists a corresponding neural network ensemble that computes the program. This provides a massively parallel model for intuitionistic modal reasoning, and sets the scene for integrated reasoning, knowledge representation, and learning of intuitionistic theories in neural networks, since the networks in the ensemble can be trained by examples using standard neural learning algorithms.

1 Introduction

Automated reasoning and learning theory have been the subject of intensive investigation since the early developments in computer science [14]. However, while (machine) learning has focused mainly on quantitative and connectionist approaches [16], the reasoning component of intelligent systems has been developed mainly by formalisms of classical and non-classical logics [7, 9]. More recently, the recognition of the need for systems that integrate reasoning and learning into the same foundation, and the evolution of the fields of cognitive and neural computation, has led to a number of proposals that attempt to integrate reasoning and learning [1, 3, 12, 13, 15].

We claim that an effective integration of reasoning and learning can be obtained by neural-symbolic learning systems [3, 4]. Such systems concern the application of problem-specific symbolic knowledge within the neurocomputing paradigm. By integrating logic and neural networks, they may provide (*i*) a sound logical characterisation of a connectionist system, (*ii*) a connectionist (parallel) implementation of a logic, or (*iii*) a hybrid learning system bringing together advantages from connectionism and symbolic reasoning.

Intuitionistic logical systems have been advocated by many as providing adequate logical foundations for computation (see [2] for a survey). We argue, therefore, that intuitionism could also play an important part in neural computation. In this paper, we follow the research path outlined in [4, 5], and develop a computational model for integrated reasoning, representation, and learning of intuitionistic modal knowledge. We concentrate on reasoning and knowledge representation issues, which set the scene for connectionist intuitionistic learning, since effective knowledge representation should precede learning [15]. Still, we base the representation on standard, simple neural network architectures, aiming at future work on experimental learning within the model proposed here.

A key contribution of this paper is the proposal to shift the notion of logical implication (and negation) in neural networks from the standard notion of implication as a partial function from input to output (and of negation as failure to activate a neuron), to an intuitionistic notion which we will see can be implemented in neural networks if we make use of network ensembles. We claim that the intuitionistic interpretation introduced here will make sense for a number of problems in neural computation in the same way that intuitionistic logic is more appropriate than classical logic in a number of computational settings. We will start by illustrating the proposed computational model in an appropriate constructive reasoning, distributed knowledge representation scenario, namely, the *wise men puzzle* [7]. Then, we will show how ensembles of *Connectionist Inductive Learning and Logic Programming* (C-ILP) networks [3] can compute intuitionistic modal knowledge. The networks are set up by an *Intuitionistic Modal Algorithm* introduced in this paper. A proof that the algorithm produces a neural network ensemble that computes a semantics of its associated intuitionistic modal theory is then given. Furthermore, the networks in the ensemble are kept simple and in a modular structure, and may be trained from examples with the use of standard learning algorithms such as *backpropagation* [11].

In Section 2, we present the basic concepts of intuitionistic reasoning used in the paper. In Section 3, we motivate the proposed model using the wise men puzzle. In Section 4, we introduce the *Intuitionistic Modal Algorithm*, which translates intuitionistic modal theories into neural network ensembles, and prove that the ensemble computes a semantics of the theory. Section 5 concludes the paper and discusses directions for future work.

2   Background

In this section, we present some basic concepts of artificial neural networks and intuitionistic programs used throughout the paper. We concentrate on ensembles of single hidden layer feedforward networks, and on recurrent networks typically with feedback only from the output to the input layer. Feedback is used with the sole purpose of denoting that the output of a neuron should serve as the input of another neuron when we run the network, i.e. the weight of any feedback connection is fixed at 1. We use *bipolar* semi-linear activation functions $h(x) = \frac{2}{1+e^{-\beta x}} - 1$ with inputs in $\{-1, 1\}$. Throughout, we will use 1 to denote truth-value $true$, and -1 to denote truth-value $false$.

Intuitionistic logic was originally developed by Brouwer, and later by Heyting and Kolmogorov [2]. In intuitionistic logics, a statement that there exists a proof of a proposition x is only made if there is a constructive method of the proof of x. One of the consequences of Brouwer's ideas is the rejection of the law of the excluded middle, namely $\alpha \vee \neg\alpha$, since one cannot always state that there is a proof of α or of its negation, as accepted in classical logic and in (classical) mathematics. The development of these ideas and applications in mathematics has led to developments in *constructive* mathematics and has influenced several lines of research on logic and computing science [2].

An intuitionistic modal language $\mathcal{L}$ includes propositional letters (atoms) $p, q, r...$, the connectives $\neg, \wedge$, an intuitionistic implication $\Rightarrow$, the *necessity* ($\square$) and *possibility* ($\Diamond$) modal operators, where an atom will be necessarily true in a possible world if it is true in every world that is related to this possible world, while it will be possibly true if it is true in some world related to this world. Formally, we interpret the language as follows, where formulas are denoted by $\alpha, \beta, \gamma...$

Definition 1 (Kripke Models for Intuitionistic Modal Logic) *Let $\mathcal{L}$ be an intuitionistic language. A model for $\mathcal{L}$ is a tuple $\mathcal{M} = \langle \Omega, \mathcal{R}, v \rangle$ where Ω is a set of worlds, v is a mapping that assigns to each $\omega \in \Omega$ a subset of the atoms of $\mathcal{L}$, and $\mathcal{R}$ is a reflexive, transitive, binary relation over Ω, such that: (a) $(\mathcal{M}, \omega) \models p$ iff $p \in v(\omega)$ (for atom p); (b) $(\mathcal{M}, \omega) \models \neg\alpha$ iff for all ω' such that $\mathcal{R}(\omega, \omega')$, $(\mathcal{M}, \omega') \not\models \alpha$; (c) $(\mathcal{M}, \omega) \models \alpha \wedge \beta$ iff $(\mathcal{M}, \omega) \models \alpha$ and $(\mathcal{M}, \omega) \models \beta$; (d) $(\mathcal{M}, \omega) \models \alpha \Rightarrow \beta$ iff for all ω' with $\mathcal{R}(\omega, \omega')$ we have $(\mathcal{M}, \omega') \models \beta$ whenever we have $(\mathcal{M}, \omega') \models \alpha$; (e) $(\mathcal{M}, \omega) \models \square\alpha$ iff for all $\omega' \in \Omega$ if $\mathcal{R}(\omega, \omega')$ then $(\mathcal{M}, \omega') \models \alpha$; (f) $(\mathcal{M}, \omega) \models \Diamond\alpha$ iff there exists $\omega' \in \Omega$ such that $\mathcal{R}(\omega, \omega')$ and $(\mathcal{M}, \omega') \models \alpha$.*

We now define *labelled intuitionistic programs* as sets of intuitionistic rules, where each rule is labelled by the world at which it holds, similarly to Gabbay's Labelled Deductive Systems [8].

Definition 2 (Labelled Intuitionistic Program) *A Labelled Intuitionistic Program is a finite set of rules C of the form $\omega_i : A_1, ..., A_n \Rightarrow A_0$ (where "," abbreviates "$\wedge$", as usual), and a finite set of relations $\mathcal{R}$ between worlds ω_i ($1 \leq i \leq m$) in C, where A_k ($0 \leq k \leq n$) are atoms and ω_i is a label representing a world in which the associated rule holds.*

To deal with intuitionistic negation, we adopt the approach of [10], as follows. We rename any negative literal $\neg A$ as an atom A' not present originally in the language. This form of renaming allows our definition of labelled intuitionistic programs above to consider atoms only. For example, given $A_1, ..., A'_k, ..., A_n \Rightarrow A_0$, where A'_k is a renaming of $\neg A_k$, an interpretation that assigns true to A'_k represents that $\neg A_k$ is true; it does not represent that A_k is false. Following Definition 1 (intuitionistic negation), A' will be true in a world ω_i if and only if A does not hold in every world ω_j such that $\mathcal{R}(\omega_i, \omega_j)$.
Finally, we extend labelled intuitionistic programs to include modalities.

Definition 3 (Labelled Intuitionistic Modal Program) *A modal atom is of the form MA where $M \in \{\square, \Diamond\}$ and A is an atom. A Labelled Intuitionistic Modal Program is a finite set of rules C of the form $\omega_i : MA_1, ..., MA_n \Rightarrow MA_0$, where MA_k ($0 \leq k \leq n$) are modal atoms and ω_i is a label representing a world in which the associated rule holds, and a finite set of (accessibility) relations $\mathcal{R}$ between worlds ω_i ($1 \leq i \leq m$) in C.*

3 Motivating Scenario

In this section, we consider an archetypal testbed for distributed knowledge representation, namely, the *wise men puzzle* [7], and model it intuitionistically in a neural network ensemble. Our aim is to illustrate the combination of neural networks and intuitionistic modal reasoning. The formalisation of our computational model will be given in Section 4.

A certain king wishes to test his three wise men. He arranges them in a circle so that they can see and hear each other. They are all perceptive, truthful and intelligent, and this is common knowledge in the group. It is also common knowledge among them that there are three red hats and two white hats, and five hats in total. The king places a hat on the head

*of each wise man in a way that they are not able to see the colour of their own hats, and
then asks each one whether they know the colour of the hats on their heads.*

The puzzle illustrates a situation in which intuitionistic implication and intuitionistic negation occur. Knowledge evolves in time, with the current knowledge persisting in time. For
example, at the first round it is known that there are at most two white hats on the wise
men's heads. Then, if the wise men get to a second round, it becomes known that there is
at most one white hat on their heads.[1] This new knowledge subsumes the previous knowl-
edge, which in turn persists. This means that if $A \Rightarrow B$ is true at a world t_1 then $A \Rightarrow B$
will be true at a world t_2 that is related to t_1 (intuitionistic implication). Now, in any situation in which a wise man knows that his hat is red, this knowledge - constructed with
the use of sound reasoning processes - cannot be refuted. In other words, in this puzzle, if
$\neg A$ is true at world t_1 then A cannot be true at a world t_2 that is related to t_1 (intuitionistic
negation).

We model the wise men puzzle by constructing the relative knowledge of each wise man
along time points. This allows us to explicitly represent the relativistic notion of knowledge, which is a principle of intuitionistic reasoning. For simplicity, we refer to wise man
1 (respectively, 2 and 3) as agent 1 (respectively, 2 and 3). The resulting model is a two-
dimensional network ensemble (agents × time), containing three networks in each dimension. In addition to p_i - denoting the fact that wise man i wears a red hat - to model each
agent's individual knowledge, we need to use a modality K_j, $j \in \{1, 2, 3\}$, which represents the relative notion of knowledge at each time point t_1, t_2, t_3. Thus, $K_j p_i$ denotes the
fact that agent j knows that agent i wears a red hat. The K modality above corresponds to
the $\square$ modality in intuitionistic modal reasoning, as customary in the logics of knowledge
[7], and as exemplified below.

First, we model the fact that each agent knows the colour of the others' hats. For example,
if wise man 3 wears a red hat (neuron p_3 is active) then wise man 1 knows that wise man
3 wears a red hat (neuron $K p_3$ is active for wise man 1). We then need to model the
reasoning process of each wise man. In this example, let us consider the case in which
neurons p_1 and p_3 are active. For agent 1, we have the rule $t_1 : K_1 \neg p_2 \wedge K_1 \neg p_3 \Rightarrow K_1 p_1$,
which states that agent 1 can deduce that he is wearing a red hat if he knows that the other
agents are both wearing white hats. Analogous rules exist for agents 2 and 3. As before,
the implication is intuitionistic, so that it persists at t_2 and t_3 as depicted in Figure 1 for
wise man 1 (represented via hidden neuron h_1 in each network). In addition, according to
the philosophy of intuitionistic negation, we may only conclude that agent 1 knows $\neg p_2$, if
in every world envisaged by agent 1, p_2 is not derived. This is illustrated with the use of
dotted lines in Figure 1, in which, e.g., if neuron $K p_2$ is not active at t_3 then neuron $K \neg p_2$
will be active at t_2. As a result, the network ensemble will never derive p_2 (as one should
expect), and thus it will derive $K_1 \neg p_2$ and $K_3 \neg p_2$.[2]

4 Connectionist Intuitionistic Modal Reasoning

The wise men puzzle example of Section 3 shows that simple, single-hidden layer neural
networks can be combined in a modular structure where each network represents a possible
world in the Kripke structure of Definition 1. The way that the networks should then be
inter-connected can be defined by following a semantics for $\Rightarrow$ and $\neg$, and for $\square$ and $\Diamond$ from
intuitionistic logic. In this section, we see how exactly we construct a network ensemble

---

[1]This is because if there were two white hats on their heads, one of them would have known (and
have said), in the first round, that his hat was red, for he would have been seeing the other two with
white hats.

[2]To complete the formalisation of the problem, the following rules should also hold at t_2 (and at
t_3): $K_1 \neg p_2 \Rightarrow K_1 p_1$ and $K_1 \neg p_3 \Rightarrow K_1 p_1$. Analogous rules exist for agents 2 and 3.

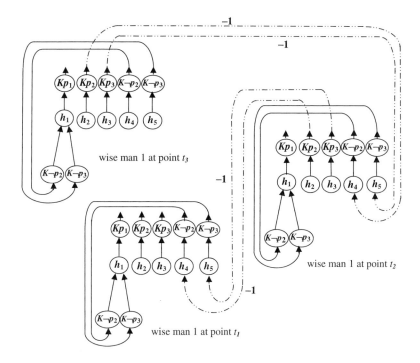

Figure 1: Wise men puzzle: Intuitionistic negation and implication.

given an intuitionistic modal program. We introduce a translation algorithm, which takes the program as input and produces the ensemble as output by setting the initial architecture, set of weights, and thresholds of the networks according to a Kripke semantics for the program. We then prove that the translation is correct, and thus that the network ensemble can be used to compute the logical consequences of the program in parallel.

Before we present the algorithm, let us illustrate informally how $\Rightarrow$, $\neg$, $\Box$, and $\Diamond$ are represented in the ensemble. We follow the key idea behind *Connectionist Modal Logics* (CML) to represent Kripke models in neural networks [6]. Each possible world is represented by a single hidden layer neural network. In each network, input and output neurons represent atoms or modal atoms of the form A, $\neg A$, $\Box A$, or $\Diamond A$, while each hidden neuron encodes a rule. For example, in Figure 1, hidden neuron h_1 encodes a rule of the form $A \wedge B \Rightarrow C$. Thresholds and weights must be such that the hidden layer computes a logical *and* of the input layer, while the output layer computes a logical *or* of the hidden layer.[3] Furthermore, in each network, each output neuron is connected to its corresponding input neuron with a weight fixed at 1.0 (as depicted in Figure 1 for $K\neg p_2$ and $K\neg p_3$), so that chains of the form $A \Rightarrow B$ and $B \Rightarrow C$ can be represented and computed. This basically characterises C-ILP networks [3]. Now, in CML, we allow for an ensemble of C-ILP networks, each network representing knowledge in a (learnable) possible world. In addition, we allow for a number of fixed feedforward and feedback connections to occur among different networks in the ensemble, as shown in Figure 1. These are defined as follows: in the case of $\Box$, if neuron $\Box A$ is activated (*true*) in network (world) ω_i then A must be activated in every network ω_j that is related to ω_i (this is analogous to the situation in which we activate $K_1 p_3$ and $K_2 p_3$ whenever p_3 is active). Dually, if A is active in every ω_j then $\Box A$ must be activated

---

[3]For example, if $A \wedge B \Rightarrow D$ and $C \Rightarrow D$ then a hidden neuron h_1 is used to connect A and B to D, and a hidden neuron h_2 is used to connect C to D such that if h_1 or h_2 is activated then D is activated.

in ω_i (this is done with the use of feedback connections and a hidden neuron that computes a logical *and*, as detailed in the algorithm below). In the case of $\Diamond$, if $\Diamond A$ is activated in network ω_i then A must be activated in at least one network ω_j that is related to ω_i (we do this by choosing an arbitrary ω_j to make A active). Dually, if A is activated in any ω_j that is related to ω_i then $\Diamond A$ must be activated in ω_i (this is done with the use of a hidden neuron that computes a logical *or*, also as detailed in the algorithm below). Now, in the case of $\Rightarrow$, according to the semantics of intuitionistic implication, $\omega_i : A \Rightarrow B$ and $\mathcal{R}(\omega_i, \omega_j)$ imply $\omega_j : A \Rightarrow B$. We implement this by copying the neural representation of $A \Rightarrow B$ from ω_i to ω_j, as done via h_1 in Figure 1. Finally, in the case of $\neg$, we need to make sure that $\neg A$ is activated in ω_i if, for every ω_j such that $\mathcal{R}(\omega_i, \omega_j)$, A is not active in ω_j. This is implemented with the use of negative weights (to account for the fact that the non-activation of a neuron needs to activate another neuron), as depicted in Figure 1 (dashed arrows), and detailed in the algorithm below.

We are now in a position to introduce the *Intuitionistic Modal Algorithm*. Let $\mathcal{P} = \{\mathcal{P}_1, ..., \mathcal{P}_n\}$ be a labelled intuitionistic modal program with rules of the form $\omega_i : MA_1, ..., MA_k \rightarrow MA_0$, where each A_j ($0 \leq j \leq k$) is an atom and $M \in \{\Box, \Diamond\}$, $1 \leq i \leq n$. Let $\mathcal{N} = \{\mathcal{N}_1, ..., \mathcal{N}_n\}$ be a neural network ensemble with each network $\mathcal{N}_i$ corresponding to program $\mathcal{P}_i$. Let q denote the number of rules occurring in $\mathcal{P}$. Consider that the atoms of $\mathcal{P}_i$ are numbered from 1 to η_i such that the input and output layers of $\mathcal{N}_i$ are vectors of length η_i, where the j-th neuron represents the j-th atom of $\mathcal{P}_i$. In addition, let A_{min} denote the minimum activation for a neuron to be considered *active* (or *true*), $A_{min} \in (0, 1)$; for each rule r_l in each program $\mathcal{P}_i$, let k_l denote the number of atoms in the body of rule r_l, and let μ_l denote the number of rules in $\mathcal{P}_i$ with the same consequent as r_l (including r_l). Let $MAX_{r_l}(k_l, \mu_l)$ denote the greater of k_l and μ_l for rule r_l, and let $MAX_{\mathcal{P}}(k_1, ..., k_q, \mu_1, ..., \mu_q)$ denote the greatest of $k_1, ..., k_q, \mu_1, ..., \mu_q$ for program $\mathcal{P}$. Below, we use $\mathbf{k}$ as a shorthand for $k_1, ..., k_q$, and μ as a shorthand for $\mu_1, ..., \mu_q$. The equations in the algorithm come from the proof of Theorem 1, given in the sequel.

Intuitionistic Modal Algorithm

1. Rename each modal atom MA_j by a new atom not occurring in $\mathcal{P}$ of the form $A_j^{\Box}$ if $M = \Box$, or $A_j^{\Diamond}$ if $M = \Diamond$;

2. For each rule r_l of the form $A_1, ..., A_k \Rightarrow A_0$ in $\mathcal{P}_i$ ($1 \leq i \leq n$) such that $\mathcal{R}(\omega_i, \omega_j)$, do: add a rule $A_1, ..., A_k \Rightarrow A_0$ to $\mathcal{P}_j$ ($1 \leq j \leq n$).

3. Calculate $A_{min} > (MAX_{\mathcal{P}}(\mathbf{k}, \mu, n) - 1)/(MAX_{\mathcal{P}}(\mathbf{k}, \mu, n) + 1)$;

4. Calculate $W \geq (2/\beta) \cdot (\ln(1 + A_{min}) - \ln(1 - A_{min}))/(MAX_{\mathcal{P}}(\mathbf{k}, \mu) \cdot (A_{min} - 1) + A_{min} + 1)$;

5. For each rule r_l of the form $A_1, ..., A_k \Rightarrow A_0$ ($k \geq 0$) in $\mathcal{P}_i$ ($1 \leq i \leq n$), do:

(a) Add a neuron N_l to the hidden layer of neural network $\mathcal{N}_i$ associated with $\mathcal{P}_i$; (b) Connect each neuron A_i ($1 \leq i \leq k$) in the input layer of $\mathcal{N}_i$ to N_l and set the connection weight to W; (c) Connect N_l to neuron A_0 in the output layer of $\mathcal{N}_i$ and set the connection weight to W; (d) Set the threshold θ_l of N_l to $\theta_l = ((1 + A_{min}) \cdot (k_l - 1)/2)W$; (e) Set the threshold θ_{A_0} of A_0 in the output layer of $\mathcal{N}_i$ to $\theta_{A_0} = ((1 + A_{min}) \cdot (1 - \mu_l)/2)W$. (f) For each atom of the form A' in r_l, do:

(i) Add a hidden neuron $N_{A'}$ to $\mathcal{N}_i$; (ii) Set the step function $s(x)$ as the activation function of $N_{A'}$;[4] (iii) Set the threshold $\theta_{A'}$ of $N_{A'}$ such that $n - (1 + A_{min}) < \theta_{A'} < n A_{min}$; (iv) For each

---

[4]Any hidden neuron created to encode negation (such as h_4 in Figure 1) shall have a non-linear activation function $s(x) = y$, where $y = 1$ if $x > 0$, and $y = 0$ otherwise. Such neurons encode (meta-level) knowledge about negation, while the other hidden neurons encode (object-level) knowledge about the problem domain. The former are not expected to be trained by examples and, as a result, the use of the step function will simplify the algorithm. The latter are to be trained, and therefore require a differentiable, semi-linear activation function.

network $\mathcal{N}_j$ corresponding to program $\mathcal{P}_j$ $(1 \leq j \leq n)$ in $\mathcal{P}$ such that $\mathcal{R}(\omega_i, \omega_j)$, do: Connect the output neuron A of $\mathcal{N}_j$ to the hidden neuron $N_{A'}$ of $\mathcal{N}_i$ and set the connection weight to -1; and Connect the hidden neuron $N_{A'}$ of $\mathcal{N}_i$ to the output neuron A' of $\mathcal{N}_i$ and set the connection weight to W^I such that $W^I > h^{-1}(A_{min}) + \mu_{A'}.W + \theta_{A'}$.

6. For each output neuron $A_j^{\Diamond}$ in network $\mathcal{N}_i$, do:

(a) Add a hidden neuron A_j^M and an output neuron A_j to an arbitrary network $\mathcal{N}_z$ such that $\mathcal{R}(\omega_i, \omega_z)$; (b) Set the step function $s(x)$ as the activation function of A_j^M, and set the semi-linear function $h(x)$ as the activation function of A_j; (c) Connect $A_j^{\Diamond}$ in $\mathcal{N}_i$ to A_j^M and set the connection weight to 1; (d) Set the threshold θ^M of A_j^M such that $-1 < \theta^M < A_{min}$; (e) Set the threshold θ_{A_j} of A_j in $\mathcal{N}_z$ such that $\theta_{A_j} = ((1 + A_{min}) \cdot (1 - \mu_{A_j})/2)W$; (f) Connect A_j^M to A_j in $\mathcal{N}_z$ and set the connection weight to $W^M > h^{-1}(A_{min}) + \mu_{A_j} W + \theta_{A_j}$.

7. For each output neuron $A_j^{\Box}$ in network $\mathcal{N}_i$, do:

(a) Add a hidden neuron A_j^M to each $\mathcal{N}_u$ $(1 \leq u \leq n)$ such that $\mathcal{R}(\omega_i, \omega_u)$, and add an output neuron A_j to $\mathcal{N}_u$ if $A_j \notin \mathcal{N}_u$; (b) Set the step function $s(x)$ as the activation function of A_j^M, and set the semi-linear function $h(x)$ as the activation function of A_j; (c) Connect $A_j^{\Box}$ in $\mathcal{N}_i$ to A_j^M and set the connection weight to 1; (d) Set the threshold θ^M of A_j^M such that $-1 < \theta^M < A_{min}$; (e) Set the threshold θ_{A_j} of A_j in each $\mathcal{N}_u$ such that $\theta_{A_j} = ((1 + A_{min}) \cdot (1 - \mu_{A_j})/2)W$; (f) Connect A_j^M to A_j in $\mathcal{N}_u$ and set the connection weight to $W^M > h^{-1}(A_{min}) + \mu_{A_j} W + \theta_{A_j}$.

8. For each output neuron A_j in network $\mathcal{N}_u$ such that $\mathcal{R}(\omega_i, \omega_u)$, do:
(a) Add a hidden neuron $A_j^{\vee}$ to $\mathcal{N}_i$; (b) Set the step function $s(x)$ as the activation function of $A_j^{\vee}$; (c) For each output neuron $A_j^{\Diamond}$ in $\mathcal{N}_i$, do:

(i) Connect A_j in $\mathcal{N}_u$ to $A_j^{\vee}$ and set the connection weight to 1; (ii) Set the threshold $\theta^{\vee}$ of $A_j^{\vee}$ such that $-nA_{min} < \theta^{\vee} < A_{min} - (n-1)$; (iii) Connect $A_j^{\vee}$ to $A_j^{\Diamond}$ in $\mathcal{N}_i$ and set the connection weight to $W^M > h^{-1}(A_{min}) + \mu_{A_j} W + \theta_{A_j}$.

9. For each output neuron A_j in network $\mathcal{N}_u$ such that $\mathcal{R}(\omega_i, \omega_u)$, do:
(a) Add a hidden neuron $A_j^{\wedge}$ to $\mathcal{N}_i$; (b) Set the step function $s(x)$ as the activation function of $A_j^{\wedge}$; (c) For each output neuron $A_j^{\Box}$ in $\mathcal{N}_i$, do:

(i) Connect A_j in $\mathcal{N}_u$ to $A_j^{\wedge}$ and set the connection weight to 1; (ii) Set the threshold $\theta^{\wedge}$ of $A_j^{\wedge}$ such that $n - (1 + A_{min}) < \theta^{\wedge} < nA_{min}$; (iii) Connect $A_j^{\wedge}$ to $A_j^{\Box}$ in $\mathcal{N}_i$ and set the connection weight to $W^M > h^{-1}(A_{min}) + \mu_{A_j} W + \theta_{A_j}$.

Finally, we prove that $\mathcal{N}$ is equivalent to $\mathcal{P}$.

Theorem 1 *(Correctness of Intuitionistic Modal Algorithm) For any intuitionistic modal program $\mathcal{P}$ there exists an ensemble of neural networks $\mathcal{N}$ such that $\mathcal{N}$ computes the intuitionistic modal semantics of $\mathcal{P}$.*
Proof *The algorithm to build each individual network in the ensemble is that of C-ILP, which we know is provably correct [3]. The algorithm to include modalities is that of CML, which is also provably correct [6]. We need to consider when modalities and intuitionistic negation are to be encoded together. Consider an output neuron A_0 with neurons M (encoding modalities) and neurons n (encoding negation) among its predecessors in a network's hidden layer. There are four cases to consider. (i) Both neurons M and neurons n are not activated: since the activation function of neurons M and n is the step function, their activation is zero, and thus this case reduces to C-ILP. (ii) Only neurons M are activated: from the algorithm above, A_0 will also be activated (with minimum input potential $W^M + \varsigma$, where $\varsigma \in \mathbb{R}$). (iii) Only neurons n are activated: as before, A_0 will also be activated (now with minimum input potential $W^I + \varsigma$). (iv) Both neurons M and neurons n are activated: the input potential of A_0 is at least $W^M + W^I + \varsigma$. Since $W^M > 0$ and $W^I > 0$, and since the activation function of A_0, $h(x)$, is monotonically increasing, A_0 will be activated whenever both M and n neurons are activated. This completes the proof.*

5 Concluding Remarks

In this paper, we have presented a new model of computation that integrates neural networks and constructive, intuitionistic modal reasoning. We have defined labelled intuitionistic modal programs, and have presented an algorithm to translate the intuitionistic theories into ensembles of C-ILP neural networks, and showed that the ensembles compute a semantics of the corresponding theories. As a result, each ensemble can be seen as a new massively parallel model for the computation of intuitionistic modal logic. In addition, since each network can be trained efficiently using, e.g., backpropagation, one can adapt the network ensemble by training possible world representations from examples. Work along these lines has been done in [4, 5], where learning experiments in possible worlds settings were investigated. As future work, we shall consider learning experiments based on the constructive model introduced in this paper. Extensions of this work also include the study of how to represent other non-classical logics such as branching time temporal logics, and conditional logics of normality, which are relevant for cognitive and neural computation.

Acknowledgments
Artur Garcez is partly supported by the Nuffield Foundation and The Royal Society. Luis Lamb is partly supported by the Brazilian Research Council CNPq and by the CAPES and FAPERGS foundations.

References

[1] A. Browne and R. Sun. Connectionist inference models. *Neural Networks*, 14(10):1331–1355, 2001.

[2] D. Van Dalen. Intuitionistic logic. In D. M. Gabbay and F. Guenthner, editors, *Handbook of Philosophical Logic*, volume 5. Kluwer, 2nd edition, 2002.

[3] A. S. d'Avila Garcez, K. Broda, and D. M. Gabbay. *Neural-Symbolic Learning Systems: Foundations and Applications*. Perspectives in Neural Computing. Springer-Verlag, 2002.

[4] A. S. d'Avila Garcez and L. C. Lamb. Reasoning about time and knowledge in neural-symbolic learning systems. In *Advances in Neural Information Processing Systems 16*, Proceedings of NIPS 2003, pages 921–928, Vancouver, Canada, 2004. MIT Press.

[5] A. S. d'Avila Garcez, L. C. Lamb, K. Broda, and D. M. Gabbay. Applying connectionist modal logics to distributed knowledge representation problems. *International Journal on Artificial Intelligence Tools*, 13(1):115–139, 2004.

[6] A. S. d'Avila Garcez, L. C. Lamb, and D. M. Gabbay. Connectionist modal logics. *Theoretical Computer Science*. Forthcoming.

[7] R. Fagin, J. Halpern, Y. Moses, and M. Vardi. *Reasoning about Knowledge*. MIT Press, 1995.

[8] D. M. Gabbay. *Labelled Deductive Systems*. Clarendom Press, Oxford, 1996.

[9] D. M. Gabbay, C. Hogger, and J. A. Robinson, editors. *Handbook of Logic in Artificial Intelligence and Logic Programming*, volume 1-5, Oxford, 1994-1999. Clarendom Press.

[10] M. Gelfond and V. Lifschitz. Classical negation in logic programs and disjunctive databases. *New Generation Computing*, 9:365–385, 1991.

[11] D. E. Rumelhart, G. E. Hinton, and R. J. Williams. Learning representations by backpropagating errors. *Nature*, 323:533–536, 1986.

[12] L. Shastri. Advances in SHRUTI: a neurally motivated model of relational knowledge representation and rapid inference using temporal synchrony. *Applied Intelligence*, 11:79–108, 1999.

[13] G. G. Towell and J. W. Shavlik. Knowledge-based artificial neural networks. *Artificial Intelligence*, 70(1):119–165, 1994.

[14] A. M. Turing. Computer machinery and intelligence. *Mind*, 59:433–460, 1950.

[15] L. G. Valiant. Robust logics. *Artificial Intelligence*, 117:231–253, 2000.

[16] V. Vapnik. *The nature of statistical learning theory*. Springer-Verlag, 1995.

Large-Scale Multiclass Transduction

Thomas Gärtner
Fraunhofer AIS.KD, 53754 Sankt Augustin, Thomas.Gaertner@ais.fraunhofer.de

Quoc V. Le, Simon Burton, Alex J. Smola, Vishy Vishwanathan
Statistical Machine Learning Program, NICTA and ANU, Canberra, ACT
{Quoc.Le, Simon.Burton, Alex.Smola, SVN.Vishwanathan}@nicta.com.au

Abstract

We present a method for performing transductive inference on very large datasets. Our algorithm is based on multiclass Gaussian processes and is effective whenever the multiplication of the kernel matrix or its inverse with a vector can be computed sufficiently fast. This holds, for instance, for certain graph and string kernels. Transduction is achieved by variational inference over the unlabeled data subject to a balancing constraint.

1 Introduction

While obtaining labeled data remains a time and labor consuming task, acquisition and storage of unlabelled data is becoming increasingly cheap and easy. This development has driven machine learning research into exploring algorithms that make extensive use of unlabelled data at training time in order to obtain better generalization performance.

A common problem of many transductive approaches is that they scale badly with the amount of unlabeled data, which prohibits the use of massive sets of unlabeled data. Our algorithm shows improved scaling behavior, both for standard Gaussian Process classification and transduction. We perform classification on a dataset consisting of a digraph with $75,888$ vertices and $508,960$ edges. To the best of our knowledge it has so far not been possible to perform transduction on graphs of this size in reasonable time (with standard hardware). On standard data our method shows competitive or better performance.

Existing Transductive Approaches for SVMs use nonlinear programming [2] or EM-style iterations for binary classification [4]. Moreover, on graphs various methods for unsupervised learning have been proposed [12, 11], all of which are mainly concerned with computing the kernel matrix on training and test set jointly. Other formulations impose that the label assignment on the test set be consistent with the assumption of confident classification [8]. Yet others impose that training and test set have similar marginal distributions [4].

The present paper uses all three properties. It is particularly efficient whenever $K\alpha$ or $K^{-1}\alpha$ can be computed in linear time, where $K \in \mathbb{R}^{m \times m}$ is the kernel matrix and $\alpha \in \mathbb{R}^m$.

- We require consistency of training and test marginals. This avoids problems with overly large majority classes and small training sets.
- Kernels (or their inverses) are computed on training and test set simultaneously. On graphs this can lead to considerable computational savings.
- Self consistency of the estimates is achieved by a variational approach. This allows us to make use of Gaussian Process multiclass formulations.

2 Multiclass Classification

We begin with a brief overview over Gaussian Process multiclass classification [10] recast in terms of exponential families. Denote by $\mathcal{X} \times \mathcal{Y}$ with $\mathcal{Y} = \{1..n\}$ the domain of observations and labels. Moreover let $X := \{x_1, \ldots, x_m\}$ and $Y := \{y_1, \ldots, y_m\}$ be the set of observations. It is our goal to estimate $y|x$ via

$$p(y|x, \theta) = \exp\left(\langle \phi(x, y), \theta \rangle - g(\theta|x)\right) \text{ where } g(\theta|x) = \log \sum_{y \in \mathcal{Y}} \exp\left(\langle \phi(x, y), \theta \rangle\right). \quad (1)$$

$\phi(x, y)$ are the joint sufficient statistics of x and y and $g(\theta|x)$ is the log-partition function which takes care of the normalization. We impose a normal prior on θ, leading to the following negative joint likelihood in θ and Y:

$$\mathcal{P} := -\log p(\theta, Y|X) = \sum_{i=1}^{m} \left[g(\theta|x_i) - \langle \phi(x_i, y_i), \theta \rangle\right] + \frac{1}{2\sigma^2} \|\theta\|^2 + \text{const.} \quad (2)$$

For transduction purposes $p(\theta, Y|X)$ will prove more useful than $p(\theta|Y, X)$. Note that a normal prior on θ with variance $\sigma^2 \mathbf{1}$ implies a Gaussian process on the random variable $t(x, y) := \langle \phi(x, y), \theta \rangle$ with covariance kernel

$$\text{Cov}\left[t(x, y), t(x', y')\right] = \sigma^2 \langle \phi(x, y), \phi(x', y') \rangle =: \sigma^2 k((x, y), (x', y')). \quad (3)$$

Parametric Optimization Problem In the following we assume isotropy among the class labels, that is $\langle \phi(x, y), \phi(x', y') \rangle = \delta_{y, y'} \langle \phi(x), \phi(x') \rangle$ (this is not a necessary requirement for the efficiency of our algorithm, however it greatly simplifies the presentation). This allows us to decompose θ into $\theta_1, \ldots, \theta_n$ such that

$$\langle \phi(x, y), \theta \rangle = \langle \phi(x), \theta_y \rangle \text{ and } \|\theta\|^2 = \sum_{y=1}^{n} \|\theta_y\|^2. \quad (4)$$

Applying the representer theorem allows us to expand θ in terms of $\phi(x_i, y_i)$ as $\theta = \sum_{i=1}^{m} \sum_{y=1}^{n} \alpha_{iy} \phi(x_i, y)$. In conjunction with (4) we have

$$\theta_y = \sum_{i=1}^{m} \alpha_{iy} \phi(x_i) \text{ where } \alpha \in \mathbb{R}^{m \times n}. \quad (5)$$

Let $\mu \in \mathbb{R}^{m \times n}$ with $\mu_{ij} = 1$ if $y_i = j$ and $\mu_{ij} = 0$ otherwise, and $K \in \mathbb{R}^{m \times m}$ with $K_{ij} = \langle \phi(x_i), \phi(x_j) \rangle$. Here joint log-likelihood (2) in terms of α and K yields

$$\sum_{i=1}^{m} \log \sum_{y=1}^{n} \exp\left([K\alpha]_{iy}\right) - \text{tr } \mu^\top K\alpha + \frac{1}{2\sigma^2} \text{tr } \alpha^\top K\alpha + \text{const.} \quad (6)$$

Equivalently we could expand (2) in terms of $t := K\alpha$. This is commonly done in Gaussian process literature and we will use both formulations, depending on the problem we need to solve: if $K\alpha$ can be computed effectively, as is the case with string kernels [9], we use the α-parameterization. Conversely, if $K^{-1}\alpha$ is cheap, as for example with graph kernels [7], we use the t-parameterization.

Derivatives Second order methods such as Conjugate Gradient require the computation of derivatives of $-\log p(\theta, Y|X)$ with respect to θ in terms of α or t. Using the shorthand $\pi \in \mathbb{R}^{m \times n}$ with $\pi_{ij} := p(y = j|x_i, \theta)$ we have

$$\partial_\alpha \mathcal{P} = K(\pi - \mu + \sigma^{-2}\alpha) \text{ and } \partial_t \mathcal{P} = \pi - \mu + \sigma^{-2} K^{-1} t. \quad (7)$$

To avoid spelling out tensors of fourth order for the second derivatives (since $\alpha \in \mathbb{R}^{m \times n}$) we state the action of the latter as bilinear forms on vectors $\beta, \gamma, u, v \in \mathbb{R}^{m \times n}$. For convenience we use the "Matlab" notation of '.∗' to denote element-wise multiplication of matrices:

$$\partial_\alpha^2 \mathcal{P}[\beta, \gamma] = \operatorname{tr}(K\gamma)^\top (\pi. * (K\beta)) - \operatorname{tr}(\pi. * K\gamma)^\top (\pi. * (K\beta)) + \sigma^{-2} \operatorname{tr} \gamma^\top K\beta \quad \text{(8a)}$$

$$\partial_t^2 \mathcal{P}[u, v] = \operatorname{tr} u^\top (\pi. * v) - \operatorname{tr}(\pi. * u)^\top (\pi. * v) + \sigma^{-2} \operatorname{tr} u^\top K^{-1} v. \quad \text{(8b)}$$

Let $L \cdot n$ be the computational time required to compute $K\alpha$ and $K^{-1}t$ respectively. One may check that $L = O(m)$ implies that each conjugate gradient (CG) descent step can be performed in $O(m)$ time. Combining this with rates of convergence for Newton-type or nonlinear CG solver strategies yields overall time costs in the order of $O(m \log m)$ to $O(m^2)$ worst case, a significant improvement over conventional $O(m^3)$ methods.

3   Transductive Inference by Variational Methods

As we are interested in transduction, the labels Y (and analogously the data X) decompose as $Y = Y_{\text{train}} \cup Y_{\text{test}}$. To directly estimate $p(Y_{\text{test}}|X, Y_{\text{train}})$ we would need to integrating out θ, which is usually intractable. Instead, we now aim at estimating the mode of $p(\theta|X, Y_{\text{train}})$ by variational means. With the KL-divergence D and an arbitrary distribution q the well-known bound (see e.g. [5])

$$-\log p(\theta|X, Y_{\text{train}}) \leq -\log p(\theta|X, Y_{\text{train}}) + D(q(Y_{\text{test}})\|p(Y_{\text{test}}|X, Y_{\text{train}}, \theta)) \quad \text{(9)}$$

$$= -\sum_{Y_{\text{test}}} (\log p(Y_{\text{test}}, \theta|X, Y_{\text{train}}) - \log q(Y_{\text{test}})) \, q(Y_{\text{test}}) \quad \text{(10)}$$

holds. This bound (10) can be minimized with respect to θ and q in an iterative fashion. The key trick is that while using a factorizing approximation for q we restrict the latter to distributions which satisfy balancing constraints. That is, we require them to yield marginals on the unlabeled data which are comparable with the labeled observations.

Decomposing the Variational Bound   To simplify (10) observe that

$$p(Y_{\text{test}}, \theta|X, Y_{\text{train}}) = p(Y_{\text{train}}, Y_{\text{test}}, \theta|X)/p(Y_{\text{train}}|X). \quad \text{(11)}$$

In other words, the first term in (10) equals (6) up to a constant independent of θ or Y_{test}. With $q_{ij} := q(y_i = j)$ we define $\mu_{ij}(q) = q_{ij}$ for all $i > m_{\text{train}}$ and $\mu_{ij}(q) = 1$ if $y_i = 1$ and 0 otherwise for all $i \leq m_{\text{train}}$. In other words, we are taking the expectation in μ over all unobserved labels Y_{test} with respect to the distribution $q(Y_{\text{test}})$. We have

$$\sum_{Y_{\text{test}}} q(Y_{\text{test}}) \log p(Y_{\text{test}}, \theta|X, Y_{\text{train}})$$

$$= \sum_{i=1}^m \log \sum_{j=1}^n \exp([K\alpha]_{ij}) - \operatorname{tr} \mu(q)^\top K\alpha + \frac{1}{2\sigma^2} \operatorname{tr} \alpha^\top K\alpha + \text{const.} \quad \text{(12)}$$

For fixed q the optimization over θ proceeds as in Section 2. Next we discuss q.

Optimization over q   The second term in (10) is the negative entropy of q. Since q factorizes we have

$$\sum_{Y_{\text{test}}} q(Y_{\text{test}}) \log q(Y_{\text{test}}) = \sum_{i=m_{\text{train}}+1}^m q_{ij} \log q_{ij}. \quad \text{(13)}$$

It is unreasonable to assume that q may be chosen freely from all factorizing distributions (the latter would lead to a straightforward EM algorithm for transductive inference): if we observe a certain distribution of labels on the training set, e.g., for binary classification we see 45% positive and 55% negative labels, then it is very unlikely that the label distribution on the test set deviates significantly. Hence we should make use of this information.

If $m \gg m_{\text{train}}$, however, a naive application of the variational bound can lead to cases where q is concentrated on one class — the increase in likelihood for a resulting very simple classifier completely outweighs any balancing constraints implicit in the data. This is confirmed by experimental results. It is, incidentally, also the reason why SVM transduction optimization codes [4] impose a balancing constraint on the assignment of test labels. We impose the following conditions:

$$r_j^- \leq \sum_{i=m_{\text{train}}+1}^{m} q_{ij} \leq r_j^+ \text{ for all } j \in \mathcal{Y} \text{ and } \sum_{j=1}^{n} q_{ij} = 1 \text{ for all } i \in \{m_{\text{train}}..m\}.$$

Here the constraints $r_j^- = p_{\text{emp}}(y = j) - \epsilon$ and $r_j^+ = p_{\text{emp}}(y = j) + \epsilon$ are chosen such as to correspond to confidence intervals given by finite sample size tail bounds. In other words we set $p_{\text{emp}}(y = j) = m_{\text{train}}^{-1} \sum_{i=1}^{m_{\text{train}}} \{y_i = j\}$ and ϵ such as to satisfy

$$\Pr\left\{\left|m_{\text{train}}^{-1} \sum_{i=1}^{m_{\text{train}}} \xi_i - m_{\text{test}}^{-1} \sum_{i=1}^{m_{\text{test}}} \xi_i'\right| > \epsilon\right\} \leq \delta \tag{14}$$

for iid $\{0,1\}$ random variables ξ_i and ξ_i' with mean p. This is a standard ghost-sample inequality. It follows directly from [3, Eq. (2.7)] after application of a union bound over the class labels that $\epsilon \leq \sqrt{\log(2n/\delta)m/(2m_{\text{train}}m_{\text{test}})}$.

4 Graphs, Strings and Vectors

We now discuss the two main applications where computational savings can be achieved: graphs and strings. In the case of graphs, the advantage arises from the fact that K^{-1} is sparse, whereas for texts we can use fast string kernels [9] to compute $K\alpha$ in linear time.

Graphs Denote by $G(V, E)$ the graph given by vertices V and edges E where each edge is a set of two vertices. Then $W \in \mathbb{R}^{|V| \times |V|}$ denotes the adjacency matrix of the graph, where $W_{ij} > 0$ only if edge $\{i, j\} \in E$. We assume that the graph G, and thus also the adjacency matrix W, is sparse. Now denote by $\mathbf{1}$ the identity matrix and by D the diagonal matrix of vertex degrees, i.e., $D_{ii} = \sum_j W_{ij}$. Then the graph Laplacian and the normalized graph Laplacian of G are given by

$$L := D - W \quad \text{and} \quad \tilde{L} := \mathbf{1} - D^{-\frac{1}{2}} W D^{-\frac{1}{2}}, \tag{15}$$

respectively. Many kernels K (or their inverse) on G are given by low-degree polynomials of the Laplacian or the adjacency matrix of G, such as the following:

$$K = \sum_{i=1}^{l} c_i W^{2i}, K = \prod_{i=1}^{l} (\mathbf{1} - c_i \tilde{L}), \text{ or } K^{-1} = \tilde{L} + \epsilon \mathbf{1}. \tag{16}$$

In all three cases we assumed $c_i, \epsilon \geq 0$ and $l \in \mathbb{N}$. The first kernel arises from an l-step random walk, the third case is typically referred to as regularized graph Laplacian. In these cases $K\alpha$ or $K^{-1}t$ can be computed using $L = l(|V| + |E|)$ operations. This means that if the average degree of the graph does not increase with the number of observations, $L = O(m)$ as $m = |V|$ for inference on graphs.

From Graphs to Graphical Models Graphs are one of the examples where transduction actually improves computational cost: Assume that we are given the inverse kernel matrix K^{-1} on training and test set and we wish to perform induction only. In this case we need to compute the kernel matrix (or its inverse) restricted to the training set. Let $K^{-1} = \begin{bmatrix} A & B \\ B^\top & C \end{bmatrix}$, then the upper left hand corner (representing the training set part only) of

K is given by the Schur complement $(A - B^\top C^{-1}B)^{-1}$. Computing the latter is costly. Moreover, neither the Schur complement nor its inverse are typically sparse.

Here we have a nice connection between graphical models and graph kernels. Assume that t is a normal random variable with conditional independence properties. In this case the inverse covariance matrix has nonzero entries only for variables with a direct dependency structure. This follows directly from an application of the Clifford-Hammersley theorem to Gaussian random variables [6]. In other words, if we are given a graphical model of normal random variables, their conditional independence structure is reflected by K^{-1}.

In the same way as in graphical models marginalization may induce dependencies, computing the kernel matrix on the training set only, may lead to dense matrices, even when the inverse kernel on training and test data combined is sparse. The bottom line is there are cases where it is computationally cheaper to take both training and test set into account and optimize over a larger set of variables rather than dealing with a smaller dense matrix.

Strings: Efficient computation of string kernels using suffix trees was described in [9]. In particular, it was observed that expansions of the form $\sum_{i=1}^{m} \alpha_i k(x_i, x)$ can be evaluated in linear time in the length of x, provided some preprocessing for the coefficients α and observations x_i is performed. This preprocessing is independent of x and can be computed in $O(\sum_i |x_i|)$ time. The efficient computation scheme covers all kernels of type

$$k(x, x') = \sum_s w_s \#_s(x) \#_s(x') \tag{17}$$

for arbitrary $w_s \geq 0$. Here, $\#_s(x)$ denotes the number of occurrences of s in x and the sum is carried out over all substrings of x. This means that computation time for evaluating $K\alpha$ is again $O(\sum_i |x_i|)$ as we need to evaluate the kernel expansion for all $x \in X$. Since the average string length is independent of m this yields an $O(m)$ algorithm for $K\alpha$.

Vectors: If $k(x, x') = \phi(x)^\top \phi(x')$ and $\phi(x) \in \mathbb{R}^d$ for $d \ll m$, it is possible to carry out matrix vector multiplications in $O(md)$ time. This is useful for cases where we have a sparse matrix with a small number of low-rank updates (e.g. from low rank dense fill-ins).

5 Optimization

Optimization in α and t: $\mathcal{P}$ is convex in α (and in t since $t = K\alpha$). This means that a combination of Conjugate-Gradient and Newton-Raphson (NR) can be used for optimization.

- Compute updates $\alpha \longleftarrow \alpha - \eta \partial_\alpha^2 \mathcal{P}^{-1} \partial_\alpha \mathcal{P}$ via
  - Solve the linear system approximately by Conjugate Gradient iterations.
  - Find optimal η by line search.
- Repeat until the norm of the gradient is sufficiently small.

Key is the fact that the arising linear system is only solved approximately, which can be done using very few CG iterations. Since each of them is $O(m)$ for fast kernel-vector computations the overall cost is a sub-quadratic function of m.

Optimization in q is somewhat less straightforward: we need to find the optimal q in terms of KL-divergence subject to the marginal constraint. Denote by τ the part of $K\alpha$ pertaining to test data, or more formally $\tau \in \mathbb{R}^{m_{\text{test}} \times n}$ with $\tau_{ij} = [K\alpha]_{i+m_{\text{train}},j}$. We have:

$$\underset{q}{\text{minimize}} \ \operatorname{tr} q^\top \tau + \sum_{i,j} q_{ij} \log q_{ij} \tag{18}$$

$$\text{subject to } q_j^- \leq \sum_i q_{ij} \leq q_j^+, q_{ij} \geq 0 \text{ and } \sum_i q_{li} = 1 \text{ for all } j \in \mathcal{Y}, l \in \{1..m_{\text{test}}\}$$

Table 1: Error rates on some benchmark datasets (mostly from UCI). The last column is the error rates reported in [1]

DATASET	#INST	#ATTR	IND. GP	TRANSD. GP	S³VMMIP
cancer	699	9	3.4%±4.1%	2.1%±4.7%	3.4%
cancer (progn.)	569	30	6.1%±3.7%	6.0%±3.7%	3.3%
heart (cleave.)	297	13	15.0%±5.6%	13.0%±6.3%	16.0%
housing	506	13	7.0%±1.0%	6.8%±0.9%	15.1%
ionosphere	351	34	8.6%±6.3%	6.1%±3.4%	10.6%
pima	769	8	19.6%±8.1%	17.6%±8.0%	22.2%
sonar	208	60	10.5%±5.1%	8.6%±3.4%	21.9%
glass	214	10	20.5%±1.6%	17.3%±4.5%	—
wine	178	13	19.4%±5.7%	15.6%±4.2%	—
tictactoe	958	9	3.9%±0.7%	3.3%±0.6%	—
cmc	1473	10	32.5%±7.1%	28.9%±7.5%	—
USPS	9298	256	5.9%	4.8%	—[1]

This is a convex optimization problem. Using Lagrange multipliers one can show that q needs to satisfy $q_{ij} = \exp(-\tau_{ij})b_i c_j$ where $b_i, c_j \geq 0$. Solving for $\sum_j^n q_{ij} = 1$ yields $q_{ij} = \frac{\exp(-\tau_{ij})c_j}{\sum_{l=1}^n \exp(-\tau_{il})c_l}$. This means that instead of an optimization problem in $m_{\text{test}} \times n$ variables we now only need to optimize over n variables subject to $2n$ constraints.

Note that the exact matching constraint where $q_i^+ = q_i^-$ amounts to a maximum likelihood problem for a shifted exponential family model where $q_{ij} = \exp(\tau_{ij})\exp(\gamma_i - g_j(\gamma_i))$. It can be shown that the approximate matching problem is equivalent to a maximum a posteriori optimization problem using the norm dual to expectation constraints on q_{ij}. We are currently working on extending this setting

In summary, the optimization now only depends on n variables. It can be solved by standard second order methods. As initialization we choose γ_i such that the per class averages match the marginal constraint while ignoring the per sample balance. After that a small number Newton steps suffices for optimization.

6 Experiments

Unfortunately, we are not aware of other multiclass transductive learning algorithms. To still be able to compare our approach to other transductive learning algorithms we performed experiments on some benchmark datasets. To investigate the performance of our algorithm in classifying vertices of a graph, we choose the WebKB dataset.

Benchmark datasets Table 1 reports results on some benchmark datasets. To be able to compare the error rates of the transductive multiclass Gaussian Process classifier proposed in this paper, we also report error rates from [2] and an inductive multiclass Gaussian Process classifier. The reported error rates are for 10-fold crossvalidations. Parameters were chosen by crossvalidation inside the training folds.

Graph Mining To illustrate the effectiveness of our approach on graphs we performed experiments on the well known WebKB dataset. This dataset consists of 8275 webpages classified into 7 classes. Each webpage contains textual content and/or links to other webpages. As we are using this dataset to evaluate our graph mining algorithm, we ignore the text on each webpage and consider the dataset as a labelled directed graph. To have the data

---

[1]In [2] only subsets of USPS were considered due to the size of this problem.

Table 2: Results on WebKB for 'inverse' 10-fold crossvalidation

DATASET	$|V|$	$|E|$	ERROR	DATASET	$|V|$	$|E|$	ERROR
Cornell	867	1793	10%	Misc	4113	4462	66%
Texas	827	1683	8%	all	8275	14370	53%
Washington	1205	2368	10%	Universities	4162	9591	12%
Wisconsin	1263	3678	15%				

set as large as possible, we did not remove any webpages, opposed to most other work.

Table 2 reports the results of our algorithm on different subsets of the WebKB data as well as on the full data. We use the co-linkage graph and report results for 'inverse' 10-fold stratified crossvalidations, i.e., we use 1 fold as training data and 9 folds as test data. Parameters are the same for all reported experiments and were found by experimenting with a few parametersets on the 'Cornell' subset only. It turned out that the class membership probabilities are not well-calibrated on this dataset. To overcome this, we predict on the test set as follows: For each class the instances that are most likely to be in this class are picked (if they haven't been picked for a class with lower index) such that the fraction of instances assigned to this class is the same on the training and test set. We will investigate the reason for this in future work.

The setting most similar to ours is probably the one described in [11]. Although a directed graph approach outperforms there an undirected approach, we resorted to kernels for undirected graphs, as those are computationally more attractive. We will investigate computationally attractive digraph kernels in future work and expect similar benefits as reported by [11]. Though we are using more training data than [11] we are also considering a more difficult learning problem (multiclass without removing various instances). To investigate the behaviour of our algorithm with less training data, we performed a 20-fold inverse crossvalidation on the 'wisconsin' subset and observed an error rate of 17% there.

To further strengthen our results and show that the runtime performance of our algorithm is sufficient for classifying the vertices of massive graphs, we also performed initial experiments on the Epinions dataset collected by Mathew Richardson and Pedro Domingos. The dataset is a social network consisting of $75,888$ people connected by $508,960$ 'trust' edges. Additionally the dataset comes with a list of 185 'topreviewers' for 25 topic areas. We tried to predict these but only got 12% of the topreviewers correct. As we are not aware of any predictive results on this task, we suppose this low accuracy is inherent to this task. However, the experiments show that the algorithm can be run on very large graph datasets.

7 Discussion and Extensions

We presented an efficient method for performing transduction on multiclass estimation problems with Gaussian Processes. It performs particularly well whenever the kernel matrix has special numerical properties which allow fast matrix vector multiplication. That said, also on standard dense problems we observed very good improvements (typically a 10% reduction of the training error) over standard induction.

Structured Labels and Conditional Random Fields are a clear area where to extend the transductive setting. The key obstacle to overcome in this context is to find a suitable marginal distribution: with increasing structure of the labels the confidence bounds per subclass decrease dramatically. A promising strategy is to use only partial marginals on maximal cliques and enforce them directly similarly to an unconditional Markov network.

417

Applications to Document Analysis require efficient small-memory-footprint suffix tree implementations. We are currently working on this, which will allow GP classification to perform estimation on large document collections. We believe it will be possible to use out-of-core storage in conjunction with annotation to work on sequences of 10^8 characters.

Other Marginal Constraints than matching marginals are worth exploring. In particular, constraints derived from exchangeable distributions such as those used by Latent Dirichlet Allocation are a promising area to consider. This may also lead to connections between GP classification and clustering.

Sparse $O(m^{1.3})$ Solvers for Graphs have recently been proposed by the theoretical computer science community. It is worthwhile exploring their use for inference on graphs.

Acknowledgements The authors thank Mathew Richardson and Pedro Domingos for collecting the Epinions data and Deepayan Chakrabarti and Christos Faloutsos for providing a preprocessed version. Parts of this work were carried out when TG was visiting NICTA. National ICT Australia is funded through the Australian Government's *Backing Australia's Ability* initiative, in part through the Australian Research Council. This work was supported by grants of the ARC and by the Pascal Network of Excellence.

References

[1] K. Bennett. Combining support vector and mathematical programming methods for classification. In *Advances in Kernel Methods - -Support Vector Learning*, pages 307 – 326. MIT Press, 1998.

[2] K. Bennett. Combining support vector and mathematical programming methods for induction. In B. Schölkopf, C. J. C. Burges, and A. J. Smola, editors, *Advances in Kernel Methods - -SV Learning*, pages 307 – 326, Cambridge, MA, 1999. MIT Press.

[3] W. Hoeffding. Probability inequalities for sums of bounded random variables. *Journal of the American Statistical Association*, 58:13 – 30, 1963.

[4] T. Joachims. *Learning to Classify Text Using Support Vector Machines: Methods, Theory, and Algorithms*. The Kluwer International Series In Engineering And Computer Science. Kluwer Academic Publishers, Boston, May 2002. ISBN 0 - 7923 - 7679-X.

[5] M. I. Jordan, Z. Ghahramani, Tommi S. Jaakkola, and L. K. Saul. An introduction to variational methods for graphical models. *Machine Learning*, 37(2):183 – 233, 1999.

[6] S. L. Lauritzen. *Graphical Models*. Oxford University Press, 1996.

[7] A. J. Smola and I. R. Kondor. Kernels and regularization on graphs. In B. Schölkopf and M. K. Warmuth, editors, *Proceedings of the Annual Conference on Computational Learning Theory*, Lecture Notes in Computer Science. Springer, 2003.

[8] V. Vapnik. *Statistical Learning Theory*. John Wiley and Sons, New York, 1998.

[9] S. V. N. Vishwanathan and A. J. Smola. Fast kernels for string and tree matching. In K. Tsuda, B. Schölkopf, and J.P. Vert, editors, *Kernels and Bioinformatics*, Cambridge, MA, 2004. MIT Press.

[10] C. K. I. Williams and D. Barber. Bayesian classification with Gaussian processes. *IEEE Transactions on Pattern Analysis and Machine Intelligence PAMI*, 20(12):1342 – 1351, 1998.

[11] D. Zhou, J. Huang, and B. Schölkopf. Learning from labeled and unlabeled data on a directed graph. In *International Conference on Machine Learning*, 2005.

[12] X. Zhu, J. Lafferty, and Z. Ghahramani. Semi-supervised learning using gaussian fields and harmonic functions. In *International Conference on Machine Learning ICML'03*, 2003.

Products of "Edge-perts"

Peter Gehler
Max Planck Institute for Biological Cybernetics
Spemannstraße 38, 72076 Tübingen, Germany
pgehler@tuebingen.mpg.de

Max Welling
Department of Computer Science
University of California Irvine
welling@ics.uci.edu

Abstract

Images represent an important and abundant source of data. Understanding their statistical structure has important applications such as image compression and restoration. In this paper we propose a particular kind of probabilistic model, dubbed the "products of edge-perts model" to describe the structure of wavelet transformed images. We develop a practical denoising algorithm based on a single edge-pert and show state-of-the-art denoising performance on benchmark images.

1 Introduction

Images, when represented as a collection of pixel values, exhibit a high degree of redundancy. Wavelet transforms, which capture most of the second order dependencies, form the basis of many successful image processing applications such as image compression (e.g. JPEG2000) or image restoration (e.g. wavelet coring). However, the higher order dependencies can not be filtered out by these linear transforms. In particular, the absolute values of neighboring wavelet coefficients (but not their signs) are mutually dependent. This kind of dependency is caused by the presence of edges that induce clustering of wavelet activity. Our philosophy is that by modelling this clustering effect we can potentially improve the performance of some important image processing tasks.

Our model builds on earlier work in the image processing literature. In particular, the PoEdges models that we discuss in this paper can be viewed as generalizations of the models proposed in [1] and [2]. The state-of-art in this area is the joint model discussed in [3] based on the "Gaussian scale mixture" model (GSM). While the GSM falls in the category of directed graphical models and has a top-down structure, the PoEdges model is best classified as an (undirected) Markov random field model and follows bottom-up semantics.

The main contributions of this paper are 1) a new model to describe the higher order statistical dependencies among wavelet coefficients (section 2), 2) an efficient estimation procedure to fit the parameters of a single edge-pert model and a new technique to estimate the wavelet coefficients that participate in each such (local) model (section 3.1) and 3) a new "iterated Wiener denoising algorithm" (section 3.2). In section 4 we report on a number of experiments to compare performance of our algorithm with several methods in the literature and with the GSM-based method in particular.

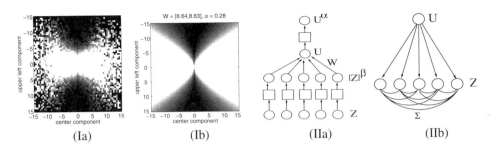

(Ia)	(Ib)	(IIa)	(IIb)

Figure 1: Estimated (Ia) and modelled (Ib) conditional distribution of a wavelet coefficient given its upper left neighbor. The statistics were collected from the vertical subband at the lowest level of a Haar filter wavelet decomposition of the "Lena" image. Note that the "bow-tie" dependencies are captured by the PoEdges model. (IIa) Bottom up network interpretation of "products of edge-perts" model. (IIb) Top-down generative Gaussian scale mixture model.

2 "Product of Edge-perts"

It has long been recognized in the image processing community that wavelet transforms form an excellent basis for representation of images. Within the class of *linear* transforms, it represents a compromise between many conflicting but desirable properties of image representation such as multi-scale and multi-orientation representation, locality both in space and frequency, and orthogonality resulting in decorrelation. A particularly suitable wavelet transform which forms the basis of the best denoising algorithms today is the over-complete steerable wavelet pyramid [4] freely downloadable from *http://www.cns.nyu.edu/~lcv/software.html*. In our experiments we have confirmed that the best results were obtained using this wavelet pyramid.

In the following we will describe a model for the statistical dependencies between wavelet coefficients. This model was inspired by recent studies of these dependencies (see e.g. [1, 5]). It also represents a generalization of the bivariate Laplacian model proposed in [2]. The probability distribution of the "product of edge-pert" model (PoEdges) over the wavelet coefficients $\mathbf{z}$ has the following form,

$$P(\mathbf{z}) = \frac{1}{Z} \exp \left[- \sum_i \left(\sum_j W_{ij} |\hat{\mathbf{a}}_j^T \mathbf{z}|^{\beta_j} \right)^{\alpha_i} \right], \quad \beta_j > 0, \ \alpha_i \in (0,1], \ W_{ij} \geq 0$$

where the normalization constant Z depends on all the parameters in the model $\{W_{ij}, \hat{\mathbf{a}}_j, \beta_j, \alpha_i\}$ and where $\hat{\mathbf{a}}$ indicates an unit-length vector.

In figure 2 we show the effect of changing some parameters for a single edge-pert model (i.e. set $i = 1$ in Eqn.1 above). The parameters $\{\beta_j\}$ control the shape of the contours: for $\beta = 2$ we have elliptical contours, for $\beta = 1$ the contours are straight lines while for $\beta < 1$ the contours curve inwards. The parameters $\{\alpha_i\}$ control the rate at which the distribution decays, i.e. the distance between iso-probability contours. The unit vectors $\{\hat{\mathbf{a}}_i\}$ determine the orientation of basis vectors. If the $\{\hat{\mathbf{a}}_i\}$ are axis-aligned (as in figure 2), the distribution is symmetric w.r.t. reflections of any subset of the $\{z_i\}$ in the origin, which implies that the wavelet coefficients are necessarily decorrelated (although higher order dependencies may still remain). Finally, the weights $\{W_{ij}\}$ model the scale (inverse variance) of the wavelet coefficients. We mention that it is possible to entertain a larger number of bases vectors than wavelet coefficients (a so-called "over-complete basis"), which seems appropriate for some of the empirical joint histograms shown in [1].

This model describes two important statistical properties which have been observed for wavelet coefficients: 1) its marginal distributions $p(z_i)$ are peaked and have heavy tails (high kurtosis) and 2) the conditional distributions $p(z_i|z_j)$ display "bow-tie" dependencies which are indicative of clustering of wavelet coefficients (neighboring wavelet coefficient

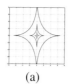 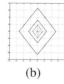 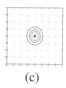

(a)   (b)   (c)   (d)

Figure 2: Contour plots for a single edge-pert model with (a) $\beta_{1,2} = 0.5$, $\alpha = 0.5$, (b) $\beta_{1,2} = 1$, $\alpha = 0.5$, (c) $\beta_{1,2} = 2$, $\alpha = 0.5$, (d) $\beta_{1,2} = 2$, $\alpha = 0.3$. For all figures $W_1 = 1$ and $W_2 = 0.8$.

are often active together). This phenomenon is shown in figure 1Ia,b. To better understand the qualitative behavior of our model we provide the following network interpretation (see figure 1IIa,b. Input to the model (i.e. the wavelet coefficients) undergo a nonlinear transformation $z_i \rightarrow |z_i|^{\beta_i} \rightarrow u = W|\mathbf{z}|^{\beta} \rightarrow u^{\alpha}$. The output of this network, u^{α}, can be interpreted as a "penalty" for the input: the larger this penalty is, the more unlikely this input becomes under the probabilistic model. This process is most naturally understood [6] as enforcing constraints of the form $u = W|\mathbf{z}|^{\beta} \approx 0$, by penalizing violations of these constraints with u^{α}.

What is the reason that the PoEdges model captures the clustering of wavelet activities? Consider a local model describing the statistical structure of a patch of wavelet coefficients and recall that the weighted sum of these activities is penalized. At a fixed position the activities are typically very small across images. However, when an edge happens to fall within the window of the model, most coefficients become active jointly. This "sparse" pattern of activity incurs less penalty than for instance the same amount[1] of activity distributed equally over all images because of the concave shape of the penalty function, i.e. $(act)^{\alpha} < (\frac{1}{2}act)^{\alpha} + (\frac{1}{2}act)^{\alpha}$ where "act" is the activity level and $\alpha < 1$.

2.1 Related Work

Early wavelet denoising techniques were based on the observation that the marginal distribution of a wavelet coefficient is highly kurtotic (peaked and heavy tails). It was found that the generalized Gaussian density represents a very good fit to the empirical histograms [1, 7],

$$p(z) = \frac{\alpha w}{2\Gamma(\frac{1}{\alpha})} \exp\left[-(w|z|)^{\alpha}\right], \quad \alpha > 0, \ w > 0. \tag{1}$$

This has lead to the successful wavelet coring and shrinkage methods. A bivariate generalization of that model describing a wavelet coefficient z_c and its "parent" z_p at a higher level in the pyramid jointly, was proposed in [2]. The probability density,

$$p(z_c, z_p) = \frac{w}{2\pi} \exp\left(-\sqrt{w(z_c^2 + z_p^2)}\right) \tag{2}$$

is easily seen to be a special case of the PoEdges model proposed here. This model, unlike the univariate model, captures the bow-tie dependencies described above resulting a significant gain in denoising performance.

"Gaussian scale mixtures" (GSM) have been proposed to model even larger neighborhoods of wavelet coefficients. In particular, very good denoising results have been obtained by including within subband neighborhoods of size 3×3 in addition to the parent of a wavelet coefficient [3]. A GSM is defined in terms of a precision variable u, the square-root of which multiplies a multivariate Gaussian variable: $\mathbf{z} = \sqrt{u}\, \mathbf{y}$, $\mathbf{y} \sim \mathcal{N}[0, \Sigma]$, resulting in the following expression for the distribution over the wavelet coefficients: $p(\mathbf{z}) = \int du\, \mathcal{N}_z[0, u\Sigma]\, p(u)$. Here, $p(u)$ is the prior distribution for the precision variable. Hence, the GSM represents an example of a generative model with top-down semantics.

---

[1] We assume the total amount of variance in wavelet activity is fixed in this comparison.

This in contrast to the PoEdges model which is better interpreted as a bottom-up network with log-probability proportional to its output. This difference is contrasted in figure 1IIa,b.

3 Edge-pert Denoising

Based on the PoEdges model discussed in the previous sections we now introduce a simplified model that forms the basis for a practical denoising algorithm. Recent progress in the field has indicated that it is important to model the higher order dependencies which exist between wavelet coefficients [2, 3]. This can be realized through the estimation of a *joint* model on a small cluster of wavelet coefficients around each coefficient. Ideally, we would like to use the full PoEdges model, but training these models from data is cumbersome. Therefore, in order to keep computations tractable, we proceed with a simplified model,

$$p(\mathbf{z}) \propto \exp\left[-\left(\sum_j w_j\left(\hat{\mathbf{a}}_j^T \mathbf{z}\right)^2\right)^\alpha\right]. \tag{3}$$

Compared to the full PoEdges model we use only one edge-pert and we have set $\beta_j = 2\,\forall j$.

3.1 Model Estimation

Our next task is to estimate the parameters of this model efficiently. We will learn separate models for each wavelet coefficient jointly with a small neighborhood of dependent coefficients. Each such model is estimated in three steps: I) determine the coefficients that participate in each model, II) transform each model into a decorrelated domain (this implicitly estimates the $\{\hat{\mathbf{a}}_j\}$) and III) estimate the remaining parameters $\mathbf{w}, \alpha$ in the decorrelated domain using moment matching. Below we will describe these steps in more detail.

By $z_i, \tilde{z}_i$ we will denote the clean and noisy wavelet coefficients respectively. With $y_i, \tilde{y}_i$ we denote the *decorrelated* clean and noisy wavelet coefficients while n_i denotes the Gaussian noise random variable in the wavelet domain, i.e. $\tilde{z}_i = z_i + n_i$. Both due to the details of the wavelet decomposition and due to the properties of the noise itself we assume the noise to be correlated and zero mean: $\mathbb{E}[n_i] = 0$, $\mathbb{E}[n_i n_j] = \Sigma_{ij}$. In this paper we further assume that we know the noise covariance in the image domain from which one can easily compute the noise covariance in the wavelet domain, however only minor changes are needed to estimate it from the noisy image itself.

Step I: We start with a 7×7 neighborhood from which we will adaptively select the best candidates to include in the model. In addition, we will always include the parent coefficient in the subband of a coarser scale if it exists (this is done by first up-sampling this band, see [3]). The coefficients that participate in a model are selected by estimating their dependencies relative to the center coefficient. Anticipating that (second order) correlations will be removed by sphering we are only interested in higher order dependencies, in particular dependencies between the variances. The following cumulant is used to obtain these estimates,

$$H_{cj} = \mathbb{E}[\tilde{z}_c^2 \tilde{z}_j^2] - 2\mathbb{E}[\tilde{z}_c \tilde{z}_j]^2 - \mathbb{E}[\tilde{z}_c^2]\mathbb{E}[\tilde{z}_j^2] \tag{4}$$

where c is the center coefficient which will be denoised. The necessary averages $\mathbb{E}[\cdot]$ are computed by collecting samples within each subband, assuming that the statistics are location invariant. It can be shown that this cumulant is invariant under addition of possibly correlated Gaussian noise, i.e. it's value is the same for $\{z_i\}$ and $\{\tilde{z}_i\}$. Effectively, we measure the (higher order) dependencies between squared wavelet coefficients after subtraction of all correlations. Finally, we select the participants of a model centered at coefficient $\tilde{z}_c$ by ranking the positive H_{cj} and picking all the ones which satisfy: $H_{ci} > 0.7 \times \max_{j \neq c} H_{cj}$.

Step II: For each model (with varying number of participants) we estimate the covariance,

$$C_{ij} = \mathbb{E}[z_i, z_j] = \mathbb{E}[\tilde{z}_i \tilde{z}_j] - \Sigma_{ij} \tag{5}$$

and correct it by setting to zero all negative eigenvalues in such a way that the sum of the eigenvalues is invariant (see [3]). Statistics are again collected by sampling within a subband. Then, we perform a linear transformation to a new basis onto which $\Sigma = \mathbf{I}$ and C are diagonal. This can be accomplished by the following procedure,

$$RR^T = \Sigma \quad \Rightarrow \quad U\Lambda U^T = R^{-1}CR^{-T} \quad \Rightarrow \quad \tilde{\mathbf{y}} = (RU)^{-1}\tilde{\mathbf{z}}. \tag{6}$$

In this new space (which is different for every wavelet coefficient) we can now assume $\hat{\mathbf{a}}_j = \mathbf{e}_j$, the axis aligned basis vector.

Step III: In the decorrelated space we estimate the single edge-pert model by moment matching. The moments of the edge-pert model in this space are easily computed using

$$\mathbb{E}\left[\left(\sum_{j=1}^{N_p} w_j y_j^2\right)^\ell\right] = \Gamma\left(\frac{N_p + 2\ell}{2\alpha}\right) / \Gamma\left(\frac{N_p}{2\alpha}\right) \tag{7}$$

where N_p is the number of participating coefficients in the model. We note that $\mathbb{E}[\tilde{y}_i^2] = 1 + \mathbb{E}[y_i^2]$. This leads to the following equation for α

$$\frac{N_p^2 \Gamma\left(\frac{N_p+4}{2\alpha}\right)\Gamma\left(\frac{N_p}{2\alpha}\right)}{\Gamma\left(\frac{N_p+2}{2\alpha}\right)^2} = \sum_{i=1}^{N_p}\frac{\mathbb{E}[\tilde{y}_i^4] - 6\mathbb{E}[\tilde{y}_i^2] + 3}{(\mathbb{E}[\tilde{y}_i^2] - 1)^2} + \sum_{i\neq j}^{N_p}\frac{\mathbb{E}[\tilde{y}_i^2\tilde{y}_j^2] - \mathbb{E}[\tilde{y}_i^2] - \mathbb{E}[\tilde{y}_j^2] + 1}{(\mathbb{E}[\tilde{y}_i^2] - 1)(\mathbb{E}[\tilde{y}_j^2] - 1)}. \tag{8}$$

Thus we can estimate α by a line search and approximate the second term on the right hand side with $N_p(N_p-1)$ to simplify the calculations. By further noting that the model (Eqn.3) is symmetric w.r.t. permutations of the variables $u_j = w_j y_j^2$ we find

$$w_j = \Gamma\left(\frac{N_p+2}{2\alpha}\right) / \left(N_p(\mathbb{E}[\tilde{y}_i^2] - 1)\ \Gamma\left(\frac{N_p}{2\alpha}\right)\right). \tag{9}$$

A common strategy in the wavelet literature is to estimate the averages $\mathbb{E}[\cdot]$ by collecting samples in a local neighborhood around the coefficient under consideration. The advantage is that the estimates are adapting to the local statistics in the image. We have adopted this strategy and used a 11×11 box around each coefficient to collect 121 samples in the decorrelated wavelet domain. Coefficients for which $\mathbb{E}[\tilde{y}_i^2] < 1$ are set to zero and removed from consideration. The estimation of α depends on the fourth moment and is thus very sensitive to outliers, which is a commonly known problem with the moment matching method. We encounter the same problem so whenever we find no estimate of α in $[0, 1]$ using Eqn.8 we simply set it to 0.5.

3.2 The Iterated Wiener Filter

To infer a wavelet coefficient given its noisy observation in the decorrelated wavelet domain, we maximize the *a posteriori* probability of our joint model. This is equivalent to,

$$\mathbf{z}^* = \underset{\mathbf{z}}{\operatorname{argmax}}\left(\log p(\tilde{\mathbf{z}}|\mathbf{z}) + \log p(\mathbf{z})\right). \tag{10}$$

When we assume Gaussian pixel noise, this translates into,

$$\mathbf{z}^* = \underset{\mathbf{z}}{\operatorname{argmin}}\left(\tfrac{1}{2}(\mathbf{z} - \tilde{\mathbf{z}})^T K(\mathbf{z} - \tilde{\mathbf{z}}) + \left(\sum_j w_j z_j^2\right)^\alpha\right) \tag{11}$$

where J is the (linear) wavelet transform $\tilde{\mathbf{z}} = J\mathbf{x}$, $K = J^{\#T}\Sigma_n^{-1}J^{\#}$ with $J^{\#} = (J^T J)^{-1}J^T$ the pseudo-inverse of J (i.e. $J^{\#}J = I$) and Σ_n the noise covariance matrix. In the decorrelated wavelet domain we simply set $K = \mathbf{I}$.

One can now construct an upper bound on this objective by using,

$$f^\alpha \leq \gamma f + (1-\alpha)\left(\frac{\gamma}{\alpha}\right)^{\frac{\alpha}{\alpha-1}} \qquad \alpha < 1. \tag{12}$$

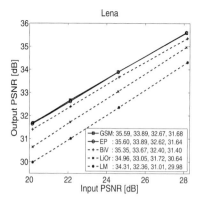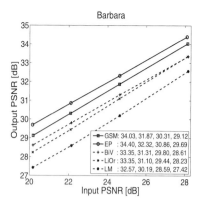

Figure 3: Output PSNR as a function of input PSNR for various methods on Lena (left) and Barbara (right) images. GSM: Gaussian scale mixture (3×3+p)[3], EP: edge-pert, BIV: Bivariate adaptive shrinkage [2], LiOr: results from [8], LM: 5×5 LAWMAP results from [9]. Dashed lines indicate results copied from the literature, while solid lines indicate that the values were (re)produced on our computer.

This bound is saturated for $\gamma = \alpha f^{\alpha-1}$, and hence we can construct the following iterative algorithm that is guaranteed to converge to a local minimum,

$$ \mathbf{z}^{t+1} = \left(K + \mathbf{Diag}[2\gamma^t \mathbf{w}]\right)^{-1} K \tilde{\mathbf{z}} \quad \Leftrightarrow \quad \gamma^{t+1} = \alpha \Big(\sum_j w_j (z_j^{t+1})^2 \Big)^{\alpha-1}. \quad (13) $$

This algorithm has a natural interpretation as an "iterated Wiener filter" (IWF), since the first step (left hand side) is an ordinary Wiener filter while the second step (right hand side) adapts the variance of the filter. A summary of the complete algorithm is provided below.

Edge-pert Denoising Algorithm

---

1. Decompose image into subbands.
2. *For each subband (except low-pass residual):*
2i.   Determine coefficients participating in joint model by using Eqn.4 (includes parent).
2ii.   Compute noise covariance Σ.
2iii. Compute signal covariance using Eqn.5.
3. *For each coefficient in a subband:*
3i.   Transform coefficients into the decorrelated domain using Eqn.6.
3ii.   Estimate parameters $\{\alpha, w_i\}$ on a local neighborhood using Eqn.8 and Eqn.9.
3iii. Denoise all wavelet coefficients in the neighborhood using IWF from section 3.2.
3iv. Transform denoised cluster back to the wavelet domain and retain the "center coefficient" only.
4. Reconstruct denoised image by inverting the wavelet transform.

---

4 Experiments

Denoising experiments were run on the steerable wavelet pyramid with oriented high-pass residual bands (FSpyr) using 8 orientations as described in [3]. Results are reported on six images: "Lena", "Barbara", "Boat", "Fingerprint", "House" and "Peppers" and averaged over 5 experiments. In each experiment an image was artificially contaminated with independent Gaussian pixel noise of some predetermined variance and denoised using 20 iterations of the proposed algorithm. To reduce artifacts at the boundaries we used "reflective boundary extensions". The images were obtained from *http://decsai.ugr.es/~javier/denoise/index.html* to ensure comparison on the same set of images.

In table 1 we compare performance between the PoEdges and GSM based denoising algorithms on six test images and ten different noise levels. In figure 3 we compare results on

σ		1	2	5	10	15	20	25	50	75	100
Lena	EP	48.65	43.53	38.51	35.60	33.89	32.62	31.64	28.58	26.74	25.53
	GSM	48.46	43.23	38.49	35.61	33.90	32.66	31.69	28.61	26.84	25.64
Barbara	EP	48.70	43.59	38.06	34.40	32.32	30.86	29.69	26.12	24.12	22.90
	GSM	48.37	43.29	37.79	34.03	31.86	30.32	29.13	25.48	23.65	22.61
Boat	EP	48.46	43.09	37.05	33.49	31.58	30.28	29.24	26.27	24.64	23.56
	GSM	48.44	42.99	36.97	33.58	31.70	30.38	29.37	26.38	24.79	23.75
Fingerprint	EP	48.44	43.02	36.66	32.35	30.02	28.42	27.31	24.15	22.45	21.28
	GSM	48.46	43.05	36.68	32.45	30.14	28.60	27.45	24.16	22.40	21.22
House	EP	49.06	44.32	39.00	35.54	33.67	32.37	31.33	28.15	26.12	24.84
	GSM	48.85	44.07	38.65	35.35	33.64	32.39	31.40	28.26	26.41	25.11
Peppers	EP	48.50	43.20	37.40	33.79	31.74	30.29	29.13	25.69	23.85	22.50
	GSM	48.38	43.00	37.31	33.77	31.74	30.31	29.21	25.90	24.00	22.66

Table 1: Comparison of image denoising results between PoEdges (EP above) and its closest competitor (GSM). All results are averaged over 5 noise samples. The GSM results are copied from [3]. Details of the PoEdges algorithm are described in main text. Note that PoEdges outperforms GSM for low noise levels while the GSM performs better at high noise levels. Also, PoEdges performs best at all noise levels on the Barbara image, while GSM is superior on the boat image.

FSpyr against various methods published in the literature [3, 2, 9] on the images "Lena" and "Barbara".

These experiments lead to some interesting conclusions. In comparing PoEdges with GSM the general trend seems to be that PoEdges performs superior at lower noise levels while the reverse is true for higher noise levels. We observe that the PoEdges give significantly better results on the "Barbara" image than any other published method (by a large magin). According to the findings of the authors of [3][2] this stems mainly from the fact that the parameters are estimated locally which is particularly suited for this image. Increasing the estimation window in step 3ii of the algorithm let the denoising results drop down to the GSM solution (not reported here). Comparing the quality of restored images in detail (as in figure 3) we conclude that the GSM produces slightly sharper edges at the expense of more artifacts. Denoising a 512×512 pixel sized image on a pentium 4 $2.8GHz$ PC for our adaptive neighborhood selection model took 26 seconds for the QMF9 and 440 seconds for the FSpyr.

We also compared GSM and EP using a separable orthonormal pyramid (QMF9). Using this simpler orthonormal decomposition we found that the EP model outperforms GSM in all experiments described above. However the results are significantly inferior because the wavelet representation plays a prominent role for denoising performance. These results and our matlab implementation of the algorithm are available online[3].

5   Discussion

We have proposed a general "product of edge-perts" model to capture the dependency structure in wavelet coefficients. This was turned into a practical denoising algorithm by simplifying to a single edge-pert and choosing $\beta_j = 2 \; \forall j$. The parameters of this model can be adapted based on the noisy observation of the image. In comparison with the closest competitor (GSM [3]) we found superior performance at low noise levels while the reverse is true for high noise levels. Also, the PoEdges model performs better than any competitor on the Barbara image, but consistency less well than GSM on the boat image.

The GSM model aims at capturing the same statistical regularities as the PoEdges but using a very different modelling paradigm: where PoEdges is best interpreted as a bottom-up constraint satisfaction model, the GSM is a causal generative model with top-down semantics. We have found that these two modelling paradigms exhibit different denoising accuracies

---

[2]Personal communication

[3]http://www.kyb.mpg.de/~pgehler

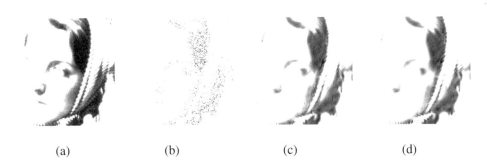

| (a) | (b) | (c) | (d) |

Figure 4: Comparison between (c) GSM with 3×3+parent [3] (PSNR 29.13) and (d) edge-pert denoiser with parameter settings as described in the text (PSNR 29.69) on Barbara image (cropped to 150×150 to enhance artifacts). Noisy image (b) has PSNR 20.17. Although the results turn out very similar, the GSM seems to be slightly less blurry at the expense of introducing more artifacts.

on some types of images implying an opportunity for further study and improvement.

The model in Eqn.3 can be extended in a number of ways. For example, we can lift the restriction on $\beta_j = 2$, allow more basis-vectors $\hat{a}_j$ than coefficients or extend the neighborhood selection to subbands of different scales and/or orientations. More substantial performance gains are expected if we can extend the single edge-pert case to a multi edge-pert model. However, approximations in the estimation of these models will become necessary to keep the denoising algorithm practical. The adaptation of α relies on empirical estimations of the fourth moment and is therefore very sensitive to outliers. We are currently investigating more robust estimators to fit α.

Further performance gains may still be expected through the development of new wavelet pyramids and through modelling of new dependency structures such as the phenomenon of phase alignment at the edges.

Acknowledgments We would like to thank the authors of [2] and [3] for making their code available online.

References

[1] J. Huang and D. Mumford. Statistics of natural images and models. In *Proc. of the Conf. on Computer Vision and Pattern Recognition*, pages 1541–1547, Ft. Collins, CO, USA, 1999.

[2] L. Sendur and I.W. Selesnick. Bivariate shrinkage with local variance estimation. *IEEE Signal Processing Letters*, 9(12):438–441, 2002.

[3] J. Portilla, V. Strela, M. Wainwright, and E. P. Simoncelli. Image denoising using scale mixtures of Gaussians in the wavelet domain. *IEEE Trans Image Processing*, 12(11):1338–1351, 2003.

[4] E.P. Simoncelli and W.T. Freeman. A flexible architecture for multi-scale derivative computation. In *IEEE Second Int'l Conf on Image Processing*, Washington DC, 1995.

[5] E.P. Simoncelli. Modeling the joint statistics of images in the wavelet domain. In *Proc SPIE, 44th Annual Meeting*, volume 3813, pages 188–195, Denver, 1999.

[6] G.E. Hinton and Y.W. Teh. Discovering multiple constraints that are frequently approximately satisfied. In *Proc. of the Conf. on Uncertainty in Artificial Intelligence*, pages 227–234, 2001.

[7] E.P. Simoncelli and E.H. Adelson. Noise removal via bayesian wavelet coring. In *3rd IEEE Int'l Conf on Image Processing*, Laussanne Switzerland, 1996.

[8] X. Li and M.T. Orchard. Spatially adaptive image denoising under over-complete expansion. In *IEEE Int'l. conf. on Image Processing*, Vancouver, BC, 2000.

[9] M. Kivanc, I. Kozintsev, K. Ramchandran, and P. Moulin. Low-complexity image denoising based on statistical modeling of wavelet coefficients. *IEEE Signal Proc. Letters*, 6:300–303, 1999.

Fast biped walking with a reflexive controller and real-time policy searching

Tao Geng[1], Bernd Porr[2] and Florentin Wörgötter[1,3]
[1] Dept. Psychology, University of Stirling, UK.
runbot05@gmail.com
[2] Dept. Electronics & Electrical Eng., University of Glasgow, UK.
b.porr@elec.gla.ac.uk
[3] Bernstein Centre for Computational Neuroscience, University of Göttingen
worgott@chaos.gwdg.de

Abstract

In this paper, we present our design and experiments of a planar biped robot ("RunBot") under pure reflexive neuronal control. The goal of this study is to combine neuronal mechanisms with biomechanics to obtain very fast speed and the on-line learning of circuit parameters. Our controller is built with biologically inspired sensor- and motor-neuron models, including local reflexes and not employing any kind of position or trajectory-tracking control algorithm. Instead, this reflexive controller allows RunBot to exploit its own natural dynamics during critical stages of its walking gait cycle. To our knowledge, this is the first time that dynamic biped walking is achieved using only a pure reflexive controller. In addition, this structure allows using a policy gradient reinforcement learning algorithm to tune the parameters of the reflexive controller in real-time during walking. This way RunBot can reach a relative speed of 3.5 leg-lengths per second after a few minutes of online learning, which is faster than that of any other biped robot, and is also comparable to the fastest relative speed of human walking. In addition, the stability domain of stable walking is quite large supporting this design strategy.

1 Introduction

Building and controlling fast biped robots demands a deeper understanding of biped walking than for slow robots. While slow robots may walk statically, fast biped walking has to be dynamically balanced and more robust as less time is available to recover from disturbances [1]. Although many biped robots have been developed using various technologies in the past 20 years, their walking speeds are still not comparable to that of their counterpart in nature, humans. Most of the successful biped robots have commonly used the ZMP (Zero Moment Point, [2]) as the criterion for stability control and motion generation. The ZMP is the point on the ground where the total moment generated by gravity and inertia equals zero. This measure has two deficiencies in the case of high-speed walking. First, the ZMP must always reside in the convex hull of the stance foot, and the stability margin is measured by the minimal distance between the ZMP and the edge of the foot. To ensure an appropriate stability margin, the foot has to be flat and large, which will deteriorate the robot's performance and pose great difficulty during fast walking. This difficulty can be shown clearly when humans try to walk with skies or swimming fins. Second, the ZMP criterion does not permit rotation of the stance foot at the heel or the toe, which, however, can amount to up to eighty percent of a normal human walking gait, and is important and inevitable in fast biped walking.

On the other hand, sometimes dynamic biped walking can be achieved without considering any stability criterion such as the ZMP. For example, passive biped robots can walk down a shallow slope without sensing or control. Some researchers have proposed approaches to equip a passive biped with actuators to improve its performance and drive it to walk on the flat ground [3] [4]. Nevertheless, these passive bipeds excessively depend on their natural dynamics for gait generation, which, while making their gaits efficient in energy, also limits their walking rate to be very slow.

In this study, we will show that, with a properly designed mechanical structure, a novel, pure reflexive controller, and an online policy gradient reinforcement learning algorithm, our biped robot can attain a fast walking speed of 3.5 leg-lengths per second. This makes it faster than any other biped robot we know. Though not a passive biped, it exploits its own natural dynamics during some stages of its walking gait, greatly simplifying the necessary control structures.

2   The robot

RunBot (Fig. 1) is 23 cm high, foot to hip joint axis. It has four joints: left hip, right hip, left knee, right knee. Each joint is driven by a modified RC servo motor. A hard mechanical stop is installed on the knee joints, preventing it from going into hyperextension. Each foot is equipped with a modified piezo transducer to sense ground contact events. Similar to other approaches [1], we constrain the robot only in the sagittal plane by a boom of one meter length freely rotating in its joints (planar robot). This assures that RunBot can still very easily trip and fall in the sagittal plane.

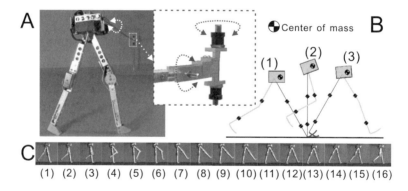

Figure 1: A): The robot, RunBot, and its boom structure. All three orthogonal axis of the boom can rotate freely. B) Illustration of a walking step of RunBot. C) A series of sequential frames of a walking gait cycle. The interval between every two adjacent frames is 33 ms. Note that, during the time between frame (8) and frame (13), which is nearly one third of the duration of a step, the motor voltage of all four joints remain to be zero, and the whole robot is moving passively. At the time of frame (13), the swing leg touches the floor and a next step begins.

Since we intended to exploit RunBot's natural dynamics during some stages of its gait cycle; similar to passive bipeds; its foot bottom is also curved with a radius equal to half the leg-length (with a too large radius, the tip of the foot may strike the ground during its swing phase). During the stance phase of such a curved foot, always only one point touches the ground, thus allowing the robot to roll passively around the contact point, which is similar to the rolling action of human feet facilitating fast walking.

The most important consideration in the mechanical design of our robot is the location of its center of mass. About seventy percent of the robot's weight is concentrated on its trunk. The parts of the trunk are assembled in such a way that its center of mass is located before the hip axis (Fig. 1 A). The effect of this design is illustrated in Fig. 1 B. As shown, one walking step includes two stages, the first from (1) to (2), the second from (2) to (3). During the first stage, the robot has to use its own momentum to rise up on the stance leg. When walking at a low speed, the robot may have not enough momentum to do this. So, the distance the center of mass has to cover in this stage should be as short as possible, which can be fulfilled by locating the center of mass of the trunk forward. In the second stage, the robot just falls forward naturally and catches itself on the next stance leg. Then the walking cycle is repeated. The figure also shows clearly the rolling movement of the curved foot of the stance leg. A stance phase begins with the heel touching ground, and terminates with the toe leaving ground.

In summary, our mechanical design of RunBot has following special features that distinguish it from other powered biped robots and facilitate high-speed walking and exploitation of natural dynamics: (a) Small curved feet allowing for rolling action; (b) Unactuated, hence, light ankles; (c) Light-weight structure; (d) Light and fast motors; (e) Proper mass distribution of the limbs; (f) Properly positioned mass center of the trunk.

3   The neural structure of our reflexive controller

The reflexive walking controller of RunBot follows a hierarchical structure (Fig. 2). The bottom level is the reflex circuit local to the joints, including motor-neurons and angle sensor neurons involved in the joint reflexes. The top level is a distributed neural network consisting of hip stretch receptors and ground contact sensor neurons, which modulate the local reflexes of the bottom level. Neurons are modelled as non-spiking neurons simulated on a Linux PC, and communicated to the robot via the DA/AD board. Though somewhat simplified, they still retain some of the prominent neuronal characteristics.

3.1   Model neuron circuit of the top level

The joint coordination mechanism in the top level is implemented with the neuron circuit illustrated in Fig. 2. While other biologically inspired locomotive models and robots use two stretch receptors on each leg to signal the attaining of the leg's AEP (Anterior Extreme Position) and PEP (Posterior Extreme Position) respectively, our robot has only one stretch receptor on each leg to signal the AEA (Anterior Extreme Angle) of its hip joint. Furthermore, the function of the stretch receptor on our robot is only to trigger the extensor reflex on the knee joint of the same leg, rather than to implicitly reset the phase relations between different legs as in the case of Cruse's model. As the hip joint approaches the AEA, the output of the stretch receptors for the left (AL) and the right hip (AR) are increased as:

$$\rho_{AL} = \left(1 + e^{\alpha_{AL}(\Theta_{AL} - \phi)}\right)^{-1} \tag{1}$$

$$\rho_{AL} = \left(1 + e^{\alpha_{AR}(\Theta_{AR} - \phi)}\right)^{-1} \tag{2}$$

Where ϕ is the real time angular position of the hip joint, Θ_{AL} and Θ_{AR} are the hip anterior extreme angles whose values are tuned by hand, α_{AL} and α_{AR} are positive constants. This

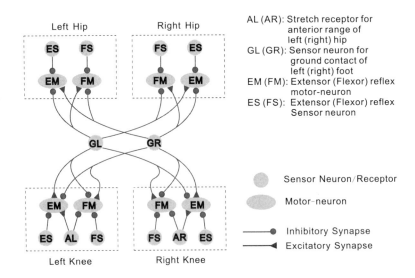

Figure 2: The neuron model of reflexive controller on RunBot.

model is inspired by a sensor neuron model presented in [5] that is thought capable of emulating the response characteristics of populations of sensor neurons in animals. Another kind of sensor neuron incorporated in the top level is the ground contact sensor neuron, which is active when the foot is in contact with the ground. Its output, similar to that of the stretch receptors, changes according to:

$$\rho_{GL} = \left(1 + e^{\alpha_{GL}(\Theta_{GL} - V_L + V_R)}\right)^{-1} \tag{3}$$

$$\rho_{GR} = \left(1 + e^{\alpha_{GR}(\Theta_{GR} - V_R + V_L)}\right)^{-1} \tag{4}$$

Where V_L and V_R are the output voltage signals from piezo sensors of the left foot and right foot respectively, Θ_{GL} and Θ_{GR} work as thresholds, α_{GL} and α_{GR} are positive constants.

3.2 Neural circuit of the bottom level

The bottom-level reflex system of our robot consists of reflexes local to each joint (Fig. 2). The neuron module for one reflex is composed of one angle sensor neuron and the motor-neuron it contacts. Each joint is equipped with two reflexes, extensor reflex and flexor reflex, both are modelled as a monosynaptic reflex, that is, whenever its threshold is exceeded, the angle sensor neuron directly excites the corresponding motor-neuron. This direct connection between angle sensor neuron and motor-neuron is inspired by a reflex described in cockroach locomotion [6]. In addition, the motor-neurons of the local reflexes also receive an excitatory synapse and an inhibitory synapse from the neurons of the top level, by which the top level can modulate the bottom-level reflexes. Each joint has two angle sensor neurons, one for the extensor reflex, and the other for the flexor reflex (Fig. 2). Their models are similar to that of the stretch receptors described above. The extensor angle sensor neuron changes its output according to:

$$\rho_{ES} = \left(1 + e^{\alpha_{ES}(\Theta_{ES} - \phi)}\right)^{-1} \tag{5}$$

where ϕ is the real time angular position obtained from the potentiometer of the joint. Θ_{ES} is the threshold of the extensor reflex and α_{ES} a positive constant. Likewise, the output of

Table 1: Parameters of neurons for hip- and knee joints. For meaning of the subscripts, see Fig. 2.

	Θ_{EM}	Θ_{FM}	α_{ES}	α_{FS}
Hip Joints	5	5	2	2
Knee Joints	5	5	2	2

Table 2: Parameters of stretch receptors and ground contact sensor neurons.

Θ_{GL} (v)	Θ_{GR} (v)	Θ_{AL} (deg)	Θ_{AR} (deg)	α_{GL}	α_{GR}	α_{AL}	α_{AR}
2	2	$= \Theta_{ES}$	$= \Theta_{ES}$	2	2	2	2

the flexor sensor neuron is modelled as:

$$\rho_{FS} = (1 + e^{\alpha_{FS}(\phi - \Theta_{FS})})^{-1} \qquad (6)$$

with Θ_{FS} and α_{FS} similar as above. The direction of extensor on both hip and knee joints is forward while that of flexors is backward.

It should be particularly noted that the thresholds of the sensor neurons in the reflex modules do not work as desired positions for joint control, because our reflexive controller does not involve any exact position control algorithms that would ensure that the joint positions converge to a desired value. The motor-neuron model is adapted from one used in the neural controller of a hexapod simulating insect locomotion [7]. The state and output of each extensor motor-neuron is governed by equations 7,8 [8] (that of flexor motor-neurons are similar):

$$\tau \frac{dy}{dt} = -y + \sum \omega_X \rho_X \qquad (7)$$

$$u_{EM} = \left(1 + e^{\Theta_{EM} - y}\right)^{-1} \qquad (8)$$

Where y represents the mean membrane potential of the neuron. Equation 8 is a sigmoidal function that can be interpreted as the neuron's short-term average firing frequency, Θ_{EM} is a bias constant that controls the firing threshold. τ is a time constant associated with the passive properties of the cell membrane [8], ω_X represents the connection strength from the sensor neurons and stretch receptors to the motor-neuron neuron (Fig. 2). ρ_X represents the output of the sensor-neurons and stretch receptors that contact this motor-neuron (e.g., $\rho_{ES}, \rho_{AL}, \rho_{GL}$, etc.)

Note that, on RunBot, the output value of the motor-neurons, after multiplication by a gain coefficient, is sent to the servo amplifier to directly drive the joint motor. The voltage of joint motor is determined by

$$Motor\ Voltage = M_{AMP} G_M (s_{EM} u_{EM} + s_{FM} u_{FM}), \qquad (9)$$

where M_{AMP} represents the magnitude of the servo amplifier, which is 3 on RunBot. G_M stands for output gain of the motor-neurons. s_{EM} and s_{FM} are signs for the motor voltage of flexor and extensor, being +1 or -1, depending on the the hardware of the robot. u_{EM} and u_{FM} are the outputs of the motor-neurons.

4 Robot walking experiments

The model neuron parameters chosen jointly for all experiments are listed in Tables 1 and 2. The time constants τ_i of all neurons take the same value of 3ms. The weights of all

Table 3: Fixed parameters of the knee joints.

	$\Theta_{ES,k}$ (deg)	$\Theta_{FS,k}$ (deg)	$G_{M,k}$
Knee Joints	175	110	$0.9G_{M,h}$

the inhibitory connections are set to -10, except those between sensor-neurons and motor-neurons, which are -30, and those between stretch receptors and flexor motor-neurons, which are -15. The weights of all excitatory connections are 10, except those between stretch receptors and extensor motor-neurons, which are 15. Because the movements of the knee joints is needed mainly for timely ground clearance without big contributions to the walking speed, we set their neuron parameters to fixed values (see Table 3). We also fix the threshold of the flexor sensor neurons of the hips ($\Theta_{FS,h}$) to $85°$. So, in the experiments described below, we only need to tune the two parameters of the hip joints, the threshold of the extensor sensor neurons ($\Theta_{ES,h}$) and the gain of the motor-neurons ($G_{M,h}$), which work together to determine the walking speed and the important gait properties of RunBot. In RunBot, $\Theta_{ES,h}$ determines roughly the stride length (not exactly, because the hip joint moves passively after passing $\Theta_{ES,h}$), while $G_{M,h}$ is proportional to the angular velocity of the motor on the hip joint.

In experiments of walking on a flat floor, surprisingly, we have found that stable gaits can appear in a considerably large range of the parameters $\Theta_{ES,h}$ and $G_{M,h}$ (Fig. 3A).

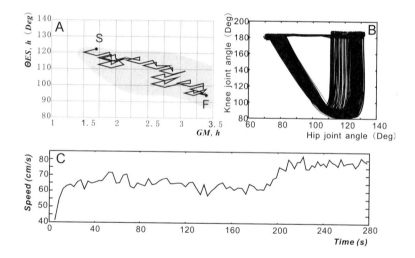

Figure 3: (A), The range of the two parameters, $G_{M,h}$ and $\Theta_{ES,h}$, in which stable gaits appear. The maximum permitted value of $G_{M,h}$ is 3.5 (higher value will destroy the motor of the hip joint). See text for more information. (B), Phase diagrams of hip joint position and knee joint position of one leg during the whole learning process. The smallest orbit is the fastest walking gait. (C), The walking speed of RunBot during the learning process.

In RunBot, passive movements appear on two levels, at the single joint level and at the whole robot level. Due to the high gear ratio of the joint motors, the passive movement of each joint is not very large. Whereas the effects of passive movements at the whole robot level can be clearly seen especially when RunBot is walking at a medium or slow speed (Fig. 1 C).

4.1 Policy gradient searching for fast walking gaits

In order to get a fast walking speed, the biped robot should have a long stride length, a short swing time, and a short double support phase [1]. In RunBot, because the phase-switching of its legs is triggered immediately by ground contact signals, its double support phase is so short (usually less than 30 ms) that it is negligible. A long stride length and a short swing time are mutually exclusive. Because there are no position or trajectory tracking control in RunBot, it is impossible to control its walking speed directly or explicitly. However, knowing that runBot's walking gait is determined by only two parameters, $\Theta_{ES,h}$ and $G_{M,h}$ (Fig. 3A), we formulate RunBot's fast walking control as a policy gradient reinforcement learning problem by considering each point in the the parameter space (Fig. 3A) as an open-loop policy that can be executed by RunBot in real-time.

Our approach is modified from [9]. It starts from an initial parameter vector $\pi = (\theta_1, \theta_2)$ (here θ_1 and θ_2 represent $G_{M,h}$ and $\Theta_{ES,h}$, respectively) and proceeds to evaluate following 5 polices near π: $(\theta_1, \theta_2), (\theta_1, \theta_2 + \epsilon_2), (\theta_1 - \epsilon_1, \theta_2), (\theta_1, \theta_2 - \epsilon_2), (\theta_1 + \epsilon_1, \theta_2)$, where each ϵ_j is a adaptive value that is small relative to θ_j. The evaluation of each policy generates a score that is a measure of the speed of the gait described by that policy. We use these scores to construct an adjustment vector A [9]. Then A is normalized and multiplied by an adaptive step-size. Finally, we add A to π, and begin the next iteration. If $A = 0$, this means a possible local minimum is encountered. In this case, we replace A with a stochastically generated vector. Although this is a very simple strategy, our experiments show that it can effectively prevent the real-time learning from trapping in the local minimums.

One experiment result is shown in Fig. 3. RunBot starts its walking with the parameters corresponding to point S in Fig. 3A whose speed is 41 cm/s (see Fig. 3C). After 240 seconds of continuous walking with the learning algorithm and no any human intervention, RunBot attains a walking speed of about 80 cm/s (see Fig. 3C, corresponding to point F in Fig. 3A), which is equivalent to 3.5 leg-lengths per second. To compare the walking speed of various biped robots whose sizes are quite different from each other, we use the relative speed, speed divided by the leg-length. We know of no other biped robot attaining such a fast relative speed. The world record of human walking race is equivalent to about $4.0 - 4.5$ leg-lengths per second. So, RunBot's highest walking speed is comparable to that of humans. To get a feeling of how fast RunBot can walk, we strongly encourage readers to watch the videos of the experiment at, http://www.cn.stir.ac.uk/~tgeng/nips

Although there is no specifically designed controller in charge of the sensing and control of the transient stages of policy changing (speed changing), the natural dynamics of the robot itself ensures the stability during the changes. By exploiting the natural dynamics, the reflexive controller is robust to its parameter variation as shown in Fig. 3A.

5   Discussions

Cruse developed a completely decentralized reflexive controller model to understand the locomotion control of walking in stick insects (Carausius morosus, [10]), which can immensely decrease the computational burden of the locomotion controller, and has been applied in many hexapod robots. Up to date, however, no real biped robot has existed that depends exclusively on reflexive controllers. This may be because of the intrinsic instability specific to biped-walking, which makes the dynamic stability of biped robots much more difficult to control than that of multi-legged robots. To our knowledge, our RunBot is the first dynamic biped exclusively controlled by a pure reflexive controller. Although such a pure reflexive controller itself involves no explicit mechanisms for the global stability control of the biped, its coupling with the properly designed mechanics of RunBot has substantially ensured the considerably large stable domain of the dynamic biped gaits.

Our reflexive controller has some evident differences from Cruse's model. Cruse's model depends on PEP, AEP and GC (Ground Contact) signals to generate the movement pattern of the individual legs. Whereas our reflexive controller presented here uses only GC and AEA signals to coordinate the movements of the joints. Moreover, the AEA signal of one hip in RunBot only acts on the knee joint belonging to the same leg, not functioning on the leg-level as the AEP and PEP did in Cruse's model. The use of fewer phasic feedback signals has further simplified the controller structure in RunBot.

In order to achieve real time walking gait in a real world, even biological inspired robots often have to depend on some kinds of position- or trajectory tracking control on their joints [6, 11, 12]. However, in RunBot, there is no exact position control implemented. The neural structure of our reflexive controller does not depend on, or ensure the tracking of, any desired position. Indeed, it is this approximate nature of our reflexive controller that allows the physical properties of the robot itself to contribute implicitly to generation of overall gait trajectories. The effectiveness of this hybrid neuro-mechanical system is also reflected in the fact that real-time learning of parameters was possible, where sometimes the speed of the robot changes quite strongly (see movie) without tripping it.

References

[1] J. Pratt. *Exploiting Inherent Robustness and Natural Dynamics in the Control of Bipedal Walking Robots*. PhD thesis, Massachusetts Institute of Technology, 2000.

[2] B. Surla D. Vukobratovic, M. Borovac and D. Stokic. *Biped locomotion: dynamics, stability, control and application*. Springer-Verlag, 1990.

[3] R. Q. V. Van der Linde. Active leg compliance for passive walking. In *Proceedings of IEEE International Conference on Robotics and Automation*, Orlando, Florida, 1998.

[4] Steve Collins and Andy Ruina. Efficient bipedal robots based on passive-dynamic walkers. *Science*, 37:1082–1085, 2005.

[5] T. Wadden and O. Ekeberg. A neuro-mechanical model of legged locomotion: Single leg control. *Biological Cybernetics*, 79:161–173, 1998.

[6] R.D. Beer, R.D. Quinn, H.J. Chiel, and R.E. Ritzmann. Biologically inspired approaches to robotics. *Communications of the ACM*, 40(3):30–38, 1997.

[7] R.D. Beer and H.J. Chiel. A distributed neural network for hexapod robot locomotion. *Neural Computation*, 4:356–365, 1992.

[8] J.C. Gallagher, R.D. Beer, K.S. Espenschied, and R.D. Quinn. Application of evolved locomotion controllers to a hexapod robot. *Robotics and Autonomous Systems*, 19:95–103, 1996.

[9] Nate Kohl and Peter Stone. Policy gradient reinforcement learning for fast quadrupedal locomotion. In *Proceedings of the IEEE International Conference on Robotics and Automation*, volume 3, pages 2619–2624, May 2004.

[10] H. Cruse, T. Kindermann, M. Schumm, and et.al. Walknet - a biologically inspired network to control six-legged walking. *Neural Networks*, 11(7-8):1435–1447, 1998.

[11] Y. Fukuoka, H. Kimura, and A.H. Cohen. Adaptive dynamic walking of a quadruped robot on irregular terrain based on biological concepts. *Int. J. of Robotics Research*, 22:187–202, 2003.

[12] M.A. Lewis. Certain principles of biomorphic robots. *Autonomous Robots*, 11:221–226, 2001.

Bayesian Sets

Zoubin Ghahramani[*] and **Katherine A. Heller**
Gatsby Computational Neuroscience Unit
University College London
London WC1N 3AR, U.K.
{zoubin,heller}@gatsby.ucl.ac.uk

Abstract

Inspired by "Google™ Sets", we consider the problem of retrieving items from a concept or cluster, given a query consisting of a few items from that cluster. We formulate this as a Bayesian inference problem and describe a very simple algorithm for solving it. Our algorithm uses a model-based concept of a cluster and ranks items using a score which evaluates the marginal probability that each item belongs to a cluster containing the query items. For exponential family models with conjugate priors this marginal probability is a simple function of sufficient statistics. We focus on sparse binary data and show that our score can be evaluated exactly using a single sparse matrix multiplication, making it possible to apply our algorithm to very large datasets. We evaluate our algorithm on three datasets: retrieving movies from EachMovie, finding completions of author sets from the NIPS dataset, and finding completions of sets of words appearing in the Grolier encyclopedia. We compare to Google™ Sets and show that Bayesian Sets gives very reasonable set completions.

1 Introduction

What do Jesus and Darwin have in common? Other than being associated with two different views on the origin of man, they also have colleges at Cambridge University named after them. If these two names are entered as a query into Google™ Sets (http://labs.google.com/sets) it returns a list of other colleges at Cambridge.

Google™ Sets is a remarkably useful tool which encapsulates a very practical and interesting problem in machine learning and information retrieval.[1] Consider a universe of items $\mathcal{D}$. Depending on the application, the set $\mathcal{D}$ may consist of web pages, movies, people, words, proteins, images, or any other object we may wish to form queries on. The user provides a query in the form of a very small subset of items $\mathcal{D}_c \subset \mathcal{D}$. The assumption is that the elements in $\mathcal{D}_c$ are examples of some concept / class / cluster in the data. The algorithm then has to provide a completion to the set $\mathcal{D}_c$—that is, some set $\mathcal{D}'_c \subset \mathcal{D}$ which presumably includes all the elements in $\mathcal{D}_c$ and other elements in $\mathcal{D}$ which are also in this concept / class / cluster[2].

---

[*]ZG is also at CALD, Carnegie Mellon University, Pittsburgh PA 15213.

[1]Google™ Sets is a large-scale clustering algorithm that uses many millions of data instances extracted from web data (Simon Tong, personal communication). We are unable to describe any details of how the algorithm works due its proprietary nature.

[2]From here on, we will use the term "cluster" to refer to the target concept.

We can view this problem from several perspectives. First, the query can be interpreted as elements of some unknown cluster, and the output of the algorithm is the completion of that cluster. Whereas most clustering algorithms are completely unsupervised, here the query provides supervised hints or constraints as to the membership of a particular cluster. We call this view *clustering on demand*, since it involves forming a cluster once some elements of that cluster have been revealed. An important advantage of this approach over traditional clustering is that the few elements in the query can give useful information as to the features which are relevant for forming the cluster. For example, the query "Bush", "Nixon", "Reagan" suggests that the features *republican* and *US President* are relevant to the cluster, while the query "Bush", "Putin", "Blair" suggests that *current* and *world leader* are relevant. Given the huge number of features in many real world data sets, such hints as to feature relevance can produce much more sensible clusters.

Second, we can think of the goal of the algorithm to be to solve a particular *information retrieval* problem [2, 3, 4]. As in other retrieval problems, the output should be relevant to the query, and it makes sense to limit the output to the top few items ranked by relevance to the query. In our experiments, we take this approach and report items ranked by relevance. Our relevance criterion is closely related to a Bayesian framework for understanding patterns of generalization in human cognition [5].

2 Bayesian Sets

Let $\mathcal{D}$ be a data set of items, and $\mathbf{x} \in \mathcal{D}$ be an item from this set. Assume the user provides a query set $\mathcal{D}_c$ which is a small subset of $\mathcal{D}$. Our goal is to rank the elements of $\mathcal{D}$ by how well they would "fit into" a set which includes $\mathcal{D}_c$. Intuitively, the task is clear: if the set $\mathcal{D}$ is the set of all movies, and the query set consists of two animated Disney movies, we expect other animated Disney movies to be ranked highly.

We use a model-based probabilistic criterion to measure how well items fit into $\mathcal{D}_c$. Having observed $\mathcal{D}_c$ as belonging to some concept, we want to know how probable it is that $\mathbf{x}$ also belongs with $\mathcal{D}_c$. This is measured by $p(\mathbf{x}|\mathcal{D}_c)$. Ranking items simply by this probability is not sensible since some items may be more probable than others, regardless of $\mathcal{D}_c$. For example, under most sensible models, the probability of a string decreases with the number of characters, the probability of an image decreases with the number of pixels, and the probability of any continuous variable decreases with the precision to which it is measured. We want to remove these effects, so we compute the ratio:

$$\text{score}(\mathbf{x}) = \frac{p(\mathbf{x}|\mathcal{D}_c)}{p(\mathbf{x})} \tag{1}$$

where the denominator is the prior probability of $\mathbf{x}$ and under most sensible models will scale exactly correctly with number of pixels, characters, discretization level, etc. Using Bayes rule, this score can be re-written as:

$$\text{score}(\mathbf{x}) = \frac{p(\mathbf{x}, \mathcal{D}_c)}{p(\mathbf{x}) \, p(\mathcal{D}_c)} \tag{2}$$

which can be interpreted as the ratio of the joint probability of observing $\mathbf{x}$ *and* $\mathcal{D}_c$, to the probability of independently observing $\mathbf{x}$ and $\mathcal{D}_c$. Intuitively, this ratio compares the probability that $\mathbf{x}$ and $\mathcal{D}_c$ were generated by the same model with the *same*, though unknown, parameters θ, to the probability that $\mathbf{x}$ and $\mathcal{D}_c$ came from models with *different* parameters θ and θ' (see figure 1). Finally, up to a multiplicative constant independent of $\mathbf{x}$, the score can be written as: $\text{score}(\mathbf{x}) = p(\mathcal{D}_c|\mathbf{x})$, which is the probability of observing the query set given $\mathbf{x}$ (i.e. the likelihood of $\mathbf{x}$).

From the above discussion, it is still not clear how one would compute quantities such as $p(\mathbf{x}|\mathcal{D}_c)$ and $p(\mathbf{x})$. A natural model-based way of defining a cluster is to assume that

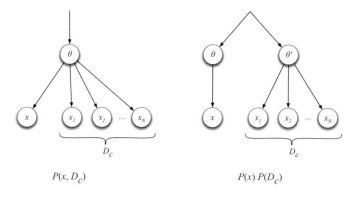

$$P(x, D_c) \qquad\qquad\qquad P(x)\, P(D_c)$$

Figure 1: Our Bayesian score compares the hypotheses that the data was generated by each of the above graphical models.

the data points in the cluster all come independently and identically distributed from some simple parameterized statistical model. Assume that the parameterized model is $p(\mathbf{x}|\theta)$ where θ are the parameters. If the data points in D_c all belong to one cluster, then under this definition they were generated from the same setting of the parameters; however, that setting is unknown, so we need to average over possible parameter values weighted by some prior density on parameter values, $p(\theta)$. Using these considerations and the basic rules of probability we arrive at:

$$p(\mathbf{x}) \;=\; \int p(\mathbf{x}|\theta)\, p(\theta)\, d\theta \tag{3}$$

$$p(D_c) \;=\; \int \prod_{\mathbf{x}_i \in D_c} p(\mathbf{x}_i|\theta)\, p(\theta)\, d\theta \tag{4}$$

$$p(\mathbf{x}|D_c) \;=\; \int p(\mathbf{x}|\theta)\, p(\theta|D_c)\, d\theta \tag{5}$$

$$p(\theta|D_c) \;=\; \frac{p(D_c|\theta)\, p(\theta)}{p(D_c)} \tag{6}$$

We are now fully equipped to describe the "Bayesian Sets" algorithm:

Bayesian Sets Algorithm
    background: a set of items D, a probabilistic model $p(\mathbf{x}|\theta)$ where
        $\mathbf{x} \in D$, a prior on the model parameters $p(\theta)$
    input: a query $D_c = \{\mathbf{x}_i\} \subset D$
    for all $\mathbf{x} \in D$ **do**
        compute $\mathrm{score}(\mathbf{x}) = \dfrac{p(\mathbf{x}|D_c)}{p(\mathbf{x})}$
    end for
    output: return elements of D sorted by decreasing score

We mention two properties of this algorithm to assuage two common worries with Bayesian methods—tractability and sensitivity to priors:

1. For the simple models we will consider, the integrals (3)-(5) are analytical. In fact, for the model we consider in section 3 computing all the scores can be reduced to a single sparse matrix multiplication.

2. Although it clearly makes sense to put some thought into choosing sensible models $p(\mathbf{x}|\theta)$ and priors $p(\theta)$, we will show in 5 that even with very simple models and almost no tuning of the prior one can get very competitive retrieval results. In practice, we use a simple empirical heuristic which sets the prior to be vague but centered on the mean of the data in $\mathcal{D}$.

3   Sparse Binary Data

We now derive in more detail the application of the Bayesian Sets algorithm to sparse binary data. This type of data is a very natural representation for the large datasets we used in our evaluations (section 5). Applications of Bayesian Sets to other forms of data (real-valued, discrete, ordinal, strings) are also possible, and especially practical if the statistical model is a member of the exponential family (section 4).

Assume each item $\mathbf{x}_i \in \mathcal{D}_c$ is a binary vector $\mathbf{x}_i = (x_{i1}, \ldots, x_{iJ})$ where $x_{ij} \in \{0, 1\}$, and that each element of $\mathbf{x}_i$ has an independent Bernoulli distribution:

$$p(\mathbf{x}_i|\theta) = \prod_{j=1}^{J} \theta_j^{x_{ij}} (1 - \theta_j)^{1-x_{ij}} \tag{7}$$

The conjugate prior for the parameters of a Bernoulli distribution is the Beta distribution:

$$p(\theta|\alpha, \beta) = \prod_{j=1}^{J} \frac{\Gamma(\alpha_j + \beta_j)}{\Gamma(\alpha_j)\Gamma(\beta_j)} \theta_j^{\alpha_j - 1} (1 - \theta_j)^{\beta_j - 1} \tag{8}$$

where α and β are hyperparameters, and the Gamma function is a generalization of the factorial function. For a query $\mathcal{D}_c = \{\mathbf{x}_i\}$ consisting of N vectors it is easy to show that:

$$p(\mathcal{D}_c|\alpha, \beta) = \prod_j \frac{\Gamma(\alpha_j + \beta_j)}{\Gamma(\alpha_j)\Gamma(\beta_j)} \frac{\Gamma(\tilde{\alpha}_j)\Gamma(\tilde{\beta}_j)}{\Gamma(\tilde{\alpha}_j + \tilde{\beta}_j)} \tag{9}$$

where $\tilde{\alpha} = \alpha + \sum_{i=1}^{N} x_{ij}$ and $\tilde{\beta} = \beta + N - \sum_{i=1}^{N} x_{ij}$. For an item $\mathbf{x} = (x_{.1} \ldots x_{.J})$ the score, written with the hyperparameters explicit, can be computed as follows:

$$\text{score}(\mathbf{x}) = \frac{p(\mathbf{x}|\mathcal{D}_c, \alpha, \beta)}{p(\mathbf{x}|\alpha, \beta)} = \prod_j \frac{\frac{\Gamma(\alpha_j+\beta_j+N)}{\Gamma(\alpha_j+\beta_j+N+1)} \frac{\Gamma(\tilde{\alpha}_j+x_{.j})\Gamma(\tilde{\beta}_j+1-x_{.j})}{\Gamma(\tilde{\alpha}_j)\Gamma(\tilde{\beta}_j)}}{\frac{\Gamma(\alpha_j+\beta_j)}{\Gamma(\alpha_j+\beta_j+1)} \frac{\Gamma(\alpha_j+x_{.j})\Gamma(\beta_j+1-x_{.j})}{\Gamma(\alpha_j)\Gamma(\beta_j)}} \tag{10}$$

This daunting expression can be dramatically simplified. We use the fact that $\Gamma(x) = (x - 1)\Gamma(x - 1)$ for $x > 1$. For each j we can consider the two cases $x_{.j} = 0$ and $x_{.j} = 1$ and separately. For $x_{.j} = 1$ we have a contribution $\frac{\alpha_j+\beta_j}{\alpha_j+\beta_j+N} \frac{\tilde{\alpha}_j}{\alpha_j}$. For $x_{.j} = 0$ we have a contribution $\frac{\alpha_j+\beta_j}{\alpha_j+\beta_j+N} \frac{\tilde{\beta}_j}{\beta_j}$. Putting these together we get:

$$\text{score}(\mathbf{x}) = \prod_j \frac{\alpha_j + \beta_j}{\alpha_j + \beta_j + N} \left(\frac{\tilde{\alpha}_j}{\alpha_j}\right)^{x_{.j}} \left(\frac{\tilde{\beta}_j}{\beta_j}\right)^{1-x_{.j}} \tag{11}$$

The log of the score is *linear* in $\mathbf{x}$:

$$\log \text{score}(\mathbf{x}) = c + \sum_j q_j x_{.j} \tag{12}$$

where

$$c = \sum_j \log(\alpha_j + \beta_j) - \log(\alpha_j + \beta_j + N) + \log \tilde{\beta}_j - \log \beta_j \tag{13}$$

and

$$q_j = \log \tilde{\alpha}_j - \log \alpha_j - \log \tilde{\beta}_j + \log \beta_j \qquad (14)$$

If we put the entire data set $\mathcal{D}$ into one large matrix $\mathbf{X}$ with J columns, we can compute the vector $\mathbf{s}$ of log scores for all points using a single matrix vector multiplication

$$\mathbf{s} = c + \mathbf{X}\mathbf{q} \qquad (15)$$

For sparse data sets this linear operation can be implemented very efficiently. Each query $\mathcal{D}_c$ corresponds to computing the vector $\mathbf{q}$ and scalar c. This can also be done efficiently if the query is also sparse, since most elements of $\mathbf{q}$ will equal $\log \beta_j - \log(\beta_j + N)$ which is independent of the query.

4 Exponential Families

We generalize the above result to models in the exponential family. The distribution for such models can be written in the form $p(\mathbf{x}|\theta) = f(\mathbf{x})g(\theta) \exp\{\theta^\top \mathbf{u}(\mathbf{x})\}$, where $\mathbf{u}(\mathbf{x})$ is a K-dimensional vector of sufficient statistics, θ are the natural parameters, and f and g are non-negative functions. The conjugate prior is $p(\theta|\eta, \nu) = h(\eta, \nu)g(\theta)^\eta \exp\{\theta^\top \nu\}$, where η and ν are hyperparameters, and h normalizes the distribution.

Given a query $\mathcal{D}_c = \{\mathbf{x}_i\}$ with N items, and a candidate $\mathbf{x}$, it is not hard to show that the score for the candidate is:

$$\text{score}(\mathbf{x}) = \frac{h(\eta + 1, \nu + \mathbf{u}(\mathbf{x}))\, h(\eta + N, \nu + \sum_i \mathbf{u}(\mathbf{x}_i))}{h(\eta, \nu)\, h(\eta + N + 1, \nu + \mathbf{u}(\mathbf{x}) + \sum_i \mathbf{u}(\mathbf{x}_i))} \qquad (16)$$

This expression helps us understand when the score can be computed efficiently. First of all, the score only depends on the size of the query (N), the sufficient statistics computed from each candidate, and from the whole query. It therefore makes sense to precompute $\mathbf{U}$, a matrix of sufficient statistics corresponding to $\mathbf{X}$. Second, whether the score is a linear operation on $\mathbf{U}$ depends on whether $\log h$ is linear in the second argument. This is the case for the Bernoulli distribution, but not for all exponential family distributions. However, for many distributions, such as diagonal covariance Gaussians, even though the score is nonlinear in $\mathbf{U}$, it can be computed by applying the nonlinearity elementwise to $\mathbf{U}$. For sparse matrices, the score can therefore still be computed in time linear in the number of non-zero elements of $\mathbf{U}$.

5 Results

We ran our Bayesian Sets algorithm on three different datasets: the Groliers Encyclopedia dataset, consisting of the text of the articles in the Encyclopedia, the EachMovie dataset, consisting of movie ratings by users of the EachMovie service, and the NIPS authors dataset, consisting of the text of articles published in NIPS volumes 0-12 (spanning the 1987-1999 conferences). The Groliers dataset is 30991 articles by 15276 words, where the entries are the number of times each word appears in each document. We preprocess (binarize) the data by column normalizing each word, and then thresholding so that a (article,word) entry is 1 if that word has a frequency of more than twice the article mean. We do essentially no tuning of the hyperparameters. We use broad empirical priors, where $\alpha = c \times \mathbf{m}$, $\beta = c \times (1 - \mathbf{m})$ where $\mathbf{m}$ is a mean vector over all articles, and $c = 2$. The analogous priors are used for both other datasets.

The EachMovie dataset was preprocessed, first by removing movies rated by less than 15 people, and people who rated less than 200 movies. Then the dataset was binarized so that a (person, movie) entry had value 1 if the person gave the movie a rating above 3 stars (from a possible 0-5 stars). The data was then column normalized to account for overall movie popularity. The size of the dataset after preprocessing was 1813 people by 1532 movies.

Finally the NIPS author dataset (13649 words by 2037 authors), was preprocessed very similarly to the Grolier dataset. It was binarized by column normalizing each author, and then thresholding so that a (word,author) entry is 1 if the author uses that word more frequently than twice the word mean across all authors.

The results of our experiments, and comparisons with Google Sets for word and movie queries are given in tables 2 and 3. Unfortunately, NIPS authors have not yet achieved the kind of popularity on the web necessary for Google Sets to work effectively. Instead we list the top words associated with the cluster of authors given by our algorithm (table 4).

The running times of our algorithm on all three datasets are given in table 1. All experiments were run in Matlab on a 2GHz Pentium 4, Toshiba laptop. Our algorithm is very fast both at pre-processing the data, and answering queries (about 1 sec per query).

	GROLIERS	EACHMOVIE	NIPS
SIZE	30991×15276	1813×1532	13649×2037
NON-ZERO ELEMENTS	2,363,514	517,709	933,295
PREPROCESS TIME	6.1s	0.56s	3.22s
QUERY TIME	1.1s	0.34s	0.47s

Table 1: For each dataset we give the size of that dataset along with the time taken to do the (one-time) preprocessing and the time taken to make a query (both in seconds).

QUERY: WARRIOR, SOLDIER		QUERY: ANIMAL		QUERY: FISH, WATER, CORAL	
GOOGLE SETS	BAYES SETS	GOOGLE SETS	BAYES SETS	GOOGLE SETS	BAYES SETS
WARRIOR	SOLDIER	ANIMAL	ANIMAL	FISH	WATER
SOLDIER	WARRIOR	PLANT	ANIMALS	WATER	FISH
SPY	MERCENARY	FREE	PLANT	CORAL	SURFACE
ENGINEER	CAVALRY	LEGAL	HUMANS	AGRICULTURE	SPECIES
MEDIC	BRIGADE	FUNGAL	FOOD	FOREST	WATERS
SNIPER	COMMANDING	HUMAN	SPECIES	RICE	MARINE
DEMOMAN	SAMURAI	HYSTERIA	MAMMALS	SILK ROAD	FOOD
PYRO	BRIGADIER	VEGETABLE	AGO	RELIGION	TEMPERATURE
SCOUT	INFANTRY	MINERAL	ORGANISMS	HISTORY POLITICS	OCEAN
PYROMANIAC	COLONEL	INDETERMINATE	VEGETATION	DESERT	SHALLOW
HWGUY	SHOGUNATE	FOZZIE BEAR	PLANTS	ARTS	FT

Table 2: Clusters of words found by Google Sets and Bayesian Sets based on the given queries. The top few are shown for each query and each algorithm. Bayesian Sets was run using Grolier Encyclopedia data.

It is very difficult to objectively evaluate our results since there is no ground truth for this task. One person's idea of a good query cluster may differ drastically from another person's. We chose to compare our algorithm to Google Sets since it was our main inspiration and it is currently the most public and commonly used algorithm for performing this task.

Since we do not have access to the Google Sets algorithm it was impossible for us to run their method on our datasets. Moreover, Google Sets relies on vast amounts of web data, which we do not have. Despite those two important caveats, Google Sets clearly "knows" a lot about movies[3] and words, and the comparison to Bayesian Sets is informative.

We found that Google Sets performed very well when the query consisted of items which can be found listed on the web (e.g. Cambridge colleges). On the other hand, for more abstract concepts (e.g. "soldier" and "warrior", see Table 2) our algorithm returned more sensible completions.

While we believe that most of our results are self-explanatory, there are a few details that we would like to elaborate on. The top query in table 3 consists of two classic romantic movies,

---

[3]In fact, one of the example queries on the Google Sets website is a query of movie titles.

QUERY: GONE WITH THE WIND, CASABLANCA	
GOOGLE SETS	BAYES SETS
CASABLANCA (1942)	GONE WITH THE WIND (1939)
GONE WITH THE WIND (1939)	CASABLANCA (1942)
ERNEST SAVES CHRISTMAS (1988)	THE AFRICAN QUEEN (1951)
CITIZEN KANE (1941)	THE PHILADELPHIA STORY (1940)
PET DETECTIVE (1994)	MY FAIR LADY (1964)
VACATION (1983)	THE ADVENTURES OF ROBIN HOOD (1938)
WIZARD OF OZ (1939)	THE MALTESE FALCON (1941)
THE GODFATHER (1972)	REBECCA (1940)
LAWRENCE OF ARABIA (1962)	SINGING IN THE RAIN (1952)
ON THE WATERFRONT (1954)	IT HAPPENED ONE NIGHT (1934)

QUERY: MARY POPPINS, TOY STORY		QUERY: CUTTHROAT ISLAND, LAST ACTION HERO	
GOOGLE SETS	BAYES SETS	GOOGLE SETS	BAYES SETS
TOY STORY	MARY POPPINS	LAST ACTION HERO	CUTTHROAT ISLAND
MARY POPPINS	TOY STORY	CUTTHROAT ISLAND	LAST ACTION HERO
TOY STORY 2	WINNIE THE POOH	GIRL	KULL THE CONQUEROR
MOULIN ROUGE	CINDERELLA	END OF DAYS	VAMPIRE IN BROOKLYN
THE FAST AND THE FURIOUS	THE LOVE BUG	HOOK	SPRUNG
PRESQUE RIEN	BEDKNOBS AND BROOMSTICKS	THE COLOR OF NIGHT	JUDGE DREDD
SPACED	DAVY CROCKETT	CONEHEADS	WILD BILL
BUT I'M A CHEERLEADER	THE PARENT TRAP	ADDAMS FAMILY I	HIGHLANDER III
MULAN	DUMBO	ADDAMS FAMILY II	VILLAGE OF THE DAMNED
WHO FRAMED ROGER RABBIT	THE SOUND OF MUSIC	SINGLES	FAIR GAME

Table 3: Clusters of movies found by Google Sets and Bayesian Sets based on the given queries. The top 10 are shown for each query and each algorithm. Bayesian Sets was run using the EachMovie dataset.

and while most of the movies returned by Bayesian Sets are also classic romances, hardly any of the movies returned by Google Sets are romances, and it would be difficult to call "Ernest Saves Christmas" either a romance or a classic. Both "Cutthroat Island" and "Last Action Hero" are action movie flops, as are many of the movies given by our algorithm for that query. All the Bayes Sets movies associated with the query "Mary Poppins" and "Toy Story" are children's movies, while 5 of Google Sets' movies are not. "But I'm a Cheerleader", while appearing to be a children's movie, is actually an R rated movie involving lesbian and gay teens.

QUERY: A.SMOLA, B.SCHOLKOPF		QUERY: L.SAUL, T.JAAKKOLA		QUERY: A.NG, R.SUTTON	
TOP MEMBERS	TOP WORDS	TOP MEMBERS	TOP WORDS	TOP MEMBERS	TOP WORDS
A.SMOLA	VECTOR	L.SAUL	LOG	R.SUTTON	DECISION
B.SCHOLKOPF	SUPPORT	T.JAAKKOLA	LIKELIHOOD	A.NG	REINFORCEMENT
S.MIKA	KERNEL	M.RAHIM	MODELS	Y.MANSOUR	ACTIONS
G.RATSCH	PAGES	M.JORDAN	MIXTURE	B.RAVINDRAN	REWARDS
R.WILLIAMSON	MACHINES	N.LAWRENCE	CONDITIONAL	D.KOLLER	REWARD
K.MULLER	QUADRATIC	T.JEBARA	PROBABILISTIC	D.PRECUP	START
J.WESTON	SOLVE	W.WIEGERINCK	EXPECTATION	C.WATKINS	RETURN
J.SHAWE-TAYLOR	REGULARIZATION	M.MEILA	PARAMETERS	R.MOLL	RECEIVED
V.VAPNIK	MINIMIZING	S.IKEDA	DISTRIBUTION	T.PERKINS	MDP
T.ONODA	MIN	D.HAUSSLER	ESTIMATION	D.MCALLESTER	SELECTS

Table 4: NIPS authors found by Bayesian Sets based on the given queries. The top 10 are shown for each query along with the top 10 words associated with that cluster of authors. Bayesian Sets was run using NIPS data from vol 0-12 (1987-1999 conferences).

The NIPS author dataset is rather small, and co-authors of NIPS papers appear very similar to each other. Therefore, many of the authors found by our algorithm are co-authors of a NIPS paper with one or more of the query authors. An example where this is not the case is Wim Wiegerinck, who we do not believe ever published a NIPS paper with Lawrence Saul or Tommi Jaakkola, though he did have a NIPS paper on variational learning and graphical models.

As part of the evaluation of our algorithm, we showed 30 naïve subjects the unlabeled results of Bayesian Sets and Google Sets for the queries shown from the EachMovie and Groliers Encyclopedia datasets, and asked them to choose which they preferred. The results of this study are given in table 5.

QUERY	% BAYES SETS	P-VALUE
WARRIOR	96.7	< 0.0001
ANIMAL	93.3	< 0.0001
FISH	90.0	< 0.0001
GONE WITH THE WIND	86.7	< 0.0001
MARY POPPINS	96.7	< 0.0001
CUTTHROAT ISLAND	81.5	0.0008

Table 5: For each evaluated query (listed by first query item), we give the percentage of respondents who preferred the results given by Bayesian Sets and the p-value rejecting the null hypothesis that Google Sets is preferable to Bayesian Sets on that particular query.

Since, in the case of binary data, our method reduces to a matrix-vector multiplication, we also came up with ten heuristic matrix-vector methods which we ran on the same queries, using the same datasets. Descriptions and results can be found in supplemental material on the authors websites.

6 Conclusions

We have described an algorithm which takes a query consisting of a small set of items, and returns additional items which belong in this set. Our algorithm computes a score for each item by comparing the posterior probability of that item given the set, to the prior probability of that item. These probabilities are computed with respect to a statistical model for the data, and since the parameters of this model are unknown they are marginalized out.

For exponential family models with conjugate priors, our score can be computed exactly and efficiently. In fact, we show that for sparse binary data, scoring all items in a large data set can be accomplished using a single sparse matrix-vector multiplication. Thus, we get a very fast and practical Bayesian algorithm without needing to resort to approximate inference. For example, a sparse data set with over 2 million nonzero entries (Grolier) can be queried in just over 1 second.

Our method does well when compared to Google Sets in terms of set completions, demonstrating that this Bayesian criterion can be useful in realistic problem domains. One of the problems we have not yet addressed is deciding on the size of the response set. Since the scores have a probabilistic interpretation, it should be possible to find a suitable threshold to these probabilities. In the future, we will incorporate such a threshold into our algorithm.

The problem of retrieving sets of items is clearly relevant to many application domains. Our algorithm is very flexible in that it can be combined with a wide variety of types of data (e.g. sequences, images, etc.) and probabilistic models. We plan to explore efficient implementations of some of these extensions. We believe that with even larger datasets the Bayesian Sets algorithm will be a very useful tool for many application areas.

Acknowledgements: Thanks to Avrim Blum and Simon Tong for useful discussions, and to Sam Roweis for some of the data. ZG was partially supported at CMU by the DARPA CALO project.

References

[1] Google ™Sets. http://labs.google.com/sets

[2] Lafferty, J. and Zhai, C. (2002) Probabilistic relevance models based on document and query generation. In *Language modeling and information retrieval*.

[3] Ponte, J. and Croft, W. (1998) A language modeling approach to information retrieval. *SIGIR*.

[4] Robertson, S. and Sparck Jones, K. (1976). Relevance weighting of search terms. *J Am Soc Info Sci*.

[5] Tenenbaum, J. B. and Griffiths, T. L. (2001). Generalization, similarity, and Bayesian inference. *Behavioral and Brain Sciences*, 24:629–641.

[6] Tong, S. (2005). Personal communication.

Query By Committee Made Real

Ran Gilad-Bachrach[†◇]   **Amir Navot**[‡]   **Naftali Tishby**[†‡]
† School of Computer Science and Engineering
‡ Interdisciplinary Center for Neural Computation
The Hebrew University, Jerusalem, Israel.
◇ Intel Research

Abstract

Training a learning algorithm is a costly task. A major goal of active learning is to reduce this cost. In this paper we introduce a new algorithm, KQBC, which is capable of actively learning large scale problems by using selective sampling. The algorithm overcomes the costly sampling step of the well known *Query By Committee* (QBC) algorithm by projecting onto a low dimensional space. KQBC also enables the use of kernels, providing a simple way of extending QBC to the non-linear scenario. Sampling the low dimension space is done using the *hit and run* random walk. We demonstrate the success of this novel algorithm by applying it to both artificial and a real world problems.

1 Introduction

Stone's celebrated theorem proves that given a large enough training sequence, even naive algorithms such as the k-nearest neighbors can be optimal. However, collecting large training sequences poses two main obstacles. First, collecting these sequences is a lengthy and costly task. Second, processing large datasets requires enormous resources. The selective sampling framework [1] suggests permitting the learner some control over the learning process. In this way, the learner can collect a short and informative training sequence. This is done by generating a large set of unlabeled instances and allowing the learner to select the instances to be labeled.

The *Query By Committee* algorithm (QBC) [2] was the inspiration behind many algorithms in the selective sampling framework [3, 4, 5]. QBC is a simple yet powerful algorithm. During learning it maintains a *version space*, the space of all the classifiers which are consistent with all the previous labeled instances. Whenever an unlabeled instance is available, QBC selects two random hypotheses from the version space and only queries for the label of the new instance if the two hypotheses disagree. Freund et al. [6] proved that when certain conditions apply, QBC will reach a generalization error of ϵ when using only $O\left(\log 1/\epsilon\right)$ labels. QBC works in an online fashion where each instance is considered only once to decide whether to query for its label or not. This is significant when there are a large number of unlabeled instances. In this scenario, batch processing of the data is unfeasible (see e.g. [7]). However, QBC was never implemented as is, since it requires the ability to sample hypotheses from the version space, a task that all known method do in an unreasonable amount of time [8].

The algorithm we present in this paper uses the same skeleton as QBC, but replaces sampling from the high dimensional version space by sampling from a low dimensional projection of it. By doing so, we obtain an algorithm which can cope with large scale problems and at the same time authorizes the use of kernels. Although the algorithm uses linear classifiers at its core, the use of kernels makes it much broader in scope. This new sampling method is presented in section 2. Section 3 gives a detailed description of the kernelized version, the *Kernel Query By Committee* (KQBC) algorithm. The last building block is a method for sampling from convex bodies. We suggest the *hit and run* [9] random walk for this purpose in section 4. A Matlab implementation of KQBC is available at http://www.cs.huji.ac.il/labs/learning/code/qbc.

The empirical part of this work is presented in section 5. We demonstrate how KQBC works on two binary classification tasks. The first is a synthetic linear classification task. The second involves differentiating male and female facial images. We show that in both cases, KQBC learns faster than Support Vector Machines (SVM) [10]. KQBC can be used to select a subsample to which SVM is applied. In our experiments, this method was superior to SVM; however, KQBC outperformed both.

Related work: Many algorithms for selective sampling have been suggested in the literature. However only a few of them have a theoretical justification. As already mentioned, QBC has a theoretical analysis. Two other notable algorithms are the greedy active learning algorithm [11] and the perceptron based active learning algorithm [12]. The greedy active learning algorithm has the remarkable property of being close to optimal in all settings. However, it operates in a batch setting, where selecting the next query point requires reevaluation of the whole set of unlabeled instances. This is problematic when the dataset is large. The perceptron based active learning algorithm, on the other hand, is extremely efficient in its computational requirements, but is restricted to linear classifiers since it requires the explicit use of the input dimension.

Graepel et al. [13] presented a *billiard walk* in the version space as a part of the Bayes Point Machine. Similar to the method presented here, the *billiard walk* is capable of sampling hypotheses from the version space when kernels are used. The method presented here has several advantages: it has better theoretical grounding and it is easier to implement.

2   A New Method for Sampling the Version-Space

The *Query By Committee* algorithm [2] provides a general framework that can be used with any concept class. Whenever a new instance is presented, QBC generates two independent predictions for its label by sampling two hypotheses from the version space[1]. If the two predictions differ, QBC queries for the label of the instance at hand (see algorithm 1). The main obstacle in implementing QBC is the need to sample from the version space (step 2b). It is not clear how to do this with reasonable computational complexity. As is the case for most research in machine learning, we first focus on the class of linear classifiers and then extend the discussion by using kernels. In the linear case, the dimension of the version space is the input dimension which is typically large for real world problems. Thus direct sampling is practically impossible. We overcome this obstacle by projecting the version space onto a low dimensional subspace.

Assume that the learner has seen the labeled sample $S = \{(x_i, y_i)\}_{i=1}^k$, where $x_i \in \mathbb{R}^d$ and $y_i \in \{\pm 1\}$. The version space is defined to be the set of all classifiers which correctly classify all the instances seen so far:

$$V = \{w \ : \ \|w\| \leq 1 \text{ and } \forall i \ y_i \,(w \cdot x_i) > 0\} \tag{1}$$

---

[1]The version space is the collection of hypotheses that are consistent with previous labels.

Algorithm 1 Query By Committee [2]

Inputs:

- A concept class $\mathcal{C}$ and a probability measure ν defined over $\mathcal{C}$.

The algorithm:

1. Let $S \leftarrow \phi, V \leftarrow \mathcal{C}$.
2. For $t = 1, 2, \dots$

    (a) Receive an instance x.

    (b) Let h_1, h_2 be two random hypotheses selected from ν restricted to V.

    (c) If $h_1(x) \neq h_2(x)$ then

        i. Ask for the label y of x.

        ii. Add the pair (x, y) to S.

        iii. Let $V \leftarrow \{c \in \mathcal{C} : \forall (x, y) \in S \ c(x) = y\}$.

QBC assumes a prior ν over the class of linear classifiers. The sample S induces a posterior over the class of linear classifiers which is the restriction of ν to V. Thus, the probability that QBC will query for the label of an instance x is exactly

$$2 \Pr_{w \sim \nu | V} [w \cdot x > 0] \Pr_{w \sim \nu | V} [w \cdot x < 0] \tag{2}$$

where $\nu | V$ is the restriction of ν to V.

From (2) we see that there is no need to explicitly select two random hypotheses. Instead, we can use any stochastic approach that will query for the label with the same probability as in (2). Furthermore, if we can sample $\hat{y} \in \{\pm 1\}$ such that

$$\Pr [\hat{y} = 1] = \Pr_{w \sim \nu | V} [w \cdot x > 0] \qquad \text{and} \tag{3}$$
$$\Pr [\hat{y} = -1] = \Pr_{w \sim \nu | V} [w \cdot x < 0] \tag{4}$$

we can use it instead, by querying the label of x with a probability of $2 \Pr [\hat{y} = 1] \Pr [\hat{y} = -1]$. Based on this observation, we introduce a stochastic algorithm which returns $\hat{y}$ with probabilities as specified in (3) and (4). This procedure can replace the sampling step in the QBC algorithm.

Let $S = \{(x_i, y_i)\}_{i=1}^{k}$ be a labeled sample. Let x be an instance for which we need to decide whether to query for its label or not. We denote by V the version space as defined in (1) and denote by T the space spanned by $x_1, \dots, x_k$ and x. QBC asks for two random hypotheses from V and queries for the label of x only if these two hypotheses predict different labels for x. Our procedure does the same thing, but instead of sampling the hypotheses from V we sample them from $V \cap T$. One main advantage of this new procedure is that it samples from a space of low dimension and therefore its computational complexity is much lower. This is true since T is a space of dimension $k + 1$ at most, where k is the number of queries for label QBC made so far. Hence, the body $V \cap T$ is a low-dimensional convex body[2] and thus sampling from it can be done efficiently. The input dimension plays a minor role in the sampling algorithm. Another important advantage is that it allows us to use kernels, and therefore gives a systematic way to extend QBC to the non-linear scenario. The use of kernels is described in detail in section 3.

The following theorem proves that indeed sampling from $V \cap T$ produces the desired results. It shows that if the prior ν (see algorithm 1) is uniform, then sampling hypotheses uniformly from V or from $V \cap T$ generates the same results.

---

[2]From the definition of the version space V it follows that it is a convex body.

Theorem 1 *Let $S = \{(x_i, y_i)\}_{i=1}^k$ be a labeled sample and x an instance. Let the version space be $V = \{w : \|w\| \leq 1 \text{ and } \forall i \ y_i (w \cdot x_i) > 0\}$ and $T = span (x, x_1, \ldots, x_k)$ then*

$$\Pr_{w \sim U(V)} [w \cdot x > 0] = \Pr_{w \sim U(V \cap T)} [w \cdot x > 0] \qquad and$$

$$\Pr_{w \sim U(V)} [w \cdot x < 0] = \Pr_{w \sim U(V \cap T)} [w \cdot x < 0]$$

where $U(\cdot)$ is the uniform distribution.

The proof of this theorem is given in the supplementary material [14].

3 Sampling with Kernels

In this section we show how the new sampling method presented in section 2 can be used together with kernel. QBC uses the random hypotheses for one purpose alone: to check the labels they predict for instances. In our new sampling method the hypotheses are sampled from $V \cap T$, where $T = span (x, x_1, \ldots, x_k)$. Hence, any hypothesis is represented by $w \in V \cap T$, that has the form

$$w = \alpha_0 x + \sum_{j=1}^k \alpha_j x_j \tag{5}$$

The label w assigns to an instance x' is

$$w \cdot x' = \left(\alpha_0 x + \sum_{j=1}^k \alpha_j x_j \right) \cdot x' = \alpha_0 x \cdot x' + \sum_{j=1}^k \alpha_j x_j \cdot x' \tag{6}$$

Note that in (6) only inner products are used, hence we can use kernels. Using these observations, we can sample a hypothesis by sampling $\alpha_0, \ldots, \alpha_k$ and define w as in (5). However, since the x_i's do not form an orthonormal basis of T, sampling the α's uniformly is not equivalent to sampling the w's uniformly. We overcome this problem by using an orthonormal basis of T. The following lemma shows a possible way in which the orthonormal basis for T can be computed when only inner products are used. The method presented here does not make use of the fact that we can build this basis incrementally.

Lemma 1 *Let $x_0, \ldots, x_k$ be a set of vectors, let $T = span (x_0, \ldots, x_k)$ and let $G = (g_{i,j})$ be the Grahm matrix such that $g_{i,j} = x_i \cdot x_j$. Let $\lambda_1, \ldots, \lambda_r$ be the non-zero eigen values of G with the corresponding eigen-vectors $\gamma_1, \ldots, \gamma_r$. Then the vectors $t_1, \ldots, t_r$ such that*

$$t_i = \sum_{l=0}^k \frac{\gamma_i (l)}{\sqrt{\lambda_i}} x_l$$

form an orthonormal basis of the space T.

The proof of lemma 1 is given in the supplementary material [14]. This lemma is significant since the basis $t_1, \ldots, t_r$ enables us to sample from $V \cap T$ using simple techniques. Note that a vector $w \in T$ can be expressed as $\sum_{i=1}^r \alpha(i) t_i$. Since the t_i's form an orthonormal basis, $\|w\| = \|\alpha\|$. Furthermore, we can check the label w assigns to x_j by

$$w \cdot x_j = \sum_i \alpha (i) t_i \cdot x_j = \sum_{i,l} \alpha (i) \frac{\gamma_i (l)}{\sqrt{\gamma_i}} x_l \cdot x_j$$

which is a function of the Grahm matrix. Therefore, sampling from $V \cap T$ boils down to the problem of sampling from convex bodies, where instead of sampling a vector directly we sample the coefficients of the orthonormal basis $t_1, \ldots, t_r$.

There are several methods for generating the final hypothesis to be used in the generalization phase. In the experiments reported in section 5 we have randomly selected a single hypothesis from $V \cap T$ and used it to make all predictions, where V is the version space at the time when the learning terminated and T is the span of all instances for which KQBC queried for label during the learning process.

4 Hit and Run

Hit and run [9] is a method of sampling from a convex body $\mathcal{K}$ using a random walk. Let $z \in \mathcal{K}$, a single step of the hit and run begins by choosing a random point u from the unit sphere. Afterwards the algorithm moves to a random point selected uniformly from $l \cap \mathcal{K}$, where l is the line passing through z and $z + u$.

Hit and run has several advantages over other random walks for sampling from convex bodies. First, its stationary distribution is indeed the uniform distribution, it mixes fast [9] and it does not require a "warm" starting point [15]. What makes it especially suitable for practical use is the fact that it does not require any parameter tuning other than the number of random steps. It is also very easy to implement.

Current proofs [9, 15] show that $O^*\left(d^3\right)$ steps are needed for the random walk to mix. However, the constants in these bounds are very large. In practice hit and run mixes much faster than that. We have used it to sample from the body $V \cap T$. The number of steps we used was very small, ranging from couple of hundred to a couple of thousands. Our empirical study shows that this suffices to obtain impressive results.

5 Empirical Study

In this section we present the results of applying our new kernelized version of the query by committee (KQBC), to two learning tasks. The first task requires classification of synthetic data while the second is a real world problem.

5.1 Synthetic Data

In our first experiment we studied the task of learning a linear classifier in a d-dimensional space. The target classifier is the vector $w^* = (1, 0, \ldots, 0)$ thus the label of an instance $x \in \mathbb{R}^d$ is the sign of its first coordinate. The instances were normally distributed $N\left(\mu = 0, \Sigma = I_d\right)$. In each trial we used 10000 unlabeled instances and let KQBC select the instances to query for the labels. We also applied Support Vector Machine (SVM) to the same data in order to demonstrate the benefit of using active learning. The linear kernel was used for both KQBC and SVM. Since SVM is a passive learner, SVM was trained on prefixes of the training data of different sizes. The results are presented in figure 1.

The difference between KQBC and SVM is notable. When both are applied to a 15-dimensional linear discrimination problem (figure 1b), SVM and KQBC have an error rate of $\sim 6\%$ and $\sim 0.7\%$ respectively after 120 labels. After such a short training sequence the difference is of an order of magnitude. The same qualitative results appear for all problem sizes.

As expected, the generalization error of KQBC decreases exponentially fast as the number of queries is increased, whereas the generalization error of SVM decreases only at an inverse-polynomial rate (the rate is $O^*\left(1/k\right)$ where k is the number of labels). This should not come as a surprise since Freund et al. [6] proved that this is the expected behavior. Note also that the bound of $50 \cdot 2^{-0.67k/d}$ over the generalization error that was proved in [6] was replicated in our experiments (figure 1c).

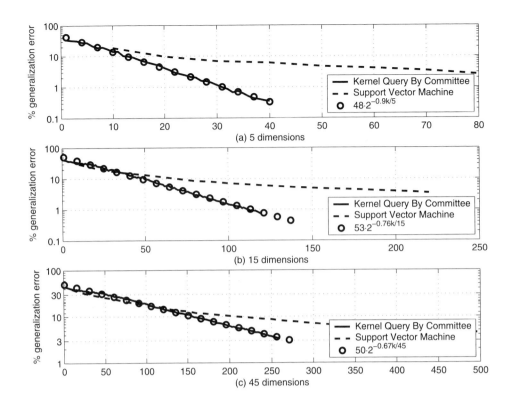

Figure 1: **Results on the synthetic data**. The generalization error (y-axis) in percents (in logarithmic scale) versus the number of queries (x-axis). Plots (a), (b) and (c) represent the synthetic task in 5, 15 and 45 dimensional spaces respectively. The generalization error of KQBC is compared to the generalization error of SVM. The results presented here are averaged over 50 trials. Note that the error rate of KQBC decreases exponentially fast. Recall that [6] proved a bound on the generalization error of $50 \cdot 2^{-0.67k/d}$ where k is the number of queries and d is the dimension.

5.2   Face Images Classification

The learning algorithm was then applied in a more realistic setting. In the second task we used the AR face images dataset [16]. The people in these images are wearing different accessories, have different facial expressions and the faces are lit from different directions. We selected a subset of 1456 images from this dataset. Each image was converted into gray-scale and re-sized to 85×60 pixels, i.e. each image was represented as a 5100 dimensional vector. See figure 2 for sample images. The task was to distinguish male and female images. For this purpose we split the data into a training sequence of 1000 images and a test sequence of 456 images. To test statistical significance we repeated this process 20 times, each time splitting the dataset into training and testing sequences.

We applied both KQBC and SVM to this dataset. We used the Gaussian kernel: $K(x_1, x_2) = \exp\left(-\|x_1 - x_2\|^2 / 2\sigma^2\right)$ where $\sigma = 3500$ which is the value favorable by SVM. The results are presented in figure 3. It is apparent from figure 3 that KQBC outperforms SVM. When the budget allows for $100 - 140$ labels, KQBC has an error rate of $2 - 3$ percent less than the error rate of SVM. When 140 labels are used, KQBC outperforms SVM by 3.6% on average. This difference is significant as in 90% of the trials

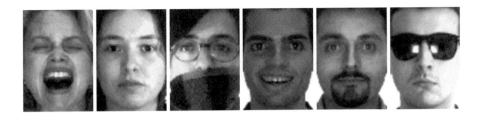

Figure 2: **Examples of face images used for the face recognition task**.

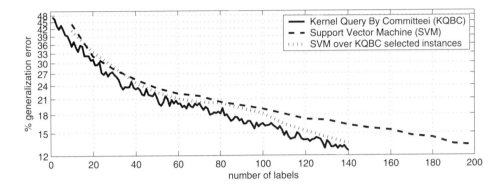

Figure 3: **The generalization error of KQBC and SVM for the faces dataset** (averaged over 20 trials). The generalization error (y-axis) vs. number of queries (x-axis) for KQBC (solid) and SVM (dashed) are compared. When SVM was applied solely to the instances selected by KQBC (dotted line) the results are better than SVM but worse than KQBC.

KQBC outperformed SVM by more than 1%. In one of the cases, KQBC was 11% better.

We also used KQBC as an active selection method for SVM. We trained SVM over the instances selected by KQBC. The generalization error obtained by this combined scheme was better than the passive SVM but worse than KQBC.

In figure 4 we see the last images for which KQBC queried for labels. It is apparent, that the selection made by KQBC is non-trivial. All the images are either highly saturated or partly covered by scarves and sunglasses. We conclude that KQBC indeed performs well even when kernels are used.

6 Summary and Further Study

In this paper we present a novel version of the QBC algorithm. This novel version is both efficient and rigorous. The time-complexity of our algorithm depends solely on the number of queries made and not on the input dimension or the VC-dimension of the class. Furthermore, our technique only requires inner products of the labeled data points - thus it can be implemented with kernels as well.

We showed a practical implementation of QBC using kernels and the hit and run random walk which is very close to the "provable" version. We conducted a couple of experiments with this novel algorithm. In all our experiments, KQBC outperformed SVM significantly. However, this experimental study needs to be extended. In the future, we would like to compare our algorithm with other active learning algorithms, over a variety of datasets.

449

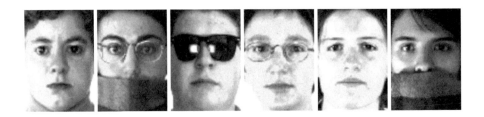

Figure 4: **Images selected by KQBC**. The last six faces for which KQBC queried for a label. Note that three of the images are saturated and that two of these are wearing a scarf that covers half of their faces.

References

[1] D. Cohn, L. Atlas, and R. Ladner. Training connectionist networks with queries and selective sampling. *Advanced in Neural Information Processing Systems 2*, 1990.

[2] H. S. Seung, M. Opper, and H. Sompolinsky. Query by committee. *Proc. of the Fifth Workshop on Computational Learning Theory*, pages 287–294, 1992.

[3] C. Campbell, N. Cristianini, and A. Smola. Query learning with large margin classifiers. In *Proc. 17'th International Conference on Machine Learning (ICML)*, 2000.

[4] S. Tong. *Active Learning: Theory and Applications*. PhD thesis, Stanford University, 2001.

[5] G. Tur, R. Schapire, and D. Hakkani-Tür. Active learning for spoken language understanding. In *Proc. IEEE International Conference on Acoustics, Speech and Signal Processing*, 2003.

[6] Y. Freund, H. Seung, E. Shamir, and N. Tishby. Selective sampling using the query by committee algorithm. *Machine Learning*, 28:133–168, 1997.

[7] H. Mamitsuka and N. Abe. Efficient data mining by active learning. In *Progress in Discovery Science*, pages 258–267, 2002.

[8] R. Bachrach, S. Fine, and E. Shamir. Query by committee, linear separation and random walks. *Theoretical Computer Science*, 284(1), 2002.

[9] L. Lovász and S. Vempala. Hit and run is fast and fun. Technical Report MSR-TR-2003-05, Microsoft Research, 2003.

[10] B. Boser, I. Guyon, and V. Vapnik. Optimal margin classifiers. In *Fifth Annual Workshop on Computational Learning Theory*, pages 144–152, 1992.

[11] S. Dasgupta. Analysis of a greedy active learning strategy. In *Neural Information Processing Systems (NIPS)*, 2004.

[12] S. Dasgupta, A. T. Kalai, and C. Monteleoni. Analysis of perceptron-based active learning. In *Proceeding of the 18th annual Conference on Learning Theory (COLT)*, 2005.

[13] R. Herbrich, T. Graepel, and C. Campbell. Bayes point machines. *Journal of Machine Learning Research*, 1:245–279, 2001.

[14] R. Gilad-Bachrach, A. Navot, and N. Tishby. Query by committee made real - supplementary material. http://www.cs.huji.ac.il/~ranb/kqcb_supp.ps.

[15] L. Lovász and S. Vempala. Hit-and-run from a corner. In *Proc. of the 36th ACM Symposium on the Theory of Computing (STOC)*, 2004.

[16] A.M. Martinez and R. Benavente. The ar face database. Technical report, CVC Tech. Rep. #24, 1998.

Metric Learning by Collapsing Classes

Amir Globerson
School of Computer Science and Engineering,
Interdisciplinary Center for Neural Computation
The Hebrew University Jerusalem, 91904, Israel
gamir@cs.huji.ac.il

Sam Roweis
Machine Learning Group
Department of Computer Science
University of Toronto, Canada
roweis@cs.toronto.edu

Abstract

We present an algorithm for learning a quadratic Gaussian metric (Mahalanobis distance) for use in classification tasks. Our method relies on the simple geometric intuition that a good metric is one under which points in the same class are simultaneously near each other and far from points in the other classes. We construct a convex optimization problem whose solution generates such a metric by trying to collapse all examples in the same class to a single point and push examples in other classes infinitely far away. We show that when the metric we learn is used in simple classifiers, it yields substantial improvements over standard alternatives on a variety of problems. We also discuss how the learned metric may be used to obtain a compact low dimensional feature representation of the original input space, allowing more efficient classification with very little reduction in performance.

1 Supervised Learning of Metrics

The problem of learning a distance measure (metric) over an input space is of fundamental importance in machine learning [10, 9], both supervised and unsupervised. When such measures are learned directly from the available data, they can be used to improve learning algorithms which rely on distance computations such as nearest neighbour classification [5], supervised kernel machines (such as GPs or SVMs) and even unsupervised clustering algorithms [10]. Good similarity measures may also provide insight into the underlying structure of data (e.g. inter-protein distances), and may aid in building better data visualizations via embedding. In fact, there is a close link between distance learning and feature extraction since whenever we construct a feature $f(x)$ for an input space X, we can measure distances between $x_1, x_2 \in X$ using a simple distance function (e.g. Euclidean) $d[f(x_1), f(x_2)]$ in feature space. Thus by fixing d, any feature extraction algorithm may be considered a metric learning method. Perhaps the simplest illustration of this approach is when the $f(x)$ is a linear projection of $\mathbf{x} \in \Re^r$ so that $f(\mathbf{x}) = W\mathbf{x}$. The Euclidean distance between $f(\mathbf{x}_1)$ and $f(\mathbf{x}_2)$ is then the Mahalanobis distance $\|f(\mathbf{x}_1) - f(\mathbf{x}_2)\|^2 = (\mathbf{x}_1 - \mathbf{x}_2)^T A(\mathbf{x}_1 - \mathbf{x}_2)$, where $A = W^T W$ is a positive semidefinite matrix. Much of the recent work on metric learning has indeed focused on learning Mahalanobis distances, i.e. learning the matrix A. This is also the goal of the current work.

A common approach to learning metrics is to assume some knowledge in the form of equivalence relations, i.e. which points should be close and which should be far (without speci-fying their exact distances). In the classification setting there is a natural equivalence rela-tion, namely whether two points are in the same class or not. One of the classical statistical methods which uses this idea for the Mahalanobis distance is Fisher's Linear Discriminant Analysis (see e.g. [6]). Other more recent methods are [10, 9, 5] which seek to minimize various separation criteria between the classes under the new metric.

In this work, we present a novel approach to learning such a metric. Our approach, the Maximally Collapsing Metric Learning algorithm (MCML), relies on the simple geometric intuition that if all points in the same class could be mapped into a single location in feature space and all points in other classes mapped to other locations, this would result in an ideal approximation of our equivalence relation. Our algorithm approximates this scenario via a stochastic selection rule, as in Neighborhood Component Analysis (NCA) [5]. However, unlike NCA, the optimization problem is convex and thus our method is completely spec-ified by our objective function. Different initialization and optimization techniques may affect the speed of obtaining the solution but the final solution itself is unique. We also show that our method approximates the local covariance structure of the data, as opposed to Linear Discriminant Analysis methods which use only global covariance structure.

2 The Approach of Collapsing Classes

Given a set of n labeled examples $(\mathbf{x}_i, y_i)$, where $\mathbf{x}_i \in \Re^r$ and $y_i \in \{1 \ldots k\}$, we seek a similarity measure between two points in X space. We focus on Mahalanobis form metrics

$$d(\mathbf{x}_i, \mathbf{x}_j | A) = d_{ij}^A = (\mathbf{x}_i - \mathbf{x}_j)^T A (\mathbf{x}_i - \mathbf{x}_j) \,, \tag{1}$$

where A is a positive semidefinite (PSD) matrix.

Intuitively, what we want from a good metric is that it makes elements of X in the same class look *close* whereas those in different classes appear *far*. Our approach starts with the ideal case when this is true in the most optimistic sense: same class points are at zero distance, and different class points are infinitely far. Alternatively this can be viewed as mapping $\mathbf{x}$ via a linear projection $W\mathbf{x}$ ($A = W^T W$), such that all points in the same class are mapped into the same point. This intuition is related to the analysis of spectral clustering [8], where the ideal case analysis of the algorithm results in all same cluster points being mapped to a single point.

To learn a metric which approximates the ideal geometric setup described above, we in-troduce, for each training point, a conditional distribution over other points (as in [5]). Specifically, for each $\mathbf{x}_i$ we define a conditional distribution over points $i \neq j$ such that

$$p^A(j|i) = \frac{1}{Z_i} e^{-d_{ij}^A} = \frac{e^{-d_{ij}^A}}{\sum_{k \neq i} e^{-d_{ik}^A}} \qquad i \neq j \,. \tag{2}$$

If all points in the same class were mapped to a single point and infinitely far from points in different classes, we would have the ideal "bi-level" distribution:

$$p_0(j|i) \propto \begin{cases} 1 & y_i = y_j \\ 0 & y_i \neq y_j \end{cases} . \tag{3}$$

Furthermore, under very mild conditions, any set of points which achieves the above distri-bution must have the desired geometry. In particular, assume there are at least $\hat{r} + 2$ points in each class, where $\hat{r} = \text{rank}[A]$ (note that $\hat{r} \leq r$). Then $p^A(j|i) = p_0(j|i)$ ($\forall i, j$) implies that under A all points in the same class will be mapped to a single point, infinitely far from other class points [1].

---

[1]Proof sketch: The infinite separation between points of different classes follows simply from

Thus it is natural to seek a matrix A such that $p^A(j|i)$ is as close as possible to $p_0(j|i)$. Since we are trying to match distributions, we minimize the KL divergence $KL[p_0|p]$:

$$\min_A \sum_i KL[p_0(j|i)|p^A(j|i)] \qquad \text{s.t. } A \in PSD \qquad (4)$$

The crucial property of this optimization problem is that it is *convex* in the matrix A. To see this, first note that any convex linear combination of feasible solutions $A = \alpha A_0 + (1 - \alpha)A_1$ s.t. $0 \le \alpha \le 1$ is still a feasible solution, since the set of PSD matrices is convex. Next, we can show that $f(A)$ alway has a greater cost than either of the endpoints. To do this, we rewrite the objective function $f(A) = \sum_i KL[p_0(j|i)|p(j|i)]$ in the form [2]:

$$f(A) = - \sum_{i,j:y_j=y_i} \log p(j|i) = \sum_{i,j:y_j=y_i} d_{ij}^A + \sum_i \log Z_i$$

where we assumed for simplicity that classes are equi-probable, yielding a multiplicative constant. To see why $f(A)$ is convex, first note that $d_{ij}^A = (\mathbf{x}_i - \mathbf{x}_j)^T A (\mathbf{x}_i - \mathbf{x}_j)$ is linear in A, and thus convex. The function $\log Z_i$ is a $\log \sum \exp$ function of affine functions of A and is therefore also convex (see [4], page 74).

2.1 Convex Duality

Since our optimization problem is convex, it has an equivalent convex dual. Specifically, the convex dual of Eq. (4) is the following entropy maximization problem:

$$\max_{p(j|i)} \sum_i H[p(j|i)] \qquad \text{s.t.} \quad \sum_i E_{p_0(j|i)}[\mathbf{v}_{ji}\mathbf{v}_{ji}^T] - \sum_i E_{p(j|i)}[\mathbf{v}_{ji}\mathbf{v}_{ji}^T] \succeq 0 \qquad (5)$$

where $\mathbf{v}_{ji} = \mathbf{x}_j - \mathbf{x}_i$, $H[\cdot]$ is the entropy function and we require $\sum_j p(j|i) = 1 \ \forall i$.

To prove this duality we start with the proposed dual and obtain the original problem in Equation 4 as its dual. Write the Lagrangian for the above problem (where λ is PSD) [3]

$$L(p, \lambda, \beta) = -\sum_i H(p(j|i)) - Tr(\lambda(\sum_i (E_{p_0}[\mathbf{v}_{ji}\mathbf{v}_{ji}^T] - E_p[\mathbf{v}_{ji}\mathbf{v}_{ji}^T]))) - \sum_i \beta_i (\sum_j p(j|i) - 1)$$

The dual function is defined as $g(\lambda, \beta) = \min_p L(p, \lambda, \beta)$. To derive it, we first solve for the minimizing p by setting the derivative of $L(p, \lambda, \beta)$ w.r.t. $p(j|i)$ equal to zero.

$$0 = 1 + \log p(j|i) + Tr(\lambda \mathbf{v}_{ji}\mathbf{v}_{ji}^T) - \beta_i \quad \Rightarrow \quad p(j|i) = e^{\beta_i - 1 - Tr(\lambda \mathbf{v}_{ji}\mathbf{v}_{ji}^T)}$$

Plugging this solution to $L(p, \lambda, \beta)$ we get $g(\lambda, \beta) = -Tr(\lambda \sum_i E_{p_0}[\mathbf{v}_{ji}\mathbf{v}_{ji}^T]) + \sum_i \beta_i - \sum_{i,j} p(j|i)$. The dual problem is to maximize $g(\lambda, \beta)$. We can do this analytically w.r.t. β_i, yielding $1 - \beta_i = \log \sum_j e^{-Tr(\lambda \mathbf{v}_{ji}\mathbf{v}_{ji}^T)}$.

Now note that $Tr(\lambda \mathbf{v}_{ji}\mathbf{v}_{ji}^T) = \mathbf{v}_{ji}^T \lambda \mathbf{v}_{ji} = d_{ji}^\lambda$, so we can write

$$g(\lambda) = - \sum_{i,j:y_i=y_j} d_{ji}^\lambda - \sum_i \log \sum_j e^{-d_{ji}^\lambda}$$

which is minus our original target function. Since $g(\lambda)$ should be maximized, and $\lambda \succeq 0$ we have the desired duality result (identifying λ with A).

$p_0(j|i) = 0$ when $y_j \ne y_i$. For a given point $\mathbf{x}_i$, all the points j in its class satisfy $p(j|i) \propto 1$. Due to the structure of $p(j|i)$ in Equation 2, and because it is obeyed for all points in $\mathbf{x}_i's$ class, this implies that all the points in that class are equidistant from each other. However, it is easy to show that the maximum number of *different* equidistant points (also known as the equilateral dimension [1]) in $\hat{r}$ dimensions is $\hat{r} + 1$. Since by assumption we have at least $\hat{r} + 2$ points in the class of $\mathbf{x}_i$, and A maps points into $\mathcal{R}^{\hat{r}}$, it follows that all points are identical.

[2] Up to an additive constant $- \sum_i H[p_0(j|i)]$.

[3] We consider the equivalent problem of minimizing minus entropy.

2.1.1 Relation to covariance based and embedding methods

The convex dual derived above reveals an interesting relation to covariance based learning methods. The sufficient statistics used by the algorithm are a set of n "spread" matrices. Each matrix is of the form $E_{p_0(j|i)}[\mathbf{v}_{ji}\mathbf{v}_{ji}^T]$. The algorithm tries to find a maximum entropy distribution which matches these matrices when averaged over the sample.

This should be contrasted with the covariance matrices used in metric learning such as Fisher's Discriminant Analysis. The latter uses the within and between class covariance matrices. The within covariance matrix is similar to the covariance matrix used here, but is calculated with respect to the class means, whereas here it is calculated separately for every point, and is centered on this point. This highlights the fact that MCML is not based on Gaussian assumptions where it is indeed sufficient to calculate a single class covariance.

Our method can also be thought of as a supervised version of the Stochastic Neighbour Embedding algorithm [7] in which the "target" distribution is p_0 (determined by the class labels) and the embedding points are not completely free but are instead constrained to be of the form $W\mathbf{x}_i$.

2.2 Optimizing the Convex Objective

Since the optimization problem in Equation 4 is convex, it is guaranteed to have only a single minimum which is the globally optimal solution[4]. It can be optimized using any appropriate numerical convex optimization machinery; all methods will yield the same solution although some may be faster than others. One standard approach is to use interior point Newton methods. However, these algorithms require the Hessian to be calculated, which would require $O(d^4)$ resources, and could be prohibitive in our case. Instead, we have experimented with using a first order gradient method, specifically the projected gradient approach as in [10]. At each iteration we take a small step in the direction of the negative gradient of the objective function[5], followed by a projection back onto the PSD cone. This projection is performed simply by taking the eigen-decomposition of A and removing the components with negative eigenvalues. The algorithm is summarized below:

Input: Set of labeled data points $(\mathbf{x}_i, y_i)$, $i = 1 \ldots n$

Output: PSD metric which optimally *collapses* classes.

Initialization: Initialize A_0 to some PSD matrix
                       (randomly or using some initialization heuristic).

Iterate:

- Set $A_{t+1} = A_t - \epsilon \triangledown f(A_t)$ where
$\triangledown f(A) = \sum_{ij}(p_0(j|i) - p(j|i))(\mathbf{x}_j - \mathbf{x}_i)(\mathbf{x}_j - \mathbf{x}_i)^T$
- Calculate the eigen-decomposition of A_{t+1}
$A_{t+1} = \sum_k \lambda_k \mathbf{u}_k \mathbf{u}_k^T$, then set $A_{t+1} = \sum_k \max(\lambda_k, 0)\mathbf{u}_k \mathbf{u}_k^T$

Of course in principle it is possible to optimize over the dual instead of the primal but in our case, if the training data consists of n points in r-dimensional space then the primal has only $O(r^2/2)$ variables while the dual has $O(n^2)$ so it will almost always be more efficient to operate on the primal A directly. One exception to this case may be the kernel version (Section 4) where the primal is also of size $O(n^2)$.

---

[4] When the data can be exactly collapsed into single class points, there will be multiple solutions at infinity. However, this is very unlikely to happen in real data.

[5] In the experiments, we used an Armijo like step size rule, as described in [3].

3   Low Dimensional Projections for Feature Extraction

The Mahalanobis distance under a metric A can be interpreted as a linear projection of the original inputs by the square root of A, followed by Euclidean distance in the projected space. Matrices A which have less than full rank correspond to Mahalanobis distances based on low dimensional projections. Such metrics and the induced distances can be advantageous for several reasons [5]. First, low dimensional projections can substantially reduce the storage and computational requirements of a supervised method since only the projections of the training points must be stored and the manipulations at test time all occur in the lower dimensional feature space. Second, low dimensional projections re-represent the inputs, allowing for a supervised embedding or visualization of the original data.

If we consider matrices A with rank at most q, we can always represent them in the form $A = W^T W$ for some projection matrix W of size $q \times r$. This corresponds to projecting the original data into a q-dimensional space specified by the rows of W. However, rank constraints on a matrix are not convex [4], and hence the rank constrained problem is not convex and is likely to have local minima which make the optimization difficult and ill-defined since it becomes sensitive to initial conditions and choice of optimization method.

Luckily, there is an alternative approach to obtaining low dimensional projections, which *does* specify a unique solution by sequentially solving two globally tractable problems. This is the approach we follow here. First we solve for a (potentially) full rank metric A using the convex program outlined above, and then obtain a low rank projection from it via spectral decomposition. This is done by diagonalizing A into the form $A = \sum_{i=1}^{r} \lambda_i \mathbf{v}_i \mathbf{v}_i^T$ where $\lambda_1 \geq \lambda_2 \ldots \lambda_r$ are eigenvalues of A and $\mathbf{v}_i$ are the corresponding eigenvectors. To obtain a low rank projection we constrain the sum above to include only the q terms corresponding to the q largest eigenvalues: $A_q = \sum_{i=1}^{q} \lambda_i \mathbf{v}_i \mathbf{v}_i^T$. The resulting projection is uniquely defined (up to an irrelevant unitary transformation) as $W = \text{diag}(\sqrt{\lambda_1}, \ldots \sqrt{\lambda_q})[\mathbf{v}_1^T; \ldots; \mathbf{v}_q^T]$.

In general, the projection returned by this approach is not guaranteed to be the same as the projection corresponding to minimizing our objective function subject to a rank constraint on A unless the optimal metric A is of rank less than or equal to q. However, as we show in the experimental results, it is often the case that for practical problems the optimal A has an eigen-spectrum which is rapidly decaying, so that many of its eigenvalues are indeed very small, suggesting the low rank solution will be close to optimal.

4   Learning Metrics with Kernels

It is interesting to consider the case where $\mathbf{x}_i$ are mapped into a high dimensional feature space $\phi(\mathbf{x}_i)$ and a Mahalanobis distance is sought in this space. We focus on the case where dot products in the feature space may be expressed via a kernel function, such that $\phi(\mathbf{x}_i) \cdot \phi(\mathbf{x}_j) = k(\mathbf{x}_i, \mathbf{x}_j)$ for some kernel k. We now show how our method can be changed to accommodate this setting, so that optimization depends only on dot products. Consider the regularized target function:

$$f_{Reg}(A) = \sum_i \text{KL}[p_0(j|i)|p(j|i)] + \lambda Tr(A), \tag{6}$$

where the regularizing factor is equivalent to the Frobenius norm of the projection matrix W since $Tr(A) = \|W\|^2$. Deriving w.r.t. W we obtain $W = UX$, where U is some matrix which specifies W as a linear combination of sample points, and the ith row of the matrix X is $\mathbf{x}_i$. Thus A is given by $A = X^T U^T U X$. Defining the PSD matrix $\hat{A} = U^T U$, we can recast our optimization as looking for a PSD matrix $\hat{A}$, where the Mahalanobis distance is $(\mathbf{x}_i - \mathbf{x}_j)^T X^T \hat{A} X (\mathbf{x}_i - \mathbf{x}_j) = (\mathbf{k}_i - \mathbf{k}_j)^T \hat{A}(\mathbf{k}_i - \mathbf{k}_j)$, where we define $\mathbf{k}_i = X \mathbf{x}_i$.

This is exactly our original distance, with $\mathbf{x}_i$ replaced by $\mathbf{k}_i$, which depends only on dot products in X space. The regularization term also depends solely on the dot products since $Tr(A) = Tr(X^T \hat{A} X) = Tr(XX^T \hat{A}) = Tr(K\hat{A})$, where K is the kernel matrix given by $K = XX^T$. Note that the trace is a linear function of $\hat{A}$, keeping the problem convex. Thus, as long as dot products can be represented via kernels, the optimization can be carried out without explicitly using the high dimensional space.

To obtain a low dimensional solution, we follow the approach in Section 3: obtain a decomposition $A = V^T DV$ [6], and take the projection matrix to be the first q rows of $D^{0.5}V$. As a first step, we calculate a matrix B such that $\hat{A} = B^T B$, and thus $A = X^T B^T BX$. Since A is a correlation matrix for the rows of BX it can be shown (as in Kernel PCA) that its (left) eigenvectors are linear combinations of the rows of BX. Denoting by $V = \alpha BX$ the eigenvector matrix, we obtain, after some algebra, that $\alpha BKB^T = D\alpha$. We conclude that α is an eigenvector of the matrix BKB^T. Denote by $\hat{\alpha}$ the matrix whose rows are orthonormal eigenvectors of BKB^T. Then V can be shown to be orthonormal if we set $V = D^{-0.5}\hat{\alpha} BX$. The final projection will then be $D^{0.5}V\mathbf{x}_i = \hat{\alpha} B\mathbf{k}_i$. Low dimensional projections will be obtained by keeping only the first q components of this projection.

5   Experimental Results

We compared our method to several metric learning algorithms on a supervised classification task. Training data was first used to learn a metric over the input space. Then this metric was used in a 1-nearest-neighbor algorithm to classify a test set. The datasets we investigated were taken from the UCI repository and have been used previously in evaluating supervised methods for metric learning [10, 5]. To these we added the USPS handwritten digits (downsampled to 8x8 pixels) and the YALE faces [2] (downsampled to 31x22).

The algorithms used in the comparative evaluation were

- Fisher's Linear Discriminant Analysis (LDA), which projects on the eigenvectors of $S_W^{-1} S_B$ where S_W, S_B are the within and between class covariance matrices.
- The method of Xing et al [10] which minimizes the mean *within class* distance, while keeping the mean *between class* distance larger than one.
- Principal Component Analysis (PCA). There are several possibilities for scaling the PCA projections. We tested several, and report results of the empirically superior one (PCAW), which scales the projection components so that the covariance matrix after projection is the identity. PCAW often performs poorly on high dimensions, but globally outperforms all other variants.

We also evaluated the kernel version of MCML with an RBF kernel (denoted by KM-CML)[7]. Since all methods allow projections to lower dimensions we compared performance for different projection dimensions [8].

The out-of sample performance results (based on 40 random splits of the data taking 70% for training and 30% for testing[9]) are shown in Figure 1. It can be seen that when used in a simple nearest-neighbour classifier, the metric learned by MCML almost always performs as well as, or significantly better than those learned by all other methods, across most dimensions. Furthermore, the kernel version of MCML outperforms the linear one on most datasets.

---

[6] Where V is orthonormal, and the eigenvalues in D are sorted in decreasing order.

[7] The regularization parameter λ and the width of the RBF kernel were chosen using 5 fold cross-validation. KMCML was only evaluated for datasets with less than 1000 training points.

[8] To obtain low dimensional mappings we used the approach outlined in Section 3.

[9] Except for the larger datasets where 1000 random samples were used for training.

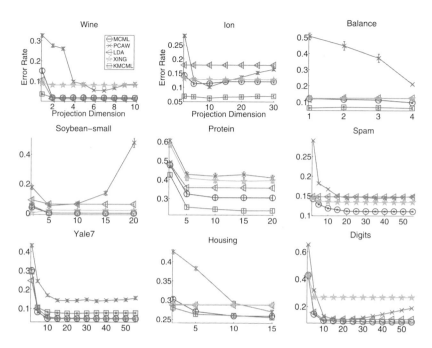

Figure 1: Classification error rate on several UCI datasets, USPS digits and YALE faces, for different projection dimensions. Algorithms are our Maximally Collapsing Metric Learning (MCML), Xing et.al.[10], PCA with whitening transformation (PCAW) and Fisher's Discriminant Analysis (LDA). Standard errors of the means shown on curves. No results given for XING on YALE and KMCML on Digits and Spam due to the data size.

5.1 Comparison to non convex procedures

The methods in the previous comparison are all well defined, in the sense that they are not susceptible to local minima in the optimization. They also have the added advantage of obtaining projections to all dimensions using one optimization run. Below, we also compare the MCML results to the results of two non-convex procedures. The first is the Non Convex variant of MCML (NMCML): The objective function of MCML can be optimized w.r.t the projection matrix W, where $A = W^T W$. Although this is no longer a convex problem, it is not constrained and is thus easier to optimize. The second non convex method is Neighbourhood Components Analysis (NCA) [5], which attempts to directly minimize the error incurred by a nearest neighbor classifier.

For both methods we optimized the matrix W by restarting the optimization separately for each size of W. Minimization was performed using a conjugate gradient algorithm, initialized by LDA or randomly. Figure 2 shows results on a subset of the UCI datasets. It can be seen that the performance of NMCML is similar to that of MCML, although it is less stable, possibly due to local minima, and both methods usually outperform NCA. The inset in each figure shows the spectrum of the MCML matrix A, revealing that it often drops quickly after a few dimensions. This illustrates the effectiveness of our two stage optimization procedure, and suggests its low dimensional solutions are close to optimal.

6 Discussion and Extensions

We have presented an algorithm for learning maximally collapsing metrics (MCML), based on the intuition of collapsing classes into single points. MCML assumes that each class

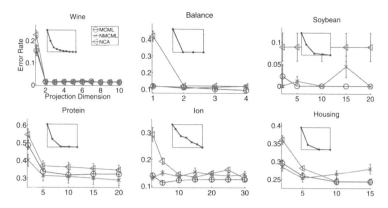

Figure 2: Classification error for non convex procedures, and the MCML method. Eigen-spectra for the MCML solution are shown in the inset.

may be collapsed to a single point, at least approximately, and thus is only suitable for unimodal class distributions (or for simply connected sets if kernelization is used). However, if points belonging to a single class appear in several disconnected clusters in input (or feature) space, it is unlikely that MCML could collapse the class into a single point. It is possible that using a mixture of distributions, an EM-like algorithm can be constructed to accommodate this scenario.

The method can also be used to learn low dimensional projections of the input space. We showed that it performs well, even across a range of projection dimensions, and consistently outperforms existing methods. Finally, we have shown how the method can be extended to projections in high dimensional feature spaces using the kernel trick. The resulting nonlinear method was shown to improve classification results over the linear version.

References

[1] N. Alon and P. Pudlak. Equilateral sets in l_p^n. *Geom. Funct. Anal.*, 13(3), 2003.

[2] P. N. Belhumeur, J. Hespanha, and D. J. Kriegman. Eigenfaces vs. Fisherfaces: Recognition using class specific linear projection. In *ECCV (1)*, 1996.

[3] D.P. Bertsekas. On the Goldstein-Levitin-Polyak gradient projection method. *IEEE Transaction on Automatic Control*, 21(2):174–184, 1976.

[4] S. Boyd and L. Vandenberghe. *Convex Optimization*. Cambridge Univ. Press, 2004.

[5] J. Goldberger, S. Roweis, G. Hinton, and R. Salakhutdinov. Neighbourhood components analysis. In *Advances in Neural Information Processing Systems (NIPS)*, 2004.

[6] T. Hastie, R. Tibshirani, and J.H. Friedman. *The elements of statistical learning: data mining, inference, and prediction*. New York: Springer-Verlag, 2001.

[7] G. Hinton and S. Roweis. Stochastic neighbor embedding. In *Advances in Neural Information Processing Systems (NIPS)*, 2002.

[8] A. Ng, M. Jordan, and Y. Weiss. On spectral clustering: Analysis and an algorithm. In *Advances in Neural Information Processing Systems (NIPS)*, 2001.

[9] N. Shental, T. Hertz, D. Weinshall, and M. Pavel. Adjustment learning and relevant component analysis. In *Proc. of ECCV*, 2002.

[10] E. Xing, A. Ng, M. Jordan, and S. Russell. Distance metric learning, with application to clustering with side-information. In *Advances in Neural Information Processing Systems (NIPS)*, 2004.

Interpolating Between Types and Tokens by Estimating Power-Law Generators *

Sharon Goldwater   **Thomas L. Griffiths**   **Mark Johnson**
Department of Cognitive and Linguistic Sciences
Brown University, Providence RI 02912, USA
{sharon_goldwater,tom_griffiths,mark_johnson}@brown.edu

Abstract

Standard statistical models of language fail to capture one of the most striking properties of natural languages: the power-law distribution in the frequencies of word tokens. We present a framework for developing statistical models that generically produce power-laws, augmenting standard generative models with an *adaptor* that produces the appropriate pattern of token frequencies. We show that taking a particular stochastic process – the Pitman-Yor process – as an adaptor justifies the appearance of type frequencies in formal analyses of natural language, and improves the performance of a model for unsupervised learning of morphology.

1   Introduction

In general it is important for models used in unsupervised learning to be able to describe the gross statistical properties of the data they are intended to learn from, otherwise these properties may distort inferences about the parameters of the model. One of the most striking statistical properties of natural languages is that the distribution of word frequencies is closely approximated by a power-law. That is, the probability that a word w will occur with frequency n_w in a sufficiently large corpus is proportional to n_w^{-g}. This observation, which is usually attributed to Zipf [1] but enjoys a long and detailed history [2], stimulated intense research in the 1950s (e.g., [3]) but has largely been ignored in modern computational linguistics. By developing models that generically exhibit power-laws, it may be possible to improve methods for unsupervised learning of linguistic structure.

In this paper, we introduce a framework for developing generative models for language that produce power-law distributions. Our framework is based upon the idea of specifying language models in terms of two components: a *generator*, an underlying generative model for words which need not (and usually does not) produce a power-law distribution, and an *adaptor*, which transforms the stream of words produced by the generator into one whose frequencies obey a power law distribution. This framework is extremely general: any generative model for language can be used as a generator, with the power-law distribution being produced as the result of making an appropriate choice for the adaptor.

In our framework, estimation of the parameters of the generator will be affected by assumptions about the form of the adaptor. We show that use of a particular adaptor, the Pitman-Yor process [4, 5, 6], sheds light on a tension exhibited by formal approaches to natural language: whether explanations should be based upon the *types* of words that languages

---
*This work was partially supported by NSF awards IGERT 9870676 and ITR 0085940 and NIMH award 1R0-IMH60922-01A2

exhibit, or the frequencies with which *tokens* of those words occur. One place where this tension manifests is in accounts of morphology, where formal linguists develop accounts of why particular words appear in the lexicon (e.g., [7]), while computational linguists focus on statistical models of the frequencies of tokens of those words (e.g., [8]). The tension between types and tokens also appears within computational linguistics. For example, one of the most successful forms of smoothing used in statistical language models, Kneser-Ney smoothing, explicitly interpolates between type and token frequencies [9, 10, 11].

The plan of the paper is as follows. Section 2 discusses stochastic processes that can produce power-law distributions, including the Pitman-Yor process. Section 3 specifies a two-stage language model that uses the Pitman-Yor process as an adaptor, and examines some properties of this model: Section 3.1 shows that estimation based on type and token frequencies are special cases of this two-stage language model, and Section 3.2 uses these results to provide a novel justification for the use of Kneser-Ney smoothing. Section 4 describes a model for unsupervised learning of the morphological structure of words that uses our framework, and demonstrates that its performance improves as we move from estimation based upon tokens to types. Section 5 concludes the paper.

2   Producing power-law distributions

Assume we want to generate a sequence of N outcomes, $\mathbf{z} = \{z_1, \ldots, z_N\}$ with each outcome z_i being drawn from a set of (possibly unbounded) size Z. Many of the stochastic processes that produce power-laws are based upon the principle of *preferential attachment*, where the probability that the ith outcome, z_i, takes on a particular value k depends upon the frequency of k in $\mathbf{z}_{-i} = \{z_1, \ldots, z_{i-1}\}$ [2]. For example, one of the earliest and most widely used preferential attachment schemes [3] chooses z_i according to the distribution

$$P(z_i = k \mid \mathbf{z}_{-i}) = a\frac{1}{Z} + (1-a)\frac{n_k^{(\mathbf{z}_{-i})}}{i-1} \tag{1}$$

where $n_k^{(\mathbf{z}_{-i})}$ is the number of times k occurs in $\mathbf{z}_{-i}$. This "rich-get-richer" process means that a few outcomes appear with very high frequency in $\mathbf{z}$ – the key attribute of a power-law distribution. In this case, the power-law has parameter $g = 1/(1-a)$.

One problem with these classical models is that they assume a fixed ordering on the outcomes $\mathbf{z}$. While this may be appropriate for some settings, the assumption of a temporal ordering restricts the contexts in which such models can be applied. In particular, it is much more restrictive than the assumption of independent sampling that underlies most statistical language models. Consequently, we will focus on a different preferential attachment scheme, based upon the two-parameter species sampling model [4, 5] known as the Pitman-Yor process [6]. Under this scheme outcomes follow a power-law distribution, but remain *exchangeable*: the probability of a set of outcomes is not affected by their ordering.

The Pitman-Yor process can be viewed as a generalization of the Chinese restaurant process [6]. Assume that N customers enter a restaurant with infinitely many tables, each with infinite seating capacity. Let z_i denote the table chosen by the ith customer. The first customer sits at the first table, $z_1 = 1$. The ith customer chooses table k with probability

$$P(z_i = k \mid \mathbf{z}_{-i}) = \begin{cases} \frac{n_k^{(\mathbf{z}_{-i})} - a}{i-1+b} & k \leq K(\mathbf{z}_{-i}) \\ \frac{K(\mathbf{z}_{-i})a+b}{i-1+b} & k = K(\mathbf{z}_{-i}) + 1 \end{cases} \tag{2}$$

where a and b are the two parameters of the process and $K(\mathbf{z}_{-i})$ is the number of tables that are currently occupied.

The Pitman-Yor process satisfies our need for a process that produces power-laws while retaining exchangeability. Equation 2 is clearly a preferential attachment scheme. When

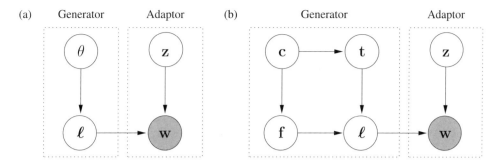

Figure 1: Graphical models showing dependencies among variables in (a) the simple two-stage model, and (b) the morphology model. Shading of the node containing **w** reflects the fact that this variable is observed. Dotted lines delimit the generator and adaptor.

$a = 0$ and $b > 0$, it reduces to the standard Chinese restaurant process [12, 4] used in Dirichlet process mixture models [13]. When $0 < a < 1$, the number of people seated at each table follows a power-law distribution with $g = 1 + a$ [5]. It is straightforward to show that the customers are exchangeable: the probability of a partition of customers into sets seated at different tables is unaffected by the order in which the customers were seated.

3 A two-stage language model

We can use the Pitman-Yor process as the foundation for a language model that generically produces power-law distributions. We will define a two-stage model by extending the restaurant metaphor introduced above. Imagine that each table k is labelled with a word ℓ_k from a vocabulary of (possibly unbounded) size W. The first stage is to generate these labels, sampling ℓ_k from a generative model for words that we will refer to as the *generator*. For example, we could choose to draw the labels from a multinomial distribution θ. The second stage is to generate the actual sequence of words itself. This is done by allowing a sequence of customers to enter the restaurant. Each customer chooses a table, producing a seating arrangement, **z**, and says the word used to label that table, producing a sequence of words, **w**. The process by which customers choose tables, which we will refer to as the *adaptor*, defines a probability distribution over the sequence of words **w** produced by the customers, determining the frequency with which tokens of the different types occur. The statistical dependencies among the variables in one such model are shown in Figure 1 (a).

Given the discussion in the previous section, the Pitman-Yor process is a natural choice for an adaptor. The result is technically a Pitman-Yor mixture model, with z_i indicating the "class" responsible for generating the ith word, and ℓ_k determining the multinomial distribution over words associated with class k, with $P(w_i = w \,|\, z_i = k, \ell_k) = 1$ if $\ell_k = w$, and 0 otherwise. Under this model the probability that the ith customer produces word w given previously produced words $\mathbf{w}_{-i}$ and current seating arrangement $\mathbf{z}_{-i}$ is

$$P(w_i = w \,|\, \mathbf{w}_{-i}, \mathbf{z}_{-i}, \theta) = \sum_k \sum_{\ell_k} P(w_i = w \,|\, z_i = k, \ell_k) P(\ell_k \,|\, \mathbf{w}_{-i}, \mathbf{z}_{-i}, \theta) P(z_i = k \,|\, \mathbf{z}_{-i})$$

$$= \sum_{k=1}^{K(\mathbf{z}_{-i})} \frac{n_k^{(\mathbf{z}_{-i})} - a}{i - 1 + b} I(\ell_k = w) + \frac{K(\mathbf{z}_{-i})a + b}{i - 1 + b} \theta_w \qquad (3)$$

where $I(\cdot)$ is an indicator function, being 1 when its argument is true and 0 otherwise. If θ is uniform over all W words, then the distribution over **w** reduces to the Pitman-Yor process as $W \to \infty$. Otherwise, multiple tables can receive the same label, increasing the frequency of the corresponding word and producing a distribution with $g < 1 + a$. Again, it is straightforward to show that words are exchangeable under this distribution.

3.1 Types and tokens

The use of the Pitman-Yor process as an adaptor provides a justification for the role of word types in formal analyses of natural language. This can be seen by considering the question of how to estimate the parameters of the multinomial distribution used as a generator, θ.[1] In general, the parameters of generators can be estimated using Markov chain Monte Carlo methods, as we demonstrate in Section 4. In this section, we will show that estimation schemes based upon type and token frequencies are special cases of our language model, corresponding to the extreme values of the parameter a. Values of a between these extremes identify estimation methods that interpolate between types and tokens.

Taking a multinomial distribution with parameters θ as a generator and the Pitman-Yor process as an adaptor, the probability of a sequence of words $\mathbf{w}$ given θ is

$$P(\mathbf{w}\,|\,\theta) = \sum_{\mathbf{z},\boldsymbol{\ell}} P(\mathbf{w},\mathbf{z},\boldsymbol{\ell}\,|\,\theta) = \sum_{\mathbf{z},\boldsymbol{\ell}} \frac{\Gamma(b)}{\Gamma(N+b)} \prod_{k=1}^{K(\mathbf{z})} \left(\theta_{\ell_k}((k-1)a+b)\frac{\Gamma(n_k^{(\mathbf{z})}-a)}{\Gamma(1-a)} \right)$$

where in the last sum $\mathbf{z}$ and $\boldsymbol{\ell}$ are constrained such that $\ell_{z_i} = w_i$ for all i. In the case where $b = 0$, this simplifies to

$$P(\mathbf{w}\,|\,\theta) = \sum_{\mathbf{z},\boldsymbol{\ell}} \left(\prod_{k=1}^{K(\mathbf{z})} \theta_{\ell_k} \right) \cdot \frac{\Gamma(K(\mathbf{z}))}{\Gamma(N)} \cdot a^{K(\mathbf{z})} \cdot \left(\prod_{k=1}^{K(\mathbf{z})} \frac{\Gamma(n_k^{(\mathbf{z})}-a)}{\Gamma(1-a)} \right) \tag{4}$$

The distribution $P(\mathbf{w}\,|\,\theta)$ determines how the data $\mathbf{w}$ influence estimates of θ, so we will consider how $P(\mathbf{w}\,|\,\theta)$ changes under different limits of a.

In the limit as a approaches 1, estimation of θ is based upon word tokens. When $a \to 1$, $\frac{\Gamma(n_k^{\mathbf{z}}-a)}{\Gamma(1-a)}$ is 1 for $n_k^{(\mathbf{z})} = 1$ but approaches 0 for $n_k^{(\mathbf{z})} > 1$. Consequently, all terms in the sum over $(\mathbf{z},\boldsymbol{\ell})$ go to zero, except that in which every word token has its own table. In this case, $K(\mathbf{z}) = N$ and $\ell_k = w_k$. It follows that $\lim_{a\to 1} P(\mathbf{w}\,|\,\theta) = \prod_{k=1}^{N} \theta_{w_k}$. Any form of estimation using $P(\mathbf{w}\,|\,\theta)$ will thus be based upon the frequencies of word tokens in $\mathbf{w}$.

In the limit as a approaches 0, estimation of θ is based upon word types. The appearance of $a^{K(\mathbf{z})}$ in Equation 4 means that as $a \to 0$, the sum over $\mathbf{z}$ is dominated by the seating arrangement that minimizes the total number of tables. Under the constraint that $\ell_{z_i} = w_i$ for all i, this minimal configuration is the one in which every word type receives a single table. Consequently, $\lim_{a\to 0} P(\mathbf{w}\,|\,\theta)$ is dominated by a term in which there is a single instance of θ_w for each word w that appears in $\mathbf{w}$.[2] Any form of estimation using $P(\mathbf{w}\,|\,\theta)$ will thus be based upon a single instance of each word type in $\mathbf{w}$.

3.2 Predictions and smoothing

In addition to providing a justification for the role of types in formal analyses of language in general, use of the Pitman-Yor process as an adaptor can be used to explain the assumptions behind a specific scheme for combining token and type frequencies: Kneser-Ney smoothing.[3] Smoothing methods are schemes for regularizing empirical estimates of the probabilities of words, with the goal of improving the predictive performance of language

---

[1] Under the interpretation of this model as a Pitman-Yor process mixture model, this is analogous to estimating the base measure G_0 in a Dirichlet process mixture model (e.g. [13]).

[2] Despite the fact that $P(\mathbf{w}\,|\,\theta)$ approaches 0 in this limit, $a^{K(\mathbf{z})}$ will be constant across all choices of θ. Consequently, estimation schemes that depend only on the non-constant terms in $P(\mathbf{w}\,|\,\theta)$, such as maximum-likelihood or Bayesian inference, will remain well defined.

[3] A similar observation was recently independently made in [14].

models. The Kneser-Ney smoother estimates the probability of a word by combining type and token frequencies, and has proven particularly effective for n-gram models [9, 10, 11].

To use an n-gram language model, we need to estimate the probability distribution over words given their *history*, i.e. the n preceding words. Assume we are given a vector of N words $\mathbf{w}$ that all share a common history, and want to predict the next word, w_{N+1}, that will occur with that history. Assume that we also have vectors of words from H other histories, $\mathbf{w}^{(1)}, \ldots, \mathbf{w}^{(H)}$. The interpolated Kneser-Ney smoother [11] makes the prediction

$$P(w_{N+1} = w \mid \mathbf{w}) = \frac{n_w^{(\mathbf{w})} - I(n_w^{(\mathbf{w})} > D)D}{N} + \frac{\sum_w I(n_w^{(\mathbf{w})} > D)D}{N} \frac{\sum_h I(w \in \mathbf{w}^{(h)})}{\sum_w \sum_h I(w \in \mathbf{w}^{(h)})} \quad (5)$$

where we have suppressed the dependence on $\mathbf{w}^{(1)}, \ldots, \mathbf{w}^{(H)}$, D is a "discount factor" specified as a parameter of the model, and the sum over h includes $\mathbf{w}$.

We can define a two-stage model appropriate for this setting by assuming that the sets of words for all histories are produced by the same adaptor and generator. Under this model, the probability of word w_{N+1} given $\mathbf{w}$ and θ is

$$P(w_{N+1} = w \mid \mathbf{w}, \theta) = \sum_{\mathbf{z}} P(w_{N+1} = w | \mathbf{w}, \mathbf{z}, \theta) P(\mathbf{z} | \mathbf{w}, \theta)$$

where $P(w_{N+1} = w | \mathbf{w}, \mathbf{z}, \theta)$ is given by Equation 3. Assuming $b = 0$, this becomes

$$P(w_{N+1} = w \mid \mathbf{w}, \theta) = \frac{n_w^{\mathbf{w}} - E_{\mathbf{z}}[K_w(\mathbf{z})] a}{N} + \frac{\sum_w E_{\mathbf{z}}[K_w(\mathbf{z})] a}{N} \theta_w \quad (6)$$

where $E_{\mathbf{z}}[K_w(\mathbf{z})] = \sum_{\mathbf{z}} K_w(\mathbf{z}) P(\mathbf{z} | \mathbf{w}, \theta)$, and $K_w(\mathbf{z})$ is the number of tables with label w under the seating assignment $\mathbf{z}$. The other histories enter into this expression via θ. Since the words associated with each history is assumed to be produced from a single set of parameters θ, the maximum-likelihood estimate of θ_w will approach

$$\theta_w = \frac{\sum_h I(w \in \mathbf{w}^{(h)})}{\sum_w \sum_h I(w \in \mathbf{w}^{(h)})}$$

as a approaches 0, since only a single instance of each word type in each context will contribute to the estimate of θ. Substituting this value of θ_w into Equation 6 reveals the correspondence to the Kneser-Ney smoother (Equation 5). The only difference is that the constant discount factor D is replaced by $a E_{\mathbf{z}}[K_w(\mathbf{z})]$, which will increase slowly as n_w increases. This difference might actually lead to an improved smoother: the Kneser-Ney smoother seems to produce better performance when D increases as a function of n_w [11].

4 Types and tokens in modeling morphology

Our attempt to develop statistical models of language that generically produce power-law distributions was motivated by the possibility that models that account for this statistical regularity might be able to learn linguistic information better than those that do not. Our two-stage language modeling framework allows us to create exactly these sorts of models, with the generator producing individual lexical items, and the adaptor producing the power-law distribution over words. In this section, we show that taking a generative model for morphology as the generator and varying the parameters of the adaptor results in an improvement in unsupervised learning of the morphological structure of English.

4.1 A generative model for morphology

Many languages contain words built up of smaller units of meaning, or *morphemes*. These units can contain lexical information (as stems) or grammatical information (as affixes).

For example, the English word *walked* can be parsed into the stem *walk* and the past-tense suffix *ed*. Knowledge of morphological structure enables language learners to understand and produce novel wordforms, and facilitates tasks such as stemming (e.g., [15]).

As a basic model of morphology, we assume that each word consists of a single stem and suffix, and belongs to some inflectional class. Each class is associated with a stem distribution and a suffix distribution. We assume that stems and suffixes are independent given the class, so we have

$$P(\ell_k = w) = \sum_{c,t,f} I(w = t.f)P(c_k = c)P(t_k = t \mid c_k = c)P(f_k = f \mid c_k = c) \quad (7)$$

where c_k, t_k, and f_k are the class, stem, and suffix associated with ℓ_k, and $t.f$ indicates the concatenation of t and f. In other words, we generate a label by first drawing a class, then drawing a stem and a suffix conditioned on the class. Each of these draws is from a multinomial distribution, and we will assume that these multinomials are in turn generated from symmetric Dirichlet priors, with parameters κ, τ, and ϕ respectively. The resulting generative model can be used as the generator in a two-stage language model, providing a more structured replacement for the multinomial distribution, θ. As before, we will use the Pitman-Yor process as an adaptor, setting $b = 0$. Figure 1 (b) illustrates the dependencies between the variables in this model.

Our morphology model is similar to that used by Goldsmith in his unsupervised morphological learning system [8], with two important differences. First, Goldsmith's model is recursive, i.e. a word stem can be further split into a smaller stem plus suffix. Second, Goldsmith's model assumes that all occurrences of each word type have the same analysis, whereas our model allows different tokens of the same type to have different analyses.

4.2 Inference by Gibbs sampling

Our goal in defining this morphology model is to be able to automatically infer the morphological structure of a language. This can be done using Gibbs sampling, a standard Markov chain Monte Carlo (MCMC) method [16]. In MCMC, variables in the model are repeatedly sampled, with each sample conditioned on the current values of all other variables in the model. This process defines a Markov chain whose stationary distribution is the posterior distribution over model variables given the input data.

Rather than sampling all the variables in our two-stage model simultaneously, our Gibbs sampler alternates between sampling the variables in the generator and those in the adaptor. Fixing the assignment of words to tables, we sample c_k, t_k, and f_k for each table from

$$\begin{aligned} P(c_k = c, t_k = t, f_k = f \mid \mathbf{c}_{-k}, \mathbf{t}_{-k}, \mathbf{f}_{-k}, \ell) \\ \propto \quad I(\ell_k = t_k.f_k) \quad P(c_k = c \mid \mathbf{c}_{-k}) \quad P(t_k = t \mid \mathbf{t}_{-k}, c) \quad P(f_k = f \mid \mathbf{f}_{-k}, c) \\ = \quad I(\ell_k = t_k.f_k) \cdot \frac{n_c + \kappa}{K(\mathbf{z}) - 1 + \kappa C} \cdot \frac{n_{c,t} + \tau}{n_c + \tau T} \cdot \frac{n_{c,f} + \phi}{n_c + \phi F} \quad (8) \end{aligned}$$

where n_c is the number of other labels assigned to class c, $n_{c,t}$ and $n_{c,f}$ are the number of other labels in class c with stem t and suffix f, respectively, and C, T, and F, are the total number of possible classes, stems, and suffixes, which are fixed. We use the notation $\mathbf{c}_{-k}$ here to indicate all members of $\mathbf{c}$ except for c_k. Equation 8 is obtained by integrating over the multinomial distributions specified in Equation 7, exploiting the conjugacy between multinomial and Dirichlet distributions.

Fixing the morphological analysis $(\mathbf{c}, \mathbf{t}, \mathbf{f})$, we sample the table z_i for each word token from

$$P(z_i = k \mid \mathbf{z}_{-i}, \mathbf{w}, \mathbf{c}, \mathbf{t}, \mathbf{f}) \propto \begin{cases} I(\ell_k = w_i)(n_k^{(\mathbf{z}_{-i})} - a) & n_k^{(\mathbf{z}_{-i})} > 0 \\ P(\ell_k = w_i)(K(\mathbf{z}_{-i})a + b) & n_k^{(\mathbf{z}_{-i})} = 0 \end{cases} \quad (9)$$

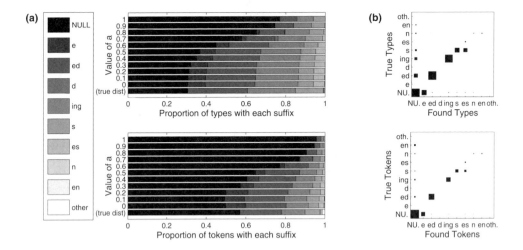

Figure 2: (a) Results for the morphology model, varying a. (b) Confusion matrices for the morphology model with $a = 0$. The area of a square at location (i, j) is proportional to the number of word types (top) or tokens (bottom) with true suffix i and found suffix j.

where $P(\ell_k = w_i)$ is found using Equation 7, with $P(c)$, $P(t)$, and $P(f)$ replaced with the corresponding conditional distributions from Equation 8.

4.3 Experiments

We applied our model to a data set consisting of all the verbs in the training section of the Penn Wall Street Journal treebank (137,997 tokens belonging to 7,761 types). This simple test case using only a single part of speech makes our results easy to analyze. We determined the true suffix of each word using simple heuristics based on the part-of-speech tag and spelling of the word.[4] We then ran a Gibbs sampler using 6 classes, and compared the results of our learning algorithm to the true suffixes found in the corpus.

As noted above, the Gibbs sampler does not converge to a single analysis of the data, but rather to a distribution over analyses. For evaluation, we used a single sample taken after 1000 iterations. Figure 2 (a) shows the distribution of suffixes found by the model for various values of a, as well as the true distribution. We analyzed the results in two ways: by counting each suffix once for each word type it was associated with, and by counting once for each word token (thus giving more weight to the results for frequent words).

The most salient aspect of our results is that, regardless of whether we evaluate on types or tokens, it is clear that low values of a are far more effective for learning morphology than higher values. With higher values of a, the system has too strong a preference for empty suffixes. This observation seems to support the linguists' view of type-based generalization.

It is also worth explaining why our morphological learner finds so many e and es suffixes. This problem is common to other morphological learning systems with similar models (e.g. [8]) and is due to the spelling rule in English that deletes stem-final e before certain suffixes. Since the system has no knowledge of spelling rules, it tends to hypothesize analyses such as {*stat.e, stat.ing, stat.ed, stat.es*}, where the e and es suffixes take the place of *NULL*

---

[4]The part-of-speech tags distinguish between past tense, past participle, progressive, 3rd person present singular, and infi nitive/unmarked verbs, and therefore roughly correlate with actual suffi xes.

and s. This effect can be seen clearly in the confusion matrices shown in Figure 2 (b). The remaining errors seen in the confusion matrices are those where the system hypothesized an empty suffix when in fact a non-empty suffix was present. Analysis of our results showed that these cases were mostly words where no other form with the same stem was present in the corpus. There was therefore no reason for the system to prefer a non-empty suffix.

5   Conclusion

We have shown that statistical language models that exhibit one of the most striking properties of natural languages – power-law distributions – can be defined by breaking the process of generating words into two stages, with a generator producing a set of words, and an adaptor determining their frequencies. Our morphology model and the Pitman-Yor process are particular choices for a generator and an adaptor. These choices produce empirical and theoretical results that justify the role of word types in formal analyses of natural language. However, the greatest strength of this framework lies in its generality: we anticipate that other choices of generators and adaptors will yield similarly interesting results.

References

[1] G. Zipf. *Selective Studies and the Principle of Relative Frequency in Language*. Harvard University Press, Cambridge, MA, 1932.

[2] M. Mitzenmacher. A brief history of generative models for power law and lognormal distributions. *Internet Mathematics*, 1(2):226–251, 2003.

[3] H.A. Simon. On a class of skew distribution functions. *Biometrika*, 42(3/4):425–440, 1955.

[4] J. Pitman. Exchangeable and partially exchangeable random partitions. *Probability Theory and Related Fields*, 102:145–158, 1995.

[5] J. Pitman and M. Yor. The two-parameter Poisson-Dirichlet distribution derived from a stable subordinator. *Annals of Probability*, 25:855–900, 1997.

[6] H. Ishwaran and L. F. James. Generalized weighted Chinese restaurant processes for species sampling mixture models. *Statistica Sinica*, 13:1211–1235, 2003.

[7] J. B. Pierrehumbert. Probabilistic phonology: discrimination and robustness. In R. Bod, J. Hay, and S. Jannedy, editors, *Probabilistic linguistics*. MIT Press, Cambridge, MA, 2003.

[8] J. Goldsmith. Unsupervised learning of the morphology of a natural language. *Computational Linguistics*, 27:153–198, 2001.

[9] H. Ney, U. Essen, and R. Kneser. On structuring probabilistic dependences in stochastic language modeling. *Computer, Speech, and Language*, 8:1–38, 1994.

[10] R. Kneser and H. Ney. Improved backing-off for n-gram language modeling. In *Proceedings of the IEEE International Conference on Acoustics, Speech and Signal Processing*, 1995.

[11] S. F. Chen and J. Goodman. An empirical study of smoothing techniques for language modeling. Technical Report TR-10-98, Center for Research in Computing Technology, Harvard University, 1998.

[12] D. Aldous. Exchangeability and related topics. In *École d'été de probabilités de Saint-Flour, XIII—1983*, pages 1–198. Springer, Berlin, 1985.

[13] R. M. Neal. Markov chain sampling methods for Dirichlet process mixture models. *Journal of Computational and Graphical Statistics*, 9:249–265, 2000.

[14] Y. W. Teh. A Bayesian interpretation of interpolated Kneser-Ney. Presentation at the NIPS Workshop on Bayesian Methods for Natural Language Processing, Dec. 2005.

[15] L. Larkey, L. Ballesteros, and M. Connell. Improving stemming for arabic information retrieval: Light stemming and co-occurrence analysis. In *Proceedings of the 25th International Conference on Research and Development in Information Retrieval (SIGIR)*, 2002.

[16] W.R. Gilks, S. Richardson, and D. J. Spiegelhalter, editors. *Markov Chain Monte Carlo in Practice*. Chapman and Hall, Suffolk, 1996.

A Probabilistic Interpretation of SVMs with an Application to Unbalanced Classification

Yves Grandvalet *
Heudiasyc, CNRS/UTC
60205 Compiègne cedex, France
grandval@utc.fr

Johnny Mariéthoz   Samy Bengio
IDIAP Research Institute
1920 Martigny, Switzerland
{marietho,bengio}@idiap.ch

Abstract

In this paper, we show that the hinge loss can be interpreted as the neg-log-likelihood of a semi-parametric model of posterior probabilities. From this point of view, SVMs represent the parametric component of a semi-parametric model fitted by a maximum a posteriori estimation procedure. This connection enables to derive a mapping from SVM scores to estimated posterior probabilities. Unlike previous proposals, the suggested mapping is interval-valued, providing a set of posterior probabilities compatible with each SVM score. This framework offers a new way to adapt the SVM optimization problem to unbalanced classification, when decisions result in unequal (asymmetric) losses. Experiments show improvements over state-of-the-art procedures.

1 Introduction

In this paper, we show that support vector machines (SVMs) are the solution of a relaxed maximum a posteriori (MAP) estimation problem. This relaxed problem results from fitting a semi-parametric model of posterior probabilities. This model is decomposed into two components: the parametric component, which is a function of the SVM score, and the non-parametric component which we call a nuisance function. Given a proper binding of the nuisance function adapted to the considered problem, this decomposition enables to concentrate on selected ranges of the probability spectrum. The estimation process can thus allocate model capacity to the neighborhoods of decision boundaries.

The connection to semi-parametric models provides a probabilistic interpretation of SVM scores, which may have several applications, such as estimating confidences over the predictions, or dealing with unbalanced losses. (which occur in domains such as diagnosis, intruder detection, etc). Several mappings relating SVM scores to probabilities have already been proposed (Sollich 2000, Platt 2000), but they are subject to arbitrary choices, which are avoided here by their integration to the nuisance function.

The paper is organized as follows. Section 2 presents the semi-parametric modeling approach; Section 3 shows how we reformulate SVM in this framework; Section 4 proposes several outcomes of this formulation, including a new method to handle unbalanced losses, which is tested empirically in Section 5. Finally, Section 6 briefly concludes the paper.

---

*This work was supported in part by the IST Programme of the European Community, under the PASCAL Network of Excellence IST-2002-506778. This publication only reflects the authors' views.

2 Semi-Parametric Classification

We address the binary classification problem of estimating a decision rule from a learning set $\mathcal{L}_n = \{(\mathbf{x}_i, y_i)\}_{i=1}^n$, where the ith example is described by the pattern $\mathbf{x}_i \in \mathcal{X}$ and the associated response $y_i \in \{-1, 1\}$. In the framework of maximum likelihood estimation, classification can be addressed either via generative models, *i.e.* models of the joint distribution $P(X, Y)$, or via discriminative methods modeling the conditional $P(Y|X)$.

2.1 Complete and Marginal Likelihood, Nuisance Functions

Let $p(1|\mathbf{x}; \boldsymbol{\theta})$ denote the model of $P(Y = 1|X = \mathbf{x})$, $p(\mathbf{x}; \boldsymbol{\psi})$ the model of $P(X)$ and t_i the binary response variable such that $t_i = 1$ when $y_i = 1$ and $t_i = 0$ when $y_i = -1$. Assuming independent examples, the complete log-likelihood can be decomposed as

$$L(\boldsymbol{\theta}, \boldsymbol{\psi}; \mathcal{L}_n) = \sum_i t_i \log(p(1|\mathbf{x}_i; \boldsymbol{\theta})) + (1 - t_i)\log(1 - p(1|\mathbf{x}_i; \boldsymbol{\theta})) + \log(p(\mathbf{x}_i; \boldsymbol{\psi})) , \quad (1)$$

where the two first terms of the right-hand side represent the marginal or conditional likelihood, that is, the likelihood of $p(1|\mathbf{x}; \boldsymbol{\theta})$.

For classification purposes, the parameter $\boldsymbol{\psi}$ is not relevant, and may thus be qualified as a nuisance parameter (Lindsay 1985). When $\boldsymbol{\theta}$ can be estimated independently of $\boldsymbol{\psi}$, maximizing the marginal likelihood provides the estimate returned by maximizing the complete likelihood with respect to $\boldsymbol{\theta}$ and $\boldsymbol{\psi}$. In particular, when no assumption whatsoever is made on $P(X)$, maximizing the conditional likelihood amounts to maximize the joint likelihood (McLachlan 1992). The density of inputs is then considered as a nuisance function.

2.2 Semi-Parametric Models

Again, for classification purposes, estimating $P(Y|X)$ may be considered as too demanding. Indeed, taking a decision only requires the knowledge of $\mathrm{sign}(2P(Y = 1|X = \mathbf{x}) - 1)$. We may thus consider looking for the decision rule minimizing the empirical classification error, but this problem is intractable for non-trivial models of discriminant functions.

Here, we briefly explore how semi-parametric models (Oakes 1988) may be used to reduce the modelization effort as compared to the standard likelihood approach. For this, we consider a two-component semi-parametric model of $P(Y = 1|X = \mathbf{x})$, defined as $p(1|\mathbf{x}; \boldsymbol{\theta}) = g(\mathbf{x}; \boldsymbol{\theta}) + \varepsilon(\mathbf{x})$, where the parametric component $g(\mathbf{x}; \boldsymbol{\theta})$ is the function of interest, and where the non-parametric component ε is a constrained nuisance function. Then, we address the maximum likelihood estimation of the semi-parametric model $p(1|\mathbf{x}; \boldsymbol{\theta})$

$$\begin{cases} \min_{\boldsymbol{\theta}, \varepsilon} & -\sum_i t_i \log(p(1|\mathbf{x}_i; \boldsymbol{\theta})) + (1 - t_i)\log(1 - p(1|\mathbf{x}_i; \boldsymbol{\theta})) \\ \text{s.t.} & p(1|\mathbf{x}; \boldsymbol{\theta}) = g(\mathbf{x}; \boldsymbol{\theta}) + \varepsilon(\mathbf{x}) \\ & 0 \leq p(1|\mathbf{x}; \boldsymbol{\theta}) \leq 1 \\ & \varepsilon^-(\mathbf{x}) \leq \varepsilon(\mathbf{x}) \leq \varepsilon^+(\mathbf{x}) \end{cases} \quad (2)$$

where ε^- and ε^+ are user-defined functions, which place constraints on the non-parametric component ε. According to these constraints, one pursues different objectives, which can be interpreted as either weakened or focused versions of the original problem of estimating precisely $P(Y|X)$ on the whole range $[0, 1]$.

At the one extreme, when $\varepsilon^- = \varepsilon^+$, one recovers a parametric maximum likelihood problem, where the estimate of posterior probabilities $p(1|\mathbf{x}; \boldsymbol{\theta})$ is simply $g(\mathbf{x}; \boldsymbol{\theta})$ shifted by the baseline function ε. At the other extreme, when $\varepsilon^-(\mathbf{x}) \leq -g(\mathbf{x})$ and $\varepsilon^+(\mathbf{x}) \geq 1 - g(\mathbf{x})$, $p(1|\cdot; \boldsymbol{\theta})$ perfectly explains (interpolates) any training sample for any $\boldsymbol{\theta}$, and the optimization problem in $\boldsymbol{\theta}$ is ill-posed. Note that the optimization problem in ε is always ill-posed, but this is not of concern as we do not wish to estimate the nuisance function.

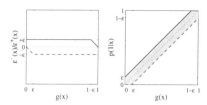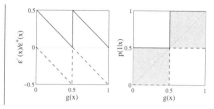

Figure 1: Two examples of $\varepsilon^-(\mathbf{x})$ (dashed) and $\varepsilon^+(\mathbf{x})$ (plain) *vs.* $g(\mathbf{x})$ and resulting ϵ-tube of possible values for the estimate of $P(Y = 1|X = \mathbf{x})$ (gray zone) *vs.* $g(\mathbf{x})$.

Generally, as ε is not estimated, the estimate of posterior probabilities $p(1|\mathbf{x}; \boldsymbol{\theta})$ is only known to lie within the interval $[g(\mathbf{x}; \boldsymbol{\theta}) + \varepsilon^-(\mathbf{x}), g(\mathbf{x}; \boldsymbol{\theta}) + \varepsilon^+(\mathbf{x})]$. In what follows, we only consider functions ε^- and ε^+ expressed as functions of the argument $g(\mathbf{x})$, for which the interval can be recovered from $g(\mathbf{x})$ alone. We also require $\varepsilon^-(\mathbf{x}) \leq 0 \leq \varepsilon^+(\mathbf{x})$, in order to ensure that $g(\mathbf{x}; \boldsymbol{\theta})$ is an admissible value of $p(1|\mathbf{x}; \boldsymbol{\theta})$.

Two simple examples are displayed in Figure 1. The two first graphs represent ε^- and ε^+ designed to estimate posterior probabilities up to precision ϵ, and the corresponding ϵ-tube of admissible estimates knowing $g(\mathbf{x})$. The two last graphs represent the same functions for ε^- and ε^+ defined to focus on the only relevant piece of information regarding decision: estimating where $P(Y|X)$ is above $1/2$. [1]

2.3 Estimation of the Parametric Component

The definitions of ε^- and ε^+ affect the estimation of the parametric component. Regarding $\boldsymbol{\theta}$, when the values of $g(\mathbf{x}; \boldsymbol{\theta}) + \varepsilon^-(\mathbf{x})$ and $g(\mathbf{x}; \boldsymbol{\theta}) + \varepsilon^+(\mathbf{x})$ lie within $[0, 1]$, problem (2) is equivalent to the following relaxed maximum likelihood problem

$$\begin{cases} \min_{\boldsymbol{\theta}, \varepsilon} & -\sum_i t_i \log(g(\mathbf{x}_i; \boldsymbol{\theta}) + \varepsilon_i) + (1 - t_i) \log(1 - g(\mathbf{x}_i; \boldsymbol{\theta}) - \varepsilon_i) \\ \text{s. t.} & \varepsilon^-(\mathbf{x}_i) \leq \varepsilon_i \leq \varepsilon^+(\mathbf{x}_i) \quad i = 1, \dots, n \end{cases} \tag{3}$$

where ε is an n-dimensional vector of slack variables. The problem is qualified as relaxed compared to the the maximum likelihood estimation of posterior probabilities by $g(\mathbf{x}_i; \boldsymbol{\theta})$, because modeling posterior probabilities by $g(\mathbf{x}_i; \boldsymbol{\theta}) + \varepsilon_i$ is a looser objective.

The monotonicity of the objective function with respect to ε_i implies that the constraints $\varepsilon^-(\mathbf{x}_i) \leq \varepsilon_i$ and $\varepsilon_i \leq \varepsilon^+(\mathbf{x}_i)$ are saturated at the solution of (3) for $t_i = 0$ or $t_i = 1$ respectively. Thus, the loss in (3) is the neg-log-likelihood of the lower or the upper bound on $p(1|\mathbf{x}_i; \boldsymbol{\theta})$ respectively. Provided that g, ε^- and ε^+ are defined such that $\varepsilon^-(\mathbf{x}) \leq \varepsilon^+(\mathbf{x})$, $0 \leq g(\mathbf{x}) + \varepsilon^-(\mathbf{x}) \leq 1$ and $0 \leq g(\mathbf{x}) + \varepsilon^+(\mathbf{x}) \leq 1$, the optimization problem with respect to $\boldsymbol{\theta}$ reduces to

$$\min_{\boldsymbol{\theta}} -\sum_i t_i \log(g(\mathbf{x}_i; \boldsymbol{\theta}) + \varepsilon^+(\mathbf{x}_i)) + (1 - t_i) \log(1 - g(\mathbf{x}_i; \boldsymbol{\theta}) - \varepsilon^-(\mathbf{x}_i)) . \tag{4}$$

Figure 2 displays the losses for positive examples corresponding to the choices of ε^- and ε^+ depicted in Figure 1 (the losses are symmetrical around 0.5 for negative examples). Note that the convexity of the objective function with respect to g depends on the choices of ε^- and ε^+. One can show that, providing ε^+ and ε^- are respectively concave and convex functions of g, then the loss (4) is convex in g.

When $\varepsilon^-(\mathbf{x}) \leq 0 \leq \varepsilon^+(\mathbf{x})$, $g(\mathbf{x})$ is an admissible estimate of $P(Y = 1|\mathbf{x})$. However, the relaxed loss (4) is optimistic, below the neg-log-likelihood of g. This optimism usually

---

[1] Of course, this naive attempt to minimize the training classification error is doomed to failure. Reformulating the problem does not affect its convexity: it remains NP-hard.

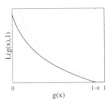
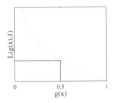

Figure 2: Losses for positive examples (plain) and neg-log-likelihood of $g(\mathbf{x})$ (dotted) *vs.* $g(\mathbf{x})$. Left: for the function ε^+ displayed on the left-hand side of Figure 1; right: for the function ε^+ displayed on the right-hand side of Figure 1.

results in a non-consistent estimation of posterior probabilities (*i.e* $g(\mathbf{x})$ does not converge towards $P(Y = 1|X = \mathbf{x})$ as the sample size goes to infinity), a common situation in semi-parametric modeling (Lindsay 1985). This lack of consistency should not be a concern here, since the non-parametric component is purposely introduced to address a looser estimation problem. We should therefore restrict consistency requirements to the primary goal of having posterior probabilities in the ϵ-tube $[g(\mathbf{x}) + \varepsilon^-(\mathbf{x}), g(\mathbf{x}) + \varepsilon^+(\mathbf{x})]$.

3   Semi-Parametric Formulation of SVMs

Several authors pointed the closeness of SVM and the MAP approach to Gaussian processes (Sollich (2000) and references therein). However, this similarity does not provide a proper mapping from SVM scores to posterior probabilities. Here, we resolve this difficulty thanks to the additional degrees of freedom provided by semi-parametric modelling.

3.1   SVMs and Gaussian Processes

In its primal Lagrangian formulation, the SVM optimization problem reads

$$\min_{f,b} \frac{1}{2}\|f\|_{\mathcal{H}}^2 + C\sum_i [1 - y_i(f(\mathbf{x}_i) + b)]_+ \ , \tag{5}$$

where $\mathcal{H}$ is a reproducing kernel Hilbert space with norm $\|\cdot\|_{\mathcal{H}}$, C is a regularization parameter and $[f]_+ = \max(f, 0)$.

The penalization term in (5) can be interpreted as a Gaussian prior on f, with a covariance function proportional to the reproducing kernel of $\mathcal{H}$ (Sollich 2000). Then, the interpretation of the hinge loss as a marginal log-likelihood requires to identify an affine function of the last term of (5) with the two first terms of (1). We thus look for two constants c_0 and $c_1 \neq 0$, such that, for all values of $f(\mathbf{x}) + b$, there exists a value $0 \leq p(1|\mathbf{x}) \leq 1$ such that

$$\begin{cases} p(1|\mathbf{x}) &= \exp-(c_0 + c_1[1 - (f(\mathbf{x}) + b)]_+) \\ 1 - p(1|\mathbf{x}) &= \exp-(c_0 + c_1[1 + (f(\mathbf{x}) + b)]_+) \end{cases} . \tag{6}$$

The system (6) has a solution over the whole range of possible values of $f(\mathbf{x}) + b$ if and only if $c_0 = \log(2)$ and $c_1 = 0$. Thus, the SVM optimization problem does not implement the MAP approach to Gaussian processes.

To proceed with a probabilistic interpretation of SVMs, Sollich (2000) proposed a normalized probability model. The normalization functional was chosen arbitrarily, and the consequences of this choice on the probabilistic interpretation was not evaluated. In what follows, we derive an imprecise mapping, with interval-valued estimates of probabilities, representing the set of all admissible semi-parametric formulations of SVM scores.

3.2   SVMs and Semi-Parametric Models

With the semi-parametric models of Section 2.2, one has to identify an affine function of the hinge loss with the two terms of (4). Compared to the previous situation, one has the

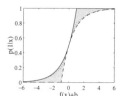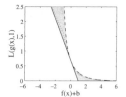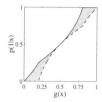

Figure 3: Left: lower (dashed) and upper (plain) posterior probabilities $[g(\mathbf{x}) + \varepsilon^-(\mathbf{x}), g(\mathbf{x}) + \varepsilon^+(\mathbf{x})]$ vs. SVM scores $f(\mathbf{x}) + b$; center: corresponding neg-log-likelihood of $g(\mathbf{x})$ for positive examples vs. $f(\mathbf{x})+b$. right: lower (dashed) and upper (plain) posterior probabilities vs. $g(\mathbf{x})$, for g defined in (8).

freedom to define the slack functions ε^- and ε^+. The identification problem is now

$$
\begin{cases}
g(\mathbf{x}) + \varepsilon^+(\mathbf{x}) = \exp-(c_0 + c_1[1 - (f(\mathbf{x}) + b)]_+) \\
1 - g(\mathbf{x}) - \varepsilon^-(\mathbf{x}) = \exp-(c_0 + c_1[1 + (f(\mathbf{x}) + b)]_+) \\
\text{s.t.} \quad 0 \le g(\mathbf{x}) + \varepsilon^-(\mathbf{x}) \le 1 \\
\qquad 0 \le g(\mathbf{x}) + \varepsilon^+(\mathbf{x}) \le 1 \\
\qquad \varepsilon^-(\mathbf{x}) \le \varepsilon^+(\mathbf{x})
\end{cases}
\tag{7}
$$

Provided $c_0 = 0$ and $0 < c_1 \le \log(2)$, there are functions g, ε^- and ε^+ such that the above problem has a solution. Hence, we obtain a set of probabilistic interpretations fully compatible with SVM scores. The solutions indexed by c_1 are nested, in the sense that, for any $\mathbf{x}$, the length of the uncertainty interval, $\varepsilon^+(\mathbf{x}) - \varepsilon^-(\mathbf{x})$, is monotonically decreasing in c_1: the interpretation of SVM scores as posterior probabilities gets tighter as c_1 increases.

The most restricted subset of admissible interpretations, with the shortest uncertainty intervals, obtained for $c_1 = \log(2)$, is represented in the left-hand side of Figure 3. The loss incurred by a positive example is represented on the central graph, where the gray zone represents the neg-log-likelihood of all admissible solutions of $g(\mathbf{x})$. Note that the hinge loss is proportional to the neg-log-likelihood of the upper posterior probability $g(\mathbf{x}) + \varepsilon^+(\mathbf{x})$, which is the loss for positive examples in the semi-parametric model in (4). Conversely, the hinge loss for negative examples is reached for $g(\mathbf{x}) + \varepsilon^-(\mathbf{x})$. An important observation, that will be useful in Section 4.2 is that the neg-log-likelihood of any admissible functions $g(\mathbf{x})$ is tangent to the hinge loss at $f(\mathbf{x}) + b = 0$.

The solution is unique in terms of the admissible interval $[g + \varepsilon^-, g + \varepsilon^+]$, but many definitions of $(\varepsilon^-, \varepsilon^+, g)$ solve (7). For example, g may be defined as

$$
g(\mathbf{x}; \boldsymbol{\theta}) = \frac{2^{-[1-(f(\mathbf{x})+b)]_+}}{2^{-[1+(f(\mathbf{x})+b)]_+} + 2^{-[1-(f(\mathbf{x})+b)]_+}} ,
\tag{8}
$$

which is essentially the posterior probability model proposed by Sollich (2000), represented dotted in the first two graphs of Figure 3.

The last graph of Figure 3 displays the mapping from $g(\mathbf{x})$ to admissible values of $p(1|\mathbf{x})$ which results from the choice described in (8). Although the interpretation of SVM scores does not require to specify g, it may worth to list some features common to all options. First, $g(\mathbf{x}) + \varepsilon^-(\mathbf{x}) = 0$ for all $g(\mathbf{x})$ below some threshold $g_0 > 0$, and conversely, $g(\mathbf{x}) + \varepsilon^+(\mathbf{x}) = 1$ for all $g(\mathbf{x})$ above some threshold $g_1 < 1$. These two features are responsible for the sparsity of the SVM solution. Second, the estimation of posterior probabilities is accurate at 0.5, and the length of the uncertainty interval on $p(1|\mathbf{x})$ monotonically increases in $[g_0, 0.5]$ and then monotonically decreases in $[0.5, g_1]$. Hence, the training objective of SVMs is intermediate between the accurate estimation of posterior probabilities on the whole range $[0, 1]$ and the minimization of the classification risk.

471

4 Outcomes of the Probabilistic Interpretation

This section gives two consequences of our probabilistic interpretation of SVMs. Further outcomes, still reserved for future research are listed in Section 6.

4.1 Pointwise Posterior Probabilities from SVM Scores

Platt (2000) proposed to estimate posterior probabilities from SVM scores by fitting a logistic function over the SVM scores. The only logistic function compatible with the most stringent interpretation of SVMs in the semi-parametric framework,

$$g(\mathbf{x}; \boldsymbol{\theta}) = \frac{1}{1 + 4^{-(f(\mathbf{x})+b)}} , \tag{9}$$

is identical to the model of Sollich (2000) (8) when $f(\mathbf{x}) + b$ lies in the interval $[-1, 1]$.

Other logistic functions are compatible with the looser interpretations obtained by letting $c_1 < \log(2)$, but their use as pointwise estimates is questionable, since the associated confidence interval is wider. In particular, the looser interpretations do not ensure that $f(\mathbf{x}) + b = 0$ corresponds to $g(\mathbf{x}) = 0.5$. Then, the decision function based on the estimated posterior probabilities by $g(\mathbf{x})$ may differ from the SVM decision function.

Being based on an arbitrary choice of $g(\mathbf{x})$, pointwise estimates of posterior probabilities derived from SVM scores should be handled with caution. As discussed by Zhang (2004), they may only be consistent at $f(\mathbf{x}) + b = 0$, where they may converge towards 0.5.

4.2 Unbalanced Classification Losses

SVMs are known to perform well regarding misclassification error, but they provide skewed decision boundaries for unbalanced classification losses, where the losses associated with incorrect decisions differ according to the true label. The mainstream approach used to address this problem consists in using different losses for positive and negative examples (Morik et al. 1999, Veropoulos et al. 1999), *i.e.*

$$\min_{f,b} \frac{1}{2}\|f\|_{\mathcal{H}}^2 + C^+ \sum_{\{i|y_i=1\}} [1 - (f(\mathbf{x}_i) + b)]_+ + C^- \sum_{\{i|y_i=-1\}} [1 + (f(\mathbf{x}_i) + b)]_+ , \tag{10}$$

where the coefficients C^+ and C^- are constants, whose ratio is equal to the ratio of the losses ℓ_{FN} and ℓ_{FP} pertaining to false negatives and false positives, respectively (Lin et al. 2002).[2] Bayes' decision theory defines the optimal decision rule by positive classification when $P(y = 1|\mathbf{x}) > P_0$, where $P_0 = \frac{\ell_{\mathrm{FP}}}{\ell_{\mathrm{FP}}+\ell_{\mathrm{FN}}}$. We may thus rewrite $C^+ = C \cdot (1 - P_0)$ and $C^- = C \cdot P_0$. With such definitions, the optimization problem may be interpreted as an upper-bound on the classification risk defined from ℓ_{FN} and ℓ_{FP}. However, the machinery of Section 3.2 unveils a major problem: the SVM decision function provided by $\mathrm{sign}(f(\mathbf{x}_i) + b)$ is not consistent with the probabilistic interpretation of SVM scores.

We address this problem by deriving another criterion, by requiring that the neg-log-likelihood of any admissible functions $g(\mathbf{x})$ is tangent to the hinge loss at $f(\mathbf{x}) + b = 0$. This leads to the following problem:

$$\min_{f,b} \frac{1}{2}\|f\|_{\mathcal{H}}^2 + C \left(\sum_{\{i|y_i=1\}} [-\log(P_0) - (1 - P_0)(f(\mathbf{x}_i) + b)]_+ + \right.$$

$$\left. \sum_{\{i|y_i=-1\}} [-\log(1 - P_0) + P_0(f(\mathbf{x}_i) + b)]_+ \right) . \tag{11}$$

---

[2] False negatives/positives respectively designate positive/negative examples incorrectly classified.

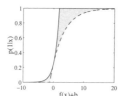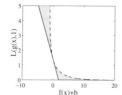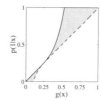

Figure 4: Left: lower (dashed) and upper (plain) posterior probabilities $[g(\mathbf{x}) + \varepsilon^-(\mathbf{x}), g(\mathbf{x}) + \varepsilon^+(\mathbf{x})]$ vs. SVM scores $f(\mathbf{x}) + b$ obtained from (11) with $P_0 = 0.25$; center: corresponding neg-log-likelihood of $g(\mathbf{x})$ for positive examples vs. $f(\mathbf{x}) + b$. right: lower (dashed) and upper (plain) posterior probabilities vs. $g(\mathbf{x})$, for g defined by $\varepsilon^+(\mathbf{x}) = 0$ for $f(\mathbf{x}) + b \leq 0$ and $\varepsilon^-(\mathbf{x}) = 0$ for $f(\mathbf{x}) + b \geq 0$.

This loss differs from (10), in the respect that the margin for positive examples is smaller than the one for negative examples when $P_0 < 0.5$. In particular, (10) does not affect the SVM solution for separable problems, while in (11), the decision boundary moves towards positive support vectors when P_0 decreases. The analogue of Figure 3, displayed on Figure 4, shows that one recovers the characteristics of the standard SVM loss, except that the focus is now on the posterior probability P_0 defined by Bayes' decision rule.

5 Experiments with Unbalanced Classifications Losses

It is straightforward to implement (11) in standard SVM packages. For experimenting with difficult unbalanced two-class problems, we used the Forest database, the largest available UCI dataset (http://kdd.ics.uci.edu/databases/covertype/). We consider the subproblem of discriminating the positive class Krummholz (20510 examples) against the negative class Spruce/Fir (211840 examples). The ratio of negative to positive examples is high, a feature commonly encountered with unbalanced classification losses.

The training set was built by random selection of size 11 000 (1000 and 10 000 examples from the positive and negative class respectively); a validation set, of size 11 000 was drawn identically among the other examples; finally, the test set, of size 99 000, was drawn among the remaining examples.

The performance was measured by the weighted risk function $R = \frac{1}{n}(N_{\mathrm{FN}}\ell_{\mathrm{FN}} + N_{\mathrm{FP}}\ell_{\mathrm{FP}})$, where N_{FN} and N_{FP} are the number of false negatives and false positives, respectively. The loss ℓ_{FP} was set to one, and ℓ_{FN} was successively set to 1, 10 and 100, in order to penalize more and more heavily errors from the under-represented class.

All approaches were tested using SVMs with a Gaussian kernel on normalized data. The hyper-parameters were tuned on the validation set for each of the ℓ_{FN} values. We additionally considered three tuning for the bias b: $\hat{b}$ is the bias returned by the algorithm; $\hat{b}_v$ the bias returned by minimizing R on the validation set, which is an optimistic estimate of the bias that could be computed by cross-validation. We also provide results for b^*, the optimal bias computed on the test set. This "crystal ball" tuning may not represent an achievable goal, but it shows how far we are from the optimum. Table 1 compares the risk R obtained with the three approaches for the different values of ℓ_{FN}.

The first line, with $\ell_{\mathrm{FN}} = 1$ corresponds to the standard classification error, where all training criteria are equivalent in theory and in practice. The bias returned by the algorithm is very close to the optimal one. For $\ell_{\mathrm{FN}} = 10$ and $\ell_{\mathrm{FN}} = 100$, the models obtained by optimizing C^+/C^- (10) and P_0 (11) achieve better results than the baseline with the crystal ball bias. While the solutions returned by C^+/C^- can be significantly improved

Table 1: Errors for 3 different criteria and for 3 different models over the Forest database

ℓ_{FN}	Baseline, problem (5)		C^+/C^-, problem (10)			P_0, problem (11)		
	$\hat{b}$	b^*	$\hat{b}$	$\hat{b}_v$	b^*	$\hat{b}$	$\hat{b}_v$	b^*
1	0.027	0.026	0.027	0.027	0.026	0.027	0.027	0.026
10	0.167	0.108	0.105	0.104	0.094	0.095	0.104	0.094
100	1.664	0.406	0.403	0.291	0.289	0.295	0.291	0.289

by tuning the bias, our criterion provides results that are very close to the optimum, in the range of the performances obtained with the bias optimized on an independant validation set. The new optimization criterion can thus outperform standard approaches for highly unbalanced problems.

6 Conclusion

This paper introduced a semi-parametric model for classification which provides an interesting viewpoint on SVMs. The non-parametric component provides an intuitive means of transforming the likelihood into a decision-oriented criterion. This framework was used here to propose a new parameterization of the hinge loss, dedicated to unbalanced classification problems, yielding significant improvements over the classical procedure.

Among other prospectives, we plan to apply the same framework to investigate hinge-like criteria for decision rules including a reject option, where the classifier abstains when a pattern is ambiguous. We also aim at defining losses encouraging sparsity in probabilistic models, such as kernelized logistic regression. We could thus build sparse probabilistic classifiers, providing an accurate estimation of posterior probabilities on a (limited) predefined range of posterior probabilities. In particular, we could derive decision-oriented criteria for multi-class probabilistic classifiers. For example, minimizing classification error only requires to find the class with highest posterior probability, and this search does not require precise estimates of probabilities outside the interval $[1/K, 1/2]$, where K is the number of classes.

References

Y. Lin, Y. Lee, and G. Wahba. Support vector machines for classification in non-standard situations. *Machine Learning*, 46:191–202, 2002.

B. G. Lindsay. Nuisance parameters. In S. Kotz, C. B. Read, and D. L. Banks, editors, *Encyclopedia of Statistical Sciences*, volume 6. Wiley, 1985.

G. J. McLachlan. *Discriminant analysis and statistical pattern recognition*. Wiley, 1992.

K. Morik, P. Brockhausen, and T. Joachims. Combining statistical learning with a knowledge-based approach - a case study in intensive care monitoring. In *Proceedings of ICML*, 1999.

D. Oakes. Semi-parametric models. In S. Kotz, C. B. Read, and D. L. Banks, editors, *Encyclopedia of Statistical Sciences*, volume 8. Wiley, 1988.

J. C. Platt. Probabilities for SV machines. In A. J. Smola, P. L. Bartlett, B. Schölkopf, and D. Schuurmans, editors, *Advances in Large Margin Classifiers*, pages 61–74. MIT Press, 2000.

P. Sollich. Probabilistic methods for support vector machines. In S. A. Solla, T. K. Leen, and K.-R. Müller, editors, *Advances in Neural Information Processing Systems 12*, pages 349–355, 2000.

K. Veropoulos, C. Campbell, and N. Cristianini. Controlling the sensitivity of support vector machines. In T. Dean, editor, *Proc. of the IJCAI*, pages 55–60, 1999.

T. Zhang. Statistical behavior and consistency of classification methods based on convex risk minimization. *Annals of Statistics*, 32(1):56–85, 2004.

Infinite Latent Feature Models and the Indian Buffet Process

Thomas L. Griffiths
Cognitive and Linguistic Sciences
Brown University, Providence RI
tom_griffiths@brown.edu

Zoubin Ghahramani
Gatsby Computational Neuroscience Unit
University College London, London
zoubin@gatsby.ucl.ac.uk

Abstract

We define a probability distribution over equivalence classes of binary matrices with a finite number of rows and an unbounded number of columns. This distribution is suitable for use as a prior in probabilistic models that represent objects using a potentially infinite array of features. We identify a simple generative process that results in the same distribution over equivalence classes, which we call the Indian buffet process. We illustrate the use of this distribution as a prior in an infinite latent feature model, deriving a Markov chain Monte Carlo algorithm for inference in this model and applying the algorithm to an image dataset.

1 Introduction

The statistical models typically used in unsupervised learning draw upon a relatively small repertoire of representations. The simplest representation, used in mixture models, associates each object with a single latent class. This approach is appropriate when objects can be partitioned into relatively homogeneous subsets. However, the properties of many objects are better captured by representing each object using multiple latent features. For instance, we could choose to represent each object as a binary vector, with entries indicating the presence or absence of each feature [1], allow each feature to take on a continuous value, representing objects with points in a latent space [2], or define a factorial model, in which each feature takes on one of a discrete set of values [3, 4].

A critical question in all of these approaches is the dimensionality of the representation: how many classes or features are needed to express the latent structure expressed by a set of objects. Often, determining the dimensionality of the representation is treated as a model selection problem, with a particular dimensionality being chosen based upon some measure of simplicity or generalization performance. This assumes that there is a single, finite-dimensional representation that correctly characterizes the properties of the observed objects. An alternative is to assume that the true dimensionality is unbounded, and that the observed objects manifest only a finite subset of classes or features [5]. This alternative is pursued in nonparametric Bayesian models, such as Dirichlet process mixture models [6, 7, 8, 9]. In a Dirichlet process mixture model, each object is assigned to a latent class, and each class is associated with a distribution over observable properties. The prior distribution over assignments of objects to classes is defined in such a way that the number of classes used by the model is bounded only by the number of objects, making Dirichlet process mixture models "infinite" mixture models [10].

The prior distribution assumed in a Dirichlet process mixture model can be specified in terms of a sequential process called the Chinese restaurant process (CRP) [11, 12]. In the CRP, N customers enter a restaurant with infinitely many tables, each with infinite seating capacity. The ith customer chooses an already-occupied table k with probability $\frac{m_k}{i-1+\alpha}$, where m_k is the number of current occupants, and chooses a new table with probability $\frac{\alpha}{i-1+\alpha}$. Customers are *exchangeable* under this process: the probability of a particular seating arrangement depends only on the number of people at each table, and not the order in which they enter the restaurant.

If we replace customers with objects and tables with classes, the CRP specifies a distribution over partitions of objects into classes. A partition is a division of the set of N objects into subsets, where each object belongs to a single subset and the ordering of the subsets does not matter. Two assignments of objects to classes that result in the same division of objects correspond to the same partition. For example, if we had three objects, the class assignments $\{c_1, c_2, c_3\} = \{1, 1, 2\}$ would correspond to the same partition as $\{2, 2, 1\}$, since all that differs between these two cases is the labels of the classes. A partition thus defines an equivalence class of assignment vectors.

The distribution over partitions implied by the CRP can be derived by taking the limit of the probability of the corresponding equivalence class of assignment vectors in a model where class assignments are generated from a multinomial distribution with a Dirichlet prior [9, 10]. In this paper, we derive an infinitely exchangeable distribution over infinite binary matrices by pursuing this strategy of taking the limit of a finite model. We also describe a stochastic process (the Indian buffet process, akin to the CRP) which generates this distribution. Finally, we demonstrate how this distribution can be used as a prior in statistical models in which each object is represented by a sparse subset of an unbounded number of features. Further discussion of the properties of this distribution, some generalizations, and additional experiments, are available in the longer version of this paper [13].

2   A distribution on infinite binary matrices

In a latent feature model, each object is represented by a vector of latent feature values $\mathbf{f}_i$, and the observable properties of that object $\mathbf{x}_i$ are generated from a distribution determined by its latent features. Latent feature values can be continuous, as in principal component analysis (PCA) [2], or discrete, as in cooperative vector quantization (CVQ) [3, 4]. In the remainder of this section, we will assume that feature values are continuous. Using the matrix $\mathbf{F} = \begin{bmatrix} \mathbf{f}_1^T & \mathbf{f}_2^T & \cdots & \mathbf{f}_N^T \end{bmatrix}^T$ to indicate the latent feature values for all N objects, the model is specified by a prior over features, $p(\mathbf{F})$, and a distribution over observed property matrices conditioned on those features, $p(\mathbf{X}|\mathbf{F})$, where $p(\cdot)$ is a probability density function. These distributions can be dealt with separately: $p(\mathbf{F})$ specifies the number of features and the distribution over values associated with each feature, while $p(\mathbf{X}|\mathbf{F})$ determines how these features relate to the properties of objects. Our focus will be on $p(\mathbf{F})$, showing how such a prior can be defined without limiting the number of features.

We can break $\mathbf{F}$ into two components: a binary matrix $\mathbf{Z}$ indicating which features are possessed by each object, with $z_{ik} = 1$ if object i has feature k and 0 otherwise, and a matrix $\mathbf{V}$ indicating the value of each feature for each object. $\mathbf{F}$ is the elementwise product of $\mathbf{Z}$ and $\mathbf{V}$, $\mathbf{F} = \mathbf{Z} \otimes \mathbf{V}$, as illustrated in Figure 1. In many latent feature models (e.g., PCA) objects have non-zero values on every feature, and every entry of $\mathbf{Z}$ is 1. In *sparse* latent feature models (e.g., sparse PCA [14, 15]) only a subset of features take on non-zero values for each object, and $\mathbf{Z}$ picks out these subsets. A prior on $\mathbf{F}$ can be defined by specifying priors for $\mathbf{Z}$ and $\mathbf{V}$, with $p(\mathbf{F}) = P(\mathbf{Z})p(\mathbf{V})$, where $P(\cdot)$ is a probability mass function. We will focus on defining a prior on $\mathbf{Z}$, since the effective dimensionality of a latent feature model is determined by $\mathbf{Z}$. Assuming that $\mathbf{Z}$ is sparse, we can define a prior for infinite latent feature models by defining a distribution over infinite binary matrices. Our discussion of the Chinese restaurant process provides two desiderata for such a distribution: objects

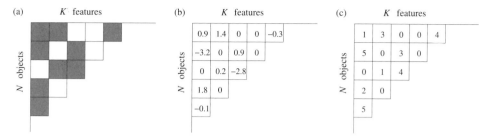

Figure 1: A binary matrix $\mathbf{Z}$, as shown in (a), indicates which features take non-zero values. Elementwise multiplication of $\mathbf{Z}$ by a matrix $\mathbf{V}$ of continuous values produces a representation like (b). If $\mathbf{V}$ contains discrete values, we obtain a representation like (c).

should be exchangeable, and posterior inference should be tractable. It also suggests a method by which these desiderata can be satisfied: start with a model that assumes a finite number of features, and consider the limit as the number of features approaches infinity.

2.1 A finite feature model

We have N objects and K features, and the possession of feature k by object i is indicated by a binary variable z_{ik}. The z_{ik} form a binary $N \times K$ feature matrix, $\mathbf{Z}$. Assume that each object possesses feature k with probability π_k, and that the features are generated independently. Under this model, the probability of $\mathbf{Z}$ given $\pi = \{\pi_1, \pi_2, \ldots, \pi_K\}$, is

$$P(\mathbf{Z}|\pi) = \prod_{k=1}^{K}\prod_{i=1}^{N} P(z_{ik}|\pi_k) = \prod_{k=1}^{K} \pi_k^{m_k}(1 - \pi_k)^{N - m_k}, \tag{1}$$

where $m_k = \sum_{i=1}^{N} z_{ik}$ is the number of objects possessing feature k. We can define a prior on π by assuming that each π_k follows a beta distribution, to give

$$\pi_k \,|\, \alpha \;\sim\; \mathrm{Beta}(\tfrac{\alpha}{K}, 1)$$

$$z_{ik} \,|\, \pi_k \sim \mathrm{Bernoulli}(\pi_k)$$

Each z_{ik} is independent of all other assignments, conditioned on π_k, and the π_k are generated independently. We can integrate out π to obtain the probability of $\mathbf{Z}$, which is

$$P(\mathbf{Z}) \;\;=\;\; \prod_{k=1}^{K} \frac{\frac{\alpha}{K}\Gamma(m_k + \frac{\alpha}{K})\Gamma(N - m_k + 1)}{\Gamma(N + 1 + \frac{\alpha}{K})}. \tag{2}$$

This distribution is exchangeable, since m_k is not affected by the ordering of the objects.

2.2 Equivalence classes

In order to find the limit of the distribution specified by Equation 2 as $K \rightarrow \infty$, we need to define equivalence classes of binary matrices – the analogue of partitions for class assignments. Our equivalence classes will be defined with respect to a function on binary matrices, $lof(\cdot)$. This function maps binary matrices to *left-ordered* binary matrices. $lof(\mathbf{Z})$ is obtained by ordering the columns of the binary matrix $\mathbf{Z}$ from left to right by the magnitude of the binary number expressed by that column, taking the first row as the most significant bit. The left-ordering of a binary matrix is shown in Figure 2. In the first row of the left-ordered matrix, the columns for which $z_{1k} = 1$ are grouped at the left. In the second row, the columns for which $z_{2k} = 1$ are grouped at the left of the sets for which $z_{1k} = 1$. This grouping structure persists throughout the matrix.

The *history* of feature k at object i is defined to be $(z_{1k}, \ldots, z_{(i-1)k})$. Where no object is specified, we will use *history* to refer to the full history of feature k, $(z_{1k}, \ldots, z_{Nk})$. We

477

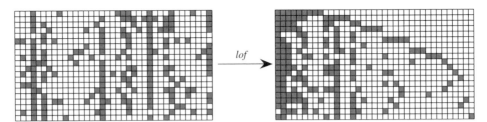

Figure 2: Left-ordered form. A binary matrix is transformed into a left-ordered binary matrix by the function $lof(\cdot)$. The entries in the left-ordered matrix were generated from the Indian buffet process with $\alpha = 10$. Empty columns are omitted from both matrices.

will individuate the histories of features using the decimal equivalent of the binary numbers corresponding to the column entries. For example, at object 3, features can have one of four histories: 0, corresponding to a feature with no previous assignments, 1, being a feature for which $z_{2k} = 1$ but $z_{1k} = 0$, 2, being a feature for which $z_{1k} = 1$ but $z_{2k} = 0$, and 3, being a feature possessed by both previous objects were assigned. K_h will denote the number of features possessing the history h, with K_0 being the number of features for which $m_k = 0$ and $K_+ = \sum_{h=1}^{2^N-1} K_h$ being the number of features for which $m_k > 0$, so $K = K_0 + K_+$.

Two binary matrices $\mathbf{Y}$ and $\mathbf{Z}$ are lof-equivalent if $lof(\mathbf{Y}) = lof(\mathbf{Z})$. The lof-equivalence class of a binary matrix $\mathbf{Z}$, denoted $[\mathbf{Z}]$, is the set of binary matrices that are lof-equivalent to $\mathbf{Z}$. lof-equivalence classes play the role for binary matrices that partitions play for assignment vectors: they collapse together all binary matrices (assignment vectors) that differ only in column ordering (class labels). lof-equivalence classes are preserved through permutation of the rows or the columns of a matrix, provided the same permutations are applied to the other members of the equivalence class. Performing inference at the level of lof-equivalence classes is appropriate in models where feature order is not identifiable, with $p(\mathbf{X}|\mathbf{F})$ being unaffected by the order of the columns of $\mathbf{F}$. Any model in which the probability of $\mathbf{X}$ is specified in terms of a linear function of $\mathbf{F}$, such as PCA or CVQ, has this property. The cardinality of the lof-equivalence class $[\mathbf{Z}]$ is $\binom{K}{K_0 \dots K_{2^N-1}} = \frac{K!}{\prod_{h=0}^{2^N-1} K_h!}$, where K_h is the number of columns with full history h.

2.3 Taking the infinite limit

Under the distribution defined by Equation 2, the probability of a particular lof-equivalence class of binary matrices, $[\mathbf{Z}]$, is

$$P([\mathbf{Z}]) = \sum_{\mathbf{Z} \in [\mathbf{Z}]} P(\mathbf{Z}) = \frac{K!}{\prod_{h=0}^{2^N-1} K_h!} \prod_{k=1}^{K} \frac{\frac{\alpha}{K}\Gamma(m_k + \frac{\alpha}{K})\Gamma(N - m_k + 1)}{\Gamma(N + 1 + \frac{\alpha}{K})}. \tag{3}$$

Rearranging terms, and using the fact that $\Gamma(x) = (x - 1)\Gamma(x - 1)$ for $x > 1$, we can compute the limit of $P([\mathbf{Z}])$ as K approaches infinity

$$\lim_{K \to \infty} \frac{\alpha^{K_+}}{\prod_{h=1}^{2^N-1} K_h!} \cdot \frac{K!}{K_0! K^{K_+}} \cdot \left(\frac{N!}{\prod_{j=1}^{N}(j + \frac{\alpha}{K})} \right)^K \cdot \prod_{k=1}^{K_+} \frac{(N - m_k)! \prod_{j=1}^{m_k-1}(j + \frac{\alpha}{K})}{N!}$$

$$= \frac{\alpha^{K_+}}{\prod_{h=1}^{2^N-1} K_h!} \cdot 1 \cdot \exp\{-\alpha H_N\} \cdot \prod_{k=1}^{K_+} \frac{(N - m_k)!(m_k - 1)!}{N!}, \tag{4}$$

where H_N is the Nth harmonic number, $H_N = \sum_{j=1}^{N} \frac{1}{j}$. This distribution is infinitely exchangeable, since neither K_h nor m_k are affected by the ordering on objects. Technical details of this limit are provided in [13].

2.4 The Indian buffet process

The probability distribution defined in Equation 4 can be derived from a simple stochastic process. Due to the similarity to the Chinese restaurant process, we will also use a culinary metaphor, appropriately adjusted for geography. Indian restaurants in London offer buffets with an apparently infinite number of dishes. We will define a distribution over infinite binary matrices by specifying how customers (objects) choose dishes (features).

In our Indian buffet process (IBP), N customers enter a restaurant one after another. Each customer encounters a buffet consisting of infinitely many dishes arranged in a line. The first customer starts at the left of the buffet and takes a serving from each dish, stopping after a Poisson(α) number of dishes. The ith customer moves along the buffet, sampling dishes in proportion to their popularity, taking dish k with probability $\frac{m_k}{i}$, where m_k is the number of previous customers who have sampled that dish. Having reached the end of all previous sampled dishes, the ith customer then tries a Poisson($\frac{\alpha}{i}$) number of new dishes. We can indicate which customers chose which dishes using a binary matrix $\mathbf{Z}$ with N rows and infinitely many columns, where $z_{ik} = 1$ if the ith customer sampled the kth dish.

Using $K_1^{(i)}$ to indicate the number of new dishes sampled by the ith customer, the probability of any particular matrix being produced by the IBP is

$$P(\mathbf{Z}) = \frac{\alpha^{K_+}}{\prod_{i=1}^N K_1^{(i)}!} \exp\{-\alpha H_N\} \prod_{k=1}^{K_+} \frac{(N - m_k)!(m_k - 1)!}{N!}. \tag{5}$$

The matrices produced by this process are generally not in left-ordered form. These matrices are also not ordered arbitrarily, because the Poisson draws always result in choices of new dishes that are to the right of the previously sampled dishes. Customers are not exchangeable under this distribution, as the number of dishes counted as $K_1^{(i)}$ depends upon the order in which the customers make their choices. However, if we only pay attention to the lof-equivalence classes of the matrices generated by this process, we obtain the infinitely exchangeable distribution $P([\mathbf{Z}])$ given by Equation 4: $\frac{\prod_{i=1}^N K_1^{(i)}!}{\prod_{h=1}^{2^N-1} K_h!}$ matrices generated via this process map to the same left-ordered form, and $P([\mathbf{Z}])$ is obtained by multiplying $P(\mathbf{Z})$ from Equation 5 by this quantity. A similar but slightly more complicated process can be defined to produce left-ordered matrices directly [13].

2.5 Conditional distributions

To define a Gibbs sampler for models using the IBP, we need to know the conditional distribution on feature assignments, $P(z_{ik} = 1 | \mathbf{Z}_{-(ik)})$. In the finite model, where $P(\mathbf{Z})$ is given by Equation 2, it is straightforward to compute this conditional distribution for any z_{ik}. Integrating over π_k gives

$$P(z_{ik} = 1 | \mathbf{z}_{-i,k}) = \frac{m_{-i,k} + \frac{\alpha}{K}}{N + \frac{\alpha}{K}}, \tag{6}$$

where $\mathbf{z}_{-i,k}$ is the set of assignments of other objects, not including i, for feature k, and $m_{-i,k}$ is the number of objects possessing feature k, not including i. We need only condition on $\mathbf{z}_{-i,k}$ rather than $\mathbf{Z}_{-(ik)}$ because the columns of the matrix are independent.

In the infinite case, we can derive the conditional distribution from the (exchangeable) IBP. Choosing an ordering on objects such that the ith object corresponds to the last customer to visit the buffet, we obtain

$$P(z_{ik} = 1 | \mathbf{z}_{-i,k}) = \frac{m_{-i,k}}{N}, \tag{7}$$

for any k such that $m_{-i,k} > 0$. The same result can be obtained by taking the limit of Equation 6 as $K \to \infty$. The number of new features associated with object i should be drawn from a Poisson($\frac{\alpha}{N}$) distribution. This can also be derived from Equation 6, using the same kind of limiting argument as that presented above.

3 A linear-Gaussian binary latent feature model

To illustrate how the IBP can be used as a prior in models for unsupervised learning, we derived and tested a linear-Gaussian latent feature model in which the features are binary. In this case the feature matrix $\mathbf{F}$ reduces to the binary matrix $\mathbf{Z}$. As above, we will start with a finite model and then consider the infinite limit.

In our finite model, the D-dimensional vector of properties of an object i, $\mathbf{x}_i$ is generated from a Gaussian distribution with mean $\mathbf{z}_i \mathbf{A}$ and covariance matrix $\Sigma_X = \sigma_X^2 \mathbf{I}$, where $\mathbf{z}_i$ is a K-dimensional binary vector, and $\mathbf{A}$ is a $K \times D$ matrix of weights. In matrix notation, $E[\mathbf{X}] = \mathbf{ZA}$. If $\mathbf{Z}$ is a feature matrix, this is a form of binary factor analysis. The distribution of $\mathbf{X}$ given $\mathbf{Z}$, $\mathbf{A}$, and σ_X is matrix Gaussian with mean $\mathbf{ZA}$ and covariance matrix $\sigma_X^2 \mathbf{I}$, where $\mathbf{I}$ is the identity matrix. The prior on $\mathbf{A}$ is also matrix Gaussian, with mean 0 and covariance matrix $\sigma_A^2 \mathbf{I}$. Integrating out $\mathbf{A}$, we have

$$p(\mathbf{X}|\mathbf{Z}, \sigma_X, \sigma_A) = \frac{1}{(2\pi)^{ND/2} \sigma_X^{(N-K)D} \sigma_A^{KD} |\mathbf{Z}^T \mathbf{Z} + \frac{\sigma_X^2}{\sigma_A^2} \mathbf{I}|^{D/2}}$$

$$\exp\{-\frac{1}{2\sigma_X^2} \mathrm{tr}(\mathbf{X}^T (\mathbf{I} - \mathbf{Z}(\mathbf{Z}^T \mathbf{Z} + \frac{\sigma_X^2}{\sigma_A^2} \mathbf{I})^{-1} \mathbf{Z}^T)\mathbf{X})\}. \quad (8)$$

This result is intuitive: the exponentiated term is the difference between the inner product of $\mathbf{X}$ and its projection onto the space spanned by $\mathbf{Z}$, regularized to an extent determined by the ratio of the variance of the noise in $\mathbf{X}$ to the variance of the prior on $\mathbf{A}$. It follows that $p(\mathbf{X}|\mathbf{Z}, \sigma_X, \sigma_A)$ depends only on the non-zero columns of $\mathbf{Z}$, and thus remains well-defined when we take the limit as $K \to \infty$ (for more details see [13]).

We can define a Gibbs sampler for this model by computing the full conditional distribution

$$P(z_{ik}|\mathbf{X}, \mathbf{Z}_{-(i,k)}, \sigma_X, \sigma_A) \propto p(\mathbf{X}|\mathbf{Z}, \sigma_X, \sigma_A) P(z_{ik}|\mathbf{z}_{-i,k}). \quad (9)$$

The two terms on the right hand side can be evaluated using Equations 8 and 7 respectively. The Gibbs sampler is then straightforward. Assignments for features for which $m_{-i,k} > 0$ are drawn from the distribution specified by Equation 9. The distribution over the number of new features for each object can be approximated by truncation, computing probabilities for a range of values of $K_1^{(i)}$ up to an upper bound. For each value, $p(\mathbf{X}|\mathbf{Z}, \sigma_X, \sigma_A)$ can be computed from Equation 8, and the prior on the number of new features is Poisson($\frac{\alpha}{N}$).

We will demonstrate this Gibbs sampler for the infinite binary linear-Gaussian model on a dataset consisting of 100 240×320 pixel images. We represented each image, $\mathbf{x}_i$, using a 100-dimensional vector corresponding to the weights of the mean image and the first 99 principal components. Each image contained up to four everyday objects – a \$20 bill, a Klein bottle, a prehistoric handaxe, and a cellular phone. Each object constituted a single latent feature responsible for the observed pixel values. The images were generated by sampling a feature vector, $\mathbf{z}_i$, from a distribution under which each feature was present with probability 0.5, and then taking a photograph containing the appropriate objects using a LogiTech digital webcam. Sample images are shown in Figure 3 (a).

The Gibbs sampler was initialized with $K_+ = 1$, choosing the feature assignments for the first column by setting $z_{i1} = 1$ with probability 0.5. σ_A, σ_X, and α were initially set to 0.5, 1.7, and 1 respectively, and then sampled by adding Metropolis steps to the MCMC algorithm. Figure 3 shows trace plots for the first 1000 iterations of MCMC for the number of features used by at least one object, K_+, and the model parameters σ_A, σ_X, and α. All of these quantities stabilized after approximately 100 iterations, with the algorithm

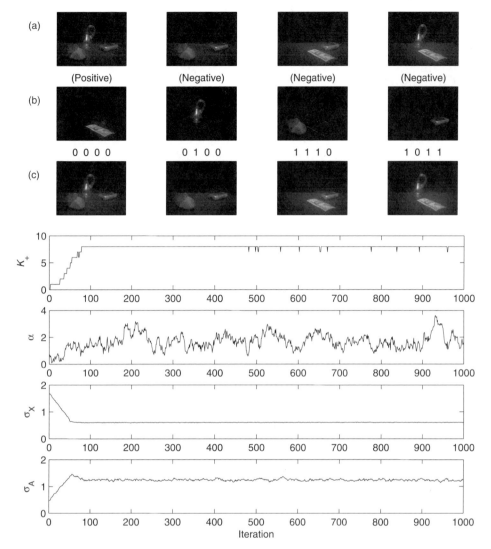

Figure 3: Data and results for the demonstration of the infinite linear-Gaussian binary latent feature model. (a) Four sample images from the 100 in the dataset. Each image had 320×240 pixels, and contained from zero to four everyday objects. (b) The posterior mean of the weights ($\mathbf{A}$) for the four most frequent binary features from the 1000th sample. Each image corresponds to a single feature. These features perfectly indicate the presence or absence of the four objects. The first feature indicates the presence of the \$20 bill, the other three indicate the absence of the Klein bottle, the handaxe, and the cellphone. (c) Reconstructions of the images in (a) using the binary codes inferred for those images. These reconstructions are based upon the posterior mean of $\mathbf{A}$ for the 1000th sample. For example, the code for the first image indicates that the \$20 bill is absent, while the other three objects are not. The lower panels show trace plots for the dimensionality of the representation (K_+) and the parameters α, σ_X, and σ_A over 1000 iterations of sampling. The values of all parameters stabilize after approximately 100 iterations.

finding solutions with approximately seven latent features. The four most common features perfectly indicated the presence and absence of the four objects (shown in Figure 3 (b)), and three less common features coded for slight differences in the locations of those objects.

4   Conclusion

We have shown that the methods that have been used to define infinite latent class models [6, 7, 8, 9, 10, 11, 12] can be extended to models in which objects are represented in terms of a set of latent features, deriving a distribution on infinite binary matrices that can be used as a prior for such models. While we derived this prior as the infinite limit of a simple distribution on finite binary matrices, we have shown that the same distribution can be specified in terms of a simple stochastic process – the Indian buffet process. This distribution satisfies our two desiderata for a prior for infinite latent feature models: objects are exchangeable, and inference remains tractable. Our success in transferring the strategy of taking the limit of a finite model from latent classes to latent features suggests that a similar approach could be applied with other representations, expanding the forms of latent structure that can be recovered through unsupervised learning.

References

[1] N. Ueda and K. Saito. Parametric mixture models for multi-labeled text. In *Advances in Neural Information Processing Systems 15*, Cambridge, 2003. MIT Press.

[2] I. T. Jolliffe. *Principal component analysis*. Springer, New York, 1986.

[3] R. S. Zemel and G. E. Hinton. Developing population codes by minimizing description length. In *Advances in Neural Information Processing Systems 6*. Morgan Kaufmann, San Francisco, CA, 1994.

[4] Z. Ghahramani. Factorial learning and the EM algorithm. In *Advances in Neural Information Processing Systems 7*. Morgan Kaufmann, San Francisco, CA, 1995.

[5] C. E. Rasmussen and Z. Ghahramani. Occam's razor. In *Advances in Neural Information Processing Systems 13*. MIT Press, Cambridge, MA, 2001.

[6] C. Antoniak. Mixtures of Dirichlet processes with applications to Bayesian nonparametric problems. *The Annals of Statistics*, 2:1152–1174, 1974.

[7] M. D. Escobar and M. West. Bayesian density estimation and inference using mixtures. *Journal of the American Statistical Association*, 90:577–588, 1995.

[8] T. S. Ferguson. Bayesian density estimation by mixtures of normal distributions. In M. Rizvi, J. Rustagi, and D. Siegmund, editors, *Recent advances in statistics*, pages 287–302. Academic Press, New York, 1983.

[9] R. M. Neal. Markov chain sampling methods for Dirichlet process mixture models. *Journal of Computational and Graphical Statistics*, 9:249–265, 2000.

[10] C. Rasmussen. The infinite Gaussian mixture model. In *Advances in Neural Information Processing Systems 12*. MIT Press, Cambridge, MA, 2000.

[11] D. Aldous. Exchangeability and related topics. In *École d'été de probabilités de Saint-Flour, XIII—1983*, pages 1–198. Springer, Berlin, 1985.

[12] J. Pitman. Combinatorial stochastic processes, 2002. Notes for Saint Flour Summer School.

[13] T. L. Griffiths and Z. Ghahramani. Infinite latent feature models and the Indian buffet process. Technical Report 2005-001, Gatsby Computational Neuroscience Unit, 2005.

[14] A. d'Aspremont, L. El Ghaoui, I. Jordan, and G. R. G. Lanckriet. A direct formulation for sparse PCA using semidefinite programming. In *Advances in Neural Information Processing Systems 17*. MIT Press, Cambridge, MA, 2005.

[15] H. Zou, T. Hastie, and R. Tibshirani. Sparse principal component analysis. *Journal of Computational and Graphical Statistics*, in press.

Computing the Solution Path for the Regularized Support Vector Regression

Lacey Gunter
Department of Statistics
University of Michigan
Ann Arbor, MI 48109
lgunter@umich.edu

Ji Zhu[*]
Department of Statistics
University of Michigan
Ann Arbor, MI 48109
jizhu@umich.edu

Abstract

In this paper we derive an algorithm that computes the entire solution path of the support vector regression, with essentially the same computational cost as fitting one SVR model. We also propose an unbiased estimate for the degrees of freedom of the SVR model, which allows convenient selection of the regularization parameter.

1 Introduction

The support vector regression (SVR) is a popular tool for function estimation problems, and it has been widely used on many real applications in the past decade, for example, time series prediction [1], signal processing [2] and neural decoding [3].

In this paper, we focus on the regularization parameter of the SVR, and propose an efficient algorithm that computes the entire regularized solution path; we also propose an unbiased estimate for the degrees of freedom of the SVR, which allows convenient selection of the regularization parameter.

Suppose we have a set of training data $(\boldsymbol{x}_1, y_1), \ldots, (\boldsymbol{x}_n, y_n)$, where the input $\boldsymbol{x}_i \in \mathbb{R}^p$ and the output $y_i \in \mathbb{R}$. Many researchers have noted that the formulation for the linear ϵ-SVR can be written in a *loss + penalty* form [4]:

$$\min_{\beta_0, \boldsymbol{\beta}} \sum_{i=1}^{n} \left| y_i - \beta_0 - \boldsymbol{\beta}^\mathsf{T} \boldsymbol{x}_i \right|_\epsilon + \frac{\lambda}{2} \boldsymbol{\beta}^\mathsf{T} \boldsymbol{\beta} \tag{1}$$

where $|\xi|_\epsilon$ is the so called ϵ-insensitive loss function:

$$|\xi|_\epsilon = \begin{cases} 0 & \text{if } |\xi| \leq \epsilon \\ |\xi| - \epsilon & \text{otherwise} \end{cases}$$

The idea is to disregard errors as long as they are less than ϵ. Figure 1 plots the loss function. Notice that it has two non-differentiable points at $\pm\epsilon$. The regularization parameter λ controls the trade-off between the ϵ-insensitive loss and the complexity of the fitted model.

---

[*]To whom the correspondence should be addressed.

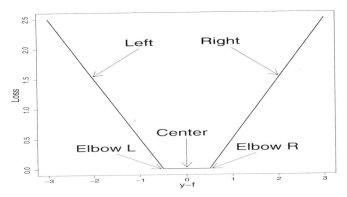

Figure 1: The ϵ-insensitive loss function.

In practice, one often maps $\boldsymbol{x}$ into a high (often infinite) dimensional reproducing kernel Hilbert space (RKHS), and fits a nonlinear *kernel* SVR model [4]:

$$\min_{\beta_0, \boldsymbol{\theta}} \sum_{i=1}^{n} |y_i - f(\boldsymbol{x}_i)|_\epsilon + \frac{1}{2\lambda} \sum_{i=1}^{n} \sum_{i'=1}^{n} \theta_i \theta_{i'} K(\boldsymbol{x}_i, \boldsymbol{x}_{i'}) \tag{2}$$

where $f(\boldsymbol{x}) = \beta_0 + \frac{1}{\lambda} \sum_{i=1}^{n} \theta_i K(\boldsymbol{x}, \boldsymbol{x}_i)$, and $K(\cdot, \cdot)$ is a positive-definite reproducing kernel that generates a RKHS. Notice that we write $f(\boldsymbol{x})$ in a way that involves λ explicitly, and we will see later that $\theta_i \in [-1, 1]$.

Both (1) and (2) can be transformed into a quadratic programming problem, hence most commercially available packages can be used to solve the SVR. In the past years, many specific algorithms for the SVR have also been developed, for example, interior point algorithms [4-5], subset selection algorithms [6–7], and sequential minimal optimization [4, 8–9]. All these algorithms solve the SVR for a pre-fixed regularization parameter λ, and it is well known that an appropriate value of λ is crucial for achieving small prediction error of the SVR.

In this paper, we show that the solution $\boldsymbol{\theta}(\lambda)$ is *piecewise linear* as a function of λ, which allows us to derive an efficient algorithm that computes the *exact entire solution path* $\{\boldsymbol{\theta}(\lambda), 0 \leq \lambda \leq \infty\}$. We acknowledge that this work was inspired by one of the authors' earlier work on the SVM setting [10].

Before delving into the technical details, we illustrate the concept of piecewise linearity of the solution path with a simple example. We generate 10 training observations using the famous $sinc(\cdot)$ function:

$$y = \frac{\sin(\pi x)}{\pi x} + e, \quad \text{where } x \sim U(-2\pi, 2\pi) \text{ and } e \sim N(0, 0.19^2)$$

We use the SVR with a 1-dimensional spline kernel

$$K(x, x') = 1 + k_1(x)k_1(x') + k_2(x)k_2(x') - k_4(|x - x'|) \tag{3}$$

where $k_1(\cdot) = \cdot - 1/2, k_2 = (k_1^2 - 1/12)/2, k_4 = (k_1^4 - k_1^2/2 + 7/240)/24$. Figure 2 shows a subset of the piecewise linear solution path $\boldsymbol{\theta}(\lambda)$ as a function of λ.

In section 2, we describe the algorithm that computes the entire solution path of the SVR. In section 3, we propose an unbiased estimate for the degrees of freedom of the SVR, which can be used to select the regularization parameter λ. In section 4, we present numerical results on simulation data. We conclude the paper with a discussion section.

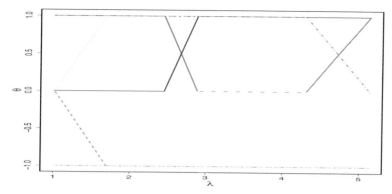

Figure 2: A subset of the solution path $\boldsymbol{\theta}(\lambda)$ as a function of λ.

2 Algorithm

For simplicity in notation, we describe the problem setup using the linear SVR, and the algorithm using the kernel SVR.

2.1 Problem Setup

The linear ϵ-SVR (1) can be re-written in an equivalent way:

$$\min_{\beta_0,\beta} \quad \sum_{i=1}^{n}(\xi_i + \delta_i) + \frac{\lambda}{2}\boldsymbol{\beta}^{\mathsf{T}}\boldsymbol{\beta}$$

$$\text{subject to} \quad -(\delta_i + \epsilon) \le y_i - f(\boldsymbol{x}_i) \le (\xi_i + \epsilon), \quad \xi_i, \delta_i \ge 0;$$

$$f(\boldsymbol{x}_i) = \beta_0 + \boldsymbol{\beta}^{\mathsf{T}}\boldsymbol{x}_i, \quad i = 1, \dots n$$

This gives us the Lagrangian primal function

$$L_P: \quad \sum_{i=1}^{n}(\xi_i + \delta_i) + \frac{\lambda}{2}\boldsymbol{\beta}^{\mathsf{T}}\boldsymbol{\beta} + \sum_{i=1}^{n}\alpha_i(y_i - f(\boldsymbol{x}_i) - \xi_i - \epsilon) -$$

$$\sum_{i=1}^{n}\gamma_i(y_i - f(\boldsymbol{x}_i) + \delta_i + \epsilon) - \sum_{i=1}^{n}\rho_i\xi_i - \sum_{i=1}^{n}\tau_i\delta_i.$$

Setting the derivatives to zero we arrive at:

$$\frac{\partial}{\partial\boldsymbol{\beta}} : \quad \boldsymbol{\beta} = \frac{1}{\lambda}\sum_{i=1}^{n}(\alpha_i - \gamma_i)\boldsymbol{x}_i \tag{4}$$

$$\frac{\partial}{\partial\beta_0} : \quad \sum_{i=1}^{n}\alpha_i = \sum_{i=1}^{n}\gamma_i \tag{5}$$

$$\frac{\partial}{\partial\xi_i} : \quad \alpha_i = 1 - \rho_i \tag{6}$$

$$\frac{\partial}{\partial\delta_i} : \quad \gamma_i = 1 - \tau_i \tag{7}$$

where the Karush-Kuhn-Tucker conditions are

$$\alpha_i(y_i - f(\boldsymbol{x}_i) - \xi_i - \epsilon) = 0 \tag{8}$$

$$\gamma_i(y_i - f(\boldsymbol{x}_i) + \delta_i + \epsilon) = 0 \tag{9}$$

$$\rho_i\xi_i = 0 \tag{10}$$

$$\tau_i\delta_i = 0 \tag{11}$$

Along with the constraint that our Lagrange multipliers must be non-negative, we can conclude from (6) and (7) that both $0 \leq \alpha_i \leq 1$ and $0 \leq \gamma_i \leq 1$. We also see from (8) and (9) that if α_i is positive, then γ_i must be zero, and vice versa. These lead to the following relationships:

$$
\begin{array}{llllll}
y_i - f(\boldsymbol{x}_i) > \epsilon & \Rightarrow & \alpha_i = 1, & \xi_i > 0, & \gamma_i = 0, & \delta_i = 0; \\
y_i - f(\boldsymbol{x}_i) < -\epsilon & \Rightarrow & \alpha_i = 0, & \xi_i = 0, & \gamma_i = 1, & \delta_i > 0; \\
y_i - f(\boldsymbol{x}_i) \in (-\epsilon, \epsilon) & \Rightarrow & \alpha_i = 0, & \xi_i = 0, & \gamma_i = 0, & \delta_i = 0; \\
y_i - f(\boldsymbol{x}_i) = \epsilon & \Rightarrow & \alpha_i \in [0,1], & \xi_i = 0, & \gamma_i = 0, & \delta_i = 0; \\
y_i - f(\boldsymbol{x}_i) = -\epsilon & \Rightarrow & \alpha_i = 0, & \xi_i = 0, & \gamma_i \in [0,1], & \delta_i = 0.
\end{array}
$$

Using these relationships, we define the following sets that will be used later on when we are calculating the regularization path of the SVR:

- $\mathcal{R} = \{i : y_i - f(\boldsymbol{x}_i) > \epsilon, \ \alpha_i = 1, \gamma_i = 0\}$ (Right of the elbows)
- $\mathcal{E_R} = \{i : y_i - f(\boldsymbol{x}_i) = \epsilon, \ 0 \leq \alpha_i \leq 1, \gamma_i = 0\}$ (Right elbow)
- $\mathcal{C} = \{i : -\epsilon < y_i - f(\boldsymbol{x}_i) < \epsilon, \ \alpha_i = 0, \gamma_i = 0\}$ (Center)
- $\mathcal{E_L} = \{i : y_i - f(\boldsymbol{x}_i) = -\epsilon, \ \alpha_i = 0, 0 \leq \gamma_i \leq 0\}$ (Left elbow)
- $\mathcal{L} = \{i : y_i - f(\boldsymbol{x}_i) < -\epsilon, \ \alpha_i = 0, \gamma_i = 1\}$ (Left of the elbows)

Notice from (4) that for every λ, $\boldsymbol{\beta}$ is fully determined by the values of α_i and γ_i. For points in $\mathcal{R}$, $\mathcal{L}$ and $\mathcal{C}$, the values of α_i and γ_i are known; therefore, the algorithm will focus on points resting at the two elbows $\mathcal{E_R}$ and $\mathcal{E_L}$.

2.2 Initialization

Initially, when $\lambda = \infty$ we can see from (4) that $\boldsymbol{\beta} = 0$. We can determine the value of β_0 via a simple 1-dimensional optimization. For lack of space, we focus on the case that all the values of y_i are distinct, and furthermore, the initial sets $\mathcal{E_R}$ and $\mathcal{E_L}$ have at most one point combined (which is the usual situation). In this case β_0 will not be unique and each of the α_i and γ_i will be either 0 or 1.

Since β_0 is not unique, we can focus on one particular solution path, for example, by always setting β_0 equal to one of its boundary values (thus keeping one point at an elbow). As λ decreases, the range of β_0 shrinks toward zero and reaches zero when we have two points at the elbows, and the algorithm proceeds from there.

2.3 The Path

The formalized setup above can be easily modified to accommodate non-linear kernels; in fact, θ_i in (2) is equal to $\alpha_i - \gamma_i$. For the remaining portion of the algorithm we will use the kernel notation.

The algorithm focuses on the sets of points $\mathcal{E_R}$ and $\mathcal{E_L}$. These points have either $f(\boldsymbol{x}_i) = y_i - \epsilon$ with $\alpha_i \in [0,1]$, or $f(\boldsymbol{x}_i) = y_i + \epsilon$ with $\gamma_i \in [0,1]$. As we follow the path we will examine these sets until one or both of them change, at which point we will say an *event* has occurred. Thus events can be categorized as:

1. The initial event, for which two points must enter the elbow(s)
2. A point from $\mathcal{R}$ has just entered $\mathcal{E_R}$, with α_i initially 1
3. A point from $\mathcal{L}$ has just entered $\mathcal{E_L}$, with γ_i initially 1
4. A point from $\mathcal{C}$ has just entered $\mathcal{E_R}$, with α_i initially 0

5. A point from $\mathcal{C}$ has just entered $\mathcal{E}_\mathcal{L}$, with γ_i initially 0

6. One or more points in $\mathcal{E}_\mathcal{R}$ and/or $\mathcal{E}_\mathcal{L}$ have just left the elbow(s) to join either $\mathcal{R}$, $\mathcal{L}$, or $\mathcal{C}$, with α_i and γ_i initially 0 or 1

Until another event has occurred, all sets will remain the same. As a point passes through $\mathcal{E}_\mathcal{R}$ or $\mathcal{E}_\mathcal{L}$, its respective α_i or γ_i must change from $0 \to 1$ or $1 \to 0$. Relying on the fact that $f(\boldsymbol{x}_i) = y_i - \epsilon$ or $f(\boldsymbol{x}_i) = y_i + \epsilon$ for all points in $\mathcal{E}_\mathcal{R}$ or $\mathcal{E}_\mathcal{L}$ respectively, we can calculate α_i and γ_i for these points.

We use the subscript ℓ to index the sets above immediately after the ℓth event has occurred, and let α_i^ℓ, γ_i^ℓ, β_0^ℓ and λ^ℓ be the parameter values immediately after the ℓth event. Also let f^ℓ be the function at this point. We define for convenience $\beta_{0,\lambda} = \lambda \cdot \beta_0$ and hence $\beta_{0,\lambda}^\ell = \lambda^\ell \cdot \beta_0^\ell$. Then since

$$f(\boldsymbol{x}) = \frac{1}{\lambda}\left(\sum_{i=1}^n (\alpha_i - \gamma_i) K(\boldsymbol{x}, \boldsymbol{x}_i) + \beta_{0,\lambda}\right)$$

for $\lambda^{\ell+1} < \lambda < \lambda^\ell$ we can write

$$
\begin{aligned}
f(\boldsymbol{x}) &= \left[f(\boldsymbol{x}) - \frac{\lambda^\ell}{\lambda}f^\ell(\boldsymbol{x})\right] + \frac{\lambda^\ell}{\lambda}f^\ell(\boldsymbol{x}) \\
&= \frac{1}{\lambda}\left[\sum_{i \in \mathcal{E}_\mathcal{R}^\ell} \nu_i K(\boldsymbol{x}, \boldsymbol{x}_i) - \sum_{j \in \mathcal{E}_\mathcal{L}^\ell} \omega_j K(\boldsymbol{x}, \boldsymbol{x}_j) + \nu_0 + \lambda^\ell f^\ell(\boldsymbol{x})\right],
\end{aligned}
$$

where $\nu_i = \alpha_i - \alpha_i^\ell$, $\omega_j = \gamma_j - \gamma_j^\ell$ and $\nu_0 = \beta_{0,\lambda} - \beta_{0,\lambda}^\ell$, and we can do the reduction in the second line since the α_i and γ_i are fixed for all points in $\mathcal{R}^\ell$, $\mathcal{L}^\ell$, and $\mathcal{C}^\ell$ and all points remain in their respective sets. Suppose $|\mathcal{E}_\mathcal{R}^\ell| = n_R^\ell$ and $|\mathcal{E}_\mathcal{L}^\ell| = n_L^\ell$, so for the $n_R^\ell + n_L^\ell$ points staying at the elbows we have (after some algebra) that

$$\frac{1}{y_k - \epsilon}\left[\sum_{i \in \mathcal{E}_\mathcal{R}^\ell} \nu_i K(\boldsymbol{x}_k, \boldsymbol{x}_i) - \sum_{j \in \mathcal{E}_\mathcal{L}^\ell} \omega_j K(\boldsymbol{x}_k, \boldsymbol{x}_j) + \nu_0\right] = \lambda - \lambda^\ell, \ \ \forall k \in \mathcal{E}_\mathcal{R}^\ell$$

$$\frac{1}{y_m + \epsilon}\left[\sum_{i \in \mathcal{E}_\mathcal{R}^\ell} \nu_i K(\boldsymbol{x}_m, \boldsymbol{x}_i) - \sum_{j \in \mathcal{E}_\mathcal{L}^\ell} \omega_j K(\boldsymbol{x}_m, \boldsymbol{x}_j) + \nu_0\right] = \lambda - \lambda^\ell, \ \ \forall m \in \mathcal{E}_\mathcal{L}^\ell$$

Also, by condition (5) we have that

$$\sum_{i \in \mathcal{E}_\mathcal{R}^\ell} \nu_i - \sum_{j \in \mathcal{E}_\mathcal{L}^\ell} \omega_j = 0$$

This gives us $n_R^\ell + n_L^\ell + 1$ linear equations we can use to solve for each of the $n_R^\ell + n_L^\ell + 1$ unknown variables ν_i, ω_j and ν_0. Notice this system is linear in $\lambda - \lambda^\ell$, which implies that α_i, γ_j and $\beta_{0,\lambda}$ change linearly in $\lambda - \lambda^\ell$. So we can write:

$$
\begin{aligned}
\alpha_i &= \alpha_i^\ell + (\lambda - \lambda^\ell)b_i & \forall i \in \mathcal{E}_\mathcal{R}^\ell & & (12) \\
\gamma_j &= \gamma_j^\ell + (\lambda - \lambda^\ell)b_j & \forall j \in \mathcal{E}_\mathcal{L}^\ell & & (13) \\
\beta_{0,\lambda} &= \beta_{0,\lambda}^\ell + (\lambda - \lambda^\ell)b_0 & & & (14) \\
f(\boldsymbol{x}) &= \frac{\lambda^\ell}{\lambda}\left[f^\ell(\boldsymbol{x}) - h^\ell(\boldsymbol{x})\right] + h^\ell(\boldsymbol{x}) & & & (15)
\end{aligned}
$$

where (b_i, b_j, b_0) is the solution when $\lambda - \lambda^\ell$ is equal to 1, and

$$h^\ell(\boldsymbol{x}) = \sum_{i \in \mathcal{E}_\mathcal{R}^\ell} b_i K(\boldsymbol{x}, \boldsymbol{x}_i) - \sum_{j \in \mathcal{E}_\mathcal{L}^\ell} b_j K(\boldsymbol{x}, \boldsymbol{x}_j) + b_0.$$

Given λ_ℓ, equations (12), (13) and (15) allow us to compute the λ at which the next event will occur, $\lambda_{\ell+1}$. This will be the largest λ less than λ_ℓ, such that either α_i for $i \in \mathcal{E}_\mathcal{R}^\ell$ reaches 0 or 1, or γ_j for $j \in \mathcal{E}_\mathcal{L}^\ell$ reaches 0 or 1, or one of the points in $\mathcal{R}$, $\mathcal{L}$ or $\mathcal{C}$ reaches an elbow.

We terminate the algorithm either when the sets $\mathcal{R}$ and $\mathcal{L}$ become empty, or when λ has become sufficiently close to zero. In the later case we must have $f^\ell - h^\ell$ sufficiently small as well.

2.4 Computational cost

The major computational cost for updating the solutions at any event ℓ involves two things: solving the system of $(n_R^\ell + n_L^\ell)$ linear equations, and computing $h^\ell(\boldsymbol{x})$. The former takes $O((n_R^\ell + n_L^\ell)^2)$ calculations by using inverse updating and downdating since the elbow sets usually differ by only one point between consecutive events, and the latter requires $O(n(n_R^\ell + n_L^\ell))$ computations.

According to our experience, the total number of steps taken by the algorithm is on average some small multiple of n. Letting m be the average size of $\mathcal{E}_\mathcal{R}^\ell \cup \mathcal{E}_\mathcal{L}^\ell$, then the approximate computational cost of the algorithm is $O\left(cn^2m + nm^2\right)$, which is comparable to a single SVR fitting algorithm that uses quadratic programming.

3   The Degrees of Freedom

The *degrees of freedom* is an informative measure of the complexity of a fitted model. In this section, we propose an unbiased estimate for the degrees of freedom of the SVR, which allows convenient selection of the regularization parameter λ.

Since the usual goal of regression analysis is to minimize the predicted squared-error loss, we study the degrees of freedom using Stein's unbiased risk estimation (SURE) theory [11]. Given $\boldsymbol{x}$, assuming y is generated according to a homoskedastic model:

$$y \sim (\mu(\boldsymbol{x}), \sigma^2)$$

where μ is the true mean and σ^2 is the common variance. Then the degrees of freedom of a fitted model $f(\boldsymbol{x})$ can be defined as

$$\mathrm{df}(f) = \sum_{i=1}^{n} \mathrm{cov}(f(\boldsymbol{x}_i), y_i)/\sigma^2$$

Stein showed that under mild conditions, $\sum_{i=1}^{n} \partial f_i/\partial y_i$ is an unbiased estimate of $\mathrm{df}(f)$. It turns out that for the SVR model, for every fixed λ, $\sum_{i=1}^{n} \partial f_i/\partial y_i$ has an extremely simple formula:

$$\widehat{\mathrm{df}} \equiv \sum_{i=1}^{n} \frac{\partial f_i}{\partial y_i} = |\mathcal{E}_\mathcal{R}| + |\mathcal{E}_\mathcal{L}| \tag{16}$$

Therefore, $|\mathcal{E}_\mathcal{R}| + |\mathcal{E}_\mathcal{L}|$ is a convenient unbiased estimate for the degrees of freedom of $f(\boldsymbol{x})$. Due to the space restriction, we omit the proof here, but make a note that the proof relies on our SVR algorithm.

In applying (16) to select the regularization parameter λ, we plug it into the GCV criterion [12] for model selection:

$$\frac{\sum_{i=1}^{n}(y_i - f(\boldsymbol{x}_i))^2}{(n - \widehat{\mathrm{df}})^2}$$

The advantages of this criterion are that it does not assume a known σ^2, and it avoids cross-validation, which is computationally intensive. In practice, we can first use our efficient algorithm to compute the entire solution path, then identify the appropriate value of λ that minimizes the GCV criterion.

4 Numerical Results

To demonstrate our algorithm and the selection of λ using the GCV criterion, we show numerical results on simulated data. We consider both additive and multiplicative kernels using the 1-dimensional spline kernel (3), which are respectively

$$K(\boldsymbol{x}, \boldsymbol{x}') = \sum_{j=1}^{p} K(x_j, x_j') \quad \text{and} \quad K(\boldsymbol{x}, \boldsymbol{x}') = \prod_{j=1}^{p} K(x_j, x_j')$$

Simulations were based on the following four functions [13]:

1. $f(x) = \frac{sin(\pi x)}{\pi x} + e_1, \quad x \in (-2\pi, 2\pi)$

2. $f(\boldsymbol{x}) = 0.1e^{4x_1} + \frac{1}{1+e^{-20(x_2-.5)}} + 3x_3 + 2x_4 + x_5 + e_2, \quad \boldsymbol{x} \in (0,1)^2$

3. $f(R, \omega, L, C) = \left[R^2 + \left(\omega L + \frac{1}{\omega C}\right)^2\right]^{1/2} + e_3,$

4. $f(R, \omega, L, C) = \tan^{-1}\left[\frac{\omega L + \frac{1}{\omega C}}{R}\right] + e_4,$

   where $(R, \omega, L, C) \in (0, 100) \times (2\pi(20, 280)) \times (0, 1) \times (1, 11)$

e_i are distributed as $N(0, \sigma_i^2)$, where $\sigma_1 = 0.19, \sigma_2 = 1, \sigma_3 = 218.5, \sigma_4 = 0.18$.

We generated 300 training observations from each function along with 10,000 validation observations and 10,000 test observations. For the first two simulations we used the additive 1-dimensional spline kernel and for the second two simulations the multiplicative 1-dimensional spline kernel. We then found the λ that minimized the GCV criterion. The validation set was used to select the *gold standard* λ which minimized the prediction MSE. Using these λ's we calculated the prediction MSE with the test data for each criterion. After repeating this for 20 times, the average MSE and standard deviation for the MSE can be seen in Table 1, which indicates the GCV criterion performs closely to optimal.

Table 1: Simulation results of λ selection for SVR

$f(\boldsymbol{x})$	MSE-Gold Standard	MSE-GCV
1	0.0385 (0.0011)	0.0389 (0.0011)
2	1.0999 (0.0367)	1.1120 (0.0382)
3	50095 (1358)	50982 (2205)
4	0.0459 (0.0023)	0.0471 (0.0028)

5 Discussion

In this paper, we have proposed an efficient algorithm that computes the entire regularization path of the SVR. We have also proposed the GCV criterion for selecting the best λ given the entire path. The GCV criterion seems to work sufficiently well on the simulation data. However, we acknowledge that according to our experience on real data sets (not shown here due to lack of the space), the GCV criterion sometimes tends to over-fit the model. We plan to explore this issue further.

Due to the difficulty of also selecting the best ϵ for the SVR, an alternate algorithm exists that automatically adjusts the value of ϵ, called the ν-SVR [4]. In this scenario, ϵ is treated as another free parameter. Using arguments similar to those for β_0 in our above algorithm, one can show that ϵ is piecewise linear in $1/\lambda$ and its path can be calculated similarly.

Acknowledgments

We would like to thank Saharon Rosset for helpful comments. Gunter and Zhu are partially supported by grant DMS-0505432 from the National Science Foundation.

References

[1] Müler K, Smola A, Rätsch G, Schölkopf B, Kohlmorgen J & Vapnik V (1997) Predicting time series with support vector machines. *Artificial Neural Networks*, 999-1004.

[2] Vapnik V, Golowich S & Smola A (1997) Support vector method for function approximation, regression estimation, and signal processing. *NIPS* **9**.

[3] Shpigelman L, Crammer K, Paz R, Vaadia E & Singer Y (2004) A temporal kernel-based model for tracking hand movements from neural activities. *NIPS* **17**, 1273-1280.

[4] Smola A & Schölkopf B (2004) A tutorial on support vector regression. *Statistics and Computing* **14**: 199-222.

[5] Vanderbei, R. (1994) LOQO: An interior point code for quadratic programming. *Technical Report SOR-94-15, Princeton University.*

[6] Osuna E, Freund R & Girosi F (1997) An improved training algorithm for support vector machines. *Neural Networks for Signal Processing*, 276-284.

[7] Joachims T (1999) Making large-scale SVM learning practical. *Advances in Kernel Methods – Support Vector Learning*, 169-184.

[8] Platt J (1999) Fast training of support vector machines using sequential minimal optimization. *Advances in Kernel Methods – Support Vector Learning*, 185-208.

[9] Keerthi S, Shevade S, Bhattacharyya C & Murthy K (1999) Improvements to Platt's SMO algorithm for SVM classifier design. *Technical Report CD-99-14, NUS.*

[10] Hastie, T., Rosset, S., Tibshirani, R. & Zhu, J. (2004) The Entire Regularization Path for the Support Vector Machine. *JMLR*, **5**, 1391-1415.

[11] Stein, C. (1981) Estimation of the mean of a multivariate normal distribution. *Annals of Statistics* **9**: 1135-1151.

[12] Craven, P. & Wahba, G. (1979) Smoothing noisy data with spline function. *Numerical Mathematics* 31: 377-403.

[13] Friedman, J. (1991) Multivariate Adaptive Regression Splines. *Annals of Statistics* **19**: 1-67.

Hot Coupling: A Particle Approach to Inference and Normalization on Pairwise Undirected Graphs of Arbitrary Topology

Firas Hamze   Nando de Freitas
Department of Computer Science
University of British Columbia

Abstract

This paper presents a new sampling algorithm for approximating functions of variables representable as undirected graphical models of arbitrary connectivity with pairwise potentials, as well as for estimating the notoriously difficult partition function of the graph. The algorithm fits into the framework of sequential Monte Carlo methods rather than the more widely used MCMC, and relies on constructing a sequence of intermediate distributions which get closer to the desired one. While the idea of using "tempered" proposals is known, we construct a novel sequence of target distributions where, rather than dropping a global temperature parameter, we sequentially couple individual pairs of variables that are, initially, sampled exactly from a spanning tree of the variables. We present experimental results on inference and estimation of the partition function for sparse and densely-connected graphs.

1 Introduction

Undirected graphical models are powerful statistical tools having a wide range of applications in diverse fields such as image analysis [1, 2], conditional random fields [3], neural models [4] and epidemiology [5]. Typically, when doing inference, one is interested in obtaining the *local beliefs*, that is the marginal probabilities of the variables given the evidence set. The methods used to approximate these intractable quantities generally fall into the categories of *Markov Chain Monte Carlo* (MCMC) [6] and *variational methods* [7]. The former, involving running a Markov chain whose invariant distribution is the distribution of interest, can suffer from slow convergence to stationarity and high correlation between samples at stationarity, while the latter is not guaranteed to give the right answer or always converge. When performing learning in such models however, a more serious problem arises: the parameter update equations involve the normalization constant of the joint model at the current value of parameters, from here on called the *partition function*. MCMC offers no obvious way of approximating this wildly intractable sum [5, 8]. Although there exists a polynomial time MCMC algorithm for simple graphs with binary nodes, ferromagnetic potentials and *uniform observations* [9], this algorithm is hardly applicable to the complex models encountered in practice. Of more interest, perhaps, are the theoretical results that show that Gibbs sampling and even Swendsen-Wang[10] can mix exponentially slowly in many situations [11]. This paper introduces a new sequential Monte Carlo method for approximating expectations of a *pairwise* graph's variables (of which beliefs are a special case) and of reasonably estimating the partition function. Intuitively, the new method uses interacting parallel chains to handle multimodal distributions,

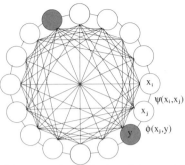

Figure 1: A small example of the type of graphical model treated in this paper. The observations correspond to the two shaded nodes.

with communicating chains distributed across the modes. In addition, there is no requirement that the chains converge to equilibrium as the bias due to incomplete convergence is corrected for by importance sampling.

Formally, given hidden variables $\mathbf{x}$ and observations $\mathbf{y}$, the model is specified on a graph $\mathcal{G}(\mathcal{V}, \mathcal{E})$, with edges $\mathcal{E}$ and M nodes $\mathcal{V}$ by:

$$\pi(\mathbf{x}, \mathbf{y}) = \frac{1}{Z} \prod_{i \in \mathcal{V}} \phi(x_i, y_i) \prod_{(i,j) \in \mathcal{E}} \psi(x_i, x_j)$$

where $\mathbf{x} = \{x_1, \ldots, x_M\}$, Z is the partition function, $\phi(\cdot)$ denotes the observation potentials and $\psi(\cdot)$ denotes the pair-wise interaction potentials, which are strictly positive but otherwise arbitrary. The partition function is: $Z = \sum_{\mathbf{x}} \prod_{i \in \mathcal{V}} \phi(x_i, y_i) \prod_{(i,j) \in \mathcal{E}} \psi(x_i, x_j)$, where the sum is over all possible system states. We make no assumption about the graph's topology or sparseness, an example is in Figure 1. We present experimental results on both *fully-connected* graphs (cases where each node neighbors every other node) and sparse graphs.

Our approach belongs to the framework of *Sequential Monte Carlo* (SMC), which has its roots in the seminal paper of [12]. Particle filters are a well-known instance of SMC methods [13]. They apply naturally to dynamic systems like tracking. Our situation is different. We introduce artificial dynamics simply as a constructive strategy for obtaining samples of a sequence of distributions converging to the distribution of interest. That is, initially we sample from and easy-to-sample distribution. This distribution is then used as a proposal mechanism to obtain samples from a slightly more complex distribution that is closer to the target distribution. The process is repeated until the sequence of distributions of increasing complexity reaches the target distribution. Our algorithm has connections to a general annealing strategy proposed in the physics [14] and statistics [15] literature, known as *Annealed Importance Sampling* (AIS). AIS is a special case of the general SMC framework [16]. The term *annealing* refers to the lowering of a "temperature parameter," the process of which makes the joint distribution more concentrated on its modes, whose number can be massive for difficult problems. The celebrated *simulated annealing* (SA) [17] algorithm is an *optimization* method relying on this phenomenon; presently, however we are interested in *integration* and so SA does not apply here.

Our approach does not use a global temperature, but sequentially introduces *dependencies* among the variables; graphically, this can be understood as "adding edges" to the graph. In this paper, we restrict ourselves to discrete state-spaces although the method applies to arbitrary continuous distributions.

For our initial distribution we choose a spanning tree of the variables, on which analytic marginalization, *exact* sampling, and computation of the partition function are easily done. After drawing a *population* of samples (*particles*) from this distribution, the sequential phase begins: an edge of the desired graph is chosen and gradually added to the current one as shown in Figure 2. The particles then follow a trajectory according to some proposal mechanism. The "fitness" of the particles is measured via their importance weights. When the set of samples has become skewed, that is with some containing high weights and many containing low ones, the particles are *resampled* according to their weights. The sequential structure is thus imposed by the propose-and-resample mechanism rather than by any property of the original system. The algorithm is formally described after an overview of SMC and recent work presenting a unifying framework of the SMC methodology outside the context of Bayesian dynamic filtering[16].

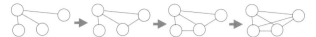

Figure 2: A graphical illustration of our algorithm. First we construct a spanning tree, of which a population of iid samples can be easily drawn using the forward filtering/backward sampling algorithm for trees. The tree then becomes the proposal mechanism for generating samples for a graph with an extra potential. The process is repeated until we obtain samples from the target distribution (defined on a fully connected graph in this case). Edges can be added "slowly" using a coupling parameter.

2 Sequential Monte Carlo

As shown in Figure 2, we consider a sequence of auxiliary distributions $\tilde{\pi}_1(\mathbf{x}_1), \tilde{\pi}_2(\mathbf{x}_{1:2}), \dots, \tilde{\pi}_n(\mathbf{x}_{1:n})$, where $\tilde{\pi}_1(\mathbf{x}_1)$ is the distribution on the weighted spanning tree. The sequence of distributions can be constructed so that it satisfies $\tilde{\pi}_n(\mathbf{x}_{1:n}) = \pi_n(\mathbf{x}_n)\tilde{\pi}_n(\mathbf{x}_{1:n-1}|\mathbf{x}_{1:n})$. Marginalizing over $\mathbf{x}_{1:n-1}$ gives us the target distribution of interest $\pi_n(\mathbf{x}_n)$ (the distribution of the graphical model that we want to sample from as illustrated in Figure 2 for $n = 4$). So we first focus on sampling from the sequence of auxiliary distributions. The joint distribution is only known up to a normalization constant: $\tilde{\pi}_n(\mathbf{x}_{1:n}) = Z_n^{-1} f_n(\mathbf{x}_{1:n})$, where $Z_n \triangleq \int f_n(\mathbf{x}_{1:n})d\mathbf{x}_{1:n}$ is the partition function. We are often interested in computing this partition function and other expectations, such as $I(g(\mathbf{x}_n)) = \int g(\mathbf{x}_n)\pi_n(\mathbf{x}_n)d\mathbf{x}_n$, where g is a function of interest (e.g. $g(\mathbf{x}) = \mathbf{x}$ if we are interested in computing the mean of $\mathbf{x}$).

If we had a set of samples $\{\mathbf{x}_{1:n}^{(i)}\}_{i=1}^{N}$ from $\tilde{\pi}$, we could approximate this integral with the following Monte Carlo estimator: $\widehat{\tilde{\pi}}_n(d\mathbf{x}_{1:n}) = \frac{1}{N}\sum_{i=1}^{N}\delta_{\mathbf{x}_{1:n}^{(i)}}(d\mathbf{x}_{1:n})$, where $\delta_{\mathbf{x}_{1:n}^{(i)}}(d\mathbf{x}_{1:n})$ denotes the delta Dirac function, and consequently approximate any expectations of interest. These estimates converge almost surely to the true expectation as N goes to infinity. It is typically hard to sample from $\tilde{\pi}$ directly. Instead, we sample from a proposal distribution q and weight the samples according to the following importance ratio

$$w_n = \frac{f_n(\mathbf{x}_{1:n})}{q_n(\mathbf{x}_{1:n})} = \frac{f_n(\mathbf{x}_{1:n})}{q_n(\mathbf{x}_{1:n})}\frac{q_{n-1}(\mathbf{x}_{1:n-1})}{f_{n-1}(\mathbf{x}_{1:n-1})}w_{n-1}$$

The proposal is constructed sequentially: $q(\mathbf{x}_{1:n}) = q_{n-1}(\mathbf{x}_{1:n-1})q_n(\mathbf{x}_n|\mathbf{x}_{1:n-1})$. Hence, the importance weights can be updated recursively

$$w_n = \frac{f_n(\mathbf{x}_{1:n})}{q_n(\mathbf{x}_n|\mathbf{x}_{1:n-1})f_{n-1}(\mathbf{x}_{1:n-1})}w_{n-1} \qquad (1)$$

Given a set of N particles $\mathbf{x}_{1:n-1}^{(i)}$, we obtain a set of particles $\mathbf{x}_n^{(i)}$ by sampling from $q_n(\mathbf{x}_n|\mathbf{x}_{1:n-1}^{(i)})$ and applying the weights of equation (1). To overcome slow drift in the particle population, a resampling (selection) step chooses the fittest particles (see the introductory chapter in [13] for a more detailed explanation). We use a state-of-the-art minimum variance resampling algorithm [18].

The ratio of successive partition functions can be easily estimated using this algorithm as follows:

$$\frac{Z_n}{Z_{n-1}} = \frac{\int f_n(\mathbf{x}_{1:n})d\mathbf{x}_{1:n}}{Z_{n-1}} = \int \widehat{w}_n \, \tilde{\pi}_{n-1}(\mathbf{x}_{1:n-1})q_n(\mathbf{x}_n|\mathbf{x}_{1:n-1})d\mathbf{x}_{1:n} \approx \sum_{i=1}^{N} \widehat{w}_n^{(i)}\widetilde{w}_{n-1}^{(i)},$$

where $\widetilde{w}_{n-1}^{(i)} = w_{n-1}^{(i)}/\sum_j w_{n-1}^{(j)}$, $\widehat{w}_n = \frac{f_n(\mathbf{x}_{1:n})}{q_n(\mathbf{x}_n|\mathbf{x}_{1:n-1})f_{n-1}(\mathbf{x}_{1:n-1})}$ and Z_1 can be easily computed as it is the partition function for a tree.

We can choose a (non-homogeneous) Markov chain with transition kernel $K_n(\mathbf{x}_{n-1}, \mathbf{x}_n)$ as the proposal distribution $q_n(\mathbf{x}_n|\mathbf{x}_{1:n-1})$. Hence, given an initial proposal distribution $q_1(\cdot)$, we have *joint* proposal distribution at step n: $q_n(\mathbf{x}_{1:n}) = q_1(\mathbf{x}_1)\prod_{k=2}^{n} K_k(\mathbf{x}_{k-1}, \mathbf{x}_k)$. It is convenient to assume that the artificial distribution $\widetilde{\pi}_n(\mathbf{x}_{1:n-1}|\mathbf{x}_n)$ is also the product of (backward) Markov kernels: $\widetilde{\pi}_n(\mathbf{x}_{1:n-1}|\mathbf{x}_n) = \prod_{k=1}^{n-1} L_k(\mathbf{x}_{k+1}, \mathbf{x}_k)$ [16]. Under these choices, the (unnormalized) incremental importance weight becomes:

$$w_n \propto \frac{f_n(\mathbf{x}_n)L_{n-1}(\mathbf{x}_n, \mathbf{x}_{n-1})}{f_{n-1}(\mathbf{x}_{n-1})K_n(\mathbf{x}_{n-1}, \mathbf{x}_n)} \tag{2}$$

Different choices of the backward Kernel L result in different algorithms [16]. For example, the choice: $L_{n-1}(\mathbf{x}_n, \mathbf{x}_{n-1}) = \frac{f_n(\mathbf{x}_{n-1})K_n(\mathbf{x}_{n-1}, \mathbf{x}_n)}{f_n(\mathbf{x}_n)}$ results in the AIS algorithm, with weights $w_n \propto \frac{f_n(\mathbf{x}_{n-1})}{f_{n-1}(\mathbf{x}_{n-1})}$. However, we should point out that this method is more general as one can carry out resampling. Note that in this case, the importance weights do not depend on $\mathbf{x}_n$ and, hence, it is possible to do resampling before the importance sampling step. This often leads to huge reduction in estimation error [19]. Also, note that if there are big discrepancies between $f_n(\cdot)$ and $f_{n-1}(\cdot)$ the method might perform poorly. To overcome this, [16] use variance results to propose a different choice of backward kernel, which results in the following incremental importance weights:

$$w_n \propto \frac{f_n(\mathbf{x}_n)}{\int f_{n-1}(\mathbf{x}_{n-1})K_n(\mathbf{x}_{n-1}, \mathbf{x}_n)d\mathbf{x}_{n-1}} \tag{3}$$

The integral in the denominator can be evaluated when dealing with Gaussian or reasonable discrete networks.

3 The new algorithm

We could try to perform traditional importance sampling by seeking some proposal distribution for the entire graph. This is very difficult and performance degrades *exponentially* in dimension if the proposal is mismatched [20]. We propose, however, to use the samples from the tree distribution (which we call π_0) as candidates to an intermediate target distribution, consisting of the tree along with a "weak" version of a potential corresponding to some edge of the original graph. Given a set of edges G_0 which form a spanning tree of the target graph, we can can use the belief propagation equations [21] and *bottom-up propagation, top-down sampling* [22], to draw a set of N *independent* samples from the tree. Computation of the normalization constant Z_1 is also straightforward and efficient in the case of trees using a sum-product recursion. From then on, however, the normalization constants of subsequent target distributions cannot be analytically computed.

We then choose a new edge e_1 from the set of "unused" edges $\mathcal{E} - G_0$ and add it to G_0 to form the new edge set $G_1 = e_1 \cup G_0$. Let the vertices of e_1 be u_1 and v_1. Then, the intermediate target distribution π_1 is proportional to $\pi_0(\mathbf{x}_1)\psi_{e_1}(x_{u_1}, x_{v_1})$. In doing straightforward importance sampling, using π_0 as a proposal for π_1, the importance weight is proportional to $\psi_{e_1}(x_{u_1}, x_{v_1})$. We adopt a slow proposal process to move the population of particles towards π_1. We gradually introduce the potential between X_{u_1} and X_{v_1} via a *coupling parameter* α which increases from 0 to 1 in order to "softly" bring the edge's potential in and allow the particles to adjust to the new environment. Formally, when adding edge e_1 to the graph, we introduce a number of coupling steps so that we have the intermediate target distribution:

$$\pi_0(\mathbf{x}_0)\left[\psi_{e_1}(x_{u_1}, x_{v_1})\right]^{\alpha_n}$$

where α_n is defined to be 0 when a new edge enters the sequence, increases to 1 as the edge is brought in, and drops back to zero when another edge is added at the following edge iteration.

At each time step, we want a proposal mechanism that is close to the target distribution. Proposals based on simple perturbations, such as random walks, are easy to implement, but can be inefficient. Metropolis-Hastings proposals are not possible because of the integral in the rejection term. We can, however, employ a single-site Gibbs sampler with random scan whose invariant distribution at each step is the *the next target density* in the sequence; this kernel is applied to each particle. When an edge has been fully added a new one is chosen and the process is repeated until the final target density is the full graph. We use an analytic expression for the incremental weights corresponding to Equation (3).

To alleviate potential confusion with MCMC, while any one particle obviously forms a correlated path, we are using a population and are making no assumption or requirement that the chains have converged as is done in MCMC as we are correcting for incomplete convergence with the weights.

4 Experiments and discussion

Four approximate inference methods were compared: our SMC method with sequential edge addition (Hot Coupling (HC)), a more typical annealing strategy with a global temperature parameter(SMCG), single-site Gibbs sampling with random scan and loopy belief propagation. SMCG can be thought of as related to HC but where all the edges and local evidence are annealed at the same time.

The majority of our experiments were performed on graphs that were small enough for exact marginals and partition functions to be exhaustively calculated. However, even in toy cases MCMC and loopy can give unsatisfactory and sometimes disastrous results. We also ran a set of experiments on a relatively large MRF.

For the small examples we examined both fully-connected (FC) and square grid (MRF) networks, with 18 and 16 nodes respectively. Each variable could assume one of 3 states. Our pairwise potentials corresponded to the well-known *Potts model*: $\psi_{i,j}(x_i, x_j) = e^{\frac{1}{T} J_{ij} \delta_{x_i, x_j}}$, $\phi_i(x_i) = e^{\frac{1}{T} J \delta_{x_i}(y_i)}$. We set $T = 0.5$ (a low temperature) and tested models with uniform and positive J_{ij}, widely used in image analysis, and models with J_{ij} drawn from a standard Gaussian; the latter is an instance of the much-studied *spin-glass* models of statistical physics which are known to be notoriously difficult to simulate at low temperatures [23]. Of course fully-connected models are known as *Boltzmann machines* [4] to the neural computation community. The output potentials were randomly selected in both the uniform and random interaction cases. The HC method used a linear coupling schedule for each edge, increasing from $\alpha = 0$ to $\alpha = 1$ over 100 iterations; our SMCG implementation used a linear global cooling schedule, whose number of steps depended on the graph in order to match those taken by SMCG.

All Monte Carlo algorithms were independently run 50 times each to approximate the variance of the estimates. Our SMC simulations used 1000 particles for each run, while each Gibbs run performed 20000 single-site updates. For these models, this was more than enough steps to settle into local minima; runs of up to 1 million iterations did not yield a difference, which is characteristic of the exponential mixing time of the sampler on these graphs. For our HC method, *spanning trees and edges in the sequential construction were randomly chosen from the full graph;* the rationale for doing so is to allay any criticism that "tweaking" the ordering may have had a crucial effect on the algorithm. The order clearly would matter to some extent, but this will be examined in later work. Also in the tables by "error" we mean the quantity $\frac{|\hat{a}-a|}{a}$ where $\hat{a}$ is an estimate of some quantity a obtained exactly (say Z).

First, we used HC, SMCG and Gibbs to approximate the expected sum of our graphs' variables, the so-called *magnetization*: $m = E[\sum_{i=1}^{M} x_i]$. We then approximated the partition functions of the graphs using HC, SMCG, and loopy.[1] We note again that there is no obvious way of estimating Z using Gibbs. Finally, we approximated the marginal probabilities using the four approximate methods. For loopy, we only kept the runs where it converged.

---

[1] Code for Bethe Z approximation kindly provided by Kevin Murphy.

Method	MRF Random Ψ		MRF Homogeneous Ψ		FC Random Ψ		FC Homogeneous Ψ	
	Error	Var	Error	Var	Error	Var	Error	Var
HC	0.0022	0.012	0.0251	0.17	0.0016	0.0522	0.0036	0.038
SMCG	0.0001	0.03	0.2789	10.09	0.127	0.570	0.331	165.61
Gibbs	0.0003	0.014	0.4928	200.95	0.02	0.32	0.3152	201.08

Figure 3: Approximate magnetization for the nodes of the graphs, as defined in the text, calculated using HC, SMCG, and Gibbs sampling and compared to the true value obtained by brute force. Observe the massive variance of Gibbs sampling in some cases.

Method	MRF Random Ψ		MRF Homogeneous Ψ		FC Random Ψ		FC Homogeneous Ψ	
	Error	Var	Error	Var	Error	Var	Err	Var
HC	0.0105	0.002	0.0227	0.001	0.0043	0.0537	0.0394	0.001
SMCG	0.004	0.005	6.47	7.646	1800	1.24	1	29.99
loopy	0.005	-	0.155	-	1	-	0.075	-

Figure 4: Approximate partition function of the graphs discussed in the text calculated using HC, SMCG, and Loopy Belief Propagation (loopy.) For HC and SMCG are shown the error of the sample average of results over 50 independent runs and the variance across those runs. loopy is of course a deterministic algorithm and has no variance. HC maintains a low error and variance in all cases.

Figure 3 shows the results of the magnetization experiments. On the MRF with random interactions, all three methods gave very accurate answers with small variance, but for the other graphs, the accuracies and variances began to diverge. On both positive-potential graphs, Gibbs sampling gives high error and huge variance; SMCG gives lower variance but is still quite skewed. On the fully-connected random-potential graph the 3 methods give good results but HC has the lowest variance. Our method experiences its worst performance on the homogeneous MRF but *it is only 2.5% error!*

Figure 4 tabulates the approximate partition function calculations. Again, for the MRF with random interactions, the 3 methods give estimates of Z of comparable quality. This example appeared to work for loopy, Gibbs, and SMCG. For the homogeneous MRF, SMCG degrades rapidly; loopy is still satisfactory at 15% error, but HC is at 2.7% with very low variance. In the fully-connected case with random potentials, HC's error is 0.43% while loopy's error is very high, having underestimated Z by a factor of 10^5. SMCG fails completely here as well. On the uniform fully-connected graph, loopy actually gives a reasonable estimate of Z at 7.5%, but is still beaten by HC.

Figure 5 shows the *variational* (L_1) distance between the exact marginal for a randomly chosen node in each graph and the approximate marginals of the 4 algorithms, a common measure of the "distance" between 2 distributions. For the Monte Carlo methods (HC, SMCG and Gibbs) the average over 50 independent runs was used to approximate the *expected* L_1 error of the estimate. All 4 methods perform well on the random Ψ MRF. On the MRF with homogeneous Ψ, both loopy and SMCG degrade, but HC maintains a low error. Among the FC graphs, HC performs extremely well on the homogeneous Ψ and surprisingly loopy does well too. In the random Ψ case, loopy's error increases dramatically.

Our final set of simulations was the classic Mean Squared reconstruction of a noisy image problem; we used a 100x100 MRF with a noisy "patch" image (consisting of shaded, rectangular regions) with an isotropic 5-state prior model. The object was to calculate the pixels' posterior marginal expectations. We chose this problem because it is a large model on which loopy is known to do well on, and can hence provide us with a measure of quality of the HC and SMCG results as larger numbers of edges are involved. From the toy examples we infer that the mechanism of HC is quite different from that of loopy as we have seen that it can work when loopy does not. Hence good performance on this problem would suggest that HC would *scale well,* which is a crucial question as in the large graph the final distribution has many more edges than the initial spanning tree. The results were promising: the mean-squared reconstruction error using loopy and using HC were virtually identical at 9.067×10^{-5} and 9.036×10^{-5} respectively, showing that HC seemed to be

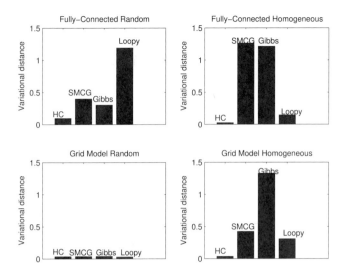

Figure 5: Variational(L_1) distance between estimated and true marginals for a randomly chosen node in each of the 4 graphs using the four approximate methods (smaller values mean less error.) The MRF-random example was again "easy" for all the methods, but the rest raise problems for all but HC.

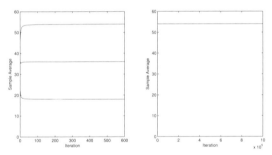

Figure 6: An example of how MCMC can get "stuck:" 3 different runs of a Gibbs sampler estimating the magnetization of FC-Homogeneous graph. At left are shown the first 600 iterations of the runs; after a brief transient behaviour the samplers settled into different minima which persisted for the entire duration (20000 steps) of the runs. Indeed for 1 million steps the local minima persist, as shown at right.

robust to the addition of around 9000 edges and many resampling stages. SMCG on the large MRF did not fare as well.

It is crucial to realize that MCMC is completely unsuited to some problems; see for example the "convergence" plots of the estimated magnetization of 3 independent Gibbs sampler runs on one of our "toy" graphs shown in Figure 6. Such behavior has been studied by Gore and Jerrum [11] and others, who discuss pessimistic theoretical results on the mixing properties of both Gibbs sampling and the celebrated Swendsen-Wang algorithm in several cases. To obtain a good estimate, MCMC requires that the process "visit" each of the target distribution's basins of energy with a frequency representative of their probability. Unfortunately, some basins take an exponential amount of time to exit, and so different finite runs of MCMC will give quite different answers, leading to tremendous variance. The methodology presented here is an attempt to sidestep the whole issue of mixing by permitting the independent particles to be stuck in modes, but then considering them *jointly* when estimating. In other words, instead of using a *time average,* we estimate using a weighted *ensemble average.* The object of the sequential phase is to address the difficult problem of constructing a suitable proposal for high-dimensional problems; to this the resampling-based methodology of particle filters was thought to be particularly suited. For the graphs we have considered, the single-edge algorithm we propose seems to be preferable to global annealing.

References

[1] S Z Li. *Markov random field modeling in image analysis.* Springer-Verlag, 2001.

[2] P Carbonetto and N de Freitas. Why can't José read? the problem of learning semantic associations in a robot environment. In *Human Language Technology Conference Workshop on Learning Word Meaning from Non-Linguistic Data*, 2003.

[3] J D Lafferty, A McCallum, and F C N Pereira. Conditional random fields: Probabilistic models for segmenting and labeling sequence data. In *International Conference on Machine Learning*, 2001.

[4] D E Rumelhart, G E Hinton, and R J Williams. Learning internal representations by error propagation. In D E Rumelhart and J L McClelland, editors, *Parallel Distributed Processing: Explorations in the Microstructure of Cognition*, pages 318–362, Cambridge, MA, 1986.

[5] P J Green and S Richardson. Hidden Markov models and disease mapping. *Journal of the American Statistical Association*, 97(460):1055–1070, 2002.

[6] C P Robert and G Casella. *Monte Carlo Statistical Methods.* Springer-Verlag, New York, 1999.

[7] M. I. Jordan, Z. Ghahramani, T. S. Jaakkola, and L. K. Saul. An introduction to variational methods for graphical models. *Machine Learning*, 37:183–233, 1999.

[8] J Moller, A N Pettitt, K K Berthelsen, and R W Reeves. An efficient Markov chain Monte Carlo method for distributions with intractable normalising constants. Technical report, The Danish National Research Foundation: Network in Mathematical Physics and Stochastics, 2004.

[9] M Jerrum and A Sinclair. The Markov chain Monte Carlo method: an approach to approximate counting and integration. In D S Hochbaum, editor, *Approximation Algorithms for NP-hard Problems*, pages 482–519. PWS Publishing, 1996.

[10] R H Swendsen and J S Wang. Nonuniversal critical dynamics in Monte Carlo simulations. *Physical Review Letters*, 58(2):86–88, 1987.

[11] V Gore and M Jerrum. The swendsen-wang process does not always mix rapidly. In *29th Annual ACM Symposium on Theory of Computing*, 1996.

[12] N Metropolis and S Ulam. The Monte Carlo method. *Journal of the American Statistical Association*, 44(247):335–341, 1949.

[13] A Doucet, N de Freitas, and N J Gordon, editors. *Sequential Monte Carlo Methods in Practice.* Springer-Verlag, 2001.

[14] C Jarzynski. Nonequilibrium equality for free energy differences. *Phys. Rev. Lett.*, 78, 1997.

[15] R M Neal. Annealed importance sampling. Technical Report No 9805, University of Toronto, 1998.

[16] P Del Moral, A Doucet, and G W Peters. Sequential Monte Carlo samplers. Technical Report CUED/F-INFENG/2004, Cambridge University Engineering Department, 2004.

[17] S Kirkpatrick, C D Gelatt, and M P Vecchi. Optimization by simulated annealing. *Science*, 220:671–680, 1983.

[18] G Kitagawa. Monte Carlo filter and smoother for non-Gaussian nonlinear state space models. *Journal of Computational and Graphical Statistics*, 5:1–25, 1996.

[19] N de Freitas, R Dearden, F Hutter, R Morales-Menendez, J Mutch, and D Poole. Diagnosis by a waiter and a mars explorer. *IEEE Proceedings*, 92, 2004.

[20] J A Bucklew. *Large Deviation Techniques in Decision, Simulation, and Estimation.* John Wiley & Sons, 1986.

[21] J Pearl. *Probabilistic reasoning in intelligent systems: networks of plausible inference.* Morgan-Kaufmann, 1988.

[22] C K Carter and R Kohn. On Gibbs sampling for state space models. *Biometrika*, 81(3):541–553, 1994.

[23] M E J Newman and G T Barkema. *Monte Carlo Methods in Statistical Physics.* Oxford University Press, 1999.

Tensor Subspace Analysis

Xiaofei He[1]   **Deng Cai**[2]   **Partha Niyogi**[1]
[1] Department of Computer Science, University of Chicago
{xiaofei, niyogi}@cs.uchicago.edu
[2] Department of Computer Science, University of Illinois at Urbana-Champaign
dengcai2@uiuc.edu

Abstract

Previous work has demonstrated that the image variations of many objects (human faces in particular) under variable lighting can be effectively modeled by low dimensional linear spaces. The typical linear subspace learning algorithms include Principal Component Analysis (PCA), Linear Discriminant Analysis (LDA), and Locality Preserving Projection (LPP). All of these methods consider an $n_1 \times n_2$ image as a high dimensional vector in $\mathbb{R}^{n_1 \times n_2}$, while an image represented in the plane is intrinsically a matrix. In this paper, we propose a new algorithm called **Tensor Subspace Analysis** (TSA). TSA considers an image as the second order tensor in $\mathcal{R}^{n_1} \otimes \mathcal{R}^{n_2}$, where $\mathcal{R}^{n_1}$ and $\mathcal{R}^{n_2}$ are two vector spaces. The relationship between the column vectors of the image matrix and that between the row vectors can be naturally characterized by TSA. TSA detects the intrinsic local geometrical structure of the tensor space by learning a lower dimensional tensor subspace. We compare our proposed approach with PCA, LDA and LPP methods on two standard databases. Experimental results demonstrate that TSA achieves better recognition rate, while being much more efficient.

1 Introduction

There is currently a great deal of interest in appearance-based approaches to face recognition [1], [5], [8]. When using appearance-based approaches, we usually represent an image of size $n_1 \times n_2$ pixels by a vector in $\mathbb{R}^{n_1 \times n_2}$. Throughout this paper, we denote by *face space* the set of all the face images. The face space is generally a low dimensional manifold embedded in the ambient space [6], [7], [10]. The typical linear algorithms for learning such a face manifold for recognition include Principal Component Analysis (PCA), Linear Discriminant Analysis (LDA) and Locality Preserving Projection (LPP) [4].

Most of previous works on statistical image analysis represent an image by a *vector* in high-dimensional space. However, an image is intrinsically a *matrix*, or the second order tensor. The relationship between the rows vectors of the matrix and that between the column vectors might be important for finding a projection, especially when the number of training samples is small. Recently, multilinear algebra, the algebra of higher-order tensors, was applied for analyzing the multifactor structure of image ensembles [9], [11], [12]. Vasilescu and Terzopoulos have proposed a novel face representation algorithm called Tensorface [9]. Tensorface represents the set of face images by a higher-order tensor and extends Singular Value Decomposition (SVD) to higher-order tensor data. In this way, the multiple factors related to expression, illumination and pose can be separated from different dimensions of the tensor.

In this paper, we propose a new algorithm for image (human faces in particular) representation based on the considerations of multilinear algebra and differential geometry. We call it *Tensor Subspace Analysis* (TSA). For an image of size $n_1 \times n_2$, it is represented as the second order tensor (or, matrix) in the tensor space $\mathcal{R}^{n_1} \otimes \mathcal{R}^{n_2}$. On the other hand, the face space is generally a submanifold embedded in $\mathcal{R}^{n_1} \otimes \mathcal{R}^{n_2}$. Given some images sampled from the face manifold, we can build an adjacency graph to model the local geometrical structure of the manifold. TSA finds a projection that respects this graph structure. The obtained tensor subspace provides an optimal linear approximation to the face manifold in the sense of local isometry. Vasilescu shows how to extend SVD(PCA) to higher order tensor data. We extend Laplacian based idea to tensor data.

It is worthwhile to highlight several aspects of the proposed approach here:

1. While traditional linear dimensionality reduction algorithms like PCA, LDA and LPP find a map from $\mathbb{R}^n$ to $\mathbb{R}^l$ ($l < n$), TSA finds a map from $\mathcal{R}^{n_1} \otimes \mathcal{R}^{n_2}$ to $\mathcal{R}^{l_1} \otimes \mathcal{R}^{l_2}$ ($l_1 < n_1, l_2 < n_2$). This leads to structured dimensionality reduction.

2. TSA can be performed in either supervised, unsupervised, or semi-supervised manner. When label information is available, it can be easily incorporated into the graph structure. Also, by preserving neighborhood structure, TSA is less sensitive to noise and outliers.

3. The computation of TSA is very simple. It can be obtained by solving two eigenvector problems. The matrices in the eigen-problems are of size $n_1 \times n_1$ or $n_2 \times n_2$, which are much smaller than the matrices of size $n \times n$ ($n = n_1 \times n_2$) in PCA, LDA and LPP. Therefore, TSA is much more computationally efficient in time and storage. There are few parameters that are independently estimated, so performance in small data sets is very good.

4. TSA explicitly takes into account the manifold structure of the image space. The local geometrical structure is modeled by an adjacency graph.

5. This paper is primarily focused on the second order tensors (or, matrices). However, the algorithm and analysis presented here can also be applied to higher order tensors.

2   Tensor Subspace Analysis

In this section, we introduce a new algorithm called *Tensor Subspace Analysis* for learning a tensor subspace which respects the geometrical and discriminative structures of the original data space.

2.1   Laplacian based Dimensionality Reduction

Problems of dimensionality reduction has been considered. One general approach is based on graph Laplacian [2]. The objective function of Laplacian eigenmap is as follows:

$$\min_f \sum_{ij} \left(f(\mathbf{x}_i) - f(\mathbf{x}_j) \right)^2 S_{ij}$$

where S is a similarity matrix. These optimal functions are nonlinear but may be expensive to compute.

A class of algorithms may be optimized by restricting problem to more tractable families of functions. One natural approach restricts to linear function giving rise to LPP [4]. In this paper we will consider a more structured subset of linear functions that arise out of tensor analysis. This provided greater computational benefits.

2.2 The Linear Dimensionality Reduction Problem in Tensor Space

The generic problem of linear dimensionality reduction in the second order tensor space is the following. Given a set of data points $X_1, \cdots, X_m$ in $\mathcal{R}^{n_1} \otimes \mathcal{R}^{n_2}$, find two transformation matrices U of size $n_1 \times l_1$ and V of size $n_2 \times l_2$ that maps these m points to a set of points $Y_1, \cdots, Y_m \in \mathcal{R}^{l_1} \otimes \mathcal{R}^{l_2} (l_1 < n_1, l_2 < n_2)$, such that Y_i "represents" X_i, where $Y_i = U^T X_i V$. Our method is of particular applicability in the special case where $X_1, \cdots, X_m \in \mathcal{M}$ and $\mathcal{M}$ is a nonlinear submanifold embedded in $\mathcal{R}^{n_1} \otimes \mathcal{R}^{n_2}$.

2.3 Optimal Linear Embeddings

As we described previously, the face space is probably a nonlinear submanifold embedded in the tensor space. One hopes then to estimate geometrical and topological properties of the submanifold from random points ("scattered data") lying on this unknown submanifold. In this section, we consider the particular question of finding a linear subspace approximation to the submanifold in the sense of local isometry. Our method is fundamentally based on LPP [4].

Given m data points $\mathcal{X} = \{X_1, \cdots, X_m\}$ sampled from the face submanifold $\mathcal{M} \in \mathcal{R}^{n_1} \otimes \mathcal{R}^{n_1}$, one can build a nearest neighbor graph $\mathcal{G}$ to model the local geometrical structure of $\mathcal{M}$. Let S be the weight matrix of $\mathcal{G}$. A possible definition of S is as follows:

$$S_{ij} = \begin{cases} e^{-\frac{\|X_i - X_j\|^2}{t}}, & \text{if } X_i \text{ is among the } k \text{ nearest} \\ & \text{neighbors of } X_j, \text{ or } X_j \text{ is among} \\ & \text{the } k \text{ nearest neighbors of } X_i; \\ 0, & \text{otherwise.} \end{cases} \qquad (1)$$

where t is a suitable constant. The function $\exp(-\|X_i - X_j\|^2/t)$ is the so called heat kernel which is intimately related to the manifold structure. $\| \cdot \|$ is the Frobenius norm of matrix, i.e. $\|A\| = \sqrt{\sum_i \sum_j a_{ij}^2}$. When the label information is available, it can be easily incorporated into the graph as follows:

$$S_{ij} = \begin{cases} e^{-\frac{\|X_i - X_j\|^2}{t}}, & \text{if } X_i \text{ and } X_j \text{ share the same label}; \\ 0, & \text{otherwise.} \end{cases} \qquad (2)$$

Let U and V be the transformation matrices. A reasonable transformation respecting the graph structure can be obtained by solving the following objective functions:

$$\min_{U,V} \sum_{ij} \|U^T X_i V - U^T X_j V\|^2 S_{ij} \qquad (3)$$

The objective function incurs a heavy penalty if neighboring points X_i and X_j are mapped far apart. Therefore, minimizing it is an attempt to ensure that if X_i and X_j are "close" then $U^T X_i V$ and $U^T X_j V$ are "close" as well. Let $Y_i = U^T X_i V$. Let D be a diagonal matrix, $D_{ii} = \sum_j S_{ij}$. Since $\|A\|^2 = tr(AA^T)$, we see that:

$$\frac{1}{2} \sum_{ij} \|U^T X_i V - U^T X_j V\|^2 S_{ij} = \frac{1}{2} \sum_{ij} tr\left((Y_i - Y_j)(Y_i - Y_j)^T\right) S_{ij}$$

$$= \frac{1}{2} \sum_{ij} tr\left(Y_i Y_i^T + Y_j Y_j^T - Y_i Y_j^T - Y_j Y_i^T\right) S_{ij}$$

$$= tr\left(\sum_i D_{ii} Y_i Y_i^T - \sum_{ij} S_{ij} Y_i Y_j^T\right)$$

$$
= tr\left(\sum_i D_{ii} U^T X_i V V^T X_i^T U - \sum_{ij} S_{ij} U^T X_i V V^T X_j^T U\right)
$$

$$
= tr\left(U^T \left(\sum_i D_{ii} X_i V V^T X_i^T - \sum_{ij} S_{ij} X_i V V^T X_j^T\right) U\right)
$$

$$
\doteq tr\left(U^T (D_V - S_V) U\right)
$$

where $D_V = \sum_i D_{ii} X_i V V^T X_i^T$ and $S_V = \sum_{ij} S_{ij} X_i V V^T X_j^T$. Similarly, $\|A\|^2 = tr(A^T A)$, so we also have

$$
\frac{1}{2} \sum_{ij} \|U^T X_i V - U^T X_j V\|^2 S_{ij}
$$

$$
= \frac{1}{2} \sum_{ij} tr\left((Y_i - Y_j)^T (Y_i - Y_j)\right) S_{ij}
$$

$$
= \frac{1}{2} \sum_{ij} tr\left(Y_i^T Y_i + Y_j^T Y_j - Y_i^T Y_j - Y_j^T Y_i\right) S_{ij}
$$

$$
= tr\left(\sum_i D_{ii} Y_i^T Y_i - \sum_{ij} S_{ij} Y_i^T Y_j\right)
$$

$$
= tr\left(V^T \left(\sum_i D_{ii} X_i^T U U^T X_i - \sum_{ij} X_i^T U U^T X_j\right) V\right)
$$

$$
\doteq tr\left(V^T (D_U - S_U) V\right)
$$

where $D_U = \sum_i D_{ii} X_i^T U U^T X_i$ and $S_U = \sum_{ij} S_{ij} X_i^T U U^T X_j$. Therefore, we should simultaneously minimize $tr\left(U^T (D_V - S_V) U\right)$ and $tr\left(V^T (D_U - S_U) V\right)$.

In addition to preserving the graph structure, we also aim at maximizing the global variance on the manifold. Recall that the variance of a random variable x can be written as follows:

$$
var(x) = \int_{\mathcal{M}} (x - \mu)^2 dP(x), \quad \mu = \int_{\mathcal{M}} x dP(x)
$$

where $\mathcal{M}$ is the data manifold, μ is the expected value of x and dP is the probability measure on the manifold. By spectral graph theory [3], dP can be discretely estimated by the diagonal matrix $D(D_{ii} = \sum_j S_{ij})$ on the sample points. Let $Y = U^T X V$ denote the random variable in the tensor subspace and suppose the data points have a zero mean. Thus, the *weighted* variance can be estimated as follows:

$$
var(Y) = \sum_i \|Y_i\|^2 D_{ii} = \sum_i tr(Y_i^T Y_i) D_{ii} = \sum_i tr(V^T X_i^T U U^T X_i V) D_{ii}
$$

$$
= tr\left(V^T \left(\sum_i D_{ii} X_i^T U U^T X_i\right) V\right) = tr\left(V^T D_U V\right)
$$

Similarly, $\|Y_i\|^2 = tr(Y_i Y_i^T)$, so we also have:

$$
var(Y) = \sum_i tr(Y_i Y_i^T) D_{ii} = tr\left(U^T \left(\sum_i D_{ii} X_i V V^T X_i^T\right) U\right) = tr\left(U^T D_V U\right)
$$

Finally, we get the following optimization problems:

$$
\min_{U,V} \frac{tr\left(U^T (D_V - S_V) U\right)}{tr\left(U^T D_V U\right)} \tag{4}
$$

$$\min_{U,V} \frac{tr\left(V^T \left(D_U - S_U\right) V\right)}{tr\left(V^T D_U V\right)} \tag{5}$$

The above two minimization problems (4) and (5) depends on each other, and hence can not be solved independently. In the following subsection, we describe a simple computational method to solve these two optimization problems.

2.4 Computation

In this subsection, we discuss how to solve the optimization problems (4) and (5). It is easy to see that the optimal U should be the generalized eigenvectors of $(D_V - S_V, D_V)$ and the optimal V should be the generalized eigenvectors of $(D_U - S_U, D_U)$. However, it is difficult to compute the optimal U and V simultaneously since the matrices D_V, S_V, D_U, S_U are not fixed. In this paper, we compute U and V iteratively as follows. We first fix U, then V can be computed by solving the following generalized eigenvector problem:

$$(D_U - S_U)\mathbf{v} = \lambda D_U \mathbf{v} \tag{6}$$

Once V is obtained, U can be updated by solving the following generalized eigenvector problem:

$$(D_V - S_V)\mathbf{u} = \lambda D_V \mathbf{u} \tag{7}$$

Thus, the optimal U and V can be obtained by iteratively computing the generalized eigenvectors of (6) and (7). In our experiments, U is initially set to the identity matrix. It is easy to show that the matrices $D_U, D_V, D_U - S_U$, and $D_V - S_V$ are all symmetric and positive semi-definite.

3 Experimental Results

In this section, several experiments are carried out to show the efficiency and effectiveness of our proposed algorithm for face recognition. We compare our algorithm with the Eigenface (PCA) [8], Fisherface (LDA) [1], and Laplacianface (LPP) [5] methods, three of the most popular linear methods for face recognition.

Two face databases were used. The first one is the PIE (Pose, Illumination, and Experience) database from CMU, and the second one is the ORL database. In all the experiments, preprocessing to locate the faces was applied. Original images were normalized (in scale and orientation) such that the two eyes were aligned at the same position. Then, the facial areas were cropped into the final images for matching. The size of each cropped image in all the experiments is 32×32 pixels, with 256 gray levels per pixel. No further preprocessing is done. For the Eigenface, Fisherface, and Laplacianface methods, the image is represented as a 1024-dimensional vector, while in our algorithm the image is represented as a (32×32)-dimensional matrix, or the second order tensor. The nearest neighbor classifier is used for classification for its simplicity.

In short, the recognition process has three steps. First, we calculate the face subspace from the training set of face images; then the new face image to be identified is projected into d-dimensional subspace (PCA, LDA, and LPP) or $(d \times d)$-dimensional tensor subspace (TSA); finally, the new face image is identified by nearest neighbor classifier. In our TSA algorithm, the number of iterations is taken to be 3.

3.1 Experiments on PIE Database

The CMU PIE face database contains 68 subjects with 41,368 face images as a whole. The face images were captured by 13 synchronized cameras and 21 flashes, under varying pose, illumination and expression. We choose the five near frontal poses (C05, C07, C09, C27,

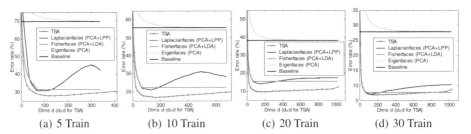

| (a) 5 Train | (b) 10 Train | (c) 20 Train | (d) 30 Train |

Figure 1: Error rate vs. dimensionality reduction on PIE database

Table 1: Performance comparison on PIE database

Method	5 Train			10 Train		
	error	dim	time(s)	error	dim	time(s)
Baseline	69.9%	1024	-	55.7%	1024	-
Eigenfaces	69.9%	338	0.907	55.7%	654	5.297
Fisherfaces	31.5%	67	1.843	22.4%	67	9.609
Laplacianfaces	30.8%	67	2.375	21.1%	134	11.516
TSA	**27.9%**	**11^2**	**0.594**	**16.9%**	**13^2**	**2.063**

	20 Train			30 Train		
Method	error	dim	time(s)	error	dim	time(s)
Baseline	38.2%	1024	-	27.9%	1024	-
Eigenfaces	38.1%	889	14.328	27.9%	990	15.453
Fisherfaces	15.4%	67	35.828	7.77%	67	38.406
Laplacianfaces	14.1%	146	39.172	7.13%	131	47.610
TSA	**9.64%**	**13^2**	**7.125**	**6.88%**	**12^2**	**15.688**

C29) and use all the images under different illuminations and expressions, thus we get 170 images for each individual. For each individual, $l(= 5, 10, 20, 30)$ images are randomly selected for training and the rest are used for testing.

The training set is utilized to learn the subspace representation of the face manifold by using Eigenface, Fisherface, Laplacianface and our algorithm. The testing images are projected into the face subspace in which recognition is then performed. For each given l, we average the results over 20 random splits. It would be important to note that the Laplacianface algorithm and our algorithm share the same graph structure as defined in Eqn. (2).

Figure 1 shows the plots of error rate versus dimensionality reduction for the Eigenface, Fisherface, Laplacianface, TSA and baseline methods. For the baseline method, the recognition is simply performed in the original 1024-dimensional image space without any dimensionality reduction. Note that, the upper bound of the dimensionality of Fisherface is $c - 1$ where c is the number of individuals. For our TSA algorithm, we only show its performance in the $(d \times d)$-dimensional tensor subspace, say, 1, 4, 9, etc. As can be seen, the performance of the Eigenface, Fisherface, Laplacianface, and TSA algorithms varies with the number of dimensions. We show the best results obtained by them in Table 1 and the corresponding face subspaces are called optimal face subspace for each method.

It is found that our method outperforms the other four methods with different numbers of training samples (5, 10, 20, 30) per individual. The Eigenface method performs the worst. It does not obtain any improvement over the baseline method. The Fisherface and Laplacianface methods perform comparatively to each each. The dimensions of the optimal subspaces are also given in Table 1.

As we have discussed, TSA can be implemented very efficiently. We show the running time in seconds for each method in Table 1. As can be seen, TSA is much faster than the

504

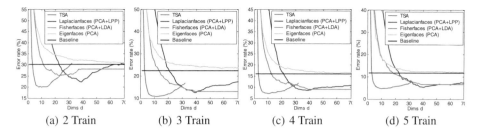

| (a) 2 Train | (b) 3 Train | (c) 4 Train | (d) 5 Train |

Figure 2: Error rate vs. dimensionality reduction on ORL database

Table 2: Performance comparison on ORL database

Method	2 Train			3 Train		
	error	dim	time	error	dim	time
Baseline	30.2%	1024	-	22.4%	1024	-
Eigenfaces	30.2%	79	38.13	22.3%	113	85.16
Fisherfaces	25.2%	23	60.32	13.1%	39	119.69
Laplacianfaces	22.2%	39	62.65	12.5%	39	136.25
TSA	**20.0%**	10^2	**65.00**	**10.7%**	11^2	**135.93**

	4 Train			5 Train		
Method	error	dim	time	error	dim	time
Baseline	16.0%	1024	-	11.7%	1024	-
Eigenfaces	15.9%	122	141.72	11.6%	182	224.69
Fisherfaces	9.17%	39	212.82	6.55%	39	355.63
Laplacianfaces	8.54%	39	248.90	5.45%	40	410.78
TSA	**7.12%**	10^2	**201.40**	**4.75%**	10^2	**302.97**

Eigenface, Fisherface and Laplacianface methods. All the algorithms were implemented in Matlab 6.5 and run on a Intel P4 2.566GHz PC with 1GB memory.

3.2 Experiments on ORL Database

The ORL (Olivetti Research Laboratory) face database is used in this test. It consists of a total of 400 face images, of a total of 40 people (10 samples per person). The images were captured at different times and have different variations including expressions (open or closed eyes, smiling or non-smiling) and facial details (glasses or no glasses). The images were taken with a tolerance for some tilting and rotation of the face up to 20 degrees. For each individual, $l(= 2, 3, 4, 5)$ images are randomly selected for training and the rest are used for testing.

The experimental design is the same as that in the last subsection. For each given l, we average the results over 20 random splits. Figure 3.2 shows the plots of error rate versus dimensionality reduction for the Eigenface, Fisherface, Laplacianface, TSA and baseline methods. Note that, the presentation of the performance of the TSA algorithm is different from that in the last subsection. Here, for a given d, we show its performance in the $(d \times d)$-dimensional tensor subspace. The reason is for better comparison, since the Eigenface and Laplacianface methods start to converge after 70 dimensions and there is no need to show their performance after that. The best result obtained in the optimal subspace and the running time (millisecond) of computing the eigenvectors for each method are shown in Table 2.

As can be seen, our TSA algorithm performed the best in all the cases. The Fisherface and Laplacianface methods performed comparatively to our method, while the Eigenface method performed poorly.

4   Conclusions and Future Work

Tensor based face analysis (representation and recognition) is introduced in this paper in order to detect the underlying nonlinear face manifold structure in the manner of tensor subspace learning. The manifold structure is approximated by the adjacency graph computed from the data points. The optimal tensor subspace respecting the graph structure is then obtained by solving an optimization problem. We call this *Tensor Subspace Analysis* method.

Most of traditional appearance based face recognition methods (i.e. Eigenface, Fisherface, and Laplacianface) consider an image as a vector in high dimensional space. Such representation ignores the spacial relationships between the pixels in the image. In our work, an image is naturally represented as a matrix, or the second order tensor. Tensor representation makes our algorithm much more computationally efficient than PCA, LDA, and LPP. Experimental results on PIE and ORL databases demonstrate the efficiency and effectiveness of our method.

TSA is linear. Therefore, if the face manifold is highly nonlinear, it may fail to discover the intrinsic geometrical structure. It remains unclear how to generalize our algorithm to nonlinear case. Also, in our algorithm, the adjacency graph is induced from the local geometry and class information. Different graph structures lead to different projections. It remains unclear how to define the optimal graph structure in the sense of discrimination.

References

[1] P.N. Belhumeur, J.P. Hepanha, and D.J. Kriegman, "Eigenfaces vs. fisherfaces: recognition using class specific linear projection,"*IEEE. Trans. Pattern Analysis and Machine Intelligence*, vol. 19, no. 7, pp. 711-720, July 1997.

[2] M. Belkin and P. Niyogi, "Laplacian Eigenmaps and Spectral Techniques for Embedding and Clustering ," *Advances in Neural Information Processing Systems 14*, 2001.

[3] Fan R. K. Chung, *Spectral Graph Theory,* Regional Conference Series in Mathematics, number 92, 1997.

[4] X. He and P. Niyogi, "Locality Preserving Projections,"*Advance in Neural Information Processing Systems 16*, Vancouver, Canada, December 2003.

[5] X. He, S. Yan, Y. Hu, P. Niyogi, and H.-J. Zhang, "Face Recognition using Laplacian-faces,"*IEEE. Trans. Pattern Analysis and Machine Intelligence*, vol. 27, No. 3, 2005.

[6] S. Roweis, and L. K. Saul, "Nonlinear Dimensionality Reduction by Locally Linear Embedding," *Science*, vol 290, 22 December 2000.

[7] J. B. Tenenbaum, V. de Silva, and J. C. Langford, "A Global Geometric Framework for Nonlinear Dimensionality Reduction," *Science*, vol 290, 22 December 2000.

[8] M. Turk and A. Pentland, "Eigenfaces for recognition," *Journal of Cognitive Neuroscience*, 3(1):71-86, 1991.

[9] M. A. O. Vasilescu and D. Terzopoulos, "Multilinear Subspace Analysis for Image Ensembles," *IEEE Conference on Computer Vision and Pattern Recognition*, 2003.

[10] K. Q. Weinberger and L. K. Saul, "Unsupervised Learning of Image Manifolds by SemiDefinite Programming," *IEEE Conference on Computer Vision and Pattern Recognition*, Washington, DC, 2004.

[11] J. Yang, D. Zhang, A. Frangi, and J. Yang, "Two-dimensional PCA: a new approach to appearance-based face representation and recognition,"*IEEE. Trans. Pattern Analysis and Machine Intelligence*, vol. 26, No. 1, 2004.

[12] J. Ye, R. Janardan, Q. Li, "Two-Dimensional Linear Discriminant Analysis ," *Advances in Neural Information Processing Systems 17*, 2004.

Laplacian Score for Feature Selection

Xiaofei He[1]   **Deng Cai**[2]   **Partha Niyogi**[1]
[1] Department of Computer Science, University of Chicago
{xiaofei, niyogi}@cs.uchicago.edu
[2] Department of Computer Science, University of Illinois at Urbana-Champaign
dengcai2@uiuc.edu

Abstract

In supervised learning scenarios, feature selection has been studied widely in the literature. Selecting features in unsupervised learning scenarios is a much harder problem, due to the absence of class labels that would guide the search for relevant information. And, almost all of previous unsupervised feature selection methods are "wrapper" techniques that require a learning algorithm to evaluate the candidate feature subsets. In this paper, we propose a "filter" method for feature selection which is independent of any learning algorithm. Our method can be performed in either supervised or unsupervised fashion. The proposed method is based on the observation that, in many real world classification problems, data from the same class are often close to each other. The importance of a feature is evaluated by its power of locality preserving, or, **Laplacian Score**. We compare our method with data variance (unsupervised) and Fisher score (supervised) on two data sets. Experimental results demonstrate the effectiveness and efficiency of our algorithm.

1   Introduction

Feature selection methods can be classified into "wrapper" methods and "filter" methods [4]. The wrapper model techniques evaluate the features using the learning algorithm that will ultimately be employed. Thus, they "wrap" the selection process around the learning algorithm. Most of the feature selection methods are wrapper methods. Algorithms based on the filter model examine intrinsic properties of the data to evaluate the features prior to the learning tasks. The filter based approaches almost always rely on the class labels, most commonly assessing correlations between features and the class label. In this paper, we are particularly interested in the filter methods. Some typical filter methods include data variance, Pearson correlation coefficients, Fisher score, and Kolmogorov-Smirnov test.

Most of the existing filter methods are supervised. Data variance might be the simplest *unsupervised* evaluation of the features. The variance along a dimension reflects its representative power. Data variance can be used as a criteria for feature selection and extraction. For example, Principal Component Analysis (PCA) is a classical feature extraction method which finds a set of mutually orthogonal basis functions that capture the directions of maximum variance in the data.

Although the data variance criteria finds features that are useful for representing data, there is no reason to assume that these features must be useful for discriminating between data in different classes. Fisher score seeks features that are efficient for discrimination. It assigns the highest score to the feature on which the data points of different classes are far from each other while requiring data points of the same class to be close to each other. Fisher criterion can be also used for feature extraction, such as Linear Discriminant Analysis (LDA).

In this paper, we introduce a novel feature selection algorithm called **Laplacian Score** (LS). For each feature, its Laplacian score is computed to reflect its locality preserving power. LS is based on the observation that, two data points are probably related to the same topic if they are close to each other. In fact, in many learning problems such as classification, the local structure of the data space is more important than the global structure. In order to model the local geometric structure, we construct a nearest neighbor graph. LS seeks those features that respect this graph structure.

2 Laplacian Score

Laplacian Score (LS) is fundamentally based on Laplacian Eigenmaps [1] and Locality Preserving Projection [3]. The basic idea of LS is to evaluate the features according to their locality preserving power.

2.1 The Algorithm

Let L_r denote the Laplacian Score of the r-th feature. Let f_{ri} denote the i-th sample of the r-th feature, $i = 1, \cdots, m$. Our algorithm can be stated as follows:

1. Construct a nearest neighbor graph G with m nodes. The i-th node corresponds to $\mathbf{x}_i$. We put an edge between nodes i and j if $\mathbf{x}_i$ and $\mathbf{x}_j$ are "close", i.e. $\mathbf{x}_i$ is among k nearest neighbors of $\mathbf{x}_j$ or $\mathbf{x}_j$ is among k nearest neighbors of $\mathbf{x}_i$. When the label information is available, one can put an edge between two nodes sharing the same label.

2. If nodes i and j are connected, put $S_{ij} = e^{-\frac{\|\mathbf{x}_i - \mathbf{x}_j\|^2}{t}}$, where t is a suitable constant. Otherwise, put $S_{ij} = 0$. The weight matrix S of the graph models the local structure of the data space.

3. For the r-th feature, we define:
$$\mathbf{f}_r = [f_{r1}, f_{r2}, \cdots, f_{rm}]^T, D = diag(S\mathbf{1}), \mathbf{1} = [1, \cdots, 1]^T, L = D - S$$
   where the matrix L is often called graph Laplacian [2]. Let
$$\widetilde{\mathbf{f}}_r = \mathbf{f}_r - \frac{\mathbf{f}_r^T D \mathbf{1}}{\mathbf{1}^T D \mathbf{1}} \mathbf{1}$$

4. Compute the Laplacian Score of the r-th feature as follows:
$$L_r = \frac{\widetilde{\mathbf{f}}_r^T L \widetilde{\mathbf{f}}_r}{\widetilde{\mathbf{f}}_r^T D \widetilde{\mathbf{f}}_r} \tag{1}$$

3 Justification

3.1 Objective Function

Recall that given a data set we construct a weighted graph G with edges connecting nearby points to each other. S_{ij} evaluates the similarity between the i-th and j-th nodes. Thus, the importance of a feature can be thought of as the degree it respects the graph structure. To be specific, a "good" feature should the one on which two data points are close to each other if and only if there is an edge between these two points. A reasonable criterion for choosing a good feature is to minimize the following object function:

$$L_r = \frac{\sum_{ij}(f_{ri} - f_{rj})^2 S_{ij}}{Var(\mathbf{f}_r)} \tag{2}$$

where $Var(\mathbf{f}_r)$ is the estimated variance of the r-th feature. By minimizing $\sum_{ij}(f_{ri} - f_{rj})^2 S_{ij}$, we prefer those features respecting the pre-defined graph structure. For a good feature, the bigger S_{ij}, the smaller $(f_{ri} - f_{rj})$, and thus the Laplacian Score tends to be small. Following some simple algebraic steps, we see that

$$\sum_{ij}(f_{ri} - f_{rj})^2 S_{ij} = \sum_{ij}(f_{ri}^2 + f_{rj}^2 - 2f_{ri}f_{rj}) S_{ij}$$

$$= 2\sum_{ij} f_{ri}^2 S_{ij} - 2\sum_{ij} f_{ri}S_{ij}f_{rj} = 2\mathbf{f}_r^T D\mathbf{f}_r - 2\mathbf{f}_r^T S\mathbf{f}_r = 2\mathbf{f}_r^T L\mathbf{f}_r$$

By maximizing $Var(\mathbf{f}_r)$, we prefer those features with large variance which have more representative power. Recall that the variance of a random variable a can be written as follows:

$$Var(a) = \int_{\mathcal{M}} (a - \mu)^2 dP(a), \quad \mu = \int_{\mathcal{M}} adP(a)$$

where $\mathcal{M}$ is the data manifold, μ is the expected value of a and dP is the probability measure. By spectral graph theory [2], dP can be estimated by the diagonal matrix D on the sample points. Thus, the *weighted* data variance can be estimated as follows:

$$Var(\mathbf{f}_r) = \sum_i (f_{ri} - \mu_r)^2 D_{ii}$$

$$\mu_r = \sum_i \left(f_{ri}\frac{D_{ii}}{\sum_i D_{ii}}\right) = \frac{1}{(\sum_i D_{ii})}\left(\sum_i f_{ri}D_{ii}\right) = \frac{\mathbf{f}_r^T D\mathbf{1}}{\mathbf{1}^T D\mathbf{1}}$$

To remove the mean from the samples, we define:

$$\tilde{\mathbf{f}}_r = \mathbf{f}_r - \frac{\mathbf{f}_r^T D\mathbf{1}}{\mathbf{1}^T D\mathbf{1}}\mathbf{1}$$

Thus,

$$Var(\mathbf{f}_r) = \sum_i \tilde{f}_{ri}^2 D_{ii} = \tilde{\mathbf{f}}_r^T D\tilde{\mathbf{f}}_r$$

Also, it is easy to show that $\tilde{\mathbf{f}}_r^T L\tilde{\mathbf{f}}_r = \mathbf{f}_r^T L\mathbf{f}_r$ (please see Proposition 1 in Section 4.2 for detials). We finally get equation (1).

It would be important to note that, if we do not remove the mean, the vector $\mathbf{f}_r$ can be a non-zero constant vector such as $\mathbf{1}$. It is easy to check that, $\mathbf{1}^T L\mathbf{1} = 0$ and $\mathbf{1}^T D\mathbf{1} > 0$. Thus, $L_r = 0$. Unfortunately, this feature is clearly of no use since it contains no information. With mean being removed, the new vector $\tilde{\mathbf{f}}_r$ is orthogonal to $\mathbf{1}$ with respect to D, i.e. $\tilde{\mathbf{f}}_r^T D\mathbf{1} = 0$. Therefore, $\tilde{\mathbf{f}}_r$ can not be any constant vector other than $\mathbf{0}$. If $\tilde{\mathbf{f}}_r = \mathbf{0}$, $\tilde{\mathbf{f}}_r^T L\tilde{\mathbf{f}}_r = \tilde{\mathbf{f}}_r^T D\tilde{\mathbf{f}}_r = 0$. Thus, the Laplacian Score L_r becomes a trivial solution and the r-th feature is excluded from selection. While computing the weighted variance, the matrix D models the importance (or local density) of the data points. We can also simply replace it by the identity matrix I, in which case the weighted variance becomes the standard variance. To be specific,

$$\tilde{\mathbf{f}}_r = \mathbf{f}_r - \frac{\mathbf{f}_r^T I\mathbf{1}}{\mathbf{1}^T I\mathbf{1}}\mathbf{1} = \mathbf{f}_r - \frac{\mathbf{f}_r^T \mathbf{1}}{n}\mathbf{1} = \mathbf{f}_r - \mu\mathbf{1}$$

where μ is the mean of f_{ri}, $i = 1, \cdots, n$. Thus,

$$Var(\mathbf{f}_r) = \tilde{\mathbf{f}}_r^T \tilde{I} \tilde{\mathbf{f}}_r = \frac{1}{n} (\mathbf{f}_r - \mu \mathbf{1})^T (\mathbf{f}_r - \mu \mathbf{1}) \tag{3}$$

which is just the *standard* variance.

In fact, the Laplacian scores can be thought of as the Rayleigh quotients for the features with respect to the graph G, please see [2] for details.

3.2 Connection to Fisher Score

In this section, we provide a theoretical analysis of the connection between our algorithm and the canonical Fisher score.

Given a set of data points with label, $\{\mathbf{x}_i, y_i\}_{i=1}^n$, $y_i \in \{1, \cdots, c\}$. Let n_i denote the number of data points in class i. Let μ_i and σ_i^2 be the mean and variance of class i, $i = 1, \cdots, c$, corresponding to the r-th feature. Let μ and σ^2 denote the mean and variance of the whole data set. The Fisher score is defined below:

$$F_r = \frac{\sum_{i=1}^c n_i (\mu_i - \mu)^2}{\sum_{i=1}^c n_i \sigma_i^2} \tag{4}$$

In the following, we show that Fisher score is equivalent to Laplacian score with a special graph structure. We define the weight matrix as follows:

$$S_{ij} = \begin{cases} \frac{1}{n_l}, & y_i = y_j = l; \\ 0, & \text{otherwise.} \end{cases} \tag{5}$$

Without loss of generality, we assume that the data points are ordered according to which class they are in, so that $\{\mathbf{x}_1, \cdots, \mathbf{x}_{n_1}\}$ are in the first class, $\{\mathbf{x}_{n_1+1}, \cdots, \mathbf{x}_{n_1+n_2}\}$ are in the second class, etc. Thus, S can be written as follows:

$$S = \begin{pmatrix} S_1 & 0 & 0 \\ 0 & \ddots & 0 \\ 0 & 0 & S_c \end{pmatrix}$$

where $S_i = \frac{1}{n_i} \mathbf{1}\mathbf{1}^T$ is an $n_i \times n_i$ matrix. For each S_i, the raw (or column) sum is equal to 1, so $D_i = diag(S_i \mathbf{1})$ is just the identity matrix. Define $\mathbf{f}_r^1 = [f_{r1}, \cdots, f_{rn_1}]^T$, $\mathbf{f}_r^2 = [f_{r,n_1+1}, \cdots, f_{r,n_1+n_2}]^T$, etc. We now make the following observations.

Observation 1 With the weight matrix S defined in (5), we have $\tilde{\mathbf{f}}_r^T \tilde{L} \tilde{\mathbf{f}}_r = \mathbf{f}_r^T L \mathbf{f}_r = \sum_i n_i \sigma_i^2$, where $L = D - S$.

To see this, define $L_i = D_i - S_i = I_i - S_i$, where I_i is the $n_i \times n_i$ identity matrix. We have

$$\mathbf{f}_r^T L \mathbf{f}_r = \sum_{i=1}^c (\mathbf{f}_r^i)^T L_i \mathbf{f}_r^i = \sum_{i=1}^c (\mathbf{f}_r^i)^T (I_i - \frac{1}{n_i} \mathbf{1}\mathbf{1}^T) \mathbf{f}_r^i = \sum_{i=1}^c n_i cov(\mathbf{f}_r^i, \mathbf{f}_r^i) = \sum_{i=1}^c n_i \sigma_i^2$$

Note that, since $\mathbf{u}^T L \mathbf{1} = \mathbf{1}^T L \mathbf{u} = 0$, $\forall \mathbf{u} \in \mathbb{R}^n$, the value of $\mathbf{f}_r^T L \mathbf{f}_r$ remains unchanged by subtracting a constant vector ($= \alpha \mathbf{1}$) from $\mathbf{f}_r$. This shows that $\tilde{\mathbf{f}}_r^T \tilde{L} \tilde{\mathbf{f}}_r = \mathbf{f}_r^T L \mathbf{f}_r = \sum_i n_i \sigma_i^2$.

Observation 2 With the weight matrix S defined in (5), we have $\tilde{\mathbf{f}}_r^T \tilde{D} \tilde{\mathbf{f}}_r = n\sigma^2$.

To see this, by the definition of S, we have $D = I$. Thus, this is a immediate result from equation (3).

Observation 3 With the weight matrix S defined in (5), we have $\sum_{i=1}^{c} n_i(\mu_i - \mu)^2 = \tilde{\mathbf{f}}_r^T D\tilde{\mathbf{f}}_r - \tilde{\mathbf{f}}_r^T L\tilde{\mathbf{f}}_r$.

To see this, notice

$$\sum_{i=1}^{c} n_i(\mu_i - \mu)^2 = \sum_{i=1}^{c} \left(n_i\mu_i^2 - 2n_i\mu_i\mu + n_i\mu^2\right)$$

$$= \sum_{i=1}^{c} \frac{1}{n_i}(n_i\mu_i)^2 - 2\mu \sum_{i=1}^{c} n_i\mu_i + \mu^2 \sum_{i=1}^{c} n_i = \sum_{i=1}^{c} \frac{1}{n_i}\left((\mathbf{f}_r^i)^T \mathbf{1}\mathbf{1}^T \mathbf{f}_r^i\right) - 2n\mu^2 + n\mu^2$$

$$= \sum_{i=1}^{c} \mathbf{f}_r^i S_i \mathbf{f}_r^i - \frac{1}{n}(n\mu)^2 = \mathbf{f}_r^T S\mathbf{f}_r - \mathbf{f}_r^T \left(\frac{1}{n}\mathbf{1}\mathbf{1}^T\right)\mathbf{f}_r$$

$$= \mathbf{f}_r^T(I - S)\mathbf{f}_r - \mathbf{f}_r^T\left(I - \frac{1}{n}\mathbf{1}\mathbf{1}^T\right)\mathbf{f}_r = \mathbf{f}_r^T L\mathbf{f}_r - n\sigma^2 = \tilde{\mathbf{f}}_r^T L\tilde{\mathbf{f}}_r - \tilde{\mathbf{f}}_r^T D\tilde{\mathbf{f}}_r$$

This completes the proof.

We therefore get the following relationship between the Laplacian score and Fisher score:

Theorem 1 *Let F_r denote the Fisher score of the r-th feature. With the weight matrix S defined in (5), we have $L_r = \frac{1}{1+F_r}$.*

Proof From observations 1,2,3, we see that

$$F_r = \frac{\sum_{i=1}^{c} n_i(\mu_i - \mu)^2}{\sum_{i=1}^{c} n_i\sigma_i^2} = \frac{\tilde{\mathbf{f}}_r^T D\tilde{\mathbf{f}}_r - \tilde{\mathbf{f}}_r^T L\tilde{\mathbf{f}}_r}{\tilde{\mathbf{f}}_r^T L\tilde{\mathbf{f}}_r} = \frac{1}{L_r} - 1$$

Thus, $L_r = \frac{1}{1+F_r}$. ∎

4 Experimental Results

Several experiments were carried out to demonstrate the efficiency and effectiveness of our algorithm. Our algorithm is a unsupervised filter method, while almost all the existing filter methods are supervised. Therefore, we compared our algorithm with data variance which can be performed in unsupervised fashion.

4.1 UCI Iris Data

Iris dataset, popularly used for testing clustering and classification algorithms, is taken from UCI ML repository. It contains 3 classes of 50 instances each, where each class refers to a type of Iris plant. Each instance is characterized by four features, i.e. sepal length, sepal width, petal length, and petal width. One class is linearly separable from the other two, but the other two are not linearly separable from each other. Out of the four features it is known that the features F3 (petal length) and F4 (petal width) are more important for the underlying clusters.

The class correlation for each feature is 0.7826, -0.4194, 0.9490 and 0.9565. We also used leave-one-out strategy to do classification by using each single feature. We simply used the nearest neighbor classifier. The classification error rates for the four features are 0.41, 0.52, 0.12 and 0.12, respectively. Our analysis indicates that F3 and F4 are better than F1 and F2 in the sense of discrimination. In figure 1, we present a 2-D visualization of the Iris data.

We compared three methods, i.e. Variance, Fisher score and Laplacian Score for feature selection. All of them are filter methods which are independent to any learning tasks. However, Fisher score is supervised, while the other two are unsupervised.

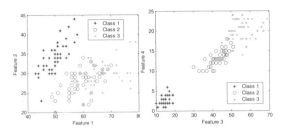

Figure 1: 2-D visualization of the Iris data.

By using variance, the four features are sorted as F3, F1, F4, F2. Laplacian score (with $k \geq 15$) sorts these four features as F3, F4, F1, F2. Laplacian score (with $3 \leq k < 15$) sorts these four features as F4, F3, F1, F2. With a larger k, we see more global structure of the data set. Therefore, the feature F3 is ranked above F4 since the variance of F3 is greater than that of F4. By using Fisher score, the four features are sorted as F3, F4, F1, F2. This indicates that Laplacian score (unsupervised) achieved the same result as Fisher score (supervised).

4.2 Face Clustering on PIE

In this section, we apply our feature selection algorithm to face clustering. By using Laplacian score, we select a subset of features which are the most useful for discrimination. Clustering is then performed in such a subspace.

4.2.1 Data Preparation

The CMU PIE face database is used in this experiment. It contains 68 subjects with 41,368 face images as a whole. Preprocessing to locate the faces was applied. Original images were normalized (in scale and orientation) such that the two eyes were aligned at the same position. Then, the facial areas were cropped into the final images for matching. The size of each cropped image is 32×32 pixels, with 256 grey levels per pixel. Thus, each image is represented by a 1024-dimensional vector. No further preprocessing is done. In this experiment, we fixed the pose and expression. Thus, for each subject, we got 24 images under different lighting conditions.

For each given number k, k classes were randomly selected from the face database. This process was repeated 20 times (except for $k = 68$) and the average performance was computed. For each test (given k classes), two algorithms, i.e. feature selection using variance and Laplacian score are used to select the features. The K-means was then performed in the selected feature subspace. Again, the K-means was repeated 10 times with different initializations and the best result in terms of the objective function of K-means was recorded.

4.2.2 Evaluation Metrics

The clustering result is evaluated by comparing the obtained label of each data point with that provided by the data corpus. Two metrics, the accuracy (AC) and the normalized mutual information metric ($\overline{MI}$) are used to measure the clustering performance [6]. Given a data point $\mathbf{x}_i$, let r_i and s_i be the obtained cluster label and the label provided by the data corpus, respectively. The AC is defined as follows:

$$AC = \frac{\sum_{i=1}^{n} \delta(s_i, map(r_i))}{n} \tag{6}$$

where n is the total number of data points and $\delta(x, y)$ is the delta function that equals one if $x = y$ and equals zero otherwise, and $map(r_i)$ is the permutation mapping function that

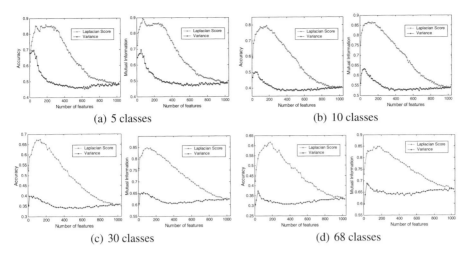

(a) 5 classes

(b) 10 classes

(c) 30 classes

(d) 68 classes

Figure 2: Clustering performance versus number of features

maps each cluster label r_i to the equivalent label from the data corpus. The best mapping can be found by using the Kuhn-Munkres algorithm [5].

Let C denote the set of clusters obtained from the ground truth and C' obtained from our algorithm. Their mutual information metric $MI(C, C')$ is defined as follows:

$$MI(C, C') = \sum_{c_i \in C, c'_j \in C'} p(c_i, c'_j) \cdot log_2 \frac{p(c_i, c'_j)}{p(c_i) \cdot p(c'_j)} \tag{7}$$

where $p(c_i)$ and $p(c'_j)$ are the probabilities that a data point arbitrarily selected from the corpus belongs to the clusters c_i and c'_j, respectively, and $p(c_i, c'_j)$ is the joint probability that the arbitrarily selected data point belongs to the clusters c_i as well as c'_j at the same time. In our experiments, we use the normalized mutual information $\overline{MI}$ as follows:

$$\overline{MI}(C, C') = \frac{MI(C, C')}{\max(H(C), H(C'))} \tag{8}$$

where $H(C)$ and $H(C')$ are the entropies of C and C', respectively. It is easy to check that $\overline{MI}(C, C')$ ranges from 0 to 1. $\overline{MI} = 1$ if the two sets of clusters are identical, and $\overline{MI} = 0$ if the two sets are independent.

4.2.3 Results

We compared Laplacian score with data variance for clustering. Note that, we did not compare with Fisher score because it is supervised and the label information is not available in the clustering experiments. Several tests were performed with different numbers of clusters (k=5, 10, 30, 68). In all the tests, the number of nearest neighbors in our algorithm is taken to be 5. The experimental results are shown in Figures 2 and Table 1. As can be seen, in all these cases, our algorithm performs much better than using variance for feature selection. The clustering performance varies with the number of features. The best performance is obtained at very low dimensionality (less than 200). This indicates that feature selection is capable of enhancing clustering performance. In Figure 3, we show the selected features in the image domain for each test (k=5, 10, 30, 68), using our algorithm, data variance and Fisher score. The brightness of the pixels indicates their importance. That is, the more bright the pixel is, the more important. As can be seen, Laplacian score provides better approximation to Fisher score than data variance. Both Laplacian score

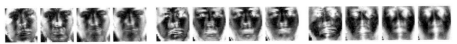

| (a) Variance | (b) Laplacian Score | (c) Fisher Score |

Figure 3: Selected features in the image domain, $k = 5, 10, 30, 68$. The brightness of the pixels indicates their importance.

Table 1: Clustering performance comparisons (k is the number of clusters)

		Accuracy						
k	Feature Number	20	50	100	200	300	500	1024
5	Laplacian Score	0.727	0.806	0.831	0.849	0.837	0.644	0.479
	Variance	0.683	0.698	0.602	0.503	0.482	0.464	0.479
10	Laplacian Score	0.685	0.743	0.787	0.772	0.711	0.585	0.403
	Variance	0.494	0.500	0.456	0.418	0.392	0.392	0.403
30	Laplacian Score	0.591	0.623	0.671	0.650	0.588	0.485	0.358
	Variance	0.399	0.393	0.390	0.365	0.346	0.340	0.358
68	Laplacian Score	0.479	0.554	0.587	0.608	0.553	0.465	0.332
	Variance	0.328	0.362	0.334	0.316	0.311	0.312	0.332
		Mutual Information						
k	Feature Number	20	50	100	200	300	500	1024
5	Laplacian Score	0.807	0.866	0.861	0.862	0.85	0.652	0.484
	Variance	0.662	0.697	0.609	0.526	0.495	0.482	0.484
10	Laplacian Score	0.811	0.849	0.865	0.842	0.796	0.705	0.538
	Variance	0.609	0.632	0.6	0.563	0.538	0.529	0.538
30	Laplacian Score	0.807	0.826	0.849	0.831	0.803	0.735	0.624
	Variance	0.646	0.649	0.649	0.624	0.611	0.608	0.624
68	Laplacian Score	0.778	0.83	0.833	0.843	0.814	0.76	0.662
	Variance	0.639	0.686	0.661	0.651	0.642	0.643	0.662

and Fisher score have the brightest pixels in the area of two eyes, nose, mouth, and face contour. This indicates that even though our algorithm is unsupervised, it can discover the most discriminative features to some extent.

5   Conclusions

In this paper, we propose a new filter method for feature selection which is independent to any learning tasks. It can be performed in either supervised or unsupervised fashion. The new algorithm is based on the observation that local geometric structure is crucial for discrimination. Experiments on Iris data set and PIE face data set demonstrate the effectiveness of our algorithm.

References

[1] M. Belkin and P. Niyogi, "Laplacian Eigenmaps and Spectral Techniques for Embedding and Clustering," *Advances in Neural Information Processing Systems*, Vol. 14, 2001.

[2] Fan R. K. Chung, *Spectral Graph Theory,* Regional Conference Series in Mathematics, number 92, 1997.

[3] X. He and P. Niyogi, "Locality Preserving Projections," *Advances in Neural Information Processing Systems*, Vol. 16, 2003.

[4] R. Kohavi and G. John, "Wrappers for Feature Subset Selection," *Artificial Intelligence*, 97(1-2):273-324, 1997.

[5] L. Lovasz and M. Plummer, *Matching Theory*, Akadémiai Kiadó, North Holland, 1986.

[6] W. Xu, X. Liu and Y. Gong, "Document Clustering Based on Non-negative Matrix Factorization ," *ACM SIGIR Conference on Information Retrieval*, 2003.

Inferring Motor Programs from Images of Handwritten Digits

Geoffrey Hinton and Vinod Nair
Department of Computer Science, University of Toronto
10 King's College Road, Toronto, M5S 3G5 Canada
{*hinton,vnair*}@*cs.toronto.edu*

Abstract

We describe a generative model for handwritten digits that uses two pairs of opposing springs whose stiffnesses are controlled by a motor program. We show how neural networks can be trained to infer the motor programs required to accurately reconstruct the MNIST digits. The inferred motor programs can be used directly for digit classification, but they can also be used in other ways. By adding noise to the motor program inferred from an MNIST image we can generate a large set of very different images of the same class, thus enlarging the training set available to other methods. We can also use the motor programs as additional, highly informative outputs which reduce overfitting when training a feed-forward classifier.

1 Overview

The idea that patterns can be recognized by figuring out how they were generated has been around for at least half a century [1, 2] and one of the first proposed applications was the recognition of handwriting using a generative model that involved pairs of opposing springs [3, 4]. The "analysis-by-synthesis" approach is attractive because the true generative model should provide the most natural way to characterize a class of patterns. The handwritten 2's in figure 1, for example, are very variable when viewed as pixels but they have very similar motor programs. Despite its obvious merits, analysis-by-synthesis has had few successes, partly because it is computationally expensive to invert non-linear generative models and partly because the underlying parameters of the generative model are unknown for most large data sets. For example, the only source of information about how the MNIST digits were drawn is the images themselves.

We describe a simple generative model in which a pen is controlled by two pairs of opposing springs whose stiffnesses are specified by a motor program. If the sequence of stiffnesses is specified correctly, the model can produce images which look very like the MNIST digits. Using a separate network for each digit class, we show that backpropagation can be used to learn a "recognition" network that maps images to the motor programs required to produce them. An interesting aspect of this learning is that the network creates its own training data, so it does not require the training images to be labelled with motor programs. Each recognition network starts with a single example of a motor program and grows an "island of competence" around this example, progressively extending the region over which it can map small changes in the image to the corresponding small changes in the motor program (see figure 2).

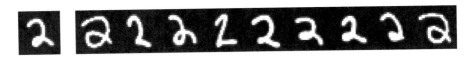

Figure 1: An MNIST image of a 2 and the additional images that can be generated by inferring the motor program and then adding random noise to it. The pixels are very different, but they are all clearly twos.

Fairly good digit recognition can be achieved by using the 10 recognition networks to find 10 motor programs for a test image and then scoring each motor program by its squared error in reconstructing the image. The 10 scores are then fed into a softmax classifier. Recognition can be improved by using PCA to model the distribution of motor trajectories for each class and using the distance of a motor trajectory from the relevant PCA hyperplane as an additional score.

Each recognition network is solving a difficult global search problem in which the correct motor program must be found by a single, "open-loop" pass through the network. More accurate recognition can be achieved by using this open-loop global search to initialize an iterative, closed-loop local search which uses the error in the reconstructed image to revise the motor program. This requires reconstruction errors in pixel space to be mapped to corrections in the space of spring stiffnesses. We cannot backpropagate errors through the generative model because it is just a hand-coded computer program. So we learn "generative" networks, one per digit class, that emulate the generator. After learning, backpropagation through these generative networks is used to convert pixel reconstruction errors into stiffness corrections.

Our final system gives 1.82% error on the MNIST test set which is similar to the 1.7% achieved by a very different generative approach [5] but worse than the 1.53% produced by the best backpropagation networks or the 1.4% produced by support vector machines [6]. It is much worse than the 0.4% produced by convolutional neural networks that use cleverly enhanced training sets [7]. Recognition of test images is quite slow because it uses ten different recognition networks followed by iterative local search. There is, however, a much more efficient way to make use of our ability to extract motor programs. They can be treated as additional output labels when using backpropagation to train a single, multi-layer, discriminative neural network. These additional labels act as a very informative regularizer that reduces the error rate from 1.53% to 1.27% in a network with two hidden layers of 500 units each. This is a new method of improving performance that can be used in conjunction with other tricks such as preprocessing the images, enhancing the training set or using convolutional neural nets [8, 7].

2   A simple generative model for drawing digits

The generative model uses two pairs of opposing springs at right angles. One end of each spring is attached to a frictionless horizontal or vertical rail that is 39 pixels from the center of the image. The other end is attached to a "pen" that has significant mass. The springs themselves are weightless and have zero rest length. The pen starts at the equilibrium position defined by the initial stiffnesses of the four springs. It then follows a trajectory that is determined by the stiffness of each spring at each of the 16 subsequent time steps in the motor program. The mass is large compared with the rate at which the stiffnesses change, so the system is typically far from equilibrium as it follows the smooth trajectory. On each time step, the momentum is multiplied by 0.9 to simulate viscosity. A coarse-grain trajectory is computed by using one step of forward integration for each time step in the motor program, so it contains 17 points. The code is at www.cs.toronto.edu/~ hinton/code.

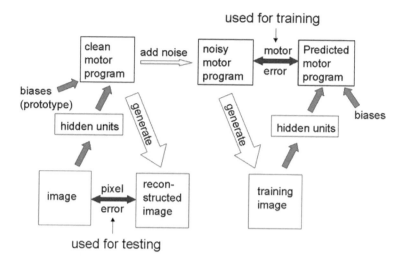

used for training

Figure 2: The training data for each class-specific recognition network is produced by adding noise to motor programs that are inferred from MNIST images using the current parameters of the recognition network. To initiate this process, the biases of the output units are set by hand so that they represent a prototypical motor program for the class.

Given a coarse-grain trajectory, we need a way of assigning an intensity to each pixel. We tried various methods until we hand-evolved one that was able to reproduce the MNIST images fairly accurately, but we suspect that many other methods would be just as good. For each point on the coarse trajectory, we share two units of ink between the the four closest pixels using bilinear interpolation. We also use linear interpolation to add three fine-grain trajectory points between every pair of coarse-grain points. These fine-grain points also contribute ink to the pixels using bilinear interpolation, but the amount of ink they contribute is zero if they are less than one pixel apart and rises linearly to the same amount as the coarse-grain points if they are more than two pixels apart. This generates a thin skeleton with a fairly uniform ink density. To flesh-out the skeleton, we use two "ink parameters", a, b, to specify a 3×3 kernel of the form $b(1+a)[\frac{a}{12}, \frac{a}{6}, \frac{a}{12}; \frac{a}{6}, 1-a, \frac{a}{6}; \frac{a}{12}, \frac{a}{6}, \frac{a}{12}]$ which is convolved with the image four times. Finally, the pixel intensities are clipped to lie in the interval [0,1]. The matlab code is at www.cs.toronto.edu/∼ hinton/code. The values of $2a$ and $b/1.5$ are additional, logistic outputs of the recognition networks[1].

3 Training the recognition networks

The obvious way to learn a recognition network is to use a training set in which the inputs are images and the target outputs are the motor programs that were used to generate those images. If we knew the distribution over motor programs for a given digit class, we could easily produce such a set by running the generator. Unfortunately, the distribution over motor programs is exactly what we want to learn from the data, so we need a way to train

---

[1] We can add all sorts of parameters to the hand-coded generative model and then get the recognition networks to learn to extract the appropriate values for each image. The global mass and viscosity as well as the spacing of the rails that hold the springs can be learned. We can even implement affine-like transformations by attaching the four springs to endpoints whose eight coordinates are given by the recognition networks. These extra parameters make the learning slower and, for the normalized digits, they do not improve discrimination, probably because they help the wrong digit models as much as the right one.

the recognition network without knowing this distribution in advance. Generating scribbles from random motor programs will not work because the capacity of the network will be wasted on irrelevant images that are far from the real data.

Figure 2 shows how a single, prototype motor program can be used to initialize a learning process that creates its own training data. The prototype consists of a sequence of 4×17 spring stiffnesses that are used to set the biases on 68 of the 70 logistic output units of the recognition net. If the weights coming from the 400 hidden units are initially very small, the recognition net will then output a motor program that is a close approximation to the prototype, whatever the input image. Some random noise is then added to this motor program and it is used to generate a training image. So initially, all of the generated training images are very similar to the one produced by the prototype. The recognition net will therefore devote its capacity to modeling the way in which small changes in these images map to small changes in the motor program. Images in the MNIST training set that are close to the prototype will then be given their correct motor programs. This will tend to stretch the distribution of motor programs produced by the network along the directions that correspond to the manifold on which the digits lie. As time goes by, the generated training set will expand along the manifold for that digit class until all of the MNIST training images of that class are well modelled by the recognition network.

It takes about 10 hours in matlab on a 3 GHz Xeon to train each recognition network. We use minibatches of size 100, momentum of 0.9, and adaptive learning rates on each connection that increase additively when the sign of the gradient agrees with the sign of the previous weight change and decrease multiplicatively when the signs disagree [9]. The net is generating its own training data, so the objective function is always changing which makes it inadvisable to use optimization methods that go as far as they can in a carefully chosen direction. Figures 3 and 4 show some examples of how well the recognition nets perform after training. Nearly all models achieve an average squared pixel error of less than 15 per image on their validation set (pixel intensities are between 0 and 1 with a preponderance of extreme values). The inferred motor programs are clearly good enough to capture the diverse handwriting styles in the data. They are not good enough, however, to give classification performance comparable to the state-of-the-art on the MNIST database. So we added a series of enhancements to the basic system to improve the classification accuracy.

4   Enhancements to the basic system

Extra strokes in ones and sevens. One limitation of the basic system is that it draws digits using only a single stroke (i.e. the trajectory is a single, unbroken curve). But when people draw digits, they often add extra strokes to them. Two of the most common examples are the dash at the bottom of ones, and the dash through the middle of sevens (see examples in figure 5). About 2.2% of ones and 13% of sevens in the MNIST training set are dashed and not modelling the dashes reduces classification accuracy significantly. We model dashed ones and sevens by augmenting their basic motor programs with another motor program to draw the dash. For example, a dashed seven is generated by first drawing an ordinary seven using the motor program computed by the seven model, and then drawing the dash with a motor program computed by a separate neural network that models only dashes.

Dashes in ones and sevens are modeled with two different networks. Their training proceeds the same way as with the other models, except now there are only 50 hidden units and the training set contains only the dashed cases of the digit. (Separating these cases from the rest of the MNIST training set is easy because they can be quickly spotted by looking at the difference between the images and their reconstructions by the dashless digit model.) The net takes the entire image of a digit as input, and computes the motor program for just the dash. When reconstructing an unlabelled image as say, a seven, we compute both

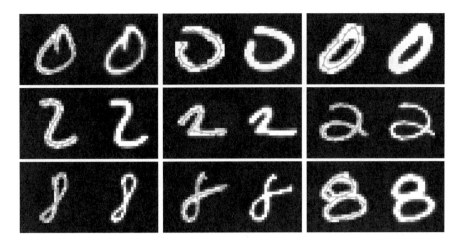

Figure 3: Examples of validation set images reconstructed by their corresponding model. In each case the original image is on the left and the reconstruction is on the right. Superimposed on the original image is the pen trajectory.

the dashed and dashless versions of seven and pick the one with the lower squared pixel error to be that image's reconstruction as a seven. Figure 5 shows examples of images reconstructed using the extra stroke.

Local search. When reconstructing an image in its own class, a digit model often produces a sensible, overall approximation of the image. However, some of the finer details of the reconstruction may be slightly wrong and need to be fixed up by an iterative local search that adjusts the motor program to reduce the reconstruction error. We first approximate the graphics model with a neural network that contains a single hidden layer of 500 logistic units. We train one such generative network for each of the ten digits and for the dashed version of ones and sevens (for a total of 12 nets). The motor programs used for training are obtained by adding noise to the motor programs inferred from the training data by the relevant, fully trained recognition network. The images produced from these motor programs by the graphics model are used as the targets for the supervised learning of each generative network. Given these targets, the weight updates are computed in the same way as for the recognition networks.

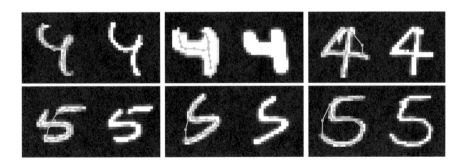

Figure 4: To model 4's we use a single smooth trajectory, but turn off the ink for timesteps 9 and 10. For images in which the pen does not need to leave the paper, the recognition net finds a trajectory in which points 8 and 11 are close together so that points 9 and 10 are not needed. For 5's we leave the top until last and turn off the ink for timesteps 13 and 14.

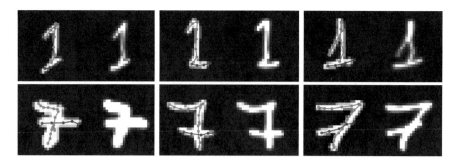

Figure 5: Examples of dashed ones and sevens reconstructed using a second stroke. The pen trajectory for the dash is shown in blue, superimposed on the original image.

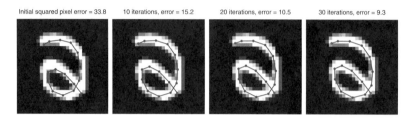

Figure 6: An example of how local search improves the detailed registration of the trajectory found by the correct model. After 30 iterations, the squared pixel error is less than a third of its initial value.

Once the generative network is trained, we can use it to iteratively improve the initial motor program computed by the recognition network for an image. The main steps in one iteration are: 1) compute the error between the image and the reconstruction generated from the current motor program by the graphics model; 2) backpropagate the reconstruction error through the generative network to calculate its gradient with respect to the motor program; 3) compute a new motor program by taking a step along the direction of steepest descent plus 0.5 times the previous step. Figure 6 shows an example of how local search improves the reconstruction by the correct model. Local search is usually less effective at improving the fits of the wrong models, so it eliminates about 20% of the classification errors on the validation set.

PCA model of the image residuals. The sum of squared pixel errors is not the best way of comparing an image with its reconstruction, because it treats the residual pixel errors as independent and zero-mean Gaussian distributed, which they are not. By modelling the structure in the residual vectors, we can get a better estimate of the conditional probability of the image given the motor program. For each digit class, we construct a PCA model of the image residual vectors for the training images. Then, given a test image, we project the image residual vector produced by each inferred motor program onto the relevant PCA hyperplane and compute the squared distance between the residual and its projection. This gives ten scores for the image that measure the quality of its reconstructions by the digit models. We don't discard the old sum of squared pixel errors as they are still useful for classifying most images correctly. Instead, all twenty scores are used as inputs to the classifier, which decides how to combine both types of scores to achieve high classification accuracy.

PCA model of trajectories. Classifying an image by comparing its reconstruction errors for the different digit models tacitly relies on the assumption that the incorrect models will reconstruct the image poorly. Since the models have only been trained on images in their

Squared error = 24.9, Shape prior score = 31.5   Squared error = 15.0, Shape prior score = 104.2

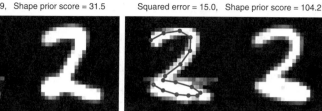

Figure 7: Reconstruction of a two image by the two model (left box) and by the three model (right box), with the pen trajectory superimposed on the original image. The three model sharply bends the bottom of its trajectory to better explain the ink, but the trajectory prior for three penalizes it with a high score. The two model has a higher squared error, but a much lower prior score, which allows the classifier to correctly label the image.

own class, they often do reconstruct images from other classes poorly, but occasionally they fit an image from another class well. For example, figure 7 shows how the three model reconstructs a two image better than the two model by generating a highly contorted three. This problem becomes even more pronounced with local search which sometimes contorts the wrong model to fit the image really well. The solution is to learn a PCA model of the trajectories that a digit model infers from images in its own class. Given a test image, the trajectory computed by each digit model is scored by its squared distance from the relevant PCA hyperplane. These 10 "prior" scores are then given to the classifier along with the 20 "likelihood" scores described above. The prior scores eliminate many classification mistakes such as the one in figure 7.

5   Classification results

To classify a test image, we apply multinomial logistic regression to the 30 scores – *i.e.* we use a neural network with no hidden units, 10 softmax output units and a cross-entropy error. The net is trained by gradient descent using the scores for the validation set images. To illustrate the gain in classification accuracy achieved by the enhancements explained above, table 1 gives the percent error on the validation set as each enhancement is added to the system. Together, the enhancements almost halve the number of mistakes.

Enhancements	Validation set % error	Test set % error
None	4.43	
1	3.84	
1, 2	3.01	
1, 2, 3	2.67	
1, 2, 3, 4	2.28	1.82

Table 1: The gain in classification accuracy on the validation set as the following enhancements are added: 1) extra stroke for dashed ones and sevens, 2) local search, 3) PCA model of image residual, and 4) PCA trajectory prior. To avoid using the test set for model selection, the performance on the official test set was only measured for the final system.

6   Discussion

After training a single neural network to output both the class label and the motor program for all classes (as described in section 1) we tried ignoring the label output and classifying the test images by using the cost, under 10 different PCA models, of the trajectory defined by the inferred motor program. Each PCA model was fitted to the trajectories extracted from the training images for a given class. This gave 1.80% errors which is as good as the 1.82% we got using the 10 separate recognition networks and local search. This is quite surprising because the motor programs produced by the single network were simplified to make them all have the same dimensionality and they produced significantly poorer reconstructions. By only using the 10 digit-specific recognition nets to create the motor programs for the *training* data, we get much faster recognition of test data because at test time we can use a single recognition network for all classes. It also means we do not need to trade-off prior scores against image residual scores because there is only one image residual.

The ability to extract motor programs could also be used to enhance the training set. [7] shows that error rates can be halved by using smooth vector distortion fields to create extra training data. They argue that these fields simulate "uncontrolled oscillations of the hand muscles dampened by inertia". Motor noise may be better modelled by adding noise to an actual motor program as shown in figure 1. Notice that this produces a wide variety of non-blurry images and it can also change the topology.

The techniques we have used for extracting motor programs from digit images may be applicable to speech. There are excellent generative models that can produce almost perfect speech if they are given the right formant parameters [10]. Using one of these generative models we may be able to train a large number of specialized recognition networks to extract formant parameters from speech without requiring labeled training data. Once this has been done, labeled data would be available for training a single feed-forward network that could recover accurate formant parameters which could be used for real-time recognition.

Acknowledgements We thank Steve Isard, David MacKay and Allan Jepson for helpful discussions. This research was funded by NSERC, CFI and OIT. GEH is a fellow of the Canadian Institute for Advanced Research and holds a Canada Research Chair in machine learning.

References

[1] D. M. MacKay. Mindlike behaviour in artefacts. *British Journal for Philosophy of Science*, 2:105–121, 1951.

[2] M. Halle and K. Stevens. Speech recognition: A model and a program for research. *IRE Transactions on Information Theory*, IT-8 (2):155–159, 1962.

[3] Murray Eden. Handwriting and pattern recognition. *IRE Transactions on Information Theory*, IT-8 (2):160–166, 1962.

[4] J.M. Hollerbach. An oscillation theory of handwriting. *Biological Cybernetics*, 39:139–156, 1981.

[5] G. Mayraz and G. E. Hinton. Recognizing hand-written digits using hierarchical products of experts. *IEEE Transactions on Pattern Analysis and Machine Intelligence*, 24:189–197, 2001.

[6] D. Decoste and B. Schoelkopf. Training invariant support vector machines. *Machine Learning*, 46:161–190, 2002.

[7] Patrice Y. Simard, Dave Steinkraus, and John Platt. Best practice for convolutional neural networks applied to visual document analysis. In *International Conference on Document Analysis and Recogntion (ICDAR), IEEE Computer Society, Los Alamitos*, pages 958–962, 2003.

[8] Y. LeCun, L. Bottou, Y. Bengio, and P. Haffner. Gradient-based learning applied to document recognition. *Proceedings of the IEEE*, 86(11):2278–2324, November 1998.

[9] A. Jacobs R. *Increased Rates of Convergence Through Learning Rate Adaptation. Technical Report: UM-CS-1987-117*. University of Massachusetts, Amherst, MA, 1987.

[10] W. Holmes, J. Holmes, and M. Judd. Extension of the bandwith of the jsru parallel-formant synthesizer for high quality synthesis of male and female speech. In *Proceedings of ICASSP 90 (1)*, pages 313–316, 1990.

Response Analysis of Neuronal Population with Synaptic Depression

Wentao Huang
Institute of Intelligent Information
Processing, Xidian University,
Xi'an 710071, China
wthuang@mail.xidian.edu.cn

Licheng Jiao
Institute of Intelligent Information
Processing, Xidian University,
Xi'an 710071, China
lchjiao@mail.xidian.edu.cn

Shan Tan
Institute of Intelligent Information
Processing, Xidian University,
Xi'an 710071, China
shtan@mail.xidian.edu.cn

Maoguo Gong
Institute of Intelligent Information
Processing, Xidian University,
Xi'an 710071, China
mggong@mail.xidian.edu.cn

Abstract

In this paper, we aim at analyzing the characteristic of neuronal population responses to instantaneous or time-dependent inputs and the role of synapses in neural information processing. We have derived an evolution equation of the membrane potential density function with synaptic depression, and obtain the formulas for analytic computing the response of instantaneous fire rate. Through a technical analysis, we arrive at several significant conclusions: The background inputs play an important role in information processing and act as a switch betwee temporal integration and coincidence detection. the role of synapses can be regarded as a spatio-temporal filter; it is important in neural information processing for the spatial distribution of synapses and the spatial and temporal relation of inputs. The instantaneous input frequency can affect the response amplitude and phase delay.

1 Introduction

Noise has an important impact on information processing of the nervous system in vivo. It is significance for us to study the stimulus-and-response behavior of neuronal populations, especially to transients or time-dependent inputs in noisy environment, viz. given this stochastic environment, the neuronal output is typically characterized by the instantaneous firing rate. It has come in for a great deal of attention in recent years[1-4]. Moreover, it is revealed recently that synapses have a more active role in information processing[5-7]. The synapses are highly dynamic and show use-dependent plasticity over a wide range of time scales. Synaptic short-term depression is one of the most common expressions of plasticity. At synapses with this type of modulation, pre-synaptic activity produces a decrease in synaptic. The present work is concerned with the processes underlying investigating the collectivity dynamics of neuronal population with synaptic depression and

523

the instantaneous response to time-dependence inputs. First, we deduce a one-dimension Fokker-Planck (FP) equation via reducing the high-dimension FP equations. Then, we derive the stationary solution and the response of instantaneous fire rate from it. Finally, the models are analyzed and discussed in theory and some conclusions are presented.

2 Models and Methods

2.1 Single Neuron Models and Density Evolution Equations

Our approach is based on the integrate-and-fire(IF) neurons. The population density based on the integrate-and-fire neuronal model is low-dimensional and thus can be computed efficiently, although the approach could be generalized to other neuron models. It is completely characterized by its membrane potential below threshold. Details of the generation of an action potential above the threshold are ignored. Synaptic and external inputs are summed until it reaches a threshold where a spike is emitted. The general form of the dynamics of the membrane potential v in IF model can be written as

$$\tau_v \frac{dv(t)}{dt} = -v(t) + S_e(t) + \tau_v \sum_{k=1}^{N} J_k(t)\delta(t - t_k^{sp}), \tag{1}$$

where $0 \leq v \leq 1$, τ_v is the membrane time constant, $S_e(t)$ is an external current directly injected in the neuron, N is the number of synaptic connections, t_k^{sp} is occurring time of the firing of a presynaptic neuron k and obeys a Poisson distribution with mean λ_k, $J_k(t)$ is the efficacy of synapse k. The transmembrane potential, v, has been normalized so that $v = 0$ marks the rest state, and $v = 1$ the threshold for firing. When the latter is achieved, v is reset to zero. $J_k(t) = AD_k(t)$, where A is a constant representing the absolute synaptic efficacy corresponding to the maximal postsynaptic response obtained if all the synaptic resources are released at once, and $D_k(t)$ act in accordance with complex dynamics rule. We use the phenomenological model by Tsodyks & Markram [7] to simulate short-term synaptic depression:

$$\frac{dD_k(t)}{dt} = \frac{(1 - D_k(t))}{\tau_d} - U_k D_k(t)\delta(t - t_k^{sp}), \tag{2}$$

where D_k is a 'depression' variable, $D_k \in [0, 1]$, τ_d is the recovery time constant, U_k is a constant determining the step decrease in D_k. Using the diffusion approximation, we can get from (1) and (2)

$$\tau_v \frac{dv(t)}{dt} = -v(t) + S_e(t) + \tau_v \sum_{k=1}^{N} AD_k(\lambda_k + \sqrt{\lambda_k}\xi_k(t)),$$

$$\frac{dD_k(t)}{dt} = \frac{(1 - D_k)}{\tau_d} - U_k D_k(\lambda_k + \sqrt{\lambda_k}\xi_k(t)). \tag{3}$$

The Fokker-Planck equation of equations (3) is

$$\frac{\partial p(t, v, \mathbf{D})}{\partial t} = -\frac{\partial}{\partial v}\left(\frac{-v + K_v}{\tau_v}p\right) - \sum_{k=1}^{N}\frac{\partial}{\partial D_k}(K_{D_k}p) - \sum_{k=1}^{N}\frac{\partial}{\partial v \partial D_k}(\lambda_k AU_k D_k^2 p)$$

$$+ \frac{1}{2}\left\{\frac{\partial^2}{\partial v^2}\left(\sum_{k=1}^{N}\lambda_k A^2 D_k^2 p\right) + \sum_{k=1}^{N}\frac{\partial^2}{\partial D_k^2}(\lambda_k U_k^2 D_k^2 p)\right\},$$

$$K_v = S_e + \sum_{k=1}^{N}\tau_v \lambda_k AD_k, \qquad K_{D_k} = \frac{(1 - D_k)}{\tau_d} - \lambda_k U_k D_k. \tag{4}$$

where $\mathbf{D} = (D_1, D_2, ...D_N)$, and

$$p(t, v, \mathbf{D}) = p_d(t, \mathbf{D}|v)p_v(t, v), \qquad \int_{-\infty}^{\infty} p_d(t, \mathbf{D}|v)d\mathbf{D} = 1. \qquad (5)$$

We assume that $D_1, D_2, ...D_N$ are uncorrelated, then we have

$$p_d(t, \mathbf{D}|v) = \prod_{k=1}^{N} \tilde{p}_d^k(t, D_k|v), \qquad (6)$$

where $\tilde{p}_d^k(t, D_k|v)$ is the conditional probability density. Moreover, we can assume

$$\tilde{p}_d^k(t, D_k|v) \approx p_d^k(t, D_k). \qquad (7)$$

Substituting (5) into (4), we get

$$p_d \frac{\partial p_v}{\partial t} + p_v \frac{\partial p_d}{\partial t} = -\frac{\partial}{\partial v}(\frac{-v + K_v}{\tau_v} p_v p_d) -$$

$$\sum_{k=1}^{N} p_v \frac{\partial}{\partial D_k}(K_{D_k} p_d) - \sum_{k=1}^{N} \frac{\partial}{\partial v \partial D_k}(A U_k D_k^2 \lambda_k p_v p_d) +$$

$$\frac{1}{2}\{\frac{\partial^2}{\partial v^2}(\sum_{k=1}^{N} \lambda_k A^2 D_k^2 p_v p_d) + \sum_{k=1}^{N} \frac{\partial^2}{\partial D_k^2}(\lambda_k U_k^2 D_k^2 p_v p_d)\}. \qquad (8)$$

Integrating Eqation (8) over $\mathbf{D}$, we get

$$\tau_v \frac{\partial p_v(t, v)}{\partial t} = -\frac{\partial}{\partial v}(-v + \tilde{K}_v)p_v(t, v) + \frac{Q_v}{2} \frac{\partial^2 p_v(t, v)}{\partial v^2}, \qquad (9)$$

where

$$\tilde{K}_v = \int K_v p_d d\mathbf{D} = S_e + \sum_{k=1}^{N} \tau_v \lambda_k A m_k, \quad Q_v = \sum_{k=1}^{N} \tau_v \lambda_k A^2 \gamma_k,$$

$$m_k = \int D_k p_d^k(t, D_k)dD_k, \qquad \gamma_k = \int D_k^2 p_d^k(t, D_k)dD_k, \qquad (10)$$

and $p_d^k(t, D_k)$ satisfies the following equation Fokker-Planck equation

$$\frac{\partial p_d^k}{\partial t} = -\frac{\partial}{\partial D_k}(K_{D_k} p_d^k) + \frac{1}{2} \frac{\partial^2}{\partial D_k^2}(U_k^2 D_k^2 \lambda_k p_d^k). \qquad (11)$$

From (10) and (11), we can get

$$\frac{dm_k}{dt} = -(\frac{1}{\tau_d} + U\lambda_k)m_k + \frac{1}{\tau_d},$$

$$\frac{d\gamma_k}{dt} = -(\frac{2}{\tau_d} + (2U - U^2)\lambda_k)\gamma_k + \frac{2m_k}{\tau_d}. \qquad (12)$$

Let

$$J_v(t, v) = (\frac{-v + \tilde{K}_v}{\tau_v})p_v(t, v) - \frac{Q_v}{2\tau_v} \frac{\partial p_v(t, v)}{\partial v},$$

$$r(t) = J_v(t, 1), \qquad (13)$$

where $J_v(t, v)$ is the probability flux of p_v, $r(t)$ is the fire rate. The boundary conditions of equation (9) are

$$p_v(t, 1) = 0, \qquad \int_0^1 p_v(t, v)dv = 1, \qquad r(t) = J_v(t, 0). \qquad (14)$$

525

2.2 Stationary Solution and Response Analysis

When the system is in the stationary states, $\partial p_v / \partial t = 0$, $dm_k/dt = 0$, $d\gamma_k/dt = 0$, $p_v(t,v) = p_v^0(v)$, $r(t) = r_0$, $m_k(t) = m_k^0$, $\gamma_k(t) = \gamma_k^0$ and $\lambda_k(t) = \lambda_k^0$. are time-independent. From (9), (12), (13) and (14), we get

$$p_v^0(v) = \frac{2\tau_v r_0}{Q_v^0} \exp[-\frac{(v - \tilde{K}_v^0)^2}{Q_v^0}] \int_v^1 \exp[\frac{(v' - \tilde{K}_v^0)^2}{Q_v^0}]dv', 0 \le v \le 1,$$

$$r_0 = \left(\tau_v \sqrt{\pi} \int_{-\frac{\tilde{K}_v^0}{\sqrt{Q_v^0}}}^{\frac{1-\tilde{K}_v^0}{\sqrt{Q_v^0}}} \exp(u^2)[\mathrm{erf}(\frac{\tilde{K}_v^0}{\sqrt{Q_v^0}}) + \mathrm{erf}(u)]du \right)^{-1},$$

$$\tilde{K}_v^0 = S_e + \sum_{k=1}^{N} \tau_v A \lambda_k^0 m_k^0, \qquad Q_v^0 = \sum_{k=1}^{N} \tau_v A^2 \lambda_k^0 \gamma_k^0,$$

$$m_k^0 = \frac{1}{1 + U_k \tau_d \lambda_k^0}, \qquad \gamma_k^0 = \frac{2m_k^0}{2 + \tau_d(2U_k - U_k^2)\lambda_k^0}. \tag{15}$$

Sometimes, we are more interested in the instantaneous response to time-dependence random fluctuation inputs. The inputs take the form:

$$\lambda_k = \lambda_k^0(1 + \varepsilon_k \lambda_k^1(t)), \tag{16}$$

where $\varepsilon_k \ll 1$. Then m_k and γ_k have the forms, i.e.,

$$m_k = m_k^0(1 + \varepsilon_k m_k^1(t) + O(\varepsilon_k^2)),$$
$$\gamma_k = \gamma_k^0(1 + \varepsilon_k \gamma_k^1(t) + O(\varepsilon_k^2)), \tag{17}$$

and $\tilde{K}_v$ and Q_v are

$$\tilde{K}_v = S_e + \sum_{k=1}^{N} \tau_v A \lambda_k^0 m_k^0 + \sum_{k=1}^{N} \varepsilon_k \tau_v A \lambda_k^0 m_k^0(\lambda_k^1 + m_k^1)) + O(\varepsilon_k^2),$$

$$Q_v = \sum_{k=1}^{N} \tau_v A^2 \lambda_k^0 \gamma_k^0 + \sum_{k=1}^{N} \varepsilon_k \tau_v A^2 \lambda_k^0 \gamma_k^0(\lambda_k^1 + \gamma_k^1) + O(\varepsilon_k^2). \tag{18}$$

Substituting (17) into (12), and ignoring the high order item, it yields:

$$\frac{dm_k^1}{dt} = -(\frac{1}{\tau_d} + U_k \lambda_k^0)m_k^1 - U_k \lambda_k^0 \lambda_k^1(t),$$

$$\frac{d\gamma_k^1}{dt} = -(\frac{2}{\tau_d} + (2U_k - U_k^2)\lambda_k^0)\gamma_k^1 + \frac{2m_k^1}{\tau_d} - (2U_k - U_k^2)\lambda_k^0 \lambda_k^1(t). \tag{19}$$

With the definitions

$$\tilde{K}_v = \tilde{K}_v^0 + \epsilon \tilde{K}_v^1(t) + O(\epsilon^2),$$
$$Q_v = Q_v^0 + \epsilon Q_v^1(t) + O(\epsilon^2),$$
$$p_v = p_v^0 + \epsilon p_1(t) + O(\epsilon^2),$$
$$r = r_0 + \epsilon r_1(t) + O(\epsilon^2), \tag{20}$$

where $\epsilon \ll 1$, and boundary conditions of p_1

$$p_1(t,1) = 0, \qquad \int_0^1 p_1(t,v)dv = 0, \tag{21}$$

using the perturbative expansion in powers of ϵ, we can get

$$0 = -\frac{\partial}{\partial v}(-v + \tilde{K}_v^0)p_v^0(v) + \frac{Q_v}{2}\frac{\partial^2 p_v^0(v)}{\partial v^2},$$

$$\tau_v \frac{\partial p_1}{\partial t} = -\frac{\partial}{\partial v}(-v + \tilde{K}_v^0)p_1 + \frac{Q_v^0}{2}\frac{\partial^2 p_1}{\partial v^2} - \frac{\partial f_0(t,v)}{\partial v},$$

$$f_0(t,v) = \tilde{K}_v^1(t)p_v^0 - \frac{Q_v^1(t)}{2}\frac{\partial p_v^0}{\partial v},$$

$$r_1 = -\frac{Q_v^0}{2\tau_v}\frac{\partial p_1(t,1)}{\partial v} - \frac{Q_v^1(t)}{2\tau_v}\frac{\partial p_v^0(1)}{\partial v}. \tag{22}$$

For the oscillatory inputs $\tilde{K}_v^1(t) = k(\omega)e^{j\omega t}$, $Q_v^1(t) = q(\omega)e^{j\omega t}$, the output has the same frequency and takes the forms $p_1(t,v) = p_\omega(\omega,v)e^{j\omega t}$, $\partial p_1/\partial t = j\omega p_1$.

For inputs that vary on a slow enough time scale, satisfy $\tau_v\omega \ll 1$, we define

$$\epsilon_l = \tau_v\omega,$$

$$p_1 = p_1^0 + \epsilon_l p_1^1 + O(\epsilon_l^2),$$

$$r_1 = r_1^0 + \epsilon_l r_1^1 + O(\epsilon_l^2). \tag{23}$$

Using the perturbative expansion in powers of ϵ_l, we get

$$\frac{\partial f_0(t,v)}{\partial v} = -\frac{\partial}{\partial v}(-v + \tilde{K}_v^0)p_1^0 + \frac{Q_v^0}{2}\frac{\partial^2 p_1^0}{\partial v^2},$$

$$jp_1^0 = -\frac{\partial}{\partial v}(-v + \tilde{K}_v^0)p_1^1 + \frac{Q_v^0}{2}\frac{\partial^2 p_1^1}{\partial v^2}. \tag{24}$$

The solutions of equtions (24) are

$$p_1^n = \frac{2}{Q_v^0}\exp[-\frac{(v - \tilde{K}_v^0)^2}{Q_v^0}]\int_v^1 (\tau_v r_1^n - F_n)\exp[\frac{(v^{'} - \tilde{K}_v^0)^2}{Q_v^0}]dv^{'},$$

$$r_1^n = \frac{2r_0}{Q_v^0}\int_0^1 \exp[-\frac{(v - \tilde{K}_v^0)^2}{Q_v^0}]\int_v^1 F_n \exp[\frac{(v^{'} - \tilde{K}_v^0)^2}{Q_v^0}]dv^{'} dv,$$

$$F_0 = f_0(t,v), \quad F_1 = j\int_0^v p_1^0(v^{'})dv^{'}, \quad n = 0,1. \tag{25}$$

In general, $Q_v^1(t) \ll \tilde{K}_v^1(t)$, then we have

$$F_0 = f_0(t,v) \approx \tilde{K}_v^1(t)p_v^0. \tag{26}$$

From (23), (25) and (26), we can get

$$r_1 \approx \frac{2r_0}{Q_v^0}\tilde{K}_v^1(t)\int_0^1 \exp[-\frac{(v - \tilde{K}_v^0)^2}{Q_v^0}]\int_v^1 p_v^0 \exp[\frac{(v^{'} - \tilde{K}_v^0)^2}{Q_v^0}]dv^{'} dv + j\omega\tau_v\times$$

$$\frac{2r_0}{Q_v^0}\int_0^1 \exp[-\frac{(v - \tilde{K}_v^0)^2}{Q_v^0}]\int_v^1 [\int_0^{v^{'}} p_1^0(v^{''})dv^{''}]\exp[\frac{(v^{'} - \tilde{K}_v^0)^2}{Q_v^0}]dv^{'} dv. \tag{27}$$

In the limit of high frequency inputs, i.e. $1/\tau_v\omega \ll 1$, with the definitions

$$\epsilon_h = \frac{1}{\tau_v\omega},$$

$$p_1 = p_h^0 + \epsilon_h p_h^1 + O(\epsilon_h^2), \tag{28}$$

527

we obtain

$$p_h^0 = 0, \qquad\qquad p_h^1 = j\frac{\partial f_0(t, v)}{\partial v},$$

$$r_1 = -\frac{Q_v^1(t)}{2\tau_v}\frac{\partial p_v^0(1)}{\partial v} - j\epsilon_h\frac{Q_v^0}{2\tau_v}\frac{\partial^2 f_0(t, 1)}{\partial v^2} + O(\epsilon_h^2)$$

$$\approx \frac{Q_v^1(t)}{Q0}r_0 - j\epsilon_h\frac{Q_v^0}{2\tau_v}\left(\tilde{K}_v^1(t)\frac{\partial^2 p_v^0(1)}{\partial v^2} - \frac{Q_v^1(t)}{2}\frac{\partial^3 p_v^0}{\partial v^3}\right)$$

$$= \frac{Q_v^1(t)r_0}{Q_v^0} - \frac{2j\epsilon_h\tilde{K}_v^1(t)r_0}{Q_v^0}\left((1 - \tilde{K}_v^0) - \frac{Q_v^1(t)}{\tilde{K}_v^1(t)Q_v^0}\left(1 - \tilde{K}_v^0 - Q_v^0\right)\right). \qquad (29)$$

When $Q_v^1(t) \ll \tilde{K}_v^1(t)$, we have

$$r_1 \approx \frac{Q_v^1(t)r_0}{Q_v^0} - \frac{2j\tilde{K}_v^1(t)r_0}{\tau_v\omega Q_v^0}(1 - \tilde{K}_v^0)(1 - \frac{Q_v^1(t)}{\tilde{K}_v^1(t)Q_v^0}), \qquad (30)$$

3   Discussion

In equation (15), $\tilde{K}_v^0$ reflects the average intensity of background inputs and Q_v^0 reflects the intensity of background noise. When $1 \ll \tau_d U_k \lambda_k^0$, we have

$$\tilde{K}_v^0 \approx S_e + \sum_{k=1}^{N}\frac{\tau_v A}{\tau_d U_k},$$

$$Q_v^0 \approx \sum_{k=1}^{N}\frac{\tau_v A^2}{\tau_d U_k(1 + \tau_d U_k \lambda_k^0(1 - U_k/2))}. \qquad (31)$$

From (31), we can know the change of background inputs λ_k^0 has little influence on $\tilde{K}_v^0$ which is dominated by parameter $\tau_v A/\tau_d U_k$, but more influence on Q_v^0 which decreases with λ_k^0 increasing.

In the low input frequency regime, from (27), we can know that the input frequency ω increasing will result in the response amplitude and the phase delay increasing. However, in the high input frequency limit regime, from (30), we can know the input frequency ω increasing will result in the response amplitude and the phase delay decreasing. More-over, from (27) and (30), we know the stationary background fire rate r_0 play an important part in response to changes in fluctuation outputs. The instantaneous response r_1 increases monotonically with background fire rate r_0. But the background fire rate r_0 is a function of the background noise Q_v^0. In equation (27), $\left\|r_1/\tilde{K}_v^1\right\|$ reflects the response amplitude, and in equation (30), r_0/Q_v^0 reflects the response amplitude. As Figure 1 (A) and (B) show that $\left\|r_1/\tilde{K}_v^1\right\|$ and r_0/Q_v^0 changes with variables Q_v^0 and $\tilde{K}_v^0$ respectively. We can know, for the subthreshold regime ($\tilde{K}_v^0 < 1$), they increase monotonically with Q_v^0 when $\tilde{K}_v^0$ is a constant. However, for the suprathreshold regime ($\tilde{K}_v^0 > 1$), they decrease monotonically with Q_v^0 when $\tilde{K}_v^0$ is a constant. When inputs remain, if the instantaneous response ampli-tude increases, then we can take for the role of neurons are more like coincidence detection than temporal integration. And from this viewpoint, it suggests that the background in-puts play an important role in information processing and act as a switch between temporal integration and coincidence detection.

In equation (16), if the inputs take the oscillatory form, $\lambda_k^1(t) = e^{j\omega t}$, according to (19),

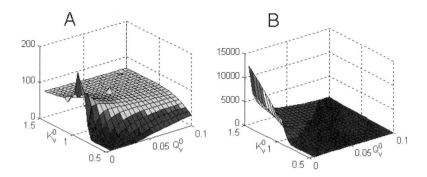

Figure 1: Response amplitude versus Q_v^0 and $\tilde{K}_v^0$. (A) $\left\| r_1/\tilde{K}_v^1 \right\|$ (for equation (27)) changes with Q_v^0 and $\tilde{K}_v^0$. (B) r_0/Q_v^0 (for equation (30)) changes with Q_v^0 and $\tilde{K}_v^0$.

we get

$$m_k^1 = -\frac{\tau_d U_k \lambda_k^0 e^{j(\omega t - \theta_m)}}{\sqrt{(\tau_d \omega)^2 + (1 + \tau_d U_k \lambda_k^0)^2}},\tag{32}$$

where $\theta_m = \arctan\left(\frac{\tau_d \omega}{1 + \tau_d U_k \lambda_k^0}\right)$ is the phase delay, $\tau_d U_k \lambda_k^0 / \sqrt{(\tau_d \omega)^2 + (1 + \tau_d U_k \lambda_k^0)^2}$ is the amplitude. The minus shows it is a 'depression' response amplitude. The phase delay increases with the input frequency ω and decreases with the background input λ_k^0. The 'depression' response amplitude decrease with the input frequency ω and increase with the background input λ_k^0. The equations (15) (18), (12), (19), (27), (30) and (32) show us a point of view that the synapses can be regarded as a time-dependent external field which impacts on the neuronal population through the time-dependent mean and variance. We assume the inputs are composed of two parts, viz. $\lambda_{k_1}^1(t) = \lambda_{k_2}^1(t) = \frac{1}{2}e^{j\omega t}$, then we can get $m_{k_1}^1$ and $m_{k_2}^1$. However, in general $m_k^1 \neq m_{k_1}^1 + m_{k_2}^1$, this suggest for us that the spatial distribution of synapses and inputs is important on neural information processing. In conclusion, the role of synapses can be regarded as a spatio-temporal filter. Figure 2 is the results of simulation of a network of 2000 neurons and the analytic solution for equation (15) and equation (27) in different conditions.

4 Summary

In this paper, we deal with the model of the integrate-and-fire neurons with synaptic current dynamics and synaptic depression. In Section 2, first, using the membrane potential equation (1) and combining the synaptic depression equation (2), we derive the evolution equation (4) of the joint distribution density function. Then, we give an approach to cut the evolution equation of the high dimensional function down to one dimension, and get equation (9). Finally, we give the stationary solution and the response of instantaneous fire rate to time-dependence random fluctuation inputs. In Section 3, the analysis and discussion of the model is given and several significant conclusions are presented. This paper can only investigate the IF neuronal model without internal connection. We can also extend to other models, such as the non-linear IF neuronal models of sparsely connected networks of excitatory and inhibitory neurons.

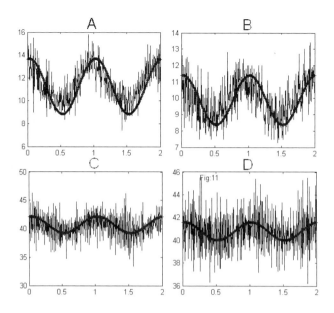

Figure 2: Simulation of a network of 2000 neurons (thin solid line) and the analytic solution (thick solid line) for equation (15) and equation (27), with $\tau_v = 15(\text{ms})$, $\tau_d = 1(\text{s})$, $A = 0.5$, $U_k = 0.5$, $N = 30$, $\omega = 6.28(\text{Hz})$, $\lambda_k^1 = \sin(\omega t)$, $\varepsilon_k \lambda_k^0 = 10(\text{Hz})$, $\lambda_k^0 = 70(\text{Hz})$ (A and C) and $100(\text{Hz})$ (B and D), $S_e = 0.5$(A and B) and 0.8(C and D). The horizontal axis is time (0-2s), and the longitudinal axis is the fire rate.

References

[1] Fourcaud N. & Brunel, N. (2005) Dynamics of the Instantaneous Firing Rate in Response to Changes in Input Statistics. *Journal of Computational Neuroscience* **18**(3):311-321.

[2] Fourcaud, N. & Brunel, N. (2002) Dynamics of the Firing Probability of Noisy Integrate-and-Fire Neurons. *Neural Computation* **14**(9):2057-2110.

[3] Gerstner, W. (2000) Population Dynamics of Spiking Neurons: Fast Transients, Asynchronous States, and Locking. *Neural Computation* **12**(1):43-89.

[4] Silberberg, G., Bethge, M., Markram, H., Pawelzik, K. & Tsodyks, M. (2004) Dynamics of Population Rate Codes in Ensembles of Neocortical Neurons. *J Neurophysiol* **91**(2):704-709.

[5] Abbott, L.F. & Regehr, W.G. (2004) Synaptic Computation. *Nature* **431**(7010):796-803.

[6] Destexhe, A. & Marder, E. (2004) Plasticity in Single Neuron and Circuit Computations. *Nature* **431**(7010):789-795.

[7] Markram, H., Wang, Y. & Tsodyks, M. (1998) Differential Signaling Via the Same Axon of Neocortical Pyramidal Neurons. *Proc Natl Acad Sci USA* **95**(9):5323-5328.

Non-iterative Estimation with Perturbed Gaussian Markov Processes

Yunsong Huang   **B. Keith Jenkins**
Signal and Image Processing Institute
Department of Electrical Engineering-Systems
University of Southern California
Los Angeles, CA 90089-2564
{yunsongh,jenkins}@sipi.usc.edu

Abstract

We develop an approach for estimation with Gaussian Markov processes that imposes a smoothness prior while allowing for discontinuities. Instead of propagating information laterally between neighboring nodes in a graph, we study the posterior distribution of the hidden nodes as a whole—how it is perturbed by invoking discontinuities, or weakening the edges, in the graph. We show that the resulting computation amounts to feed-forward fan-in operations reminiscent of V1 neurons. Moreover, using suitable matrix preconditioners, the incurred matrix inverse and determinant can be approximated, without iteration, in the same computational style. Simulation results illustrate the merits of this approach.

1 Introduction

Two issues, (i) efficient representation, and (ii) efficient inference, are of central importance in the area of statistical modeling of vision problems. For generative models, often the ease of generation and the ease of inference are two conflicting features. Factor Analysis [1] and its variants, for example, model the input as a linear superposition of basis functions. While the generation, or synthesis, of the input is immediate, the inference part is usually not. One may apply a set of filters, *e.g.*, Gabor filters, to the input image. In so doing, however, the statistical modeling is only deferred, and further steps, either implicit or explicit, are needed to capture the 'code' carried by those filter responses. By characterizing mutual dependencies among adjacent nodes, Markov Random Field (MRF) [2] and graphical models [3] are other powerful ways for modeling the input, which, when continuous, is often conveniently assumed to be Gaussian. In vision applications, it's suitable to employ smoothness priors admitting discontinuities [4]. Examples include *weak membranes* and *plates* [5], formulated in the context of variational energy minimization. Typically, the inference for MRF or graphical models would incur lateral propagation of information between neighboring units [6]. This is appealing in the sense that it consists of only simple, local operations carried out in parallel. However, the resulting latency could undermine the plausibility that such algorithms are employed in human early vision inference tasks [7].

In this paper we take the weak membrane and plate as instances of Gaussian processes (GP). We show that the effect of marking each discontinuity (hereafter termed as "bond-breaking") is to perturb the inverse of covariance matrix of the hidden nodes x by a matrix of rank 1. When multiple bonds are broken, the computation of the posterior mean and covariance of x would involve the inversion of a matrix, which typically has large condition number, implying very slow convergence in straight-forward iterative approaches. We show that there exists a family of preconditioners that can bring the condition number close to 1, thereby greatly speeding up the iteration—to the extent that a single step would suffice in practice. Therefore, the predominant computation employed in our approach is noniterative, of fan-in and fan-out style. We also devise ways to learn the parameters regarding state and observation noise non-iteratively. Finally, we report experimental results of applying the proposed algorithm to image-denoising.

2 Perturbing a Gaussian Markov Process (GMP)

Consider a spatially invariant GMP defined on a torus, $x \sim \mathcal{N}(0, Q_0)$, whose energy— defined as $x^T Q_0^{-1} x$—is the sum of energies of all edges[1] in the graph, due to the Markovian property. In what follows, we perturb the potential matrix Q_0^{-1} by reducing the coupling energy of certain bonds[2]. This relieves the smoothness constraint on the nodes connected via those bonds.

Suppose the energy reduction of a bond connecting node i and j (whose state vectors are x_i and x_j, respectively) can be expressed as $(x_i^T f_i + x_j^T f_j)^2$, where f_i and f_j are coefficient vectors. This becomes $(x^T f)^2$, if f is constructed to be a vector of same size as x, with the only non-zero entries f_i and f_j corresponding to node i and j. This manipulation can be identified with a rank-1 perturbation of Q_0^{-1}, as $Q_1^{-1} \leftarrow Q_0^{-1} - f f^T$, which is equivalent to $x^T Q_1^{-1} x \leftarrow x^T Q_0^{-1} x - (x^T f)^2, \forall x$. We call this an elementary perturbation of Q_0^{-1}, and f an elementary perturbation vector associated with the particular bond.

When L such perturbations have taken place (cf. Fig. 1), we form the L perturbation vectors into a matrix $F_1 = [f^1, \ldots, f^L]$, and then the collective perturbations yield

$$Q_1^{-1} = Q_0^{-1} - F_1 F_1^T \tag{1}$$

$$\text{and thus} \quad Q_1 = Q_0 + Q_0 F_1 (I - F_1^T Q_0 F_1)^{-1} F_1^T Q_0, \tag{2}$$

which follows from the Sherman-Morrison-Woodbury Formula (SMWF).

2.1 Perturbing a membrane and a plate

In a membrane model [5], x_i is scalar and the energy of the bond connecting x_i and x_j is $(x_i - x_j)^2/q$, where q is a parameter denoting the variance of state noise. Upon perturbation, this energy is reduced to $\eta^2 (x_i - x_j)^2/q$, where $0 < \eta \ll 1$ ensures positivity of the energy. Then, the energy reduction is $(1 - \eta^2)(x_i - x_j)^2/q$, from which we can identify $f_i = \sqrt{(1 - \eta^2)/q}$ and $f_j = -f_i$.

In the case of a plate [5], $x_i = [u_i, u_{hi}, u_{vi}]^T$, in which u_i represents the intensity, while u_{hi} and u_{vi} represent its gradient in the horizontal and vertical direction, respectively. We define the energy of a horizontal bond connecting node j and i as $E_0^{(-, i)} = (u_{vi} - u_{vj})^2/q + d^{(-,i)^T} O^{-1} d^{(-,i)}$, where

$$d^{(-,i)} = \begin{bmatrix} u_i \\ u_{hi} \end{bmatrix} - \begin{bmatrix} 1 & 1 \\ 0 & 1 \end{bmatrix} \begin{bmatrix} u_j \\ u_{hj} \end{bmatrix} \quad \text{and} \quad O = q \begin{bmatrix} 1/3 & 1/2 \\ 1/2 & 1 \end{bmatrix},$$

---

[1]Henceforth called *bonds*, as *edge* will refer to intensity discontinuity in an image.
[2]The bond energy remains positive. This ensures the positive definiteness of the potential matrix.

the superscript $(-, i)$ representing horizontal bond to the left of node i. The first and second term of $E^{(-,i)}$ would correspond to $(\partial^2 u(h,v)/\partial h \partial v)^2/q$ and $(\partial^2 u(h,v)/\partial h^2)^2/q$, respectively, if $u(h,v)$ is a continuous function of h and v (cf. [5]). If $E_0^{(-,i)}$ is reduced to $E_1^{(-,i)} = [(u_{vi} - u_{vj})^2 + (u_{hi} - u_{hj})^2]/q$, i.e., coupling between node i and j exists only through their gradient values, one can show that the energy reduction $E_0^{(-,i)} - E_1^{(-,i)} = [u_i - u_j - (u_{hi} + u_{hj})/2]^2 \cdot 12/q$. Taking the actual energy reduction to be $(1 - \eta^2)(E_0^{(-,i)} - E_1^{(-,i)})$, we can identify $f_i^{(-,i)} = \sqrt{12(1 - \eta^2)/q}[1, -1/2, 0]^T$ and $f_j^{(-,i)} = \sqrt{12(1 - \eta^2)/q}[-1, -1/2, 0]^T$, where $0 < \eta \ll 1$ ensures the positive definiteness of the resulting potential matrix. A similar procedure can be applied to a vertical bond in the plate, producing a perturbation vector $f^{(|,i)}$, whose components are zero everywhere except for $f_i^{(|,i)} = \sqrt{12(1 - \eta^2)/q}[1, 0, -1/2]^T$ and $f_j^{(|,i)} = \sqrt{12(1 - \eta^2)/q}[-1, 0, -1/2]^T$, for which node j is the lower neighbor of node i.

One can verify that $x^T f = 0$ when the plate assumes the shape of a linear slope, meaning that this perturbation produces no energy difference in such a case. $(x^T f)^2$ becomes significant when the perturbed, or broken, bond associated with f straddles across a step discontinuity of the image. Such an f is thus related to edge detection.

2.2 Hidden state estimation

Standard formulae exist for the posterior covariance K and mean $\hat{x}$ of x, given a noisy observation[3] $y = Cx + n$, where $n \sim \mathcal{N}(0, rI)$.

$$\hat{x}^\alpha = K_\alpha C^T y/r, \quad \text{and} \quad K_\alpha = [Q_\alpha^{-1} + C^T C/r]^{-1}, \tag{3}$$

for either the unperturbed ($\alpha = 0$) or perturbed ($\alpha = 1$) process. Thus,

$$
\begin{aligned}
K_1 &= [Q_0^{-1} + C^T C/r - F_1 F_1^T]^{-1}, \quad \text{following Eq. 3 and 1} \\
&= [K_0^{-1} - F_1 F_1^T]^{-1}, \\
&= K_0 + W_1 H_1^{-1} W_1^T, \quad \text{applying SMWF,}
\end{aligned}
\tag{4}
$$

$$\text{where} \quad H_1 \triangleq I - F_1^T K_0 F_1, \quad \text{and} \quad W_1 \triangleq K_0 F_1 \tag{5}$$

$$
\begin{aligned}
\therefore \hat{x}^1 &= K_1 C^T y/r \\
&= K_0 C^T y/r + W_1 H_1^{-1} W_1^T C^T y/r = \hat{x}^0 + \hat{x}^c,
\end{aligned}
\tag{6}
$$

$$\text{where} \quad \hat{x}^c \triangleq W_1 H_1^{-1} W_1^T C^T y/r,$$

$$\quad = W_1 H_1^{-1} z^1, \quad \text{where} \quad z^1 = W_1^T C^T y/r \tag{7}$$

On a digital computer, the above computation can be efficiently implemented in the Fourier domain, despite the huge size of K_α and Q_α. For example, K_1 equals K_0—a circulant matrix—plus a rank-L perturbation (cf. Eq. 4). Since each column of W_1 is a spatially shifted copy of a prototypical vector, arising from breaking either a horizontal or a vertical bond, convolution can be utilized in computing $W_1^T C^T y$. The computation of H_1^{-1} is deferred to Section 3. On a neural substrate, however, the computation can be implemented by inner-products in parallel. For instance, $z^1 r$ is the result of inner-products between the input y and the feed-forward fan-in weights CW, coded by the dendrites of identical neurons, each situated at a broken bond. Let $v^1 = H_1^{-1} z^1$ be the responses of another layer of neurons. Then $C\hat{x}^c = CWv^1$ amounts to the back-projection of layer v^1 to the input plane with fan-out weights identical to the fan-in counterpart.

We can also apply the above procedure incrementally[4], i.e., apply F_1 and then F_2, both consisting of a set of perturbation vectors. Quantities resulting from the α'th perturba-

---

[3] The observation matrix $C = I$ for a membrane, and $C = I \otimes [1, 0, 0]$ for a plate.

[4] Latency considerations, however, preclude the practicability of *fully* incremental computation.

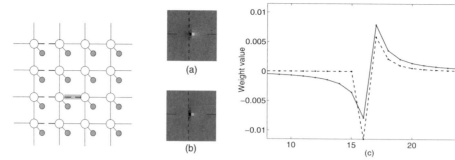

Figure 1: A portion of MRF. Solid and broken lines denote intact and broken bonds, respectively. Open circles denote hidden nodes x_i and filled circles denote observed nodes y_i.

Figure 2: The resulting receptive field of the edge detector produced by breaking the shaded bond shown in Fig. 1. The central vertical dashed line in (a) and (b) marks the location of the vertical streak of bonds shown as broken in Fig. 1. In (a), those bonds are not actually broken; in (b), they are. In (c), a central horizontal slice of (a) is plotted as a solid curve and the counterpart of (b) as a dashed curve.

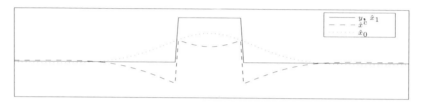

Figure 3: Estimation of x given input y. $\hat{x}_0$: by unperturbed rod; $\hat{x}_1$: coinciding perfectly with y, is obtained by a rod whose two bonds at the step edges of y are broken; $\hat{x}^c$: correction term, engendered by the perturbed rod.

tion step can be obtained from those of the $(\alpha - 1)$'th step, simply by replacing the subscript/superscript '1' and '0' with α and $\alpha - 1$, respectively, in Eqs. 1 to 6. In particular,

$$W_2 = K_1 F_2 = \underbrace{K_0 F_2}_{\widetilde{W_2}} + \underbrace{W_1 H_1^{-1} W_1^T F_2}_{\delta W_2}, \tag{8}$$

where $\widetilde{W}_2$ refers to the weights due to F_2 in the absence of perturbation F_1, which, when indeed existent, would exert a contextual effect on F_2, thereby contributing to the term δW_2.

Figure 2 illustrates this effect on one perturbation vector (termed 'edge detector') in a membrane model, wherein 'receptive field' refers to $\widetilde{W}_2$ and W_2 in the case of panel (a) and (b), respectively. Evidently, the receptive field of W_2 across the contextual boundary is pinched off. Figure 3 shows the estimation of x, cf. Eq. 6 and 7, using a 1D plate, *i.e.*, rod. We stress that once the relevant edges are detected, $\hat{x}^c$ is computed almost instantly, without the need of iterative refinement via lateral propagation. This could be related to the brightness filling-in signal[8].

2.3 Parameter estimation

As edge inference/detection is outside the scope of this paper, we limit our attention to finding optimal values for the parameters r and q. Although the EM algorithm is possible for that purpose, we strive for a non-iterative alternative. To that end, we reparameterize r and q into r and $\varrho = q/r$. Given a possibly perturbed model M_α, in which $x \sim \mathcal{N}(0, Q_\alpha)$, we have $y \sim \mathcal{N}(0, S_\alpha)$, where $S_\alpha = rI + CQ_\alpha C^T$. Note that $\widetilde{S_\alpha} \triangleq S_\alpha/r$ does not depend on r when ϱ is fixed, as $Q_\alpha \propto q \propto r \Longrightarrow S_\alpha \propto r$. Next, we aim to maximize the log-probability of y, which is a vector of N components (or pixels).

$$
\begin{aligned}
\tilde{J}_\alpha \triangleq \mathrm{Ln} p(y|M_\alpha) &= -(N\mathrm{Ln}(2\pi) + \mathrm{Ln}|S_\alpha| + y^T S_\alpha^{-1} y)/2 \\
&= -(N\mathrm{Ln}(2\pi) + N\mathrm{Ln}r + \mathrm{Ln}|\widetilde{S_\alpha}| + (y^T \widetilde{S_\alpha}^{-1} y)/r)/2
\end{aligned}
$$

$$
\text{Setting} \quad \partial \tilde{J}_\alpha/\partial r = 0 \quad \Rightarrow \quad \hat{r} = E_\alpha/N, \quad \text{where} \quad E_\alpha \triangleq y^T \widetilde{S_\alpha}^{-1} y \tag{9}
$$

$$
\text{Define} \quad J \triangleq N\mathrm{Ln}E_\alpha + \mathrm{Ln}|\widetilde{S_\alpha}| = \text{const.} - 2\tilde{J}_\alpha|_{\hat{r}} \tag{10}
$$

J is a function of ϱ only, and we locate the $\hat{\varrho}$ that minimizes J as follows. Prompted by the fact that ϱ governs the *spatial scale* of the process [5] and scale channels exist in primate visual system, we compute $J(\varrho)$ for a preselected set of ϱ, corresponding to spatial scales half-octave apart, and then fit the resulting J's with a cubic polynomial, whose location of minimum suggests $\hat{\varrho}$. We use this approach in Section 4.

Computing J in Eq. 10 needs two identities, which are included here without proof (the second can be proven by using SMWF and its associated determinant identity): $E_\alpha = y^T(y - C\hat{x}^\alpha)$ (cf. Appendix A of [5]), and $|S_0|/|S_\alpha| = |B_\alpha|/|H_\alpha|$, where

$$
H_\alpha = I - F_\alpha^T K_0 F_\alpha, \quad \text{and} \quad B_\alpha \triangleq I - F_\alpha^T Q_0 F_\alpha \tag{11}
$$

That is, E_α can be readily obtained once $\hat{x}^\alpha$ has been estimated, and $|\widetilde{S_\alpha}| = |\widetilde{S_0}||H_\alpha|/|B_\alpha|$, in which $|\widetilde{S_0}|$ can be calculated in the spectral domain, as S_0 is circulant. The computation of $|H_\alpha|$ and $|B_\alpha|$ is dealt with in the next section.

3 Matrix Preconditioning

Some of the foregoing computation necessitates matrix determinant and matrix inverse, e.g., $H^{-1}z^1$ (cf. Eq. 7). Because H is typically poorly conditioned, plain iterative means to evaluate $H^{-1}z^a$ would converge very slowly. Methods exist in the literature for finding a matrix P ([9] and references therein) satisfying the following two criteria: (1) inverting P is easy; (2) the condition number $\kappa(P^{-1}H)$ approaches 1. Ideally, $\kappa(P^{-1}H) = 1$ implies $P = H$. Here we summarize our findings regarding the best class of preconditioners when H arises from some prototypical configurations of bond breaking. We call the following procedure Approximate Diagonalization (AD).

(1) 'DFT'. When a streak of broken bonds forms a closed contour, with a consistent polarity convention (*e.g.*, the excitatory region of the receptive field of the edge detector associated with each bond lies inside the enclosed region), H and B (cf. Eq. 11) are approximately circulant. Let X be the unitary Fourier matrix of same size as H, then $H^e = X^\dagger H X$ would be approximately diagonal. Let Λ_H be diagonal: $\Lambda_{Hij} = \delta_{ij} H^e_{ii}$, then $\widetilde{H} = X\Lambda_H X^\dagger$ is a circulant matrix approximating H; $\prod_i \Lambda_{Hii}$ approximates $|H|$; $X\Lambda_H^{-1}X^\dagger$ approximates H^{-1}. In this way, a computation such as $H^{-1}z^1$ becomes $X\Lambda_H^{-1}X^\dagger z^1$, which amounts to simple fan-in and fan-out operations, if we regard each column of X as a fan-in weight vector. The quality of this preconditioner $\widetilde{H}$ can be evaluated by both the condition number $\kappa(\widetilde{H}^{-1}H)$ and the relative error between the inverse matrices:

$$
\epsilon \triangleq \|\widetilde{H}^{-1} - H^{-1}\|_F / \|H^{-1}\|_F, \tag{12}
$$

where $\| . \|_F$ denotes Frobenius norm. The same X can approximately diagonalize B, and the product of the diagonal elements of the resulting matrix approximates $|B|$.

(2) 'DCST'. One end of the streak of broken bonds (target contour) abuts another contour, and the other end is open (*i.e.*, line-end). Imagine a vibrational mode of the membrane/plate given the configuration of broken bonds. The vibrational contrast of the nodes across the broken bond at a line-end has to be small, since in the immediate vicinity there exist paths of intact bonds linking the two nodes. This suggests a Dirichlet boundary condition at the line-end. At the abutting end (*i.e.*, a T-junction), however, the vibrational contrast can be large, since the nodes on different sides of the contour are practically decoupled. This suggests a von Neumann boundary condition. This analysis leads to using a transform (termed 'HSWA' in [10]) which we call 'DCST', denoting sine phase at the open end and cosine phase at the abutting end. The unitary transform matrix X is given by: $X_{i,j} = 2\sqrt{2L+1}\cos(\pi(i-1/2)(j-1/2)/(L+1/2))$, $1 \leq i,j \leq L$, where L is the number of broken bonds in the target contour.

(3) 'DST'. When the streak of broken bonds form an open-ended contour, H can be approximately diagonalized by Sine Transform (cf. the intuitive rationale stated in case (2)), of which the unitary transform matrix X is given by: $X_{i,j} = \sqrt{2/(L+1)}\sin(\pi ij/(L+1))$, $1 \leq i,j \leq L$.

For a 'clean' prototypical contour, the performance of such preconditioners is remarkable, typically producing $1 \leq \kappa < 1.2$ and $\epsilon < 0.05$. When contours in the image are interconnected in a complex way, we first parse the image domain into non-overlapping enclosed regions, and then treat each region independently. A contour segment dividing two regions is shared between them, and thus would contribute two copies, each belonging to one region[11].

4   Experiment

We test our approach on a real image (Fig. 4a), which is corrupted with three increasing levels of white Gaussian noise: SNR = 4.79db (Fig. 4b), 3.52db, and 2.34db. Our task is to estimate the original image, along with finding optimal q and r. We used both membrane and plate models, and in each case we used both the 'direct' method, which directly computes H^{-1} in Eq. 7 and $|H|/|B|$ required in Eq. 10, and the 'AD' method, as described in Section 3, to compute those quantities in approximation.

We first apply a Canny detector to generate an edge map (Fig. 4g) for each noisy image, which is then converted to broken bonds. The large number (over 10^4) of broken bonds makes the direct method impractical. In order to attain a 'direct' result, we partition the image domain into a 5×5 array of blocks (one such block is delineated by the inner square in Fig. 4g), and focus on each of them in turn by retaining edges not more than 10 pixels from the target block (this block's outer scope is delineated with the outer square in Fig. 4g). When $\hat{x}$ is inferred given this partial edge map, only its pixels within the block are considered valid and are retained. We mosaic up $\hat{x}$ from all those blocks to get the complete inferred image. In 'AD', we parse the contours in each block and apply different diagonalizers accordingly, as summarized in Section 3. The performance of the three types of AD is plotted in Fig. 5, from which it is evident that in majority of cases $\kappa < 1.5$ and $\epsilon \leq 10\%$. Fig. 4e and f illustrate the procedure to find optimal q/r for a membrane and a plate, respectively, as explained in Section 2.3. Note how good the cubic polynomial fit is, and that the results of AD do not deviate much from those of the direct (rigorous) method. Fig. 4c and 4d show $\hat{x}$ by a perturbed and intact membrane model, respectively. Notice that the edges, for instance around Lena's shoulder and her hat, in Fig. 4d are more smeared than those in Fig. 4c (cf. Fig. 3). Table 1 summarizes the value of optimal q/r and Mean-Squared-Error (MSE). Our results compare favorably with those listed in the last column of the table, which is excerpted from [12].

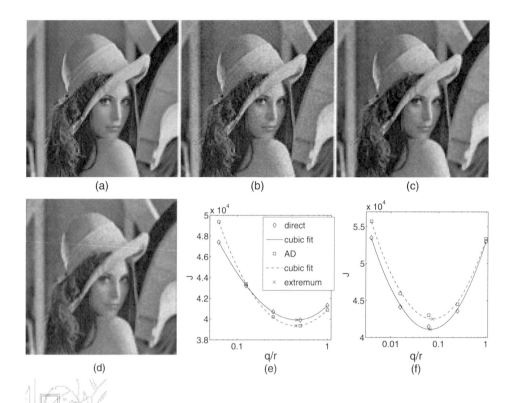

(a)   (b)   (c)

(d)   (e)   (f)

(g)

Figure 4: (a) Original image, (b) noisy image. Estimation by (c) a perturbed membrane, and (d) an intact membrane. The criterion function of varying q/r for (e) perturbed membrane, and (f) perturbed plate, which shares the same legend as in (e). (g) Canny edge map.

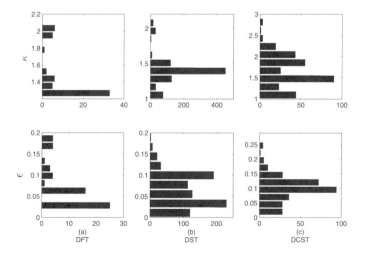

Figure 5: Histograms of condition number κ after preconditioning, and relative error ϵ as defined in Eq. 12, illustrating the performance of preconditioners, DFT, DST, and DCST, on their respective datasets. Horizontal axes indicate the number of occurrences in each bin.

Table 1: Optimal q/r and MSE.

SNR	membrane model				plate model				Improved Entropic [12]
	direct		AD		direct		AD		
	q/r	MSE	q/r	MSE	q/r	MSE	q/r	MSE	MSE
4.79	0.456	92	0.444	92	0.067	100	0.075	98	121
3.52	0.299	104	0.311	104	0.044	111	0.049	108	138
2.34	0.217	115	0.233	115	0.033	119	0.031	121	166

5 Conclusions

We have shown how the estimation with perturbed Gaussian Markov processes—hidden state and parameter estimation—can be carried out in non-iterative way. We have adopted a holistic viewpoint. Instead of focusing on each individual hidden node, we have taken each process as an entity under scrutiny. This paradigm shift changes the way information is stored and represented—from the scenario where the global pattern of the process is embodied entirely by local couplings to the scenario where fan-in and fan-out weigths, in addition to local couplings, reflect the patterns of larger scales.

Although edge detection has not been treated in this paper, our formulation is capable of doing so, and our preliminary results are encouraging. It may be premature at this stage to translate the operations of our model to neural substrate; we speculate nevertheless that our approach may have relevance to understanding biological visual systems.

Acknowledgments

This work was supported in part by the TRW Foundation, ARO (Grant Nos. DAAG55-98-1-0293 and DAAD19-99-1-0057), and DARPA (Grant No. DAAD19-0010356).

References

[1] Z. Ghahramani and M.J. Beal. Variational inference for Bayesian mixtures of factor analysers. In *Advances in Neural Information Processing Systems*, volume 12. MIT Press, 2000.

[2] S.Z. Li. *Markov Random Field Modeling in Computer Vision*. Springer-Verlag, 1995.

[3] M.I. Jordan, Z. Ghahramani, T.S. Jaakkola, and L.K. Saul. An introduction to variational methods for graphical models. *Machine Learning*, 37:183–233, 1999.

[4] F. C. Jeng and J. W. Woods. Compound Gauss-Markov random fields for image estimation. *IEEE Trans. on Signal Processing*, 39(3):683–697, 1991.

[5] A. Blake and A. Zisserman. *Visual Reconstruction*. MIT Press, 1987.

[6] J.S. Yedidia, W.T. Freeman, and Y. Weiss. Bethe free energy, kikuchi approximations, and belief propagation algorithms. Technical Report TR2001-16, MERL, May 2001.

[7] S. Thorpe, D. Fize, and C. Marlot. Speed of processing in the human visual system. *Nature*, 381:520–522, 1996.

[8] L. Pessoa and P. De Weerd, editors. *Filling-in: From Perceptual Completion to Cortical Reorganization*. Oxford: Oxford University Press, 2003.

[9] R. Chan, M. Ng, and C. Wong. Sine transform based preconditioners for symmetric toeplitz systems. *Linear Algebra and its Applications*, 232:237–259, 1996.

[10] S. A. Martucci. Symmetric convolution and the discrete sine and cosine transforms. *IEEE Trans. on Signal Processing*, 42(5):1038–1051, May 1994.

[11] H. Zhou, H. Friedman, and R. von der Heydt. Coding of border ownership in monkey visual cortex. *J. Neuroscience*, 20(17):6594–6611, 2000.

[12] A. Ben Hamza, H. Krim, and G. B. Unal. Unifying probabilistic and variational estimation. *IEEE Signal Processing Magazine*, pages 37–47, September 2002.

Learning Cue-Invariant Visual Responses

Jarmo Hurri
HIIT Basic Research Unit, University of Helsinki
P.O.Box 68, FIN-00014 University of Helsinki, Finland

Abstract

Multiple visual cues are used by the visual system to analyze a scene; achromatic cues include luminance, texture, contrast and motion. Single-cell recordings have shown that the mammalian visual cortex contains neurons that respond similarly to scene structure (e.g., orientation of a boundary), regardless of the cue type conveying this information. This paper shows that cue-invariant response properties of simple- and complex-type cells can be learned from natural image data in an unsupervised manner. In order to do this, we also extend a previous conceptual model of cue invariance so that it can be applied to model simple- and complex-cell responses. Our results relate cue-invariant response properties to natural image statistics, thereby showing how the statistical modeling approach can be used to model processing beyond the elemental response properties visual neurons. This work also demonstrates how to learn, from natural image data, more sophisticated feature detectors than those based on changes in mean luminance, thereby paving the way for new data-driven approaches to image processing and computer vision.

1 Introduction

When segmenting a visual scene, the brain utilizes a variety of visual cues. Spatiotemporal variations in the mean luminance level – which are also called *first-order* cues – are computationally the simplest of these; the name 'first-order' comes from the idea that a single linear filtering operation can detect these cues. Other types of visual cues include contrast, texture and motion; in general, cues related to variations in other characteristics than mean luminance are called *higher-order* (also called non-Fourier) cues; the analysis of these is thought to involve more than one level of processing/filtering. Single-cell recordings have shown that the mammalian visual cortex contains neurons that are selective to both first- and higher-order cues. For example, a neuron may exhibit similar selectivity to the orientation of a boundary, regardless of whether the boundary is a result of spatial changes in mean luminance or contrast [1]. Monkey cortical areas V1 and V2, and cat cortical areas 17 and 18, contain both simple- (orientation-, frequency- and phase-selective) and complex-type (orientation- and frequency-selective, phase-invariant) cells that exhibit such *cue-invariant* response properties [2, 1, 3, 4, 5]. Previous research has been unable to pinpoint the connectivity that gives rise to cue-invariant responses.

Recent computational modeling of the visual system has produced fundamental results relating stimulus statistics to first-order response properties of simple and complex cells (see, e.g., [6, 7, 8, 9]). The contribution of this paper is to introduce a similar, natural image

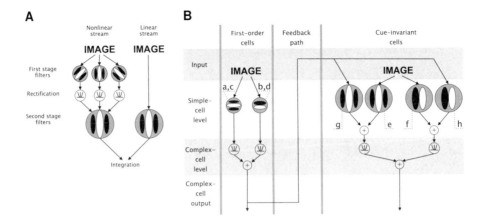

Figure 1: (**A**) The two-stream model [1], with a linear stream (on the right) and a nonlinear stream (on the left). The linear stream responds to first-order cues, while the nonlinear stream responds to higher-order cues. In the nonlinear stream, the stimulus (image) is first filtered with multiple high-frequency filters, whose outputs are transformed nonlinearly (rectified), and subsequently used as inputs for a second-stage filter. Cue-invariant responses are obtained when the outputs of these two streams are integrated. (**B**) Our model of cue-invariant responses. The model consists of simple cells, complex cells and a feedback path leading from a population of high-frequency first-order complex cells to low-frequency cue-invariant simple cells. In a cue-invariant simple cell, the feedback is filtered with a filter that has similar spatial characteristics as the feedforward filter of the cell. The output of a cue-invariant simple cell is given by the sum of the linearly filtered input and the filtered feedback. Note that while our model results in cue-invariant response properties, it is not a model of cue *integration*, because in the sum the two paths can cancel out. However, this simplification does *not* affect our results, that is, learning, since the summed output is not used in learning (see Section 3), or measurements, which excite only one of the paths significantly and do not consider integration effects (see Figures 3 and 4). In this instance of the model, the high-frequency cells prefer horizontal stimuli, while the low-frequency cue-invariant cells prefer vertical stimuli; in other instances, this relationship can be different. For actual filters used in an implementation of this model, see Figure 2. Lowercase letters a–g refer to the corresponding subfigures in Figure 2.

statistics -based framework for cue-invariant responses of both simple and complex cells. In order to achieve this, we also extend the two-stream model of cue-invariant responses (Figure 1A) to account for cue-invariant responses at both simple- and complex-cell levels.

The rest of this paper is organized as follows. In Section 2 we describe our version of the two-stream model of cue-invariant responses, which is based on feedback from complex cells to simple cells. In Section 3 we formulate an unsupervised learning rule for learning these feedback connections. We apply our learning rule to natural image data, and show that this results in the emergence of connections that give rise to cue-invariant responses at both simple- and complex-cell levels. We end this paper with conclusions in Section 4.

2 A model of cue-invariant responses

The most prominent model of cue-invariant responses introduced in previous research is the two-stream model (see, e.g., [1]), depicted in Figure 1A. In this research we have extended this model so that it can be applied directly to model the cue-invariant responses of simple and complex cells. Our model, shown in Figure 1B, employs standard linear-filter

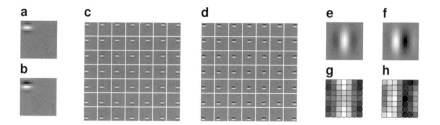

Figure 2: The filters used in an implementation of our model. The reader is referred to Figure 1B for the correspondence between subfigures (a)–(h) and the schematic model of Figure 1B. (**a**) The feedforward filter (Gabor function [10]) of a high-frequency first-order simple cell; the filter has size 19×19 pixels, which is the size of the image data in our experiments. (**b**) The feedforward filter of another first-order simple cell. This feedforward filter is otherwise similar to the one in (a), except that there is a phase difference of $\pi/2$ between the two; together, the feedforward filters in (a) and (b) are used to implement an energy model of a complex cell. (**c**) A lattice of size 7×7 of high-frequency filters of the type shown in (a); these filters are otherwise identical, except that their spatial locations vary. (**d**) A lattice of filters of the type shown in (b). Together, the lattices shown in (c) and (d) are used to implement a 7×7 lattice of energy-model complex cells with different spatial positions; the output of this lattice is the feedback relayed to the low-frequency cue-invariant cells. (**e,f**) Feedforward filters of low-frequency simple cells. (**g**) A feedback filter of size 7×7 for the simple cell whose feedforward filter is shown in (e); in order to avoid confusion between feedforward filters and feedback filters, the latter are visualized as lattices of slightly rounded rectangles. (**h**) A feedback filter for the simple cell whose feedforward filter is shown in (f). The feedback filters in (g) and (h) have been obtained by applying the learning algorithm introduced in this paper (see Section 3 for details).

models of simple cells and energy models of complex cells [10], and a feedback path from the complex-cell level to the simple-cell level. This feedback path introduces a second, nonlinear input stream to cue-invariant cells, and gives rise to cue-invariant responses in these cells. To avoid confusion between the two types of filters – one type operating on the input image and the other on the feedback – we will use the term 'feedforward filter' for the former and the term 'feedback filter' for the latter. Figure 2 shows the feedforward and feedback filters of a concrete instance (implementation) of our model. Gabor functions [10] are used to model simple-cell feedforward filters.

Figure 3 illustrates the design of higher-order gratings, and shows how the complex-cell lattice of the model transforms higher-order cues into feedback activity patterns that resemble corresponding first-order cues. A quantitative evaluation of the model is given in Figure 4. These measurements show that our model possesses the fundamental cue-invariant response properties: in our model, a cue-invariant neuron has similar selectivity to the orientation, frequency and phase of a grating stimulus, regardless of cue type (see figure caption for details). We now proceed to show how the feedback filters of our model (Figures 2g and h) can be learned from natural image data.

3   Learning feedback connections in an unsupervised manner

3.1   The objective function and the learning algorithm

In this section we introduce an unsupervised algorithm for learning feedback connection weights from complex cells to simple cells. When this learning algorithm is applied to natural image data, the resulting feedback filters are those shown in Figures 2g and h – as

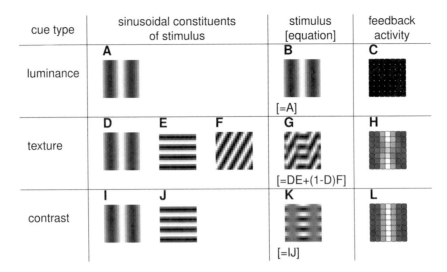

cue type	sinusoidal constituents of stimulus			stimulus [equation]	feedback activity
luminance	**A**			**B**	**C**
				[=A]	
texture	**D**	**E**	**F**	**G**	**H**
				[=DE+(1-D)F]	
contrast	**I**	**J**		**K**	**L**
				[=IJ]	

Figure 3: The design of grating stimuli with different cues, and the feedback activity for these gratings. **Design of grating stimuli:** Each row illustrates how, for a particular cue, a grating stimulus is composed of sinusoidal constituents; the equation of each stimulus (B, G, K) as a function of the constituents is shown under the stimulus. Note that the orientation, frequency and phase of each grating is determined by the first sinusoidal constituent (A, D, I); here these parameters are the same for all stimuli. Here (E) and (F) are two different textures, and (I) is called the *envelope* and (J) the *carrier* of a contrast-defined stimulus. **Feedback activity:** The rightmost column shows the feedback activity – that is, response of the complex-cell lattice (see Figures 2c and d) – for the three types of stimuli. (**C**) There is no response to the luminance stimuli, since the orientation and frequency of the stimulus are different from those of the high-frequency feedforward filters. (**H, L**) For other cue types, the lattice detects the locations of energy of the vertical high-frequency constituent (E, J), thereby resulting in feedback activity that has a spatial pattern similar to a corresponding luminance pattern (A). Thus, the complex-cell lattice transforms higher-order cues into activity patterns that resemble first-order cues, and these can subsequently produce a strong response in a feedback filter (compare (H) and (L) with the feedback filter in Figure 2g). For a quantitative evaluation of the model with these stimuli, see Figure 4.

was shown in Figure 4, these feedback filters give rise to cue-invariant response properties.

The intuitive idea behind the learning algorithm is the following: in natural images, higher-order cues tend to coincide with first-order cues. For example, when two different textures are adjacent, there is often also a luminance border between them; two examples of this phenomenon are shown in Figure 5. Therefore, cue-invariant response properties could be a result of learning in which large responses in the feedforward channel (first-order responses) have become associated with large responses in the feedback channel (higher-order responses). Previous research has demonstrated the importance of such energy dependencies in modeling the visual system (see, e.g., [11, 9, 12, 13, 14]).

To turn this idea into equations, let us introduce some notation. Let vector $c(n) = [c_1(n)\ c_2(n)\ \cdots\ c_K(n)]^T$ denote the responses of a set of K first-order high-frequency complex cells for the input image with index n. In our case the number of these complex cells is $K = 7 \times 7 = 49$ (see Figures 2c and d), so the dimension of this vector is 49. This vectorization can be done in a standard manner [15] by scanning values from the 2D lattice column-wise into a vector; when the learned feedback filter is visualized, the filter is "unvectorized" with a reverse procedure. Let $s(n)$ denote the response of a single low-

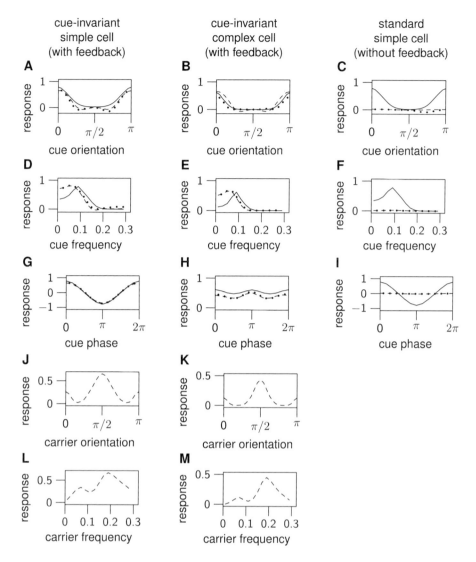

Figure 4: Our model fulfills the fundamental properties of cue-invariant responses. The plots show tuning curves for a cue-invariant simple cell – corresponding to the filters of Figures 2e and g – and complex cell of our new model (two leftmost columns), and a standard simple-cell model without feedback processing (rightmost column). Solid lines show responses to luminance-defined gratings (Figure 3B), dotted lines show responses to texture-defined gratings (Figure 3G), and dashed lines show responses to contrast-defined gratings (Figure 3K). (**A–I**) In our model, a neuron has similar selectivity to the orientation, frequency and phase of a grating stimulus, regardless of cue type; in contrast, a standard simple-cell model, without the feedback path, is only selective to the parameters of a luminance-defined grating. The preferred frequency is lower for higher-order gratings than for first-order gratings; similar observations have been made in single-cell recordings [4]. (**J–M**) In our model, the neurons are also selective to the orientation and frequency of the carrier (Figure 3J) of a contrast-defined grating (Figure 3K), thus conforming with single-cell recordings [1]. Note that these measurements were made with the feedback filters learned by our unsupervised algorithm (see Section 3); thus, these measurements confirm that learning results in cue-invariant response properties.

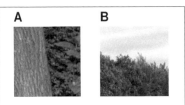

A   **B**

Figure 5: Two examples of co-inciding first- and higher-order boundary cues. Image in (A) contains a near-vertical lumi-nance boundary across the im-age; the boundary in (B) is near-horizontal. In both (A) and (B), texture is different on different sides of the luminance border. (For image source, see [8].)

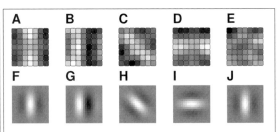

Figure 6: (**A-D, F-I**) Feedback filters (top row) learned from natural image data by using our un-supervised learning algorithm; the bottom row shows the corresponding feedforward filters. For a quantitative evaluation of the cue-invariant re-sponse properties resulting from the learned fil-ters (A) and (B), see Figure 4. (**E, J**) The result of a control experiment, in which Gaussian white noise was used as input data; (J) shows the feed-forward filter used in this control experiment.

frequency simple cell for the input image with index n. In our learning algorithm all the feedforward filters are fixed and only a feedback filter is learned; this means that $c(n)$ and $s(n)$ can be computed for all n (all images) prior to applying the learning algorithm.

Let us denote the K-dimensional feedback filter with w; this filter is learned by our algo-rithm. Let $b(n) = w^T c(n)$, that is, $b(n)$ is the signal obtained when the feedback activity from the complex-cell lattice is filtered with the feedback filter; the overall activity of a cue-invariant simple cell is then $s(n) + b(n)$. Our objective function measures the correlation of energies of the feedforward response $s(n)$ and the feedback response $b(n)$:

$$f(w) = \mathrm{E}\left\{s^2(n)b^2(n)\right\} = w^T \mathrm{E}\left\{s^2(n)c(n)c(n)^T\right\} w = w^T M w, \tag{1}$$

where $M = \mathrm{E}\left\{s^2(n)c(n)c(n)^T\right\}$ is a positive-semidefinite matrix that can be computed from samples prior to learning. To keep the output of the feedback filter $b(n)$ bounded, we enforce a unit energy constraint on $b(n)$, leading into constraint

$$h(w) = \mathrm{E}\left\{b^2(n)\right\} = w^T \mathrm{E}\left\{c(n)c(n)^T\right\} w = w^T C w = 1, \tag{2}$$

where $C = \mathrm{E}\left\{c(n)c(n)^T\right\}$ is also positive-semidefinite and can be computed prior to learning. The problem of maximizing objective (1) with constraint (2) is a well-known quadratic optimization problem with a norm constraint, the solution of which is given by an eigenvalue-eigenvector problem (see below). However, in order to handle the case where C is not invertible – which will be the case below in our experiments – and to attenuate the noise in the data, we first use a technique called dimensionality reduction (see, e.g., [15]). Let $C = EDE^T$ be the eigenvalue decomposition of C; in the decomposition, the eigenvectors corresponding to the r smallest eigenvalues (subspaces with smallest energy; the exact value for r is given in Section 3.2) have been dropped out, so E is a $K \times (K - r)$ matrix of $K - r$ eigenvectors and D is a $(K - r) \times (K - r)$ diagonal matrix containing the largest eigenvalues. Now let $v = D^{1/2}E^T w$. A one-to-one correspondence between v and w can be formed by using the pseudoinverse solution $w = ED^{-1/2}v$. Now let $z(n) = D^{-1/2}E^T c(n)$. Using these definitions of v and $z(n)$, it is straightforward to show that the objective and constraint become $f(v) = v^T \mathrm{E}\left\{s^2(n)z(n)z(n)^T\right\} v$ and $h(v) = \|v\|^2 = 1$. The global maximum v_{opt} is the eigenvector of $\mathrm{E}\left\{s^2(n)z(n)z(n)^T\right\}$ that corresponds to the largest eigenvalue.

In practice learning from sampled data $s(n)$ and $c(n)$ proceeds as follows. First the eigenvalue decomposition of C is computed. Then the transformed data set $z(n)$ is computed, and v_{opt} is calculated from the eigenvalue-eigenvector problem. Finally, the optimal filter w_{opt} is obtained from the pseudoinverse relationship. In learning from sampled data, all expectations are replaced with sample averages.

3.2 Experiments

The algorithm described above was applied to natural image data, which was sampled from a set of over 4,000 natural images [8]. The size of the sampled image patches was 19×19 pixels, and the number of samples was 250,000. The local mean (DC component) was removed from each image sample.

Simple-cell feedforward responses $s(n)$ were computed using the filter shown in Figure 2e, and the set of high-frequency complex-cell lattice activities $c(n)$ was computed using the filters shown in Figures 2c and d. A form of contrast gain control [16], which can be used to compensate for the large variation in contrast in natural images, was also applied to the natural image data: prior to filtering a natural image sample with a feedforward filter, the energy of the image was normalized inside the Gaussian modulation window of the Gabor function [10] of the feedforward filter. This preprocessing tends to weaken contrast borders, implying that in our experiments, learning higher-order responses is mostly based on texture boundaries that coincide with luminance boundaries. It should be noted, however, that in spite of this preprocessing step, the resulting feedback filters produce cue-invariant responses to both texture- and contrast-defined cues (see Figure 4). In order to make the components of $c(n)$ have zero mean, and focus on the structure of feedback activity patterns instead of overall constant activation, the local mean (DC component) was removed from each $c(n)$. To attenuate the noise in the data, the dimensionality of $c(n)$ was reduced to 16 (see Section 3.1); this retains 85% of original signal energy.

The algorithm described in Section 3.1 was then applied to this data. The resulting feedback filter is shown in Figure 6A (see also Figure 2g). Data sampling, preprocessing and the learning algorithm were then repeated, but this time using the feedforward filter shown in Figure 2f; the feedback filter obtained from this run is shown in Figure 6B (see also Figure 2h). The measurements in Figure 4 show that these feedback filters result in cue-invariant response properties at both simple- and complex-cell levels. Thus, our unsupervised algorithm learns cue-invariant response properties from natural image data. The results shown in Figures 6C and D were obtained with feedforward filters whose orientation was different from vertical, demonstrating that the observed phenomenon applies to other orientations also (in these experiments, the orientation of the high-frequency filters was orthogonal to that of the low-frequency feedforward filter).

To make sure that the results shown in Figures 6A–D are not a side effect of the preprocessing or the structure of our model, but truly reflect the statistical properties of natural image data, we ran a control experiment by repeating our first experiment, but using Gaussian white noise as input data (instead of natural image data). All other steps, including preprocessing and dimensionality reduction, were the same as in the original experiment. The result is shown in Figure 6E; as can be seen, the resulting filter lacks any spatial structure. This verifies that our original results do reflect the statistics of natural image data.

4 Conclusions

This paper has shown that cue-invariant response properties can be learned from natural image data in an unsupervised manner. The results were based on a model in which there is a feedback path from complex cells to simple cells, and an unsupervised algorithm which maximizes the correlation of the energies of the feedforward and filtered feedback signals.

The intuitive idea behind the algorithm is that in natural visual stimuli, higher-order cues tend to coincide with first-order cues. Simulations were performed to validate that the learned feedback filters give rise to in cue-invariant response properties.

Our results are important for three reasons. First, for the first time it has been shown that cue-invariant response properties of simple and complex cells emerge from the statistical properties of natural images. Second, our results suggest that cue invariance can result from feedback from complex cells to simple cells; no feedback from higher cortical areas would thus be needed. Third, our research demonstrates how higher-order feature detectors can be learned from natural data in an unsupervised manner; this is an important step towards general-purpose data-driven approaches to image processing and computer vision.

Acknowledgments

The author thanks Aapo Hyvärinen and Patrik Hoyer for their valuable comments. This research was supported by the Academy of Finland (project #205742).

References

[1] I. Mareschal and C. Baker, Jr. A cortical locus for the processing of contrast-defined contours. *Nature Neuroscience* 1(2):150–154, 1998.

[2] Y.-X. Zhou and C. Baker, Jr. A processssing stream in mammalian visual cortex neurons for non-Fourier responses. *Science* 261(5117):98–101, 1993.

[3] A. G. Leventhal, Y. Wang, M. T. Schmolesky, and Y. Zhou. Neural correlates of boundary perception. *Visual Neuroscience* 15(6):1107–1118, 1998.

[4] I. Mareschal and C. Baker, Jr. Temporal and spatial response to second-order stimuli in cat area 18. *Journal of Neurophysiology* 80(6):2811–2823, 1998.

[5] J. A. Bourne, R. Tweedale, and M. G. P. Rosa. Physiological responses of New World monkey V1 neurons to stimuli defined by coherent motion. *Cerebral Cortex* 12(11):1132–1145, 2002.

[6] B. A. Olshausen and D. Field. Emergence of simple-cell receptive field properties by learning a sparse code for natural images. *Nature* 381(6583):607–609, 1996.

[7] A. Bell and T. J. Sejnowski. The independent components of natural scenes are edge filters. *Vision Research* 37(23):3327–3338, 1997.

[8] J. H. van Hateren and A. van der Schaaf. Independent component filters of natural images compared with simple cells in primary visual cortex. *Proceedings of the Royal Society of London B* 265(1394):359–366, 1998.

[9] A. Hyvärinen and P. O. Hoyer. A two-layer sparse coding model learns simple and complex cell receptive fields and topography from natural images. *Vision Research* 41(18):2413–2423, 2001.

[10] P. Dayan and L. F. Abbott. *Theoretical Neuroscience*. The MIT Press, 2001.

[11] O. Schwartz and E. P. Simoncelli. Natural signal statistics and sensory gain control. *Nature Neuroscience* 4(8):819–825, 2001.

[12] J. Hurri and A. Hyvärinen. Simple-cell-like receptive fields maximize temporal coherence in natural video. *Neural Computation* 15(3):663–691, 2003.

[13] J. Hurri and A. Hyvärinen. Temporal and spatiotemporal coherence in simple-cell responses: a generative model of natural image sequences. *Network: Computation in Neural Systems* 14(3):527–551, 2003.

[14] Y. Karklin and M. S. Lewicki. Higher-order structure of natural images. *Network: Computation in Neural Systems* 14(3):483–499, 2003.

[15] A. Hyvärinen, J. Karhunen, and E. Oja. *Independent Component Analysis*. John Wiley & Sons, 2001.

[16] D. J. Heeger. Normalization of cell responses in cat striate cortex. *Visual Neuroscience* 9(2):181–197, 1992.

Bayesian Surprise Attracts Human Attention

Laurent Itti
Department of Computer Science
University of Southern California
Los Angeles, California 90089-2520, USA
itti@usc.edu

Pierre Baldi
Department of Computer Science
University of California, Irvine
Irvine, California 92697-3425, USA
pfbaldi@ics.uci.edu

Abstract

The concept of surprise is central to sensory processing, adaptation, learning, and attention. Yet, no widely-accepted mathematical theory currently exists to quantitatively characterize surprise elicited by a stimulus or event, for observers that range from single neurons to complex natural or engineered systems. We describe a formal Bayesian definition of surprise that is the only consistent formulation under minimal axiomatic assumptions. Surprise quantifies how data affects a natural or artificial observer, by measuring the difference between posterior and prior beliefs of the observer. Using this framework we measure the extent to which humans direct their gaze towards surprising items while watching television and video games. We find that subjects are strongly attracted towards surprising locations, with 72% of all human gaze shifts directed towards locations more surprising than the average, a figure which rises to 84% when considering only gaze targets simultaneously selected by all subjects. The resulting theory of surprise is applicable across different spatio-temporal scales, modalities, and levels of abstraction.

Life is full of surprises, ranging from a great christmas gift or a new magic trick, to wardrobe malfunctions, reckless drivers, terrorist attacks, and tsunami waves. Key to survival is our ability to rapidly attend to, identify, and learn from surprising events, to decide on present and future courses of action [1]. Yet, little theoretical and computational understanding exists of the very essence of surprise, as evidenced by the absence from our everyday vocabulary of a quantitative unit of surprise: Qualities such as the "wow factor" have remained vague and elusive to mathematical analysis.

Informal correlates of surprise exist at nearly all stages of neural processing. In sensory neuroscience, it has been suggested that only the unexpected at one stage is transmitted to the next stage [2]. Hence, sensory cortex may have evolved to adapt to, to predict, and to quiet down the expected statistical regularities of the world [3, 4, 5, 6], focusing instead on events that are unpredictable or surprising. Electrophysiological evidence for this early sensory emphasis onto surprising stimuli exists from studies of adaptation in visual [7, 8, 4, 9], olfactory [10, 11], and auditory cortices [12], subcortical structures like the LGN [13], and even retinal ganglion cells [14, 15] and cochlear hair cells [16]: neural response greatly attenuates with repeated or prolonged exposure to an initially novel stimulus. Surprise and novelty are also central to learning and memory formation [1], to the point that surprise is believed to be a necessary trigger for associative learning [17, 18], as supported by mounting evidence for a role of the hippocampus as a novelty detector [19, 20, 21]. Finally, seeking novelty is a well-identified human character trait, with possible association with the dopamine D4 receptor gene [22, 23, 24].

In the Bayesian framework, we develop the only consistent theory of surprise, in terms of the difference between the posterior and prior distributions of beliefs of an observer over the available class of models or hypotheses about the world. We show that this definition derived from first principles presents key advantages over more *ad-hoc* formulations, typically relying on detecting outlier stimuli. Armed with this new framework, we provide direct experimental evidence that surprise best characterizes what attracts human gaze in large amounts of natural video stimuli. We here extend a recent pilot study [25], adding more comprehensive theory, large-scale human data collection, and additional analysis.

1 Theory

Bayesian Definition of Surprise. We propose that surprise is a general concept, which can be derived from first principles and formalized across spatio-temporal scales, sensory modalities, and, more generally, data types and data sources. Two elements are essential for a principled definition of surprise. First, surprise can exist only in the presence of uncertainty, which can arise from intrinsic stochasticity, missing information, or limited computing resources. A world that is purely deterministic and predictable in real-time for a given observer contains no surprises. Second, surprise can only be defined in a relative, subjective, manner and is related to the expectations of the observer, be it a single synapse, neuronal circuit, organism, or computer device. The same data may carry different amount of surprise for different observers, or even for the same observer taken at different times.

In probability and decision theory it can be shown that the only consistent and optimal way for modeling and reasoning about uncertainty is provided by the Bayesian theory of probability [26, 27, 28]. Furthermore, in the Bayesian framework, probabilities correspond to subjective degrees of beliefs in hypotheses or models which are updated, as data is acquired, using Bayes' theorem as the fundamental tool for transforming prior belief distributions into posterior belief distributions. Therefore, within the same optimal framework, the only consistent definition of surprise must involve: (1) probabilistic concepts to cope with uncertainty; and (2) prior and posterior distributions to capture subjective expectations.

Consistently with this Bayesian approach, the background information of an observer is captured by his/her/its prior probability distribution $\{P(M)\}_{M \in \mathcal{M}}$ over the hypotheses or models M in a model space $\mathcal{M}$. Given this prior distribution of beliefs, the fundamental effect of a new data observation D on the observer is to change the prior distribution $\{P(M)\}_{M \in \mathcal{M}}$ into the posterior distribution $\{P(M|D)\}_{M \in \mathcal{M}}$ via Bayes theorem, whereby

$$\forall M \in \mathcal{M}, \qquad P(M|D) = \frac{P(D|M)}{P(D)} P(M). \qquad (1)$$

In this framework, the new data observation D carries no surprise if it leaves the observer beliefs unaffected, that is, if the posterior is identical to the prior; conversely, D is surprising if the posterior distribution resulting from observing D significantly differs from the prior distribution. Therefore we formally measure surprise elicited by data as some distance measure between the posterior and prior distributions. This is best done using the relative entropy or Kullback-Leibler (KL) divergence [29]. Thus, surprise is defined by the average of the log-odd ratio:

$$S(D, \mathcal{M}) = KL(P(M|D), P(M)) = \int_{\mathcal{M}} P(M|D) \log \frac{P(M|D)}{P(M)} dM \qquad (2)$$

taken with respect to the posterior distribution over the model class $\mathcal{M}$. Note that KL is not symmetric but has well-known theoretical advantages, including invariance with respect to

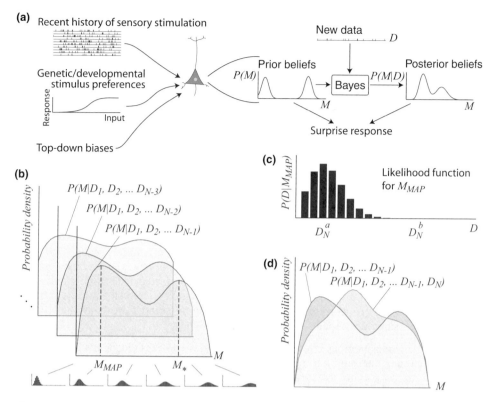

Figure 1: Computing surprise in early sensory neurons. (**a**) Prior data observations, tuning prefer-ences, and top-down influences contribute to shaping a set of "prior beliefs" a neuron may have over a class of internal models or hypotheses about the world. For instance, $\mathcal{M}$ may be a set of Poisson processes parameterized by the rate λ, with $\{P(M)\}_{M \in \mathcal{M}} = \{P(\lambda)\}_{\lambda \in \mathbb{R}^{+*}}$ the prior distribution of beliefs about which Poisson models well describe the world as sensed by the neuron. New data D updates the prior into the posterior using Bayes' theorem. Surprise quantifies the difference be-tween the posterior and prior distributions over the model class $\mathcal{M}$. The remaining panels detail how surprise differs from conventional model fitting and outlier-based novelty. (**b**) In standard it-erative Bayesian model fitting, at every iteration N, incoming data D_N is used to update the prior $\{P(M|D_1, D_2, ..., D_{N-1})\}_{M \in \mathcal{M}}$ into the posterior $\{P(M|D_1, D_2, ..., D_N)\}_{M \in \mathcal{M}}$. Freezing this learning at a given iteration, one then picks the currently best model, usually using either a maxi-mum likelihood criterion, or a maximum a posteriori one (yielding M_{MAP} shown). (**c**) This best model is used for a number of tasks at the current iteration, including outlier-based novelty detec-tion. New data is then considered novel at that instant if it has low likelihood for the best model (e.g., D_N^b is more novel than D_N^a). This focus onto the single best model presents obvious limita-tions, especially in situations where other models are nearly as good (e.g., M_* in panel (b) is entirely ignored during standard novelty computation). One palliative solution is to consider mixture mod-els, or simply $P(D)$, but this just amounts to shifting the problem into a different model class. (**d**) Surprise directly addresses this problem by simultaneously considering all models and by measuring how data changes the observer's distribution of beliefs from $\{P(M|D_1, D_2, ..., D_{N-1})\}_{M \in \mathcal{M}}$ to $\{P(M|D_1, D_2, ..., D_N)\}_{M \in \mathcal{M}}$ over the entire model class $\mathcal{M}$ (orange shaded area).

reparameterizations. A unit of surprise — a *"wow"* — may then be defined for a single model M as the amount of surprise corresponding to a two-fold variation between $P(M|D)$ and $P(M)$, i.e., as $\log P(M|D)/P(M)$ (with $\log$ taken in base 2), with the total number of wows experienced for all models obtained through the integration in eq. 2.

Surprise and outlier detection. Outlier detection based on the likelihood $P(D|M_{\text{best}})$ of D given a single best model M_{best} is at best an approximation to surprise and, in some cases, is misleading. Consider, for instance, a case where D has very small probability both for a model or hypothesis M and for a single alternative hypothesis $\overline{M}$. Although D is a strong outlier, it carries very little information regarding whether M or $\overline{M}$ is the better model, and therefore very little surprise. Thus an outlier detection method would strongly focus attentional resources onto D, although D is a false positive, in the sense that it carries no useful information for discriminating between the two alternative hypotheses M and $\overline{M}$. Figure 1 further illustrates this disconnect between outlier detection and surprise.

2   Human experiments

To test the surprise hypothesis — that surprise attracts human attention and gaze in natural scenes — we recorded eye movements from eight naïve observers (three females and five males, ages 23-32, normal or corrected-to-normal vision). Each watched a subset from 50 videoclips totaling over 25 minutes of playtime (46,489 video frames, 640×480, 60.27 Hz, mean screen luminance 30 cd/m^2, room 4 cd/m^2, viewing distance 80cm, field of view $28° \times 21°$). Clips comprised outdoors daytime and nighttime scenes of crowded environments, video games, and television broadcast including news, sports, and commercials. Right-eye position was tracked with a 240 Hz video-based device (ISCAN RK-464), with methods as previously [30]. Two hundred calibrated eye movement traces (10,192 saccades) were analyzed, corresponding to four distinct observers for each of the 50 clips. Figure 2 shows sample scanpaths for one videoclip.

To characterize image regions selected by participants, we process videoclips through computational metrics that output a topographic dynamic master response map, assigning in real-time a response value to every input location. A good master map would highlight, more than expected by chance, locations gazed to by observers. To score each metric we hence sample, at onset of every human saccade, master map activity around the saccade's future endpoint, and around a uniformly random endpoint (random sampling was repeated 100 times to evaluate variability). We quantify differences between histograms of master

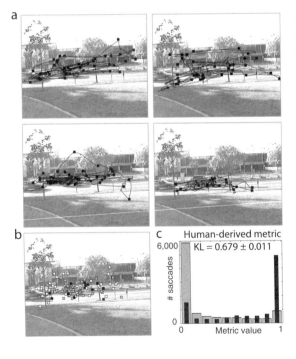

Figure 2: **(a)** Sample eye movement traces from four observers (squares denote saccade endpoints). **(b)** Our data exhibits high inter-individual overlap, shown here with the locations where one human saccade endpoint was nearby ($\approx 5°$) one (white squares), two (cyan squares), or all three (black squares) other humans. **(c)** A metric where the master map was created from the three eye movement traces other than that being tested yields an upper-bound KL score, computed by comparing the histograms of metric values at human (narrow blue bars) and random (wider green bars) saccade targets. Indeed, this metric's map was very sparse (many random saccades landing on locations with near-zero response), yet humans preferentially saccaded towards the three active hotspots corresponding to the eye positions of three other humans (many human saccades landing on locations with near-unity responses).

map samples collected from human and random saccades using again the Kullback-Leibler (KL) distance: metrics which better predict human scanpaths exhibit higher distances from random as, typically, observers non-uniformly gaze towards a minority of regions with highest metric responses while avoiding a majority of regions with low metric responses. This approach presents several advantages over simpler scoring schemes [31, 32], including agnosticity to putative mechanisms for generating saccades and the fact that applying any continuous nonlinearity to master map values would not affect scoring.

Experimental results. We test six computational metrics, encompassing and extending the state-of-the-art found in previous studies. The first three quantify static image properties (local intensity variance in 16×16 image patches [31]; local oriented edge density as measured with Gabor filters [33]; and local Shannon entropy in 16×16 image patches [34]). The remaining three metrics are more sensitive to dynamic events (local motion [33]; outlier-based saliency [33]; and surprise [25]).

For all metrics, we find that humans are significantly attracted by image regions with higher metric responses. However, the static metrics typically respond vigorously at numerous visual locations (Figure 3), hence they are poorly specific and yield relatively low KL scores between humans and random. The metrics sensitive to motion, outliers, and surprising events, in comparison, yield sparser maps and higher KL scores.

The surprise metric of interest here quantifies low-level surprise in image patches over space and time, and at this point does not account for high-level or cognitive beliefs of our human observers. Rather, it assumes a family of simple models for image patches, each processed through 72 early feature detectors sensitive to color, orientation, motion, etc., and computes surprise from shifts in the distribution of beliefs about which models better describe the patches (see [25] and [35] for details). We find that the surprise metric significantly outperforms all other computational metrics ($p < 10^{-100}$ or better on t-tests for equality of KL scores), scoring nearly 20% better than the second-best metric (saliency) and 60% better than the best static metric (entropy). Surprising stimuli often substantially differ from simple feature outliers; for example, a continually blinking light on a static background elicits sustained flicker due to its locally outlier temporal dynamics but is only surprising for a moment. Similarly, a shower of randomly-colored pixels continually excites all low-level feature detectors but rapidly becomes unsurprising.

Strongest attractors of human attention. Clearly, in our and previous eye-tracking experiments, in some situations potentially interesting targets were more numerous than in others. With many possible targets, different observers may orient towards different locations, making it more difficult for a single metric to accurately predict all observers. Hence we consider (Figure 4) subsets of human saccades where at least two, three, or all four observers simultaneously agreed on a gaze target. Observers could have agreed based on bottom-up factors (e.g., only one location had interesting visual appearance at that time), top-down factors (e.g., only one object was of current cognitive interest), or both (e.g., a single cognitively interesting object was present which also had distinctive appearance). Irrespectively of the cause for agreement, it indicates consolidated belief that a location was attractive. While the KL scores of all metrics improved when progressively focusing onto only those locations, dynamic metrics improved more steeply, indicating that stimuli which more reliably attracted all observers carried more motion, saliency, and surprise. Surprise remained significantly the best metric to characterize these agreed-upon attractors of human gaze ($p < 10^{-100}$ or better on t-tests for equality of KL scores).

Overall, surprise explained the greatest fraction of human saccades, indicating that humans are significantly attracted towards surprising locations in video displays. Over 72% of all human saccades were targeted to locations predicted to be more surprising than on average. When only considering saccades where two, three, or four observers agreed on a common gaze target, this figure rose to 76%, 80%, and 84%, respectively.

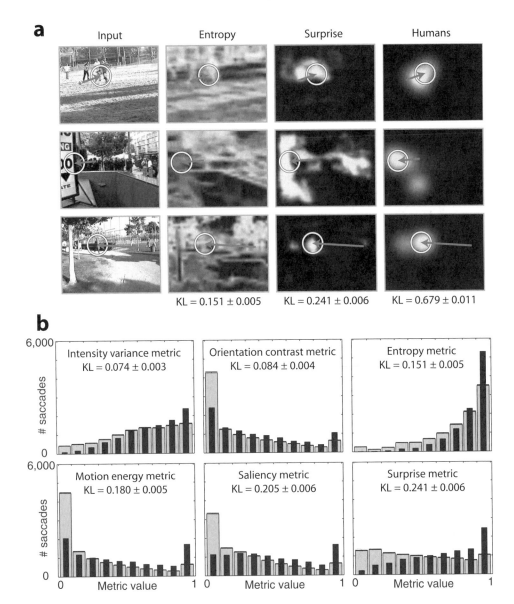

Figure 3: **(a)** Sample video frames, with corresponding human saccades and predictions from the entropy, surprise, and human-derived metrics. Entropy maps, like intensity variance and orientation maps, exhibited many locations with high responses, hence had low specificity and were poorly discriminative. In contrast, motion, saliency, and surprise maps were much sparser and more specific, with surprise significantly more often on target. For three example frames (first column), saccades from one subject are shown (arrows) with corresponding apertures over which master map activity at the saccade endpoint was sampled (circles). **(b)** KL scores for these metrics indicate significantly different performance levels, and a strict ranking of variance < orientation < entropy < motion < saliency < surprise < human-derived. KL scores were computed by comparing the number of human saccades landing onto each given range of master map values (narrow blue bars) to the number of random saccades hitting the same range (wider green bars). A score of zero would indicate equality between the human and random histograms, i.e., humans did not tend to hit various master map values any differently from expected by chance, or, the master map could not predict human saccades better than random saccades. Among the six computational metrics tested in total, surprise performed best, in that surprising locations were relatively few yet reliably gazed to by humans.

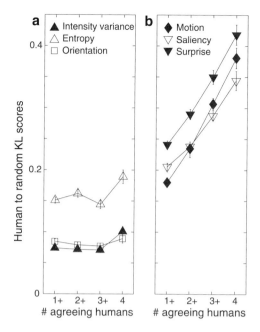

Figure 4: KL scores when considering only saccades where at least one (all 10,192 saccades), two (7,948 saccades), three (5,565 saccades), or all four (2,951 saccades) humans agreed on a common gaze location, for the static (a) and dynamic metrics (b). Static metrics improved substantially when progressively focusing onto saccades with stronger inter-observer agreement (average slope 0.56 ± 0.37 percent KL score units per 1,000 pruned saccades). Hence, when humans agreed on a location, they also tended to be more reliably predicted by the metrics. Furthermore, dynamic metrics improved 4.5 times more steeply (slope 2.44 ± 0.37), suggesting a stronger role of dynamic events in attracting human attention. Surprising events were significantly the strongest (t-tests for equality of KL scores between surprise and other metrics, $p < 10^{-100}$).

3 Discussion

While previous research has shown with either static scenes or dynamic synthetic stimuli that humans preferentially fixate regions of high entropy [34], contrast [31], saliency [32], flicker [36], or motion [37], our data provides direct experimental evidence that humans fixate surprising locations even more reliably. These conclusions were made possible by developing new tools to quantify what attracts human gaze over space and time in dynamic natural scenes. Surprise explained best where humans look when considering all saccades, and even more so when restricting the analysis to only those saccades for which human observers tended to agree. Surprise hence represents an inexpensive, easily computable approximation to human attentional allocation.

In the absence of quantitative tools to measure surprise, most experimental and modeling work to date has adopted the approximation that novel events are surprising, and has focused on experimental scenarios which are simple enough to ensure an overlap between informal notions of novelty and surprise: for example, a stimulus is novel during testing if it has not been seen during training [9]. Our definition opens new avenues for more sophisticated experiments, where surprise elicited by different stimuli can be precisely compared and calibrated, yielding predictions at the single-unit as well as behavioral levels.

The definition of surprise — as the distance between the posterior and prior distributions of beliefs over models — is entirely general and readily applicable to the analysis of auditory, olfactory, gustatory, or somatosensory data. While here we have focused on behavior rather than detailed biophysical implementation, it is worth noting that detecting surprise in neural spike trains does not require semantic understanding of the data carried by the spike trains, and thus could provide guiding signals during self-organization and development of sensory areas. At higher processing levels, top-down cues and task demands are known to combine with stimulus novelty in capturing attention and triggering learning [1, 38], ideas which may now be formalized and quantified in terms of priors, posteriors, and surprise. Surprise, indeed, inherently depends on uncertainty and on prior beliefs. Hence surprise theory can further be tested and utilized in experiments where the prior is biased, for example by top-down instructions or prior exposures to stimuli [38]. In addition, simple surprise-based behavioral measures such as the eye-tracking one used here may prove useful for early diagnostic of human conditions including autism and attention-deficit hyperactive disorder, as well as for quantitative comparison between humans and animals which may have lower or different priors, including monkeys, frogs, and flies. Beyond sensory biology, computable surprise could guide the development of data mining and compression systems (giving more bits to surprising regions of interest), to find surprising agents in crowds, surprising sentences in books or speeches, surprising sequences in genomes, surprising medical symptoms, surprising odors in airport luggage racks, surprising documents on the world-wide-web, or to design surprising advertisements.

Acknowledgments: *Supported by HFSP, NSF and NGA (L.I.), NIH and NSF (P.B.). We thank UCI's Institute for Genomics and Bioinformatics and USC's Center High Performance Computing and Communications (www.usc.edu/hpcc) for access to their computing clusters.*

References

[1] Ranganath, C. & Rainer, G. *Nat Rev Neurosci* **4**, 193–202 (2003).

[2] Rao, R. P. & Ballard, D. H. *Nat Neurosci* **2**, 79–87 (1999).

[3] Olshausen, B. A. & Field, D. J. *Nature* **381**, 607–609 (1996).

[4] Müller, J. R., Metha, A. B., Krauskopf, J. & Lennie, P. *Science* **285**, 1405–1408 (1999).

[5] Dragoi, V., Sharma, J., Miller, E. K. & Sur, M. *Nat Neurosci* **5**, 883–891 (2002).

[6] David, S. V., Vinje, W. E. & Gallant, J. L. *J Neurosci* **24**, 6991–7006 (2004).

[7] Maffei, L., Fiorentini, A. & Bisti, S. *Science* **182**, 1036–1038 (1973).

[8] Movshon, J. A. & Lennie, P. *Nature* **278**, 850–852 (1979).

[9] Fecteau, J. H. & Munoz, D. P. *Nat Rev Neurosci* **4**, 435–443 (2003).

[10] Kurahashi, T. & Menini, A. *Nature* **385**, 725–729 (1997).

[11] Bradley, J., Bonigk, W., Yau, K. W. & Frings, S. *Nat Neurosci* **7**, 705–710 (2004).

[12] Ulanovsky, N., Las, L. & Nelken, I. *Nat Neurosci* **6**, 391–398 (2003).

[13] Solomon, S. G., Peirce, J. W., Dhruv, N. T. & Lennie, P. *Neuron* **42**, 155–162 (2004).

[14] Smirnakis, S. M., Berry, M. J. & et al. *Nature* **386**, 69–73 (1997).

[15] Brown, S. P. & Masland, R. H. *Nat Neurosci* **4**, 44–51 (2001).

[16] Kennedy, H. J., Evans, M. G. & et al. *Nat Neurosci* **6**, 832–836 (2003).

[17] Schultz, W. & Dickinson, A. *Annu Rev Neurosci* **23**, 473–500 (2000).

[18] Fletcher, P. C., Anderson, J. M., Shanks, D. R. et al. *Nat Neurosci* **4**, 1043–1048 (2001).

[19] Knight, R. *Nature* **383**, 256–259 (1996).

[20] Stern, C. E., Corkin, S., Gonzalez, R. G. et al. *Proc Natl Acad Sci U S A* **93**, 8660–8665 (1996).

[21] Li, S., Cullen, W. K., Anwyl, R. & Rowan, M. J. *Nat Neurosci* **6**, 526–531 (2003).

[22] Ebstein, R. P., Novick, O., Umansky, R. et al. *Nat Genet* **12**, 78–80 (1996).

[23] Benjamin, J., Li, L. & et al. *Nat Genet* **12**, 81–84 (1996).

[24] Lusher, J. M., Chandler, C. & Ball, D. *Mol Psychiatry* **6**, 497–499 (2001).

[25] Itti, L. & Baldi, P. In *Proc. IEEE CVPR*. San Siego, CA (2005 in press).

[26] Cox, R. T. *Am. J. Phys.* **14**, 1–13 (1964).

[27] Savage, L. J. *The foundations of statistics* (Dover, New York, 1972). (First Edition in 1954).

[28] Jaynes, E. T. *Probability Theory. The Logic of Science* (Cambridge University Press, 2003).

[29] Kullback, S. *Information Theory and Statistics* (Wiley, New York:New York, 1959).

[30] Itti, L. *Visual Cognition* (2005 in press).

[31] Reinagel, P. & Zador, A. M. *Network* **10**, 341–350 (1999).

[32] Parkhurst, D., Law, K. & Niebur, E. *Vision Res* **42**, 107–123 (2002).

[33] Itti, L. & Koch, C. *Nat Rev Neurosci* **2**, 194–203 (2001).

[34] Privitera, C. M. & Stark, L. W. *IEEE Trans Patt Anal Mach Intell* **22**, 970–982 (2000).

[35] All source code for all metrics is freely available at http://iLab.usc.edu/toolkit/.

[36] Theeuwes, J. *Percept Psychophys* **57**, 637–644 (1995).

[37] Abrams, R. A. & Christ, S. E. *Psychol Sci* **14**, 427–432 (2003).

[38] Wolfe, J. M. & Horowitz, T. S. *Nat Rev Neurosci* **5**, 495–501 (2004).

Efficient Estimation of OOMs

Herbert Jaeger, Mingjie Zhao, Andreas Kolling
International University Bremen
Bremen, Germany
h.jaeger|m.zhao|a.kolling@iu-bremen.de

Abstract

A standard method to obtain stochastic models for symbolic time series is to train state-emitting hidden Markov models (SE-HMMs) with the Baum-Welch algorithm. Based on observable operator models (OOMs), in the last few months a number of novel learning algorithms for similar purposes have been developed: (1,2) two versions of an "efficiency sharpening" (ES) algorithm, which iteratively improves the statistical efficiency of a sequence of OOM estimators, (3) a constrained gradient descent ML estimator for transition-emitting HMMs (TE-HMMs). We give an overview on these algorithms and compare them with SE-HMM/EM learning on synthetic and real-life data.

1 Introduction

Stochastic symbol sequences with memory effects are frequently modelled by training hidden Markov models with the Baum-Welch variant of the EM algorithm. More specifically, state-emitting HMMs (SE-HMMs) are standardly employed, which emit observable events from hidden states. Known weaknesses of HMM training with Baum-Welch are long runtimes and proneness to getting trapped in local maxima.

Over the last few years, an alternative to HMMs has been developed, *observable operator models* (OOMs). The class of processes that can be described by (finite-dimensional) OOMs properly includes the processes that can be described by (finite-dimensional) HMMs. OOMs identify the observable events a of a process with linear *observable operators* τ_a acting on a real vector space of *predictive states* w [1]. A basic learning algorithm for OOMs [2] estimates the observable operators τ_a by solving a linear system of *learning equations*. The learning algorithm is constructive, fast and yields asymptotically correct estimates. Two problems that so far prevented OOMs from practical use were (i) poor statistical efficiency, (ii) the possibility that the obtained models might predict negative "probabilities" for some sequences. Since a few months the first problem has been very satisfactorily solved [2]. In this novel approach to learning OOMs from data we iteratively construct a sequence of estimators whose statistical efficiency increases, which led us to call the method *efficiency sharpening* (ES).

Another, somewhat neglected class of stochastic models is transition-emitting HMMs (TE-HMMs). TE-HMMs fall in between SE-HMMs and OOMs w.r.t. expressiveness. TE-HMMs are equivalent to OOMs whose operator matrices are non-negative. Because TE-HMMs are frequently referred to as Mealy machines (actually a misnomer because originally Mealy machines are not probabilistic but only non-deterministic), we have started to call non-negative OOMs "Mealy OOMs" (MOOMs). We use either name according to the way the models are represented. A variant of Baum-Welch has recently been described for TE-HMMs [3]. We have derived an alternative learning constrained log gradient (CLG) algorithm for MOOMs which performs a constrained gradient descent on the log likelihood surface in the log model parameter space of MOOMs.

In this article we give a compact introduction to the basics of OOMs (Section 2), outline the new ES and CLG algorithms (Sections 3 and 4), and compare their performance on a variety of datasets (Section 5). In the conclusion (Section 6) we also provide a pointer to a Matlab toolbox.

2 Basics of OOMs

Let $(\Omega, \mathfrak{A}, P, (X_n)_{n\geq 0})$ or (X_n) for short be a discrete-time stochastic process with values in a finite symbol set $O = \{a_1, \ldots, a_M\}$. We will consider only stationary processes here for notational simplicity; OOMs can equally model nonstationary processes. An m-dimensional OOM for (X_n) is a structure $\mathcal{A} = (\mathbb{R}^m, (\tau_a)_{a\in O}, w_0)$, where each *observable operator* τ_a is a real-valued $m \times m$ matrix and $w_0 \in \mathbb{R}^m$ is the *starting state*, provided that for any finite sequence $a_{i_0} \ldots a_{i_n}$ it holds that

$$P(X_0 = a_{i_0}, \ldots X_n = a_{i_n}) = \mathbf{1}_m \tau_{a_{i_n}} \cdots \tau_{a_{i_0}} w_0, \tag{1}$$

where $\mathbf{1}_m$ always denotes a row vector of units of length m (we drop the subscript if it is clear from the context). We will use the shorthand notation $\bar{a}$ to denote a generic sequence and $\tau_{\bar{a}}$ to denote a concatenation of the corresponding operators in reverse order, which would condense (1) into $P(\bar{a}) = \mathbf{1}\tau_{\bar{a}}w_0$.

Conversely, if a structure $\mathcal{A} = (\mathbb{R}^m, (\tau_a)_{a\in O}, w_0)$ satisfies

$$\text{(i) } \mathbf{1}w_0 = 1, \quad \text{(ii) } \mathbf{1}(\sum_{a\in O} \tau_a) = \mathbf{1}, \quad \text{(iii) } \forall \bar{a} \in O^* : \mathbf{1}\tau_{\bar{a}}w_0 \geq 0, \tag{2}$$

(where O^* denotes the set of all finite sequences over O), then there exists a process whose distribution is described by $\mathcal{A}$ via (1). The process is stationary iff $(\sum_{a\in O} \tau_a)w_0 = w_0$. Conditions (i) and (ii) are easy to check, but no efficient criterium is known to decide whether the non-negativity criterium (iii) holds for a structure $\mathcal{A}$ (for recent progress in this problem, which is equivalent to a problem of general interest in linear algebra, see [4]). Models $\mathcal{A}$ learnt from data tend to marginally violate (iii) – this is the unresolved non-negativity problem in the theory of OOMs.

The *state* $w_{\bar{a}}$ of an OOM after an initial history $\bar{a}$ is obtained by normalizing $\tau_{\bar{a}}w_0$ to unit component sum via $w_{\bar{a}} = \tau_{\bar{a}}w_0/\mathbf{1}\tau_{\bar{a}}w_0$.

A fundamental (and nontrivial) theorem for OOMs characterizes equivalence of two OOMs. Two m-dimensional OOms $\mathcal{A} = (\mathbb{R}^m, (\tau_a)_{a\in O}, w_0)$ and $\tilde{\mathcal{A}} = (\mathbb{R}^m, (\tilde{\tau}_a)_{a\in O}, \tilde{w}_0)$ are defined to be equivalent if they generate the same probability distribution according to (1). By the equivalence theorem, $\mathcal{A}$ is equivalent to $\tilde{\mathcal{A}}$ if and only if there exists a transformation matrix ϱ of size $m \times m$, satisfying $\mathbf{1}\varrho = \mathbf{1}$, such that $\tilde{\tau}_a = \varrho\tau_a\varrho^{-1}$ for all symbols a.

We mentioned in the Introduction that OOM states represent the future probability distribution of the process. This can be algebraically captured in the notion of *characterizers*. Let $\mathcal{A} = (\mathbb{R}^m, (\tau_a)_{a\in O}, w_0)$ be an OOM for (X_n) and choose k such that $\kappa = |O|^k \geq m$. Let

$\bar{b}_1, \ldots, \bar{b}_\kappa$ be the alphabetical enumeration of O^k. Then a $m \times \kappa$ matrix C is a *characterizer of length* k for $\mathcal{A}$ iff $\mathbf{1}C = \mathbf{1}$ (that is, C has unit column sums) and

$$\forall \bar{a} \in O^* : \quad w_{\bar{a}} = C(P(\bar{b}_1|\bar{a}) \cdots P(\bar{b}_\kappa|\bar{a}))', \tag{3}$$

where $'$ denotes the transpose and $P(\bar{b}|\bar{a})$ is the conditional probability that the process continues with $\bar{b}$ after an initial history $\bar{a}$. It can be shown [2] that every OOM has characterizers of length k for suitably large k. Intuitively, a characterizer "bundles" the length k future distribution into the state vector by projection.

If two equivalent OOMs $\mathcal{A}, \tilde{\mathcal{A}}$ are related by $\tilde{\tau}_a = \varrho \tau_a \varrho^{-1}$, and C is a characterizer for $\mathcal{A}$, it is easy to check that ϱC is a characterizer for $\tilde{\mathcal{A}}$.

We conclude this section by explaining the basic learning equations. An analysis of (1) reveals that for any state $w_{\bar{a}}$ and operator τ_b from an OOM it holds that

$$\tau_a w_{\bar{a}} = P(a|\bar{a})w_{\bar{a}a}, \tag{4}$$

where $\bar{a}a$ is the concatenation of $\bar{a}$ with a. The vectors $w_{\bar{a}}$ and $P(a|\bar{a})w_{\bar{a}a}$ thus form an argument-value pair for τ_a. Let $\bar{a}_1, \ldots, \bar{a}_l$ be a finite sequence of finite sequences over O, and let $V = (w_{\bar{a}_1} \cdots w_{\bar{a}_l})$ be the matrix containing the corresponding state vectors. Let again C be a $m \times \kappa$ sized characterizer of length k and $\bar{b}_1, \ldots, \bar{b}_\kappa$ be the alphabetical enumeration of O^k. Let $\underline{V} = (P(\bar{b}_i|\bar{a}_j))$ be the $\kappa \times l$ matrix containing the conditional continuation probabilities of the initial sequences $\bar{a}_j$ by the sequences $\bar{b}_i$. It is easy to see that $V = C\underline{V}$. Likewise, let $W_a = (P(a|\bar{a}_1)w_{\bar{a}_1 a} \cdots P(a|\bar{a}_l)w_{\bar{a}_l a})$ contain the vectors corresponding to the rhs of (4), and let $\underline{W}_a = (P(a\bar{b}_i|\bar{a}_j))$ be the analog of $\underline{V}$. It is easily verified that $W_a = C\underline{W}_a$. Furthermore, by construction it holds that $\tau_a V = W_a$.

A linear operator on $\mathbb{R}^m$ is uniquely determined by $l \geq m$ argument-value pairs provided there are at least m linearly independent argument vectors in these pairs. Thus, if a characterizer C is found such that $V = C\underline{V}$ has rank m, the operators τ_a of an OOM characterized by C are uniquely determined by $\underline{V}$ and the matrices $\underline{W}_a$ via $\tau_a = W_a V^\dagger = C\underline{W}_a(C\underline{V})^\dagger$, where $\dagger$ denotes the pseudo-inverse. Now, given a training sequence S, the conditional continuation probabilities $P(\bar{b}_i|\bar{a}_j), P(a\bar{b}_i|\bar{a}_j)$ that make up $\underline{V}, \underline{W}_a$ can be estimated from S by an obvious counting scheme, yielding estimates $\hat{P}(\bar{b}_i|\bar{a}_j), \hat{P}(a\bar{b}_i|\bar{a}_j)$ for making up $\hat{\underline{V}}$ and $\hat{\underline{W}}_a$, respectively. This leads to the general form of OOM learning equations:

$$\hat{\tau}_a = C\hat{\underline{W}}_a(C\hat{\underline{V}})^\dagger. \tag{5}$$

In words, to learn an OOM from S, first fix a model dimension m, a characterizer C, *indicative sequences* $\bar{a}_1, \ldots, \bar{a}_l$, then construct estimates $\hat{\underline{V}}$ and $\hat{\underline{W}}_a$ by frequency counting, and finally use (5) to obtain estimates of the operators. This estimation procedure is asymptotically correct in the sense that, if the training data were generated by an m-dimensional OOM in the first place, this generator will almost surely be perfectly recovered as the size of training data goes to infinity. The reason for this is that the estimates $\hat{\underline{V}}$ and $\hat{\underline{W}}_a$ converge almost surely to $\underline{V}$ and $\underline{W}_a$. The starting state can be recovered from the estimated operators by exploiting $(\sum_{a \in O} \tau_a)w_0 = w_0$ or directly from C and $\hat{\underline{V}}$ (see [2] for details).

3 The ES Family of Learning Algorithms

All learning algorithms based on (5) are asymptotically correct (which EM algorithms are not, by the way), but their statistical efficiency (model variance) depends crucially on (i) the choice of indicative sequences $\bar{a}_1, \ldots, \bar{a}_l$ and (ii) the characterizer C (assuming that the model dimension m is determined by other means, e.g. by cross-validation). We will first address (ii) and describe an iterative scheme to obtain characterizers that lead to a low model variance.

The choice of C has a twofold impact on model variance. First, the pseudoinverse operation in (5) blows up variation in $C\hat{V}$ depending on the matrix condition number of this matrix. Thus, C should be chosen such that the condition of $C\hat{V}$ gets close to 1. This strategy was pioneered in [5], who obtained the first halfway statistically satisfactory learning procedures. In contrast, here we set out from the second mechanism by which C influences model variance, namely, choose C such that the variance of $C\hat{V}$ itself is minimized.

We need a few algebraic preparations. First, observe that if some characterizer C is used with (5), obtaining a model $\hat{A}$, and ϱ is an OOM equivalence transformation, then if $\tilde{C} = \varrho C$ is used with (5), the obtained model $\tilde{\hat{A}}$ is an equivalent version of $\hat{A}$ via ϱ.

Furthermore, it is easy to see [2] that two characterizers C_1, C_2 characterize the same OOM iff $C_1 \underline{V} = C_2 \underline{V}$. We call two characterizers *similar* if this holds, and write $C_1 \sim C_2$. Clearly $C_1 \sim C_2$ iff $C_2 = C_1 + G$ for some G satisfying $G\underline{V} = 0$ and $1G = 0$. That is, the similarity equivalence class of some characterizer C is the set $\{C + G | G\underline{V} = 0, 1G = 0\}$. Together with the first observation this implies that we may confine our search for "good" characterizers to a single (and arbitrary) such equivalence class of characterizers. Let C_0 in the remainder be a representative of an arbitrarily chosen similarity class whose members all characterize $\mathcal{A}$.

In [2] it is explained that the variance of $C\hat{V}$ is monotonically tied to $\sum_{i=1,\ldots,\kappa; j=1,\ldots,l} P(\bar{a}_j \bar{b}_i) \|w_{\bar{a}_j} - C(:,i)\|^2$, where $C(:,i)$ is the i-th column of C. This observation allows us to determine an optimal (minimal variance of $C\hat{V}$ within the equivalence class of C_0) characterizer C_{opt} as the solution to the following minimization problem:

$$
\begin{aligned}
C_{\text{opt}} &= C_0 + G_{\text{opt}}, \quad \text{where} \\
G_{\text{opt}} &= \arg\min_{G} \sum_{i=1,\ldots,\kappa; j=1,\ldots,l} P(\bar{a}_j \bar{b}_i) \|w_{\bar{a}_j} - (C_0 + G)(:,i)\|^2
\end{aligned}
\tag{6}
$$

under the constraints $G\underline{V} = 0$ and $1G = 0$. This problem can be analytically solved [2] and has a surprising and beautiful solution, which we now explain. In a nutshell, C_{opt} is composed column-wise by certain states of a time-reversed version of $\mathcal{A}$. We describe in more detail time-reversal of OOMs. Given an OOM $\mathcal{A} = (\mathbb{R}^m, (\tau_a)_{a \in O}, w_0)$ with an induced probability distribution P_A, its *reverse* OOM $\mathcal{A}^r = (\mathbb{R}^m, (\tau_a^r)_{a \in O}, w_0^r)$ is characterized by a probability distribution P_{A^r} satisfying

$$
\forall \, a_0 \cdots a_n \in O^* : \quad P_A(a_0 \cdots a_n) = P_{A^r}(a_n \cdots a_0).
\tag{7}
$$

A reverse OOM can be easily computed from the "forward" OOM as follows. If $\mathcal{A} = (\mathbb{R}^m, (\tau_a)_{a \in O}, w_0)$ is an OOM for a stationary process, and w_0 has no zero entry, then

$$
\mathcal{A}^r = (\mathbb{R}^m, (D\tau_a' D^{-1})_{a \in O}, w_0)
\tag{8}
$$

is a reverse OOM to $\mathcal{A}$, where $D = \text{diag}(w_0)$ is a diagonal matrix with w_0 on its diagonal.

Now let $\bar{b}_1, \ldots, \bar{b}_\kappa$ again be the sequences employed in $\underline{V}$. Let $\mathcal{A}^r = (\mathbb{R}^m, (\tau_a^r)_{a \in O}, w_0)$ be the reverse OOM to $\mathcal{A}$, which was characterized by C_0. Furthermore, for $\bar{b}_i = b_1 \ldots b_k$ let

$w_{\tilde{b}_i}^r = \tau_{\tilde{b}_1}^r \cdots \tau_{\tilde{b}_k}^r w_0 / \mathbf{1}\tau_{\tilde{b}_1}^r \cdots \tau_{\tilde{b}_k}^r w_0$. Then it holds that $C = (w_{\tilde{b}_1}^r \cdots w_{\tilde{b}_\kappa}^r)$ is a characterizer for an OOM equivalent to $\mathcal{A}$. C can effectively be transformed into a characterizer C^r for $\mathcal{A}$ by $C^r = \varrho^r C$, where

$$\varrho^r = (C \begin{pmatrix} \mathbf{1}\tau_{\tilde{b}_1} \\ \vdots \\ \mathbf{1}\tau_{\tilde{b}_\kappa} \end{pmatrix})^{-1}. \tag{9}$$

We call C^r the *reverse characterizer* of $\mathcal{A}$, because it is composed from the states of a reverse OOM to $\mathcal{A}$. The analytical solution to (6) turns out to be [2]

$$C_{\text{opt}} = C^r. \tag{10}$$

To summarize, within a similarity class of characterizers, the one which minimizes model variance is the (unique) reverse characterizer in this class. It can be cheaply computed from the "forward" OOM via (8) and (9). This analytical finding suggests the following generic, iterative procedure to obtain characterizers that minimize model variance:

1. **Setup.** Choose a model dimension m and a characterizer length k. Compute $\underline{V}, \underline{W}_a$ from the training string S.

2. **Initialization.** Estimate an initial model $\hat{\mathcal{A}}^{(0)}$ with some "classical" OOM estimation method (a refined such method is detailed out in [2]).

3. **Efficiency sharpening iteration.** Assume that $\hat{\mathcal{A}}^{(n)}$ is given. Compute its reverse characterizer $\hat{C}^{r(n+1)}$. Use this in (5) to obtain a new model estimate $\hat{\mathcal{A}}^{(n+1)}$.

4. **Termination**. Terminate when the training log-likelihood of models $\hat{\mathcal{A}}^{(n)}$ appear to settle on a plateau.

The rationale behind this scheme is that the initial model $\hat{\mathcal{A}}^{(0)}$ is obtained essentially from an uninformed, ad hoc characterizer, for which one has to expect a large model variation and thus (on the average) a poor $\hat{\mathcal{A}}^{(0)}$. However, the characterizer $\hat{C}^{r(1)}$ obtained from the reversed $\hat{\mathcal{A}}^{(0)}$ is not uninformed any longer but shaped by a reasonable reverse model. Thus the estimator producing $\hat{\mathcal{A}}^{(1)}$ can be expected to produce a model closer to the correct one due to its improved efficiency, etc. Notice that this does not guarantee a convergence of models, nor any monotonic development of any performance parameter in the obtained model sequence. In fact, the training log likelihood of the model sequence typically shoots to a plateau level in about 2 to 5 iterations, after which it starts to jitter about this level, only slowly coming to rest – or even not stabilizing at all; it is sometimes observed that the log likelihood enters a small-amplitude oscillation around the plateau level. An analytical understanding of the asymptotic learning dynamics cannot currently be offered.

We have developed two specific instantiations of the general ES learning scheme, differentiated by the set of indicative sequences used. The first simply uses $l = \kappa, \bar{a}_1, \ldots, \bar{a}_l = \bar{b}_1, \ldots, \bar{b}_\kappa$, which leads to a computationally very cheap iterated recomputation of (5) with updated reverse characterizers. We call this the "poor man's" ES algorithm.

The statistical efficiency of the poor man's ES algorithm is impaired by the fact that only the counting statistics of subsequences of length $2k$ are exploited. The other ES instantiation exploits the statistics of *all* subsequences in the original training string. It is technically rather involved and rests on a suffix tree (ST) representation of S. We can only give a coarse sketch here (details in [2]). In each iteration, the current reverse model is run backwards through S and the obtained reverse states are additively collected bottom-up in the nodes of the ST. From the ST nodes the collected states are then harvested into matrices corresponding directly to $C\hat{\underline{V}}$ and $C\hat{\underline{W}}_a$, that is, an explicit computation of the reverse characterizer is not required. This method incurs a computational load per iteration which is somewhat lower than Baum-Welch for SE-HMMs (because only a backward pass of the current model has to be computed), plus the required initial ST construction which is linear in the size of S.

4   The CLG Algorithm

We must be very brief here due to space limitations. The CLG algorithm will be detailed out in a future paper. It is an iterative update scheme for the matrix parameters $[\hat{\tau}_a]_{ij}$ of a MOOM. This scheme is analytically derived as gradient descent in the model log likelihood surface over the log space of these matrix parameters, observing constraints of non-negativity of these parameters and the general OOM constraints (i) and (ii) from Eqn. (2). Note that the constraint (iii) from (2) is automatically satisfied in MOOMs.

We skip the derivation of the CLG scheme and describe only its "mechanics". Let $S = s_1 \ldots s_N$ be the training string and for $1 \leq k \leq N$ define $\bar{a}_k = s_1 \ldots s_k, \bar{b}_k = s_{k+1} \ldots s_N$. Define for some m-dimensional OOM and $a \in O$

$$
\sigma_k = \frac{1 \tau_{\bar{b}_k}}{1 \tau_{\bar{b}_k} w_{\bar{a}_k}}, \quad y_a = \sum_{s_k = a} \frac{\sigma'_k w'_{\bar{a}_{k-1}}}{1 \tau_{s_k} w_{\bar{a}_{k-1}}}, \quad y_0 = \max_{i,j,a}\{[y_a]_{ij}\}, \quad [y_{a0}]_{i,j} = [y_a]_{i,j}/y_0.
$$

$$\tag{11}$$

Then the update equation is

$$
[\hat{\tau}_a^+]_{ij} = \eta_j \cdot [\hat{\tau}_a]_{ij} \cdot [y_{a0}]_{ij}^\lambda,
\tag{12}
$$

where $\hat{\tau}_a^+$ is the new estimate of τ_a, η_j's are normalization parameters determined by the constraint (ii) from Eqn. (2), and λ is a learning rate which here unconventionally appears in the exponent because the gradient descent is carried out in the log parameter space. Note that by (12) $[\hat{\tau}_a^+]_{ij}$ remains non-negative if $[\hat{\tau}_a]_{ij}$ is. This update scheme is derived in a way that is unrelated to the derivation of the EM algorithm; to our surprise we found that for $\lambda = 1$ (12) is equivalent to the Baum-Welch algorithm for TE-HMMs. However, significantly faster convergence is achieved with non-unit λ; in the experiments carried out so far a value close to 2 was heuristically found to work best.

5   Numerical Comparisons

We compared the poor man's ES algorithm, the suffix-tree based algorithm, the CLG algorithm and the standard SE-HMM/Baum-Welch method on four different types of data, which were generated by (a) randomly constructed, 10-dimensional, 5-symbol SE-HMMs, (b) randomly constructed, 10-dimensional, 5-symbol MOOMs, (c) a 3-dimensional, 2-symbol OOM which is not equivalent to any HMM nor MOOM (the "probability clock" process [2]), (d) a belletristic text (Mark Twain's short story "The 1,000,000 Pound Note"). For each of (a) and (b), 40 experiments were carried out with freshly constructed generators per experiment; a training string of length 1000 and a test string of length 10000 was produced from each generator. For (c), likewise 40 experiments were carried out with freshly generated training/testing sequences of same lengthes as before; here however the generator was identical for all experiments. For (a) – (c), the results reported below are averaged numbers over the 40 experiments. For the (d) dataset, after preprocessing which shrunk the number of different symbols to 27, the original string was sorted sentence-wise into a training and a testing string, each of length ~ 21000 (details in [2]).

The following settings were used with the various training methods. (i) The poor man's ES algorithm was used with a length $k = 2$ of indicative sequences on all datasets. Two ES iterations were carried out and the model of the last iteration was used to compute the reported log likelihoods. (ii) For the suffix-tree based ES algorithm, on datasets (a) – (c), likewise two ES iterations were done and the model from the iteration with the lowest (reverse) training LL was used for reporting. On dataset (d), 4 ES iterations were called and similarly the model with the best reverse training LL was chosen. (iii) In the MOOM studies, a learning rate of $\lambda = 1.85$ was used. Iterations were stopped when two consecutive training LL's differed by less than 5e-5% or after 100 iterations. (iv) For HMM/Baum-Welch training, the public-domain implementation provided by Kevin Murphy was used. Iterations were stopped after 100 steps or if LL's differed by less than 1e-5%. All computations were done in Matlab on 2 GHz PCs except the HMM training on dataset (d) which was done on a 330 MHz machine (the reported CPU times were scaled by 330/2000 to make them comparable with the other studies). Figure 1 shows the training and testing loglikelihoods as well as the CPU times for all methods and datasets.

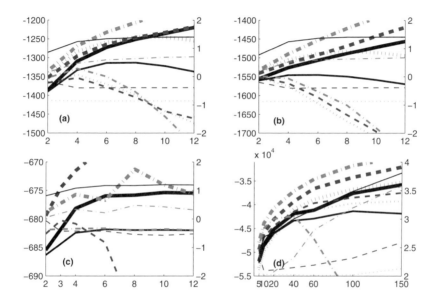

Figure 1: Findings for datasets (a)–(d). In each panel, the left y-axis shows log likelihoods for training and testing (testing LL normalized to training stringlength) and the right y-axis measures the log 10 of CPU times. HMM models are documented in solid/black lines, poor man's ES models in dotted/magenta lines, suffix-tree ES models in broken/blue, and MOOMs in dash-dotted/red lines. The thickest lines in each panel show training LL, the thinnest CPU time, and intermediate testing LL. The x-axes indicate model dimension. On dataset (c), no results of the poor man's algorithm are given because the learning equations became ill-conditioned for all but the lowest dimensions.

Some comments on Fig. 1. (1) The CPU times roughly exhibit an even log spread over almost 2 orders of magnitude, in the order poor man's (fastest) – suffix-tree ES – CLG – Baum-Welch. (2) CLG has the lowest training LL throughout, which needs an explanation because the proper OOMs trained by ES are more expressive. Apparently the ES algorithm does not lead to local ML optima; otherwise suffix-tree ES models should show the lowest training LL. (3) On HMM-generated data (a), Baum-Welch HMMs can play out their natural bias for this sort of data and achieve a lower test error than the other methods. (4) On the MOOM data (b), the test LL of MOOM/CLG and OOM/poor man models of dimension 2 equals the best HMM/Baum-Welch test LL which is attained at a dimension of 4; the OOM/suffix-tree test LL at dimension 2 is superior to the best HMM test LL. (5) On the "probability clock" data (c), the suffix-tree ES trained OOMs surpassed the non-OOM models in test LL, with the optimal value obtained at the (correct) model dimension 3. This comes as no surprise because these data come from a generator that is incommensurable with either HMMs or MOOMs. (6) On the large empirical dataset (d) the CLG/MOOMs have by a fair margin the highest training LL, but the test LL quickly drops to unacceptable lows. It is hard to explain this by overfitting, considering the complexity and the size of the training string. The other three types of models are evenly ordered in both training and testing error from HMMs (poorest) to suffix-tree ES trained OOMs. Overfitting does not occur up to the maximal dimension investigated. Depending on whether one wants a very fast algorithm with good, or a fast algorithm with very good train/test LL, one here would choose the poor man's or the suffix-tree ES algorithm as the winner. (7) One detail in panel (d) needs an explanation. The CPU time for the suffix-tree ES has an isolated peak for the smallest dimension. This is earned by the construction of the suffix tree, which was built only for the smallest dimension and re-used later.

6   Conclusion

We presented, in a sadly condensed fashion, three novel learning algorithms for symbol dynamics. A detailed treatment of the Efficiency Sharpening algorithm is given in [2], and a Matlab toolbox for it can be fetched from http://www.faculty.iu-bremen.de/hjaeger/OOM/OOMTool.zip. The numerical investigations reported here were done using this toolbox. Our numerical simulations demonstrate that there is an altogether new world of faster and often statistically more efficient algorithms for sequence modelling than Baum-Welch/SE-HMMs. The topics that we will address next in our research group are (i) a mathematical analysis of the asymptotic behaviour of the ES algorithms, (ii) online adaptive versions of these algorithms, and (iii) versions of the ES algorithms for nonstationary time series.

References

[1] M. L. Littman, R. S. Sutton, and S. Singh. Predictive representation of state. In *Advances in Neural Information Processing Systems 14 (Proc. NIPS 01)*, pages 1555–1561, 2001. http://www.eecs.umich.edu/~baveja/Papers/psr.pdf.

[2] H. Jaeger, M. Zhao, K. Kretzschmar, T. Oberstein, D. Popovici, and A. Kolling. Learning observable operator models via the es algorithm. In S. Haykin, J. Principe, T. Sejnowski, and J. McWhirter, editors, *New Directions in Statistical Signal Processing: from Systems to Brains*, chapter 20. MIT Press, to appear in 2005.

[3] H. Xue and V. Govindaraju. Stochastic models combining discrete symbols and continuous attributes in handwriting recognition. In *Proc. DAS 2002*, 2002.

[4] R. Edwards, J.J. McDonald, and M.J. Tsatsomeros. On matrices with common invariant cones with applications in neural and gene networks. *Linear Algebra and its Applications*, in press, 2004 (online version). http://www.math.wsu.edu/math/faculty/tsat/files/emt.pdf.

[5] K. Kretzschmar. Learning symbol sequences with Observable Operator Models. GMD Report 161, Fraunhofer Institute AIS, 2003. http://omk.sourceforge.net/files/OomLearn.pdf.

Representing Part-Whole Relationships in Recurrent Neural Networks

Viren Jain[2], Valentin Zhigulin[1,2], and H. Sebastian Seung[1,2]
[1]Howard Hughes Medical Institute and
[2]Brain & Cog. Sci. Dept., MIT
viren@mit.edu, valentin@mit.edu, seung@mit.edu

Abstract

There is little consensus about the computational function of top-down synaptic connections in the visual system. Here we explore the hypothesis that top-down connections, like bottom-up connections, reflect part-whole relationships. We analyze a recurrent network with bidirectional synaptic interactions between a layer of neurons representing parts and a layer of neurons representing wholes. Within each layer, there is lateral inhibition. When the network detects a whole, it can rigorously enforce part-whole relationships by ignoring parts that do not belong. The network can complete the whole by filling in missing parts. The network can refuse to recognize a whole, if the activated parts do not conform to a stored part-whole relationship. Parameter regimes in which these behaviors happen are identified using the theory of permitted and forbidden sets [3, 4]. The network behaviors are illustrated by recreating Rumelhart and McClelland's "interactive activation" model [7].

In neural network models of visual object recognition [2, 6, 8], patterns of synaptic connectivity often reflect part-whole relationships between the features that are represented by neurons. For example, the connections of Figure 1 reflect the fact that feature B both contains simpler features A1, A2, and A3, and is contained in more complex features C1, C2, and C3. Such connectivity allows neurons to follow the rule that existence of the part is evidence for existence of the whole. By combining synaptic input from multiple sources of evidence for a feature, a neuron can "decide" whether that feature is present. [1]

The synapses shown in Figure 1 are purely bottom-up, directed from simple to complex features. However, there are also top-down connections in the visual system, and there is little consensus about their function. One possibility is that top-down connections also reflect part-whole relationships. They allow feature detectors to make decisions using the rule that existence of the whole is evidence for existence of its parts.

In this paper, we analyze the dynamics of a recurrent network in which part-whole relationships are stored as bidirectional synaptic interactions, rather than the unidirectional interactions of Figure 1. The network has a number of interesting computational capabilities. When the network detects a whole, it can rigorously enforce part-whole relationships

---

[1]Synaptic connectivity may reflect other relationships besides part-whole. For example, invariances can be implemented by connecting detectors of several instances of the same feature to the same target, which is consequently an invariant detector of the feature.

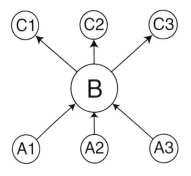

Figure 1: The synaptic connections (arrows) of neuron B represent part-whole relationships. Feature B both contains simpler features and is contained in more complex features. The synaptic interactions are drawn one-way, as in most models of visual object recognition. Existence of the part is regarded as evidence for existence of the whole. This paper makes the interactions bidirectional, allowing the existence of the whole to be evidence for the existence of its parts.

by ignoring parts that do not belong. The network can complete the whole by filling in missing parts. The network can refuse to recognize a whole, if the activated parts do not conform to a stored part-whole relationship. Parameter regimes in which these behaviors happen are identified using the recently developed theory of permitted and forbidden sets [3, 4].

Our model is closely related to the interactive activation model of word recognition, which was proposed by McClelland and Rumelhart to explain the word superiority effect studied by visual psychologists [7]. Here our concern is not to model a psychological effect, but to characterize mathematically how computations involving part-whole relationships can be carried out by a recurrent network.

1 Network model

Suppose that we are given a set of part-whole relationships specified by

$$
\xi_i^a = \begin{cases} 1, & \text{if part } i \text{ is contained in whole } a \\ 0, & \text{otherwise} \end{cases}
$$

We assume that every whole contains at least one part, and every part is contained in at least one whole.

The stimulus drives a layer of neurons that detect parts. These neurons also interact with a layer of neurons that detect wholes. We will refer to part-detectors as "P-neurons" and whole-detectors as "W-neurons."

The part-whole relationships are directly stored in the synaptic connections between P and W neurons. If $\xi_i^a = 1$, the ith neuron in the P layer and the ath neuron in the W layer have an excitatory interaction of strength γ. If $\xi_i^a = 0$, the neurons have an inhibitory interaction of strength σ. Furthermore, the P-neurons inhibit each other with strength β, and the W-neurons inhibit each other with strength α. All of these interactions are symmetric, and all activation functions are the rectification nonlinearity $[z]^+ = \max\{z, 0\}$.

Then the dynamics of the network takes the form

$$
\dot{W}_a + W_a = \left[\gamma \sum_i P_i \xi_i^a - \sigma \sum_i (1 - \xi_i^a) P_i - \alpha \sum_{b \neq a} W_b \right]^+ , \tag{1}
$$

$$
\dot{P}_i + P_i = \left[\gamma \sum_a W_a \xi_i^a - \sigma \sum_a (1 - \xi_i^a) W_a - \beta \sum_{j \neq i} P_j + B_i \right]^+ . \tag{2}
$$

where B_i is the input to the P layer from the stimulus. Figure 2 shows an example of a network with two wholes. Each whole contains two parts. One of the parts is contained in both wholes.

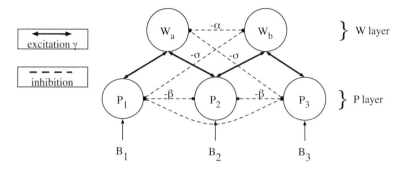

Figure 2: Model in example configuration: $\xi = \{(1, 1, 0), (0, 1, 1)\}$.

When a stimulus is presented, it activates some of the P-neurons, which activate some of the W-neurons. The network eventually converges to a stable steady state. We will assume that $\alpha > 1$. In the Appendix, we prove that this leads to unconditional winner-take-all behavior in the W layer. In other words, no more than one W-neuron can be active at a stable steady state.

If a single W-neuron is active, then a whole has been detected. Potentially there are also many P-neurons active, indicating detection of parts. This representation may have different properties, depending on the choice of parameters β, γ, and σ. As discussed below, these include rigorous enforcement of part-whole relationships, completion of wholes by "filling in" missing parts, and non-recognition of parts that do not conform to a whole.

2 Enforcement of part-whole relationships

Suppose that a single W-neuron is active at a stable steady state, so that a whole has been detected. Part-whole relationships are said to be enforced if the network always ignores parts that are not contained in the detected whole, despite potentially strong bottom-up evidence for them. It can be shown that enforcement follows from the inequality

$$\sigma^2 + \beta^2 + \gamma^2 + 2\sigma\beta\gamma > 1. \tag{3}$$

which guarantees that neuron i in the P layer is inactive, if neuron a in the W layer is active and $\xi_i^a = 0$. When part-whole relations are enforced, prior knowledge about legal combinations of parts strictly constrains what may be perceived. This result is proven in the Appendix, and only an intuitive explanation is given here.

Enforcement is easiest to understand when there is interlayer inhibition ($\sigma > 0$). In this case, the active W-neuron directly inhibits the forbidden P-neurons. The case of $\sigma = 0$ is more subtle. Then enforcement is mediated by lateral inhibition in the P layer. Excitatory feedback from the W-neuron has the effect of counteracting the lateral inhibition between the P-neurons that belong to the whole. As a result, these P-neurons become strongly activated enough to inhibit the rest of the P layer.

3 Completion of wholes by filling in missing parts

If a W-neuron is active, it excites the P-neurons that belong to the whole. As a result, even if one of these P-neurons receives no bottom-up input ($B_i = 0$), it is still active. We call this phenomenon "completion," and it is guaranteed to happen when

$$\gamma > \sqrt{\beta} \tag{4}$$

The network may thus "imagine" parts that are consistent with the recognized whole, but are not actually present in the stimulus. As with enforcement, this condition depends on top-down connections.

In the special case $\gamma = \sqrt{\beta}$, the interlayer excitation between a W-neuron and its P-neurons exactly cancels out the lateral inhibition between the P-neurons at a steady state. So the recurrent connections effectively vanish, letting the activity of the P-neurons be determined by their feedforward inputs. When the interlayer excitation is stronger than this, the inequality (4) holds, and completion occurs.

4 Non-recognition of a whole

If there is no interlayer inhibition ($\sigma = 0$), then a single W-neuron is always active, assuming that there is some activity in the P layer. To see this, suppose for the sake of contradiction that all the W-neurons are inactive. Then they receive no inhibition to counteract the excitation from the P layer. This means some of them must be active, which contradicts our assumption. This means that the network always recognizes a whole, even if the stimulus is very different from any part-whole combination that is stored in the network.

However, if interlayer inhibition is sufficiently strong (large σ), the network may refuse to recognize a whole. Neurons in the P layer are activated, but there is no activity in the W layer. Formal conditions on σ can be derived, but are not given here because of space limitations.

In case of non-recognition, constraints on the P-layer are not enforced. It is possible for the network to detect a configuration of parts that is not consistent with any stored whole.

5 Example: Interactive Activation model

To illustrate the computational capabilities of our network, we use it to recreate the interactive activation (IA) model of McClelland and Rumelhart. Figure 3 shows numerical simulations of a network containing three layers of neurons representing strokes, letters, and words, respectively. There are 16 possible strokes in each of four letter positions. For each stroke, there are two neurons, one signaling the presence of the stroke and the other signaling its absence. Letter neurons represent each letter of the alphabet in each of four positions. Word neurons represent each of 1200 common four letter words.

The letter and word layers correspond to the P and W layers that were introduced previously. There are bidirectional interactions between the letter and word layers, and lateral inhibition within the layers. The letter neurons also receive input from the stroke neurons, but this interaction is unidirectional.

Our network differs in two ways from the original IA model. First, all interactions involving letter and word neurons are symmetric. In the original model, the interactions between the letter and word layers were asymmetric. In particular, inhibitory connections only ran from letter neurons to word neurons, and not vice versa. Second, the only nonlinearity in our model is rectification. These two aspects allow us to apply the full machinery of the theory of permitted and forbidden sets.

Figure 3 shows the result of presenting the stimulus "MO M" for four different settings of parameters. In each of the four cases, the word layer of the network converges to the same result, detecting the word "MOON", which is the closest stored word to the stimulus. However, the activity in the letter layer is different in the four cases.

566

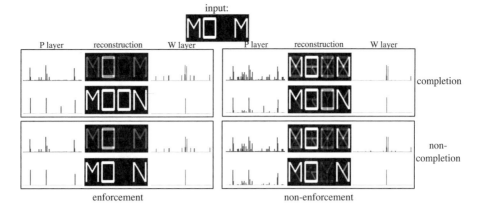

Figure 3: Simulation of 4 different parameter regimes in a letter-word recognition network. Within each panel, the middle column presents a feature-layer reconstruction based on the letter activity shown in the left column. W layer activity is shown in the right column. The top row shows the network state after 10 iterations of the dynamics. The bottom row shows the steady state.

In the left column, the parameters obey the inequality (3), so that part-whole relationships are enforced. The activity of the letter layer is visualized by activating the strokes corresponding to each active letter neuron. The activated letters are part of the word "MOON". In the top left, the inequality (4) is satisfied, so that the missing "O" in the stimulus is filled in. In the bottom left, completion does not occur.

In the simulations of the right column, parameters are such that part-whole relationships are not enforced. Consequently, the word layer is much more active. Bottom-up input provides evidence for several other letters, which is not suppressed. In the top right, the inequality (4) is satisfied, so that the missing "O" in the stimulus is filled in. In the bottom right, the "O" neuron is not activated in the third position, so there is no completion. However, some letter neurons for the third position are activated, due to the input from neurons that indicate the absence of strokes.

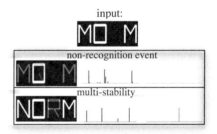

Figure 4: Simulation of a non-recognition event and example of multistability.

Figure 4 shows simulations for large σ, deep in the enforcement regime where non-recognition is a possibility. From one initial condition, the network converges to a state in which no W neurons are active, a non-recognition. From another initial condition, the network detects the word "NORM". Deep in the enforcement regime, the top-down feedback can be so strong that the network has multiple stable states, many of which bear little resemblance to the stimulus at all. This is a problematic aspect of this network. It can be prevented by setting parameters at the edge of the enforcement regime.

6 Discussion

We have analyzed a recurrent network that performs computations involving part-whole relationships. The network can fill in missing parts and suppress parts that do not belong.

These two computations are distinct and can be dissociated from each other, as shown in Figure 3.

While these two computations can also be performed by associative memory models, they are not typically dissociable in these models. For example, in the Hopfield model pattern completion and noise suppression are both the result of recall of one of a finite number of stereotyped activity patterns.

We believe that our model is more appropriate for perceptual systems, because its behavior is piecewise linear, due its reliance on rectification nonlinearity. Therefore, analog aspects of computation are able to coexist with the part-whole relationships. Furthermore, in our model the stimulus is encoded in maintained synaptic input to the network, rather than as an initial condition of the dynamics.

A   Appendix: Permitted and forbidden sets

Our mathematical results depend on the theory of permitted and forbidden sets [3, 4], which is summarized briefly here. The theory is applicable to neural networks with rectification nonlinearity, of the form $\dot{x}_i + x_i = [b_i + \sum_j W_{ij} x_j]^+$. Neuron i is said to be active when $x_i > 0$. For a network of N neurons, there are 2^N possible sets of active neurons. For each active set, consider the submatrix of W_{ij} corresponding to the synapses between active neurons. If all eigenvalues of this submatrix have real parts less than or equal to unity, then the active set is said to be *permitted*. Otherwise the active set is said to be *forbidden*. A set is permitted if and only if there exists an input vector b such that those neurons are active at a stable steady state. Permitted sets can be regarded as memories stored in the synaptic connections W_{ij}. If W_{ij} is a symmetric matrix, the *nesting property* holds: every subset of a permitted set is permitted, and every superset of a forbidden set is forbidden.

The present model can be seen as a general method for storing permitted sets in a recurrent network. This method introduces a neuron for each permitted set, relying on a unary or "grandmother cell" representation. In contrast, Xie et al.[9] used lateral inhibition in a single layer of neurons to store permitted sets. By introducing extra neurons, the present model achieves superior storage capacity, much as unary models of associative memory [1] surpass distributed models [5].

A.1   Unconditional winner-take-all in the W layer

The synapses between two W-neurons have strengths

$$\begin{pmatrix} 0 & -\alpha \\ -\alpha & 0 \end{pmatrix}$$

The eigenvalues of this matrix are $\pm \alpha$. Therefore two W-neurons constitute a forbidden set if $\alpha > 1$. By the nesting property, it follows more than two W-neurons is also a forbidden set, and that the W layer has the unconditional winner-take-all property.

A.2   Part-whole combinations as permitted sets

Theorem 1. *Suppose that $\beta < 1$. If $\gamma^2 < \beta + (1 - \beta)/k$ then any combination of $k \geq 1$ parts consistent with a whole corresponds to a permitted set.*

Proof. Consider k parts belonging to a whole. They are represented by one W-neuron and k P-neurons, with synaptic connections given by the $(k + 1) \times (k + 1)$ matrix

$$M = \begin{pmatrix} -\beta(\mathbf{1}\mathbf{1}^T - I) & \gamma\mathbf{1} \\ \gamma\mathbf{1}^T & 0 \end{pmatrix}, \tag{5}$$

where $\mathbf{1}$ is the k-dimensional vector whose elements are all equal to one. Two eigenvectors of M are of the form $(\mathbf{1}^T c)$, and have the same eigenvalues as the 2×2 matrix

$$\begin{pmatrix} -\beta(k-1) & \gamma \\ \gamma k & 0 \end{pmatrix}$$

This matrix has eigenvalues less than one when $\gamma^2 < \beta + (1 - \beta)/k$ and $\beta(k-1) + 2 > 0$. The other $k - 1$ eigenvectors are of the form $(d^T, 0)$, where $d^T \mathbf{1} = 0$. These have eigenvalues β. Therefore all eigenvalues of W are less than one if the condition of the theorem is satisfied. $\square$

A.3 Constraints on combining parts

Here, we derive conditions under which the network can enforce the constraint that steady state activity be confined to parts that constitute a whole.

Theorem 2. *Suppose that $\beta > 0$ and $\sigma^2 + \beta^2 + \gamma^2 + 2\sigma\beta\gamma > 1$ If a W-neuron is active, then only P-neurons corresponding to parts contained in the relevant whole can be active at a stable steady state.*

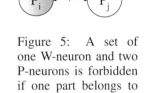

Figure 5: A set of one W-neuron and two P-neurons is forbidden if one part belongs to the whole and the other does not.

Proof. Consider P-neurons P_i, P_j, and W-neuron W_a. Suppose that $\xi_i^a = 1$ but $\xi_j^a = 0$. As shown in Figure 5, the matrix of connections is given by:

$$W = \begin{pmatrix} 0 & -\beta & \gamma \\ -\beta & 0 & -\sigma \\ \gamma & -\sigma & 0 \end{pmatrix} \tag{6}$$

This set is permitted if all eigenvalues of $W - I$ have negative real parts. The characteristic equation of $I - W$ is $\lambda^3 + b_1\lambda^2 + b_2\lambda + b_3 = 0$, where $b_1 = 3$, $b_2 = 3 - \sigma^2 - \beta^2 - \gamma^2$ and $b_3 = 1 - 2\sigma\beta\gamma - \sigma^2 - \beta^2 - \gamma^2$. According to the Routh-Hurwitz theorem, all the eigenvalues have negative real parts if and only if $b_1 > 0$, $b_3 > 0$ and $b_1 b_2 > b_3$. Clearly, the first condition is always satisfied. The second condition is more restrictive than the third. It is satisfied only when $\sigma^2 + \beta^2 + \gamma^2 + 2\sigma\beta\gamma < 1$. Hence, one of the eigenvalues has a positive real part when this condition is broken, i.e., when $\sigma^2 + \beta^2 + \gamma^2 + 2\sigma\beta\gamma > 1$. By the nesting property, any larger set of P-neurons inconsistent with the W-neuron is also forbidden. $\square$

A.4 Completion of wholes

Theorem 3. *If $\gamma > \sqrt{\beta}$ and a single W-neuron a is active at a steady state, then $P_i > 0$ for all i such that $\xi_i^a = 1$.*

Proof. Suppose that the detected whole has k parts. At the steady state

$$P_i = \frac{\xi_i^a}{1 - \beta} \left[B_i - (\beta - \gamma^2) P_{tot} \right]^+$$

where

$$P_{tot} = \sum_i P_i = \frac{1}{1 - \beta + (\beta - \gamma^2)k} \sum_{i=1}^{k} B_i \xi_i^a \tag{7}$$

$\square$

A.5 Preventing runaway

If feedback loops cause the network activity to diverge, then the preceding analyses are not relevant. Here we give a sufficient condition guaranteeing that runaway instability does not happen. It is not a necessary condition. Interestingly, the condition implies the condition of Theorem 1.

Theorem 4. *Suppose that P and W obey the dynamics of Eqs. (1) and (2), and define the objective function*

$$
\begin{aligned}
E &= \frac{1-\alpha}{2} \sum_a W_a^2 + \frac{\alpha}{2} \left(\sum_a W_a \right)^2 + \frac{1-\beta}{2} \sum_i P_i^2 + \frac{\beta}{2} \left(\sum_i P_i \right)^2 \\
&\quad - \sum_i B_i P_i - \gamma \sum_{ia} P_i W_a \xi_i^a + \sigma \sum_{ia} (1 - \xi_i^a) P_i W_a.
\end{aligned}
\tag{8}
$$

Then E is a Lyapunov like function that, given $\beta > \gamma^2 - \frac{1-\gamma^2}{N-1}$, ensures convergence of the dynamics to a stable steady state.

Proof. (sketch) Differentiation of E with respect to time shows that that E is nonincreasing in the nonnegative orthant and constant only at steady states of the network dynamics. We must also show that E is radially unbounded, which is true if the quadratic part of E is copositive definite. Note that the last term of E is lower-bounded by zero and the previous term is upper bounded by $\gamma \sum_{ia} P_i W_a$. We assume $\alpha > 1$. Thus, we can use Cauchy's inequality, $\sum_i P_i^2 \geq \left(\sum_i P_i \right)^2 / N$, and the fact that $\sum_a W_a^2 \leq \left(\sum_a W_a \right)^2$ for $W_a \geq 0$, to derive

$$
E \geq \frac{1}{2} \left(\left(\sum_a W_a \right)^2 + \frac{1-\beta+\beta N}{N} \left(\sum_i P_i \right)^2 - 2\gamma \left(\sum_a W_a \sum_i P_i \right) \right) - \sum_i B_i P_i.
\tag{9}
$$

If $\beta > \gamma^2 - \frac{1-\gamma^2}{N-1}$, the quadratic form in the inequality is positive definite and E is radially unbounded. □

References

[1] E. B. Baum, J. Moody, and F. Wilczek. Internal representations for associative memory. *Biol. Cybern.*, 59:217–228, 1988.

[2] K. Fukushima. Neocognitron: a self organizing neural network model for a mechanism of pattern recognition unaffected by shift in position. *Biol Cybern*, 36(4):193–202, 1980.

[3] R.H. Hahnloser, R. Sarpeshkar, M.A. Mahowald, R.J. Douglas, and H.S. Seung. Digital selection and analogue amplification coexist in a cortex-inspired silicon circuit. *Nature*, 405(6789):947–51, Jun 22 2000.

[4] R.H. Hahnloser, H.S. Seung, and J.-J. Slotine. Permitted and forbidden sets in symmetric threshold-linear networks. *Neural Computation*, 15:621–638, 2003.

[5] J.J. Hopfield. Neural networks and physical systems with emergent collective computational abilities. *Proc Natl Acad Sci U S A*, 79(8):2554–8, Apr 1982.

[6] Y. LeCun, B. Boser, J. S. Denker, D. Henderson, R. E. Howard, W. Hubbard, and L. D. Jackel. Backpropagation applied to handwritten zip code recognition. *Neural Comput.*, 1:541–551, 1989.

[7] J. L. McClelland and D. E. Rumelhart. An interactive activation model of context effects in letter perception: Part i. an account of basic findings. *Psychological Review*, 88(5):375–407, Sep 1981.

[8] M Riesenhuber and T Poggio. Hierarchical models of object recognition in cortex. *Nat Neurosci*, 2(11):1019–25, Nov 1999.

[9] X. Xie, R.H. Hahnloser, and H. S. Seung. Selectively grouping neurons in recurrent networks of lateral inhibition. *Neural Computation*, 14:2627–2646, 2002.

A Probabilistic Approach for Optimizing Spectral Clustering

Rong Jin[*], **Chris Ding**[†], **Feng Kang**[*]
[*]Lawrence Berkeley National Laboratory, Berkeley, CA 94720
[†]Michigan State University, East Lansing , MI 48824

Abstract

Spectral clustering enjoys its success in both data clustering and semi-supervised learning. But, most spectral clustering algorithms cannot handle multi-class clustering problems directly. Additional strategies are needed to extend spectral clustering algorithms to multi-class clustering problems. Furthermore, most spectral clustering algorithms employ hard cluster membership, which is likely to be trapped by the local optimum. In this paper, we present a new spectral clustering algorithm, named "Soft Cut". It improves the normalized cut algorithm by introducing soft membership, and can be efficiently computed using a bound optimization algorithm. Our experiments with a variety of datasets have shown the promising performance of the proposed clustering algorithm.

1 Introduction

Data clustering has been an active research area with a long history. Well-known clustering methods include the K-means methods (Hartigan & Wong., 1994), Gaussian Mixture Model (Redner & Walker, 1984), Probabilistic Latent Semantic Indexing (PLSI) (Hofmann, 1999), and Latent Dirichlet Allocation (LDA) (Blei et al., 2003). Recently, spectral clustering methods (Shi & Malik, 2000; Ng et al., 2001; Zha et al., 2002; Ding et al., 2001; Bach & Jordan, 2004)have attracted more and more attention given their promising performance in data clustering and simplicity in implementation. They treat the data clustering problem as a graph partitioning problem. In its simplest form, a minimum cut algorithm is used to minimize the weights (or similarities) assigned to the removed edges. To avoid unbalanced clustering results, different objectives have been proposed, including the ratio cut (Hagen & Kahng, 1991), normalized cut (Shi & Malik, 2000) and min-max cut (Ding et al., 2001).

To reduce the computational complexity, most spectral clustering algorithms use the relaxation approach, which maps discrete cluster memberships into continuous real numbers. As a result, it is difficult to directly apply current spectral clustering algorithms to multi-class clustering problems. Various strategies (Shi & Malik, 2000; Ng et al., 2001; Yu & Shi, 2003) have been used to extend spectral clustering algorithms to multi-class clustering problems. One common approach is to first construct a low-dimension space for data representation using the smallest eigenvectors of a graph Laplacian that is constructed based on the pair wise similarity of data. Then, a standard clustering algorithm, such as the K-means method, is applied to cluster data points in the low-dimension space.

One problem with the above approach is how to determine the appropriate number of eigen-vectors. A too small number of eigenvectors will lead to an insufficient representation of data, and meanwhile a too large number of eigenvectors will bring in a significant amount of noise to the data representation. Both cases will degrade the quality of clustering. Although it has been shown in (Ng et al., 2001) that the number of required eigenvectors is generally equal to the number of clusters, the analysis is valid only when data points of different clusters are well separated. As will be shown later, when data points are not well separated, the optimal number of eigenvectors can be different from the number of clusters.

Another problem with the existing spectral clustering algorithms is that they are based on binary cluster membership and therefore are unable to express the uncertainty in data clustering. Compared to hard cluster membership, probabilistic membership is advantageous in that it is less likely to be trapped by local minimums. One example is the Bayesian clustering method (Redner & Walker, 1984), which is usually more robust than the K-means method because of its soft cluster memberships. It is also advantageous to use probabilistic memberships when the cluster memberships are the intermediate results and will be used for other processes, for example selective sampling in active learning (Jin & Si, 2004).

In this paper, we present a new spectral clustering algorithm, named "Soft Cut", that explicitly addresses the above two problems. It extends the normalized cut algorithm by introducing probabilistic membership of data points. By encoding membership of multiple clusters into a set of probabilities, the proposed clustering algorithm can be applied directly to multi-class clustering problems. Our empirical studies with a variety of datasets have shown that the soft cut algorithm can substantially outperform the normalized cut algorithm for multi-class clustering.

The rest paper is arranged as follows. Section 2 presents the related work. Section 3 describes the soft cut algorithm. Section 4 discusses the experimental results. Section 5 concludes this study with the future work.

2 Related Work

The key idea of spectral clustering is to convert a clustering problem into a graph partitioning problem.

Let n be the number of data points to be clustered. Let $\mathbf{W} = [w_{i,j}]_{n \times n}$ be the weight matrix where each $w_{i,j}$ is the similarity between two data points. For the convenience of discussion, $w_{i,i} = 0$ for all data points. Then, a clustering problem can be formulated into the minimum cut problem, i.e.,

$$\mathbf{q}^* = \arg \min_{\mathbf{q} \in \{-1,1\}^n} \sum_{i,j=1}^{n} w_{i,j}(q_i - q_j)^2 = \mathbf{q}^T \mathbf{L} \mathbf{q} \qquad (1)$$

where $\mathbf{q} = (q_1, q_2, ..., q_n)$ is a vector for binary memberships and each q_i can be either -1 or 1. $\mathbf{L}$ is the Laplacian matrix. It is defined as $\mathbf{L} = \mathbf{D} - \mathbf{W}$, where $\mathbf{D} = [d_{i,i}]_{n \times n}$ is a diagonal matrix with each element $d_{i,i} = \delta_{i,j} \sum_{j=1}^{n} w_{i,j}$. Directly solving the problem in (1) requires combinatorial optimization, which is computationally expensive. Usually, a relaxation approach (Chung, 1997) is used to replace the vector $\mathbf{q} \in \{-1,1\}^n$ with a vector $\hat{\mathbf{q}} \in \mathbf{R}^n$ under the constraint $\sum_{i=1}^{n} \hat{q}_i^2 = n$. As a result of the relaxation, the approximate solution to (1) is the second smallest eigenvector of Laplacian L.

One problem with the minimum cut approach is that it does not take into account the size of clusters, which can lead to clusters of unbalanced sizes. To resolve this problem, several different criteria are proposed, including the ratio cut (Hagen & Kahng, 1991), normalized cut (Shi & Malik, 2000) and min-max cut (Ding et al., 2001). For example, in the normalized cut algorithm, the following objective is used:

$$J_n(\mathbf{q}) = \frac{C_{+,-}(\mathbf{q})}{D_+(\mathbf{q})} + \frac{C_{+,-}(\mathbf{q})}{D_-(\mathbf{q})} \tag{2}$$

where $C_{+,-}(\mathbf{q}) = \sum_{i,j=1}^{n} w_{i,j}\delta(q_i, +)\delta(q_j, -)$ and $D_{\pm} = \sum_{i=1}^{n}\delta(q_i, \pm)\sum_{j=1}^{n} w_{i,j}$. In the above objective, the size of clusters, i.e., $D_{\pm}$, is used as the denominators to avoid clusters of too small size. Similar to the minimum cut approach, a relaxation approach is used to convert the problem in (2) into a eigenvector problem. For multi-class clustering, we can extend the objective in (2) into the following form:

$$J_{norm\_mc}(\mathbf{q}) = \sum_{z=1}^{K}\sum_{z' \neq z} \frac{C_{z,z'}(\mathbf{q})}{D_z(\mathbf{q})} \tag{3}$$

where K is the number of clusters, vector $\mathbf{q} \in \{1, 2, ..., K\}^n$, $C_{z,z'} = \sum_{i,j=1}^{n}\delta(q_i, z)\delta(q_j, z')w_{i,j}$, and $D_z = \sum_{i=1}^{n}\sum_{j=1}^{n}\delta(q_i, z)w_{i,j}$. However, efficiently finding the solution that minimizes (3) is rather difficult. In particular, a simple relaxation method cannot be applied directly here. In the past, several heuristic approaches (Shi & Malik, 2000; Ng et al., 2001; Yu & Shi, 2003) have been proposed for finding approximate solutions to (3). One common strategy is to first obtain the K smallest (excluding the one with zero eigenvalue) eigenvectors of Laplacian $\mathbf{L}$, and project data points onto the low-dimension space that is spanned by the K eigenvectors. Then, a standard clustering algorithm, such as the K-means method, is applied to cluster data points in this low-dimension space. In contrast to these approaches, the proposed spectral clustering algorithm deals with the multi-class clustering problem directly. It estimates the probabilities for each data point be in different clusters simultaneously. Through the probabilistic cluster memberships, the proposed algorithm will be less likely to be trapped by local minimums, and therefore will be more robust than the existing spectral clustering algorithms.

3 Spectral Clustering with Soft Membership

In this section, we describe a new spectral clustering algorithm, named "**Soft Cut**", which extends the normalized cut algorithm by introducing probabilistic cluster membership. In the following, we will present a formal description of the soft cut algorithm, followed by the procedure that efficiently optimizes the related optimization problem.

3.1 Algorithm Description

First, notice that D_z in (3) can be expanded as $D_z = \sum_{j=1}^{K} C_{i,j}$. Thus, the objective function for multi-class clustering in (3) can be rewritten as:

$$J_{n\_mc}(\mathbf{q}) = \sum_{z=1}^{K}\sum_{z' \neq z} \frac{C_{z,z'}(\mathbf{q})}{D_z(\mathbf{q})} = K - \sum_{z=1}^{K} \frac{C_{z,z}(\mathbf{q})}{D_z(\mathbf{q})} \tag{4}$$

Let $J'_{n\_mc} = \sum_{z=1}^{K} \frac{C_{z,z}(\mathbf{q})}{D_z(\mathbf{q})}$. Thus, instead of minimizing J_{n_mc}, we can maximize J'_{n_mc}.

To extend the above objective function to a probabilistic framework, we introduce the probabilistic cluster membership. Let $q_{z,i}$ denote the probability for the i-th data point to be in the z-th cluster. Let matrix $\mathbf{Q} = [q_{z,i}]_{K \times n}$ include all probabilities $q_{z,i}$. Using the probabilistic notations, we can rewrite $C_{z,z'}$ and D_z as follows:

$$C_{z,z'}(\mathbf{Q}) = \sum_{i,j=1}^{n} q_{z,i}q_{z',j}w_{i,j}, \quad D_z(\mathbf{Q}) = \sum_{i,j=1}^{n} q_{z,i}w_{i,j} \tag{5}$$

Substituting the probabilistic expression for $C_{z,z'}$ and D_z into J'_{n_mc}, we have the following optimization problem for probabilistic spectral clustering:

$$\mathbf{Q}^* = \arg \min_{\mathbf{Q} \in \mathbb{R}^{K \times n}} J_{prob}(\mathbf{Q}) = \arg \max_{\mathbf{Q} \in \mathbb{R}^{K \times n}} \sum_{z=1}^{K} \frac{\sum_{i,j=1}^{n} q_{z,i} q_{z,j} w_{i,j}}{\sum_{i,j=1}^{n} q_{z,i} w_{i,j}}$$

$$\text{s.t.} \forall i \in [1..n], z \in [1..K] : q_{z,i} \geq 0, \sum_{z=1}^{K} q_{z,i} = 1 \qquad (6)$$

3.2 Optimization Procedure

In this subsection, we present a bound optimization algorithm (Salakhutdinov & Roweis, 2003) for efficiently finding the solution to (6). It maximizes the objective function in (6) iteratively. In each iteration, a concave lower bound is first constructed for the objective function based on the solution obtained from the previous iteration. Then, a new solution for the current iteration is obtained by maximizing the lower bound. The same procedure is repeated until the solution converges to a local maximum.

Let $\mathbf{Q}' = [q'_{i,j}]_{K \times n}$ be the probabilities obtained in the previous iteration, and $\mathbf{Q} = [q_{i,j}]_{K \times n}$ be the probabilities for current iteration. Define

$$\Delta(\mathbf{Q}, \mathbf{Q}') = \log \frac{J_{prob}(\mathbf{Q})}{J_{prob}(\mathbf{Q}')}$$

which is the logarithm of the ratio of the objective functions between two consecutive iterations. Using the convexity of logarithm function, i.e., $\log(\sum_i p_i q_i) \geq \sum_i p_i \log(q_i)$ for a pdf $\{p_i\}$, we have $\Delta(\mathbf{Q}, \mathbf{Q}')$ lower bound by the following expression:

$$\Delta(\mathbf{Q}, \mathbf{Q}') = \log \left(\sum_{z=1}^{K} \frac{C_{z,z}(\mathbf{Q})}{D_z(\mathbf{Q})} \right) - \log \left(\sum_{z=1}^{K} \frac{C_{z,z}(\mathbf{Q}')}{D_z(\mathbf{Q}')} \right)$$

$$\geq \sum_{z=1}^{K} t_z \left(\log \frac{C_{z,z}(\mathbf{Q})}{C_{z,z}(\mathbf{Q}')} - \log \frac{D_z(\mathbf{Q})}{D_z(\mathbf{Q}')} \right) \qquad (7)$$

where t_z is defined as:

$$t_z = \frac{\frac{C_{z,z}(\mathbf{Q}')}{D_z(\mathbf{Q}')}}{\sum_{z'=1}^{K} \frac{C_{z',z'}(\mathbf{Q}')}{D_{z'}(\mathbf{Q}')}} \qquad (8)$$

Now, the first term within the big bracket in (7), i.e., $\log \frac{C_{z,z}(\mathbf{Q})}{C_{z,z}(\mathbf{Q}')}$, can be further relaxed as:

$$\log \frac{C_{z,z}(\mathbf{Q})}{C_{z,z}(\mathbf{Q}')} = \log \left(\sum_{i,j=1}^{n} \frac{q'_{z,i} q'_{z,j} w_{i,j}}{C_{z,z}(\mathbf{Q}')} \frac{q_{z,i} q_{z,j}}{q'_{z,i} q'_{z,j}} \right)$$

$$\geq 2 \sum_{i=1}^{n} \left(\sum_{j=1}^{n} s_z^{i,j} \right) \log(q_{z,i}) - \sum_{i,j=1}^{n} s_z^{i,j} \log(q'_{z,i} q'_{z,j}) \qquad (9)$$

where $s_z^{i,j}$ is defined as:

$$s_z^{i,j} = \frac{q'_{z,i} q'_{z,j} w_{i,j}}{C_{z,z}(\mathbf{Q}')} \qquad (10)$$

Meanwhile, using the inequality $\log x \leq x - 1$, we have $\log \frac{D_z(\mathbf{Q})}{D_z(\mathbf{Q'})}$ upper bounded by the following expression:

$$\log \frac{D_z(\mathbf{Q})}{D_z(\mathbf{Q'})} \leq \frac{D_z(\mathbf{Q})}{D_z(\mathbf{Q'})} - 1 = \sum_{i=1}^{n} q_{z,i} \sum_{j=1}^{n} \frac{w_{i,j}}{D_z(\mathbf{Q'})} - 1 \tag{11}$$

Putting together (7), (9), and (11), we have a concave lower bound for the objective function in (6), i.e.,

$$\log J_{prob}(\mathbf{Q}) \geq$$

$$\log J_{prob}(\mathbf{Q'}) + \Delta_0(\mathbf{Q'}) + 2 \sum_{z=1}^{K} \sum_{i,j=1}^{n} t_z s_z^{i,j} \log q_{z,i} - \sum_{z=1}^{K} \sum_{i,j=1}^{n} \frac{q_{z,i} w_{i,j}}{D_z(\mathbf{Q'})} \tag{12}$$

where $\Delta_0(\mathbf{Q'})$ is defined as:

$$\Delta_0(\mathbf{Q'}) = - \sum_{z=1}^{K} t_z \sum_{i,j=1}^{n} s_z^{i,j} w_{i,j} \log(q'_{z,i} q'_{z,j}) + 1$$

The optimal solution that maximizes the lower bound in (12) can be computed by setting its derivative to zero, which leads to the following solution:

$$q_{z,i} = \frac{2 t_z \sum_{j=1}^{n} s_z^{i,j}}{t_z \sum_{j=1}^{n} \frac{w_{i,j}}{D_z(\mathbf{Q'})} + \lambda_i} \tag{13}$$

where λ_i is a Lagrangian multiplier that ensure $\sum_{z=1}^{K} q_{z,i} = 1$. It can be acquired by maximizing the following objective function:

$$l(\lambda_i) = -\lambda_i + 2 \sum_{z=1}^{K} \left(t_z \sum_{j=1}^{n} s_z^{i,j} \right) \log \left(t_z \sum_{j=1}^{n} \frac{w_{i,j}}{D_z(\mathbf{Q'})} + \lambda_i \right) \tag{14}$$

Since the above objective function is concave, we can apply a standard numerical procedure, such as the Newton's method, to efficiently find the value for λ_i.

4 Experiment

In this section, we focus on examining the effectiveness of the proposed soft cut algorithm for multi-class clustering. In particular, we will address the following two research questions:

1. *How effective is the proposed algorithm for data clustering?* We compare the proposed soft cut algorithm to the normalized cut algorithm with various numbers of eigenvectors.

2. *How robust is the proposed algorithm for data clustering?* We evaluate the robustness of clustering algorithms by examining their variance across multiple trials.

4.1 Experiment Design

Datasets In order to extensively examine the effectiveness of the proposed soft cut algorithm, a variety of datasets are used in this experiment. They are:

- *Text documents* that are extracted from the 20 newsgroups to form two five-class datasets, named as "M5" and "L5". Each class contain 100 document and there are totally 500 documents.

Table 1: Datasets Description

Dataset	Description	#Class	#Instance	#Features
M5	Text documents	5	500	1000
L5	Text documents	5	500	1000
Pendigit	Pen-based handwritting	10	2000	16
Ribosome	Ribosome rDNA sequences	8	1907	27617

- *Pendigit* that comes from the UCI data repository. It contains 2000 examples that belong to 10 different classes.

- *Ribosomal sequences* that are from RDP project (http://rdp.cme.msu.edu/index.jsp). It contains annotated rRNA sequences of ribosome for 2000 different bacteria that belong to 10 different phylum (e.g., classes). Table 1 provides the detailed information regarding each dataset.

Evaluation metrics To evaluate the performance of different clustering algorithms, two different metrics are used:

- *Clustering accuracy.* For the datasets that have no more than five classes, clustering accuracy is used as the evaluation metric. To compute clustering accuracy, each automatically generated cluster is first aligned with a true class. The classification accuracy based on the alignment is then computed, and the clustering accuracy is defined as the maximum classification accuracy among all possible alignments.

- *Normalized mutual information.* For the datasets that have more than five classes, due to the expensive computation involved in finding the optimal alignment, we use the normalized mutual information (Banerjee et al., 2003) as the alternative evaluation metric. If T_u and T_l denote the cluster labels and true class labels assigned to data points, the normalized mutual information "nmi" is defined as

$$\text{nmi} = \frac{2I(T_u, T_l)}{(H(T_u) + H(T_l))}$$

where $I(T_u, T_l)$ stands for the mutual information between clustering labels T_u and true class labels T_l. $H(T_u)$ and $H(T_l)$ are the entropy functions for T_u and T_l, respectively.

Each experiment was run 10 times with different initialization of parameters. The averaged results together with their variance are used as the final evaluation metric.

Implementation We follow the paper (Ng et al., 2001) for implementing the normalized cut algorithm. A cosine similarity is used to measure the affinity between any two data points. Both the EM algorithm and the Kmeans methods are used to cluster the data points that are projected into the low-dimension space spanned by the smallest eigenvectors of a graph Laplacian.

4.2   Experiment (I): Effectiveness of The Soft Cut Algorithm

The clustering results of both the soft cut algorithm and the normalized cut algorithm are summarized in Table 2. In addition to the Kmeans algorithm, we also apply the EM clustering algorithm to the normalized cut algorithm. In this experiment, the number of eigenvectors used for the normalized cut algorithms is equal to the number of clusters.

First, comparing to both normalized cut algorithms, we see that the proposed clustering algorithm substantially outperform the normalized cut algorithms for all datasets. Second,

Table 2: Clustering results for different clustering methods. Clustering accuracy is used for dataset "L5" and "M5" as the evaluation metric, and normalized mutual information is used for "Pendigit" and "Ribosome" .

	Soft Cut	Normalized Cut (Kmeans)	Normalized Cut (EM)
M5	89.2 ± 1.3	83.2 ± 8.8	62.4 ± 5.6
L5	69.2 ± 2.7	64.2 ± 4.9	45.1 ± 4.8
Pendigit	56.3 ± 3.8	46.0 ± 6.4	52.8 ± 2.0
Ribosome	69.7 ± 2.9	62.2 ± 9.1	63.2 ± 3.8

Table 3: Clustering accuracy for normalized cut with embedding in eigenspace with K eigenvectors. K-means is used.

#Eigenvector	M5	L5	Pendigit	Ribosome
K	$\mathbf{83.2 \pm 8.8}$	64.1 ± 4.9	46.0 ± 6.4	62.2 ± 9.1
$K+1$	77.6 ± 8.6	$\mathbf{69.6 \pm 6.7}$	43.3 ± 9.1	65.9 ± 5.8
$K+2$	79.7 ± 8.5	64.1 ± 5.7	41.6 ± 9.3	63.4 ± 4.8
$K+3$	80.2 ± 6.6	61.4 ± 5.8	42.9 ± 9.6	$\mathbf{67.2 \pm 7.6}$
$K+4$	74.9 ± 9.2	59.1 ± 4.7	47.5 ± 3.7	60.7 ± 8.4
$K+5$	70.5 ± 5.7	66.1 ± 4.7	39.2 ± 9.3	63.9 ± 8.2
$K+6$	75.5 ± 8.6	61.9 ± 4.7	43.4 ± 8.3	63.5 ± 10.4
$K+7$	75.8 ± 7.5	59.7 ± 5.6	46.8 ± 7.3	56.6 ± 10.7
$K+8$	73.5 ± 6.6	61.2 ± 4.7	$\mathbf{49.8 \pm 8.9}$	54.3 ± 7.2

comparing to the normalized cut algorithm using the Kmeans method, we see that the soft cut algorithm has smaller variance in its clustering results. This can be explained by the fact that the Kmeans algorithm uses binary cluster membership and therefore is likely to be trapped by local optimums. As indicated in Table 2, if we replace the Kmeans algoirthm with the EM algorithm in the normalized cut algorithm, the variance in clustering results is generally reduced but at the price of degradation in the performance of clustering. Based on the above observation, we conclude that the soft cut algorithm appears to be effective and robust for multi-class clustering.

4.3 Experiment (II): Normalized Cut using Different Numbers of Eigenvectors

One potential reason why the normalized cut algorithm perform worse than the proposed algorithm is that the number of clusters may not be the optimal number of eigenvectors. To examine this issue, we test the normalized cut algorithm with different number of eigenvectors. The Kmeans method is used for clustering the eigenvectors. The results of the normalized cut algorithm using different number of eigenvectors are summarized in Table 3. The best performance is highlighted by the bold fold.

First, we clearly see that the best clustering results may not necessarily happen when the number of eigenvectors is exactly equal to the number of clusters. In fact, for three out of four cases, the best performance is achieved when the number of eigenvectors is larger than the number of clusters. This result indicates that the choice of numbers of eigenvectors can have a significant impact on the performance of clustering. Second, comparing the results in Table 3 to the results in Table 2, we see that the soft cut algorithm is still able to outperform the normalized cut algorithm even with the optimal number of eigenvectors. In general, since spectral clustering is originally designed for binary-class classification, it requires an extra step when it is extended to multi-class clustering problems. Hence, the resulting solutions are usually suboptimal. In contrast, the soft cut algorithm directly targets on multi-class clustering problems, and thus is able to achieve better performance than the normalized cut algorithm.

5 Conclusion

In this paper, we proposed a novel probabilistic algorithm for spectral clustering, called "soft cut" algorithm. It introduces probabilistic membership into the normalized cut algorithm and directly targets on the multi-class clustering problems. Our empirical studies with a number of datasets have shown that the proposed algorithm outperforms the normalized cut algorithm considerably. In the future, we plan to extend this work to other applications such as image segmentation.

References

Bach, F. R., & Jordan, M. I. (2004). Learning spectral clustering. *Advances in Neural Information Processing Systems 16*.

Banerjee, A., Dhillon, I., Ghosh, J., & Sra, S. (2003). Generative model-based clustering of directional data. *Proceedings of the Ninth ACM SIGKDD International Conference on Knowledge Discovery and Data Mining (KDD-2003)*.

Blei, D. M., Ng, A. Y., & Jordan, M. I. (2003). Latent dirichlet allocation. *J. Mach. Learn. Res., 3*, 993–1022.

Chung, F. (1997). *Spectral graph theory*. Amer. Math. Society.

Ding, C., He, X., Zha, H., Gu, M., & Simon, H. (2001). A min-max cut algorithm for graph partitioning and data clustering. *Proc. IEEE Int'l Conf. Data Mining*.

Hagen, L., & Kahng, A. (1991). Fast spectral methods for ratio cut partitioning and clustering. *Proceedings of IEEE International Conference on Computer Aided Design* (pp. 10–13).

Hartigan, J., & Wong., M. (1994). A k-means clustering algorithm. *Appl. Statist., 28*, 100–108.

Hofmann, T. (1999). Probabilistic latent semantic indexing. *Proceedings of the 22nd Annual ACM Conference on Research and Development in Information Retrieval* (pp. 50–57). Berkeley, California.

Jin, R., & Si, L. (2004). A bayesian approach toward active learning for collaborative filtering. *Proceedings of the 20th conference on Uncertainty in artificial intelligence* (pp. 278–285). Banff, Canada: AUAI Press.

Ng, A., Jordan, M., & Weiss, Y. (2001). On spectral clustering: Analysis and an algorithm. *Advances in Neural Information Processing Systems 14*.

Redner, R. A., & Walker, H. F. (1984). Mixture densities, maximum likelihood and the em algorithm. *SIAM Review, 26*, 195–239.

Salakhutdinov, R., & Roweis, S. T. (2003). Adaptive overrelaxed bound optimization methods. *Proceedings of the Twentieth International Conference (ICML 2003)* (pp. 664–671).

Shi, J., & Malik, J. (2000). Normalized cuts and image segmentation. *IEEE Transactions on Pattern Analysis and Machine Intelligence, 22*, 888–905.

Yu, S. X., & Shi, J. (2003). Multiclass spectral clustering. *Proceedings of Ninth IEEE International Conference on Computer Vision*. Nice, France.

Zha, H., He, X., Ding, C., Gu, M., & Simon, H. (2002). Spectral relaxation for k-means clustering. *Advances in Neural Information Processing Systems 14*.

Walk-Sum Interpretation and Analysis of Gaussian Belief Propagation

Jason K. Johnson, Dmitry M. Malioutov and Alan S. Willsky
Department of Electrical Engineering and Computer Science
Massachusetts Institute of Technology
Cambridge, MA 02139
{jasonj,dmm,willsky}@mit.edu

Abstract

This paper presents a new framework based on walks in a graph for analysis and inference in Gaussian graphical models. The key idea is to decompose correlations between variables as a sum over all walks between those variables in the graph. The weight of each walk is given by a product of edgewise partial correlations. We provide a walk-sum interpretation of Gaussian belief propagation in trees and of the approximate method of loopy belief propagation in graphs with cycles. This perspective leads to a better understanding of Gaussian belief propagation and of its convergence in loopy graphs.

1 Introduction

We consider multivariate Gaussian distributions defined on graphs. The nodes of the graph denote random variables and the edges indicate statistical dependencies between variables. The family of all Gauss-Markov models defined on a graph is naturally represented in the *information form* of the Gaussian density which is parameterized by the inverse covariance matrix, i.e., the *information matrix*. This information matrix is sparse, reflecting the structure of the defining graph such that only the diagonal elements and those off-diagonal elements corresponding to edges of the graph are non-zero.

Given such a model, we consider the problem of computing the mean and variance of each variable, thereby determining the marginal densities as well as the mode. In principle, these can be obtained by inverting the information matrix, but the complexity of this computation is cubic in the number of variables. More efficient recursive calculations are possible in graphs with very sparse structure – e.g., in chains, trees and in graphs with "thin" junction trees. For these models, belief propagation (BP) or its junction tree variants efficiently compute the marginals [1]. In more complex graphs, even this approach can become computationally prohibitive. Then, approximate methods such as loopy belief propagation (LBP) provide a tractable alternative to exact inference [1, 2, 3, 4].

We develop a "walk-sum" formulation for computation of means, variances and correlations that holds in a wide class of Gauss-Markov models which we call *walk-summable*. In particular, this leads to a new interpretation of BP in trees and of LBP in general. Based on this interpretation we are able to extend the previously known sufficient conditions for convergence of LBP to the class of walk-summable models (which includes all of the following: trees, attractive models, and pairwise-normalizable models). Our sufficient condition is tighter than that given in [3] as the class of diagonally-dominant models is a strict subset of the class of pairwise-normalizable models. Our results also explain why no examples were found in [3] where LBP did not converge. The reason is that they presume a pairwise-normalizable model. We also explain why, in walk-summable models, LBP converges to the correct means but not to the correct variances (proving "walk-sum" analogs of results in [3]). In general, walk-summability is not necessary for LBP convergence. Hence, we also provide a tighter (essentially necessary) condition for convergence of LBP variances based on walk-summability of the LBP computation tree. This provides deeper insight into why LBP can fail to converge – because the LBP computation tree is not always well-posed – which suggests connections to [5]. This paper presents the key ideas and outlines proofs of the main results. A more detailed presentation will appear in a technical report [6].

2   Preliminaries

A Gauss-Markov model (GMM) is defined by a graph $\mathcal{G} = (V, \mathcal{E})$ with edge set $\mathcal{E} \subset \binom{V}{2}$, i.e., some set of two-element subsets of V, and a collection of random variables $x = (x_i, i \in V)$ with probability density given in *information form*[1]:

$$p(x) \propto \exp\{-\frac{1}{2}x'Jx + h'x\} \tag{1}$$

where J is a symmetric positive definite ($J \succ 0$) matrix which is sparse so as to respect the graph $\mathcal{G}$: if $\{i,j\} \notin \mathcal{E}$ then $J_{i,j} = 0$. We call J the *information matrix* and h the *potential vector*. Let $N(i) = \{j | \{i, j\} \in \mathcal{E}\}$ denote the *neighbors* of i in the graph. The mean $\mu \equiv \mathbb{E}\{x\}$ and covariance $P \equiv \mathbb{E}\{(x - \mu)(x - \mu)'\}$ are given by:

$$\mu = J^{-1}h \quad \text{and} \quad P = J^{-1} \tag{2}$$

The *partial correlation coefficients* are given by:

$$\rho_{i,j} \equiv \frac{\operatorname{cov}(x_i; x_j | x_{V \setminus \{i,j\}})}{\sqrt{\operatorname{var}(x_i | x_{V \setminus \{i,j\}}) \operatorname{var}(x_j | x_{V \setminus \{i,j\}})}} = -\frac{J_{i,j}}{\sqrt{J_{i,i} J_{j,j}}} \tag{3}$$

Thus, $J_{ij} = 0$ if and only if x_i and x_j are independent given the other variables $x_{V \setminus \{i,j\}}$. We say that this model is *attractive* if all partial correlations are non-negative. It is *pairwise-normalizable* if there exists a diagonal matrix $D \succ 0$ and a collection of non-negative definite matrices $\{J_e \succeq 0, e \in \mathcal{E}\}$, where $(J_e)_{i,j}$ is zero unless $i, j \in e$, such that:

$$J = D + \sum_{e \in \mathcal{E}} J_e \tag{4}$$

It is *diagonally-dominant* if for all $i \in V : \sum_{j \neq i} |J_{i,j}| < J_{i,i}$. The class of diagonally-dominant models is a strict subset of the class of pairwise-normalizable models [6].

Gaussian Elimination and Belief Propagation   Integrating (1) over all possible values of x_i reduces to *Gaussian elimination* (GE) in the information form (see also [7]), i.e.,

$$p(x_{\setminus i}) \equiv \int p(x_{\setminus i}, x_i) dx_i \propto \exp\{-\frac{1}{2}x'_{\setminus i}\hat{J}_{\setminus i}x_{\setminus i} + \hat{h}'_{\setminus i}x_{\setminus i}\} \tag{5}$$

where $\setminus i \equiv V \setminus \{i\}$, i.e. all variables except i, and

$$\hat{J}_{\setminus i} = J_{\setminus i, \setminus i} - J_{\setminus i, i}J_{i,i}^{-1}J_{i, \setminus i} \quad \text{and} \quad \hat{h}_{\setminus i} = h_{\setminus i} - J_{\setminus i, i}J_{i,i}^{-1}h_i \tag{6}$$

---

[1]The work also applies to $p(x|y)$, i.e. where some variables y are observed. However, the observations y are fixed, and we redefine $p(x) \triangleq p(x|y)$ (conditioning on y is implicit throughout). With local observations $p(x|y) \propto p(x) \prod_i p(y_i|x_i)$, conditioning does not change the graph structure.

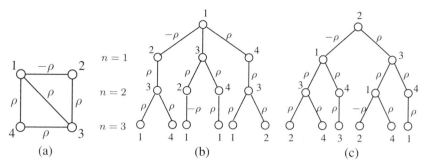

Figure 1: (a) Graph of a GMM with nodes $\{1, 2, 3, 4\}$ and with edge weights (partial correlations) as shown. In (b) and (c) we illustrate the first three levels of the LBP computation tree rooted at nodes 1 and 2. After 3 iterations of LBP in (a), the marginals at nodes 1 and 2 are identical to the marginals at the root of (b) and (c) respectively.

In trees, the marginal of any given node can be efficiently computed by sequentially eliminating leaves of the tree until just that node remains. BP may be seen as a message-passing form of GE in which a message passed from node i to node $j \in N(i)$ captures the effect of eliminating the subtree rooted at i. Thus, by a two-pass procedure, BP efficiently computes the marginals at *all* nodes of the tree. The equations for LBP are identical except that messages are updated iteratively and in parallel. There are two messages per edge, one for each ordered pair $(i, j) \in \mathcal{E}$. We specify each message in information form with parameters: $\Delta h_{i \to j}^{(n)}, \Delta J_{i \to j}^{(n)}$ (initialized to zero for $n = 0$). These are iteratively updated as follows. For each $(i, j) \in \mathcal{E}$, messages from $N(i) \setminus j$ are fused at node i:

$$\hat{h}_{i \setminus j}^{(n)} = h_i + \sum_{k \in N(i) \setminus j} \Delta h_{k \to i}^{(n)} \quad \text{and} \quad \hat{J}_{i \setminus j}^{(n)} = J_{i,i} + \sum_{k \in N(i) \setminus j} \Delta J_{k \to i}^{(n)} \tag{7}$$

This fused information at node i is predicted to node j:

$$\Delta h_{i \to j}^{(n+1)} = -J_{j,i} (\hat{J}_{i \setminus j}^{(n)})^{-1} \hat{h}_{i \setminus j}^{(n)} \quad \text{and} \quad \Delta J_{i \to j}^{(n+1)} = -J_{j,i} (\hat{J}_{i \setminus j}^{(n)})^{-1} J_{i,j} \tag{8}$$

After n iterations, the marginal of node i is obtained by fusing all incoming messages:

$$\hat{h}_i^{(n)} = h_i + \sum_{k \in N(i)} \Delta h_{k \to i}^{(n)} \quad \text{and} \quad \hat{J}_i^{(n)} = J_{i,i} + \sum_{k \in N(i)} \Delta J_{k \to i}^{(n)} \tag{9}$$

The mean and variance are given by $(\hat{J}_i^{(n)})^{-1} \hat{h}_i^{(n)}$ and $(\hat{J}_i^{(n)})^{-1}$. In trees, this is the marginal at node i conditioned on zero boundary conditions at nodes $(n + 1)$ steps away and LBP converges to the correct marginals after a finite number of steps equal to the diameter of the tree. In graphs with cycles, LBP may not converge and only yields approximate marginals when it does. A useful fact about LBP is the following [2, 3, 5]: the marginal computed at node i after n iterations is identical to the marginal at the root of the n-step *computation tree* rooted at node i. This tree is obtained by "unwinding" the loopy graph for n steps (see Fig. 1). Note that each node of the graph may be replicated many times in the computation tree. Also, neighbors of a node in the computation tree correspond exactly with neighbors of the associated node in the original graph (except at the last level of the tree where some neighbors are missing). The corresponding J matrix defined on the computation tree has the same node and edge values as in the original GMM.

3 Walk-Summable Gauss-Markov Models

In this section we present the walk-sum formulation of inference in GMMs. Let $\varrho(A)$ denote the *spectral radius* of a symmetric matrix A, defined to be the maximum of the absolute values of the eigenvalues of A. The geometric series $(I + A + A^2 + \dots)$ converges if and only if $\varrho(A) < 1$. If it converges, it converges to $(I - A)^{-1}$. Now, consider a GMM with information matrix J. Without loss of generality, let J be normalized (by rescaling variables) to have $J_{i,i} = 1$ for all i. Then, $\rho_{i,j} = -J_{i,j}$ and the (zero-diagonal) matrix of partial correlations is given by $R = I - J$. If $\varrho(R) < 1$, then we have a geometric series for the covariance matrix:

$$\sum_{l=0}^{\infty} R^l = (I - R)^{-1} = J^{-1} = P \tag{10}$$

Let $\bar{R} = (|r_{ij}|)$ denote the matrix of element-wise absolute values. We say that the model is *walk-summable* if $\varrho(\bar{R}) < 1$. Walk-summability implies $\varrho(R) < 1$ and $J \succ 0$.

Example 1. Consider a 5-node cycle with normalized information matrix J, which has all partial correlations on the edges set to ρ. If $\rho = -.45$, then the model is valid (i.e. positive definite) with minimum eigenvalue $\lambda_{\min}(J) \approx .2719 > 0$, and walk-summable with $\varrho(\bar{R}) = .9 < 1$. However, when $\rho = -.55$, then the model is still valid with $\lambda_{\min}(J) \approx .1101 > 0$, but no longer walk-summable with $\varrho(\bar{R}) = 1.1 > 1$.

Walk-summability allows us to interpret (10) as computing walk-sums in the graph. Recall that the matrix R reflects graph structure: $\rho_{i,j} = 0$ if $\{i,j\} \notin \mathcal{E}$. These act as weights on the edges of the graph. A *walk* $w = (w_0, w_1, ..., w_l)$ is a sequence of nodes $w_i \in V$ connected by edges $\{w_i, w_{i+1}\} \in \mathcal{E}$ where l is the *length* of the walk. The *weight* $\rho(w)$ of walk w is the product of edge weights along the walk:

$$\rho(w) = \prod_{s=1}^{l} \rho_{w_{s-1}, w_s} \tag{11}$$

At each node $i \in V$, we also define a zero-length walk $w = (i)$ for which $\rho(w) = 1$.

Walk-Sums. Given a set of walks $\mathcal{W}$, we define the *walk-sum* over $\mathcal{W}$ by

$$\rho(\mathcal{W}) = \sum_{w \in \mathcal{W}} \rho(w) \tag{12}$$

which is well-defined (i.e., independent of summation order) because $\varrho(\bar{R}) < 1$ implies absolute convergence. Let $\mathcal{W}_{i \xrightarrow{l} j}$ denote the set of l-length walks from i to j and let $\mathcal{W}_{i \to j} = \cup_{l=0}^{\infty} \mathcal{W}_{i \xrightarrow{l} j}$. The relation between walks and the geometric series (10) is that the entries of R^l correspond to walk-sums over l-length walks from i to j in the graph, i.e., $(R^l)_{i,j} = \rho(\mathcal{W}_{i \xrightarrow{l} j})$. Hence,

$$P_{i,j} = \sum_{l=0}^{\infty} (R^l)_{i,j} = \sum_l \rho(\mathcal{W}_{i \xrightarrow{l} j}) = \rho(\cup_l \mathcal{W}_{i \xrightarrow{l} j}) = \rho(\mathcal{W}_{i \to j}) \tag{13}$$

In particular, the variance $\sigma_i^2 \equiv P_{i,i}$ of variable i is the walk-sum taken over the set $\mathcal{W}_{i \to i}$ of *self-return walks* that begin and end at i (defined so that $(i) \in \mathcal{W}_{i \to i}$). The means can be computed as reweighted walk-sums, i.e., where each walk is scaled by the potential at the start of the walk: $\rho(w; h) = h_{w_0} \rho(w)$, and $\rho(\mathcal{W}; h) = \sum_{w \in \mathcal{W}} \rho(w; h)$. Then,

$$\mu_i = \sum_{j \in V} P_{i,j} h_j = \sum_j \rho(\mathcal{W}_{j \to i}) h_j = \rho(\mathcal{W}_{* \to i}; h) \tag{14}$$

where $\mathcal{W}_{* \to i} \equiv \cup_{j \in V} \mathcal{W}_{j \to i}$ is the set of all walks which end at node i.

We have found that a wide class of GMMs are walk-summable:

Proposition 1 (Walk-Summable GMMs) *All of the following classes of GMMs are walk-summable:[2] (i) attractive models, (ii) trees and (iii) pairwise-normalizable[3] models.*

---

[2] That is if we take a valid model (with $J \succ 0$) in these classes then it automatically has $\varrho(\bar{R}) < 1$.
[3] In [6], we also show that walk-summability is actually equivalent to pairwise-normalizability.

Proof Outline. (i) $R = \bar{R}$ and $J = I - \bar{R} \succ 0$ implies $\lambda_{\max}(\bar{R}) < 1$. Because $\bar{R}$ has non-negative elements, $\varrho(\bar{R}) = \lambda_{\max}(\bar{R}) < 1$. In (ii) & (iii), negating any ρ_{ij}, it still holds that $J = I - R \succ 0$: (ii) negating ρ_{ij} doesn't affect the eigenvalues of J (remove edge $\{i,j\}$ and, in each eigenvector, negate all entries in one subtree); (iii) negating ρ_{ij} preserves $J_{\{i,j\}} \succeq 0$ in (4) so $J \succ 0$. Thus, making all $\rho_{ij} > 0$, we find $I - \bar{R} \succ 0$ and $\bar{R} \prec I$. Similarly, making all $\rho_{ij} < 0$, $-\bar{R} \prec I$. Therefore, $\varrho(\bar{R}) < 1$. ◇

4 Recursive Walk-Sum Calculations on Trees

In this section we derive a recursive algorithm which accrues the walk-sums (over infinite sets of walks) necessary for exact inference on trees and relate this to BP. Walk-summability guarantees correctness of this algorithm which reorders walks in a non-trivial way.

We start with a chain of N nodes: its graph $\mathcal{G}$ has nodes $V = \{1, \ldots, N\}$ and edges $\mathcal{E} = \{e_1, \ldots, e_{N-1}\}$ where $e_i = \{i, i+1\}$. The variance at node i is $\sigma_i^2 = \rho(\mathcal{W}_{i \to i})$. The set $\mathcal{W}_{i \to i}$ can be partitioned according to the number of times that walks return to node i: $\mathcal{W}_{i \to i} = \cup_{r=0}^{\infty} \mathcal{W}_{i \to i}^{(r)}$ where $\mathcal{W}_{i \to i}^{(r)}$ is the set of all self-return walks which return to i exactly r times. In particular, $\mathcal{W}_{i \to i}^{(0)} = \{(i)\}$ for which $\rho(\mathcal{W}_{i \to i}^{(0)}) = 1$. A walk which starts at node i and returns r times is a concatenation of r single-revisit self-return walks, so $\rho(\mathcal{W}_{i \to i}^{(r)}) = \rho(\mathcal{W}_{i \to i}^{(1)})^r$. This means:

$$\rho(\mathcal{W}_{i \to i}) = \rho(\cup_{r=0}^{\infty} \mathcal{W}_{i \to i}^{(r)}) = \sum_{r=0}^{\infty} \rho(\mathcal{W}_{i \to i}^{(r)}) = \sum_{r=0}^{\infty} \rho(\mathcal{W}_{i \to i}^{(1)})^r = \frac{1}{1 - \rho(\mathcal{W}_{i \to i}^{(1)})} \quad (15)$$

This geometric series converges since the model is walk-summable. Hence, calculating the single-revisit self-return walk-sum $\rho(\mathcal{W}_{i \to i}^{(1)})$ determines the variance σ_i^2. The single-revisit walks at node i consist of walks in the left subchain, and walks in the right subchain. Let $\mathcal{W}_{i \to i \backslash j}$ be the set of self-return walks of i which never visit j, so e.g. all $w \in \mathcal{W}_{i \to i \backslash i+1}$ are contained in the subgraph $\{1, \ldots, i\}$. With this notation:

$$\rho(\mathcal{W}_{i \to i}^{(1)}) = \rho(\mathcal{W}_{i \to i \backslash i+1}^{(1)}) + \rho(\mathcal{W}_{i \to i \backslash i-1}^{(1)}) \quad (16)$$

The left single-revisit self-return walk-sums $\rho(\mathcal{W}_{i \to i \backslash i+1}^{(1)})$ can be computed recursively starting from node 1. At node 1, $\rho(\mathcal{W}_{1 \to 1 \backslash 2}^{(1)}) = 0$ and $\rho(\mathcal{W}_{1 \to 1 \backslash 2}) = 1$. A single-revisit self-return walk from node i in the left subchain consists of a step to node $i-1$, then some number of self-return walks in the subgraph $\{1, \ldots, i-1\}$, and a step from $i-1$ back to i:

$$\rho(\mathcal{W}_{i \to i \backslash i+1}^{(1)}) = \rho_{i,i-1}^2 \rho(\mathcal{W}_{i-1 \to i-1 \backslash i}) = \frac{\rho_{i,i-1}^2}{1 - \rho(\mathcal{W}_{i-1 \to i-1 \backslash i}^{(1)})} \quad (17)$$

Thus single-revisit (and multiple revisit) walk-sums in the left subchain of every node i can be calculated in one forward pass through the chain. The same can be done for the right subchain walk-sums at every node i, by starting at node N, and going backwards. Using equations (15) and (16) these quantities suffice to calculate the variances at *all* nodes of the chain. A similar forwards-backwards procedure computes the means as reweighted walk-sums over the left and right single-visit walks for node i, which start at an arbitrary node (in the left or right subchain) and end at i, never visiting i before that [6]. In fact, these recursive walk-sum calculations map exactly to operations in BP – e.g., in a normalized chain $\Delta J_{i-1 \to i} = -\rho(\mathcal{W}_{i \to i \backslash i+1}^{(1)})$ and $\Delta h_{i-1 \to i} = -\rho(\mathcal{W}_{* \to i \backslash i+1}^{(1)}; h)$. The same strategy applies for trees: both single-revisit and single-visit walks at node i can be partitioned according to which subtree (rooted at a neighbor $j \in N(i)$ of i) the walk lives in. This leads to a two-pass walks-sum calculation on trees (from the leaves to the root, and back) to calculate means and variances at all nodes.

5   Walk-sum Analysis of Loopy Belief Propagation

First, we analyze LBP in the case that the model is walk-summable and show that LBP converges and includes all the walks for the means, but only a subset of the walks for the variances. Then, we consider the case of non-walksummable models and relate convergence of the LBP variances to walk-summability of the computation tree.

5.1   LBP in walk-summable models

To compute means and variances in a walk-summable model, we need to calculate walk-sums for certain sets of walks in the graph $\mathcal{G}$. Running LBP in $\mathcal{G}$ is equivalent to exact inference in the computation tree for $\mathcal{G}$, and hence calculating walk-sums for certain walks in the computation tree. In the computation tree rooted at node i, walks ending at the root have a one-to-one correspondence with walks ending at node i in $\mathcal{G}$. Hence, LBP captures all of the walks necessary to calculate the means. For variances, the walks captured by LBP have to start and end at the root in the computation tree. However, some of the self-return walks in $\mathcal{G}$ translate to walks in the computation tree that end at the root but start at a replica of the root, rather than at the root itself. These walks are not captured by the LBP variances. For example, in Fig. 1(a), the walk $(1, 2, 3, 1)$ is a self-return walk in the original graph $\mathcal{G}$ but is *not* a self-return walk in the computation tree shown in Fig. 1(b). LBP variances capture only those self-return walks of the original graph $\mathcal{G}$ which also are self-return walks in the computation tree – e.g., the walk $(1, 3, 2, 3, 4, 3, 1)$ is a self-return walk in both Figs. 1(a) and (b). We call these *backtracking walks*. These simple observations lead to our main result:

Proposition 2 (Convergence of LBP for walk-summable GMMs) *If the model is walk-summable, then LBP converges: the means converge to the true means and the LBP variances converge to walk-sums over just the backtracking self-return walks at each node.*

Proof Outline. All backtracking walks have positive weights, since each edge is traversed an even number of times. For a walk-summable model, LBP variances are walks-sums over the backtracking walks and are therefore monotonically increasing with the iterations. They also are bounded above by the absolute self-return walk-sums (diagonal elements of $\sum_l \bar{R}^l$) and hence converge. For the means: the series $\sum_{l=0}^{\infty} R^l h$ converges absolutely since $|R^l h| \leq \bar{R}^l |h|$, and the series $\sum_l \bar{R}^l |h|$ is a linear combination of terms of the absolutely convergent series $\sum_l \bar{R}^l$. The LBP means are a rearrangement of the absolutely convergent series $\sum_{l=0}^{\infty} R^l h$, so they converge to the same values. $\diamond$

As a corollary, LBP converges for all of the model classes listed in Proposition 1. Also, in attractive models, the LBP variances are less than or equal to the true variances. Correctness of the means was also shown in [3] for pairwise-normalizable models.[4] They also show that LBP variances omit some terms needed for the correct variances. These terms correspond to correlations between the root and its replicas in the computation tree. In our framework, each such correlation is a walk-sum over the subset of non-backtracking self-return walks in $\mathcal{G}$ which, in the computation tree, begin at a particular replica of the root.

Example 2. Consider the graph in Fig. 1(a). For $\rho = .39$, the model is walk-summable with $\varrho(\bar{R}) \approx .9990$. For $\rho = .395$ and $\rho = .4$, the model is still valid but is not walk-summable, with $\varrho(\bar{R}) \approx 1.0118$ and 1.0246 respectively. In Fig. 2(a) we show LBP variances for node 1 (the other nodes are similar) vs. the iteration number. As ρ increases, first the model is walk-summable and LBP converges, then for a small interval the model is not walk-summable but LBP still converges,[5] and for larger ρ LBP does not converge. Also,

---

[4] However, they only prove convergence for the subset of diagonally dominant models.
[5] Hence, walk-summability is sufficient but not necessary for convergence of LBP.

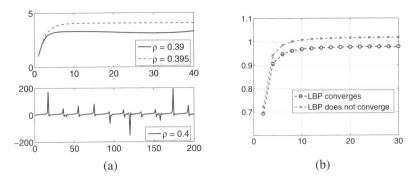

Figure 2: (a) LBP variances vs. iteration. (b) $\varrho(R_n)$ vs. iteration.

for $\rho = .4$, we note that $\varrho(R) = .8 < 1$ and the series $\sum_l R^l$ converges (but $\sum_l \bar{R}^l$ does not) and LBP does not converge. Hence, $\varrho(R) < 1$ is *not* sufficient for LBP convergence showing the importance of the stricter walk-summability condition $\varrho(\bar{R}) < 1$.

5.2 LBP in non-walksummable models

We extend our analysis to develop a tighter condition for convergence of LBP variances based on walk-summability of the computation tree (rather than walk-summability on $\mathcal{G}$).[6] For trees, walk-summability and validity are equivalent, i.e. $J \succ 0 \Leftrightarrow \varrho(\bar{R}) < 1$, hence our condition is equivalent to validity of the computation tree.

First, we note that when a model on $\mathcal{G}$ is valid (J is positive-definite) but not walk-summable, then some finite computation trees may be invalid (indefinite). This turns out to be the reason why LBP variances can fail to converge. Walk-summability of the original GMM implies walk-summability (and hence validity) of all of its computation trees. But if the GMM is not walk-summable, then its computation tree may or may not be walk-summable. In Example 2, for $\rho = .395$ the computation tree is still walk-summable (even though the model on $\mathcal{G}$ is not) and LBP converges. For $\rho = .4$, the computation tree is not walk-summable and LBP does not converge. Indeed, LBP is not even well-posed in this case (because the computation tree is indefinite) which explains its strange behavior seen in the bottom plot of Fig. 2(a) (e.g., non-monotonicity and negative variances).

We characterize walk-summability of the computation tree as follows. Let T_n be the n-step computation tree rooted at some node i and define $R_n \triangleq I_n - J_n$ where J_n is the normalized information matrix on T_n and I_n is the $n \times n$ identity matrix. The n-step computation tree T_n is walk-summable (valid) if and only if $\varrho(R_n) < 1$ (in trees, $\varrho(\bar{R}_n) = \varrho(R_n)$). The sequence $\{\varrho(R_n)\}$ is monotonically increasing and bounded above by $\varrho(\bar{R})$ (see [6]) and hence converges. We are interested in the quantity $\varrho_\infty \equiv \lim_{n\to\infty} \varrho(R_n)$.

Proposition 3 (LBP validity/variance convergence) *(i) If $\varrho_\infty < 1$, then all finite computation trees are valid and the LBP variances converge. (ii) If $\varrho_\infty > 1$, then the computation tree eventually becomes invalid and LBP is ill-posed.*

Proof Outline. (i) For some $\delta > 0$, $\varrho(R_n) \leq 1 - \delta$ for all n which implies: all computation trees are walk-summable and variances monotonically increase; $\lambda_{\max}(R_n) \leq 1 - \delta$, $\lambda_{\min}(J_n) \geq \delta$, and $(P_n)_{i,i} \leq \lambda_{\max}(P_n) \leq \frac{1}{\delta}$. The variances are monotonically increasing

---

[6]We can focus on one tree: if the computation tree rooted at node i is walk-summable, then so is the computation tree rooted at any node j. Also, if a finite computation tree rooted at node i is not walk-summable, then some finite tree at node j also becomes non-walksummable for n large enough.

and bounded above, hence they converge. (ii) If $\lim_{n\to\infty} \varrho(R_n) > 1$, then there exists an m for which $\varrho(R_n) > 1$ for all $n \geq m$ and the computation tree is invalid. $\diamond$

As discussed in [6], LBP is well-posed if and only if the information numbers computed on the right in (7) and (9) are strictly positive for all n. Hence, it is easily detected if the LBP computation tree becomes invalid. In this case, continuing to run LBP is not meaningful and will lead to division by zero and/or negative variances.

Example 3. Consider a 4-node cycle with edge weights $(-\rho, \rho, \rho, \rho)$. In Fig. 2(b), for $\rho = .49$ we plot $\varrho(R_n)$ vs. n (lower curve) and observe that $\lim_{n\to\infty} \varrho(R_n) \approx .98 < 1$, and LBP converges (similar to the upper plot of Fig. 2(a)). For $\rho = .51$ (upper curve), the model defined on the 4-node cycle is still valid but $\lim_{n\to\infty} \varrho(R_n) \approx 1.02 > 1$ so LBP is ill-posed and does not converge (similar to the lower plot of Fig. 2(a)).

In non-walksummable models, the series LBP computes for the means is not absolutely convergent and may diverge even when variances converge (e.g., in Example 2 with $\rho = .39867$). However, in all cases where variances converge we have observed that with enough damping of BP messages[7] we also obtain convergence of the means. Apparently, it is the validity of the computation tree that is critical for convergence of Gaussian LBP.

6   Conclusion

We have presented a walk-sum interpretation of inference in GMMs and have applied this framework to analyze convergence of LBP extending previous results. In future work, we plan to develop extended walk-sum algorithms which gather more walks than LBP. Another approach is to estimate variances by sampling random walks in the graph. We also are interested to explore possible connections between results in [8] – based on self-avoiding walks in Ising models – and sufficient conditions for convergence of discrete LBP [9] which have some parallels to our walk-sum analysis in the Gaussian case.

Acknowledgments   This research was supported by the Air Force Office of Scientific Research under Grant FA9550-04-1, the Army Research Office under Grant W911NF-05-1-0207 and by a grant from MIT Lincoln Laboratory.

References

[1] J. Pearl. *Probabilistic inference in intelligent systems*. Morgan Kaufmann, 1988.

[2] J. Yedidia, W. Freeman, and Y. Weiss. Understanding belief propagation and its generalizations. *Exploring AI in the new millennium*, pages 239–269, 2003.

[3] Y. Weiss and W. Freeman. Correctness of belief propagation in Gaussian graphical models of arbitrary topology. *Neural Computation*, 13:2173–2200, 2001.

[4] P. Rusmevichientong and B. Van Roy. An analysis of belief propagation on the turbo decoding graph with Gaussian densities. *IEEE Trans. Information Theory*, 48(2):745–765, Feb. 2001.

[5] S. Tatikonda and M. Jordan. Loopy belief propagation and Gibbs measures. *UAI*, 2002.

[6] J. Johnson, D. Malioutov, and A. Willsky. Walk-Summable Gaussian Networks and Walk-Sum Interpretation of Gaussian Belief Propagation. TR-2650, LIDS, MIT, 2005.

[7] K. Plarre and P. Kumar. Extended message passing algorithm for inference in loopy Gaussian graphical models. *Ad Hoc Networks*, 2004.

[8] M. Fisher. Critical temperatures of anisotropic Ising lattices II, general upper bounds. *Physical Review*, 162(2), 1967.

[9] A. Ihler, J. Fisher III, and A. Willsky. Message Errors in Belief Propagation. *NIPS*, 2004.

---

[7]Modify (8) as follows: $\Delta h_{i\to j}^{(n+1)} = (1-\alpha)\Delta h_{i\to j}^{(n)} + \alpha(-J_{i,j}(\hat{J}_{i\backslash j}^{(n)})^{-1}\hat{h}_{i\backslash j}^{(n)})$ with $0 < \alpha \leq 1$. In Example 2, with $\rho = .39867$ and $\alpha = .9$ the means converge.

Using "epitomes" to model genetic diversity: Rational design of HIV vaccine cocktails

Nebojsa Jojic, Vladimir Jojic, Brendan Frey, Chris Meek and David Heckerman
Microsoft Research

Abstract

We introduce a new model of genetic diversity which summarizes a large input dataset into an epitome, a short sequence or a small set of short sequences of probability distributions capturing many overlapping subsequences from the dataset. The epitome as a representation has already been used in modeling real-valued signals, such as images and audio. The discrete sequence model we introduce in this paper targets applications in genetics, from multiple alignment to recombination and mutation inference. In our experiments, we concentrate on modeling the diversity of HIV where the epitome emerges as a natural model for producing relatively small vaccines covering a large number of immune system targets known as epitopes. Our experiments show that the epitome includes more epitopes than other vaccine designs of similar length, including cocktails of consensus strains, phylogenetic tree centers, and observed strains. We also discuss epitome designs that take into account uncertainty about T-cell cross reactivity and epitope presentation. In our experiments, we find that vaccine optimization is fairly robust to these uncertainties.

1 Introduction

Within and across instances of a certain class of a natural signal, such as a facial image, a bird song recording, or a certain type of a gene, we find many repeating fragments. The repeating fragments can vary slightly and can have arbitrary (and usually unknown) sizes. For instance, in cropped images of human faces, a small patch capturing an eye appears in an image twice (with a symmetry transformation applied), and across different facial images many times, as humans have a limited number of eye types. Another repeating structure across facial images is the nose, which occupies a larger patch. In mammalian DNA sequences, we find repeating regulatory elements within a single sequence, and repeating larger structures (genes, or gene fragments) across species. Instead of defining size, variability and typical relative locations of repeating fragments manually, in an application-driven way, the 'epitomic analysis' [5] is an unsupervised approach to estimating repeating fragment models, and simultaneously aligning the data to them. This is achieved by considering data in terms of randomly selected overlapping fragments, or patches, of various sizes and mapping them onto an 'epitome,' a learned structure which is considerably larger than any of the fragments, and yet much smaller than the total size of the dataset.

We first introduced this model for image analysis [5], and it has since been used for video and audio analysis [2, 6], as well. This paper introduces a new form of the epitome as a sequence of multinomial distributions (Fig. 1), and describe its applications to HIV diversity modeling and rational vaccine design. We show that the vaccines optimized using our algorithms are likely to have broader predicted coverage of immune targets in HIV than the previous rational designs.

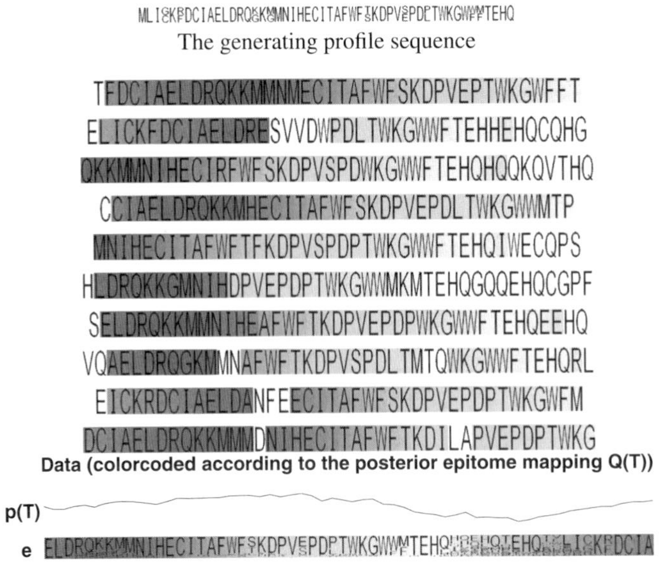

MLI?K?DCIAELDRQ?K?MNIHECITAFWF?KDPV?PDETWKGW?^TEHQ
The generating profile sequence

TFDCIAELDRQKKMMNMECITAFWFSKDPVEPTWKGWFFT
ELICKFDCIAELDRESVVDWPDLTWKGWWFTEHHEHQCQHG
QKKMMNIHECIRFWFSKDPVSPDWKGWWFTEHQHQQKQVTHQ
CCIAELDRQKKMHECITAFWFSKDPVEPDLTWKGWWMTP
MNIHECITAFWFTFKDPVSPDPTWKGWWFTEHQIWECQPS
HLDRQKKGMNIHDPVEPDPTWKGWWMKMTEHQGQQEHQCGPF
SELDRQKKMMNIHEAFWFTKDPVEPDPWKGWWFTEHQEEHQ
VQAELDRQGKMMNAFWFTKDPVSPDLTMTQWKGWWFTEHQRL
EICKRDCIAELDANFEECITAFWFSKDPVEPDPTWKGWFM
DCIAELDRQKKMMMDNIHECITAFWFTKDILAPVEPDPTWKG

Data (colorcoded according to the posterior epitome mapping Q(T))

p(T)

e ELDRQKKMMNIHECITAFWFSKDPVEPDPTWKGWW^TEHQ...EHQ...CICKFDCIA

Figure 1: The epitome (e) learned from data synthesized from the generating profile sequence (Section 5). A color coding in the epitome and data sequences is used to show the mapping between epitome and data positions. A white color indicates that the letter was likely generated from the garbage component of the epitome. The distribution $p(\mathcal{T})$ shows which 9mers from the epitome were more likely to generate patches of the data.

2 Sequence epitome

The central part of Fig. 1 illustrates a small set of amino acid sequences $X = \{x_{ij}\}$ of size MN (with i indexing a sequence, and j indexing a letter within a sequence, and $M = \max i$, $N = \max j$). The sequences share patterns (although sometimes with discrepancies in isolated amino-acids) but one sequence may be similar to other sequences in different regions. The sequences are generated synthetically by combining the pieces of the profile sequence given in the first line of the figure, with occasional insertions of random sequence fragments, as discussed in Section 5. Sequence variability in this synthetic example is slightly higher than that found in the NEF protein of the human immunodeficiency virus (HIV) [7], while the envelope proteins of the same virus exhibit more variability. Examples of high genetic diversity can also be found in higher-level organisms, for example in the regions coding for immune system's pattern recognition molecules.

The last row in the figure illustrates an epitome optimized to represent the variability in the sequences above. In general, the epitome is a smaller array $E = \{e_{mn}\}$ of size $M_e \times N_e$, where $M_e N_e \ll MN$. In the figure, $M_e = 1$. An epitome can be parameterized in different ways, but in the figure, each epitome element e_{mn} is a multinomial distribution with the probability of each letter represented by its height. The epitome's summarization quality is defined by a simple generative model which considers the data X in terms of shorter subsequences, X_S. A subsequence X_S is defined as an ordered subset of letters from X taken from positions listed in the ordered index set S. For instance, the set $S = \{(4,8),(4,9),(4,10),(4,11)\}$ points to a contiguous patch of letters in the fourth sequence $X_S = RQKK$. Similarly, set $S = \{(6,2),(6,3),(6,4),(6,5),(6,6)\}$ points to the patch $X_S = LDRQK$ in the sixth sequence. A number of such patches[1] of various lengths can be taken randomly (and with overlap). The quality of the epitome is then defined as the total likelihood of these patches under the generative model which generates each patch from a set of distributions $E_\mathcal{T}$, where $\mathcal{T}$ is an ordered set of indices into the epitome (In the figure, the epitome is defined on a circle, so that the index progression continues from N_e to 1. (This reduces local minima problems in the EM algorithm for epitome learning as discussed in Sections 4 and 5). For each data patch, the mapping $\mathcal{T}$ is considered a hidden variable,

---

[1] In principal, noncontiguous patches can be taken as well, if the application so requires.

and the generative process is assumed to consist of the following two steps

- Sample a patch $E_{\mathcal{T}}$ from E according to $p(\mathcal{T})$. To illustrate $p(\mathcal{T})$ in Fig. 1, we consider only the set of of all 9-long contiguous patches. For such patches, which are sometimes called nine-mers, we can index different sets $\mathcal{T}$ by their first elements and plot $p(\mathcal{T})$ as a curve with the domain $\{1, ..., N_e - 8\}$.

- Generate a patch $X_{\mathcal{S}}$ from $E_{\mathcal{T}}$ according to $p(X_{\mathcal{S}}|E_{\mathcal{T}}) = \prod_{k=1}^{|\mathcal{T}|} e_{\mathcal{T}(k)}(X_{\mathcal{S}(k)})$, with $\mathcal{T}(k)$ and $\mathcal{S}(k)$ denoting the k-th element in the epitome and data patches.

Each execution of these two steps can, in principle, generate any pattern. The probability (likelihood) of generating a particular pattern indicated by $\mathcal{S}$ is

$$p(X_{\mathcal{S}}) = \sum_{\mathcal{T}} p(X_{\mathcal{S}}|E_{\mathcal{T}})p(\mathcal{T}). \tag{1}$$

Given the epitome, we can perform inference in this model and compute the posterior distribution over mappings $\mathcal{T}$ for a particular model. For instance, for $X_{\mathcal{S}} = RQKK$, the most probable mapping is $\mathcal{T} = \{(1,4), (1,5), (1,6), (1,7)\}$. In Section 4, we discuss algorithms for estimating the epitome distributions.

Our illustration points to possible applications of epitomes to multiple sequence alignment, and therefore requires a short discussion on similarity to other biological sequence models [3]. While the epitome is a fully probabilistic model and thus defines a precise cost function for optimization, as was the case with HMM-based models, or dynamic programming solutions to sequence alignment, the main novelty in our approach is the consideration of both the data and the model parameters in terms of overlapping patches. This leads to the alignment of different parts of the sequences to the joint representation without explicit constraints on contiguity of the mappings or temporal models used in HMMs. Also, as we discuss in the next section, our goal is diversity modeling, and *not* multiple alignment. The epitome's robustness to the length, position and variability of repeating sequence fragments allows us to bypass both the task of optimal global alignment, and the problem of *defining* the notion of global alignment. In addition, consideration of overlapping patches in a biological sequence can be viewed as modeling independent binding processes, making the patch independence assumption of our generative model biologically relevant. We illustrate these properties of the epitome on the problem of HIV diversity modeling and rational vaccine design.

3   HIV evolution and rational vaccine design

Recent work on the rational design of HIV vaccines has turned to cocktail approaches with the intention of protecting a person against many possible variants of the HIV virus. One of the potential difficulties with cocktail design is vaccine size. Vaccines with a large number of nucleotides or amino acids are expensive to manufacture and more difficult to deliver. In this section, we will show that epitome modeling can overcome this limitation by providing a means for generating smaller vaccines representing a wide diversity of HIV in an immunologically relevant way. We focus on the problem of constructing an optimal cellular vaccine in terms of its coverage of MHC-I epitopes, short contiguous patterns of 8-11 aminoacids in HIV proteins [8].

Major histocompatibility complex (MHC) molecules are responsible for presentation of short segments of internal proteins, called "epitopes," on the surface of a cell. These peptides (protein segments) can then be observed from outside the cell by killer T-cells, which normally react only to foreign peptides, instructing the cell to self-distruct. The killer cells and their offspring have the opportunity to bind to multiple infected cells, and so their first binding to a particular foreign epitope is used to accelerate an immune reaction to other infected cells exposing the same epitope. Such responses are called memory responses and can persist for a long time after the infection has been cleared, providing longer-term immunity to the disease. The goal of vaccine design is to create artifical means to produce such immunological memory of a particular virus without the danger of developing the disease.

In the case of a less variable virus, the vaccination may be possible by delivering a foreign protein similar to the viral protein into a patient's cells, triggering the immune response. However, HIV is capable of assuming many different forms, and immunization against a single strain is largely expected to be insufficient. In fact, without appropriate optimization, the number of different proteins needed to cover the viral diversity would be too large for the known vaccine delivery mechanisms. It is well known that epitopes within and across the strains in a population overlap [7]. The epitome model naturally exploits this overlap to construct a vaccine that can prime the immune system to attack as many potential epitopes as possible. For instance, if the sequences in Fig 1 were HIV fragments from different strains of the virus, then the epitome would contain many potential epitopes of lengths 8-11 from these sequences. Furthermore, the context of the captured epitopes in the epitome is similar to the context in the epitomized sequences, which increases the chances of equivalent presentation of the epitome and data epitopes.

MHC molecules are encoded within the most diverse region of the human genome. This gives our species a diversity advantage in numerous clashes with viruses. Each individual has a slightly different set of MHC molecules which bind to different motifs in the proteins expressed and cleaved in the cell. Due to the limitation in MHC binding, each person's cells are capable of presenting only a small number of epitopes from the invading virus, but an entire human population attacks a diverse set of epitopes. The MHC molecule selects the protein fragments for presentation through a binding process which is loosely motif-specific. There are several other processes that precede or follow the MHC binding, and the combination of all of these processes can be characterized either by the concentration of presented epitopes, or by the combination of the binding energies involved in these processes[2]. Some of these processes can be influenced by a context of the epitope (short amino acid fragments in the regions on either side of the epitope).

Another issue to be considered in HIV evolution and vaccine design is the T-cell cross reactivity: The killer cells primed with one epitope may be capable of binding to other related epitopes, and therefore a small set of priming epitopes may induce a broader immunity. As in the case of MHC binding, the likelihood of priming a T-cell, as well as cross-reaction with a different epitope, can be linked to the binding energies.

The epitome model maps directly to these immunity variables. If the epitome content is to be delivered to a cell in the vaccination phase, then each patch $E_{\mathcal{T}}$ indexed by data index set $\mathcal{T}$ corresponds either to an epitope or to a longer contiguous patch (e.g. 12 amino acids or more) containing both an epitope and its context that influences presentation. The prior $p(\mathcal{T})$ reflects the probability of presentation of the epitome fragments, and should reflect processes invloved in presentation, including MHC binding. The presented epitome fragments $E_{\mathcal{T}}$ in different patients' cells may prime T-cells capable of cross-reacting with some of the epitopes $\mathbf{X}_S$ presented by the infected cells infected by one of the known strains in the dataset $\mathbf{X}$. The cross-reaction distribution corresponds to the epitome distribution $p(\mathbf{X}_S|E_{\mathcal{T}})$. Vaccination is successful if the vaccine primes the immune system to attack targets found in the known circulating strains. A natural criterion to optimize is the similarity between the distribution over the epitopes learned by the immune systems of patients vaccinated with the epitome (taking into account the cross-reactivity) and the distribution over the epitopes from circulating strains. Therefore, the vaccine quality directly depends on the likelihood of the designated epitopes $p(X_S)$ under the epitome. To see this, consider directly optimizing the KL divergence between the distribution $p_d(\mathbf{X}_s)$ over epitopes found in the data and the distribution over the targets for which the T-cells are primed according to $p(\mathbf{X}_s)$. This KL distance differs from the log likelihood of all the data patches weighted by $p_d(\mathbf{X}_s)$,

$$\log p(\{X_S\}_d) = \sum_S p_d(X_S) \log \sum_{\mathcal{T}} p(X_S|E_{\mathcal{T}})p(\mathcal{T}), \tag{2}$$

only by a constant (the entropy of $p_d(\mathbf{X}_s)$). The distribution $p_d(\mathbf{X}_s)$ can serve as the indicator of epitopes and be equal to either zero or a constant for all patches, and then the above weighted likelihood is equivalent to the total likelihood of selected patches. This

---

[2]The probabilities of physical events are often modeled as having an exponential relationship with the energy changes.

distribution can also reflect the probability of presentation of epitopes X_S, or the uncertainty of the experiment or the prediction algorithm used to predict which parts of the circulating strains correspond to MHC epitopes.

While the epitome can serve as a diversity model and be used to construct evolutionary models and peptides for experimental epitope discovery, it can also serve as as an actual immungen (the pattern containing the immunologically important message to the cell) in vaccine. The most general version of epitome as a sequence of mutlinomial distributions could be relevant for sequence classification, recombination modeling, and design of peptides for binding essays. In some of these applications, the distribution $p(X_S|E_T)$ may have a semantics different than cross-reactivity, and could for instance represent mutations dependent on the immune type of the host, or the subtype of the virus. On the other hand, when the epitome is used for immunogen design, then cross-reactivity $p(X_S|E_T)$ can be conveniently captured by constraining each distribution e_{mn} to have probabilities for the twenty aminoacids from the set $\{\frac{\epsilon}{19}, 1 - \epsilon\}$. The mode of the epitome can then be used as a deterministic vaccine immunogen[3], and the probability of cross-reaction will then directly depend on the number of letters in $\mathbf{X}_S$ that are different from the mode of E_T.

While the epitome model components are mapped here to the elements of the interaction between HIV and the immune system of the host, other applications in biology would probably be based on a different semantics for the epitome components. We would expect that the epitome would map to biological sequence analysis problems more naturally than to image and audio modeling tasks, where the issue of the partition function arises. Epitome as a generative model over-generates - generated patches overlap, and so each data element is generated multiple times. In the image applications, we have avoided this problem through constraints on the posterior distributions, while the traditional approach would be to deal with the partition function (perhaps through sampling). However, the strains of a virus are observed by the immune system through overlapping patches, independently sampled from the viral proteins by biological processes. This fits epitome as a vaccination model. More generally, epitome is compatible with the evolutionary forces that act independently on overlapping patches of a biological sequence.

4 Epitome learning

Since epitomes can have multiple applications, we provide a general discussion of optimization of all parameters of the epitome, although in some applications, some of the parameters may be known a priori. As a unified optimization criterion we use the free energy [9] of the model (2),

$$F(\{X_S\}_d|E) = \sum_S p_d(X_S) \sum_T q(T|S) \log \frac{q(T|S)}{p(X_S|E_T)\,p(T)}, \qquad (3)$$

where $q(T|S)$ is an variational distribution, where

$$-\log p(\{X_S\}_d|E) = \arg\min_q F(\{X_S\}_d|E). \qquad (4)$$

The model can be learned by iteratively reducing F, varying in each iteration either q or the model parameters. When modeling biological sequences, the free energy *may* be associated with real physical events, such as molecular binding processes, where log probabilities correspond to molecular binding energies.

Setting to zero the derivatives of F with respect to the q distributions, the distribution $p(T)$, and the distributions $e_m(\ell)$ for all positions m, we obtain the EM algorithm [5]:

- For each X_S, compute the posterior distribution over patches $q(T|S)$:

$$q(T|S) \leftarrow \frac{p(X_S|E_T)\,p(T)}{\sum_T p(X_S|E_T)\,p(T)}. \qquad (5)$$

---

[3]To our knowledge, there is no effective way of delivering epitome as a distribution over proteins or fragments into the cell

- Using these q distributions, update the profile sequence:

$$e_m(\ell) \leftarrow \frac{\sum_{\mathcal{S}} p_d(X_{\mathcal{S}}) \sum_k \sum_{\mathcal{T}|\mathcal{T}(k)=m} q(\mathcal{T}|\mathcal{S})[X_{\mathcal{S}(k)} = \ell]}{\sum_{\mathcal{S}} p_d(X_{\mathcal{S}}) \sum_k \sum_{\mathcal{T}|\mathcal{T}(k)=m} q(\mathcal{T}|\mathcal{S})}, \tag{6}$$

where $[\cdot]$ is the indicator function ($[true] = 1$; $[false] = 0$). If desired, also update $p(\mathcal{T})$:

$$p(\mathcal{T}) \leftarrow \frac{\sum_{\mathcal{S}} p_d(X_{\mathcal{S}}) \, q(\mathcal{T}|\mathcal{S})}{\sum_{\mathcal{S}} p_d(X_{\mathcal{S}})}. \tag{7}$$

The E step assigns a responsibility for $\mathcal{S}$ to each possible epitome patch. The M step re-estimates the epitome multinomials using these responsibilities. As mentioned, this step can re-estimate the usage probabilities of patches in the epitome, or this distribution can be kept constant. It is often useful to construct the index sets $\mathcal{T}$ such that they wrap around from one end to another. Such circular topologies can deter the EM algorithm from settling in a poor local maximum of log likelihood. It is also sometimes useful to include a garbage component (a component that generates patches containing random letters) in the model.

In general, the EM algorithm is prone to problems of local maxima. For example, if we allowed the epitome to be longer, then some of the sites with two equally likely letters could be split into two separate regions of the epitome (and in some applications, such as vaccine optimization, this is preferred, as the epitomes need to become deterministic). Epitomes situated at different local maxima, however, often define similar probability distributions $p(\{X_{\mathcal{S}}\}|E)$, and can be used for various inference tasks such as sequence recognition/classification, noise removal, and context-dependent mutation prediction.

Of course, there are optimization algorithms other than EM that can learn a profile sequence by minimizing the free energy, $E = \arg\min_E \min_q F(\{X_{\mathcal{S}}\}_d|E)$. In some situations, such as vaccine design, it is desirable to produce deterministic epitomes (containing point-mass probability distributions). Such profile sequences can be obtained by annealing the parameter ϵ that controls the amount of probability allowed to be distributed to the letter different from the most likely letter $\hat{\ell}_m = \arg\max_\ell e_m(\ell)$:

$$E = \lim_{\epsilon \to 0} \arg\min_E \min_q F(\{X_{\mathcal{S}}\}_d|E). \tag{8}$$

Finally, in cases when the probability mass is uniformly spread over the letters other than the modes of the epitome distributions, i.e., $e_{mn}(\ell) \in \{\frac{\epsilon}{19}, 1 - \epsilon\}$, the myopic optimization is a faster way of creating epitomes of high fragment (epitope) coverage than the EM with multiple initializations. The myopic optimization consists of iteratively increasing the length of the epitome by appending a patch (possibly with overlap) from the data which maximally reduces the free energy. The process stops once the desired length is achieved (rather than when the entire set of patches is included as in the superstring problem).

5 Experiments

To illustrate the EM algorithm for epitome learning, we created the synthetic data shown (in part) in Figure 1. The data, eighty sequences in all, were synthesized from the generating profile sequence of length fifty shown on the top line of the figure. In particular, each data sequence was created by extracting one to four (mean two) patches from the generating sequence of length three to thirty (mean sixteen), sampling from these patches to produce corresponding patches of amino acids in the data sequence, and then filling in the gaps in the data sequence with amino acids sampled from a uniform distribution over amino acids. In addition, five percent of the sites in the each data sequence were subsequently replaced with an amino acid sampled from a uniform distribution. The resulting data sequences ranged in length from 38 to 43; and on average 80% of aminoacids in each sequence come from the generating sequence. Thus, the synthesized data roughly simulates genetic diversity resulting from a combination of mutation, insertion, deletion, and recombination.

We learned an epitome model using the EM algorithm applied to all 9mer patches from the data, equally weighted. We used a two-component epitome mixture, where the first component is an (initially unknown) sequence of probability distributions, and the second component is a garbage component, useful for representing the random insertions and mutations. Each site in the first component was initialized to a distribution slightly (and randomly) perturbed from uniform. The length of this component was set to be slightly longer than the original generating sequence. In previous experiments, we have found that a longer length helps to prevent the EM algorithm from settling in a poor local maximum of log likelihood, and it is subsequently possible to cut out unnecessary parts which can be detected in the learned prior $p(\mathcal{T})$. Also, we used an epitome with a circular topology. The first (non-garbage) component of the epitome learned after sixty iterations, shown in Figure 1, closely resembels the generating sequence even though it never saw this generating sequence during learning. (Roughly, the generating sequence starts near the end of the epitome with the patch "LIC" coded in red, and wraps around to the patch "EHQ" coded in yellow. The portion of the epitome between yellow and red is not responsible for many patches, as reflected in the distribution $p(\mathcal{T})$.) The sixty iterations of EM are illustrated in the video available at www.research.microsoft.com/~jojic/pEpitome.mpg. For each iteration, we show the first (non-garbage) component of the epitome E, the distribution $p(\mathcal{T})$, and the first ten sequences in the dataset, color-coded according to the mode of $q(\mathcal{T}|\mathcal{S})$, as in Figure 1. The video illustrates how the EM algorithm simultaneously learns the epitome model and aligns the data sequences.

When used for vaccine optimization, some epitome parameters can be preset based on biological knowledge. In particular, in the experiments we report on 176 gag HIV proteins from the WA cohort [8], we assume no cross reactivity (i.e., we set $\epsilon = 0$) and we consider two different possibilities for the patch data distribution $p_d(\mathbf{X}_\mathcal{S})$. The first parameter setting we consider is that $p_d(\mathbf{X}_\mathcal{S})$ is uniform for all ten amino-acid blocks found in the sequence data. The advantage of the uniform data distribution is that we only need sequence data for vaccine optimization, and not the epitome identities. The free energy criterion can be easily shown to be proportional (with a negative constant) to the coverage - the percentage of all 10mers from the data covered by the epitome, where the 10mer is considered covered if it can be found as a contiguous patch in the epitome's mode. Another advantage of this approach is that it can not miss epitopes due to errors in prediction algorithms or experimental epitope discovery, as long as sufficient coverage can be guaranteed for the given vaccine length.

The second setting of the parameters $p_d(\mathbf{X}_\mathcal{S})$ we consider is based the SYFPEITHI database [10] of known epitopes. We trained $p_d(\mathbf{X}_\mathcal{S})$ on this data using a decision tree model to represent the probability that an observed 10mer contains a presentable epitope. The advantage of this approach is that we can potentially focus our modeling power only to immunologically important variability, as long as the known epitope dataset is sufficient to capture properly the epitope distribution for at least the most frequent MHC-I molecules. Thus, for a given epitome length, we may obtain more potent vaccines than using the first parameter setting. Since $\epsilon = 0$, the resulting optimization reduces to optimizing *expected* epitope coverage, i.e., the sum of all probabilities

For both epitome settings, we epitomized the 176 gag proteins in the dataset, using the myopic algorithm, and compared the expected epitope coverage of our vaccine candidates with those of other designs, including cocktails of tree centers, consensus, and actual strains (Fig. 2). Phylogenies were constructed using neighbor joining, as is used in Phylip [4]. Clusters were generated using a mixture model of independent multinomials [1]. Observed sequences in the sequence cocktails were chosen at random. Both epitome models yield better coverage and the expected epitope coverage than other designs for any fixed length. Results are similar for the pol, nef, and env proteins. An interesting finding to note is that the epitome optimized for coverage (using uniform distribution $p_d(\mathbf{X}_\mathcal{S})$) provides essentially equally good expected coverage as the epitome directly optimized for the expected coverage. This is less surprising than it may seem - both true and predicted epitopes overlap in the sequence data, and so epitomizing all 10mers leads to similar epitomes as optimizing for coverage of the select few, but frequently overlapping epitopes. This is a direct consequence of the epitome representation, which was found appealing in previous applications for the same robustness to the number and sizes of the overlapping patches. It also indicates the possibility that an effective vaccine can be optimized without precise knowledge of all HIV epitopes.

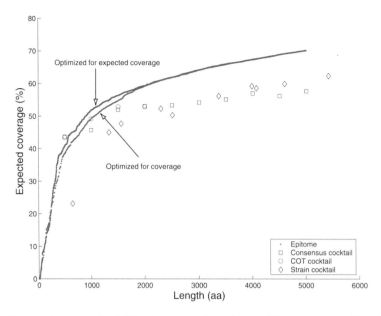

Figure 2: Expected coverage for 176 Perth gag proteins using candidate sequences of length ten. For comparison, we show expected coverage for the epitome optimized to cover all 10mers.

6 Conclusions

We have introduced the epitome as a new model of genetic diversity, especially well suited to highly variable biological sequences. We show that our model can be used to optimize HIV vaccines with larger predicted coverage of MHC-I epitopes than other constructs of similar lengths and so epitome can be used to create vaccines that cover a large fraction of HIV diversity. We also show that epitome optimization leads to good vaccines even when all subsequence of length 10 are considered epitopes. This suggests that the vaccines could be optimized directly from sequence data, which are technologically much easier to obtain than epitope data. Our analysis of cross-reactivity which provided similar empirical evidence of epitome robustness to cross-reactivity assumptions (see www.research.microsoft.com/~jojic/HIVepitome.html for the full set of results).

References and Notes

[1] P. Cheeseman and J. Stutz. Bayesian classification (AutoClass): Theory and results. In *Advances in Knowledge Discovery and Data Mining,* Fayyad, U., Piatesky-Shapiro, G., Smyth, P., and Uthurusamy, R., eds. (AAAI Press, 1995).

[2] V. Cheung, B. Frey, and N. Jojic. Video epitome. *CVPR* 2005.

[3] R. Durbin et al. *Biological Sequence Analysis : Probabilistic Models of Proteins and Nucleic Acids.* Cambridge University Press, 1998.

[4] J. Felsenstein. Phylip (phylogeny inference package) version 3.6, 2004.

[5] N. Jojic, B. Frey, and A. Kannan. Epitomic analysis of appearance and shape. In *Proceedings of the Ninth International Conference on Computer Vision,* Nice (2003). Video available at http://www.robots.ox.ac.uk/ awf/iccv03videos/.

[6] A. Kapoor and S. Basu. The audio epitome: A new representation for modeling and classifying auditory phenomena. *ICASSP* 2004.

[7] B.T.M. Korber, C. Brander, B.F. Haynes, R. Koup, C. Kuiken, J.P. Moore, B.D. Walker, and D.I. Watkins. *HIV Molecular Immunology.* Los Alamos National Laboratory, Theoretical Biology and Biophysics, Los Alamos, NM, 2002.

[8] C. Moore, M. John, I. James, F. Christiansen, C. Witt, and S. Mallal. Evidence of HIV-1 adaptation to HLA-restricted immune responses at a population level. *Science*, 296:1439–1443, 2002.

[9] R. Neal and G. Hinton. A view of the EM algorithm that justifies incremental, sparse, and other variants. In *Learning in graphical models*, M. Jordan ed. (MIT Press,1999).

[10] H Rammensee, J Bachmann, N P Emmerich, O A Bachor, and S Stevanovic. SYFPEITHI: database for MHC ligands and peptide motifs. *Immunogenetics*, 50(3-4):213–219, Nov 1999.

Integrate-and-Fire models with adaptation are good enough: predicting spike times under random current injection

Renaud Jolivet*
Brain Mind Institute, EPFL
CH-1015 Lausanne, Switzerland
renaud.jolivet@epfl.ch

Alexander Rauch
MPI for Biological Cybernetics
D-72012 Tübingen, Germany
alexander.rauch@tuebingen.mpg.de

Hans-Rudolf Lüscher
Institute of Physiology
CH-3012 Bern, Switzerland
luescher@pyl.unibe.ch

Wulfram Gerstner
Brain Mind Institute, EPFL
CH-1015 Lausanne, Switzerland
wulfram.gerstner@epfl.ch

Abstract

Integrate-and-Fire-type models are usually criticized because of their simplicity. On the other hand, the Integrate-and-Fire model is the basis of most of the theoretical studies on spiking neuron models. Here, we develop a sequential procedure to quantitatively evaluate an equivalent Integrate-and-Fire-type model based on intracellular recordings of cortical pyramidal neurons. We find that the resulting effective model is sufficient to predict the spike train of the real pyramidal neuron with high accuracy. In in vivo-like regimes, predicted and recorded traces are almost indistinguishable and a significant part of the spikes can be predicted at the correct timing. Slow processes like spike-frequency adaptation are shown to be a key feature in this context since they are necessary for the model to connect between different driving regimes.

1 Introduction

In a recent paper, Feng [1] was questioning the "goodness" of the Integrate-and-Fire model (I&F). This is a question of importance since the I&F model is one of the most commonly used spiking neuron model in theoretical studies as well as in the machine learning community (see [2-3] for a review). The I&F model is usually criticized in the biological community because of its simplicity. It is believed to be much too simple to capture the firing dynamics of real neurons beyond a very rough and conceptual description of input integration and spikes initiation.

Nevertheless, recent years have seen several groups reporting that this type of model yields quantitative predictions of the activity of real neurons. Rauch and colleagues have shown that I&F-type models (with adaptation) reliably predict the mean firing rate of cortical

---

* homepage: http://icwww.epfl.ch/~rjolivet

pyramidal cells [4]. Keat and colleagues have shown that a similar model is able to predict almost exactly the timing of spikes of neurons in the visual pathway [5]. However, the question is still open of how the predictions of I&F-type models compare to the precise structure of spike trains in the cortex. Indeed, cortical pyramidal neurons are known to produce spike trains whose reliability highly depends on the input scenario [6].

The aim of this paper is twofold. Firstly, we will show that there exists a systematic way to extract relevant parameters of an I&F-type model from intracellular recordings. To do so, we will follow the method exposed in [7] and which is based on optimal filtering techniques. Alternative approaches like maximum-likelihood methods exist and have been explored recently by Paninski and colleagues [8]. Note that both approaches had already been mentioned by Brillinger and Segundo [9]. Secondly, we will show by a quantitative evaluation of the model performances that the quality of simple threshold models is surprisingly good and is close to the intrinsic reliability of real neurons. We will try to convince the reader that, given the addition of a slow process, the I&F model is in fact a model that can be considered good enough for pyramidal neurons of the neocortex under random current injection.

2 Model and Methods

We started by collecting recordings. Layer 5 pyramidal neurons of the rat neocortex were recorded intracellularly in vitro while stimulated at the soma by a randomly fluctuating current generated by an Ornstein-Uhlenbeck (OU) process with a 1 ms autocorrelation time. Both the mean μ_I and the variance σ_I^2 of the OU process were varied in order to sample the response of the neurons to various levels of tonic and noisy inputs. Details of the experimental procedure can be found in [4]. A subset of these recordings was used to construct, separately for each recorded neuron, a generalized I&F-type model that we formulated in the framework of the Spike Response Model [3].

2.1 Definition of the model

The Spike Response Model (SRM) is written

$$u(t) = \eta(t - \hat{t}) + \int_0^{+\infty} \kappa(s)\, I(t - s)\mathrm{d}s \tag{1}$$

with u the membrane voltage of the neuron and I the external driving current. The kernel κ models the integrative properties of the membrane. The kernel η acts as a template for the shape of spikes (usually highly stereotyped). Like in the I&F model, the model neuron fires each time that the membrane voltage u crosses the threshold ϑ from below

$$\text{if } u(t) \geq \vartheta(t) \text{ and } \frac{d}{dt}u(t) \geq \frac{d}{dt}\vartheta(t), \text{ then } \hat{t} = t \tag{2}$$

Here, the threshold includes a mechanism of spike-frequency adaptation. ϑ is given by the following equation

$$\frac{\mathrm{d}\vartheta}{\mathrm{d}t} = -\frac{\vartheta - \vartheta_0}{\tau_\vartheta} + A_\vartheta \sum_k \delta(t - t_k) \tag{3}$$

Each time that a spike is fired, the threshold ϑ is increased by a fixed amount A_ϑ. It then decays back to its resting value ϑ_0 with time constant τ_ϑ. t_k denote the past firing times of the model neuron. During discharge at rate f, the threshold fluctuates around the average value

$$\bar{\vartheta} \approx \vartheta_0 + \alpha f \tag{4}$$

where $\alpha = A_\vartheta \tau_\vartheta$. This type of adaptation mechanism has been shown to constitute a universal model for spike-frequency adaptation [10] and has already been applied in a similar context [11]. During the model estimation, we use as a first step a traditional constant threshold denoted by $\vartheta(t) = \vartheta_{\text{cst}}$ which is then transformed in the adaptive threshold of Equation (3) by a procedure to be detailed below.

2.2 Mapping technique

The mapping technique itself is extensively described in [7,12-13] and we refer interested readers to these publications. In short, it is a systematic step-by-step evaluation and optimization procedure based on intracellular recordings. It consists in sequentially evaluating kernels (η and κ) and parameters [A_ϑ, ϑ_0 and τ_ϑ in Equation (3)] that characterize a specific instance of the model. The consecutive steps of the procedure are as follows

1. Extract the kernel η from a sample voltage recording by spike triggered averaging. For the sake of simplicity, we assume that the mean drive $\mu_I = 0$.

2. Subtract η from the voltage recording to isolate the subthreshold fluctuations.

3. Extract the kernel κ by the Wiener-Hopf optimal filtering technique [7,14]. This step involves a comparison between the subthreshold fluctuations and the corresponding input current.

4. Find the optimal constant threshold ϑ_{cst}. The optimal value of ϑ_{cst} is the one that maximizes the coefficient Γ (see subsection 2.3 below for the definition of Γ). The parameter ϑ_{cst} depends on the specific set of input parameters (mean μ_I and variance σ_I^2) used during stimulation.

5. Plot the threshold ϑ_{cst} as a function of the firing frequency f of the neuron and run a linear regression. ϑ_0 is identified with the value of the fit at $f = 0$ and α with the slope [see Equation (4) and Figure 1C].

6. Optimize A_ϑ for the best performances (again measured with Γ), τ_ϑ is defined as $\tau_\vartheta = \alpha/A_\vartheta$.

Figure 1A and B show kernels η (step 1) and κ (step 3) for a typical neuron. The double exponential shape of κ is due to the coupling between somatic and dendritic compartments [15]. Figure 1C shows the optimal constant ϑ_{cst} plotted versus f. It is very well fitted by a simple linear function and allows to determine the parameters ϑ_0 and α (steps 4 and 5).

2.3 Evaluation of performances

The performances of the model are evaluated with the coincidence factor Γ [16]. It is defined by

$$\Gamma = \frac{N_{\text{coinc}} - \langle N_{\text{coinc}} \rangle}{\frac{1}{2}(N_{\text{data}} + N_{\text{SRM}})} \frac{1}{\mathcal{N}} \tag{5}$$

where N_{data} is the number of spikes in the reference spike train, N_{SRM} is the number of spikes in the predicted spike train S_{SRM}, N_{coinc} is the number of coincidences with precision Δ between the two spike trains, and $\langle N_{\text{coinc}} \rangle = 2\nu\Delta N_{\text{data}}$ is the expected number of coincidences generated by a homogeneous Poisson process with the same rate ν as the spike train S_{SRM}. The factor $\mathcal{N} = 1 - 2\nu\Delta$ normalizes Γ to a maximum value $\Gamma = 1$ which is reached if and only if the spike train of the SRM reproduces exactly that of the cell. A homogeneous Poisson process with the same number of spikes as the SRM would yield $\Gamma = 0$. We compute the coincidence factor Γ by comparing the two complete spike trains as in [7]. Throughout the paper, we use $\Delta = 2\,\text{ms}$. Results do depend on Δ but the exact value of Δ is not critical as long as it is chosen in a reasonable range $1 \leq \Delta \leq 4\,\text{ms}$ [17]. The coincidence factor Γ is similar to the "reliability" as defined in [6]. All measures of Γ

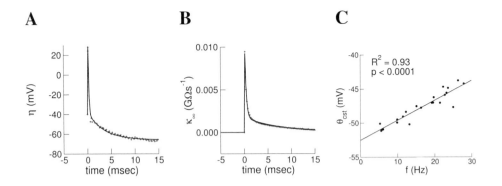

Figure 1: Kernels η (**A**) and κ (**B**) as extracted by the method exposed in this paper. Raw data (symbols) and fit by double exponential functions (solid line). **C.** The optimal constant threshold ϑ_{cst} is plotted versus the output frequency f (symbols). It is very neatly fitted by a linear function (line).

reported in this paper are given for new stimuli, independent of those used for parameter optimization during the model estimation procedure.

3   Results

Figure 2 shows a direct comparison between predicted and recorded spike train for a typical neuron. Both spike trains are almost indistinguishable (A). Even when zooming on the subthreshold regime, differences are in the range of a few millivolts only (B). The spike dynamics is correctly predicted apart from a short period of time just after a spike is emitted (C). This is due to the fact that the kernel η was extracted for a mean drive $\mu_I = 0$. Here, the mean is much larger than 0 and the neuron has already adapted to this new regime. It produces slightly different after-spike effects. This can be corrected easily in our framework by taking a time-dependent time constant in the kernel κ, i.e. $\kappa(s) \rightarrow \kappa(t - \hat{t}, s)$. This dependence is of importance to account for spike-to-spike interactions [18]. The mapping procedure discussed above allows, in principle, to compute $\kappa(t - \hat{t}, s)$ for any $t - \hat{t}$ (see [7] for further details). However, it requires longer recordings than the ones provided by our experiments and was dropped here.

Before moving to a quantitative estimate of the quality of the predictions of our model, we need to understand what kind of limits are imposed on predictions by the modelled neurons themselves. It is well known that pyramidal neurons of the cortex respond with very different reliability depending on the type of stimulation they receive [6]. Neurons tend to fire regularly but without conserving the exact timing of spikes in response to constant or quasi constant input current. On the other hand, they fire irregularly but reliably in terms of spike timing in response to fluctuating current. We do not expect our model to yield better predictions than the intrinsic reliability of the modelled neuron. To evaluate the intrinsic reliability of the pyramidal neurons, we repeated injection of the same OU process, i.e. injection of processes with the same seed, and computed Γ between the repeated spike trains obtained in response to this procedure. Figure 3A shows a surface plot of the intrinsic reliability $\Gamma_{n \rightarrow n}$ of a typical neuron (the subscript $n \rightarrow n$ is written for *neuron to itself*). It is plotted versus the parameters of the stimulation, the current mean drive μ_I and its standard deviation σ_I. We find that the mean drive μ_I has almost no impact on $\Gamma_{n \rightarrow n}$ (measured cross-correlation coefficient $r = 0.04$ with a p-value $p = 0.81$). On the other hand, σ_I has a strong impact on the reliability of the neuron ($r = 0.93$ with $p < 10^{-4}$). When σ_I is large ($\sigma_I \gtrsim 300\,\mathrm{pA}$), $\Gamma_{n \rightarrow n}$ reaches a plateau at about 0.84 ± 0.05 (mean $\pm$ s.d.).

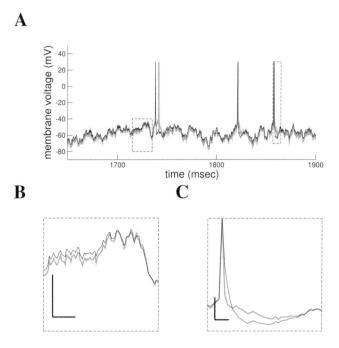

Figure 2: Performances of the SRM constructed by the method presented in this paper. **A.** The prediction of the model (black line) is compared to the spike train of the corresponding neuron (thick grey line). **B.** Zoom on the subthreshold regime. This panel corresponds to the first dotted zone in A (horizontal bar is 5 ms; vertical bar is 5 mV) **C.** Zoom on a correctly predicted spike. This panel corresponds to the second dotted zone in A (horizontal bar is 1 ms; vertical bar is 20 mV). The model slightly undershoots during about 4 ms after the spike (see text for further details).

When σ_I decreases to $100 \leq \sigma_I \leq 300$ pA, $\Gamma_{n \to n}$ quickly drops to an intermediate value of 0.65 ± 0.1 and finally for $\sigma_I \leq 100$ pA drops down to 0.09 ± 0.05. These findings are stable across the different neurons that we recorded and repeat the findings of Mainen and Sejnowski [6].

In order to connect model predictions to these findings, we evaluate the Γ coincidence factor between the predicted spike train and the recorded spike trains (this Γ is labelled $m \to n$ for *model to neuron*). Figure 3B shows a plot of $\Gamma_{m \to n}$ versus $\Gamma_{n \to n}$. We find that the predictions of our minimal model are close to the natural upper bound set by the intrinsic reliability of the pyramidal neuron. On average, the minimal model achieves a quality $\Gamma_{m \to n}$ which is 65% ($\pm 3\%$ s.e.m.) of the upper bound, i.e. $\Gamma_{m \to n} = 0.65 \Gamma_{n \to n}$. Furthermore, let us recall that due to the definition of the coincidence factor Γ, the threshold for statistical significance here is $\Gamma_{m \to n} = 0$. All the points are well above this value, hence highly significant. Finally, we compare the predictions of our minimal model in terms of two other indicators, the mean rate and the coefficient of variation of the interspike interval distribution (C_v). The mean rate is usually correctly predicted by our minimal model (see Figure 3C) in agreement with the findings of Rauch and colleagues [4]. The C_v is predicted in the correct range as well but may vary due to missed or extra spikes added in the prediction (data not shown). It is also noteworthy that available spike trains are not very long (a few seconds) and the number of spikes is sometimes too low to yield a reliable estimate of the C_v.

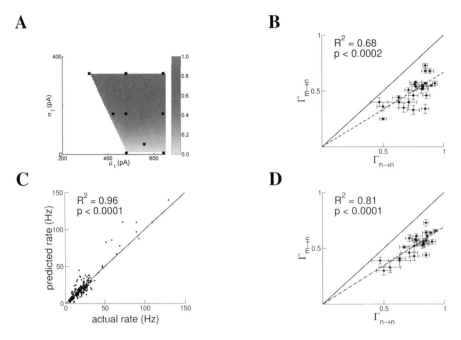

Figure 3: Quantitative performances of the model. **A.** Intrinsic reliability $\Gamma_{n \to n}$ of a typical pyramidal neuron in function of the mean drive μ_I and its standard deviation σ_I. **B.** Performances of the SRM in correct spike timing prediction $\Gamma_{m \to n}$ are plotted versus the cells intrinsic reliability $\Gamma_{n \to n}$ (symbols) for the very same stimulation parameters. The diagonal line (solid) denotes the "natural" upper bound limit imposed by the neurons intrinsic reliability. **C.** Predicted frequency versus actual frequency (symbols). **D.** Same as in A but in a model without adaptation where the threshold has been optimized separately for each set of stimulation parameters (see text for further details.)

Previous model studies had shown that a model with a threshold simpler than the one used here is able to reliably predict the spike train of more detailed neuron models [7,12]. Here, we used a threshold including an adaptation mechanism. Without adaptation, i.e. when the sum over all preceding spikes in Equation (3) is replaced by the contribution of the last emitted spike only, it is still possible to reach the same quality of predictions for each driving regime (Figure 3D) under the condition that the three threshold parameters (A_ϑ, ϑ_0 and τ_ϑ) are chosen differently for each set of input parameters μ_I and σ_I. In contrast to this, our I&F model with adaptation achieves the same level of predictive quality (Figure 3B) with one single set of threshold parameters. This illustrates the importance of adaptation to I&F models or SRM.

4 Discussion

Mapping real neurons to simplified neuronal models has benefited from many developments in recent years [4-5,7-8,11-13,19-22] and was applied to both in vitro [4,9,13,22] and in vivo recordings [5]. We have shown here that a simple estimation procedure allows to build an equivalent I&F-type model for a collection of cortical neurons. The model neuron is built sequentially from intracellular recordings. The resulting model is very efficient in the sense that it allows a quantitative and accurate prediction of the spike train of the real neuron. Most of the time, the predicted subthreshold membrane voltage differs from the recorded one by a few millivolts only. The mean firing rate of the minimal model corresponds to that of the real neuron. The statistical structure of the spike train is approximately conserved since we observe that the coefficient of variation (C_v) of the interspike interval distribution is predicted in the correct range by our minimal model. But most important, our minimal model has the ability to predict spikes with the correct timing ($\pm 2\,\mathrm{ms}$) and the level of prediction that is reached is close to the intrinsic reliability of the real neuron in terms of spike timing [6]. The adapting threshold has been found to play an important role. It allows the model to tune to variable input characteristics and to extend its predictions beyond the input regimes used for model evaluation.

This work suggests that L5 neocortical pyramidal neurons under random current injection behave very much like I&F neurons including a spike-frequency adaptation process. This is a result of importance. Indeed, the I&F-type models are extremely popular in large scale network studies. Our results can be viewed as a strong *a posteriori* justification to the use of this class of model neurons. They also indicate that the picture of a neuron combining a linear summation in the subthreshold regime with a threshold criterion for spike initiation is good enough to account for much of the behavior in an in vivo-like lab setting. This should however be moderated since several important aspects were neglected in this study.

First, we used random current injection rather than a more realistic random conductance protocol [23]. In a previous report [12], we had checked the consequences of random conductance injection with simulated data. We found that random conductance injection mainly changes the effective membrane time constant of the neuron and can be accounted for by making the time course of the optimal linear filter (κ here) depend on the mean input to the neuron. The minimal model reached the same quality level of predictions when driven by random conductance injection [12] as the level it reaches when driven by random current injection [7]. Second, a largely fluctuating current generated by a random process can only be seen as a poor approximation to the input a neuron would receive in vivo. Our input has stationary statistics with a spectrum that is close to white (cut-off at $1\,\mathrm{kHz}$), but a lower cut-off frequency could be used as well. Whether random input is a reasonable model of the input a neuron would receive in vivo is highly controversial [24-26], but from a purely practical point of view random stimulation provides at least a well-defined experimental paradigm for in vitro experiments that mimics some aspects of synaptic bombardment [27]. Third, all transient effects have been excluded since neuronal data is analyzed in the adapted state. Finally, our experimental paradigm used *somatic* current injection. Thus, all dendritic non-linearities, including backpropagating action potentials and dendritic spikes are excluded.

In summary, simple threshold models will never be able to account for all the variety of neuronal responses that can be probed in an artificial laboratory setting. For example, effects of delayed spike initiation cannot be reproduced by simple threshold models that combine linear subthreshold behavior with a strict threshold criterion (but could be reproduced by quadratic or exponential I&F models). For this reason, we are currently studying exponential I&F models with adaptation that allow us to relate our approach with other known models [21,28]. However, for random current injection that mimics synaptic bombardment, the picture of a neuron that combines linear summation with a threshold criterion is not too wrong. Moreover, in contrast to more complicated neuron models, the simple threshold model allows rapid parameter extraction from experimental traces; efficient numerical simulation; and rigorous mathematical analysis. Our results also suggest that, if any elaborated computation is taking place in single neurons, it is likely to happen at dendritic level rather than at somatic level. In absence of a clear understanding of dendritic computation, the I&F neuron with adaptation thus appears as a model that we consider "good enough".

Acknowledgments

This work was supported by *Swiss National Science Foundation* grants number FN 200020-103530/1 to WG and number 3100-061335.00 to HRL.

References

[1] Feng J. *Neural Net.* **14**: 955–975, 2001.

[2] Maass W & Bishop C. *Pulsed Neural Networks.* MIT Press, Cambridge, 1998.

[3] Gerstner W & Kistler W. *Spiking neurons models: single neurons, populations, plasticity.* Cambridge Univ. Press, Cambridge, 2002.

[4] Rauch A, La Camera G, Lüscher H, Senn W & Fusi S. *J. Neurophysiol.* **90**: 1598–1612, 2003.

[5] Keat J, Reinagel P, Reid R & Meister M. *Neuron* **30**: 803-817, 2001.

[6] Mainen Z and Sejnowski T. *Science* **268**: 1503–1506, 1995.

[7] Jolivet R, Lewis TJ & Gerstner W. *J. Neurophysiol.* **92**: 959–976, 2004.

[8] Paninski L, Pillow J & Simoncelli E. *Neural Comp.* **16**: 2533-2561, 2004.

[9] Brillinger D & Segundo J. *Biol. Cyber.* **35**: 213-220, 1979.

[10] Benda J & Herz A. *Neural Comp.* **15**: 2523-2564, 2003.

[11] La Camera G, Rauch A, Lüscher H, Senn W & Fusi S. *Neural Comp.* **16**: 2101-2124, 2004.

[12] Jolivet R & Gerstner W. *J. Physiol.-Paris* **98**: 442-451, 2004.

[13] Jolivet R, Rauch A, Lüscher H & Gerstner W. *Accepted in J. Comp. Neuro.*

[14] Wiener N. *Nonlinear problems in random theory.* MIT Press, Cambridge, 1958.

[15] Roth A & Häusser M. *J. Physiol.* **535**: 445-472, 2001.

[16] Kistler W, Gerstner W & van Hemmen J. *Neural Comp.* **9**: 1015-1045, 1997.

[17] Jolivet R (2005). *Effective minimal threshold models of neuronal activity.* PhD thesis, EPFL, Lausanne.

[18] Arcas B & Fairhall A. *Neural Comp.* **15**: 1789-1807, 2003.

[19] Brillinger D. *Ann. Biomed. Engineer.* **16**: 3-16, 1988.

[20] Arcas B, Fairhall A & Bialek W. *Neural Comp.* **15**: 1715-1749, 2003.

[21] Izhikevich E. *IEEE Trans. Neural Net.* **14**: 1569-1572, 2003.

[22] Paninski L, Pillow J & Simoncelli E. *Neurocomp.* **65-66**: 379-385, 2005.

[23] Robinson H & Kawai N. *J. Neurosci. Meth.* **49**: 157-165, 1993.

[24] Arieli A, Sterkin A, Grinvald A & Aertsen A. *Science* **273**: 1868–1871, 1996.

[25] De Weese M & Zador A. *J. Neurosci.* **23**: 7940–7949, 2003.

[26] Stevens C & Zador A. In *Proc. of the 5th Joint Symp. on Neural Comp.*, Inst. for Neural Comp., La Jolla, 1998.

[27] Destexhe A, Rudolph M & Paré D. *Nat. Rev. Neurosci.* **4**: 739-751, 2003.

[28] Fourcaud-Trocmé N, Hansel D, van Vreeswijk C & Brunel N. *J. Neurosci.* **23**: 11628-11640, 2003.

Generalization Error Bounds for Aggregation by Mirror Descent with Averaging

Anatoli Juditsky
Laboratoire de Modélisation et Calcul - Université Grenoble I
B.P. 53, 38041 Grenoble, France
anatoli.iouditski@imag.fr

Alexander Nazin
Institute of Control Sciences - Russian Academy of Science
65, Profsoyuznaya str., GSP-7, Moscow, 117997, Russia
nazine@ipu.rssi.ru

Alexandre Tsybakov
Laboratoire de Probabilités et Modèles Aléatoires - Université Paris VI
4, place Jussieu, 75252 Paris Cedex, France
tsybakov@ccr.jussieu.fr

Nicolas Vayatis
Laboratoire de Probabilités et Modèles Aléatoires - Université Paris VI
4, place Jussieu, 75252 Paris Cedex, France
vayatis@ccr.jussieu.fr

Abstract

We consider the problem of constructing an aggregated estimator from a finite class of base functions which approximately minimizes a convex risk functional under the ℓ_1 constraint. For this purpose, we propose a stochastic procedure, the mirror descent, which performs gradient descent in the dual space. The generated estimates are additionally averaged in a recursive fashion with specific weights. Mirror descent algorithms have been developed in different contexts and they are known to be particularly efficient in high dimensional problems. Moreover their implementation is adapted to the online setting. The main result of the paper is the upper bound on the convergence rate for the generalization error.

1 Introduction

We consider the aggregation problem (cf. [16]) where we have at hand a *finite* class of M predictors which are to be combined linearly under an ℓ_1 constraint $\|\theta\|_1 = \lambda$ on the vector $\theta \in \mathbb{R}^M$ that determines the coefficients of the linear combination. In order to exhibit such a combination, we focus on the strategy of penalized convex risk minimization which is motivated by recent statistical studies of boosting and SVM algorithms [11, 14, 18]. Moreover, we take a stochastic approximation approach which is particularly relevant in the online setting since it leads to recursive algorithms where the update uses a single data observation per iteration step. In this paper, we consider a general setting for which we propose a novel stochastic gradient algorithm and show tight upper bounds on its expected accuracy. Our algorithm builds on the ideas of mirror descent methods, first introduced by Nemirovski and Yudin [12], which consider updates of the gradient in the dual space. The mirror descent algorithm has been successfully applied in high dimensional problems both in deterministic and stochastic settings [2, 7]. In the present work, we describe a partic- ular instance of the algorithm with an entropy-like proxy function. This method presents similarities with the exponentiated gradient descent algorithm which was derived under dif- ferent motivations in [10]. A crucial distinction between the two is the additional averaging step in our version which guarantees statistical performance. The idea of averaging recur- sive procedures is well-known (see e.g. [13] and the references therein) and it has been invoked recently by Zhang [19] for the standard stochastic gradient descent (taking place in the initial parameter space). Also it is worth noticing that most of the existing online methods are evaluated in terms of relative loss bounds which are related to the empirical risk while we focus on generalization error bounds (see [4, 5, 10] for insights on connec- tions between the two types of criteria). The rest of the paper is organized as follows. We first introduce the setup (Section 2), then we describe the algorithm and state the main convergence result (Section 3). Further we provide the intuition underlying the proposed algorithm, and compare it to other methods (Section 4). We end up with a technical section dedicated to the proof of our main result (Section 5).

2 Setup and notations

Let Z be a random variable with values in a measurable space $(\mathcal{Z}, \mathcal{A})$. We set a parameter $\lambda > 0$, and an integer $M \geq 2$. The unknown parameter is a vector $\theta \in \mathbb{R}^M$ which is compelled to stay in the decision set $\Theta = \Theta_{M,\lambda}$ defined by:

$$\Theta_{M,\lambda} = \left\{ \theta = (\theta^{(1)}, \ldots, \theta^{(M)})^T \in \mathbb{R}_+^M : \sum_{i=1}^M \theta^{(i)} = \lambda \right\} . \tag{1}$$

Now we introduce the loss function $Q : \Theta \times \mathcal{Z} \to \mathbb{R}_+$ such that the random function $Q(\cdot, Z) : \Theta \to \mathbb{R}_+$ is convex for almost all Z and define the convex risk function $A : \Theta \to \mathbb{R}_+$ to be minimized as follows:

$$A(\theta) = \mathbb{E}\, Q(\theta, Z) . \tag{2}$$

Assume a training sample is given in the form of a sequence $(Z_1, \ldots, Z_{t-1})$, where each Z_i has the same distribution as Z. We assume for simplicity that the training sequence is i.i.d. though this assumption can be weakened.

We propose to minimize the convex target function A over the decision set Θ on the basis of the stochastic sub-gradients of Q:

$$u_i(\theta) = \nabla_\theta Q(\theta, Z_i), \quad i = 1, 2, \ldots, \tag{3}$$

Note that the expectations $\mathbb{E}\, u_i(\cdot)$ belong to the sub-differential of $A(\cdot)$.

In the sequel, we will characterize the accuracy of an estimate $\widehat{\theta}_t = \widehat{\theta}_t(Z_1, \ldots, Z_{t-1}) \in \Theta$ of the minimizer of A by the excess risk:

$$\mathbb{E}\, A(\widehat{\theta}_t) - \min_{\theta \in \Theta} A(\theta) \tag{4}$$

where the expectation is taken over the sample $(Z_1, \ldots, Z_{t-1})$.

We now introduce the notation that is necessary to present the algorithm in the next section.

For a vector $z = \left(z^{(1)}, \ldots, z^{(M)} \right)^T \in \mathbb{R}^M$, define the norms

$$\|z\|_1 \overset{\text{def}}{=} \sum_{j=1}^M \left| z^{(j)} \right|, \quad \|z\|_\infty \overset{\text{def}}{=} \max_{\|\theta\|_1 = 1} z^T \theta = \max_{j=1,\ldots,M} \left| z^{(j)} \right|.$$

The space $\mathbb{R}^M$ equipped with the norm $\| \cdot \|_1$ is called the primal space E and the same space equipped with the dual norm $\| \cdot \|_\infty$ is called the dual space E^*.

Introduce a so-called entropic proxy function:

$$\forall \theta \in \Theta, \quad V(\theta) = \lambda \ln (M/\lambda) + \sum_{j=1}^M \theta^{(j)} \ln \theta^{(j)}, \tag{5}$$

which has its minimum at $\theta_0 = (\lambda/M, \ldots, \lambda/M)^T$. It is easy to check that this function is α-strongly convex with respect to the norm $\| \cdot \|_1$ with parameter $\alpha = 1/\lambda$, i.e.,

$$V(sx + (1-s)y) \leq sV(x) + (1-s)V(y) - \frac{\alpha}{2} s(1-s)\|x - y\|_1^2 \tag{6}$$

for all $x, y \in \Theta$ and any $s \in [0, 1]$.

Let $\beta > 0$ be a parameter. We call β-*conjugate* of V the following convex transform:

$$\forall z \in \mathbb{R}^M, \quad W_\beta(z) \overset{\text{def}}{=} \sup_{\theta \in \Theta} \left\{ -z^T \theta - \beta V(\theta) \right\}.$$

As it straightforwardly follows from (5), the β-conjugate is given here by:

$$W_\beta(z) = \lambda \beta \ln \left(\frac{1}{M} \sum_{k=1}^M e^{-z^{(k)}/\beta} \right), \quad \forall z \in \mathbb{R}^M, \tag{7}$$

which has a Lipschitz-continuous gradient w.r.t. $\| \cdot \|_1$, namely,

$$\|\nabla W_\beta(z) - \nabla W_\beta(\tilde z)\|_1 \leq \frac{\lambda}{\beta} \|z - \tilde z\|_\infty, \quad \forall z, \tilde z \in \mathbb{R}^M. \tag{8}$$

Though we will focus on a particular algorithm based on the entropic proxy function, our results apply for a generic algorithmic scheme which takes advantage of the general properties of convex transforms (see [8] for details). The key property in the proof is the inequality (8).

3   Algorithm and main result

The mirror descent algorithm is a stochastic gradient algorithm in the dual space. At each iteration i, a new data point (X_i, Y_i) is observed and there are two updates: one is the value ζ_i as the result of the stochastic gradient descent in the dual space, the other is the update of the parameter θ_i which is the "mirror image" of ζ_i. In order to tune the algorithm properly, we need two fixed positive sequences $(\gamma_i)_{i \geq 1}$ (stepsize) and $(\beta_i)_{i \geq 1}$ (temperature) such that $\beta_i \geq \beta_{i-1}$. The *mirror descent algorithm with averaging* is as follows:

Algorithm.

- *Fix the initial values $\theta_0 \in \Theta$ and $\zeta_0 = 0 \in \mathbb{R}^M$.*
- *For $i = 1, \ldots, t - 1$, do*

$$\begin{aligned} \zeta_i &= \zeta_{i-1} + \gamma_i u_i(\theta_{i-1}), \\ \theta_i &= -\nabla W_{\beta_i}(\zeta_i). \end{aligned} \tag{9}$$

- Output at iteration t the following convex combination:

$$\hat{\theta}_t = \sum_{i=1}^{t} \gamma_i \theta_{i-1} \bigg/ \sum_{j=1}^{t} \gamma_j \,. \tag{10}$$

At this point, we actually have described a class of algorithms. Given the observations of the stochastic sub-gradient (3), particular choices of the proxy function V, of the stepsize and temperature parameters, will determine the algorithm completely. We discuss these choices with more details in [8]. In this paper, we focus on the entropic proxy function and consider a nearly optimal choice for the stepsize and temperature parameters which is the following:

$$\gamma_i \equiv 1, \quad \beta_i = \beta_0 \sqrt{i+1}, \quad i = 1, 2, \ldots, \quad \beta_0 > 0 \,. \tag{11}$$

We can now state our rate of convergence result.

Theorem. *Assume that the loss function Q satisfies the following boundedness condition:*

$$\sup_{\theta \in \Theta} \mathbb{E} \, \|\nabla_\theta Q(\theta, Z)\|_\infty^2 \leq L^2 < \infty \,. \tag{12}$$

Fix also $\beta_0 = L/\sqrt{\ln M}$.

Then, for any integer $t \geq 1$, the excess risk of the estimate $\hat{\theta}_t$ described above satisfies the following bound:

$$\mathbb{E} \, A(\hat{\theta}_t) - \min_{\theta \in \Theta} A(\theta) \leq 2 \, L\lambda \, (\ln M)^{1/2} \frac{\sqrt{t+1}}{t} \,. \tag{13}$$

Example. Consider the setting of supervised learning where the data are modelled by a pair (X, Y) with $X \in \mathcal{X}$ being an observation vector and Y a label, either integer (classification) or real-valued (regression). Boosting and SVM algorithms are related to the minimization of a functional

$$R(f) = \mathbb{E}\varphi(Y f(X))$$

where φ is a convex non-negative cost function (typically exponential, logit or hinge loss) and f belongs to a given class of combined predictors. The aggregation problem consists in finding the best linear combination of elements from a finite set of predictors $\{h_1, \ldots, h_M\}$ with $h_j : \mathcal{X} \to [-K, K]$. Taking compact notations, it means that we search for f of the form $f = \theta^T H$ with H denoting the vector-valued function whose components are these base predictors:

$$H(x) = (h_1(x), \ldots, h_M(x))^T \,,$$

and θ belonging in a decision set $\Theta = \Theta_{M,\lambda}$. Take for instance φ to be non-increasing. It is easy to see that this problem can be interpreted in terms of our general setting with $Z = (X, Y)$, $Q(Z, \theta) = \varphi(Y \theta^T H(X))$ and $L = K\varphi'(K\lambda)$. ∎

4 Discussion

In this section, we provide some insights on the method and the result of the previous section.

4.1 Heuristics

Suppose that we want to minimize a convex function $\theta \mapsto A(\theta)$ over a convex set Θ. If $\theta_0, \ldots, \theta_{t-1}$ are the available search points at iteration t, we can provide the affine approximations ϕ_i of the function A defined, for $\theta \in \Theta$, by

$$\phi_i(\theta) = A(\theta_{i-1}) + (\theta - \theta_{i-1})^T \nabla A(\theta_{i-1}), \quad i = 1, \ldots, t \,.$$

Here $\theta \mapsto \nabla A(\theta)$ is a vector function belonging to the sub-gradient of $A(\cdot)$. Taking a convex combination of the ϕ_i's, we obtain an averaged approximation of $A(\theta)$:

$$\bar{\phi}_t(\theta) = \frac{\sum_{i=1}^{t} \gamma_i \left(A(\theta_{i-1}) + (\theta - \theta_{i-1})^T \nabla A(\theta_{i-1}) \right)}{\sum_{i=1}^{t} \gamma_i}.$$

At first glance, it would seem reasonable to choose as the next search point a vector $\theta \in \Theta$ minimizing the approximation $\bar{\phi}_t$, i.e.,

$$\theta_t = \arg\min_{\theta \in \Theta} \bar{\phi}_t(\theta) = \arg\min_{\theta \in \Theta} \theta^T \left(\sum_{i=1}^{t} \gamma_i \nabla A(\theta_{i-1}) \right). \tag{14}$$

However, this does not make any progress, because our approximation is "good" only in the vicinity of search points $\theta_0, \ldots, \theta_{t-1}$. Therefore, it is necessary to modify the criterion, for instance, by adding a special penalty $B_t(\theta, \theta_{t-1})$ to the target function in order to keep the next search point θ_t in the desired region. Thus, one chooses the point:

$$\theta_t = \arg\min_{\theta \in \Theta} \left[\theta^T \left(\sum_{i=1}^{t} \gamma_i \nabla A(\theta_{i-1}) \right) + B_t(\theta, \theta_{t-1}) \right]. \tag{15}$$

Our algorithm corresponds to a specific type of penalty $B_t(\theta, \theta_{t-1}) = \beta_t V(\theta)$, where V is the proxy function. Also note that in our problem the vector-function $\nabla A(\cdot)$ is not available. Therefore, we replace in (15) the unknown gradients $\nabla A(\theta_{i-1})$ by the observed stochastic sub-gradients $u_i(\theta_{i-1})$. This yields a new definition of the t-th search point:

$$\theta_t = \arg\min_{\theta \in \Theta} \left[\theta^T \left(\sum_{i=1}^{t} \gamma_i u_i(\theta_{i-1}) \right) + \beta_t V(\theta) \right] = \arg\max_{\theta \in \Theta} \left[-\zeta_t^T \theta - \beta_t V(\theta) \right], \tag{16}$$

where $\zeta_t = \sum_{i=1}^{t} \gamma_i u_i(\theta_{i-1})$. By a standard result of convex analysis (see e.g. [3]), the solution to this problem reads as $-\nabla W_{\beta_t}(\zeta_t)$ and it is now easy to deduce the iterative scheme (9) of the mirror descent algorithm.

4.2 Comparison with previous work

The versions of mirror descent method proposed in [12] are somewhat different from our iterative scheme (9). One of them, closest to ours, is studied in detail in [3]. It is based on the recursive relation

$$\theta_i = -\nabla W_1 \left(-\nabla V(\theta_{i-1}) + \gamma_i u_i(\theta_{i-1}) \right), \quad i = 1, 2, \ldots, \tag{17}$$

where the function V is strongly convex with respect to the norm of initial space E (which is not necessarily the space ℓ_1^M) and W_1 is the 1-conjugate function to V.

If $\Theta = \mathbb{R}^M$ and $V(\theta) = \frac{1}{2}\|\theta\|_2^2$, the scheme of (17) coincides with the ordinary gradient method.

For the unit simplex $\Theta = \Theta_{M,1}$ and the entropy type proxy function V from (5) with $\lambda = 1$, the coordinates $\theta_i^{(j)}$ of vector θ_i from (17) are:

$$\forall j = 1, \ldots, M, \quad \theta_i^{(j)} = \frac{\theta_0^{(j)} \exp\left(-\sum_{m=1}^{i} \gamma_m u_{m,j}(\theta_{m-1}) \right)}{\sum_{k=1}^{M} \theta_0^{(k)} \exp\left(-\sum_{m=1}^{i} \gamma_m u_{m,k}(\theta_{m-1}) \right)}. \tag{18}$$

The algorithm is also known as the exponentiated gradient (EG) method [10]. The differences between the algorithm (17) and ours are the following:

- the initial iterative scheme of the Algorithm is different than that of (17), particularly, it includes the second tuning parameter β_i; moreover, the algorithm (18) uses initial value θ_0 in a different manner;

- our algorithm contains the additional averaging step of the updates (10).

The convergence properties of the EG method (18) have been studied in a deterministic setting [6]. Namely, it has been shown that, under some assumptions, the difference $A_t(\theta_t) - \min_{\theta \in \Theta_{M,1}} A_t(\theta)$, where A_t is the empirical risk, is bounded by a constant depending on M and t. If this constant is small enough, these results show that the EG method provides good numerical minimizers of the empirical risk A_t. The averaging step allows the use of the results provided in [5] to derive generalization error bounds from relative loss bounds. This technique leads to rates of convergence of the order $\sqrt{(\ln M)/t}$ as well but with suboptimal multiplicative factor in λ.

Finally, we point out that the algorithm (17) may be deduced from the ideas mentioned in Subsection 4.1 and which are studied in the literature on proximal methods within the field of convex optimization (see, e.g., [9, 1] and the references therein). Namely, under rather general conditions, the variable θ_i from (17) solves the the minimization problem

$$\theta_i = \arg\min_{\theta \in \Theta} \left(\theta^T \gamma_i u_i(\theta_{i-1}) + B(\theta, \theta_{i-1})\right), \tag{19}$$

where the penalty $B(\theta, \theta_{i-1}) = V(\theta) - V(\theta_{i-1}) - (\theta - \theta_{i-1})^T \nabla V(\theta_{i-1})$ represents the Bregman divergence between θ and θ_{i-1} related to the function V.

4.3 General comments

Performance and efficiency. The rate of convergence of order $\sqrt{\ln M}/\sqrt{t}$ is typical without low noise assumptions (as they are introduced in [17]). Batch procedures based on minimization of the empirical convex risk functional present a similar rate. From the statistical point of view, there is no remarkable difference between batch and our mirror-descent procedure. On the other hand, from the computational point of view, our procedure is quite comparable with the direct stochastic gradient descent. However, the mirror-descent algorithm presents two major advantages as compared both to batch and to direct stochastic gradient: (i) its behavior with respect to the cardinality of the base class is better than for direct stochastic gradient descent (of the order of $\sqrt{\ln M}$ in the Theorem, instead of M or $\sqrt{M}$ for direct stochastic gradient); (ii) mirror-descent presents a higher efficiency especially in high-dimensional problems as its algorithmic complexity and memory requirements are of strictly smaller order than for corresponding batch procedures (see [7] for a comparison).

Optimality of the rate of convergence. Using the techniques of [7] and [16] it is not hard to prove minimax lower bound on the excess risk $\mathbb{E}\, A(\widehat{\theta}_t) - \min_{\theta \in \Theta_{M,\lambda}} A(\theta)$ having the order $(\ln M)^{1/2}/\sqrt{t}$ for $M \geq t^{1/2+\delta}$ with some $\delta > 0$. This indicates that the upper bound of the Theorem is rate optimal for such values of M.

Choice of the base class. We point out that the good behaviour of this method crucially relies on the choice of the base class of functions $\{h_j\}_{1 \leq j \leq M}$. As far as theory is concerned, in order to provide a complete statistical analysis, one should establish approximation error bounds on the quantity $\inf_{f \in \mathcal{F}_{M,\lambda}} A(f) - \inf_f A(f)$ showing that the richness of the base class is reflected both by diversity (orthogonality or independence) of the h_j's and by its cardinality M. For example, one can take h_j's as the eigenfunctions associated to some positive definite kernel. We refer to [14], [15], for related results. The choice of λ can be motivated by similar considerations. In fact, to minimize the approximation error it might be useful to take λ depending on the sample size t and tending to infinity with some slow rate as in [11]. A balance between the stochastic error as given in the Theorem and the approximation error would then determine the optimal choice of λ.

5 Proof of the Theorem

Introduce the notation $\nabla A(\theta) = \mathbb{E}u_i(\theta)$ and $\xi_i(\theta) = u_i(\theta) - \nabla A(\theta)$. Put $v_i = u_i(\theta_{i-1})$ which gives $\zeta_i - \zeta_{i-1} = \gamma_i v_i$. By continuous differentiability of $W_{\beta_{t-1}}$ and by (8) we have:

$$
\begin{aligned}
W_{\beta_{i-1}}(\zeta_i) &= W_{\beta_{i-1}}(\zeta_{i-1}) + \gamma_i v_i^T \nabla W_{\beta_{i-1}}(\zeta_{i-1}) \\
&\quad + \gamma_i \int_0^1 v_i^T \left[\nabla W_{\beta_{i-1}}(\tau\zeta_i + (1-\tau)\zeta_{i-1}) - \nabla W_{\beta_{i-1}}(\zeta_{i-1}) \right] d\tau \\
&\leq W_{\beta_{i-1}}(\zeta_{i-1}) + \gamma_i v_i^T \nabla W_{\beta_{i-1}}(\zeta_{i-1}) + \frac{\lambda \gamma_i^2 \|v_i\|_\infty^2}{2\beta_{i-1}} .
\end{aligned}
$$

Then, using the fact that $(\beta_i)_{i \geq 1}$ is a non-decreasing sequence and that, for z fixed, $\beta \mapsto W_\beta(z)$ is a non-increasing function, we get

$$
W_{\beta_i}(\zeta_i) \leq W_{\beta_{i-1}}(\zeta_i) \leq W_{\beta_{i-1}}(\zeta_{i-1}) - \gamma_i \theta_{i-1}^T v_i + \frac{\lambda \gamma_i^2 \|v_i\|_\infty^2}{2\beta_{i-1}} .
$$

Summing up over the i's and using the representation $\zeta_t = \sum_{i=1}^t \gamma_i v_i$, we get:

$$
\forall \theta \in \Theta, \quad \sum_{i=1}^t \gamma_i(\theta_{i-1} - \theta)^T v_i \leq -W_{\beta_t}(\zeta_t) - \zeta_t^T \theta + \sum_{i=1}^t \frac{\lambda \gamma_i^2 \|v_i\|_\infty^2}{2\beta_{i-1}}
$$

since $W_{\beta_0}(\zeta_0) = 0$. From definition of W_β, we have, $\forall \zeta \in \mathbb{R}^M$ and $\forall \theta \in \Theta$, $-W_{\beta_t}(\zeta) - \zeta^T \theta \leq \beta_t V(\theta)$. Finally, since $v_i = \nabla A(\theta_{i-1}) + \xi_i(\theta_{i-1})$, we get

$$
\sum_{i=1}^t \gamma_i(\theta_{i-1} - \theta)^T \nabla A(\theta_{i-1}) \leq \beta_t V(\theta) - \sum_{i=1}^t \gamma_i(\theta_{i-1} - \theta)^T \xi_i(\theta_{i-1}) + \sum_{i=1}^t \frac{\lambda \gamma_i^2 \|v_i\|_\infty^2}{2\beta_{i-1}} .
$$

As we are to take expectations, we note that, conditioning on θ_{i-1} and using the independence between θ_{i-1} and (X_i, Y_i), we have: $\mathbb{E}\left((\theta_{i-1} - \theta)^T \xi_i(\theta_{i-1})\right) = 0$. Now, convexity of A and the previous display lead to:

$$
\begin{aligned}
\forall \theta \in \Theta, \quad \mathbb{E} A(\widehat{\theta}_t) - A(\theta) &\leq \frac{\sum_{i=1}^t \gamma_i \mathbb{E}\left[(\theta_{i-1} - \theta)^T \nabla A(\theta_{i-1})\right]}{\sum_{i=1}^t \gamma_i} \\
&= \frac{1}{t} \sum_{i=1}^t \mathbb{E}\left[(\theta_{i-1} - \theta)^T \nabla A(\theta_{i-1})\right] \\
&\leq \frac{\sqrt{t+1}}{t}\left(\beta_0 V^* + \frac{\lambda L^2}{\beta_0}\right),
\end{aligned}
$$

where we have set $V^* = \max_{\theta \in \Theta} V(\theta)$ and made use of the boundedness assumption $\mathbb{E}\|u_i(\theta)\|_\infty^2 \leq L^2$ and of the particular choice for the stepsize and temperature parameters. Noticing that $V^* = \lambda \ln M$ and optimizing this bound in $\beta_0 > 0$, we obtain the result.

Acknowledgments

We thank Nicolò Cesa-Bianchi for sharing with us his expertise on relative loss bounds.

References

[1] Beck, A. & Teboulle, M. (2003) Mirror descent and nonlinear projected subgradient methods for convex optimization. *Operations Research Letters*, 31:167–175.

[2] Ben-Tal, A., Margalit, T. & Nemirovski, A. (2001) The Ordered Subsets Mirror Descent optimization method and its use for the Positron Emission Tomography reconstruction problem. *SIAM J. on Optimization*, 12:79–108.

[3] Ben-Tal, A. & Nemirovski, A.S. (1999) The conjugate barrier mirror descent method for non-smooth convex optimization. MINERVA Optimization Center Report, Technion Institute of Technology.
Available at http://iew3.technion.ac.il/Labs/Opt/opt/Pap/CP_MD.pdf

[4] Cesa-Bianchi, N. & Gentile, C. (2005) Improved risk tail bounds for on-line algorithms. Submitted.

[5] Cesa-Bianchi, N., Conconi, A. & Gentile, C. (2004) On the generalization ability of on-line learning algorithms. *IEEE Transactions on Information Theory*, 50(9):2050–2057.

[6] Helmbold, D.P., Kivinen, J. & Warmuth, M.K. (1999) Relative loss bounds for single neurons. *IEEE Trans. on Neural Networks*, 10(6):1291–1304.

[7] Juditsky, A. & Nemirovski, A. (2000) Functional aggregation for nonparametric estimation. Annals of Statistics, 28(3): 681–712.

[8] Juditsky, A.B., Nazin, A.V., Tsybakov, A.B. & Vayatis N. (2005) Recursive Aggregation of Estimators via the Mirror Descent Algorithm with Averaging. Technical Report LPMA, Université Paris 6.
Available at http://www.proba.jussieu.fr/pageperso/vayatis/publication.html

[9] Kiwiel, K.C. (1997) Proximal minimization methods with generalized Bregman functions. *SIAM J. Control Optim.*, 35:1142–1168.

[10] Kivinen J. & Warmuth M.K. (1997) Additive versus exponentiated gradient updates for linear prediction. *Information and Computation*, Vol.132(1): 1–64.

[11] Lugosi, G. & Vayatis, N. (2004) On the Bayes-risk consistency of regularized boosting methods (with discussion). *Annals of Statistics*, 32(1): 30–55.

[12] Nemirovski, A.S. & Yudin, D.B. (1983) *Problem Complexity and Method Efficiency in Optimization*. Wiley-Interscience.

[13] Polyak, B.T. & Juditsky, A.B. (1992) Acceleration of stochastic approximation by averaging. *SIAM J. Control Optim.*, 30:838–855.

[14] Scovel, J.C. & Steinwart, I. (2005) Fast Rates for Support Vector Machines. In Proceedings of the 18th Conference on Learning Theory (COLT 2005), Bertinoro, Italy.

[15] Tarigan, B. & van de Geer, S. (2004) Adaptivity of Support Vector Machines with ℓ_1 Penalty. Preprint, University of Leiden.

[16] Tsybakov, A. (2003) Optimal Rates of Aggregation. Proceedings of COLT'03, LNCS, Springer, Vol. 2777:303–313.

[17] Tsybakov, A. (2004) Optimal aggregation of classifiers in statistical learning. *Annals of Statistics*, 32(1):135–166.

[18] Zhang, T. (2004) Statistical behavior and consistency of classification methods based on convex risk minimization (with discussion). *Annals of Statistics*, 32(1):56–85.

[19] Zhang, T. (2004) Solving large scale linear prediction problems using stochastic gradient descent algorithms. In Proceedings of ICML'04.

From Batch to Transductive Online Learning

Sham Kakade
Toyota Technological Institute
Chicago, IL 60637
sham@tti-c.org

Adam Tauman Kalai
Toyota Technological Institute
Chicago, IL 60637
kalai@tti-c.org

Abstract

It is well-known that everything that is learnable in the difficult online setting, where an arbitrary sequences of examples must be labeled one at a time, is also learnable in the batch setting, where examples are drawn independently from a distribution. We show a result in the opposite direction. We give an efficient conversion algorithm from batch to online that is transductive: it uses future unlabeled data. This demonstrates the equivalence between what is properly and *efficiently* learnable in a batch model and a transductive online model.

1 Introduction

There are many striking similarities between results in the standard batch learning setting, where labeled examples are assumed to be drawn independently from some distribution, and the more difficult online setting, where labeled examples arrive in an arbitrary sequence. Moreover, there are simple procedures that convert any online learning algorithm to an equally good batch learning algorithm [8]. This paper gives a procedure going in the opposite direction.

It is well-known that the online setting is strictly harder than the batch setting, even for the simple one-dimensioanl class of threshold functions on the interval $[0, 1]$. Hence, we consider the online transductive model of Ben-David, Kushilevitz, and Mansour [2]. In this model, an arbitrary but unknown sequence of n examples $(x_1, y_1), \ldots, (x_n, y_n) \in \mathcal{X} \times \{-1, 1\}$ is fixed in advance, for some instance space $\mathcal{X}$. The set of unlabeled examples is then presented to the learner, $\Sigma = \{x_i | 1 \leq i \leq n\}$. The examples are then revealed, in an online manner, to the learner, for $i = 1, 2, \ldots, n$. The learner observes example x_i (along with all previous labeled examples $(x_1, y_1), \ldots, (x_{i-1}, y_{i-1})$ and the unlabeled example set Σ) and must predict y_i. The true label y_i is then revealed to the learner. After this occurs, the learner compares its number of mistakes to the minimum number of mistakes of any of a *target class* $\mathcal{F}$ of functions $f : \mathcal{X} \to \{-1, 1\}$ (such as linear threshold functions). Note that our results are in this type of *agnostic* model [7], where we allow for arbitrary labels, unlike the *realizable* setting, i.e., noiseless or PAC models, where it is assumed that the labels are consistent with some $f \in \mathcal{F}$.

With this simple *transductive* knowledge of what unlabeled examples are to come, one can use existing expert algorithms to *inefficiently* learn any class of finite VC dimension, similar to the batch setting. How does one use unlabeled examples *efficiently* to guarantee good online performance?

Our efficient algorithm A_2 converts a proper[1] batch algorithm to a proper online algorithm (both in the agnostic setting). At any point in time, it has observed some labeled examples. It then "hallucinates" random examples by taking some number of unlabeled examples and labeling them randomly. It appends these examples to those observed so far and predicts according to the batch algorithm that finds the hypothesis of minimum empirical error on the combined data.

The idea of "hallucinating" and optimizing has been used for designing efficient online algorithms [6, 5, 1, 10, 4] in situations where exponential weighting schemes were inefficient. The hallucination analogy was suggested by Blum and Hartline [4]. In the context of transductive learning, it seems to be a natural way to try to use the unlabeled examples in conjunction with a batch learner. Let #mistakes(f, σ_n) denote the number of mistakes of a function $f \in \mathcal{F}$ on a particular sequence $\sigma_n \in (\mathcal{X} \times \{-1, 1\})^n$, and #mistakes$(A, \sigma_n)$ denote the same quantity for a transductive online learning algorithm A. Our main theorem is the following.

Theorem 1. *Let $\mathcal{F}$ be a class of functions $f : \mathcal{X} \to \{-1, 1\}$ of VC dimension d. There is an* efficient *randomized transductive online algorithm that, for any $n > 1$ and $\sigma_n \in (\mathcal{X} \times \{-1, 1\})^n$,*

$$\mathbf{E}[\#mistakes(A_2, \sigma_n)] \leq \min_{f \in \mathcal{F}} \#mistakes(f, \sigma_n) + 2.5n^{3/4}\sqrt{d \log n}.$$

The algorithm is computationally efficient in the sense that it runs in time $\mathrm{poly}(n)$, *given an efficient proper batch learning algorithm.*

One should note that the bound on the error *rate* is the same as that of the best $f \in \mathcal{F}$ plus $O(n^{-1/4}\sqrt{d \log(n)})$, approaching 0 at a rate related to the standard VC bound.

It is well-known that, without regard to computational efficiency, the learnable classes of functions are exactly those with finite VC dimension. Consequently, the classes of functions learnable in the batch and transductive online settings are the same. The classes of functions properly learnable by computationally efficient algorithms in the proper batch and transductive online settings are identical, as well.

In addition to the new algorithm, this is interesting because it helps justify a long line of work suggesting that whatever can be done in a batch setting can also be done online. Our result is surprising in light of earlier work by Blum showing that a slightly different online model is harder than its batch analog for *computational reasons* and not information-theoretic reasons [3].

In Section 2, we define the transductive online model. In Section 3, we analyze the easier case of data that is realizable with respect to some function class, i.e., when there is some function of zero error in the class. In Section 4, we present and analyze the hallucination algorithm. In Section 5, we discuss open problems such as extending the results to improper learning and the efficient realizable case.

2 Models and definitions

The *transductive online model* considered by Ben-David, Kushlevitz, and Mansour [2], consists of an instance space $\mathcal{X}$ and label set $\mathcal{Y}$ which we will always take to be binary $\mathcal{Y} = \{-1, 1\}$. An arbitrary $n > 0$ and arbitrary sequence of labeled examples $(x_1, y_1), \ldots, (x_n, y_n)$ is fixed. One can think of these as being chosen by an adversary who knows the (possibly randomized) learning algorithm but not the realization of its random coin flips. For notational convenience, we define σ_i to be the subsequence of first i

---

[1]A *proper* learning algorithm is one that always outputs a hypothesis $h \in \mathcal{F}$.

labeled examples,

$$\sigma_i = (x_1, y_1), (x_2, y_2), \ldots, (x_i, y_i),$$

and Σ to be the set of all unlabeled examples in σ_n,

$$\Sigma = \{x_i \mid i \in \{1, 2, \ldots, n\}\}.$$

A transductive online learner A is a function that takes as input n (the number of examples to be predicted), $\Sigma \subseteq \mathcal{X}$ (the set of unlabeled examples, $|\Sigma| \leq n$), $x_i \in \Sigma$ (the example to be tested), and $\sigma_{i-1} \in (\Sigma \times \mathcal{Y})^{i-1}$ (the previous $i-1$ labeled examples) and outputs a prediction $\in \mathcal{Y}$ of y_i, for any $1 \leq i \leq n$. The number of mistakes of A on the sequence $\sigma_n = (x_1, y_1), \ldots, (x_n, y_n)$ is,

$$\#\text{mistakes}(A, \sigma_n) = |\{i \mid A(n, \Sigma, x_i, \sigma_{i-1}) \neq y_i\}|.$$

If A is computed by a randomized algorithm, then we similarly define $\mathbf{E}[\#\text{mistakes}(A, \sigma_n)]$ where the expectation is taken over the random coin flips of A. In order to speak of the learnability of a set $\mathcal{F}$ of functions $f : \mathcal{X} \to \mathcal{Y}$, we define

$$\#\text{mistakes}(f, \sigma_n) = |\{i \mid f(x_i) \neq y_i\}|.$$

Formally, paralleling agnostic learning [7],[2] we define an *efficient* transductive online learner A for class $\mathcal{F}$ to be one for which the learning algorithm runs in time poly(n) and achieves, for any $\epsilon > 0$,

$$\mathbf{E}[\#\text{mistakes}(A, \sigma_n)] \leq \min_{f \in \mathcal{F}} \#\text{mistakes}(f, \sigma_n) + \epsilon n,$$

for $n = \text{poly}(1/\epsilon)$.[3]

2.1 Proper learning

Proper batch learning requires one to output a hypothesis $h \in \mathcal{F}$. An efficient proper batch learning algorithm for $\mathcal{F}$ is a batch learning algorithm B that, given any $\epsilon > 0$, with $n = \text{poly}(1/\epsilon)$ many examples from any distribution $\mathcal{D}$, outputs an $h \in \mathcal{F}$ of expected error $\mathbf{E}[\Pr_{\mathcal{D}}[h(x) \neq y]] \leq \min_{f \in \mathcal{F}} \Pr_{\mathcal{D}}[f(x) \neq y] + \epsilon$ and runs in time poly(n).

Observation 1. *Any efficient proper batch learning algorithm B can be converted into an efficient empirical error minimizer M that, for any n, given any data set $\sigma_n \in (\mathcal{X} \times \mathcal{Y})^n$, outputs an $f \in \mathcal{F}$ of minimal empirical error on σ_n.*

Proof. Running B only on σ_n, B is not guaranteed to output a hypothesis of minimum empirical error. Instead, we set an error tolerance of B to $\epsilon = 1/(4n)$, and give it examples drawn uniformly from the distribution $\mathcal{D}$ which is uniform over the data σ_n (a type of bootstrap). If B indeed returns a hypothesis h of error less than $1/n$ more than the best $f \in \mathcal{F}$, it must be a hypothesis of minimum empirical error on σ_n. By Markov's inequality, with probability at most $1/4$, the generalization error is more than $1/n$. By repeating several times and take the best hypothesis, we get a success probability exponentially close to 1. The runtime is polynomial in n. $\qquad\square$

To define *proper* learning in an online setting, it is helpful to think of the following alternative definition of transductive online learning. In this variation, the learner must output a sequence of hypotheses $h_1, h_2, \ldots, h_n : \mathcal{X} \to \{-1, 1\}$. After the ith hypothesis h_i is output, the example (x_i, y_i) is revealed, and it is clear whether the learner made an error. Formally, the (possibly randomized) algorithm A' still takes as input n, Σ, and σ_{i-1} (but

---

[2]It is more common in online learning to bound the total number of mistakes of an online algorithm on an arbitrary sequence. We bound its error rate, as is usual for batch learning.

[3]The results in this paper could be replaced by high-probability $1 - \delta$ bounds at a cost of $\log 1/\delta$.

no longer x_i), and outputs $h_i : \mathcal{X} \to \{-1, 1\}$ and errs if $h_i(x_i) \neq y_i$. To see that this model is equivalent to the previous definition, note that any algorithm A' that outputs hypotheses h_i can be used to make predictions $h_i(x_i)$ on example i (it errs if $h_i(x_i) \neq y_i$). It is equally true but less obvious than any algorithm A in the previous model can be converted to an algorithm A' in this model. This is because A' can be viewed as outputting $h_i : \mathcal{X} \to \{-1, 1\}$, where the function h_i is defined by setting $h_i(x)$ equal to be the prediction of algorithm A on the sequence σ_{i-1} followed by the example x, for each $x \in \mathcal{X}$, i.e., $h_i(x) = A(n, \Sigma, x, \sigma_{i-1})$. (The same coins can be used if A and A' are randomized.) A (possibly randomized) transductive online algorithm in this model is defined to be *proper* for family of functions $\mathcal{F}$ if it always outputs $h_i \in \mathcal{F}$.

3   Warmup: the realizable case

In this section, we consider the *realizable* special case in which there is some $f \in \mathcal{F}$ which correctly labels all examples. In particular, this means that we only consider sequences σ_n for which there is an $f \in \mathcal{F}$ with #mistakes$(f, \sigma_n) = 0$. This case will be helpful to analyze first as it is easier.

Fix arbitrary $n > 0$ and $\Sigma = \{x_1, x_2, \ldots, x_n\} \subseteq \mathcal{X}$, $|\Sigma| \leq n$. Say there are at most L different ways to label the examples in Σ according to functions $f \in \mathcal{F}$, so $1 \leq L \leq 2^{|\Sigma|}$. In the transductive online model, L is determined by Σ and $\mathcal{F}$ only. Hence, as long as prediction occurs only on examples $x \in \Sigma$, there are effectively only L different functions in $\mathcal{F}$ that matter, and we can thus pick L such functions that give rise to the L different labelings. On the ith example, one could simply take majority vote of $f_j(x_i)$ over consistent labelings f_j (the so-called *halving algorithm*), and this would easily ensure at most $\log_2(L)$ mistakes, because each mistake eliminates at least half of the consistent labelings. One can also use the following proper learning algorithm.

Proper transductive online learning algorithm in the realizable case:

- Preprocessing: Given the set of unlabeled examples Σ, take L functions $f_1, f_2, \ldots, f_L \in \mathcal{F}$ that give rise to the L different labelings of $x \in \Sigma$.[4]
- ith prediction: Output a uniformly random function f from the f_j consistent with σ_{i-1}.

The above algorithm, while possibly very inefficient, is easy to analyze.

Theorem 2. *Fix a class of binary functions $\mathcal{F}$ of VC dimension d. The above randomized proper learning algorithm makes an expected $d \log(n)$ mistakes on any sequence of examples of length $n \geq 2$, provided that there is some mistake-free $f \in \mathcal{F}$.*

Proof. Let V_i be the number of labelings f_j consistent with the first i examples, so that $L = V_0 \geq V_1 \geq \cdots \geq V_n \geq 1$ and $L \leq n^d$, by Sauer's lemma [11] for $n \geq 2$, where d is the VC dimension of $\mathcal{F}$. Observe that the number of consistent labelings that make a mistake on the ith example are exactly $V_{i-1} - V_i$. Hence, the total expected number of mistakes is,

$$\sum_{i=1}^{n} \frac{V_{i-1} - V_i}{V_{i-1}} \leq \sum_{i=1}^{n} \left(\frac{1}{V_{i-1}} + \frac{1}{V_{i-1} - 1} + \cdots + \frac{1}{V_i + 1} \right) \leq \sum_{i=2}^{V_n} \frac{1}{i} \leq \log(L). \qquad \square$$

---

[4]More formally, take L functions with the following properties: for each pair $1 \leq j, k \leq L$ with $j \neq k$, there exists $x \in \Sigma$ such that $f_j(x) \neq f_k(x)$, and for every $f \in \mathcal{F}$, there exists a $1 \leq j \leq L$ with $f(x) = f_j(x)$ for all $x \in \Sigma$.

Hence the above algorithm achieves an error rate of $O(d \log(n)/n)$, which quickly approaches zero for large n. Note that, this closely matches what one achieves in the batch setting. Like the batch setting, no better bounds can be given up to a constant factor.

4 General setting

We now consider the more difficult unrealizable setting where we have an unconstrained sequence of examples (though we still work in a transductive setting). We begin by presenting an known (inefficnet) extension to the halving algorithm of the previous section, that works in the agnostic (unrealizable) setting that is similar to the previous algorithm.

Inefficient proper transductive online learning algorithm A_1:

- Preprocessing: Given the set of unlabeled examples Σ, take L functions $f_1, f_2, \ldots, f_L$ that give rise to the L different labelings of $x \in \Sigma$. Assign an initial *weight* $w_1 = w_2 = \ldots = w_L = 1$ to each function.
- Output f_j, where $1 \leq j \leq L$ is chosen with probability $\frac{w_j}{w_1 + \ldots + w_L}$.
- Update: for each j for which $f_j(x_i) \neq y_i$, reduce w_j,

$$ w_j := w_j \left(1 - \sqrt{\frac{\log L}{n}} \right). $$

Using an analysis very similar to that of Weighted Majority [9], one can show that, for any $n > 1$ and sequence of examples $\sigma_n \in (\mathcal{X} \times \{-1, 1\})^n$,

$$ \mathbf{E}[\#\text{mistakes}(A_1, \sigma_n)] = \min_{f \in \mathcal{F}} \#\text{mistakes}(f, \sigma_n) + 2\sqrt{dn \log n}, $$

where d is the VC dimension of $\mathcal{F}$. Note the similarity to the standard VC bound.

4.1 Efficient algorithm

We can only hope to get an efficient proper online algorithm when there is an efficient proper batch algorithm. As mentioned in section 2.1, this means that there is a batch algorithm M that, given any data set, efficiently finds a hypothesis $h \in \mathcal{F}$ of minimum empirical error. (In fact, most proper learning algorithms work this way to begin with.) Using this, our efficient algorithm is as follows.

Efficient transductive online learning algorithm A_2:

- Preprocessing: Given the set of unlabeled examples Σ, create a hallucinated data set τ as follows.
  1. For each example $x \in \Sigma$, choose integer r_x uniformly at random such that $-\sqrt[4]{n} \leq r_x \leq \sqrt[4]{n}$.
  2. Add $|r_x|$ copies of the example x labeled by the sign of r_x, $(x, \text{sgn}(r_x))$, to τ.
- To predict on x_i: output hypothesis $M(\tau \sigma_{i-1}) \in \mathcal{F}$, where $\tau \sigma_{i-1}$ is the concatenation of the hallucinated examples and the observed labeled examples so far.

The current algorithm predicts $f(x_i)$ based on $f = M(\tau \sigma_{i-1})$. We first begin by analyzing the hypothetical algorithm that used the function chosen on the next iteration, i.e. predict $f(x_i)$ based on $f = M(\tau \sigma_i)$. (Of course, this is impossible to implement because we do not know σ_i when predicting $f(x_i)$.)

Lemma 1. *Fix any $\tau \in (\mathcal{X} \times \mathcal{Y})^*$ and $\sigma_n \in (\mathcal{X} \times \mathcal{Y})^n$. Let A_2' be the algorithm that, for each i, predicts $f(x_i)$ based on $f \in \mathcal{F}$ which is any empirical minimizer on the concate-nated data $\tau\sigma_i$, i.e., $f = M(\tau\sigma_i)$. Then the total number of mistakes of A_2' is,*

$$\textit{\#mistakes}(A_2', \sigma_n) \le \min_{f \in \mathcal{F}} \textit{\#mistakes}(f, \tau\sigma_n) - \min_{f \in \mathcal{F}} \textit{\#mistakes}(f, \tau).$$

It is instructive to first consider the case where τ is empty, i.e., there are no hallucinated examples. Then, our algorithm that predicts according to $M(\sigma_{i-1})$ could be called "follow the leader," as in [6]. The above lemma means that if one could use the hypothetical "be the leader" algorithm then one would make no more mistakes than the best $f \in \mathcal{F}$. The proof of this case is simple. Imagine starting with the offline algorithm that uses $M(\sigma_n)$ on each example $x_1, \ldots, x_n$. Now, on the first $n - 1$ examples, replace the use of $M(\sigma_n)$ by $M(\sigma_{n-1})$. Since $M(\sigma_{n-1})$ is an error-minimizer on σ_{n-1}, this can only reduce the number of mistakes. Next replace $M(\sigma_{n-1})$ by $M(\sigma_{n-2})$ on the first $n - 2$ examples, and so on. Eventually, we reach the hypothetical algorithm above, and we have only decreased our number of mistakes. The proof of the above lemma follows along these lines.

Proof of Lemma 1. Fix empirical minimizers g_i on $\tau\sigma_i$ for $i = 0, 1, \ldots, n$, i.e., $g_i = M(\tau\sigma_i)$. For $i \ge 1$, let m_i be 1 if $g_i(x_j) \ne y_j$ and 0 otherwise. We argue by induc-tion on t that,

$$\textit{\#mistakes}(g_0, \tau) + \sum_{i=1}^{t} m_i \le \textit{\#mistakes of } g_t \textit{ on } \tau\sigma_t. \tag{1}$$

For $t = 0$, the two are trivially equal. Assuming it holds for t, we have,

$$\textit{\#mistakes}(g_0, \tau) + \sum_{i=1}^{t+1} m_i \le \textit{\#mistakes}(g_t, \tau\sigma_t) + m_{t+1}$$
$$\le \textit{\#mistakes}(g_{t+1}, \tau\sigma_t) + m_{t+1}$$
$$= \textit{\#mistakes}(g_{t+1}, \tau\sigma_{t+1}).$$

The first inequality above holds by induction hypothesis, and the second follows from the fact that g_t is an empirical minimizer of $\tau\sigma_t$. The equality establishes (1) for $t + 1$ and thus completes the induction. The total mistakes of the hypothetical algorithm proposed in the lemma is $\sum_{i=1}^{n} m_i$, which gives the lemma by rearranging (1) for $t = n$. $\square$

Lemma 2. *For any σ_n,*

$$\mathbf{E}_\tau[\min_{f \in \mathcal{F}} \textit{\#mistakes}(f, \tau\sigma_n)] \le \mathbf{E}_\tau[|\tau|/2] + \min_{f \in \mathcal{F}} \textit{\#mistakes}(f, \sigma_n).$$

For any $\mathcal{F}$ of VC dimension d,

$$\mathbf{E}_\tau[\min_{f \in \mathcal{F}} \textit{\#mistakes}(f, \tau)] \ge \mathbf{E}_\tau[|\tau|/2] - 1.5n^{3/4}\sqrt{d \log n}.$$

Proof. For the first part of the lemma, let $g = M(\sigma_n)$ be an empirical minimizer on σ_n. Then,

$$\mathbf{E}_\tau[\min_{f \in \mathcal{F}} \textit{\#mistakes}(f, \tau\sigma_n)] \le \mathbf{E}_\tau[\textit{\#mistakes}(g, \tau\sigma_n)] = \mathbf{E}_\tau[|\tau|/2] + \textit{\#mistakes}(g, \sigma_n).$$

The last inequality holds because, since each example in τ is equally likely to have a $\pm$ label, the expected number of mistakes of any fixed $g \in \mathcal{F}$ on τ is $\mathbf{E}[|\tau|/2]$.

Fix any $f \in \mathcal{F}$. For the second part of the lemma, observe that we can write the number of mistakes of f on τ as,

$$\textit{\#mistakes}(f, \tau) = \frac{|\tau| - \sum_{i=1}^{n} f(x_i)r_i}{2}.$$

616

Hence it suffices to show that, $\max_{f \in \mathcal{F}} \sum_{i=1}^{n} f(x_i) r_i \leq 3 n^{3/4} \sqrt{\log(L)}$.

Now $\mathbf{E}_{r_i}[f(x_i) r_i] = 0$ and $|f(x_i) r_i| \leq n^{1/4}$. Next, Chernoff bounds (on the scaled random variables $f(x_i) r_i n^{-1/4}$) imply that, for any $\alpha \leq 1$, with probability at most $e^{-n\alpha^2/2}$, $\sum_{i=1}^{n} f(x_i) r_i n^{-1/4} \geq n\alpha$. Put another way, for any $\beta < n$, with probability at most $e^{-n^{-3/2}\beta^2/2}$, $\sum f(x_i) r_i n^{-1/4} \geq \beta$. As observed before, we can reduce the problem to the L different labelings. In other words, we can assume that there are only L different functions. By the union bound, the probability that $\sum f(x_i) r_i \geq \beta$ for any $f \in \mathcal{F}$ is at most $L e^{-n^{-3/2}\beta^2/2}$. Now the expectation of a non-negative random variable X is $\mathbf{E}[X] = \int_0^\infty \Pr[X \geq x] dx$. Let $X = \max_{f \in \mathcal{F}} \sum_{i=1}^{n} f(x_i) r_i$. In our case,

$$\mathbf{E}[X] \leq \sqrt{2 \log(L)} n^{3/4} + \int_{\sqrt{2 \log(L)} n^{3/4}}^{\infty} L e^{-n^{-3/4} x^2/2} dx$$

By Mathematica, the above is at most $\sqrt{2 \log(L)} n^{3/4} + 1.254 n^{3/4} \leq 3 \sqrt{\log(L)} n^{3/4}$. Finally, we use the fact that $L \leq n^d$ by Sauer's lemma. $\qquad\square$

Unfortunately, we cannot use the algorithm A_2'. However, due to the randomness we have added, we argue that algorithm A_2 is quite close:

Lemma 3. *For any σ_n, for any i, with probability at least $1 - n^{-1/4}$ over τ, $M(\tau \sigma_{i-1})$ is an empirical minimizer of $\tau \sigma_i$.*

Proof. Define, $\mathcal{F}_+ = \{f \in \mathcal{F} \mid f(x_i) = 1\}$ and $\mathcal{F}_- = \{f \in \mathcal{F} \mid f(x_i) = -1\}$. WLOG, we may assume that $\mathcal{F}_+$ and $\mathcal{F}_-$ are both nonempty. For if not, i.e., if all $f \in \mathcal{F}$ predict the same sign $f(x_i)$, then the sets of empirical minimizers of $\tau \sigma_{i-1}$ and $\tau \sigma_i$ are equal and the lemma holds trivially. For any sequence $\pi \in (\mathcal{X} \times \mathcal{Y})^*$, define,

$$s_+(\pi) = \min_{f \in \mathcal{F}_+} \#\text{mistakes}(f, \pi) \text{ and } s_-(\pi) = \min_{f \in \mathcal{F}_-} \#\text{mistakes}(f, \pi).$$

Next observe that, if $s_+(\pi) < s_-(\pi)$ then $M(\pi) \in \mathcal{F}_+$. Similarly if $s_-(\pi) < s_+(\pi)$ then $M(\pi) \in \mathcal{F}_-$. If they are equal then $f(x_i)$ can be an empirical minimizer in either. WLOG let us say that the ith example is $(x_i, 1)$, i.e., it is labeled positively. This implies that $s_+(\tau \sigma_{i-1}) = s_+(\tau \sigma_i)$ and $s_-(\tau \sigma_{i-1}) = s_-(\tau \sigma_i) + 1$. It is now clear that if $M(\tau \sigma_{i-1})$ is not also an empirical minimizer of $\tau \sigma_i$ then $s_+(\tau \sigma_{i-1}) = s_-(\tau \sigma_{i-1})$.

Now the quantity $\Delta = s_+(\tau \sigma_{i-1}) - s_-(\tau \sigma_{i-1})$ is directly related to r_{x_i}, the signed random number of times that example x_i is hallucinated. If we fix σ_n and the random choices r_x for each $x \in \Sigma \setminus \{x_i\}$, as we increase or decrease r_i by 1, Δ correspondingly increases or decreases by 1. Since r_i was chosen from a range of size $2\lfloor n^{1/4} \rfloor + 1 \geq n^{1/4}$, $\Delta = 0$ with probability at most $n^{-1/4}$. $\qquad\square$

We are now ready to prove the main theorem.

Proof of Theorem 1. Combining Lemmas 1 and 2, if on each period i, we used any minimizer of empirical error on the data $\tau \sigma_i$, we would have a total number of mistakes of at most $\min_{f \in \mathcal{F}} \#\text{mistakes}(f, \sigma_n) + 1.5 n^{3/4} \sqrt{d \log n}$. Suppose A_2 does end up using such a minimizer on all but p periods. Then, its total number of mistakes can only be p larger than this bound. By Lemma 3, the expected number p of periods i in which an empirical minimizer of $\tau \sigma_i$ is not used is $\leq n^{3/4}$. Hence, the expected total number of mistakes of A_2 is at most,

$$\mathbf{E}_\tau[\#\text{mistakes}(A_2, \sigma_n)] \leq \min_{f \in \mathcal{F}} \#\text{mistakes}(f, \sigma_n) + 1.5 n^{3/4} \sqrt{d \log n} + n^{3/4}.$$

The above implies the theorem. $\qquad\square$

Remark 1. The above algorithm is still costly in the sense that we must re-run the batch error minimizer for each prediction we would like to make. Using an idea quite similar to the "follow the lazy leader" algorithm in [6], we can achieve the same expected error while only needing to call M with probability $n^{-1/4}$ on each example.

Remark 2. The above analysis resembles previous analysis of hallucination algorithms. However, unlike previous analyses, there is no exponential distribution in the hallucination here yet the bounds still depend only logarithmically on the number of labelings.

5 Conclusions and open problems

We have given an algorithm for learning in the transductive online setting and established several results between efficient proper batch and transductive online learnability. In the realizable case, however, we have not given a computationally efficient algorithm. Hence, it is an open question as to whether *efficient* learnability in the batch and transductive online settings are the same in the realizable case. In addition, our computationally efficient algorithm requires polynomially more examples than its inefficient counterpart. It would be nice to have the best of both worlds, namely a computationally efficient algorithm that achieves a number of mistakes that is at most $O(\sqrt{dn \log n})$. Additionally, it would be nice to remove the restriction to proper algorithms.

Acknowledgements. We would like to thank Maria-Florina Balcan, Dean Foster, John Langford, and David McAllester for helpful discussions.

References

[1] B. Awerbuch and R. Kleinberg. Adaptive routing with end-to-end feedback: Distributed learning and geometric approaches. In *Proc. of the 36th ACM Symposium on Theory of Computing*, 2004.

[2] S. Ben-David, E. Kushilevitz, and Y. Mansour. Online learning versus offline learning. *Machine Learning* 29:45-63, 1997.

[3] A. Blum. Separating Distribution-Free and Mistake-Bound Learning Models over the Boolean Domain. *SIAM Journal on Computing* 23(5): 990-1000, 1994.

[4] A. Blum, J. Hartline. Near-Optimal Online Auctions. In *Proceedings of the Proceedings of the Sixteenth Annual ACM-SIAM Symposium on Discrete Algorithms* (SODA), 2005.

[5] J. Hannan. Approximation to Bayes Risk in Repeated Plays. In M. Dresher, A. Tucker, and P. Wolfe editors, *Contributions to the Theory of Games, Volume 3*, p. 97-139, Princeton University Press, 1957.

[6] A. Kalai and S. Vempala. Efficient algorithms for the online decision problem. In *Proceedings of the 16th Conference on Computational Learning Theory*, 2003.

[7] M. Kearns, R. Schapire, and L. Sellie. Toward Efficient Agnostic Learning. *Machine Learning*, 17(2/3):115–141, 1994.

[8] N. Littlestone. From On-Line to Batch Learning. In *Proceedings of the 2nd Workshop on Computational Learning Theory*, p. 269-284, 1989.

[9] N. Littlestone and M. Warmuth. The Weighted Majority Algorithm. *Information and Computation*, 108:212-261, 1994.

[10] H. Brendan McMahan and Avrim Blum. Online Geometric Optimization in the Bandit Setting Against an Adaptive Adversary. In *Proceedings of the 17th Annual Conference on Learning Theory*, COLT 2004.

[11] N. Sauer. On the Densities of Families of Sets. *Journal of Combinatorial Theory, Series A*, 13, p 145-147, 1972.

[12] V. N. Vapnik. *Estimation of Dependencies Based on Empirical Data*, New York: Springer Verlag, 1982.

[13] V. N. Vapnik. *Statistical Learning Theory*, New York: Wiley Interscience, 1998.

Worst-Case Bounds for Gaussian Process Models

Sham M. Kakade
University of Pennsylvania

Matthias W. Seeger
UC Berkeley

Dean P. Foster
University of Pennsylvania

Abstract

We present a competitive analysis of some non-parametric Bayesian algorithms in a worst-case online learning setting, where no probabilistic assumptions about the generation of the data are made. We consider models which use a Gaussian process prior (over the space of all functions) and provide bounds on the regret (under the log loss) for commonly used non-parametric Bayesian algorithms — including Gaussian regression and logistic regression — which show how these algorithms can perform favorably under rather general conditions. These bounds explicitly handle the infinite dimensionality of these non-parametric classes in a natural way. We also make formal connections to the minimax and *minimum description length* (MDL) framework. Here, we show precisely how Bayesian Gaussian regression is a minimax strategy.

1 Introduction

We study an online (sequential) prediction setting in which, at each timestep, the learner is given some input from the set $\mathcal{X}$, and the learner must predict the output variable from the set $\mathcal{Y}$. The sequence $\{(x_t, y_t) \mid t = 1, \dots, T\}$ is chosen by Nature (or by an adversary), and importantly, we do not make any statistical assumptions about its source: our statements hold for *all* sequences. Our goal is to sequentially code the next label y_t, given that we have observed $\boldsymbol{x}_{\leq t}$ and $\boldsymbol{y}_{<t}$ (where $\boldsymbol{x}_{\leq t}$ and $\boldsymbol{y}_{<t}$ denote the sequences $\{x_1, \dots x_t\}$ and $\{y_1, \dots y_{t-1}\}$). At each time t, we have a conditional distribution $P(\cdot | \boldsymbol{x}_{\leq t}, \boldsymbol{y}_{<t})$ over $\mathcal{Y}$, which is our prediction strategy that is used to predict the next variable y_t. We then incur the instantaneous loss $-\log P(y_t | \boldsymbol{x}_{\leq t}, \boldsymbol{y}_{<t})$ (referred to as *log loss*), and the cumulative loss is the sum of these instantaneous losses over $t = 1, \dots, T$.

Let Θ be a parameter space indexing elementary prediction rules in some model class, where $P(y|x, \theta)$ for $\theta \in \Theta$ is a conditional distribution over $\mathcal{Y}$ called the *likelihood*. An *expert* is a single atom $\theta \in \Theta$, or, more precisely, the algorithm which outputs the predictive distribution $P(\cdot | x_t, \theta)$ for every t. We are interested in bounds on the *regret* — the difference in the cumulative loss of a given adaptive prediction strategy and the the cumulative loss of the best possible expert chosen in hindsight from a subset of Θ.

Kakade and Ng [2004] considered a parametric setting where $\Theta = \mathbb{R}^d$, $\mathcal{X} = \mathbb{R}^d$, and the prediction rules were generalized linear models, in which $P(y|x, \theta) = P(y|\theta \cdot x)$. They derived regret bounds for the Bayesian strategy (assuming a Gaussian prior over Θ), which showed that many simple Bayesian algorithms (such as Gaussian linear regression and logistic regression) perform favorably when compared, in retrospect, to the best $\theta \in \Theta$. Importantly, these regret bounds have a time and dimensionality dependence of the form $\frac{d}{2} \log T$ — a dependence common in in most MDL procedures (see Grunwald [2005]). For Gaussian linear regression, the bounds of Kakade and Ng [2004] are comparable to the best bounds in the literature, such as those of Foster [1991], Vovk [2001], Azoury and Warmuth

[2001] (though these latter bounds are stated in terms of the closely related square loss).

In this paper, we provide worst-case regret bounds on Bayesian non-parametric methods, which show how these algorithms can have low regret. In particular, we examine the case where the prior (over functions) is a Gaussian process — thereby extending the work of Kakade and Ng [2004] to infinite-dimensional spaces of experts. There are a number of important differences between this and the parametric setting. First, it turns out that the natural competitor class is the *reproducing kernel Hilbert space (RKHS)* $\mathcal{H}$. Furthermore, the notion of dimensionality is more subtle, since the space $\mathcal{H}$ may be infinite dimensional. In general, there is no apriori reason that any strategy (including the Bayesian one) should be able to compete favorably with the complex class $\mathcal{H}$. However, for some input sequences $\boldsymbol{x}_{\leq T}$ and kernels, we show that it is possible to compete favorably. Furthermore, the relation of our results to Kakade and Ng [2004] is made explicit in Section 3.2.

Our second contribution is in making formal connections to minimax theory, where we show precisely how Bayesian Gaussian regression is a minimax algorithm. In a general setting, Shtarkov [1987] showed that a certain *normalized maximum likelihood* (NML) distribution minimizes the regret in the worst case. Unfortunately, for some "complex" model classes, there may exist no strategy which achieves finite regret, and so the NML distribution may not exist.[1] Gaussian density estimation (formally described in Example 4.2) is one such case where this NML distribution does not exist. If one makes further restrictions (on $\mathcal{Y}$), then minimax results can be derived, such as in Takimoto and Warmuth [2000], Barron et al. [1998], Foster and Stine [2001].

Instead of making further restrictions, we propose minimizing a form of a *penalized regret*, where one penalizes more "complex" experts as measured by their cost under a prior $q(\theta)$. This penalized regret essentially compares our cumulative loss to the loss of a two part code (common in MDL, see Grunwald [2005]), where one first codes the model θ under a prior q and then codes the data using this θ. Here, we show that a certain *normalized maximum a posteriori* distribution is the corresponding minimax strategy, in general. Our main result here is in showing that for Gaussian regression, the Bayesian strategy is precisely this minimax strategy. The differences between this result and that of Takimoto and Warmuth [2000] are notable. In the later, they assume $\mathcal{Y} \subset \mathbb{R}$ is bounded and derive (near) minimax algorithms which hold the variance of their predictions *constant* at each timestep (so they effectively deal with the square loss). Under Bayes rule, the variance of the predictions adapts, which allows the minimax property to hold with $\mathcal{Y} = \mathbb{R}$ being unbounded.

Other minimax results have been considered in the non-parametric setting. The work of Opper and Haussler [1998] and Cesa-Bianchi and Lugosi [2001] provide minimax bounds in some non-parametric cases (in terms of a covering number of the comparator class), though they do not consider input sequences.

The rest of the paper is organized as follows: Section 2 summarizes our model, Section 3 presents and discusses our bounds, and Section 4 draws out the connections to the minimax and MDL framework. All proofs are available in a forthcoming longer version of this paper.

2 Bayesian Methods with Gaussian Process Priors

With a Bayesian prior distribution $P_{\text{bayes}}(\theta)$ over Θ, the Bayesian predicts y_t using the rule

$$P_{\text{bayes}}(y_t|\boldsymbol{x}_{\leq t}, \boldsymbol{y}_{<t}) = \int P(y_t|x_t, \theta) P_{\text{bayes}}(\theta|\boldsymbol{x}_{<t}, \boldsymbol{y}_{<t})\, d\theta$$

where the posterior is given by

$$P_{\text{bayes}}(\theta|\boldsymbol{x}_{<t}, \boldsymbol{y}_{<t}) \propto P(\boldsymbol{y}_{<t}|\boldsymbol{x}_{<t}, \theta) P_{\text{bayes}}(\theta).$$

---

[1] For these cases, the normalization constant of the NML distribution is not finite.

620

Assuming the Bayesian learner models the data to be independent given θ, then

$$P(\boldsymbol{y}_{<t}|\boldsymbol{x}_{<t}, \theta) = \prod_{t'=1}^{t-1} P(y_{t'}|x_{t'}, \theta).$$

It is important to stress that these are "working assumptions" in the sense that they lead to a prediction strategy (the Bayesian one), but the analysis does *not* make any probabilistic assumptions about the generation of the data. The cumulative loss of the Bayesian strategy is then

$$-\sum_{t=1}^{T} \log P_{\text{bayes}}(y_t|\boldsymbol{x}_{\leq t}, \boldsymbol{y}_{<t}) = -\log P_{\text{bayes}}(\boldsymbol{y}_{\leq T}|\boldsymbol{x}_{\leq T}).$$

which follows form the chain rule of conditional probabilities.

In this paper, we are interested in non-parametric prediction, which can be viewed as working with an infinite-dimensional function space Θ — assume Θ consists of real-valued functions $u(x)$. The likelihood $P(y|x, u(\cdot))$ is thus a distribution over y given x and the function $u(\cdot)$. Similar to Kakade and Ng [2004] (where they considered generalized linear models), we make the natural restriction that $P(y|x, u(\cdot)) = P(y|u(x))$. We can think of u as a latent function and of $P(y|u(x))$ as a noise distribution. Two particularly important cases are that of Gaussian regression and logistic regression. In *Gaussian regression*, we have that $\mathcal{Y} = \mathbb{R}$ and that $P(y|u(x)) = \mathcal{N}(y|u(x), \sigma^2)$ (so y is distributed as a Gaussian with mean $u(x)$ and fixed variance σ^2). In *logistic regression*, $\mathcal{Y} = \{-1, 1\}$ and $P(y|u(x)) = (1 + e^{-yu(x)})^{-1}$.

In this paper, we consider the case in which the prior $dP_{\text{bayes}}(u(\cdot))$ is a zero-mean *Gaussian process (GP)* with covariance function K, *i.e.* a real-valued random process which has the property that for every finite set $x_1, \ldots, x_n$ the random vector $(u(x_1), \ldots, u(x_n))^T$ is multivariate Gaussian, distributed as $\mathcal{N}(\boldsymbol{0}, \boldsymbol{K})$, where $\boldsymbol{K} \in \mathbb{R}^{n,n}$ is the covariance (or kernel) matrix with $\boldsymbol{K}_{i,j} = K(x_i, x_j)$. Note that K has to be a positive semidefinite function in that for all finite sets $x_1, \ldots, x_n$ the corresponding kernel matrices $\boldsymbol{K}$ are positive semidefinite.

Finally, we specify the subset of experts we would like the Bayesian prediction strategy to compete against. Every positive semidefinite kernel K is associated with a unique *reproducing kernel Hilbert space (RKHS)* $\mathcal{H}$, defined as follows: consider the linear space of all finite kernel expansions (over any $x_1, \ldots, x_n$) of the form $f(x) = \sum_{i=1}^{n} \alpha_i K(x, x_i)$ with the inner product

$$\left(\sum_i \alpha_i K(\cdot, x_i), \sum_j \beta_j K(\cdot, y_j) \right)_K = \sum_{i,j} \alpha_i \beta_j K(x_i, y_j).$$

and define the RKHS $\mathcal{H}$ as the completion of this space. By construction, $\mathcal{H}$ contains all finite kernel expansions $f(x) = \sum_{i=1}^{n} \alpha_i K(x, x_i)$ with

$$\|f\|_K^2 = \boldsymbol{\alpha}^T \boldsymbol{K} \boldsymbol{\alpha}, \quad \boldsymbol{K}_{i,j} = K(x_i, x_j). \tag{1}$$

The characteristic property of $\mathcal{H}$ is that all (Dirac) evaluation functionals are *represented* in $\mathcal{H}$ itself by the functions $K(\cdot, x_i)$, meaning $(f, K(\cdot, x_i))_K = f(x_i)$. The RKHS $\mathcal{H}$ turns out to be the largest subspace of experts for which our results are meaningful.

3 Worst-Case Bounds

In this section, we present our worst-case bounds, give an interpretation, and relate the results to the parametric case of Kakade and Ng [2004]. The proofs are available in a forthcoming longer version.

Theorem 3.1: *Let $(\boldsymbol{x}_{\leq T}, \boldsymbol{y}_{\leq T})$ be a sequence from $(\mathcal{X} \times \mathcal{Y})^T$. For all functions f in the RKHS $\mathcal{H}$ associated with the prior covariance function K, we have*

$$-\log P_{bayes}(\boldsymbol{y}_{\leq T}|\boldsymbol{x}_{\leq T}) \leq -\log P(\boldsymbol{y}_{\leq T}|\boldsymbol{x}_{\leq T}, f(\cdot)) + \frac{1}{2}\|f\|_K^2 + \frac{1}{2}\log|\boldsymbol{I} + c\boldsymbol{K}|,$$

where $\|f\|_K$ is the RKHS norm of f, $\boldsymbol{K} = (K(x_t, x_{t'})) \in \mathbb{R}^{T,T}$ is the kernel matrix over the input sequence $\boldsymbol{x}_{\leq T}$, and $c > 0$ is a constant such that for all $y_t \in \boldsymbol{y}_{\leq T}$,

$$-\frac{d^2}{du^2}\log P(y_t|u) \leq c$$

for all $u \in \mathbb{R}$.

The proof of this theorem parallels that provided by Kakade and Ng [2004], with a number of added complexities for handling GP priors. For the special case of Gaussian regression where $c = \sigma^{-2}$, the following theorem shows the stronger result that the bound is satisfied with an equality for all sequences.

Theorem 3.2: *Assume $P(y_t|u(x_t)) = \mathcal{N}(y_t|u(x_t), \sigma^2)$ and that $\mathcal{Y} = \mathbb{R}$. Let $(\boldsymbol{x}_{\leq T}, \boldsymbol{y}_{\leq T})$ be a sequence from $(\mathcal{X} \times \mathcal{Y})^T$. Then,*

$$-\log P_{bayes}(\boldsymbol{y}_{\leq T}|\boldsymbol{x}_{\leq T}) = \min_{f \in \mathcal{H}}\left\{-\log P(\boldsymbol{y}_{\leq T}|\boldsymbol{x}_{\leq T}, f(\cdot)) + \frac{1}{2}\|f\|_K^2\right\} \tag{2}$$

$$+ \frac{1}{2}\log|\boldsymbol{I} + \sigma^{-2}\boldsymbol{K}|$$

and the minimum is attained for a kernel expansion over $\boldsymbol{x}_{\leq T}$.

This equality has important implications in our minimax theory (in Corollary 4.4, we make this precise). It is not hard to see that the equality does not hold for other likelihoods.

3.1 Interpretation

The regret bound depends on two terms, $\|f\|_K^2$ and $\log|\boldsymbol{I} + c\boldsymbol{K}|$. We discuss each in turn. The dependence on $\|f\|_K^2$ states the intuitive fact that a meaningful bound can only be obtained under smoothness assumptions on the set of experts. The more complicated f is (as measured by $\|\cdot\|_K$), the higher the regret may be. The equality shows in Theorem 3.2 shows this dependence is unavoidable. We come back to this dependence in Section 4.

Let us now interpret the $\log|\boldsymbol{I} + c\boldsymbol{K}|$ term, which we refer to as the regret term. The constant c, which bounds the curvature of the likelihood, exists for most commonly used exponential family likelihoods. For logistic regression, we have $c = 1/4$, and for the Gaussian regression, we have $c = \sigma^{-2}$. Also, interestingly, while f is an arbitrary function in $\mathcal{H}$, this regret term depends on K only at the sequence points $\boldsymbol{x}_{\leq T}$.

For most infinite-dimensional kernels and without strong restrictions on the inputs, the regret term can be as large as $\Omega(T)$ — the sequence can be chosen s.t. $\boldsymbol{K} \approx c'\boldsymbol{I}$, which implies that $\log|\boldsymbol{I} + c\boldsymbol{K}| \approx T\log(1 + cc')$. For example, for an isotropic kernel (which is a function of the norm $\|x - x'\|_2$) we can choose the x_t to be mutually far from each other. For kernels which barely enforce smoothness — e.g. the Ornstein-Uhlenbeck kernel $\exp(-b\|x - x'\|_1)$ — the regret term can easily $\Omega(T)$. The cases we are interested in are those where the regret term is $o(T)$, in which case the average regret tends to 0 with time.

A spectral interpretation of this term helps us understand the behavior. If we let $\lambda_1, \lambda_2, \ldots \lambda_T$ be the eigenvalues of $\boldsymbol{K}$, then

$$\log|\boldsymbol{I} + c\boldsymbol{K}| = \sum_{t=1}^{T}\log(1 + c\lambda_t) \leq c\operatorname{tr}\boldsymbol{K}$$

where $\operatorname{tr} \mathbf{K}$ is the trace of $\mathbf{K}$. This last quantity is closely related to the "degrees of freedom" in a system (see Hastie et al. [2001]). Clearly, if the sum of the eigenvalues has a sublinear growth rate of $o(T)$, then the average regret tends to 0. Also, if one assumes that the input sequence, $\mathbf{x}_{\leq T}$, is i.i.d. then the above eigenvalues are essentially the *process* eigenvalues. In a forthcoming longer version, we explore this spectral interpretation in more detail and provide a case using the exponential kernel in which the regret grows as $O(\operatorname{poly}(\log T))$. We now review the parametric case.

3.2 The Parametric Case

Here we obtain a slight generalization of the result in Kakade and Ng [2004] as a special case. Namely, the familiar linear model — with $u(x) = \theta \cdot x$, $\theta, x \in \mathbb{R}^d$ and Gaussian prior $\theta \sim \mathcal{N}(\mathbf{0}, \mathbf{I})$ — can be seen as a GP model with the linear kernel: $K(x, x') = x \cdot x'$.

With $\mathbf{X} = (x_1, \ldots x_T)^{\mathsf{T}}$ we have that a kernel expansion $f(x) = \sum_i \alpha_i x_i \cdot x = \theta \cdot x$ with $\theta = \mathbf{X}^{\mathsf{T}} \boldsymbol{\alpha}$, and $\|f\|_K^2 = \boldsymbol{\alpha}^{\mathsf{T}} \mathbf{X} \mathbf{X}^{\mathsf{T}} \boldsymbol{\alpha} = \|\theta\|_2^2$, so that $\mathcal{H} = \{\theta \cdot x \,|\, \theta \in \mathbb{R}^d\}$, and so

$$\log |\mathbf{I} + c\mathbf{K}| = \log |\mathbf{I} + c\mathbf{X}^{\mathsf{T}}\mathbf{X}|$$

Therefore, our result gives an input-dependent version of the result of Kakade and Ng [2004]. If we make the further assumption that $\|x\|_2 \leq 1$ (as done in Kakade and Ng [2004]), then we can obtain exactly their regret term:

$$\log |\mathbf{I} + c\mathbf{K}| \leq d \log \left(1 + \frac{cT}{d}\right)$$

which can seen by rotating K into an diagonal matrix and maximizing the expression subject to the constraint that $\|x\|_2 \leq 1$ (i.e. that the eigenvalues must sum to 1).

In general, this example shows that if K is a finite-dimension kernel such as the linear or the polynomial kernel, then the regret term is only $O(\log T)$.

4 Relationships to Minimax Procedures and MDL

This section builds the framework for understanding the minimax property of Gaussian regression. We start by reviewing Shtarkov's theorem, which shows that a certain normalized maximum likelihood density is the minimax strategy (when using the log loss). In many cases, this minimax strategy does not exist — in those cases where the minimax regret is infinite. We then propose a different, penalized notion of regret, and show that a certain *normalized maximum a posteriori* density is the minimax strategy here. Our main result (Corollary 4.4) shows that for Gaussian regression the Bayesian strategy is precisely this minimax strategy

4.1 Normalized Maximum Likelihood

Here, let us assume that there are no inputs — sequences consist of only $y_t \in \mathcal{Y}$. Given a measurable space with base measure μ, we employ a countable number of random variables y_t in $\mathcal{Y}$. Fix the sequence length T and define the model class $\mathcal{F} = \{Q(\cdot|\theta) \,|\, \theta \in \Theta)\}$, where $Q(\cdot|\theta)$ denotes a joint probability density over $\mathcal{Y}^T$ with respect to μ.

We assume that for our model class there exists a parameter, $\theta_{\mathrm{ml}}(\mathbf{y}_{\leq T})$, maximizing the likelihood $Q(\mathbf{y}_{\leq T}|\theta)$ over Θ for all $\mathbf{y}_{\leq T} \in \mathcal{Y}^T$. We make this assumption to make the connections to maximum likelihood (and, later, MAP) estimation clear. Define the regret of a joint density P on $\mathbf{y}_{\leq T}$ as:

$$R(\mathbf{y}_{\leq T}, P, \Theta) \;=\; -\log P(\mathbf{y}_{\leq T}) - \inf_{\theta \in \Theta} \{-\log Q(\mathbf{y}_{\leq T}|\theta)\} \qquad (3)$$

$$=\; -\log P(\mathbf{y}_{\leq T}) + \log Q(\mathbf{y}_{\leq T}|\theta_{\mathrm{ml}}(\mathbf{y}_{\leq T}).) \qquad (4)$$

where the latter step uses our assumption on the existence of $\theta_{ml}(\boldsymbol{y}_{\leq T})$.

Define the minimax regret with respect to Θ as:

$$R(\Theta) = \inf_P \sup_{\boldsymbol{y}_{\leq T} \in \mathcal{Y}^T} R(\boldsymbol{y}_{\leq T}, P, \Theta)$$

where the inf is over all probability densities on $\mathcal{Y}^T$.

The following theorem due to Shtarkov [1987] characterizes the minimax strategy.

Theorem 4.1: *[Shtarkov, 1987]If the following density exists (i.e. if it has a finite normalization constant), then define it to be the* normalized maximum likelihood *(NML) density.*

$$P_{ml}(\boldsymbol{y}_{\leq T}) = \frac{Q(\boldsymbol{y}_{\leq T}|\theta_{ml}(\boldsymbol{y}_{\leq T}))}{\int Q(\boldsymbol{y}_{\leq T}|\theta_{ml}(\boldsymbol{y}_{\leq T}))d\mu(\boldsymbol{y}_{\leq T})} \tag{5}$$

If P_{ml} exists, it is a minimax strategy, i.e. for all $\boldsymbol{y}_{\leq T}$, the regret $R(\boldsymbol{y}_{\leq T}, P_{ml}, \Theta)$ does not exceed $R(\Theta)$.

Note that this density exists only if the normalizing constant is finite, which is not the case in general. The proof is straightforward using the fact that the NML density is an *equalizer* — meaning that it has *constant* regret on all sequences.

Proof: First note that the regret $R(\boldsymbol{y}_{\leq T}, P_{ml}, \Theta)$ is the constant $\log \int Q(\boldsymbol{y}_{\leq T}|\theta_{ml}(\boldsymbol{y}_{\leq T}))d\mu(\boldsymbol{y}_{\leq T})$. To see this, simply substitute Eq. 5 into Eq. 4 and simplify.

For convenience, define the regret of any P as $R(P, \Theta) = \sup_{\boldsymbol{y}_{\leq T} \in \mathcal{Y}^T} R(\boldsymbol{y}_{\leq T}, P, \Theta)$. For any $P \neq P_{ml}$ (differing on a set with positive measure), there exists some $\boldsymbol{y}_{\leq T}$ such that $P(\boldsymbol{y}_{\leq T}) < P_{ml}(\boldsymbol{y}_{\leq T})$, since the densities are normalized. This implies that

$$R(P, \Theta) \geq R(\boldsymbol{y}_{\leq T}, P, \Theta) > R(\boldsymbol{y}_{\leq T}, P_{ml}, \Theta) = R(P_{ml}, \Theta)$$

where the first step follows from the definition of $R(P, \Theta)$, the second from $-\log P(\boldsymbol{y}_{\leq T}) > -\log P_{ml}(\boldsymbol{y}_{\leq T})$, and the last from the fact that P_{ml} is an equalizer (its regret is constant on all sequences). Hence, P has a strictly larger regret, implying that P_{ml} is the unique minimax strategy. $\square$

Unfortunately, in many important model classes, the minimax regret $R(\Theta)$ is not finite, and the NML density does not exist. We now provide one example (see Grunwald [2005] for further discussion).

Example 4.2: Consider a model which assumes the sequence is generated i.i.d. from a Gaussian with unknown mean and unit variance. Specifically, let $\Theta = \mathbb{R}$, $\mathcal{Y} = R$, and $P(\boldsymbol{y}_{\leq T}|\theta)$ be the product $\Pi_{t=1}^T \mathcal{N}(y_t; \theta, 1)$. It is easy to see that for this class the minimax regret is infinite and P_{ml} does not exist (see Grunwald [2005]). This example can be generalized to the Gaussian regression model (if we know the sequence $x_{\leq T}$ in advance). For this problem, if one modifies the space of allowable sequences (i.e. $\mathcal{Y}^T$ is modified), then one can obtain finite regret, such as those in Barron et al. [1998], Foster and Stine [2001]. This technique may not be appropriate in general.

4.2 Normalized Maximum a Posteriori

To remedy this problem, consider placing some structure on the model class $\mathcal{F} = \{Q(\cdot|\theta)|\theta \in \Theta\}$. The idea is to penalize $Q(\cdot|\theta) \in \mathcal{F}$ based on this structure. The motivation is similar to that of structural risk minimization [Vapnik, 1998]. Assume that Θ is a measurable space and place a prior distribution with density function q on Θ. Define the *penalized regret* of P on $\boldsymbol{y}_{\leq T}$ as:

$$R_q(\boldsymbol{y}_{\leq T}, P, \Theta) = -\log P(\boldsymbol{y}_{\leq T}) - \inf_{\theta \in \Theta} \{-\log Q(\boldsymbol{y}_{\leq T}|\theta) - \log q(\theta)\}.$$

Note that $-\log Q(\boldsymbol{y}_{\leq T}|\theta) - \log q(\theta)$ can be viewed as a "two part" code, in which we first code θ under the prior q and then code $\boldsymbol{y}_{\leq T}$ under the likelihood $Q(\cdot|\theta)$. Unlike the standard regret, the penalized regret can be viewed as a comparison to an actual code. These two part codes are common in the MDL literature (see Grunwald [2005]). However, in MDL, they consider using minimax schemes (via P_{ml}) for the likelihood part of the code, while we consider minimax schemes for this penalized regret.

Again, for clarity, assume there exists a parameter, $\theta_{\mathrm{map}}(\boldsymbol{y}_{\leq T})$ maximizing $\log Q(\boldsymbol{y}_{\leq T}|\theta) + \log q(\theta)$. Notice that this is just the maximum aposteriori (MAP) parameter, if one were to use a Bayesian strategy with the prior q (since the posterior density would be proportional to $Q(\boldsymbol{y}_{\leq T}|\theta)q(\theta)$). Here,

$$R_q(\boldsymbol{y}_{\leq T}, P, \Theta) = -\log P(\boldsymbol{y}_{\leq T}) + \log Q(\boldsymbol{y}_{\leq T}|\theta_{\mathrm{map}}(\boldsymbol{y}_{\leq T})) + \log q(\theta_{\mathrm{map}}(\boldsymbol{y}_{\leq T}))$$

Similarly, with respect to Θ, define the minimax penalized regret as:

$$R_q(\Theta) = \inf_P \sup_{\boldsymbol{y}_{\leq T} \in \mathcal{Y}^T} R_q(\boldsymbol{y}_{\leq T} P, \Theta)$$

where again the inf is over all densities on $\mathcal{Y}^T$. If Θ is finite or countable and $Q(\cdot|\theta) > 0$ for all θ, then the Bayes procedure has the desirable property of having penalized regret which is non-positive.[2] However, in general, the Bayes procedure does not achieve the minimax penalized regret, $R_q(\Theta)$, which is what we desire — though, for one case, we show that it does (in the next section).

We now characterize this minimax strategy in general.

Theorem 4.3: *Define the* normalized maximum a posteriori *(NMAP) density, if it exists, as:*

$$P_{map}(\boldsymbol{y}_{\leq T}) = \frac{Q(\boldsymbol{y}_{\leq T}|\theta_{map}(\boldsymbol{y}_{\leq T}))q(\theta_{map}(\boldsymbol{y}_{\leq T}))}{\int Q(\boldsymbol{y}_{\leq T}|\theta_{map}(\boldsymbol{y}_{\leq T}))q(\theta_{map}(\boldsymbol{y}_{\leq T}))\, d\mu(\boldsymbol{y}_{\leq T})}. \tag{6}$$

If P_{map} exists, it is a minimax strategy for the penalized regret, i.e. for all $\boldsymbol{y}_{\leq T}$, the penalized regret $R_q(\boldsymbol{y}_{\leq T}, P_{map}, \Theta)$ does not exceed $R_q(\Theta)$.

The proof relies on P_{map} being an *equalizer* for the penalized regret and is identical to that of Theorem 4.1 — just replace all quantities with their penalized equivalents.

4.3 Bayesian Gaussian Regression as a Minimax Procedure

We now return to the setting with inputs and show how the Bayesian strategy for the Gaussian regression model is a minimax strategy *for all input sequences* $\boldsymbol{x}_{\leq T}$. If we fix the input sequence $\boldsymbol{x}_{\leq T}$, we can consider the competitor class to be $\mathcal{F} = \{P(\boldsymbol{y}_{\leq T}|\boldsymbol{x}_{\leq T}, \theta) \,|\, \theta \in \Theta)\}$. In other words, we make the more stringent comparison against a model class which has *full knowledge* of the input sequence in advance. Importantly, note that the learner only observes the past inputs $\boldsymbol{x}_{<t}$ at time t.

Consider the Gaussian regression model, with likelihood $P(\boldsymbol{y}_{\leq T}|\boldsymbol{x}_{\leq T}, u(\cdot)) = \mathcal{N}(\boldsymbol{y}_{\leq T}|u(\boldsymbol{x}_{\leq T}), \sigma^2 \boldsymbol{I})$, where $u(\cdot)$ is some function and $\boldsymbol{I}$ is the $T \times T$ identity. For

---

[2]To see this, simply observe that $P_{\mathrm{bayes}}(\boldsymbol{y}_{\leq T}) = \sum_\theta Q(\boldsymbol{y}_{\leq T}|\theta)q(\theta) \geq Q(\boldsymbol{y}_{\leq T}|\theta_{\mathrm{map}}(\boldsymbol{y}_{\leq T}))q(\theta_{\mathrm{map}}(\boldsymbol{y}_{\leq T}))$ and take the $-\log$ of both sides.

625

technical reasons, we do *not* define the class of competitor functions Θ to be the RKHS $\mathcal{H}$, but instead define $\Theta = \{u(\cdot) \mid u(x) = \sum_{t=1}^{T} \alpha_t K(x, x_t), \, \boldsymbol{\alpha} \in \mathbb{R}^T\}$ — the set of kernel expansions over $\boldsymbol{x}_{\leq T}$. The model class is then $\mathcal{F} = \{P(\cdot \mid \boldsymbol{x}_{\leq T}, u(\cdot)) \mid u \in \Theta\}$. The representer theorem implies that competing against Θ is equivalent to competing against the RKHS.

It is easy to see that for this case, the NML density does not exist (recall Example 4.2) — the comparator class Θ contains very complex functions. However, the case is quite different for the penalized regret. Now let us consider using a GP prior. We choose q to be the corresponding density over Θ, which means that $q(u)$ is proportional to $\exp(-\|u\|_K^2/2)$, where $\|u\|_K^2 = \boldsymbol{\alpha}^T \boldsymbol{K} \boldsymbol{\alpha}$ with $\boldsymbol{K}_{i,j} = K(x_i, x_j)$ (recall Eq. 1). Now note that the penalty $-\log q(u)$ is just the RKHS norm $\|u\|_K^2/2$, up to an additive constant.

Using Theorem 4.3 and the equality in Theorem 3.2, we have the following corollary, which shows that the Bayesian strategy is precisely the NMAP distribution (for Gaussian regression).

Corollary 4.4: *For any $\boldsymbol{x}_{\leq T}$, in the Gaussian regression setting described above — where $\mathcal{F}$ and Θ are defined with respect to $\boldsymbol{x}_{\leq T}$ and where q is the GP prior over Θ — we have that P_{bayes} is a minimax strategy for the penalized regret, i.e. for all $\boldsymbol{y}_{\leq T}$, the regret $R_q(\boldsymbol{y}_{\leq T}, P_{bayes}, \Theta)$ does not exceed $R_q(\Theta)$. Furthermore, P_{bayes} and P_{map} are densities of the same distribution.*

Importantly, note that, while the competitor class $\mathcal{F}$ is constructed with full knowledge of $\boldsymbol{x}_{\leq T}$ in advance, the Bayesian strategy, P_{bayes}, can be implemented in an online manner in that it only needs to know $\boldsymbol{x}_{<t}$ for prediction at time t.

Acknowledgments

We thank Manfred Opper and Manfred Warmuth for helpful discussions.

References

K. S. Azoury and M. Warmuth. Relative loss bounds for on-line density estimation with the exponential family of distributions. *Machine Learning*, 43(3), 2001.

A. Barron, J. Rissanen, and B. Yu. The minimum description length principle in coding and modeling. *IEEE Trans. Information Theory*, 44, 1998.

Nicolo Cesa-Bianchi and Gabor Lugosi. Worst-case bounds for the logarithmic loss of predictors. *Machine Learning*, 43, 2001.

D. P. Foster. Prediction in the worst case. *Annals of Statistics*, 19, 1991.

D. P. Foster and R. A. Stine. The competitive complexity ratio. *Proceedings of 2001 Conf on Info Sci and Sys*, WP8, 2001.

P.D. Grunwald. A tutorial introduction to the minimum description length principle. *Advances in MDL: Theory and Applications*, 2005.

T. Hastie, R. Tibshirani, , and J. Friedman. *The Elements of Statistical Learning*. Springer, 2001.

S. M. Kakade and A. Y. Ng. Online bounds for bayesian algorithms. *Proceedings of Neural Information Processing Systems*, 2004.

M. Opper and D. Haussler. Worst case prediction over sequences under log loss. *The Mathematics of Information Coding, Extraction and Distribution*, 1998.

Y. Shtarkov. Universal sequential coding of single messages. *Problems of Information Transmission*, 23, 1987.

E. Takimoto and M. Warmuth. The minimax strategy for Gaussian density estimation. *Proc. 13th Annu. Conference on Comput. Learning Theory*, 2000.

Vladimir N. Vapnik. *Statistical Learning Theory*. Wiley, 1st edition, 1998.

V. Vovk. Competitive on-line statistics. *International Statistical Review*, 69, 2001.

Hyperparameter and Kernel Learning for Graph Based Semi-Supervised Classification

Ashish Kapoor[†], Yuan (Alan) Qi[‡], Hyungil Ahn[†] and Rosalind W. Picard[†]
[†]MIT Media Laboratory, Cambridge, MA 02139
{kapoor, hiahn, picard}@media.mit.edu
[‡]MIT CSAIL, Cambridge, MA 02139
alanqi@csail.mit.edu

Abstract

There have been many graph-based approaches for semi-supervised classification. One problem is that of hyperparameter learning: performance depends greatly on the hyperparameters of the similarity graph, transformation of the graph Laplacian and the noise model. We present a Bayesian framework for learning hyperparameters for graph-based semi-supervised classification. Given some labeled data, which can contain inaccurate labels, we pose the semi-supervised classification as an inference problem over the unknown labels. Expectation Propagation is used for approximate inference and the mean of the posterior is used for classification. The hyperparameters are learned using EM for evidence maximization. We also show that the posterior mean can be written in terms of the kernel matrix, providing a Bayesian classifier to classify new points. Tests on synthetic and real datasets show cases where there are significant improvements in performance over the existing approaches.

1 Introduction

A lot of recent work on semi-supervised learning is based on regularization on graphs [5]. The basic idea is to first create a graph with the labeled and unlabeled data points as the vertices and with the edge weights encoding the similarity between the data points. The aim is then to obtain a labeling of the vertices that is both smooth over the graph and compatible with the labeled data. The performance of most of these algorithms depends upon the edge weights of the graph. Often the smoothness constraints on the labels are imposed using a transformation of the graph Laplacian and the parameters of the transformation affect the performance. Further, there might be other parameters in the model, such as parameters to address label noise in the data. Finding a right set of parameters is a challenge, and usually the method of choice is cross-validation, which can be prohibitively expensive for real-world problems and problematic when we have few labeled data points.

Most of the methods ignore the problem of learning hyperparameters that determine the similarity graph and there are only a few approaches that address this problem. Zhu et al. [8] propose learning non-parametric transformation of the graph Laplacians using semidefinite programming. This approach assumes that the similarity graph is already provided; thus, it does not address the learning of edge weights. Other approaches include label entropy minimization [7] and evidence-maximization using the Laplace approximation [9].

This paper provides a new way to learn the kernel and hyperparameters for graph based semi-supervised classification, while adhering to a Bayesian framework. The semi-supervised classification is posed as a Bayesian inference. We use the evidence to simultaneously tune the hyperparameters that define the structure of the similarity graph, the parameters that determine the transformation of the graph Laplacian, and any other parameters of the model. Closest to our work is Zhu et al. [9], where they proposed a Laplace approximation for learning the edge weights. We use Expectation Propagation (EP), a technique for approximate Bayesian inference that provides better approximations than Laplace. An additional contribution is a new EM algorithm to learn the hyperparameters for the edge weights, the parameters of the transformation of the graph spectrum. More importantly, we explicitly model the level of label noise in the data, while [9] does not do. We provide what may be the first comparison of hyperparameter learning with cross-validation on state-of-the-art algorithms (LLGC [6] and harmonic fields [7]).

2 Bayesian Semi-Supervised Learning

We assume that we are given a set of data points $\mathbf{X} = \{\mathbf{x}_1, .., \mathbf{x}_{n+m}\}$, of which $\mathbf{X}_L = \{\mathbf{x}_1, .., \mathbf{x}_n\}$ are labeled as $\mathbf{t}_L = \{t_1, .., t_n\}$ and $\mathbf{X}_U = \{\mathbf{x}_{n+1}, .., \mathbf{x}_{n+m}\}$ are unlabeled. Throughout this paper we limit ourselves to two-way classification, thus $t \in \{-1, 1\}$. Our model assumes that the hard labels t_i depend upon hidden soft-labels y_i for all i. Given the dataset $D = [\{\mathbf{X}_L, \mathbf{t}_L\}, \mathbf{X}_U]$, the task of semi-supervised learning is then to infer the posterior $p(\mathbf{t}_U | D)$, where $\mathbf{t}_U = [t_{n+1}, .., t_{n+m}]$. The posterior can be written as:

$$p(\mathbf{t}_U | D) = \int_{\mathbf{y}} p(\mathbf{t}_U | \mathbf{y}) p(\mathbf{y} | D) \tag{1}$$

In this paper, we propose to first approximate the posterior $p(\mathbf{y}|D)$ and then use (1) to classify the unlabeled data. Using the Bayes rule we can write:

$$p(\mathbf{y}|D) = p(\mathbf{y}|\mathbf{X}, \mathbf{t}_L) \propto p(\mathbf{y}|\mathbf{X})p(\mathbf{t}_L|\mathbf{y})$$

The term, $p(\mathbf{y}|\mathbf{X})$ is the prior. It enforces a smoothness constraint and depends upon the underlying data manifold. Similar to the spirit of graph regularization [5] we use similarity graphs and their transformed Laplacian to induce priors on the soft labels $\mathbf{y}$. The second term, $p(\mathbf{t}_L|\mathbf{y})$ is the likelihood that incorporates the information provided by the labels.

In this paper, $p(\mathbf{y}|D)$ is inferred using Expectation Propagation, a technique for approximate Bayesian inference [3]. In the following subsections first we describe the prior and the likelihood in detail and then we show how evidence maximization can be used to learn hyperparameters and other parameters in the model.

2.1 Priors and Regularization on Graphs

The prior plays a significant role in semi-supervised learning, especially when there is only a small amount of labeled data. The prior imposes a smoothness constraint and should be such that it gives higher probability to the labelings that respect the similarity of the graph.

The prior, $p(\mathbf{y}|\mathbf{X})$, is constructed by first forming an undirected graph over the data points. The data points are the nodes of the graph and edge-weights between the nodes are based on similarity. This similarity is usually captured using a kernel. Examples of kernels include RBF, polynomial etc. Given the data points and a kernel, we can construct an $(n + m) \times (n + m)$ kernel matrix K, where $K_{ij} = k(\mathbf{x_i}, \mathbf{x_j})$ for all $i \in \{1, .., n + m\}$.

Lets consider the matrix $\tilde{K}$, which is same as the matrix K, except that the diagonals are set to zero. Further, if G is a diagonal matrix such that $G_{ii} = \sum_j \tilde{K}_{ij}$, then we can construct the combinatorial Laplacian ($\Delta = G - \tilde{K}$) or the normalized Laplacian ($\tilde{\Delta} = I - G^{-\frac{1}{2}}\tilde{K}G^{-\frac{1}{2}}$) of the graph. For brevity, in the text we use Δ as a notation for both the Laplacians. Both the Laplacians are symmetric and positive semidefinite. Consider the eigen decomposition of Δ where $\{v_i\}$ denote the eigenvectors and $\{\lambda_i\}$ the corresponding eigenvalues; thus, we can write $\Delta = \sum_{i=1}^{n+m} \lambda_i v_i v_i^T$. Usually, a transformation $r(\Delta) = \sum_{i=1}^{n+m} r(\lambda_i) v_i v_i^T$ that modifies the spectrum of Δ is used as a regularizer. Specifically, the smoothness imposed by this regularizer prefers soft labeling for which the norm $y^T r(\Delta) y$ is small. Equivalently, we can interpret this probabilistically as following:

$$p(\mathbf{y}|\mathbf{X}) \propto e^{-\frac{1}{2}\mathbf{y}^T r(\Delta)\mathbf{y}} = N(0, r(\Delta)^{-1}) \tag{2}$$

Where $r(\Delta)^{-1}$ denotes the pseudo-inverse if the inverse does not exist. Equation (2) suggests that the labelings with the small value of $y^T r(\Delta) y$ are more probable than the others. Note, that when $r(\Delta)$ is not invertible the prior is improper. The fact that the prior can be written as a Gaussian is advantageous as techniques for approximate inference can be easily applied. Also, different choices of transformation functions lead to different semi-supervised learning algorithms. For example, the approach based on Gaussian fields and harmonic functions (Harmonic) [7] can be thought of as using the transformation $r(\lambda) = \lambda$ on the combinatorial Laplacian without any noise model. Similarly, the approach based in local and global consistency (LLGC) [6] can be thought of as using the same transformation but on the normalized Laplacian and a Gaussian likelihood. Therefore, it is easy to see that most of these algorithms can exploit the proposed evidence maximization framework. In the following we focus only on the parametric linear transformation $r(\lambda) = \lambda + \delta$. Note that this transformation removes zero eigenvalues from the spectrum of Δ.

2.2 The Likelihood

Assuming conditional independence of the observed labels given the hidden soft labels, the likelihood $p(\mathbf{t}_L|\mathbf{y})$ can be written as $p(\mathbf{t}_L|\mathbf{y}) = \prod_{i=1}^{n} p(t_i|y_i)$. The likelihood models the probabilistic relation between the observed label t_i and the hidden label y_i. Many real-world datasets contain hand-labeled data and can often have labeling errors. While most people tend to model label errors with a linear or quadratic slack in the likelihood, it has been noted that such an approach does not address the cases where label errors are far from the decision boundary [2]. The flipping likelihood can handle errors even when they are far from the decision boundary and can be written as:

$$p(t_i|y_i) = \epsilon(1 - \Phi(y_i \cdot t_i)) + (1 - \epsilon)\Phi(y_i \cdot t_i) = \epsilon + (1 - 2\epsilon)\Phi(y_i \cdot t_i) \tag{3}$$

Here, Φ is the step function, ϵ is the labeling error rate and the model admits possibility of errors in labeling with a probability ϵ. This likelihood has been earlier used in the context of Gaussian process classification [2][4]. The above described likelihood explicitly models the labeling error rate; thus, the model should be more robust to the presence of label noise in the data. The experiments in this paper use the flipping noise likelihood shown in (3).

2.3 Approximate Inference

In this paper, we use EP to obtain a Gaussian approximation of the posterior $p(\mathbf{y}|D)$. Although, the prior derived in section 2.1 is a Gaussian distribution, the exact posterior is not a Gaussian due to the form of the likelihood. We use EP to approximate the posterior as a Gaussian and then equation (1) can be used to classify unlabeled data points. EP has been previously used [3] to train a Bayes Point Machine, where EP starts with a Gaussian prior over the classifiers and produces a Gaussian posterior. Our task is very similar and we use the same algorithm. In our case, EP starts with the prior defined in (2) and incorporates likelihood to approximate the posterior $p(\mathbf{y}|D) \sim N(\bar{\mathbf{y}}, \Sigma_{\mathbf{y}})$.

2.4 Hyperparameter Learning

We use evidence maximization to learn the hyperparameters. Denote the parameters of the kernel as Θ_K and the parameters of transformation of the graph Laplacian as Θ_T. Let $\Theta = \{\Theta_K, \Theta_T, \epsilon\}$, where ϵ is the noise hyperparameter. The goal is to solve $\hat{\Theta} = \arg\max_\Theta \log[p(\mathbf{t_L}|\mathbf{X}, \Theta)]$.

Non-linear optimization techniques, such as gradient descent or Expectation Maximization (EM) can be used to optimize the evidence. When the parameter space is small then the Matlab function fminbnd, based on golden section search and parabolic interpolation, can be used. The main challenge is that the gradient of evidence is not easy to compute.

Previously, an EM algorithm for hyperparameter learning [2] has been derived for Gaussian Process classification. Using similar ideas we can derive an EM algorithm for semi-supervised learning. In the E-step EP is used to infer the posterior $q(\mathbf{y})$ over the soft labels. The M-step consists of maximizing the lower bound:

$$F = \int_\mathbf{y} q(\mathbf{y}) \log \frac{p(\mathbf{y}|\mathbf{X}, \Theta)p(\mathbf{t_L}|\mathbf{y}, \Theta)}{q(\mathbf{y})}$$

$$= -\int_\mathbf{y} q(\mathbf{y}) \log q(\mathbf{y}) + \int_\mathbf{y} q(\mathbf{y}) \log N(\mathbf{y}; 0, r(\Delta)^{-1})$$

$$+ \sum_{i=1}^{n} \int_{y_i} q(y_i) \log(\epsilon + (1 - 2\epsilon)\Phi(y_i \cdot t_i)) \leq p(\mathbf{t_L}|\mathbf{X}, \Theta)$$

The EM procedure alternates between the E-step and the M-step until convergence.

- **E-Step**: Given the current parameters Θ^i, approximate the posterior $q(\mathbf{y}) \sim N(\bar{\mathbf{y}}, \Sigma_\mathbf{y})$ by EP.
- **M-Step**: Update
$$\Theta^{i+1} = \arg\max_\Theta \int_\mathbf{y} q(\mathbf{y}) \log \frac{p(\mathbf{y}|\mathbf{X}, \Theta)p(\mathbf{t_L}|\mathbf{y}, \Theta)}{q(\mathbf{y})}$$

In the M-step the maximization with respect to the Θ cannot be computed in a closed form, but can be solved using gradient descent. For maximizing the lower bound, we used gradient based projected BFGS method using Armijo rule and simple line search. When using the linear transformation $r(\lambda) = \lambda + \delta$ on the Laplacian Δ, the prior $p(\mathbf{y}|\mathbf{X}, \Theta)$ can be written as $N(0, (\Delta + \delta I)^{-1})$. Define $\mathbf{Z} = \Delta + \delta I$ then, the gradients of the lower bound with respect to the parameters are as follows:

$$\frac{\partial F}{\partial \Theta_K} = \frac{1}{2} tr(\mathbf{Z}^{-1} \frac{\partial \Delta}{\partial \Theta_K}) - \frac{1}{2} \bar{\mathbf{y}}^T \frac{\partial \Delta}{\partial \Theta_K} \bar{\mathbf{y}} - \frac{1}{2} tr(\frac{\partial \Delta}{\partial \Theta_K} \Sigma_\mathbf{y})$$

$$\frac{\partial F}{\partial \Theta_T} = \frac{1}{2} tr(\mathbf{Z}^{-1}) - \frac{1}{2} \bar{\mathbf{y}}^T \bar{\mathbf{y}} - \frac{1}{2} tr(\Sigma_\mathbf{y})$$

$$\frac{\partial F}{\partial \epsilon} \approx \sum_{i=1}^{n} \frac{1 - 2\Phi(t_i \cdot \bar{y}_i)}{\epsilon + (1 - 2\epsilon)\Phi(t_i \cdot \bar{y}_i)} \quad \text{where: } \bar{y}_i = \int_\mathbf{y} y_i q(\mathbf{y})$$

It is easy to show that the provided approximation of the derivative $\frac{\partial F}{\partial \epsilon}$ equals zero, when $\epsilon = \frac{k}{n}$, where k is the number of labeled data points differing in sign from their posterior means. The EM procedure described here is susceptible to local minima and in a few cases might be too slow to converge. Especially, when the evidence curve is flat and the initial values are far from the optimum, we found that the EM algorithm provided very small steps, thus, taking a long time to converge.

Whenever we encountered this problem in the experiments, we used an approximate gradient search to find a good value of initial parameters for the EM algorithm. Essentially as the gradients of the evidence are hard to compute, they can be approximated by the gradients of the lower bound and can be used in any gradient ascent procedure.

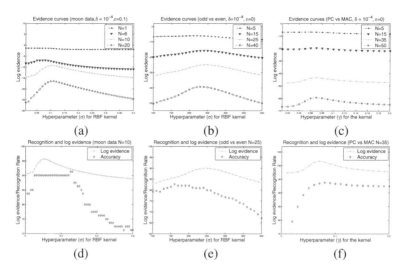

(a)	(b)	(c)

(d)	(e)	(f)

Figure 1: Evidence curves showing similar properties across different datasets (half-moon, odd vs even and PC vs MAC). The top row figures (a), (b) and (c) show the evidence curves for different amounts of labeled data per class. The bottom row figures (d), (e) and (f) show the correlation between recognition accuracy on unlabeled points and the evidence.

2.5 Classifying New Points

Since we compute a posterior distribution over the soft-labels of the labeled and unlabeled data points, classifying a new point is tricky. Note, that from the parameterization lemma for Gaussian Processes [1] it follows that given a prior distribution $p(\mathbf{y}|\mathbf{X}) \sim N(0, r(\Delta)^{-1})$, the mean of the posterior $p(\mathbf{y}|D)$ is a linear combination of the columns of $r(\Delta)^{-1}$. That is:

$$\bar{\mathbf{y}} = r(\Delta)^{-1}\mathbf{a} \quad \text{where,} \quad \mathbf{a} \in I\!R^{(n+m)\times 1}$$

Further, if the similarity matrix K is a valid kernel matrix[1] then we can write the mean directly in terms of the linear combination of the columns of K:

$$\bar{\mathbf{y}} = KK^{-1}r(\Delta)^{-1}\mathbf{a} = K\mathbf{b} \tag{4}$$

Here, $\mathbf{b} = [b_1, .., b_{n+m}]^T$ is a column vector and is equal to $K^{-1}r(\Delta)^{-1}\mathbf{a}$. Thus, we have that $\bar{y}_i = \sum_{j=1}^{n+m} b_j \cdot K(\mathbf{x}_i, \mathbf{x}_j)$. This provides a natural extension of the framework to classify new points.

3 Experiments

We performed experiments to evaluate the three main contributions of this work: Bayesian hyperparameter learning, classification of unseen data points, and robustness with respect to noisy labels. For all the experiments we use the linear transformation $r(\lambda) = \lambda + \delta$ either on normalized Laplacian (EP-NL) or the combinatorial Laplacian (EP-CL). The experiments were performed on one synthetic (Figure 4(a)) and on three real-world datasets. Two real-world datasets were the handwritten digits and the newsgroup data from [7]. We evaluated the task of classifying odd vs even digits (15 labeled, 485 unlabeled and rest new

---

[1]The matrix K is the adjacency matrix of the graph and depending upon the similarity criterion might not always be positive semi-definite. For example, discrete graphs induced using K-nearest neighbors might result in K that is not positive semi-definite.

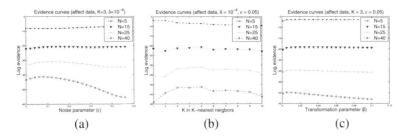

(a)   (b)   (c)

Figure 2: Evidence curves showing similar properties across different parameters of the model. The figures (a), (b) and (c) show the evidence curves for different amount of labeled data per class for the three different parameters in the model.

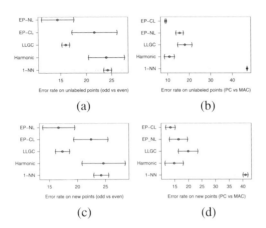

(a)   (b)

(c)   (d)

Figure 3: Error rates for different algorithms on digits (first column, (a) and (c)) and newsgroup dataset (second column (b) and (d)). The figures in the top row (a) and (b) show error rates on unlabeled points and the bottom row figures (c) and (d) on the new points. The results are averaged over 5 runs. Non-overlapping of error bars, the standard error scaled by 1.64, indicates 95% significance of the performance difference.

(unseen) points per class) and classifying PC vs MAC (5 labeled, 895 unlabeled and rest as new (unseen) points per class). An RBF kernel was used for handwritten digits, whereas kernel $K(\mathbf{x_i}, \mathbf{x_j}) = exp[-\frac{1}{\gamma}(1 - \frac{\mathbf{x_i}^T \mathbf{x_j}}{|\mathbf{x_i}||\mathbf{x_j}|})]$ was used on 10-NN graph to determine similarity. The third real-world dataset labels the level of interest (61 samples of high interest and 75 samples of low interest) of a child solving a puzzle on the computer. Each data point is a 19 dimensional real vector summarizing 8 seconds of activity from the face, posture and the puzzle. The labels in this database are suspected to be noisy because of human labeling. All the experiments on this data used K-nearest neighbor to determine the kernel matrix.

Hyperparameter learning: Figure 1 (a), (b) and (c) plots log evidence versus kernel parameters that determine the similarity graphs for the different datasets with varying size of the labeled set per class. The value of δ and ϵ were fixed to the values shown in the plots. Figure 2 (a), (b) and (c) plots the log evidence versus the noise parameter (ϵ), the kernel parameter (k in k-NN) and the transformation parameter (δ) for the affect dataset. First, we see that the evidence curves generated with very little data are flat and as the number of labeled data points increases we see the curves become peakier. When there is very little labeled data, there is not much information available for the evidence maximization framework to prefer one parameter value over the other. With more labeled data, the evidence curves become more informative. Figure 1 (d), (e) and (f) show the correlation between the evidence curves and the recognition rate on the unlabeled data and reveal that the recognition over the unlabeled data points is highly correlated with the evidence. Note that both of these effects are observed across all the datasets as well as all the different parameters, justifying evidence maximization for hyperparameter learning.

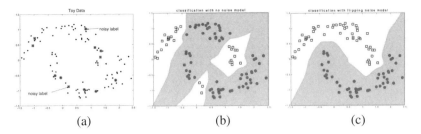

(a)   (b)   (c)

Figure 4: Semi-supervised classification in presence of label noise. (a) Input data with label noise. Classification (b) without flipping noise model and with (c) flipping noise model.

How good are the learnt parameters? We performed experiments on the handwritten digits and on the newsgroup data and compared with 1-NN, LLGC and Harmonic approach. The kernel parameters for both LLGC and Harmonic were estimated using leave one out cross validation[2]. Note that both the approaches can be interpreted in terms of the new proposed Bayesian framework (see sec 2.1). We performed experiments with both the normalized (EP-NL) and the combinatorial Laplacian (EP-CL) with the proposed framework to classify the digits and the newsgroup data. The approximate gradient descent was first used to find an initial value of the kernel parameter for the EM algorithm. All three parameters were learnt and the top row in figure 3 shows the average error obtained for 5 different runs on the unlabeled points. On the task of classifying odd vs even the error rate for EP-NL was 14.46±4.4%, significantly outperforming the Harmonic (23.98±4.9%) and 1-NN (24.23±1.1%). Since the prior in EP-NL is determined using the normalized Laplacian and there is no label noise in the data, we expect EP-NL to at least work as well as LLGC (16.02 ± 1.1%). Similarly for the newsgroup dataset EP-CL (9.28±0.7%) significantly beats LLGC (18.03±3.5%) and 1-NN (46.88±0.3%) and is better than Harmonic (10.86±2.4%). Similar, results are obtained on new points as well. The unseen points were classified using eq. (4) and the nearest neighbor rule was used for LLGC and Harmonic.

Handling label noise: Figure 4(a) shows a synthetic dataset with noisy labels. We performed semi-supervised classification both with and without the likelihood model given in (3) and the EM algorithm was used to tune all the parameters including the noise (ϵ). Besides modifying the spectrum of the Laplacian, the transformation parameter δ can also be considered as latent noise and provides a quadratic slack for the noisy labels [2]. The results are shown in figure 4 (b) and (c). The EM algorithm can correctly learn the noise parameter resulting in a perfect classification. The classification without the flipping model, even with the quadratic slack, cannot handle the noisy labels far from the decision boundary.

Is there label noise in the data? It was suspected that due to the manual labeling the affect dataset might have some label noise. To confirm this and as a sanity check, we first plotted evidence using *all* the available data. For all the semi-supervised methods in these experiments, we use 3-NN to induce the adjacency graph. Figure 5(a) shows the plot for the evidence against the noise parameter (ϵ). From the figure, we see that the evidence peaks at $\epsilon = 0.05$ suggesting that the dataset has around 5% of labeling noise. Figure 5(b) shows comparisons with other semi-supervised (LLGC and SVM with graph kernel) and supervised methods (SVM with RBF kernel) for different sizes of the labeled dataset. Each point in the graph is the average error on 20 random splits of the data, where the error bars represent the standard error. EM was used to tune ϵ and δ in every run. We used the same transformation $r(\lambda) = \lambda + \delta$ on the graph kernel in the semi-supervised SVM. The hyperparameters in both the SVMs (including δ for the semi-supervised case) were estimated using leave one out. When the number of labeled points are small, both

---

[2]Search space for σ (odd vs even) was 100 to 400 with increments of 10 and for γ (PC vs MAC) was 0.01 to 0.2 with increments of 0.1

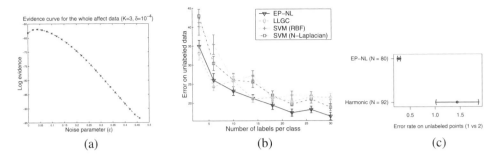

(a)　　　　　　　　　　　(b)　　　　　　　　　　　(c)

Figure 5: (a) Evidence vs noise parameter plotted using all the available data in the affect dataset. The maximum at $\epsilon = 0.05$ suggests that there is around 5% label noise in the data. (b) Performance comparison of the proposed approach with LLGC, SVM using graph kernel and the supervised SVM (RBF kernel) on the affect dataset which has label noise. The error bars represent the standard error. (c) Comparison of the proposed EM method for hyperparameter learning with the result reported in [7] using label entropy minimization. The plotted error bars represent the standard deviation.

LLGC and EP-NL perform similarly beating both the SVMs, but as the size of the labeled data increases we see a significant improvement of the proposed approach over the other methods. One of the reasons is when you have few labels the probability of the labeled set of points containing a noisy label is low. As the size of the labeled set increases the labeled data has more noisy labels. And, since LLGC has a Gaussian noise model, it cannot handle flipping noise well. As the number of labels increase, the evidence curve turns informative and EP-NL starts to learn the label noise correctly, outperforming the other Both the SVMs show competitive performance with more labels but still are worse than EP-NL. Finally, we also test the method on the task of classifying "1" vs "2" in the handwritten digits dataset. With 40 labeled examples per class (80 total labels and 1800 unlabeled), EP-NL obtained an average recognition accuracy of $99.72 \pm 0.04\%$ and figure 5(c) graphically shows the gain over the accuracy of $98.56 \pm 0.43\%$ reported in [7], where the hyperparameter were learnt by minimizing label entropy with 92 labeled and 2108 unlabeled examples.

4   Conclusion

We presented and evaluated a Bayesian framework for learning hyperparameters for graph-based semi-supervised classification. The results indicate that evidence maximization works well for learning hyperparameters, including the amount of label noise in the data.

References

[1] Csato, L. (2002) Gaussian processes-iterative sparse approximation. *PhD Thesis*, Aston Univ.

[2] Kim, H. & Ghahramani, Z. (2004) The EM-EP algorithm for Gaussian process classification. *ECML*.

[3] Minka, T. P. (2001) Expectation propagation for approximate Bayesian inference. *UAI*.

[4] Opper, M. & Winther, O. (1999) Mean field methods for classification with Gaussian processes. *NIPS*.

[5] Smola, A. & Kondor, R. (2003) Kernels and regularization on graphs. *COLT*.

[6] Zhou et al. (2004) Learning with local and global consistency. *NIPS*.

[7] Zhu, X., Ghahramani, Z. & Lafferty, J. (2003) Semi-supervised learning using Gaussian fields and harmonic functions. *ICML*.

[8] Zhu, X., Kandola, J., Ghahramani, Z. & Lafferty, J. (2004) Nonparametric transforms of graph kernels for semi-supervised learning. *NIPS*.

[9] Zhu, X., Lafferty, J. & Ghahramani, Z. (2003) Semi-supervised learning: From Gaussian fields to Gaussian processes. CMU Tech Report:CMU-CS-03-175.

Is Early Vision Optimized for Extracting Higher-order Dependencies?

Yan Karklin
`yan+@cs.cmu.edu`

Michael S. Lewicki[*]
`lewicki@cnbc.cmu.edu`

Computer Science Department &
Center for the Neural Basis of Cognition
Carnegie Mellon University

Abstract

Linear implementations of the efficient coding hypothesis, such as independent component analysis (ICA) and sparse coding models, have provided functional explanations for properties of simple cells in V1 [1, 2]. These models, however, ignore the non-linear behavior of neurons and fail to match individual and population properties of neural receptive fields in subtle but important ways. Hierarchical models, including Gaussian Scale Mixtures [3, 4] and other generative statistical models [5, 6], can capture higher-order regularities in natural images and explain non-linear aspects of neural processing such as normalization and context effects [6, 7]. Previously, it had been assumed that the lower level representation is independent of the hierarchy, and had been fixed when training these models. Here we examine the optimal lower-level representations derived in the context of a hierarchical model and find that the resulting representations are strikingly different from those based on linear models. Unlike the the basis functions and filters learned by ICA or sparse coding, these functions individually more closely resemble simple cell receptive fields and collectively span a broad range of spatial scales. Our work unifies several related approaches and observations about natural image structure and suggests that hierarchical models might yield better representations of image structure throughout the hierarchy.

1 Introduction

Efficient coding hypothesis has been proposed as a guiding computational principle for the analysis of early visual system and motivates the search for good statistical models of natural images. Early work revealed that image statistics are highly non-Gaussian [8, 9], and models such as independent component analysis (ICA) and sparse coding have been developed to capture these statistics to form efficient representations of natural images. It has been suggested that these models explain the basic computational goal of early visual cortex, as evidenced by the similarity between the learned parameters and the measured receptive fields of simple cells in V1.

---

[*]To whom correspondence should be addressed

In fact, it is not clear exactly how well these methods predict the shapes of neural receptive fields. There has been no thorough characterization of ICA and sparse coding results for different datasets, pre-processing methods, and specific learning algorithms employed, although some of these factors clearly affect the resulting representation [10]. When ICA or sparse coding is applied to natural images, the resulting basis functions resemble Gabor functions [1, 2] — 2D sine waves modulated by Gaussian envelopes — which also accurately model the shapes of simple cell receptive fields [11]. Often, these results are visualized in a transformed space, by taking the logarithm of the pixel intensities, sphering (whitening) the image space, or filtering the images to flatten their spectrum. When analyzed in the *original* image space, the learned filters (the models' analogues of neural receptive fields) do not exhibit the multi-scale properties of the visual system, as they tend to cluster at high spatial frequencies [10, 12]. Neural receptive fields, on the other hand, span a broad range of spatial scales, and exhibit distributions of spatial phase and other parameters unmatched by ICA and SC results [13, 14]. Therefore, as models of early visual processing, these models fail to predict accurately either the individual or the population properties of cortical visual neurons.

Linear efficient coding methods are also limited in the type of statistical structure they can capture. Applied to natural images, their coefficients contain significant residual dependencies that cannot be accounted for by the linear form of the models. Several solutions have been proposed, including multiplicative Gaussian Scale Mixtures [4] and generative hierarchical models [5, 6]. These models capture some of the observed dependencies; but their analysis so far has been focused on the higher-order structure learned by the model. Meanwhile, the lower-level representation is either chosen *a priori* [4] or adapted separately, in the absence of the hierarchy [6] or with a fixed hierarchical structure specified in advance [5].

Here we examine whether the optimal lower-level representation of natural images is different when trained in the context of such non-linear hierarchical models. We also illustrate how the model not only describes sparse marginal densities and magnitude dependencies, but captures a variety of joint density functions that are consistent with previous observations and theoretical conjectures. We show that learned lower-level representations are strikingly different from those learned by the linear models: they are more multi-scale, spanning a wide range of spatial scales and phases of the Gabor sinusoid relative to the Gaussian envelope. Finally, we place these results in the context of whitening, gain control, and non-linear neural processing.

2 Fully adaptable scale mixture model

A simple and scalable model for natural image patches is a linear factor model, in which the data $\mathbf{x}$ are assumed to be generated as a linear combination of basis functions with additive noise

$$\mathbf{x} = \mathbf{A}\mathbf{u} + \boldsymbol{\epsilon}. \tag{1}$$

Typically, the noise is assumed to be Gaussian with variance σ_ϵ^2, thus

$$P(\mathbf{x}|\mathbf{A}, \mathbf{u}) \propto \exp\left(-\sum_i \frac{1}{2\sigma_\epsilon^2} |\mathbf{x} - \mathbf{A}\mathbf{u}|_i^2\right). \tag{2}$$

The coefficients $\mathbf{u}$ are assumed to be mutually independent, and often modeled with sparse distributions (e.g. Laplacian) that reflect the non-Gaussian statistics of natural scenes [8, 9],

$$P(\mathbf{u}) = \prod_i P(u_i) \propto \exp(-\sum_i |u_i|). \tag{3}$$

We can then adapt the basis functions $\mathbf{A}$ to maximize the expected log-likelihood of the data $L = \langle \log P(\mathbf{x}|\mathbf{A}) \rangle$ over the data ensemble, thereby learning a compact, efficient representation of structure in natural images. This is the model underlying the sparse coding algorithm [2] and closely related to independent component analysis (ICA) [1].

An alternative to fixed sparse priors for $\mathbf{u}$ (3) is to use a Gaussian Scale Mixture (GSM) model [3]. In these models, each observed coefficient u_i is modeled as a product of random Gaussian variable y_i and a multiplier λ_i,

$$u_i = \sqrt{\lambda_i} y_i \qquad (4)$$

Conditional on the value of the multiplier λ_i, the probability $P(u_i|\lambda_i)$ is Gaussian with variance λ_i, but the form of the marginal distribution

$$P(u_i) = \int \mathcal{N}(0, \lambda_i) P(\lambda_i) d\lambda_i \qquad (5)$$

depends on the probability function of λ_i and can assume a variety of shapes, including sparse heavy-tailed functions that fit the observed distributions of wavelet and ICA coefficients [4]. This type of model can also account for the observed dependencies among coefficients $\mathbf{u}$, for example, by expressing them as pair-wise dependencies among the multiplier variables $\boldsymbol{\lambda}$ [4, 15].

A more general model, proposed in [6, 16], employs a hierarchical prior for $P(\mathbf{u})$ with adapted parameters tuned to the global patterns in higher-order dependencies. Specifically, the logarithm of the variances of $P(\mathbf{u})$ is assumed to be a linear function of the higher-order random variables $\mathbf{v}$,

$$\log \sigma_u^2 = \mathbf{B}\mathbf{v} . \qquad (6)$$

Conditional on the higher-order variables, the joint distribution of coefficients is factorisable, as in GSM. In fact, if the conditional density $P(\mathbf{u}|\mathbf{v})$ is Gaussian, this *Hierarchical Scale Mixture* (HSM) is equivalent to a GSM model, with $\boldsymbol{\lambda} = \sigma_u^2$ and $P(\mathbf{u}|\boldsymbol{\lambda}) = P(\mathbf{u}|\mathbf{v}) = \mathcal{N}(0, \exp(\mathbf{B}\mathbf{v}))$, with the added advantage of a more flexible representation of higher-order statistical regularities in $\mathbf{B}$. Whereas previous GSM models of natural images focused on modeling local relationships between coefficients of fixed linear transforms, this general hierarchical formulation is fully adaptable, allowing us to recover the optimal lower-level representation $\mathbf{A}$, as well as the higher-order components $\mathbf{B}$.

Parameter estimation in the HSM involves adapting model parameters $\mathbf{A}$ and $\mathbf{B}$ to maximize data log-likelihood $L = \langle \log P(\mathbf{x}|\mathbf{A}, \mathbf{B}) \rangle$. The gradient descent algorithm for the estimation of $\mathbf{B}$ has been previously described (see [6]). The optimal lower-level basis $\mathbf{A}$ is computed similarly to the sparse coding algorithm — the goal is to minimize reconstruction error of the inferred MAP estimate $\hat{\mathbf{u}}$. However, $\hat{\mathbf{u}}$ is estimated not with a fixed sparsifying prior, but with a concurrently adapted hierarchical prior. If we assume a Gaussian conditional density $P(\mathbf{u}|\mathbf{v})$ and a standard-Normal prior $P(\mathbf{v})$, the MAP estimates are computed as

$$\{\hat{\mathbf{u}}, \hat{\mathbf{v}}\} = \arg \min_{\mathbf{u}, \mathbf{v}} P(\mathbf{u}, \mathbf{v}|\mathbf{x}, \mathbf{A}, \mathbf{B}) \qquad (7)$$

$$= \arg \min_{\mathbf{u}, \mathbf{v}} P(\mathbf{x}|\mathbf{A}, \mathbf{B}, \mathbf{u}, \mathbf{v}) P(\mathbf{u}|\mathbf{v}) P(\mathbf{v}) \qquad (8)$$

$$= \arg \min_{\mathbf{u}, \mathbf{v}} \left(\frac{1}{2\sigma_\epsilon^2} \sum_i |\mathbf{x} - \mathbf{A}\mathbf{u}|_i^2 + \sum_j \left(\frac{[\mathbf{B}\mathbf{v}]_j}{2} + \frac{u_j^2}{2e^{[\mathbf{B}\mathbf{v}]_j}} \right) + \sum_k \frac{v_k^2}{2} \right) . \qquad (9)$$

Marginalizing over the latent higher-order variables in the hierarchical models leads to sparse distributions similar to the Laplacian and other density functions assumed in ICA.

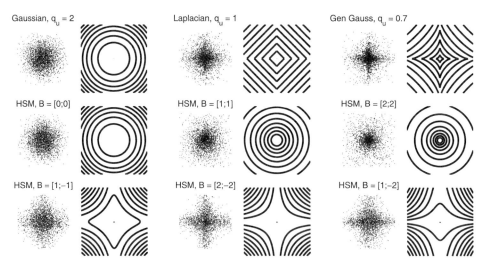

Figure 1: This model can describe a variety of joint density functions for coefficients **u**. Here we show example scatter plots and contour plots of some bivariate densities. Top row: Gaussian, Laplacian, and generalized Gaussian densities of the form $p(u) \propto \exp(-|u|^q)$. Middle and bottom row: Hierarchical Scale Mixtures with different sets of parameters **B**. For illustration, in the hierarchical models the dimensionality of **v** is 1, and the matrix **B** is simply a *column* vector. These densities are computed by marginalizing over the latent variables **v**, here assumed to follow a standard normal distribution. Even with this simple hierarchy, the model can generate sparse star-shaped (bottom row) or radially symmetric (middle row) densities, as well as more complex non-symmetric densities (bottom right). In higher dimensions, it is possible to describe more complex joint distributions, with different marginals along different projections.

However, although the model distribution for individual coefficients is similar to the fixed sparse priors of ICA and sparse coding, the model is fundamentally non-linear and might yield a different lower-level representation; the coefficients **u** are no longer mutually independent, and the optimal set of basis functions must account for this.

Also, the shape of the *joint* marginal distribution in the space of all the coefficients is more complex than the i.i.d. joint density of the linear models. Bi-variate joint distributions of GSM coefficients can capture non-linear dependencies in wavelet coefficients [4]. In the fully adaptable HSM, however, the joint density can take a variety of shapes that depend on the learned parameters **B** (figure 1). Note that this model can produce sparse, star-shaped distributions as in the linear models, or radially symmetric distributions that cannot be described by the linear models. Such joint density profiles have been observed empirically in the responses of phase-offset wavelet coefficients to natural images and have inspired polar transformation and quadrature pair models [17] (as well as connections to phase-invariant neural responses). The model described here can capture these joint densities and others, but rather than assume this structure *a priori*, it learns it automatically from the data.

3   Methods

To examine how the lower-level representation is affected by the hierarchical model structure, we compared **A** learned by the sparse coding algorithm [2] and the HSM described above. The models were trained on 20×20 image patches sampled from 40 images of outdoor scenes in the Kyoto dataset [12]. We applied a low-pass radially symmetric filter to the full images to eliminate high corner frequencies (artifacts of the square sampling lattice), and removed the DC component from each image patch, but did no further pre-processing. All the results and analyses are reported in the original data space. Noise variance σ_ϵ^2 was set to 0.1, and the basis functions were initialized to small random values and adapted on stochastically sampled batches of 300 patches. We ran the algorithm for 10,000 iterations with a step size of 0.1 (tapered for the last 1,000 iterations, once model parameters were relatively unchanging).

The parameters of the hierarchical model were estimated in a similar fashion. Gradient descent on $\mathbf{A}$ and $\mathbf{B}$ was performed in parallel using MAP estimates $\hat{\mathbf{u}}$ and $\hat{\mathbf{v}}$. The step size for adapting $\mathbf{B}$ was gradually increased from .0001 to .01, because emergence of the variance patterns requires some stabilization in the basis functions in $\mathbf{A}$.

Because encoding in the sparse coding and in the hierarchical model is a non-linear process, it is not possible to compare the inverse of $\mathbf{A}$ to physiological data. Instead, we estimated the corresponding *filters* using reverse correlation to derive a linear approximation to a non-linear system, which is also a common method for characterizing V1 simple cells. We analyzed the resulting filters by fitting them with 2D Gabor functions, then examining the distribution of their frequencies, phase, and orientation parameters.

4   Results

The shapes of basis functions and filters obtained with sparse coding have been previously analyzed and compared to neural receptive fields [10, 14]. However, some of the reported results were in the whitened space or obtained by training on filtered images. In the original space, sparse coding basis functions have very particular shapes: except for a few large, low frequency functions, all are localized, odd-symmetric, and span only a single period of the sinusoid (figure 2, top left). The estimated filters are similar but smaller (figure 2, bottom left), with peak spatial frequencies clustered at higher frequencies (figure 3).

In the hierarchical model, the learned representation is strikingly different (figure 2, right panels). Both the basis and the filters span a wider range of spatial scales, a result previously unobserved for models trained on non-preprocessed images, and one that is more consistent with physiological data [13, 14]. Also, the shapes of the basis functions are different — they more closely resemble Gabor functions, although they tend to be less smooth than the sparse coding basis functions. Both SC- and HSM-derived filters are well fit with Gabor functions.

We also compared the distributions of spatial phases for filters obtained with sparse coding and the hierarchical model (figure 4). While sparse coding filters exhibit a strong tendency for odd-symmetric phase profiles, the hierarchical model results in a much more uniform distribution of spatial phases. Although some phase asymmetry has been observed in simple cell receptive fields, their phase properties tend to be much more uniform than sparse coding filters [14].

In the hierarchical model, the higher-order representation $\mathbf{B}$ is also adapted to the statistical structure of natural images. Although the choice of the prior density for $\mathbf{v}$ (e.g. sparse or Gaussian) can determine the type of structure captured in $\mathbf{B}$, we discovered that it does not affect the nature of the lower-level representation. For the results reported here, we assumed a Gaussian prior on $\mathbf{v}$. Thus, as in other multi-variate Gaussian models, the precise directions of $\mathbf{B}$ are not important; the learned vectors only serve to collectively describe the volume of the space. In this case, they capture the *principal components of the log-variances*. Because we were interested specifically in the lower-level representation, we did not analyze the matrix $\mathbf{B}$ in detail, though the principal components of this space seem to

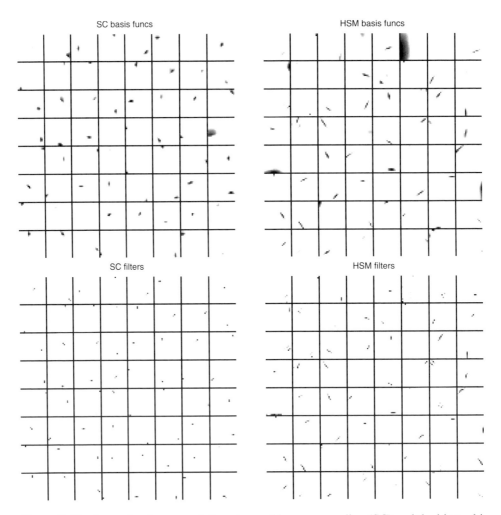

Figure 2: The lower-level representations learned by sparse coding (SC) and the hierarchical scale model (HSM). Shown are subsets of the learned basis functions and the estimates for the filters obtained with reverse correlation. These functions are displayed in the original image space.

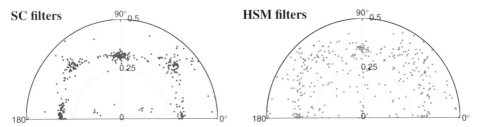

Figure 3: Scatter plots of peak frequencies and orientations of the Gabor functions fitted to the estimated filters. The units on the radial scale are cycles/pixel and the solid line is the Nyquist limit. Although both SC and HSM filters exhibit predominantly high spatial frequencies, the hierarchical model yields a representation that tiles the spatial frequency space much more evenly.

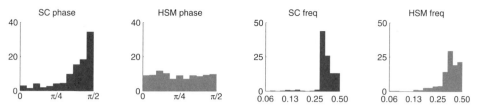

Figure 4: The distributions of phases and frequencies for Gabor functions fitted to sparse coding (SC) and hierarchical scale model (HSM) filters. The phase units specify the phase of the sinusoid in relation to the peak of the Gaussian envelope of the Gabor function; 0 is even-symmetric, $\pi/2$ is odd-symmetric. The frequency axes are in cycles/pixel.

group co-localized lower-level basis functions and separately represent spatial contrast and oriented image structure. As reported previously [6, 16], with a sparse prior on $\mathbf{v}$, the model learns higher-order components that individually capture complex spatial, orientation, and scale regularities in image data.

5 Discussion

We have demonstrated that adapting a general hierarchical model yields lower-level representations that are significantly different than those obtained using fixed priors and linear generative models. The resulting basis functions and filters are multi-scale and more consistent with several observed characteristics of neural receptive fields.

It is interesting that the learned representations are similar to the results obtained when ICA or sparse coding is applied to whitened images (i.e. with a flattened power spectrum). This might be explained by the fact that whitening "spheres" the input space, normalizing the scale of different directions in the space. The hierarchical model is performing a similar scaling operation through the inference of higher-order variables $\mathbf{v}$ that scale the priors on basis function coefficients $\mathbf{u}$. Thus the model can rely on a generic "white" lower level representation, while employing an *adaptive* mechanism for normalizing the space, which accounts for non-stationary statistics on an image-by-image basis [6]. A related phenomenon in neural processing is gain control, which might be one specific type of a general adaptation process.

The flexibility of the hierarchical model allows us to learn a lower-level representation that is optimal in the context of the hierarchy. Thus, we expect the learned parameters to define a better statistical model for natural images than other approaches in which the lower-level representation or the higher-order dependencies are fixed in advance. For example, the flexible marginal distributions, illustrated in figure 1, should be able to capture a wider range of statistical structure in natural images. One way to quantify the benefit of an adapted lower-level representation is to apply the model to problems like image de-noising and filling-in missing pixels. Related models have achieved state-of-the-art performance [15, 18], and we are currently investigating whether the added flexibility of the model discussed here confers additional advantages.

Finally, although the results presented here are more consistent with the observed properties of neural receptive fields, several discrepancies remain. For example, our results, as well as those of other statistical models, fail to account for the prevalence of low spatial frequency receptive fields observed in V1. This could be a result of the specific choice of the distribution assumed by the model, although the described hierarchical framework makes few assumptions about the joint distribution of basis function coefficients. More likely, the non-stationary statistics of the natural scenes play a role in determining the properties of the learned representation. As suggested by previous results [10], different image data-sets can lead to different parameters. This provides a strong motivation for training models with an "over-complete" basis, in which the number of basis functions is greater than the dimensionality of the input data [19]. In this case, different subsets of the basis functions can adapt to optimally represent different image contexts, and the population properties of such over-complete representations could be significantly different. It would be particularly interesting to investigate representations learned in these models in the context of a hierarchical model.

References

[1] A. J. Bell and T. J. Sejnowski. The 'independent components' of natural scenes are edge filters. *Vision Research*, 37(23):3327–3338, 1997.

[2] B. A. Olshausen and D. J. Field. Emergence of simple-cell receptive-field properties by learning a sparse code for natural images. *Nature*, 381:607–609, 1996.

[3] D. F. Andrews and C. L. Mallows. Scale mixtures of normal distributions. *Journal of the Royal Statistical Society B*, 36(1):99–102, 1974.

[4] M. J. Wainwright, E. P. Simoncelli, and A. S. Willsky. Random cascades on wavelet trees and their use in analyzing and modeling natural images. *Applied Computational and Harmonic Analysis*, 11:89–123, 2001.

[5] A. Hyvärinen, P. O. Hoyer, and M. Inki. Topographic independent component analysis. *Neural Computation*, 13:1527–1558, 2001.

[6] Y. Karklin and M.S. Lewicki. A hierarchical bayesian model for learning non-linear statistical regularities in non-stationary natural signals. *Neural Computation*, 17:397–423, 2005.

[7] O. Schwartz and E. P. Simoncelli. Natural signal statistics and sensory gain control. *Nat. Neurosci.*, 4:819–825, 2001.

[8] D. Field. What is the goal of sensory coding. *Neural Computation*, 6:559–601, 1994.

[9] D. R. Ruderman and W. Bialek. Statistics of natural images: Scaling in the woods. *Physical Review Letters*, 73(6):814–818, 1994.

[10] J. H. van Hateren and A. van der Schaaf. Independent component filters of natural images compared with simple cells in primary visual cortex. *Proceedings of the Royal Society, London B*, 265:359–366, 1998.

[11] J. P. Jones and L. A. Palmer. An evaluation of the two-dimensional gabor filter model of simple receptive fields in cat striate cortex. *Journal of Neurophysiology*, 58(6):1233–1258, 1987.

[12] E. Doi and M. S. Lewicki. Sparse coding of natural images using an overcomplete set of limited capacity units. In *Advances in Neural Processing Information Systems 18*, 2004.

[13] R. L. De Valois, D. G. Albrecht, and L. G. Thorell. Spatial frequency selectivity of cells in macaque visual cortex. *Vision Research*, 22:545–559, 1982.

[14] D. L. Ringach. Spatial structure and symmetry of simple-cell receptive fields in macaque primary visual cortex. *Journal of Neurophysiology*, 88:455–463, 2002.

[15] J. Portilla, V. Strela, M. J. Wainwright, and E.P. Simoncelli. Image denoising using Gaussian scale mixtures in the wavelet domain. *IEEE Transactions on Image Processing*, 12:1338–1351, 2003.

[16] Y. Karklin and M.S. Lewicki. Learning higher-order structures in natural images. *Network: Computation in Neural Systems*, 14:483–499, 2003.

[17] C. Zetzsche and G. Krieger. Nonlinear neurons and highorder statistics: New approaches to human vision and electronic image processing. In B. Rogowitz and T.V. Pappas, editors, *Proc. SPIE on Human Vision and Electronic Imaging IV*, volume 3644, pages 2–33, 1999.

[18] M. S. Lewicki and B. A. Olshausen. A probabilistic framework for the adaptation and comparison of image codes. *Journal of the Optical Society of America A*, 16(7):1587–1601, 1999.

[19] B. A. Olshausen and D. J. Field. Sparse coding with an overcomplete basis set: A strategy employed by V1? *Vision Research*, 37(23), 1997.

A Matching Pursuit Approach to Sparse Gaussian Process Regression

S. Sathiya Keerthi
Yahoo! Research Labs
210 S. DeLacey Avenue
Pasadena, CA 91105
selvarak@yahoo-inc.com

Wei Chu
Gatsby Computational Neuroscience Unit
University College London
London, WC1N 3AR, UK
chuwei@gatsby.ucl.ac.uk

Abstract

In this paper we propose a new basis selection criterion for building sparse GP regression models that provides promising gains in accuracy as well as efficiency over previous methods. Our algorithm is much faster than that of Smola and Bartlett, while, in generalization it greatly outperforms the information gain approach proposed by Seeger et al, especially on the quality of predictive distributions.

1 Introduction

Bayesian Gaussian processes provide a promising probabilistic kernel approach to supervised learning tasks. The advantage of Gaussian process (GP) models over non-Bayesian kernel methods, such as support vector machines, comes from the explicit probabilistic formulation that yields predictive distributions for test instances and allows standard Bayesian techniques for model selection. The cost of training GP models is $\mathcal{O}(n^3)$ where n is the number of training instances, which results in a huge computational cost for large data sets. Furthermore, when predicting a test case, a GP model requires $\mathcal{O}(n)$ cost for computing the mean and $\mathcal{O}(n^2)$ cost for computing the variance. These heavy scaling properties obstruct the use of GPs in large scale problems.

Recently, sparse GP models which bring down the complexity of training as well as testing have attracted considerable attention. Williams and Seeger (2001) applied the Nyström method to calculate a reduced rank approximation of the original $n \times n$ kernel matrix. Csató and Opper (2002) developed an on-line algorithm to maintain a sparse representation of the GP models. Smola and Bartlett (2001) proposed a forward selection scheme to approximate the log posterior probability. Candela (2004) suggested a promising alternative criterion by maximizing the approximate model evidence. Seeger et al. (2003) presented a very fast greedy selection method for building sparse GP regression models. All of these methods make efforts to select an informative subset of the training instances for the predictive model. This subset is usually referred to as the set of *basis vectors*, denoted as $\mathcal{I}$. The maximal size of $\mathcal{I}$ is usually limited by a value $d_{\max}$. As $d_{\max} \ll n$, the sparseness greatly alleviates the computational burden in both training and prediction of the GP models. The performance of the resulting sparse GP models crucially depends on the criterion used in the basis vector selection. Motivated by the ideas of Matching Pursuit (Vincent and Bengio, 2002), we propose a new criterion of greedy forward selection for sparse GP models.

Our algorithm is closely related to that of Smola and Bartlett (2001), but the criterion we propose is much more efficient. Compared with the information gain method of Seeger et al. (2003) our approach yields clearly better generalization performance, while essentially having the same algorithm complexity. We focus only on regression in this paper, but the main ideas are applicable to other supervised learning tasks.

The paper is organized as follows: in Section 2 we present the probabilistic framework for sparse GP models; in Section 3 we describe our method of greedy forward selection after motivating it via the previous methods; in Section 4 we discuss some issues in model adaptation; in Section 5 we report results of numerical experiments that demonstrate the effectiveness of our new method.

2 Sparse GPs for regression

In regression problems, we are given a training data set composed of n samples. Each sample is a pair of an input vector $x_i \in \mathbb{R}^m$ and its corresponding target $y_i \in \mathbb{R}$. The true function value at x_i is represented as an unobservable latent variable $f(x_i)$ and the target y_i is a noisy measurement of $f(x_i)$. The goal is to construct a predictive model that estimates the relationship $x \mapsto f(x)$.

Gaussian process regression. In standard GPs for regression, the latent variables $\{f(x_i)\}$ are random variables in a zero mean Gaussian process indexed by $\{x_i\}$. The prior distribution of $\{f(x_i)\}$ is a multivariate joint Gaussian, denoted as $\mathcal{P}(f) = \mathcal{N}(f; 0, \mathbf{K})$, where $f = [f(x_1), \ldots, f(x_n)]^T$ and $\mathbf{K}$ is the $n \times n$ covariance matrix whose ij-th element is $\mathcal{K}(x_i, x_j)$, $\mathcal{K}$ being the kernel function. The likelihood is essentially a model of the measurement noise, which is usually evaluated as a product of independent Gaussian noises, $\mathcal{P}(y|f) = \mathcal{N}(y; f, \sigma^2 \mathbf{I})$, where $y = [y_1, \ldots, y_n]^T$ and σ^2 is the noise variance. The posterior distribution $\mathcal{P}(f|y) \propto \mathcal{P}(y|f)\mathcal{P}(f)$ is also exactly a Gaussian:

$$\mathcal{P}(f|y) = \mathcal{N}(f; \mathbf{K}\alpha^\star, \sigma^2 \mathbf{K}(\mathbf{K} + \sigma^2 \mathbf{I})^{-1})$$ (1)

where $\alpha^\star = (\mathbf{K} + \sigma^2 \mathbf{I})^{-1} y$. For any test instance x, the predictive distribution is $\mathcal{N}(f(x); \mu_x, \sigma_x^2)$ where $\mu_x = k^T (\mathbf{K} + \sigma^2 \mathbf{I})^{-1} y = k^T \alpha^\star$, $\sigma_x^2 = \mathcal{K}(x, x) - k^T (\mathbf{K} + \sigma^2 \mathbf{I})^{-1} k$, and $k = [\mathcal{K}(x_1, x), \ldots, \mathcal{K}(x_n, x)]^T$. The computational cost of training is $\mathcal{O}(n^3)$, which mainly comes from the need to invert the matrix $(\mathbf{K} + \sigma^2 \mathbf{I})$ and obtain the vector $\alpha^\star$. For doing predictions of a test instance the cost is $\mathcal{O}(n)$ to compute the mean and $\mathcal{O}(n^2)$ for computing the variance. This heavy scaling with respect to n makes the use of standard GP computationally prohibitive on large datasets.

Projected latent variables. Seeger et al. (2003) gave a neat method for working with a reduced number of latent variables, laying the foundation for forming sparse GP models. In this section we review their ideas. Instead of assuming n latent variables for all the training instances, sparse GP models assume only d latent variables placed at some chosen basis vectors $\{\tilde{x}_i\}$, denoted as a column vector $f_{\mathcal{I}} = [f(\tilde{x}_1), \ldots, f(\tilde{x}_d)]^T$. The prior distribution of the sparse GP is a joint Gaussian over $f_{\mathcal{I}}$ only, i.e.,

$$\mathcal{P}(f_{\mathcal{I}}) = \mathcal{N}(f_{\mathcal{I}}; 0, \mathbf{K}_{\mathcal{I}})$$ (2)

where $\mathbf{K}_{\mathcal{I}}$ is the $d \times d$ covariance matrix of the basis vectors whose ij-th element is $\mathcal{K}(\tilde{x}_i, \tilde{x}_j)$.

These latent variables are then projected to all the training instances. Under the imposed joint Gaussian prior, the conditional mean at the training instances is $\mathbf{K}_{\mathcal{I},.}^T \mathbf{K}_{\mathcal{I}}^{-1} f_{\mathcal{I}}$, where $\mathbf{K}_{\mathcal{I},.}$ is a $d \times n$ matrix of the covariance functions between the basis vectors and all the training instances. The likelihood can be evaluated by these projected latent variables as follows

$$\mathcal{P}(y|f_{\mathcal{I}}) = \mathcal{N}(y; \mathbf{K}_{\mathcal{I},.}^T \mathbf{K}_{\mathcal{I}}^{-1} f_{\mathcal{I}}, \sigma^2 \mathbf{I})$$ (3)

The posterior is $\mathcal{P}(\boldsymbol{f}_\mathcal{I}|\boldsymbol{y}) = \mathcal{N}(\boldsymbol{f}_\mathcal{I}; \mathbf{K}_\mathcal{I}\, \boldsymbol{\alpha}_\mathcal{I}^\star, \sigma^2 \mathbf{K}_\mathcal{I}(\sigma^2 \mathbf{K}_\mathcal{I} + \mathbf{K}_{\mathcal{I},\cdot}\, \mathbf{K}_{\mathcal{I},\cdot}^T)^{-1}\mathbf{K}_\mathcal{I})$, where $\boldsymbol{\alpha}_\mathcal{I}^\star = (\sigma^2 \mathbf{K}_\mathcal{I} + \mathbf{K}_{\mathcal{I},\cdot}\, \mathbf{K}_{\mathcal{I},\cdot}^T)^{-1}\mathbf{K}_{\mathcal{I},\cdot}\, \boldsymbol{y}$. The predictive distribution at any test instance $\boldsymbol{x}$ is $\mathcal{N}(f(\boldsymbol{x}); \tilde{\mu}_{\boldsymbol{x}}, \tilde{\sigma}_{\boldsymbol{x}}^2)$, where $\tilde{\mu}_{\boldsymbol{x}} = \tilde{\boldsymbol{k}}^T \boldsymbol{\alpha}_\mathcal{I}^\star$, $\tilde{\sigma}_{\boldsymbol{x}}^2 = \mathcal{K}(\boldsymbol{x}, \boldsymbol{x}) - \tilde{\boldsymbol{k}}^T \mathbf{K}_\mathcal{I}^{-1} \tilde{\boldsymbol{k}}^T + \sigma^2 \tilde{\boldsymbol{k}}^T (\sigma^2 \mathbf{K}_\mathcal{I} + \mathbf{K}_{\mathcal{I},\cdot}\, \mathbf{K}_{\mathcal{I},\cdot}^T)^{-1}\tilde{\boldsymbol{k}}$, and $\tilde{\boldsymbol{k}}$ is a column vector of the covariance functions between the basis vectors and the test instance $\boldsymbol{x}$, i.e. $\tilde{\boldsymbol{k}} = [\mathcal{K}(\tilde{\boldsymbol{x}}_1, \boldsymbol{x}), \ldots, \mathcal{K}(\tilde{\boldsymbol{x}}_d, \boldsymbol{x})]^T$.

While the cost of training the full GP model is $\mathcal{O}(n^3)$, the training complexity of sparse GP models is only $\mathcal{O}(nd_{\max}^2)$. This corresponds to the cost of forming $\mathbf{K}_\mathcal{I}^{-1}$, $(\sigma^2 \mathbf{K}_\mathcal{I} + \mathbf{K}_{\mathcal{I},\cdot}\, \mathbf{K}_{\mathcal{I},\cdot}^T)^{-1}$ and $\boldsymbol{\alpha}_\mathcal{I}^\star$. Thus, if $d_{\max}$ is not big, learning on large datasets is feasible via sparse GP models. Also, for these sparse models, prediction for each test instance costs $\mathcal{O}(d_{\max})$ for the mean and $\mathcal{O}(d_{\max}^2)$ for the variance.

Generally the basis vectors can be placed anywhere in the input space $\mathbb{R}^m$. Since training instances usually cover the input space of interest quite well, it is quite reasonable to select basis vectors from just the set of training instances. For a given problem $d_{\max}$ is chosen to be as large as possible subject to constraints on computational time in training and/or testing. Then we use some basis selection method to find $\mathcal{I}$ of size $d_{\max}$. This important step is taken up in section 3.

A Useful optimization formulation. As pointed out by Smola and Bartlett (2001), it is useful to view the determination of the mean of the posterior as coming from an optimization problem. This viewpoint helps in the selection of basis vectors. The mean of the posterior distribution is exactly the maximum a posteriori (MAP) estimate, and it is possible to give an equivalent parametric representation of the latent variables as $\boldsymbol{f} = \mathbf{K}\boldsymbol{\alpha}$, where $\boldsymbol{\alpha} = [\alpha_1, \ldots, \alpha_n]^T$. The MAP estimate of the full GP is equivalent to minimizing the negative logarithm of the posterior (1):

$$\min_{\boldsymbol{\alpha}} \pi(\boldsymbol{\alpha}) := \frac{1}{2}\boldsymbol{\alpha}^T(\sigma^2 \mathbf{K} + \mathbf{K}^T \mathbf{K})\boldsymbol{\alpha} - \boldsymbol{y}^T \mathbf{K}\boldsymbol{\alpha} \quad (4)$$

Similarly, using $\boldsymbol{f}_\mathcal{I} = \mathbf{K}_\mathcal{I}\boldsymbol{\alpha}_\mathcal{I}$ for sparse GP models, the MAP estimate of the sparse GP is equivalent to minimizing the negative logarithm of the posterior, $\mathcal{P}(\boldsymbol{f}_\mathcal{I}|\boldsymbol{y})$:

$$\min_{\boldsymbol{\alpha}_\mathcal{I}} \tilde{\pi}(\boldsymbol{\alpha}_\mathcal{I}) := \frac{1}{2}\boldsymbol{\alpha}_\mathcal{I}^T(\sigma^2 \mathbf{K}_\mathcal{I} + \mathbf{K}_{\mathcal{I},\cdot}\mathbf{K}_{\mathcal{I},\cdot}^T)\boldsymbol{\alpha}_\mathcal{I} - \boldsymbol{y}^T \mathbf{K}_{\mathcal{I},\cdot}^T\, \boldsymbol{\alpha}_\mathcal{I} \quad (5)$$

Suppose $\boldsymbol{\alpha}$ in (4) is composed of two parts, $\boldsymbol{\alpha} = [\boldsymbol{\alpha}_\mathcal{I}; \boldsymbol{\alpha}_\mathcal{R}]$ where $\mathcal{I}$ denotes the set of basis vectors and $\mathcal{R}$ denotes the remaining instances. Interestingly, as pointed out by Seeger et al. (2003), the optimization problem (5) is same as minimizing $\pi(\boldsymbol{\alpha})$ in (4) using $\boldsymbol{\alpha}_\mathcal{I}$ only, i.e., with the constraint, $\boldsymbol{\alpha}_\mathcal{R} = 0$. In other words, the basis vectors of the sparse GPs can be selected to minimize the negative log-posterior of the full GPs, $\pi(\boldsymbol{\alpha})$ defined as in (4).

3 Selection of basis functions

The most crucial element of the sparse GP approach of the previous section is the choice of $\mathcal{I}$, the set of basis vectors, which we take to be a subset of the training vectors. The cheapest method is to select the basis vectors at *random* from the training data set. But, such a choice will not work well when $d_{\max}$ is much smaller than n. A principled approach is to select $\mathcal{I}$ that makes the corresponding sparse GP approximate well, the posterior distribution of the full GP. The optimization formulation of the previous section is useful here. It would be ideal to choose, among all subsets, $\mathcal{I}$ of size $d_{\max}$, the one that gives the best value of $\tilde{\pi}$ in (5). But, this requires a combinatorial search that is infeasible for large problems. A practical approach is to do greedy forward selection. This is the approach used in previous methods as well as in our method of this paper.

Before we go into the details of the methods, let us give a brief discussion of the time complexities associated with forward selection. There are two costs involved. (1) There is a basic cost associated with updating of the sparse GP solution, given a sequence of chosen basis functions. Let us refer to this cost as T_{basic}. This cost is the same for all forward selection methods, and is $\mathcal{O}(nd_{\max}^2)$. (2) Then, depending on the basis selection method, there is the cost associated with basis selection. We will refer to the accumulated value of this cost for choosing all $d_{\max}$ basis functions as $T_{\mathrm{selection}}$. Forward basis selection methods differ in the way they choose effective basis functions while keeping $T_{\mathrm{selection}}$ small. It is useful to note that the total cost associated with the *random* basis selection method mentioned earlier is just $T_{\mathrm{basic}} = \mathcal{O}(nd_{\max}^2)$. This cost forms a baseline for comparison.

Smola and Bartlett's method. Consider the typical situation in forward selection where we have a current working set $\mathcal{I}$ and we are interested in choosing the next basis vector, x_i. The method of Smola and Bartlett (2001) evaluates each given $x_i \notin \mathcal{I}$ by trying its complete inclusion, i.e., set $\mathcal{I}' = \mathcal{I} \cup \{x_i\}$ and optimize $\pi(\alpha)$ using $\alpha_{\mathcal{I}'} = [\alpha_{\mathcal{I}}; \alpha_i]$. Thus, their selection criterion for the instance $x_i \notin \mathcal{I}$ is the decrease in $\pi(\alpha)$ that can be obtained by allowing both $\alpha_{\mathcal{I}}$ and α_i as variables to be non-zero. The minimal value of $\pi(\alpha)$ can be obtained by solving $\min_{\alpha_{\mathcal{I}'}} \tilde{\pi}(\alpha_{\mathcal{I}'})$ defined in (5). This costs $\mathcal{O}(nd)$ time for each candidate, x_i, where d is the size of the current set, $\mathcal{I}$. If all $x_i \notin \mathcal{I}$ need to be tried, it will lead to $\mathcal{O}(n^2 d)$ cost. Accumulated till $d_{\max}$ basis functions are added, this leads to a $T_{\mathrm{selection}}$ that has $\mathcal{O}(n^2 d_{\max}^2)$ complexity, which is disproportionately higher than T_{basic}. Therefore, Smola and Bartlett (2001) resorted to a randomized scheme by considering only κ basis elements randomly chosen from outside $\mathcal{I}$ during one basis selection. They used a value of $\kappa = 59$. For this randomized method, the complexity of $T_{\mathrm{selection}}$ is $\mathcal{O}(\kappa nd_{\max}^2)$. Although, from a complexity viewpoint, T_{basic} and $T_{\mathrm{selection}}$ are same, it should be noted that the overall cost of the method is about 60 times that of T_{basic}.

Seeger et al's information gain method. Seeger et al. (2003) proposed a novel and very cheap heuristic criterion for basis selection. The "informativeness" of an input vector $x_i \notin \mathcal{I}$ is scored by the information gain between the true posterior distribution, $\mathcal{P}(f_{\mathcal{I}'}|y)$ and a posterior approximation, $\mathcal{Q}(f_{\mathcal{I}'}|y)$, where $\mathcal{I}'$ denotes the new set of basis vectors after including a new element x_i into the current set $\mathcal{I}$. The posterior approximation $\mathcal{Q}(f_{\mathcal{I}'}|y)$ ignores the dependencies between the latent variable $f(x_i)$ and the targets other than y_i. Due to this simplification, this value of information gain is computed in $\mathcal{O}(1)$ time, given the current predictive model represented by $\mathcal{I}$. Thus, the scores of all instances outside $\mathcal{I}$ can be efficiently evaluated in $\mathcal{O}(n)$ time, which makes this algorithm almost as fast as using random selection! The potential weakness of this algorithm might be the non-use of the correlation in the remaining instances $\{x_i : x_i \notin \mathcal{I}\}$.

Post-backfitting approach. The two methods presented above are extremes in efficiency: in Smola and Bartlett's method $T_{\mathrm{selection}}$ is disproportionately larger than T_{basic} while, in Seeger et al's method $T_{\mathrm{selection}}$ is very much smaller than T_{basic}. In this section we introduce a moderate method that is effective and whose complexity is in between the two earlier methods. Our method borrows an idea from kernel matching pursuit.

Kernel Matching Pursuit (Vincent and Bengio, 2002) is a sparse method for ordinary least squares that consists of two general greedy sparse approximation schemes, called *pre-backfitting* and *post-backfitting*. It is worth pointing out that the same methods were also considered much earlier in Adler et al. (1996). Both methods can be generalized to select the basis vectors for sparse GPs. The *pre-backfitting* approach is very similar in spirit to Smola and Bartlett's method. Our method is an efficient selection criterion that is based on the *post-backfitting* idea. Recall that, given the current $\mathcal{I}$, the minimal value of $\pi(\alpha)$ when it is optimized using only $\alpha_{\mathcal{I}}$ as variables is equivalent to $\min_{\alpha_{\mathcal{I}}} \tilde{\pi}(\alpha_{\mathcal{I}})$ as in (5). The minimizer, denoted as $\alpha_{\mathcal{I}}^{\star}$, is given by

$$\alpha_{\mathcal{I}}^{\star} = (\sigma^2 \mathbf{K}_{\mathcal{I}} + \mathbf{K}_{\mathcal{I},\cdot} \mathbf{K}_{\mathcal{I},\cdot}^T)^{-1} \mathbf{K}_{\mathcal{I},\cdot}\, y \qquad (6)$$

Our scoring criterion for an instance $x_i \notin \mathcal{I}$ is based on optimizing $\pi(\alpha)$ by fixing $\alpha_{\mathcal{I}} = \alpha_{\mathcal{I}}^{\star}$ and changing α_i only. The one-dimensional minimizer can be easily found as

$$\alpha_i^* = \frac{\mathbf{K}_{i,\cdot}^T (\boldsymbol{y} - \mathbf{K}_{\mathcal{I},\cdot}^T \boldsymbol{\alpha}_{\mathcal{I}}^\star) - \sigma^2 \tilde{\boldsymbol{k}}_i^T \boldsymbol{\alpha}_{\mathcal{I}}^\star}{\sigma^2 \mathcal{K}(\boldsymbol{x}_i, \boldsymbol{x}_i) + \mathbf{K}_{i,\cdot}^T \mathbf{K}_{i,\cdot}} \tag{7}$$

where $\mathbf{K}_{i,\cdot}$ is the $n \times 1$ matrix of covariance functions between $\boldsymbol{x}_i$ and all the training data, and $\tilde{\boldsymbol{k}}_i$ is a d dimensional vector having $\mathcal{K}(\boldsymbol{x}_j, \boldsymbol{x}_i)$, $\boldsymbol{x}_j \in \mathcal{I}$. The selection score of the instance $\boldsymbol{x}_i$ is the decrease in $\pi(\boldsymbol{\alpha})$ achieved by the one dimensional optimization of α_i, which can be written in closed form as

$$\Delta_i = \frac{1}{2} (\alpha_i^*)^2 \left(\sigma^2 \mathcal{K}(\boldsymbol{x}_i, \boldsymbol{x}_i) + \mathbf{K}_{i,\cdot}^T \mathbf{K}_{i,\cdot} \right) \tag{8}$$

where α_i^* is defined as in (7). Note that a full kernel column $\mathbf{K}_{i,\cdot}$ is required and so it costs $\mathcal{O}(n)$ time to compute (8). In contrast, for scoring one instance, Smola and Bartlett's method requires $\mathcal{O}(nd)$ time and Seeger et al's method requires $\mathcal{O}(1)$ time.

Ideally we would like to run over all $\boldsymbol{x}_i \notin \mathcal{I}$ and choose the instance which gives the largest decrease. This will need $\mathcal{O}(n^2)$ effort. Summing the cost till $d_{\max}$ basis vectors are selected, we get an overall complexity of $\mathcal{O}(n^2 d_{\max})$, which is much higher than T_{basic}. To restrict the overall complexity of $T_{\text{selection}}$ to $\mathcal{O}(n d_{\max}^2)$, we resort to a randomization scheme that selects a relatively good one rather than the best. Since it costs only $\mathcal{O}(n)$ time to evaluate our selection criterion in (8) for one instance, we can choose the next basis vector from a set of $d_{\max}$ instances randomly selected from outside of $\mathcal{I}$. Such a scheme keeps the overall complexity of $T_{\text{selection}}$ to $\mathcal{O}(n d_{\max}^2)$. But, from a practical point of view the scheme is expensive because the selection criterion (8) requires computing a full kernel row $\mathbf{K}_{i,\cdot}$ for each instance to be evaluated. As kernel evaluations could be very expensive, we propose a modified scheme to keep the number of such evaluations small.

Let us maintain a matrix cache, $\mathcal{C}$ of size $c \times n$, that contains c rows of the full kernel matrix $\mathbf{K}$. At the beginning of the algorithm (when $\mathcal{I}$ is empty) we initialize $\mathcal{C}$ by randomly choosing c training instances, computing the full kernel row, $\mathbf{K}_{i,\cdot}$ for the chosen i's and putting them in the rows of $\mathcal{C}$. Each step corresponding to a new basis vector selection proceeds as follows. First we compute Δ_i for the c instances corresponding to the rows of $\mathcal{C}$ and select the instance with the highest score for inclusion in $\mathcal{I}$. Let x_j denote the chosen basis vector. Then we sort the remaining instances (that define $\mathcal{C}$) according to their Δ_i values. Finally, we randomly select κ fresh instances (from outside of $\mathcal{I}$ and the vectors that define $\mathcal{C}$) to replace x_j and the $\kappa - 1$ cached instances with the lowest score. Thus, in each basis selection step, we compute the criterion scores for c instances, but evaluate full kernel rows only for κ fresh instances. An important advantage of the above scheme is that, those basis elements which have very good scores, but are overtaken by another better element in a particular step, continue to remain in $\mathcal{C}$ and probably get to be selected in future basis selection steps. Like in Smola and Bartlett's method we use $\kappa = 59$. The value of c can be set to be any integer between κ and $d_{\max}$. For any c in this range, the complexity of $T_{\text{selection}}$ remains at most $\mathcal{O}(n d_{\max}^2)$. The above cache scheme is special to our method and cannot be used with Smola and Bartlett's method without unduly increasing its complexity. If available, it is also useful to have an extra cache for storing kernel rows of instances which get discarded in one step, but which get to be considered again in a future step. Smola and Bartlett's method can also gain from such a cache.

4 Model adaptation

In this section we address the problem of model adaptation for a given number of basis functions, $d_{\max}$. Seeger (2003) and Seeger et al. (2003) give the details together with a very good discussion of various issues associated with gradient based model adaptation. Since the same ideas hold for all basis selection methods, we will not discuss them in detail. The sparse GP model is conditional on the parameters in the kernel function and the Gaussian noise level σ^2, which can all be collected together in θ, the hyperparameter vector. The optimal values of θ can be inferred by minimizing the negative log of the marginal likelihood, $\phi(\theta) = -\log P(y|\theta)$ using gradient based techniques, where $P(y|\theta) = \int P(y|f_{\mathcal{I}})P(f_{\mathcal{I}})df_{\mathcal{I}} = \mathcal{N}(y|0, \sigma^2 \mathbf{I} + \mathbf{K}_{\mathcal{I},\cdot}^T \mathbf{K}_{\mathcal{I}}^{-1} \mathbf{K}_{\mathcal{I},\cdot})$. One of the problems in doing this is the dependence of $\mathcal{I}$ on θ that makes ϕ a non-differentiable function. This problem can be handled by repeating the following alternating steps: (1) fix θ and select $\mathcal{I}$ by the given basis selection algorithm; and (2) fix $\mathcal{I}$ and do a (short) gradient based adaptation of θ. For the cache-based post-backfitting method of basis selection we also do the following for adding some stability to the model adaptation process. After we do step (2) using some $\mathcal{I}$ and obtain a θ we set the initial kernel cache, $\mathcal{C}$ using the rows of $\mathbf{K}_{\mathcal{I},\cdot}$ at θ.

5   Numerical experiments

In this section, we compare our method against other sparse GP methods to verify the usefulness of our algorithm. To evaluate generalization performance, we utilize *Normalized Mean Square Error* (NMSE) given by $\frac{1}{t}\sum_{i=1}^{t} \frac{(y_i - \mu_i)^2}{\text{Var}(y)}$ and *Negative Logarithm of Predictive Distribution* (NLPD) defined as $\frac{1}{t}\sum_{i=1}^{t} -\log P(y_i|\mu_i, \sigma_i^2)$ where t is the number of test cases, y_i, μ_i and σ_i^2 are, respectively, the target, the predictive mean and the predictive variance of the i-th test case. NMSE uses only the mean while NLPD measures the quality of predictive distributions as it penalizes over-confident predictions as well as under-confident ones. For all experiments, we use the ARD Gaussian kernel defined by $\mathcal{K}(x_i, x_j) = v_0 \exp\left(\sum_{\ell=1}^{m} v_\ell (x_i^\ell - x_j^\ell)^2\right) + v_b$ where $v_0, v_\ell, v_b > 0$ and x_i^ℓ denotes the ℓ-th element of x_i. The ARD parameters $\{v_\ell\}$ give variable weights to input features that leads to a type of feature selection.

Quality of Basis Selection in KIN40K Data Set. We use the KIN40K data set,[1] composed of 40,000 samples, to evaluate and compare the performance of the various basis selection criteria. We first trained a full GPR model with the ARD Gaussian kernel on a subset of 2000 samples randomly selected in the dataset. The optimal values of the hyperparameters that we obtained were fixed and used for all the sparse GP models in this experiment. We compare the following five basis selection methods:

1. the baseline algorithm (RAND) that selects $\mathcal{I}$ at random;
2. the information gain algorithm (INFO) proposed by Seeger et al. (2003);
3. our algorithm described in Section 3 with cache size $c = \kappa = 59$ (KAPPA) in which we evaluate the selection scores of κ instances at each step;
4. our algorithm described in Section 3 with cache size $c = d_{\max}$ (DMAX);
5. the algorithm (SB) proposed by Smola and Bartlett (2001) with $\kappa = 59$.

We randomly selected 10,000 samples for training, and kept the remaining 30,000 samples as test cases. For the purpose of studying variability the methods were run on ten such random partitions. We varied $d_{\max}$ from 100 to 1200. The test performances of the five methods are presented in Figure 1. From the upper plot of Figure 1 we can see that INFO yields much worse NMSE results than KAPPA, DMAX and SB, when $d_{\max}$ is less than 600. When the size is around 100, INFO is even worse than RAND. DMAX is always better than KAPPA. Interestingly, DMAX is even slightly better than SB when $d_{\max}$ is less than 200. This is probably because DMAX has a bigger set of basis functions to choose from, than SB. SB generally yields slightly better results than KAPPA. From the middle plot of Figure 1 we can note that INFO always gives poor NLPD results, even worse than RAND. The performances of KAPPA, DMAX and SB are close.

The lower plot of Figure 1 gives the CPU time consumed by the five algorithms for training, as a function of $d_{\max}$, in $\log - \log$ scale. The scaling exponents of RAND, INFO and SB are

---

[1] The dataset is available at http://www.igi.tugraz.at/aschwaig/data.html.

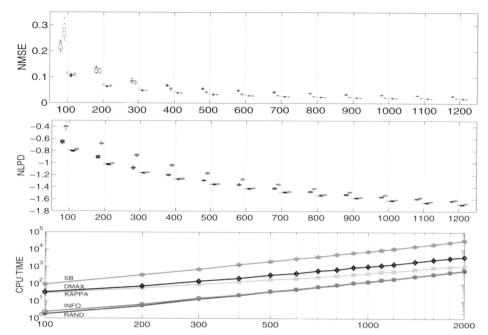

Figure 1: The variations of test set NMSE, test set NLPD and CPU time (in seconds) for training of the five algorithms as a function of $d_{\max}$. In the NMSE and NLPD plots, at each value of $d_{\max}$, the results of the five algorithms are presented as a boxplot group. From left to right, they are RAND(blue), INFO(red), KAPPA(green), DMAX(black), and SB(magenta). Note that the CPU time plot is on a $\log - \log$ scale.

around 2.0 (i.e., cost is proportional to $d_{\max}^2$), which is consistent with our analysis. INFO is almost as fast as RAND, while SB is about 60 times slower than INFO. The gap between KAPPA and INFO is the $\mathcal{O}(\kappa n d_{\max})$ time in computing the score (8) for κ candidates.[2] As $d_{\max}$ increases, the cost of KAPPA asymptotically gets close to INFO. The gap between DMAX and KAPPA is the $\mathcal{O}(n d_{\max}^2 - \kappa n d_{\max})$ cost in computing the score (8) for the additional $(d_{\max} - \kappa)$ instances. Thus, as $d_{\max}$ increases, the curve of DMAX asymptotically becomes parallel to the curve of INFO. Asymptotically, the ratio of the computational times of DMAX and INFO is only about 3. Thus, unlike SB, which is about 60 times slower than INFO, DMAX is only about 3 times slower than INFO. Thus DMAX is an excellent method for achieving excellent generalization while also being quite efficient.

Model Adaptation on Benchmark Data Sets. Next, we compare model adaptation abilities of the following three algorithms for $d_{\max} = 500$.

1. The SB algorithm is applied to build a sparse GPR model with fixed hyperparameters (FIXED-SB). The values of these hyperparameters were obtained by training via a standard full GPR model on a manageable subset of 2000 samples randomly selected from the training data. FIXED-SB serves as a baseline.

2. The model adaptation scheme is coupled with the INFO basis selection algorithm (ADAPT-INFO).

3. The model adaptation scheme is coupled with our DMAX basis selection algorithm (ADAPT-DMAX).

---

[2]If we want to take kernel evaluations also into account, the cost of KAPPA is $\mathcal{O}(m\kappa n d_{\max})$ where m is the number of input variables. Note that INFO does not require any kernel evaluations for computing its selection criterion.

Table 1: Test results of the three algorithms on the seven benchmark regression datasets. The results are the averages over 20 trials, along with the standard deviation. d denotes the number of input features, n_{trg} denotes the training data size and n_{tst} denotes the test data size. We use bold face to indicate the lowest average value among the results of the three algorithms. The symbol $\star$ is used to indicate the cases significantly worse than the winning entry; a p-value threshold of 0.01 in Wilcoxon rank sum test was used to decide this.

				NMSE			NLPD		
DATASET	d	n_{trg}	n_{tst}	FIXED-SB	ADAPT-INFO	ADAPT-DMAX	FIXED-SB	ADAPT-INFO	ADAPT-DMAX
BANK8FM	8	4500	3692	$\mathbf{3.52 \pm 0.08}$	3.54 ± 0.08	3.56 ± 0.09	$3.11 \pm 0.65^\star$	$1.37 \pm 0.34^\star$	$\mathbf{0.67 \pm 0.53}$
BANK32NH	32	4500	3692	48.08 ± 2.92	$49.04 \pm 1.34^\star$	$\mathbf{47.41 \pm 1.35}$	-1.02 ± 0.21	$-0.79 \pm 0.06^\star$	$-0.88 \pm 0.03^\star$
CPUSMALL	12	4500	3692	2.45 ± 0.16	$\mathbf{2.45 \pm 0.15}$	2.46 ± 0.14	$5.18 \pm 0.61^\star$	$3.70 \pm 0.46^\star$	$\mathbf{3.04 \pm 0.17}$
CPUACT	21	4500	3692	$\mathbf{1.58 \pm 0.13}$	1.61 ± 0.14	1.61 ± 0.11	$4.49 \pm 0.26^\star$	$3.68 \pm 0.40^\star$	$\mathbf{3.09 \pm 0.20}$
CALHOUSE	8	10000	10640	$22.58 \pm 0.34^\star$	$22.82 \pm 0.46^\star$	$\mathbf{20.02 \pm 0.88}$	$31.83 \pm 3.35^\star$	$21.20 \pm 1.47^\star$	$\mathbf{13.03 \pm 0.30}$
HOUSE8L	8	10000	12784	$42.27 \pm 2.14^\star$	$37.30 \pm 1.29^\star$	$\mathbf{35.87 \pm 0.94}$	12.06 ± 0.67	$12.06 \pm 0.07^\star$	$\mathbf{11.71 \pm 0.03}$
HOUSE16H	16	10000	12784	$53.45 \pm 7.05^\star$	$45.72 \pm 1.15^\star$	$\mathbf{44.29 \pm 0.76}$	12.72 ± 1.69	$12.48 \pm 0.06^\star$	$\mathbf{12.13 \pm 0.04}$

We selected seven large regression datasets.[3] Each of them is randomly partitioned into training/test splits. For the purpose of analyzing statistical significance, the partition was repeated 20 times independently. Test set performances (NMSE and NLPD) of the three methods on the seven datasets are presented in Table 1. On the four datasets with 4500 training instances, the NMSE results of the three methods are quite comparable. ADAPT-DMAX yields significantly better NLPD results on three of those four datasets. On the three larger datasets with 10,000 training instances, ADAPT-DMAX is significantly better than ADAPT-INFO on both NMSE and NLPD.

We also tested our algorithm on the Outaouais dataset, which consists of 29000 training samples and 20000 test cases whose targets are held by the organizers of the "Evaluating Predictive Uncertainty Challenge".[4] The results of NMSE and NLPD we obtained in this blind test are 0.014 and -1.037 respectively, which are much better than the results of other participants.

References

Adler, J., B. D. Rao, and K. Kreutz-Delgado. Comparison of basis selection methods. In *Proceedings of the 30th Asilomar conference on signals, systems and computers*, pages 252–257, 1996.

Candela, J. Q. *Learning with uncertainty - Gaussian processes and relevance vector machines*. PhD thesis, Technical University of Denmark, 2004.

Csató, L. and M. Opper. Sparse online Gaussian processes. *Neural Computation, The MIT Press*, 14:641–668, 2002.

Seeger, M. *Bayesian Gaussian process models: PAC-Bayesian generalisation error bounds and sparse approximations*. PhD thesis, University of Edinburgh, July 2003.

Seeger, M., C. K. I. Williams, and N. Lawrence. Fast forward selection to speed up sparse Gaussian process regression. In *Workshop on AI and Statistics 9*, 2003.

Smola, A. J. and P. Bartlett. Sparse greedy Gaussian process regression. In Leen, T. K., T. G. Dietterich, and V. Tresp, editors, *Advances in Neural Information Processing Systems 13*, pages 619–625. MIT Press, 2001.

Vincent, P. and Y. Bengio. Kernel matching pursuit. *Machine Learning*, 48:165–187, 2002.

Williams, C. K. I. and M. Seeger. Using the Nyström method to speed up kernel machines. In Leen, T. K., T. G. Dietterich, and V. Tresp, editors, *Advances in Neural Information Processing Systems 13*, pages 682–688. MIT Press, 2001.

---

[3]These datasets are vailable at http://www.liacc.up.pt/~ltorgo/Regression/DataSets.html.

[4]The dataset and the results contributed by other participants can be found at the web site of the challenge http://predict.kyb.tuebingen.mpg.de/.

Benchmarking Non-Parametric Statistical Tests

Mikaela Keller[*]
IDIAP Research Institute
1920 Martigny
Switzerland
mkeller@idiap.ch

Samy Bengio
IDIAP Research Institute
1920 Martigny
Switzerland
bengio@idiap.ch

Siew Yeung Wong
IDIAP Research Institute
1920 Martigny
Switzerland
sywong@idiap.ch

Abstract

Although non-parametric tests have already been proposed for that purpose, statistical significance tests for non-standard measures (different from the classification error) are less often used in the literature. This paper is an attempt at empirically verifying how these tests compare with more classical tests, on various conditions. More precisely, using a very large dataset to estimate the whole "population", we analyzed the behavior of several statistical test, varying the class unbalance, the compared models, the performance measure, and the sample size. The main result is that providing big enough evaluation sets non-parametric tests are relatively reliable in all conditions.

1 Introduction

Statistical tests are often used in machine learning in order to assess the performance of a new learning algorithm or model over a set of benchmark datasets, with respect to the state-of-the-art solutions. Several researchers (see for instance [4] and [9]) have proposed statistical tests suited for 2-class classification tasks where the performance is measured in terms of the classification error (ratio of the number of errors and the number of examples), which enables the use of assumptions based on the fact that the error can be seen as a sum of random variables over the evaluation examples. On the other hand, various research domains prefer to measure the performance of their models using different indicators, such as the F_1 measure, used in information retrieval [11], described in Section 2.1. Most classical statistical tests cannot cope directly with such measure as the usual necessary assumptions are no longer correct, and non-parametric bootstrap-based methods are then used [5].

Since several papers already use these non-parametric tests [2, 1], we were interested in verifying empirically how reliable they were. For this purpose, we used a very large text categorization database (the extended Reuters dataset [10]), composed of more than 800000 examples, and concerning more than 100 categories (each document was labelled with one or more of these categories). We purposely set aside the largest part of the dataset and considered it as the whole population, while a much smaller part of it was used as a training set for the models. Using the large set aside dataset part, we *tested* the statistical test in the

[*]This work was supported in part by the Swiss NSF through the NCCR on IM2 and in part by the European PASCAL Network of Excellence, IST-2002-506778, through the Swiss OFES.

same spirit as was done in [4], by sampling evaluation sets over which we observed the performance of the models and the behavior of the significance test.

Following the taxonomy of questions of interest defined by Dietterich in [4], we can differentiate between statistical tests that analyze learning algorithms and statistical tests that analyze classifiers. In the first case, one intends to be robust to possible variations of the train and evaluation sets, while in the latter, one intends to only be robust to variations of the evaluation set. While the methods discussed in this paper can be applied alternatively to both approaches, we concentrate here on the second one, as it is more tractable (for the empirical section) while still corresponding to real life situations where the training set is fixed and one wants to compare two solutions (such as during a competition).

In order to conduct a thorough analysis, we tried to vary the evaluation set size, the class unbalance, the error measure, the statistical test itself (with its associated assumptions), and even the *closeness* of the compared learning algorithms. This paper, and more precisely Section 3, is a detailed account of this analysis. As it will be seen empirically, the *closeness* of the compared learning algorithms seems to have an effect on the resulting quality of the statistical tests: comparing an MLP and an SVM yields less reliable statistical tests than comparing two SVMs with a different kernel. To the best of our knowledge, this has never been considered in the literature of statistical tests for machine learning.

2   A Statistical Significance Test for the Difference of F_1

Let us first remind the basic classification framework in which statistical significance tests are used in machine learning. We consider comparing two models A and B on a two-class classification task where the goal is to classify input examples x_i into the corresponding class $y_i \in \{-1, 1\}$, using already trained models $f_A(x_i)$ or $f_B(x_i)$. One can estimate their respective performance on some test data by counting the number of utterances of each possible outcome: either the obtained class corresponds to the desired class, or not. Let $N_{e,A}$ (resp. $N_{e,B}$) be the number of errors of model A (resp. B) and N the total number of test examples; The difference between models A and B can then be written as

$$D = \frac{N_{e,A} - N_{e,B}}{N} . \tag{1}$$

The usual starting point of most statistical tests is to define the so-called *null hypothesis* H_0 which considers that the two models are equivalent, and then verifies how probable this hypothesis is. Hence, assuming that D is an instance of some random variable $\mathbf{D}$ which follows some distribution, we are interested in

$$p\left(|\mathbf{D}| < |D|\right) < \alpha \tag{2}$$

where α represents the risk of selecting the *alternate hypothesis* (the two models are different) while the *null hypothesis* is in fact true. This can in general be estimated easily when the distribution of $\mathbf{D}$ is known. In the simplest case, known as the *proportion test*, one assumes (reasonably) that the decision taken by each model on each example can be modeled by a Bernoulli, and further assumes that the errors of the models are independent. This is in general wrong in machine learning since the evaluation sets are the same for both models. When N is large, this leads to estimate $\mathbf{D}$ as a Normal distribution with zero mean and standard deviation σ_D

$$\sigma_D = \sqrt{\frac{2\bar{C}(1 - \bar{C})}{N}} \tag{3}$$

where $\bar{C} = \frac{N_{e,A} + N_{e,B}}{2N}$ is the average classification error. In order to get rid of the wrong independence assumption between the errors of the models, the McNemar test [6] concentrates on examples which were differently classified by the two compared models. Following the notation of [4], let N_{01} be the number of examples misclassified by model A but not by model B and N_{10} the number of examples misclassified by model B but not by model A. It can be shown that the following statistics is approximatively distributed as a χ^2 with 1 degree of freedom:

$$z = \frac{(|N_{01} - N_{10}| - 1)^2}{N_{01} + N_{10}}. \tag{4}$$

More recently, several other statistical tests have been proposed, such as the 5x2cv method [4] or the variance estimate proposed in [9], which both claim to better estimate the distribution of the errors (and hence the confidence on the statistical significance of the results). Note however that these solutions assume that the error of one model is the average of some random variable (the error) estimated on each example. Intuitively, it will thus tend to be Normally distributed as N grows, following the central limit theorem.

2.1 The F_1 Measure

Text categorization is the task of assigning one or several categories, among a predefined set of K categories, to textual documents. As explained in [11], text categorization is usually solved as K 2-class classification problems, in a one-against-the-others approach. In this field two measures are considered of importance:

$$\text{Precision} = \frac{N_{tp}}{N_{tp} + N_{fp}}, \quad \text{and} \quad \text{Recall} = \frac{N_{tp}}{N_{tp} + N_{fn}},$$

where for each category N_{tp} is the number of true positives (documents belonging to the category that were classified as such), N_{fp} the number of false positives (documents out of this category but classified as being part of it) and N_{fn} the number of false negatives (documents from the category classified as out of it). Precision and Recall are effectiveness measures, i.e. inside $[0, 1]$ interval, the closer to 1 the better. For each category k, Precision_k measures the proportion of documents of the class among the ones considered as such by the classifier and Recall_k the proportion of documents of the class correctly classified.

To summarize these two values, it is common to consider the so-called F_1 measure [12], often used in domains such as information retrieval, text categorization, or vision processing. F_1 can be described as the inverse of the harmonic mean of Precision and Recall:

$$F_1 = \left(\frac{1}{2} \left[\frac{1}{\text{Recall}} + \frac{1}{\text{Precision}} \right] \right)^{-1} = \frac{2 \cdot \text{Precision} \cdot \text{Recall}}{\text{Precision} + \text{Recall}} = \frac{2 N_{tp}}{2 N_{tp} + N_{fn} + N_{fp}}. \tag{5}$$

Let us consider two models A and B, which achieve a performance measured by $F_{1,A}$ and $F_{1,B}$ respectively. The difference $dF_1 = F_{1,A} - F_{1,B}$ does not fit the assumptions of the tests presented earlier. Indeed, it cannot be decomposed into a sum over the documents of independent random variables, since the numerator and the denominator of dF_1 are non constant sums over documents of independent random variables. For the same reason F_1, while being a proportion, cannot be considered as a random variable following a Normal distribution for which we could easily estimate the variance.

An alternative solution to measure the statistical significance of dF_1 is based on the Bootstrap Percentile Test proposed in [5]. The idea of this test is to approximate the unknown distribution of dF_1 by an estimate based on bootstrap replicates of the data.

2.2 Bootstrap Percentile Test

Given an evaluation set of size N, one draws, *with replacement*, N samples from it. This gives the first bootstrap replicate B_1, over which one can compute the statistics of interest,

dF_{1,B_1}. Similarly, one can create as many bootstrap replicates B_n as needed, and for each, compute dF_{1,B_n}. The higher n is, the more precise should be the statistical test. Literature [3] suggests to create at least $\frac{50}{\alpha}$ replicates where α is the level of the test; for the smallest α we considered (0.01), this amounts to 5000 replicates. These 5000 estimates dF_{1,B_i} represent the non-parametric distribution of the random variable $\mathbf{dF_1}$. From it, one can for instance consider an interval $[a, b]$ such that $p(a < \mathbf{dF_1} < b) = 1 - \alpha$ centered around the mean of $p(\mathbf{dF_1})$. If 0 lies outside this interval, one can say that $dF_1 = 0$ is not among the most probable results, and thus reject the null hypothesis.

3   Analysis of Statistical Tests

We report in this section an analysis of the bootstrap percentile test, as well as other more classical statistical tests, based on a real large database. We first describe the database itself and the protocol we used for this analysis, and then provide results and comments.

3.1   Database, Models and Protocol

All the experiments detailed in this paper are based on the very large RCV1 Reuters dataset [10], which contains up to 806,791 documents. We divided it as follows: 798,809 documents were kept aside and any statistics computed over this set D_{true} was considered as being the *truth* (*ie* a very good estimate of the actual value); the remaining 7982 documents were used as a training set D_{tr} (to train models A and B). There was a total of 101 categories and each document was labeled with one or more of these categories.

We first extracted the dictionary from the training set, removed stop-words and applied stemming to it, as normally done in text categorization. Each document was then represented as a bag-of-words using the usual $tfidf$ coding. We trained three different models: a linear Support Vector Machine (SVM), a Gaussian kernel SVM, and a multi-layer perceptron (MLP). There was one model for each category for the SVMs, and a single MLP for the 101 categories. All models were properly tuned using cross-validation on the training set.

Using the notation introduced earlier, we define the following competing hypotheses: $H_0 : |dF_1| = 0$ and $H_1 : |dF_1| > 0$. We further define the level of the test $\alpha = p(\text{Reject } H_0 | H_0)$, where α takes on values 0.01, 0.05 and 0.1. Table 1 summarizes the possible outcomes of a statistical test. With that respect, rejecting H_0 means that one is confident with $(1 - \alpha) \cdot 100\%$ that H_0 is really false.

Table 1: Various outcomes of a statistical test, with $\alpha = p(\text{Type I error})$.

Truth	Decision	
	Reject H_0	Accept H_0
H_0	Type I error	OK
H_1	OK	Type II error

In order to assess the performance of the statistical tests on their Type I error, also called Size of the test, and on their Power $= 1-$ Type II error, we used the following protocol.

For each category C_i, we sampled over D_{true}, S (500) evaluation sets D_{te}^s of N documents, ran the significance test over each D_{te}^s and computed the proportion of sets for which H_0 was rejected given that H_0 was true over D_{true} (*resp.* H_0 was false over D_{true}), which we note α_{true} (*resp.* π).

We used α_{true} as an estimate of the significance test's probability of making a Type I error and π as an estimate of the significance test's Power. When α_{true} is higher than the α fixed by the statistical test, the test underestimates Type I error, which means we should not rely on its decision regarding the superiority of one model over the other. Thus, we consider that the significance test fails. On the contrary, $\alpha_{true} < \alpha$ yields a pessimistic statistical test that decides correctly H_0 more often than predicted.

Furthermore we would like to favor significance tests with a high π, since the Power of the test reflects its ability to reject H_0 when H_0 is false.

3.2 Summary of Conditions

In order to verify the sensitivity of the analyzed statistical tests to several conditions, we varied the following parameters:

- the value of α: it took on values in $\{0.1, 0.05, 0.01\}$;
- the two compared models: there were three models, two of them were of the same family (SVMs), hence optimizing the same criterion, while the third one was an MLP. Most of the times the two SVMs gave very similar results, (probably because the optimal capacity for this problem was near linear), while the MLP gave poorer results on average. The point here was to verify whether the test was sensitive to the *closeness* of the tested models (although a more formal definition of *closeness* should certainly be devised);
- the evaluation sample size: we varied it from small sizes (100) up to larger sizes (6000) to see the robustness of the statistical test to it;
- the class unbalance: out of the 101 categories of the problem, most of them resulted in highly unbalanced tasks, often with a ratio of 10 to 100 between the two classes. In order to experiment with more balanced tasks, we artificially created *meta-categories*, which were random aggregations of normal categories that tended to be more balanced;
- the tested measure: our initial interest was to directly test dF_1, the difference of F_1, but given poor initial results, we also decided to assess $dCerr$, the difference of classification errors, in order to see whether the tests were sensitive to the measure itself;
- the statistical test: on top of the bootstrap percentile test, we also analyzed the more classical *proportion test* and *McNemar test*, both of them only on $dCerr$ (since they were not adapted to dF_1).

3.3 Results

Figure 1 summarizes the results for the Size of the test estimates. All graphs show α_{true}, the number of times the test rejected H_0 while H_0 was true, for a fixed $\alpha = 0.05$, with respect to the sample size, for various statistical tests and tested measures.

Figure 2 shows the obtained results for the Power of the test estimates. The proportion of evaluation sets over which the significance test (with $\alpha = 0.05$) rejected H_0 when indeed H_0 was false, is plotted against the evaluation set size.

Figures 1(a) and 2(a) show the results for balanced data (where the positive and negative examples were approximatively equally present in the evaluation set) when comparing two different models (an SVM and an MLP).

Figures 1(b) and 2(b) show the results for unbalanced data when comparing two different models.

Figures 1(c) and 2(c) show the results for balanced data when comparing two similar models (a linear SVM and a Gaussian SVM) for balanced data, and finally Figures 1(d) and 2(d) show the results for unbalanced data and two similar models.

Note that each point in the graphs was computed over a different number of samples, since *eg* over the (500 evaluation sets $\times$ 101 categories) experiments only those for which H_0 was true in D_{true} were taken into account in the computation of α_{true}.

When the proportion of H_0 true in D_{true} equals 0 (*resp.* the proportion of H_0 false in D_{true} equals 0), α_{true} (*resp.* π) is set to -1. Hence, for instance the first points ($\{100, \ldots, 1000\}$) of Figures 2(c) and 2(d) were computed over only 500 evaluation sets on which respectively the same categorization task was performed. This makes these points unreliable. See [8] for more details.

For each of the Size's graphs, when the curves are over the 0.05 line, we can state that the statistical test is optimistic, while when it is below the line, the statistical test is pessimistic. As already explained, a pessimistic test should be favored whenever possible.

Several interesting conclusions can be drawn from the analysis of these graphs. First of all, as expected, most of the statistical tests are positively influenced by the size of the evaluation set, in the sense that their α_{true} value converges to α for large sample sizes [1].

On the available results, the McNemar test and the bootstrap test over $dCerr$ have a similar performance. They are always pessimistic even for small evaluation set sizes, and tend to the expected α values when the models compared on balanced tasks are dissimilar. They have also a similar performance in Power over all the different conditions, higher in general when comparing very different models.

When the compared models are similar, the bootstrap test over dF_1 has a pessimistic behavior even on quite small evaluation sets. However, when the models are really different the bootstrap test over dF_1 is on average always optimistic. Note nevertheless that most of the points in Figures 1(a) and 1(b) have a standard deviation std, over the categories, such that $\alpha_{true} - std < \alpha$ (see [8] for more details). Another interesting point is that in the available results for the Power, the dF_1's bootstrap test have relatively high values with respect to the other tests.

The proportion test have in general, on the available results, a more conservative behavior than the McNemar test and the $dCerr$ bootstrap test. It has more pessimistic results and less Power. It is too often prone to "Accept H_0", *ie* to conclude that the compared models have an equivalent performance, whether it is true or not. This results seem to be consistent with those of [4] and [9]. However, when comparing *close* models in a small unbalanced evaluation set (Figure 1(d)), this conservative behavior is not present.

To summarize the findings, the bootstrap-based statistical test over $dCerr$ obtained a good performance in Size comparable to the one of the McNemar test in all conditions. However both significance test performances in Power are low even for big evaluation sets in particular when the compared models are close. The bootstrap-based statistical test over dF_1 has higher Power than the other compared tests, however it must be emphasized that it is slightly over-optimistic in particular for small evaluation sets. Finally, when applying the proportion test over unbalanced data for *close* models we obtained an optimistic behavior, untypical of this usually conservative test.

4   Conclusion

In this paper, we have analyzed several parametric and non-parametric statistical tests for various conditions often present in machine learning tasks, including the class balancing, the performance measure, the size of the test sets, and the *closeness* of the compared mod-

---

[1]Note that the same is true for the variance of $\alpha_{true} (\to 0)$, and this for any of the α values tested.

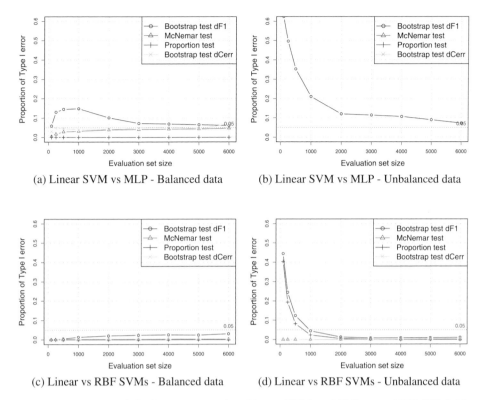

(a) Linear SVM vs MLP - Balanced data (b) Linear SVM vs MLP - Unbalanced data

(c) Linear vs RBF SVMs - Balanced data (d) Linear vs RBF SVMs - Unbalanced data

Figure 1: Several statistical tests comparing Linear SVM vs MLP or vs RBF SVM. The proportion of Type I error equals -1, in Figure 1(b), when there was no data to compute the proportion (*ie* H_0 was always false).

els. More particularly, we were concerned by the quality of non-parametric tests since in some cases (when using more complex performance measures such as F_1), they are the only available statistical tests.

Fortunately, most statistical tests performed reasonably well (in the sense that they were more often pessimistic than optimistic in their decisions) and larger test sets always improved their performance. Note however that for dF_1 the only available statistical test was too optimistic although consistant for different levels. An unexpected result was that the rather conservative proportion test used over unbalanced data for *close* models yielded an optimistic behavior.

It has to be noted that recently, a probabilistic interpretation of F_1 was suggested in [7], and a comparison with bootstrap-based tests should be worthwhile.

References

[1] M. Bisani and H. Ney. Bootstrap estimates for confidence intervals in ASR performance evaluation. In *Proceedings of ICASSP*, 2004.

[2] R. M. Bolle, N. K. Ratha, and S. Pankanti. Error analysis of pattern recognition systems - the subsets bootstrap. *Computer Vision and Image Understanding*, 93:1–33, 2004.

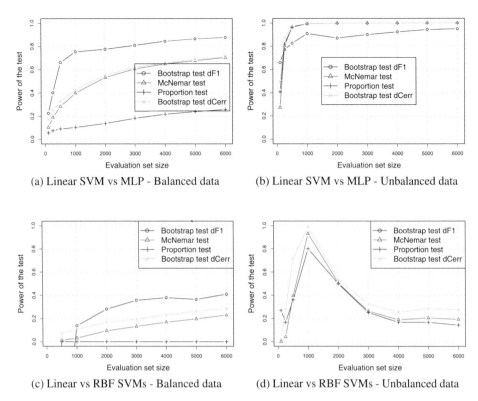

(a) Linear SVM vs MLP - Balanced data   (b) Linear SVM vs MLP - Unbalanced data

(c) Linear vs RBF SVMs - Balanced data   (d) Linear vs RBF SVMs - Unbalanced data

Figure 2: Power of several statistical tests comparing Linear SVM vs MLP or vs RBF SVM. The power equals -1, in Figures 2(c) and 2(d), when there was not data to compute the proportion (*ie* H_1 was never true).

[3] A. C. Davison and D. V. Hinkley. *Bootstrap methods and their application.* Cambridge University Press, 1997.

[4] T.G. Dietterich. Approximate statistical tests for comparing supervised classification learning algorithms. *Neural Computation*, 10(7):1895–1924, 1998.

[5] B. Efron and R. Tibshirani. *An Introduction to the Bootstrap.* Chapman and Hall, 1993.

[6] B. S. Everitt. *The analysis of contingency tables.* Chapman and Hall, 1977.

[7] C. Goutte and E. Gaussier. A probabilistic interpretation of precision, recall and F-score, with implication for evaluation. In *Proceedings of ECIR*, pages 345–359, 2005.

[8] M. Keller, S. Bengio, and S. Y. Wong. Surprising Outcome While Benchmarking Statistical Tests. IDIAP-RR 38, IDIAP, 2005.

[9] Claude Nadeau and Yoshua Bengio. Inference for the generalization error. *Machine Learning*, 52(3):239–281, 2003.

[10] T.G. Rose, M. Stevenson, and M. Whitehead. The Reuters Corpus Volume 1 - from yesterday's news to tomorrow's language resources. In *Proceedings of the 3rd Int. Conf. on Language Resources and Evaluation*, 2002.

[11] F. Sebastiani. Machine learning in automated text categorization. *ACM Computing Surveys*, 34(1):1–47, 2002.

[12] C. J. van Rijsbergen. *Information Retrieval.* Butterworths, London, UK, 1975.

Robust Fisher Discriminant Analysis

Seung-Jean Kim   Alessandro Magnani   Stephen P. Boyd
Information Systems Laboratory
Electrical Engineering Department, Stanford University
Stanford, CA 94305-9510
`sjkim@stanford.edu     alem@stanford.edu     boyd@stanford.edu`

Abstract

Fisher linear discriminant analysis (LDA) can be sensitive to the problem data. Robust Fisher LDA can systematically alleviate the sensitivity problem by explicitly incorporating a model of data uncertainty in a classification problem and optimizing for the worst-case scenario under this model. The main contribution of this paper is show that with general convex uncertainty models on the problem data, robust Fisher LDA can be carried out using convex optimization. For a certain type of product form uncertainty model, robust Fisher LDA can be carried out at a cost comparable to standard Fisher LDA. The method is demonstrated with some numerical examples. Finally, we show how to extend these results to robust kernel Fisher discriminant analysis, *i.e.*, robust Fisher LDA in a high dimensional feature space.

1   Introduction

Fisher linear discriminant analysis (LDA), a widely-used technique for pattern classification, finds a linear discriminant that yields optimal discrimination between two classes which can be identified with two random variables, say $\mathbf{X}$ and $\mathbf{Y}$ in $\mathbb{R}^n$. For a (linear) discriminant characterized by $w \in \mathbb{R}^n$, the degree of discrimination is measured by the Fisher discriminant ratio

$$f(w, \mu_x, \mu_y, \Sigma_x, \Sigma_y) = \frac{w^T(\mu_x - \mu_y)(\mu_x - \mu_y)^T w}{w^T(\Sigma_x + \Sigma_y)w} = \frac{(w^T(\mu_x - \mu_y))^2}{w^T(\Sigma_x + \Sigma_y)w},$$

where μ_x and Σ_x (μ_y and Σ_y) denote the mean and covariance of $\mathbf{X}$ ($\mathbf{Y}$). A discriminant that maximizes the Fisher discriminant ratio is given by

$$w^{\mathrm{nom}} = (\Sigma_x + \Sigma_y)^{-1}(\mu_x - \mu_y),$$

which gives the maximum Fisher discriminant ratio

$$(\mu_x - \mu_y)^T(\Sigma_x + \Sigma_y)^{-1}(\mu_x - \mu_y) = \max_{w \neq 0} f(w, \mu_x, \mu_y, \Sigma_x, \Sigma_y).$$

In applications, the problem data μ_x, μ_y, Σ_x, and Σ_y are not known but are estimated from sample data. Fisher LDA can be sensitive to the problem data: the discriminant w^{nom} computed from an estimate of the parameters μ_x, μ_y, Σ_x, and Σ_y can give very poor discrimination for another set of problem data that is also a reasonable estimate of the parameters. In this paper, we attempt to systematically alleviate this sensitivity problem by explicitly incorporating a model of data uncertainty in the classification problem and optimizing for the worst-case scenario under this model.

We assume that the problem data μ_x, μ_y, Σ_x, and Σ_y are uncertain, but known to belong to a convex compact subset $\mathcal{U}$ of $\mathbb{R}^n \times \mathbb{R}^n \times \mathbb{S}^n_{++} \times \mathbb{S}^n_{++}$. Here we use $\mathbb{S}^n_{++}$ ($\mathbb{S}^n_+$) to denote the set of all $n \times n$ symmetric positive definite (semidefinite) matrices. We make one technical assumption: for each $(\mu_x, \mu_y, \Sigma_x, \Sigma_y) \in \mathcal{U}$, we have $\mu_x \neq \mu_y$. This assumption simply means that for each possible value of the means and covariances, the classes are distinguishable via Fisher LDA.

The *worst-case analysis problem* of finding the worst-case means and covariances for a given discriminant w can be written as

$$
\begin{aligned}
\text{minimize} \quad & f(w, \mu_x, \mu_y, \Sigma_x, \Sigma_y) \\
\text{subject to} \quad & (\mu_x, \mu_y, \Sigma_x, \Sigma_y) \in \mathcal{U},
\end{aligned}
\tag{1}
$$

with variables μ_x, μ_y, Σ_x, and Σ_y. The optimal value of this problem is the *worst-case Fisher discriminant ratio* (over the class $\mathcal{U}$ of possible means and covariances), and any optimal points for this problem are called *worst-case means and covariances*. These depend on w.

We will show in §2 that (1) is a convex optimization problem, since the Fisher discriminant ratio is a convex function of μ_x, μ_y, Σ_x, Σ_y for a given discriminant w. As a result, it is computationally tractable to find the worst-case performance of a discriminant w over the set of possible means and covariances.

The *robust Fisher LDA problem* is to find a discriminant that maximizes the worst-case Fisher discriminant ratio. This can be cast as the optimization problem

$$
\begin{aligned}
\text{maximize} \quad & \min_{(\mu_x, \mu_y, \Sigma_x, \Sigma_y) \in \mathcal{U}} f(w, \mu_x, \mu_y, \Sigma_x, \Sigma_y) \\
\text{subject to} \quad & w \neq 0,
\end{aligned}
\tag{2}
$$

with variable w. We denote any optimal w for this problem as $w^\star$. Here we choose a linear discriminant that maximizes the Fisher discrimination ratio, with the worst possible means and covariances that are consistent with our data uncertainty model.

The main result of this paper is to give an effective method for solving the robust Fisher LDA problem (2). We will show in §2 that the robust optimal Fisher discriminant $w^\star$ can be found as follows. First, we solve the (convex) optimization problem

$$
\begin{aligned}
\text{minimize} \quad & \max_{w \neq 0} f(w, \mu_x, \mu_y, \Sigma_x, \Sigma_y) = (\mu_x - \mu_y)^T (\Sigma_x + \Sigma_y)^{-1} (\mu_x - \mu_y) \\
\text{subject to} \quad & (\mu_x, \mu_y, \Sigma_x, \Sigma_y) \in \mathcal{U},
\end{aligned}
\tag{3}
$$

with variables $(\mu_x, \mu_y, \Sigma_x, \Sigma_y)$. Let $(\mu_x^\star, \mu_y^\star, \Sigma_x^\star, \Sigma_y^\star)$ denote any optimal point. Then the discriminant

$$
w^\star = \left(\Sigma_x^\star + \Sigma_y^\star\right)^{-1} \left(\mu_x^\star - \mu_y^\star\right)
\tag{4}
$$

is a robust optimal Fisher discriminant, *i.e.*, it is optimal for (2). Moreover, we will see that $\mu_x^\star, \mu_y^\star$ and $\Sigma_x^\star, \Sigma_y^\star$ are worst-case means and covariances for the robust optimal Fisher discriminant $w^\star$. Since convex optimization problems are tractable, this means that we have a *tractable general method* for computing a robust optimal Fisher discriminant.

A robust Fisher discriminant problem of modest size can be solved by standard convex optimization methods, *e.g.*, interior-point methods [3]. For some special forms of the uncertainty model, the robust optimal Fisher discriminant can be solved more efficiently than by a general convex optimization formulation. In §3, we consider an important special form for $\mathcal{U}$ for which a more efficient formulation can be given.

In comparison with the 'nominal' Fisher LDA, which is based on the means and covariances estimated from the sample data set without considering the estimation error, the robust Fisher LDA performs well even when the sample size used to estimate the means and covariances is small, resulting in estimates which are not accurate. This will be demonstrated with some numerical examples in §4.

Recently, there has been a growing interest in kernel Fisher discriminant analysis *i.e.*, Fisher LDA in a higher dimensional feature space, *e.g.*, [7]. Our results can be extended to robust kernel Fisher discriminant analysis under certain uncertainty models. This will be briefly discussed in §5.

Various types of robust classification problems have been considered in the prior literature, *e.g.*, [2, 5, 6]. Most of the research has focused on formulating robust classification problems that can be efficiently solved via convex optimization. In particular, the robust classification method developed in [6] is based on the criterion

$$g(w, \mu_x, \mu_y, \Sigma_x, \Sigma_y) = \frac{|w^T(\mu_x - \mu_y)|}{(w^T \Sigma_x w)^{1/2} + (w^T \Sigma_y w)^{1/2}},$$

which is similar to the Fisher discriminant ratio f. With a specific uncertainty model on the means and covariances, the robust classification problem with discrimination criterion g can be cast as a second-order cone program, a special type of convex optimization problem [5]. With general uncertainty models, however, it is not clear whether robust discriminant analysis with g can be performed via convex optimization.

2 Robust Fisher LDA

We first consider the worst-case analysis problem (1). Here we consider the discriminant w as fixed, and the parameters μ_x, μ_y, Σ_x, and Σ_y are variables, constrained to lie in the convex uncertainty set $\mathcal{U}$. To show that (1) is a convex optimization problem, we must show that the Fisher discriminant ratio is a convex function of μ_x, μ_y, Σ_x, and Σ_y. To show this, we express the Fisher discriminant ratio f as the composition

$$f(w, \mu_x, \mu_y, \Sigma_x, \Sigma_y) = g(H(\mu_x, \mu_y, \Sigma_x, \Sigma_y)),$$

where $g(u, t) = u^2/t$ and H is the function

$$H(\mu_x, \mu_y, \Sigma_x, \Sigma_y) = (w^T(\mu_x - \mu_y), w^T(\Sigma_x + \Sigma_y)w).$$

The function H is linear (as a mapping from μ_x, μ_y, Σ_x, and Σ_y into $\mathbb{R}^2$), and the function g is convex (provided $t > 0$, which holds here). Thus, the composition f is a convex function of μ_x, μ_y, Σ_x, and Σ_y. (See [3].)

Now we turn to the main result of this paper. Consider a function of the form

$$R(w, a, B) = \frac{(w^T a)^2}{w^T B w}, \tag{5}$$

which is the Rayleigh quotient for the matrix pair $aa^T \in \mathbb{S}_+^n$ and $B \in \mathbb{S}_{++}^n$, evaluated at w. The robust Fisher LDA problem (2) is equivalent to a problem of the form

$$\begin{array}{ll} \text{maximize} & \min_{(a,B) \in \mathcal{V}} R(w, a, B) \\ \text{subject to} & w \neq 0, \end{array} \tag{6}$$

where

$$a = \mu_x - \mu_y, \quad B = \Sigma_x + \Sigma_y, \quad \mathcal{V} = \{(\mu_x - \mu_y, \Sigma_x + \Sigma_y) \mid (\mu_x, \mu_y, \Sigma_x, \Sigma_y) \in \mathcal{U}\}. \tag{7}$$

(This equivalence means that robust FLDA is a special type of robust matched filtering problem studied in the 1980s; see, *e.g.*, [8] for more on robust matched filtering.)

We will prove a 'nonconventional' minimax theorem for a Rayleigh quotient of the form (5), which will establish the main result described in §1. To do this, we consider a problem of the form

$$
\begin{array}{ll}
\text{minimize} & a^T B^{-1} a \\
\text{subject to} & (a, B) \in \mathcal{V},
\end{array}
\tag{8}
$$

with variables $a \in \mathbb{R}^n$, $B \in \mathbb{S}^n_{++}$, and $\mathcal{V}$ is a convex compact subset of $\mathbb{R}^n \times \mathbb{S}^n_{++}$ such that for each $(a, B) \in \mathcal{V}$, a is not zero. The objective of this problem is a matrix fractional function and so is convex on $\mathbb{R}^n \times \mathbb{S}^n_{++}$; see [3, §3.1.7]. Our problem (3) is the same as (8), with (7). It follows that (3) is a convex optimization problem.

The following theorem states the minimax theorem for the function R. While R is convex in (a, B) for fixed w, it is *not* concave in w for fixed (a, B), so conventional convex-concave minimax theorems do not apply here.

Theorem 1. *Let $(a^\star, B^\star)$ be an optimal solution to the problem (8), and let $w^\star = B^{\star-1} a^\star$. Then $(w^\star, a^\star, B^\star)$ satisfies the minimax property*

$$
R(w^\star, a^\star, B^\star) = \max_{w \neq 0} \min_{(a,B) \in \mathcal{V}} R(w, a, B) = \min_{(a,B) \in \mathcal{V}} \max_{w \neq 0} R(w, a, B),
\tag{9}
$$

and the saddle point property

$$
R(w, a^\star, B^\star) \leq R(w^\star, a^\star, B^\star) \leq R(w^\star, a, B), \quad \forall w \in \mathbb{R}^n \setminus \{0\}, \ \forall (a, B) \in \mathcal{V}.
\tag{10}
$$

Proof. It suffices to prove (10), since the saddle point property (10) implies the minimax property (9) [1, §2.6]. We start by observing that $R(w, a^\star, B^\star)$ is maximized over nonzero $w \neq 0$ by $w^\star = B^{\star-1} a^\star$ (by the Cauchy-Schwartz inequality). What remains is to show

$$
\min_{(a,B) \in \mathcal{V}} R(w^\star, a, B) = R(w^\star, a^\star, B^\star).
\tag{11}
$$

Since $a^\star$ and $B^\star$ are optimal for the convex problem (8) (by definition), they must satisfy the optimality condition

$$
\left\langle \nabla_a (a^T B^{-1} a)\big|_{(a^\star, B^\star)}, (a - a^\star) \right\rangle + \left\langle \nabla_B (a^T B^{-1} a)\big|_{(a^\star, B^\star)}, (B - B^\star) \right\rangle \\
\geq 0, \quad \forall (a, B) \in \mathcal{V}
$$

(see [3, §4.2.3]). Using $\nabla_a (a^T B^{-1} a) = 2B^{-1} a$, $\nabla_B (a^T B^{-1} a) = -B^{-1} a a^T B^{-1}$, and $\langle X, Y \rangle = \mathbf{Tr}(XY)$ for $X, Y \in \mathbb{S}^n$, where $\mathbf{Tr}$ denotes trace, we can express the optimality condition as

$$
2 a^{\star T} B^{\star-1} (a - a^\star) - \mathbf{Tr} B^{\star-1} a^\star a^{\star T} B^{\star-1} (B - B^\star) \geq 0, \quad \forall (a, B) \in \mathcal{V},
$$

or equivalently,

$$
2 w^{\star T} (a - a^\star) - w^{\star T} (B - B^\star) w^\star \geq 0, \quad \forall (a, B) \in \mathcal{V}.
\tag{12}
$$

Now we turn to the convex optimization problem

$$
\begin{array}{ll}
\text{minimize} & R(w^\star, a, B) \\
\text{subject to} & (a, B) \in \mathcal{V},
\end{array}
\tag{13}
$$

with variables (a, B). We will show that $(a^\star, B^\star)$ is optimal for this problem, which will establish (11).

A pair $(\bar{a}, \bar{B})$ is optimal for (13) if and only if

$$\left\langle \nabla_a \frac{(w^{\star T} a)^2}{w^T B w^\star}\bigg|_{(\bar{a}, \bar{B})}, (a - \bar{a}) \right\rangle + \left\langle \nabla_B \frac{(w^{\star T} a)^2}{w^T B w^\star}\bigg|_{(\bar{a}, \bar{B})}, (B - \bar{B}) \right\rangle \geq 0, \quad \forall (a, B) \in \mathcal{V}.$$

Using

$$\nabla_a \frac{(w^{\star T} a)^2}{w^{\star T} B w^\star} = 2 \frac{a^T w^\star}{w^\star B w^\star} w^\star, \qquad \nabla_B \frac{(w^{\star T} a)^2}{w^{\star T} B w^\star} = -\frac{(a^T w^\star)^2}{(w^{\star T} B w^\star)^2} w^\star w^{\star T},$$

the optimality condition can be written as

$$2 \frac{\bar{a}^T w^\star}{w^{\star T} \bar{B} w^\star} w^{\star T} (a - \bar{a}) - \mathbf{Tr} \frac{(\bar{a}^T w^\star)^2}{(w^{\star T} \bar{B} w^\star)^2} w^\star w^{\star T} (B - \bar{B})$$

$$= \quad 2 \frac{\bar{a}^T w^\star}{w^{\star T} \bar{B} w^\star} w^{\star T} (a - \bar{a}) - \frac{(\bar{a}^T w^\star)^2}{(w^{\star T} \bar{B} w^\star)^2} w^{\star T} (B - \bar{B}) w^\star$$

$$\geq \quad 0, \quad \forall (a, B) \in \mathcal{V}.$$

Substituting $\bar{a} = a^\star$, $\bar{B} = B^\star$, and noting that $a^{\star T} w^\star / w^{\star T} B^\star w^\star = 1$, the optimality condition reduces to

$$2 w^{\star T} (a - a^\star) - w^{\star T} (B - B^\star) w^\star \geq 0, \quad \forall (a, B) \in \mathcal{V},$$

which is precisely (12). Thus, we have shown that $(a^\star, B^\star)$ is optimal for (13), which in turn establishes (11). $\qquad\qquad\square$

3 Robust Fisher LDA with product form uncertainty models

In this section, we focus on robust Fisher LDA with the product form uncertainty model

$$\mathcal{U} = \mathcal{M} \times \mathcal{S}, \tag{14}$$

where $\mathcal{M}$ is the set of possible means and $\mathcal{S}$ is the set of possible covariances. For this model, the worst-case Fisher discriminant ratio can be written as

$$\min_{(\mu_x, \mu_y, \Sigma_x, \Sigma_y) \in \mathcal{U}} f(a, \mu_x, \mu_y, \Sigma_x, \Sigma_y) = \min_{(\mu_x, \mu_y) \in \mathcal{M}} \frac{(w^T(\mu_x - \mu_y))^2}{\max_{(\Sigma_x, \Sigma_y) \in \mathcal{S}} w^T(\Sigma_x + \Sigma_y) w}.$$

If we can find an analytic expression for $\max_{(\Sigma_x, \Sigma_y) \in \mathcal{S}} w^T(\Sigma_x + \Sigma_y) w$ (as a function of w), we can simplify the robust Fisher LDA problem.

As a more specific example, we consider the case in which $\mathcal{S}$ is given by

$$\begin{aligned}
\mathcal{S} &= \mathcal{S}_x \times \mathcal{S}_y, \\
\mathcal{S}_x &= \{\Sigma_x \mid \Sigma_x \succeq 0, \|\Sigma_x - \bar{\Sigma}_x\|_F \leq \delta_x\}, \\
\mathcal{S}_y &= \{\Sigma_y \mid \Sigma_y \succeq 0, \|\Sigma_y - \bar{\Sigma}_y\|_F \leq \delta_y\},
\end{aligned} \tag{15}$$

where δ_x, δ_y are positive constants, $\bar{\Sigma}_x, \bar{\Sigma}_y \in \mathbb{S}_{++}^n$, and $\|A\|_F$ denotes the Frobenius norm of A, i.e., $\|A\|_F = (\sum_{i,j=1}^n A_{ij}^2)^{1/2}$. For this case, we have

$$\max_{(\Sigma_x, \Sigma_y) \in \mathcal{S}} w^T(\Sigma_x + \Sigma_y) w = w^T(\bar{\Sigma}_x + \bar{\Sigma}_y + (\delta_x + \delta_y) I) w. \tag{16}$$

Here we have used the fact that for given $\bar{\Sigma} \in \mathbb{S}_{++}^n$, $\max_{\|\Sigma - \bar{\Sigma}\|_F \leq \delta} x^T \Sigma x = x^T(\bar{\Sigma} + \delta I) x$ (see, e.g., [6]). The worst-case Fisher discriminant ratio can be expressed as

$$\min_{(\mu_x, \mu_y) \in \mathcal{M}} \frac{(w^T(\mu_x - \mu_y))^2}{w^T(\bar{\Sigma}_x + \bar{\Sigma}_y + (\delta_x + \delta_y) I) w}.$$

This is the same worst-case Fisher discriminant ratio obtained for a problem in which the covariances are certain, *i.e.*, fixed to be $\bar{\Sigma}_x + \delta_x I$ and $\bar{\Sigma}_y + \delta_y I$, and the means lie in the set $\mathcal{M}$. We conclude that a robust optimal Fisher discriminant with the uncertainty model (14) in which S has the form (15) can be found by solving a robust Fisher LDA problem with these fixed values for the covariances. From the general solution method described in §1, it is given by

$$w^\star = \left(\bar{\Sigma}_x + \bar{\Sigma}_y + (\delta_x + \delta_y)I\right)^{-1}(\mu_x^\star - \mu_y^\star),$$

where $\mu_x^\star$ and $\mu_y^\star$ solve the convex optimization problem

$$\begin{array}{ll}
\text{minimize} & (\mu_x - \mu_y)^T \left(\bar{\Sigma}_x + \bar{\Sigma}_y + (\delta_x + \delta_y)I\right)^{-1}(\mu_x - \mu_y) \\
\text{subject to} & (\mu_x, \mu_y) \in \mathcal{M},
\end{array} \tag{17}$$

with variables μ_x and μ_y.

The problem (17) is relatively simple: it involves minimizing a convex quadratic function over the set of possible μ_x and μ_y. For example, if $\mathcal{M}$ is a product of two ellipsoids, (*e.g.*, μ_x and μ_y each lie in some confidence ellipsoid) the problem (17) is to minimize a convex quadratic subject to two convex quadratic constraints. Such a problem is readily solved in $O(n^3)$ flops, since the dual problem has two variables, and evaluating the dual function and its derivatives can be done in $O(n^3)$ flops [3]. Thus, the effort to solve the robust is the same order (*i.e.*, n^3) as solving the nominal Fisher LDA (but with a substantially larger constant).

4   Numerical results

To demonstrate robust Fisher LDA, we use the sonar and ionosphere benchmark problems from the UCI repository (www.ics.uci.edu/~mlearn/MLRepository.html). The two benchmark problems have 208 and 351 points, respectively, and the dimension of each data point is 60 and 34, respectively. Each data set is randomly partitioned into a training set and a test set. We use the training set to compute the optimal discriminant and then test its performance using the test set. A larger training set typically gives better test performance. We let α denote the size of the training set, as a fraction of the total number of data points. For example, $\alpha = 0.3$ means that 30% of the data points are used for training, and 70% are used to test the resulting discriminant. For various values of α, we generate 100 random partitions of the data (for each of the two benchmark problems), and collect the results.

We use the following uncertainty models for the means μ_x, μ_y and the covariances Σ_x, Σ_y:

$$\begin{array}{ll}
(\mu_x - \bar{\mu}_x)^T P_x (\mu_x - \bar{\mu}_x) \leq 1, & \|\Sigma_x - \bar{\Sigma}_x\|_F \leq \rho_x, \\
(\mu_y - \bar{\mu}_y)^T P_y (\mu_y - \bar{\mu}_y) \leq 1, & \|\Sigma_y - \bar{\Sigma}_y\|_F \leq \rho_y,
\end{array}$$

Here the vectors $\bar{\mu}_x, \bar{\mu}_y$ represent the nominal means and the matrices $\bar{\Sigma}_x, \bar{\Sigma}_y$ represent the nominal covariances, and the matrices P_x, P_y and the constants ρ_x and ρ_y represent the confidence regions. The parameters are estimated through a resampling technique [4] as follows. For a given training set we create 100 new sets by resampling the original training set with a uniform distribution over all the data points. For each of these sets we estimate its mean and covariance and then take their average values as the nominal mean and covariance. We also evaluate the covariance Σ_μ of all the means obtained with the resampling. We then take $P_x = \Sigma_\mu^{-1}/n$ and $P_y = \Sigma_\mu^{-1}/n$. This choice corresponds to a 50% confidence ellipsoid in the case of a Gaussian distribution. The parameters ρ_x and ρ_y are taken to be the maximum deviations between the covariances and the average covariances in the Frobenius norm sense, over the resampling of the training set.

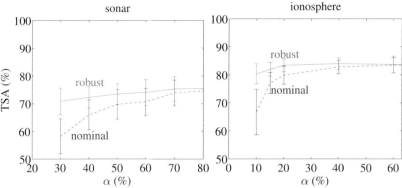

Figure 1: Test-set accuracy (TSA) for sonar and ionosphere benchmark versus size of the training set. The solid line represents the robust Fisher LDA results and the dotted line the nominal Fisher LDA results. The vertical bars represent the standard deviation.

Figure 1 summarizes the classification results. For each of our two problems, and for each value of α, we show the average test set accuracy (TSA), as well as the standard deviation (over the 100 instances of each problem with the given value of α). The plots show the robust Fisher LDA performs substantially better than the nominal Fisher LDA for small training sets, but this performance gap disappears as the training set becomes larger.

5   Robust kernel Fisher discriminant analysis

In this section we show how to 'kernelize' the robust Fisher LDA. We will consider only a specific class of uncertainty models; the arguments we develop here can be extended to more general cases. In the kernel approach we map the problem to an higher dimensional space $\mathbb{R}^f$ via a mapping $\phi : \mathbb{R}^n \to \mathbb{R}^f$ so that the new decision boundary is more general and possibly nonlinear. Let the data be mapped as

$$x \to \phi(x) \sim (\bar{\mu}_{\phi(x)}, \bar{\Sigma}_{\phi(x)}), \quad y \to \phi(y) \sim (\bar{\mu}_{\phi(y)}, \bar{\Sigma}_{\phi(y)}).$$

The uncertainty model we consider has the form

$$\mu_{\phi(x)} - \mu_{\phi(y)} = \bar{\mu}_{\phi(x)} - \bar{\mu}_{\phi(y)} + Pu_f, \quad \|u_f\| \le 1,$$
$$\|\Sigma_{\phi(x)} - \bar{\Sigma}_{\phi(x)}\|_F \le \rho_x, \quad \|\Sigma_{\phi(y)} - \bar{\Sigma}_{\phi(y)}\|_F \le \rho_y. \tag{18}$$

Here the vectors $\bar{\mu}_{\phi(x)}, \bar{\mu}_{\phi(y)}$ represent the nominal means, the matrices $\bar{\Sigma}_{\phi(x)}, \bar{\Sigma}_{\phi(y)}$ represent the nominal covariances, and the (positive semidefinite) matrix P and the constants ρ_x and ρ_y represent the confidence regions in the feature space. The worst-case Fisher discriminant ratio in the feature space is then given by

$$\min_{\|u_f\| \le 1, \|\Sigma_{\phi(x)} - \bar{\Sigma}_{\phi(x)}\|_F \le \rho_x, \|\Sigma_{\phi(y)} - \bar{\Sigma}_{\phi(y)}\|_F \le \rho_y} \frac{(w_f^T(\bar{\mu}_{\phi(x)} - \bar{\mu}_{\phi(y)} + Pu_f))^2}{w_f^T(\Sigma_{\phi(x)} + \Sigma_{\phi(y)})w_f}.$$

The robust kernel Fisher discriminant analysis problem is to find the discriminant in the feature space that maximizes this ratio.

Using the technique described in §3, we can see that the robust kernel Fisher discriminant analysis problem can be cast as

$$\begin{aligned} \text{maximize} \quad & \min_{\|u_f\| \le 1} \frac{(w_f^T(\bar{\mu}_{\phi(x)} - \bar{\mu}_{\phi(y)} + Pu_f))^2}{w_f^T(\bar{\Sigma}_{\phi(x)} + \bar{\Sigma}_{\phi(y)} + (\rho_x + \rho_y)I)w_f} \\ \text{subject to} \quad & w_f \neq 0, \end{aligned} \tag{19}$$

where the discriminant $w_f \in \mathbb{R}^f$ is defined in the new feature space.

To apply the kernel trick to the problem (19), the nonlinear decision boundary should be entirely expressed in terms of inner products of the mapped data only. The following proposition tells us a set of conditions to do so.

Proposition 1. *Given the sample points $\{x_i\}_{i=1}^{N_x}$ and $\{y_i\}_{i=1}^{N_y}$, suppose that $\bar{\mu}_{\phi(x)}, \bar{\mu}_{\phi(y)}$, $\bar{\Sigma}_{\phi(x)}, \bar{\Sigma}_{\phi(y)}$, and P can be written as*

$$\bar{\mu}_{\phi(x)} = \sum_{i=1}^{N_x} \lambda_i \phi(x_i), \quad \bar{\mu}_{\phi(y)} = \sum_{i=1}^{N_y} \lambda_{i+N_x} \phi(y_i), \quad P = U \Upsilon U^T,$$

$$\bar{\Sigma}_{\phi(x)} = \sum_{i=1}^{N_x} \Lambda_{i,i} (\phi(x_i) - \bar{\mu}_{\phi(x)})(\phi(x_i) - \bar{\mu}_{\phi(x)})^T,$$

$$\bar{\Sigma}_{\phi(y)} = \sum_{i=1}^{N_y} \Lambda_{i+N_x, i+N_x} (\phi(y_i) - \bar{\mu}_{\phi(y)})(\phi(y_i) - \bar{\mu}_{\phi(y)})^T,$$

where $\lambda \in \mathbb{R}^{N_x+N_y}$, $\Upsilon \in \mathbb{S}_+^{N_x+N_y}$, $\Lambda \in \mathbb{S}_+^{N_x+N_y}$ is a diagonal matrix, and U is a matrix whose columns are the vectors $\{\phi(x_i) - \bar{\mu}_{\phi(x)}\}_{i=1}^{N_x}$ and $\{\phi(y_i) - \bar{\mu}_{\phi(y)}\}_{i=1}^{N_y}$. Denote as Φ the matrix whose columns are the vectors $\{\phi(x_i)\}_{i=1}^{N_x}, \{\phi(y_i)\}_{i=1}^{N_y}$ and define

$$D_1 = K\beta, \quad D_2 = K(I - \lambda 1_N^T)\Upsilon(I - \lambda 1_N^T)K^T,$$

$$D_3 = K(I - \lambda 1_N^T)\Lambda(I - \lambda 1_N^T)K^T + (\rho_x + \rho_y)K, \quad D_4 = K,$$

where K is the kernel matrix $K_{ij} = (\Phi^T\Phi)_{ij}$, 1_N is a vector of ones of length $N_x + N_y$, and $\beta \in \mathbb{R}^{N_x+N_y}$ is such that $\beta_i = \lambda_i$ for $i = 1, \ldots, N_x$ and $\beta_i = -\lambda_i$ for $i = N_x + 1, \ldots, N_x + N_y$. Let $\nu^\star$ be an optimal solution of the problem

$$\begin{array}{ll}
\text{maximize} & \min_{\xi^T D_4 \xi \le 1} \dfrac{\nu^T(D_1 + D_2\xi)(D_1 + D_2\xi)^T \nu}{\nu^T D_3 \nu} \\
\text{subject to} & \nu \ne 0.
\end{array} \tag{20}$$

Then, $w_f^\star = \Phi\nu^\star$ is an optimal solution of the problem (19). Moreover, for every point $z \in \mathbb{R}^n$,

$$w_f^{\star T}\phi(z) = \sum_{i=1}^{N_x} \nu_i^\star K(z, x_i) + \sum_{i=1}^{N_y} \nu_{i+N_x}^\star K(z, y_i). \tag{21}$$

Along the lines of the proofs of Corollary 5 in [6], we can prove this proposition.

References

[1] D. Bertsekas, A. Nedić, and A. Ozdaglar. *Convex Analysis and Optimization*. Athena Scientific, 2003.

[2] C. Bhattacharyya. Second order cone programming formulations for feature selection. *Journal of Machine Learning Research*, 5:1417–1433, 2004.

[3] S. Boyd and L. Vandenberghe. *Convex Optimization*. Cambridge University Press, 2004.

[4] B. Efron and R.J. Tibshirani. *An Introduction to Bootstrap*. Chapman and Hall, London UK, 1993.

[5] K. Huang, H. Yang, I. King, M. Lyu, and L. Chan. The minimum error minimax probability machine. *Journal of Machine Learning Research*, 5:1253–1286, 2004.

[6] G. Lanckriet, L. El Ghaoui, C. Bhattacharyya, and M. Jordan. A robust minimax approach to classification. *Journal of Machine Learning Research*, 3:555–582, 2002.

[7] S. Mika, G. Rätsch, and K. Müller. A mathematical programming approach to the kernel Fisher algorithm, 2001. In *Advances in Neural Information Processing Systems*, 13, pp. 591-597, MIT Press.

[8] S. Verdú and H. Poor. On minimax robustness: A general approach and applications. *IEEE Transactions on Information Theory*, 30(2):328–340, 1984.

Measuring Shared Information and Coordinated Activity in Neuronal Networks

Kristina Lisa Klinkner
Statistics Department
University of Michigan
Ann Arbor, MI 48109
kshalizi@umich.edu

Cosma Rohilla Shalizi
Statistics Department
Carnegie Mellon University
Pittsburgh, PA 15213
cshalizi@stat.cmu.edu

Marcelo F. Camperi
Physics Department
University of San Francisco
San Francisco, CA 94118
camperi@usfca.edu

Abstract

Most nervous systems encode information about stimuli in the responding activity of large neuronal networks. This activity often manifests itself as dynamically coordinated sequences of action potentials. Since multiple electrode recordings are now a standard tool in neuroscience research, it is important to have a measure of such network-wide behavioral coordination and information sharing, applicable to multiple neural spike train data. We propose a new statistic, *informational coherence*, which measures how much better one unit can be predicted by knowing the dynamical state of another. We argue informational coherence is a measure of association and shared information which is superior to traditional pairwise measures of synchronization and correlation. To find the dynamical states, we use a recently-introduced algorithm which reconstructs effective state spaces from stochastic time series. We then extend the pairwise measure to a multivariate analysis of the network by estimating the network multi-information. We illustrate our method by testing it on a detailed model of the transition from gamma to beta rhythms.

Much of the most important information in neural systems is shared over multiple neurons or cortical areas, in such forms as population codes and distributed representations [1]. On behavioral time scales, neural information is stored in temporal patterns of activity as opposed to static markers; therefore, as information is shared between neurons or brain regions, it is physically instantiated as coordination between entire sequences of neural spikes. Furthermore, neural systems and regions of the brain often require coordinated neural activity to perform important functions; acting in concert requires multiple neurons or cortical areas to share information [2]. Thus, if we want to measure the dynamic network-wide behavior of neurons and test hypotheses about them, we need reliable, practical methods to detect and quantify behavioral coordination and the associated information sharing across multiple neural units. These would be especially useful in testing ideas about how particular forms of coordination relate to distributed coding (e.g., that of [3]). Current techniques to analyze relations among spike trains handle only pairs of neurons, so we further need a method which is extendible to analyze the coordination in the network, system, or region as a whole. Here we propose a new measure of behavioral coordination and information sharing, *informational coherence*, based on the notion of dynamical state.

Section 1 argues that coordinated behavior in neural systems is often not captured by exist-

667

ing measures of synchronization or correlation, and that something sensitive to nonlinear, stochastic, predictive relationships is needed. Section 2 defines informational coherence as the (normalized) mutual information between the dynamical states of two systems and explains how looking at the states, rather than just observables, fulfills the needs laid out in Section 1. Since we rarely know the right states *a prori*, Section 2.1 briefly describes how we reconstruct effective state spaces from data. Section 2.2 gives some details about how we calculate the informational coherence and approximate the global information stored in the network. Section 3 applies our method to a model system (a biophysically detailed conductance-based model) comparing our results to those of more familiar second-order statistics. In the interest of space, we omit proofs and a full discussion of the existing literature, giving only minimal references here; proofs and references will appear in a longer paper now in preparation.

1 Synchrony or Coherence?

Most hypotheses which involve the idea that information sharing is reflected in coordinated activity across neural units invoke a very specific notion of coordinated activity, namely strict synchrony: the units should be doing exactly the same thing (e.g., spiking) at exactly the same time. Investigators then measure coordination by measuring how close the units come to being strictly synchronized (e.g., variance in spike times).

From an informational point of view, there is no reason to favor strict synchrony over other kinds of coordination. One neuron consistently spiking 50 ms after another is just as informative a relationship as two simultaneously spiking, but such stable phase relations are missed by strict-synchrony approaches. Indeed, whatever the exact nature of the neural code, it uses temporally extended patterns of activity, and so information sharing should be reflected in coordination of those patterns, rather than just the instantaneous activity.

There are three common ways of going beyond strict synchrony: cross-correlation and related second-order statistics, mutual information, and topological generalized synchrony.

The cross-correlation function (the normalized covariance function; this includes, for present purposes, the joint peristimulus time histogram [2]), is one of the most widespread measures of synchronization. It can be efficiently calculated from observable series; it handles statistical as well as deterministic relationships between processes; by incorporating variable lags, it reduces the problem of phase locking. Fourier transformation of the covariance function $\gamma_{XY}(h)$ yields the cross-spectrum $F_{XY}(\nu)$, which in turn gives the spectral coherence $c_{XY}(\nu) = F_{XY}^2(\nu)/F_X(\nu)F_Y(\nu)$, a normalized correlation between the Fourier components of X and Y. Integrated over frequencies, the spectral coherence measures, essentially, the degree of linear cross-predictability of the two series. ([4] applies spectral coherence to coordinated neural activity.) However, such second-order statistics *only* handle linear relationships. Since neural processes are known to be strongly nonlinear, there is little reason to think these statistics adequately measure coordination and synchrony in neural systems.

Mutual information is attractive because it handles both nonlinear and stochastic relationships and has a very natural and appealing interpretation. Unfortunately, it often seems to fail in practice, being disappointingly small even between signals which are known to be tightly coupled [5]. The major reason is that the neural codes use distinct patterns of activity over time, rather than many different instantaneous actions, and the usual approach misses these extended patterns. Consider two neurons, one of which drives the other to spike 50 ms after it does, the driving neuron spiking once every 500 ms. These are very tightly coordinated, but whether the first neuron spiked at time t conveys little information about what the second neuron is doing at t — it's not spiking, but it's not spiking most of the time anyway. Mutual information calculated from the direct observations conflates the "no spike" of the second neuron preparing to fire with its just-sitting-around "no spike". Here, mutual information could find the coordination if we used a 50 ms lag, but that won't work in general. Take two rate-coding neurons with base-line firing rates of 1 Hz, and suppose that a stimulus excites one to 10 Hz and suppresses the other to 0.1 Hz. The spiking rates thus share a lot of information, but whether the one neuron spiked at t is uninformative about what the other neuron did then, and lagging won't help.

Generalized synchrony is based on the idea of establishing relationships between the states of the various units. "State" here is taken in the sense of physics, dynamics and control theory: the state at time t is a variable which fixes the distribution of observables at all times $\geq t$, rendering the past of the system irrelevant [6]. Knowing the state allows us to predict, as well as possible, how the system will evolve, and how it will respond to external forces [7]. Two coupled systems are said to exhibit generalized synchrony if the state of one system is given by a mapping from the state of the other. Applications to data employ state-space reconstruction [8]: if the state $x \in \mathcal{X}$ evolves according to smooth, d-dimensional deterministic dynamics, and we observe a generic function $y = f(x)$, then the space $\mathcal{Y}$ of time-delay vectors $[y(t), y(t - \tau), ...y(t - (k - 1)\tau)]$ is diffeomorphic to $\mathcal{X}$ if $k > 2d$, for generic choices of lag τ. The various versions of generalized synchrony differ on how, precisely, to quantify the mappings between reconstructed state spaces, but they all appear to be empirically equivalent to one another and to notions of phase synchronization based on Hilbert transforms [5]. Thus all of these measures accommodate nonlinear relationships, and are potentially very flexible. Unfortunately, there is essentially no reason to believe that neural systems have deterministic dynamics at experimentally-accessible levels of detail, much less that there are deterministic relationships among such states for different units.

What we want, then, but none of these alternatives provides, is a quantity which measures predictive relationships among states, but allows those relationships to be nonlinear and stochastic. The next section introduces just such a measure, which we call "informational coherence".

2 States and Informational Coherence

There are alternatives to calculating the "surface" mutual information between the sequences of observations themselves (which, as described, fails to capture coordination). If we know that the units are phase oscillators, or rate coders, we can estimate their instantaneous phase or rate and, by calculating the mutual information between those variables, see how coordinated the units' patterns of activity are. However, phases and rates do not exhaust the repertoire of neural patterns and a more general, common scheme is desirable. The most general notion of "pattern of activity" is simply that of the dynamical state of the system, in the sense mentioned above. We now formalize this.

Assuming the usual notation for Shannon information [9], the information content of a state variable X is $H[X]$ and the mutual information between X and Y is $I[X;Y]$. As is well-known, $I[X;Y] \leq \min H[X], H[Y]$. We use this to normalize the mutual state information to a $0 - 1$ scale, and this is the *informational coherence* (IC).

$$\psi(X, Y) \quad = \quad \frac{I[X;Y]}{\min H[X], H[Y]} , \quad \text{with } 0/0 = 0 . \tag{1}$$

ψ can be interpreted as follows. $I[X;Y]$ is the Kullback-Leibler divergence between the joint distribution of X and Y, and the product of their marginal distributions [9], indicating the error involved in ignoring the dependence between X and Y. The mutual information between predictive, dynamical states thus gauges the error involved in assuming the two systems are independent, i.e., how much predictions could improve by taking into account the dependence. Hence it measures the amount of *dynamically-relevant* information shared between the two systems. ψ simply normalizes this value, and indicates the degree to which two systems have coordinated *patterns* of behavior (cf. [10], although this only uses directly observable quantities).

2.1 Reconstruction and Estimation of Effective State Spaces

As mentioned, the state space of a deterministic dynamical system can be reconstructed from a sequence of observations. This is the main tool of experimental nonlinear dynamics [8]; but the assumption of determinism is crucial and false, for almost any interesting neural system. While classical state-space reconstruction won't work on stochastic processes, such processes *do* have state-space representations [11], and, in the special case of discrete-valued, discrete-time series, there are ways to reconstruct the state space.

Here we use the CSSR algorithm, introduced in [12] (code available at `http://bactra.org/CSSR`). This produces *causal state models*, which are stochastic automata capable of statistically-optimal nonlinear prediction; the state of the machine is a minimal sufficient statistic for the future of the observable process[13].[1] The basic idea is to form a set of states which should be (1) Markovian, (2) sufficient statistics for the next observable, and (3) have deterministic transitions (in the automata-theory sense). The algorithm begins with a minimal, one-state, IID model, and checks whether these properties hold, by means of hypothesis tests. If they fail, the model is modified, generally but not always by adding more states, and the new model is checked again. Each state of the model corresponds to a distinct distribution over future events, i.e., to a statistical pattern of behavior. Under mild conditions, which do not involve prior knowledge of the state space, CSSR converges in probability to the unique causal state model of the data-generating process [12]. In practice, CSSR is quite fast (linear in the data size), and generalizes at least as well as training hidden Markov models with the EM algorithm and using cross-validation for selection, the standard heuristic [12].

One advantage of the causal state approach (which it shares with classical state-space reconstruction) is that state estimation is greatly simplified. In the general case of nonlinear state estimation, it is necessary to know not just the form of the stochastic dynamics in the state space and the observation function, but also their precise parametric values and the distribution of observation and driving noises. Estimating the state from the observable time series then becomes a computationally-intensive application of Bayes's Rule [17].

Due to the way causal states are built as statistics of the data, with probability 1 there is a finite time, t, at which the causal state at time t is certain. This is not just with some degree of belief or confidence: because of the way the states are constructed, it is impossible for the process to be in any other state at that time. Once the causal state has been established, it can be updated recursively, i.e., the causal state at time $t + 1$ is an explicit function of the causal state at time t and the observation at $t + 1$. The causal state model can be automatically converted, therefore, into a finite-state transducer which reads in an observation time series and outputs the corresponding series of states [18, 13]. (Our implementation of CSSR filters its training data automatically.) The result is a new time series of states, from which all non-predictive components have been filtered out.

2.2 Estimating the Coherence

Our algorithm for estimating the matrix of informational coherences is as follows. For each unit, we reconstruct the causal state model, and filter the observable time series to produce a series of causal states. Then, for each pair of neurons, we construct a joint histogram of

---

[1]Causal state models have the same expressive power as observable operator models [14] or predictive state representations [7], and greater power than variable-length Markov models [15, 16].

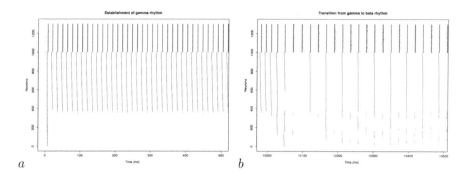

a b

Figure 1: Rastergrams of neuronal spike-times in the network. Excitatory, pyramidal neurons (numbers 1 to 1000) are shown in green, inhibitory interneurons (numbers 1001 to 1300) in red. During the first 10 seconds (a), the current connections among the pyramidal cells are suppressed and a gamma rhythm emerges (left). At $t = 10$s, those connections become active, leading to a beta rhythm (b, right).

the state distribution, estimate the mutual information between the states, and normalize by the single-unit state informations. This gives a symmetric matrix of ψ values.

Even if two systems are independent, their estimated IC will, on average, be positive, because, while they should have zero mutual information, the empirical estimate of mutual information is non-negative. Thus, the significance of IC values must be assessed against the null hypothesis of system independence. The easiest way to do so is to take the reconstructed state models for the two systems and run them forward, independently of one another, to generate a large number of simulated state sequences; from these calculate values of the IC. This procedure will approximate the sampling distribution of the IC under a null model which preserves the dynamics of each system, but not their interaction. We can then find p-values as usual. We omit them here to save space.

2.3 Approximating the Network Multi-Information

There is broad agreement [2] that analyses of networks should not just be an analysis of pairs of neurons, averaged over pairs. Ideally, an analysis of information sharing in a network would look at the over-all structure of statistical dependence between the various units, reflected in the complete joint probability distribution P of the states. This would then allow us, for instance, to calculate the n-fold multi-information, $I[X_1, X_2, \ldots X_n] \equiv D(P\|Q)$, the Kullback-Leibler divergence between the joint distribution P and the product of marginal distributions Q, analogous to the pairwise mutual information [19]. Calculated over the predictive states, the multi-information would give the total amount of shared dynamical information in the system. Just as we normalized the mutual information $I[X_1, X_2]$ by its maximum possible value, $\min H[X_1], H[X_2]$, we normalize the multi-information by its maximum, which is the smallest sum of $n - 1$ marginal entropies:

$$I[X_1; X_2; \ldots X_n] \leq \min_k \sum_{i \neq k} H[X_n]$$

Unfortunately, P is a distribution over a very high dimensional space and so, hard to estimate well without strong parametric constraints. We thus consider approximations.

The lowest-order approximation treats all the units as independent; this is the distribution Q. One step up are tree distributions, where the global distribution is a function of the joint distributions of pairs of units. Not every pair of units needs to enter into such a distribution,

671

though every unit must be part of some pair. Graphically, a tree distribution corresponds to a spanning tree, with edges linking units whose interactions enter into the global probability, and conversely spanning trees determine tree distributions. Writing E_T for the set of pairs (i, j) and abbreviating $X_1 = x_1, X_2 = x_2, \ldots X_n = x_n$ by $\mathbf{X} = \mathbf{x}$, one has

$$T(\mathbf{X} = \mathbf{x}) = \prod_{(i,j) \in E_T} \frac{T(X_i = x_i, X_j = x_j)}{T(X_i = x_i)T(X_j = x_j)} \prod_{i=1}^{n} T(X_i = x_i) \tag{2}$$

where the marginal distributions $T(X_i)$ and the pair distributions $T(X_i, X_j)$ are estimated by the empirical marginal and pair distributions.

We must now pick edges E_T so that T best approximates the true global distribution P. A natural approach is to minimize $D(P\|T)$, the divergence between P and its tree approximation. Chow and Liu [20] showed that the maximum-weight spanning tree gives the divergence-minimizing distribution, taking an edge's weight to be the mutual information between the variables it links.

There are three advantages to using the Chow-Liu approximation. (1) Estimating T from empirical probabilities gives a consistent maximum likelihood estimator of the ideal Chow-Liu tree [20], with reasonable rates of convergence, so T can be reliably known even if P cannot. (2) There are efficient algorithms for constructing maximum-weight spanning trees, such as Prim's algorithm [21, sec. 23.2], which runs in time $O(n^2 + n \log n)$. Thus, the approximation is computationally tractable. (3) The KL divergence of the Chow-Liu distribution from Q gives a lower bound on the network multi-information; that bound is just the sum of the mutual informations along the edges in the tree:

$$I[X_1; X_2; \ldots X_n] \geq D(T\|Q) = \sum_{(i,j) \in E_T} I[X_i; X_j] \tag{3}$$

Even if we knew P exactly, Eq. 3 would be useful as an alternative to calculating $D(P\|Q)$ directly, evaluating $\log P(\mathbf{x})/Q(\mathbf{x})$ for all the exponentially-many configurations $\mathbf{x}$.

It is natural to seek higher-order approximations to P, e.g., using three-way interactions not decomposable into pairwise interactions [22, 19]. But it is hard to do so effectively, because finding the optimal approximation to P when such interactions are allowed is NP [23], and analytical formulas like Eq. 3 generally do not exist [19]. We therefore confine ourselves to the Chow-Liu approximation here.

3 Example: A Model of Gamma and Beta Rhythms

We use simulated data as a test case, instead of empirical multiple electrode recordings, which allows us to try the method on a system of over 1000 neurons and compare the measure against expected results. The model, taken from [24], was originally designed to study episodes of gamma (30–80Hz) and beta (12–30Hz) oscillations in the mammalian nervous system, which often occur successively with a spontaneous transition between them. More concretely, the rhythms studied were those displayed by *in vitro* hippocampal (CA1) slice preparations and by *in vivo* neocortical EEGs.

The model contains two neuron populations: excitatory (AMPA) pyramidal neurons and inhibitory (GABA$_A$) interneurons, defined by conductance-based Hodgkin-Huxley-style equations. Simulations were carried out in a network of 1000 pyramidal cells and 300 interneurons. Each cell was modeled as a one-compartment neuron with all-to-all coupling, endowed with the basic sodium and potassium spiking currents, an external applied current, and some Gaussian input noise.

The first 10 seconds of the simulation correspond to the gamma rhythm, in which only a group of neurons is made to spike via a linearly increasing applied current. The beta rhythm

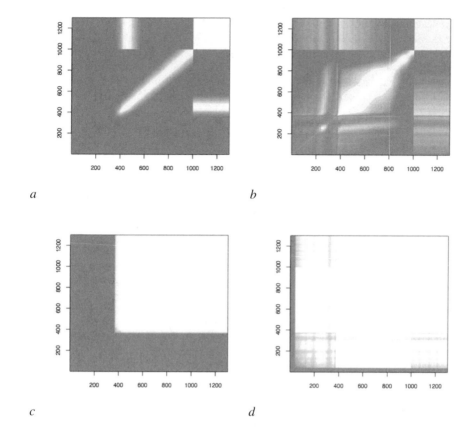

a   *b*

c   *d*

Figure 2: Heat-maps of coordination for the network, as measured by zero-lag cross-correlation (top row) and informational coherence (bottom), contrasting the gamma rhythm (left column) with the beta (right). Colors run from red (no coordination) through yellow to pale cream (maximum).

(subsequent 10 seconds) is obtained by activating pyramidal-pyramidal recurrent connections (potentiated by Hebbian preprocessing as a result of synchrony during the gamma rhythm) and a slow outward after-hyper-polarization (AHP) current (the M-current), suppressed during gamma due to the metabotropic activation used in the generation of the rhythm. During the beta rhythm, pyramidal cells, silent during gamma rhythm, fire on a subset of interneurons cycles (Fig. 1).

Fig. 2 compares zero-lag cross-correlation, a second-order method of quantifying coordination, with the informational coherence calculated from the reconstructed states. (In this simulation, we could have calculated the actual states of the model neurons directly, rather than reconstructing them, but for purposes of testing our method we did not.) Cross-correlation finds some of the relationships visible in Fig. 1, but is confused by, for instance, the phase shifts between pyramidal cells. (Surface mutual information, not shown, gives similar results.) Informational coherence, however, has no trouble recognizing the two populations as effectively coordinated blocks. The presence of dynamical noise, problematic for ordinary state reconstruction, is not an issue. The average IC is 0.411 (or 0.797 if the inactive, low-numbered neurons are excluded). The tree estimate of the global informational multi-information is 3243.7 bits, with a global coherence of 0.777. The right half of

Fig. 2 repeats this analysis for the beta rhythm; in this stage, the average IC is 0.614, and the tree estimate of the global multi-information is 7377.7 bits, though the estimated global coherence falls very slightly to 0.742. This is because low-numbered neurons which were quiescent before are now active, contributing to the global information, but the over-all pattern is somewhat weaker and more noisy (as can be seen from Fig. 1*b*.) So, as expected, the total information content is higher, but the overall coordination across the network is lower.

4 Conclusion

Informational coherence provides a measure of neural information sharing and coordinated activity which accommodates nonlinear, stochastic relationships between extended patterns of spiking. It is robust to dynamical noise and leads to a genuinely multivariate measure of global coordination across networks or regions. Applied to data from multi-electrode recordings, it should be a valuable tool in evaluating hypotheses about distributed neural representation and function.

Acknowledgments

Thanks to R. Haslinger, E. Ionides and S. Page; and for support to the Santa Fe Institute (under grants from Intel, the NSF and the MacArthur Foundation, and DARPA agreement F30602-00-2-0583), the Clare Booth Luce Foundation (KLK) and the James S. McDonnell Foundation (CRS).

References

[1] L. F. Abbott and T. J. Sejnowski, eds. *Neural Codes and Distributed Representations*. MIT Press, 1998.

[2] E. N. Brown, R. E. Kass, and P. P. Mitra. *Nature Neuroscience*, 7:456–461, 2004.

[3] D. H. Ballard, Z. Zhang, and R. P. N. Rao. In R. P. N. Rao, B. A. Olshausen, and M. S. Lewicki, eds., *Probabilistic Models of the Brain*, pp. 273–284, MIT Press, 2002.

[4] D. R. Brillinger and A. E. P. Villa. In D. R. Brillinger, L. T. Fernholz, and S. Morgenthaler, eds., *The Practice of Data Analysis*, pp. 77–92. Princeton U.P., 1997.

[5] R. Quian Quiroga et al. *Physical Review E*, 65:041903, 2002.

[6] R. F. Streater. *Statistical Dynamics*. Imperial College Press, London.

[7] M. L. Littman, R. S. Sutton, and S. Singh. In T. G. Dietterich, S. Becker, and Z. Ghahramani, eds., *Advances in Neural Information Processing Systems 14*, pp. 1555–1561. MIT Press, 2002.

[8] H. Kantz and T. Schreiber. *Nonlinear Time Series Analysis*. Cambridge U.P., 1997.

[9] T. M. Cover and J. A. Thomas. *Elements of Information Theory*. Wiley, 1991.

[10] M. Palus et al. *Physical Review E*, 63:046211, 2001.

[11] F. B. Knight. *Annals of Probability*, 3:573–596, 1975.

[12] C. R. Shalizi and K. L. Shalizi. In M. Chickering and J. Halpern, eds., *Uncertainty in Artificial Intelligence: Proceedings of the Twentieth Conference*, pp. 504–511. AUAI Press, 2004.

[13] C. R. Shalizi and J. P. Crutchfield. *Journal of Statistical Physics*, 104:817–819, 2001.

[14] H. Jaeger. *Neural Computation*, 12:1371–1398, 2000.

[15] D. Ron, Y. Singer, and N. Tishby. *Machine Learning*, 25:117–149, 1996.

[16] P. Bühlmann and A. J. Wyner. *Annals of Statistics*, 27:480–513, 1999.

[17] N. U. Ahmed. *Linear and Nonlinear Filtering for Scientists and Engineers*. World Scientific, 1998.

[18] D. R. Upper. PhD thesis, University of California, Berkeley, 1997.

[19] E. Schneidman, S. Still, M. J. Berry, and W. Bialek. *Physical Review Letters*, 91:238701, 2003.

[20] C. K. Chow and C. N. Liu. *IEEE Transactions on Information Theory*, IT-14:462–467, 1968.

[21] T. H. Cormen et al. *Introduction to Algorithms*. 2nd ed. MIT Press, 2001.

[22] S. Amari. *IEEE Transacttions on Information Theory*, 47:1701–1711, 2001.

[23] S. Kirshner, P. Smyth, and A. Robertson. Tech. Rep. 04-04, UC Irvine, Information and Computer Science, 2004.

[24] M. S. Olufsen et al. *Journal of Computational Neuroscience*, 14:33–54, 2003.

Inference with Minimal Communication: a Decision-Theoretic Variational Approach

O. Patrick Kreidl and Alan S. Willsky
Department of Electrical Engineering and Computer Science
MIT Laboratory for Information and Decision Systems
Cambridge, MA 02139
{opk,willsky}@mit.edu

Abstract

Given a directed graphical model with binary-valued hidden nodes and real-valued noisy observations, consider deciding upon the maximum a-posteriori (MAP) or the maximum posterior-marginal (MPM) assignment under the restriction that each node broadcasts only to its children exactly one single-bit message. We present a variational formulation, viewing the processing rules local to all nodes as degrees-of-freedom, that minimizes the loss in expected (MAP or MPM) performance subject to such online communication constraints. The approach leads to a novel message-passing algorithm to be executed *offline*, or before observations are realized, which mitigates the performance loss by iteratively coupling all rules in a manner implicitly driven by global statistics. We also provide (i) illustrative examples, (ii) assumptions that guarantee convergence and efficiency and (iii) connections to active research areas.

1 Introduction

Given a probabilistic model with discrete-valued hidden variables, Belief Propagation (BP) and related graph-based algorithms are commonly employed to solve for the Maximum A-Posteriori (MAP) assignment (i.e., the mode of the joint distribution of all hidden variables) and Maximum-Posterior-Marginal (MPM) assignment (i.e., the modes of the marginal distributions of every hidden variable) [1]. The established "message-passing" interpretation of BP extends naturally to a distributed network setting: associating to each node and edge in the graph a distinct processor and communication link, respectively, the algorithm is equivalent to a sequence of purely-local computations interleaved with only nearest-neighbor communications. Specifically, each computation event corresponds to a node evaluating its local *processing rule*, or a function by which all messages received in the preceding communication event map to messages sent in the next communication event.

Practically, the viability of BP appears to rest upon an implicit assumption that network communication resources are abundant. In a general network, because termination of the algorithm is in question, the required communication resources are a-priori unbounded. Even when termination can be guaranteed, transmission of exact messages presumes communication channels with infinite capacity (in bits per observation), or at least of sufficiently high bandwidth such that the resulting finite message precision is essentially error-free. In

675

some distributed settings (e.g., energy-limited wireless sensor networks), it may be prohibitively costly to justify such idealized online communications. While recent evidence suggests substantial but "small-enough" message errors will not alter the behavior of BP [2], [3], it also suggests BP may perform poorly when communication is very constrained.

Assuming communication constraints are severe, we examine the extent to which alternative processing rules can avoid a loss in (MAP or MPM) performance. Specifically, given a directed graphical model with binary-valued hidden variables and real-valued noisy observations, we assume each node may broadcast only to its children a single binary-valued message. We cast the problem within a variational formulation [4], seeking to minimize a decision-theoretic penalty function subject to such online communication constraints. The formulation turns out to be an extension of the optimization problem underlying the decentralized detection paradigm [5], [6], which advocates a team-theoretic [7] relaxation of the original problem to both justify a particular finite parameterization for all local processing rules and obtain an iterative algorithm to be executed *offline* (i.e., before observations are realized). To our knowledge, that this relaxation permits analytical progress given any directed acyclic network is new. Moreover, for MPM assignment in a tree-structured network, we discover an added convenience with respect to the envisioned distributed processor setting: the offline computation itself admits an efficient message-passing interpretation.

This paper is organized as follows. Section 2 details the decision-theoretic variational formulation for discrete-variable assignment. Section 3 summarizes the main results derived from its connection to decentralized detection, culminating in the offline message-passing algorithm and the assumptions that guarantee convergence and maximal efficiency. We omit the mathematical proofs [8] here, focusing instead on intuition and illustrative examples. Closing remarks and relations to other active research areas appear in Section 4.

2 Variational Formulation

In abstraction, the basic ingredients are (i) a joint distribution $p(x, y)$ for two length-N random vectors X and Y, taking hidden and observable values in the sets $\{0, 1\}^N$ and $\mathbb{R}^N$, respectively; (ii) a decision-theoretic penalty function $J : \Gamma \to \mathbb{R}$, where Γ denotes the set of all candidate strategies $\gamma : \mathbb{R}^N \to \{0, 1\}^N$ for posterior assignment; and (iii) the set $\Gamma^{\mathcal{G}} \subset \Gamma$ of strategies that also respect stipulated communication constraints in a given N-node directed acyclic network $\mathcal{G}$. The ensuing optimization problem is expressed by

$$J(\gamma^*) = \min_{\gamma \in \Gamma} J(\gamma) \quad \text{subject to } \gamma \in \Gamma^{\mathcal{G}}, \tag{1}$$

where γ^* then represents an *optimal network-constrained strategy* for discrete-variable assignment. The following subsections provide details unseen at this level of abstraction.

2.1 Decision-Theoretic Penalty Function

Let $U = \gamma(Y)$ denote the decision process induced from the observation process Y by any candidate assignment strategy $\gamma \in \Gamma$. If we associate a numeric "cost" $c(u, x)$ to every possible joint realization of (U, X), then the expected cost is a well-posed penalty function:

$$J(\gamma) = E\left[c\left(\gamma(Y), X\right)\right] = E\left[E\left[c(\gamma(Y), X) \mid Y\right]\right]. \tag{2}$$

Expanding the inner expectation and recognizing $p(x|y)$ to be proportional to $p(x)p(y|x)$ for every y such that $p(y) > 0$, it follows that $\bar{\gamma}^*$ minimizes (2) over Γ if and only if

$$\bar{\gamma}^*(Y) = \arg\min_{u \in \{0,1\}^N} \sum_{x \in \{0,1\}^N} p(x)c(u, x)p(Y|x) \quad \text{with probability one.} \tag{3}$$

Of note are (i) the likelihood function $p(Y|x)$ is a finite-dimensional sufficient statistic of Y, (ii) real-valued coefficients $\bar{b}(u, x)$ provide a finite parameterization of the function space Γ and (iii) optimal coefficient values $\bar{b}^*(u, x) = p(x)c(u, x)$ are computable offline.

Before introducing communication constraints, we illustrate by examples how the decision-theoretic penalty function relates to familiar discrete-variable assignment problems.

Example 1: Let $c(u, x)$ indicate whether $u \neq x$. Then (2) and (3) specialize to, respectively, the *word error rate* (viewing each x as an N-bit word) and the MAP strategy:

$$\bar{\gamma}^*(Y) = \arg \max_{x \in \{0,1\}^N} p(x|Y) \quad \text{with probability one.}$$

Example 2: Let $c(u, x) = \sum_{n=1}^{N} c_n(u_n, x_n)$, where each c_n indicates whether $u_n \neq x_n$. Then (2) and (3) specialize to, respectively, the *bit error rate* and the MPM strategy:

$$\bar{\gamma}^*(Y) = \left(\arg \max_{x_1 \in \{0,1\}} p(x_1|Y), \ldots, \arg \max_{x_N \in \{0,1\}} p(x_N|Y) \right) \quad \text{with probability one.}$$

2.2 Network Communication Constraints

Let $\mathcal{G}(\mathcal{V}, \mathcal{E})$ be any directed acyclic graph with vertex set $\mathcal{V} = \{1, \ldots, N\}$ and edge set

$$\mathcal{E} = \{(i, j) \in \mathcal{V} \times \mathcal{V} \mid i \in \pi(j) \Leftrightarrow j \in \chi(i)\},$$

where index sets $\pi(n) \subset \mathcal{V}$ and $\chi(n) \subset \mathcal{V}$ indicate, respectively, the parents and children of each node $n \in \mathcal{V}$. Without loss-of-generality, we assume the node labels respect the natural partial-order implied by the graph $\mathcal{G}$; specifically, we assume every node n has parent nodes $\pi(n) \subset \{1, \ldots, n-1\}$ and child nodes $\chi(n) \subset \{n+1, \ldots, N\}$. Local to each node $n \in \mathcal{V}$ are the respective components X_n and Y_n of the joint process (X, Y). Under best-case assumptions on $p(x, y)$ and $\mathcal{G}$, Belief Propagation methods (e.g., max-product in Example 1, sum-product in Example 2) require at least $2|\mathcal{E}|$ real-valued messages per observation $Y = y$, one per direction along each edge in $\mathcal{G}$. In contrast, we insist upon a single forward-pass through $\mathcal{G}$ where each node n broadcasts to its children (if any) a single binary-valued message. This yields communication overhead of only $|\mathcal{E}|$ bits per observation $Y = y$, but also renders the minimizing strategy of (3) infeasible.

Accepting that performance-communication tradeoffs are inherent to distributed algorithms, we proceed with the goal of minimizing the *loss* in performance relative to $J(\bar{\gamma}^*)$. Specifically, we now translate the stipulated restrictions on communication into explicit constraints on the function space Γ over which to minimize (2). The simplest such translation assumes the binary-valued message produced by node n also determines the respective component u_n in decision vector $u = \gamma(y)$. Recognizing that every node n receives the messages $u_{\pi(n)}$ from its parents (if any) as side information to y_n, any function of the form $\gamma_n : \mathbb{R} \times \{0,1\}^{|\pi(n)|} \rightarrow \{0,1\}$ is a feasible *processing rule*; we denote the set of all such rules by Γ_n. Then, every strategy in the set $\Gamma^{\mathcal{G}} = \Gamma_1 \times \cdots \times \Gamma_N$ respects the constraints.

3 Summary of Main Results

As stated in Section 1, the variational formulation presented in Section 2 can be viewed as an extension of the optimization problem underlying decentralized Bayesian detection [5], [6]. Even for specialized network structures (e.g., the N-node chain), it is known that exact solution to (1) is NP-hard, stemming from the absence of a guarantee that $\gamma^* \in \Gamma^{\mathcal{G}}$ possesses a finite parameterization. Also known is that analytical progress can be made for a relaxation of (1), which is based on the following intuition: if strategy $\gamma^* = (\gamma_1^*, \ldots, \gamma_N^*)$ is optimal over $\Gamma^{\mathcal{G}}$, then for each n and assuming all components $i \in \mathcal{V} \backslash n$ are fixed at rules γ_i^*, the component rule γ_n^* must be optimal over Γ_n. Decentralized detection has roots in team decision theory [7], a subset of game theory, in which the relaxation is named *person-by-person* (pbp) optimality. While global optimality always implies pbp-optimality, the converse is false—in general, there can be multiple pbp-optimal solutions with varying penalty. Nonetheless, pbp-optimality (along with a specialized observation process) justifies a particular finite parameterization for the function space $\Gamma^{\mathcal{G}}$, leading to a nonlinear fixed-point equation and an iterative algorithm with favorable convergence properties. Before presenting the general algorithm, we illustrate its application in two simple examples.

Example 3: Consider the MPM assignment problem in Example 2, assuming $N = 2$ and distribution $p(x, y)$ is defined by positive-valued parameters α, β_1 and β_2 as follows:

$$p(x) \propto \begin{cases} 1 & , & x_1 = x_2 \\ \alpha & , & x_1 \neq x_2 \end{cases} \quad \text{and} \quad p(y|x) = \prod_{n=1}^{N} \frac{1}{\sqrt{2\pi}} \exp\left[-\frac{(y_n - \beta_n x_n)^2}{2}\right].$$

Note that X_1 and X_2 are marginally uniform and α captures their correlation (positive, zero, or negative when α is less than, equal to, or greater than unity, respectively), while Y captures the presence of additive white Gaussian noise with signal-to-noise ratio at node n equal to β_n. The (unconstrained) MPM strategy $\bar{\gamma}^*$ simplifies to a pair of threshold rules

$$L_1(y_1) \underset{u_1=0}{\overset{u_1=1}{\gtrless}} \bar{\eta}_1^* = \frac{1 + \alpha L_2(y_2)}{\alpha + L_2(y_2)} \quad \text{and} \quad L_2(y_2) \underset{u_2=0}{\overset{u_2=1}{\gtrless}} \bar{\eta}_2^* = \frac{1 + \alpha L_1(y_1)}{\alpha + L_1(y_1)},$$

where $L_n(y_n) = \exp\left[\beta_n\left(y_n - \beta_n/2\right)\right]$ denotes the *likelihood-ratio* local to node n. Let $\mathcal{E} = \{(1, 2)\}$ and define two network-constrained strategies: *myopic* strategy γ^0 employs thresholds $\eta_1^0 = \eta_2^0 = 1$, meaning each node n acts to minimize $\Pr[U_n \neq X_n]$ as if in isolation, whereas *heuristic* strategy γ^h employs thresholds $\eta_1^h = \eta_1^0$ and $\eta_2^h = \alpha^{2u_1 - 1}$, meaning node 2 adjusts its threshold as if $X_1 = u_1$ (i.e., as if the myopic decision by node 1 is always correct). Figure 1 compares these strategies and a pbp-optimal strategy γ^k—only γ^k is both feasible and consistently "hedging" against all uncertainty i.e., $J(\gamma^0) \geq J(\gamma^k) \geq J(\bar{\gamma}^*)$.

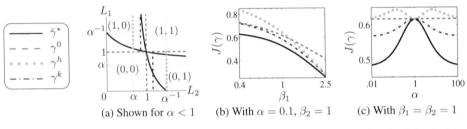

(a) Shown for $\alpha < 1$ (b) With $\alpha = 0.1$, $\beta_2 = 1$ (c) With $\beta_1 = \beta_2 = 1$

Figure 1. Comparison of the four alternative strategies in Example 3: (a) sketch of the decision regions in likelihood-ratio space, showing that network-constrained threshold rules cannot exactly reproduce $\bar{\gamma}^*$ (unless $\alpha = 1$); (b) bit-error-rate versus β_1 with α and β_2 fixed, showing γ^h performs comparably to γ^k when Y_1 is accurate relative to Y_2 but otherwise performs worse than even γ^0 (which requires no communication); (c) bit-error-rate versus α with β_1 and β_2 fixed, showing γ^k uses the allotted bit of communication such that roughly 35% of the loss $J(\gamma^0) - J(\bar{\gamma}^*)$ is recovered.

Example 4: Extend Example 3 to $N > 2$ nodes, but assuming X is equally-likely to be all zeros or all ones (i.e., the extreme case of positive correlation) and Y has identically-accurate components with $\beta_n = 1$ for all n. The MPM strategy employs thresholds $\bar{\eta}_n^* = \prod_{i \in V \setminus n} 1/L_i(y_i)$ for all n, leading to $U = \bar{\gamma}^*(Y)$ also being all zeros or all ones; thus, its *cost distribution*, or the probability mass function for $c(\bar{\gamma}^*(Y), X)$, has mass only on the values 0 and N. The myopic strategy employs thresholds $\eta_n^0 = 1$ for all n, leading to independent and identically-distributed (binary-valued) random variables $c_n(\gamma_n^0(Y_n), X_n)$; thus, its cost distribution, approaching a normal shape as N gets large, has mass on all values $0, 1, \ldots, N$. Figure 2 considers a particular directed network $\mathcal{G}$ and, initializing to γ^0, shows the sequence of cost distributions resulting from the iterative offline algorithm—note the shape progression towards the cost distribution of the (infeasible) MPM strategy and the successive reduction in bit-error-rate $J(\gamma^k)$. Also noteworthy is the rapid convergence and the successive reduction in word-error-rate $\Pr[c(\gamma^k(Y), X) \neq 0]$.

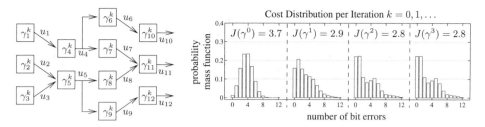

Figure 2. Illustration of the iterative offline computation given $p(x, y)$ as described in Example 4 and the directed network shown ($N = 12$). A Monte-Carlo analysis of $\bar{\gamma}^*$ yields an estimate for its bit-error-rate of $J(\bar{\gamma}^*) \approx 0.49$ (with standard deviation of 0.05)—thus, with a total of just $|\mathcal{E}| = 11$ bits of communication, the pbp-optimal strategy γ^3 recovers roughly 28% of the loss $J(\gamma^0) - J(\bar{\gamma}^*)$.

3.1 Necessary Optimality Conditions

We start by providing an explicit probabilistic interpretation of the general problem in (1).

Lemma 1 *The minimum penalty $J(\gamma^*)$ defined in (1) is, firstly, achievable by a deterministic[1] strategy and, secondly, equivalently defined by*

$$J(\gamma^*) = \min_{p(u|y)} \sum_{x \in \{0,1\}^N} p(x) \sum_{u \in \{0,1\}^N} c(u, x) \int_{y \in \mathbb{R}^N} p(u|y)p(y|x)\, dy$$

$$\text{subject to} \quad p(u|y) = \prod_{n \in \mathcal{V}} p(u_n|y_n, u_{\pi(n)}).$$

Lemma 1 is primarily of conceptual value, establishing a correspondence between fixing a component rule $\gamma_n \in \Gamma_n$ and inducing a decision process U_n from the information $(Y_n, U_{\pi(n)})$ local to node n. The following assumption permits analytical progress towards a finite parameterization for each function space Γ_n and the basis of an offline algorithm.

Assumption 1 *The observation process Y satisfies $p(y|x) = \prod_{n \in \mathcal{V}} p(y_n|x)$.*

Lemma 2 *Let Assumption 1 hold. Upon fixing a deterministic rule $\gamma_n \in \Gamma_n$ local to node n (in correspondence with $p(u_n|y_n, u_{\pi(n)})$ by virtue of Lemma 1), we have the identity*

$$p(u_n|x, u_{\pi(n)}) = \int_{y_n \in \mathbb{R}} p(u_n|y_n, u_{\pi(n)})p(y_n|x)\, dy_n. \tag{4}$$

Moreover, upon fixing a deterministic strategy $\gamma \in \Gamma^{\mathcal{G}}$, we have the identity

$$p(u|x) = \prod_{n \in \mathcal{V}} p(u_n|x, u_{\pi(n)}). \tag{5}$$

Lemma 2 implies fixing component rule $\gamma_n \in \Gamma_n$ is in correspondence with inducing the conditional distribution $p(u_n|x, u_{\pi(n)})$, now a probabilistic description that persists local to node n no matter the rule γ_i at any other node $i \in \mathcal{V} \backslash n$. Lemma 2 also introduces further structure in the constrained optimization expressed by Lemma 1: recognizing the integral over $\mathbb{R}^N$ to equal $p(u|x)$, (4) and (5) together imply it can be expressed as a product of

---

[1]A randomized (or mixed) strategy, modeled as a probabilistic selection from a finite collection of deterministic strategies, takes more inputs than just the observation process Y. That deterministic strategies suffice, however, justifies "post-hoc" our initial abuse of notation for elements in the set Γ.

component integrals, each over $\mathbb{R}$. We now argue that, despite these simplifications, the component rules of γ^* continue to be globally coupled.

Starting with any deterministic strategy $\gamma \in \Gamma^{\mathcal{G}}$, consider optimizing the nth component rule γ_n over Γ_n assuming all other components stay fixed. With γ_n a degree-of-freedom, decision process U_n is no longer well-defined so each $u_n \in \{0,1\}$ merely represents a candidate decision local to node n. Online, each local decision will be made only upon receiving both the local observation $Y_n = y_n$ and all parents' local decisions $U_{\pi(n)} = u_{\pi(n)}$. It follows that node n, upon deciding a particular u_n, may assert that random vector U is restricted to values in the subset $\mathcal{U}[u_{\pi(n)}, u_n] = \{u' \in \{0,1\}^N \mid u'_{\pi(n)} = u_{\pi(n)}, u'_n = u_n\}$. Then, viewing $(Y_n, U_{\pi(n)})$ as a composite local observation and proceeding in the manner by which (3) is derived, the pbp-optimal relaxation of (1) reduces to the following form.

Proposition 1 *Let Assumption 1 hold. In an optimal network-constrained strategy $\gamma^* \in \Gamma^{\mathcal{G}}$, for each n and assuming all components $i \in \mathcal{V} \backslash n$ are fixed at rules γ_i^* (each in correspondence with $p^*(u_i|x, u_{\pi(i)})$ by virtue of Lemma 2), the rule γ_n^* satisfies*

$$\gamma_n^*(Y_n, U_{\pi(n)}) = \arg \min_{u_n \in \{0,1\}} \sum_{x \in \{0,1\}^N} b_n^*(u_n, x; U_{\pi(n)}) p(Y_n|x) \quad \text{with probability one}$$

(6)

where, for each $u_{\pi(n)} \in \{0,1\}^{|\pi(n)|}$,

$$b_n^*(u_n, x; u_{\pi(n)}) = p(x) \sum_{u \in \mathcal{U}[u_{\pi(n)}, u_n]} c(u, x) \prod_{i \in \mathcal{V} \backslash n} p^*(u_i|x, u_{\pi(i)}).$$

(7)

Of note are (i) the likelihood function $p(Y_n|x)$ is a finite-dimensional sufficient statistic of Y_n, (ii) real-valued coefficients b_n provide a finite parameterization of the function space Γ_n and (iii) the pbp-optimal coefficient values b_n^*, while still computable offline, also depend on the distributions $p^*(u_i|x, u_{\pi(i)})$ in correspondence with all fixed rules γ_i^*.

3.2 Offline Message-Passing Algorithm

Let f_n map from coefficients $\{b_i; i \in \mathcal{V} \backslash n\}$ to coefficients b_n by the following operations:

1. for each $i \in \mathcal{V} \backslash n$, compute $p(u_i|x, u_{\pi(i)})$ via (4) and (6) given b_i and $p(y_i|x)$;

2. compute b_n via (7) given $p(x)$, $c(u, x)$ and $\{p(u_i|x, u_{\pi(i)}); i \in \mathcal{V} \backslash n\}$.

Then, the simultaneous satisfaction of Proposition 1 at all N nodes can be viewed as a system of $2^{N+1} \sum_{n \in \mathcal{V}} 2^{|\pi(n)|}$ nonlinear equations in as many unknowns,

$$b_n = f_n(b_1, \ldots, b_{n-1}, b_{n+1}, \ldots, b_N), \quad n = 1, \ldots, N,$$

(8)

or, more concisely, $b = f(b)$. The connection between each f_n and Proposition 1 affords an equivalence between solving the fixed-point equation f via a Gauss-Seidel iteration and minimizing $J(\gamma)$ via a coordinate-descent iteration [9], implying an algorithm guaranteed to terminate and achieve penalty no greater than that of an arbitrary initial strategy $\gamma^0 \leftrightarrow b^0$.

Proposition 2 *Initialize to any coefficients $b^0 = (b_1^0, \ldots, b_N^0)$ and generate the sequence $\{b^k\}$ using a component-wise iterative application of f in (8) i.e., for $k = 1, 2, \ldots,$*

$$b_n^k := f_n(b_1^{k-1}, \ldots, b_{n-1}^{k-1}, b_{n+1}^k, \ldots, b_N^k), \quad n = N, N-1, \ldots, 1.$$

(9)

If Assumption 1 holds, the associated sequence $\{J(\gamma^k)\}$ is non-increasing and converges:

$$J(\gamma^0) \geq J(\gamma^1) \geq \cdots \geq J(\gamma^k) \to J^* \geq J(\gamma^*) \geq J(\bar{\gamma}^*).$$

Direct implementation of (9) is clearly imprudent from a computational perspective, because the transformation from fixed coefficients b_n^k to the corresponding distribution $p^k(u_n|x, u_{\pi(n)})$ need not be repeated within every component evaluation of f. In fact, assuming every node n stores in memory its own likelihood function $p(y_n|x)$, this transformation can be accomplished locally (cf. (4) and (6)) and, also assuming the resulting distribution is broadcast to all other nodes before they proceed with their subsequent component evaluation of f, the termination guarantee of Proposition 2 is retained. Requiring every node to perform a network-wide broadcast within every iteration k makes (9) a decidedly global algorithm, not to mention that each node n must also store in memory $p(x, y_n)$ and $c(u, x)$ to carry forth the supporting local computations.

Assumption 2 *The cost function satisfies $c(u, x) = \sum_{n \in \mathcal{V}} c_n(u_n, x)$ for some collection of functions $\{c_n : \{0, 1\}^{N+1} \to \mathbb{R}\}$ and the directed graph $\mathcal{G}$ is tree-structured.*

Proposition 3 *Under Assumption 2, the following two-pass procedure is identical to (9):*

- *Forward-pass at node n: upon receiving messages from all parents $i \in \pi(n)$, store them for use in the next reverse-pass and send to each child $j \in \chi(n)$ the following messages:*

$$P_{n \to j}^k(u_n|x) := \sum_{u_{\pi(n)} \in \{0,1\}^{|\pi(n)|}} p^{k-1}\left(u_n|x, u_{\pi(n)}\right) \prod_{i \in \pi(n)} P_{i \to n}^k(u_i|x). \qquad (10)$$

- *Reverse-pass at node n: upon receiving messages from all children $j \in \chi(n)$, update*

$$b_n^k\left(u_n, x; u_{\pi(n)}\right) := p(x) \prod_{i \in \pi(n)} P_{i \to n}^k(u_i|x) \left(c_n(u_n, x) + \sum_{j \in \chi(n)} C_{j \to n}^k(u_n, x)\right) \qquad (11)$$

and the corresponding distribution $p^k(u_n|x, u_{\pi(n)})$ via (4) and (6), store the distribution for use in the next forward pass and send to each parent $i \in \pi(n)$ the following messages:

$$C_{n \to i}^k(u_i, x) := \sum_{u_n \in \{0,1\}} p(u_n|x, u_i) \left(c_n(u_n, x) + \sum_{j \in \chi(n)} C_{j \to n}^k(u_n, x)\right), \qquad (12)$$

$$p(u_n|x, u_i) = \sum_{u_{\pi(n)} \in \{u' \in \{0,1\}^{|\pi(n)|} | u'_i = u_i\}} p^k\left(u_n|x, u_{\pi(n)}\right) \prod_{\ell \in \pi(n) \setminus i} P_{\ell \to n}^k(u_\ell|x).$$

An intuitive interpretation of Proposition 3, from the perspective of node n, is as follows. From (10) in the forward pass, the messages received from each parent define what, during subsequent online operation, that parent's local decision means (in a likelihood sense) about its ancestors' outputs and the hidden process. From (12) in the reverse pass, the messages received from each child define what the local decision will mean (in an expected cost sense) to that child and its descendants. From (11), both types of incoming messages impact the local rule update and, in turn, the outgoing messages to both types of neighbors. While Proposition 3 alleviates the need for the iterative global broadcast of distributions $p^k(u_n|x, u_{\pi(n)})$, the explicit dependence of (10)-(12) on the full vector x implies the memory and computation requirements local to each node can still be exponential in N.

Assumption 3 *The hidden process X is Markov on $\mathcal{G}$, or $p(x) = \prod_{n \in \mathcal{V}} p(x_n|x_{\pi(n)})$, and all component likelihoods/costs satisfy $p(y_n|x) = p(y_n|x_n)$ and $c_n(u_n, x) = c_n(u_n, x_n)$.*

Proposition 4 *Under Assumption 3, the iterates in Proposition 3 specialize to the form of*

$$b_n^k(u_n, x_n; u_{\pi(n)}), \quad P_{n \to j}^k(u_n|x_n) \quad and \quad C_{n \to i}^k(u_i, x_i), \qquad k = 0, 1, \ldots$$

and each node n need only store in memory $p(x_{\pi(n)}, x_n, y_n)$ and $c_n(u_n, x_n)$ to carry forth the supporting local computations. (The actual equations can be found in [8].)

Proposition 4 implies the convergence properties of Proposition 2 are upheld with maximal efficiency (linear in N) when $\mathcal{G}$ is tree-structured and the global distribution and costs satisfy $p(x, y) = \prod_{n \in \mathcal{V}} p(x_n | x_{\pi(n)}) p(y_n | x_n)$ and $c(u, x) = \sum_{n \in \mathcal{V}} c_n(u_n, x_n)$, respectively. Note that these conditions hold for the MPM assignment problems in Examples 3 & 4.

4 Discussion

Our decision-theoretic variational approach reflects several departures from existing methods for communication-constrained inference. Firstly, instead of imposing the constraints on an algorithm derived from an ideal model, we explicitly model the constraints and derive a different algorithm. Secondly, our penalty function drives the approximation by the desired application of inference (e.g., posterior assignment) as opposed to a generic error measure on the result of inference (e.g., divergence in true and approximate marginals). Thirdly, the necessary offline computation gives rise to a downside, namely less flexibility against time-varying statistical environments, decision objectives or network conditions.

Our development also evokes principles in common with other research areas. Similar to the sum-product version of Belief Propagation (BP), our message-passing algorithm originates assuming a tree structure, an additive cost and a synchronous message schedule. It is thus enticing to claim that the maturation of BP (e.g., max-product, asynchronous schedule, cyclic graphs) also applies, but unique aspects to our development (e.g., directed graph, weak convergence, asymmetric messages) merit caution. That we solve for correlated equilibria and depend on probabilistic structure commensurate with cost structure for efficiency is in common with graphical games [10], which distinctly are formulated on undirected graphs and absent of hidden variables. Finally, our offline computation resembles learning a conditional random field [11], in the sense that factors of $p(u|x)$ are iteratively modified to reduce penalty $J(\gamma)$; online computation via strategy $u = \gamma(y)$, repeated per realization $Y = y$, is then viewed as sampling from this distribution. Along the learning thread, a special case of our formulation appears in [12], but assuming $p(x, y)$ is unknown.

Acknowledgments

This work supported by the Air Force Office of Scientific Research under contract FA9550-04-1 and by the Army Research Office under contract DAAD19-00-1-0466. We are grateful to Professor John Tsitsiklis for taking time to discuss the correctness of Proposition 1.

References

[1] J. Pearl. *Probabilistic Reasoning in Intelligent Systems*. Morgan Kaufmann, 1988.

[2] L. Chen, et al. Data association based on optimization in graphical models with application to sensor networks. *Mathematical and Computer Modeling*, 2005. To appear.

[3] A. T. Ihler, et al. Message errors in belief propagation. *Advances in NIPS 17*, MIT Press, 2005.

[4] M. I. Jordan, et al. An introduction to variational methods for graphical models. *Learning in Graphical Models*, pp. 105–161, MIT Press, 1999.

[5] J. N. Tsitsiklis. Decentralized detection. *Adv. in Stat. Sig. Proc.*, pp. 297–344, JAI Press, 1993.

[6] P. K. Varshney. *Distributed Detection and Data Fusion*. Springer-Verlag, 1997.

[7] J. Marschak and R. Radner. *The Economic Theory of Teams*. Yale University Press, 1972.

[8] O. P. Kreidl and A. S. Willsky. Posterior assignment in directed graphical models with minimal online communication. Available: http://web.mit.edu/opk/www/res.html

[9] D. P. Bertsekas. *Nonlinear Programming*. Athena Scientific, 1995.

[10] S. Kakade, et al. Correlated equilibria in graphical games. *ACM-CEC*, pp. 42–47, 2003.

[11] J. Lafferty, et al. Conditional random fields: Probabilistic models for segmenting and labeling sequence data. *ICML*, 2001.

[12] X. Nguyen, et al. Decentralized detection and classification using kernel methods. *ICML*, 2004.

Generalization in Clustering with Unobserved Features

Eyal Krupka and **Naftali Tishby**
School of Computer Science and Engineering,
Interdisciplinary Center for Neural Computation
The Hebrew University Jerusalem, 91904, Israel
{eyalkr,tishby}@cs.huji.ac.il

Abstract

We argue that when objects are characterized by many attributes, clustering them on the basis of a relatively small *random* subset of these attributes can capture information on the unobserved attributes as well. Moreover, we show that under mild technical conditions, clustering the objects on the basis of such a random subset performs almost as well as clustering with the full attribute set. We prove a finite sample generalization theorems for this novel learning scheme that extends analogous results from the supervised learning setting. The scheme is demonstrated for collaborative filtering of users with movies rating as attributes.

1 Introduction

Data clustering is unsupervised classification of objects into groups based on their similarity [1]. Often, it is desirable to have the clusters to match some labels that are unknown to the clustering algorithm. In this context, a good data clustering is expected to have homogeneous labels in each cluster, under some constraints on the number or complexity of the clusters. This can be quantified by mutual information (see e.g. [2]) between the objects' cluster identity and their (unknown) labels, for a given complexity of clusters. Since the clustering algorithm has no access to the labels, it is unclear how the algorithm can optimize the quality of the clustering. Even worse, the clustering quality depends on the specific choice of the unobserved labels. For example a good documents clustering with respect to topics is very different from a clustering with respect to authors.

In our setting, instead of trying to cluster by some "arbitrary" labels, we try to predict unobserved features from observed ones. In this sense our target "labels" are yet other features that "happened" to be unobserved. For example, when clustering fruits based on their observed features, such as shape, color and size, the target of clustering is to match unobserved features, such as nutritional value and toxicity.

In order to theoretically analyze and quantify this new learning scheme, we make the following assumptions. Consider an infinite set of features, and assume that we observe only a *random* subset of n features, called *observed features*. The other features are called *unobserved features*. We assume that the random selection of features is done uniformly and independently.

Table 1: Analogy with supervised learning

Training set	n randomly selected features (observed features)
Test set	Unobserved features
Learning algorithm	Cluster the *instances* into k clusters
Hypothesis class	All possible partitions of m instances into k clusters
Min generalization error	Max expected information on *unobserved* features
ERM	Observed Information Maximization (OIM)
Good generalization	Mean *observed* and *unobserved* information are similar

The clustering algorithm has access only to the observed features of m instances. After the clustering, one of the *unobserved* features is randomly and uniformly selected to be a target label, i.e. clustering performance is measured with respect to this feature. Obviously, the clustering algorithm cannot be directly optimized for this specific feature.

The question is whether we can optimize the *expected* performance on the unobserved feature, based on the observed features alone. The expectation is over the *random* selection of the target feature. In other words, can we find clusters that match as many unobserved features as possible? Perhaps surprisingly, for large enough number of observed features, the answer is yes. We show that for any clustering algorithm, the average performance of the clustering with respect to the observed and unobserved features, is similar. Hence we can indirectly optimize clustering performance with respect to the unobserved features, in analogy to generalization in supervised learning. These results are universal and do not require any additional assumptions such as underling model or a distribution that created the instances.

In order to quantify these results, we define two terms: the average observed information and the expected unobserved information. Let T be the variable which represents the cluster for each instance, and $\{X_1, ..., X_\infty\}$ the set of random variables which denotes the features. The average observed information, denoted by I_{ob}, is the average mutual information between T and each of the observed features. In other words, if the observed features are $\{X_1, ..., X_n\}$ then $I_{ob} = \frac{1}{n}\sum_{j=1}^{n} I(T; X_j)$. The expected unobserved information, denoted by I_{un}, is the *expected* value of the mutual information between T and a *randomly* selected unobserved feature, i.e. $E_j\{I(T; X_j)\}$. Note that whereas I_{ob} can be measured directly, this paper deals with the question of how to infer and maximize I_{un}.

Our main results consist of two theorems. The first is a generalization theorem. It gives an upper bound on the probability of large difference between I_{ob} and I_{un} for all possible clusterings. It also states a *uniform convergence in probability* of $|I_{ob} - I_{un}|$ as the number of observed features increases. Conceptually, the observed mean information, I_{ob}, is analogous to the training error in standard supervised learning [3], whereas the unobserved information, I_{un}, is similar to the generalization error.

The second theorem states that under constraint on the number of clusters, and large enough number of observed features, one can achieve nearly the best possible performance, in terms of I_{un}. Analogous to the principle of Empirical Risk Minimization (ERM) in statistical learning theory [3], this is done by maximizing I_{ob}.

Table 1 summarizes the correspondence of our setting to that of supervised learning. The key difference is that in supervised learning, the set of features is fixed and the training instances (samples) are assumed to be randomly drawn from some distribution. In our setting, the set of instances is fixed, but the set of observed features is assumed to be randomly selected.

Our new theorems are evaluated empirically in section 3, on a data set of movie ratings.

This empirical test also suggests one future research direction: use the framework suggested in this paper for collaborative filtering. Our main point in this paper, however, is the new conceptual framework and not a specific algorithm or experimental performance.

Related work The idea of an information tradeoff between complexity and information on target variables is similar to the idea of the information bottleneck [4]. But unlike the bottleneck method, here we are trying to maximize information on *unobserved* variables, using finite samples.

In the framework of learning with labeled and unlabeled data [5], a fundamental issue is the link between the marginal distribution $P(\mathbf{x})$ over examples $\mathbf{x}$ and the conditional $P(y|\mathbf{x})$ for the label y [6]. From this point of view our approach assumes that y is a feature in itself.

2 Mathematical Formulation and Analysis

Consider a set of discrete random variables $\{X_1, ..., X_L\}$, where L is very large ($L \rightarrow \infty$). We randomly, uniformly and independently select $n << \sqrt{L}$ variables from this set. These variables are the observed features and their indexes are denoted by $\{q_1, ..., q_n\}$. The remaining $L - n$ variables are the *unobserved features*. A clustering algorithm has access only to the *observed* features over m instances $\{\mathbf{x}[1], ..., \mathbf{x}[m]\}$. The algorithm assigns a cluster label $t_i \in \{1, ..., k\}$ for each instance $\mathbf{x}[i]$, where k is the number of clusters. Let T denote the cluster label assigned by the algorithm.

Shannon's mutual information between two variables is a function of their joint distribution, defined as $I(T; X_j) = \sum_{t, x_j} P(t, x_j) \log \left(\frac{P(t, x_j)}{P(t) P(x_j)} \right)$. Since we are dealing with a finite number of samples, m, the distribution P is taken as the *empirical* joint distribution of (T, X_j), for every j. For a random j, this empirical mutual information is a random variable on its own.

The average observed information, I_{ob}, is now defined as $I_{ob} = \frac{1}{n} \sum_{i=1}^{n} I(T; X_{q_i})$. In general, I_{ob} is higher when clusters are more coherent, i.e. elements within each cluster have many similar attributes. The expected unobserved information, I_{un}, is defined as $I_{un} = E_j \{I(T; X_j)\}$. We can assume that the unobserved feature is with high probability from the unobserved set. Equivalently, I_{un} can be the mean mutual information between the clusters and each of the unobserved features, $I_{un} = \frac{1}{L-n} \sum_{j \notin \{q_1, ..., q_n\}} I(T; X_j)$.

The goal of the clustering algorithm is to find cluster labels $\{t_1, ..., t_m\}$, that maximize I_{un}, subject to a constraint on their complexity - henceforth considered as the number of clusters ($k \leq D$) for simplicity, where D is an integer bound.

Before discussing how to maximize I_{un}, we consider first the problem of estimating it. Similar to the generalization error in supervised learning, I_{un} cannot be estimated directly in the learning algorithm, but we may be able to bound the difference between the observed information I_{ob} - our "training error" - and I_{un} - the "generalization error". To obtain generalization this bound should be *uniform over all possible clusterings* with a high probability over the randomly selected features. The following lemma argues that such *uniform convergence in probability* of I_{ob} to I_{un} always occurs.

Lemma 1 *With the definitions above,*

$$\Pr \left\{ \sup_{\{t_1, ..., t_m\}} |I_{ob} - I_{un}| > \epsilon \right\} \leq 2e^{-2n\epsilon^2/(\log k)^2 + m \log k} \quad \forall \epsilon > 0$$

where the probability is over the random selection of the observed features.

Proof: For fixed cluster labels, $\{t_1, ..., t_m\}$, and a random feature j, the mutual information $I(T; X_j)$ is a function of the random variable j, and hence $I(T; X_j)$ is a random variable in itself. I_{ob} is the average of n such independent random variables and I_{un} is its expected value. Clearly, for all j, $0 \leq I(T; X_j) \leq \log k$. Using Hoeffding's inequality [7], $\Pr\{|I_{ob} - I_{un}| > \epsilon\} \leq 2e^{-2n\epsilon^2/(\log k)^2}$. Since there are at most k^m possible partitions, the union bound is sufficient to prove the lemma 1. $\square$

Note that for any $\epsilon > 0$, the probability that $|I_{ob} - I_{un}| > \epsilon$ goes to zero, as $n \to \infty$. The convergence rate of I_{ob} to I_{un} is bounded by $O(\log n/\sqrt{n})$. As expected, this upper bound decreases as the number of clusters, k, decreases.

Unlike the standard bounds in supervised learning, this bound increases with the number of instances (m), and decreases with increasing number of observed features (n). This is because in our scheme the training size is not the number of instances, but rather the number of observed features (See Table 1). However, in the next theorem we obtain an upper bound that is independent of m, and hence is tighter for large m.

Theorem 1 *(Generalization Theorem) With the definitions above,*

$$\Pr\left\{\sup_{\{t_1,...,t_m\}} |I_{ob} - I_{un}| > \epsilon\right\} \leq 8(\log k)e^{-\frac{n\epsilon^2}{8(\log k)^2} + \frac{4k \max_j |\mathcal{X}_j|}{\epsilon} \log k - \log \epsilon} \quad \forall \epsilon > 0$$

where $|\mathcal{X}_j|$ denotes the alphabet size of X_j (i.e. the number of different values it can obtain). Again, the probability is over the random selection of the observed features.

The convergence rate here is bounded by $O(\log n/^3\sqrt{n})$. However, for relatively large n one can use the bound in lemma 1, which converge faster.

A detailed proof of theorem 1 can be found in [8]. Here we provide the outline of the proof.

Proof outline: From the given m instances and any given cluster labels $\{t_1, ..., t_m\}$, draw uniformly and independently m' instances (repeats allowed) and denote their indexes by $\{i_1, ..., i_{m'}\}$. We can estimate $I(T; X_j)$ from the empirical distribution of (T, X_j) over the m' instances. This distribution is denoted by $\hat{P}(t, x_j)$ and the corresponding mutual information is denoted by $I_{\hat{P}}(T; X_j)$. Theorem 1 is build up from the following upper bounds, which are independent of m, but depend on the choice of m'. The first bound is on $E\{|I(T; X_j) - I_{\hat{P}}(T; X_j)|\}$, where the expectation is over random selection of the m' instances. From this bound we derive upper bounds on $|I_{ob} - E(\hat{I}_{ob})|$ and $|I_{un} - E(\hat{I}_{un})|$, where $\hat{I}_{ob}$, $\hat{I}_{un}$ are the estimated values of I_{ob}, I_{un} based on the subset of m' instances. The last required bound is on the probability that $\sup_{\{t_1,...,t_m\}} |E(\hat{I}_{ob}) - E(\hat{I}_{un})| > \epsilon_1$, for any $\epsilon_1 > 0$. This bound is obtained from lemma 1. The choice of m' is independent on m. Its value should be large enough for the estimations $\hat{I}_{ob}$, $\hat{I}_{un}$ to be accurate, but not too large, so as to limit the number of possible clusterings over the m' instances.

We now describe the above mentioned upper bounds in more details. Using Paninski [9] (proposition 1) it is easy to show that the bias between $I(T; X_j)$ and its maximum likelihood estimation, based on $\hat{P}(t, x_j)$ is bounded as follows.

$$E_{\{i_1,...,i_{m'}\}}\left\{|I(T; X_j) - I_{\hat{P}}(T; X_j)|\right\} \leq \log\left(1 + \frac{k|\mathcal{X}_j| - 1}{m'}\right) \leq \frac{k|\mathcal{X}_j|}{m'} \quad (1)$$

From this equation we obtain,

$$|I_{ob} - E_{\{i_1,...,i_{m'}\}}(\hat{I}_{ob})|, \ |I_{un} - E_{\{i_1,...,i_{m'}\}}(\hat{I}_{un})| \leq k \max_j |\mathcal{X}_j|/m' \quad (2)$$

Using lemma 1 we have an upper bound on the probability that $\sup_{\{t_1,\ldots,t_m\}}|\hat{I}_{ob}-\hat{I}_{un}|>\epsilon$ over the random selection of *features*, as a function of m'. However, the upper bound we need is on the probability that $\sup_{\{t_1,\ldots,t_m\}}|E(\hat{I}_{ob})-E(\hat{I}_{un})|>\epsilon_1$. Note that the expectations $E(\hat{I}_{ob})$, $E(\hat{I}_{un})$ are done over random selection of the subset of m' *instances*, for a set of features that were randomly selected *once*. In order to link between these two probabilities, we need the following lemma.

Lemma 2 *Consider a function f of two independent random variables (Y,Z). We assume that $f(y,z)\le c$, $\forall y,z$, where c is some constant. If $\Pr\{f(Y,Z)>\tilde{\epsilon}\}\le\delta$, then*

$$\Pr_Z\{E_y\left(f(y,Z)\right)\ge\epsilon\}\le\frac{c-\tilde{\epsilon}}{\epsilon-\tilde{\epsilon}}\delta\quad\forall\epsilon>\tilde{\epsilon}$$

The proof of this lemma is rather standard and is given in [8]. From lemmas 1 and 2 it is easy to show that

$$\Pr\left\{E_{\{i_1,\ldots,i_{m'}\}}\left(\sup_{\{t_1,\ldots,t_m\}}\left|\hat{I}_{ob}-\hat{I}_{un}\right|\right)>\epsilon_1\right\}\le\frac{4\log k}{\epsilon_1}e^{-\frac{n\epsilon_1^2}{2(\log k)^2}+m'\log k}\quad(3)$$

Lemma 2 is used, where Z represents the random selection of features, Y represents the random selection of m' instances, $f(y,z)=\sup_{\{t_1,\ldots,t_m\}}|\hat{I}_{ob}-\hat{I}_{un}|$, $c=\log k$, and $\tilde{\epsilon}=\epsilon_1/2$. From eq. 2 and 3 it can be shown that

$$\Pr\left\{\sup_{\{t_1,\ldots,t_m\}}|I_{ob}-I_{un}|>\epsilon_1+\frac{2k\max_j|\mathcal{X}_j|}{m'}\right\}\le\frac{4\log k}{\epsilon_1}e^{-\frac{n\epsilon_1^2}{2(\log k)^2}+m'\log k}$$

By selecting $\epsilon_1=\epsilon/2$, $m'=4k\max_j|\mathcal{X}_j|/\epsilon$, we obtain theorem 1. $\qquad\square$

Note that the selection of m' depends on $k\max_j|\mathcal{X}_j|$. This reflects the fact that in order to accurately estimate $I(T,X_j)$, we need a number of instances, m', which is much larger than the product of the alphabet sizes of T, X_j.

We can now return to the problem of specifying a clustering that maximizes I_{un}, using only the observed features. For a reference, we will first define I_{un} of the best possible clusters.

Definition 1 *Maximally achievable unobserved information: Let $I_{un,D}^*$ be the maximum value of I_{un} that can be achieved by any clustering $\{t_1,\ldots,t_m\}$, subject to the constraint $k\le D$, for some constant D*

$$I_{un,D}^*=\sup_{\{\{t_1,\ldots,t_m\}:k\le D\}}I_{un}$$

*The clustering that achieves this value is called **the best clustering**. The average observed information of this clustering is denoted by $I_{ob,D}^*$.*

Definition 2 *Observed information maximization algorithm: Let **IobMax** be any clustering algorithm that, based on the values of observed features alone, selects the cluster labels $\{t_1,\ldots,t_m\}$ having the maximum possible value of I_{ob}, subject to the constraint $k\le D$.*

Let $\tilde{I}_{ob,D}$ be the average observed information achieved by IobMax algorithm. Let $\tilde{I}_{un,D}$ be the expected unobserved information achieved by the IobMax algorithm.

The next theorem states that *IobMax* not only maximizes I_{ob}, but also I_{un}.

Theorem 2 *With the definitions above,*

$$\Pr\left\{\tilde{I}_{un,D} \le I^*_{un,D} - \epsilon\right\} \le 8(\log k)e^{-\frac{n\epsilon^2}{32(\log k)^2} + \frac{8k\max_j |\mathcal{X}_j|}{\epsilon}\log k - \log(\epsilon/2)} \quad \forall \epsilon > 0 \quad (4)$$

where the probability is over the random selection of the observed features.

Proof: We now define a *bad clustering* as a clustering whose expected unobserved information satisfies $I_{un} \le I^*_{un,D} - \epsilon$. Using Theorem 1, the probability that $|I_{ob} - I_{un}| > \epsilon/2$ for any of the clusterings is upper bounded by the right term of equation 4. If for all clusterings $|I_{ob} - I_{un}| \le \epsilon/2$, then surely $I^*_{ob,D} \ge I^*_{un,D} - \epsilon/2$ (see Definition 1) and I_{ob} of all bad clusterings satisfies $I_{ob} \le I^*_{un,D} - \epsilon/2$. Hence the probability that a bad clustering has a higher average observed information than the best clustering is upper bounded as in Theorem 2. □

As a result of this theorem, when n is large enough, even an algorithm that knows the value of *all* the features (observed and unobserved) cannot find a clustering with the same complexity (k) which is significantly better than the clustering found by $IobMax$ algorithm.

3 Empirical Evaluation

In this section we describe an experimental evaluation of the generalization properties of the *IobMax* algorithm for a finite large number of features. We examine the difference between I_{ob} and I_{un} as function of the number of observed features and the number of clusters used. We also compare the value of I_{un} achieved by *IobMax* algorithm to the maximum achievable $I^*_{un,D}$ (See definition 1).

Our evaluation uses a data set typically used for collaborative filtering. Collaborative filtering refers to methods of making predictions about a user's preferences, by collecting preferences of many users. For example, collaborative filtering for movie ratings could make predictions about rating of movies by a user, given a partial list of ratings from this user and many other users. Clustering methods are used for collaborative filtering by cluster users based on the similarity of their ratings (see e.g. [10]).

In our setting, each user is described as a vector of movie ratings. The rating of each movie is regarded as a feature. We cluster users based on the set of observed features, i.e. rated movies. In our context, the goal of the clustering is to maximize the information between the clusters and unobserved features, i.e. movies that have not yet been rated by any of the users. By Theorem 2, given large enough number of rated movies, we can achieve the best possible clustering of users with respect to unseen movies. In this region, no additional information (such as user age, taste, rating of more movies) beyond the observed features can improve I_{un} by more than some small ϵ.

The purpose of this section is *not* to suggest a new algorithm for collaborative filtering or compare it to other methods, but simply to illustrate our new theorems on empirical data.

Dataset. We used MovieLens (www.movielens.umn.edu), which is a movie rating data set. It was collected distributed by GroupLens Research at the University of Minnesota. It contains approximately 1 million ratings for 3900 movies by 6040 users. Ratings are on a scale of 1 to 5. We used only a subset consisting of 2400 movies by 4000 users. In our setting, each instance is a vector of ratings $(x_1, ..., x_{2400})$ by specific user. Each movie is viewed as a feature, where the rating is the value of the feature.

Experimental Setup. We randomly split the 2400 movies into two groups, denoted by "A" and "B", of 1200 movies (features) each. We used a subset of the movies from group "A" as observed features and all movies from group "B" as the unobserved features. The experiment was repeated with 10 random splits and the results averaged. We estimated I_{un} by the mean information between the clusters and ratings of movies from group "B".

688

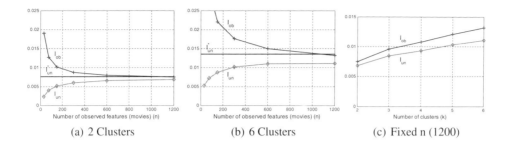

| (a) 2 Clusters | (b) 6 Clusters | (c) Fixed n (1200) |

Figure 1: I_{ob}, I_{un} and I_{un}^* per number of training movies and clusters. In (a) and (b) the number of movies is variable, and the number of clusters is fixed. In (c) The number of observed movies is fixed (1200), and the number of clusters is variable. The overall mean information is low, since the rating matrix is sparse.

Handling Missing Values. In this data set, most of the values are missing (not rated). We handle this by defining the feature variable as 1,2,...,5 for the ratings and 0 for missing value. We maximize the mutual information based on the empirical distribution of values that are present, and weight it by the probability of presence for this feature. Hence, $I_{ob} = \sum_{j=1}^{n} P(X_j \neq 0) I(T; X_j | X_j \neq 0)$ and $I_{un} = E_j \{P(X_j \neq 0) I(T; X_j | X_j \neq 0)\}$. The weighting prevents 'overfitting' to movies with few ratings. Since the observed features were selected at random, the statistics of missing values of the observed and unobserved features are the same. Hence, all theorems are applicable to these definitions of I_{ob} and I_{un} as well.

Greedy *IobMax* Algorithm

We cluster the users using a simple greedy clustering algorithm . The input to the algorithm is all users, represented solely by the observed features. Since this algorithm can only find a local maximum of I_{ob}, we ran the algorithm 10 times (each used a different random initialization) and selected the results that had a maximum value of I_{ob}. More details about this algorithm can be found in [8].

In order to estimate $I_{un,D}^*$ (see definition 1), we also ran the same algorithm, where all the features are available to the algorithm (i.e. also features from group "B"). The algorithm finds clusters that maximize the mean mutual information on features from group "B".

Results

The results are shown in Figure 1. As n increases, I_{ob} decreases and I_{un} increases, until they converge to each other. For small n, the clustering 'overfits' to the observed features. This is similar to training and test errors in supervised learning. For large n, I_{un} approaches to $I_{un,D}^*$, which means the $IobMax$ algorithm found nearly the best possible clustering - as expected from the theorem 2. As the number of clusters increases, both I_{ob} and I_{un} increase, but the difference between them also increases.

4 Discussion and Summary

We introduce a new learning paradigm: clustering based on observed features that generalizes to unobserved features. Our results are summarized by two theorems that tell us how, without knowing the value of the unobserved features, one can estimate and maximize information between the clusters and the unobserved features.

The key assumption that enables us to prove the theorems is the *random independent* selection of the observed features. Another interpretation of the generalization theorem, without using this assumption, might be combinatorial. The difference between the observed and unobserved information is large only for a small portion of all possible partitions into observed and unobserved features. This means that almost any arbitrary partition generalizes well.

The importance of clustering which preserves information on unobserved features is that it enables us to learn new - previously unobserved - attributes from a small number of examples. Suppose that after clustering fruits based on their observed features, we eat a chinaberry[1] and thus, we "observe" (by getting sick), the previously unobserved attribute of toxicity. Assuming that in each cluster, all fruits have similar unobserved attributes, we can conclude that all fruits in the same cluster, i.e. all chinaberries, are likely to be poisonous.

We can even relate the *IobMax* principle to cognitive clustering in sensory information processing. In general, a symbolic representation (e.g. assigning object names in language) may be based on a similar principle - find a representation (clusters) that contain significant information on as many observed features as possible, while still remaining simple. Such representations are expected to contain information on other rarely viewed salient features.

Acknowledgments

We thank Amir Globerson, Ran Bachrach, Amir Navot, Oren Shriki, Avner Dor and Ilan Sutskover for helpful discussions. We also thank the GroupLens Research Group at the University of Minnesota for use of the MovieLens data set. Our work is partly supported by grant from the Israeli Academy of Science.

References

[1] A. K. Jain, M. N. Murty, and P. J. Flynn. Data clustering: a review. *ACM Computing Surveys*, 31(3):264–323, September 1999.

[2] T. M. Cover and J. A. Thomas. *Elements Of Information Theory*. Wiley Interscience, 1991.

[3] V. N. Vapnik. *Statistical Learning Theory*. Wiley, 1998.

[4] N. Tishby, F. Pereira, and W. Bialek. The information bottleneck method. *Proc. 37th Allerton Conf. on Communication and Computation*, 1999.

[5] M. Seeger. Learning with labeled and unlabeled data. Technical report, University of Edinburgh, 2002.

[6] M. Szummer and T. Jaakkola. Information regularization with partially labeled data. In *NIPS*, 2003.

[7] W. Hoeffding. Probability inequalities for sums of bounded random variables. *Journal of the American Statistical Association*, 58:13–30, 1963.

[8] E. Krupka and N. Tishby. Generalization in clustering with unobserved features. Technical report, Hebrew University, 2005. http://www.cs.huji.ac.il/~tishby/nips2005tr.pdf.

[9] L. Paninski. Estimation of entropy and mutual information. *Neural Computation*, 15:1101–1253, 2003.

[10] B. Marlin. Collaborative filtering: A machine learning perspective. Master's thesis, University of Toronto, 2004.

---

[1]Chinaberries are the fruits of the Melia azedarach tree, and are poisonous.

Variable KD-Tree Algorithms for Spatial Pattern Search and Discovery

Jeremy Kubica
Robotics Institute
Carnegie Mellon University
Pittsburgh, PA 15213
jkubica@ri.cmu.edu

Joseph Masiero
Institute for Astronomy
University of Hawaii
Honolulu, HI 96822
masiero@ifa.hawaii.edu

Andrew Moore
Robotics Institute
Carnegie Mellon University
Pittsburgh, PA 15213
awm@cs.cmu.edu

Robert Jedicke
Institute for Astronomy
University of Hawaii
Honolulu, HI 96822
jedicke@ifa.hawaii.edu

Andrew Connolly
Physics & Astronomy Department
University of Pittsburgh
Pittsburgh, PA 15213
ajc@phyast.pitt.edu

Abstract

In this paper we consider the problem of finding sets of points that conform to a given underlying model from within a dense, noisy set of observations. This problem is motivated by the task of efficiently linking faint asteroid detections, but is applicable to a range of spatial queries. We survey current tree-based approaches, showing a trade-off exists between single tree and multiple tree algorithms. To this end, we present a new type of multiple tree algorithm that uses a variable number of trees to exploit the advantages of both approaches. We empirically show that this algorithm performs well using both simulated and astronomical data.

1 Introduction

Consider the problem of detecting faint asteroids from a series of images collected on a single night. Inherently, the problem is simply one of connect-the-dots. Over a single night we can treat the asteroid's motion as linear, so we want to find detections that, up to observational errors, lie along a line. However, as we consider very faint objects, several difficulties arise. First, objects near our brightness threshold may oscillate around this threshold, blinking into and out-of our images and providing only a small number of actual detections. Second, as we lower our detection threshold we will begin to pick up more spurious noise points. As we look for really dim objects, the number of noise points increases greatly and swamps the number of detections of real objects.

The above problem is one example of a model based spatial search. The goal is to identify sets of points that fit some given underlying model. This general task encompasses a wide range of real-world problems and spatial models. For example, we may want to detect a specific configuration of corner points in an image or search for multi-way structure in scientific data. We focus our discussion on problems that have a high density of both true

691

and noise points, but which may have only a few points actually from the model of interest. Returning to the asteroid linking example, this corresponds to finding a handful of points that lie along a line within a data set of millions of detections.

Below we survey several tree-based approaches for efficiently solving this problem. We show that both single tree and conventional multiple tree algorithms can be inefficient and that a trade-off exists between these approaches. To this end, we propose a new type of multiple tree algorithm that uses a *variable* number of tree nodes. We empirically show that this new algorithm performs well using both simulated and real-world data.

2 Problem Definition

Our problem consists of finding sets of points that fit a given underlying spatial model. In doing so, we are effectively looking for known types of structure buried within the data. In general, we are interested in finding sets with k or more points, thus providing a sufficient amount of support to confirm the discovery. Finding this structure within the data may either be our end goal, such as in asteroid linkage, or may just be a preprocessor for a more sophisticated statistical test, such as renewal strings [1]. We are particularly interested in high-density, low-support domains where there may be many hundreds of thousands of points, but only a handful actually support our model.

Formally, the data consists of N unique D-dimensional points. We assume that the underlying model can be estimated from c unique points. Since $k \geq c$, the model may over-constrained. In these cases we divide the points into two sets: *Model Points* and *Support Points*. Model points are the c points used to fully define the underlying model. Support points are the remaining points used to confirm the model. For example, if we are searching for sets of k linear points, we could use a set's endpoints as model points and treat the middle $k - 2$ as support points. Or we could allow any two points to serve as model points, providing an exhaustive variant of the RANSAC algorithm [2].

The prototypical example used in this paper is the (linear) asteroid linkage problem:

> For each pair of points find the $k - 2$ best support points for the line that they define (such that we use at most one point at each time step).

In addition, we place restrictions on the validity of the initial pairs by providing velocity bounds. It is important to note that although we use this problem as a running example, the techniques described can be applied to a range of spatial problems.

3 Overview of Previous Approaches

3.1 Constructive Algorithms

Constructive algorithms "build up" valid sets of points by repeatedly finding additional points that are compatible with the current set. Perhaps the simplest approach is to perform a two-tiered *brute force* search. First, we exhaustively test all sets of c points to determine if they define a valid model. Then, for each valid set we test all of the remaining points for support. For example in the asteroid linkage problem, we can initially search over all $O(N^2)$ pairs of points and for each of the resulting lines test all $O(N)$ points to determine if they support that line. A similar approach within the domain of target tracking is sequential tracking (for a good introduction see [3]), where points at early time steps are used to estimate a track that is then projected to later time steps to find additional support points.

In large-scale domains, these approaches can often be made tractable by using spatial structure in the data. Again returning to our asteroid example, we can place the points in a

KD-tree [4]. We can then limit the number of initial pairs examined by using this tree to find points compatible with our velocity constraints. Further, we can use the KD-tree to only search for support points in localized regions around the line, ignoring large numbers of obviously infeasible points. Similarly, trees have been used in tracking algorithms to efficiently find points near predicted track positions [5]. We call these adaptations *single tree* algorithms, because at any given time the algorithm is searching at most one tree.

3.2 Parameter Space Methods

Another approach is to search for valid sets of points by searching the model's parameter space, such as in the Hough transform [6]. The idea behind these approaches is that we can test whether each point is compatible with a small set of model parameters, allowing us to search parameter space to find the valid sets. However, this method can be expensive in terms of both computation and memory, especially for high dimensional parameter spaces. Further, if the model's total support is low, the true model occurrences may be effectively washed out by the noise. For these reasons we do not consider parameter space methods.

3.3 Multiple Tree Algorithms

The primary benefit of tree-based algorithms is that they are able to use spatial structure within the data to limit the cost of the search. However, there is a clear potential to push further and use structure from multiple aspects of the search *at the same time*. In doing so we can hopefully avoid many of the dead ends and wrong turns that may result from exploring bad initial associations in the first few points in our model. For example, in the domain of asteroid linkage we may be able to limit the number of short, initial associations that we have to consider by using information from later time steps. This idea forms the basis of multiple tree search algorithms [7, 8, 9].

Multiple tree methods explicitly search for the entire set of points at once by searching over *combinations* of tree nodes. In standard single tree algorithms, the search tries to find individual points satisfying some criteria (e.g. the next point to add) and the search state is represented by a single node that *could* contain such a point. In contrast, multiple tree algorithms represent the current search state with multiple tree nodes that *could* contain points that together conform to the model. Initially, the algorithm begins with k root nodes from either the same or different tree data structures, representing the k different points that must be found. At each step in the search, it narrows in on a set of mutually compatible spatial regions and thus a set of individual points that fit the model by picking one of the model nodes and recursively exploring its children. As with a standard "single tree" search, we constantly check for opportunities to prune the search.

There are several important drawbacks to multiple tree algorithms. First, additional trees introduce a higher branching factor in the search and increase the potential for taking deep "wrong turns." Second, care must be taken in order to deal with missing or a variable number of support points. Kubica *et. al.* discuss the use of an additional "missing" tree node to handle these cases [9]. However, this approach can effectively make repeated searches over subsets of trees, making it more expensive both in theory and practice.

4 Variable Tree Algorithms

In general we would like to exploit structural information from all aspects of our search problem, but do so while branching the search on just the parameters of interest. To this end we propose a new type of search that uses a *variable* number of tree nodes. Like a standard multiple tree algorithm, the variable tree algorithm searches combinations of tree nodes to find valid sets of points. However, we limit this search to just those points required

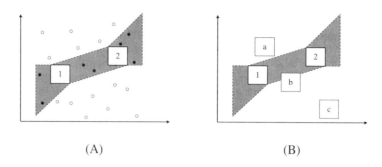

(A)   (B)

Figure 1: The model nodes' bounds (1 and 2) define a region of feasible support (shaded) for *any* combination of model points from those nodes (A). As shown in (B), we can classify entire support tree nodes as feasible (node b) or infeasible (nodes a and c).

to define, and thus bound, the models currently under consideration. Specifically, we use M model tree nodes,[1] which guide the recursion and thus the search. In addition, throughout the search we maintain information about other potential *supporting* points that can be used to confirm the final track or prune the search due to a lack of support.

For example in the asteroid linking problem each line is defined by only 2 points, thus we can efficiently search through the models using a multiple tree search with 2 *model trees*. As shown in Figure 1.A, the spatial bounds of our current model nodes immediately limit the set of feasible support points for *all* line segments compatible with these nodes. If we track which support points are feasible, we can use this information to prune the search due to a lack of support for *any* model defined by the points in those nodes.

The key idea behind the variable tree search is that we can use a *dynamic* representation of the potential support. Specifically, we can place the support points in trees and maintain a dynamic *list* of currently valid support nodes. As shown in Figure 1.B, by only testing entire nodes (instead of individual points), we are using spatial coherence of the support points to remove the expense of testing each support point at each step in the search. And by maintaining a list of support tree nodes, we are no longer branching the search over these trees. Thus we remove the need to make a hard "left or right" decision. Further, using a combination of a list and a tree for our representation allows us to refine our support representation on the fly. If we reach a point in the search where a support node is no longer valid, we can simply drop it off the list. And if we reach a point where a support node provides too coarse a representation of the current support space, we can simply remove it and add both of its children to the list.

This leaves the question of when to split support nodes. If we split them too soon, we may end up with many support nodes in our list and mitigate the benefits of the nodes' spatial coherence. If we wait too long to split them, then we may have a few large support nodes that cannot efficiently be pruned. Although we are still investigating splitting strategies, the experiments in this paper use a heuristic that seeks to provide a small number of support nodes that are a reasonable fit to the feasible region. We effectively split a support node if doing so would allow one of its two children to be pruned. For KD-trees this roughly means checking whether the split value lies outside the feasible region.

The full variable tree algorithm is given in Figure 2. A simple example of finding *linear* tracks while using the track's endpoints (earliest and latest in time) as model points and

---

[1]Typically $M = c$, although in some cases it may be beneficial to use a different number of model nodes.

	Variable Tree Model Detection
	Input: A set of M current model tree nodes $\mathbf{M}$
	A set of current support tree nodes $\mathbf{S}$
	Output: A list $\mathbf{Z}$ of feasible sets of points
1.	$\mathbf{S}' \leftarrow \{\}$ and $\mathbf{S}_{curr} \leftarrow \mathbf{S}$
2.	IF we cannot prune based on the mutual compatibility of $\mathbf{M}$:
3.	FOR each $\mathbf{s} \in \mathbf{S}_{curr}$
4.	IF $\mathbf{s}$ is compatible with $\mathbf{M}$:
5.	IF $\mathbf{s}$ is "too wide":
6.	Add $\mathbf{s}$'s left and right child to the end of $\mathbf{S}_{curr}$.
7.	ELSE
8.	Add $\mathbf{s}$ to $\mathbf{S}'$.
9.	IF we have enough valid support points:
10.	IF all of $\mathbf{m} \in \mathbf{M}$ are leaves:
11.	Test all combinations of points owned by the model nodes, using the support nodes' points as potential support. Add valid sets to $\mathbf{Z}$.
12.	ELSE
13.	Let $\mathbf{m}^*$ be the non-leaf model tree node that owns the most points.
14.	Search using $\mathbf{m}^*$'s left child in place of $\mathbf{m}^*$ and $\mathbf{S}'$ instead of $\mathbf{S}$.
15.	Search using $\mathbf{m}^*$'s right child in place of $\mathbf{m}^*$ and $\mathbf{S}'$ instead of $\mathbf{S}$.

Figure 2: A simple variable tree algorithm for spatial structure search. This algorithm shown uses simple heuristics such as: searching the model node with the most points and splitting a support node if it is too wide. These heuristics can be replaced by more accurate, problem-specific ones.

using all other points for support is illustrated in Figure 3. The first column shows all the tree nodes that are currently part of the search. The second and third columns show the search's position on the two model trees and the current set of valid support nodes respectively. Unlike the pure multiple tree search, the variable tree search does not "branch off" on the support trees, allowing us to consider multiple support nodes from the same time step at any point in the search. Again, it is important to note that by testing the support points as we search, we are both incorporating support information into the pruning decisions and "pruning" the support points for entire sets of models at once.

5 Results on the Asteroid Linking Domain

The goal of the single-night asteroid linkage problem is to find sets of 2-dimensional point detections that correspond to a roughly linear motion model. In the below experiments we are interested in finding sets of at least 7 detections from a sequence of 8 images. The movements were constrained to have a speed between 0.05 and 0.5 degrees per day and were allowed an observational error threshold of 0.0003 degrees. All experiments were run on a dual 2.5 GHz Apple G5 with 4 GB of RAM.

The asteroid detection data consists of detections from 8 images of the night sky separated by half-hour intervals. The images were obtained with the MegaCam instrument on the 3.6-meter Canada-France-Hawaii Telescope. The detections, along with confidence levels, were automatically extracted from the images. We can pre-filter the data to pull out only those observations above a given confidence threshold σ. This allows us to examine how the algorithms perform as we begin to look for increasingly faint asteroids. It should be noted that only limited preprocessing was done to the data, resulting in a very high level

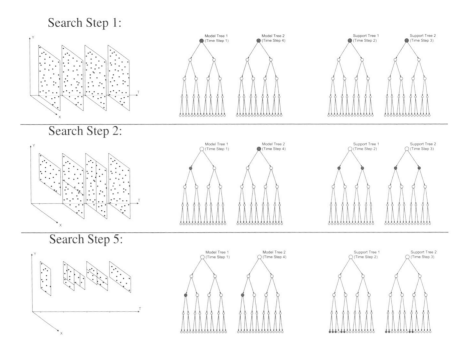

Figure 3: The variable tree algorithm performs a depth first search over the model nodes. At each level of the search the model nodes are checked for mutual compatibility and each support node on the list is check for compatibility with the *set* of model nodes. Since we are not branching on the support nodes, we can split a support node and add *both* children to our list. This figure shows the current model and support nodes and their spatial regions.

Table 1: The running times (in seconds) for the asteroid linkers with different detection thresholds σ and thus different numbers N and density of observations.

σ	10.0	8.0	6.0	5.0	4.0
N	3531	5818	12911	24068	48646
Single Tree	2	7	61	488	2442
Multiple Tree	1	3	30	607	4306
Variable Tree	< 1	1	4	40	205

of false detections. While future data sets will contain significantly reduced noise, it is interesting to examine the performance of the algorithms on this real-world high noise, high density data.

The results on the intra-night asteroid tracking domain, shown in Table 1, illustrate a clear advantage to using a variable tree approach. As the significance threshold σ decreases, the number and density of detections increases, allowing the support tree nodes to capture feasibility information for a large number of support points. In contrast, neither the full multiple tree algorithm nor the single-tree algorithm performed well. For the multiple tree algorithm, this decrease in performance is likely due to a combination of the high number of time steps, the allowance of a missing observation, and the high density. In particular, the increased density can reduce opportunities for pruning, causing the algorithm to explore deeper before backtracking.

Table 2: Average running times (in seconds) for a 2-dimensional rectangle search with different numbers of points N. The brute force algorithm was only run to $N = 2500$.

N	500	1000	2000	2500	5000	10000	25000	50000
Brute Force	0.37	2.73	21.12	41.03	n/a	n/a	n/a	n/a
Single Tree	0.02	0.07	0.30	0.51	2.15	10.05	66.24	293.10
Multi-Tree	0.01	0.02	0.06	0.09	0.30	1.11	6.61	27.79
Variable-Tree	0.01	0.02	0.05	0.07	0.22	0.80	4.27	16.30

Table 3: Average running times (in seconds) for a rectangle search with different numbers of required corners k. For this experiment $N = 10000$ and $D = 3$.

k	8	7	6	5	4
Single Tree	4.71	4.72	4.71	4.71	4.71
Multi-Tree	3.96	19.45	45.02	67.50	78.81
Variable-Tree	0.65	0.75	0.85	0.92	1.02

6 Experiments on the Simulated Rectangle Domain

We can apply the above techniques to a range of other model-based spatial search problems. In this section we consider a toy template matching problem, finding axis-aligned hyper-rectangles in D-dimensional space by finding k or more *corners* that fit a rectangle. We use this simple, albeit artificial, problem both to demonstrate potential pattern recognition applications and to analyze the algorithms as we vary the properties of the data.

Formally, we restrict the model to use the upper and lower corners as the two model points. Potential support points are those points that fall within some threshold of the other $2^D - 2$ corners. In addition, we restrict the allowable bounds of the rectangles by providing a maximum width.

To evaluate the algorithms' relative performance, we used random data generated from a uniform distribution on a unit hyper-cube. The threshold and maximum width were fixed for all experiments at 0.0001 and 0.2 respectively. All experiments were run on a dual 2.5 GHz Apple G5 with 4 GB of RAM.

The first factor that we examined was how each algorithm scales with the number of points. We generated random data with 5 known rectangles and N additional random points and computed the average wall-clock running time (over ten trials) for each algorithm. The results, shown in Table 2, show a graceful scaling of all of the multiple tree algorithms. In contrast, the brute force and single tree algorithms run into trouble as the number of points becomes moderately large. The variable tree algorithm consistently performs the best, as it is able to avoid significant amounts of redundant computation.

One potential drawback of the full multiple tree algorithm is that since it branches on all points, it may become inefficient as the allowable number of missing support points grows. To test this we looked at 3-dimensional data and varied the minimum number of required support points k. As shown in Table 3, all multiple tree methods become *more* expensive as the number of required support points decreases. This is especially the case for the multi-tree algorithm, which has to perform several almost identical searches to account for missing points. However, the variable-tree algorithm's performance degrades gracefully and is the best for all trials.

7 Conclusions

Tree-based spatial algorithms provide the potential for significant computational savings with multiple tree algorithms providing further opportunities to exploit structure in the data. However, a distinct trade-off exists between ignoring structure from all aspects of the problem and increasing the combinatorics of the search. We presented a variable tree approach that exploits the advantages of both single tree and multiple tree algorithms. A combinatorial search is carried out over just the minimum number of model points, while still tracking the feasibility of the various support points. As shown in the above experiments, this approach provides significant computational savings over both the traditional single tree and and multiple tree searches. Finally, it is interesting to note that the dynamic support technique described in this paper is general and may be applied to a range of other algorithms, such as the Fast Hough Transform [10], that maintain information on which points support a given model.

Acknowledgments

Jeremy Kubica is supported by a grant from the Fannie and John Hertz Foundation. Andrew Moore and Andrew Connolly are supported by a National Science Foundation ITR grant (CCF-0121671).

References

[1] A.J. Storkey, N.C. Hambly, C.K.I. Williams, and R.G. Mann. Renewal Strings for Cleaning Astronomical Databases. In *UAI 19*, 559-566, 2003.

[2] M.A. Fischler and R.C. Bolles. Random Sample Consensus: A Paradigm for Model Fitting with Applications to Image Analysis and Automated Cartography. *Comm. of the ACM*, 24:381–395, 1981.

[3] S. Blackman and R. Popoli. *Design and Analysis of Modern Tracking Systems*. Artech House, 1999.

[4] J.L. Bentley . Multidimensional Binary Search Trees Used for Associative Searching. *Comm. of the ACM*, 18 (9), 1975.

[5] J. K. Uhlmann. Algorithms for multiple-target tracking. *American Scientist*, 80(2):128–141, 1992.

[6] P. V. C. Hough. Machine analysis of bubble chamber pictures. In *International Conference on High Energy Accelerators and Instrumentation*. CERN, 1959.

[7] A. Gray and A. Moore. N-body problems in statistical learning. In T. K. Leen and T. G. Dietterich, editors, *Advances in Neural Information Processing Systems*. MIT Press, 2001.

[8] G. R. Hjaltason and H. Samet. Incremental distance join algorithms for spatial databases. In *Proc. of the 1998 ACM-SIGMOD Conference*, 237–248, 1998.

[9] J. Kubica, A. Moore, A. Connolly, and R. Jedicke. A Multiple Tree Algorithm for the Efficient Association of Asteroid Observations. In *KDD'05*. August 2005.

[10] H. Li, M.A. Lavin, and R.J. Le Master. Fast Hough Transform: A Hierarchical Approach. In *Computer Vision, Graphics, and Image Processing*, 36(2-3):139–161, November 1986.

Assessing Approximations for Gaussian Process Classification

Malte Kuss and **Carl Edward Rasmussen**
Max Planck Institute for Biological Cybernetics
Spemannstraße 38, 72076 Tübingen, Germany
{kuss,carl}@tuebingen.mpg.de

Abstract

Gaussian processes are attractive models for probabilistic classification but unfortunately exact inference is analytically intractable. We compare Laplace's method and Expectation Propagation (EP) focusing on marginal likelihood estimates and predictive performance. We explain theoretically and corroborate empirically that EP is superior to Laplace. We also compare to a sophisticated MCMC scheme and show that EP is surprisingly accurate.

In recent years models based on Gaussian process (GP) priors have attracted much attention in the machine learning community. Whereas inference in the GP regression model with Gaussian noise can be done analytically, probabilistic classification using GPs is analytically intractable. Several approaches to approximate Bayesian inference have been suggested, including Laplace's approximation, Expectation Propagation (EP), variational approximations and Markov chain Monte Carlo (MCMC) sampling, some of these in conjunction with generalisation bounds, online learning schemes and sparse approximations.

Despite the abundance of recent work on probabilistic GP classifiers, most experimental studies provide only anecdotal evidence, and no clear picture has yet emerged, as to when and why which algorithm should be preferred. Thus, from a practitioners point of view probabilistic GP classification *remains a jungle*. In this paper, we set out to understand and compare two of the most wide-spread approximations: Laplace's method and Expectation Propagation (EP). We also compare to a sophisticated, but computationally demanding MCMC scheme to examine how close the approximations are to *ground truth*.

We examine two aspects of the approximation schemes: Firstly the accuracy of approximations to the marginal likelihood which is of central importance for model selection and model comparison. In any practical application of GPs in classification (usually multiple) parameters of the covariance function (hyperparameters) have to be handled. Bayesian model selection provides a consistent framework for setting such parameters. Therefore, it is essential to evaluate the accuracy of the marginal likelihood approximations as a function of the hyperparameters, in order to assess the practical usefulness of the approach

Secondly, we need to assess the quality of the approximate probabilistic predictions. In the past, the probabilistic nature of the GP predictions have not received much attention, the focus being mostly on classification error *rates*. This unfortunate state of affairs is caused primarily by typical benchmarking problems being considered outside of a realistic context. The ability of a classifier to produce class probabilities or confidences, have obvious relevance in most areas of application, eg. medical diagnosis. We evaluate the predictive distributions of the approximate methods, and compare to the MCMC gold standard.

1 The Gaussian Process Model for Binary Classification

Let $y \in \{-1, 1\}$ denote the class label of an input $\mathbf{x}$. Gaussian process classification (GPC) is discriminative in modelling $p(y|\mathbf{x})$ for given $\mathbf{x}$ by a Bernoulli distribution. The probability of success $p(y = 1|\mathbf{x})$ is related to an unconstrained latent function $f(\mathbf{x})$ which is mapped to the unit interval by a sigmoid transformation, eg. the *logit* or the *probit*. For reasons of analytic convenience we exclusively use the probit model $p(y = 1|\mathbf{x}) = \Phi(f(\mathbf{x}))$, where Φ denotes the cumulative density function of the standard Normal distribution.

In the GPC model Bayesian inference is performed about the latent function f in the light of observed data $\mathcal{D} = \{(y_i, \mathbf{x}_i)|i = 1, \ldots, m\}$. Let $f_i = f(\mathbf{x}_i)$ and $\mathbf{f} = [f_1, \ldots, f_m]^\top$ be shorthand for the values of the latent function and $\mathbf{y} = [y_1, \ldots, y_m]^\top$ and $\mathbf{X} = [\mathbf{x}_1, \ldots, \mathbf{x}_m]^\top$ collect the class labels and inputs respectively. Given the latent function the class labels are independent Bernoulli variables, so the joint likelihood factories:

$$p(\mathbf{y}|\mathbf{f}) = \prod_{i=1}^{m} p(y_i|f_i) = \prod_{i=1}^{m} \Phi(y_i f_i),$$

and depends on f only through its value at the observed inputs. We use a zero-mean Gaussian process prior over the latent function f with a covariance function $k(\mathbf{x}, \mathbf{x}'|\boldsymbol{\theta})$, which may depend on *hyperparameters* $\boldsymbol{\theta}$ [1]. The functional form and parameters of the covariance function encodes assumptions about the latent function, and adaptation of these is part of the inference. The posterior distribution over latent function values $\mathbf{f}$ at the observed $\mathbf{X}$ for given hyperparameters $\boldsymbol{\theta}$ becomes:

$$p(\mathbf{f}|\mathcal{D}, \boldsymbol{\theta}) = \frac{\mathcal{N}(\mathbf{f}|\mathbf{0}, \mathbf{K})}{p(\mathcal{D}|\boldsymbol{\theta})} \prod_{i=1}^{m} \Phi(y_i f_i), \quad \text{where} \quad p(\mathcal{D}|\boldsymbol{\theta}) = \int p(\mathbf{y}|\mathbf{f}) p(\mathbf{f}|\mathbf{X}, \boldsymbol{\theta}) d\mathbf{f},$$

denotes the marginal likelihood. Unfortunately neither the marginal likelihood, nor the posterior itself, or predictions can be computed analytically, so approximations are needed.

2 Approximate Bayesian Inference

For the GPC model approximations are either based on a Gaussian approximation to the posterior $p(\mathbf{f}|\mathcal{D}, \boldsymbol{\theta}) \approx q(\mathbf{f}|\mathcal{D}, \boldsymbol{\theta}) = \mathcal{N}(\mathbf{f}|\mathbf{m}, \mathbf{A})$ or involve Markov chain Monte Carlo (MCMC) sampling [2]. We compare Laplace's method and Expectation Propagation (EP) which are two alternative approaches to finding parameters $\mathbf{m}$ and $\mathbf{A}$ of the Gaussian $q(\mathbf{f}|\mathcal{D}, \boldsymbol{\theta})$. Both methods also allow approximate evaluation of the marginal likelihood, which is useful for ML-II hyperparameter optimisation.

Laplace's approximation (LA) is found by making a second order Taylor approximation of the (un-normalised) log posterior [3]. The mean $\mathbf{m}$ is placed at the mode (MAP) and the covariance $\mathbf{A}$ equals the negative inverse Hessian of the log posterior density at $\mathbf{m}$.

The EP approximation [4] also gives a Gaussian approximation to the posterior. The parameters $\mathbf{m}$ and $\mathbf{A}$ are found in an iterative scheme by matching the approximate marginal moments of $p(f_i|\mathcal{D}, \boldsymbol{\theta})$ by the marginals of the approximation $\mathcal{N}(f_i|\mathbf{m}_i, \mathbf{A}_{ii})$. Although we cannot *prove* the convergence of EP, we conjecture that it always converges for GPC with probit likelihood, and have never encountered an exception.

A key insight is that a Gaussian approximation to the GPC posterior is equivalent to a GP approximation to the posterior distribution over latent functions. For a test input $\mathbf{x}_*$ the

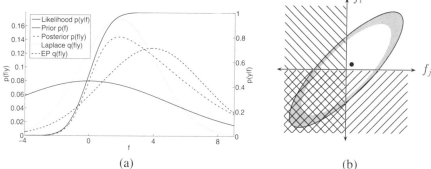

(a)   (b)

Figure 1: Panel (a) provides a one-dimensional illustration of the approximations. The prior $\mathcal{N}(f|0, 5^2)$ combined with the probit likelihood $(y = 1)$ results in a skewed posterior. The likelihood uses the right axis, all other curves use the left axis. Laplace's approximation peaks at the posterior mode, but places far too much mass over negative values of f and too little at large positive values. The EP approximation matches the first two posterior moments, which results in a larger mean and a more accurate placement of probability mass compared to Laplace's approximation. In Panel (b) we caricature a high dimensional zero-mean Gaussian prior as an ellipse. The gray shadow indicates that for a high dimensional Gaussian most of the mass lies in a thin shell. For large latent signals (large entries in $\mathbf{K}$), the likelihood essentially cuts off regions which are incompatible with the training labels (hatched area), leaving the upper right orthant as the posterior. The dot represents the mode of the posterior, which remains close to the origin.

approximate predictive latent and class probabilities are:

$$q(f_*|\mathcal{D}, \boldsymbol{\theta}, \mathbf{x}_*) = \mathcal{N}(\mu_*, \sigma_*^2), \quad \text{and} \quad q(y_* = 1|\mathcal{D}, \mathbf{x}_*) = \Phi(\mu_*/\sqrt{1 + \sigma_*^2}),$$

where $\mu_* = \mathbf{k}_*^\top \mathbf{K}^{-1}\mathbf{m}$ and $\sigma_*^2 = k(\mathbf{x}_*, \mathbf{x}_*) - \mathbf{k}_*^\top (\mathbf{K}^{-1} - \mathbf{K}^{-1}\mathbf{A}\mathbf{K}^{-1})\mathbf{k}_*$, where the vector $\mathbf{k}_* = [k(\mathbf{x}_1, \mathbf{x}_*), \ldots, k(\mathbf{x}_m, \mathbf{x}_*)]^\top$ collects covariances between $\mathbf{x}_*$ and training inputs $\mathbf{X}$.

MCMC sampling has the advantage that it becomes exact in the limit of long runs and so provides a *gold standard* by which to measure the two analytic methods described above. Although MCMC methods can in principle be used to do inference over $\mathbf{f}$ and $\boldsymbol{\theta}$ *jointly* [5], we compare to methods using ML-II optimisation over $\boldsymbol{\theta}$, thus we use MCMC to integrate over $\mathbf{f}$ only. Good marginal likelihood estimates are notoriously difficult to obtain; in our experiments we use Annealed Importance Sampling (AIS) [6], combining several Thermo-dynamic Integration runs into a single (unbiased) estimate of the marginal likelihood.

Both analytic approximations have a computational complexity which is cubic $\mathcal{O}(m^3)$ as common among non-sparse GP models due to inversions $m \times m$ matrices. In our imple-mentations LA and EP need similar running times, on the order of a few minutes for several hundred data-points. Making AIS work efficiently requires some fine-tuning and a single estimate of $p(\mathcal{D}|\boldsymbol{\theta})$ can take several hours for data sets of a few hundred examples, but this could conceivably be improved upon.

3   Structural Properties of the Posterior and its Approximations

Structural properties of the posterior can best be understood by examining its construction. The prior is a correlated m-dimensional Gaussian $\mathcal{N}(\mathbf{f}|0, \mathbf{K})$ centred at the origin. Each likelihood term $p(y_i|f_i)$ *softly* truncates the half-space from the prior that is incompatible with the observed label, see Figure 1. The resulting posterior is *unimodal* and *skewed*, similar to a multivariate Gaussian truncated to the orthant containing $\mathbf{y}$. The mode of

701

the posterior remains close to the origin, while the mass is placed in accordance with the observed class labels. Additionally, high dimensional Gaussian distributions exhibit the property that most probability mass is contained in a thin ellipsoidal shell – depending on the covariance structure – away from the mean [7, ch. 29.2]. Intuitively this occurs since in high dimensions the volume grows extremely rapidly with the radius. As an effect the mode becomes less representative (typical) for the prior distribution as the dimension increases. For the GPC posterior this property persists: the mode of the posterior distribution stays relatively close to the origin, still being unrepresentative for the posterior distribution, while the mean moves to the mass of the posterior making mean and mode differ significantly.

We cannot generally assume the posterior to be close to Gaussian, as in the often studied limit of low-dimensional parametric models with large amounts of data. Therefore in GPC we must be aware of making a Gaussian approximation to a non-Gaussian posterior. From the properties of the posterior it can be expected that Laplace's method places $\mathbf{m}$ in the right orthant but too close to the origin, such that the approximation will overlap with regions having practically zero posterior mass. As an effect the amplitude of the approximate latent posterior GP will be underestimated systematically, leading to overly cautious predictive distributions. The EP approximation does not rely on a local expansion, but assumes that the marginal distributions can be well approximated by Gaussians. This assumption will be examined empirically below.

4 Experiments

In this section we compare and inspect approximations for GPC using various benchmark data sets. The primary focus is not to optimise the absolute performance of GPC models but to compare the relative accuracy of approximations and to validate the arguments given in the previous section. In all experiments we use a covariance function of the form:

$$k(\mathbf{x}, \mathbf{x}'|\boldsymbol{\theta}) = \sigma^2 \exp\left(-\tfrac{1}{2}\|\mathbf{x} - \mathbf{x}'\|^2/\ell^2\right), \tag{1}$$

such that $\boldsymbol{\theta} = [\sigma, \ell]$. We refer to σ^2 as the signal variance and to ℓ as the characteristic length-scale. Note that for many classification tasks it may be reasonable to use an individual length scale parameter for every input dimension (ARD) or a different kind of covariance function. Nevertheless, for the sake of presentability we use the above covariance function and we believe the conclusions about the accuracy of approximations to be independent of this choice, since it relies on arguments which are independent of the form of the covariance function.

As measure of the accuracy of predictive probabilities we use the average information in bits of the predictions about the test targets in excess of that of random guessing. Let $p^* = p(y_* = 1|\mathcal{D}, \boldsymbol{\theta}, \mathbf{x}_*)$ be the model's prediction, then we average:

$$I(p_i^*, y_i) = \tfrac{y_i+1}{2} \log_2(p_i^*) + \tfrac{1-y_i}{2} \log_2(1 - p_i^*) + H \tag{2}$$

over all test cases, where H is the entropy of the training labels. The error rate E is equal to the percentage of erroneous class assignments if prediction is understood as a decision problem with symmetric costs.

For the first set of experiments presented here the well-known USPS digits and the Ionosphere data set were used. A binary sub-problem from the USPS digits is defined by only considering 3's vs. 5's (which is probably the hardest of the binary sub-problems) and dividing the data into 767 cases for training and 773 for testing. The Ionosphere data is split into 200 training and 151 test cases. We do an exhaustive investigation on a fine regular grid of values for the log hyperparameters. For each $\boldsymbol{\theta}$ on the grid we compute the approximated log marginal likelihood by LA, EP and AIS. Additionally we compute the respective predictive performance (2) on the test set. Results are shown in Figure 2.

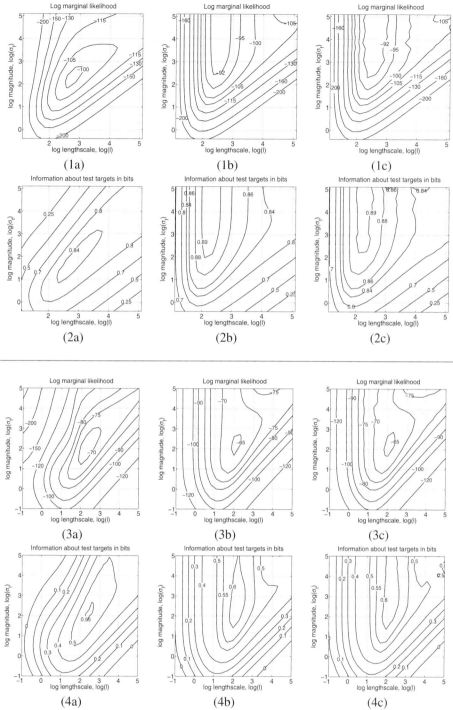

Figure 2: Comparison of marginal likelihood approximations and predictive performances of different approximation techniques for USPS 3s vs. 5s (upper half) and the Ionosphere data (lower half). The columns correspond to LA (a), EP (b), and MCMC (c). The rows show estimates of the log marginal likelihood (rows 1 & 3) and the corresponding predictive performance (2) on the test set (rows 2 & 4) respectively.

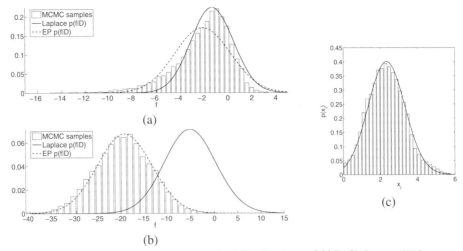

(a)

(b)

(c)

Figure 3: Panel (a) and (b) show two marginal distributions $p(f_i|\mathcal{D}, \boldsymbol{\theta})$ from a GPC posterior and its approximations. The true posterior is approximated by a normalised histogram of 9000 samples of f_i obtained by MCMC sampling. Panel (c) shows a histogram of samples of a marginal distribution of a truncated high-dimensional Gaussian. The line describes a Gaussian with mean and variance estimated from the samples.

For all three approximation techniques we see an agreement between marginal likelihood estimates and test performance, which justifies the use of ML-II parameter estimation. But the shape of the contours and the values differ between the methods. The contours for Laplace's method appear to be *slanted* compared to EP. The marginal likelihood estimates of EP and AIS agree surprisingly well[1], given that the marginal likelihood comes as a 767 respectively 200 dimensional integral. The EP predictions contain as much information about the test cases as the MCMC predictions and significantly more than for LA. Note that for small signal variances (roughly $\ln(\sigma^2) < 1$) LA and EP give very similar results. A possible explanation is that for small signal variances the likelihood does not *truncate* the prior but only *down-weights* the tail that disagrees with the observation. As an effect the posterior will be less skewed and both approximations will lead to similar results.

For the USPS 3's vs. 5's we now inspect the marginal distributions $p(f_i|\mathcal{D}, \boldsymbol{\theta})$ of single latent function values under the posterior approximations for a given value of $\boldsymbol{\theta}$. We have chosen the values $\ln(\sigma) = 3.35$ and $\ln(\ell) = 2.85$ which are between the ML-II estimates of EP and LA. Hybrid MCMC was used to generate 9000 samples from the posterior $p(\mathbf{f}|\mathcal{D}, \boldsymbol{\theta})$. For LA and EP the approximate marginals are $q(f_i|\mathcal{D}, \boldsymbol{\theta}) = \mathcal{N}(f_i|\mathbf{m}_i, \mathbf{A}_{ii})$ where $\mathbf{m}$ and $\mathbf{A}$ are found by the respective approximation techniques.

In general we observe that the marginal distributions of MCMC samples agree very well with the respective marginal distributions of the EP approximation. For Laplace's approximation we find the mean to be underestimated and the marginal distributions to overlap with zero far more than the EP approximations. Figure (3a) displays the marginal distribution and its approximations for which the MCMC samples show maximal skewness. Figure (3b) shows a typical example where the EP approximation agrees very well with the MCMC samples. We show this particular example because under the EP approximation $p(y_i = 1|\mathcal{D}, \boldsymbol{\theta}) < 0.1\%$ but LA gives a wrong $p(y_i = 1|\mathcal{D}, \boldsymbol{\theta}) \approx 18\%$.

In the experiment we saw that the marginal distributions of the posterior often agree very

---

[1]Note that the agreement between the two seems to be limited by the accuracy of the MCMC runs, as judged by the regularity of the contour lines; the tolerance is less than one unit on a (natural) log scale.

well with a Gaussian approximation. This seems to contradict the description given in the previous section were we argued that the posterior is skewed by construction. In order to inspect the marginals of a truncated high-dimensional multivariate Gaussian distribution we made an additional synthetic experiment. We constructed a 767 dimensional Gaussian $\mathcal{N}(\mathbf{x}|\mathbf{0}, \mathbf{C})$ with a covariance matrix having one eigenvalue of 100 with eigenvector $\mathbf{1}$, and all other eigenvalues are 1. We then truncate this distribution such that all $\mathbf{x}_i \geq 0$. Note that the mode of the truncated Gaussian is still at zero, whereas the mean moves towards the remaining mass. Figure (3c) shows a normalised histogram of samples from a marginal distribution of one $\mathbf{x}_i$. The samples agree very well with a Gaussian approximation. In the previous section we described the somewhat surprising property, that for a truncated high-dimensional Gaussian, resembling the posterior, the mode (used by LA) may not be particularly representative of the distribution. Although the marginal is also truncated, it is still exceptionally well modelled by a Gaussian – however, the Laplace approximation centred on the origin would be completely inappropriate.

In a second set of experiments we compare the predictive performance of LA and EP for GPC on several well known benchmark problems. Each data set is randomly split into 10 folds of which one at a time is left out as a test set to measure the predictive performance of a model trained (or selected) on the remaining nine folds. All performance measures are averages over the 10 folds. For GPC we implement model selection by ML-II hyperparameter estimation, reporting results given the $\boldsymbol{\theta}$ that maximised the respective approximate marginal likelihoods $p(\mathcal{D}|\boldsymbol{\theta})$.

In order to get a better picture of the absolute performance we also compare to results obtained by C-SVM classification. The kernel we used is equivalent to the covariance function (1) without the signal variance parameter. For each fold the parameters C and ℓ are found in an inner loop of 5-fold cross-validation, in which the parameter grids are refined until the performance stabilises. Predictive probabilities for test cases are obtained by mapping the unthresholded output of the SVM to $[0, 1]$ using a sigmoid function [8].

Results are summarised in Table 1. Comparing Laplace's method to EP the latter shows to be more accurate both in terms of error rate and information. While the error rates are relatively similar the predictive distribution obtained by EP shows to be more informative about the test targets. Note that for GPC the error rate only depends of the sign of the mean μ_* of the approximated posterior over latent functions and not the entire posterior predictive distribution. As to be expected, the length of the mean vector $\|\mathbf{m}\|$ shows much larger values for the EP approximations. Comparing EP and SVMs the results are mixed. For the Crabs data set all methods show the same error rate but the information content of the predictive distributions differs dramatically. For some test cases the SVM predicts the wrong class with large certainty.

5 Summary & Conclusions

Our experiments reveal serious differences between Laplace's method and EP when used in GPC models. From the structural properties of the posterior we described why LA systematically underestimates the mean $\mathbf{m}$. The resulting posterior GP over latent functions will have too small amplitude, although the sign of the mean function will be mostly correct. As an effect LA gives over-conservative predictive probabilities, and diminished information about the test labels. This effect has been show empirically on several real world examples. Large resulting discrepancies in the actual posterior probabilities were found, even at the training locations, which renders the predictive class probabilities produced under this approximation grossly inaccurate. Note, the difference becomes less dramatic if we only consider the classification error rates obtained by thresholding p^* at $1/2$. For this particular task, we've seen the the sign of the latent function tends to be correct (at least at the training locations).

Data Set	m	n	Laplace			EP			SVM	
			E%	I	$\|\mathbf{m}\|$	E%	I	$\|\mathbf{m}\|$	E%	I
Ionosphere	351	34	8.84	0.591	49.96	7.99	0.661	124.94	5.69	0.681
Wisconsin	683	9	3.21	0.804	62.62	3.21	0.805	84.95	3.21	0.795
Pima Indians	768	8	22.77	0.252	29.05	22.63	0.253	47.49	23.01	0.232
Crabs	200	7	2.0	0.682	112.34	2.0	0.908	2552.97	2.0	0.047
Sonar	208	60	15.36	0.439	26.86	13.85	0.537	15678.55	11.14	0.567
USPS 3 vs 5	1540	256	2.27	0.849	163.05	2.21	0.902	22011.70	2.01	0.918

Table 1: Results for benchmark data sets. The first three columns give the name of the data set, number of observations m and dimension of inputs n. For Laplace's method and EP the table reports the average error rate E%, the average information I (2) and the average length $\|\mathbf{m}\|$ of the mean vector of the Gaussian approximation. For SVMs the error rate and the average information about the test targets are reported. Note that for the Crabs data set we use the sex (not the colour) of the crabs as class label.

The EP approximation has shown to give results very close to MCMC both in terms of predictive distributions and marginal likelihood estimates. We have shown and explained why the marginal distributions of the posterior can be well approximated by Gaussians.

Further, the marginal likelihood values obtained by LA and EP differ systematically which will lead to different results of ML-II hyperparameter estimation. The discrepancies are similar for different tasks. Using AIS we were able to show the accuracy of marginal likelihood estimates, which to the best of our knowledge has never been done before.

In summary, we found that EP is the method of choice for approximate inference in binary GPC models, when the computational cost of MCMC is prohibitive. In contrast, the Laplace approximation is so inaccurate that we advise against its use, especially when predictive probabilities are to be taken seriously. Further experiments and a detailed description of the approximation schemes can be found in [2].

Acknowledgements   Both authors acknowledge support by the German Research Foundation (DFG) through grant RA 1030/1. This work was supported in part by the IST Programme of the European Community, under the PASCAL Network of Excellence, IST-2002-506778. This publication only reflects the authors' views.

References

[1] C. K. I. Williams and C. E. Rasmussen. Gaussian processes for regression. In David S. Touretzky, Michael C. Mozer, and Michael E. Hasselmo, editors, *NIPS 8*, pages 514–520. MIT Press, 1996.

[2] M. Kuss and C. E. Rasmussen. Assessing approximate inference for binary Gaussian process classification. *Journal of Machine Learning Research*, 6:1679–1704, 2005.

[3] C. K. I. Williams and D. Barber. Bayesian classification with Gaussian processes. *IEEE Transactions on Pattern Analysis and Machine Intelligence*, 20(12):1342–1351, 1998.

[4] T. P. Minka. *A Family of Algorithms for Approximate Bayesian Inference*. PhD thesis, Department of Electrical Engineering and Computer Science, MIT, 2001.

[5] R. M. Neal. Regression and classification using Gaussian process priors. In J. M. Bernardo, J. O. Berger, A. P. Dawid, and A. F. M. Smith, editors, *Bayesian Statistics 6*, pages 475–501. Oxford University Press, 1998.

[6] R. M. Neal. Annealed importance sampling. *Statistics and Computing*, 11:125–139, 2001.

[7] D. J. C. MacKay. *Information Theory, Inference and Learning Algorithms*. CUP, 2003.

[8] J. C. Platt. Probabilities for SV machines. In *Advances in Large Margin Classifiers*, pages 61–73. The MIT Press, 2000.

Rodeo: Sparse Nonparametric Regression in High Dimensions

John Lafferty
School of Computer Science
Carnegie Mellon University

Larry Wasserman
Department of Statistics
Carnegie Mellon University

Abstract

We present a method for nonparametric regression that performs bandwidth selection and variable selection simultaneously. The approach is based on the technique of incrementally decreasing the bandwidth in directions where the gradient of the estimator with respect to bandwidth is large. When the unknown function satisfies a sparsity condition, our approach avoids the curse of dimensionality, achieving the optimal minimax rate of convergence, up to logarithmic factors, as if the relevant variables were known in advance. The method—called *rodeo* (regularization of derivative expectation operator)—conducts a sequence of hypothesis tests, and is easy to implement. A modified version that replaces hard with soft thresholding effectively solves a sequence of lasso problems.

1 Introduction

Estimating a high dimensional regression function is notoriously difficult due to the "curse of dimensionality." Minimax theory precisely characterizes the curse. Let $Y_i = m(X_i) + \epsilon_i$, $i = 1, \ldots, n$ where $X_i = (X_i(1), \ldots, X_i(d)) \in \mathbb{R}^d$ is a d-dimensional covariate, $m : \mathbb{R}^d \to \mathbb{R}$ is the unknown function to estimate, and $\epsilon_i \sim N(0, \sigma^2)$. Then if m is in $W_2(c)$, the d-dimensional Sobolev ball of order two and radius c, it is well known that

$$\liminf_{n \to \infty} n^{4/(4+d)} \inf_{\widehat{m}_n} \sup_{m \in W_2(c)} \mathcal{R}(\widehat{m}_n, m) > 0, \tag{1}$$

where $\mathcal{R}(\widehat{m}_n, m) = \mathbb{E}_m \int (\widehat{m}_n(x) - m(x))^2 \, dx$ is the risk of the estimate $\widehat{m}_n$ constructed on a sample of size n (Györfi et al. 2002). Thus, the best rate of convergence is $n^{-4/(4+d)}$, which is impractically slow if d is large.

However, for some applications it is reasonable to expect that the true function only depends on a small number of the total covariates. Suppose that m satisfies such a sparseness condition, so that $m(x) = m(x_R)$ where $x_R = (x_j : j \in R)$, $R \subset \{1, \ldots, d\}$ is a subset of the d covariates, of size $r = |R| \ll d$. We call $\{x_j\}_{j \in R}$ the *relevant variables*. Under this sparseness assumption we can hope to achieve the better minimax convergence rate of $n^{-4/(4+r)}$ if the r relevant variables can be isolated. Thus, we are faced with the problem of variable selection in nonparametric regression.

A large body of previous work has addressed this fundamental problem, which has led to a variety of methods to combat the curse of dimensionality. Many of these are based on very clever, though often heuristic techniques. For additive models of the form $f(x) = \sum_j f_j(x_j)$, standard methods like stepwise selection, C_p and AIC can be used (Hastie et al. 2001). For spline models, Zhang et al. (2005) use likelihood basis pursuit, essentially the lasso adapted to the spline setting. CART (Breiman et al. 1984) and MARS (Friedman 1991) effectively perform variable selection as part of their function fitting. More recently, Li et al. (2005) use independence testing for variable selection and Bühlmann and Yu (2005) introduced a boosting approach. While these methods have met with varying degrees of empirical success, they can be challenging to implement and demanding computationally. Moreover, these methods are typically difficult to analyze theoretically, and so often come with no formal guarantees. Indeed, the theoretical analysis of sparse *parametric* estimators such as the lasso (Tibshirani 1996) is difficult, and only recently has significant progress been made on this front (Donoho 2004; Fu and Knight 2000).

In this paper we present a new approach to sparse nonparametric function estimation that is both computationally simple and amenable to theoretical analysis. We call the general framework *rodeo*, for regularization of derivative expectation operator. It is based on the idea that bandwidth and variable selection can be simultaneously performed by computing the infinitesimal change in a nonparametric estimator as a function of the smoothing parameters, and then thresholding these derivatives to effectively get a sparse estimate. As a simple version of this principle we use hard thresholding, effectively carrying out a sequence of hypothesis tests. A modified version that replaces testing with soft thresholding effectively solves a sequence of lasso problems. The potential appeal of this approach is that it can be based on relatively simple and theoretically well understood nonparametric techniques such as local linear smoothing, leading to methods that are simple to implement and can be used in high dimensional problems. Moreover, we show that the rodeo can achieve near optimal minimax rates of convergence, and therefore circumvents the curse of dimensionality when the true function is indeed sparse. When applied in one dimension, our method yields a locally optimal bandwidth. We present experiments on both synthetic and real data that demonstrate the effectiveness of the new approach.

2   Rodeo: The Main Idea

The key idea in our approach is as follows. Fix a point x and let $\widehat{m}_h(x)$ denote an estimator of $m(x)$ based on a vector of smoothing parameters $h = (h_1, \ldots, h_d)$. If c is a scalar, then we write $h = c$ to mean $h = (c, \ldots, c)$. Let $M(h) = \mathbb{E}(\widehat{m}_h(x))$ denote the mean of $\widehat{m}_h(x)$. For now, assume that x_i is one of the observed data points and that $\widehat{m}_0(x) = Y_i$. In that case, $m(x) = M(0) = \mathbb{E}(Y_i)$. If $P = (h(t) : 0 \leq t \leq 1)$ is a smooth path through the set of smoothing parameters with $h(0) = 0$ and $h(1) = 1$ (or any other fixed, large bandwidth) then

$$m(x) = M(0) = M(1) - \int_0^1 \frac{dM(h(s))}{ds} \, ds = M(1) - \int_0^1 \langle D(s), \dot{h}(s) \rangle ds$$

where $D(h) = \nabla M(h) = \left(\frac{\partial M}{\partial h_j}, \ldots, \frac{\partial M}{\partial h_j} \right)^T$ is the gradient of $M(h)$ and $\dot{h}(s) = \frac{dh(s)}{ds}$ is the derivative of $h(s)$ along the path. A biased, low variance estimator of $M(1)$ is $\widehat{m}_1(x)$. An unbiased estimator of $D(h)$ is

$$Z(h) = \left(\frac{\partial \widehat{m}_h(x)}{\partial h_1}, \ldots, \frac{\partial \widehat{m}_h(x)}{\partial h_d} \right)^T. \tag{2}$$

The naive estimator

$$\widehat{m}(x) = \widehat{m}_1(x) - \int_0^1 \langle Z(s), \dot{h}(s) \rangle ds \tag{3}$$

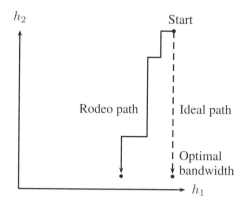

Figure 1: The bandwidths for the relevant variables (h_2) are shrunk, while the bandwidths for the irrelevant variables (h_1) are kept relatively large. The simplest rodeo algorithm shrinks the bandwidths in discrete steps $1, \beta, \beta^2, \ldots$ for some $0 < \beta < 1$.

is identically equal to $\widehat{m}_0(x) = Y_i$, which has poor risk since the variance of $Z(h)$ is large for small h. However, our sparsity assumption on m suggests that there should be paths for which $D(h)$ is also sparse. Along such a path, we replace $Z(h)$ with an estimator $\widehat{D}(h)$ that makes use of the sparsity assumption. Our estimate of $m(x)$ is then

$$\widetilde{m}(x) = \widehat{m}_1(x) - \int_0^1 \langle \widehat{D}(s), \dot{h}(s) \rangle ds. \tag{4}$$

To implement this idea we need to do two things: (i) we need to find a sparse path and (ii) we need to take advantage of this sparseness when estimating D along that path.

The key observation is that if x_j is irrelevant, then we expect that changing the bandwidth h_j for that variable should cause only a small change in the estimator $\widehat{m}_h(x)$. Conversely, if x_j is relevant, then we expect that changing the bandwidth h_j for that variable should cause a large change in the estimator. Thus, $Z_j = \partial \widehat{m}_h(x)/\partial h_j$ should discriminate between relevant and irrelevant covariates. To simplify the procedure, we can replace the continuum of bandwidths with a discrete set where each $h_j \in \mathcal{B} = \{h_0, \beta h_0, \beta^2 h_0, \ldots\}$ for some $0 < \beta < 1$. Moreover, we can proceed in a greedy fashion by estimating $D(h)$ sequentially with $h_j \in \mathcal{B}$ and setting $\widehat{D}_j(h) = 0$ when $h_j < \widehat{h}_j$, where $\widehat{h}_j$ is the first h such that $|Z_j(h)| < \lambda_j(h)$ for some threshold λ_j. This greedy version, coupled with the hard threshold estimator, yields $\widetilde{m}(x) = \widehat{m}_{\widehat{h}}(x)$. A conceptual illustration of the idea is shown in Figure 1. This idea can be implemented using a greedy algorithm, coupled with the hard threshold estimator, to yield a bandwidth selection procedure based on testing.

This approach to bandwidth selection is similar to that of Lepski et al. (1997), which uses a more refined test leads to estimators that achieve good spatial adaptation over large function classes. Our approach is also similar to a method of Ruppert (1997) that uses a sequence of decreasing bandwidths and then estimates the optimal bandwidth by estimating the mean squared error as a function of bandwidth. Our greedy approach tests whether an infinitesimal change in the bandwidth from its current setting leads to a significant change in the estimate, and is more easily extended to a practical method in higher dimensions. Related work of Hristache et al. (2001) focuses on variable selection in multi-index models rather than on bandwidth estimation.

3   Rodeo using Local Linear Regression

We now present the multivariate case in detail, using local linear smoothing as the basic method since it is known to have many good properties. Let $x = (x(1), \ldots, x(d))$ be some point at which we want to estimate m. Let $\widehat{m}_H(x)$ denote the local linear estimator of

$m(x)$ using bandwidth matrix H. Thus,

$$\widehat{m}_H(x) = e_1^T (X_x^T W_x X_x)^{-1} X_x^T W_x Y, \qquad X_x = \begin{pmatrix} 1 & (X_1 - x)^T \\ \vdots & \vdots \\ 1 & (X_n - x)^T \end{pmatrix} \tag{5}$$

where $e_1 = (1, 0, \ldots, 0)^T$, and W_x is the diagonal matrix with (i, i) element $K_H(X_i - x)$ and $K_H(u) = |H|^{-1} K(H^{-1}u)$. The estimator $\widehat{m}_H$ can be written as $\widehat{m}_H(x) = \sum_{i=1}^n G(X_i, x, h) Y_i$ where

$$G(u, x, h) = e_1^T (X_x^T W_x X_x)^{-1} \begin{pmatrix} 1 \\ (u - x)^T \end{pmatrix} K_H(u - x) \tag{6}$$

is called the *effective kernel*. We assume that the covariates are random with sampling density $f(x)$, and make the same assumptions as Ruppert and Wand (1994) in their analysis of the bias and variance of local linear regression. In particular, (i) the kernel K has compact support with zero odd moments and $\int u u^\top K(u)\, du = \nu_2(K) I$ and (ii) the sampling density $f(x)$ is continuously differentiable and strictly positive. In the version of the algorithm that follows, we take K to be a product kernel and H to be diagonal with elements $h = (h_1, \ldots, h_d)$.

Our method is based on the statistic

$$Z_j = \frac{\partial \widehat{m}_h(x)}{\partial h_j} = \sum_{i=1}^n G_j(X_i, x, h) Y_i \tag{7}$$

where $G_j(u, x, h) = \frac{\partial G(u,x,h)}{\partial h_j}$. Straightforward calculations show that

$$Z_j = \frac{\partial \widehat{m}_h(x)}{\partial h_j} = = e_1^\top (X_x^\top W_x X_x)^{-1} X_x^\top \frac{\partial W_x}{\partial h_j} (Y - X_x \widehat{\alpha}) \tag{8}$$

where $\widehat{\alpha} = (X_x^\top W_x X_x)^{-1} X_x^\top W_x Y$ is the coefficient vector for the local linear fit. Note that the factor $|H|^{-1} = \prod_{i=1}^d 1/h_i$ in the kernel cancels in the expression for $\widehat{m}$, and therefore we can ignore it in our calculation of Z_j. Assuming a product kernel we have

$$W_x = \operatorname{diag}\left(\prod_{j=1}^d K((X_{1j} - x_j)/h_j), \ldots, \prod_{j=1}^d K((X_{nj} - x_j)/h_j) \right) \tag{9}$$

and $\partial W_x / \partial h_j = W_x D_j$ where

$$D_j = \operatorname{diag}\left(\frac{\partial \log K((X_{1j} - x_j)/h_j)}{\partial h_j}, \ldots, \frac{\partial \log K((X_{nj} - x_j)/h_j)}{\partial h_j} \right) \tag{10}$$

and thus $Z_j = e_1^\top (X_x^\top W_x X_x)^{-1} X_x^\top W_x D_j (Y - X_x \widehat{\alpha})$. For example, with the Gaussian kernel $K(u) = \exp(-u^2/2)$ we have $D_j = \frac{1}{h_j^3} \operatorname{diag}\left((X_{1j} - x_j)^2, \ldots, (X_{nj} - x_j)^2 \right)$.

Let

$$\mu_j \equiv \mu_j(h) = \mathbb{E}(Z_j | X_1, \ldots, X_n) = \sum_{i=1}^n G_j(X_i, x, h) m(X_i) \tag{11}$$

$$s_j^2 \equiv s_j^2(h) = \mathbb{V}(Z_j | X_1, \ldots, X_n) = \sigma^2 \sum_{i=1}^n G_j(X_i, x, h)^2. \tag{12}$$

Then the hard thresholding version of the rodeo algorithm is given in Figure 2.

The algorithm requires that we insert an estimate $\widehat{\sigma}$ of σ in (12). One estimate of σ can be obtained by generalizing a method of Rice (1984). For $i < \ell$, let $d_{i\ell} = \|X_i - X_\ell\|$. Fix an integer J and let $\mathcal{E}$ denote the set of pairs (i, ℓ) corresponding to the J smallest values of $d_{i\ell}$. Now define $\widehat{\sigma}^2 = \frac{1}{2J} \sum_{i,\ell \in \mathcal{E}} (Y_i - Y_\ell)^2$. Then $\mathbb{E}(\widehat{\sigma}^2) = \sigma^2 + \text{bias}$ where

1. *Select* parameter $0 < \beta < 1$ and initial bandwidth h_0 slowly decreasing to zero, with $h_0 = \Omega\left(1/\sqrt{\log\log n}\right)$. Let $c_n = \Omega(1)$ be a sequence satisfying $dc_n = \Omega(\log n)$.

2. *Initialize* the bandwidths, and activate all covariates:
   (a) $h_j = h_0, j = 1, 2, \ldots, d$.
   (b) $\mathcal{A} = \{1, 2, \ldots, d\}$

3. *While $\mathcal{A}$ is nonempty*, do for each $j \in \mathcal{A}$:
   (a) Compute the estimated derivative expectation: Z_j (equation 7) and s_j (equation 12).
   (b) Compute the threshold $\lambda_j = s_j \sqrt{2\log(dc_n)}$.
   (c) If $|Z_j| \geq \lambda_j$, then set $h_j \leftarrow \beta h_j$, otherwise remove j from $\mathcal{A}$.

4. *Output* bandwidths $h^\star = (h_1, \ldots, h_d)$ and estimator $\tilde{m}(x) = \hat{m}_{h^\star}(x)$.

Figure 2: The hard thresholding version of the rodeo, which can be applied using the derivatives Z_j of any nonparametric smoother.

bias $\leq D \sup_x \sum_{j \in R} \left|\frac{\partial f(x)}{\partial x_j}\right|$ with $D = \max_{i,\ell \in \mathcal{E}} \|X_i - X_\ell\|$. There is a bias-variance tradeoff: large J makes $\hat{\sigma}^2$ positively biased, and small J makes $\hat{\sigma}^2$ highly variable. Note however that the bias is mitigated by sparsity (small r). This is the estimator used in our examples.

4 Analysis

In this section we present some results on the properties of the resulting estimator. Formally, we use a triangular array approach so that $f(x)$, $m(x)$, d and r can all change as n changes. For convenience of notation we assume that the covariates are numbered such that the relevant variables x_j correspond to $1 \leq j \leq r$, and the irrelevant variables to $j > r$. To begin, we state the following technical lemmas on the mean and variance of Z_j.

Lemma 4.1. *Suppose that K is a product kernel with bandwidth vector $h = (h_1, \ldots, h_d)$. If the sampling density f is uniform, then $\mu_j = 0$ for all $j \in R^c$. More generally, assuming that r is bounded, we have the following when $h_j \to 0$: If $j \in R^c$ the derivative of the bias is*

$$\mu_j = \frac{\partial}{\partial h_j} \mathbb{E}[\hat{m}_H(x) - m(x)] = -\text{tr}(H_R \mathcal{H}_R) \, \nu_2^2 \, (\nabla_j \log f(x))^2 \, h_j + o_P(h_j) \quad (13)$$

where the Hessian of $m(x)$ is $\mathcal{H} = \begin{pmatrix} \mathcal{H}_R & 0 \\ 0 & 0 \end{pmatrix}$ and $H_R = \text{diag}(h_1^2, \ldots, h_r^2)$. For $j \in R$ we have

$$\mu_j = \frac{\partial}{\partial h_j} \mathbb{E}[\hat{m}_H(x) - m(x)] = h_j \nu_2 m_{jj}(x) + o_P(h_j). \quad (14)$$

Lemma 4.2. *Let $C = \left(\frac{\sigma^2 R(K)}{4m(x)}\right)$ where $R(K) = \int K(u)^2 \, du$. Then, if $h_j = o(1)$,*

$$s_j^2 = \mathbb{V}\text{ar}(Z_j | X_1, \ldots, X_n) = \frac{C}{nh_j^2} \left(\prod_{k=1}^d \frac{1}{h_k}\right) \left(1 + o_P(1)\right). \quad (15)$$

These lemmas parallel the calculations of Ruppert and Wand (1994) except for the difference that the irrelevant variables have different leading terms in the expansions than relevant variables.

Our main theoretical result characterizes the asymptotic running time, selected bandwidths, and risk of the algorithm. In order to get a practical algorithm, we need to make assumptions on the functions m and f.

(A1) For some constant $k > 0$, each $j > r$ satisfies

$$\nabla_j \log f(x) = O\left(\frac{\log^k n}{n^{1/4}}\right) \tag{16}$$

(A2) For each $j \leq r$,

$$m_{jj}(x) \neq 0. \tag{17}$$

Explanation of the Assumptions. To give the intuition behind these assumptions, recall from Lemma 4.1 that

$$\mu_j = \begin{cases} A_j h_j + o_P(h_j) & j \leq r \\ B_j h_j + o_P(h_j) & j > r \end{cases} \tag{18}$$

where

$$A_j = \nu_2 m_{jj}(x), \quad B_j = -\text{tr}(H\mathcal{H})\nu_2^2(\nabla_j \log f(x))^2. \tag{19}$$

Moreover, $\mu_j = 0$ when the sampling density f is uniform or the data are on a regular grid. Consider assumption (A1). If f is uniform then this assumption is automatically satisfied since then $\mu_j(s) = 0$ for $j > r$. More generally, μ_j is approximately proportional to $(\nabla_j \log f(x))^2$ for $j > r$ which implies that $|\mu_j| \approx 0$ for irrelevant variables if f is sufficiently smooth in the variable x_j. Hence, assumption (A1) can be interpreted as requiring that f is sufficiently smooth in the irrelevant dimensions.

Now consider assumption (A2). Equation (18) ensures that μ_j is proportional to $h_j|m_{jj}(x)|$ for small h_j. Since we take the initial bandwidth h_0 to be decreasing slowly with n, (A2) implies that $|\mu_j(h)| \geq ch_j|m_{jj}(x)|$ for some constant $c > 0$, for sufficiently large n.

In the following we write $Y_n = \widetilde{O}_P(a_n)$ to mean that $Y_n = O_P(b_n a_n)$ where b_n is logarithmic in n; similarly, $a_n = \widetilde{\Omega}(b_n)$ if $a_n = \Omega(b_n c_n)$ where c_n is logarithmic in n.

Theorem 4.3. *Suppose assumptions (A1) and (A2) hold. In addition, suppose that* $d_{min} = \min_{j \leq r} |m_{jj}(x)| = \widetilde{\Omega}(1)$ *and* $d_{max} = \max_{j \leq r} |m_{jj}(x)| = \widetilde{O}(1)$. *Then the number of iterations* T_n *until the rodeo stops satisfies*

$$\mathbb{P}\left(\frac{1}{4+r}\log_{1/\beta}(na_n) \leq T_n \leq \frac{1}{4+r}\log_{1/\beta}(nb_n)\right) \longrightarrow 1 \tag{20}$$

where $a_n = \widetilde{\Omega}(1)$ *and* $b_n = \widetilde{O}(1)$. *Moreover, the algorithm outputs bandwidths* $h^\star$ *that satisfy*

$$\mathbb{P}\left(h_j^\star \geq \frac{1}{\log^k n} \text{ for all } j > r\right) \longrightarrow 1 \tag{21}$$

and

$$\mathbb{P}\left(h_0(nb_n)^{-1/(4+r)} \leq h_j^\star \leq h_0(na_n)^{-1/(4+r)} \text{ for all } j \leq r\right) \longrightarrow 1. \tag{22}$$

Corollary 4.4. *Under the conditions of Theorem 4.3, the risk* $\mathcal{R}(h^\star)$ *of the rodeo estimator satisfies*

$$\mathcal{R}(h^\star) = \widetilde{O}_P\left(n^{-4/(4+r)}\right). \tag{23}$$

In the one-dimensional case, this result shows that the algorithm recovers the locally optimal bandwidth, giving an adaptive estimator, and in general attains the optimal (up to logarithmic factors) minimax rate of convergence.

The proofs of these results are given in the full version of the paper.

5 Some Examples and Extensions

Figure 3 illustrates the rodeo on synthetic and real data. The left plot shows the bandwidths obtained on a synthetic dataset with $n = 500$ points of dimension $d = 20$. The covariates are generated as $x_i \sim \text{Uniform}(0, 1)$, the true function is $m(x) = 2(x_1 + 1)^2 + 2\sin(10x_2)$, and $\sigma = 1$. The results are averaged over 50 randomly generated data sets; note that the displayed bandwidth paths are not monotonic because of this averaging. The plot shows how the bandwidths of the relevant variables shrink toward zero, while the bandwidths of the irrelevant variables remain large. Simulations on other synthetic data sets, not included here, are similar and indicate that the algorithm's performance is consistent with our theoretical analysis.

The framework introduced here has many possible generalizations. While we have focused on estimation of m locally at a point x, the idea can be extended to carry out global bandwidth and variable selection by averaging over multiple evaluation points $x_1, \ldots, x_k$. These could be points interest for estimation, could be randomly chosen, or could be taken to be identical to the observed X_is. In addition, it is possible to consider more general paths, for example using soft thresholding or changing only the bandwidth corresponding to the largest $|Z_j|/\lambda_j$.

Such a version of the rodeo can be seen as a nonparametric counterpart to least angle regression (LARS) (Efron et al. 2004), a refinement of forward stagewise regression in which one adds the covariate most correlated with the residuals of the current fit, in small, incremental steps. Note first that Z_j is essentially the correlation between the Y_is and the $G_j(X_i, x, h)$s (the change in the effective kernel). Reducing the bandwidth is like adding in more of that variable. Suppose now that we make the following modifications to the rodeo: (i) change the bandwidths one at a time, based on the largest $Z_j^* = |Z_j|/\lambda_j$, (ii) reduce the bandwidth continuously, rather than in discrete steps, until the largest Z_j^* is equal to the next largest Z_j^*. Figure 3 (right) shows the result of running this greedy version of the rodeo on the diabetes dataset used to illustrate LARS. The algorithm averages Z_j^* over a randomly chosen set of $k = 100$ data points. The resulting variable ordering is seen to be very similar to, but different from, the ordering obtained from the parametric LARS fit.

Acknowledgments

We thank the reviewers for their helpful comments. Research supported in part by NSF grants IIS-0312814, IIS-0427206, and DMS-0104016, and NIH grants R01-CA54852-07 and MH57881.

References

L. Breiman, J. H. Friedman, R. A. Olshen, and C. J. Stone. *Classification and regression trees.* Wadsworth Publishing Co Inc, 1984.

P. Bühlmann and B. Yu. Boosting, model selection, lasso and nonnegative garrote. Technical report, Berkeley, 2005.

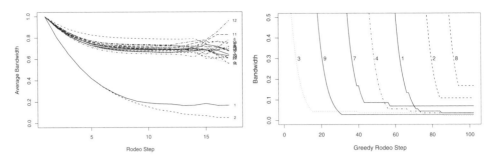

Figure 3: Left: Average bandwidth output by the rodeo for a function with $r = 2$ relevant variables in $d = 20$ dimensions ($n = 500$, with 50 trials). Covariates are generated as $x_i \sim \text{Uniform}(0, 1)$, the true function is $m(x) = 2(x_1 + 1)^3 + 2\sin(10x_2)$, and $\sigma = 1$, fit at the test point $x = (\frac{1}{2}, \ldots, \frac{1}{2})$. The variance is greater for large step sizes since the rodeo runs that long for fewer data sets. Right: Greedy rodeo on the diabetes data, used to illustrate LARS (Efron et al. 2004). A set of $k = 100$ of the total $n = 442$ points were sampled ($d = 10$), and the bandwidth for the variable with largest average $|Z_j|/\lambda_j$ was reduced in each step. The variables were selected in the order 3 (body mass index), 9 (serum), 7 (serum), 4 (blood pressure), 1 (age), 2 (sex), 8 (serum), 5 (serum), 10 (serum), 6 (serum). The parametric LARS algorithm adds variables in the order 3, 9, 4, 7, 2, 10, 5, 8, 6, 1. One notable difference is in the position of the age variable.

D. Donoho. For most large underdetermined systems of equations, the minimal ℓ^1-norm near-solution approximates the sparest near-solution. Technical report, Stanford, 2004.

B. Efron, T. Hastie, I. Johnstone, and R. Tibshirani. Least angle regression. *The Annals of Statistics*, 32:407–499, 2004.

J. H. Friedman. Multivariate adaptive regression splines. *The Annals of Statistics*, 19:1–67, 1991.

W. Fu and K. Knight. Asymptotics for lasso type estimators. *The Annals of Statistics*, 28:1356–1378, 2000.

L. Györfi, M. Kohler, A. Krzyżak, and H. Walk. *A Distribution-Free Theory of Nonparametric Regression*. Springer-Verlag, 2002.

T. Hastie, R. Tibshirani, and J. H. Friedman. *The Elements of Statistical Learning: Data Mining, Inference, and Prediction*. Springer-Verlag, 2001.

M. Hristache, A. Juditsky, J. Polzehl, and V. Spokoiny. Structure adaptive approach for dimension reduction. *Ann. Statist.*, 29:1537–1566, 2001.

O. V. Lepski, E. Mammen, and V. G. Spokoiny. Optimal spatial adaptation to inhomogeneous smoothness: An approach based on kernel estimates with variable bandwidth selectors. *The Annals of Statistics*, 25:929–947, 1997.

L. Li, R. D. Cook, and C. Nachsteim. Model-free variable selection. *J. R. Statist. Soc. B.*, 67:285–299, 2005.

J. Rice. Bandwidth choice for nonparametric regression. *The Annals of Statistics*, 12:1215–1230, 1984.

D. Ruppert. Empirical-bias bandwidths for local polynomial nonparametric regression and density estimation. *Journal of the American Statistical Association*, 92:1049–1062, 1997.

D. Ruppert and M. P. Wand. Multivariate locally weighted least squares regression. *The Annals of Statistics*, 22:1346–1370, 1994.

R. Tibshirani. Regression shrinkage and selection via the lasso. *Journal of the Royal Statistical Society, Series B, Methodological*, 58:267–288, 1996.

H. Zhang, G. Wahba, Y. Lin, M. Voelker, R. K. Ferris, and B. Klein. Variable selection and model building via likelihood basis pursuit. *J. of the Amer. Stat. Assoc.*, 99(467):659–672, 2005.

Fixing two weaknesses of the Spectral Method

Kevin J. Lang
Yahoo Research
3333 Empire Ave, Burbank, CA 91504
langk@yahoo-inc.com

Abstract

We discuss two intrinsic weaknesses of the spectral graph partitioning method, both of which have practical consequences. The first is that spectral embeddings tend to hide the best cuts from the commonly used hyperplane rounding method. Rather than cleaning up the resulting sub-optimal cuts with local search, we recommend the adoption of flow-based rounding. The second weakness is that for many "power law" graphs, the spectral method produces cuts that are highly unbalanced, thus decreasing the usefulness of the method for visualization (see figure 4(b)) or as a basis for divide-and-conquer algorithms. These balance problems, which occur even though the spectral method's quotient-style objective function does encourage balance, can be fixed with a stricter balance constraint that turns the spectral mathematical program into an SDP that can be solved for million-node graphs by a method of Burer and Monteiro.

1 Background

Graph partitioning is the NP-hard problem of finding a small graph cut subject to the constraint that neither side of the resulting partitioning of the nodes is "too small". We will be dealing with several versions: the graph bisection problem, which requires perfect $\frac{1}{2} : \frac{1}{2}$ balance; the β-balanced cut problem (with β a fraction such as $\frac{1}{3}$), which requires at least $\beta : (1 - \beta)$ balance; and the quotient cut problem, which requires the small side to be large enough to "pay for" the edges in the cut. The quotient cut metric is $c/\min(a, b)$, where c is the cutsize and a and b are the sizes of the two sides of the cut. All of the well-known variants of the quotient cut metric (e.g. normalized cut [15]) have similar behavior with respect to the issues discussed in this paper.

The spectral method for graph partitioning was introduced in 1973 by Fiedler and Donath & Hoffman [6]. In the mid-1980's Alon & Milman [1] proved that spectral cuts can be at worst quadratically bad; in the mid 1990's Guattery & Miller [10] proved that this analysis is tight by exhibiting a family of n-node graphs whose spectral bisections cut $O(n^{2/3})$ edges versus the optimal $O(n^{1/3})$ edges. On the other hand, Spielman & Teng [16] have proved stronger performance guarantees for the special case of spacelike graphs.

The spectral method can be derived by relaxing a quadratic integer program which encodes the graph bisection problem (see section 3.1). The solution to this relaxation is the "Fiedler vector", or second smallest eigenvector of the graph's discrete Laplacian matrix, whose elements x_i can be interpreted as an embedding of the graph on the line. To obtain a

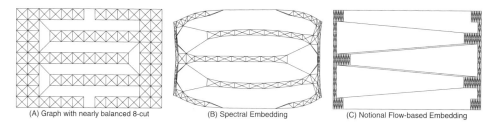

| (A) Graph with nearly balanced 8-cut | (B) Spectral Embedding | (C) Notional Flow-based Embedding |

Figure 1: The spectral embedding hides the best solution from hyperplane rounding.

specific cut, one must apply a "rounding method" to this embedding. The hyperplane rounding method chooses one of the $n-1$ cuts which separate the nodes whose x_i values lie above and below some split value $\hat{x}$.

2   Using flow to find cuts that are hidden from hyperplane rounding

Theorists have long known that the spectral method cannot distinguish between deep cuts and long paths, and that this confusion can cause it to cut a graph in the wrong direction thereby producing the spectral method's worst-case behavior [10]. In this section we will show by example that even when the spectral method is not fooled into cutting in the wrong direction, the resulting embedding can hide the best cuts from the hyperplane rounding method. This is a possible explanation for the frequently made empirical observation (see e.g. [12]) that hyperplane roundings of spectral embeddings are noisy and therefore benefit from cleanup with a local search method such as Fiduccia-Matheyses [8].

Consider the graph in figure 1(a), which has a near-bisection cutting 8 edges. For this graph the spectral method produces the embedding shown in figure 1(b), and recommends that we make a vertical cut (across the horizontal dimension which is based on the Fiedler vector). This is correct in a generalized sense, but it is obvious that no hyperplane (or vertical line in this picture) can possibly extract the optimal 8-edge cut.

Some insight into why spectral embeddings tend to have this problem can be obtained from the spectral method's electrical interpretation. In this view the graph is represented by a resistor network [7]. Current flowing in this network causes voltage drops across the resistors, thus determining the nodes' voltages and hence their positions. When current flows through a long series of resistors, it induces a progressive voltage drop. This is what causes the excessive length of the embeddings of the horizontal girder-like structures which are blocking all vertical hyperplane cuts in figure 1(b).

If the embedding method were somehow not based on current, but rather on flow, which does not distinguish between a pipe and a series of pipes, then the long girders could retract into the two sides of the embedding, as suggested by figure 1(c), and the best cut would be revealed. Because theoretical flow-like embedding methods such as [14] are currently not practical, we point out that in cases like figure 1(b), where the spectral method has not chosen an incorrect direction for the cut, one can use an S-T max flow problem with the flow running in the recommended direction (horizontally for this embedding) to extract the good cut even though it is hidden from all hyperplanes.

We currently use two different flow-based rounding methods. A method called MQI looks for quotient cuts, and is already described in [13]. Another method, that we shall call Midflow, looks for β-balanced cuts. The input to Midflow is a graph and an ordering of its nodes (obtained e.g. from a spectral embedding or from the projection of any embedding onto a line). We divide the graph's nodes into 3 sets F, L, and U. The sets F and L respectively contain the first βn and last βn nodes in the ordering, and U contains the remaining

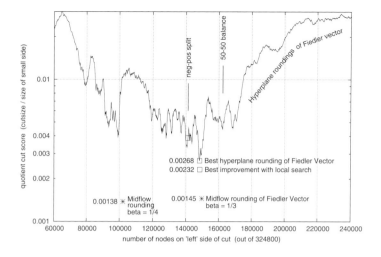

Figure 2: A typical example (see section 2.1) where flow-based rounding beats hyperplane rounding, even when the hyperplane cuts are improved with Fiduccia-Matheyses search. Note that for this spacelike graph, the best quotient cuts have reasonably good balance.

$U = n - 2\beta n$ nodes, which are "up for grabs". We set up an S-T max flow problem with one node for every graph node plus 2 new nodes for the source and sink. For each graph edge there are two arcs, one in each direction, with unit capacity. Finally, the nodes in F are pinned to the source and the nodes in L are pinned to sink by infinite capacity arcs. This max-flow problem can be solved by a good implementation of the push-relabel algorithm (such as Goldberg and Cherkassky's hi_pr [4]) in time that empirically is nearly linear with a very good constant factor. Figure 6 shows that solving a MidFlow problem with hi_pr can be 1000 times cheaper than finding a spectral embedding with ARPACK.

When the goal is finding good β-balanced cuts, MidFlow rounding is strictly more powerful than hyperplane rounding; from a given node ordering hyperplane rounding chooses the best of $U + 1$ candidate cuts, while MidFlow rounding chooses the best of 2^U candidates, including all of those considered by hyperplane rounding. [Similarly, MQI rounding is strictly more powerful than hyperplane rounding for the task of finding good quotient cuts.]

2.1 A concrete example

The plot in figure 2 shows a number of cuts in a 324,800 node nearly planar graph derived from a 700x464 pixel downward-looking view of some clouds over some mountains.[1] The y-axis of the plot is quotient cut score; smaller values are better. We note in passing that the commonly used split point $\hat{x} = 0$ does *not* yield the best hyperplane cut. Our main point is that the two cuts generated by MidFlow rounding of the Fiedler vector (with $\beta = \frac{1}{3}$ and $\beta = \frac{1}{4}$) are nearly twice as good as the best hyperplane cut. Even after the best hyperplane cut has been improved by taking the best result of 100 runs of a version of Fiduccia-Matheyses local search, it is still much worse than the cuts obtained by flow-based rounding.

---

[1]The graph's edges are unweighted but are chosen by a randomized rule which is more likely to include an edge between two neighboring pixels if they have a similar grey value. Good cuts in the graph tend to run along discontinuities in the image, as one would expect.

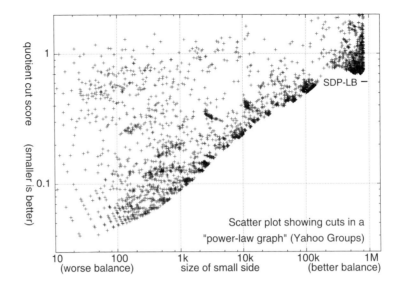

Figure 3: This scatter plot of cuts in a 1.6 million node collaborative filtering graph shows a surprising relationship between cut quality and balance (see section 3). The SDP lower bound proves that *all* balanced cuts are worse than the unbalanced cuts seen on the left.

2.2 Effectiveness on real graphs and benchmarks

We have found the flow-based Midflow and MQI rounding methods to be highly effective in practice on diverse classes of graphs including space-like graphs and power law graphs. Results for real-world power law graphs are shown in figure 5. Results for a number of FE meshes can be found on the Graph Partitioning Archive website `http://staffweb.cms.gre.ac.uk/~c.walshaw/partition`, which keeps track of the best nearly balanced cuts ever found for a number of classic benchmarks. Using flow-based rounding to extract cuts from spectral-type embeddings, we have found new record cuts for the majority of the largest graphs on the site, including `fe_body`, `t60k`, `wing`, `brack2`, `fe_tooth`, `fe_rotor`, `598a`, `144`, `wave`, `m14b`, and `auto`. It is interesting to note that the spectral method previously did not own any of the records for these classic benchmarks, although it could have if flow-based rounding had been used instead of hyperplane rounding.

3 Finding balanced cuts in "power law" graphs

The spectral method does not require cuts to have perfect balance, but the denominator in its quotient-style objective function does reward balance and punish imbalance. Thus one might expect the spectral method to produce cuts with fairly good balance, and this is what does happen for the class of spacelike graphs that inform much of our intuition.

However, there are now many economically important "power law" [5] graphs whose best quotient cuts have extremely bad balance. Examples at Yahoo include the web graph, social graphs based on DLBP co-authorship and Yahoo IM buddy lists, a music similarity graph, and bipartite collaborative filtering graphs relating Yahoo Groups with users, and advertisers with search phrases. To save space we show one scatter plot (figure 3) of quotient cut scores versus balance that is typical for graphs from this class. We see that apparently there is a tradeoff between these two quantities, and in fact the quotient cut score gets better as

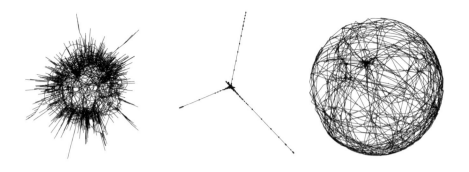

Figure 4: Left: a social graph with octopus structure as predicted by Chung and Lu [5]. Center: a "normalized cut" Spectral embedding chops off one tentacle per dimension. Right: an SDP embedding looks better and is more useful for finding balanced cuts.

balance gets worse, which is exactly the opposite of what one would expect.

When run on graphs of this type, the spectral method (and other quotient cut methods such as Metis+MQI [13]) wants to chop off tiny pieces. This has at least two bad practical effects. First, cutting off a tiny piece after paying for a computation on the whole graph kills the scalability of divide and conquer algorithms by causing their overall run time to increase e.g. from $n \log n$ to n^2. Second, low-dimensional spectral embeddings of these graphs (see e.g. figure 4(b) are nearly useless for visualization, and are also very poor inputs for clustering schemes that use a small number of eigenvectors.

These problems can be avoided by solving a semidefinite relaxation of graph bisection that has a much stronger balance constraint. This SDP (explained in the next section) has a long history, with connections to papers going all the way back to Donath and Hoffman [6] (via the concept of "eigenvalue optimization"). In 2004, Arora, Rao, and Vazirani [14] proved the best-ever approximation guarantee for graph partitioning by analysing a version of this SDP which was augmented with certain triangle inequalities that serve much the same purpose as flow (but which are too expensive to solve for large graphs).

3.1 A semidefinite program which strengthens the balance requirement

The graph bisection problem can be expressed as a Quadratic Integer Program as follows. There is an n-element column vector x of indicator variables x_i, each of which assigns one node to a particular side of the cut by assuming a value from the set $\{-1, 1\}$. With these indicator values, the objective function $\frac{1}{4}x^T L x$ (where L is the graph's discrete Laplacian matrix) works out to be equal to the number of edges crossing the cut. Finally, the requirement of perfect balance is expressed by the constraint $x^T e = 0$, where e is a vector of all ones. Since this QIP exactly encodes the graph bisection problem, solving it is NP-hard.

The spectral relaxation of this QIP attains solvability by allowing the indicator variables to assume arbitrary real values, provided that their average squared magnitude is 1.0. After this change, the objective function $\frac{1}{4}x^T L x$ is now just a lower bound on the cutsize. More interestingly for the present discussion, the balance constraint $x^T e = 0$ now permits a qualitatively different kind of balance where a tiny group of nodes moves a long way out from the origin where the nodes acquire enough leverage to counterbalance everyone else. For graphs where the best quotient cut has good balance (e.g. meshes) this does not actually happen, but for graphs whose best quotient cut has bad balance, it does happen, as can be seen in figure 4(b).

719

These undesired solutions could be ruled out by requiring the squared magnitudes of the indicator values to be 1.0 individually instead of on average. However, in one dimension that would require picking values from the set $\{-1, 1\}$, which would once again cause the problem to be NP-hard. Fortunately, there is a way to escape from this dilemma which was brought to the attention of the CS community by the Max Cut algorithm of Goemans and Williamson [9]: if we allow the indicator variables to assume values that are r-dimensional unit vectors for some sufficiently large r,[2] then the program is solvable even with the strict requirement that every vector has squared length 1.0. After a small change of notation to reflect the fact that the collected indicator variables now form an n by r matrix X rather than a vector, this idea results in the nonlinear program

$$min\left\{\frac{1}{4}L \bullet (XX^T) : diag(XX^T) = e, e^T(XX^T)e = 0\right\} \qquad (1)$$

which becomes an SDP by a change of variables from XX^T to the "Gram matrix" G:

$$min\left\{\frac{1}{4}L \bullet G : diag(G) = e, e^T Ge = 0, G \succeq 0\right\} \qquad (2)$$

The added constraint $G \succeq 0$ requires G to be positive semidefinite, so that it can be factored to get back to the desired matrix of indicator vectors X.

3.2 Methods for solving the SDP for large graphs

Interior point methods cannot solve (2) for graphs with more than a few thousand nodes, but newer methods achieve better scaling by ensuring that all dense n by n matrices have only an implicit (and approximate) existence. A good example is Helmberg and Rendl's program SBmethod [11], which can solve the dual of (2) for graphs with about 50,000 nodes by converting it to an equivalent "eigenvalue optimization" problem. The output of SBmethod is a low-rank approximate spectral factorization of the Gram matrix, consisting of an estimated rank r, plus an n by r matrix X whose rows are the nodes' indicator vectors. SBmethod typically produces r-values that are much smaller than n or even $\sqrt{2n}$. Moreover they seem to match the true dimensionality of simple spacelike graphs. For example, for a 3-d mesh we get $r = 4$, which is 3 dimensions for the manifold plus one more dimension for the hypersphere that it is wrapped around.

Burer and Monteiro's direct low-rank solver SDP-LR scales even better [2]. Surprisingly, their approach is to essentially forget about the SDP (2) and instead use non-linear programming techniques to solve (1). Specifically, they use an augmented Lagrangian approach to move the constraints into the objective function, which they then minimize using limited memory BFGS. A follow-up paper [3] provides a theoretical explanation of why the method does not fall into bad local minima despite the apparent non-convexity of (1). We have successfully run Burer and Monteiro's code on large graphs containing more than a million nodes. We typically run it several times with different small fixed values of r, and then choose the smallest r which allows the objective function to reach its best known value. On medium-size graphs this produces estimates for r which are in rough agreement with those produced by SBmethod. The run time scaling of SDP-LR is compared with that of ARPACK and hi_pr in figure 6.

---

[2]In the original work $r = n$, but there are theoretical reasons for believing that $r \sim \sqrt{2n}$ is big enough [3], plus there is empirical evidence that much smaller values work in practice.

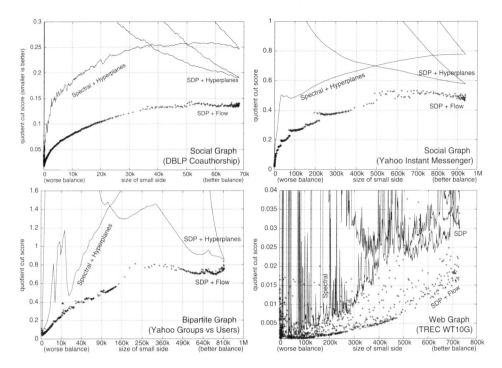

Figure 5: Each of these four plots contains two lines showing the results of sweeping a hyperplane through a spectral embedding and through one dimension of an SDP embedding. In all four cases, the spectral line is lower on the left, and the SDP line is lower on the right, which means that Spectral produces better unbalanced cuts and the SDP produces better balanced cuts. Cuts obtained by rounding random 1-d projections of the SDP embedding using Midflow (to produce β-balanced cuts) followed by MQI (to improve the quotient cut score) are also shown; these flow-based cuts are consistently better than hyperplane cuts.

3.3 Results

We have used the `minbis` program from Burer and Monteiro's `SDP-LR_v0.130301` package (with $r < 10$) to approximately solve (1) for several large graphs including: a 130,000 node social graph representing co-authorship in DBLP; a 1.9 million node social graph built from the buddy lists of a subset of the users of Yahoo Instant Messenger; a 1.6 million node bipartite graph relating Yahoo Groups and users; and a 1.5 million node graph made by symmetrizing the TREC WT10G web graph. It is clear from figure 5 that in all four cases the SDP embedding leads to better balanced cuts, and that flow-based rounding works better hyperplane rounding. Also, figures 4(b) and 4(c) show 3-d Spectral and SDP embeddings of a small subset of the Yahoo IM social graph; the SDP embedding is qualitatively different and arguably better for visualization purposes.

Acknowledgments

We thank Satish Rao for many useful discussions.

References

[1] N. Alon and V.D. Milman. λ_1, isoperimetric inequalities for graphs, and superconcentrators. *Journal of Combinatorial Theory, Series B*, 38:73–88, 1985.

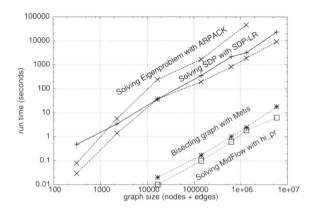

Figure 6: Run time scaling on subsets of the Yahoo IM graph. Finding Spectral and SDP embeddings with ARPACK and SDP-LR requires about the same amount of time, while MidFlow rounding with hi_pr is about 1000 times faster.

[2] Samuel Burer and Renato D.C. Monteiro. A nonlinear programming algorithm for solving semidefinite programs via low-rank factorization. *Mathematical Programming (series B)*, 95(2):329–357, 2003.

[3] Samuel Burer and Renato D.C. Monteiro. Local minima and convergence in low-rank semidefinite programming. Technical report, Department of Management Sciences, University of Iowa, September 2003.

[4] Boris V. Cherkassky and Andrew V. Goldberg. On implementing the push-relabel method for the maximum flow problem. *Algorithmica*, 19(4):390–410, 1997.

[5] F. Chung and L. Lu. Average distances in random graphs with given expected degree sequences. *Proceedings of National Academy of Science*, 99:15879–15882, 2002.

[6] W.E. Donath and A. J. Hoffman. Lower bounds for partitioning of graphs. *IBM J. Res. Develop.*, 17:420–425, 1973.

[7] Peter G. Doyle and J. Laurie Snell. Random walks and electric networks, 1984. Mathematical Association of America; now available under the GPL.

[8] C.M. Fiduccia and R.M. Mattheyses. A linear time heuristic for improving network partitions. In *Design Automation Conference*, pages 175–181, 1982.

[9] Michel X. Goemans and David P. Williamson. Improved Approximation Algorithms for Maximum Cut and Satisfiability Problems Using Semidefinite Programming. *J. Assoc. Comput. Mach.*, 42:1115–1145, 1995.

[10] Stephen Guattery and Gary L. Miller. On the quality of spectral separators. *SIAM Journal on Matrix Analysis and Applications*, 19(3):701–719, 1998.

[11] C. Helmberg. Numerical evaluation of sbmethod. *Math. Programming*, 95(2):381–406, 2003.

[12] Bruce Hendrickson and Robert W. Leland. A multi-level algorithm for partitioning graphs. In *Supercomputing*, 1995.

[13] Kevin Lang and Satish Rao. A flow-based method for improving the expansion or conductance of graph cuts. In *Integer Programming and Combinatorial Optimization*, pages 325–337, 2003.

[14] Umesh V. Vazirani Sanjeev Arora, Satish Rao. Expander flows, geometric embeddings and graph partitioning. In *STOC*, pages 222–231, 2004.

[15] Jianbo Shi and Jitendra Malik. Normalized cuts and image segmentation. *IEEE Transactions on Pattern Analysis and Machine Intelligence*, 22(8):888–905, 2000.

[16] Daniel A. Spielman and Shang-Hua Teng. Spectral partitioning works: Planar graphs and finite element meshes. In *FOCS*, pages 96–105, 1996.

Fusion of Similarity Data in Clustering

Tilman Lange and Joachim M. Buhmann
(langet,jbuhmann)@inf.ethz.ch
Institute of Computational Science, Dept. of Computer Sience,
ETH Zurich, Switzerland

Abstract

Fusing multiple information sources can yield significant benefits to successfully accomplish learning tasks. Many studies have focussed on fusing information in *supervised* learning contexts. We present an approach to utilize multiple information sources in the form of similarity data for *unsupervised* learning. Based on similarity information, the clustering task is phrased as a non-negative matrix factorization problem of a mixture of similarity measurements. The tradeoff between the informativeness of data sources and the sparseness of their mixture is controlled by an entropy-based weighting mechanism. For the purpose of model selection, a stability-based approach is employed to ensure the selection of the most self-consistent hypothesis. The experiments demonstrate the performance of the method on toy as well as real world data sets.

1 Introduction

Clustering has found increasing attention in the past few years due to the enormous information flood in many areas of information processing and data analysis. The ability of an algorithm to determine an interesting partition of the set of objects under consideration, however, heavily depends on the available information. It is, therefore, reasonable to equip an algorithm with as much information as possible and to endow it with the capability to distinguish between *relevant* and *irrelevant* information sources. How to reasonably identify a weighting of the different information sources such that an interesting group structure can be successfully uncovered, remains, however, a largely unresolved issue.

Different sources of information about the same objects naturally arise in many application scenarios. In computer vision, for example, information sources can consist of plain intensity measurements, edge maps, the similarity to other images or even human similarity assessments. Similarly in bio-informatics: the similarity of proteins,e.g., can be assessed in different ways, ranging from the comparison of gene profiles to direct comparisons at the sequence level using alignment methods.

In this work, we use a non-negative matrix factorization approach (nmf) to *pairwise* clustering of similarity data that is extended in a second step in order to incorporate a suitable weighting of multiple information sources, leading to a *mixture* of similarities. The latter represents the main contribution of this work. Algorithms for nmf have recently found a lot of attention. Our proposal is inspired by the work in [11] and [5]. Only recently, [18] have also employed a nmf to perform clustering. For the purpose of model selection, we employ a stability-based approach that has already been successfully applied to model selection problems in clustering (e.g. in [9]). Instead of following the strategy to first embed the similarities into a space with Euclidean geometry and then to perform clustering and, where required, feature selection/weighting on the stacked feature vector, we advocate an approach that is closer to the original similarity data by performing nmf.

Some work has been devoted to feature selection and weighting in clustering problems. In [13] a variant of the k-means algorithm has been studied that employs the Fisher criterion to assess the importance of individual features. In [14, 10], Gaussian mixture model-based approaches to feature selection are introduced. The more general problem of learning a suitable metric has also been investigated, e.g. in [17]. Similarity measurements represent a particularly generic form of providing input to a clustering algorithm. Fusing such representations has only recently been studied in the context of kernel-based *supervised* learning, e.g. in [7] using semi-definite programming and in [3] using a boosting procedure. In [1], an approach to learning the bandwidth parameter of an rbf-kernel for spectral clustering is studied.

The paper is organized as follows: section 2 introduces the nmf-based clustering method combined with a data-source weighting (section 3). Section 4 discusses an out-of-sample extension allowing us to *predict* assignments and to employ the *stability principle* for model selection. Experimental evidence in favor of our approach is given in section 5.

2   Clustering by Non-Negative Matrix Factorization

Suppose we want to group a finite set of objects $\mathcal{O}_n := \{o_1, \ldots, o_n\}$. Usually, there are multiple ways of measuring the similarity between different objects. Such relations give rise to similarities $s_{ij} := s(o_i, o_j)$ [1] where we assume non-negativity $s_{ij} \geq 0$, symmetry $s_{ji} = s_{ij}$, and boundedness $s_{ij} < \infty$. For n objects, we summarize the similarity data in a $n \times n$ matrix $\mathbf{S} = (s_{ij})$ which is re-normalized to $\mathbf{P} = \mathbf{S}/\mathbf{1}_n^t \mathbf{S} \mathbf{1}_n$, where $\mathbf{1}_n := (1, \ldots, 1)^t$. The re-normalized similarities can be interpreted as the probability of the *joint* occurrence of objects i, j.

We aim now at finding a non-negative matrix factorization of $\mathbf{P} \in [0, 1]^{n \times n}$ into a product $\mathbf{W}\mathbf{H}^t$ of the $n \times k$ matrices $\mathbf{W}$ and $\mathbf{H}$ with non-negative entries for which additionally holds $\mathbf{1}_n^t \mathbf{W} \mathbf{1}_k = 1$ and $\mathbf{H}^t \mathbf{1}_n = \mathbf{1}_k$, where k denotes the number of clusters. That is, one aims at explaining the overall probability for a co-occurrence by a latent cause, the unobserved classes. The constraints ensure, that the entries of both, $\mathbf{W}$ and $\mathbf{H}$, can be considered as probabilities: the entry $w_{i\nu}$ of $\mathbf{W}$ is the joint probability $q(i, \nu)$ of object i and class ν whereas h_{jk} in $\mathbf{H}$ is the probability $q(j|\nu)$. This model implicitly assumes independence of object i and j conditioned on ν. Given a factorization of $\mathbf{P}$ in $\mathbf{W}$ and $\mathbf{H}$, we can use the maximum a posteriori estimate, $\arg\max_\nu h_{i\nu} \sum_j w_{j\nu}$, to arrive at a *hard* assignment of objects to classes.

In order to obtain a factorization, we *minimize the cross-entropy*

$$C(\mathbf{P}\|\mathbf{W}\mathbf{H}^t) := -\sum_{i,j} p_{ij} \log \sum_\nu w_{i\nu} h_{j\nu} \tag{1}$$

which becomes minimal *iff* $\mathbf{P} = \mathbf{W}\mathbf{H}^t$ [2] and is not convex in $\mathbf{W}$ and $\mathbf{H}$ together. Note, that the factorization is not necessarily unique. We resort to a local optimization scheme, which is inspired by the Expectation-Maximization (EM) algorithm: Let $\tau_{\nu ij} \geq 0$ with $\sum_\nu \tau_{\nu ij} = 1$. Then, by the convexity of $-\log x$, we obtain $-\log \sum_\nu w_{i\nu} h_{j\nu} \leq -\sum_\nu \tau_{\nu ij} \log \frac{w_{i\nu} h_{j\nu}}{\tau_{\nu ij}}$,

---

[1] In the following, we represent objects by their indices.

[2] The Kullback-Leibler divergence is $D(\mathbf{P}\|\mathbf{W}\mathbf{H}^t) = -H(\mathbf{P}) + C(\mathbf{P}\|\mathbf{W}\mathbf{H}^t) \geq 0$ with equality *iff* $\mathbf{P} = \mathbf{W}\mathbf{H}^t$.

which yields the relaxed objective function:

$$\tilde{C}(\mathbf{P}\|\mathbf{W}\mathbf{H}^t) := -\sum_{i,j,\nu} p_{ij}\tau_{\nu ij} \log w_{i\nu}h_{j\nu} + \tau_{\nu ij} \log \tau_{\nu ij} \geq C(\mathbf{P}\|\mathbf{W}\mathbf{H}^t). \quad (2)$$

With this relaxation, we can employ an *alternating minimization* scheme for minimizing the bound on C. As in EM, one iterates

1. Given $\mathbf{W}$ and $\mathbf{H}$, minimize $\tilde{C}$ w.r.t. $\tau_{\nu ij}$

2. Given the values $\tau_{\nu ij}$, find estimates for $\mathbf{W}$ and $\mathbf{H}$ by minimizing $\tilde{C}$.

until convergence, which produces a sequence of estimates

$$\tau_{\nu ij}^{(t)} = \frac{w_{i\nu}^{(t)}h_{j\nu}^{(t)}}{\sum_\mu w_{i\mu}^{(t)}h_{j\mu}^{(t)}}, \quad w_{i\nu}^{(t+1)} = \sum_j p_{ij}\tau_{\nu ij}^{(t)}, \quad h_{j\nu}^{(t+1)} = \frac{\sum_i p_{ij}\tau_{\nu ij}^{(t)}}{\sum_{a,b} p_{ab}\tau_{\nu ab}^{(t)}} \quad (3)$$

that converges to a local minimum of $\tilde{C}$. This is an instance of an MM algorithm [8]. We use the convention $h_{j\nu} = 0$ whenever $\sum_{i,j} p_{ij}\tau_{\nu ij} = 0$. The per-iteration complexity is $O(n^2)$.

3 Fusing Multiple Data Sources

Measuring the similarity of objects in, say, L different ways results in L normalized similarity matrices $\mathbf{P}_1, \ldots, \mathbf{P}_L$. We introduce now weights α_l, $1 \leq l \leq L$, with $\sum_l \alpha_l = 1$. For fixed $\boldsymbol{\alpha} = (\alpha_l) \in [0,1]^L$, the aggregated and normalized similarity becomes the convex combination $\bar{\mathbf{P}} = \sum_l \alpha_l \mathbf{P}_l$. Hence, $\bar{p}_{ij}$ is a *mixture* of individual similarities $p_{ij}^{(l)}$, i.e. a mixture of different explanations. Again, we seek a good factorization of $\bar{\mathbf{P}}$ by minimizing the cross-entropy, which then becomes

$$\min_{\boldsymbol{\alpha},\mathbf{W},\mathbf{H}} \mathbb{E}_{\boldsymbol{\alpha}}\left[C(\mathbf{P}_l\|\mathbf{W}\mathbf{H}^t)\right] \quad (4)$$

where $\mathbb{E}_{\boldsymbol{\alpha}}[f_l] = \sum_l \alpha_l f_l$ denotes the expectation w.r.t. the discrete distribution $\boldsymbol{\alpha}$. The same relaxation as in the last section can be used, i.e. for all $\boldsymbol{\alpha}$, $\mathbf{W}$ and $\mathbf{H}$, we have $\mathbb{E}_{\boldsymbol{\alpha}}\left[C(\mathbf{P}_l\|\mathbf{W}\mathbf{H}^t)\right] \leq \mathbb{E}_{\boldsymbol{\alpha}}[\tilde{C}(\mathbf{P}_l\|\mathbf{W}\mathbf{H}^t)]$. Hence, we can employ a slightly modified, *nested* alternating minimization approach: Given fixed $\boldsymbol{\alpha}$, obtain estimates $\mathbf{W}$ and $\mathbf{H}$ using the relaxation of the last section. The update equations change to

$$w_{i\nu}^{(t+1)} = \sum_l \alpha_l \sum_j p_{ij}^{(l)}\tau_{\nu ij}^{(t)}, \quad h_{j\nu}^{(t+1)} = \frac{\sum_l \alpha_l \sum_i p_{ij}^{(l)}\tau_{\nu ij}^{(t)}}{\sum_l \alpha_l \sum_{i,j} p_{ij}^{(l)}\tau_{\nu ij}^{(t)}}. \quad (5)$$

Given the current estimates of $\mathbf{W}$ and $\mathbf{H}$, we could minimize the objective in equation (4) w.r.t. $\boldsymbol{\alpha}$ subject to the constraint $\|\boldsymbol{\alpha}\|_1 = 1$. To this end, set $c_l := C(\mathbf{P}_l\|\mathbf{W}\mathbf{H}^t)$ and let $\mathbf{c} = (c_l)_l$. Minimizing the expression in equation (4) subject to the constraints $\sum_l \alpha_l = 1$ and $\boldsymbol{\alpha} \succeq 0$, therefore, becomes a *linear program (LP)* $\min_{\boldsymbol{\alpha}} \mathbf{c}^t\boldsymbol{\alpha}$ such that $\mathbf{1}_L^t\boldsymbol{\alpha} = 1$, $\boldsymbol{\alpha} \succeq 0$, where $\succeq$ denotes the element-wise $\geq$-relation. The LP solution is very sparse since the optimal solutions for the linear program lie on the corners of the simplex in the positive orthant spanned by the constraints. In particular, it lacks a means to control the *sparseness* of the coefficients $\boldsymbol{\alpha}$. We, therefore, use a maximum entropy approach ([6]) for sparseness control: the entropy is upper bounded by $\log L$ and measures the sparseness of the vector $\boldsymbol{\alpha}$, since the lower the entropy the more peaked the distribution $\boldsymbol{\alpha}$ can be. Hence, by *lower bounding* the entropy, we specify the maximal admissible sparseness. This approach is reasonable as we actually want to combine *multiple* (not only identify one) information sources but the best fit in an unsupervised problem will be usually obtained by choosing only a single source. Thus, we modify the objective originally given in eq. (4) to the entropy-regularized problem $\mathbb{E}_{\boldsymbol{\alpha}}[\tilde{C}(\mathbf{P}_l \| \mathbf{W}\mathbf{H}^t)] - \eta H(\boldsymbol{\alpha})$, so that the mathematical program given above becomes

$$\min_{\boldsymbol{\alpha}} \mathbf{c}^t \boldsymbol{\alpha} - \eta H(\boldsymbol{\alpha}) \qquad \text{s.t.} \ \mathbf{1}_L^t \boldsymbol{\alpha} = 1, \ \boldsymbol{\alpha} \succeq 0, \tag{6}$$

where H denotes the (discrete) entropy and $\eta \in \mathbb{R}_+$ is a positive Lagrange parameter. The optimization problem in eq. (6) has an analytical solution, namely the Gibbs distribution

$$\alpha_l \propto \exp(-c_l/\eta) \tag{7}$$

For $\eta \to \infty$ one obtains $\alpha_l = 1/L$, while for $\eta \to 0$, the LP solution is recovered and the estimates become the sparser the more the individual c_l differ. Put differently, the parameter η enables us to explore the space of different similarity combinations. The issue of selecting a reasonable value for the parameter η will be discussed in the next section.

Iterating this nested procedure will yield a *locally* optimal solution to the problem of minimizing the entropy-constrained objective, since (i) we obtain a local minimum of the modified objective function and (ii) solving the outer optimization problem can only further *decrease* the entropy-constrained objective function.

4   Generalization and Model Selection

In this section, we introduce an out-of-sample extension that allows us to classify objects, that have not been used for learning the parameters $\boldsymbol{\alpha}$, $\mathbf{W}$ and $\mathbf{H}$. The extension mechanism can be seen as in spirit of the Nyström extension (c.f. [16]). Introducing such a generalization mechanism is worthwhile for two reasons: (i) To speed-up the computation if the number n of objects under consideration is very large: By selecting a small subset of $m \ll n$ objects for the initial fit followed by the application of a computationally less expensive prediction step, one can realize such a speed-up. (ii) The free parameters of the approach, the number of clusters k as well as the sparseness control parameter η, can be estimated using a re-sampling-based stability assessment that relies on the ability of an algorithm to generalize to previously unseen objects.

Out-of-Sample Extension: Suppose we have to predict class memberships for $r \ (= n - m$ in the hold-out case) additional objects in the $r \times m$ matrix $\tilde{\mathbf{S}}_l$. Given the decomposition into $\mathbf{W}$ and $\mathbf{H}$, let z_{ik} be the "posterior" estimated for the i-th object in the data set used for the original fit, i.e. $z_{i\nu} \propto h_{i\nu} \sum_j w_{j\nu}$. We can express the weighted, normalized similarity between a new object o and object i as $\hat{p}_{io} := \sum_l \alpha_l \tilde{s}_{oi}^{(l)} / \sum_{l,j} \alpha_l \tilde{s}_{oj}^{(l)}$. We *approximate* now $z_{o\nu}$ for a new object o by

$$\hat{z}_{o\nu} = \sum_i z_{i\nu} \hat{p}_{io}, \tag{8}$$

which amounts to an *interpolation* of the $z_{o\nu}$. These values can be obtained using the originally computed $z_{i\nu}$ which are weighted according to their similarity between object i and o. In the analogy to the Nyström approximation, the $(z_{i\nu})$ play the role of basis elements while the $\hat{p}_{io}$ amount to coefficients in the basis approximation. The prediction procedure requires $O(mr(l + r + k))$ steps.

Model Selection: The approach presented so far has two free parameters, the number of classes k and the sparseness penalty η. In [9], a method for determining the number of classes has been introduced, that assesses the variability of clustering solutions. Thus, we focus on selecting η using stability. The assessment can be regarded as a generalization of cross-validation, as it relies on the dissimilarity of solutions generated from multiple sub-samples. In a second step, the solutions obtained from these samples are extended to the complete data set by an appropriate predictor. Multiple classifications of the same data

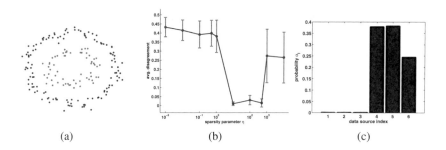

| (a) | (b) | (c) |

Figure 1: Results on the toy data set (1(a)): The stability assessment (1(b)) suggests the range $\eta \in \{10^1, 10^2, 5 \cdot 10^2\}$, which yield solutions matching the ground-truth. In 1(c), the α_l are depicted for a sub-sample and η in this range.

set are obtained, whose similarity can be measured. For two clustering solutions $\mathbf{Y}, \mathbf{Y}' \in \{1, \ldots, k\}^n$, we define their disagreement as

$$d(\mathbf{Y}, \mathbf{Y}') = \min_{\pi \in \mathfrak{S}_k} \frac{1}{n} \sum_{i=1}^{n} \mathbb{I}_{\{y_i \neq \pi(y_i')\}} \qquad (9)$$

where $\mathfrak{S}_k$ denotes the set of all permutation on sets of size k and $\mathbb{I}_A$ is the indicator function on the expression A. The measure quantifies the 0-1 loss after the labels have been permuted, so that the two clustering solutions are in the best possible agreement. Perfect agreement up to a permutation of the labels implies $d(\mathbf{Y}, \mathbf{Y}') = 0$. The optimal permutation can be determined in $O(k^3)$ by phrasing the problem as a weighted bipartite matching problem. Following the approach in [9], we select the η, given a pre-specified range of admissible values, such that the *average* disagreement observed on B sub-samples is minimal. In this sense, the entropy regularization mechanism guides the search for similarity combinations leading to stable grouping solutions. Note that, multiple minima can occur and may yield solutions emphasizing different aspects of the data.

5   Experimental Results and Discussion

The performance of our proposal is explored by analyzing toy and real world data. For the model selection (sec. 4), we have used $B = 20$ sub-samples with the proposed out-of-sample extension for prediction. For the stability assessment, different η have been chosen by $\eta \in \{10^{-3}, 10^{-2}, 10^{-1}, .5, 1, 10^1, 10^2, 5 \cdot 10^2, 10^3, 10^4\}$. We compared our results with NCut [15] and Lee and Seung's two NMF algorithms [11] (which measure the approximation error of the factorization with (i) the KL divergence and (ii) the squared Frobenius norm) applied to the uniform combination of similarities.

Toy Experiment: Figure 1(a) depicts a data set consisting of two nested rings, where the clustering task consists of identifying each ring as a class. We used rbf-kernels $k(\mathbf{x}, \mathbf{y}) = \exp(-\|\mathbf{x} - \mathbf{y}\|^2 / 2\sigma^2)$ for σ varying in $\{10^{-4}, 10^{-3}, 10^{-2}, 10^0, 10^1\}$ as well as the path kernel introduced in [4]. All methods *fail* when used with the individual kernels except for the path-kernel. The non-trivial problem is to detect the correct structure despite the disturbing influence of 5 un-informative kernels. Data sets of size $\lceil n/5 \rceil$ have been generated by sub-sampling. Figure 1(b) depicts the stability assessment, where we see very small disagreements for $\eta \in \{10^1, 10^2, 5 \cdot 10^2\}$. At the minimum, the solution almost perfectly matches the ground-truth (1 error). A plot of the resulting $\boldsymbol{\alpha}$-coefficients is given in figure 1(c). NCut as well as the other nmf-methods lead to an error rate of ≈ 0.5 when applied to the uniformly combined similarities.

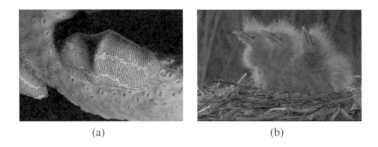

(a)

(b)

Figure 2: Images for the segmentation experiments.

Image segmentation example:[3] The next task consists of finding a reasonable segmentation of the images depicted in figures 2(b) and 2(a). For both images, we measured localized intensity histograms and additionally computed Gabor filter responses (e.g. [12]) on 3 scales for 4 different orientations. For each response image, the same histogramming procedure has been used. For all the histograms, we computed the pairwise Jensen-Shannon divergence (e.g. [2]) for all pairs (i, j) of image sites and took the element-wise exponential of the negative Jensen-Shannon divergences. The resulting similarity matrices have been used as input for the nmf-based data fusion. For the sub-sampling, $m = 500$ objects have been employed. Figures 3(a) (for the shell image) and 3(b) (for the bird image) show the stability curves for these examples which exhibit minima for non-trivial η resulting in non-uniform $\boldsymbol{\alpha}$. Figure 3(c) depicts the resulting segmentation generated using $\boldsymbol{\alpha}$ indicated by the stability assessment, while 3(d) shows a segmentation result, where $\boldsymbol{\alpha}$ is closer to the uniform distribution but the stability score for the corresponding η is low. Again, we can see that weighting the different similarity measurements has a beneficial effect, since it leads to improved results. The comparison with the NCut result on the uniformly weighted data (fig. 3(e)) confirms that a non-trivial weighting is desirable here. Note that we have used the full data set with NCut. For, the image in fig. 2(b), we observe similar behavior: the stability selected solution (fig. 3(f)) is more meaningful than the NCut solution (fig. 3(g)) obtained on the uniformly weighted data. In this example, the intensity information dominates the solution obtained on the uniformly combined similarities. However, the texture information alone does *not* yield a sensible segmentation. Only the non-trivial combination, where the influence of intensity information is decreased and that of the texture information is increased, gives rise to the desired result. It is additionally noteworthy, that the prediction mechanism employed works rather well: In both examples, it has been able to generalize the segmentation from $m = 500$ to more than 3500 objects. However, artifacts resulting from the subsampling-and-prediction procedure cannot always be avoided, as can be seen in 3(f). They vanish, however, once the algorithm is re-applied to the full data (fig. 3(h)).

Clustering of Protein Sequences: Our final application is about the functional categorization of yeast proteins. We partially adopted the data used in [7] [4]. Since several of the 3588 proteins belong to *more than one* category, we extracted a subset of 1579 proteins exclusively belonging to one of the three categories *cell cycle + DNA processing*,*transcription* and *protein fate*. This step ensures a clear ground-truth for comparison. Of the matrices used in [7], we employed a Gauss Kernel derived from gene expression profiles, one derived from Swiss-Waterman alignments, one obtained from comparisons of protein domains as well as two diffusion kernels derived from protein-protein interaction data. Although the data is not very discriminative for the 3-class problem, the solutions generated on the data combined using the $\boldsymbol{\alpha}$ for the most stable η lead to more than 10% improvement w.r.t. the

---

[3]Only comparisons with NCut reported. The nmf results are slightly worse than those of NCut.

[4]The data is available at http://noble.gs.washington.edu/proj/yeast/.

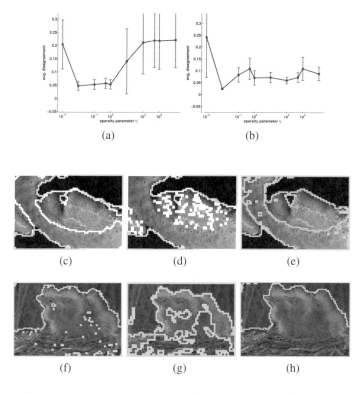

Figure 3: Stability plots and segmentation results for the images in 2(a) and 2(b) (see text).

ground-truth (the disagreement measure of section 4 is used) in comparison with the solution obtained using the least stable η-parameter. The latter, however, was hardly better than random guessing by having an overall disagreement of more than 0.60 (more precisely, 0.6392 ± 0.0455) on this data. For the most stable η, we observed a disagreement around 0.52 depending on the sub-sample (best 0.5267 ± 0.0403). In this case, the largest weight was assigned to the protein-protein interaction data. NCut and the two nmf methods proposed in [11] lead to rates 0.5953, 0.6080 and 0.6035, respectively, when applied to the naive combination. Note, that the clustering results are comparable with some of those obtained in [7], where the protein-protein interaction data has been used to construct a (supervised) classifier.

6 Conclusion

This work introduced an approach to combining similarity data originating from multiple sources for grouping a set of objects. Adopting a pairwise clustering perspective enables a smooth integration of multiple similarity measurements. To be able to distinguish between desired and distractive information, a weighting mechanism is introduced leading to a potentially sparse convex combination of the measurements. Here, an entropy constraint is employed to control the amount of sparseness actually allowed. A stability-based model selection mechanism is used to select this free parameter. We emphasize, that this procedure represents a completely unsupervised model selection strategy. The experimental evaluation on toy and real world data demonstrates that our proposal yields meaningful partitions and is able to distinguish between desired and spurious structure in data.

Future work will focus on (i) improving the optimization of the proposed model, (ii) the integration of additional constraints and (iii) the introduction of a *cluster-specific* weighting mechanism. The proposed method as well as its relation to other approaches discussed in the literature is currently under further investigation.

References

[1] F. R. Bach and M. I. Jordan. Learning spectral clustering. In *NIPS*, volume 16. MIT Press, 2004.

[2] J. Burbea and C. R. Rao. On the convexity of some divergence measures based on entropy functions. *IEEE Trans. Inform. Theory*, 28(3), 1982.

[3] K. Crammer, J. Keshet, and Y. Singer. Kernel design using boosting. In *NIPS*, volume 15. MIT Press, 2003.

[4] B. Fischer, V. Roth, and J. M. Buhmann. Clustering with the connectivity kernel. In *NIPS*, volume 16. MIT Press, 2004.

[5] Thomas Hofmann. Unsupervised learning by probabilistic latent semantic analysis. *Mach. Learn.*, 42(1-2):177–196, 2001.

[6] E. T. Jaynes. Information theory and statistical mechanics, I and II. *Physical Reviews*, 106 and 108:620–630 and 171–190, 1957.

[7] G. R. G. Lanckriet, M. Deng, N. Cristianini, M. I. Jordan, and W. S. Noble. Kernel-based data fusion and its application to protein function prediction in yeast. In *Pacific Symposium on Biocomputing*, pages 300–311, 2004.

[8] Kenneth Lange. *Optimization*. Springer Texts in Statistics. Springer, 2004.

[9] T. Lange, M. Braun, V. Roth, and J.M. Buhmann. Stability-based model selection. In *NIPS*, volume 15. MIT Press, 2003.

[10] M. H. C. Law, M. A. T. Figueiredo, and A. K. Jain. Simultaneous feature selection and clustering using mixture models. *IEEE Trans. Pattern Anal. Mach. Intell.*, 26(9):1154–1166, 2004.

[11] Daniel D. Lee and H. Sebastian Seung. Algorithms for non-negative matrix factorization. In *NIPS*, volume 13, pages 556–562, 2000.

[12] B. S. Manjunath and W. Y. Ma. Texture features for browsing and retrieval of image data. *IEEE Trans. Pattern Anal. Mach. Intell.*, 18(8):837–842, 1996.

[13] D. S. Modha and W. S. Spangler. Feature weighting in k-means clustering. *Mach. Learn.*, 52(3):217–237, 2003.

[14] V. Roth and T. Lange. Feature selection in clustering problems. In *NIPS*, volume 16. MIT Press, 2004.

[15] Jianbo Shi and Jitendra Malik. Normalized cuts and image segmentation. *IEEE Trans. Pattern Anal. Mach. Intell.*, 22(8):888–905, 2000.

[16] C. K. I. Williams and M. Seeger. Using the Nystrï¿½m method to speed up kernel machines. In *NIPS*, volume 13. MIT Press, 2001.

[17] E. Xing, A. Ng, M. Jordan, and S. Russell. Distance metric learning with application to clustering with side-information. In *NIPS*, volume 15, 2003.

[18] W. Xu, X. Liu, and Y. Gong. Document clustering based on non-negative matrix factorization. In *SIGIR '03*, pages 267–273. ACM Press, 2003.

A PAC-Bayes approach to the Set Covering Machine

François Laviolette, Mario Marchand
IFT-GLO, Université Laval
Sainte-Foy (QC) Canada, G1K-7P4
given_name.surname@ift.ulaval.ca

Mohak Shah
SITE, University of Ottawa
Ottawa, Ont. Canada,K1N-6N5
mshah@site.uottawa.ca

Abstract

We design a new learning algorithm for the Set Covering Machine from a PAC-Bayes perspective and propose a PAC-Bayes risk bound which is minimized for classifiers achieving a non trivial margin-sparsity trade-off.

1 Introduction

Learning algorithms try to produce classifiers with small prediction error by trying to optimize some function that can be computed from a training set of examples and a classifier. We currently do not know exactly what function should be optimized but several forms have been proposed. At one end of the spectrum, we have the set covering machine (SCM), proposed by Marchand and Shawe-Taylor (2002), that tries to find the sparsest classifier making few training errors. At the other end, we have the support vector machine (SVM), proposed by Boser et al. (1992), that tries to find the maximum soft-margin separating hyperplane on the training data. Since both of these learning machines can produce classifiers having small prediction error, we have recently investigated (Laviolette et al., 2005) if better classifiers could be found by learning algorithms that try to optimize a non-trivial function that depends on both the sparsity of a classifier and the magnitude of its separating margin. Our main result was a general data-compression risk bound that applies to any algorithm producing classifiers represented by two complementary sources of information: a subset of the training set, called the *compression set*, and a *message string* of additional information. In addition, we proposed a new algorithm for the SCM where the information string was used to encode radius values for data-dependent balls and, consequently, the location of the decision surface of the classifier. Since a small message string is sufficient when large regions of equally good radius values exist for balls, the data compression risk bound applied to this version of the SCM exhibits, *indirectly*, a non-trivial margin-sparsity trade-off. Moreover, this version of the SCM currently suffers from the fact that the radius values, used in the final classifier, depends on a *a priori* chosen distance scale R. In this paper, we use a new PAC-Bayes approach, that applies to the sample-compression setting, and present a new learning algorithm for the SCM that does not suffer from this scaling problem. Moreover, we propose a risk bound that depends more explicitly on the margin and which is also minimized by classifiers achieving a non-trivial margin-sparsity trade-off.

2 Definitions

We consider binary classification problems where the input space $\mathcal{X}$ consists of an arbitrary subset of $\mathbb{R}^n$ and the output space $\mathcal{Y} = \{0, 1\}$. An example $\mathbf{z} \stackrel{\text{def}}{=} (\mathbf{x}, y)$ is an input-output pair where $\mathbf{x} \in \mathcal{X}$ and $y \in \mathcal{Y}$. In the probably approximately correct (PAC) setting, we assume that each example $\mathbf{z}$ is generated independently according to the same (but unknown) distribution D. The (true) *risk* $R(f)$ of a classifier $f : \mathcal{X} \to \mathcal{Y}$ is defined to be the probability that f misclassifies $\mathbf{z}$ on a random draw according to D:

$$R(f) \stackrel{\text{def}}{=} \Pr_{(\mathbf{x}, y) \sim D} (f(\mathbf{x}) \neq y) = \mathbf{E}_{(\mathbf{x}, y) \sim D} I(f(\mathbf{x}) \neq y)$$

where $I(a) = 1$ if predicate a is true and 0 otherwise. Given a training set $S = (\mathbf{z}_1, \ldots, \mathbf{z}_m)$ of m examples, the task of a learning algorithm is to construct a classifier with the smallest possible risk without any information about D. To achieve this goal, the learner can compute the *empirical risk* $R_S(f)$ of any given classifier f according to:

$$R_S(f) \stackrel{\text{def}}{=} \frac{1}{m} \sum_{i=1}^{m} I(f(\mathbf{x}_i) \neq y_i) \stackrel{\text{def}}{=} \mathbf{E}_{(\mathbf{x}, y) \sim S} I(f(\mathbf{x}) \neq y)$$

We focus on learning algorithms that construct a *conjunction (or disjunction)* of features called *data-dependent balls* from a training set. Each *data-dependent ball* is defined by a *center* and a *radius* value. The center is an input example $\mathbf{x}_i$ chosen among the training set S. For any test example $\mathbf{x}$, the output of a ball h, of radius ρ and centered on example $\mathbf{x}_i$, and is given by

$$h_{i,\rho}(\mathbf{x}) \stackrel{\text{def}}{=} \begin{cases} y_i & \text{if } d(\mathbf{x}, \mathbf{x}_i) \leq \rho \\ \bar{y}_i & \text{otherwise} \end{cases},$$

where $\bar{y}_i$ denotes the boolean complement of y_i and $d(\mathbf{x}, \mathbf{x}_i)$ denotes the distance between the two points. Note that any metric can be used for the distance here.

To specify a *conjunction of balls* we first need to list all the examples that participate as centers for the balls in the conjunction. For this purpose, we use a vector $\mathbf{i} \stackrel{\text{def}}{=} (i_1, \ldots, i_{|\mathbf{i}|})$ of indices $i_j \in \{1, \ldots, m\}$ such that $i_1 < i_2 < \ldots < i_{|\mathbf{i}|}$ where $|\mathbf{i}|$ is the number of indices present in $\mathbf{i}$ (and thus the number of balls in the conjunction).

To complete the specification of a conjunction of balls, we need a vector $\boldsymbol{\rho} = (\rho_{i_1}, \rho_{i_2}, \ldots, \rho_{i_{|\mathbf{i}|}})$ of radius values where $i_j \in \{1, \ldots, m\}$ for $j \in \{1, \ldots, |\mathbf{i}|\}$.

On any input example $\mathbf{x}$, the output $C_{\mathbf{i}, \boldsymbol{\rho}}(\mathbf{x})$ of a conjunction of balls is given by:

$$C_{\mathbf{i}, \boldsymbol{\rho}}(\mathbf{x}) \stackrel{\text{def}}{=} \begin{cases} 1 & \text{if } h_{j, \rho_j}(\mathbf{x}) = 1 \quad \forall j \in \mathbf{i} \\ 0 & \text{if } \exists j \in \mathbf{i} : h_{j, \rho_j}(\mathbf{x}) = 0 \end{cases}$$

Finally, any algorithm that builds a conjunction can be used to build a disjunction just by exchanging the role of the positive and negative labelled examples. Due to lack of space, we describe here only the case of a conjunction.

3 A PAC-Bayes Risk Bound

The PAC-Bayes approach, initiated by McAllester (1999a), aims at providing PAC guarantees to "Bayesian" learning algorithms. These algorithms are specified in terms of a *prior distribution* P over a space of classifiers that characterizes our prior belief about good classifiers (before the observation of the data) and a *posterior distribution* Q (over the same space of classifiers) that takes into account the additional information provided by the training data. A remarkable result that came out from this line of research, known as the "PAC-Bayes theorem", provides a tight upper bound on the risk of a stochastic classifier called the *Gibbs classifier*. Given an input example $\mathbf{x}$, the label $G_Q(\mathbf{x})$ assigned to $\mathbf{x}$ by the Gibbs classifier is defined by the following process. We first choose a classifier h according to the posterior distribution Q and then use h to assign the label $h(\mathbf{x})$ to $\mathbf{x}$. The PAC-Bayes theorem was first proposed by McAllester (1999b) and later improved by others (see Langford (2005) for a survey). However, for all these versions of the PAC-Bayes theorem, the prior P must be defined without reference to the training data. Consequently, these theorems cannot be applied to the sample-compression setting where classifiers are partly described by a subset of the training data (as for the case of the SCM).

In the sample compression setting, each classifier is described by a subset $S_\mathbf{i}$ of the training data, called the *compression set*, and a *message string* σ that represents the additional information needed to obtain a classifier. In other words, in this setting, there exists a reconstruction function $\mathcal{R}$ that outputs a classifier $\mathcal{R}(\sigma, S_\mathbf{i})$ when given an arbitrary compression set $S_\mathbf{i}$ and a message string σ.

Given a training set S, the compression set $S_\mathbf{i} \subseteq S$ is defined by a vector of indices $\mathbf{i} \overset{\text{def}}{=} (i_1, \ldots, i_{|\mathbf{i}|})$ that points to individual examples in S. For the case of a conjunction of balls, each $j \in \mathbf{i}$ will point to a training example that is used for a ball center and the message string σ will be the vector $\boldsymbol{\rho}$ of radius values (defined above) that are used for the balls. Hence, given $S_\mathbf{i}$ and $\boldsymbol{\rho}$, the classifier obtained from $\mathcal{R}(\boldsymbol{\rho}, S_\mathbf{i})$ is just the conjunction $C_{\mathbf{i}, \boldsymbol{\rho}}$ defined previously.[1]

Recently, Laviolette and Marchand (2005) have extended the PAC-Bayes theorem to the sample-compression setting. Their proposed risk bound depends on a data-independent prior P and a data-dependent posterior Q that are both defined on $\mathcal{I} \times \mathcal{M}$ where $\mathcal{I}$ denotes the set of the 2^m possible index vectors $\mathbf{i}$ and $\mathcal{M}$ denotes, in our case, the set of possible radius vectors $\boldsymbol{\rho}$. The posterior Q is used by a stochastic classifier, called the *sample-compressed Gibbs classifier* G_Q, defined as follows. Given a training set S and given a new (testing) input example $\mathbf{x}$, a sample-compressed Gibbs classifier G_Q chooses randomly $(\mathbf{i}, \boldsymbol{\rho})$ according to Q to obtain classifier $\mathcal{R}(\boldsymbol{\rho}, S_\mathbf{i})$ which is then used to determine the class label of $\mathbf{x}$.

In this paper we focus on the case where, given any training set S, the learner returns a Gibbs classifier defined with a posterior distribution Q having all its weight on a single vector $\mathbf{i}$. Hence, a single compression set $S_\mathbf{i}$ will be used for the final classifier. However, the radius ρ_i for each $i \in \mathbf{i}$ will be chosen stochastically according to the posterior Q. Hence we consider posteriors Q such that $Q(\mathbf{i}', \boldsymbol{\rho}) = I(\mathbf{i} = \mathbf{i}') Q_\mathbf{i}(\boldsymbol{\rho})$ where $\mathbf{i}$ is the vector of indices chosen by the learner. Hence, given a training set S, the true risk $R(G_{Q_\mathbf{i}})$ of $G_{Q_\mathbf{i}}$ and its empirical risk $R_S(G_{Q_\mathbf{i}})$ are defined by

$$R(G_{Q_\mathbf{i}}) \overset{\text{def}}{=} \underset{\boldsymbol{\rho} \sim Q_\mathbf{i}}{\mathbf{E}} R(\mathcal{R}(\boldsymbol{\rho}, S_\mathbf{i})) \quad ; \quad R_S(G_{Q_\mathbf{i}}) \overset{\text{def}}{=} \underset{\boldsymbol{\rho} \sim Q_\mathbf{i}}{\mathbf{E}} R_{S_{\bar{\mathbf{i}}}}(\mathcal{R}(\boldsymbol{\rho}, S_\mathbf{i})) ,$$

where $\bar{\mathbf{i}}$ denotes the set of indices not present in $\mathbf{i}$. Thus, $\bar{\mathbf{i}} \cap \mathbf{i} = \emptyset$ and $\mathbf{i} \cup \bar{\mathbf{i}} = (1, \ldots, m)$.

In contrast with the posterior Q, the prior P assigns a non zero weight to several vectors $\mathbf{i}$. Let $P_\mathcal{I}(\mathbf{i})$ denote the prior probability P assigned to vector $\mathbf{i}$ and let $P_\mathbf{i}(\boldsymbol{\rho})$

---

[1]We assume that the examples in $S_\mathbf{i}$ are ordered as in S so that the kth radius value in $\boldsymbol{\rho}$ is assigned to the kth example in $S_\mathbf{i}$.

denote the probability density function associated with prior P given $\mathbf{i}$. The risk bound depends on the Kullback-Leibler divergence $\mathrm{KL}(Q\|P)$ between the posterior Q and the prior P which, in our case, gives

$$\mathrm{KL}(Q_{\mathbf{i}}\|P) = \mathop{\mathbf{E}}_{\boldsymbol{\rho} \sim Q_{\mathbf{i}}} \ln \frac{Q_{\mathbf{i}}(\boldsymbol{\rho})}{P_{\mathcal{I}}(\mathbf{i})P_{\mathbf{i}}(\boldsymbol{\rho})} .$$

For these classes of posteriors Q and priors P, the PAC-Bayes theorem of Laviolette and Marchand (2005) reduces to the following simpler version.

Theorem 1 (Laviolette and Marchand (2005)) *Given all our previous definitions, for any prior P and for any $\delta \in (0, 1]$*

$$\mathop{\mathrm{Pr}}_{S \sim D^m} \left(\forall Q_{\mathbf{i}} : \mathrm{kl}(R_S(G_{Q_{\mathbf{i}}})\|R(G_{Q_{\mathbf{i}}})) \le \tfrac{1}{m-|\mathbf{i}|} \left[\mathrm{KL}(Q_{\mathbf{i}}\|P) + \ln \tfrac{m+1}{\delta} \right] \right) \ge 1 - \delta ,$$

where

$$\mathrm{kl}(q\|p) \stackrel{\mathrm{def}}{=} q \ln \frac{q}{p} + (1-q) \ln \frac{1-q}{1-p} .$$

To obtain a bound for $R(G_{Q_{\mathbf{i}}})$ we need to specify $Q_{\mathbf{i}}(\boldsymbol{\rho})$, $P_{\mathcal{I}}(\mathbf{i})$, and $P_{\mathbf{i}}(\boldsymbol{\rho})$.

Since all vectors $\mathbf{i}$ having the same size $|\mathbf{i}|$ are, *a priori*, equally "good", we choose

$$P_{\mathcal{I}}(\mathbf{i}) = \frac{1}{\binom{m}{|\mathbf{i}|}} p(|\mathbf{i}|)$$

for any $p(\cdot)$ such that $\sum_{d=0}^{m} p(d) = 1$. We could choose $p(d) = 1/(m+1)$ for $d \in \{0, 1, \ldots, m\}$ if we have complete ignorance about the size $|\mathbf{i}|$ of the final classifier. But since the risk bound will deteriorate for large $|\mathbf{i}|$, it is generally preferable to choose, for $p(d)$, a slowly decreasing function of d.

For the specification of $P_{\mathbf{i}}(\boldsymbol{\rho})$, we assume that each radius value, in some predefined interval $[0, R]$, is equally likely to be chosen for each ρ_i such that $i \in \mathbf{i}$. Here R is some "large" distance specified *a priori*. For $Q_{\mathbf{i}}(\boldsymbol{\rho})$, a margin interval $[a_i, b_i] \subseteq [0, R]$ of equally good radius values is chosen by the learner for each $i \in \mathbf{i}$. Hence, we choose

$$P_{\mathbf{i}}(\boldsymbol{\rho}) = \prod_{i \in \mathbf{i}} \frac{1}{R} = \left(\frac{1}{R}\right)^{|\mathbf{i}|} \quad ; \quad Q_{\mathbf{i}}(\boldsymbol{\rho}) = \prod_{i \in \mathbf{i}} \frac{1}{b_i - a_i} .$$

Therefore, the Gibbs classifier returned by the learner will draw each radius ρ_i uniformly in $[a_i, b_i]$. A deterministic classifier is then specified by fixing each radius values $\rho_i \in [a_i, b_i]$. It is tempting at this point to choose $\rho_i = (a_i + b_i)/2 \; \forall i \in \mathbf{i}$ (*i.e.*, in the middle of each interval). However, we will see shortly that the PAC-Bayes theorem offers a better guarantee for another type of deterministic classifier.

Consequently, with these choices for $Q_{\mathbf{i}}(\boldsymbol{\rho})$, $P_{\mathcal{I}}(\mathbf{i})$, and $P_{\mathbf{i}}(\boldsymbol{\rho})$, the KL divergence between $Q_{\mathbf{i}}$ and P is given by

$$KL(Q_{\mathbf{i}}\|P) = \ln \binom{m}{|\mathbf{i}|} + \ln \left(\frac{1}{p(|\mathbf{i}|)}\right) + \sum_{i \in \mathbf{i}} \ln \left(\frac{R}{b_i - a_i}\right) .$$

Notice that the KL divergence is small for small values of $|\mathbf{i}|$ (whenever $p(|\mathbf{i}|)$ is not too small) and for large margin values $(b_i - a_i)$. Hence, the KL divergence term in Theorem 1 favors both sparsity (small $|\mathbf{i}|$) and large margins. Hence, in practice, the minimum might occur for some $G_{Q_{\mathbf{i}}}$ that sacrifices sparsity whenever larger margins can be found.

Since the posterior Q is identified by $\mathbf{i}$ and by the intervals $[a_i, b_i]$ $\forall i \in \mathbf{i}$, we will now refer to the Gibbs classifier G_{Q_i} by $G_{\mathbf{ab}}^{\mathbf{i}}$ where $\mathbf{a}$ and $\mathbf{b}$ are the vectors formed by the unions of a_is and b_is respectively. To obtain a risk bound for $G_{\mathbf{ab}}^{\mathbf{i}}$, we need to find a closed-form expression for $R_S(G_{\mathbf{ab}}^{\mathbf{i}})$. For this task, let $U[a, b]$ denote the uniform distribution over $[a, b]$ and let $\sigma_{a,b}^i(\mathbf{x})$ be the probability that a ball with center $\mathbf{x}_i$ assigns to $\mathbf{x}$ the class label y_i when its radius ρ is drawn according to $U[a, b]$:

$$\sigma_{a,b}^i(\mathbf{x}) \stackrel{\text{def}}{=} \Pr_{\rho \sim U[a,b]} (h_{i,\rho}(\mathbf{x}) = y_i) = \begin{cases} 1 & \text{if } d(\mathbf{x}, \mathbf{x}_i) \leq a \\ \frac{b - d(\mathbf{x}, \mathbf{x}_i)}{b-a} & \text{if } a \leq d(\mathbf{x}, \mathbf{x}_i) \leq b \\ 0 & \text{if } d(\mathbf{x}, \mathbf{x}_i) \geq b_i \; . \end{cases}$$

Therefore,

$$\zeta_{a,b}^i(\mathbf{x}) \stackrel{\text{def}}{=} \Pr_{\rho \sim U[a,b]} (h_{i,\rho}(\mathbf{x}) = 1) = \begin{cases} \sigma_{a,b}^i(\mathbf{x}) & \text{if } y_i = 1 \\ 1 - \sigma_{a,b}^i(\mathbf{x}) & \text{if } y_i = 0 \; . \end{cases}$$

Now let $G_{\mathbf{ab}}^{\mathbf{i}}(\mathbf{x})$ denote the probability that $C_{\mathbf{i},\rho}(\mathbf{x}) = 1$ when each $\rho_i \in \boldsymbol{\rho}$ are drawn according to $U[a_i, b_i]$. We then have

$$G_{\mathbf{ab}}^{\mathbf{i}}(\mathbf{x}) = \prod_{i \in \mathbf{i}} \zeta_{a_i,b_i}^i(\mathbf{x}) \; .$$

Consequently, the risk $R_{(\mathbf{x},y)}(G_{\mathbf{ab}}^{\mathbf{i}})$ on a single example $(\mathbf{x}, y)$ is given by $G_{\mathbf{ab}}^{\mathbf{i}}(\mathbf{x})$ if $y = 0$ and by $1 - G_{\mathbf{ab}}^{\mathbf{i}}(\mathbf{x})$ otherwise. Therefore

$$R_{(\mathbf{x},y)}(G_{\mathbf{ab}}^{\mathbf{i}}) = y(1 - G_{\mathbf{ab}}^{\mathbf{i}}(\mathbf{x})) + (1 - y)G_{\mathbf{ab}}^{\mathbf{i}}(\mathbf{x}) = (1 - 2y)(G_{\mathbf{ab}}^{\mathbf{i}}(\mathbf{x}) - y) \; .$$

Hence, the empirical risk $R_S(G_{\mathbf{ab}}^{\mathbf{i}})$ of the Gibbs classifier $G_{\mathbf{ab}}^{\mathbf{i}}$ is given by

$$R_S(G_{\mathbf{ab}}^{\mathbf{i}}) = \frac{1}{m - |\mathbf{i}|} \sum_{j \in \bar{\mathbf{i}}} (1 - 2y_j)(G_{\mathbf{ab}}^{\mathbf{i}}(\mathbf{x}_j) - y_j) \; .$$

From this expression we see that $R_S(G_{\mathbf{ab}}^{\mathbf{i}})$ is small when $G_{\mathbf{ab}}^{\mathbf{i}}(\mathbf{x}_j) \to y_j$ $\forall j \in \bar{\mathbf{i}}$. Training points where $G_{\mathbf{ab}}^{\mathbf{i}}(\mathbf{x}_j) \approx 1/2$ should therefore be avoided.

The PAC-Bayes theorem below provides a risk bound for the Gibbs classifier $G_{\mathbf{ab}}^{\mathbf{i}}$. Since the Bayes classifier $B_{\mathbf{ab}}^{\mathbf{i}}$ just performs a majority vote under the same posterior distribution as the one used by $G_{\mathbf{ab}}^{\mathbf{i}}$, we have that $B_{\mathbf{ab}}^{\mathbf{i}}(\mathbf{x}) = 1$ iff $G_{\mathbf{ab}}^{\mathbf{i}}(\mathbf{x}) > 1/2$. From the above definitions, note that the decision surface of the Bayes classifier, given by $G_{\mathbf{ab}}^{\mathbf{i}}(\mathbf{x}) = 1/2$, differs from the decision surface of classifier $C_{\mathbf{i}\rho}$ when $\rho_i = (a_i + b_i)/2$ $\forall i \in \mathbf{i}$. In fact there does not exists any classifier $C_{\mathbf{i}\rho}$ that has the same decision surface as Bayes classifier $B_{\mathbf{ab}}^{\mathbf{i}}$. From the relation between $B_{\mathbf{ab}}^{\mathbf{i}}$ and $G_{\mathbf{ab}}^{\mathbf{i}}$, it also follows that $R_{(\mathbf{x},y)}(B_{\mathbf{ab}}^{\mathbf{i}}) \leq 2R_{(\mathbf{x},y)}(G_{\mathbf{ab}}^{\mathbf{i}})$ for any $(\mathbf{x}, y)$. Consequently, $R(B_{\mathbf{ab}}^{\mathbf{i}}) \leq 2R(G_{\mathbf{ab}}^{\mathbf{i}})$. Hence, we have the following theorem.

Theorem 2 *Given all our previous definitions, for any $\delta \in (0, 1]$, for any p satisfying $\sum_{d=0}^{m} p(d) = 1$, and for any fixed distance value R, we have:*

$$\Pr_{S \sim D^m} \left(\forall \mathbf{i}, \mathbf{a}, \mathbf{b} \colon R(G_{\mathbf{ab}}^{\mathbf{i}}) \leq \sup \left\{ \epsilon \colon \mathrm{kl}(R_S(G_{\mathbf{ab}}^{\mathbf{i}}) \| \epsilon) \leq \frac{1}{m - |\mathbf{i}|} \left[\ln \binom{m}{|\mathbf{i}|} + \right. \right. \right.$$

$$\left. \left. \left. + \ln \left(\frac{1}{p(|\mathbf{i}|)} \right) + \sum_{i \in \mathbf{i}} \ln \left(\frac{R}{b_i - a_i} \right) + \ln \frac{m+1}{\delta} \right] \right\} \right) \geq 1 - \delta \; .$$

Furthermore: $R(B_{\mathbf{ab}}^{\mathbf{i}}) \leq 2R(G_{\mathbf{ab}}^{\mathbf{i}})$ $\forall \mathbf{i}, \mathbf{a}, \mathbf{b}$.

Recall that the KL divergence is small for small values of $|\mathbf{i}|$ (whenever $p(|\mathbf{i}|)$ is not too small) and for large margin values $(b_i - a_i)$. Furthermore, the Gibbs empirical risk $R_S(G_{\mathbf{ab}}^{\mathbf{i}})$ is small when the training points are located far away from the Bayes decision surface $G_{\mathbf{ab}}^{\mathbf{i}}(\mathbf{x}) = 1/2$ (with $G_{\mathbf{ab}}^{\mathbf{i}}(\mathbf{x}_j) \to y_j \ \forall j \in \bar{\mathbf{i}}$). *Consequently, the Gibbs classifier with the smallest guarantee of risk should perform a non trivial margin-sparsity tradeoff.*

4 A Soft Greedy Learning Algorithm

Theorem 2 suggests that the learner should try to find the Bayes classifier $B_{\mathbf{ab}}^{\mathbf{i}}$ that uses a small number of balls (*i.e.*, a small $|\mathbf{i}|$), each with a large separating margin $(b_i - a_i)$, while keeping the empirical Gibbs risk $R_S(G_{\mathbf{ab}}^{\mathbf{i}})$ at a low value. To achieve this goal, we have adapted the greedy algorithm for the set covering machine (SCM) proposed by Marchand and Shawe-Taylor (2002). It consists of choosing the (Boolean-valued) feature i with the largest *utility* U_i defined as $U_i = |N_i| - p\,|P_i|$, where N_i is the set of negative examples covered (classified as 0) by feature i, P_i is the set of positive examples misclassified by this feature, and p is a learning parameter that gives a penalty p for each misclassified positive example. Once the feature with the largest U_i is found, we remove N_i and P_i from the training set S and then repeat (on the remaining examples) until either no more negative examples are present or that a maximum number of features has been reached.

In our case, however, we need to keep the Gibbs risk on S low instead of the risk of a deterministic classifier. Since the Gibbs risk is a "soft measure" that uses the piece-wise linear functions $\sigma_{a,b}^i$ instead of "hard" indicator functions, we need a "softer" version of the utility function U_i. Indeed, a negative example that falls in the linear region of a $\sigma_{a,b}^i$ is in fact partly covered. Following this observation, let $\mathbf{k}$ be the vector of indices of the examples that we have used as ball centers so far for the construction of the classifier. Let us first define the *covering value* $\mathcal{C}(G_{\mathbf{ab}}^{\mathbf{k}})$ of $G_{\mathbf{ab}}^{\mathbf{k}}$ by the "amount" of negative examples assigned to class 0 by $G_{\mathbf{ab}}^{\mathbf{k}}$:

$$\mathcal{C}(G_{\mathbf{ab}}^{\mathbf{k}}) \overset{\text{def}}{=} \sum_{j \in \bar{\mathbf{k}}} (1 - y_j) \left[1 - G_{\mathbf{ab}}^{\mathbf{k}}(\mathbf{x}_j) \right] .$$

We also define the *positive-side error* $\mathcal{E}(G_{\mathbf{ab}}^{\mathbf{k}})$ of $G_{\mathbf{ab}}^{\mathbf{k}}$ as the "amount" of positive examples assigned to class 0 :

$$\mathcal{E}(G_{\mathbf{ab}}^{\mathbf{k}}) \overset{\text{def}}{=} \sum_{j \in \bar{\mathbf{k}}} y_j \left[1 - G_{\mathbf{ab}}^{\mathbf{k}}(\mathbf{x}_j) \right] .$$

We now want to add another ball, centered on an example with index i, to obtain a new vector $\mathbf{k}'$ containing this new index in addition to those present in $\mathbf{k}$. Hence, we now introduce the *covering contribution* of ball i (centered on $\mathbf{x}_i$) as

$$\mathcal{C}_{\mathbf{ab}}^{\mathbf{k}}(i) \overset{\text{def}}{=} \mathcal{C}(G_{\mathbf{a}'\mathbf{b}'}^{\mathbf{k}'}) - \mathcal{C}(G_{\mathbf{ab}}^{\mathbf{k}})$$

$$= (1 - y_i) \left[1 - \zeta_{a_i,b_i}^i(\mathbf{x}_i)\, G_{\mathbf{ab}}^{\mathbf{k}}(\mathbf{x}_i) \right] + \sum_{j \in \bar{\mathbf{k}'}} (1 - y_j) \left[1 - \zeta_{a_i,b_i}^i(\mathbf{x}_j) \right] G_{\mathbf{ab}}^{\mathbf{k}}(\mathbf{x}_j) ,$$

and the *positive-side error contribution* of ball i as

$$\mathcal{E}_{\mathbf{ab}}^{\mathbf{k}}(i) \overset{\text{def}}{=} \mathcal{E}(G_{\mathbf{a}'\mathbf{b}'}^{\mathbf{k}'}) - \mathcal{E}(G_{\mathbf{ab}}^{\mathbf{k}})$$

$$= y_i \left[1 - \zeta_{a_i,b_i}^i(\mathbf{x}_i)\, G_{\mathbf{ab}}^{\mathbf{k}}(\mathbf{x}_i) \right] + \sum_{j \in \bar{\mathbf{k}'}} y_j \left[1 - \zeta_{a_i,b_i}^i(\mathbf{x}_j) \right] G_{\mathbf{ab}}^{\mathbf{k}}(\mathbf{x}_j) .$$

Typically, the covering contribution of ball i should increase its "utility" and its positive-side error should decrease it. Hence, we define the *utility $U_{\mathbf{ab}}^{\mathbf{k}}(i)$ of adding ball i to $G_{\mathbf{ab}}^{\mathbf{k}}$* as

$$U_{\mathbf{ab}}^{\mathbf{k}}(i) \quad \stackrel{\text{def}}{=} \quad \mathcal{C}_{\mathbf{ab}}^{\mathbf{k}}(i) - p\mathcal{E}_{\mathbf{ab}}^{\mathbf{k}}(i) \,,$$

where parameter p represents the *penalty* of misclassifying a positive example. For a fixed value of p, the "soft greedy" algorithm simply consists of adding, to the current Gibbs classifier, a ball with maximum added utility until either the maximum number of possible features (balls) has been reached or that all the negative examples have been (totally) covered. It is understood that, during this soft greedy algorithm, we can remove an example $(\mathbf{x}_j, y_j)$ from S whenever it is totally covered. This occurs whenever $G_{\mathbf{ab}}^{\mathbf{k}}(\mathbf{x}_j) = 0$.

The term $\sum_{i \in \mathbf{i}} \ln(R/(b_i - a_i))$, present in the risk bound of Theorem 2, favors "soft balls" having large margins $b_i - a_i$. Hence, we introduce a *margin parameter $\gamma \geq 0$* that we use as follows. At each greedy step, we first search among balls having $b_i - a_i = \gamma$. Once such a ball, of center $\mathbf{x}_i$, having maximum utility has been found, we try to increase further its utility be searching among all possible values of a_i and $b_i > a_i$ while keeping its center $\mathbf{x}_i$ fixed[2]. Both p and γ will be chosen by cross validation on the training set.

We conclude this section with an analysis of the running time of this soft greedy learning algorithm for fixed p and γ. For each potential ball center, we first sort the $m-1$ other examples with respect to their distances from the center in $O(m \log m)$ time. Then, for this center $\mathbf{x}_i$, the set of a_i values that we examine are those specified by the distances (from $\mathbf{x}_i$) of the $m-1$ sorted examples[3]. Since the examples are sorted, it takes time $\in O(km)$ to compute the covering contributions and the positive-side error *for all* the $m-1$ values of a_i. Here k is the largest number of examples falling into the margin. We are always using small enough γ values to have $k \in O(\log m)$ since, otherwise, the results are terrible. It therefore takes time $\in O(m \log m)$ to compute the utility values of all the $m-1$ different balls of a given center. This gives a time $\in O(m^2 \log m)$ to compute the utilities for all the possible m centers. Once a ball with a largest utility value has been chosen, we then try to increase further its utility by searching among $O(m^2)$ pair values for (a_i, b_i). We then remove the examples covered by this ball and repeat the algorithm on the remaining examples. It is well known that greedy algorithms of this kind have the following guarantee: if there exist r balls that covers all the m examples, the greedy algorithm will find at most $r \ln(m)$ balls. Since we almost always have $r \in O(1)$, the running time of the whole algorithm will almost always be $\in O(m^2 \log^2(m))$.

5   Empirical Results on Natural Data

We have compared the new PAC-Bayes learning algorithm (called here SCM-PB), with the old algorithm (called here SCM). Both of these algorithms were also compared with the SVM equipped with a RBF kernel of variance σ^2 and a soft margin parameter C. Each SCM algorithm used the L_2 metric since this is the metric present in the argument of the RBF kernel. However, in contrast with Laviolette et al. (2005), each SCM was constrained to use only balls having centers of the same class (negative for conjunctions and positive for disjunctions).

---

[2]The possible values for a_i and b_i are defined by the location of the training points.

[3]Recall that for each value of a_i, the value of b_i is set to $a_i + \gamma$ at this stage.

Table 1: SVM and SCM results on UCI data sets.

Data Set			SVM results				SCM		SCM-PB		
Name	train	test	C	σ^2	SVs	errs	b	errs	b	γ	errs
breastw	343	340	1	5	38	15	1	12	4	.08	10
bupa	170	175	2	.17	169	66	5	62	6	.1	67
credit	353	300	100	2	282	51	3	58	11	.09	55
glass	107	107	10	.17	51	29	5	22	16	.04	19
heart	150	147	1	.17	64	26	1	23	1	0	28
haberman	144	150	2	1	81	39	1	39	1	.2	38
USvotes	235	200	1	25	53	13	10	27	18	.14	12

Each algorithm was tested the UCI data sets of Table 1. Each data set was randomly split in two parts. About half of the examples was used for training and the remaining set of examples was used for testing. The corresponding values for these numbers of examples are given in the "train" and "test" columns of Table 1. The learning parameters of all algorithms were determined from the training set *only*. The parameters C and γ for the SVM were determined by the 5-fold cross validation (CV) method performed on the training set. The parameters that gave the smallest 5-fold CV error were then used to train the SVM on the whole training set and the resulting classifier was then run on the testing set. Exactly the same method (with the same 5-fold split) was used to determine the learning parameters of both SCM and SCM-PB.

The SVM results are reported in Table 1 where the "SVs" column refers to the number of support vectors present in the final classifier and the "errs" column refers to the number of classification errors obtained on the testing set. This notation is used also for all the SCM results reported in Table 1. In addition to this, the "b" and "γ" columns refer, respectively, to the number of balls and the margin parameter (divided by the average distance between the positive and the negative examples). The results reported for SCM-PB refer to the Bayes classifier only. The results for the Gibbs classifier are similar. We observe that, except for bupa and heart, the generalization error of SCM-PB was always smaller than SCM. However, the only significant difference occurs on USvotes. We also observe that SCM-PB generally sacrifices sparsity (compared to SCM) to obtain some margin $\gamma > 0$.

References

B. E. Boser, I. M. Guyon, and V. N. Vapnik. A training algorithm for optimal margin classifiers. In *Proceedings of the 5th Annual ACM Workshop on Computational Learning Theory*, pages 144–152. ACM Press, 1992.

John Langford. Tutorial on practical prediction theory for classification. *Journal of Machine Learning Research*, 6:273–306, 2005.

François Laviolette and Mario Marchand. PAC-Bayes risk bounds for sample-compressed Gibbs classifiers. *Proceedings of the 22nth International Conference on Machine Learning (ICML 2005)*, pages 481–488, 2005.

François Laviolette, Mario Marchand, and Mohak Shah. Margin-sparsity trade-off for the set covering machine. *Proceedings of the 16th European Conference on Machine Learning (ECML 2005); Lecture Notes in Artificial Intelligence*, 3720:206–217, 2005.

Mario Marchand and John Shawe-Taylor. The set covering machine. *Journal of Machine Learning Reasearch*, 3:723–746, 2002.

David McAllester. Some PAC-Bayesian theorems. *Machine Learning*, 37:355–363, 1999a.

David A. McAllester. Pac-bayesian model averaging. In *COLT*, pages 164–170, 1999b.

Off-Road Obstacle Avoidance through End-to-End Learning

Yann LeCun
Courant Institute of Mathematical Sciences
New York University,
New York, NY 10004, USA
http://yann.lecun.com

Urs Muller
Net-Scale Technologies
Morganville, NJ 07751, USA
urs@net-scale.com

Jan Ben
Net-Scale Technologies
Morganville, NJ 07751, USA

Eric Cosatto
NEC Laboratories,
Princeton, NJ 08540

Beat Flepp
Net-Scale Technologies
Morganville, NJ 07751, USA

Abstract

We describe a vision-based obstacle avoidance system for off-road mobile robots. The system is trained from end to end to map raw input images to steering angles. It is trained in supervised mode to predict the steering angles provided by a human driver during training runs collected in a wide variety of terrains, weather conditions, lighting conditions, and obstacle types. The robot is a 50cm off-road truck, with two forward-pointing wireless color cameras. A remote computer processes the video and controls the robot via radio. The learning system is a large 6-layer convolutional network whose input is a single left/right pair of unprocessed low-resolution images. The robot exhibits an excellent ability to detect obstacles and navigate around them in real time at speeds of 2 m/s.

1 Introduction

Autonomous off-road vehicles have vast potential applications in a wide spectrum of domains such as exploration, search and rescue, transport of supplies, environmental management, and reconnaissance. Building a fully autonomous off-road vehicle that can reliably navigate and avoid obstacles at high speed is a major challenge for robotics, and a new domain of application for machine learning research.

The last few years have seen considerable progress toward that goal, particularly in areas such as mapping the environment from active range sensors and stereo cameras [11, 7], simultaneously navigating and building maps [6, 15], and classifying obstacle types.

Among the various sub-problems of off-road vehicle navigation, obstacle detection and avoidance is a subject of prime importance. The wide diversity of appearance of potential obstacles, and the variability of the surroundings, lighting conditions, and other factors, make the problem very challenging.

Many recent efforts have attacked the problem by relying on a multiplicity of sensors, including laser range finder and radar [11]. While active sensors make the problem considerably simpler, there seems to be an interest from potential users for purely passive systems that rely exclusively on camera input. Cameras are considerably less expensive, bulky, power hungry, and detectable than active sensors, allowing levels of miniaturization that are not otherwise possible. More importantly, active sensors can be slow, limited in range, and easily confused by vegetation, despite rapid progress in the area [2].

Avoiding obstacles by relying solely on camera input requires solving a highly complex vision problem. A time-honored approach is to derive range maps from multiple images through multiple cameras or through motion [6, 5]. Deriving steering angles to avoid obstacles from the range maps is a simple matter. A large number of techniques have been proposed in the literature to construct range maps from stereo images. Such methods have been used successfully for many years for navigation in indoor environments where edge features can be reliably detected and matched [1], but navigation in outdoors environment, despite a long history, is still a challenge [14, 3]: real-time stereo algorithms are considerably less reliable in unconstrained outdoors environments. The extreme variability of lighting conditions, and the highly unstructured nature of natural objects such as tall grass, bushes and other vegetation, water surfaces, and objects with repeating textures, conspire to limit the reliability of this approach. In addition, stereo-based methods have a rather limited range, which dramatically limits the maximum driving speed.

2 End-To-End Learning for Obstacle Avoidance

In general, computing depth from stereo images is an ill-posed problem, but the depth map is only a means to an end. Ultimately, the output of an obstacle avoidance system is a set of possible steering angles that direct the robot toward traversable regions.

Our approach is to view the entire problem of mapping input stereo images to possible steering angles as a single indivisible task to be learned *from end to end*. Our learning system takes raw color images from two forward-pointing cameras mounted on the robot, and maps them to a set of possible steering angles through a single trained function.

The training data was collected by recording the actions of a human driver together with the video data. The human driver remotely drives the robot straight ahead until the robot encounters a non-traversable obstacle. The human driver then avoids the obstacle by steering the robot in the appropriate direction. The learning system is trained in supervised mode. It takes a single pair of heavily-subsampled images from the two cameras, and is trained to predict the steering angle produced by the human driver at that time.

The learning architecture is a 6-layer convolutional network [9]. The network takes the left and right 149×58 color images and produces two outputs. A large value on the first output is interpreted as a left steering command while a large value on the second output indicates a right steering command. Each layer in a convolutional network can be viewed as a set of trainable, shift-invariant linear filters with local support, followed by a point-wise non-linear saturation function. All the parameters of all the filters in the various layers are trained simultaneously. The learning algorithm minimizes the discrepancy between the desired output vector and the output vector produced by the output layer.

The approach is somewhat reminiscent of the ALVINN and MANIAC systems [13, 4]. The main differences with ALVINN are: (1) our system uses stereo cameras; (2) it is trained for off-road obtacle avoidance rather than road following; (3) Our trainable system uses a convolutional network rather than a traditional fully-connected neural net.

Convolutional networks have two considerable advantages for this applications. Their local and sparse connection scheme allows us to handle images of higher resolution than ALVINN while keeping the size of the network within reasonnable limits. Convolutional nets are particularly well suited for our task because local feature detectors that combine inputs from the left and right images can be useful for estimating distances to obstacles (possibly by estimating disparities). Furthermore, the local and shift-invariant property of the filters allows the system to learn relevant local features with a limited amount of training data.

They key advantage of the approach is that the entire function from raw pixels to steering angles is trained from data, which completely eliminates the need for feature design and selection, geometry, camera calibration, and hand-tuning of parameters. The main motivation for the use of end-to-end learning is, in fact, to eliminate the need for hand-crafted heuristics. Relying on automatic global optimization of an objective function from massive amounts for data may produce systems that are more robust to the unpredictable variability of the real world. Another potential benefit of a pure learning-based approach is that the system may use other cues than stereo disparity to detect obstacles, possibly alleviating the short-sightedness of methods based purely on stereo matching.

3 Vehicle Hardware

We built a small and light-weight vehicle which can be carried by a single person so as to facilitate data collection and testing in a wide variety of environments. Using a small, rugged and low-cost robot allowed us to drive at relatively high speed without fear of causing damage to people, property or the robot itself. The downside of this approach is the limited payload, too limited for holding the computing power necessary for the visual processing. Therefore, the robot has no significant on-board computing power. It is remotely controlled by an off-board computer. A wireless link is used to transmit video and sensor readings to the remote computer. Throttle and steering controls are sent from the computer to the robot through a regular radio control channel.

The robot chassis was built around a customized 1/10-th scale remote-controlled, electric-powered, four-wheel-drive truck which was roughly 50cm in length. The typical speed of the robot during data collection and testing sessions was roughly 2 meters per second. Two forward-pointing low-cost 1/3-inch CCD cameras were mounted 110mm apart behind a clear lexan window. With 2.5mm lenses, the horizontal field of view of each camera was about 100 degrees.

A pair of 900MHz analog video transmitters was used to send the camera outputs to the remote computer. The analog video links were subject to high signal noise, color shifts, frequent interferences, and occasional video drop-outs. But the small size, light weight, and low cost provided clear advantages. The vehicle is shown in Figure 1. The remote control station consisted of a 1.4GHz Athlon PC running Linux with video capture cards, and an interface to an R/C transmitter.

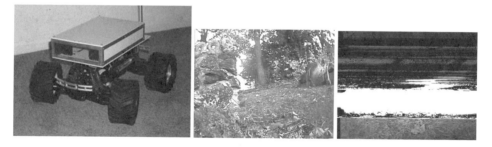

Figure 1: Left: The robot is a modified 50 cm-long truck platform controled by a remote computer. Middle: sample images images from the training data. Right: poor reception occasionally caused bad quality images.

4 Data Collection

During a data collection session, the human operator wears video goggles fed with the video signal from one the robot's cameras (no stereo), and controls the robot through a joystick connected to the PC. During each run, the PC records the output of the two video cameras at 15 frames per second, together with the steering angle and throttle setting from the operator.

A crucially important requirement of the data collection process was to collect large amounts of data with enough diversity of terrain, obstacles, and lighting conditions. Tt was necessary for the human driver to adopt a *consistent* obstacle avoidance behaviour. To ensure this, the human driver was to drive the vehicle straight ahead whenever no obstacle was present within a threatening distance. Whenever the robot approached an obstacle, the human driver had to steer left or right so as to avoid the obstacle. The general strategy for collecting training data was as follows: (a) Collecting data from as large a variety of off-road training grounds as possible. Data was collected from a large number of parks, playgrounds, frontyards and backyards of a number of suburban homes, and heavily cluttered construction areas; (b) Collecting data with various lighting conditions, i. e., different weather conditions and different times of day; (c) Collecting sequences where the vehicle starts driving straight and then is steered left or right as the robot approached an obstacle; (d) Avoiding turns when no obstacles were present; (e) Including straight runs with no obstacles and no turns as part of the training set; (f) Trying to be consistent in the turning behavior, i. e., always turning at approximately the same distance from an obstacle.

Even though great care was taken in collecting the highest quality training data, there were a number of imperfections in the training data that could not be avoided: (a) The small-form-factor, low-cost cameras presented significant differences in their default settings. In particular, the white balance of the two cameras were somewhat different; (b) To maximize image quality, the automatic gain control and automatic exposure were activated. Because of differences in fabrication, the left and right images had slightly different brightness and contrast characteristics. In particular, the AGC adjustments seem to react at different speeds and amplitudes; (c) Because of AGC, driving into the sunlight caused the images to become very dark and obstacles to become hard to detect; (d) The wireless video connection caused dropouts and distortions of some frames. Approximately 5 % of the frames were affected. An example is shown in Figures 1; (e) The cameras were mounted rigidly on the vehicle and were exposed to vibration, despite the suspension. Despite these difficult conditions, the system managed to learn the task quite well as will be shown later.

The data was recorded and archived at a resolution of $320 \times 240 \times$ pixels at 15 frames per second. The data was collected on 17 different days during the Winter of 2003/2004 (the sun was very low on the horizon). A total of 1,500 clips were collected with an average length of about 85 frames each. This resulted in a total of about 127,000 individual pairs of frames. Segments during which the robot was driven into position in preparation for a run were edited out. No other manual data cleaning took place. In the end, 95,000 frame pairs were used for training and 32,000 for validation/testing. The training pairs and testing pairs came from different sequences (and often different locations).

Figure 1 shows example snapshots from the training data, including an image with poor reception. Note that only one of the two (stereo) images is shown. High noise and frame dropouts occurred in approximately 5 % of the frames. It was decided to leave them in the training set and test set so as to train the system under realistic conditions.

5 The Learning System

The entire processing consists of a single convolutional network. The architecture of convolutional nets is somewhat inspired by the structure of biological visual systems. Convolutional nets have been used successfully in a number of vision applications such as handwriting recognition [9], object recognition [10], and face detection [12].

The input to the convolutional net consists of 6 planes of size 149×58 pixels. The six planes respectively contain the Y, U and V components for the left camera and the right camera. The input images were obtained by cropping the 320×240 images, and through $2\times$ horizontal low-pass filtering and subsampling, and $4\times$ vertical low-pass filtering and subsampling. The horizontal resolution was set higher so as to preserve more accurate image disparity information.

Each layer in a convolutional net is composed of units organized in planes called feature maps. Each unit in a feature map takes inputs from a small neighborhood within the feature maps of the previous layer. Neighborhing units in a feature map are connected to neighboring (possibly overlapping) windows. Each unit computes a weighted sum of its inputs and passes the result through a sigmoid saturation function. All units within a feature map share the same weights. Therefore, each feature map can be seen as convolving the feature maps of the previous layers with small-size kernels, and passing the sum of those convolutions through sigmoid functions. Units in a feature map detect local features at all locations on the previous layer.

The first layer contains 6 feature maps of size 147×56 connected to various combinations of the input maps through 3×3 kernels. The first feature map is connected to the YUV planes of the left image, the second feature map to the YUV planes of the right image, and the other 4 feature maps to all 6 input planes. Those 4 feature maps are binocular, and can learn filters that compare the location of features in the left and right images. Because of the weight sharing, the first layer merely has 276 free parameters (30 kernels of size 3×3 plus 6 biases). The next layer is an averaging/subsampling layer of size 49×14 whose purpose is to reduce the spatial resolution of the feature maps so as to build invariances to small geometric distortions of the input. The subsampling ratios are 3 horizontally and 4 vertically. The 3-rd layer contains 24 feature maps of size 45×12. Each feature map is connected to various subsests of maps in the previous layer through a total of 96 kernels of size 5×3. The 4-th layer is an averaging/subsampling layer of size 9×4 with 5×3 subsampling ratios. The 5-th layer contains 100 feature maps of size 1×1 connected to the 4-th layer through 2400 kernels of size 9×4 (full connection). finally, the output layer contains two units fully-connected to the 100 units in the 5-th layer. The two outputs respectively code for "turn left" and "turn right" commands. The network has 3.15 Million connections and about 72,000 trainable parameters.

The bottom half of figure 2 shows the states of the six layers of the convolutional net. the size of the input, 149×58, was essentially limited by the computing power of the remote computer (a 1.4GHz Athlon). The network as shown runs in about 60ms per image pair on the remote computer. Including all the processing, the driving system ran at a rate of 10 cycles per second.

The system's output is computed on a frame by frame basis with no memory of the past and no time window. Using multiple successive frames as input would seem like a good idea since the multiple views resulting from ego-motion facilitates the segmentation and detection of nearby obstacles. Unfortunately, the supervised learning approach precludes the use of multiple frames. The reason is that since the steering is fairly smooth in time (with long, stable periods), the current rate of turn is an excellent predictor of the next desired steering angle. But the current rate of turn is easily derived from multiple successive frames. Hence, a system trained with multiple frames would merely predict a steering angle equal to the current rate of turn as observed through the camera. This would lead to catastrophic behavior in test mode. The robot would simply turn in circles.

The system was trained with a stochastic gradient-based method that automatically sets the relative step sizes of the parameters based on the local curvature of the loss surface [8]. Gradients were computed using the variant of back-propagation appropriate for convolutional nets.

6 Results

Two performance measurements were recorded, the average loss, and the percentage of "correctly classified" steering angles. The average loss is the sum of squared differences between outputs produced by the system and the target outputs, averaged over all samples. The percentage of correctly classified steering angles measures the number of times the predicted steering angle, quantized into three bins (left, straight, right), agrees with steering angle provided by the human driver. Since the thresholds for deciding whether an angle counted as left, center, or right were somewhat arbitrary, the percentages cannot be intepreted in absolute terms, but merely as a relative figure of merit for comparing runs and architectures.

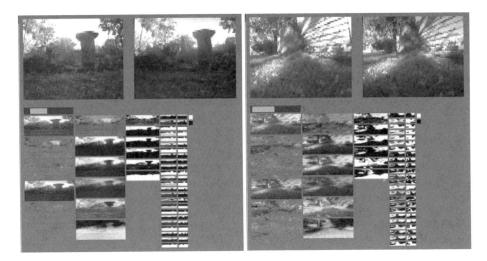

Figure 2: Internal state of the convolutional net for two sample frames. The top row shows left/right image pairs extracted from the test set. The light-blue bars below show the steering angle produced by the system. The bottom halves show the state of the layers of the network, where each column is a layer (the penultimate layer is not shown). Each rectangular image is a feature map in which each pixel represents a unit activation. The YUV components of the left and right input images are in the leftmost column.

With 95,000 training image pairs, training took 18 epochs through the training set. No significant improvements in the error rate occurred thereafter. After training, the error rate was 25.1% on the training set, and 35.8% on the test set. The average loss (mean-sqaured error) was 0.88 on the training set and 1.24 on the test set. A complete training session required about four days of CPU time on a 3.0GHz Pentium/Xeon-based server. Naturally, a classification error rate of 35.8% doesn't mean that the vehicle crashes into obstacles 35.8% of the time, but merely that the prediction of the system was in a different bin than that of the human drivers for 35.8% of the frames. The seemingly high error rate is not an accurate reflection of the actual effectiveness of the robot in the field. There are several reasons for this. First, there may be several legitimate steering angles for a given image pair: turning left or right around an obstacle may both be valid options, but our performance measure would record one of those options as incorrect. In addition, many illegitimate errors are recorded when the system starts turning at a different time than the human driver, or when the precise values of the steering angles are different enough to be in different bins, but close enough to cause the robot to avoid the obstacle. Perhaps more informative is diagram in figure 3. It shows the steering angle produced by the system and the steering angle provided by the human driver for 8000 frames from the test set. It is clear for the plot that only a small number of obstacles would not have been avoided by the robot.

The best performance measure is a set of actual runs through representative testing grounds. Videos of typical test runs are available at **http://www.cs.nyu.edu/˜yann/research/dave/index.html**.

Figure 2 shows a snapshot of the trained system in action. The network was presented with a scene that was not present in the training set. This figure shows that the system can detect obstacles and predict appropriate steering angles in the presence of back-lighting and with wild difference between the automatics gain settings of the left and right cameras.

Another visualization of the results can be seen in Figures 4. They are snapshots of video clips recorded from the vehicle's cameras while the vehicle was driving itself autonomously. Only one of the two camera outputs is shown here. Each picture also shows

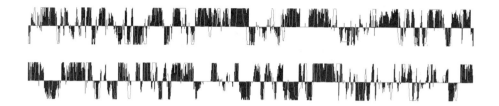

Figure 3: The steering angle produced by the system (black) compared to the steering angle provided by the human operator (red line) for 8000 frames from the test set. Very few obstacles would not have been avoided by the system.

the steering angle produced by the system for that particular input.

7 Conclusion

We have demonstrate the applicability of end-to-end learning methods to the task of obstacle avoidance for off-road robots.

A 6-layer convolutional network was trained with massive amounts of data to emulate the obstacle avoidance behavior of a human driver. the architecture of the system allowed it to learn low-level and high-level features that reliably predicted the bearing of traversible areas in the visual field.

The main advantage of the system is its robustness to the extreme diversity of situations in off-road environments. Its main design advantage is that it is trained from raw pixels to directly produce steering angles. The approach essentially eliminates the need for manual calibration, adjustments, parameter tuning etc. Furthermore, the method gets around the need to design and select an appropriate set of feature detectors, as well as the need to design robust and fast stereo algorithms.

The construction of a fully autonomous driving system for ground robots will require several other components besides the purely-reactive obstacle detection and avoidance system described here. The present work is merely one component of a future system that will include map building, visual odometry, spatial reasoning, path finding, and other strategies for the identification of traversable areas.

Acknowledgment

This project was a preliminary study for the DARPA project "Learning Applied to Ground Robots" (LAGR). The material presented is based upon work supported by the Defense Advanced Research Project Agency Information Processing Technology Office, ARPA Order No. Q458, Program Code No. 3D10, Issued by DARPA/CMO under Contract #MDA972-03-C-0111.

References

[1] N. Ayache and O. Faugeras. Maintaining representations of the environment of a mobile robot. *IEEE Trans. Robotics and Automation*, 5(6):804–819, 1989.

[2] C. Bergh, B. Kennedy, L. Matthies, and Johnson A. A compact, low power two-axis scanning laser rangefinder for mobile robots. In *The 7th Mechatronics Forum International Conference*, 2000.

[3] S. B. Goldberg, M. Maimone, and L. Matthies. Stereo vision and rover navigation software for planetary exploration. In *IEEE Aerospace Conference Proceedings*, March 2002.

[4] T. Jochem, D. Pomerleau, and C. Thorpe. Vision-based neural network road and intersection detection and traversal. In *Proc. IEEE Conf. Intelligent Robots and Systems*, volume 3, pages 344–349, August 1995.

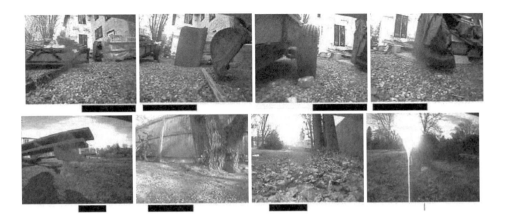

Figure 4: Snapshots from the left camera while the robots drives itself through various environment. The black bar beneath each image indicates the steering angle produced by the system. Top row: four successive snapshots showing the robot navigating through a narrow passageway between a trailer, a backhoe, and some construction material. Bottom row, left: narrow obstacles such as table legs and poles (left), and solid obstacles such as fences (center-left) are easily detected and avoided. Higly textured objects on the ground do not detract the system from the correct response (center-right). One scenario where the vehicle occasionally made wrong decisions is when the sun is in the field of view: the system seems to systematically drive towards the sun, whenever the sun is low on the horizon (right). Videos of these sequences are available at **http://www.cs.nyu.edu/~yann/research/dave/index.html**.

[5] A. Kelly and A. Stentz. Stereo vision enhancements for low-cost outdoor autonomous vehicles. In *International Conference on Robotics and Automation, Workshop WS-7, Navigation of Outdoor Autonomous Vehicles, (ICRA '98)*, May 1998.

[6] D.J. Kriegman, E. Triendl, and T.O. Binford. Stereo vision and navigation in buildings for mobile robots. *IEEE Trans. Robotics and Automation*, 5(6):792–803, 1989.

[7] E. Krotkov and M. Hebert. Mapping and positioning for a prototype lunar rover. In *Proc. IEEE Int'l Conf. Robotics and Automation*, pages 2913–2919, May 1995.

[8] Y. LeCun, L. Bottou, G. Orr, and K. Muller. Efficient backprop. In G. Orr and Muller K., editors, *Neural Networks: Tricks of the trade*. Springer, 1998.

[9] Yann LeCun, Leon Bottou, Yoshua Bengio, and Patrick Haffner. Gradient-based learning applied to document recognition. *Proceedings of the IEEE*, 86(11):2278–2324, November 1998.

[10] Yann LeCun, Fu-Jie Huang, and Leon Bottou. Learning methods for generic object recognition with invariance to pose and lighting. In *Proceedings of CVPR'04*. IEEE Press, 2004.

[11] L. Matthies, E. Gat, R. Harrison, B. Wilcox, R. Volpe, and T. Litwin. Mars microrover navigation: Performance evaluation and enhancement. In *Proc. IEEE Int'l Conf. Intelligent Robots and Systems*, volume 1, pages 433–440, August 1995.

[12] R. Osadchy, M. Miller, and Y. LeCun. Synergistic face detection and pose estimation with energy-based model. In *Advances in Neural Information Processing Systems (NIPS 2004)*. MIT Press, 2005.

[13] Dean A. Pomerleau. Knowledge-based training of artificial neural netowrks for autonomous robot driving. In J. Connell and S. Mahadevan, editors, *Robot Learning*. Kluwer Academic Publishing, 1993.

[14] C. Thorpe, M. Herbert, T. Kanade, and S Shafer. Vision and navigation for the carnegie-mellon navlab. *IEEE Trans. Pattern Analysis and Machine Intelligence*, 10(3):362–372, May 1988.

[15] S. Thrun. Learning metric-topological maps for indoor mobile robot navigation. *Artificial Intelligence*, 99(1):21–71, February 1998.

Dual-Tree Fast Gauss Transforms

Dongryeol Lee
Computer Science
Carnegie Mellon Univ.
dongryel@cmu.edu

Alexander Gray
Computer Science
Carnegie Mellon Univ.
agray@cs.cmu.edu

Andrew Moore
Computer Science
Carnegie Mellon Univ.
awm@cs.cmu.edu

Abstract

In previous work we presented an efficient approach to computing kernel summations which arise in many machine learning methods such as kernel density estimation. This approach, dual-tree recursion with finite-difference approximation, generalized existing methods for similar problems arising in computational physics in two ways appropriate for statistical problems: toward distribution sensitivity and general dimension, partly by avoiding series expansions. While this proved to be the fastest practical method for multivariate kernel density estimation at the optimal bandwidth, it is much less efficient at larger-than-optimal bandwidths. In this work, we explore the extent to which the dual-tree approach can be integrated with multipole-like Hermite expansions in order to achieve reasonable efficiency across all bandwidth scales, though only for low dimensionalities. In the process, we derive and demonstrate the first truly hierarchical fast Gauss transforms, effectively combining the best tools from discrete algorithms and continuous approximation theory.

1 Fast Gaussian Summation

Kernel summations are fundamental in both statistics/learning and computational physics. This paper will focus on the common form $G(x_q) = \sum_{r=1}^{N_R} e^{\frac{-||x_q - x_r||^2}{2h^2}}$ *i.e.* where the kernel is the Gaussian kernel with scaling parameter, or *bandwidth h*, there are N_R *reference points* x_r, and we desire the sum for N_Q different *query points* x_q. Such kernel summations appear in a wide array of statistical/learning methods [5], perhaps most obviously in kernel density estimation [11], the most widely used distribution-free method for the fundamental task of density estimation, which will be our main example. Understanding kernel summation algorithms from a recently developed unified perspective [5] begins with the picture of Figure 1, then separately considers the discrete and continuous aspects.

Discrete/geometric aspect. In terms of discrete algorithmic structure, the dual-tree framework of [5], in the context of kernel summation, generalizes all of the well-known algorithms. [1] It was applied to the problem of kernel density estimation in [7] using a simple

---

[1] These include the Barnes-Hut algorithm [2], the Fast Multipole Method [8], Appel's algorithm [1], and the WSPD [4]: the dual-tree method is a node-node algorithm (considers query regions rather than points), is fully recursive, can use distribution-sensitive data structures such as *kd*-trees, and is bichromatic (can specialize for differing query and reference sets).

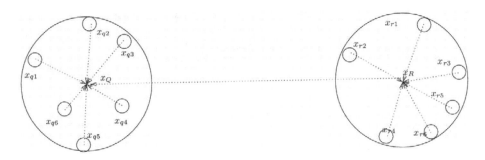

Figure 1: The basic idea is to approximate the kernel sum contribution of some subset of the reference points X_R, lying in some compact region of space R with centroid x_R, to a query point. In more efficient schemes a query region is considered, *i.e.* the approximate contribution is made to an entire subset of the query points X_Q lying in some region of space Q, with centroid x_Q.

finite-difference approximation, which is tantamount to a centroid approximation. Partially by avoiding series expansions, which depend explicitly on the dimension, the result was the fastest such algorithm for general dimension, when operating at the optimal bandwidth. Unfortunately, when performing cross-validation to determine the (initially unknown) optimal bandwidth, both suboptimally small and large bandwidths must be evaluated. The finite-difference-based dual-tree method tends to be efficient at or below the optimal bandwidth, and at very large bandwidths, but for intermediately-large bandwidths it suffers.

Continuous/approximation aspect. This motivates investigating a multipole-like series approximation which is appropriate for the Gaussian kernel, as introduced by [9], which can be shown the generalize the centroid approximation. We define the Hermite functions $h_n(t)$ by $h_n(t) = e^{-t^2} H_n(t)$, where the Hermite polynomials $H_n(t)$ are defined by the Rodrigues formula: $H_n(t) = (-1)^n e^{t^2} D^n e^{-t^2}, t \in \mathbb{R}^1$. After scaling and shifting the argument t appropriately, then taking the product of univariate functions for each dimension, we obtain the multivariate *Hermite expansion*

$$G(x_q) = \sum_{r=1}^{N_R} e^{\frac{-||x_q - x_r||^2}{2h^2}} = \sum_{r=1}^{N_R} \sum_{\alpha \geq 0} \frac{1}{\alpha!} \left(\frac{x_r - x_R}{\sqrt{2h^2}} \right)^\alpha h_\alpha \left(\frac{x_q - x_R}{\sqrt{2h^2}} \right) \qquad (1)$$

where we've adopted the usual multi-index notation as in [9]. This can be re-written as

$$G(x_q) = \sum_{r=1}^{N_R} e^{\frac{-||x_q - x_r||^2}{2h^2}} = \sum_{r=1}^{N_R} \sum_{\alpha \geq 0} \frac{1}{\alpha!} h_\alpha \left(\frac{x_r - x_Q}{\sqrt{2h^2}} \right) \left(\frac{x_q - x_Q}{\sqrt{2h^2}} \right)^\alpha \qquad (2)$$

to express the sum as a *Taylor (local) expansion* about a nearby representative centroid x_Q in the query region. We will be using both types of expansions simultaneously.

Since series approximations only hold locally, Greengard and Rokhlin [8] showed that it is useful to think in terms of a set of three 'translation operators' for converting between expansions centered at different points, in order to create their celebrated hierarchical algorithm. This was done in the context of the Coulombic kernel, but the Gaussian kernel has importantly different mathematical properties. The original Fast Gauss Transform (FGT) [9] was based on a flat grid, and thus provided only one operator ("H2L" of the next section), with an associated error bound (which was unfortunately incorrect). The Improved Fast Gauss Transform (IFGT) [14] was based on a flat set of clusters and provided no operators with a rearranged series approximation, which intended to be more favorable in higher dimensions but had an incorrect error bound. We will show the derivations of all the translation operators and associated error bounds needed to obtain, for the first time, a *hierarchical* algorithm for the Gaussian kernel.

2 Translation Operators and Error Bounds

The first operator converts a multipole expansion of a reference node to form a local expansion centered at the centroid of the query node, and is our main approximation workhorse.

Lemma 2.1. Hermite-to-local (H2L) translation operator for Gaussian kernel (*as presented in Lemma 2.2 in [9, 10]*): *Given a reference node X_R, a query node X_Q, and the Hermite expansion centered at a centroid x_R of X_R: $G(x_q) = \sum_{\alpha \geq 0} A_\alpha h_\alpha \left(\frac{x_q - x_R}{\sqrt{2h^2}} \right)$, the Taylor expansion of the Hermite expansion at the centroid x_Q of the query node X_Q is given by $G(x_q) = \sum_{\beta \geq 0} B_\beta \left(\frac{x_q - x_Q}{\sqrt{2h^2}} \right)^\beta$ where $B_\beta = \frac{(-1)^{|\beta|}}{\beta!} \sum_{\alpha \geq 0} A_\alpha h_{\alpha+\beta} \left(\frac{x_Q - x_R}{\sqrt{2h^2}} \right)$.*

Proof. (sketch) The proof consists of replacing the Hermite function portion of the expansion with its Taylor series. □

Note that we can rewrite $G(x_q) = \sum_{\alpha \geq 0} \left[\sum_{r=1}^{N_R} \frac{1}{\alpha!} \left(\frac{x_r - x_R}{\sqrt{2h^2}} \right)^\alpha \right] h_\alpha \left(\frac{x_q - x_R}{\sqrt{2h^2}} \right)$ by interchanging the summation order, such that the term in the brackets depends only on the reference points, and can thus be computed indepedent of any query location – we will call such terms Hermite moments. The next operator allows the efficient pre-computation of the Hermite moments in the reference tree in a bottom-up fashion from its children.

Lemma 2.2. Hermite-to-Hermite (H2H) translation operator for Gaussian kernel: *Given the Hermite expansion centered at a centroid $x_{R'}$ in a reference node $X_{R'}$: $G(x_q) = \sum_{\alpha \geq 0} A'_\alpha h_\alpha \left(\frac{x_q - x_{R'}}{\sqrt{2h^2}} \right)$, this same Hermite expansion shifted to a new location x_R of the parent node of X_R is given by $G(x_q) = \sum_{\gamma \geq 0} A_\gamma h_\gamma \left(\frac{x_q - x_R}{\sqrt{2h^2}} \right)$ where $A_\gamma = \sum_{0 \leq \alpha \leq \gamma} \frac{1}{(\gamma - \alpha)!} A'_\alpha \left(\frac{x_{R'} - x_R}{\sqrt{2h^2}} \right)^{\gamma - \alpha}$.*

Proof. We simply replace the Hermite function part of the expansion by a new Taylor series, as follows:

$$G(x_q) = \sum_{\alpha \geq 0} A'_\alpha h_\alpha \left(\frac{x_q - x_{R'}}{\sqrt{2h^2}} \right)$$

$$= \sum_{\alpha \geq 0} A'_\alpha \sum_{\beta \geq 0} \frac{1}{\beta!} \left(\frac{x_R - x_{R'}}{\sqrt{2h^2}} \right)^\beta (-1)^{|\beta|} h_{\alpha+\beta} \left(\frac{x_q - x_R}{\sqrt{2h^2}} \right)$$

$$= \sum_{\alpha \geq 0} \sum_{\beta \geq 0} A'_\alpha \frac{1}{\beta!} \left(\frac{x_R - x_{R'}}{\sqrt{2h^2}} \right)^\beta (-1)^{|\beta|} h_{\alpha+\beta} \left(\frac{x_q - x_R}{\sqrt{2h^2}} \right)$$

$$= \sum_{\alpha \geq 0} \sum_{\beta \geq 0} A'_\alpha \frac{1}{\beta!} \left(\frac{x_{R'} - x_R}{\sqrt{2h^2}} \right)^\beta h_{\alpha+\beta} \left(\frac{x_q - x_R}{\sqrt{2h^2}} \right)$$

$$= \sum_{\gamma \geq 0} \left[\sum_{0 \leq \alpha \leq \gamma} \frac{1}{(\gamma - \alpha)!} A'_\alpha \left(\frac{x_{R'} - x_R}{\sqrt{2h^2}} \right)^{\gamma - \alpha} \right] h_\gamma \left(\frac{x_q - x_R}{\sqrt{2h^2}} \right)$$

where $\gamma = \alpha + \beta$. □

The next operator acts as a "clean-up" routine in a hierarchical algorithm. Since we can approximate at different scales in the query tree, we must somehow combine all the approximations at the end of the computation. By performing a breadth-first traversal of the query tree, the L2L operator shifts a node's local expansion to the centroid of each child.

Lemma 2.3. Local-to-local (L2L) translation operator for Gaussian kernel: *Given a Taylor expansion centered at a centroid $x_{Q'}$ of a query node*

$$X_{Q'}: \quad G(x_q) = \sum_{\beta \geq 0} B_\beta \left(\frac{x_q - x_{Q'}}{\sqrt{2h^2}} \right)^\beta, \quad \text{the Taylor expansion obtained by shift-}$$

ing this expansion to the new centroid x_Q of the child node X_Q is $G(x_q) =$

$$\sum_{\alpha \geq 0} \left[\sum_{\beta \geq \alpha} \frac{\beta!}{\alpha!(\beta-\alpha)!} B_\beta \left(\frac{x_Q - x_{Q'}}{\sqrt{2h^2}} \right)^{\beta - \alpha} \right] \left(\frac{x_q - x_Q}{\sqrt{2h^2}} \right)^\alpha.$$

Proof. Applying the multinomial theorem to to expand about the new center x_Q yields:

$$G(x_q) = \sum_{\beta \geq 0} B_\beta \left(\frac{x_q - x_{Q'}}{\sqrt{2h^2}} \right)^\beta$$

$$= \sum_{\beta \geq 0} \sum_{\alpha \leq \beta} B_\beta \frac{\beta!}{\alpha!(\beta - \alpha)!} \left(\frac{x_Q - x_{Q'}}{\sqrt{2h^2}} \right)^{\beta - \alpha} \left(\frac{x_q - x_Q}{\sqrt{2h^2}} \right)^\alpha.$$

whose summation order can be interchanged to achieve the result. □

Because the Hermite and the Taylor expansion are truncated after taking p^D terms, we incur an error in approximation. The original error bounds for the Gaussian kernel in [9, 10] were wrong and corrections were shown in [3]. Here, we will present all necessary three error bounds incurred in performing translation operators. We note that these error bounds place limits on the size of the query node and the reference node. [2]

Lemma 2.4. Error Bound for Truncating an Hermite Expansion *(as presented in [3]):* *Suppose we are given an Hermite expansion of a reference node X_R about its centroid x_R:*

$$G(x_q) = \sum_{\alpha \geq 0} A_\alpha h_\alpha \left(\frac{x_q - x_R}{\sqrt{2h^2}} \right) \text{ where } A_\alpha = \sum_{r=1}^{N_R} \frac{1}{\alpha!} \left(\frac{x_r - x_R}{\sqrt{2h^2}} \right)^\alpha. \text{ For any query point } x_q, \text{ the}$$

error due to truncating the series after the first p^D term is $|\epsilon_M(p)| \leq \frac{N_R}{(1-r)^D} \sum_{k=0}^{D-1} \binom{D}{k} (1 -$

$r^p)^k \left(\frac{r^p}{\sqrt{p!}} \right)^{D-k}$ *where $\forall x_r \in X_R$ satisfies $||x_r - x_R||_\infty < rh$ for $r < 1$.*

Proof. (sketch) We expand the Hermite expansion as a product of one-dimensional Hermite functions, and utilize a bound on one-dimensional Hermite functions due to [13]:
$\frac{1}{n!} |h_n(x)| \leq \frac{2^{\frac{n}{2}}}{\sqrt{n!}} e^{\frac{-x^2}{2}}, n \geq 0, x \in \mathbb{R}^1.$ □

Lemma 2.5. Error Bound for Truncating a Taylor Expansion Converted from an Hermite Expansion of Infinite Order: *Suppose we are given the following Taylor expansion about the centroid x_Q of a query node $G(x_q) = \sum_{\beta \geq 0} B_\beta \left(\frac{x_q - x_Q}{\sqrt{2h^2}} \right)^\beta$ where*

---

[2] Strain [12] proposed the interesting idea of using Stirling's formula (for any non-negative integer n: $\left(\frac{n+1}{e} \right)^n \leq n!$) to lift the node size constraint; one might imagine that this could allow approximation of larger regions in a tree-based algorithm. Unfortunately, the error bounds developed in [12] were also incorrect. We have derived the three necessary corrected error bounds based on the techniques in [3]. However, due to space, and because using these bounds actually degraded performance slightly, we do not include those lemmas here.

$B_\beta = \frac{(-1)^{|\beta|}}{\beta!} \sum_{\alpha \geq 0} A_\alpha h_{\alpha+\beta} \left(\frac{x_Q - x_R}{\sqrt{2h^2}} \right)$ and A_α's are the coefficients of the Hermite ex-

pansion centered at the reference node centroid x_R. Then, truncating the series after

p^D terms satisfies the error bound $|\epsilon_L(p)| \leq \frac{N_R}{(1-r)^D} \sum_{k=0}^{D-1} \binom{D}{k} (1 - r^p)^k \left(\frac{r^p}{\sqrt{p!}} \right)^{D-k}$ where

$||x_q - x_Q||_\infty < rh$ for $r < 1$, $\forall x_q \in X_Q$.

Proof. Taylor expansion of the Hermite function yields

$$e^{\frac{-||x_q - x_r||^2}{2h^2}} = \sum_{\beta \geq 0} \frac{(-1)^{|\beta|}}{\beta!} \sum_{\alpha \geq 0} \frac{1}{\alpha!} \left(\frac{x_r - x_R}{\sqrt{2h^2}} \right)^\alpha h_{\alpha+\beta} \left(\frac{x_Q - x_R}{\sqrt{2h^2}} \right) \left(\frac{x_q - x_Q}{\sqrt{2h^2}} \right)^\beta$$

$$= \sum_{\beta \geq 0} \frac{(-1)^{|\beta|}}{\beta!} \sum_{\alpha \geq 0} \frac{1}{\alpha!} \left(\frac{x_R - x_r}{\sqrt{2h^2}} \right)^\alpha (-1)^{|\alpha|} h_{\alpha+\beta} \left(\frac{x_Q - x_R}{\sqrt{2h^2}} \right) \left(\frac{x_q - x_Q}{\sqrt{2h^2}} \right)^\beta$$

$$= \sum_{\beta \geq 0} \frac{(-1)^{|\beta|}}{\beta!} h_\beta \left(\frac{x_Q - x_r}{\sqrt{2h^2}} \right) \left(\frac{x_q - x_Q}{\sqrt{2h^2}} \right)^\beta$$

Use $e^{\frac{-||x_q - x_r||^2}{2h^2}} = \prod_{i=1}^{D} \left(u_p(x_{q_i}, x_{r_i}, x_{Q_i}) + v_p(x_{q_i}, x_{r_i}, x_{Q_i}) \right)$ for $1 \leq i \leq D$, where

$$u_p(x_{q_i}, x_{r_i}, x_{Q_i}) = \sum_{n_i=0}^{p-1} \frac{(-1)^{n_i}}{n_i!} h_{n_i} \left(\frac{x_{Q_i} - x_{r_i}}{\sqrt{2h^2}} \right) \left(\frac{x_{q_i} - x_{Q_i}}{\sqrt{2h^2}} \right)^{n_i}$$

$$v_p(x_{q_i}, x_{r_i}, x_{Q_i}) = \sum_{n_i=p}^{\infty} \frac{(-1)^{n_i}}{n_i!} h_{n_i} \left(\frac{x_{Q_i} - x_{r_i}}{\sqrt{2h^2}} \right) \left(\frac{x_{q_i} - x_{Q_i}}{\sqrt{2h^2}} \right)^{n_i}.$$

These univariate functions respectively satisfy $u_p(x_{q_i}, x_{r_i}, x_{Q_i}) \leq \frac{1-r^p}{1-r}$ and
$v_p(x_{q_i}, x_{r_i}, x_{Q_i}) \leq \frac{1}{\sqrt{p!}} \frac{r^p}{1-r}$, for $1 \leq i \leq D$, achieving the multivariate bound. $\qquad\square$

Lemma 2.6. Error Bound for Truncating a Taylor Expansion Converted from an Already Truncated Hermite Expansion: *A truncated Hermite expansion centered about the centroid x_R of a reference node $G(x_q) = \sum_{\alpha < p} A_\alpha h_\alpha \left(\frac{x_q - x_R}{\sqrt{2h^2}} \right)$ has the following*

Taylor expansion about the centroid x_Q of a query node: $G(x_q) = \sum_{\beta \geq 0} C_\beta \left(\frac{x_q - x_Q}{\sqrt{2h^2}} \right)^\beta$

where the coefficients C_β are given by $C_\beta = \frac{(-1)^{|\beta|}}{\beta!} \sum_{\alpha < p} A_\alpha h_{\alpha+\beta} \left(\frac{x_Q - x_R}{\sqrt{2h^2}} \right)$. Truncat-

ing the series after p^D terms satisfies the error bound $|\epsilon_L(p)| \leq \frac{N_R}{(1-2r)^{2D}} \sum_{k=0}^{D-1} \binom{D}{k} ((1 -$

$(2r)^p)^2)^k \left(\frac{((2r)^p)(2 - (2r)^p)}{\sqrt{p!}} \right)^{D-k}$ *for a query node X_Q for which $||x_q - x_Q||_\infty < rh$, and a reference node X_R for which $||x_r - x_R||_\infty < rh$ for $r < \frac{1}{2}$, $\forall x_q \in X_Q$, $\forall x_r \in X_R$.*

Proof. We define $u_{pi} = u_p(x_{q_i}, x_{r_i}, x_{Q_i}, x_{R_i})$, $v_{pi} = v_p(x_{q_i}, x_{r_i}, x_{Q_i}, x_{R_i})$, $w_{pi} = w_p(x_{q_i}, x_{r_i}, x_{Q_i}, x_{R_i})$ for $1 \leq i \leq D$:

$$u_{pi} = \sum_{n_i=0}^{p-1} \frac{(-1)^{n_i}}{n_i!} \sum_{n_j=0}^{p-1} \frac{1}{n_j!} \left(\frac{x_{R_i} - x_{r_i}}{\sqrt{2h^2}} \right)^{n_j} (-1)^{n_j} h_{n_i+n_j} \left(\frac{x_{Q_i} - x_{R_i}}{\sqrt{2h^2}} \right) \left(\frac{x_{q_i} - x_{Q_i}}{\sqrt{2h^2}} \right)^{n_i}$$

$$v_{pi} = \sum_{n_i=0}^{p-1} \frac{(-1)^{n_i}}{n_i!} \sum_{n_j=p}^{\infty} \frac{1}{n_j!} \left(\frac{x_{R_i} - x_{r_i}}{\sqrt{2h^2}} \right)^{n_j} (-1)^{n_j} h_{n_i+n_j} \left(\frac{x_{Q_i} - x_{R_i}}{\sqrt{2h^2}} \right) \left(\frac{x_{q_i} - x_{Q_i}}{\sqrt{2h^2}} \right)^{n_i}$$

751

$$w_{pi} = \sum_{n_i=p}^{\infty} \frac{(-1)^{n_i}}{n_i!} \sum_{n_j=0}^{\infty} \frac{1}{n_j!} \left(\frac{x_{R_i} - x_{r_i}}{\sqrt{2h^2}} \right)^{n_j} (-1)^{n_j} h_{n_i+n_j} \left(\frac{x_{Q_i} - x_{R_i}}{\sqrt{2h^2}} \right) \left(\frac{x_{q_i} - x_{Q_i}}{\sqrt{2h^2}} \right)^{n_i}$$

Note that $e^{\frac{-||x_q - x_r||^2}{2h^2}} = \prod_{i=1}^{D} (u_{pi} + v_{pi} + w_{pi})$ for $1 \le i \le D$. Using the bound for Hermite functions and the property of geometric series, we obtain the following upper bounds:

$$u_{pi} \le \sum_{n_i=0}^{p-1} \sum_{n_j=0}^{p-1} (2r)^{n_i} (2r)^{n_j} = \left(\frac{1 - (2r)^p}{1 - 2r} \right)^2$$

$$v_{pi} \le \frac{1}{\sqrt{p!}} \sum_{n_i=0}^{p-1} \sum_{n_j=p}^{\infty} (2r)^{n_i} (2r)^{n_j} = \frac{1}{\sqrt{p!}} \left(\frac{1 - (2r)^p}{1 - 2r} \right) \left(\frac{(2r)^p}{1 - 2r} \right)$$

$$w_{pi} \le \frac{1}{\sqrt{p!}} \sum_{n_i=p}^{\infty} \sum_{n_j=0}^{\infty} (2r)^{n_i} (2r)^{n_j} = \frac{1}{\sqrt{p!}} \left(\frac{1}{1 - 2r} \right) \left(\frac{(2r)^p}{1 - 2r} \right)$$

Therefore,

$$\left| e^{\frac{-||x_q - x_r||^2}{2h^2}} - \prod_{i=1}^{D} u_{pi} \right| \le (1 - 2r)^{-2D} \sum_{k=0}^{D-1} \binom{D}{k} ((1 - (2r)^p)^2)^k \left(\frac{((2r)^p)(2 - (2r)^p)}{\sqrt{p!}} \right)^{D-k}$$

$$\left| G(x_q) - \sum_{\beta < p} C_\beta \left(\frac{x_q - x_Q}{\sqrt{2h^2}} \right)^\beta \right| \le \frac{N_R}{(1 - 2r)^{2D}} \sum_{k=0}^{D-1} \binom{D}{k} ((1 - (2r)^p)^2)^k \left(\frac{((2r)^p)(2 - (2r)^p)}{\sqrt{p!}} \right)^{D-k}$$

$\square$

3 Algorithm and Results

Algorithm. The algorithm mainly consists of making the function call **DFGT**(Q.root, R.root), *i.e.* calling the recursive function **DFGT**() with the root nodes of the query tree and reference tree. After the **DFGT**() routine is completed, the pre-order traversal of the query tree implied by the L2L operator is performed. Before the **DFGT**() routine is called, the reference tree could be initialized with Hermite coefficients stored in each node using the H2H translation operator, but instead we will compute them as needed on the fly. It adaptively chooses among three possible methods for approximating the summation contribution of the points in node R to the queries in node Q, which are self-explanatory, based on crude operation count estimates. G_Q^{min}, a running lower bound on the kernel sum $G(x_q)$ for any $x_q \in X_Q$, is used to ensure locally that the global relative error is ϵ or less. This automatic mechanism allows the user to specify only an error tolerance ϵ rather than other tweak parameters. Upon approximation, the upper and lower bounds on G for Q and all its children are updated; the latter can be done in an $O(1)$ delayed fashion as in [7]. The remainder of the routine implements the characteristic four-way dual-tree recursion. We also tested a hybrid method (DFGTH) which approximates if either of the DFD or DFGT approximation criteria are met.

Experimental results. We empirically studied the runtime [3] performance of five algorithms on five real-world datasets for kernel density estimation at every query point with a range of bandwidths, from 3 orders of magnitude smaller than optimal to three orders larger than optimal, according to the standard least-squares cross-validation score [11]. The naive

---

[3] All times include all preprocessing costs including any data structure construction. Times are measured in CPU seconds on a dual-processor AMD Opteron 242 machine with 8 Gb of main memory and 1 Mb of CPU cache. All the codes that we have written and obtained are written in C and C++, and was compiled under -06 $-funroll-loops$ flags on Linux kernel 2.4.26.

algorithm computes the sum explicitly and thus exactly. We have limited all datasets to 50K points so that true relative error, *i.e.* $\left(|\widehat{G}(x_q) - G_{true}(x_q)|\right)/G_{true}(x_q)$, can be evaluated, and set the tolerance at 1% relative error for all query points. When any method fails to achieve the error tolerance in less time than twice that of the naive method, we give up. Codes for the FGT [9] and for the IFGT [14] were obtained from the authors' websites. Note that both of these methods require the user to tweak parameters, while the others are automatic. [4] DFD refers to the depth-first dual-tree finite-difference method [7].

DFGT(Q, R)

$p_{DH} = p_{DL} = p_{H2L} = \infty$

`if` R.maxside $< 2h$, $p_{DH} =$ the smallest $p \geq 1$ such that

$$\frac{N_R}{(1-r)^D} \sum_{k=0}^{D-1} \binom{D}{k}(1-r^p)^k \left(\frac{r^p}{\sqrt{p!}}\right)^{D-k} < \epsilon G_Q^{min}.$$

`if` Q.maxside $< 2h$, $p_{DL} =$ the smallest $p \geq 1$ such that

$$\frac{N_R}{(1-r)^D} \sum_{k=0}^{D-1} \binom{D}{k}(1-r^p)^k \left(\frac{r^p}{\sqrt{p!}}\right)^{D-k} < \epsilon G_Q^{min}.$$

`if` $\max(Q$.maxside,R.maxside$) < h$, $p_{H2L} =$ the smallest $p \geq 1$ such that

$$\frac{N_R}{(1-2r)^{2D}} \sum_{k=0}^{D-1} \binom{D}{k}((1-(2r)^p)^2)^k \left(\frac{((2r)^p)(2-(2r)^p)}{\sqrt{p!}}\right)^{D-k} < \epsilon G_Q^{min}.$$

$c_{DH} = p_{DH}^D N_Q.$ $c_{DL} = p_{DL}^D N_R.$ $c_{H2L} = D p_{H2L}^{D+1}.$ $c_{Direct} = D N_Q N_R.$

`if` no Hermite coefficient of order p_{DH} exists for X_R,
   Compute it. $c_{DH} = c_{DH} + p_{DH}^D N_R.$
`if` no Hermite coefficient of order p_{H2L} exists for X_R,
   Compute it. $c_{H2L} = c_{H2L} + p_{H2L}^D N_R.$

$c = \min(c_{DH}, c_{DL}, c_{H2L}, c_{Direct}).$
`if` $c = c_{DH} < \infty$, (Direct Hermite)
   Evaluate each x_q at the Hermite series of order p_{DH} centered about x_R of X_R
   using Equation 1.
`if` $c = c_{DL} < \infty$, (Direct Local)
   Accumulate each $x_r \in X_R$ as the Taylor series of order p_{DL} about the center
   x_Q of X_Q using Equation 2.
`if` $c = c_{H2L} < \infty$, (Hermite-to-Local)
   Convert the Hermite series of order p_{H2L} centered about x_R of X_R to the Taylor
   series of the same order centered about x_Q of X_Q using Lemma 2.1.
`if` $c \neq c_{Direct}$,
   Update G^{min} and G^{max} in Q and all its children. `return`.

`if` leaf(Q) and leaf(R),
   Perform the naive algorithm on every pair of points in Q and R.
`else`
   DFGT$(Q$.left, R.left). **DFGT**$(Q$.left, R.right).
   DFGT$(Q$.right, R.left). **DFGT**$(Q$.right, R.right).

---

[4]For the FGT, note that the algorithm only ensures: $\left|\widehat{G}(x_q) - G_{true}(x_q)\right| \leq \tau$. Therefore, we first set $\tau = \epsilon$, halving τ until the error tolerance ϵ was met. For the IFGT, which has multiple parameters that must be tweaked simultaneously, an automatic scheme was created, based on the recommendations given in the paper and software documentation: For $D = 2$, use $p = 8$; for $D = 3$, use $p = 6$; set $\rho_x = 2.5$; start with $K = \sqrt{N}$ and double K until the error tolerance is met. When this failed to meet the tolerance, we resorted to additional trial and error by hand. The costs of parameter selection for these methods in both computer and human time is not included in the table.

Algorithm \ scale	0.001	0.01	0.1	1	10	100	1000
sj2-50000-2 (astronomy: positions), $D = 2$, $N = 50000$, $h^* = 0.00139506$							
Naive	301.696	301.696	301.696	301.696	301.696	301.696	301.696
FGT	out of RAM	out of RAM	out of RAM	3.892312	2.01846	0.319538	0.183616
IFGT	$> 2 \times$ Naive	$> 2 \times$ Naive	$> 2 \times$ Naive	$> 2 \times$ Naive	$> 2 \times$ Naive	$> 2 \times$ Naive	7.576783
DFD	0.837724	1.087066	1.658592	6.018158	62.077669	151.590062	1.551019
DFGT	0.849935	1.11567	4.599235	72.435177	18.450387	2.777454	2.532401
DFGTH	**0.846294**	**1.10654**	**1.683913**	**6.265131**	**5.063365**	**1.036626**	**0.68471**
colors50k (astronomy: colors), $D = 2$, $N = 50000$, $h^* = 0.0016911$							
Naive	301.696	301.696	301.696	301.696	301.696	301.696	301.696
FGT	out of RAM	out of RAM	out of RAM	$> 2 \times$ Naive	$> 2 \times$ Naive	0.475281	0.114430
IFGT	$> 2 \times$ Naive	$> 2 \times$ Naive	$> 2 \times$ Naive	$> 2 \times$ Naive	$> 2 \times$ Naive	$> 2 \times$ Naive	7.55986
DFD	1.095838	1.469454	2.802112	30.294007	280.633106	81.373053	3.604753
DFGT	1.099828	1.983888	29.231309	285.719266	12.886239	5.336602	3.5638
DFGTH	**1.081216**	**1.47692**	**2.855083**	**24.598749**	**7.142465**	**1.78648**	**0.627554**
edsgc-radec-rnd (astronomy: angles), $D = 2$, $N = 50000$, $h^* = 0.00466204$							
Naive	301.696	301.696	301.696	301.696	301.696	301.696	301.696
FGT	out of RAM	out of RAM	out of RAM	2.859245	1.768738	0.210799	0.059664
IFGT	$> 2 \times$ Naive	$> 2 \times$ Naive	$> 2 \times$ Naive	$> 2 \times$ Naive	$> 2 \times$ Naive	$> 2 \times$ Naive	7.585585
DFD	0.812462	1.083528	1.682261	5.860172	63.849361	357.099354	0.743045
DFGT	0.84023	1.120015	4.346061	73.036687	21.652047	3.424304	1.977302
DFGTH	**0.821672**	**1.104545**	**1.737799**	**6.037217**	**5.7398**	**1.883216**	**0.436596**
mockgalaxy-D-1M-rnd (cosmology: positions), $D = 3$, $N = 50000$, $h^* = 0.000768201$							
Naive	354.868751	354.868751	354.868751	354.868751	354.868751	354.868751	354.868751
FGT	out of RAM	out of RAM	out of RAM	out of RAM	$> 2 \times$ Naive	$> 2 \times$ Naive	$> 2 \times$ Naive
IFGT	$> 2 \times$ Naive	$> 2 \times$ Naive	$> 2 \times$ Naive	$> 2 \times$ Naive	$> 2 \times$ Naive	$> 2 \times$ Naive	$> 2 \times$ Naive
DFD	0.70054	0.701547	0.761524	0.843451	1.086608	42.022605	383.12048
DFGT	0.73007	0.733638	0.799711	0.999316	50.619588	125.059911	109.353701
DFGTH	**0.724004**	**0.719951**	**0.789002**	**0.877564**	**1.265064**	**22.6106**	**87.488392**
bio5-rnd (biology: drug activity), $D = 5$, $N = 50000$, $h^* = 0.000567161$							
Naive	364.439228	364.439228	364.439228	364.439228	364.439228	364.439228	364.439228
FGT	out of RAM	out of RAM	out of RAM	out of RAM	out of RAM	out of RAM	out of RAM
IFGT	$> 2 \times$ Naive	$> 2 \times$ Naive	$> 2 \times$ Naive	$> 2 \times$ Naive	$> 2 \times$ Naive	$> 2 \times$ Naive	$> 2 \times$ Naive
DFD	2.249868	2.4958865	4.70948	12.065697	94.345003	412.39142	107.675935
DFGT	$> 2 \times$ Naive	$> 2 \times$ Naive	$> 2 \times$ Naive	$> 2 \times$ Naive	$> 2 \times$ Naive	$> 2 \times$ Naive	$> 2 \times$ Naive
DFGTH	$> 2 \times$ Naive	$> 2 \times$ Naive	$> 2 \times$ Naive	$> 2 \times$ Naive	$> 2 \times$ Naive	$> 2 \times$ Naive	$> 2 \times$ Naive

Discussion. The experiments indicate that the DFGTH method is able to achieve reasonable performance across all bandwidth scales. Unfortunately none of the series approximation-based methods do well on the 5-dimensional data, as expected, highlighting the main weakness of the approach presented. Pursuing corrections to the error bounds necessary to use the intriguing series form of [14] may allow an increase in dimensionality.

References

[1] A. W. Appel. An Efficient Program for Many-Body Simulations. *SIAM Journal on Scientific and Statistical Computing*, 6(1):85–103, 1985.

[2] J. Barnes and P. Hut. A Hierarchical $O(N \log N)$ Force-Calculation Algorithm. *Nature*, 324, 1986.

[3] B. Baxter and G. Roussos. A new error estimate of the fast gauss transform. *SIAM Journal on Scientific Computing*, 24(1):257–259, 2002.

[4] P. Callahan and S. Kosaraju. A decomposition of multidimensional point sets with applications to k-nearest-neighbors and n-body potential fields. *Journal of the ACM*, 62(1):67–90, January 1995.

[5] A. Gray and A. W. Moore. N-Body Problems in Statistical Learning. In T. K. Leen, T. G. Dietterich, and V. Tresp, editors, *Advances in Neural Information Processing Systems 13 (December 2000)*. MIT Press, 2001.

[6] A. G. Gray. *Bringing Tractability to Generalized N-Body Problems in Statistical and Scientific Computation*. PhD thesis, Carnegie Mellon University, 2003.

[7] A. G. Gray and A. W. Moore. Rapid Evaluation of Multiple Density Models. In *Artificial Intelligence and Statistics 2003*, 2003.

[8] L. Greengard and V. Rokhlin. A Fast Algorithm for Particle Simulations. *Journal of Computational Physics*, 73, 1987.

[9] L. Greengard and J. Strain. The fast gauss transform. *SIAM Journal on Scientific and Statistical Computing*, 12(1):79–94, 1991.

[10] L. Greengard and X. Sun. A new version of the fast gauss transform. *Documenta Mathematica*, Extra Volume ICM(III):575–584, 1998.

[11] B. W. Silverman. *Density Estimation for Statistics and Data Analysis*. Chapman and Hall, 1986.

[12] J. Strain. The fast gauss transform with variable scales. *SIAM Journal on Scientific and Statistical Computing*, 12:1131–1139, 1991.

[13] O. Szász. On the relative extrema of the hermite orthogonal functions. *J. Indian Math. Soc.*, 15:129–134, 1951.

[14] C. Yang, R. Duraiswami, N. A. Gumerov, and L. Davis. Improved fast gauss transform and efficient kernel density estimation. *International Conference on Computer Vision*, 2003.

CMOL CrossNets: Possible Neuromorphic Nanoelectronic Circuits

Jung Hoon Lee Xiaolong Ma Konstantin K. Likharev

Stony Brook University
Stony Brook, NY 11794-3800
klikharev@notes.cc.sunysb.edu

Abstract

Hybrid "CMOL" integrated circuits, combining CMOS subsystem with nanowire crossbars and simple two-terminal nanodevices, promise to extend the exponential Moore-Law development of microelectronics into the sub-10-nm range. We are developing neuromorphic network ("CrossNet") architectures for this future technology, in which neural cell bodies are implemented in CMOS, nanowires are used as axons and dendrites, while nanodevices (bistable latching switches) are used as elementary synapses. We have shown how CrossNets may be trained to perform pattern recovery and classification despite the limitations imposed by the CMOL hardware. Preliminary estimates have shown that CMOL CrossNets may be extremely dense ($\sim 10^7$ cells per cm^2) and operate approximately a million times faster than biological neural networks, at manageable power consumption. In Conclusion, we discuss in brief possible short-term and long-term applications of the emerging technology.

1 Introduction: CMOL Circuits

Recent results [1, 2] indicate that the current VLSI paradigm based on CMOS technology can be hardly extended beyond the 10-nm frontier: in this range the sensitivity of parameters (most importantly, the gate voltage threshold) of silicon field-effect transistors to inevitable fabrication spreads grows exponentially. This sensitivity will probably send the fabrication facilities costs skyrocketing, and may lead to the end of Moore's Law some time during the next decade.

There is a growing consensus that the impending Moore's Law crisis may be preempted by a radical paradigm shift from the purely CMOS technology to hybrid CMOS/nanodevice circuits, e.g., those of "CMOL" variety (Fig. 1). Such circuits (see, e.g., Ref. 3 for their recent review) would combine a level of advanced CMOS devices fabricated by the lithographic patterning, and two-layer nanowire crossbar formed, e.g., by nanoimprint, with nanowires connected by simple, similar, two-terminal nanodevices at each crosspoint. For such devices, molecular single-electron latching switches [4] are presently the leading candidates, in particular because they may be fabricated using the self-assembled monolayer (SAM) technique which already gave reproducible results for simpler molecular devices [5].

755

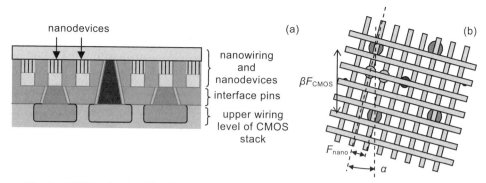

Fig. 1. CMOL circuit: (a) schematic side view, and (b) top-view zoom-in on several adjacent interface pins. (For clarity, only two adjacent nanodevices are shown.)

In order to overcome the CMOS/nanodevice interface problems pertinent to earlier proposals of hybrid circuits [6], in CMOL the interface is provided by pins that are distributed all over the circuit area, on the top of the CMOS stack. This allows to use advanced techniques of nanowire patterning (like nanoimprint) which do not have nanoscale accuracy of layer alignment [3]. The vital feature of this interface is the tilt, by angle $\alpha = \arcsin(F_{\mathrm{nano}}/\beta F_{\mathrm{CMOS}})$, of the nanowire crossbar relative to the square arrays of interface pins (Fig. 1b). Here F_{nano} is the nanowiring half-pitch, F_{CMOS} is the half-pitch of the CMOS subsystem, and β is a dimensionless factor larger than 1 that depends on the CMOS cell complexity. Figure 1b shows that this tilt allows the CMOS subsystem to address each nanodevice even if $F_{\mathrm{nano}} \ll \beta F_{\mathrm{CMOS}}$.

By now, it has been shown that CMOL circuits can combine high performance with high defect tolerance (which is necessary for any circuit using nanodevices) for several digital applications. In particular, CMOL circuits with defect rates below a few percent would enable terabit-scale memories [7], while the performance of FPGA-like CMOL circuits may be several hundred times above that of overcome purely CMOL FPGA (implemented with the same F_{CMOS}), at acceptable power dissipation and defect tolerance above 20% [8].

In addition, the very structure of CMOL circuits makes them uniquely suitable for the implementation of more complex, mixed-signal information processing systems, including ultradense and ultrafast neuromorphic networks. The objective of this paper is to describe in brief the current status of our work on the development of so-called Distributed Crossbar Networks ("CrossNets") that could provide high performance despite the limitations imposed by CMOL hardware. A more detailed description of our earlier results may be found in Ref. 9.

2 Synapses

The central device of CrossNet is a two-terminal latching switch [3, 4] (Fig. 2a) which is a combination of two single-electron devices, a transistor and a trap [3]. The device may be naturally implemented as a single organic molecule (Fig. 2b). Qualitatively, the device operates as follows: if voltage $V = V_j - V_k$ applied between the external electrodes (in CMOL, nanowires) is low, the trap island has no net electric charge, and the single-electron transistor is closed. If voltage V approaches certain threshold value $V_+ > 0$, an additional electron is inserted into the trap island, and its field lifts the Coulomb blockade of the single-electron transistor, thus connecting the nanowires. The switch state may be reset (e.g., wires disconnected) by applying a lower voltage $V < V_- < V_+$.

Due to the random character of single-electron tunneling [2], the quantitative description of the switch is by necessity probabilistic: actually, V determines only the rates $\Gamma_{\uparrow\downarrow}$ of device

756

switching between its ON and OFF states. The rates, in turn, determine the dynamics of probability p to have the transistor opened (i.e. wires connected):

$$dp/dt = \Gamma_\uparrow (1 - p) - \Gamma_\downarrow p. \qquad (1)$$

The theory of single-electron tunneling [2] shows that, in a good approximation, the rates may be presented as

$$\Gamma_{\uparrow\downarrow} = \Gamma_0 \exp\{\pm e(V - S)/k_B T\} , \qquad (2)$$

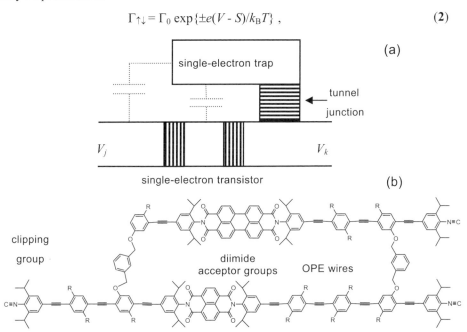

Fig. 2. (a) Schematics and (b) possible molecular implementation of the two-terminal single-electron latching switch

where Γ_0 and S are constants depending on physical parameters of the latching switches. Note that despite the random character of switching, the strong nonlinearity of Eq. (2) allows to limit the degree of the device "fuzziness".

3 CrossNets

Figure 3a shows the generic structure of a CrossNet. CMOS-implemented somatic cells (within the Fire Rate model, just nonlinear differential amplifiers, see Fig. 3b,c) apply their output voltages to "axonic" nanowires. If the latching switch, working as an elementary synapse, on the crosspoint of an axonic wire with the perpendicular "dendritic" wire is open, some current flows into the latter wire, charging it. Since such currents are injected into each dendritic wire through several (many) open synapses, their addition provides a natural passive analog summation of signals from the corresponding somas, typical for all neural networks. Examining Fig. 3a, please note the open-circuit terminations of axonic and dendritic lines at the borders of the somatic cells; due to these terminations the somas do not communicate directly (but only via synapses).

The network shown on Fig. 3 is evidently feedforward; recurrent networks are achieved in the evident way by doubling the number of synapses and nanowires per somatic cell (Fig. 3c). Moreover, using dual-rail (bipolar) representation of the signal, and hence doubling the number of nanowires and elementary synapses once again, one gets a CrossNet with somas coupled by compact 4-switch groups [9]. Using Eqs. (1) and (2), it is straightforward to show that that the average synaptic weight w_{jk} of the group obeys the "quasi-Hebbian" rule:

$$\frac{d}{dt}\langle w_{jk} \rangle = -4\Gamma_0 \sinh\left(\gamma S\right)\sinh\left(\gamma V_j\right)\sinh\left(\gamma V_k\right). \qquad (3)$$

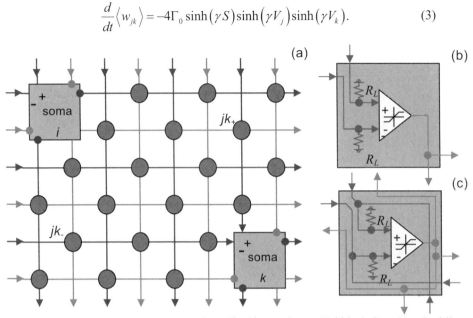

Fig. 3. (a) Generic structure of the simplest, (feedforward, non-Hebbian) CrossNet. Red lines show "axonic", and blue lines "dendritic" nanowires. Gray squares are interfaces between nanowires and CMOS-based somas (b, c). Signs show the dendrite input polarities. Green circles denote molecular latching switches forming elementary synapses. Bold red and blue points are open-circuit terminations of the nanowires, that do not allow somas to interact in bypass of synapses

In the simplest cases (e.g., quasi-Hopfield networks with finite connectivity), the tri-level synaptic weights of the generic CrossNets are quite satisfactory, leading to just a very modest (~30%) network capacity loss. However, some applications (in particular, pattern classification) may require a larger number of weight quantization levels L (e.g., $L \approx 30$ for a 1% fidelity [9]). This may be achieved by using compact square arrays (e.g., 4×4) of latching switches (Fig. 4).

Various species of CrossNets [9] differ also by the way the somatic cells are distributed around the synaptic field. Figure 5 shows feedforward versions of two CrossNet types most explored so far: the so-called FlossBar and InBar. The former network is more natural for the implementation of multilayered perceptrons (MLP), while the latter system is preferable for recurrent network implementations and also allows a simpler CMOS design of somatic cells.

The most important advantage of CrossNets over the hardware neural networks suggested earlier is that these networks allow to achieve enormous density combined with large cell connectivity $M \gg 1$ in quasi-2D electronic circuits.

4   CrossNet training

CrossNet training faces several hardware-imposed challenges:

(i) The synaptic weight contribution provided by the elementary latching switch is binary, so that for most applications the multi-switch synapses (Fig. 4) are necessary.

(ii) The only way to adjust any particular synaptic weight is to turn ON or OFF the corresponding latching switch(es). This is only possible to do by applying certain voltage $V = V_j - V_k$ between the two corresponding nanowires. At this procedure, other nanodevices attached to the same wires should not be disturbed.

(iii) As stated above, synapse state switching is a statistical progress, so that the degree of its "fuzziness" should be carefully controlled.

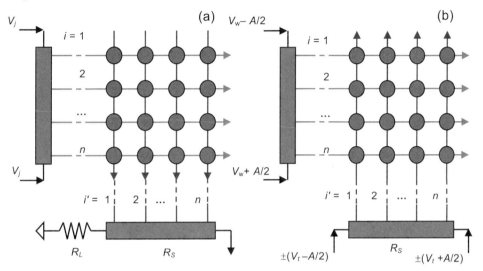

Fig. 4. Composite synapse for providing $L = 2n^2+1$ discrete levels of the weight in (a) operation and (b) weight adjustment modes. The dark-gray rectangles are resistive metallic strips at soma/nanowire interfaces

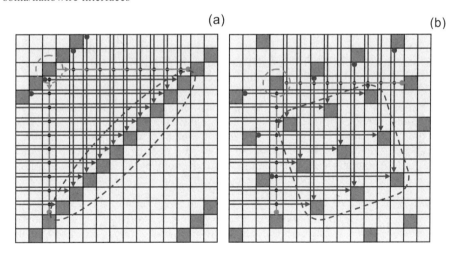

Fig. 5. Two main CrossNet species: (a) FlossBar and (b) InBar, in the generic (feedforward, non-Hebbian, ternary-weight) case for the connectivity parameter $M = 9$. Only the nanowires and nanodevices coupling one cell (indicated with red dashed lines) to M post-synaptic cells (blue dashed lines) are shown; actually all the cells are similarly coupled

We have shown that these challenges may be met using (at least) the following training methods [9]:

(i) *Synaptic weight import.* This procedure is started with training of a homomorphic "precursor" artificial neural network with continuous synaptic weighs w_{jk}, implemented in software, using one of established methods (e.g., error backpropagation). Then the synaptic weights w_{jk} are transferred to the CrossNet, with some "clipping" (rounding) due to the binary nature of elementary synaptic weights. To accomplish the transfer, pairs of somatic cells are sequentially selected via CMOS-level wiring. Using the flexibility of CMOS circuitry, these cells are reconfigured to apply external voltages $\pm V_W$ to the axonic and dendritic nanowires leading to a particular synapse, while all other nanowires are grounded. The voltage level V_W is selected so that it does not switch the synapses attached to only one of the selected nanowires, while voltage $2V_W$ applied to the synapse at the crosspoint of the selected wires is sufficient for its reliable switching. (In the composite synapses with quasi-continuous weights (Fig. 4), only a part of the corresponding switches is turned ON or OFF.)

(ii) *Error backpropagation.* The synaptic weight import procedure is straightforward when w_{jk} may be simply calculated, e.g., for the Hopfield-type networks. However, for very large CrossNets used, e.g., as pattern classifiers the precursor network training may take an impracticably long time. In this case the direct training of a CrossNet may become necessary. We have developed two methods of such training, both based on "Hebbian" synapses consisting of 4 elementary synapses (latching switches) whose average weight dynamics obeys Eq. (3). This quasi-Hebbian rule may be used to implement the backpropagation algorithm either using a periodic time-multiplexing [9] or in a continuous fashion, using the simultaneous propagation of signals and errors along the same dual-rail channels.

As a result, presently we may state that CrossNets may be taught to perform virtually all major functions demonstrated earlier with the usual neural networks, including the corrupted pattern restoration in the recurrent quasi-Hopfield mode and pattern classification in the feedforward MLP mode [11].

5   CrossNet performance estimates

The significance of this result may be only appreciated in the context of unparalleled physical parameters of CMOL CrossNets. The only fundamental limitation on the half-pitch F_{nano} (Fig. 1) comes from quantum-mechanical tunneling between nanowires. If the wires are separated by vacuum, the corresponding specific leakage conductance becomes uncomfortably large ($\sim 10^{-12}$ $\Omega^{-1}m^{-1}$) only at $F_{nano} = 1.5$ nm; however, since realistic insulation materials (SiO_2, etc.) provide somewhat lower tunnel barriers, let us use a more conservative value $F_{nano} = 3$ nm. Note that this value corresponds to 10^{12} elementary synapses per cm^2, so that for $4M = 10^4$ and $n = 4$ the areal density of neural cells is close to 2×10^7 cm^{-2}. Both numbers are higher than those for the human cerebral cortex, despite the fact that the quasi-2D CMOL circuits have to compete with quasi-3D cerebral cortex.

With the typical specific capacitance of 3×10^{-10} F/m $= 0.3$ aF/nm, this gives nanowire capacitance $C_0 \approx 1$ aF per working elementary synapse, because the corresponding segment has length $4F_{nano}$. The CrossNet operation speed is determined mostly by the time constant τ_0 of dendrite nanowire capacitance recharging through resistances of open nanodevices. Since both the relevant conductance and capacitance increase similarly with M and n, $\tau_0 \approx R_0 C_0$.

The possibilities of reduction of R_0, and hence τ_0, are limited mostly by acceptable power dissipation per unit area, that is close to $V_s^2/(2F_{nano})^2 R_0$. For room-temperature operation, the voltage scale $V_0 \approx V_t$ should be of the order of at least 30 $k_B T/e \approx 1$ V to avoid thermally-induced errors [9]. With our number for F_{nano}, and a relatively high but acceptable power consumption of 100 W/cm^2, we get $R_0 \approx 10^{10} \Omega$ (which is a very realistic value for single-molecule single-electron devices like one shown in Fig. 3). With this number, τ_0 is as small as ~10 ns. This means that the CrossNet speed may be approximately six orders of magnitude (!) higher than that of the biological neural networks. Even scaling R_0 up by a factor of 100 to bring power consumption to a more comfortable level of 1 W/cm^2, would still leave us at least a four-orders-of-magnitude speed advantage.

6 Discussion: Possible applications

These estimates make us believe that that CMOL CrossNet chips may revolutionize the neuromorphic network applications. Let us start with the example of relatively small (1-cm^2-scale) chips used for recognition of a face in a crowd [11]. The most difficult feature of such recognition is the search for face location, i.e. optimal placement of a face on the image relative to the panel providing input for the processing network. The enormous density and speed of CMOL hardware gives a possibility to time-and-space multiplex this task (Fig. 6). In this approach, the full image (say, formed by CMOS photodetectors on the same chip) is divided into P rectangular panels of $h{\times}w$ pixels, corresponding to the expected size and approximate shape of a single face. A CMOS-implemented communication channel passes input data from each panel to the corresponding CMOL neural network, providing its shift in time, say using the TV scanning pattern (red line in Fig. 6). The standard methods of image classification require the network to have just a few hidden layers, so that the time interval Δt necessary for each mapping position may be so short that the total pattern recognition time $T = hw\Delta t$ may be acceptable even for online face recognition.

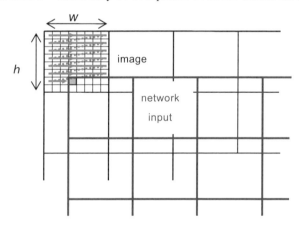

Fig. 6. Scan mapping of the input image on CMOL CrossNet inputs. Red lines show the possible time sequence of image pixels sent to a certain input of the network processing image from the upper-left panel of the pattern

Indeed, let us consider a 4-Megapixel image partitioned into 4K 32×32-pixel panels ($h = w = 32$). This panel will require an MLP net with several (say, four) layers with 1K cells each in order to compare the panel image with ~10^3 stored faces. With the feasible 4-nm nanowire half-pitch, and 65-level synapses (sufficient for better than 99% fidelity [9]), each interlayer crossbar would require chip area about $(4K{\times}64\text{ nm})^2 = 64{\times}64$ μm^2, fitting 4×4K of them on a ~0.6 cm^2 chip. (The CMOS somatic-layer and communication-system overheads are negligible.) With the acceptable power consumption of the order of 10 W/cm^2, the input-to-output signal propagation in such a network will take only about 50 ns, so that Δt may be of the order of 100 ns and the total time $T = hw\Delta t$ of processing one frame of the order of 100 microseconds, much shorter than the typical TV frame time of ~10 milliseconds. The remaining two-orders-of-magnitude time gap may be used, for example, for double-checking the results via stopping the scan mapping (Fig. 6) at the most promising position. (For this, a simple feedback from the recognition output to the mapping communication system is necessary.)

It is instructive to compare the estimated CMOL chip speed with that of the implementation of a similar parallel network ensemble on a CMOS signal processor (say, also combined on the same chip with an array of CMOS photodetectors). Even assuming an extremely high performance of 30 billion additions/multiplications per second, we would need $\sim 4 \times 4K \times 1K \times (4K)^2/(30 \times 10^9) \approx 10^4$ seconds $\sim$ 3 hours per frame, evidently incompatible with the online image stream processing.

Let us finish with a brief (and much more speculative) discussion of possible long-term prospects of CMOL CrossNets. Eventually, large-scale ($\sim 30 \times 30$ cm^2) CMOL circuits may become available. According to the estimates given in the previous section, the integration scale of such a system (in terms of both neural cells and synapses) will be comparable with that of the human cerebral cortex. Equipped with a set of broadband sensor/actuator interfaces, such (necessarily, hierarchical) system may be capable, after a period of initial supervised training, of further self-training in the process of interaction with environment, with the speed several orders of magnitude higher than that of its biological prototypes. Needless to say, the successful development of such self-developing systems would have a major impact not only on all information technologies, but also on the society as a whole.

Acknowledgments

This work has been supported in part by the AFOSR, MARCO (via FENA Center), and NSF. Valuable contributions made by Simon Fölling, Özgür Türel and Ibrahim Muckra, as well as useful discussions with P. Adams, J. Barhen, D. Hammerstrom, V. Protopopescu, T. Sejnowski, and D. Strukov are gratefully acknowledged.

References

[1] Frank, D. J. et al. (2001) Device scaling limits of Si MOSFETs and their application dependencies. Proc. IEEE **89**(3): 259-288.

[2] Likharev, K. K. (2003) Electronics below 10 nm, in J. Greer et al. (eds.), Nano and Giga Challenges in Microelectronics, pp. 27-68. Amsterdam: Elsevier.

[3] Likharev, K. K. and Strukov, D. B. (2005) CMOL: Devices, circuits, and architectures, in G. Cuniberti et al. (eds.), Introducing Molecular Electronics, Ch. 16. Springer, Berlin.

[4] Fölling, S., Türel, Ö. & Likharev, K. K. (2001) Single-electron latching switches as nanoscale synapses, in Proc. of the 2001 Int. Joint Conf. on Neural Networks, pp. 216-221. Mount Royal, NJ: Int. Neural Network Society.

[5] Wang, W. et al. (2003) Mechanism of electron conduction in self-assembled alkanethiol monolayer devices. Phys. Rev. B **68**(3): 035416 1-8.

[6] Stan M. et al. (2003) Molecular electronics: From devices and interconnect to circuits and architecture, Proc. IEEE **91**(11): 1940-1957.

[7] Strukov, D. B. & Likharev, K. K. (2005) Prospects for terabit-scale nanoelectronic memories. Nanotechnology **16**(1): 137-148.

[8] Strukov, D. B. & Likharev, K. K. (2005) CMOL FPGA: A reconfigurable architecture for hybrid digital circuits with two-terminal nanodevices. Nanotechnology **16**(6): 888-900.

[9] Türel, Ö. et al. (2004) Neuromorphic architectures for nanoelectronic circuits", Int. J. of Circuit Theory and Appl. **32**(5): 277-302.

[10] See, e.g., Hertz J. et al. (1991) Introduction to the Theory of Neural Computation. Cambridge, MA: Perseus.

[11] Lee, J. H. & Likharev, K. K. (2005) CrossNets as pattern classifiers. Lecture Notes in Computer Sciences **3575**: 434-441.

A Criterion for the Convergence of Learning with Spike Timing Dependent Plasticity

Robert Legenstein and Wolfgang Maass
Institute for Theoretical Computer Science
Technische Universitaet Graz
A-8010 Graz, Austria
{legi,maass}@igi.tugraz.at

Abstract

We investigate under what conditions a neuron can learn by experimentally supported rules for spike timing dependent plasticity (STDP) to predict the arrival times of strong "teacher inputs" to the same neuron. It turns out that in contrast to the famous Perceptron Convergence Theorem, which predicts convergence of the perceptron learning rule for a simplified neuron model whenever a stable solution exists, no equally strong convergence guarantee can be given for spiking neurons with STDP. But we derive a criterion on the statistical dependency structure of input spike trains which characterizes exactly when learning with STDP will converge on average for a simple model of a spiking neuron. This criterion is reminiscent of the linear separability criterion of the Perceptron Convergence Theorem, but it applies here to the rows of a correlation matrix related to the spike inputs. In addition we show through computer simulations for more realistic neuron models that the resulting analytically predicted positive learning results not only hold for the common interpretation of STDP where STDP changes the weights of synapses, but also for a more realistic interpretation suggested by experimental data where STDP modulates the initial release probability of dynamic synapses.

1 Introduction

Numerous experimental data show that STDP changes the value w_{old} of a synaptic weight after pairing of the firing of the presynaptic neuron at time t^{pre} with a firing of the postsynaptic neuron at time $t^{post} = t^{pre} + \Delta t$ to $w_{new} = w_{old} + \Delta w$ according to the rule

$$
w_{new} = \begin{cases} \min\{w_{max}, \ w_{old} + W_+ \cdot e^{-\Delta t/\tau_+}\} & , \quad \text{if } \Delta t > 0 \\ \max\{0, \ w_{old} - W_- \cdot e^{\Delta t/\tau_-}\} & , \quad \text{if } \Delta t \leq 0, \end{cases} \tag{1}
$$

with some parameters $W_+, W_-, \tau_+, \tau_- > 0$ (see [1]). If during training a teacher induces firing of the postsynaptic neuron, this rule becomes somewhat analogous to the well-known perceptron learning rule for McCulloch-Pitts neurons (= "perceptrons"). The Perceptron Convergence Theorem states that this rule enables a perceptron to learn, starting from any initial weights, after finitely many errors *any* transformation that it could possibly implement. However, we have constructed examples of input spike trains and teacher spike trains (omitted in this abstract) such that although a weight vector exists which produces the desired firing and which is stable under STDP, learning with STDP does not converge to a stable solution. On the other hand experiments in vivo have shown that neurons can be taught by suitable teacher input to adopt a given firing response [2, 3] (although the spike-timing dependence is not exploited there). We show in section 2 that such convergence of learning can be explained by STDP in the average case, provided that a certain criterion is met for the statistical dependence among Poisson spike inputs. The validity of the proposed criterion is tested in section 3 for more realistic models for neurons and synapses.

2   An analytical criterion for the convergence of STDP

The average case analysis in this section is based on the linear Poisson neuron model (see [4, 5]). This neuron model outputs a spike train $S^{post}(t)$ which is a realization of a Poisson process with the underlying instantaneous firing rate $R^{post}(t)$. We represent a spike train $S(t)$ as a sum of Dirac-δ functions $S(t) = \sum_k \delta(t - t_k)$, where t_k is the kth spike time of the spike train. The effect of an input spike at input i at time t' is modeled by an increase in the instantaneous firing rate of an amount $w_i(t')\epsilon(t - t')$, where ϵ is a response kernel and $w_i(t')$ is the synaptic efficacy of synapse i at time t'. We assume $\epsilon(s) = 0$ for $s < 0$ (causality), $\int_0^\infty ds\, \epsilon(s) = 1$ (normalization of the response kernel), and $\epsilon(s) \geq 0$ for all s as well as $w_i \geq 0$ for all i (excitatory inputs). In the linear model, the contributions of all inputs are summed up linearly:

$$R^{post}(t) = \sum_{j=1}^n \int_0^\infty ds\, w_j(t - s)\, \epsilon(s)\, S_j(t - s)\,, \tag{2}$$

where $S_1, \ldots, S_n$ are the n presynaptic spike trains. Note that in this spike generation process, the generation of an output spike is independent of previous output spikes.

The STDP-rule (1) avoids the growth of weights beyond bounds 0 and w_{max} by simple clipping. Alternatively one can make the weight update dependent on the actual weight value. In [5] a general rule is suggested where the weight dependence has the form of a power law with a non-negative exponent μ. This weight update rule is defined by

$$\Delta w = \begin{cases} W_+ \cdot (1 - w)^\mu \cdot e^{-\Delta t/\tau_+} & , \quad \text{if } \Delta t > 0 \\ -W_- \cdot w^\mu \cdot e^{\Delta t/\tau_-} & , \quad \text{if } \Delta t \leq 0 \,, \end{cases} \tag{3}$$

where we assumed for simplicity that $w_{max} = 1$. Instead of looking at specific input spike trains, we consider the average behavior of the weight vector for (possibly correlated) homogeneous Poisson input spike trains. Hence, the change Δw_i is a random variable with a mean drift and fluctuations around it. We will in the following focus on the drift by assuming that individual weight changes are very small and only averaged quantities enter the learning dynamics, see [6]. Let S_i be the spike train of input i and let S^* be the output spike train of the neuron. The mean drift of synapse i at time t can be approximated as

$$\dot{w}_i(t) = W_+(1 - w_i)^\mu \int_0^\infty ds\, e^{-s/\tau} C_i(s; t) - W_- w_i^\mu \int_{-\infty}^0 ds\, e^{s/\tau} C_i(s; t)\,, \tag{4}$$

where $C_i(s; t) = \langle S_i(t)S^*(t+s) \rangle_E$ is the ensemble averaged correlation function between input i and the output of the neuron (see [5, 6]). For the linear Poisson neuron model, input-output correlations can be described by means of correlations in the inputs. We define the normalized cross correlation between input spike trains S_i and S_j with a common rate $r > 0$ as

$$C_{ij}^0(s) = \frac{\langle S_i(t)\, S_j(t + s) \rangle_E}{r^2} - 1\,, \tag{5}$$

which assumes value 0 for uncorrelated Poisson spike trains. We assume in this article that C_{ij}^0 is constant over time. In our setup, the output of the neuron during learning is clamped to the teacher spike train S^* which is the output of a neuron with the target weight vector $\mathbf{w}^*$. Therefore, the input-output correlations $C_i(s;t)$ are also constant over time and we denote them by $C_i(s)$ in the following. In our neuron model, correlations are shaped by the response kernel $\epsilon(s)$ and they enter the learning equation (4) with respect to the learning window. This motivates the definition of *window correlations* c_{ij}^+ and c_{ij}^- for the positive and negative learning window respectively:

$$c_{ij}^\pm = 1 + \frac{1}{\tau} \int_0^\infty ds\, e^{-s/\tau} \int_0^\infty ds'\, \epsilon(s') C_{ij}^0(\pm s - s') \quad . \tag{6}$$

We call the matrices $C^\pm = \{c_{ij}^\pm\}_{i,j=1,\ldots,n}$ the window correlation matrices. Note that window correlations are non-negative and that for homogeneous Poisson input spike trains and for a non-negative response kernel, they are positive. For soft weight bounds and $\mu > 0$, a synaptic weight can converge to a value arbitrarily close to 0 or 1, but not to one of these values directly. This motivates the following definition of learnability.

Definition 2.1 *We say that a target weight vector $\mathbf{w}^* \in \{0,1\}^n$ can approximately be learned in a supervised paradigm by STDP with soft weight bounds on homogeneous Poisson input spike trains (short: "$\mathbf{w}^*$ can be learned") if and only if there exist $W_+, W_- > 0$, such that for $\mu \to 0$ the ensemble averaged weight vector $\langle \mathbf{w}(t) \rangle_E$ with learning dynamics given by Equation 4 converges to $\mathbf{w}^*$ for any initial weight vector $\mathbf{w}(0) \in [0,1]^n$.*

We are now ready to formulate an analytical criterion for learnability:

Theorem 2.1 *A weight vector $\mathbf{w}^*$ can be learned (when being taught with S^*) for homogeneous Poisson input spike trains with window correlation matrices C^+ and C^- to a linear Poisson neuron with non-negative response kernel if and only if $\mathbf{w}^* \neq \mathbf{0}$ and*

$$\frac{\sum_{k=1}^n w_k^* c_{ik}^+}{\sum_{k=1}^n w_k^* c_{ik}^-} > \frac{\sum_{k=1}^n w_k^* c_{jk}^+}{\sum_{k=1}^n w_k^* c_{jk}^-}$$

for all pairs $\langle i,j \rangle \in \{1,\ldots,n\}^2$ with $w_i^* = 1$ and $w_j^* = 0$.

Proof idea: The correlation between an input and the teacher induced output is (by Eq. 2):

$$C_i(s) = \langle S_i(t)\, S^*(t+s) \rangle_E = \sum_{j=1}^n w_j^* \int_0^\infty ds'\, \epsilon(s')\, \langle S_i(t)\, S_j(t+s-s') \rangle_E .$$

Substitution of this equation into Eq. 4 yields the synaptic drift

$$\dot{w}_i = \tau r^2 \left[W_+ (1-w_i)^\mu \sum_{j=1}^n w_j^* c_{ij}^+ - W_- w_i^\mu \sum_{j=1}^n w_j^* c_{ij}^- \right] . \tag{7}$$

We find the equilibrium points $w_{\mu i}$ of synapse i by setting $\dot{w}_i = 0$ in Eq. 7. This yields $w_{\mu i} = \left(1 + \frac{1}{\Lambda_i^{1/\mu}} \right)^{-1}$, where Λ_i denotes $\frac{W_+}{W_-} \frac{\sum_{j=1}^n w_j^* c_{ij}^+}{\sum_{j=1}^n w_j^* c_{ij}^-}$. Note that the drift is zero if $\mathbf{w}^* = \mathbf{0}$ which implies that $\mathbf{w}^* = \mathbf{0}$ cannot be learned. For $\mathbf{w}^* \neq \mathbf{0}$, one can show that $\mathbf{w}_\mu = (w_{\mu 1}, \ldots, w_{\mu n})$ is the only equilibrium point of the system and that it is stable. Since the system decomposes into n independent one-dimensional systems, convergence to $\mathbf{w}^*$ is guaranteed for all initial conditions. Furthermore, one sees that $\lim_{\mu \to 0} w_{\mu i} = 1$ if and only if $\Lambda_i > 1$, and $\lim_{\mu \to 0} w_{\mu i} = 0$ if and only if $\Lambda_i < 1$. Therefore, $\lim_{\mu \to 0} \mathbf{w}_\mu = \mathbf{w}^*$ holds if and only if $\Lambda_i > 1$ for all i with $w_i^* = 1$ and $\Lambda_i < 1$ for all i with $w_i^* = 0$. The theorem follows from the definition of Λ_i. ∎

For a wide class of cross-correlation functions, one can establish a relationship between learnability by STDP and the well-known concept of linear separability from linear algebra.[1] Because of synaptic delays, the response of a spiking neuron to an input spike is delayed by some time t_0. One can model such a delay in the response kernel by the restriction $\epsilon(s) = 0$ for all $s \leq t_0$. In the following Corollary we consider the case where input correlations $C_{ij}^0(s)$ appear only in a time window smaller than the delay:

Corollary 2.1 *If there exists a $t_0 \geq 0$ such that $\epsilon(s) = 0$ for all $s \leq t_0$ and $C_{ij}^0(s) = 0$ for all $s < -t_0$, $i, j \in \{1, \ldots, n\}$, then the following holds for the case of homogeneous Poisson input spike trains to a linear Poisson neuron with positive response kernel ϵ:*

A weight vector $\mathbf{w}^*$ can be learned if and only if $\mathbf{w}^* \neq \mathbf{0}$ and $\mathbf{w}^*$ linearly separates the list $L = \langle \langle \mathbf{c}_1^+, w_1^* \rangle, \ldots, \langle \mathbf{c}_n^+, w_n^* \rangle \rangle$, where $\mathbf{c}_1^+, \ldots, \mathbf{c}_n^+$ are the rows of C^+.

Proof idea: From the assumptions of the corollary it follows that $c_{ij}^- = 1$. In this case, the condition in Theorem 2.1 is equivalent to the statement that $\mathbf{w}^*$ linearly separates the list $L = \langle \langle \mathbf{c}_1^+, w_1^* \rangle, \ldots, \langle \mathbf{c}_n^+, w_n^* \rangle \rangle$. ∎

Corollary 2.1 can be viewed as an analogon of the Perceptron Convergence Theorem for the average case analysis of STDP. Its formulation is tight in the sense that linear separability of the list L alone (as opposed to linear separability by the target vector $\mathbf{w}^*$) is not sufficient to imply learnability. For uncorrelated input spike trains of rate $r > 0$, the normalized cross correlation functions are given by $C_{ij}^0(s) = \frac{\delta_{ij}}{r}\delta(s)$, where δ_{ij} is the Kronecker delta function. The positive window correlation matrix C^+ is therefore essentially a scaled version of the identity matrix. The following corollary then follows from Corollary 2.1:

Corollary 2.2 *A target weight vector $\mathbf{w}^* \in \{0, 1\}^n$ can be learned in the case of uncorrelated Poisson input spike trains to a linear Poisson neuron with positive response kernel ϵ such that $\epsilon(s) = 0$ for all $s \leq 0$ if and only if $\mathbf{w}^* \neq \mathbf{0}$.*

3   Computer simulations of supervised learning with STDP

In order to make a theoretical analysis feasible, we needed to make in section 2 a number of simplifying assumptions on the neuron model and the synapse model. In addition a number of approximations had to be used in order to simplify the estimates. We consider in this section the more realistic integrate-and-fire model[2] for neurons and a model for synapses which are subject to paired-pulse depression and paired-pulse facilitation, in addition to the long term plasticity induced by STDP [7]. This model describes synapses with parameters U (initial release probability), D (depression time constant), and F (facilitation time constant) in addition to the synaptic weight w. The parameters U, D, and F were randomly

---

[1] Let $\mathbf{c}_1, \ldots, \mathbf{c}_m \in \mathbb{R}^n$ and $y_1, \ldots, y_m \in \{0, 1\}$. We say that a vector $\mathbf{w} \in \mathbb{R}^n$ linearly separates the list $\langle \langle \mathbf{c}_1, y_1 \rangle, \ldots, \langle \mathbf{c}_m, y_m \rangle \rangle$ if there exists a threshold Θ such that $y_i = \text{sign}(\mathbf{c}_i \cdot \mathbf{w} - \Theta)$ for $i = 1, \ldots, m$. We define $\text{sign}(z) = 1$ if $z \geq 0$ and $\text{sign}(z) = 0$ otherwise.

[2] The membrane potential V_m of the neuron is given by $\tau_m \frac{dV_m}{dt} = -(V_m - V_{resting}) + R_m \cdot (I_{syn}(t) + I_{background} + I_{inject}(t))$ where $\tau_m = C_m \cdot R_m = 30ms$ is the membrane time constant, $R_m = 1M\Omega$ is the membrane resistance, $I_{syn}(t)$ is the current supplied by the synapses, $I_{background}$ is a constant background current, and $I_{inject}(t)$ represents currents induced by a 'teacher'. If V_m exceeds the threshold voltage V_{thresh} it is reset to $V_{reset} = 14.2mV$ and held there for the length $T_{refract} = 3ms$ of the absolute refractory period. *Neuron parameters:* $V_{resting} = 0V$, $I_{background}$ randomly chosen for each trial from the interval $[13.5nA, 14.5nA]$. V_{thresh} was set such that each neuron spiked at a rate of about 25 Hz. This resulted in a threshold voltage slightly above $15mV$. *Synaptic parameters:* Synaptic currents were modeled as exponentially decaying currents with decay time constants $\tau_S = 3ms$ ($\tau_S = 6ms$) for excitatory (inhibitory) synapses.

chosen from Gaussian distributions that were based on empirically found data for such connections. We also show that in some cases a less restrictive teacher forcing suffices, that tolerates undesired firing of the neuron during training. The results of section 2 predict that the temporal structure of correlations has a strong influence on the outcome of a learning experiment. We used input spike trains with cross correlations that decay exponentially with a correlation decay constant τ_{cc}.[3] In experiment 1 we consider temporal correlations with $\tau_{cc}=10$ms. Since such "broader" correlations are not problematic for STDP, sharper correlations ($\tau_{cc}=6$ms) are considered in experiment 2.

Experiment 1 (correlated input with $\tau_{cc}=10$ms): In this experiment, a leaky integrate-and-fire neuron received inputs from 100 dynamic synapses. 90% of these synapses were excitatory and 10% were inhibitory. For each excitatory synapse, the maximal efficacy w_{max} was chosen from a Gaussian distribution with mean 54 and SD 10.8, bounded by $54 \pm 3SD$. The 90 excitatory inputs were divided into 9 groups of 10 synapses per group. Spike trains were correlated within groups with correlation coefficients between 0 and 0.8, whereas there were virtually no correlations between spike trains of different groups.[4] Target weight vectors $\mathbf{w}^*$ were chosen in the most adverse way: half of the weights of $\mathbf{w}^*$ within each group was set to 0, the other half to its maximal value w_{max} (see Fig. 1C).

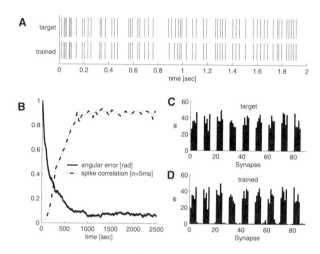

Figure 1: Learning a target weight vector $\mathbf{w}^*$ on correlated Poisson inputs. **A)** Output spike train on test data after one hour of training (trained) compared to the target output (target). **B)** Evolution of the angle between weight vector $\mathbf{w}(t)$ and the vector $\mathbf{w}^*$ that implements F in radiant (angular error, solid line), and spike correlation (dashed line). **C)** Target weight vector $\mathbf{w}^*$ consisting of elements with value 0 or the value w_{max} assigned to that synapse. **D)** Corresponding weights of the learned vector $\mathbf{w}(t)$ after 40 minutes of training. (All time data refer to simulated biological time)

Before training, the weights of all excitatory synapses were initialized by randomly chosen small values. Weights of inhibitory synapses remained fixed throughout the experiment. Information about the target weight vector $\mathbf{w}^*$ was given to the neuron only in the form of short current injections (1 μA for 0.2 ms) at those times when the neuron with the weight vector $\mathbf{w}^*$ would have produced a spike. Learning was implemented as standard STDP (see rule 1) with parameters $\tau_+ = \tau_- = 20ms$, $W_+ = 0.45$, $W_-/W_+ = 1.05$. Additional inhibitory input was given to the neuron during training that reduced the occurrence of non-

---

[3]We constructed input spike trains with normalized cross correlations (see Equation 5) approximately given by $C_{ij}^0(s) = \frac{cc_{ij}}{2\tau_{cc}r}e^{-|s|/\tau_{cc}}$ between inputs i and j for a mean input rate of $r = 20$Hz, a correlation coefficient c_{ij}, and a correlation decay constant of $\tau_{cc} = 10$ms.

[4]The correlation coefficient c_{ij} for spike trains within group k consisting of 10 spike trains was set to $c_{ij} = cc_k = 0.1 * (k - 1)$ for $k = 1, \ldots, 9$.

teacher-induced firing of the neuron (see text below).[5] Two different performance measures were used for analyzing the learning progress. The "spike correlation" measures for test inputs that were not used for training (but had been generated by the same process) the deviation between the output spike train produced by the target weight vector $\mathbf{w}^*$ for this input, and the output spike train produced for the same input by the neuron with the current weight vector $\mathbf{w}(t)$[6]. The *angular error* measures the angle between the current weight vector $\mathbf{w}(t)$ and the target weight vector $\mathbf{w}^*$. The results are shown in Fig. 1. One can see that the deviation of the learned weight vector shown in panel D from the target weight vector $\mathbf{w}^*$ (panel C) is very small, even for highly correlated groups of synapses with heterogeneous target weights. No significant changes in the results were observed for longer simulations (4 hours simulated biological time), showing stability of learning. On 20 trials (each with a new random distribution of maximal weights w_{max}, different initializations $\mathbf{w}(0)$ of the weight vector before learning, and new Poisson spike trains), a spike correlation of 0.83 ± 0.06 was achieved (angular error 6.8 ± 4.7 degrees). Note that learning is not only based on teacher spikes but also on non teacher-induced firing. Therefore, strongly correlated groups of inputs tend to cause autonomous (i.e., not teacher-induced) firing of the neuron which results in weight increases for *all* weights within the corresponding group of synapses according to well-known results for STDP [8, 5]. Obviously this effect makes it quite hard to learn a target weight vector $\mathbf{w}^*$ where half of the weights for each correlated group have value 0. The effect is reduced by the additional inhibitory input during training which reduces undesired firing. However, without this input a spike correlation of 0.79 ± 0.09 could still be achieved (angular error 14.1 ± 10 degrees).

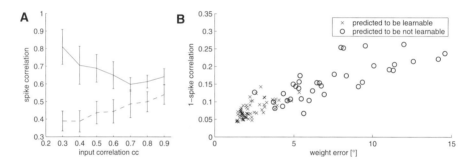

Figure 2: **A)** Spike correlation achieved for correlated inputs (solid line). Some inputs were correlated with cc plotted on the x-axis. Also, as a control the spike correlation achieved by randomly drawn weight vectors is shown (dashed line, where half of the weights were set to w_{max} and the other weights were set to 0). **B)** Comparison between theory and simulation results for a leaky integrate-and-fire neuron and input correlations between 0.1 and 0.5 ($\tau_{cc} = 6ms$). Each cross (open circle) marks a trial where the target vector was learnable (not learnable) according to Theorem 2.1. The actual learning performance of STDP is plotted for each trial in terms of the weight error (x-axis) and 1 minus the spike correlation (y-axis).

Experiment 2 (testing the theoretical predictions for τ_{cc}=6ms): In order to evaluate the dependence of correlation among inputs we proceeded in a setup similar to experiment 1. 4 input groups consisting each of 10 input spike trains were constructed for which the correlations within each group had the same value cc while the input spike train to the other 50 excitatory synapses were uncorrelated. Again, half of the weights of $\mathbf{w}^*$ within

---

[5]We added 30 inhibitory synapses with weights drawn from a gamma distribution with mean 25 and standard deviation 7.5, that received additional 30 uncorrelated Poisson spike trains at 20 Hz.

[6]For that purpose each spike in these two output spike trains was replaced by a Gaussian function with an SD of 5 ms. The *spike correlation* between both output spike trains was defined as the correlation between the resulting smooth functions of time (for segments of length 100 s).

each correlated group (and within the uncorrelated group) was set to 0, the other half to a randomly chosen maximal value. The learning performance after 1 hour of training for 20 trials is plotted in Fig. 2A for 7 different values of the correlation cc ($\tau_{cc} = 6$ms) that is applied in 4 of the input groups (solid line).

In order to test the approximate validity of Theorem 2.1 for leaky integrate-and-fire neurons and dynamic synapses, we repeated the above experiment for input correlations $cc = 0.1, 0.2, 0.3, 0.4$, and 0.5. For each correlation value, 20 learning trials (with different target vectors) were simulated. For each trial we first checked whether the (randomly chosen) target vector $\mathbf{w}^*$ was learnable according to the condition given in Theorem 2.1 (65% of the 100 learning trials were classified as being learnable).[7] The actual performance of learning with STDP was evaluated after 50 minutes of training.[8] The result is shown in Fig. 2B. It shows that the theoretical prediction of learnability or non-learnability for the case of simpler neuron models and synapses from Theorem 2.1 translates in a biologically more realistic scenario into a quantitative grading of the learning performance that can ultimately be achieved with STDP.

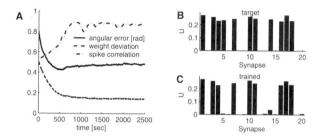

Figure 3: Results of modulation of initial release probabilities U. **A)** Performance of U-learning for a generic learning task (see text). **B)** Twenty values of the target U vector (each component assumes its maximal possible value or the value 0). **C)** Corresponding U values after 42 minutes of training.

Experiment 3 (Modulation of initial release probabilities U by STDP): Experimental data from [9] suggest that synaptic plasticity does not change the uniform scaling of the amplitudes of EPSPs resulting from a presynaptic spike train (i.e., the parameter w), but rather redistributes the sum of their amplitudes. If one assumes that STDP changes the parameter U that determines the synaptic release probability for the first spike in a spike train, whereas the weight w remains unchanged, then the same experimental data that support the classical rule for STDP, support the following rule for changing U:

$$U_{new} = \begin{cases} min\{U_{max}, U_{old} + U_+ \cdot e^{-\Delta t/\tau_+}\} &, \quad \text{if } \Delta t > 0 \\ max\{0, U_{old} - U_- \cdot e^{\Delta t/\tau_-}\} &, \quad \text{if } \Delta t \le 0 \end{cases} \quad (8)$$

with suitable nonnegative parameters $U_{max}, U_+, U_-, \tau_+, \tau_-$.

Fig. 3 shows results of an experiment where U was modulated with rule (8) (similar to experiment 1, but with uncorrelated inputs). 20 repetitions of this experiment yielded after 42 minutes of training the following results: spike correlation 0.88 ± 0.036, angular error 27.9 ± 3.7 degrees, for $U_+ = 0.0012$, $U_-/U_+ = 1.055$. Apparently the output spike train is less sensitive to changes in the values of U than to changes in w. Consequently, since

---

[7]We had chosen a response kernel of the form $\epsilon(s) = \frac{1}{\tau_1 - \tau_2}(e^{-s/\tau_1} - e^{-s/\tau_2})$ with $\tau_1 = 2ms$ and $\tau_2 = 1ms$ (Least mean squares fit of the double exponential to the peri-stimulus-time histogram (PSTH) of the neuron, which reflects the probability of spiking as a function of time s since an input spike), and calculated the window correlations c_{ij}^+ and c_{ij}^- numerically.

[8]To guarantee the best possible performance for each learning trial, training was performed on 27 different values for W_-/W_+ between 1.02 and 1.15.

only the behavior of a neuron with vector $\mathbf{U}^*$ but not the vector $\mathbf{U}^*$ is made available to the neuron during training, the resulting correlation between target- and actual output spike trains is quite high, whereas angular error between $\mathbf{U}^*$ and $\mathbf{U}(t)$, as well as the average deviation in U, remain rather large.

We also repeated experiment 1 (correlated Poisson inputs) with rule (8) for U-learning. 20 repetitions with different target weights and different initial conditions yielded after 35 minutes of training: spike correlation 0.75 ± 0.08, angular error 39.3 ± 4.8 degrees, for $U_+ = 8 \cdot 10^{-4}, U_-/U_+ = 1.09$.

4 Discussion

The main conclusion of this article is that for many common distributions of input spikes a spiking neuron can learn with STDP and teacher-induced input currents any map from input spike trains to output spike trains that it could possibly implement in a stable manner.

We have shown in section 2 that a mathematical average case analysis can be carried out for supervised learning with STDP. This theoretical analysis produces the first criterion that allows us to predict whether supervised learning with STDP will succeed in spite of correlations among Poisson input spike trains. For the special case of "sharp correlations" (i.e. when the cross correlations vanish for time shifts larger than the synaptic delay) this criterion can be formulated in terms of linear separability of the rows of a correlation matrix related to the spike input, and its mathematical form is therefore reminiscent of the well-known condition for learnability in the case of perceptron learning. In this sense Corollary 2.1 can be viewed as an analogon of the Perceptron Convergence Theorem for spiking neurons with STDP.

Furthermore we have shown that an alternative interpretation of STDP where one assumes that it modulates the initial release probabilities U of dynamic synapses, rather than their scaling factors w, gives rise to very satisfactory convergence results for learning.

Acknowledgment: We would like to thank Yves Fregnac, Wulfram Gerstner, and especially Henry Markram for inspiring discussions.

References

[1] L. F. Abbott and S. B. Nelson. Synaptic plasticity: taming the beast. *Nature Neurosci.*, 3:1178–1183, 2000.

[2] Y. Fregnac, D. Shulz, S. Thorpe, and E. Bienenstock. A cellular analogue of visual cortical plasticity. *Nature*, 333(6171):367–370, 1988.

[3] D. Debanne, D. E. Shulz, and Y. Fregnac. Activity dependent regulation of on- and off-responses in cat visual cortical receptive fields. *Journal of Physiology*, 508:523–548, 1998.

[4] R. Kempter, W. Gerstner, and J. L. van Hemmen. Intrinsic stabilization of output rates by spike-based hebbian learning. *Neural Computation*, 13:2709–2741, 2001.

[5] R. Gütig, R. Aharonov, S. Rotter, and H. Sompolinsky. Learning input correlations through non-linear temporally asymmetric hebbian plasticity. *Journal of Neurosci.*, 23:3697–3714, 2003.

[6] R. Kempter, W. Gerstner, and J. L. van Hemmen. Hebbian learning and spiking neurons. *Phys. Rev. E*, 59(4):4498–4514, 1999.

[7] H. Markram, Y. Wang, and M. Tsodyks. Differential signaling via the same axon of neocortical pyramidal neurons. *PNAS*, 95:5323–5328, 1998.

[8] S. Song, K. D. Miller, and L. F. Abbott. Competitive hebbian learning through spike-timing dependent synaptic plasticity. *Nature Neuroscience*, 3:919–926, 2000.

[9] H. Markram and M. Tsodyks. Redistribution of synaptic efficacy between neocortical pyramidal neurons. *Nature*, 382:807–810, 1996.

Dynamical Synapses Give Rise to a Power-Law Distribution of Neuronal Avalanches

Anna Levina[3,4]**, J. Michael Herrmann**[1,2]**, Theo Geisel**[1,2,4]
[1] Bernstein Center for Computational Neuroscience Göttingen
[2] Georg-August University Göttingen, Institute for Nonlinear Dynamics
[3] Graduate School Identification in Mathematical Models
[4] Max Planck Institute for Dynamics and Self-Organization
Bunsenstr. 10, 37073 Göttingen, Germany
anna|michael|geisel@chaos.gwdg.de

Abstract

There is experimental evidence that cortical neurons show avalanche activity with the intensity of firing events being distributed as a power-law. We present a biologically plausible extension of a neural network which exhibits a power-law avalanche distribution for a wide range of connectivity parameters.

1 Introduction

Power-law distributions of event sizes have been observed in a number of seemingly diverse systems such as piles of granular matter [8], earthquakes [9], the game of life [1], friction [7], and sound generated in the lung during breathing. Because it is unlikely that the specific parameter values at which the critical behavior occurs are assumed by chance, the question arises as to what mechanisms may tune the parameters towards the critical state. Furthermore it is known that criticality brings about optimal computational capabilities [10], improves mixing or enhances the sensitivity to unpredictable stimuli [5]. Therefore, it is interesting to search for mechanisms that entail criticality in biological systems, for example in the nervous tissue.

In [6] a simple model of a fully connected neural network of non-leaky integrate-and-fire neurons was studied. This study not only presented the first example of a globally coupled system that shows criticality, but also predicted the critical exponent as well as some extra-critical dynamical phenomena, which were later observed in experimental researches. Recently, Beggs and Plenz [3] studied the propagation of spontaneous neuronal activity in slices of rat cortex and neuronal cultures using multi-electrode arrays. Thereby, they found avalanche-like activity where the avalanche sizes were distributed according to a power-law with an exponent of -3/2. This distribution was stable over a long period of time. The authors suggested that such a distribution is optimal in terms of transmission and storage of the information.

The network in [6] consisted of a set of N identical threshold elements characterized by the membrane potential $u \geq 0$ and was driven by a slowly delivered random input. When the potential exceeds a threshold $\theta = 1$, the neuron spikes and relaxes. All connections in the network are described by a single parameter α representing the evoked synaptic potential which a spiking neuron transmits to the all postsynaptic neurons. The system is driven by a slowly delivered random input. The simplicity of that model allows analytical consideration: an explicit formula for probability distribution of avalanche size depending on the parameter α was derived. A major drawback of the model was the lack of any true self-organization. Only at an externally well-tuned critical value of $\alpha = \alpha_{cr}$ did the distribution take a form of a power-law, although with an exponent of precisely -3/2 (in the limit of a large system). The term *critical* will be applied here also to finite systems. True criticality requires a thermodynamic limit $N \longrightarrow \infty$, we consider approximate power-law behavior characterized by an exponent and an error that describes the remaining deviation from the best-matching exponent. The model in [6] is displayed for comparison in Fig. 3. In Fig. 1 (a-c) it is visible that the system may also exhibit other types of behavior such as small avalanches with a finite mean (even in the thermodynamic limit) at $\alpha < \alpha_{cr}$. On the other hand at $\alpha > \alpha_{cr}$ the distribution becomes non-monotonous, which indicates that avalanches of the size of the system are occurring frequently. Generally speaking, in order to drive the system towards criticality it therefore suffices to decrease the large avalanches and to enhance the small ones. Most interestingly, synaptic connections among real neurons show a similar tendency which thus deserves further study. We will consider the standard model of a short-term dynamics in synaptic efficacies [11, 13] and thereafter discuss several numerically determined quantities. Our studies imply that dynamical synapses indeed may support the criticalization of the neural activity in a small homogeneous neural system.

2 The model

We are considering a network of integrate-and-fire neurons with dynamical synapses. Each synapse is described by two parameters: amount of available neurotransmitters and a fraction of them which is ready to be used at the next synaptic event. Both parameters change in time depending on the state of the presynaptic neuron. Such a system keeps a long memory of the previous events and is known to exert a regulatory effect to the network dynamics, which will turnout to be beneficial.

Our approach is based on the model of dynamical synapses, which was shown by Tsodyks and Markram to reliably reproduce the synaptic responses between pyramidal neurons [11, 13]. Consider a set of N integrate-and-fire neurons characterized by a membrane potential $h_i \geq 0$, and two connectivity parameters for each synapse: $J_{i,j} \geq 0$, $u_{i,j} \in [0, 1]$. The parameter $J_{i,j}$ characterizes the number of available vesicles on the presynaptic side of the connection from neuron j to neuron i. Each spike leads to the usage of a portion of the resources of the presynaptic neuron, hence, at the next synaptic event less transmitters will be available i.e. activity will be depressed. Between spikes vesicles are slowly recovering on a timescale τ_1. The parameter $u_{i,j}$ denotes the actual fraction of vesicles on the presynaptic side of the connection from neuron j to neuron i, which will be used in the synaptic transmission. When a spike arrives at the presynaptic side j, it causes an increase of $u_{i,j}$. Between spikes, $u_{i,j}$ slowly decrease to zero on a timescale τ_2. The combined effect of $J_{i,j}$ and $u_{i,j}$ results in the facilitation or depression of the synapse. The dynamics of a membrane potential h_i consists of the integration of excitatory postsynaptic currents over all synapses of the neuron and the slowly delivered random input. When the membrane potential exceeds threshold, the neuron emits a spike and h_i resets to a smaller value. The

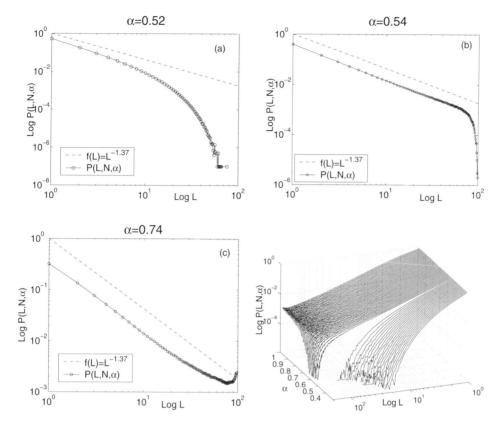

Figure 1: Probability distributions of avalanche sizes $P(L, N, \alpha)$. (a) in the subcritical, $\alpha = 0.52$, (b) the critical, $\alpha = 0.53$, and (c) supra-critical regime, $\alpha = 0.74$. In (a-c) the solid lines and symbols denote the numerical results for the avalanche size distributions, dashed lines show the best matching power-law. Here the curves are temporal averages over 10^6 avalanches with $N = 100$, $u_0 = 0.1$, $\tau_1 = \tau_2 = 0.1$. Sub-figure (d) displays $P(L, N, \alpha)$ as a function of L for α varying from 0.34 to 0.98 with step 0.01. The presented curves are temporal averages over 10^6 avalanches with $N = 200$, $u_0 = 0.1$, $\tau_1 = \tau_2 = 0.1$.

joint dynamics can be written as a system of differential equations

$$\dot{J}_{i,j} = \frac{1}{\tau_1 \tau_s}(J_0 - J_{i,j}) - u_{i,j} J_{i,j} \delta(t - t_{\mathrm{sp}}^j), \tag{1}$$

$$\dot{u}_{i,j} = -\frac{1}{\tau_2 \tau_s} u_{i,j} + u_0(1 - u_{i,j}) \delta(t - t_{\mathrm{sp}}^j), \tag{2}$$

$$\dot{h}_i = \frac{1}{\tau_s} \delta(r(t) - i) c \xi + \sum_{j=1}^{N} u_{i,j} J_{i,j} \delta(t - t_{\mathrm{sp}}^j) \tag{3}$$

Here $\delta(t)$ is the Dirac delta-function, t_{sp}^j is the spiking time of neuron j, J_0 is the resting value of $J_{i,j}$, u_0 is the minimal value of $u_{i,j}$, and τ_s is a parameter separating time-scales of random input and synaptic events. In the following study we will use the discrete version of equations (1-3).

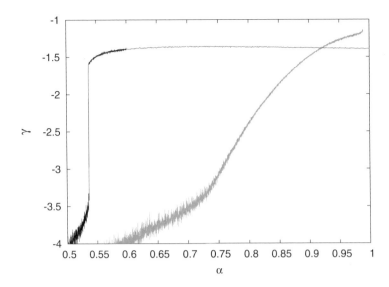

Figure 2: The best matching power-law exponent. The black line represents the present model, while the grey stands for model [6]. Average synaptic efficiency α varies from 0.3 to 1.0 with step 0.001. Presented curves are temporal averages over 10^7 avalanches with $N = 200$, $u_0 = 0.1$, $\tau_1 = \tau_2 = 10$. Note that for a network of 200 units, the absolute critical exponent is smaller than the large system limit $\gamma = -1.5$ and that the step size has been drastically reduced in the vicinity of the phase transition.

3   Discrete version of the model

We consider time being measured in discrete steps, $t = 0, 1, 2, \ldots$. Because synaptic values are essentially determined presynaptically, we assume that all synapses of a neuron are identical, i.e. J_j, u_j are used instead of $J_{i,j}$ and $u_{i,j}$ respectively. The system is initialized with arbitrary values $h_i \in [0, 1)$, $i = 1, \ldots, N$, where the threshold θ is fixed at 1. Depending on the state of the system at time t, the i-th element receives external input $I_i^{\text{ext}}(t)$ or internal input $I_i^{\text{int}}(t)$ from other neural elements. The two effects result in an activation $\tilde{h}$ at time $t + 1$,

$$\tilde{h}_i(t + 1) = h_i(t) + I_i^{\text{ext}}(t) + I_i^{\text{int}}(t) \tag{4}$$

From the activation $\tilde{h}_i(t + 1)$, the membrane potential of the i-th element at time $t + 1$ is computed as

$$h_i(t + 1) = \begin{cases} \tilde{h}_i(t + 1) & \text{if } \tilde{h}_i(t + 1) < 1, \\ \tilde{h}_i(t + 1) - 1 & \text{if } \tilde{h}_i(t + 1) \geq 1, \end{cases} \tag{5}$$

i.e. if the activation exceeds the threshold, it is reset but retains the supra-threshold portion $\tilde{h}_i(t + 1) - 1$ of the membrane potential.

The external input $I_i^{\text{ext}}(t)$ is a random amount $c\xi$, received by a randomly chosen neuron. Here, c is input strength scale, parameter of the model, ξ is uniformly distributed on $[0, 1]$ and independent of i. The external input is considered to be delivered slowly compared to the internal relaxation dynamics (which corresponds to $\tau_{\text{sep}} \gg 1$), i.e. it occurs only if no element has exceeded the threshold in the previous time step. This corresponds to an infinite separation of the time scales of external driving and avalanche dynamics discussed in the literature on self-organized criticality [12, 14]. The present results, however, are not affected by a continuous external input even during the avalanches. The external input

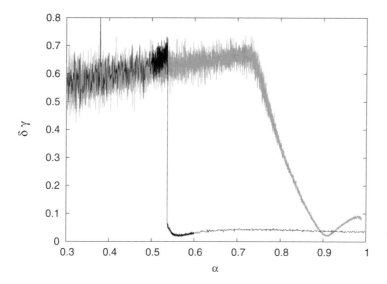

Figure 3: The mean squared deviation from the best fit power-law. The grey code and parameters are the same as in Fig. 2 For the fit, avalanches of a size larger than 1 and smaller than $N/2$ have been used. Clearly, an error levels above 0.1 indicates that the fitted curve is far from being a candidate for a power law. Near to $\alpha = 1$, when the non-dynamical model develops a supercritical behavior, the range of the power-law is quite limited. Interesting is again the sharp transition of the dynamical model, which is due to the facilitation strength surpassing a critical level.

can formally be written as $I_i^{\text{ext}}(t) = c\,\delta_{r,i}(t)\,|\delta_{M(t-1)|,0}\,\xi$, where r is an integer random variable between 1 and N indicating the chosen element, $M(t-1)$ is the set of indices of supra-threshold elements in the previous time step i.e. $M(t) = \{i|\tilde{h}_i(t) \geq 1\}$, and $\delta_{..}$ is the Kronecker delta. We will consider $c = J_0$, thus an external input is comparable with the typical internal input.

The internal input $I_i^{\text{int}}(t)$ is given by

$$I_i^{\text{int}}(t) = \sum_{j \in M(t-1)} J_j(t)\,u_j(t).$$

The system is initialized with $u_i = u_0, J_i = J_0$, where $J_0 = \alpha/(Nu_0)$ and α is the connection strength parameter. Similar to the membrane potentials dynamics, we can distinguish two situations: either there were supra-threshold neurons at the previous moment of time or not.

$$u_j(t+1) = \begin{cases} u_j(t) - \frac{1}{\tau_2}u_0u_j(t)) \cdot \delta_{|M(t)|,0} & \text{if } \tilde{h}_i(t) < 1, \\ u_j(t) + (1 - u_j(t))u_0(t) & \text{if } \tilde{h}_i(t) \geq 1, \end{cases} \tag{6}$$

$$J_j(t+1) = \begin{cases} J_j(t) + \frac{1}{\tau_1}(J_0 - J_j(t)) \cdot \delta_{|M(t)|,0} & \text{if } \tilde{h}_i(t) < 1, \\ J_j(t)(1 - u_j(t)) & \text{if } \tilde{h}_i(t) \geq 1, \end{cases} \tag{7}$$

Thus, we have a model with parameters α, u_0, τ_1, τ_2 and N. Our main focus will be on the influence of α on the cumulative dynamics of the network. The dependence on N has been studied in [6], where it was found that the critical parameter of the distribution scales as $\alpha_{\text{cr}} = 1 - N^{-1/2}$. In the same way, the exponent will be smaller in modulus than -3/2 for finite systems.

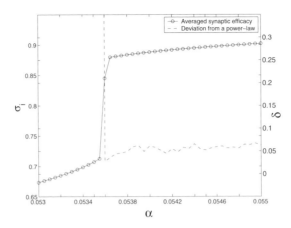

Figure 4: Average synaptic efficacy for the parameter α varied from 0.53 to 0.55 with step 0.0005 (left axis). Dashed line depicts deviation from a power-law (right axis).

If at time t_0 an element receives an external input and fires, then an avalanche starts and $|M(t_0)| = 1$. The system is globally coupled, such that during an avalanche all elements receive internal input including the unstable elements themselves. The avalanche duration $D \geq 0$ is defined to be the smallest integer for which the stopping condition $|M(t_0+D)| = 0$ is satisfied. The avalanche size L is given by $L = \sum_{k=0}^{D-1} |M(t_0 + k)|$. The subject of our interest is the probability distribution of avalanche size $P(L, N, \alpha)$ depending on the parameter α.

4 Results

Similarly, as in model [6] we considered the avalanche size distribution for different values of α, cf. Fig. 1. Three qualitatively different regimes can be distinguished: subcritical, critical, and supra-critical. For small values of α, subcritical avalanche-size distributions are observed. The subcriticality is characterized by the neglible number of avalanches of a size close to the system size. For α_{cr}, the system has an avalanche distribution with an approximate power-law behavior for L, inside a range from 1 almost up to the size of the system, where the exponential cut-off is observed (Fig. 1b). Above the critical value α_{cr}, avalanche size distributions become non-monotonous (Fig. 1c). Such supra-critical curves have a minimum at an intermediate avalanche size.

There is the sharp transition from subcritical to critical regime and then a long *critical region*, where the distribution of avalanche size stays close to the power-law. For a system of 200 neurons this transition is shown in Fig. 2. To characterize this effect we used the least-squares estimate of the closest power-law parameters C_{norm} and γ.

$$p(L, N, \alpha) \approx C_{\mathrm{norm}} L^{\gamma}$$

The mean squared deviation from the estimated power-law undergoes a fast change Fig. 3 (bottom) near $\alpha_{cr} = 0.54$. At this point the transition from the subcritical to the critical regime occurs. Then there is a long interval of parameters for which the deviation from the power-law is about 2%. Also, the parameters of the power-law approximately stay constant. For different system-sizes different values of α_{cr} and γ are observed. At large system sizes γ is close to -1.5

In order to develop more extensive analysis we considered also a number of additional sta-

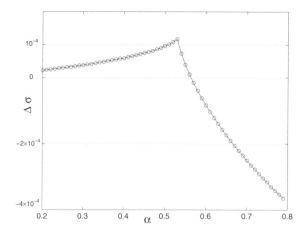

Figure 5: Difference between synaptic efficacy after and before avalanche averaged over all synapses . Values larger than zero mean facilitation, smaller ones mean depression. Presented curves are temporal averages over 10^6 avalanches with $N = 100$, $u_0 = 0.1$, $\tau_1 = \tau_2 = 10$.

tistical quantities at the beginning and after the avalanche. The average synaptic efficacy $\sigma = \langle \sigma_i \rangle = \langle J_i u_i \rangle$ is determined by taking the average over all neurons participating in an avalanche. This average shows the mean input, which neurons receive at each step of avalanche. This characteristic quantity undergoes a sharp transition together with the avalanches distribution, cf. Fig. 4. The meaning of the quantity σ in the present model is similar to the coupling strength α/N in the model discussed in [6]. It is equal to the average EPSP which all postsynaptic neurons will receive after presynaptic neuron spikes. The transition from a subcritical to a critical regime happens when σ jumps into the vicinity of α_{cr}/N of the previous model (for $N = 100$ and $\alpha_{cr} = 0.9$). This points to the correspondence between the two models.

When α is large, then the synaptic efficacy is high and, hence, avalanches are large and intervals between them are small. The depression during the avalanche dominates facilitation and decrease synaptic efficacy and vise versa. When avalanches are small, facilitation dominates depression. Thus, the synaptic dynamics stabilizes the network to remain near the critical value for a large interval of parameters α. In Fig. 4 shown the averaged effect of an avalanche for different values of parameter α. For $\alpha > \alpha_{cr}$, depression during the avalanche is stronger than facilitation and avalanches on average decrease synaptic efficacy. When α is very small, the effect of facilitation is washed out during the inter-avalanche period where synaptic parameters return to the resting state. To illustrate this, Fig. 5 shows the difference, $\Delta\sigma = \langle \sigma_{\mathrm{after}} \rangle - \langle \sigma_{\mathrm{before}} \rangle$, between the average synaptic efficacies after and before the avalanche depending on the parameter α. If this difference is larger than zero, synapses are facilitated by avalanche. If it is smaller than zero, synapses are depressed. For small values of the parameter α avalanches lead to facilitation, while, for large values of α avalanches depress synapses.

In the limit $N \to \infty$, the synaptic dynamics should be rescaled such that the maximum of transmitter available at a time t divided by the average avalanche size converges to a value which scales as $1 - N^{-1/2}$. In this way, if the average avalanche size is smaller than critical, synapses will essentially be enhanced, or they will otherwise experience depression. The necessary parameters for the model (such as the time-scales) have shown to be easily achievable in the small (although time-consuming) simulations presented here.

5 Conclusion

We presented a simple biologically plausible complement to a model of a non-leaky integrate-and-fire neurons network which exhibits a power-law avalanche distribution for a wide range of connectivity parameters. In previous studies [6] we showed, that the simplest model with only one parameter α, characterizing synaptic efficacy of all synapses exhibits subcritical, critical and supra critical regimes with continuous transition from one to another, depending on parameter α. These main classes are also present here but the region of critical behavior is immensely enlarged. Both models have a power-law distribution with an exponent approximately equal to -3/2, although the exponent is somewhat smaller for small network sizes. For network sizes close to those in the experiments described in [3] the result is indistinguishable from the limiting value.

References

[1] P. Bak, K. Chen, and M. Creutz. Self-organized criticality in the 'Game of Life. *Nature*, 342:780–782, 1989.

[2] P. Bak, C. Tang, and K. Wiesenfeld. Self-organized criticality: an explanation of $1/f$ noise. *Phys. Rev. Lett.*, 59:381–384, 1987.

[3] J. Beggs and D. Plenz. Neuronal avalanches in neocortical circuits. *J Neurosci*, 23:11167–11177, 2003.

[4] J. Beggs and D. Plenz. Neuronal Avalanches Are Diverse and Precise Activity Patterns That Are Stable for Many Hours in Cortical Slice Cultures. *J Neurosci*, 24(22):5216-5229, 2004.

[5] R. Der, F. Hesse, R. Liebscher (Contingent robot behavior from self-referential dynamical systems. Submitted to *Autonomous Robots*, 2005.

[6] C. W. Eurich, M. Herrmann, and U. Ernst. Finite-size effects of avalanche dynamics. *Phys. Rev. E*, 66, 2002.

[7] H. J. S. Feder and J. Feder. Self-organized criticality in a stick-slip process. *Phys. Rev. bibtLett.*, 66:2669–2672, 1991.

[8] V. Frette, K. Christensen, A. M. Malthe-Sørenssen, J. Feder, T. Jøssang, and P. Meakin. Avalanche dynamics in a pile of rice. *Nature*, 397:49, 1996.

[9] B. Gutenberg and C. F. Richter. Magnitude and energy of earthquakes. *Ann. Geophys.*, 9:1, 1956.

[10] R. A. Legenstein, W. Maass. Edge of chaos and prediction of computational power for neural microcircuit models. Submitted, 2005.

[11] H. Markram and M. Tsodyks. Redistribution of synaptic efficacy between pyramidal neurons. *Nature*, 382:807–810, 1996.

[12] D. Sornette, A. Johansen, and I. Dornic. Mapping self-organized criticality onto criticality. *J. Phys. I*, 5:325–335, 1995.

[13] M. Tsodyks, K. Pawelzik, and H. Markram. Neural networks with dynamic synapses. *Neural Computations*, 10:821–835, 1998.

[14] A. Vespignani and S. Zapperi. Order parameter and scaling fields in self-organized criticality. *Phys. Rev. Lett.*, 78:4793–4796, 1997.

From Lasso regression to Feature vector machine

Fan Li[1], Yiming Yang[1] and Eric P. Xing[1,2]
[1] LTI and [2]CALD, School of Computer Science, Carnegie Mellon University,
Pittsburgh, PA USA 15213
{hustlf,yiming,epxing}@cs.cmu.edu

Abstract

Lasso regression tends to assign zero weights to most irrelevant or redundant features, and hence is a promising technique for feature selection. Its limitation, however, is that it only offers solutions to linear models. Kernel machines with feature scaling techniques have been studied for feature selection with non-linear models. However, such approaches require to solve hard non-convex optimization problems. This paper proposes a new approach named the Feature Vector Machine (FVM). It reformulates the standard Lasso regression into a form isomorphic to SVM, and this form can be easily extended for feature selection with non-linear models by introducing kernels defined on feature vectors. FVM generates sparse solutions in the nonlinear feature space and it is much more tractable compared to feature scaling kernel machines. Our experiments with FVM on simulated data show encouraging results in identifying the small number of dominating features that are non-linearly correlated to the response, a task the standard Lasso fails to complete.

1 Introduction

Finding a small subset of most predictive features in a high dimensional feature space is an interesting problem with many important applications, e.g. in bioinformatics for the study of the genome and the proteome, and in pharmacology for high throughput drug screening.

Lasso regression ([Tibshirani *et al.*, 1996]) is often an effective technique for shrinkage and feature selection. The loss function of Lasso regression is defined as:

$$L = \sum_i (y_i - \sum_p \beta_p x_{ip})^2 + \lambda \sum_p ||\beta_p||_1$$

where x_{ip} denotes the pth predictor (feature) in the ith datum, y_i denotes the value of the response in this datum, and β_p denotes the regression coefficient of the pth feature. The norm-1 regularizer $\sum_p ||\beta_p||_1$ in Lasso regression typically leads to a sparse solution in the feature space, which means that the regression coefficients for most irrelevant or redundant features are shrunk to zero. Theoretical analysis in [Ng *et al.*, 2003] indicates that Lasso regression is particularly effective when there are many irrelevant features and only a few training examples.

One of the limitations of standard Lasso regression is its assumption of linearity in the feature space. Hence it is inadequate to capture non-linear dependencies from features to responses (output variables). To address this limitation, [Roth, 2004] proposed "generalized Lasso regressions" (GLR) by introducing kernels. In GLR, the loss function is defined as

$$L = \sum_i (y_i - \sum_j \alpha_j k(x_i, x_j))^2 + \lambda \sum_i ||\alpha_i||_1$$

where α_j can be regarded as the regression coefficient corresponding to the jth basis in an *instance space* (more precisely, a kernel space with its basis defined on all examples), and $k(x_i, x_j)$ represents some kernel function over the "argument" instance x_i and the "basis" instance x_j. The non-linearity can be captured by a non-linear kernel. This loss function typically yields a sparse solution in the instance space, but not in feature space where data was originally represented. Thus GLR does not lead to compression of data in the feature space.

[Weston *et al.*, 2000], [Canu *et al.*, 2002] and [Krishnapuram *et al.*, 2003] addressed the limitation from a different angle. They introduced *feature scaling kernels* in the form of:

$$K_\theta(x_i, x_j) = \phi(x_i * \theta)\phi(x_j * \theta) = K(x_i * \theta, x_j * \theta)$$

where $x_i * \theta$ denotes the component-wise product between two vectors: $x_i * \theta = (x_{i1}\theta_1, ..., x_{ip}\theta_p)$. For example, [Krishnapuram *et al.*, 2003] used a feature scaling polynomial kernel:

$$K_\gamma(x_i, x_j) = (1 + \sum_p \gamma_p x_{ip} x_{jp})^k,$$

where $\gamma_p = \theta_p^2$. With a norm-1 or norm-0 penalizer on γ in the loss function of a feature scaling kernel machine, a sparse solution is supposed to identify the most influential features. Notice that in this formalism the feature scaling vector θ is inside the kernel function, which means that the solution space of θ could be non-convex. Thus, estimating θ in feature scaling kernel machines is a much harder problem than the convex optimization problem in conventional SVM of which the weight parameters to be estimated are outside of the kernel functions.

What we are seeking for here is an alternative approach that guarantees a sparse solution in the feature space, that is sufficient for capturing both linear and non-linear relationships between features and the response variable, and that does not involve parameter optimization inside of kernel functions. The last property is particularly desirable in the sense that it will allow us to leverage many existing works in kernel machines which have been very successful in SVM-related research.

We propose a new approach where the key idea is to re-formulate and extend Lasso regression into a form that is similar to SVM except that it generates a sparse solution in the feature space rather than in the instance space. We call our newly formulated and extended Lasso regression "Feature Vector Machine" (FVM). We will show (in Section 2) that FVM has many interesting properties that mirror SVM. The concepts of support vectors, kernels and slack variables can be easily adapted in FVM. Most importantly, all the parameters we need to estimate for FVM are outside of the kernel functions, ensuring the convexity of the solution space, which is the same as in SVM. [1] When a linear kernel is put to use with no slack variables, FVM reduces to the standard Lasso regression.

---

[1]Notice that we can not only use FVM to select important features from training data, but also use it to predict the values of response variables for test data (see section 5). We have shown that we only need convex optimization in the training phase of FVM. In the test phase, FVM makes a prediction for each test example independently. This only involves with a one-dimensional optimization problem with respect to the response variable for the test example. Although the optimization in the test phase may be non-convex, it will be relatively easy to solve because it is only one-dimensional. This is the price we pay for avoiding the high dimensional non-convex optimization in the training phase, which may involve thousands of model parameters.

We notice that [Hochreiter *et al.*, 2004] has recently developed an interesting feature selection technique named "potential SVM", which has the same form as the basic version of FVM (with linear kernel and no slack variables). However, they did not explore the relationship between "potential SVM" and Lasso regression. Furthermore, their method does not work for feature selection tasks with non-linear models since they did not introduce the concepts of kernels defined on feature vectors.

In section 2, we analyze some geometric similarities between the solution hyper-planes in the standard Lasso regression and in SVM. In section 3, we re-formulate Lasso regression in a SVM style form. In this form, all the operations on the training data can be expressed by dot products between feature vectors. In section 4, we introduce kernels (defined for feature vectors) to FVM so that it can be used for feature selection with non-linear models. In section 5, we give some discussions on FVM. In section 6, we conduct experiments and in section 7 we give conclusions.

2 Geometric parity between the solution hyper-planes of Lasso regression and SVM

Formally, let $\mathbf{X} = [x_1, \ldots, x_N]$ denote a sample matrix, where each column $x_i = (x_1, \ldots, x_K)^T$ represents a *sample vector* defined on K features. A *feature vector* can be defined as a transposed row in the sample matrix, i.e., $f_q = (x_{1q}, \ldots, x_{Nq})^T$ (corresponding to the q row of $\mathbf{X}$). Note that we can write $\mathbf{X}^T = [f_1, \ldots, f_K] = \mathbf{F}$. For convenience, let $y = (y_1, \ldots, y_n)^T$ denote a *response vector* containing the responses corresponding to all the samples.

Now consider an *example space* of which each basis is represented by an x_i in our sample matrix (note that this is different from the space "spanned" by the sample vectors). Under the example space, both the features f_q and the response vector y can be regarded as a point in this space. It can be shown that the solution of Lasso regression has a very intuitive meaning in the example space: the regression coefficients can be regarded as the weights of feature vectors in the example space; moreover, all the non-zero weighted feature vectors are on two parallel hyper-planes in the example space. These feature vectors, together with the response variable, determine the directions of these two hyper-planes. This geometric view can be drawn from the following recast of the Lasso regression due to [Perkins *et al.*, 2003]:

$$|\sum_i (y_i - \sum_p \beta_p x_{ip}) x_{iq}| \le \frac{\lambda}{2}, \quad \forall q$$

$$\Rightarrow \quad |f_q(y - [f_1, \ldots, f_K]\beta)| \le \frac{\lambda}{2}, \quad \forall q. \tag{1}$$

It is apparent from the above equation that $y - [f_1, \ldots, f_K]\beta$ defines the orientation of a separation hyper-plane. It can be shown that equality only holds for non-zero weighted features, and all the zero weighted feature vectors are between the hyper-planes with $\lambda/2$ margin (Fig. 1a).

The separating hyper-planes due to (hard, linear) SVM have similar properties as those of the regression hyper-planes described above, although the former are now defined in the feature space (in which each axis represents a feature and each point represents a sample) instead of the example space. In an SVM, all the non-zero weighted samples are also on the two $\lambda/2$-margin separating hyper-planes (as is the case in Lasso regression), whereas all the zero-weighted samples are now *outside* the pair of hyper-planes (Fig 1b). It's well known that the classification hyper-planes in SVM can be extended to hyper-surfaces by introducing kernels defined for *example vectors*. In this way, SVM can model non-linear dependencies between samples and the classification boundary. Given the similarity of the

781

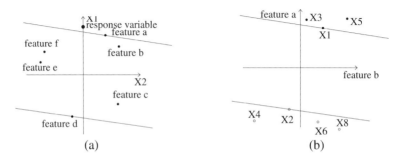

(a)   (b)

Figure 1: Lasso regression vs. SVM. (a) The solution of Lasso regression in the example space. $X1$ and $X2$ represent two examples. Only feature a and d have non-zero weights, and hence the *support features*. (b)The solution of SVM in the feature space. Sample $X1$, $X3$ and $X5$ are in one class and $X2$, $X4$, $X6$ and $X8$ are in the other. $X1$ and $X2$ are the *support vectors* (i.e., with non-zero weights).

geometric structures of Lasso regression and SVM, it is nature to pursue in parallel how one can apply similar "kernel tricks" to the *feature vectors* in Lasso regression, so that its feature selection power can be extended to non-linear models. This is the intension of this paper, and we envisage full leverage of much of the computational/optimization techniques well-developed in the SVM community in our task.

3 A re-formulation of Lasso regression akin to SVM

[Hochreiter *et al.*, 2004] have proposed a "potential SVM" as follows:

$$\begin{cases} \min_\beta & \frac{1}{2}\sum_i(\sum_p \beta_p x_{ip})^2 \\ \text{s.t.} & |\sum_i(y_i - \sum_p \beta_p x_{ip})x_{iq}| \le \frac{\lambda}{2} \quad \forall q. \end{cases} \tag{2}$$

To clean up a little bit, we rewrite Eq. (2) in linear algebra format:

$$\begin{cases} \min_\beta & \frac{1}{2}\|[f_1^T,\ldots,f_K^T]\beta\|^2 \\ \text{s.t.} & |f_q(y - [f_1,\ldots,f_K]\beta)| \le \frac{\lambda}{2}, \quad \forall q. \end{cases} \tag{3}$$

A quick eyeballing of this formulation reveals that it shares the same constrain function needed to be satisfied in Lasso regression. Unfortunately, this connection was not further explored in [Hochreiter *et al.*, 2004], e.g., to relate the objection function to that of the Lasso regression, and to extend the objective function using kernel tricks in a way similar to SVM. Here we show that the solution to Eq. (2) is exactly the same as that of a standard Lasso regression. In other words, Lasso regression can be re-formulated as Eq. (2). Then, based on this re-formulation, we show how to introduce kernels to allow feature selection under a non-linear Lasso regression. We refer to the optimization problem defined by Eq. (3), and its kernelized extensions, as *feature vector machine* (FVM).

Proposition 1: For a Lasso regression problem $min_\beta \sum_i(\sum_p x_{ip}\beta_p - y_i)^2 + \lambda \sum_p |\beta_p|$, if we have β such that: if $\beta_q = 0$, then $|\sum_i(\sum_p \beta_p x_{ip} - y_i)x_{iq}| < \frac{\lambda}{2}$; if $\beta_q < 0$, then $\sum_i(\sum_p \beta_p x_{ip} - y_i)x_{iq} = \frac{\lambda}{2}$; and if $\beta_q > 0$, then $\sum_i(\sum_p \beta_p x_{ip} - y_i)x_{iq} = -\frac{\lambda}{2}$, then β is the solution of the Lasso regression defined above. For convenience, we refer to the aforementioned three conditions on β as the *Lasso sandwich*.

Proof: see [Perkins *et al.*, 2003].   ■

Proposition 2: For Problem (3), its solution β satisfies the *Lasso sandwich*

Sketch of proof: Following the equivalence between feature matrix $\mathbf{F}$ and sample matrix $\mathbf{X}$ (see the begin of §2), Problem (3) can be re-written as:

$$
\begin{cases}
\min_{\beta} & \frac{1}{2}\|X^T\beta\|^2 \\
\text{s.t.} & X(X^T\beta - y) - \frac{\lambda}{2}e \le 0 \\
& X(X^T\beta - y) + \frac{\lambda}{2}e \ge 0
\end{cases}
\tag{4}
$$

where e is a one-vector of K dimensions. Following the standard constrained optimization procedure, we can derive the dual of this optimization problem. The Lagrange L is given by

$$
L = \frac{1}{2}\beta^T X X^T \beta - \alpha_+^T(X(X^T\beta - y) + \frac{\lambda}{2}e) + \alpha_-^T(X(X^T\beta - y) + \frac{\lambda}{2}e)
$$

where α_+ and α_- are $K \times 1$ vectors with positive elements. The optimizer satisfies:

$$
\nabla_\beta L = X X^T \beta - X X^T(\alpha_+ - \alpha_-) = 0
$$

Suppose the data matrix $\mathbf{X}$ has been pre-processed so that the feature vectors are centered and normalized. In this case the elements of $X X^T$ reflect the correlation coefficients of feature pairs and $X X^T$ is non-singular. Thus we know $\beta = \alpha_+ - \alpha_-$ is the solution of this loss function. For any element $\beta_q > 0$, obviously α_{+q} should be larger than zero. From the KKT condition, we know $\sum_i (y_i - \sum_p \beta_p x_{ip}) x_{iq} = -\frac{\lambda}{2}$ holds at this time. For the same reason we can get when $\beta_q < 0$, α_{-q} should be larger than zero thus $\sum_i (y_i - \sum_p \beta_p x_{ip}) x_{iq} = \frac{\lambda}{2}$ holds. When $\beta_q = 0$, α_{+q} and α_{-q} must both be zero (it's easy to see they can not be both non-zero from KKT condition), thus from KKT condition, both $\sum_i (y_i - \sum_p \beta_p x_{ip}) x_{iq} > -\frac{\lambda}{2}$ and $\sum_i (y_i - \sum_p \beta_p x_{ip}) x_{iq} < \frac{\lambda}{2}$ hold now, which means $|\sum_i (y_i - \sum_p \beta_p x_{ip}) x_{iq}| < \frac{\lambda}{2}$ at this time. ∎

Theorem 3: Problem (3) $\equiv$ Lasso regression.

Proof. Follows from proposition 1 and proposition 2. ∎

4 Feature kernels

In many cases, the dependencies between feature vectors are non-linear. Analogous to the SVM, here we introduce kernels that capture such non-linearity. Note that unlike SVM, our kernels are defined on feature vectors instead of the sampled vectors (i.e., the rows rather than the columns in the data matrix). Such kernels can also allow us to easily incorporate certain domain knowledge into the classifier.

Suppose that two feature vectors f_p and f_q have a non-linear dependency relationship. In the absence of linear interaction between f_p and f_q in the the original space, we assume that they can be mapped to some (higher dimensional, possibly infinite-dimensional) space via transformation $\phi(\cdot)$, so that $\phi(f_q)$ and $\phi(f_q)$ interact linearly, i.e., via a dot product $\phi(f_p)^T\phi(f_q)$. We introduce kernel $K(f_q, f_p) = \phi(f_p)^T\phi(f_q)$ to represent the outcome of this operation.

Replacing f with $\phi(f)$ in Problem (3), we have

$$
\begin{cases}
\min_{\beta} & \frac{1}{2}\sum_{p,q} \beta_p \beta_q K(f_p, f_p) \\
\text{s.t.} & \forall q, \quad |\sum_p \beta_p K(f_q, f_p) - K(f_q, y)| \le \frac{\lambda}{2}
\end{cases}
\tag{5}
$$

Now, in Problem 5, we no longer have $\phi(\cdot)$, which means we do not have to work in the transformed feature space, which could be high or infinite dimensional, to capture non-linearity of features. The kernel $K(\cdot, \cdot)$ can be any symmetric semi-positive definite matrix.

When domain knowledge from experts is available, it can be incorporated into the choice of kernel (e.g., based on the distribution of feature values). When domain knowledge is not available, we can use some general kernels that can detect non-linear dependencies without any distribution assumptions. In the following we give one such example.

One possible kernel is the mutual information [Cover *et al.*, 1991] between two feature vectors: $K(f_p, f_q) = MI(f_p, f_q)$. This kernel requires a pre-processing step to discritize the elements of features vectors because they are continuous in general. In this paper, we discritize the continuous variables according to their ranks in different examples. Suppose we have N examples in total. Then for each feature, we sort its values in these N examples. The first m values (the smallest m values) are assigned a scale 1. The $m + 1$ to $2m$ values are assigned a scale 2. This process is iterated until all the values are assigned with corresponding scales. It's easy to see that in this way, we can guarantee that for any two features p and q, $K(f_p, f_p) = K(f_q, f_q)$, which means the feature vectors are normalized and have the same length in the ϕ space (residing on a unit sphere centered at the origin).

Mutual information kernels have several good properties. For example, it is symmetric (i.e., $K(f_p, f_q) = K(f_q, f_p)$, non-negative, and can be normalized. It also has intuitive interpretation related to the redundancy between features. Therefore, a non-linear feature selection using generalized Lasso regression with this kernel yields human interpretable results.

5 Some extensions and discussions about FVM

As we have shown, FVM is a straightforward feature selection algorithm for nonlinear features captured in a kernel; and the selection can be easily done by solving a standard SVM problem in the feature space, which yield an optimal vector β of which most elements are zero. It turns out that the same procedure also seemlessly leads to a Lasso-style regularized nonlinear regression capable of predicting the response given data in the original space.

In the prediction phase, all we have to do is to keep the trained β fixed, and turn the optimization problem (5) into an analogous one that optimizes over the response y. Specifically, given a new sample x_t of unknown response, our sample matrix $\mathbf{X}$ grows by one column $\mathbf{X} \rightarrow [\mathbf{X}, x_t]$, which means all our feature vectors gets one more dimension. We denote the newly elongated features by $F' = \{f'_q\}_{q \in A}$ (note that A is the pruned index set corresponding to features whose weight β_q is non-zero). Let y' denote the elongated response vector due to the newly given sample: $y' = (y_1, ..., y_N, y_t)^T$, it can be shown that the optimum response y_t can be obtained by solving the following optimization problem [2]:

$$\min_{y_t} K(y', y') - 2 \sum_{p \in A} \beta_p K(y', f'_p) \tag{6}$$

When we replace the kernel function K with a linear dot product, FVM reduces to Lasso regression. Indeed, in this special case, it is easy to see from Eq. (6) that $y_t = \sum_{p \in A} \beta_p x_{tp}$, which is exactly how Lasso regression would predict the response. In this case one predicts y_t according to β and x_t without using the training data $\mathbf{X}$. However, when a more complex kernel is used, solving Eq. (6) is not always trivial. In general, to predict y_t, we need not only x_t and β, but also the non-zero weight features extracted from the training data.

---

[2]For simplicity we omit details here, but as a rough sketch, note that Eq. (5) can be reformed as

$$min_\beta ||\phi(y') - \sum_p \beta_p \phi(f'_p)||^2 + \sum_p ||\beta_p||_1.$$

Replacing the opt. argument β with y and dropping terms irrelevant to y_t, we will arrive at Eq. (6).

As in SVM, we can introduce slack variables into FVM to define a "soft" feature surface. But due to space limitation, we omit details here. Essentially, most of the methodologies developed for SVM can be easily adapted to FVM for nonlinear feature selection.

6 Experiments

We test FVM on a simulated dataset with 100 features and 500 examples. The response variable y in the simulated data is generated by a highly nonlinear rule:

$$y = sin(10 * f_1 - 5) + 4 * \sqrt{1 - f_2^2} - 3 * f_3 + \xi.$$

Here feature f_1 and f_3 are random variables following a uniform distribution in $[0, 1]$; feature f_2 is a random variable uniformly distributed in $[-1, 1]$; and ξ represents Gaussian noise. The other 97 features $f_4, f_5, ..., f_{100}$ are conditionally independent of y given the three features f_1, f_2 and f_3. In particular, $f_4, ..., f_{33}$ are all generated by the rule $f_j = 3 * f_1 + \xi$; $f_{34}, ..., f_{72}$ are all generated by the rule $f_j = sin(10 * f_2) + \xi$; and the remaining features ($f_{73}, ..., f_{100}$) simply follow a uniform distribution in $[0, 1]$. Fig. 2 shows our data projected in a space spanned by f_1 and f_2 and y.

We use a mutual information kernel for our FVM. For each feature, we sort its value in different examples and use the rank to discritize these values into 10 scales (thus each scale corresponds to 50 data points). An FVM can be solved by quadratic programming, but more efficient solutions exist. [Perkins *et al.*, 2003] has proposed a fast grafting algorithm to solve Lasso regression, which is a special case of FVM when linear kernel is used. In our implementation, we extend the idea of fast grafting algorithm to FVM with more general kernels. The only difference is that, each time when we need to calculate $\sum_i x_{pi} x_{qi}$, we calculate $K(f_p, f_q)$ instead. We found that fast grafting algorithm is very efficient in our case because it uses the sparse property of the solution of FVM.

We apply both standard Lasso regression and FVM with mutual information kernel on this dataset. The value of the regularization parameter λ can be tuned to control the number of non-zero weighted features. In our experiment, we tried two choices of the λ, for both FVM and the standard Lasso regression. In one case, we set λ such that only 3 non-zero weighted features are selected; in another case, we relaxed a bit and allowed 10 features.

The results are very encouraging. As shown in Fig. (3), under stringent λ, FVM successfully identified the three correct features, f_1, f_2 and f_3, whereas Lasso regression has missed f_1 and f_2, which are non-linearly correlated with y. Even when λ was relaxed, Lasso regression still missed the right features, whereas FVM was very robust.

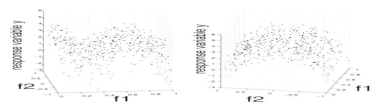

Figure 2: The responses y and the two features f_1 and f_2 in our simulated data. Two graphs from different angles are plotted to show the distribution more clearly in 3D space.

7 Conclusions

In this paper, we proposed a novel non-linear feature selection approach named FVM, which extends standard Lasso regression by introducing kernels on feature vectors. FVM

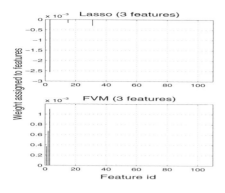
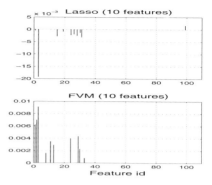

Figure 3: Results of FVM and the standard Lasso regression on this dataset. The X axis represents the feature IDs and the Y axis represents the weights assigned to features. The two left graphs show the case when 3 features are selected by each algorithm and the two right graphs show the case when 10 features are selected. From the down left graph, we can see that FVM successfully identified f_1, f_2 and f_3 as the three non-zero weighted features. From the up left graph, we can see that Lasso regression missed f_1 and f_2, which are non-linearly correlated with y. The two right graphs show similar patterns.

has many interesting properties that mirror the well-known SVM, and can therefore leverage many computational advantages of the latter approach. Our experiments with FVM on highly nonlinear and noisy simulated data show encouraging results, in which it can correctly identify the small number of dominating features that are non-linearly correlated to the response variable, a task the standard Lasso fails to complete.

References

[Canu *et al.*, 2002] Canu, S. and Grandvalet, Y. Adaptive Scaling for Feature Selection in SVMs NIPS 15, 2002

[Hochreiter *et al.*, 2004] Hochreiter, S. and Obermayer, K. Gene Selection for Microarray Data. In Kernel Methods in Computational Biology, pp. 319-355, MIT Press, 2004.

[Krishnapuram *et al.*, 2003] Krishnapuram, B. et al. Joint classifier and feature optimization for cancer diagnosis using gene expression data. The Seventh Annual International Conference on Research in Computational Molecular Biology (RECOMB) 2003, ACM press, April 2003

[Ng *et al.*, 2003] Ng, A. Feature selection, L1 vs L2 regularization, and rotational invariance. ICML 2004

[Perkins *et al.*, 2003] Perkins, S., Lacker, K. & Theiler, J. Grafting: Fast,Incremental Feature Selection by gradient descent in function space JMLR 2003 1333-1356

[Roth, 2004] Roth, V. The Generalized LASSO. IEEE Transactions on Neural Networks (2004), Vol. 15, NO. 1.

[Tibshirani *et al.*, 1996] Tibshirani, R. Optimal Reinsertion:Regression shrinkage and selection via the lasso. J.R.Statist. Soc. B(1996), 58,No.1, 267-288

[Cover *et al.*, 1991] Cover, TM. and Thomas, JA. Elements in Information Theory. New York: John Wiley & Sons Inc (1991).

[Weston *et al.*, 2000] Weston, J., Mukherjee, S., Chapelle, O., Pontil, M., Poggio, T. and Vapnik V. Feature Selection for SVMs NIPS 13, 2000

Location-based Activity Recognition

Lin Liao, Dieter Fox, and Henry Kautz
Computer Science & Engineering
University of Washington
Seattle, WA 98195

Abstract

Learning patterns of human behavior from sensor data is extremely important for high-level activity inference. We show how to extract and label a person's activities and significant places from traces of GPS data. In contrast to existing techniques, our approach simultaneously detects and classifies the significant locations of a person and takes the high-level context into account. Our system uses relational Markov networks to represent the hierarchical activity model that encodes the complex relations among GPS readings, activities and significant places. We apply FFT-based message passing to perform efficient summation over large numbers of nodes in the networks. We present experiments that show significant improvements over existing techniques.

1 Introduction

The problem of learning patterns of human behavior from sensor data arises in many areas and applications of computer science, including intelligent environments, surveillance, and assistive technology for the disabled. A focus of recent interest is the use of data from wearable sensors, and in particular, GPS (global positioning system) location data. Such data is used to recognize the high-level activities in which a person is engaged and to determine the relationship between activities and locations that are important to the user [1, 6, 8, 3]. Our goal is to segment the user's day into everyday activities such as "working," "visiting," "travel," and to recognize and label significant locations that are associated with one or more activity, such as "work place," "friend's house," "user's bus stop." Such activity logs can be used, for instance, for automated diaries or long-term health monitoring. Previous approaches to location-based activity recognition suffer from design decisions that limit their accuracy and flexibility:

First, previous work decoupled the subproblem of determining whether or not a geographic location is significant and *should* be assigned a label, from that of labeling places and activities. The first problem was handled by simply assuming that a location is significant if and only if the user spends at least N minutes there, for some fixed threshold N [1, 6, 8, 3]. Some way of restricting the enormous set of all locations recorded for the user to a meaningful subset is clearly necessary. However, in practice, any fixed threshold leads to many errors. Some significant locations, for example, the place where the user drops off his children at school, may be visited only briefly, and so would be excluded by a high threshold. A lower threshold, however, would include too many insignificant locations, for example, a place where the user briefly waited at a traffic light. The inevitable errors cannot be resolved because information cannot flow from the label assignment process back to the one that determines the domain to be labeled.

Second, concerns for computational efficiency prevented previous approaches from tackling the problem of activity and place labeling in full generality. [1] does not distinguish between places and activities; although [8] does, the implementation limited places to a single activity. Neither approaches model or label the user's activities when moving between places. [6] and [3] learn transportation patterns, but not place labels.

The third problem is one of the underlying causes of the other limitations. The representations and algorithms used in previous work make it difficult to learn and reason with the kinds of *non-local features* that are useful in disambiguating human activity. For a simple example, if a system could learn that a person rarely went to a restaurant more than once a day, then it could correctly give a low probability to an interpretation of a day's data under which the user went to three restaurants. Our previous work [8] used *clique templates* in relational Markov networks for concisely expressing global features, but the MCMC inference algorithm we used made it costly to reason with aggregate features, such as statistics on the number of times a given activity occurs. The ability to *efficiently* leverage global features of the data stream could enhance the scope and accuracy of activity recognition.

This paper presents a unified approach to automated activity and place labeling which overcomes these limitations. Contributions of this work include the following:

- We show how to simultaneously solve the tasks of identifying significant locations and labeling both places and activities from raw GPS data, all in a conditionally trained relational Markov network. Our approach is notable in that nodes representing significant places are dynamically added to the graph during inference. No arbitrary thresholds regarding the time spent at a location or the number of significant places are employed.

- Our model creates a complete interpretation of the log of a user's data, including transportation activities as well as activities performed at particular places. It allows different kinds of activities to be performed at the same location.

- We extend our work on using clique templates for global features to support efficient inference by belief propagation. We introduce, in particular, specialized *Fast Fourier Transform* (FFT) templates for belief propagation over aggregate (counting) features, which reduce computation time by an exponential amount. Although [9] introduced the use of the FFT to compute probability distributions over summations, our work appears to be the first to employ it for full bi-directional belief propagation.

This paper is organized as follows. We begin with a discussion of relational Markov networks and a description of an FFT belief propagation algorithm for aggregate statistical features. Then we explain how to apply RMNs to the problem of location-based activity recognition. Finally, we present experimental results on real-world data that demonstrate significant improvement in coverage and accuracy over previous work.

2 Relational Markov Networks and Aggregate Features

2.1 Preliminaries

Relational Markov Networks (RMNs) [10] are extensions of Conditional Random Fields (CRFs), which are undirected graphical models that were developed for labeling sequence data [5]. CRFs have been shown to produce excellent results in areas such as natural language processing [5] and computer vision [4]. RMNs extend CRFs by providing a relational language for describing clique structures and enforcing parameter sharing at the template level. Thereby RMNs provide a very flexible and concise framework for defining the features we use in our activity recognition context.

A key concept of RMNs are *relational clique templates*, which specify the structure of a CRF in a concise way. In a nutshell, a clique template $C \in \mathcal{C}$ is similar to a database query (*e.g.*, SQL) in that it selects tuples of nodes from a CRF and connects them into cliques. Each clique template C is additionally associated with a potential function $\phi_C(\mathbf{v}_C)$ that maps values of variables to a non-negative real number. Using a log-linear combination of feature functions, we get $\phi_C(\mathbf{v}_C) = \exp\{\mathbf{w}_C^T \cdot \mathbf{f}_C(\mathbf{v}_C)\}$, where $\mathbf{f}_C()$ defines a feature vector for C and $\mathbf{w}_C^T$ is the transpose of the corresponding weight vector.

An RMN defines a conditional distribution $p(\mathbf{y}|\mathbf{x})$ over labels $\mathbf{y}$ given observations $\mathbf{x}$. To compute such a conditional distribution, the RMN generates a CRF with the cliques specified by the clique templates. All cliques that originate from the same template must share the same weight vector $\mathbf{w}_C$. The resulting cliques factorize the conditional distribution as

$$p(\mathbf{y} \mid \mathbf{x}) = \frac{1}{Z(\mathbf{x})} \prod_{C \in \mathcal{C}} \prod_{\mathbf{v}_C \in C} \exp\{\mathbf{w}_C^T \cdot \mathbf{f}_C(\mathbf{v}_C)\}, \tag{1}$$

where $Z(\mathbf{x})$ is the normalizing partition function.

The weights $\mathbf{w}$ of an RMN can be learned discriminatively by maximizing the log-likelihood of labeled training data [10, 8]. This requires running an inference procedure at each iteration of the optimization and can be very expensive. To overcome this problem, we instead maximize the pseudo-log-likelihood of the training data:

$$L(\mathbf{w}) \equiv \sum_{i=1}^{n} \log p(\mathbf{y}_i \mid \mathrm{MB}(\mathbf{y}_i), \mathbf{w}) - \frac{\mathbf{w}^T \mathbf{w}}{2\sigma^2} \tag{2}$$

where $\mathrm{MB}(\mathbf{y}_i)$ is the Markov Blanket of variable $\mathbf{y}_i$. The rightmost term avoids overfitting by imposing a zero-mean, Gaussian shrinkage prior on each component of the weights [10]. In the context of place labeling, [8] showed how to use non-zero mean priors in order to transfer weights learned for one person to another person. In our experiments, learning the weights using pseudo-log-likelihood is very efficient and performs well in our tests.

In our previous work [8] we used MCMC for inference. While this approach performed well for the models considered in [8], it does not scale to more complex activity models such as the one described here. Taskar and colleagues [10] relied on belief propagation (BP) for inference. The BP (sum-product) algorithm converts a CRF to a pairwise representation and performs message passing, where the message from node i to its neighbor j is computed as

$$m_{ij}(\mathbf{y}_j) = \sum_{\mathbf{y}_i} \phi(\mathbf{y}_i)\phi(\mathbf{y}_i, \mathbf{y}_j) \prod_{k \in n(i) \setminus j} m_{ki}(\mathbf{y}_i), \tag{3}$$

where $\phi(\mathbf{y}_i)$ is a local potential, $\phi(\mathbf{y}_i, \mathbf{y}_j)$ is a pairwise potential, and $\{n(i) \setminus j\}$ denotes i's neighbors other than j. All messages are updated iteratively until they (possibly) converge. However, our model takes into account aggregate features, such as summation. Performing aggregation would require the generation of cliques that contain all nodes over which the aggregation is performed. Since the complexity of standard BP is exponential in the number of nodes in the largest clique, aggregation can easily make BP intractable.

2.2 Efficient summation templates

In our model, we address the inference of aggregate cliques at the template level within the framework of BP. Each type of aggregation function is associated with a *computation template* that specifies how to propagate messages through the clique. In this section, we discuss an efficient computation template for summation.

To handle summation cliques with potentially large numbers of addends, our summation template dynamically builds a *summation tree*, which is a pairwise Markov network as shown in Fig. 1(a). In a summation tree, the leaves are the original addends and each

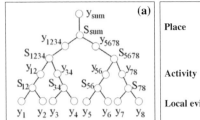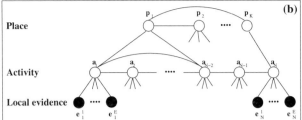

Figure 1: (a) Summation tree that represents $\mathbf{y}_{sum} = \sum_{i=1}^{8} \mathbf{y}_i$, where the S_i's are auxiliary nodes to ensure the summation relation. (b) CRF for labeling activities and places. Each activity node a_i is connected to E observed local evidence nodes e_i^1 to e_i^E. Place nodes p_i are generated based on the inferred activities and each place is connected to all activity nodes that are within a certain distance.

internal node $\mathbf{y}_{jk}$ represents the sum of its two children $\mathbf{y}_j$ and $\mathbf{y}_k$, and this sum relation is encoded by an auxiliary node S_{jk} and its potential. The state space of S_{jk} consists of the joint (cross-product) state of its neighbors $\mathbf{y}_j$, $\mathbf{y}_k$, and $\mathbf{y}_{jk}$. It is easy to see that the summation tree guarantees that the root represents $\mathbf{y}_{sum} = \sum_{i=1}^{n} \mathbf{y}_i$, where $\mathbf{y}_1$ to $\mathbf{y}_n$ are the leaves of the tree. To define the BP protocol for summation trees, we need to specify two types of messages: an *upward message* from an auxiliary node to its parent (*e.g.*, $m_{S_{12}\mathbf{y}_{12}}$), and a *downward message* from an auxiliary node to one of its two children (*e.g.*, $m_{S_{12}\mathbf{y}_1}$).

Upward message update: Starting with Equation (3), we can update an upward message $m_{S_{ij}\mathbf{y}_{ij}}$ as follows.

$$
\begin{aligned}
m_{S_{ij}\mathbf{y}_{ij}}(\mathbf{y}_{ij}) &= \sum_{\mathbf{y}_i, \mathbf{y}_j} \phi_S(\mathbf{y}_i, \mathbf{y}_j, \mathbf{y}_{ij}) \, m_{\mathbf{y}_i S_{ij}}(\mathbf{y}_i) \, m_{\mathbf{y}_j S_{ij}}(\mathbf{y}_j) \\
&= \sum_{\mathbf{y}_i} m_{\mathbf{y}_i S_{ij}}(\mathbf{y}_i) \, m_{\mathbf{y}_j S_{ij}}(\mathbf{y}_{ij} - \mathbf{y}_i) \quad (4) \\
&= \mathcal{F}^{-1} \left(\mathcal{F}(m_{\mathbf{y}_i S_{ij}}(\mathbf{y}_i)) \cdot \mathcal{F}(m_{\mathbf{y}_j S_{ij}}(\mathbf{y}_j)) \right) \quad (5)
\end{aligned}
$$

where $\phi_S(\mathbf{y}_i, \mathbf{y}_j, \mathbf{y}_{ij})$ is the local potential of S_{ij} encoding the equality $\mathbf{y}_{ij} = \mathbf{y}_i + \mathbf{y}_j$. (4) follows because all terms not satisfying the equality disappear. Therefore, message $m_{S_{ij}\mathbf{y}_{ij}}$ is the *convolution* of $m_{\mathbf{y}_i S_{ij}}$ and $m_{\mathbf{y}_j S_{ij}}$. (5) follows from the *convolution theorem*, which states that the Fourier transform of a convolution is the point-wise product of Fourier transforms [2], where $\mathcal{F}$ and $\mathcal{F}^{-1}$ represent the Fourier transform and its inverse, respectively. When the messages are discrete functions, the Fourier transform and its inverse can be computed efficiently using the Fast Fourier Transform (FFT) [2, 9]. The computational complexity of one summation using FFT is $O(k \log k)$, where k is the maximum number of states in $\mathbf{y}_i$ and $\mathbf{y}_j$.

Downward message update: We also allow messages to pass from sum variables downward to its children. This is necessary if we want to use the belief on sum variables (*e.g.*, knowledge on the number of homes) to change the distribution of individual variables (*e.g.*, place labels). From Equation (3) we get the downward message $m_{S_{ij}\mathbf{y}_i}$ as

$$
\begin{aligned}
m_{S_{ij}\mathbf{y}_i}(\mathbf{y}_i) &= \sum_{\mathbf{y}_j, \mathbf{y}_{ij}} \phi_S(\mathbf{y}_i, \mathbf{y}_j, \mathbf{y}_{ij}) m_{\mathbf{y}_j S_{ij}}(\mathbf{y}_j) m_{\mathbf{y}_{ij} S_{ij}}(\mathbf{y}_{ij}) \\
&= \sum_{\mathbf{y}_j} m_{\mathbf{y}_j S_{ij}}(\mathbf{y}_j) m_{\mathbf{y}_{ij} S_{ij}}(\mathbf{y}_i + \mathbf{y}_j) \quad (6) \\
&= \mathcal{F}^{-1} \left(\overline{\mathcal{F}}(m_{\mathbf{y}_j S_{ij}}(\mathbf{y}_j)) \cdot \mathcal{F}(m_{\mathbf{y}_{ij} S_{ij}}(\mathbf{y}_{ij})) \right) \quad (7)
\end{aligned}
$$

where (6) again follows from the sum relation. Note that the downward message $m_{S_{ij}\mathbf{y}_i}$ turns out to be the *correlation* of messages $m_{\mathbf{y}_j S_{ij}}$ and $m_{\mathbf{y}_{ij} S_{ij}}$. (7) follows from the *correlation theorem* [2], which is similar to the convolution theorem except, for correlation, we must compute the *complex conjugate* of the first Fourier transform, denoted as $\overline{\mathcal{F}}$. Again, for discrete messages, (7) can be evaluated efficiently using FFT.

At each level of a summation tree, the number of messages (nodes) is reduced by half and the size of each message is doubled. Suppose the tree has n upward messages at the bottom and the maximum size of a message is k . For large summation trees where $n \gg k$, the total complexity of updating the upward messages at all the $\log n$ levels follows now as

$$\sum_{i=1}^{\log n} \frac{n}{2^i} \cdot O\left(2^{i-1} k \log 2^{i-1} k\right) \;=\; O\left(\frac{n}{2} \sum_{i=1}^{\log n} \log 2^{i-1}\right) \;=\; O(n \log^2 n) \qquad (8)$$

Similar reasoning shows that the complexity of the downward pass is $O(n \log^2 n)$ as well. Therefore, updating all messages in a summation clique takes $O(n \log^2 n)$ instead of time exponential in n, as would be the case for a non-specialized implementation of aggregation.

3   Location-based Activity Model

3.1   Overview

To recognize activities and places, we first segment raw GPS traces by grouping consecutive GPS readings based on their spatial relationship. This segmentation can be performed by simply combining all consecutive readings that are within a certain distance from each other (10m in our implementation). However, it might be desirable to associate GPS traces to a street map, for example, in order to relate locations to addresses in the map. To jointly estimate the GPS to street association and trace segmentation, we construct an RMN that takes into account the spatial relationship and temporal consistency between the measurements and their associations (see [7] for more details). In this section, we focus on inferring activities and types of significant places after segmentation. To do so, we construct a hierarchical RMN that explicitly encodes the relations between activities and places. A CRF instantiated from the RMN is shown in Fig. 1(b). At the lower level of the hierarchy, each activity node is connected to various features, summarizing information resulting from the GPS segmentation. These features include:

- Temporal information such as time of day, day of week, and duration of the stay;
- Average speed through a segment, for discriminating transportation modes;
- Information extracted from geographic databases, such as whether a location is close to a bus route or bus stop, and whether it is near a restaurant or store;
- Additionally, each activity node is connected to its neighbors. These features measure compatibility between types of activities at neighboring nodes in the trace.

Our model also aims at determining those places that play a significant role in the activities of a person, such as home, work place, friend's home, grocery stores, restaurants, and bus stops. Such *significant places* comprise the upper level of the CRF shown in Fig. 1(b). However, since these places are not known a priori, we must additionally *detect* a person's significant places. To incorporate place detection into our system, we use an iterative algorithm that re-estimates activities and places. Before we describe this algorithm, let us first look at the features that are used to determine the types of significant places under the assumption that the locations and number of these places are known.

- The activities that occur at a place strongly indicate the type of the place. For example, at a friends' home people either visit or pick up / drop off someone. Our features consider the *frequencies* of the different activities at a place. This is done by generating a clique for each place that contains all activity nodes in its vicinity. For example, the nodes p_1, a_1, and a_{N-2} in Fig. 1(b) form such a clique.
- A person usually has only a limited number of different homes or work places. We add two additional summation cliques that count the number of homes and work places. These counts provide soft constraints that bias the system to generate interpretations with reasonable numbers of homes and work places.

1.	**Input:** GPS trace $\langle g_1, g_2, \ldots, g_T \rangle$ and iteration counter $i := 0$
2.	$\left(\langle a_1, \ldots, a_N \rangle, \langle e_1^1, \ldots, e_1^E, \ldots \rangle \right) :=$ trace_segmentation $\left(\langle g_1, g_2, \ldots, g_T \rangle \right)$
3.	*// Generate CRF containing activity and local evidence (lower two levels in Fig. 1(b))* $\mathrm{CRF}_0 :=$ instantiate_crf$\left(\langle \, \rangle, \langle a_1, \ldots, a_N \rangle, \langle e_1^1, \ldots, e_1^E, \ldots \rangle \right)$
4.	$\mathbf{a}^*{}_0 :=$ BP_inference(CRF_0) *// infer sequence of activities*
5.	**do**
6.	$\quad i := i + 1$
7.	$\quad \langle p_1, \ldots, p_K \rangle_i :=$ generate_places($\mathbf{a}^*{}_{i-1}$) *// Instantiate places*
8.	$\quad \mathrm{CRF}_i :=$ instantiate_crf$\left(\langle p_1, \ldots, p_K \rangle_i, \langle a_1, \ldots, a_N \rangle, \langle e_1^1, \ldots, e_1^E, \ldots \rangle \right)$
9	$\quad \langle \mathbf{a}_i^*, \mathbf{p}_i^* \rangle :=$ BP_inference(CRF_i) *// inference in complete CRF*
10.	**until** $\mathbf{a}_i^* = \mathbf{a}_{i-1}^*$
11.	**return** $\langle \mathbf{a}_i^*, \mathbf{p}_i^* \rangle$

Table 1: Algorithm for extracting and labeling activities and significant places.

Note that the above two types of aggregation features can generate large cliques in the CRF, which could make standard inference intractable. In our inference, we use the optimized summation templates discussed in Section 2.2.

3.2 Place Detection and Labeling Algorithm

Table 1 summarizes our algorithm for efficiently constructing a CRF that jointly estimates a person's activities and the types of his significant places. The algorithm takes as input a GPS trace. In Step 2 and 3, this trace is segmented into activities a_i and their local evidence e_i^j, which are then used to generate CRF_0 *without significant places*. BP inference is first performed in this CRF so as to determine the activity estimate $\mathbf{a}^*{}_0$, which consists of a sequence of locations and the most likely activity performed at that location (Step 4). Within each iteration of the loop starting at Step 5, such an activity estimate is used to extract a set of significant places. This is done by classifying individual activities in the sequence according to whether or not they belong to a significant place. For instance, while walking, driving a car, or riding a bus are not associated with significant places, working or getting on or off the bus indicate a significant place. All instances at which a *significant activity* occurs generate a place node. Because a place can be visited multiple times within a sequence, we perform clustering and merge duplicate places into the same place node. This classification and clustering is performed by the algorithm generate_places() in Step 7. These places are added to the model and BP is performed in this complete CRF. Since a CRF_i can have a different structure than the previous CRF_{i-1}, it might generate a different activity sequence. If this is the case, the algorithm returns to Step 5 and re-generates the set of places using the improved activity sequence. This process is repeated until the activity sequence does not change. In our experiments we observed that this algorithm converges very quickly, typically after three or four iterations.

4 Experimental Results

In our experiments, we collected GPS data traces from four different persons, approximately seven days of data per person. The data from each person consisted of roughly 40,000 GPS measurements, resulting in about 10,000 10m segments. We used leave-one-out cross-validation for evaluation. Learning from three persons' data took about one minute and BP inference on the last person's data converged within one minute.

Extracting significant places

We compare our model with a widely-used approach that uses a time threshold to determine whether or not a location is significant [1, 6, 8, 3]. We use four different thresholds from

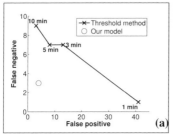
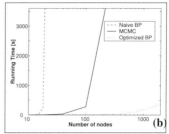

Figure 2: (a) Accuracy of extracting places. (b) Computation times for summation cliques.

Truth	Inferred labels							FN
	Work	Sleep	Leisure	Visit	Pickup	On/off car	Other	
Work	12 / 11	0	0 / 1	0	0	0	1	0
Sleep	0	21	1	2	0	0	0	0
Leisure	2	0	20 / 17	1 / 4	0	0	3	0
Visiting	0	0	0 / 2	7 / 5	0	0	2	0
Pickup	0	0	0	0	1	0	0	2
On/Off car	0	0	0	0	1	13 / 12	0	2 / 3
Other	0	0	0	0	0	0	37	1
FP	0	0	0	0	2	2	3	-

Table 2: Activity confusion matrix of cross-validation data with (left values) and without (right values) considering places for activity inference (FN and FP are false negatives and false positives).

1 minute to 10 minutes, and we measure the false positive and false negative locations extracted from the GPS traces. As shown in Fig. 2(a), any fixed threshold is not satisfactory: low thresholds have many false positives, and high thresholds result in many false negatives. In contrast, our model performs much better: it only generates 4 false positives and 3 false negative. This experiment shows that using high-level context information drastically improves the extraction of significant places.

Labeling places and activities

In our system the labels of activities generate instances of places, which then help to better estimate the activities occurring in their spatial area. The confusion matrix given in Table 2 summarizes the activity estimation results achieved with our system on the cross-validation data. The results are given with and without taking the detected places into account. More specifically, without places are results achieved by CRF_0 generated by Step 4 of the algorithm in Table 1, and results with places are those achieved after model convergence. When the results of both approaches are identical, only one number is given, otherwise, the first number gives the result achieved with the complete model. The table shows two main results. First, the accuracy of our approach is quite high, especially when considering that the system was evaluated on only one week of data and was trained on only three weeks of data collected by different persons. Second, performing joint inference over activities and places increases the quality of inference. The reason for this is that a place node connects all the activities occurring in its spatial area so that these activities can be labeled in a more consistent way. A further evaluation of the detected places showed that our system achieved 90.6% accuracy in place detection and labeling (see [7] for more results).

Efficiency of inference

We compared our optimized BP algorithm using FFT summation cliques with inference based on MCMC and regular BP, using the model and data from [8]. Note that a naive implementation of BP is exponential in the number of nodes in a clique. In our experiments, the test accuracies resulting from using the different algorithms are almost identical. Therefore, we only focus on comparing the efficiency and scalability of summation aggregations. The running times for the different algorithms are shown in Fig. 2(b). As can be seen, naive

BP becomes extremely slow for only 20 nodes, MCMC only works for up to 500 nodes, while our algorithm can perform summation for $2,000$ variables within a few minutes.

5   Conclusions

We provided a novel approach to performing location-based activity recognition. In contrast to existing techniques, our approach uses one consistent framework for both low-level inference and the extraction of a person's significant places. Thereby, our model is able to take high-level context into account in order to detect the significant locations of a person. Furthermore, once these locations are determined, they help to better detect low-level activities occurring in their vicinity.

Summation cliques are extremely important to introduce long-term, soft constraints into activity recognition. We show how to incorporate such cliques into belief propagation using bi-directional FFT computations. The clique templates of RMNs are well suited to specify such clique-specific inference mechanisms and we are developing additional techniques, including clique-specific MCMC and local dynamic programming.

Our experiments based on traces of GPS data show that our system significantly outperforms existing approaches. We demonstrate that the model can be trained from a group of persons and then applied successfully to a different person, achieving more than 85% accuracy in determining low-level activities and above 90% accuracy in detecting and labeling significant places. In future work, we will add more sensor data, including accelerometers, audio signals, and barometric pressure. Using the additional information provided by these sensors, we will be able to perform more fine-grained activity recognition.

Acknowledgments

The authors would like to thank Jeff Bilmes for useful comments. This work has partly been supported by DARPA's ASSIST and CALO Programme (contract numbers: NBCH-C-05-0137, SRI subcontract 27-000968) and by the NSF under grant number IIS-0093406.

References

[1] D. Ashbrook and T. Starner. Using GPS to learn significant locations and predict movement across multiple users. *Personal and Ubiquitous Computing*, 7(5), 2003.

[2] E. Oran Brigham. *Fast Fourier Transform and Its Applications*. Prentice Hall, 1988.

[3] V. Gogate, R. Dechter, C. Rindt, and J. Marca. Modeling transportation routines using hybrid dynamic mixed networks. In *Proc. of the Conference on Uncertainty in Artificial Intelligence*, 2005.

[4] S. Kumar and M. Hebert. Discriminative random fields: A discriminative framework for contextual interaction in classification. In *Proc. of the International Conference on Computer Vision*, 2003.

[5] J. Lafferty, A. McCallum, and F. Pereira. Conditional random fields: Probabilistic models for segmenting and labeling sequence data. In *Proc. of the International Conference on Machine Learning*, 2001.

[6] L. Liao, D. Fox, and H. Kautz. Learning and inferring transportation routines. In *Proc. of the National Conference on Artificial Intelligence*, 2004.

[7] L. Liao, D. Fox, and H. Kautz. Hierarchical conditional random fields for GPS-based activity recognition. In *Proc. of the 12th International Symposium of Robotics Research (ISRR)*, 2005.

[8] L. Liao, D. Fox, and H. Kautz. Location-based activity recognition using relational Markov networks. In *Proc. of the International Joint Conference on Artificial Intelligence*, 2005.

[9] Yongyi Mao, Frank R. Kschischang, and Brendan J. Frey. Convolutional factor graphs as probabilistic models. In *Proc. of the Conference on Uncertainty in Artificial Intelligence*, 2004.

[10] B. Taskar, P. Abbeel, and D. Koller. Discriminative probabilistic models for relational data. In *Proc. of the Conference on Uncertainty in Artificial Intelligence*, 2002.

Radial Basis Function Network for Multi-task Learning

Xuejun Liao
Department of ECE
Duke University
Durham, NC 27708-0291, USA
xjliao@ee.duke.edu

Lawrence Carin
Department of ECE
Duke University
Durham, NC 27708-0291, USA
lcarin@ee.duke.edu

Abstract

We extend radial basis function (RBF) networks to the scenario in which multiple correlated tasks are learned simultaneously, and present the corresponding learning algorithms. We develop the algorithms for learning the network structure, in either a supervised or unsupervised manner. Training data may also be actively selected to improve the network's generalization to test data. Experimental results based on real data demonstrate the advantage of the proposed algorithms and support our conclusions.

1 Introduction

In practical applications, one is frequently confronted with situations in which multiple tasks must be solved. Often these tasks are not independent, implying what is learned from one task is transferable to another correlated task. By making use of this transferability, each task is made easier to solve. In machine learning, the concept of explicitly exploiting the transferability of expertise between tasks, by learning the tasks simultaneously under a unified representation, is formally referred to as "multi-task learning" [1].

In this paper we extend radial basis function (RBF) networks [4,5] to the scenario of multi-task learning and present the corresponding learning algorithms. Our primary interest is to learn the regression model of several data sets, where any given data set may be correlated with some other sets but not necessarily with all of them. The advantage of multi-task learning is usually manifested when the training set of each individual task is weak, i.e., it does not generalize well to the test data. Our algorithms intend to enhance, in a mutually beneficial way, the weak training sets of multiple tasks, by learning them simultaneously. Multi-task learning becomes superfluous when the data sets all come from the same generating distribution, since in that case we can simply take the union of them and treat the union as a single task. In the other extreme, when all the tasks are independent, there is no correlation to utilize and we learn each task separately.

The paper is organized as follows. We define the structure of multi-task RBF network in Section 2 and present the supervised learning algorithm in Section 3. In Section 4 we show how to learn the network structure in an unsupervised manner, and based on this we demonstrate how to actively select the training data, with the goal of improving the generalization to test data. We perform experimental studies in Section 5 and conclude the paper in Section 6.

2   Multi-Task Radial Basis Function Network

Figure 1 schematizes the radial basis function (RBF) network structure customized to multitask learning. The network consists of an input layer, a hidden layer, and an output layer. The input layer receives a data point $\mathbf{x} = [x_1, \cdots, x_d]^T \in \mathbb{R}^d$ and submits it to the hidden layer. Each node at the hidden layer has a localized activation $\phi^n(\mathbf{x}) = \phi(||\mathbf{x} - \mathbf{c}_n||, \sigma_n)$, $n = 1, \cdots, N$, where $|| \cdot ||$ denotes the vector norm and $\phi^n(\cdot)$ is a radial basis function (RBF) localized around $\mathbf{c}_n$ with the degree of localization parameterized by σ_n. Choosing $\phi(z, \sigma) = \exp(-\frac{z^2}{2\sigma^2})$ gives the Gaussian RBF. The activations of all hidden nodes are weighted and sent to the output layer. Each output node represents a unique task and has its own hidden-to-output weights. The weighted activations of the hidden nodes are summed at each output node to produce the output for the associated task. Denoting $\mathbf{w}_k = [w_{0k}, w_{1k}, \cdots, w_{Nk}]^T$ as the weights connecting hidden nodes to the k-th output node, then the output for the k-th task, in response to input $\mathbf{x}$, takes the form

$$f_k(\mathbf{x}) = \mathbf{w}_k^T \boldsymbol{\phi}(\mathbf{x}) \tag{1}$$

where $\boldsymbol{\phi}(\mathbf{x}) = \left[\phi^0(\mathbf{x}), \phi^1(\mathbf{x}), \ldots, \phi^N(\mathbf{x})\right]^T$ is a column containing $N + 1$ basis functions with $\phi^0(\mathbf{x}) \equiv 1$ a dummy basis accounting for the bias in Figure 1.

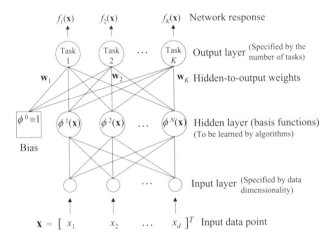

Figure 1: A multi-task structure of RBF Network. Each of the output nodes represents a unique task. Each task has its own hidden-to-output weights but all the tasks share the same hidden nodes. The activation of hidden node n is characterized by a basis function $\phi_n(\mathbf{x}) = \phi(||\mathbf{x} - \mathbf{c}_n||, \sigma_n)$. A typical choice of ϕ is $\phi(z, \sigma) = \exp(-\frac{z^2}{2\sigma^2})$, which gives the Gaussian RBF.

3   Supervised Learning

Suppose we have K tasks and the data set of the k-th task is $\mathcal{D}_k = \{(\mathbf{x}_{1k}, y_{1k}), \cdots, (\mathbf{x}_{J_k k}, y_{J_k k})\}$, where y_{ik} is the target (desired output) of $\mathbf{x}_{ik}$. By definition, a given data point $\mathbf{x}_{ik}$ is said to be supervised if the associated target y_{ik} is provided and unsupervised if y_{ik} is not provided. The definition extends similarly to a set of data

Table 1: Learning Algorithm of Multi-Task RBF Network

Input: $\{(\mathbf{x}_{1k}, y_{2k}), \cdots, (\mathbf{x}_{J_k,k}, y_{J_k,k})\}_{k=1:K}$, $\phi(\cdot, \sigma)$, σ, and ρ;   Output: $\phi(\cdot)$ and $\{\mathbf{w}_k\}_{k=1}^K$.

1. **For** $m = 1:K$, **For** $n = 1:J_m$, **For** $k = 1:K$, **For** $i = 1:J_k$
   Compute $\widehat{\phi}_{ik}^{nm} = \phi(||\mathbf{x}_{nm} - \mathbf{x}_{ik}||, \sigma)$;
2. **Let** $N = 0$, $\phi(\cdot) = 1$, $e_0 = \sum_{k=1}^K \left[\sum_{i=1}^{J_k} y_{ik}^2 - (J_k + \rho)^{-1} (\sum_{i=1}^{J_k} y_{ik})^2 \right]$;
   For $k = 1:K$, compute $\mathbf{A}_k = J_k + \rho$, $\mathbf{w}_k = (J_k + \rho)^{-1} \sum_{i=1}^{J_k} y_{ik}$;
3. **For** $m = 1:K$, **For** $n = 1:J_m$
   If $\widehat{\phi}^{nm}$ is not marked as "deleted"
   For $k = 1:K$, compute
   $$\mathbf{c}_k = \sum_{i=1}^{J_k} \phi_{ik} \widehat{\phi}_{ik}^{nm}, \quad q_k = \sum_{i=1}^{J_k} (\widehat{\phi}_{ik}^{nm})^2 + \rho - \mathbf{c}_k^T \mathbf{A}_k^{-1} \mathbf{c}_k;$$
   If there exists k such that $q_k = 0$, mark $\widehat{\phi}^{nm}$ as "deleted";
   else, compute $\delta e(\phi, \widehat{\phi}^{nm})$ using (5).
4. **If** $\{\widehat{\phi}^{ik}\}_{i=1:J_k, k=1:K}$ are all marked as "deleted", go to 10.
5. **Let** $(n^*, m^*) = \arg\max_{\widehat{\phi}^{nm} \text{ not marked as "deleted"}} \delta e(\phi, \widehat{\phi}^{nm})$; Mark $\widehat{\phi}^{n^*m^*}$ as "deleted".
6. Tune RBF parameter $\sigma_{N+1} = \arg\max_\sigma \delta e(\phi, \phi(|| \cdot -\mathbf{x}_{n^*m^*}||, \sigma))$
7. **Let** $\phi^{N+1}(\cdot) = \phi(|| \cdot -\mathbf{x}_{n^*m^*}||, \sigma_{N+1})$; Update $\phi(\cdot) \leftarrow [\phi^T(\cdot), \phi^{N+1}(\cdot)]^T$;
8. **For** $k = 1:K$
   Compute $\mathbf{A}_k^{new}$ and $\mathbf{w}_k^{new}$ respectively by (A-1) and (A-3) in the appendix; Update $\mathbf{A}_k \leftarrow \mathbf{A}_k^{new}$, $\mathbf{w}_k \leftarrow \mathbf{w}_k^{new}$
9. **Let** $e_{N+1} = e_N - \delta e(\phi, \phi^{N+1})$;   **If** the sequence $\{e_n\}_{n=0:(N+1)}$ is converged, go to 10, **else** update $N \leftarrow N + 1$ and go back to 3.
10. **Exit** and output $\phi(\cdot)$ and $\{\mathbf{w}_k\}_{k=1}^K$.

points. We are interested in learning the functions $f_k(\mathbf{x})$ for the K tasks, based on $\cup_{k=1}^K \mathcal{D}_k$. The learning is based on minimizing the squared error

$$e(\phi, \mathbf{w}) = \sum_{k=1}^K \left\{ \sum_{i=1}^{J_k} \left(\mathbf{w}_k^T \phi_{ik} - y_{ik} \right)^2 + \rho ||\mathbf{w}_k||^2 \right\} \tag{2}$$

where $\phi_{ik} = \phi(\mathbf{x}_{ik})$ for notational simplicity. The regularization terms $\rho ||\mathbf{w}_k||^2$, $k = 1, \cdots, K$, are used to prevent singularity of the $\mathbf{A}$ matrices defined in (3), and ρ is typically set to a small positive number. For fixed ϕ's, the $\mathbf{w}$'s are solved by minimizing $e(\phi, \mathbf{w})$ with respect to $\mathbf{w}$, yielding

$$\mathbf{w}_k = \mathbf{A}_k^{-1} \sum_{i=1}^{J_k} y_{ik} \phi_{ik} \quad \text{and} \quad \mathbf{A}_k = \sum_{i=1}^{J_k} \phi_{ik} \phi_{ik}^T + \rho \mathbf{I}, \quad k = 1, \cdots, K \tag{3}$$

In a multi-task RBF network, the input layer and output layer are respectively specified by the data dimensionality and the number of tasks. We now discuss how to determine the hidden layer (basis functions ϕ). Substituting the solutions of the $\mathbf{w}$'s in (3) into (2) gives

$$e(\phi) = \sum_{k=1}^K \sum_{i=1}^{J_k} \left(y_{ik}^2 - y_{ik} \mathbf{w}_k^T \phi_{ik} \right) \tag{4}$$

where $e(\phi)$ is a function of ϕ only because $\mathbf{w}$'s are now functions of ϕ as given by (3). By minimizing $e(\phi)$, we can determine ϕ. Recalling that ϕ_{ik} is an abbreviation of $\phi(\mathbf{x}_{ik}) = [1, \phi^1(\mathbf{x}_{ik}), \ldots, \phi^N(\mathbf{x}_{ik})]^T$, this amounts to determining N, the number of basis functions, and the functional form of each basis function $\phi^n(\cdot)$, $n = 1, \ldots, N$. Consider the candidate functions $\{\phi^{nm}(\mathbf{x}) = \phi(||\mathbf{x} - \mathbf{x}_{nm}||, \sigma) : n = 1, \cdots, J_m, m = 1, \cdots, K\}$. We learn the RBF network structure by selecting $\phi(\cdot)$ from these candidate functions such that $e(\phi)$ in (4) is minimized. The following theorem tells us how to perform the selection in a sequential way; the proof is given in the Appendix.

797

Theorem 1 *Let $\phi(\mathbf{x}) = [1, \phi^1(\mathbf{x}), \ldots, \phi^N(\mathbf{x})]^T$ and $\phi^{N+1}(\mathbf{x})$ be a single basis function. Assume the $\mathbf{A}$ matrices corresponding to ϕ and $[\phi, \phi^{N+1}]^T$ are all non-degenerate. Then*

$$\delta e(\phi, \phi^{N+1}) = e(\phi) - e([\phi, \phi^{N+1}]^T) = \sum_{k=1}^{K} \left(\mathbf{c}_k^T \mathbf{w}_k - \sum_{i=1}^{J_k} y_{ik} \phi_{ik}^{N+1} \right)^2 q_k^{-1} \quad (5)$$

where $\phi_{ik}^{N+1} = \phi^{N+1}(\phi_{ik})$, $\mathbf{w}_k$ and $\mathbf{A}$ are the same as in (3), and

$$\mathbf{c}_k = \sum_{i=1}^{J_k} \phi_{ik} \phi_{ik}^{N+1}, \quad d_k = \sum_{i=1}^{J_k} (\phi_{ik}^{N+1})^2 + \rho, \quad q_k = d_k - \mathbf{c}_k^T \mathbf{A}_k^{-1} \mathbf{c}_k \quad (6)$$

By the conditions of the theorem $\mathbf{A}_k^{new}$ is full rank and hence it is positive definite by construction. By (A-2) in the Appendix, q_k^{-1} is a diagonal element of $(\mathbf{A}_k^{new})^{-1}$, therefore q_k^{-1} is positive and by (5) $\delta e(\phi, \phi^{N+1}) > 0$, which means adding ϕ^{N+1} to ϕ generally makes the squared error decrease. The decrease $\delta e(\phi, \phi^{N+1})$ depends on ϕ^{N+1}. By sequentially selecting basis functions that bring the maximum error reduction, we achieve the goal of maximizing $e(\phi)$. The details of the learning algorithm are summarized in Table 1.

4 Active Learning

In the previous section, the data in D_k are supervised (provided with the targets). In this section, we assume the data in D_k are initially unsupervised (only $\mathbf{x}$ is available without access to the associated y) and we select a subset from $\mathcal{D}_k$ to be supervised (targets acquired) such that the resulting network generalizes well to the remaining data in $\mathcal{D}_k$. The approach is generally known as active learning [6]. We first learn the basis functions ϕ from the unsupervised data, and based on ϕ select data to be supervised. Both of these steps are based on the following theorem, the proof of which is given in the Appendix.

Theorem 2 *Let there be K tasks and the data set of the k-th task is $\mathcal{D}_k \cup \widetilde{\mathcal{D}}_k$ where $\mathcal{D}_k = \{(\mathbf{x}_{ik}, y_{ik})\}_{i=1}^{J_k}$ and $\widetilde{\mathcal{D}}_k = \{(\mathbf{x}_{ik}, y_{ik})\}_{i=J_k+1}^{J_k+\widetilde{J}_k}$. Let there be two multi-task RBF networks, whose output nodes are characterized by $f_k(\cdot)$ and $f_k^{\sim}(\cdot)$, respectively, for task $k = 1, \ldots, K$. The two networks have the same given basis functions (hidden nodes) $\phi(\cdot) = [1, \phi^1(\cdot), \cdots, \phi^N(\cdot)]^T$, but different hidden-to-output weights. The weights of $f_k(\cdot)$ are trained with $\mathcal{D}_k \cup \widetilde{\mathcal{D}}_k$, while the weights of $f_k^{\sim}(\cdot)$ are trained using $\widetilde{\mathcal{D}}_k$. Then for $k = 1, \cdots, K$, the square errors committed on $\mathcal{D}_k$ by $f_k(\cdot)$ and $f_k^{\sim}(\cdot)$ are related by*

$$0 \leq [det\,\mathbf{\Gamma}_k]^{-1} \leq \lambda_{max,k}^{-1} \leq \left[\sum_{i=1}^{J_k}(y_{ik} - f_k^{\sim}(\mathbf{x}_{ik}))^2\right]^{-1} \sum_{i=1}^{J_k}(y_{ik} - f_k(\mathbf{x}_{ik}))^2 \leq \lambda_{min,k}^{-1} \leq 1 \quad (7)$$

where $\mathbf{\Gamma}_k = \left[\mathbf{I} + \mathbf{\Phi}_k^T(\rho\,\mathbf{I} + \widetilde{\mathbf{\Phi}}_k\widetilde{\mathbf{\Phi}}_k^T)^{-1}\mathbf{\Phi}_k\right]^2$ with $\mathbf{\Phi} = \left[\phi(\mathbf{x}_{1k}), \ldots, \phi(\mathbf{x}_{J_k k})\right]$ and $\widetilde{\mathbf{\Phi}} = \left[\phi(\mathbf{x}_{J_k+1,k}), \ldots, \phi(\mathbf{x}_{J_k+\widetilde{J}_k,k})\right]$, and $\lambda_{max,k}$ and $\lambda_{min,k}$ are respectively the largest and smallest eigenvalues of $\mathbf{\Gamma}_k$.

Specializing Theorem 2 to the case $\widetilde{J}_k = 0$, we have

Corollary 1 *Let there be K tasks and the data set of the k-th task is $\mathcal{D}_k = \{(\mathbf{x}_{ik}, y_{ik})\}_{i=1}^{J_k}$. Let the RBF network, whose output nodes are characterized by $f_k(\cdot)$ for task $k = 1, \ldots, K$, have given basis functions (hidden nodes) $\phi(\cdot) = [1, \phi^1(\cdot), \cdots, \phi^N(\cdot)]^T$ and the hidden-to-output weights of task k be trained with $\mathcal{D}_k$. Then for $k = 1, \cdots, K$, the squared error committed on $\mathcal{D}_k$ by $f_k(\cdot)$ is bounded as $0 \leq [det\,\mathbf{\Gamma}_k]^{-1} \leq \lambda_{max,k}^{-1} \leq \left[\sum_{i=1}^{J_k} y_{ik}^2\right]^{-1} \sum_{i=1}^{J_k}(y_{ik} - f_k(\mathbf{x}_{ik}))^2 \leq \lambda_{min,k}^{-1} \leq 1$, where $\mathbf{\Gamma}_k = \left(\mathbf{I} + \rho^{-1}\mathbf{\Phi}_k^T\mathbf{\Phi}_k\right)^2$ with $\mathbf{\Phi} = \left[\phi(\mathbf{x}_{1,k}), \ldots, \phi(\mathbf{x}_{J_k,k})\right]$, and $\lambda_{max,k}$ and $\lambda_{min,k}$ are respectively the largest and smallest eigenvalues of $\mathbf{\Gamma}_k$.*

It is evident from the properties of matrix determinant [7] and the definition of $\mathbf{\Phi}$ that $\det\mathbf{\Gamma}_k = \left[\det(\rho\mathbf{I} + \mathbf{\Phi}_k\mathbf{\Phi}_k^T)\right]^2[\det(\rho\,\mathbf{I})]^{-2} = \left[\det(\rho\mathbf{I} + \sum_{i=1}^{J_k}\phi_{ik}\phi_{ik}^T)\right]^2[\det(\rho\,\mathbf{I})]^{-2}$.

Using (3) we write succinctly $\det \mathbf{\Gamma}_k = [\det \mathbf{A}_k^2][\det(\rho \mathbf{I})]^{-2}$. We are interested in selecting the basis functions ϕ that minimize the error, before seeing y's. By Corollary 1 and the equation $\det \mathbf{\Gamma}_k = [\det \mathbf{A}_k^2][\det(\rho \mathbf{I})]^{-2}$, the squared error is lower bounded by $\sum_{i=1}^{J_k} y_{ik}^2 [\det(\rho \mathbf{I})]^2 [\det \mathbf{A}_k]^{-2}$. Instead of minimizing the error directly, we minimize its lower bound. As $[\det(\rho \mathbf{I})]^2 \sum_{i=1}^{L_k} y_{ik}^2$ does not depend on ϕ, this amounts to selecting ϕ to minimize $(\det \mathbf{A}_k)^{-2}$. To minimize the errors for all tasks $k = 1 \cdots, K$, we select ϕ to minimize $\prod_{k=1}^{K} (\det \mathbf{A}_k)^{-2}$.

The selection proceeds in a sequential manner. Suppose we have selected basis functions $\phi = [1, \phi^1, \cdots, \phi^N]^T$. The associated $\mathbf{A}$ matrices are $\mathbf{A}_k = \sum_{i=1}^{J_k} \phi_{ik} \phi_{ik}^T + \rho \mathbf{I}_{(N+1) \times (N+1)}$, $k = 1, \cdots, K$. Augmenting basis functions to $[\phi^T, \phi^{N+1}]^T$, the $\mathbf{A}$ matrices change to $\mathbf{A}_k^{new} = \sum_{i=1}^{J_k} [\phi_{ik}^T, \phi_{ik}^{N+1}]^T [\phi_{ik}^T, \phi_{ik}^{N+1}] + \rho \mathbf{I}_{(N+2) \times (N+2)}$. Using the determinant formula of block matrices [7], we get $\prod_{k=1}^{K} (\det \mathbf{A}_k^{new})^{-2} = \prod_{k=1}^{K} (q_k \det \mathbf{A}_k)^{-2}$, where q_k is the same as in (6). As $\mathbf{A}_k$ does not depend on ϕ^{N+1}, the left-hand side is minimized by maximizing $\prod_{k=1}^{K} q_k^2$. The selection is easily implemented by making the following two minor modifications in Table 1: (a) in step 2, compute $e_0 = \sum_{k=1}^{K} \ln(J_k + \rho)^{-2}$; in step 3, compute $\delta e(\phi, \widehat{\phi}^{nm}) = \sum_{k=1}^{K} \ln q_k^2$. Employing the logarithm is for gaining additivity and it does not affect the maximization.

Based on the basis functions ϕ determined above, we proceed to selecting data to be supervised and determining the hidden-to-output weights $\mathbf{w}$ from the supervised data using the equations in (3). The selection of data is based on an iterative use of the following corollary, which is a specialization of Theorem 2 and was originally given in [8].

Corollary 2 *Let there be K tasks and the data set of the k-th task is $\mathcal{D}_k = \{(\mathbf{x}_{ik}, y_{ik})\}_{i=1}^{J_k}$. Let there be two RBF networks, whose output nodes are characterized by $f_k(\cdot)$ and $f_k^+(\cdot)$, respectively, for task $k = 1, \ldots, K$. The two networks have the same given basis functions $\phi(\cdot) = [1, \phi^1(\cdot), \cdots, \phi^N(\cdot)]^T$, but different hidden-to-output weights. The weights of $f_k(\cdot)$ are trained with $\mathcal{D}_k$, while the weights of $f_k^+(\cdot)$ are trained using $\mathcal{D}_k^+ = \mathcal{D}_k \cup \{(\mathbf{x}_{J_k+1,k}, y_{J_k+1,k})\}$. Then for $k = 1, \cdots, K$, the squared errors committed on $(\mathbf{x}_{J_k+1,k}, y_{J_k+1,k})$ by $f_k(\cdot)$ and $f_k^+(\cdot)$ are related by $[f_k^+(\mathbf{x}_{J_k+1,k}) - y_{J_k+1,k}]^2 = [\gamma(\mathbf{x}_{J_k+1,k})]^{-1} [f_k(\mathbf{x}_{J_k+1,k}) - y_{J_k+1,k}]^2$, where $\gamma(\mathbf{x}_{J_k+1,k}) = [1 + \phi^T(\mathbf{x}_{J_k+1,k}) \mathbf{A}_k^{-1} \phi(\mathbf{x}_{J_k+1,k})]^2 \geq 1$ and $\mathbf{A}_k = \sum_{i=1}^{J_k} [\rho \mathbf{I} + \phi(\mathbf{x}_{ik}) \phi^T(\mathbf{x}_{ik})]$ is the same as in (3).*

Two observations are made from Corollary 2. First, if $\gamma(\mathbf{x}_{J_k+1,k}) \approx 1$, seeing $y_{J_k+1,k}$ does not effect the error on $\mathbf{x}_{J_k+1,k}$, indicating $\mathcal{D}_k$ already contain sufficient information about $(\mathbf{x}_{J_k+1,k}, y_{J_k+1,k})$. Second, if $\gamma(\mathbf{x}_i) \gg 1$, seeing $y_{J_k+1,k}$ greatly decrease the error on $\mathbf{x}_{J_k+1,k}$, indicating $\mathbf{x}_{J_k+1,k}$ is significantly dissimilar (novel) to $\mathcal{D}_k$ and $\mathbf{x}_{J_k+1,k}$ must be supervised to reduce the error. Based on Corollary 2, the selection proceeds sequentially. Suppose we have selected data $\mathcal{D}_k = \{(\mathbf{x}_{ik}, y_{ik})\}_{i=1}^{J_k}$, from which we compute $\mathbf{A}_k$. We select the next data point as $\mathbf{x}_{J_k+1,k} = \arg \max_{i > J_k, k=1, \cdots, K} \gamma(\mathbf{x}_{ik}) = \arg \max_{i > J_k, k=1, \cdots, K} [1 + \phi^T(\mathbf{x}_{ik}) \mathbf{A}_k^{-1} \phi(\mathbf{x}_{ik})]^2$. After $\mathbf{x}_{J_k+1,k}$ is selected, the $\mathbf{A}_k$ is updated and the next selection begins. As the iteration advances γ will decrease until it reaches convergence. We use (3) to compute $\mathbf{w}$ from the selected $\mathbf{x}$ and their associated targets y, completing learning of the RBF network.

5 Experimental Results

In this section we compare the multi-task RBF network against single-task RBF networks via experimental studies. We consider three types of RBF networks to learn K tasks, each with its data set $\mathcal{D}_k$. In the first, which we call "one RBF network", we let the K tasks share both basis functions ϕ (hidden nodes) and hidden-to output weights $\mathbf{w}$, thus we do not distinguish the K tasks and design a single RBF network to learn a union of them. The second is the multi-task RBF network, where the K tasks share the same ϕ but each has its own $\mathbf{w}$. In the third, we have K independent networks, each designed for a single task.

We use a school data set from the Inner London Education Authority, consisting of examination records of 15362 students from 139 secondary schools. The data are available at http://multilevel.ioe.ac.uk/intro/datasets.html. This data set was originally used to study the effectiveness of schools and has recently been used to evaluate multi-task algorithms [2,3]. The goal is to predict the exam scores of the students based on 9 variables: year of exam (1985, 1986, or 1987), school code (1-139), FSM (percentage of students eligible for free school meals), VR1 band (percentage of students in school in VR band one), gender, VR band of student (3 categories), ethnic group of student (11 categories), school gender (male, female, or mixed), school denomination (3 categories). We consider each school a task, leading to 139 tasks in total. The remaining 8 variables are used as inputs to the RBF network. Following [2,3], we converted each categorical variable to a number of binary variables, resulting in a total number of 27 input variables, i.e., $\mathbf{x} \in \mathbb{R}^{27}$. The exam score is the target to be predicted.

The three types of RBF networks as defined above are designed as follows. The multi-task RBF network is implemented as the structure as shown in Figure 1 and trained with the learning algorithm in Table 1. The "one RBF network" is implemented as a special case of Figure 1, with a single output node and trained using the union of supervised data from all 139 schools. We design 139 independent RBF networks, each of which is implemented with a single output node and trained using the supervised data from a single school. We use the Gaussian RBF $\phi^n(\mathbf{x}) = \exp(-\frac{\|\mathbf{x}-\mathbf{c}_n\|^2}{2\sigma^2})$, where the $\mathbf{c}_n$'s are selected from training data points and σ_n's are initialized as 20 and optimized as described in Table 1. The main role of the regularization parameter ρ is to prevent the $\mathbf{A}$ matrices from being singular and it does not affect the results seriously. In the results reported here, ρ is set to 10^{-6}.

Following [2-3], we randomly take 75% of the 15362 data points as training (supervised) data and the remaining 25% as test data. The generalization performance is measured by the squared error $(f_k(\mathbf{x}_{ik}) - y_{ik})^2$ averaged over all test data $\mathbf{x}_{ik}$ of tasks $k = 1, \cdots, K$. We made 10 independent trials to randomly split the data into training and test sets and the squared error averaged over the test data of all the 139 schools and the trials are shown in Table 2, for the three types of RBF networks.

Table 2: Squared error averaged over the test data of all 139 schools and the 10 independent trials for randomly splitting the school data into training (75%) and testing (25%) sets.

Multi-task RBF network	Independent RBF networks	One RBF network
109.89 ± 1.8167	136.41 ± 7.0081	149.48 ± 2.8093

Table 2 clearly shows the multi-task RBF network outperforms the other two types of RBF networks by a considerable margin. The "one RBF network" ignores the difference between the tasks and the independent RBF networks ignore the tasks' correlations, therefore they both perform inferiorly. The multi-task RBF network uses the shared hidden nodes (basis functions) to capture the common internal representation of the tasks and meanwhile uses the independent hidden-to-output weights to learn the statistics specific to each task.

We now demonstrate the results of active learning. We use the method in Section 4 to actively split the data into training and test sets using a two-step procedure. First we learn the basis functions ϕ of multi-task RBF network using all 15362 data (unsupervised). Based on the ϕ, we then select the data to be supervised and use them as training data to learn the hidden-to-output weights **w**. To make the results comparable, we use the same training data to learn the other two types of RBF networks (including learning their own ϕ and **w**). The networks are then tested on the remaining data.

Figure 2 shows the results of active learning. Each curve is the squared error averaged over the test data of all 139 schools, as a function of number of training data. It is clear that the multi-task RBF network maintains its superior performance all the way down to 5000 training data points, whereas the independent RBF networks have their performances degraded seriously as the training data diminish. This demonstrates the increasing advantage of multi-task learning as the number of training data decreases. The "one RBF network" seems also insensitive to the number of training data, but it ignores the inherent dissimilarity between the tasks, which makes its performance inferior.

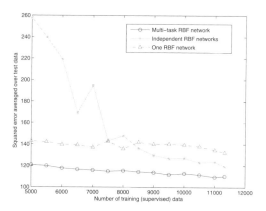

Figure 2: Squared error averaged over the test data of all 139 schools, as a function of the number of training (supervised) data. The data are split into training and test sets via active learning.

6   Conclusions

We have presented the structure and learning algorithms for multi-task learning with the radial basis function (RBF) network. By letting multiple tasks share the basis functions (hidden nodes) we impose a common internal representation for correlated tasks. Exploiting the inter-task correlation yields a more compact network structure that has enhanced generalization ability. Unsupervised learning of the network structure enables us to actively split the data into training and test sets. As the data novel to the previously selected ones are selected next, what finally remain unselected and to be tested are all similar to the selected data which constitutes the training set. This improves the generalization of the resulting network to the test data. These conclusions are substantiated via results on real multi-task data.

References

[1] R. Caruana. (1997) Multitask learning. *Machine Learning*, 28, p. 41-75, 1997.

[2] B. Bakker and T. Heskes (2003). Task clustering and gating for Bayesian multitask learning. *Journal of Machine Learning Research*, 4: 83-99, 2003

[3] T. Evgeniou, C. A. Micchelli, and M. Pontil (2005). Learning Multiple Tasks with Kernel Methods. *Journal of Machine Learning Research*, 6: 615637, 2005

[4] Powell M. (1987), Radial basis functions for multivariable interpolation : A review, J.C. Mason and M.G. Cox, eds, *Algorithms for Approximation*, pp.143-167.

[5] Chen, F. Cowan, and P. Grant (1991), Orthogonal least squares learning algorithm for radial basis function networks, *IEEE Transactions on Neural Networks*, Vol. 2, No. 2, 302-309, 1991

[6] Cohn, D. A., Ghahramani, Z., and Jordan, M. I. (1995). Active learning with statistical models. *Advances in Neural Information Processing Systems*, 7, 705-712.

[7] V. Fedorov (1972), *Theory of Optimal Experiments*, Academic Press, 1972

[8] M. Stone (1974), Cross-validatory choice and assessment of statistical predictions, *Journal of the Royal Statistical Society, Series B*, 36, pp. 111-147, 1974.

Appendix

Proof of Theorem 1:. Let $\phi^{new} = [\phi, \phi^{N+1}]^T$. By (3), the $\mathbf{A}$ matrices corresponding to ϕ^{new} are

$$\mathbf{A}_k^{new} = \sum_{i=1}^{J_k} \begin{bmatrix} \phi_{ik} \\ \phi_{ik}^{N+1} \end{bmatrix} \begin{bmatrix} \phi_{ik}^T & \phi_{ik}^{N+1} \end{bmatrix} + \rho \, \mathbf{I}_{(N+2)\times(N+2)} = \begin{bmatrix} \mathbf{A}_k & \mathbf{c}_k \\ \mathbf{c}_k^T & d_k \end{bmatrix} \qquad \text{(A-1)}$$

where $\mathbf{c}_k$ and d_k are as in (6). By the conditions of the theorem, the matrices $\mathbf{A}_k$ and $\mathbf{A}_k^{new}$ are all non-degenerate. Using the block matrix inversion formula [7] we get

$$(\mathbf{A}_k^{new})^{-1} = \begin{bmatrix} \mathbf{A}_k^{-1} + \mathbf{A}_k^{-1}\mathbf{c}_k q_k^{-1}\mathbf{c}_k^T \mathbf{A}_k^{-1} & -\mathbf{A}_k^{-1}\mathbf{c}_k q_k^{-1} \\ -q_k^{-1}\mathbf{c}_k^T \mathbf{A}_k^{-1} & q_k^{-1} \end{bmatrix} \qquad \text{(A-2)}$$

where q_k is as in (6). By (3), the weights $\mathbf{w}_k^{new}$ corresponding to $[\phi^T, \phi^{N+1}]^T$ are

$$\mathbf{w}_k^{new} = (\mathbf{A}_k^{new})^{-1} \begin{bmatrix} \sum_{i=1}^{J_k} y_{ik}\phi_{ik} \\ \sum_{i=1}^{J_k} y_{ik}\phi_{ik}^{N+1} \end{bmatrix} = \begin{bmatrix} \mathbf{w}_k + \mathbf{A}_k^{-1}\mathbf{c}_k q_k^{-1} g_k \\ -q_k^{-1} g_k \end{bmatrix} \qquad \text{(A-3)}$$

with $g_k = \mathbf{c}_k^T \mathbf{w}_k - \sum_{i=1}^{J_k} y_{ik}\phi_{ik}^{N+1}$. Hence, $(\phi_{ik}^{new})^T \mathbf{w}_k^{new} = \phi_{ik}^T \mathbf{w}_k + (\phi_{ik}^T \mathbf{A}_k^{-1}\mathbf{c}_k - \phi_{ik}^{N+1})g_k q_k^{-1}$, which is put into (4) to get $e(\phi^{new}) = \sum_{k=1}^{K}\sum_{i=1}^{J_k} [y_{ik}^2 - y_{ik}(\phi_{ik}^{new})^T \mathbf{w}_k^{new}] = \sum_{k=1}^{K}\sum_{i=1}^{J_k} [y_{ik}^2 - y_{ik}\phi_{ik}^T \mathbf{w}_k - y_{ik}(\phi_{ik}^T \mathbf{A}_k^{-1}\mathbf{c}_k - \phi_{ik}^{N+1})g_k q_k^{-1}] = e(\phi) - \sum_{k=1}^{K}(\mathbf{c}_k^T \mathbf{w}_k - \sum_{i=1}^{J_k} y_{ik}\phi_{ik}^{N+1})^2 q_k^{-1}$, where in arriving the last equality we have used (3) and (4) and $g_k = \mathbf{c}_k^T \mathbf{w}_k - \sum_{i=1}^{J_k} y_{ik}\phi_{ik}^{N+1}$. The theorem is proved. $\square$

Proof of Theorem 2: The proof applies to $k = 1, \cdots, K$. For any given k, define $\mathbf{\Phi} = [\phi(\mathbf{x}_{1k}), \ldots, \phi(\mathbf{x}_{J_kk})]$, $\widetilde{\mathbf{\Phi}} = [\phi(\mathbf{x}_{J_k+1,k}), \ldots, \phi(\mathbf{x}_{J_k+\tilde{J}_k,k})]$, $\mathbf{y}_k = [y_{1k}, \ldots, y_{J_kk}]^T$, $\widetilde{\mathbf{y}}_k = [y_{J_k+1,k}, \ldots, y_{J_k+\tilde{J}_k,k}]^T$, $\mathbf{f}_k = [f(\mathbf{x}_{1k}), \ldots, f(\mathbf{x}_{J_kk})]^T$, $\mathbf{f}_{\tilde{k}} = [f_{\tilde{k}}(\mathbf{x}_{1k}), \ldots, f_{\tilde{k}}(\mathbf{x}_{J_kk})]^T$, and $\widetilde{\mathbf{A}}_k = \rho\mathbf{I} + \widetilde{\mathbf{\Phi}}_k \widetilde{\mathbf{\Phi}}_k^T$. By (1), (3), and the conditions of the theorem, $\mathbf{f}_k = \mathbf{\Phi}_k^T (\widetilde{\mathbf{A}}_k + \mathbf{\Phi}_k \mathbf{\Phi}_k^T)^{-1}(\mathbf{\Phi}_k \mathbf{y}_k + \widetilde{\mathbf{\Phi}}_k \widetilde{\mathbf{y}}_k) \overset{(a)}{=} [\mathbf{\Phi}_k^T \widetilde{\mathbf{A}}_k^{-1} - (\mathbf{\Phi}_k^T \widetilde{\mathbf{A}}_k^{-1}\mathbf{\Phi}_k + \mathbf{I} - \mathbf{I})(\mathbf{I} + \mathbf{\Phi}_k^T \widetilde{\mathbf{A}}_k^{-1}\mathbf{\Phi}_k)^{-1}\mathbf{\Phi}_k^T \widetilde{\mathbf{A}}_k^{-1}][\mathbf{\Phi}_k \mathbf{y}_k + \widetilde{\mathbf{\Phi}}_k \widetilde{\mathbf{y}}_k] = [(\mathbf{I} + \mathbf{\Phi}_k^T \widetilde{\mathbf{A}}_k^{-1}\mathbf{\Phi}_k)^{-1}\mathbf{\Phi}_k^T \widetilde{\mathbf{A}}_k^{-1}][\widetilde{\mathbf{\Phi}}_k \widetilde{\mathbf{y}}_k + \mathbf{\Phi}_k \mathbf{y}_k] \overset{(b)}{=} (\mathbf{I} + \mathbf{\Phi}_k^T \widetilde{\mathbf{A}}_k^{-1}\mathbf{\Phi}_k)^{-1}\mathbf{f}_{\tilde{k}} + (\mathbf{I} + \mathbf{\Phi}_k^T \widetilde{\mathbf{A}}_k^{-1}\mathbf{\Phi}_k)^{-1}(\mathbf{\Phi}_k^T \widetilde{\mathbf{A}}_k^{-1}\mathbf{\Phi}_k + \mathbf{I} - \mathbf{I})\mathbf{y}_k = \mathbf{y}_k + (\mathbf{I} + \mathbf{\Phi}_k^T \widetilde{\mathbf{A}}_k^{-1}\mathbf{\Phi}_k)^{-1}(\mathbf{f}_{\tilde{k}} - \mathbf{y}_k)$, where equation (a) is due to the Sherman-Morrison-Woodbury formula and equation (b) results because $\mathbf{f}_{\tilde{k}} = \mathbf{\Phi}_k^T \widetilde{\mathbf{A}}_k^{-1}\widetilde{\mathbf{\Phi}}_k \widetilde{\mathbf{y}}_k$. Hence, $\mathbf{f}_k - \mathbf{y}_k = (\mathbf{I} + \mathbf{\Phi}_k^T \widetilde{\mathbf{A}}_k^{-1}\mathbf{\Phi}_k)^{-1}(\mathbf{f}_{\tilde{k}} - \mathbf{y}_k)$, which gives

$$\sum_{i=1}^{J_k} (y_{ik} - f_k(\mathbf{x}_{ik}))^2 = (\mathbf{f}_k - \mathbf{y}_k)^T (\mathbf{f}_k - \mathbf{y}_k) = (\mathbf{f}_{\tilde{k}} - \mathbf{y}_k)^T \mathbf{\Gamma}_k^{-1}(\mathbf{f}_{\tilde{k}} - \mathbf{y}_k) \qquad \text{(A-4)}$$

where $\mathbf{\Gamma}_k = [\mathbf{I} + \mathbf{\Phi}_k^T \widetilde{\mathbf{A}}_k^{-1}\mathbf{\Phi}_k]^2 = [\mathbf{I} + \mathbf{\Phi}_k^T (\rho\,\mathbf{I} + \widetilde{\mathbf{\Phi}}_k \widetilde{\mathbf{\Phi}}_k^T)^{-1}\mathbf{\Phi}_k]^2$.

By construction, $\mathbf{\Gamma}_k$ has all its eigenvalues no less than 1, i.e., $\mathbf{\Gamma}_k = \mathbf{E}_k^T \text{diag}[\lambda_{1k}, \cdots, \lambda_{J_kk}]\mathbf{E}_k$ with $\mathbf{E}_k^T \mathbf{E}_k = \mathbf{I}$ and $\lambda_{1k}, \cdots, \lambda_{J_kk} \geq 1$, which makes the first, second, and last inequality in (7) hold. Using this expansion of $\mathbf{\Gamma}_k$ in (A-4) we get

$$\sum_{i=1}^{J_k} (f_k(\mathbf{x}_{ik}) - y_{ik})^2 = (\mathbf{f}_{\tilde{k}} - \mathbf{y}_k)^T \mathbf{E}_k^T \text{diag}[\sigma_{1k}^{-1}, \ldots, \sigma_{J_kk}^{-1}](\mathbf{f}_{\tilde{k}} - \mathbf{y}_k)$$

$$\leq (\mathbf{f}_{\tilde{k}} - \mathbf{y}_k)^T \mathbf{E}_k^T [\lambda_{min,k}^{-1}\mathbf{I}]\mathbf{E}_k (\mathbf{f}_{\tilde{k}} - \mathbf{y}_k) = \lambda_{min,k}^{-1}\sum_{i=1}^{J_k}(f_{\tilde{k}}(\mathbf{x}_{ik}) - y_{ik})^2 \qquad \text{(A-5)}$$

where the inequality results because $\lambda_{min,k} = \min(\lambda_{1,k}, \cdots, \lambda_{J_k,k})$. From (A-5) follows the fourth inequality in (7). The third inequality in (7) can be proven in in a similar way. $\square$

Asymptotics of Gaussian Regularized Least-Squares

Ross A. Lippert
M.I.T., Department of Mathematics
77 Massachusetts Avenue
Cambridge, MA 02139-4307
lippert@math.mit.edu

Ryan M. Rifkin
Honda Research Institute USA, Inc.
145 Tremont Street
Boston, MA 02111
rrifkin@honda-ri.com

Abstract

We consider regularized least-squares (RLS) with a Gaussian kernel. We prove that if we let the Gaussian bandwidth $\sigma \to \infty$ while letting the regularization parameter $\lambda \to 0$, the RLS solution tends to a polynomial whose order is controlled by the rielative rates of decay of $\frac{1}{\sigma^2}$ and λ: if $\lambda = \sigma^{-(2k+1)}$, then, as $\sigma \to \infty$, the RLS solution tends to the kth order polynomial with minimal empirical error. We illustrate the result with an example.

1 Introduction

Given a data set $(x_1, y_1), (x_2, y_2), \ldots, (x_n, y_n)$, the inductive learning task is to build a function $f(x)$ that, given a new x point, can predict the associated y value. We study the Regularized Least-Squares (RLS) algorithm for finding f, a common and popular algorithm [2, 5] that can be used for either regression or classification:

$$\min_{f \in \mathcal{H}} \frac{1}{n} \sum_{i=1}^{n} (f(x_i) - y_i)^2 + \lambda ||f||_K^2.$$

Here, $\mathcal{H}$ is a Reproducing Kernel Hilbert Space (RKHS) [1] with associated kernel function K, $||f||_K^2$ is the squared norm in the RKHS, and λ is a regularization constant controlling the tradeoff between fitting the training set accurately and forcing smoothness of f.

The Representer Theorem [7] proves that the RLS solution will have the form $f(x) = \sum_{i=1}^{n} c_i K(x_i, x)$, and it is easy to show [5] that we can find the coefficients c by solving the linear system

$$(K + \lambda n I)c = y, \tag{1}$$

where K is the n by n matrix satisfying $K_{ij} = K(x_i, x_j)$. We focus on the Gaussian kernel $K(x_i, x_j) = \exp(-||x_i - x_j||^2 / 2\sigma^2)$.

Our work was originally motivated by the empirical observation that on a range of benchmark classification tasks, we achieved surprisingly accurate classification using a Gaussian kernel with a very large σ and a very small λ (Figure 1; additional examples in [6]). This prompted us to study the large-σ asymptotics of RLS. As $\sigma \to \infty, K(x_i, x_j) \to 1$ for arbitrary x_i and x_j. Consider a single test point x_0. RLS will first find c using Equation 1,

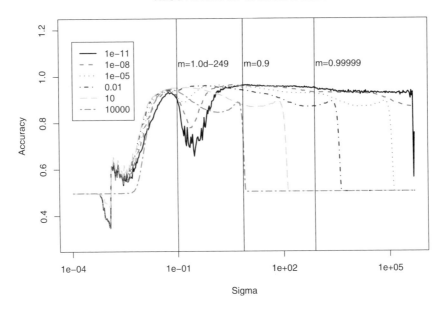

Fig. 1. RLS classification accuracy results for the UCI Galaxy dataset over a range of σ (along the x-axis) and λ (different lines) values. The vertical labelled lines show m, the smallest entry in the kernel matrix for a given σ. We see that when $\lambda = 1e - 11$, we can classify quite accurately when the smallest entry of the kernel matrix is .99999.

then compute $f(x_0) = c^t k$ where k is the kernel vector, $k_i = K(x_i, x_0)$. Combining the training and testing steps, we see that $f(x_0) = y^t (K + \lambda n I)^{-1} k$.

Both K and k are close to 1 for large σ, i.e. $K_{ij} = 1 + \epsilon_{ij}$ and $k_i = 1 + \epsilon_i$. If we directly compute $c = (K + \lambda n I)^{-1} y$, we will tend to wash out the effects of the ϵ_{ij} term as σ becomes large. If, instead, we compute $f(x_0)$ by associating to the right, first computing *point affinities* $(K + \lambda n I)^{-1} k$, then the ϵ_{ij} and ϵ_j interact meaningfully; this interaction is crucial to our analysis.

Our approach is to Taylor expand the kernel elements (and thus K and k) in $1/\sigma$, noting that as $\sigma \to \infty$, consecutive terms in the expansion differ enormously. In computing $(K + \lambda n I)^{-1} k$, these scalings cancel each other out, and result in finite point affinities even as $\sigma \to \infty$. The asymptotic affinity formula can then be "transposed" to create an alternate expression for $f(x_0)$. Our main result is that if we set $\sigma^2 = s^2$ and $\lambda = s^{-(2k+1)}$, then, as $s \to \infty$, the RLS solution tends to the kth order polynomial with minimal empirical error.

The main theorem is proved in full. Due to space restrictions, the proofs of supporting lemmas and corollaries are omitted; an expanded version containing all proofs is available [4].

2 Notation and definitions

Definition 1. *Let x_i be a set of $n + 1$ points $(0 \leq i \leq n)$ in a d dimensional space. The scalar x_{ia} denotes the value of the ath vector component of the ith point.*

The $n \times d$ matrix, X is given by $X_{ia} = x_{ia}$.

We think of X as the matrix of training data $x_1, \ldots, x_n$ and x_0 as an $1 \times d$ matrix consisting of the test point.

Let $1_m, 1_{lm}$ denote the m dimensional vector and $l \times m$ matrix with components all 1, similarly for $0_m, 0_{lm}$. We will dispense with such subscripts when the dimensions are clear from context.

Definition 2 (Hadamard products and powers). *For two $l \times m$ matrices, N, M, $N \odot M$ denotes the $l \times m$ matrix given by $(N \odot M)_{ij} = N_{ij}M_{ij}$. Analogously, we set $(N^{\odot c})_{ij} = N_{ij}^c$.*

Definition 3 (polynomials in the data). *Let $I \in \mathbb{Z}_{\geq 0}^d$ (non-negative multi-indices) and Y be a $k \times d$ matrix. Y^I is the k dimensional vector given by $\left(Y^I\right)_i = \prod_{a=1}^d Y_{ia}^{I_a}$. If $h : \mathbb{R}^d \to \mathbb{R}$ then $h(Y)$ is the k dimensional vector given by $(h(Y))_i = h(Y_{i1}, \ldots, Y_{id})$.*

The d canonical vectors, $e_a \in \mathbb{Z}_{\geq 0}^d$, are given by $(e_a)_b = \delta_{ab}$.

Any scalar function, $f : \mathbb{R} \to \mathbb{R}$, applied to any matrix or vector, A, will be assumed to denote the elementwise application of f. We will treat $y \to e^y$ as a scalar function (we have no need of matrix exponentials in this work, so the notation is unambiguous).

We can re-express the kernel matrix and kernel vector in this notation:

$$K = e^{\frac{1}{2\sigma^2} \sum_{a=1}^d 2X^{e_a}(X^{e_a})^t - X^{2e_a}1_n^t - 1_n(X^{2e_a})^t} \tag{2}$$

$$= \operatorname{diag}\left(e^{-\frac{1}{2\sigma^2}||X||^2}\right) e^{\frac{1}{\sigma^2}XX^t} \operatorname{diag}\left(e^{-\frac{1}{2\sigma^2}||X||^2}\right) \tag{3}$$

$$k = e^{\frac{1}{2\sigma^2} \sum_{a=1}^d 2X^{e_a}x_0^{e_a} - X^{2e_a}1_1 - 1_n x_0^{2e_a}} \tag{4}$$

$$= \operatorname{diag}\left(e^{-\frac{1}{2\sigma^2}||X||^2}\right) e^{\frac{1}{\sigma^2}Xx_0^t} e^{-\frac{1}{2\sigma^2}||x_0||^2}. \tag{5}$$

3 Orthogonal polynomial bases

Let $V_c = \operatorname{span}\{X^I : |I| = c\}$ and $V_{\leq c} = \bigcup_{a=0}^c V_c$ which can be thought of as the set of all d variable polynomials of degree c, evaluated on the training data. Since the data are finite, there exists b such that $V_{\leq c} = V_{\leq b}$ for all $c \geq b$. Generically, b is the smallest c such that $\binom{c+d}{d} \geq n$.

Let Q be an orthonormal matrix in $\mathbb{R}^{n \times n}$ whose columns progressively span the $V_{\leq c}$ spaces, i.e. $Q = (\begin{array}{cccc} B_0 & B_1 & \cdots & B_b \end{array})$ where $Q^t Q = I$ and $\operatorname{colspan}\{(\begin{array}{ccc} B_0 & \cdots & B_c \end{array})\} = V_{\leq c}$. We might imagine building such a Q via the Gramm-Schmidt process on the vectors $X^0, X^{e_1}, \ldots, X^{e_d}, \ldots X^I, \ldots$ taken in order of non-decreasing $|I|$.

Letting $C_I = \begin{pmatrix} |I| \\ I_1 \ldots I_d \end{pmatrix}$ be multinomial coefficients, the following relations between Q, X, and x_0 are easily proved.

$$(Xx_0^t)^{\odot c} = \sum_{|I|=c} C_I X^I (x_0^I)^t \quad \text{hence} \quad (Xx_0^t)^{\odot c} \in V_c$$

$$(XX^t)^{\odot c} = \sum_{|I|=c} C_I X^I (X^I)^t \quad \text{hence} \quad \operatorname{colspan}\{(XX^t)^{\odot c}\} = V_c$$

and thus, $B_i^t(Xx_0^t)^{\odot c} = 0$ if $i > c$, $B_i^t(XX^t)^{\odot c}B_j = 0$ if $i > c$ or $j > c$, and $B_c^t(XX^t)^{\odot c}B_c$ is non-singular.

Finally, we note that $\mathrm{argmin}_{v \in V_{\leq c}}\{||y - v||\} = \sum_{a \leq c} B_a(B_a^t y)$.

4 Taking the $\sigma \to \infty$ limit

We will begin with a few simple lemmas about the limiting solutions of linear systems. At the end of this section we will arrive at the limiting form of suitably modified RLSC equations.

Lemma 1. *Let $i_1 < \cdots < i_q$ be positive integers. Let $A(s), y(s)$ be a block matrix and block vector given by*

$$A(s) = \begin{pmatrix} A_{00}(s) & s^{i_1}A_{01}(s) & \cdots & s^{i_q}A_{0q}(s) \\ s^{i_1}A_{10}(s) & s^{i_1}A_{11}(s) & \cdots & s^{i_q}A_{1q}(s) \\ \cdots & \cdots & \cdots & \cdots \\ s^{i_q}A_{q0}(s) & s^{i_q}A_{q1}(s) & \cdots & s^{i_q}A_{qq}(s) \end{pmatrix}, \quad y(s) = \begin{pmatrix} b_0(s) \\ s^{i_1}b_1(s) \\ \cdots \\ s^{i_q}b_q(s) \end{pmatrix}$$

where $A_{ij}(s)$ and $b_i(s)$ are continuous matrix-valued and vector-valued functions of s with $A_{ii}(0)$ non-singular for all i.

$$\lim_{s \to 0} A^{-1}(s)y(s) = \begin{pmatrix} A_{00}(0) & 0 & \cdots & 0 \\ A_{10}(0) & A_{11}(0) & \cdots & 0 \\ \cdots & \cdots & \cdots & \cdots \\ A_{q0}(0) & A_{q1}(0) & \cdots & A_{qq}(0) \end{pmatrix}^{-1} \begin{pmatrix} b_0(0) \\ b_1(0) \\ \cdots \\ b_q(0) \end{pmatrix}$$

We are now ready to state and prove the main result of this section, characterizing the limiting large-σ solution of Gaussian RLS.

Theorem 1. *Let q be an integer satisfying $q < b$, and let $p = 2q + 1$. Let $\lambda = C\sigma^{-p}$ for some constant C. Define $A_{ij}^{(c)} = \frac{1}{c!}B_i^t(XX^t)^{\odot c}B_j$, and $b_i^{(c)} = \frac{1}{c!}B_i^t(Xx_0^t)^{\odot c}$.*

$$\lim_{\sigma \to \infty} \left(K + nC\sigma^{-p}I\right)^{-1}k = v$$

where

$$v = (\; B_0 \quad \cdots \quad B_q \;)\, w \tag{6}$$

$$\begin{pmatrix} b_0^{(0)} \\ b_1^{(1)} \\ \cdots \\ b_q^{(q)} \end{pmatrix} = \begin{pmatrix} A_{00}^{(0)} & 0 & \cdots & 0 \\ A_{10}^{(1)} & A_{11}^{(1)} & \cdots & 0 \\ \cdots & \cdots & \cdots & \cdots \\ A_{q0}^{(q)} & A_{q1}^{(q)} & \cdots & A_{qq}^{(q)} \end{pmatrix} w \tag{7}$$

We first manipulate the equation $(K + n\lambda I)y = k$ according to the factorizations in (3) and (5).

$$K = \mathrm{diag}\left(e^{-\frac{1}{2\sigma^2}||X||^2}\right)e^{\frac{1}{\sigma^2}XX^t}\mathrm{diag}\left(e^{-\frac{1}{2\sigma^2}||X||^2}\right) = NPN$$

$$k = \mathrm{diag}\left(e^{-\frac{1}{2\sigma^2}||X||^2}\right)e^{\frac{1}{\sigma^2}Xx_0^t}e^{-\frac{1}{2\sigma^2}||x_0||^2} = Nw\alpha$$

Noting that $\lim_{\sigma\to\infty} e^{-\frac{1}{2\sigma^2}\|x_0\|^2}\text{diag}\left(e^{\frac{1}{2\sigma^2}\|X\|^2}\right) = \lim_{\sigma\to\infty}\alpha N^{-1} = I$, we have

$$v \equiv \lim_{\sigma\to\infty}(K + nC\sigma^{-p}I)^{-1}k$$
$$= \lim_{\sigma\to\infty}(NPN + \beta I)^{-1}Nw\alpha$$
$$= \lim_{\sigma\to\infty}\alpha N^{-1}(P + \beta N^{-2})^{-1}w$$
$$= \lim_{\sigma\to\infty}\left(e^{\frac{1}{\sigma^2}XX^t} + nC\sigma^{-p}\text{diag}\left(e^{\frac{1}{\sigma^2}\|X\|^2}\right)\right)^{-1}e^{\frac{1}{\sigma^2}Xx_0^t}.$$

Changing bases with Q,

$$Q^t v = \lim_{\sigma\to\infty}\left(Q^t e^{\frac{1}{\sigma^2}XX^t}Q + nC\sigma^{-p}Q^t\text{diag}\left(e^{\frac{1}{\sigma^2}\|X\|^2}\right)Q\right)^{-1}Q^t e^{\frac{1}{\sigma^2}Xx_0^t}.$$

Expanding via Taylor series and writing in block form (in the $b\times b$ block structure of Q),

$$Q^t e^{\frac{1}{\sigma^2}XX^t}Q = Q^t(XX^t)^{\odot 0}Q + \frac{1}{1!\sigma^2}Q^t(XX^t)^{\odot 1}Q + \frac{1}{2!\sigma^4}Q^t(XX^t)^{\odot 2}Q + \cdots$$

$$= \begin{pmatrix} A_{00}^{(0)} & 0 & \cdots & 0 \\ 0 & 0 & \cdots & 0 \\ \cdots & \cdots & \cdots & \cdots \\ 0 & 0 & \cdots & 0 \end{pmatrix} + \frac{1}{\sigma^2}\begin{pmatrix} A_{00}^{(1)} & A_{01}^{(1)} & \cdots & 0 \\ A_{10}^{(1)} & A_{11}^{(1)} & \cdots & 0 \\ \cdots & \cdots & \cdots & \cdots \\ 0 & 0 & \cdots & 0 \end{pmatrix} + \cdots$$

$$Q^t e^{\frac{1}{\sigma^2}Xx_0^t} = Q^t(Xx_0^t)^{\odot 0} + \frac{1}{\sigma^2}Q^t(Xx_0^t)^{\odot 1} + \frac{1}{\sigma^4}Q^t(Xx_0^t)^{\odot 2} + \cdots$$

$$= \begin{pmatrix} b_0^{(0)} \\ 0 \\ \cdots \\ 0 \end{pmatrix} + \frac{1}{\sigma^2}\begin{pmatrix} b_0^{(1)} \\ b_1^{(1)} \\ \cdots \\ 0 \end{pmatrix} + \cdots$$

$$nC\sigma^{-p}Q^t\text{diag}\left(e^{\frac{1}{\sigma^2}\|X\|^2}\right)Q = nC\sigma^{-p}I + \cdots.$$

Since the $A_{cc}^{(c)}$ are non-singular, Lemma 3 applies, giving our result. $\qquad\square$

5 The classification function

When performing RLS, the actual prediction of the limiting classifier is given via

$$f_\infty(x_0) \equiv \lim_{\sigma\to\infty}y^t(K + nC\sigma^{-p}I)^{-1}k.$$

Theorem 1 determines $v = \lim_{\sigma\to\infty}(K + nC\sigma^{-p}I)^{-1}k$, showing that $f_\infty(x_0)$ is a polynomial in the training data X. In this section, we show that $f_\infty(x_0)$ is, in fact, a polynomial in the test point x_0. We continue to work with the orthonormal vectors B_i as well as the auxilliary quantities $A_{ij}^{(c)}$ and $b_i^{(c)}$ from Theorem 1.

Theorem 1 shows that $v \in V_{\leq q}$: the point affinity function is a polynomial of degree q in the training data, determined by (7).

$$\sum_{i,j\leq c}c!B_i A_{ij}^{(c)}B_j^t = (XX^t)^{\odot c} \quad \text{hence} \quad \sum_{j\leq c}c!B_c A_{cj}^{(c)}B_j^t = B_c B_c^t(XX^t)^{\odot c}$$

$$\sum_{i\leq c}c!B_i b_i^{(c)} = (Xx_0^t)^{\odot c} \quad \text{hence} \quad c!B_c b_c^{(c)} = B_c B_c^t(Xx_0^t)^{\odot c}$$

807

we can restate Equation 7 in an equivalent form:

$$
\begin{pmatrix} B_0^t \\ \cdots \\ B_q^t \end{pmatrix}^t \left(\begin{pmatrix} 0!b_0^{(0)} \\ 1!b_1^{(1)} \\ \cdots \\ q!b_q^{(q)} \end{pmatrix} - \begin{pmatrix} 0!A_{00}^{(0)} & 0 & \cdots & 0 \\ 1!A_{10}^{(1)} & 1!A_{11}^{(1)} & \cdots & 0 \\ \cdots & \cdots & \cdots & \cdots \\ q!A_{q0}^{(q)} & q!A_{q1}^{(q)} & \cdots & q!A_{qq}^{(q)} \end{pmatrix} \begin{pmatrix} B_0^t \\ \cdots \\ B_q^t \end{pmatrix} v \right) = 0 \quad (8)
$$

$$
\sum_{c \leq q} c! B_c b_c^{(c)} - \sum_{c \leq q} \sum_{j \leq c} c! B_c A_{cj}^{(c)} B_j^t v = 0 \quad (9)
$$

$$
\sum_{c \leq q} B_c B_c^t \left((X x_0^t)^{\odot c} - (X X^t)^{\odot c} v \right) = 0. \quad (10)
$$

Up to this point, our results hold for arbitrary training data X. To proceed, we require a mild condition on our training set.

Definition 4. *X is called* generic *if $X^{I_1}, \ldots, X^{I_n}$ are linearly independent for any distinct multi-indices $\{I_i\}$.*

Lemma 2. *For generic X, the solution to Equation 7 (or equivalently, Equation 10) is determined by the conditions $\forall I : |I| \leq q, (X^I)^t v = x_0^I$, where $v \in V_{\leq q}$.*

Theorem 2. *For generic data, let v be the solution to Equation 10. For any $y \in \mathbb{R}^n$, $f(x_0) = y^t v = h(x_0)$, where $h(x) = \sum_{|I| \leq q} a_I x^I$ is a multivariate polynomial of degree q minimizing $\|y - h(X)\|$.*

We see that as $\sigma \to \infty$, the RLS solution tends to the minimum empirical error kth order polynomial.

6 Experimental Verification

In this section, we present a simple experiment that illustrates our results. We consider a fith-degree polynomial function. Figure 2 plots f, along with a 150 point dataset drawn by choosing x_i uniformly in $[0, 1]$, and choosing $y = f(x) + \epsilon_i$, where ϵ_i is a Gaussian random variable with mean 0 and standard deviation .05. Figure 2 also shows (in red) the best polynomial approximations to the data (not to the ideal f) of various orders. (We omit third order because it is nearly indistinguishable from second order.)

According to Theorem 1, if we parametrize our system by a variable s, and solve a Gaussian regularized least-squares problem with $\sigma^2 = s^2$ and $\lambda = Cs^{-(2k+1)}$ for some integer k, then, as $s \to \infty$, we expect the solution to the system to tend to the kth-order data-based polynomial approximation to f. Asymptotically, the value of the constant C does not matter, so we (arbitrarily) set it to be 1. Figure 3 demonstrates this result.

We note that these experiments frequently require setting λ much smaller than machine-ϵ. As a consequence, we need more precision than IEEE double-precision floating-point, and our results cannot be obtained via many standard tools (e.g., MATLAB(TM)) We performed our experiments using CLISP, an implementation of Common Lisp that includes arithmetic operations on arbitrary-precision floating point numbers.

7 Discussion

Our result provides insight into the asymptotic behavior of RLS, and (partially) explains Figure 1: in conjunction with additional experiments not reported here, we believe that

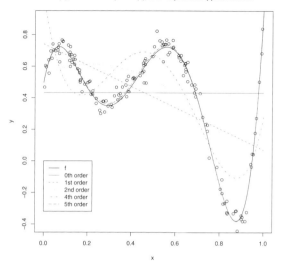

Fig. 2. $f(x) = .5(1 - x) + 150x(x - .25)(x - .3)(x - .75)(x - .95)$, a random dataset drawn from $f(x)$ with added Gaussian noise, and data-based polynomial approximations to f.

we are recovering second-order polynomial behavior, with the drop-off in performance at various λ's occurring at the transition to third-order behavior, which cannot be accurately recovered in IEEE double-precision floating-point. Although we used the specific details of RLS in deriving our solution, we expect that in practice, a similar result would hold for Support Vector Machines, and perhaps for Tikhonov regularization with convex loss more generally.

An interesting implication of our theorem is that for very large σ, we can obtain various order polynomial classifications by sweeping λ. In [6], we present an algorithm for solving for a wide range of λ for essentially the same cost as using a single λ. This algorithm is not currently practical for large σ, due to the need for extended-precision floating point.

Our work also has implications for approximations to the Gaussian kernel. Yang et al. use the Fast Gauss Transform (FGT) to speed up matrix-vector multiplications when performing RLS [8]. In [6], we studied this work; we found that while Yang et al. used moderate-to-small values of σ (and did not tune λ), the FGT sacrificed substantial accuracy compared to the best achievable results on their datasets. We showed empirically that the FGT becomes much more accurate at larger values of σ; however, at large-σ, it seems likely we are merely recovering low-order polynomial behavior. We suggest that approximations to the Gaussian kernel must be checked carefully, to show that they produce sufficiently good results are moderate values of σ; this is a topic for future work.

References

1. Aronszajn. Theory of reproducing kernels. *Transactions of the American Mathematical Society*, 68:337–404, 1950.

2. Evgeniou, Pontil, and Poggio. Regularization networks and support vector machines. *Advances In Computational Mathematics*, 13(1):1–50, 2000.

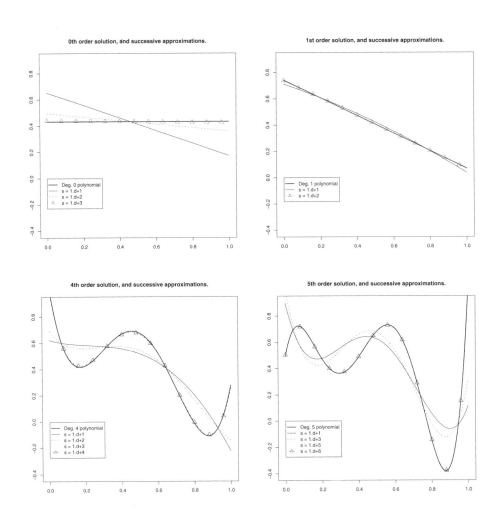

Fig. 3. As $s \to \infty$, $\sigma^2 = s^2$ and $\lambda = s^{-(2k+1)}$, the solution to Gaussian RLS approaches the kth order polynomial solution.

3. Keerthi and Lin. Asymptotic behaviors of support vector machines with gaussian kernel. *Neural Computation*, 15(7):1667–1689, 2003.

4. Ross Lippert and Ryan Rifkin. Asymptotics of gaussian regularized least-squares. Technical Report MIT-CSAIL-TR-2005-067, MIT Computer Science and Artificial Intelligence Laboratory, 2005.

5. Rifkin. *Everything Old Is New Again: A Fresh Look at Historical Approaches to Machine Learning*. PhD thesis, Massachusetts Institute of Technology, 2002.

6. Rifkin and Lippert. Practical regularized least-squares: λ-selection and fast leave-one-out computation. In preparation, 2005.

7. Wahba. *Spline Models for Observational Data*, volume 59 of *CBMS-NSF Regional Conference Series in Applied Mathematics*. Society for Industrial & Applied Mathematics, 1990.

8. Yang, Duraiswami, and Davis. Efficient kernel machines using the improved fast Gauss transform. In *Advances in Neural Information Processing Systems*, volume 16, 2004.

Efficient Unsupervised Learning for Localization and Detection in Object Categories

Nicolas Loeff, Himanshu Arora
ECE Department
University of Illinois at
Urbana-Champaign
{loeff,harora1}@uiuc.edu

Alexander Sorokin, David Forsyth
Computer Science Department
University of Illinois at
Urbana-Champaign
{sorokin2,daf}@uiuc.edu

Abstract

We describe a novel method for learning templates for recognition and localization of objects drawn from categories. A generative model represents the configuration of multiple object parts with respect to an object coordinate system; these parts in turn generate image features. The complexity of the model in the number of features is low, meaning our model is much more efficient to train than comparative methods. Moreover, a variational approximation is introduced that allows learning to be orders of magnitude faster than previous approaches while incorporating many more features. This results in both accuracy and localization improvements. Our model has been carefully tested on standard datasets; we compare with a number of recent template models. In particular, we demonstrate state-of-the-art results for detection and localization.

1 Introduction

Building appropriate object models is central to object recognition, which is a fundamental problem in computer vision. Desirable characteristics of a model include good representation of objects, fast and efficient learning algorithms that require as little supervised information as possible. We believe an appropriate representation of an object should allow for both detection of its presence and localization ('where is it?'). So far the quality of object recognition in the literature has been measured by its detection performance only. Viola and Jones [1] present a fast object detection system boosting Haar filter responses. Another effective discriminative approach is that of a *bag of keypoints* [2, 3]. It is based on clustering image patches using appearance only, disregarding geometric information. The performance for detection in this algorithm is among the state of the art. However as no geometry cues are used during training, features that do not belong to the object can be incorporated into the object model. This is similar to classic *overfitting* and typically leads to problems in object localization.

Weber *et. al.* [4] represent an object as a constellation of parts. Fergus *et. al.* [5] extend the model to account for variability in appearance. The model encodes a template as a set of feature-generating parts. Each part generates at most one feature. As a result the complexity is determined by hardness of part-feature assignment. Heuristic search is used to approximate the solution, but feasible problems are limited to 7 parts with 30 features.

Agarwal and Roth [6] learn using SNoW a classifier on a sparse representation of patches extracted around interesting points in the image. In [7], Leibe and Schiele use a voting scheme to predict object configuration from locations of individual patches. Both approaches provide localization, but require manually localizing the objects in training images. Hillel et. al. [8] independently proposed an approach similar to ours. Their model however has higher learning complexity and inferior detection performance despite being of discriminative nature.

In this paper, we present a generative probabilistic model for detection and localization of objects that can be efficiently learnt with minimal supervision. The first crucial property of the model is that it represents the configuration of multiple object parts with respect to an unobserved, *abstract* object root (unlike [9, 10], where an "object root" is chosen as one of the visible parts of the object). This simplifies localization and allows our model to overcome occlusion and errors in feature extraction. The model also becomes symmetric with respect to visible parts. The second crucial assumption of the model is that a single part can generate multiple features in the image (or none). This may seem counterintuitive, but keypoint detectors generally detects several features around *interesting* areas. This hypothesis also makes an explicit model for part occlusion unnecessary: instead occlusion of a part means implicitly that no feature in the image is produced by it.

These assumptions allow us to model all features in the image as being emitted independently conditioned on the object center. As a result the complexity of inference in our model is **linear** in the number of parts of the model and the number of features in the image, obviating the exponential complexity of combinatoric assignments in other approaches [4, 5, 11]. This means our model is much easier than constellation models to train using Expectation Maximization (EM), which enables the use of more features and more complex models with resulting improvements in both accuracy and localization. Furthermore we introduce a variational (mean-field) approximation during learning that allows it to be hundreds of times faster than previous approaches, with no substantial loss of accuracy.

2 Model

Our model of an object category is a template that generates features in the image. Each image is represented as a set $\{f_j\}$ of F features extracted with the scale-saliency point detector [13]. Each feature is described by its location and appearance. Feature extraction and representation will be detailed in section 3. As described in the introduction, we hypothesize that given the object center all features are generated *independently*: $p^{obj}(f_1, .., f_F) = \sum_{o_c} P(o_c) \prod_j p(f_j | o_c)$. The abstract object center - which does not generate any features - is represented by a *hidden* random variable o_c. For simplicity it takes values in a discrete grid of size $N_x \times N_y$ inside the image and o_c is assumed to be a priori uniformly distributed in its domain.

Conditioned on the object center, each feature is generated by a mixture of P parts plus a background part. A set of *hidden* variables $\{\omega_{ij}\}$ represents which part (i) produced feature f_j. These variables ω_{ij} then take values $\{0, 1\}$ restricted to $\sum_{i=1}^{P+1} \omega_{ij} = 1$. In other words, $\omega_{ij} = 1$ means feature j was produced by part i; each part can produce multiple features, each feature is produced by only one part. The distribution of a feature conditioned on the object center is then $p(f_j | o_c) = \sum_i p(f_j, \omega_{ij} = 1 | o_c) = \sum_i p(f_j | \omega_{ij} = 1, o_c) \pi_i$, where π_i is the prior emission probability of part i. π_i is subject to $\sum_{i=1}^{P+1} \pi_i = 1$.

Each part has a location distribution with respect to the object center corresponding to a two dimensional full covariance Gaussian, $p_L^i(x | o_c)$. The appearance (see section 3 for details) of a part does not depend on the configuration of the object; we consider two models :

Gaussian Model (G) Appearance p_A^i is modeled as a k dimensional diagonal covariance Gaussian distribution.

Local Topic Model (LT) Appearance p_A^i is modeled as a multinomial distribution on a previously learnt k-word image patch dictionary. This can be considered as a local topic model.

Let θ denote the set of parameters. The complete data likelihood (joint distribution) for image n in the object model is then,

$$P_\theta^{obj}\left(\{\omega_{ij}\}, o_c, \{f_j\}\right) = \prod_{o_c'} \left\{ \prod_{j,i} \left\{ p_L^i(f_j|o_c')p_A^i(f_j)\pi_i \right\}^{[\omega_{ij}=1]} P(o_c') \right\}^{[o_c=o_c']} \quad (1)$$

where $[expr]$ is one if $expr$ is true and zero otherwise. Marginalizing, the probability of the observed image in the object model is then,

$$P_\theta^{obj}\left(\{f_j\}\right) = \sum_{o_c} P(o_c) \prod_{j'} \left\{ \sum_i P(f_{j'}, \omega_{ij'} = 1|o_c) \right\} \quad (2)$$

The background model assumes all features are produced independently, with uniform location on the image. In the G model of appearance, the appearance is modeled with a k dimensional full covariance matrix Gaussian distribution. In the LT model, we use a multinomial distribution on the k-word image patch dictionary to model the appearance.

2.1 Learning

The maximum-likelihood solution for the parameters of the above model does not have a closed form. In order to train the model the parameters are computed numerically using the approach of [14], minimizing a free-energy F_e associated with the model that is an upper bound on the negative log-likelihood. Following [14], we denote $v = \{f_j\}$ as the set of visible and $h = \{o_c, \omega_{ij}\}$ as the set of hidden variables. Let D_{KL} be the K-L divergence:

$$F_e(Q, \theta) = D_{KL}\left\{Q(h) \| P_\theta(h|v)\right\} - \log P_\theta(v) = \int_h Q(h) \log \frac{Q(h)}{P_\theta(h, v)} dh \quad (3)$$

In this bound, $Q(h)$ can be a *simpler* approximation of the posterior probability $P_\theta(h|v)$, that is used to compute estimates and update parameters. Minimizing eq. 3 with respect to Q and θ under different restrictions, produces a range of algorithms including exact EM, variational learning and others [14]. Table 2.1 shows sample updates and complexity of these algorithms and comparison to other relevant work.

The background model is learnt before the object model is trained. As assumed earlier, for Gaussian appearance model the background appearance model is a single gaussian, whose mean and variance are estimated as the sample mean and covariance. For the Local Topic model, the multinomial distribution is estimated as the sample histogram. The model for background feature location is uniform and does not have any parameters.

EM Learning for the Object model: In the E-step, the set of parameters θ is fixed and F_e is minimized with respect to $Q(h)$ without restrictions. This is equivalent to computing the actual posteriors in EM [14, 15]. In this case the optimal solution factorizes as $Q(h) = Q(o_c)Q(\omega_{ij}|o_c) = P(o_c|v)P(\omega_{ij}|o_c, v)$. In the M-step, F_e is minimized with respect to the parameters θ using the current estimate of Q. Due to the conditional independence introduced in the model, inference is tractable and thus the E-step can be computed efficiently. The overall complexity of inference is $O(FP \cdot N_x N_y)$.

Model	Update for μ_L^i	Complexity	Time (F,P)
Fergus *et al.*	N/A	F^P	36 hrs (30, 7)
Model (EM)	$\mu_L^i \leftarrow \dfrac{\sum_n \sum_{o_c} Q(o_c) \sum_j Q(\omega_{ji}\mid o_c)\{x_L^j - o_c\}}{\sum_n \sum_{o_c} Q(o_c) \sum_j Q(\omega_{ji}\mid o_c)}$	$FP \cdot N_x N_y$	3 hrs (50, 30)
(Variational)	$\mu_L^i \leftarrow \dfrac{\sum_n \{\sum_j Q(\omega_{ji}) x_L^j - \sum_{o_c} Q(o_c) o_c\}}{\sum_n \sum_{o_c} Q(o_c) \sum_j Q(\omega_{ji})}$	$FP + N_x N_y$	3 mins (100, 30)

Table 1: An example of an update, overall complexity and convergence time for our models and [5], for different number of features per image (F) and number of parts in the object model (P). There is an increase in speed of several orders of magnitude with respect to [5] on similar hardware.

Variational Learning: In this approach a mean field approximation of Q is considered; in the E-step the parameters θ are fixed and F is minimized with respect to Q under the restriction that it factorizes as $Q(h) = Q(o_c)Q(w_{ij})$. This corresponds to a decoupling of location (o_c) and part-feature assignment (w_{ij}) in the approximation (Q) of the posterior $P_\theta(h\mid v)$. In the M-step θ is fixed and the free energy F_e is minimized with respect to this (mean field) version of Q. A comparison between EM and Variational updates of the mean in location μ_L^i of a part is shown in table 2.1. The overall complexity of inference is now $O(FP) + O(N_x N_y)$; this represents orders of magnitude of speedup with respect to the already efficient EM learning. The impact on performance of the variational approximation is discussed in section 4.

2.2 Detection and localization

For detection of object presence, a natural decision rule is the likelihood ratio test. After the models are learnt, for each test image $P_\theta^{obj}(\{f_j\})/P^{bg}(\{f_j\})$ is compared to a threshold to make the decision. Once the presence of the object is established, the most likely location is given by the MAP estimate of o_c. We assign parts in the model to the object if they exhibit consistent appearance and location. To remove model parts representing background we use a threshold on the entropy of the appearance distribution for the LT model (the determinant of the covariance in location for the G model). The MAP estimate of which features in the image are assigned (marginalizing over the object center) to parts in the model determines the support of the object. Bounding boxes include all keypoints assigned to the object and means of all model parts belonging to the object even if no keypoint is observed to be produced by such part. This explicitly handles occlusion (fig. 1).

3 Experimental setup

The performance of the method depends on the feature detector making consistent extraction in different instances of objects of the same type. We use the scale-saliency interest point detector proposed in [13]. This method selects regions exhibiting unpredictable characteristics over both location and scale. The F regions with highest saliency over the image provide the features for learning and recognition. After the keypoints are detected, patches are extracted around this points and scale-normalized. A SIFT descriptor [16] (without orientation) is obtained from these patches. For model G, due to the high dimensionality of resulting space, PCA is performed choosing $k = 15$ components to represent the appearance of a feature. For model LT, we instead cluster the appearance of features in the original SIFT space with a gaussian mixture model with $k = 250$ components and use the most likely cluster as feature appearance representation.

For all experiments we use $P = 30$ parts. The number of features is $F = 50$ for G model and $F = 100$ for LT model, $N_x \times N_y = 238$. We test our approach on the Caltech 5 dataset: faces, motorbikes, airplanes, spotted cats vs. Caltech background and cars rear 2001 vs. cars background [5]. We initialize appearance and location of the parts with P randomly chosen features from the training set. The stopping criterion is the change in F_e.

814

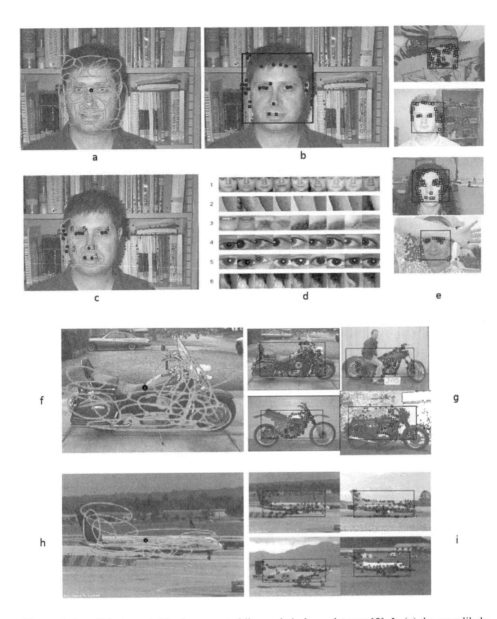

Figure 1: Local Topic model for faces, motorbikes and airplanes datasets [5]. In **(a)** the most likely location of the object center is plotted as a black circle. With respect to this reference, the spatial distribution (2D gaussian) of each part associated with the object is plotted in green. In **(b)** the centers of all features extracted are depicted. Blue ones are assigned by the model to the object, and red ones to the background. The bounding box is plotted in blue. Image **(c)** shows how many features in the image are assigned to the same part (a property of our model, not shared by [5]): six parts are chosen, their spatial distribution is plotted (green), and the features assigned to them are depicted in blue. Eyes (4,5), mouth (3) and left ear (6) have multiple assignments each. For each these parts, image **(d)** image shows the best matches in features extracted from the dataset. Note that the local topic model can learn parts uniform in appearance (i.e. eyes) but also more complex parts (i.e. the mouth part includes moustaches, beards and chins). The G appearance model and [5] do not have this property. The images **(e)** show the robustness of the method in cases with occlusion, missed detections and one caricature of a face. Images **(f)** and **(g)** show plots for motorbikes, and **(h)** and **(i)** for airplanes.

4 Results

Detection: Although we believe that localization is an essential performance criterion, it is useless if the approach cannot detect objects. Figure 2 depicts equal error rate detection performance for our models and [5, 3, 8]. We can not compare our range of performance (for train/test splits), shown on the plot, because this data is not available for other approaches. Our method is robust to initialization (the variance for starting points is negligible compared to train/test split variance). The results show higher detection performance of all our algorithms compared to the generative model presented in [5]. The local topic (LT) model performs better than the model presented in [8]. The purely discriminative approach presented in [3] shows higher detection performance with different ("optimal combination") features, but performs worse for the features we are using. The LT model showed consistently higher detection performance than the Gaussian (G) model. For both LT and G models the variational approximations showed similar discriminative power to that of the respective exact models. Unlike [5, 3], our model currently is not scale invariant. Nevertheless the probabilistic nature of the model allows for some tolerance to scale changes.

In datasets of manageable size, it is inevitable that the background is correlated with the object. The result is that most modern methods that infer the template form partially supervised data can tend to model some background parts as lying on the object (see figure 4). Doing so tends to *increase* detection performance. It is reasonable to expect this increase will not persist in the face of a dramatic change in background. One symptom of this phenomenon (as in classical overfitting) is that methods that detect very well may be bad at localization, because they cannot separate the object from background. We are able to avoid this difficulty by predicting object extent conditioned on detection using only a subset of parts known to have relatively low variance in location or appearance, given the object center. We do not yet have an estimate of the increase in detection rate resulting from *overfitting*. This is a topic of ongoing research. In our opinion, if a method can detect but performs poorly at localization, the reason may be overfitting.

Localization: Previous work on localization required aligned images (bounding boxes) or segmentation masks [7, 6]. A novel property of our model is that it learns to localize the object and determine its spatial extent without supervision. Figure 1 shows learned models and examples of localization. There is no standard measure to evaluate localization performance in an unsupervised setting. In such a case, the object center can be learnt at any position in the image, provided that this position is consistent across all images. We thus use as our performance measure, the standard deviation of estimated object centers and bounding boxes (obtained as in §2.2), after normalizing the estimates of each image to a coordinate system in which the ground truth bounding box is a unit square $(0,0) - (1,1)$.

As a baseline we use the rectified center of the image. All objects of interest in both airplane and motorbike datasets are centered in the image. As a result the baseline is a good predictor of the object center and is hard to beat. However in the faces dataset there is much more variation in location; then the advantage of our approach becomes clear. Figure 3 shows the scatterplot of normalized object centers and bounding boxes. The table in figure 2 shows the localization performance results using the proposed metric.

Variational approximation comparison: Unusually for a variational approximation it is possible to compare it to the exact model; the results are excellent especially for the G model. This is consistent with our observation that during learning the variational approximation is good in this case (the free energy bound appears tight). On the other hand, for the LT model, the variational bound is loose during learning and localization performance is equivalent, but slightly lower than that of exact LT model. This may be explained by the fact that gaussian appearance model is less flexible then the topic model and thus G model can better tolerate decoupling of location and appearance.

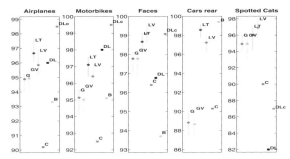

Model	Bbox(%)		Obj. center(%)	
	vert	horz	vert	horz
Faces				
G	8.88	21.88	4.58	16.59
GV	8.64	16.10	4.47	16.10
LT	**8.17**	**13.16**	**3.92**	**6.45**
LV	7.86	18.62	3.76	11.04
BL	-	-	4.50	24.71
Airplanes				
LT	19.30	9.09	10.06	4.42
BL	-	-	10.37	4.47
Motorbikes				
LT	8.41	7.33	4.93	4.65
BL	-	-	5.11	2.01

Figure 2: Plots on the left show detection performance on Caltech 5 datasets [5]. Equal error rate is reported. The original performance of constellation model [5] is denoted by C. We denote by DLc the performance (best in literature) reported by [3] using an optimal combination of feature types, and by DL the performance using our features. The performance of [8] is denoted by B. We show performance for our G model (G), LT model (L) and their variational approximations (GV) and (LV) respectively. We report median performance ($\times$) over 20 runs and performance range excluding 10% best and 10% worst runs. On the right we show localization performance for all models on Faces dataset and performance of the best model (LT) on all datasets. Standard deviation is reported in percentage units with respect to the ground truth bounding box. For bounding boxes we average the standard deviation in each direction. BL denotes baseline performance.

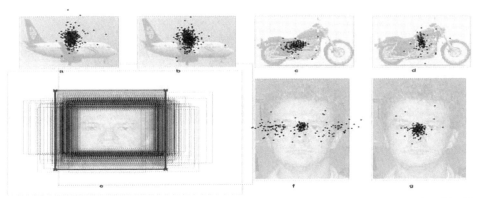

Figure 3: The airplane and motorbike datasets are aligned. Thus the image center baseline (**b**), (**d**) performs well there. Our localization performs similarly (**a**), (**c**). There is more variation in location in faces dataset. Scatterplot (**f**) shows the baseline performance and (**g**) shows the performance of our model. (**e**) shows the bounding boxes computed by our approach (LT model). Object centers and bounding boxes are rectified using the ground truth bounding boxes (blue). No information about location or spatial extent of the object is given to the algorithm.

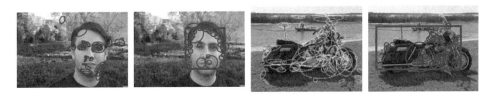

Figure 4: Approaches like [3] do not use geometric constraints during learning. Therefore, correlation between background and object in the dataset is incorporated into the object model. In this case the ellipses represent the features that are used by the algorithm in [3] to decide the presence of a face and motorbike (**left** images taken from [3]). On the other hand, our model (**right** images) can estimate the location and support of the object, even though no information about it is provided during learning. Blue circles represent the features assigned by the model to the face, the red points are centers of features assigned to background (plot for Local Topic Model).

817

5 Conclusions and future work

We have presented a novel model for object categories. Our model allows efficient unsupervised learning, bringing the learning time to a few hours for full models and to minutes for variational approximations. The significant reduction in complexity allows to handle many more parts and features than comparable algorithms. The detection performance of our approach compares favorably to the state of the art even when compared to purely discriminative approaches. Also our model is capable of learning the spatial extent of the objects without supervision, with good results.

This combination of fast learning and ability to localize is required to tackle challenging problems in computer vision. Among the most interesting applications we see unsupervised segmentation, learning, detection and localization of multiple object categories, deformable objects and objects with varying aspects.

References

[1] P. Viola and M. Jones. Rapid object detection using a boosted cascade of simple features. *Proc. of CVPR*, pages 511–518, 2001.

[2] G. Csurka, C. Dance, L. Fan, and C. Bray. Visual Categorization with Bags of Keypoints. In *Workshop on Stat. Learning in Comp. Vision, ECCV*, pages 1–22, 2004.

[3] G. Dorkó and C. Schmid. Object class recognition using discriminative local features. Submitted to *IEEE trans. on PAMI*, 2004.

[4] M. Weber, M. Welling, and P. Perona. Unsupervised Learning of Models for Recognition. *Proc. of ECCV (1)*, pages 18–32, 2000.

[5] R. Fergus, P. Perona, and A. Zisserman. Object Class Recognition by Unsupervised Scale-Invariant Learning. *Proc. of CVPR*, pages 264–271, 2003.

[6] S. Agarwal and D. Roth. Learning a sparse representation for object detection. In *Proc. of ECCV*, volume 4, pages 113–130, Copenhagen, Denmark, May 2002.

[7] B. Leibe, A. Leonardis, and B. Schiele. Combined object categorization and segmentation with an implicit shape model. In *Workshop on Stat. Learning in Comp. Vision*, pages 17–32, May 2004.

[8] A. B. Hillel, T. Hertz, and D. Weinshall. Efficient learning of relational object class models. In *Proc. of ICCV*, pages 1762–1769, October 2005.

[9] R. Fergus, P. Perona, and A. Zisserman. A sparse object category model for efficient learning and exhaustive recognition. In *Proc. of CVPR*, pages 380–387, june 2005.

[10] D. Crandall, P. Felzenszwalb, and D. Huttenlocher. Spatial Priors for Part-Based Recognition using Statistical Models. In *Proc. of CVPR*, pages 10–17, 2005.

[11] L. Fei-Fei, R. Fergus, and P. Perona. Learning generative visual models from few training examples an incremental bayesian approach tested on 101 object categories. In *Workshop on Generative-Model Based Vision*, Washington, DC, June 2004.

[12] A. Opelt, M. Fussenegger, A. Pinz, and P. Auer. Generic object recognition with boosting. Technical Report TR-EMT-2004-01, EMT, TU Graz, Austria, 2004. Submitted to the *IEEE Trans. on PAMI*.

[13] T. Kadir and M. Brady. Saliency, Scale and Image Description. *IJCV*, 45(2):83–105, 2001.

[14] B. Frey and N. Jojic. A Comparison of Algorithms for Inference and Learning in Probabilistic Graphical Models. *IEEE Trans. on PAMI*, 27(9):1392–1416, 2005.

[15] R. Neal and G. Hinton. A view of the EM algorithm that justifies incremental, sparse, and other variants. In M. I. Jordan, editor, *Learning in graphical models*, pages 355–368. MIT Press, Cambridge, MA, USA, 1999.

[16] D. Lowe. Distinctive image features from scale-invariant keypoints. *IJCV*, 60(2):91–110, 2004.

Convergence and Consistency of Regularized Boosting Algorithms with Stationary β-Mixing Observations

Aurélie C. Lozano
Department of Electrical Engineering
Princeton University
Princeton, NJ 08544
alozano@princeton.edu

Sanjeev R. Kulkarni
Department of Electrical Engineering
Princeton University
Princeton, NJ 08544
kulkarni@princeton.edu

Robert E. Schapire
Department of Computer Science
Princeton University
Princeton, NJ 08544
schapire@cs.princeton.edu

Abstract

We study the statistical convergence and consistency of regularized Boosting methods, where the samples are not independent and identically distributed (i.i.d.) but come from empirical processes of stationary β-mixing sequences. Utilizing a technique that constructs a sequence of independent blocks close in distribution to the original samples, we prove the consistency of the composite classifiers resulting from a regularization achieved by restricting the 1-norm of the base classifiers' weights. When compared to the i.i.d. case, the nature of sampling manifests in the consistency result only through generalization of the original condition on the growth of the regularization parameter.

1   Introduction

A significant development in machine learning for classification has been the emergence of boosting algorithms [1]. Simply put, a boosting algorithm is an iterative procedure that combines weak prediction rules to produce a composite classifier, the idea being that one can obtain very precise prediction rules by combining rough ones. It was shown in [2] that AdaBoost, the most popular Boosting algorithm, can be seen as stage-wise fitting of additive models under the exponential loss function and it effectively minimizes an empirical loss function that differs from the probability of incorrect prediction. From this perspective, boosting can be seen as performing a greedy stage-wise minimization of various loss functions empirically. The question of whether boosting achieves Bayes-consistency then arises, since minimizing an empirical loss function does not necessarily imply minimizing the generalization error. When run a very long time, the AdaBoost algorithm, though resistant to overfitting, is not immune to it [2, 3]. There also exist cases where running Adaboost forever leads to a prediction error larger than the Bayes error in the limit of infinite sample size. Consequently, one approach for the study of consistency is to modify the original Adaboost algorithm by imposing some constraints on the weights of the composite classifier to avoid overfitting. In this regularized version of Adaboost, the 1-norm of the weights of the base classifiers is restricted to a fixed value. The minimization of the loss function is performed over the restricted class [4, 5].

In this paper, we examine the convergence and consistency of regularized boosting algorithms with samples that are no longer i.i.d. but come from empirical processes of stationary weakly dependent sequences. A practical motivation for our study of non i.i.d. sampling is that in many learning applications observations are intrinsically temporal and hence often weakly dependent. Ignoring this dependency could seriously undermine the performance of the learning process (for instance, information related to the time-dependent ordering of samples would be lost). Recognition of this issue has led to several studies of non i.i.d. sampling [6, 7, 8, 9, 10, 11, 12].

To cope with weak dependence we apply mixing theory which, through its definition of mixing coefficients, offers a powerful approach to extend results for the traditional i.i.d. observations to the case of weakly dependent or mixing sequences. We consider the β-mixing coefficients, whose mathematical definition is deferred to Sec. 2.1. Intuitively, they provide a "measure" of how fast the dependence between the observations diminishes as the distance between them increases. If certain conditions on the mixing coefficients are satisfied to reflect a sufficiently fast decline in the dependence between observations as their distance grows, counterparts to results for i.i.d. random processes can be established. A comprehensive review of mixing theory results is provided in [13].

Our principal finding is that consistency of regularized Boosting methods can be established in the case of non-i.i.d. samples coming from empirical sequences of stationary β-mixing sequences. Among the conditions that guarantee consistency, the mixing nature of sampling appears only through a generalization of the one on the growth of the regularization parameter originally stated for the i.i.d. case [4].

2 Background and Setup

2.1 Mixing Sequences

Let $\underline{W} = (W_i)_{i \geq 1}$ be a strictly stationary sequence of random variables, each having the same distribution P on $\mathcal{D} \subset R^d$. Let $\sigma_1^l = \sigma(W_1, W_2, \ldots, W_l)$ be the σ-field generated by $W_1, \ldots, W_l$. Similarly, let $\sigma_{l+k}^\infty = \sigma(W_{l+k}, W_{l+k+1}, \ldots,)$. The following mixing coefficients characterize how close to independent a sequence $\underline{W}$ is.

Definition 1. *For any sequence $\underline{W}$, the β-mixing[1] coefficient is defined by*
$$\beta_W(n) = \sup_k \mathbb{E} \sup \left\{ |P(A|\sigma_1^k) - P(A)| : A \in \sigma_{k+n}^\infty \right\},$$
where the expectation is taken w.r.t. σ_1^k.

Hence $\beta_W(n)$ quantifies the degree of dependence between 'future' observations and 'past' ones separated by a distance of at least n. In this study, we will assume that the sequences

---

[1]To gain insight into the notion of β-mixing, it is useful to think of the σ-field generated by a random variable X as the "body of information" carried by X. This leads to the following interpretation of β-mixing. Suppose that the index i in W_i is the time index. Let A be an event happening in the future within the period of time between $t = k + n$ and $t = \infty$. $|P(A|\sigma_1^k) - P(A)|$ is the absolute difference between the probability that event A occurs, given the knowledge of the information generated by the past up to $t = k$, and the probability of event A occurring without this knowledge. Then, the greater the dependence between σ_1^k (the information generated by $(W_1, \ldots, W_k)$) and σ_{k+n}^∞ (the information generated by $(W_{k+n}, \ldots, W_\infty)$), the larger the coefficient $\beta_W(n)$.

we consider are algebraically β-mixing. This property implies that the dependence between observations decreases fast enough as the distance between them increases.

Definition 2. *A sequence $\underline{W}$ is called β-mixing if $\lim_{n \to \infty} \beta_W (n) = 0$. Further, it is algebraically β-mixing if there is a positive constant r_β such that $\beta_W (n) = O (n^{-r_\beta})$.*

The choice of β-mixing appears appropriate given previous results that showed "uniform convergence of empirical means uniformly in probability" and "probably approximately correct" properties to be preserved for β-mixing inputs [11]. Some examples of β-mixing sequences that fit naturally in a learning scenario are certain Markov processes and Hidden Markov Models [11]. In practice, if the mixing properties are unknown, they need to be estimated. Although it is difficult to find them in general, there exist simple methods to determine the mixing rates for various classes of random processes (e.g. Gaussian, Markov, ARMA, ARCH, GARCH). Hence the assumption of a known mixing rate is reasonable and has been adopted by many studies [6, 7, 8, 9, 10, 12].

2.2 Classification with Stationary β-Mixing Training Data

In the standard binary classification problem, the training data consist of a set $S_n = \{(X_1, Y_1), \ldots, (X_n, Y_n)\}$, where X_k belongs to some measurable space $\mathcal{X}$, and Y_k is in $\{-1, 1\}$. Using S_n, a classifier $h_n : \mathcal{X} \to \{-1, 1\}$ is built to predict the label Y of an unlabeled observation X. Traditionally, the samples are assumed to be i.i.d., and to our knowledge, this assumption is made by all the studies on boosting consistency. In this paper, we suppose that the sampling is no longer i.i.d. but corresponds to an empirical process of stationary β-mixing sequences. More precisely, let $\mathcal{D} = \mathcal{X} \times \mathcal{Y}$, where $\mathcal{Y} = \{-1, +1\}$. Let $W_i = (X_i, Y_i)$. We suppose that $\underline{W} = (W_i)_{i \geq 1}$ is a strictly stationary sequence of random variables, each having the same distribution P on $\mathcal{D}$ and that $\underline{W}$ is β-mixing (see Definition 2). This setup is in line with [7]. We assume that the unlabeled observation is such that (X, Y) is independent of S_n but with the same marginal.

3 Statistical Convergence and Consistency of Regularized Boosting for Stationary β-Mixing Sequences

3.1 Regularized Boosting

We adopt the framework of [4] which we now recall. Let $\mathcal{H}$ denote the class of base classifiers $h : \mathcal{X} \to \{-1, 1\}$, which usually consists of simple rules (for instance decision stumps). This class is required to have finite VC-dimension. Call $\mathcal{F}$, the class of functions $f : \mathcal{X} \to [-1, 1]$ obtained as convex combinations of the classifiers in $\mathcal{H}$:

$$\mathcal{F} = \left\{ f (X) = \sum_{j=1}^{t} \alpha_j h_j (X) : t \in \mathbb{N}, \alpha_1, \ldots, \alpha_t \geq 0, \sum_{j=1}^{t} \alpha_j = 1, h_1, \ldots, h_t \in \mathcal{H} \right\}. \tag{1}$$

Each $f_n \in \mathcal{F}$ defines a classifier $h_{f_n} = \text{sign} (f_n)$ and for simplicity the generalization error $L (h_{f_n})$ is denoted by $L (f_n)$. Then the training error is denoted by $L_n (f_n) = 1/n \sum_{i=1}^{n} \mathbf{I}_{[h_{f_n} (X_i) \neq Y_i]}$. Define $Z (f) = -f (X) Y$ and $Z_i (f) = -f (X_i) Y_i$. Instead of minimizing the indicator of misclassification ($\mathbf{I}_{[-f(X)Y>0]}$), boosting methods are shown to effectively minimize a smooth convex cost function of $Z(f)$. For instance, Adaboost is based on the exponential function. Consider a positive, differentiable, strictly increasing, and strictly convex function $\phi : \mathbb{R} \to \mathbb{R}^+$ and assume that $\phi (0) = 1$ and that $\lim_{x \to -\infty} \phi (x) = 0$. The corresponding cost function and empirical cost function are respectively $C (f) = \mathbb{E}\phi (Z (f))$ and $C_n (f) = 1/n \sum_{i=1}^{n} \phi (Z_i (f))$. Note that $L (f) \leq C (f)$, since $\mathbb{I}_{[x>0]} \leq \phi (x)$.

The iterative aspect of boosting methods is ignored to consider only their performing an (approximate) minimization of the empirical cost function or, as we shall see, a series of cost functions. To avoid overfitting, the following regularization procedure is developed for the choice of the cost functions. Define ϕ_λ such that $\forall \lambda > 0 \ \phi_\lambda(x) = \phi(\lambda x)$. The corresponding empirical and expected cost functions become $C_n^\lambda(f) = \frac{1}{n} \sum_{i=1}^n \phi_\lambda(Z_i(f))$ and $C^\lambda(f) = \mathbb{E}\phi_\lambda(Z(f))$. The minimization of a series of cost functions C^λ over the convex hull of $\mathcal{H}$ is then analyzed.

3.2 Statistical Convergence

The nature of the sampling intervenes in the following two lemmas that relate the empirical cost $C_n^\lambda(f)$ and true cost $C^\lambda(f)$.

Lemma 1. *Suppose that for any n, the training data $(X_1, Y_1), \ldots (X_n, Y_n)$ comes from a stationary algebraically β-mixing sequence with β-mixing coefficients $\beta(m)$ satisfying $\beta(m) = O(m^{-r_\beta})$, $m \in \mathbb{N}$ and r_β a positive constant. Then for any $\lambda > 0$ and $b \in [0, 1)$,*

$$\mathbb{E} \sup_{f \in \mathcal{F}} |C^\lambda(f) - C_n^\lambda(f)| \leq 4\lambda\phi'(\lambda) \frac{c_1}{n^{(1-b)/2}} + 2\phi(\lambda) \left(\frac{1}{n^{b(1+r_\beta)-1}} + \frac{2}{n^{1-b}} \right). \quad (2)$$

Lemma 2. *Let the training data be as in Lemma 1. For any $b \in [0, 1)$, and $\alpha \in (0, 1-b)$, let $\epsilon_n = 3(2c_1 + n^{\alpha/2})\lambda\phi'(\lambda)/n^{(1-b)/2}$. Then for any $\lambda > 0$*

$$\mathbb{P}\left(\sup_{f \in \mathcal{F}} |C^\lambda(f) - C_n^\lambda(f)| > \epsilon_n \right) \leq \exp(-4c_2 n^\alpha) + O(n^{1-b(r_\beta+1)}). \quad (3)$$

The constants c_1 and c_2 in the above lemmas are given in the proofs of Lemma 1 (Section 4.2) and Lemma 2 (Section 4.3) respectively.

3.3 Consistency Result

The following summarizes the assumptions that are made to prove consistency.

Assumption 1.
I- Properties of the sample sequence: The samples $(X_1, Y_1), \ldots, (X_n, Y_n)$ are assumed to come from a stationary algebraically β-mixing sequence with β-mixing coefficients $\beta_{X,Y}(n) = O(n^{-r_X})$, r_β being a positive constant.
II- Properties of the cost function ϕ: ϕ is assumed to be a differentiable, strictly convex, strictly increasing cost function such that $\phi(0) = 1$ and $\lim_{x \to -\infty} \phi(x) = 0$.
III- Properties of the base hypothesis space: $\mathcal{H}$ has finite VC dimension. The distribution of (X, Y) and the class $\mathcal{H}$ are such that $\lim_{\lambda \to \infty} \inf_{f \in \lambda\mathcal{F}} C(f) = C^*$, where $\lambda\mathcal{F} = \{\lambda f : f \in \mathcal{F}\}$ and $C^* = \inf C(f)$ over all measurable functions $f : \mathcal{X} \to \mathbb{R}$.
IV- Properties of the smoothing parameter: We assume that $\lambda_1, \lambda_2, \ldots$ is a sequence of positive numbers satisfying $\lambda_n \to \infty$ as $n \to \infty$, and that there exists a constant $c \in \left(\frac{1}{1+r_\beta}, 1 \right)$ such that $\lambda_n \phi'(\lambda_n)/n^{(1-c)/2} \to 0$ as $n \to \infty$.

Call $\hat{f}_n^\lambda$ the function in $\mathcal{F}$ which approximatively minimizes $C_n^\lambda(f)$, i.e. $\hat{f}_n^\lambda$ is such that $C_n^\lambda(\hat{f}_n^\lambda) \leq \inf_{f \in \mathcal{F}} C_n^\lambda(f) + \epsilon_n = \inf_{f \in \mathcal{F}} \frac{1}{n} \sum_{i=1}^n \phi_\lambda(Z_i(f)) + \epsilon_n$, with $\epsilon_n \to 0$ as $n \to \infty$. The main result is the following.

Theorem 1. *Consistency of regularized boosting methods for stationary β-mixing sequences. Let $f_n = \hat{f}_n^{\lambda_n} \in \mathcal{F}$, where $\hat{f}_n^{\lambda_n}$ (approximatively) minimizes $C_n^{\lambda_n}(f)$. Under Assumption 1, $\lim_{n \to \infty} L(h_{f_n} = \text{sign}(f_n)) = L^*$ almost surely and h_{f_n} is strongly Bayes-risk consistent.*

Cost functions satisfying Assumption 1.II include the exponential function and the logit function $\log_2(1 + e^x)$. Regarding Assumption 1.II, the reader is referred to [4](Remark on (denseness assumption)). In Assumption 1.IV, notice that the nature of sampling leads to a generalization of the condition on the growth of $\lambda_n \phi'(\lambda_n)$ already present in the i.i.d. setting [4]. More precisely, the nature of sampling manifests through parameter c, which is limited by r_β. The assumption that r_β is known is quite strict but cannot be avoided (for instance this assumption is widely made in the field of time series analysis). On a positive note, if unknown, r_β can be determined for various classes of processes as mentioned Section 2.1.

4 Proofs

4.1 Preparation to the Proofs: the Blocking Technique

The key issue resides in upper bounding

$$\sup_{f \in \mathcal{F}} \left| C_n^\lambda(f) - C^\lambda(f) \right| = \sup_{f \in \mathcal{F}} \left| 1/n \sum_{i=1}^n \phi(-\lambda f(X_i) Y_i) - \mathbb{E}\phi(-\lambda f(X_1) Y_1) \right|, \quad (4)$$

where $\mathcal{F}$ is given by (1). Let $W = (X, Y)$, $W_i = (X_i, Y_i)$. Define the function g_λ by $g_\lambda(W) = g_\lambda(X, Y) = \phi(-\lambda f(X) Y)$ and the class $\mathcal{G}_\lambda$ by $\mathcal{G}_\lambda = \{g_\lambda : g_\lambda(X, Y) = \phi(-\lambda f(X) Y), f \in \mathcal{F}\}$. Then (4) can be rewritten as

$$\sup_{f \in \mathcal{F}} \left| C_n^\lambda(f) - C^\lambda(f) \right| = \sup_{g_\lambda \in \mathcal{G}_\lambda} \left| n^{-1} \sum_{i=1}^n g_\lambda(W_i) - \mathbb{E}g_\lambda(W_1) \right|.$$

Note that the class $\mathcal{G}_\lambda$ is uniformly bounded by $\phi(\lambda)$. Besides, if $\mathcal{H}$ is a class of measurable functions, then $\mathcal{G}_\lambda$ is also a class of measurable functions, by measurability of $\mathcal{F}$.

As the W_i's are not i.i.d, we propose to use the blocking technique developed in [12, 14] to construct i.i.d blocks of observations which are close in distribution to the original sequence $W_1, \ldots, W_n$. This enables us to work on the sequence of independent blocks instead of the original sequence. We use the same notation as in [12]. The protocol is the following. Let (b_n, μ_n) be a pair of integers, such that

$$(n - 2b_n) \le 2b_n \mu_n \le n. \quad (5)$$

Divide the segment $W_1 = (X_1, Y_1), \ldots, W_n = (X_n, Y_n)$ of the mixing sequence into $2\mu_n$ blocks of size b_n, followed by a remaining block (of size at most $2b_n$). Consider the odd blocks only. If their size b_n is large enough, the dependence between them is weak, since two odd blocks are separated by an even block of the same size b_n. Therefore, the odd blocks can be approximated by a sequence of independent blocks with the same within-block structure. The same holds if we consider the even blocks. Let $(\xi_1, \ldots, \xi_{b_n}), (\xi_{b_n+1}, \ldots, \xi_{2b_n}), \ldots, (\xi_{(2\mu_n-1)b_n}, \ldots, \xi_{2\mu_n b_n})$ be independent blocks such that $(\xi_{jb_n+1}, \ldots, \xi_{(j+1)b_n}) =_{\mathcal{D}} (W_{jb_n+1}, \ldots, W_{(j+1)b_n})$, for $j = 0, \ldots, \mu_n - 1$. For $j = 1, \ldots, 2\mu_n$, and any $g \in \mathcal{G}_\lambda$, define $Z_{j,g} := \sum_{i=(j-1)b_n+1}^{jb_n} g(\xi_i) - b_n \mathbb{E}g(\xi_1)$, $\tilde{Z}_{j,g} := \sum_{i=(j-1)b_n+1}^{jb_n} g(W_i) - b_n \mathbb{E}g(W_1)$. Let $\mathcal{O}_{\mu_n} = \{1, 3, \ldots, 2\mu_n - 1\}$ and $\mathcal{E}_{\mu_n} = \{2, 4, \ldots, 2\mu_n\}$. Define $Z_{i,j}(f)$ as $Z_{i,j}(f) := -f(\xi_{(2j-2)b_n+i,1}) \cdot \xi_{(2j-2)b_n+i,2}$, where $\xi_{k,1}$ and $\xi_{k,2}$ are respectively the 1st and 2nd coordinate of the vector ξ_k. These correspond to the $Z_k(f) = -f(X_k) Y_k$ for k in the odd blocks $1, \ldots, b_n, 2b_n + 1, \ldots, 3bn, \ldots$.

4.2 Proof sketch of Lemma 1

A. Working with Independent Blocks. We show that

$$\mathbb{E} \sup_{g \in \mathcal{G}_\lambda} \left| \frac{1}{n} \sum_{i=1}^n g(W_i) - \mathbb{E}g(W_1) \right| \le 2\mathbb{E} \sup_{g \in \mathcal{G}_\lambda} \left| \frac{1}{n} \sum_{j \in \mathcal{O}_{\mu_n}} Z_{j,g} \right| + \phi(\lambda) \left(\mu_n \beta_W(b_n) + \frac{2b_n}{n} \right).$$

$$(6)$$

Proof. Without loss of generality, assume that $\mathbb{E}g\left(W_1\right) = \mathbb{E}g\left(\xi_1\right) = 0$.

Then, $\mathbb{E}\sup_g \left|\frac{1}{n}\sum_{i=1}^{n} g\left(W_i\right)\right| = \mathbb{E}\sup_g \left|\frac{1}{n}\left(\sum_{\mathcal{O}_{\mu_n}} \tilde{Z}_{j,g} + \sum_{\mathcal{E}_{\mu_n}} \tilde{Z}_{j,g} + R\right)\right|$, where R is the remainder term consisting of a sum of at most $2b_n$ terms. Noting that $\forall g \in \mathcal{G}_\lambda$, $|g| \le \phi\left(\lambda\right)$, it follows that $\mathbb{E}\sup_g \left|\frac{1}{n}\sum_{i=1}^{n} g\left(W_i\right)\right| \le \mathbb{E}(\sup_g \left|\frac{1}{n}\sum_{\mathcal{O}_{\mu_n}} \tilde{Z}_{j,g}\right|) + \mathbb{E}(\sup_g \left|\frac{1}{n}\sum_{\mathcal{E}_{\mu_n}} \tilde{Z}_{j,g}\right|) + \frac{\phi(\lambda)(2b_n)}{n}$. We use the following intermediary lemma.

Lemma 3 (adapted from [15], Lemma 4.1). *Call* $\mathbf{Q}$ *the distribution of* $\left(W_1, \ldots, W_{b_n}, W_{2b_n+1}, \ldots, W_{3b_n}, \ldots\right)$ *and* $\widetilde{\mathbf{Q}}$ *the distribution of* $\left(\xi_1, \ldots, \xi_{b_n}, \xi_{2b_n+1}, \ldots, \xi_{3b_n}, \ldots\right)$. *For any measurable function* h *on* $\mathbb{R}^{b_n \mu_n}$ *with bound* H, $\left|\mathbf{Q}h\left(W_1, \ldots\right) - \widetilde{\mathbf{Q}}h\left(\xi_1, \ldots\right)\right| \le H\left(\mu_n - 1\right)\beta_W\left(b_n\right)$. *The same result holds for* $\left(W_{b_n+1}, \ldots, W_{2b_n}, W_{3b_n+1}, \ldots, W_{4b_n} \ldots\right)$.

Using this with $h(W_1, \ldots) = \sup_g \left|\frac{1}{n}\sum_{\mathcal{O}_{\mu_n}} \tilde{Z}_{j,g}\right|$ and $h(W_{b_n+1}, \ldots) = \sup_g \left|\frac{1}{n}\sum_{\mathcal{E}_{\mu_n}} \tilde{Z}_{j,g}\right|$ respectively, and noting that $H = \phi\left(\lambda\right)/2$, we have $\mathbb{E}\sup_g \left|\frac{1}{n}\sum_{i=1}^{n} g\left(W_i\right)\right| \le \mathbb{E}\sup_g \left|\frac{1}{n}\sum_{\mathcal{O}_{\mu_n}} Z_{j,g}\right| + \frac{\phi(\lambda)}{2}\mu_n\beta_W\left(b_n\right) + \mathbb{E}\sup_g \left|\frac{1}{n}\sum_{\mathcal{E}_{\mu_n}} Z_{j,g}\right| + \frac{\phi(\lambda)}{2}\mu_n\beta_W\left(b_n\right) + \frac{\phi(\lambda)(2b_n)}{n}$. As the $Z_{j,g}$'s from odd and even blocks have the same distribution, we obtain (6). $\qquad\square$

B. Symmetrization. The odd blocks $Z_{j,g}$'s being independent, we can use the standard symmetrization techniques. Let $Z'_{j,g}$'s be i.i.d. copies of the $Z_{j,g}$'s. Let $Z'_{i,j}(f)$'s be the corresponding copies of the $Z_{i,j}(f)$. Let (σ_i) be a Rademacher sequence, i.e. a sequence of independent random variables taking the values ± 1 with probability $1/2$. Then by [16], Lemma 6.3 (Proof is omitted due to space constraints), we have

$$\mathbb{E}\sup_g \left|\frac{1}{n}\sum_{j\in\mathcal{O}_{\mu_m}} Z_{j,g}\right| \le \mathbb{E}\sup_g \left|\frac{1}{n}\sum_{j\in\mathcal{O}_{\mu_n}} \sigma_j\left(Z_{j,g} - Z'_{j,g}\right)\right|. \tag{7}$$

C. Contraction Principle. We now show that

$$\mathbb{E}\sup_{g\in\mathcal{G}_\lambda} \left|\frac{1}{n}\sum_{j\in\mathcal{O}_{\mu_n}} Z_{j,g}\right| \le 2 \cdot b_n\lambda\phi'\left(\lambda\right)\mathbb{E}\sup_{f\in\mathcal{F}} \left|\frac{1}{n}\sum_{j=1}^{\mu_n} \sigma_j Z_{1,j}(f)\right|. \tag{8}$$

Proof. As $Z_{j,g} = \sum_{i=1}^{b_n} \phi_\lambda(Z_{i,j}(f))$, and the $Z_{i,j}(f)$'s and $Z'_{i,j}(f)$'s are i.i.d., with (7) $\mathbb{E}\sup_g \left|\frac{1}{n}\sum_{j\in\mathcal{O}_{\mu_n}} Z_{j,g}\right| \le \mathbb{E}\sup_g \left|\frac{1}{n}\sum_{j=1}^{\mu_n} \sigma_j \sum_{i=1}^{b_n} \left(\phi_\lambda\left(Z_{i,j}(f)\right) - \phi_\lambda\left(Z'_{i,j}(f)\right)\right)\right| \le 2b_n\mathbb{E}\sup_g \left|\frac{1}{n}\sum_{j=1}^{\mu_n} \sigma_j\left(\phi_\lambda\left(Z_{1,j}(f)\right) - 1\right)\right|$. By applying the "Comparison Theorem", Theorem 7 in [17], to the contraction $\psi\left(x\right) = \left(1/\lambda\phi'\left(\lambda\right)\right)\left(\phi_\lambda\left(x\right) - 1\right)$, we obtain (8). $\qquad\square$

D. Maximal Inequality. We show that there exists a constant $c_1 > 0$ such that

$$\mathbb{E}\sup_{f\in\mathcal{F}} \left|\frac{1}{n}\sum_{j=1}^{\mu_n} \sigma_j Z_{1,j}(f)\right| \le \frac{c_1\sqrt{\mu_n}}{n}. \tag{9}$$

Proof. Denote $\left(h_1, \ldots, h_N\right)$ by h_1^N. One can write $\mathbb{E}\sup_{f\in\mathcal{F}} \left|\frac{1}{n}\sum_{j=1}^{\mu_n} \sigma_j Z_{1,j}(f)\right| = \frac{1}{n}\mathbb{E}\sup_{N\ge 1}\sup_{h_1^N\in\mathcal{H}^N}\sup_{\alpha_1,\ldots,\alpha_N} \left|\sum_{j=1}^{\mu_n}\sum_{k=1}^{N} \alpha_k\sigma_j\xi_{(1,j),2}h_k\left(\xi_{(2j-2)b_n+1,1}\right)\right|$. Since $\xi_{(2j-2)b_n+1,2}$ and $\xi_{(2j'-2)b_n+1,2}$ are i.i.d. for all $j \ne j'$ (they come from different blocks), and (σ_j) is a Rademacher sequence, then $\left(\sigma_j\xi_{(2j-2)b_n+1,2}h_k\left(\xi_{(2j-2)b_n+1,1}\right)\right)_{j=1,\ldots,\mu_n}$ has the same distribution as $\left(\sigma_j h_k\left(\xi_{(2j-2)b_n+1,1}\right)\right)_{j=1,\ldots,\mu_n}$. Hence

$$\mathbb{E}\sup_{f\in\mathcal{F}} \left|\frac{1}{n}\sum_{j=1}^{\mu_n} \sigma_j Z_{1,j}(f)\right| = \frac{1}{n}\mathbb{E}\sup_{N\ge 1}\sup_{h_1^N\in\mathcal{H}^N}\sup_{\alpha_1,\ldots,\alpha_N} \left|\sum_{j=1}^{\mu_n}\sum_{k=1}^{N} \sigma_j\alpha_k h_k\left(\xi_{(2j-2)b_n+1,1}\right)\right|.$$

By the same argument as used in [4], p.53 on the maximum of a linear function over a convex polygon, the supremum is achieved when $\alpha_k = 1$ for some k. Hence we get

$\mathbb{E} \sup_{f \in \mathcal{F}} \left| \frac{1}{n} \sum_{j=1}^{\mu_n} \sigma_j Z_{1,j}(f) \right| = \frac{1}{n} \mathbb{E} \sup_{h \in \mathcal{H}} \left| \sum_{j=1}^{\mu_n} \sigma_j h\left(\xi_{(1,j),1}\right) \right|$. Noting that for all $j \neq j'$, $h(\xi_{(2j-2)b_n+1,1})$ and $h(\xi_{(2j'-2)b_n+1,1})$ are i.i.d. and that Rademacher processes are sub-gaussian, we have by [18], Corollary 2.2.8

$$\frac{1}{n} \mathbb{E} \sup_{h \in \mathcal{H}} \left| \sum_{j=1}^{\mu_n} \sigma_j h\left(\xi_{(2j-2)b_n+1,1}\right) \right| \leq \frac{1}{n} \mathbb{E} \sup_{h \in \mathcal{H} \cup \{0\}} \left| \sum_{j=1}^{\mu_n} \sigma_j h\left(\xi_{(2j-2)b_n+1,1}\right) \right|$$

$$\leq \frac{c' \sqrt{\mu_n}}{n} \int_0^\infty \left(\log \sup_P N\left(\epsilon, \rho_{2,P_n}, \mathcal{H} \cup \{0\}\right)\right)^{1/2} d\epsilon,$$

where c' is a constant and $N\left(\epsilon, \rho_{2,P_n}, \mathcal{H} \cup \{0\}\right)$ is the empirical $\mathcal{L}_2$ covering number. As $\mathcal{H}$ has finite VC-dimension (see Assumption 1.III), there exists a positive constant w such that $\sup_P N(\epsilon, \rho_{2,P_n}, \mathcal{H} \cup \{0\}) = O_P(\epsilon^{-w})$ (see [18], Theorem 2.6.1). Hence $\int_0^\infty \left(\log \sup_{P_n} N\left(\epsilon, \rho_{2,P_n}, \mathcal{H} \cup \{0\}\right)\right)^{1/2} d\epsilon < \infty$. and (9) follows. $\quad\square$

E. Establishing (2). Combining (6),(8), and (9), we have

$\mathbb{E} \sup_{g \in \mathcal{G}_\lambda} \left| \frac{1}{n} \sum_{i=1}^n g(W_i) - \mathbb{E} g(W_1) \right| \leq 4 b_n \lambda \phi'(\lambda) \frac{c_1 \sqrt{\mu_n}}{n} + \phi(\lambda) \left(\mu_n \beta_W(b_n) + \frac{2b_n}{n}\right).$

Take $b_n = n^b$, with $0 \leq b < 1$. By (5), we obtain $\mu_n \leq n^{1-b}/2$. Besides, as we assumed that the sequence $\underline{W}$ is algebraically β-mixing (see Definition 2), $\beta_W(n) = O(n^{-r_\beta})$. Then $\mu_n \beta_W(b_n) = O\left(n^{1-b(1+r_\beta)}\right)$, and we arrive at (2). $\quad\blacksquare$

4.3 Proof Sketch of Lemma 2

A. Working with Independent Blocks and Symmetrization. For any $b \in [0,1), \alpha \in (0, 1-b)$, let

$$\epsilon_n = 3(2c_1 + n^{\alpha/2})\lambda \phi'(\lambda)/n^{(1-b)/2}. \tag{10}$$

We show

$$\mathbb{P}\left(\sup_{g \in \mathcal{G}_\lambda} \left| \frac{1}{n} \sum_{i=1}^n g(W_i) - \mathbb{E} g(W_1) \right| > \epsilon_n\right) \leq 2 \mathbb{P}\left(\sup_{g \in \mathcal{G}_\lambda} \left| \frac{1}{n} \sum_{j \in \mathcal{O}_{\mu_n}} Z_{j,g} \right| > \epsilon_n/3\right) + O(n^{1-b(1+r_\beta)}). \tag{11}$$

Proof. By [12], Lemma 3.1, we have that for any ϵ_n such that $\phi(\lambda)b_n = o(n\epsilon_n)$, $\mathbb{P}\left(\sup_{g \in \mathcal{G}_\lambda} \left| \frac{1}{n} \sum_{i=1}^n g(W_i) - \mathbb{E} g(W_1) \right| > \epsilon_n\right) \leq 2 \mathbb{P}\left(\sup_{g \in \mathcal{G}_\lambda} \left| \frac{1}{n} \sum_{j \in \mathcal{O}_{\mu_n}} Z_{j,g} \right| > \epsilon_n/3\right) + 4\mu_n \beta_W(b_n)$. Set $b_n = n^b$, with $0 \leq b < 1$. Then $\mu_n \beta_W(b_n) = O(n^{1-b(1+r_\beta)})$ (for the same reasons as in Section 4.2 E.). With ϵ_n as in (10), and since Assumption 1.II implies that $\lambda \phi'(\lambda) \geq \phi(\lambda) - 1$, we automatically obtain $\phi(\lambda)b_n = o(n\epsilon_n)$. $\quad\square$

B. McDiarmid's Bounded Difference Inequality. For ϵ_n as in (10), there exists a constant $c_2 > 0$ such that,

$$\mathbb{P}\left(\sup_{g \in \mathcal{G}_\lambda} \left| \frac{1}{n} \sum_{j \in \mathcal{O}_{\mu_n}} Z_{j,g} \right| > \epsilon_n/3\right) \leq \exp(-4c_2 n^\alpha). \tag{12}$$

Proof. The $Z_{j,g}$'s of the odd block being independent, we can apply McDiarmid's bounded difference inequality ([19], Theorem 9.2 p.136) on the function $\sup_{g \in \mathcal{G}_\lambda} \left| \frac{1}{n} \sum_{j \in \mathcal{O}_{\mu_n}} Z_{j,g} \right|$ which depends of $Z_{1,g}, Z_{3,g} \ldots, Z_{2\mu_n-1,g}$. Noting that changing the value of one variable does not change the value of the function by more that $b_n \phi(\lambda)/n$, we obtain with $b_n = n^b$ that for all $\epsilon > 0$,

$\mathbb{P}\left(\sup_{g \in \mathcal{G}_\lambda} \left| \frac{1}{n} \sum_{j \in \mathcal{O}_{\mu_n}} Z_{j,g} \right| > \mathbb{E} \sup_{g \in \mathcal{G}_\lambda} \left| \frac{1}{n} \sum_{j \in \mathcal{O}_{\mu_n}} Z_{j,g} \right| + \epsilon\right) \leq \exp\left(\frac{-4\epsilon^2 n^{1-b}}{\phi(\lambda)^2}\right).$

Combining (8) and (9) from the proof of Lemma 1, and with $b_n = n^b$, we have $\mathbb{E} \sup_{g \in \mathcal{G}_\lambda} \left| \frac{1}{n} \sum_{j \in \mathcal{O}_{\mu_n}} Z_{j,g} \right| \leq 2\lambda \phi'(\lambda) C/n^{(1-b)/2}$. With $\epsilon = n^{\alpha/2} \lambda \phi'(\lambda)/n^{(1-b)/2}$, we obtain ϵ_n as in (10). Pick λ_0 such that $0 < \lambda_0 < \lambda$. Then, since $\lambda \phi'(\lambda) \geq \phi(\lambda) - 1$, (12) follows with $c_2 = (1 - 1/\phi(\lambda_0))^2$. $\quad\square$

C. Establishing (3). Combining (11) and (12) we obtain (3). ∎

4.4 Proof Sketch of Theorem 1

Let $\bar{f}_\lambda$ a function in $\mathcal{F}$ minimizing C^λ. With $f_n = \hat{f}_n^{\lambda_n}$, we have

$$C\left(\lambda_n f_n\right) - C^* = \left(C^{\lambda_n}(\hat{f}_n^{\lambda_n}) - C^{\lambda_n}(\bar{f}_{\lambda_n})\right) + \left(\inf_{f \in \lambda_n \mathcal{F}} C(f) - C^*\right).$$

Since $\lambda_n \to \infty$, the second term on the right-hand side converges to zero by Assumption 1.III. By [19], Lemma 8.2, we have $C^{\lambda_n}(\hat{f}_n^{\lambda_n}) - C^{\lambda_n}(\bar{f}_{\lambda_n}) \leq 2 \sup_{f \in \mathcal{F}} |C^{\lambda_n}(f) - C_n^{\lambda_n}(f)|$. By Lemma 2, $\sup_{f \in \mathcal{F}} |C^{\lambda_n}(f) - C_n^{\lambda_n}(f)| \to 0$ with probability 1 if, as $n \to \infty$, $\lambda_n \phi'(\lambda_n) n^{(a+b-1)/2} \to 0$ and $b > 1/(1 + r_\beta)$. Hence if Assumption 1.IV holds, $C(\lambda_n f_n) \to C^*$ with probability 1. By [4], Lemma 5, the theorem follows. ∎

References

[1] Schapire, R.E.: The Boosting Approach to Machine Learning An Overview. In Proc. of the MSRI Workshop on Nonlinear Estimation and Classification (2002)

[2] Friedman, J., Hastie T., Tibshirani, R.: Additive logistic regression: A statistical view of boosting. Ann. Statist. **38** (2000) 337–374

[3] Jiang, W.: Does Boosting Overfit:Views From an Exact Solution. Technical Report **00-03** Department of Statistics, Northwestern University (2000)

[4] Lugosi, G., Vayatis, N.: On the Bayes-risk consistency of boosting methods. Ann. Statist. **32** (2004) 30–55

[5] Zhang, T.: Statistical Behavior and Consistency of Classification Methods based on Convex Risk Minimization. Ann. Statist. **32** (2004) 56–85

[6] Györfi, L., Härdle, W., Sarda, P., and Vieu, P.: Nonparametric Curve Estimation from Time Series. Lecture Notes in Statistics. Springer-Verlag, Berlin. (1989)

[7] Irle, A.: On the consistency in nonparametric estimation under mixing assumptions. J. Multivariate Anal. **60** (1997) 123–147

[8] Meir, R.: Nonparametric Time Series Prediction Through Adaptive Model Selection. Machine Learning **39** (2000) 5–34

[9] Modha, D., Masry, E.: Memory-Universal Prediction of Stationary Random Processes. IEEE Trans. Inform. Theory **44** (1998) 117–133

[10] Roussas, G.G.: Nonparametric estimation in mixing sequences of random variables. J. Statist. Plan. Inference. **18** (1988) 135–149

[11] Vidyasagar, M.: A Theory of Learning and Generalization: With Applications to Neural Networks and Control Systems. Second Edition. Springer-Verlag, London (2002)

[12] Yu, B.: Density estimation in the L^∞ norm for dependent data with applications. Ann. Statist. **21** (1993) 711–735

[13] Doukhan, P.: Mixing Properties and Examples. Springer-Verlag, New York (1995)

[14] Yu, B.: Some Results on Empirical Processes and Stochastic Complexity. Ph.D. Thesis, Dept of Statistics, U.C. Berkeley (Apr. 1990)

[15] Yu, B.: Rate of convergence for empirical processes of stationary mixing sequences. Ann. Probab. **22** (1994) 94–116.

[16] Ledoux, M., Talagrand, N.: Probability in Banach Spaces. Springer, New York (1991)

[17] Meir, R., Zhang, T.:Generalization error bounds for Bayesian mixture algorithms. J. Machine Learning Research (2003)

[18] van der Vaart, A.W., Wellner, J.A.: Weak convergence and empirical processes. Springer Series in Statistics. Springer-Verlag, New York (1996)

[19] Devroye, L., Györfi L., Lugosi, G.: A Probabilistic Theory of Pattern Recognition. Springer, New York (1996)

Ideal Observers for Detecting Motion: Correspondence Noise

Hongjing Lu
Department of Psychology, UCLA
Los Angeles, CA 90095
hongjing@psych.ucla.edu

Alan Yuille
Department of Statistics, UCLA
Los Angeles, CA 90095
yuille@stat.ucla.edu

Abstract

We derive a Bayesian Ideal Observer (BIO) for detecting motion and solving the correspondence problem. We obtain Barlow and Tripathy's classic model as an approximation. Our psychophysical experiments show that the trends of human performance are similar to the Bayesian Ideal, but overall human performance is far worse. We investigate ways to degrade the Bayesian Ideal but show that even extreme degradations do not approach human performance. Instead we propose that humans perform motion tasks using generic, general purpose, models of motion. We perform more psychophysical experiments which are consistent with humans using a Slow-and-Smooth model and which rule out an alternative model using Slowness.

1 Introduction

Ideal Observers give fundamental limits for performing visual tasks (somewhat similar to Shannon's limits on information transfer). They give benchmarks against which to evaluate human performance. This enables us to determine objectively what visual tasks humans are good at, and may help point the way to underlying neuronal mechanisms. For a recent review, see [1].

In an influential paper, Barlow and Tripathy [2] tested the ability of human subjects to detect dots moving coherently in a background of random dots. They derived an "ideal observer" model using techniques from Signal Detection theory [3]. They showed that their model predicted the trends of the human performance as properties of the stimuli changed, but that humans performed far worse than their model. They argued that degrading their model, by lowering the spatial resolution, would give predictions closer to human performance. Barlow and Tripathy's model has generated considerable interest, see [4,5,6,7].

We formulate this motion problem in terms of Bayesian Decision Theory and derive a Bayesian Ideal Observer (BIO) model. We describe why Barlow and Tripathy's (BT) model is not fully ideal, show that it can be obtained as an approximation to the BIO, and determine conditions under which it is a good approximation. We perform psychophysical experiments under a range of conditions and show that the trends of human subjects are more similar to those of the BIO. We investigate whether degrading the Bayesian Ideal enables us to reach human performance, and conclude that it does not (without implausibly large

827

deformations). We comment that Barlow and Tripathy's degradation model is implausible due to the nature of the approximations used.

Instead we show that a generic motion detection model which uses a slow-and-smooth assumption about the motion field [8,9] gives similar performance to human subjects under a range of experimental conditions. A simpler approach using a slowness assumption alone does not match new experimental data that we present. We conclude that human observers are not ideal, in the sense that they do not perform inference using the model that the experimenter has chosen to generate the data, but may instead use a general purpose model perhaps adapted to the motion statistics of natural images.

2 Bayes Decision Theory and Ideal Observers

We now give the basic elements of Bayes Decision Theory. The input data is D and we seek to estimate a binary state W (e.g. coherent or incoherent motion, horizontal motion to right or to left). We assume models $P(D|W)$ and $P(W)$. We define a decision rule $\alpha(D)$ and a loss function $L(\alpha(I), W) = 1 - \delta_{\alpha(D),W}$. The risk is $R(\alpha) = \sum_{D,W} L(\alpha(D), W) P(D|W) P(W)$.

Optimal performance is given by the Bayes rule: $\alpha^* = \arg \min R(\alpha)$. The fundamental limits are given by Bayes Risk: $R^* = R(\alpha^*)$. Bayes risk is the best performance that can be achieved. It corresponds to ideal performance.

Barlow and Tripathy's (BT) model does not achieve Bayes risk. This is because they used simplification to derive it using concepts from Signal Detection theory (SDT). SDT is essentially the application of Bayes Decision Theory to the task of signal detection but, for historical reasons, SDT restricts itself to a limited class of probability models and is unable to capture the complexity of the motion problem.

3 Experimental Setup and Correspondence Noise

We now give the details of Barlow and Tripathy's stimuli, their model, and their experiments. The stimuli consist of two image frames with N dots in each frame. The dots in the first frame are at random positions. For coherent stimuli, see figure (1), a proportion CN of dots move coherently left or right horizontally with a fixed translation motion with displacement T. The remaining $N(1 - C)$ dots in the second frame are generated at random. For incoherent stimuli, the dots in both frames are generated at random.

Estimating motion for these stimuli requires solving the correspondence problem to match dots between frames. For coherent motion, the noise dots act as *correspondence noise* and make the matching harder, see the rightmost panel in figure (1).

Barlow and Tripathy perform two types of binary forced choice experiments. In *detection experiments*, the task is to determine whether the stimuli is coherent or incoherent motion. For *discrimination experiments*, the goal is to determine if the motion is to the right or the left.

The experiments are performed by adjusting the fraction C of coherently moving dots until the human subject's performance is at threshold (i.e. 75 percent correct). Barlow and Tripathy's (BT) model gives the proportion of dots at threshold to be $C_\theta = 1/\sqrt{Q - N}$ where Q is the size of the image lattice. This is approximately $1/\sqrt{Q}$ (because $N << Q$) and so is independent of the density of dots. Barlow and Tripathy compare the thresholds of the human subjects with those of their model for a range of experimental conditions which we will discuss in later sections.

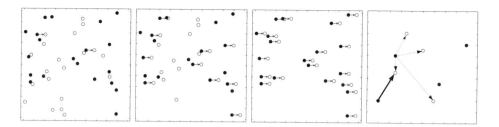

Figure 1: The left three panels show coherent stimuli with $N = 20, C = 0.1, N = 20, C = 0.5$ and $N = 20, C = 1.0$ respectively. The closed and open circles denote dots in the first and second frame respectively. The arrows show the motion of those dots which are moving coherently. Correspondence noise is illustrated by the far right panel showing that a dot in the first frame has many candidate matches in the second frame.

4 The Bayesian Ideal Model

We now compute the Bayes rule and Bayes risk by taking into account exactly how the data is generated. We denote the dot positions in the first and second frame by $D = \{x_i : i = 1, ..., N\}, \{y_a : a = 1, ..., N\}$. We define correspondence variables $V_{ia} : V_{ia} = 1$ if $x_i \rightarrow y_a$, $V_{ia} = 0$ otherwise.

The generative model for the data is given by:

$$P(D|\text{Coh}, T) = \sum_{V_{ia}} P(\{y_a\}|\{x_i\}, \{V_{ia}\}, T)P(\{V_{ia}\})P(\{x_i\}) \text{ coherent,}$$

$$P(D|\text{Incoh}) = P(\{y_a\})P(\{x_i\}), \text{ incoherent.} \tag{1}$$

The prior distributions for the dot positions $P(\{x_i\}), P(\{y_a\})$ allow all configurations of the dots to be equally likely. They are therefore of form $P(\{x_i\}) = P(\{y_a\}) = \frac{(Q-N)!}{Q!}$ where Q is the number of lattice points. The model $P(\{y_a\}|\{x_i\}, \{V_{ia}\}, T)$ for coherent motion is $P(\{y_a\}|\{x_i\}, \{V_{ia}\}, T) = \frac{(Q-N)!}{(Q-CN)!} \prod_{ia} \left(\delta_{y_a, x_i+T}\right)^{V_{ia}}$. We set the priors $P(\{V_{ia}\}$ to be the uniform distribution. There is a constraint $\sum_{ia} V_{ia} = CN$ (since only CN dots move coherently).

This gives:

$$P(D|\text{Incoh}) = \frac{(Q-N)!}{Q!}\frac{(Q-N)!}{Q!},$$

$$P(D|\text{Coh}, T) = \{\frac{(N-CN)!}{(N)!}\frac{(N-CN)!}{(N)!}\}^2(CN)! \sum_{V_{ia}} \prod_{ia} \left(\delta_{y_a+T, x_i}\right)^{V_{ia}}.$$

These can be simplified further by observing that $\sum_{V_{ia}} \prod_{ia} \left(\delta_{y_a, x_i+T}\right)^{V_{ia}} = \frac{\Psi!}{(\Psi-M)!M!}$, where Ψ is the total number of matches – i.e. the number of dots in the first frame that have a corresponding dot at displacement T in the second frame (this includes "fake" matches due to change alignment of noise dots in the two frames).

The Bayes rule for performing the tasks are given by testing the log-likelihood ratios: (i) $\log \frac{P(D|\text{Incoh})}{P(D|\text{Coh}, T)}$ for detection (i.e. coherent versus incoherent), and (ii) $\log \frac{P(D|\text{Coh}, -T)}{P(D|\text{Coh}, T)}$ for discrimination (i.e. motion to right or to left). For detection, the log-likelihood ratio is a function of Ψ. For discrimination, the log-likelihood ratio is a function of the number of matches to the right Ψ_r and to the left Ψ_l. It is straightforward to calculate the Bayes risk and determine coherence thresholds.

We can rederive Barlow and Tripathy's model as an approximation to the Bayesian Ideal. They make two approximations: (i) they model the distribution of ψ as Binomial, (ii) they use d'. Both approximations are very good near threshold, except for small N. The use of d' can be justified if $P(\Psi|\text{Coh}, T)$ and $P(\Psi|\text{Incoh})$ are Gaussians with similar variance. This is true for large $N = 1000$ and a range of C but not so good for small $N = 100$, see figure (2).

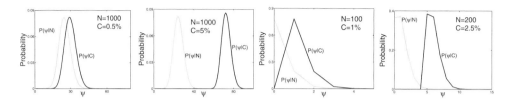

Figure 2: We plot $P(\Psi|\text{Coh}, T)$ and $P(\Psi|\text{Incoh})$, shown as $P(\Psi|C)$ and $P(\Psi|N)$ respectively, for a range of N and C. One of Barlow and Tripathy's two approximations are justified if the distributions are Gaussian with the same variance. This is true for large N (left two panels) but fails for small N (right two panels). Note that human thresholds are roughly 30 times higher than for BIO (the scales on graphs differ).

We computed the coherence threshold for the BIO and the BT models for $N = 100$ to $N = 1000$, see the second and fourth panels in figure (3). As described earlier, the BT threshold is approximately independent of the number N of dots. Our computations showed that the BIO threshold is also roughly constant except for small N (this is not surprising in light of figure (2). This motivated psychophysics experiments to determine how humans performed for small N (this range of dots was not explored in Barlow and Tripathy's experiments).

All our data points are from 300 trials using QUEST, so errors bars are so small that we do not include them.

We performed the detection and discrimination tasks with translation motion $T = 16$ (as in Barlow and Tripathy). For detection and discrimation, the human subject's thresholds showed similar trends to the thresholds for BIO and BT. But human performance at small N are more consistent with BIO, see figure (3).

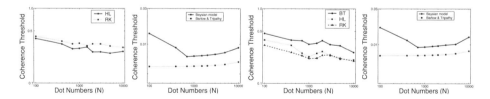

Figure 3: The left two panels show detection thresholds – human subjects (far left) and BIO and BT thresholds (left). The right two panels show discrimination thresholds – human subjects (right) and BIO and BT (far right).

But probably the most striking aspect of figure (3) is how poorly humans perform compared to the models. The thresholds for BIO are always higher than those for BT, but these differences are almost negligible compared to the differences with the human subjects. The experiments also show that the human subject trends differ from the models at large N. But these are extreme conditions where there are dots on most points on the image lattice.

5 Degradating the Ideal Observer Models

We now degrade the Bayes Ideal model to see if we can obtain human performance. We consider two mechanisms: (A) Humans do not know the precise value of the motion translation T. (B) Humans have poor spatial uncertainty. We will also combine both mechanisms.

For (A), we model lack of knowledge of the velocity T by summing over different motions. We generate the stimuli as before from $P(D|\text{Incoh})$ or $P(D|\text{Coh}, T)$, but we make the decision by thresholding: $\log \frac{\sum_T P(D|\text{Coh},T)P(T)}{P(D|\text{Incoh})}$.

For (B), we model lack of spatial resolution by replacing $P(\{y_a\}|\{x_i\}, \{V_{ia}\}, T) = \frac{(Q-N)!}{(Q-CN)!} \prod_{ia} V_{ia} \delta_{y_a, x_i+t}$ by $P(\{y_a\}|\{x_i\}, \{V_{ia}\}, T) = \frac{(Q-N)!}{(Q-CN)!} \prod_{ia} V_{ia} f_W(y_a, x_i + t)$. Here W is the width of a spatial window, so that $f_W(a,b) = 1/W^2$, if $|a - b| < W$; $f_W(a,b) = 0$, otherwise.

Our calculations, see figure (4), show that neither (A) nor (B) not their combination are sufficient to account for the poor performance of human subjects. Lack of knowledge of the correct motion (and consequently summing over several models) does little to degrade performance. Decreasing spatial resolution does degrade performance but even huge degradations are insufficient to reach human levels. Barlow and Tripathy [2] argue that they can degrade their model to reach human performance but the degradations are huge and they occur in conditions (e.g. $N = 50$ or $N = 100$) where their model is not a good approximation to the true Bayesian Ideal Observer.

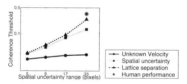

Figure 4: Comparing the degraded models to human performance. We use a log-log plot because the differences between humans and model thresholds is very large.

6 Slowness and Slow-and-Smooth

We now consider an alternative explanation for why human performance differs so greatly from the Bayesian Ideal Observer. Perhaps human subjects do not use the ideal model (which is only known to the designer of the experiments) and instead use a general purpose motion model. We now consider two possible models: (i) a slowness model, and (ii) a slow and smooth model.

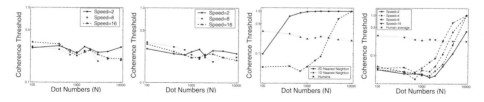

Figure 5: The coherence threshold as a function of N for different translation motions T. From left to right, human subject (HL), human subject (RK), 2DNN (shown for $T = 16$ only), and 1DNN. In the two right panels we have drawn the average human performance for comparision.

The slowness model is partly motivated by Ullman's minimal mapping theory [10] and partly by the design of practical computer vision tracking systems. This model solves the correspondence problem by simply matching a dot in the first frame to the closest dot in the second frame. We consider a 2D nearest neighbour model (2DNN) and a 1D nearest neighbour model (1DNN), for which the matching is constrained to be in horizontal directions only. After the motion has been calculated we perform a log-likelihood test to solve the discrimination and detection tasks. This enables us to calculate coherence thresholds, see figure (5). Both 1DNN and 2DNN predict that correspondence will be easy for small translation motions even when the number of dots is very large. This motivates a new class of experiments where we vary the translation motion.

Our experiments show that 1DNN and 2DNN are poor fits to human performance. Human performance thresholds are relatively insensitive to the number N of dots and the translation motion T, see the two left panels in figure (5). By contrast, the 1DNN and 2DNN thresholds are either far lower than humans for small N or far higher at large N with a transition that depends on T. We conclude that the 1DNN and 2DNN models do not match human performance.

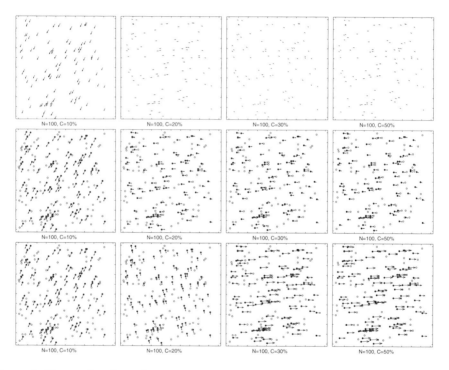

Figure 6: The motion flows from Slow-and-Smooth for $N = 100$ as functions of C and T. From left to right, $C = 0.1, C = 0.2, C = 0.3, C = 0.5$. From top to bottom, $T = 4, T = 8, T = 16$. The closed and open circles denote dots in the first and second frame respectively. The arrows indicate the motion flow specified by the Slow-and-Smooth model.

We now consider the Slow-and-Smooth model [8,9] which has been shown to account for a range of motion phenomena. We use a formulation [8] that was specifically designed for dealing with the correspondence problem.

This gives a model of form $P(V, v|\{x_i\}, \{y_a\}) = (1/Z)e^{-E[V,v]/T_m}$, where

$$E[V, v] = \sum_{i=1}^{N} \sum_{a=1}^{N} V_{ia}(y_a - x_i - v(x_i))^2 + \lambda||Lv||^2 + \zeta \sum_{i=1}^{N} V_{i0}, \qquad (2)$$

L is an operator that penalizes slow-and-smooth motion and depends on a paramters σ, see Yuille and Grzywacz for details [8]. We impose the constraint that $\sum_{i=a}^{N} V_{ia} = 1$, $\forall i$, which enforces that each point i in the first frame is either unmatched, if $V_{i0} = 1$, or is matched to a point a in the second frame.

We implemented this model using an EM algorithm to estimate the motion field $v(x)$ that maximizes $P(v|\{x_i\}, \{y_a\}) = \sum_V P(V, v|\{x_i\}, \{y_a\})$. The parameter settings are $T_m = 0.001$, $\lambda = 0.5$, $\zeta = 0.01$, $\sigma = 0.2236$. (The size of the units of length are normalized by the size of the image). The size of σ determines the spatial scale of the interaction between dots [8]. This parameter settings estimate correct motion directions in the condition that all dots move coherently, $C = 1.0$.

The following results, see figure (6), show that for 100 dots ($N = 100$) the results of the slow-and-smooth model are similar to those of the human subjects for a range of different translation motions. Slow-and-Smooth starts giving coherence thresholds between $C = 0.2$ and $C = 0.3$ consistent with human performance. Lower thresholds occurred for slower coherent translations in agreement with human performance.

Slow-and-Smooth also gives thresholds similar to human performance when we alter the number N of dots, see figure (7). Once again, Slow-and-Smooth starts giving the correct horizontal motion between $c = 0.2$ and $c = 0.3$.

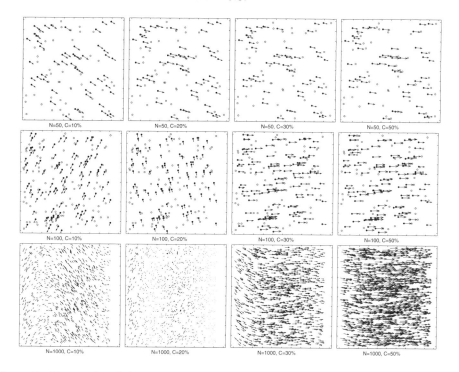

Figure 7: The motion fields of Slow-and-Smooth for $T = 16$ as a function of c and N. From left to right, $C = 0.1, C = 0.2, C = 0.3, C = 0.5$. From top to bottom, $N = 50, N = 100, N = 1000$. Same conventions as for previous figure.

7 Summary

We defined a Bayes Ideal Observer (BIO) for correspondence noise and showed that Barlow and Tripathy's (BT) model [2] can be obtained as an approximation. We performed psychophysical experiments which showed that the trends of human performance were more similar to those of BIO (when it differed from BT). We attempted to account for human's poor performance (compared to BIO) by allowing for degradations of the model such as poor spatial resolution and uncertainty about the precise translation velocity. We concluded that these degradation had to be implausibly large to account for the poorness of human performance. We noted that Barlow and Tripathy's degradation model [2] takes them into a regime where their model is a bad approximation to the BIO. Instead, we investigated the possibility that human observers perform these motion tasks using generic probability models for motion possibly adapted to the statistics of motion in the natural world. Further psychophysical experiments showed that human performance was inconsistent with a model than prefers slow motion. But human performance was consistent with the Slow-and-Smooth model [8,9].

We conclude with two metapoints. Firstly, it is possible to design ideal observer models for complex stimuli using techniques from Bayes decision theory. There is no need to restrict oneself to the traditional models described in classic signal detection books such as Green and Swets [3]. Secondly, human performance at visual tasks may be based on *generic models*, such as Slow-and-Smooth, rather than the ideal models for the experimental tasks (known only to the experimenter).

Acknowledgements

We thank Zili Liu for helpful discussions. We gratefully acknowledge funding support from the American Association of University Women (HL), NSF0413214 and W.M. Keck Foundation (ALY).

References

[1] Geisler, W.S. (2002) "Ideal Observer Analysis". In L. Chalupa and J. Werner (Eds). The Visual Neuroscienes. Boston. MIT Press. 825-837.

[2] Barlow, H., and Tripathy, S.P. (1997) Correspondence noise and signal pooling in the detection of coherent visual motion. Journal of Neuroscience, 17(20), 7954-7966.

[3] Green, D.M., and Swets, J.A. (1966) Signal detection theory and psychophysics. New York: Wiley.

[4] Morrone, M.C., Burr, D. C., and Vaina, L. M. (1995) Two stages of visual processing for radial and circular motion. Nature, 376(6540), 507-509.

[5] Neri, P., Morrone, M.C., and Burr, D.C. (1998) Seeing biological motion. Nature, 395(6705), 894-896.

[6] Song, Y., and Perona, P. (2000) A computational model for motion detection and direction discrimination in humans. IEEE computer society workshop on Human Motion, Austin, Texas.

[7] Wallace, J.M and Mamassian, P. (2004) The efficiency of depth discrimination for non-transparent and transparent stereoscopic surfaces. Vision Research, 44, 2253-2267.

[8] Yuille, A.L. and Grzywacz, N.M. (1988) A computational theory for the perception of coherent visual motion. Nature, 333,71-74,

[9] Weiss, Y., and Adelson, E.H. (1998) Slow and smooth: A Bayesian theory for the combination of local motion signals in human vision Technical Report 1624. Massachusetts Institute of Technology.

[10] Ullman, S. (1979) The interpretation of Visual Motion. MIT Press, Cambridge, MA, 1979.

Principles of real-time computing with feedback applied to cortical microcircuit models

Wolfgang Maass, Prashant Joshi
Institute for Theoretical Computer Science
Technische Universitaet Graz
A-8010 Graz, Austria
maass,joshi@igi.tugraz.at

Eduardo D. Sontag
Department of Mathematics
Rutgers, The State University of New Jersey
Piscataway, NJ 08854-8019, USA
sontag@cs.rutgers.edu

Abstract

The network topology of neurons in the brain exhibits an abundance of feedback connections, but the computational function of these feedback connections is largely unknown. We present a computational theory that characterizes the gain in computational power achieved through feedback in dynamical systems with fading memory. It implies that many such systems acquire through feedback universal computational capabilities for analog computing with a non-fading memory. In particular, we show that feedback enables such systems to process time-varying input streams in diverse ways according to rules that are implemented through internal states of the dynamical system. In contrast to previous attractor-based computational models for neural networks, these flexible internal states are *high-dimensional* attractors of the circuit dynamics, that still allow the circuit state to absorb new information from online input streams. In this way one arrives at novel models for working memory, integration of evidence, and reward expectation in cortical circuits. We show that they are applicable to circuits of conductance-based Hodgkin-Huxley (HH) neurons with high levels of noise that reflect experimental data on in-vivo conditions.

1 Introduction

Quite demanding real-time computations with fading memory[1] can be carried out by generic cortical microcircuit models [1]. But many types of computations in the brain, for

---

[1] A map (or filter) F from input- to output streams is defined to have fading memory if its current output at time t depends (up to some precision ε) only on values of the input $\mathbf{u}$ during some finite time interval $[t - T, t]$. In formulas: F has fading memory if there exists for every $\varepsilon > 0$ some $\delta > 0$ and $T > 0$ so that $|(F\mathbf{u})(t) - (F\tilde{\mathbf{u}})(t)| < \varepsilon$ for any $t \in \mathbb{R}$ and any input functions $\mathbf{u}, \tilde{\mathbf{u}}$ with

example computations that involve memory or persistent internal states, cannot be modeled by such fading memory systems. On the other hand concrete examples of artificial neural networks [2] and cortical microcircuit models [3] suggest that their computational power can be enlarged through feedback from trained readouts. Furthermore the brain is known to have an abundance of feedback connections on several levels: within cortical areas, where pyramidal cells typically have in addition to their long projecting axon a number of local axon collaterals, between cortical areas, and between cortex and subcortical structures. But the computational role of these feedback connections has remained open. We present here a computational theory which characterizes the gain in computational power that a fading memory system can acquire through feedback from trained readouts, both in the idealized case without noise and in the case with noise. This theory simultaneously characterizes the potential gain in computational power resulting from training a few neurons *within* a generic recurrent circuit for a specific task. Applications of this theory to cortical microcircuit models provide a new way of explaining the possibility of real-time processing of afferent input streams in the light of learning-induced internal circuit states that might represent for example working memory or rules for the timing of behavior. Further details to these results can be found in [4].

2 Computational Theory

Recurrent circuits of neurons are from a mathematical perspective special cases of dynamical systems. The subsequent mathematical results show that a large variety of dynamical systems, in particular also neural circuits, can overcome in the presence of feedback the computational limitations of a fading memory – without necessarily falling into the chaotic regime. In fact, feedback endows them with *universal* capabilities for *analog computing*, in a sense that can be made precise in the following way (see Fig. 1A-C for an illustration):

Theorem 2.1 *A large class $\mathcal{S}_n$ of systems of differential equations of the form*

$$x_i'(t) = f_i(x_1(t), \ldots, x_n(t)) + g_i(x_1(t), \ldots, x_n(t)) \cdot v(t), \quad i = 1, \ldots, n \tag{1}$$

are in the following sense universal for analog computing:

It can respond to an external input $u(t)$ with the dynamics of any n^{th} order differential equation of the form

$$z^{(n)}(t) = G(z(t), z'(t), z''(t), \ldots, z^{(n-1)}(t)) + u(t) \tag{2}$$

(for arbitrary smooth functions $G : \mathbb{R}^n \to \mathbb{R}$) if the input term $v(t)$ is replaced by a suitable memoryless feedback function $K(x_1(t), \ldots, x_n(t), u(t))$, and if a suitable memoryless readout function $h(x_1(t), \ldots, x_n(t))$ is applied to its internal state $\langle x_1(t), \ldots, x_n(t) \rangle$.

Also the dynamic responses of all systems consisting of several higher order differential equations of the form (2) can be simulated by fixed systems of the form (1) with a corresponding number of feedbacks.

The class $\mathcal{S}_n$ of dynamical systems that become through feedback universal for analog computing subsumes[2] systems of the form

$$x_i'(t) = -\lambda_i x_i(t) + \sigma \left(\sum_{j=1}^{n} a_{ij} \cdot x_j(t) \right) + b_i \cdot v(t), \quad i = 1, \ldots, n \tag{3}$$

$\|\mathbf{u}(\tau) - \tilde{\mathbf{u}}(\tau)\| < \delta$ for all $\tau \in [t - T, t]$. This is a characteristic property of all filters that can be approximated by an integral over the input stream $\mathbf{u}$, or more generally by Volterra- or Wiener series.

[2]for example if the λ_i are pairwise different and $a_{ij} = 0$ for all i, j, and all b_i are nonzero; fewer restrictions are needed if more then one feedback to the system (3) can be used

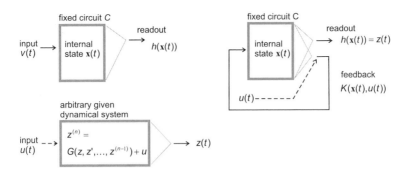

Figure 1: Universal computational capability acquired through feedback according to Theorem 2.1. **(A)** A fixed circuit C with dynamics (1). **(B)** An arbitrary given n^{th} order dynamical system (2) with external input $u(t)$. **(C)** If the input $v(t)$ to circuit C is replaced by a suitable feedback $K(\mathbf{x}(t), u(t))$, then this fixed circuit C can simulate the dynamic response $z(t)$ of the arbitrarily given system shown in B, for any input stream $u(t)$.

that are commonly used to model the temporal evolution of firing rates in neural circuits (σ is some standard activation function). If the activation function σ is also applied to the term $v(t)$ in (3), the system (3) can still simulate arbitrary differential equations (2) with bounded inputs $u(t)$ and bounded responses $z(t), \ldots, z^{(n-1)}(t)$.

Note that according to [5] all Turing machines can be simulated by systems of differential equations of the form (2). Hence the systems (1) become through feedback also universal for digital computing. A proof of Theorem 2.1 is given in [4].

It has been shown that additive noise, even with an arbitrarily small bounded amplitude, reduces the non-fading memory capacity of any recurrent neural network to some finite number of bits [6, 7]. Hence such network can no longer simulate arbitrary Turing machines. But feedback can still endow noisy fading memory systems with the maximum possible computational power within this a-priori limitation. The following result shows that in principle any finite state machine (= deterministic finite automaton), in particular any Turing machine with tapes of some arbitrary but fixed finite length, can be emulated by a fading memory system with feedback, in spite of noise in the system.

Theorem 2.2 *Feedback allows linear and nonlinear fading memory systems, even in the presence of additive noise with bounded amplitude, to employ the computational capability and non-fading states of any given finite state machine (in addition to their fading memory) for real-time processing of time varying inputs.*

The precise formalization and the proof of this result (see [4]) are technically rather involved, and cannot be given in this abstract. A key method of the proof, which makes sure that noise does not get amplified through feedback, is also applied in the subsequent computer simulations of cortical microcircuit models. There the readout functions K that provide feedback values $K(\mathbf{x}(t))$ are trained to assume values which cancel the impact of errors or imprecision in the values $K(\mathbf{x}(s))$ of this feedback for immediately preceding time steps $s < t$.

3   Application to Generic Circuits of Noisy Neurons

We tested this computational theory on circuits consisting of 600 integrate-and-fire (I&F) neurons and circuits consisting of 600 conductance-based HH neurons, in either case with a rather high level of noise that reflects experimental data on in-vivo conditions [8]. In addition we used models for dynamic synapses whose individual mixture of paired-pulse depression and facilitation is based on experimental data [9, 10]. Sparse connectivity between neurons with a biologically realistic bias towards short connections was generated by a probabilistic rule, and synaptic parameters were randomly chosen, depending on the type of pre-and postsynaptic neurons, in accordance with these empirical data (see [1] or [4] for details). External inputs and feedback from readouts were connected to populations of neurons within the circuit, with randomly varying connection strengths. The current circuit state $\mathbf{x}(t)$ was modeled by low-pass filtered spike trains from all neurons in the circuit (with a time constant of 30 ms, modeling time constants of receptors and membrane of potential readout neurons). Readout functions $K(\mathbf{x}(t))$ were modeled by weighted sums $\mathbf{w} \cdot \mathbf{x}(t)$

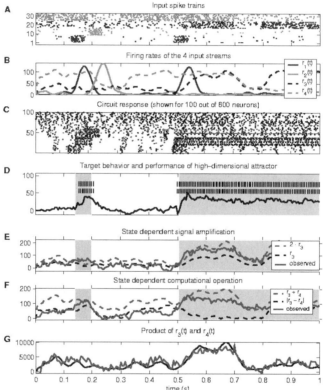

Figure 2: State-dependent real-time processing of 4 independent input streams in a generic cortical microcircuit model. (**A**) 4 input streams, consisting each of 8 spike trains generated by Poisson processes with randomly varying rates $r_i(t), i = 1, \ldots, 4$ (rates plotted in (**B**); all rates are given in Hz). The 4 input streams and the feedback were injected into disjoint but densely interconnected subpopulations of neurons in the circuit. (**C**) Resulting firing activity of 100 out of the 600 I&F neurons in the circuit. Spikes from inhibitory neurons marked in gray. (**D**) Target activation times of the high-dimensional attractor (gray shading), spike trains of 2 of the 8 I&F neurons that were trained to create the high-dimensional attractor by sending their output spike trains back into the circuit, and average firing rate of all 8 neurons (lower trace). (**E and F**) Performance of linear readouts that were trained to switch their real-time computation task depending on the current state of the high-dimensional attractor: output $2 \cdot r_3(t)$ instead of $r_3(t)$ if the high-dimensional attractor is on (E), output $r_3(t) + r_4(t)$ instead of $|r_3(t) - r_4(t)|$ if the high-dimensional attractor is on (F). (**G**) Performance of linear readout that was trained to output $r_3(t) \cdot r_4(t)$, showing that another linear readout from the same circuit can simultaneously carry out nonlinear computations that are invariant to the current state of the high-dimensional attractor.

whose weights **w** were trained during 200 s of simulated biological time to minimize the mean squared error with regard to desired target output functions K. After training these weights **w** were fixed, and the performance of the otherwise generic circuit was evaluated for new input streams **u** (with new input rates drawn from the same distribution) that had not been used for training. It was sufficient to use just linear functions K that transformed the current circuit state $\mathbf{x}(t)$ into a feedback $K(\mathbf{x}(t))$, confirming the predictions of [1] and [2] that the recurrent circuit automatically assumes the role of a kernel (in the sense of machine learning) that creates nonlinear combinations of recent inputs.

We found that computer simulations of such generic cortical microcircuit models confirm the theoretical prediction that feedback from suitably trained readouts enables complex state-dependent real-time processing of a fairly large number of diverse input spike trains within a single circuit (all results shown are for test inputs that had not been used for training). Readout neurons could be trained to turn a high-dimensional attractor on or off in response to particular signals in 2 of the 4 independent input streams (Fig. 2D). The target value for $K(\mathbf{x}(t))$ during training was the currently desired activity-state of the high-dimensional attractor, where $\mathbf{x}(t)$ resulted from giving already tentative spike trains that matched this target value as feedback into the circuit. These neurons were trained to represent in their firing activity at any time the information in which of input streams 1 or 2 a burst had most recently occurred. If it occurred most recently in stream 1, they were trained to fire at 40 Hz, and not to fire otherwise. Thus these neurons were required to represent the non-fading state of a very simple finite state machine, demonstrating in a simple example the validity of Theorem 2.2.

The weights **w** of these readout neurons were determined by a sign-constrained linear regression, so that weights from excitatory (inhibitory) presynaptic neurons were automatically positive (negative). Since these readout neurons had the same properties as neurons within the circuit, this computer simulation also provided a first indication of the gain in real-time processing capability that can be achieved by suitable training of a few spiking neurons *within* an otherwise randomly connected recurrent circuit. Fig. 2 shows that other readouts from the same circuit (that do not provide feedback) can be trained to amplify their response to one of the input streams (Fig. 2E), or even switch their computational function (Fig. 2F) if the high-dimensional attractor is in the on-state, thereby providing a model for the way in which internal circuit states can change the "program" for its online processing.

Continuous high-dimensional attractors that hold a time-varying analog value (instead of a discrete state) through globally distributed activity within the circuit can be created in the same way through feedback. In fact, several such high-dimensional attractors can co-exist within the same circuit, see Fig. 3B,C,D. This gives rise to a model (Fig. 3) that could explain how timing of behavior and reward expectation are learnt and controlled by neural microcircuits on a behaviorally relevant large time scale. In addition Fig. 4 shows that a continuous high-dimensional attractor that is created through feedback provides a new model for a neural integrator, and that the current value of this neural integrator can be combined within the same circuit and in real-time with variables extracted from time-varying analog input streams.

This learning-induced generation of high-dimensional attractors through feedback provides a new model for the emergence of persistent firing in cortical circuits that does not rely on especially constructed circuits, neurons, or synapses, and which is consistent with high noise (see Fig. 4G for the quite realistic trial-to-trial variability in this circuit of HH neurons with background noise according to [8]). This learning based model is also consistent with the surprising plasticity that has recently been observed even in quite specialized neural integrators [11]. Its robustness can be traced back to the fact that readouts can be trained to correct errors in their previous feedback. Furthermore such error correction is not restricted to linear computational operations, since the inherent kernel property of generic recurrent circuits allows even linear readouts to carry out nonlinear computations on firing rates

(Fig. 2G). Whereas previous models for discrete or continuous attractors in recurrent neural circuits required that the whole dynamics of such circuit was entrained by the attractor, our new model predicts that persistent firing states can co-exist with other high-dimensional attractors and with responses to time-varying afferent inputs within the same circuit. Note that such attractors can equivalently be generated by training (instead of readouts) a few neurons *within* an otherwise generic cortical microcircuit model.

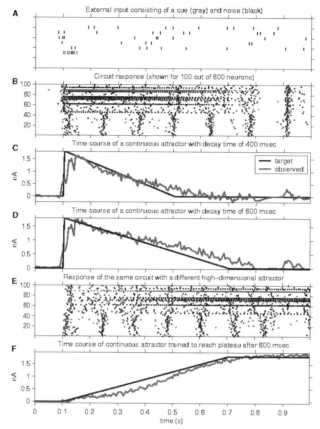

Figure 3: Representation of time for behaviorally relevant time spans in a generic cortical microcircuit model. (**A**) Afferent circuit input, consisting of a cue in one channel (gray) and random spikes (freshly drawn for each trial) in the other channels. (**B**) Response of 100 neurons from the same circuit as in Fig. 2, which has here two co-existing high-dimensional attractors. The autonomously generated periodic bursts with a periodic frequency of about 8 Hz are not related to the task, and readouts were trained to become invariant to them. (**C and D**) Feedback from two linear readouts that were simultaneously trained to create and control two high-dimensional attractors. One of them was trained to decay in 400 ms (C), and the other in 600 ms (D) (scale in nA is the average current injected by feedback into a randomly chosen subset of neurons in the circuit). (**E**) Response of the same neurons as in (B), for the same circuit input, but with feedback from a different linear readout that was trained to create a high-dimensional attractor that increases its activity and reaches a plateau 600 ms after the occurrence of the cue in the input stream. (**F**) Feedback from the linear readout that creates this continuous high-dimensional attractor.

4 Discussion

We have demonstrated that persistent memory and online switching of real-time processing can be implemented in generic cortical microcircuit models by training a few neurons

840

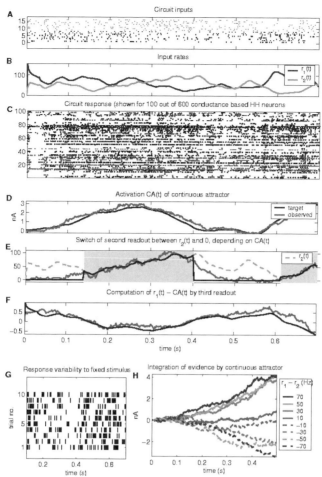

Figure 4: A model for analog real-time computation on external and internal variables in a generic cortical microcircuit (consisting of 600 conductance-based HH neurons). (**A and B**) Two input streams as in Fig. 2; their firing rates $r_1(t), r_2(t)$ are shown in (B). (**C**) Resulting firing activity of 100 neurons in the circuit. (**D**) Performance of a neural integrator, generated by feedback from a linear readout that was trained to output at any time t an approximation $CA(t)$ of the integral $\int_0^t (r_1(s) - r_2(s))ds$ over the difference of both input rates. Feedback values were injected as input currents into a randomly chosen subset of neurons in the circuit. Scale in nA shows average strength of feedback currents (also in panel H). (**E**) Performance of linear readout that was trained to output 0 as long as $CA(t)$ stayed below 1.35 nA, and to output then $r_2(t)$ until the value of $CA(t)$ dropped below 0.45 nA (i.e., in this test run during the shaded time periods). (**F**) Performance of linear readout trained to output $r_1(t) - CA(t)$, i.e. a combination of external and internal variables, at any time t (both r_1 and CA normalized into the range $[0, 1]$). (**G**) Response of a randomly chosen neuron in the circuit for 10 repetitions of the same experiment (with input spike trains generated by Poisson processes with the same time-course of firing rates), showing biologically realistic trial-to-trial variability. (**H**) Activity traces of a continuous attractor as in (D), but in 8 different trials for 8 different fixed values of r_1 and r_2 (shown on the right). The resulting traces are very similar to the temporal evolution of firing rates of neurons in area LIP that integrate sensory evidence (see Fig.5A in [12]).

(within or outside of the circuit) through very simple learning processes (linear regression, or alternatively – with some loss in performance – perceptron learning). The resulting high-dimensional attractors can be made noise-robust through training, thereby overcoming the inherent brittleness of constructed attractors. The high dimensionality of these attractors, which is caused by the small number of synaptic weights that are fixed for their creation, allows the circuit state to move in or out of other attractors, and to absorb new information from online inputs, while staying within such high-dimensional attractor. The resulting virtually unlimited computational capability of fading memory circuits with feedback can be explained on the basis of the theoretical results that were presented in section 2.

Acknowledgments

Helpful comments from Wulfram Gerstner, Stefan Haeusler, Herbert Jaeger, Konrad Koerding, Henry Markram, Gordon Pipa, Misha Tsodyks, and Tony Zador are gratefully acknowledged. Written under partial support by the Austrian Science Fund FWF, project # S9102-N04, project # IST2002-506778 (PASCAL) and project # FP6-015879 (FACETS) of the European Union.

References

[1] W. Maass, T. Natschläger, and H. Markram. Real-time computing without stable states: A new framework for neural computation based on perturbations. *Neural Computation*, 14(11):2531–2560, 2002.

[2] H. Jäger and H. Haas. Harnessing nonlinearity: predicting chaotic systems and saving energy in wireless communication. *Science*, 304:78–80, 2004.

[3] P. Joshi and W. Maass. Movement generation with circuits of spiking neurons. *Neural Computation*, 17(8):1715–1738, 2005.

[4] W. Maass, P. Joshi, and E. D. Sontag. Computational aspects of feedback in neural circuits. *submitted for publication*, 2005. Online available as #168 from http://www.igi.tugraz.at/maass/.

[5] M. S. Branicky. Universal computation and other capabilities of hybrid and continuous dynamical systems. *Theoretical Computer Science*, 138:67–100, 1995.

[6] M. Casey. The dynamics of discrete-time computation with application to recurrent neural networks and finite state machine extraction. *Neural Computation*, 8:1135–1178, 1996.

[7] W. Maass and P. Orponen. On the effect of analog noise in discrete-time analog computations. *Neural Computation*, 10:1071–1095, 1998.

[8] A. Destexhe, M. Rudolph, and D. Pare. The high-conductance state of neocortical neurons in vivo. *Nat. Rev. Neurosci.*, 4(9):739–751, 2003.

[9] H. Markram, Y. Wang, and M. Tsodyks. Differential signaling via the same axon of neocortical pyramidal neurons. *PNAS*, 95:5323–5328, 1998.

[10] A. Gupta, Y. Wang, and H. Markram. Organizing principles for a diversity of GABAergic interneurons and synapses in the neocortex. *Science*, 287:273–278, 2000.

[11] G. Major, R. Baker, E. Aksay, B. Mensh, H. S. Seung, and D. W. Tank. Plasticity and tuning by visual feedback of the stability of a neural integrator. *Proc Natl Acad Sci*, 101(20):7739–7744, 2004.

[12] M. E. Mazurek, J. D. Roitman, J. Ditterich, and M. N. Shadlen. A role for neural integrators in perceptual decision making. *Cerebral Cortex*, 13(11):1257–1269, 2003.

Value Function Approximation with Diffusion Wavelets and Laplacian Eigenfunctions

Sridhar Mahadevan
Department of Computer Science
University of Massachusetts
Amherst, MA 01003
mahadeva@cs.umass.edu

Mauro Maggioni
Program in Applied Mathematics
Department of Mathematics
Yale University
New Haven, CT 06511
mauro.maggioni@yale.edu

Abstract

We investigate the problem of automatically constructing efficient representations or basis functions for approximating value functions based on analyzing the structure and topology of the state space. In particular, two novel approaches to value function approximation are explored based on automatically constructing basis functions on state spaces that can be represented as graphs or manifolds: one approach uses the eigenfunctions of the Laplacian, in effect performing a global Fourier analysis on the graph; the second approach is based on diffusion wavelets, which generalize classical wavelets to graphs using multiscale dilations induced by powers of a diffusion operator or random walk on the graph. Together, these approaches form the foundation of a new generation of methods for solving large Markov decision processes, in which the underlying representation and policies are simultaneously learned.

1 Introduction

Value function approximation (VFA) is a well-studied problem: a variety of linear and nonlinear architectures have been studied, which are not automatically derived from the geometry of the underlying state space, but rather handcoded in an *ad hoc* trial-and-error process by a human designer [1]. A new framework for VFA called *proto-reinforcement learning* (PRL) was recently proposed in [7, 8, 9]. Instead of learning task-specific value functions using a handcoded parametric architecture, agents learn proto-value functions, or global basis functions that reflect intrinsic large-scale geometric constraints that all value functions on a manifold [11] or graph [3] adhere to, using spectral analysis of the self-adjoint Laplace operator. This approach also yields new control learning algorithms called *representation policy iteration* (RPI) where both the underlying representations (basis functions) and policies are simultaneously learned. Laplacian eigenfunctions also provide ways of automatically decomposing state spaces since they reflect *bottlenecks* and other global geometric invariants.

In this paper, we extend the earlier Laplacian approach in a new direction using the recently proposed *diffusion wavelet transform* (DWT), which is a compact multi-level representation of Markov diffusion processes on manifolds and graphs [4, 2]. Diffusion wavelets provide an interesting alternative to global Fourier eigenfunctions for value function approximation, since they encapsulate all the traditional advantages of wavelets: basis functions have compact support, and the representation is inherently hierarchical since it is based on multi-resolution modeling of processes at different spatial and temporal scales.

2 Technical Background

This paper uses the framework of spectral graph theory [3] to build basis representations for smooth (value) functions on graphs induced by Markov decision processes. Given any graph G, an obvious but poor choice of representation is the "table-lookup" orthonormal encoding, where $\phi(i) = [0 \ldots i \ldots 0]$ is the encoding of the ith node in the graph. This representation does not reflect the topology of the specific graph under consideration. Polynomials are another popular choice of orthonormal basis functions [5], where $\phi(s) = [1 \ s \ldots s^k]$ for some fixed k. This encoding has two disadvantages: it is numerically unstable for large graphs, and is dependent on the ordering of vertices. In this paper, we outline a new approach to the problem of building basis functions on graphs using Laplacian eigenfunctions and diffusion wavelets.

A finite Markov decision process (MDP) $M = (S, A, P^a_{ss'}, R^a_{ss'})$ is defined as a finite set of states S, a finite set of actions A, a transition model $P^a_{ss'}$ specifying the distribution over future states s' when an action a is performed in state s, and a corresponding reward model $R^a_{ss'}$ specifying a scalar cost or reward [10]. A state value function is a mapping $S \to \mathcal{R}$ or equivalently a vector in $\mathcal{R}^{|S|}$. Given a policy $\pi : S \to A$ mapping states to actions, its corresponding value function V^π specifies the expected long-term discounted sum of rewards received by the agent in any given state s when actions are chosen using the policy. Any optimal policy π^* defines the same unique optimal value function V^* which satisfies the nonlinear constraints

$$V^*(s) = \max_a \sum_{s'} P^a_{ss'} \left(R^a_{ss'} + \gamma V^*(s') \right)$$

For any MDP, any policy induces a Markov chain that partitions the states into classes: transient states are visited initially but not after a finite time, and recurrent states are visited infinitely often. In *ergodic* MDPs, the set of transient states is empty. The construction of basis functions below assumes that the Markov chain induced by a policy is a reversible random walk on the state space. While some policies may not induce such Markov chains, the set of basis functions learned from a reversible random walk can still be useful in approximating value functions for (reversible or non-reversible) policies. In other words, the construction of the basis functions can be considered an *off-policy* method: just as in Q-learning where the exploration policy differs from the optimal learned policy, in the proposed approach the actual MDP dynamics may induce a different Markov chain than the one analyzed to build representations. Reversible random walks greatly simplify spectral analysis since such random walks are similar to a symmetric operator on the state space.

2.1 Smooth Functions on Graphs and Value Function Representation

We assume the state space can be modeled as a finite undirected weighted graph (G, E, W), but the approach generalizes to Riemannian manifolds. We define $x \sim y$ to mean an edge between x and y, and the degree of x to be $d(x) = \sum_{x \sim y} w(x, y)$. D will denote the diagonal matrix defined by $D_{xx} = d(x)$, and W the matrix defined by $W_{xy} = w(x, y) = w(y, x)$. The $\mathcal{L}^2$ norm of a function on G is $||f||_2^2 = \sum_{x \in G} |f(x)|^2 d(x)$. The gradient of a function is $\nabla f(i, j) = w(i, j)(f(i) - f(j))$ if there is an edge e connecting i to j, 0 otherwise. The smoothness of a function on a graph, can be measured by the Sobolev norm

$$||f||_{\mathcal{H}^2}^2 = ||f||_2^2 + ||\nabla f||_2^2 = \sum_x |f(x)|^2 d(x) + \sum_{x \sim y} |f(x) - f(y)|^2 w(x, y). \quad (1)$$

The first term in this norm controls the size (in terms of $\mathcal{L}^2$-norm) for the function f, and the second term controls the size of the gradient. The smaller $||f||_{\mathcal{H}^2}$, the smoother is f. We will assume that the value functions we consider have small $\mathcal{H}^2$ norms, except at a few points, where the gradient may be large. Important variations exist, corresponding to different measures on the vertices and edges of G.

Classical techniques, such as *value iteration* and *policy iteration* [10], represent value functions using an orthonormal basis $(e_1, \ldots, e_{|S|})$ for the space $\mathcal{R}^{|S|}$ [1]. For a fixed precision ϵ, a value function V^π can be approximated as

$$||V^\pi - \sum_{i \in S(\epsilon)} \alpha_i^\pi e_i|| \leq \epsilon$$

with $\alpha_i = <V^\pi, e_i>$ since the e_i's are orthonormal, and the approximation is measured in some norm, such as $\mathcal{L}^2$ or $\mathcal{H}^2$. The goal is to obtain representations in which the index set $S(\epsilon)$ in the summation is as small as possible, for a given approximation error ϵ. This hope is well founded at least when V^π is smooth or piecewise smooth, since in this case it should be compressible in some well chosen basis $\{e_i\}$.

3   Function Approximation using Laplacian Eigenfunctions

The combinatorial Laplacian L [3] is defined as

$$Lf(x) = \sum_{y \sim x} w(x, y)(f(x) - f(y)) = (D - W)f .$$

Often one considers the *normalized* Laplacian $\mathcal{L} = D^{-\frac{1}{2}}(D-W)D^{-\frac{1}{2}}$ which has spectrum in $[0, 2]$. This Laplacian is related to the notion of smoothness as above, since $\langle f, \mathcal{L}f \rangle = \sum_x f(x)\mathcal{L}f(x) = \sum_{x,y} w(x, y)(f(x) - f(y))^2 = ||\nabla f||_2^2$, which should be compared with (1). Functions that satisfy the equation $\mathcal{L}f = 0$ are called *harmonic*. The Spectral Theorem can be applied to $\mathcal{L}$ (or L), yielding a discrete set of eigenvalues $0 \leq \lambda_0 \leq \lambda_1 \leq \ldots \lambda_i \leq \ldots$ and a corresponding orthonormal basis of eigenfunctions $\{\xi_i\}_{i \geq 0}$, solutions to the eigenvalue problem $\mathcal{L}\xi_i = \lambda_i \xi_i$.

The eigenfunctions of the Laplacian can be viewed as an orthonormal basis of global Fourier smooth functions that can be used for approximating any value function on a graph. These basis functions capture large-scale features of the state space, and are particularly sensitive to "bottlenecks", a phenomenon widely studied in Riemannian geometry and spectral graph theory [3]. Observe that ξ_i satisfies $||\nabla \xi_i||_2^2 = \lambda_i$. In fact, the variational characterization of eigenvectors shows that ξ_i is the normalized function orthogonal to $\xi_0, \ldots, \xi_{i-1}$ with minimal $||\nabla \xi_i||_2$. Hence the projection of a function f on S onto the top k eigenvectors of the Laplacian is the smoothest approximation to f, in the sense of the norm in $\mathcal{H}^2$. A potential drawback of Laplacian approximation is that it detects only global smoothness, and may poorly approximate a function which is not globally smooth but only piecewise smooth, or with different smoothness in different regions. These drawbacks are addressed in the context of analysis with diffusion wavelets, and in fact partly motivated their construction.

4   Function Approximation using Diffusion Wavelets

Diffusion wavelets were introduced in [4, 2], in order to perform a fast multiscale analysis of functions on a manifold or graph, generalizing wavelet analysis and associated signal processing techniques (such as compression or denoising) to functions on manifolds and graphs. They allow the fast and accurate computation of high powers of a Markov chain

845

```
DiffusionWaveletTree (H_0, Φ_0, J, ε):
```

// H_0: symmetric conjugate to random walk matrix, represented on the basis Φ_0
// Φ_0 : initial basis (usually Dirac's δ-function basis), one function per column
// J : number of levels to compute
// ϵ: precision

for j from 0 to J do,

    1. Compute sparse factorization $H_j \sim_\epsilon Q_j R_j$, with Q_j orthogonal.

    2. $\Phi_{j+1} \leftarrow Q_j = H_j R_j^{-1}$ and $[H_0^{2^j}]_{\Phi_{j+1}}^{\Phi_{j+1}} \sim_{j\epsilon} H_{j+1} \leftarrow R_j R_j^*$.

    3. Compute sparse factorization $I - \Phi_{j+1}\Phi_{j+1}^* = Q_j' R_j'$, with Q_j' orthogonal.

    4. $\Psi_{j+1} \leftarrow Q_j'$.

end

Figure 1: Pseudo-code for constructing a Diffusion Wavelet Tree

P on the manifold or graph, including direct computation of the Green's function (or fundamental matrix) of the Markov chain, $(I - P)^{-1}$, which can be used to solve Bellman's equation. Here, "fast" means that the number of operations required is $\mathcal{O}(|S|)$, up to logarithmic factors.

Space constraints permit only a brief description of the construction of diffusion wavelet trees. More details are provided in [4, 2]. The input to the algorithm is a "precision" parameter $\epsilon > 0$, and a weighted graph (G, E, W). We can assume that G is connected, otherwise we can consider each connected component separately. The construction is based on using the natural random walk $P = D^{-1}W$ on a graph and its powers to "dilate", or "diffuse" functions on the graph, and then defining an associated coarse-graining of the graph. We symmetrize P by conjugation and take powers to obtain

$$H^t = D^{\frac{1}{2}}P^t D^{-\frac{1}{2}} = (D^{-\frac{1}{2}}WD^{-\frac{1}{2}})^t = (I - \mathcal{L})^t = \sum_{i \geq 0}(1 - \lambda_i)^t \xi_i(\cdot)\xi_i(\cdot) \quad (2)$$

where $\{\lambda_i\}$ and $\{\xi_i\}$ are the eigenvalues and eigenfunctions of the Laplacian as above. Hence the eigenfunctions of H^t are again ξ_i and the ith eigenvalue is $(1 - \lambda_i)^t$. We assume that H^1 is a sparse matrix, and that the spectrum of H^1 has rapid decay.

A diffusion wavelet tree consist of orthogonal diffusion scaling functions Φ_j that are smooth bump functions, with some oscillations, at scale roughly 2^j (measured with respect to geodesic distance, for small j), and orthogonal wavelets Ψ_j that are smooth localized oscillatory functions at the same scale. The scaling functions Φ_j span a subspace V_j, with the property that $V_{j+1} \subseteq V_j$, and the span of Ψ_j, W_j, is the orthogonal complement of V_j into V_{j+1}. This is achieved by using the dyadic powers H^{2^j} as "dilations", to create smoother and wider (always in a geodesic sense) "bump" functions (which represent densities for the symmetrized random walk after 2^j steps), and orthogonalizing and downsampling appropriately to transform sets of "bumps" into orthonormal scaling functions.

Computationally (Figure 1), we start with the basis $\Phi_0 = I$ and the matrix $H_0 := H^1$, sparse by assumption, and construct an orthonormal basis of well-localized functions for its range (the space spanned by the columns), up to precision ϵ, through a variation of the Gram-Schmidt orthonormalization scheme, described in [4]. In matrix form, this is a sparse factorization $H_0 \sim_\epsilon Q_0 R_0$, with Q_0 orthonormal. Notice that H_0 is $|G| \times |G|$, but in general Q_0 is $|G| \times |G^{(1)}|$ and R_0 is $|G^{(1)}| \times |G|$, with $|G^{(1)}| \leq |G|$. In fact $|G^{(1)}|$ is approximately equal to the number of singular values of H_0 larger than ϵ. The columns of Q_0 are an orthonormal basis of scaling functions Φ_1 for the range of H_0, written as a linear combination of the initial basis Φ_0. We can now write H_0^2 on the basis Φ_1: $H_1 := [H^2]_{\Phi_1}^{\Phi_1} = Q_0^* H_0 H_0 Q_0 = R_0 R_0^*$, where we used $H_0 = H_0^*$. This is a compressed representation of H_0^2 acting on the range of H_0, and it is a $|G^{(1)}| \times |G^{(1)}|$ matrix. We proceed by induction: at scale j we have an orthonormal basis Φ_j for the rank of H^{2^j-1} up to precision $j\epsilon$, represented as a linear combination of elements in Φ_{j-1}. This basis contains $|G^{(j)}|$ functions, where $|G^{(j)}|$ is comparable with the number of eigenvalues λ_j of H_0 such that $\lambda_j^{2^j-1} \geq \epsilon$. We have the operator $H_0^{2^j}$ represented on Φ_j by a $|G^{(j)}| \times |G^{(j)}|$ matrix H_j, up to precision $j\epsilon$. We compute a sparse decomposition of $H_j \sim_\epsilon Q_j R_j$, and obtain the next basis $\Phi_{j+1} = Q_j = H_j R_j^{-1}$ and represent $H^{2^{j+1}}$ on this basis by the matrix $H_{j+1} := [H^{2^j}]_{\Phi_{j+1}}^{\Phi_{j+1}} = Q_j^* H_j H_j Q_j = R_j R_j^*$.

Wavelet bases for the spaces W_j can be built analogously by factorizing $I_{V_j} - Q_{j+1} Q_{j+1}^*$, which is the orthogonal projection on the complement of V_{j+1} into V_j. The spaces can be further split to obtain wavelet packets [2]. A Fast Diffusion Wavelet Transform allows expanding in $\mathcal{O}(n)$ (where n is the number of vertices) computations any function in the wavelet, or wavelet packet, basis, and efficiently search for the most suitable basis set. Diffusion wavelets and wavelet packets are a very efficient tool for representation and approximation of functions on manifolds and graphs [4, 2], generalizing to these general spaces the nice properties of wavelets that have been so successfully applied to similar tasks in Euclidean spaces.

Diffusion wavelets allow computing $H^{2^k} f$ for any fixed f, in order $\mathcal{O}(kn)$. This is non-trivial because while the matrix H is sparse, large powers of it are not, and the computation $H \cdot H \ldots \cdot (H(Hf)) \ldots)$ involves 2^k matrix-vector products. As a notable consequence, this yields a fast algorithm for computing the Green's function, or fundamental matrix, associated with the Markov process H, via $(I-H^1)^{-1} f = \sum_{k\geq 0} H^k = \prod_{k\geq 0} (I+H^{2^k})f$. In a similar way one can compute $(I - P)^{-1}$. For large classes of Markov chains we can perform this computation in time $\mathcal{O}(n)$, in a direct (as opposed to iterative) fashion. This is remarkable since in general the matrix $(I-H^1)^{-1}$ is full and only writing down the entries would take time $\mathcal{O}(n^2)$. It is the multiscale compression scheme that allows to efficiently represent $(I-H^1)^{-1}$ in compress form, taking advantage of the smoothness of the entries of the matrix. This is discussed in general in [4]. We use this approach to develop a faster policy evaluation step for solving MDPs described in [6]

5 Experiments

Figure 2 contrasts Laplacian eigenfunctions and diffusion wavelet basis functions in a three room grid world environment. Laplacian eigenfunctions were produced by solving $Lf = \lambda f$, where L is the combinatorial Laplacian, whereas diffusion wavelet basis functions were produced using the algorithm described in Figure 1. The input to both methods is an undirected graph, where edges connect states reachable through a single (reversible) action. Such graphs can be easily learned from a sample of transitions, such as that generated by RL agents while exploring the environment in early phases of policy learning. Note how the intrinsic multi-room environment is reflected in the Laplacian eigenfunctions. The Laplacian eigenfunctions are globally defined over the entire state space, whereas diffusion wavelet basis functions are progressively more compact at higher levels, beginning at the lowest level with the table-lookup representation, and converging at the highest level to basis functions similar to Laplacian eigenfunctions. Figure 3 compares the approximations produced in a two-room grid world MDP with 630 states. These experiments illustrate the superiority of diffusion wavelets: in the first experiment (top row), diffusion wavelets handily outperform Laplacian eigenfunctions because the function is highly nonlinear near

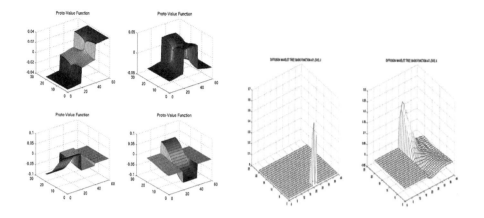

Figure 2: Examples of Laplacian eigenfunctions (left) and diffusion wavelet basis functions (right) computed using the graph Laplacian on a complete undirected graph of a deterministic grid world environment with reversible actions.

the goal, but mostly linear elsewhere. The eigenfunctions contain a lot of ripples in the flat region causing a large residual error. In the second experiment (bottom row), Laplacian eigenfunctions work significantly better because the value function is globally smooth. Even here, the superiority of diffusion wavelets is clear.

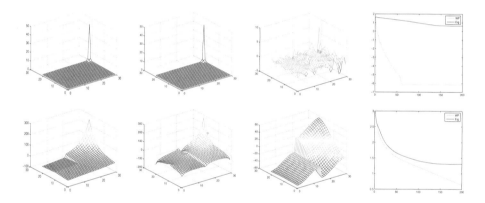

Figure 3: Left column: value functions in a two room grid world MDP, where each room has 21×15 states connected by a door in the middle of the common wall. Middle two columns: approximations produced by 5 diffusion wavelet bases and Laplacian eigenfunctions. Right column: least-squares approximation error (log scale) using up to 200 basis functions (bottom curve: diffusion wavelets; top curve: Laplacian eigenfunctions). In the top row, the value function corresponds to a random walk. In the bottom row, the value function corresponds to the optimal policy.

5.1 Control Learning using Representation Policy Iteration

This section describes results of using the automatically generated basis functions inside a control learning algorithm, in particular the Representation Policy Iteration (RPI) algorithm [8]. RPI is an approximate policy iteration algorithm where the basis functions

$\phi(s, a)$ handcoded in other methods, such as LSPI [5] are learned from a random walk of transitions by computing the graph Laplacian and then computing the eigenfunctions or the diffusion wavelet bases as described above. One striking property of the eigenfunction and diffusion wavelet basis functions is their ability to reflect nonlinearities arising from "bottlenecks" in the state space. Figure 4 contrasts the value function approximation produced by RPI using Laplacian eigenfunctions with that produced by a polynomial approximator. The polynomial approximator yields a value function that is "blind" to the nonlinearities produced by the walls in the two room grid world MDP.

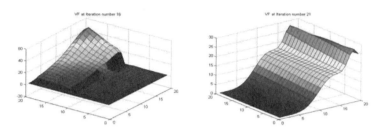

Figure 4: This figures compares the value functions produced by RPI using Laplacian eigenfunctions with that produced by LSPI using a polynomial approximator in a two room grid world MDP with a "bottleneck" region representing the door connecting the two rooms. The Laplacian basis functions on the left clearly capture the nonlinearity arising from the bottleneck, whereas the polynomial approximator on the right smooths the value function across the walls as it is "blind" to the large-scale geometry of the environment.

Table 1 compares the performance of diffusion wavelets and Laplacian eigenfunctions using RPI on the classic chain MDP from [5]. Here, an initial random walk of 5000 steps was carried out to generate the basis functions in a 50 state chain. The chain MDP is a sequential open (or closed) chain of varying number of states, where there are two actions for moving left or right along the chain. In the experiments shown, a reward of 1 was provided in states 10 and 41. Given a fixed k, the encoding $\phi(s)$ of a state s for Laplacian eigenfunctions is the vector comprised of the values of the kth lowest-order eigenfunctions on state k. For diffusion wavelets, all the basis functions at level k were evaluated at state s to produce the encoding.

Method	#Trials	Error	Method	#Trials	Error
RPI DF (5)	4.4	2.4	LSPI RBF (6)	3.8	20.8
RPI DF (14)	6.8	4.8	LSPI RBF (14)	4.4	2.8
RPI DF (19)	8.2	0.6	LSPI RBF (26)	6.4	2.8
RPI Lap (5)	4.2	3.8	LSPI Poly (5)	4.2	4
RPI Lap (15)	7.2	3	LSPI Poly (15)	1	34.4
RPI Lap (25)	9.4	2	LSPI Poly (25)	1	36

Table 1: This table compares the performance of RPI using diffusion wavelets and Laplacian eigenfunctions with LSPI using handcoded polynomial and radial basis functions on a 50 state chain graph MDP.

Each row reflects the performance of either RPI using learned basis functions or LSPI with a handcoded basis function (values in parentheses indicate the number of basis functions used for each architecture). The two numbers reported are steps to convergence and the error in the learned policy (number of incorrect actions), averaged over 5 runs. Laplacian and diffusion wavelet basis functions provide a more stable performance at both the low end and at the higher end, as compared to the handcoded basis functions. As the number of basis functions are increased, RPI with Laplacian basis functions takes longer to converge, but learns a more accurate policy. Diffusion wavelets converge slower as the number of basis functions is increased, giving the best results overall with 19 basis functions. Unlike Laplacian eigenfunctions, the policy error is not monotonically decreasing as the number of bases functions is increased. This result is being investigated. LSPI with RBF is unstable at the low end, converging to a very poor policy for 6 basis functions. LSPI with a 5 degree polynomial approximator works reasonably well, but its performance noticeably degrades at higher degrees, converging to a very poor policy in one step for $k = 15$ and $k = 25$.

6 Future Work

We are exploring many extensions of this framework, including extensions to factored MDPs, approximating action value functions as well as large state spaces by exploiting symmetries defined by a group of automorphisms of the graph. These enhancements will facilitate efficient construction of eigenfunctions and diffusion wavelets. For large state spaces, one can randomly subsample the graph, construct the eigenfunctions of the Laplacian or the diffusion wavelets on the subgraph, and then interpolate these functions using the Nyström approximation and related low-rank linear algebraic methods. In experiments on the classic inverted pendulum control task, the Nyström approximation yielded excellent results compared to radial basis functions, learning a more stable policy with a smaller number of samples.

Acknowledgements

This research was supported in part by a grant from the National Science Foundation IIS-0534999.

References

[1] D. P. Bertsekas and J. N. Tsitsiklis. *Neuro-Dynamic Programming*. Athena Scientific, Belmont, Massachusetts, 1996.

[2] J. Bremer, R. Coifman, M. Maggioni, and A. Szlam. Diffusion wavelet packets. Technical Report Tech. Rep. YALE/DCS/TR-1304, Yale University, 2004. to appear in Appl. Comp. Harm. Anal.

[3] F. Chung. *Spectral Graph Theory*. American Mathematical Society, 1997.

[4] R. Coifman and M Maggioni. Diffusion wavelets. Technical Report Tech. Rep. YALE/DCS/TR-1303, Yale University, 2004. to appear in Appl. Comp. Harm. Anal.

[5] M. Lagoudakis and R. Parr. Least-squares policy iteration. *Journal of Machine Learning Research*, 4:1107–1149, 2003.

[6] M. Maggioni and S. Mahadevan. Fast direct policy evaluation using multiscale Markov Diffusion Processes. Technical Report Tech. Rep.TR-2005-39, University of Massachusetts, 2005.

[7] S. Mahadevan. Proto-value functions: Developmental reinforcement learning. In *Proceedings of the 22nd International Conference on Machine Learning*, 2005.

[8] S. Mahadevan. Representation policy iteration. In *Proceedings of the 21st International Conference on Uncertainty in Artificial Intelligence*, 2005.

[9] S. Mahadevan. Samuel meets Amarel: Automating value function approximation using global state space analysis. In *National Conference on Artificial Intelligence (AAAI)*, 2005.

[10] M. L. Puterman. *Markov decision processes*. Wiley Interscience, New York, USA, 1994.

[11] S Rosenberg. *The Laplacian on a Riemannian Manifold*. Cambridge University Press, 1997.

Noise and the two-thirds power law

Uri Maoz[1,2,3], Elon Portugaly[3], Tamar Flash[2] and Yair Weiss[3,1]

[1] Interdisciplinary Center for Neural Computation, The Hebrew University of Jerusalem, Edmond Safra Campus, Givat Ram Jerusalem 91904, Israel; [2] Department of Computer Science and Applied Mathematics, The Weizmann Institute of Science, PO Box 26 Rehovot 76100, Israel; [3] School of Computer Science and Engineering, The Hebrew University of Jerusalem, Edmond Safra Campus, Givat Ram Jerusalem 91904, Israel

Abstract

The two-thirds power law, an empirical law stating an inverse non-linear relationship between the tangential hand speed and the curvature of its trajectory during curved motion, is widely acknowledged to be an invariant of upper-limb movement. It has also been shown to exist in eye-motion, locomotion and was even demonstrated in motion perception and prediction. This ubiquity has fostered various attempts to uncover the origins of this empirical relationship. In these it was generally attributed either to smoothness in hand- or joint-space or to the result of mechanisms that damp noise inherent in the motor system to produce the smooth trajectories evident in healthy human motion.

We show here that white Gaussian noise also obeys this power-law. Analysis of signal and noise combinations shows that trajectories that were synthetically created not to comply with the power-law are transformed to power-law compliant ones after combination with low levels of noise. Furthermore, there exist colored noise types that drive non-power-law trajectories to power-law compliance and are not affected by smoothing. These results suggest caution when running experiments aimed at verifying the power-law or assuming its underlying existence without proper analysis of the noise. Our results could also suggest that the power-law might be derived not from smoothness or smoothness-inducing mechanisms operating on the noise inherent in our motor system but rather from the correlated noise which is inherent in this motor system.

1 Introduction

A number of regularities have been empirically observed for the motion of the end-point of the human upper-limb during curved and drawing movements. One of these has been termed "the two-thirds power law" ([1]). It can be formulated as:

$$v(t) = \text{const} \cdot \kappa(t)^{\beta} \tag{1}$$

or, in log-space

$$\log\left(v(t)\right) = \text{const} + \beta \log\left(\kappa(t)\right) \tag{2}$$

851

where v is the tangential end-point speed, κ is the instantaneous curvature of the path, and β is approximately $-\frac{1}{3}$. The various studies that lend support to this power-law go beyond its simple verification. There are those that suggest it as a tool to extract natural segmentation into primitives of complex movements ([2], [3]). Others show the development of the power-law with age for children ([4]). There is also research that suggests it appears for three-dimensional (3D) drawings under isometric force conditions ([5]). It was even found in neural population coding in the monkey motor brain area controlling the hand ([6]). Other studies have located the power-law elsewhere than the hand. It was found to apply in eye-motion ([7]) and even in motion perception ([8],[9]) and movement prediction based on biological motion ([10]). Recent studies have also found it in locomotion ([11]). This power-law has thus been widely accepted as an important invariant in biological movement trajectories, so much so that it has become an evaluation criterion for the quality of models (e.g. [12]).

This has motivated various attempts to find some deeper explanation that supposedly underlies this regularity. The power-law was shown to possibly be a result of minimization of jerk ([13],[14]), jerk along a predefined path ([15]), or endpoint variability due to noise inherent in the motor system ([12]). Others have claimed that it stems from forward kinematics of sinusoidal movements at the joints ([16]). Another explanation has to do with the mathematically interesting fact that motion according to the power-law maintains constant affine velocity ([17],[18]).

We were thus very much surprised by the following:

Observation: Given a time series $(x_i, y_i)_{i=1}^n$ in which $x_i, y_i \sim N(0,1)$ i.i.d.(x_i, x_j, y_i, y_j) for $i \neq j$, and assuming that the series is of equal time intervals, calculate κ and v in order to obtain β from the linear regression of $\log(v)$ versus $\log(\kappa)$. The linear regression plot of $\log(v)$ versus $\log(\kappa)$ is within range both in its regression coefficient and R^2 value to what experimentalists consider as compliance with the power-law (see figure 1b). *Therefore this white Gaussian noise trajectory seems to fit the two-thirds power law model in equation (1) above.*

1.1 Problem formulation

For any regular planar curve parameterized with t, we get from the Frenet-Serret formulas (see [19])[1]:

$$\kappa(t) = \frac{|\ddot{x}\dot{y} - \dot{x}\ddot{y}|}{(\dot{x}^2 + \dot{y}^2)^{\frac{3}{2}}} = \frac{|\ddot{x}\dot{y} - \dot{x}\ddot{y}|}{v^3(t)} \tag{3}$$

where $v(t) = \sqrt{\dot{x}^2 + \dot{y}^2}$. Denoting $\alpha(t) = |\ddot{x}\dot{y} - \dot{x}\ddot{y}|$ we obtain:

$$v(t) = \alpha(t)^{\frac{1}{3}} \cdot \kappa(t)^{-\frac{1}{3}} \tag{4}$$

or, in log-space[2]:

$$\log(v(t)) = \frac{1}{3}\log(\alpha(t)) - \frac{1}{3}\log(\kappa(t)) \tag{5}$$

Given a trajectory for which α is constant, the power-law in equation (1) above is obtained exactly (the term α is in fact the affine velocity of [17],[18], and thus a trajectory that yields a constant α would mean movement at constant affine velocity).

---

[1]Though there exists a definition for signed curvature for planar curves (i.e. without the absolute value in the numerator of equation 3), we refer to the absolute value of the curvature, as done in the power-law. Therefore, in our case, $\kappa(t)$ is the absolute value of the instantaneous curvature.

[2]Non-linear regression in (4) should naturally be performed instead of log-space linear regression in (5). However, this linear regression in log-space is the method of choice in the motor-control literature, despite the criticism of [16]. We therefore opted for it here as well.

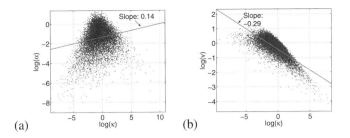

Figure 1: Given a trajectory composed of normally distributed position data with constant time intervals, we calculate and plot: **(a)** $\log(\alpha)$ versus $\log(\kappa)$ and **(b)** $\log(v)$ versus $\log(\kappa)$ with their linear regression lines. The correlation coefficient in (a) is 0.14, entailing the one in (b) to be -0.29 (see text). Moreover, the R^2 value in (a) is 0.04, much smaller than in the 0.57 value in (b).

Denoting the linear regression coefficient of $\log(v)$ versus $\log(\kappa)$ by β and the linear regression coefficient of $\log(\alpha)$ versus $\log(\kappa)$ by ξ, it can be easily shown that (5) entails:

$$\beta = -\frac{1}{3} + \frac{\xi}{3} \tag{6}$$

Hence, if $\log(\alpha)$ and $\log(\kappa)$ are statistically uncorrelated, the linear regression coefficient between them, which we termed ξ, would be 0, and thus from (6) the linear regression coefficient of $\log(v)$ versus $\log(\kappa)$, which we named β, would be exactly $-\frac{1}{3}$. Therefore, any trajectory that produces $\log(\alpha)$ and $\log(\kappa)$ that are statistically uncorrelated would precisely conform to the power-law in (1)[3].

If $\log(\alpha)$ and $\log(\kappa)$ are weakly correlated, such that ξ (the linear regression coefficient of $\log(\alpha)$ versus $\log(\kappa)$) is small, the effect on β (the linear regression coefficient of $\log(v)$ versus $\log(\kappa)$) would result in a positive offset of $\frac{\xi}{3}$ from the $-\frac{1}{3}$ value of the power-law. Below, we analyze ξ for random position data, and show that it is indeed small and that β takes values close to $-\frac{1}{3}$. Figure 1 portrays a typical $\log(v)$ versus $\log(\kappa)$ linear regression plot for the case of a trajectory composed of random data sampled from an i.i.d. normal distribution.

2 Power-law analysis for trajectories composed of normally distributed samples

Let us take the time-series $(x_i, y_i)_{i=1}^n$ where $x_i, y_i \sim N(0,1)$, i.i.d. Let t_i denote the time at sample i and for all i let $t_{i+1} - t_i = 1$. From this time series we calculate α, κ and v by central finite differences[4]. Again, we denote the linear regression coefficient of $\log(\alpha)$ versus $\log(\kappa)$ by ξ, and thus $\widehat{\log(\alpha)} = \text{const} + \xi \log(\kappa)$, where $\xi = \frac{\text{Covariance}[\log(\kappa),\log(\alpha)]}{\text{Variance}[\log(\kappa)]}$. And from (6) we know that a linear regression of $\log(v)$ versus $\log(\kappa)$ would result in $\beta = -\frac{1}{3} + \frac{\xi}{3}$.

The fact that ξ is scaled down three-fold to give the offset of β from $-\frac{1}{3}$ is significant. It means that for β to achieve values far from $-\frac{1}{3}$, ξ would need to be very big. For example,

---

[3]α being constant is naturally a special case of uncorrelated $\log(\alpha)$ and $\log(\kappa)$.

[4]We used the central finite differencing technique here mainly for ease of use and analysis. Other differentiation techniques, either utilizing more samples (e.g. the Lagrange 5-point method) or analytic differentiation of smoothing functions (e.g. smoothing splines), yielded similar results. In a more general sense, smoothing techniques introduce local correlations (between neighboring samples in time) into the trajectory. Yet globally, for large time series, the correlation remains weak.

in order for β to be 0 (i.e. motion at constant tangential speed), ξ would need to be 1, which requires perfect correlation between $\log(\alpha)$, which is a time-dependant variable, and $\log(\kappa)$, which is a geometric one. This could be taken to suggest that for a control system to maintain movement at β values that are remote from $-\frac{1}{3}$ would require some non-trivial control of the correlation between $\log(\alpha)$ and $\log(\kappa)$.

Running 100 Monte-Carlo simulations[5], each drawing a time series of 1,000,000 normally distributed points, we estimated $\xi = 0.1428 \pm 0.0013$ ($R^2 = 0.0357 \pm 0.0006$). ξ's magnitude and its corresponding R^2 value suggest that $\log(\alpha)$ and $\log(\kappa)$ are only weakly correlated (hence the ball-like shape in Figure 1a). The same type of simulations gave $\beta = -0.2857 \pm 0.0004$ ($R^2 = 0.5715 \pm 0.0011$), as expected. Both β and its R^2 magnitudes are within what is considered by experimentalists to be the range of applicable values for the power-law. Moreover, standard outlier detection and removal techniques as well as robust linear regression make β approach closer to $-\frac{1}{3}$ and increase the R^2 value.

Measurements of human drawing movements in 3D also exhibit the power-law ([20],[16]). We therefore decided to repeat the same analysis procedure for 3D data (i.e. drawing time-series $(x_i, y_i, z_i)_{i=1}^{n}$ i.i.d. from $N(0,1)$, and extracting v, α and κ according to their 3D definitions). This time we obtained $\xi = -0.0417 \pm 0.0009$ ($R^2 = 0.0036 \pm 0.0002$) and as expected $\beta = -0.3472 \pm 0.0003$ ($R^2 = 0.6944 \pm 0.0006$). This is even closer to the power-law values, as defined in (1).

This phenomenon also occurs when we repeat the procedure for trajectories composed of uniformly distributed samples with constant time intervals. The linear regression of $\log(v)$ versus $\log(\kappa)$ for planar trajectories gives $\beta = -0.2859 \pm 0.0004$ ($R^2 = 0.5724 \pm 0.0009$). 3D trajectories of uniformly distributed samples give us $\beta = -0.3475 \pm 0.0003$ ($R^2 = 0.6956 \pm 0.0007$) under the same simulation procedure. In both cases the parameters obtained for the uniform distribution are very close to those of the normal distribution.

3 Analysis of signal and noise combinations

3.1 Original (Non-filtered) signal and noise combinations

Another interesting question has to do with the combination of signal and noise. Every ex-perimentally measured signal has some noise incorporated in it, be it measurement-device noise or noise internal to the human motor system. But how much noise must be present to transform a signal that does not conform to the power-law to one that does? We took a planar ellipse with a major axis of 0.35m and minor axis of 0.13m (well within the standard range of dimensions used as templates for measuring the power-law for humans, see fig-ure 2b), and spread 120 equispaced samples over its perimeter (a typical number of samples for the sampling rate given below). The time intervals were constant at 0.01s (100 Hz is of the order of magnitude of contemporary measurement equipment). This elliptic trajec-tory is thus traversed at constant speed, despite not having constant curvature. It therefore does not obey the power-law (a "sanity check" of our simulations gave $\beta = -0.0003$, $R^2 = 0.0028$).

At this stage, normally distributed noise with various standard-deviations was added to this ellipse. We ran 100 simulations for every noise magnitude and averaged the power-law parameters β and R^2 obtained from $\log(v)$ versus $\log(\kappa)$ linear regressions for each noise magnitude (see figure 2a). The level of noise required to drive the non-power-law-compliant trajectory to obey the power-law is rather small; a standard deviation of about

---

[5]The Matlab code for this simple simulation can be found at:

http://www.cs.huji.ac.il/~urim/NIPS_2005/Monte_Carlo.m

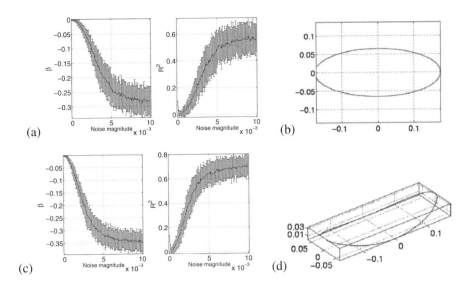

Figure 2: (a) β and R^2 values of the power-law fit for trajectories composed of the non-power-law planar ellipse given in (b) combined with various magnitudes of noise (portrayed as the standard deviations of the normally distributed noise that was added). (c) β and R^2 values for the non-power-law 3D bent ellipse given in (d). All distances are measured in meters.

0.005m is sufficient[6].

The same procedure was performed for a 3D bent-ellipse of similar proportions and perimeter in order to test the effects of noise on spatial trajectories (see figure 2c and d). We placed the samples on this bent ellipse in an equispaced manner, so that it would be traversed at constant speed (and indeed $\beta = -0.0042$, $R^2 = 0.1411$). This time the standard deviation of the noise which was required for power-law-like behavior in 3D was 0.003m or so, a bit smaller than in the planar case. Naturally, had we chosen smaller ellipses, less noise would have been required to make them obey the power-law (for instance, if we take a 0.1 by 0.05m ellipse, the same effect would be obtained with noise of about 0.002m standard deviation for the planar case and 0.0015m for a 3D bent ellipse of the same magnitude). Note that both for the planar and spatial shapes, the noise-level that drives the non-power-law signal to conform to the power-law is in the order of magnitude of the average displacement between consecutive samples.

3.2 Does filtering solve the problem?

All the analysis above was for raw data, whereas it is common practice to low-pass filter experimentally obtained trajectories before extracting κ and v. If we take a non-power-law signal, contaminate it with enough noise for it to comply with the power-law and then filter it, would the resulting signal obey the power-law or not? We attempted to answer this question by contaminating the constant-speed bent-ellipse of the previous subsection (reminder: $\beta = -0.0003$, $R^2 = 0.0028$) with Gaussian noise of standard deviation 0.005m. This resulted in a trajectory with $\beta = -0.3154 \pm 0.0323$ ($R^2 = 0.6303 \pm 0.0751$) for 100 simulation runs (actually a bit closer to the power-law than the noise alone). We then low-pass filtered each trajectory with a zero-lag second-order Butterworth filter with 10

---

[6]0.005m is about half the distance between consecutive samples in this trajectory and sampling rate.

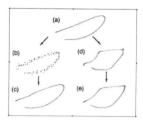

Figure 3: a graphical outline of Procedure 1 (from the top to the bottom left) and Procedure 2 (from the top to the bottom right). **(a)** The original non-power-law signal **(b)** Signal in (a) plus white noise **(c)** Signal in (b) after smoothing. **(d)** Signal in (a) with added correlated noise **(e)** Signal in (d) after smoothing. All signals but (a) and (c) obey the power-law.

Hz cutoff frequency. This returned a signal essentially without power-law compliance, i.e. $\beta = -0.0472 \pm 0.0209$ ($R^2 = 0.1190 \pm 0.0801$). Let us name this process *Procedure 1*.

But what if the noise at hand is more resistant to smoothing? Taking 3D Gaussian noise and smoothing it (using the same type of Butterworth filtering as above) does not make the resulting signal any less compliant to the power-law. Monte-Carlo simulations of smoothed random trajectories (100 repetitions of 1,000,000 samples each) resulted in $\beta = -0.3473 \pm 0.0003$ ($R^2 = 0.6945 \pm 0.0007$), which is the same as the original noise (which had $\beta = -0.3472 \pm 0.0003$, $R^2 = 0.6944 \pm 0.0006$)[7]. We therefore ran the signal plus noise simulations again, this time adding smoothed-noise (increasing its magnitude five-fold to compensate for the loss of energy of this noise due to the filtering) to the constant-speed bent-ellipse. This time the combined signal yielded a power-law fit of $\beta = -0.3175 \pm 0.0414$ ($R^2 = 0.6260 \pm 0.0798$), leaving it power-law compliant. However, this time the same filtering procedure as above left us with a signal that could still be considered to obey the power-law, with $\beta = -0.2747 \pm 0.0481$ ($R^2 = 0.5498 \pm 0.0698$). We name this process *Procedure 2*. Procedures 1 and 2 are portrayed graphically in figure 3. If we continue and increase the noise magnitude the effect of the smoothing at the end of Procedure 2 becomes less apparent, with the smoothed trajectories sometimes conforming to the power-law (mainly in terms of R^2) better than before the smoothing.

3.3   Levels of noise inherent to upper limb movement in human data

We conducted a preliminary experiment to explore the level of noise intrinsic to the human motor system. Subjects were instructed to repetitively and continuously trace ellipses in 3D while seated with their trunk restrained to the back of a rigid chair and their eyes closed (to avoid spatial cues in the room, see [16]). They were to suppose that there exists a spatial elliptical pattern before them, which they were to traverse with their hand. The 3D hand position was recorded at 100 Hz using NDI's Optotrak 2010. Given their goal, it is reasonable to assume that the variance between the trajectories in the different iterations is composed of measurement noise as well as noise internal to the subject's motor systems (since the inter-repetition drift was removed by PCA alignment after segmenting the continuous motion into underlying iterations). We thus analyzed the recorded time series in order to find that variance (see figure 4a) and compared this to the average variance of the synthetic equispaced bent ellipse combined with correlated noise (see figure 4b). While more careful experiments may be needed to extract the exact SNR of human limb movements, it appears that the level of noise in human limb movement is comparable to the level of noise that can cause power-law behavior even for non power-law signals.

---

[7]This result goes hand in hand with what was said before. Introducing local correlations between samples does not alter the power-law-from-noise phenomenon.

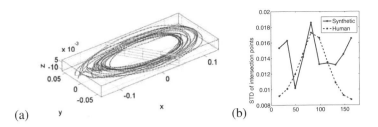

(a) y   (b)

Figure 4: Noise level in repetitive upper limb movement. The variance of the different iterations was measured at 10 different positions along the ellipse, defined by a plane passing through the origin, perpendicular to the first two principle components of the ellipses. The angles between every two neighboring planes were equal. (a) For each position, the intersection of each iteration of the trajectory with the plane was calculated. (b) The standard deviation of the different intersections of each plane was measured, and is depicted for synthetic and human data.

4 Discussion

We do not suggest that the power-law, which stems from analysis of human data, is a bogus phenomenon, resulting only from measurement noise. Yet our results do suggest caution when carrying out experiments that either aim to verify the power-law or assume its existence. When performing such experimentation, one should always be sure to verify that the signal-to-noise ratio in the system is well within the bounds where it does not drive the results toward the power-law. It might further be wise to conduct Monte-Carlo simulations with the specific parameters of the problem to ascertain this. If we focus on the measurement device noise alone, it should be noted that whereas many modern devices for planar motion measurement tend to have a measurement accuracy superior to the 0.002m or so (which we have shown to be enough to produce power-law from noise), the same cannot be said for contemporary 3D measurement devices. There, errors of magnitudes in the order of about 0.002m can certainly occur. In addition, one should keep in mind that even for smaller noise magnitudes some drift toward the power-law does occur. This must be taken into consideration when analyzing the results. Last, muscle-tremor must also be borne in mind as another source of noise, especially when dealing with pathologies.

Moreover, following the results above, it is clear that when a significant amount of noise is incorporated into the system, simply applying an off-the-shelf smoothing procedure would not necessarily satisfactorily remove it, especially if it is correlated (i.e. not white). Moreover, the smoothing procedure will most likely distort the signal to some degree, even if the noise is white. Therefore smoothing is not an easy "magic cure" for the power-law-from-noise phenomenon.

Another interesting aspect of our results has to do with the light they shed on the origins of the power-law. Previous works showed that the power-law can be derived from smoothness criteria for human trajectories, be it the assumption that these minimize the end-point's jerk ([14]), jerk along a predefined path ([15]) or variability due to noise inherent in the motor system itself ([12]), or that the power law is due to smoothing inherent in the human motor system (especially the muscles, [21]) or to smooth joint oscillations ([16]). The results presented here suggest the opposite might be true as well. The power-law can be derived from the noise itself, which is inherent in our motor system (and which is likely to be correlated noise), rather than from any smoothing mechanisms which damp it.

Acknowledgements

This research was supported in part by the HFSPO grant to T.F.; E.P. is supported by an Eshkol

857

fellowship of the Israeli Ministry of Science.

References

[1] F. Lacquaniti, C. Terzuolo, and P. Viviani. The law relating kinematic and figural aspects of drawing movements. *Acta Psychologica*, 54:115–130, 1983.

[2] P. Viviani. Do units of motor action really exist. *Experimental Brain Research*, 15:201–216, 1986.

[3] P. Viviani and M. Cenzato. Segmentation and coupling in complex movements. *Journal of Experimental Psychology: Human Perception and Performance*, 11(6):828–845, 1985.

[4] P. Viviani and R. Schneider. A developmental study of the relationship between geometry and kinematics in drawing movements. *Journal of Experimental Psychology*, 17:198–218, 1991.

[5] J. T. Massey, J. T. Lurito, G. Pellizzer, and A. P. Georgopoulos. Three-dimensional drawings in isometric conditions: relation between geometry and kinematics. *Experimental Brain Research*, 88(3):685–690, 1992.

[6] A. B. Schwartz. Direct cortical representation of drawing. *Science*, 265(5171):540–542, 1994.

[7] C. deSperati and P. Viviani. The relationship between curvature and velocity in two dimensional smooth pursuit eye movement. *The Journal of Neuroscience*, 17(10):3932–3945, 1997.

[8] P. Viviani and N. Stucchi. Biological movements look uniform: evidence of motor perceptual interactions. *Journal of Experimental Psychology: Human Perception and Performance*, 18(3):603–626, 1992.

[9] P. Viviani, G. Baud Bovoy, and M. Redolfi. Perceiving and tracking kinesthetic stimuli: further evidence of motor perceptual interactions. *Journal of Experimental Psychology: Human Perception and Performance*, 23(4):1232–1252, 1997.

[10] S. Kandel, J. Orliaguet, and P. Viviani. Perceptual anticipation in handwriting: The role of implicit motor competence. *Perception and Psychophysics*, 62(4):706–716, 2000.

[11] S. Vieilledent, Y. Kerlirzin, S. Dalbera, and A. Berthoz. Relationship between velocity and curvature of a human locomotor trajectory. *Neuroscience Letters*, 305(1):65–69, 2001.

[12] C. M. Harris and D. M. Wolpert. Signal-dependent noise determines motor planning. *Nature*, 394(6695):780–784, 1998.

[13] P. Viviani and T. Flash. Minimum-jerk, two-thirds power law, and isochrony: converging approaches to movement planning. *Journal of Experimental Psychology: Human Perception and Performance*, 21(1):32–53, 1995.

[14] M. J. Richardson and T. Flash. Comparing smooth arm movements with the two-thirds power law and the related segmented-control hypothesis. *Journal of Neuroscience*, 22(18):8201–8211, 2002.

[15] E. Todorov and M. Jordan. Smoothness maximization along a predefined path accurately predicts the speed profiles of complex arm movements. *Journal of Neurophysiology*, 80(2):696–714, 1998.

[16] S. Schaal and D. Sternad. Origins and violations of the 2/3 power law in rhythmic three-dimensional arm movements. *Experimental Brain Research*, 136(1):60–72, 2001.

[17] A. A. Handzel and T. Flash. Geometric methods in the study of human motor control. *Cognitive Studies*, 6:1–13, 1999.

[18] F. E. Pollick and G. Sapiro. Constant affine velocity predicts the 1/3 power law of planar motion perception and generation. *Vision Research*, 37(3):347–353, 1997.

[19] J. Oprea. Differential geometry and its applications. *Prentice-Hall*, 1997.

[20] U. Maoz and T. Flash. Power-laws of three-dimensional movement. *Unpublished manuscript*.

[21] P. L. Gribble and D. J. Ostry. Origins of the power law relation between movement velocity and curvature: modeling the effects of muscle mechanics and limb dynamics. *Journal of Neurophysiology*, 76:2853–2860, 1996.

858

Modeling Memory Transfer and Savings in Cerebellar Motor Learning

Naoki Masuda
RIKEN Brain Science Institute
Wako, Saitama 351-0198, Japan
masuda@brain.riken.jp

Shun-ichi Amari
RIKEN Brain Science Institute
Wako, Saitama 351-0198, Japan
amari@brain.riken.jp

Abstract

There is a long-standing controversy on the site of the cerebellar motor learning. Different theories and experimental results suggest that either the cerebellar flocculus or the brainstem learns the task and stores the memory. With a dynamical system approach, we clarify the mechanism of transferring the memory generated in the flocculus to the brainstem and that of so-called savings phenomena. The brainstem learning must comply with a sort of Hebbian rule depending on Purkinje-cell activities. In contrast to earlier numerical models, our model is simple but it accommodates explanations and predictions of experimental situations as qualitative features of trajectories in the phase space of synaptic weights, without fine parameter tuning.

1 Introduction

The cerebellum is involved in various types of motor learning. As schematically shown in Fig. 1, the cerebellum is composed of the cerebellar cortex and the cerebellar nuclei (we depict the vestibular nucleus VN in Fig. 1). There are two main pathways linking external input from the mossy fibers (mf) to motor outputs, which originate from the cerebellar nuclei. The pathway that relays the mossy fibers directly to the cerebellar nuclei is called the direct pathway. Each nucleus cell receives about 10^4 mossy fiber synapses.

The pathway involving the mossy fibers, the granule cells (gr), the parallel fibers (pl), and the Purkinje cells (Pr) in the flocculo-nodular lobes of the cerebellar cortex, is called the indirect pathway. Because the Purkinje cells, which are the sole source of output from the cerebellar cortex, are GABAergic, firing rates of the nuclei are suppressed when this pathway is active. The indirect pathway also includes recurrent collaterals terminating on various types of inhibitory cells. Another anatomical feature of the indirect pathway is that climbing fibers (Cm in Fig. 1) from the inferior olive (IO) innervate on Purkinje cells. Taking into account the huge mass of intermediate computational units in the indirect pathway, or the granule cells, Marr conjectured that the cerebellum operates as a perceptron with high computational power [8]. The climbing fibers were thought to induce long-term potentiation (LTP) of pl-Pr synapses to reinforce the signal transduction. Albus claimed that long-term depression (LTD) rather than LTP should occur so that the Purkinje cells inhibit the nuclei [2]. The climbing fibers were thought to serve as teaching lines that convey error-correcting signals.

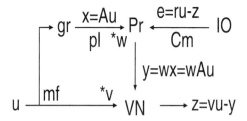

Figure 1: Architecture of the VOR model.

The vestibulo-ocular reflex (VOR) is a standard benchmark for exploring synaptic substrates of cerebellar motor learning. The VOR is a short-latency reflex eye movement that stabilizes images on the retina during head movement. Motion of the head drives eye movements in the opposite direction. When a subject wears a prism, adaptation of the VOR gain occurs for image stabilization. In this context, *in vivo* experiments confirmed that the LTD hypothesis is correct (reviewed in [6]). However, the cerebellum is not the only site of convergence of visual and vestibular signals. The learning scheme depending only on the indirect pathway is called the flocculus hypothesis. An alternative is the brainstem hypothesis in which synaptic plasticity is assumed to occur in the direct pathway ($mf \rightarrow VN$) [12]. This idea is supported by experimental evidence that flocculus shutdown after 3 days of VOR adaptation does not impair the motor memory [7]. Moreover, in other experiments, plasticity of the Purkinje cells in response to vestibular inputs, as required in the flocculus hypothesis, really occurs but in the direction opposite to that predicted by the flocculus hypothesis [5, 12]. Also, LTP of the mf-VN synapses, which is necessary to implement the brainstem hypothesis [3], has been suggested in experiments [14].

Relative contributions of the flocculus mechanism and the brainstem mechanism to motor learning remain illusive [3, 5, 9]. The same controversy exists regarding the mechanism of associative eyelid conditioning [9, 10, 11]. Related is the distinction between short-term and long-term plasticities. Many of the experiments in favor of the flocculus hypothesis are concerned with short-term learning, whereas plasticity involving the vestibular nuclei is suggested to be functional in the long term. Short-term motor memory in the flocculus may eventually be transferred to the brainstem. This is termed the memory transfer hypothesis [9]. Medina and Mauk proposed a numerical model and examined what types of brainstem learning rules are compatible with memory transfer [10]. They concluded that the brainstem plasticity should be driven by coincident activities of the Purkinje cells and the mossy fibers. The necessity of Hebbian type of learning in the direct pathway is also supported by another numerical model [13]. We propose a much simpler model to understand the essential mechanism of memory transfer without fine parameter manipulations.

Another goal of this work is to explain savings of learning. Savings are observed in natural learning tasks. Because animals can be trained just for a limited amount of time per day, the task period and the rest period, of e.g. 1 day, alternate. Performance is improved during the task period, and it degrades during the rest period (in the dark). However, when the alternation is repeated, the performance is enhanced more rapidly and progressively in later sessions [7] (also, S. Nagao, private communication). The flocculus may be responsible for daily rapid learning and forgetting, and the brainstem may underlie gradual memory consolidation [11]. While our target phenomenon of interest is the VOR, the proposed model is fairly general.

2 Model

Looking at Fig. 1, let us denote by $\mathbf{u} \in \mathbf{R}^m$ the external input to the mossy fibers. It is propagated to the granule cells via synaptic connectivity represented by an n by m matrix A, where presumably $n \gg m$. The output of the granule cells, or $\mathbf{x} \equiv A\mathbf{u} \in \mathbf{R}^n$, is received by the Purkinje-cell layer. For simplicity, we assume just one Purkinje cell whose output is written as $y \equiv \mathbf{w}x$, where $\mathbf{w} \in \mathbf{R} \times \mathbf{R}^m$. Since pl-Pr synapses are excitatory, the elements of $\mathbf{w}$ are positive. The direct pathway $(mf \to VN)$ is defined by a plastic connection matrix $\mathbf{v} \in \mathbf{R} \times \mathbf{R}^m$. The output to the VOR actuator is given by $z = \mathbf{v}\mathbf{u} - y = \mathbf{v}\mathbf{u} - \mathbf{w}A\mathbf{u}$, which is the output of the sole neuron of the cerebellar nuclei. This form of z takes into account that the contribution of the indirect pathway is inhibitory and that of the direct pathway is excitatory.

The animal learns to adapt z as close as possible to the desirable motor output $\mathbf{r}\mathbf{u}$. For a large (resp. small) desirable gain $\mathbf{r}$, the correct direction of synaptic changes is the decrease (resp. increase) in $\mathbf{w}$ and the increase (resp. decrease) in $\mathbf{v}$ [5]. The learning error $e \equiv \mathbf{r}\mathbf{u} - z$ is carried by the climbing fibers and projects onto the Purkinje cell, which enables supervised learning [6]. The LTD of $\mathbf{w}$ occurs when the parallel-fiber input and the climbing-fiber input are simultaneously large [6, 9]. Since we can write

$$\dot{\mathbf{w}} = -\eta_1 e\mathbf{x} = -\frac{1}{2}\eta_1 \frac{\partial e^2}{\partial \mathbf{w}}, \tag{1}$$

where η_1 is the learning rate, $\mathbf{w}$ evolves to minimize e^2. Equation (1) is a type of Widrow-Hoff rule [4, p. 320]. With spontaneous inputs only, or in the presence of $\mathbf{x}$ and the absence of e, $\mathbf{w}$ experiences LTP [6, 9]. We model this effect by adding $\eta_2 \mathbf{x}$ to Eq. (1). This term provides subtractive normalization that counteracts the use-dependent LTD [4, p. 290]. However, subtractive normalization cannot prohibit $\mathbf{w}$ from running away when the error signal is turned off. Therefore, we additionally assume multiplicative normalization term $\eta_3 \mathbf{w}$ to limit the magnitude of $\mathbf{w}$ [4, p. 290, 314]. In the end, Eq. (1) is modified to

$$\dot{\mathbf{w}} = -\eta_1(\mathbf{r}\mathbf{u} - \mathbf{v}\mathbf{u} + \mathbf{w}A\mathbf{u})A\mathbf{u} + \eta_2 A\mathbf{u} - \eta_3 \mathbf{w}, \tag{2}$$

where η_2 and η_3 are rates of memory decay satisfying $\eta_2, \eta_3 \ll \eta_1$.

In the dark, the VOR gain, which might have changed via adaptation, tends back to a value close to unity [5]. Let us represent this reference gain by $\mathbf{r} = \mathbf{r}_0$. With the synaptic strengths in this null condition denoted by $(\mathbf{w}, \mathbf{v}) = (\mathbf{w}_0, \mathbf{v}_0)$, we obtain $\mathbf{r}_0\mathbf{u} = \mathbf{v}_0\mathbf{u} - \mathbf{w}_0 A\mathbf{u}$. By setting $\dot{\mathbf{w}} = 0$ in Eq. (2), we derive

$$\eta_2 A\mathbf{u} = \eta_1(\mathbf{r}_0\mathbf{u} - \mathbf{v}_0\mathbf{u} + \mathbf{w}_0 A\mathbf{u})A\mathbf{u} + \eta_3 \mathbf{w}_0 = \eta_3 \mathbf{w}_0. \tag{3}$$

Substituting Eq. (3) into Eq. (2) results in

$$\dot{\mathbf{w}} = -\eta_1(\mathbf{r}\mathbf{u} - \mathbf{v}\mathbf{u} + \mathbf{w}A\mathbf{u})A\mathbf{u} - \eta_3(\mathbf{w} - \mathbf{w}_0). \tag{4}$$

Experiments show that $\mathbf{v}$ can be potentiated [14]. Enhancement of the excitability of the nucleus output (z) in response to tetanic stimulation, or sustained $\mathbf{u}$, is also in line with the LTP of v [1]. In contrast, LTD of $\mathbf{v}$ is biologically unknown. Numerical models suggest that LTP in the nuclei should be driven by y [10, 11]. However, the mechanism and the specificity underlying plasticity of $\mathbf{v}$ are not well understood [9]. Therefore, we assume that both LTP and LTD of $\mathbf{v}$ occur in an associative manner, and we represent the LTP effect by a general function F. In parallel to the learning rule of $\mathbf{w}$, we assume a subtractive normalization term $-\eta_5 \mathbf{u}$ [10]. We also add a multiplicative normalization term $\eta_6 \mathbf{v}$ to constrain $\mathbf{v}$. Finally, we obtain

$$\dot{\mathbf{v}} = \eta_4 \mathbf{F}(\mathbf{u}, y, z, e) - \eta_5 \mathbf{u} - \eta_6 \mathbf{v}. \tag{5}$$

Presumably, $\mathbf{v}$ changes much more slowly (on a time scale of 8–12 hr) than $\mathbf{w}$ changes (0.5 hr) [10, 13]. Therefore, we assume $\eta_1 \gg \eta_4 \gg \eta_5, \eta_6$.

861

3 Analysis of Memory Transfer

Let us examine a couple of learning rules in the direct pathway to identify robust learning mechanisms.

3.1 Supervised learning

Although the climbing fibers carrying e send excitatory collaterals to the cerebellar nuclei, supervised learning there has very little experimental support [5]. Here we show that supervised learning in the direct pathway is theoretically unlikely. Let us assume that modification of $\mathbf{v}$ decreases $|e|$. Accordingly, we set $\mathbf{F} = -\partial e^2 / \partial \mathbf{v} = e\mathbf{u}$. Then, Eq. (5) becomes

$$\dot{\mathbf{v}} = \eta_4(r\mathbf{u} - v\mathbf{u} + \mathbf{w}A\mathbf{u})\mathbf{u} - \eta_5\mathbf{u} - \eta_6\mathbf{v}. \tag{6}$$

In the natural situation, $\mathbf{r} = \mathbf{r}_0$. Hence,

$$\eta_5\mathbf{u} = \eta_4(r_0\mathbf{u} - v_0\mathbf{u} + \mathbf{w}_0A\mathbf{u})\mathbf{u} - \eta_6\mathbf{v}_0 = -\eta_6\mathbf{v}_0. \tag{7}$$

Inserting Eq. (7) into Eq. (6) yields

$$\dot{\mathbf{v}} = \eta_4\left(r\mathbf{u} - v\mathbf{u} + \mathbf{w}A\mathbf{u}\right)\mathbf{u} - \eta_6(\mathbf{v} - \mathbf{v}_0). \tag{8}$$

For further analysis, let us assume $m = n = 1$ (for which we quit bold notations) and perform the slow-fast analysis based on $\eta_1 \gg \eta_3, \eta_4 \gg \eta_6$. Equations (4) and (8) define the nullclines $\dot{w} = 0$ and $\dot{v} = 0$, which are represented respectively by

$$v = v_0 + r - r_0 + \frac{\eta_1 A^2 u^2 + \eta_3}{\eta_1 A u^2}(w - w_0), \quad \text{and} \tag{9}$$

$$v = v_0 + \frac{\eta_4 u^2}{\eta_4 u^2 + \eta_6}(r - r_0) + \frac{\eta_4 A u^2}{\eta_4 u^2 + \eta_6}(w - w_0). \tag{10}$$

Since $\dot{w} = O(\eta_1) \gg O(\eta_4) = \dot{v}$ in an early stage, a trajectory in the w-v plane initially approaches the fast manifold (Eq. (9)) and moves along it toward the equilibrium given by

$$w^* = w_0 - \frac{\eta_1\eta_6 A u^2(r - r_0)}{\eta_1\eta_6 A^2 u^2 + \eta_3\eta_4 u^2 + \eta_3\eta_6}, \quad v^* = v_0 + \frac{\eta_3\eta_4 u^2(r - r_0)}{\eta_1\eta_6 A^2 u^2 + \eta_3\eta_4 u^2 + \eta_3\eta_6}. \tag{11}$$

LTD of w and LTP of v are expected for adaptation to a larger gain ($r > r_0$), and LTP of w and LTD of v are expected for $r < r_0$. The results are consistent with both the flocculus hypothesis and the brainstem hypothesis as far as the direction of learning is concerned [5]. When $r > r_0$ (resp. $r < r_0$), LTD (resp. LTP) of w first occurs to decrease the learning error. Then, the motor memory stored in w is gradually transferred by LTP (resp. LTD) of v replacing LTD (resp. LTP) of w. In the long run, the memory is stored mainly in v, not in w.

However, the memory transfer based on supervised learning has fundamental deficiencies. First, since $\eta_1 \gg \eta_3$ and $\eta_4 \gg \eta_6$, both nullclines Eqs. (9) and (10) have a slope close to A in the w-v plane. This means that the relative position of the equilibrium depends heavily on the parameter values, especially on the learning rates, the choice of which is rather arbitrary. Then, (w^*, v^*) may be located so that, for example, the LTP of w or LTD of v results from $r > r_0$. Also, the degree of transfer, or $|w^* - w_0| / |v^* - v_0|$, is not robust against parameter changes. This may underlie the fact that LTD of w was not followed by partial LTP in the numerical simulations in [10]. Even if the position of (w^*, v^*) happens to support LTD of w and LTP of v, memory transfer takes a long time. This is because Eqs. (9) and (10) are fairly close, which means that $\dot{v}$ is small on the fast manifold ($\dot{w} = 0$).

We can also imagine a type of Hebbian rule with $F = \partial z^2 / \partial \mathbf{v} = z\mathbf{u}$. Similar calculations show that this rule also realizes memory transfer only in an unreliable manner.

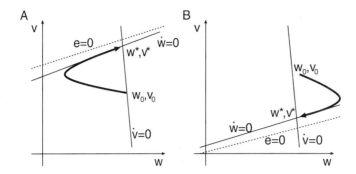

Figure 2: Dynamics of the synaptic weights in the Purkinje cell-dependent learning. (A) $r > r_0$ and (B) $r < r_0$.

3.2 Purkinje cell-dependent learning

Results of numerical studies support that $\mathbf{v}$ should be subject to a type of Hebbian learning depending on two afferents to the vestibular nuclei, namely, $\mathbf{u}$ and y [10, 11, 13]. Changes in the VOR gain are signaled by y. Since LTP should logically occur when y is small and $\mathbf{u}$ is large, we set $\mathbf{F} = (y_{max} - y)\mathbf{u}$, where y_{max} is the maximum firing rate of the Purkinje cell. Then, we obtain

$$\dot{\mathbf{v}} = \eta_4(y_{max} - \mathbf{w}A\mathbf{u})\mathbf{u} - \eta_5\mathbf{u} - \eta_6\mathbf{v}. \tag{12}$$

The subtraction normalization is determined from the equilibrum condition:

$$\eta_5\mathbf{u} = \eta_4(y_{max} - \mathbf{w}_0 A\mathbf{u}) - \eta_6\mathbf{v}_0. \tag{13}$$

Substituting Eq. (13) into Eq. (12) yields

$$\dot{\mathbf{v}} = \eta_4(\mathbf{w}_0 - \mathbf{w})A\mathbf{u}^2 + \eta_6(\mathbf{v}_0 - \mathbf{v}). \tag{14}$$

When $m = n = 1$, the nullclines are given by Eq. (9) and

$$v = v_0 - \frac{\eta_4 A u^2}{\eta_6}(w - w_0), \tag{15}$$

which are depicted in Fig. 2(A) and (B) for $r > r_0$ and $r < r_0$, respectively. As shown by arrows in Fig. 2, trajectories in the w-v space first approach the fast manifold Eq. (9) and then move along it toward the equilibrium given by

$$w^* = w_0 - \frac{\eta_1\eta_6 A u^2(r - r_0)}{\eta_1\eta_4 A^2 u^4 + \eta_1\eta_6 A^2 u^2 + \eta_3\eta_6}, \quad v^* = v_0 + \frac{\eta_1\eta_4 A^2 u^4(r - r_0)}{\eta_1\eta_4 A^2 u^4 + \eta_1\eta_6 A^2 u^2 + \eta_3\eta_6}. \tag{16}$$

Equation (15) has a large negative slope because $\eta_4 \gg \eta_6$. Consequently, setting $r > r_0$ (resp. $r < r_0$) duly results in LTD (resp. LTP) of w and LTP (resp. LTD) of v. At the same time, LTD (resp. LTP) of w in an early stage of learning is partially compensated by subsequent LTP (resp. LTD) of w, which agrees with previously reported numerical results [10]. In contrast to the supervised and Hebbian learning rules, this learning is robust against parameter changes since the positions and the slopes of the two nullclines are apart from each other. Owing to this property, in the long term, the memory is transferred more rapidly along the w-nullcline than for the other two learning rules. Another benefit of the large negative slope of Eq. (15) is that $|v^* - v_0| \gg |w^* - w_0|$ holds, which means efficient memory transfer from w to v.

The error at the equilibrum state is

$$e^* = \frac{\eta_3 \eta_6 (r - r_0) u}{\eta_1 \eta_4 A^2 u^4 + \eta_1 \eta_6 A^2 u^2 + \eta_3 \eta_6}. \tag{17}$$

Equation (17) guarantees that the $e = 0$ line is located as shown in Fig. 2, and the learning proceeds so as to decrease $|e|$. The performance overshoot, which is unrealistic, does not occur.

4   Numerical Simulations of Savings

The learning rule proposed in Sec. 3.2 explains savings as well. To show this, we mimic a situation of savings by periodically alternating the task period and the rest period. Specifically, we start with $r = r_0 = 1$, $w = w_0$, $v = v_0$, and the learning condition ($r = 2$ or $r = 0.5$) is applied for 4 hours a day. During the rest of the day (20 hours), the dark condition is simulated by giving no teaching signal to the model. Changes in the VOR gains for 8 consecutive days are shown in Fig. 3(A) and (C) for $r = 2$ and $r = 0.5$, respectively. The numerical results are consistent with the savings found in other reported experiments [7] and models [11]; the animal forgets much of the acquired gain in the dark, while a small fraction is transferred each day to the cerebellar nuclei. The time-dependent synaptic weights are shown in Fig. 3(B) ($r = 2$) and (D) ($r = 0.5$) and suggest that v is really responsible for savings and that its plasticity needs guidance under the short-term learning of w. The memory transfer occurs even in the dark condition, as indicated by the increase (resp. decrease) of v in the dark shown in Fig. 3(B) (resp. (D)). This happens because ruin of the short-term memory of w drives the learning of v for some time even after the daily training has finished. For the indirect pathway, a dark condition defines an off-task period during which w gradually loses its associations.

For comparison, let us deal with the case in which v is fixed. Then, the learning rule Eq. (4) is reduced to

$$\dot{w} = -\eta_1 \left[(r - r_0) u + (w - w_0) Au \right] Au - \eta_3 (w - w_0). \tag{18}$$

The VOR adaptation with this rule is shown in Fig. 4(A) ($r = 2$) and (B) ($r = 0.5$). Long-term retention of the acquired gain is now impossible, whereas the short-term learning, or the adaptation within a day, deteriorates little. Since savings do not occur, the ultimate learning error is larger than when v is plastic.

However, if w is fixed and v is plastic, the VOR gain is not adaptive, since y does not carry teaching signals any longer. In this case, we must implement supervised learning of v for learning to occur. Then, r adapts only gradually on the slow time scale of η_4, and the short-term learning is lost.

5   Discussion

Our model explains how the flocculus and the brainstem cooperate in motor learning. Presumably, the indirect pathway involving the flocculus is computationally powerful because of a huge number of intermediate granule cells, but its memory is of short-term nature. The direct pathway bypassing the mossy fibers to the cerebellar nuclei is likely to have less computational power but stores motor memory for a long period. A part of the motor memory is expected to be passed from the flocculus to the nuclei. This happens in a robust manner if the direct pathway is equipped with the learning rule dependent on correlation between the Purkinje-cell firing and the mossy-fiber firing. To explore whether associative LTP/LTD in the cerebellar nuclei really exists will be a subject of future experimental work. Our model is also applicable to savings.

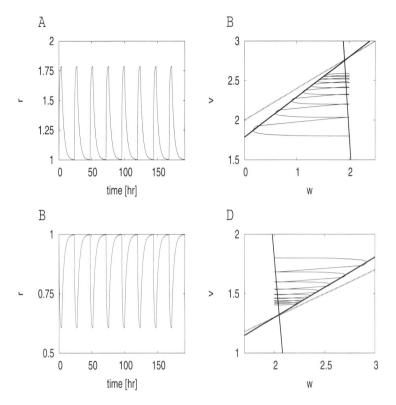

Figure 3: Numerical simulations of savings with the Purkinje cell-dependent learning rule. We set $A = 0.4$, $u = 1$, $w_0 = 2$, $r_0 = 1$, $v_0 = r_0 + Aw_0$, $\eta_1 = 7$, $\eta_3 = 0.3$, $\eta_4 = 0.05$, $\eta_6 = 0.002$. The target gains are (A, B) $r = 2$ and (C, D) $r = 0.5$. (A) and (C) show VOR gains. (B) and (D) show trajectories in the w-v space (thin solid lines) together with the nullclines (thick solid lines) and $e = 0$ (thick dotted lines).

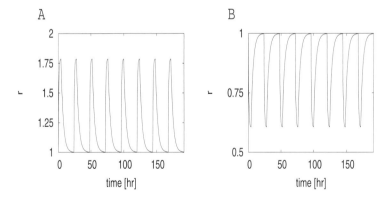

Figure 4: Numerical simulations of savings with fixed v. The parameter values are the same as those used in Fig. 3. The target gains are (A) $r = 2$ and (B) $r = 0.5$.

In the earlier models [10, 11], quantitative meanings were given to the equilibrium synaptic weights. Actually, they are solely determined from non-experimentally determined parameters, namely, the balance between the learning rates (in our terminology, η_1, η_2, η_4 and η_5). Also, the balance seems to play a role in preventing runaway of synaptic weights. In contrast, our model uses the ratio of learning rates (and values of other parameters) just for qualitative purposes and is capable of explaning and predicting experimental settings without parameter tuning. For example, the earlier arguments negating the flocculus hypothesis are based on the fact that the plasticity of the flocculus (**w**) responding to vestibular inputs occurs but in the direction opposite to the expectation of the flocculus hypothesis [5, 12]. However, this experimental observation is not necessarily contradictory to either the flocculus hypothesis or the two-site hypothesis. As shown in Fig. 2(A), when adapting to a large VOR gain, **w** experiences LTD in the initial stage [6]. Then, partial LTP ensues as the motor memory is transferred to the nuclei. Another prediction is about adaptation to a small gain. Figure 2(B) predicts that, in this case, LTP in the indirect pathway is gradually transferred to LTD in the direct pathway. Partial LTD following LTP is anticipated in the flocculus. This implies savings in unlearning.

Acknowledgments

We thank S. Nagao for helpful discussions. This work was supported by the Special Postdoctoral Researchers Program of RIKEN.

References

[1] C. D. Aizenman, D. J. Linden. Rapid, synaptically driven increases in the intrinsic excitability of cerebellar deep nuclear neurons. *Nat. Neurosci., 3*, 109–111 (2000).

[2] J. S. Albus. A theory of cerebellar function. *Math. Biosci., 10*, 25–61 (1971).

[3] E. S. Boyden, A. Katoh, J. L. Raymond. Cerebellum-dependent learning: the role of multiple plasticity mechanisms. *Annu. Rev. Neurosci., 27*, 581–609 (2004).

[4] P. Dayan, L. F. Abbott. Theoretial Neuroscience — Computational and Mathematical Modeling of Neural Systems. MIT (2001).

[5] S. du Lac, J. L. Raymond, T. J. Sejnowski, S. G. Lisberger. Learning and memory in the vestibulo-ocular reflex. *Annu. Rev. Neurosci., 18*, 409–441 (1995).

[6] M. Ito. Long-term depression. *Ann. Rev. Neurosci., 12*, 85–102 (1989).

[7] A. E. Luebke, D. A. Robinson. Gain changes of the cat's vestibulo-ocular reflex after flocculus deactivation. *Exp. Brain Res., 98*, 379–390 (1994).

[8] D. Marr. A theory of cerebellar cortex. *J. Physiol., 202*, 437–470 (1969).

[9] M. D. Mauk. Roles of cerebellar cortex and nuclei in motor learning: contradictions or clues? *Neuron, 18*, 343–346 (1997).

[10] J. F. Medina, M. D. Mauk. Simulations of cerebellar motor learning: computational analysis of plasticity at the mossy fi ber to deep nucleus synapse. *J. Neurosci., 19*, 7140–7151 (1999).

[11] J. F. Medina, K. S. Garcia, M. D. Mauk. A mechanism for savings in the cerebellum. *J. Neurosci., 21*, 4081–4089 (2001).

[12] F. A. Miles, D. J. Braitman, B. M. Dow. Long-term adaptive changes in primate vestibulooptvocular reflex. IV. Electrophysiological observations in flocculus of adapted monkeys. *J. Neurophysiol., 43*, 1477–1493 (1980).

[13] B. W. Peterson, J. F. Baker, J. C. Houk. A model of adaptive control of vestibuloocular reflex based on properties of cross-axis adaptation. *Ann. New York Acad. Sci. 627*, 319–337 (1991).

[14] R. J. Racine, D. A. Wilson, R. Gingell, D. Sunderland. Long-term potentiation in the interpositus and vestibular nuclei in the rat. *Exp. Brain Res., 63*, 158–162 (1986).

An exploration-exploitation model based on norepinepherine and dopamine activity

Samuel M. McClure[*], **Mark S. Gilzenrat**, and **Jonathan D. Cohen**
Center for the Study of Brain, Mind, and Behavior
Princeton University
Princeton, NJ 08544
smcclure@princeton.edu; mgilzen@princeton.edu; jdc@princeton.edu

Abstract

We propose a model by which dopamine (DA) and norepinepherine (NE) combine to alternate behavior between relatively exploratory and exploitative modes. The model is developed for a target detection task for which there is extant single neuron recording data available from locus coeruleus (LC) NE neurons. An exploration-exploitation trade-off is elicited by regularly switching which of the two stimuli are rewarded. DA functions within the model to change synaptic weights according to a reinforcement learning algorithm. Exploration is mediated by the state of LC firing, with higher tonic and lower phasic activity producing greater response variability. The opposite state of LC function, with lower baseline firing rate and greater phasic responses, favors exploitative behavior. Changes in LC firing mode result from combined measures of response conflict and reward rate, where response conflict is monitored using models of anterior cingulate cortex (ACC). Increased long-term response conflict and decreased reward rate, which occurs following reward contingency switch, favors the higher tonic state of LC function and NE release. This increases exploration, and facilitates discovery of the new target.

1 Introduction

A central problem in reinforcement learning is determining how to adaptively move between exploitative and exploratory behaviors in changing environments. We propose a set of neurophysiologic mechanisms whose interaction may mediate this behavioral shift. Empirical work on the midbrain dopamine (DA) system has suggested that this system is particularly well suited for guiding exploitative behaviors. This hypothesis has been reified by a number of studies showing that a temporal difference (TD) learning algorithm accounts for activity in these neurons in a wide variety of behavioral tasks [1,2]. DA release is believed to encode a reward prediction error signal that acts to change synaptic weights relevant for producing behaviors [3]. Through learning, this allows neural pathways to predict future expected reward through the relative strength of their synaptic connections

[1]. Decision-making procedures based on these value estimates are necessarily greedy. Including reward bonuses for exploratory choices supports non-greedy actions [4] and accounts for additional data derived from DA neurons [5]. We show that combining a DA learning algorithm with models of response conflict detection [6] and NE function [7] produces an effective annealing procedure for alternating between exploration and exploitation.

NE neurons within the LC alternate between two firing modes [8]. In the first mode, known as the phasic mode, NE neurons fire at a low baseline rate but have relatively robust phasic responses to behaviorally salient stimuli. The second mode, called the tonic mode, is associated with a higher baseline firing and absent or attenuated phasic responses. The effects of NE on efferent areas are modulatory in nature, and are well captured as a change in the gain of efferent inputs so that neuronal responses are potentiated in the presence of NE [9]. Thus, in phasic mode, the LC provides transient facilitation in processing, time-locked to the presence of behaviorally salient information in motor or decision areas. Conversely, in tonic mode, higher overall LC discharge rate increases gain generally and hence increases the probability of arbitrary responding. Consistent with this account, for periods when NE neurons are in the phasic mode, monkey performance is nearly perfect. However, when NE neurons are in the tonic mode, performance is more erratic, with increased response times and error rate [8]. These findings have led to a recent characterization of the LC as a dynamic temporal filter, adjusting the system's relative responsivity to salient and irrelevant information [8]. In this way, the LC is ideally positioned to mediate the shift between exploitative and exploratory behavior.

The parameters that underlie changes in LC firing mode remain largely unexplored. Based on data from a target detection task by Aston-Jones and colleagues [10], we propose that LC firing mode is determined in part by measures of response conflict and reward rate as calculated by the ACC and OFC, respectively [8]. Together, the ACC and OFC are the principle sources of cortical input to the LC [8]. Activity in the ACC is known, largely through human neuroimaging experiments, to change in accord with response conflict [6]. In brief, relatively equal activity in competing behavioral responses (reflecting uncertainty) produces high conflict. Low conflict results when one behavioral response predominates. We propose that increased long-term response conflict biases the LC towards a tonic firing mode. Increased conflict necessarily follows changes in reward contingency. As the previously rewarded target no longer produces reward, there will be a relative increase in response ambiguity and hence conflict. This relationship between conflict and LC firing is analogous to other modeling work [11], which proposes that increased tonic firing reflects increased environmental uncertainty.

As a final component to our model, we hypothesize that the OFC maintains an ongoing estimate in reward rate, and that this estimate of reward rate also influences LC firing mode. As reward rate increases, we assume that the OFC tends to bias the LC in favor of phasic firing to target stimuli.

We have aimed to fix model parameters based on previous work using simpler networks. We use parameters derived primarily from a previous model of the LC by Gilzenrat and colleagues [7]. Integration of response conflict by the ACC and its influence on LC firing was borrowed from unpublished work by Gilzenrat and colleagues in which they fit human behavioral data in a diminishing utilities task. Given this approach, we interpret our observed improvement in model performance with combined NE and DA function as validation of a mechanism for automatically switching between exploitative and exploratory action selection.

2 Go-No-Go Task and Core Model

We have modeled an experiment in which monkeys performed a target detection task [10]. In the task, monkeys were shown either a vertical bar or a horizontal bar and were required to make or omit a motor response appropriately. Initially, the vertical bar was the target stimulus and correctly responding was rewarded with a squirt of fruit juice ($r=1$ in the model). Responding to the non-target horizontal stimulus resulted in time out punishment ($r=-.1$; Figure 1A). No responses to either the target or non-target gave zero reward.

After the monkeys had fully acquired the task, the experimenters periodically switched the reward contingency such that the previously rewarded stimulus (target) became the distractor, and vice versa. Following such reversals, LC neurons were observed to change from emitting phasic bursts of firing to the target, to tonic firing following the switch, and slowly back to phasic firing for the new target as the new response criteria was obtained [10].

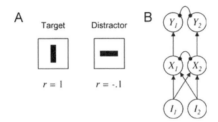

Figure 1: Task and model design. (A) Responses were required for targets in order to obtain reward. Responses to distractors resulted in a minor punishment. No responses gave zero reward. (B) In the model, vertical and horizontal bar inputs (I_1 and I_2) fed to integrator neurons (X_1 and X_2) which then drove response units (Y_1 and Y_2). Responses were made if Y_1 or Y_2 crossed a threshold while input units were active.

We have previously modeled this task [7,12] with a three-layer connectionist network in which two input units, I_1 and I_2, corresponding to the vertical and horizontal bars, drive two mutually inhibitory integrator units, X_1 and X_2. The integrator units subsequently feed two response units, Y_1 and Y_2 (Figure 1B). Responses are made whenever output from Y_1 or Y_2 crosses a threshold level of activity, θ. Relatively weak cross connections from each input unit to the opposite integrator unit (I_1 to X_2 and I_2 to X_1) are intended to model stimulus similarity.

Both the integrator and response units were modeled as noisy, leaky accumulators:

$$\dot{X}_i = -X_i + w_{X_i I_i} I_i + w_{X_i I_j} I_j - w_{X_i X_j} f(X_j) + \xi_i \tag{1}$$

$$\dot{Y}_i = -Y_i + w_{Y_i X_i} f(X_i) - w_{Y_i Y_j} f(Y_j) + \xi_i. \tag{2}$$

The ξ_i terms represent stochastic noise variables. The response function for each unit is sigmoid with gain, g_t, determined by current LC activity (Eq. 9, below)

$$f(X) = \left(1 + e^{-g_t(X-b)}\right)^{-1}. \tag{3}$$

Response units, Y, were given a positive bias, b, and integrator units were unbiased. All weight values, biases, and variance of noise are as reported in [7].

Integration was done with a Euler method at time steps of 0.02. Simulation of stimulus presentations involved setting one of the input units to a value of 1.0 for 20 units of model time. Activation of I_1 and I_2 were alternated and 20 units of model time were allowed between presentations for the integrator and response units to relax to baseline levels of activity. Input 1 was initially set to be the target and input 2 the distractor. After 50 presentations of I_1 and I_2 the reward contingencies were switched; the model was run through 6 such blocks and reversals. The response during each stimulus presentation was determined by which of the two response units first crossed a threshold of output activity (i.e. $f(Y_1) > \theta$), or was a no response if neither unit crossed threshold.

3 Performance of model with DA-mediated learning

In order to obtain a benchmark level of performance to compare against, we first determined how learning progresses with DA-mediated reinforcement learning alone. A reward unit, r, was included that had activity 0 except at the end of each stimulus presentation when its activity was set equal to the obtained reward outcome. Inhibitory inputs from the response units served as measures of expected reward. At the end of every trial, the DA unit, δ, obtained a value given by

$$\delta(t) = r(t) - w_{\delta Y_1} Z(Y_1(t)) - w_{\delta Y_2} Z(Y_2(t)) \qquad (4)$$

where $Z(Y)$ is a threshold function that is 1 if $f(Y) \geq \theta$ and is 0 otherwise.

The output of dopamine neurons was used to update the weights along the pathway that lead to the response. Thus, at the end of every stimulus presentation, the weights between response units and DA neurons were updated according to

$$w_{\delta Y_i}(t+1) = w_{\delta Y_i}(t) + \lambda \delta(t) Z(Y_i) \qquad (5)$$

where the learning rate, λ, was set to 0.3 for all simulations. This learning rule allowed the weights to converge to the expected reward for selecting each of the two actions. Weights between integrator and response units were updated using the same rule as in Eq. 5, except the weights were restricted to a minimum value of 0.8. When the weight values were allowed to decrease below 0.8, sufficient activity never accumulated in the response units to allow discovery to new reward contingencies.

As the model learned, the weights along the target pathway obtained a maximum value while those along the distractor pathway obtained a minimum value. After reversals, the model initially adapted by reducing the weights along the pathway associated with the previous target. The only way the model was able to obtain the new target was by noise pushing the new target response unit above threshold. Because of this, the performance of the model was greatly dependent of the value of the threshold used in the simulation (Figure 2B). When the threshold was low relative to noise, the model was able to quickly adapt to reversals. However, this also resulted in a high rate of responding to non-target stimuli even after learning. In order to reduce responding to the distractor, the threshold had to be raised, which also increased the time required to adapt following reward reversals.

The network was initialized with equal preference for responding to input 1 or 2, and generally acquired the initial target faster than after reversals (see Figure 2B). Because of this, all subsequent analyses ignore this first learning period. For each value of threshold studied, we ran the model 100 times. Plots shown in Figures 2 and 3 show the probability that the model responded, when each input was activated, as a function of trial number (i.e. $P(f(Y_i) \geq \theta \mid I_i = 1)$).

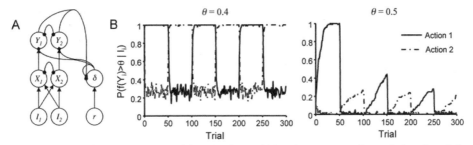

Figure 2: Model performance with DA alone. (A) DA neurons, δ, modulated weights from integrator to response units in order to modulate the probability of responding to each input. (B) The model successfully increases and decreases responding to inputs 1 and 2 as reward contingencies reverse. However, the model is unable to simultaneously obtain the new response quickly and maintain a low error rate once the response is learned. When threshold is relatively low (left plot), the model adapts quickly but makes frequent responses to the distractor. At higher threshold, responses are correctly omitted to the distractor, but the model acquires the new response slowly.

4   Improvement with NE-mediated annealing

We used the FitzHugh-Nagumo set of differential equations to model LC activity. (These equations are generally used to model individual neurons, but we use them to model the activity in the nucleus as a whole.) Previous work has shown that these equations, with simple modifications, capture the fundamental aspects of tonic and phasic mode activity in the LC [7]. The FitzHugh-Nagumo equations involve two interacting variables v and u, where v is an activity term and u is an inhibitory dampening term. The output of the LC is given by the value of u, which conveniently captures the fact that the LC is self-inhibitory and that the post-synaptic effect of NE release is somewhat delayed [7].

The model included two inputs to the LC from the integrator units (X_1 and X_2) with modifiable weights. The state of the LC is then given by

$$\tau_v \dot{v} = v(\alpha - v)(v - 1) - u + w_{vX_1} f(X_1) + w_{vX_2} f(X_2) \tag{6}$$

$$\tau_u \dot{u} = h(v) - u \tag{7}$$

where the function h is defined by

$$h(v) = Cv + (1 - C)d \tag{8}$$

and governs the firing mode of the LC. In order to change firing mode, h can be modified so that the dynamics of u depend entirely on the state of the LC or so that the dynamics are independent of state. This alternation is governed by the parameter C. When C is equal to 1.0, the model is appropriately dampened and can burst sharply and return to a relatively low baseline level of activity (phasic mode). When C is small, the LC receives a fixed level of inhibition, which simultaneously reduces bursting activity and increases baseline activity (tonic mode) [7].

The primary function of the LC in the model is to modify the gain, g, of the response function of the integrator and response units as in equation 3. We let gain be a linear function of u with base value G and dependency on u given by k

$$g_t = G + ku_t. \tag{9}$$

871

The value of C was updated after every trial by measures of response conflict and reward rate. Response conflict was calculated as a normalized measure of the energy in the response units during the trial. For convenience, define $\mathbf{Y_1}$ to be a vector of the activity in unit Y_1 at each point of time during a trial, $f(Y_1(t))$. Let $\mathbf{Y_2}$ be defined similarly. The conflict during the trial is

$$K = \frac{\mathbf{Y_1} \cdot \mathbf{Y_2}}{|\mathbf{Y_1}||\mathbf{Y_2}|} \qquad (10)$$

which correctly measures energy since Y_1 and Y_2 are connected with weight -1. This normalization procedure was necessary to account for changes in the magnitude of Y_1 and Y_2 activity due to learning.

Based on previous work [8], we let conflict modify C separately based on a short-term, K_S, and long-term, K_L, measure. The variable K_S was updated at the end of every Tth trial according to

$$K_S(T+1) = (1 - \varepsilon_S)K_S(T) + \varepsilon_S K(T). \qquad (11)$$

where ε_S was 0.2 and $K_S(T+1)$ was used to calculate the value of C used for the $T+1$th trial. K_L was update with the same rule as K_S except ε_L was 0.05. We let short- and long-term conflict have opposing effect on the firing mode of the LC. This was developed previously to capture human behavior in a diminishing utilities task. When short-term conflict increases, the LC is biased towards phasic firing (increased C). This allows the model to recover from occasional errors. However, when long-term conflict increases this is taken to indicate that the current decision strategy is not working. Therefore, increased long-term conflict biases the LC to the tonic mode so as to increase response volatility.

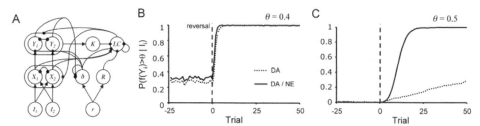

Figure 3: Model performance with DA and NE. (A) The full model includes a conflict detection unit, K, and a reward rate measure, R, which combine to modify activity in the LC. The LC modifies the gain in the integrator and response units. (B) The benefit of including the LC in the model is insignificant when the response threshold is regularly crossed by noise alone, and hence when the error rate is high. (C) However, when the threshold is greater and error rate lower, NE dramatically improves the rate at which the new reward contingencies are learned after reversal.

Reward rate, R, was updated at the end of every trial according to

$$R(T+1) = (1 - \varepsilon_R)R(T) + \varepsilon_R r \qquad (12)$$

where r is the reward earned on the Tth trial. Increased reward rate was assumed to bias the LC to phasic firing.

Reward rate, short-term conflict, and long-term conflict updated C according to

$$C = \sigma(K_S)(1 - \sigma(K_L))\sigma(R) \qquad (13)$$

872

where each σ is a sigmoid function with a gain of 6.0 and no bias as determined by fitting to behavior with previous models.

As with the model with DA alone, the effect of NE depended significantly on the value of the threshold θ. When θ was small, the improvement afforded by the LC was negligible (Figure 3B). However, when the threshold was significantly greater than noise, the improvement was substantial (Figure 3C).

Monkeys were able to perform this task with accuracy greater than 90% and simultaneously were able to adapt to reversals within 50 trials [10]. While it is impossible to compare the output of our model with monkey behavior, we can make the qualitative assertion that, as with monkeys, our NE-based annealing model allows for high accuracy (and high threshold) decision-making while preserving adaptability to changes in reward contingencies. In order to better demonstrate this improvement, we fit single exponential curves to the plots of probability of accurately responding to the new target by trial number (as in Figure 3B,C). Shown in Figure 4 is the time constant for these exponential fits, which we term the discovery time constant, for different values of the threshold. As can be seen, the model with NE-mediated annealing maintains a relatively fast discovery time even as the threshold becomes relatively large.

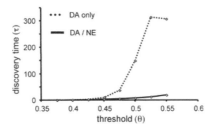

Figure 4: Summary of model performance with and without NE.

5 Discussion

We have demonstrated that a model incorporating behavioral and learning effects previously ascribed to DA and NE produces an adaptive mechanism for switching between exploratory and exploitative decision-making. Our model uses measures of response conflict and reward rate to modify LC firing mode, and hence to change network dynamics in favor of more or less volatile behavior. In essence, combining previous models of DA and NE function produces a performance-based auto-annealing algorithm.

There are several limitations to this model that can be remedied by greater sophistication in the learning algorithm. The primary limitation is that the model varies between more or less volatile action selection only over the range of reward relevant to our studied task. Model parameters could be altered on a task-by-task basis to correct this; however, a more general scheme may be accomplished with a mean reward learning algorithm [13]. It has previously been argued that DA neurons may actually emit an average reward TD error [14]. This change may require allowing both short- and long-term reward rate control the LC firing mode (Eq. 13).

Another limitation of this model is that, while exploration is increased as performance measures wane, exploration is not managed intelligently. This does not significantly affect the performance of our model since there are only two available actions. As the number of alternatives increases, rapid learning may require something akin to reward bonuses [4,5].

Understanding the interplay between DA and NE function in learning and decision-making is also relevant for understanding disease. Numerous psychiatric disorders are known to involve dysregulation of NE and DA release. Furthermore, hallmark features of ADHD and schizophrenia include cognitive disorders in which behavior appears either too volatile (ADHD) or too inflexible (schizophrenia) [15,16]. Improved models of DA-NE interplay during learning and decision-making, coupled with empirical data, may simultaneously improve knowledge of how the brain handles the exploration-exploitation dilemma and how this goes awry in disease.

Acknowledgments

This work was supported by NIH grants P50 MH62196 and MH065214.

References

[1] Montague, P.R. Dayan, P., Sejnowski, T.J. (1996) A framework for mesencephalic dopamine systems based on predictive Hebbian learning. *J. Neurosci.* **16**: 1936-1947.

[2] Schultz, W. Dayan, P. & Montague, P.R. (1997) A neural substrate for prediction and reward. *Science* **275**: 1593-1599.

[3] Reynolds, J.N., Hyland, B.I., Wickens, J.R. (2001) A cellular mechanism of reward-related learning. *Nature* **413**: 67-70.

[4] Sutton, R.S. (1990) Integrated architectures for learning, planning, and reacting based on approximated dynamic programming. *Mach. Learn., Proc. 7th International Conf.* 216-224.

[5] Kakade, S., Dayan, P. (2002) Dopamine: generalization and bonuses. *Neural Networks* **15**: 549-559.

[6] Botvinick, M.M., Braver, T.S., Barch, D.M., Carter, C.S., Cohen, J.D. (2001) Conflict monitoring and cognitive control. *Psychol. Rev.* **108**: 624-652.

[7] Gilzenrat, M.S., Holmes, B.D., Rajkowski, J., Aston-Jones, G., Cohen, J.D. (2002) Simplified dynamics in a model of noradrenergic modulation of cognitive performance. *Neural Networks* **15**: 647-663.

[8] Aston-Jones, G., Cohen, J.D. (2005) An integrative theory of locus coeruleus-norepinepherine function. *Ann. Rev. Neurosci.* **28**: 403-450.

[9] Servan-Schreiber, D., Printz, H., Cohen, J.D. (1990) A network model of catecholamine effects: gain, signal-to-noise ratio and behavior. *Science* **249**: 892-895.

[10] Aston-Jones, G., Rajkowski, J., Kubiak, P. (1997) Conditioned responses of monkey locus coeruleus neurons anticipate acquisition of discriminative behavior in a vigilance task. *Neuroscience* **80**: 697-715.

[11] Yu, A., Dayan, P. (2005) Uncertainty, neuromodulation and attention. *Neuron* **46**: 681-92.

[11] Usher, M., Cohen, J.D., Rajkowski, J., Aston-Jones, G. (1999) The role of the locus coeruleus in the regulation of cognitive performance. *Science* **283**: 549-554.

[12] Schwartz, A. (1993) A reinforcement learning method for maximizing undiscounted rewards. In: *Proc. 10th International Conf. Mach. Learn.* (pp. 298-305). San Mateo, CA: Morgan Kaufmann.

[13] Daw, N.D., Touretzky, D.S. (2002) Long-term reward prediction in TD models of the dopamine system. *Neural Computation* **14**: 2567-2583.

[14] Goldberg, T.E., Weinberger, D.R., Berman, K.F., Pliskin, N.H., Podd, M.H. (1987) Further evidence for dementia of the prefrontal type in schizophrenia? A controlled study teaching the Wisconsin Card Sorting Test. *Arch. Gen. Psychiatry* **44**: 1008-1014.

[15] Barkley, R.A. (1997) Behavioural inhibition, sustained attention, and executive functions: constructing a unified theory of AD/HD. *Psychol. Bull.* **121**: 65-94.

Online Discovery and Learning of Predictive State Representations

Peter McCracken
Department of Computing Science
University of Alberta
Edmonton, Alberta
Canada, T6G 2E8
peterm@cs.ualberta.ca

Michael Bowling
Department of Computing Science
University of Alberta
Edmonton, Alberta
Canada, T6G 2E8
bowling@cs.ualberta.ca

Abstract

Predictive state representations (PSRs) are a method of modeling dynamical systems using only observable data, such as actions and observations, to describe their model. PSRs use predictions about the outcome of future tests to summarize the system state. The best existing techniques for discovery and learning of PSRs use a Monte Carlo approach to explicitly estimate these outcome probabilities. In this paper, we present a new algorithm for discovery and learning of PSRs that uses a gradient descent approach to compute the predictions for the current state. The algorithm takes advantage of the large amount of structure inherent in a valid prediction matrix to constrain its predictions. Furthermore, the algorithm can be used online by an agent to constantly improve its prediction quality; something that current state of the art discovery and learning algorithms are unable to do. We give empirical results to show that our constrained gradient algorithm is able to discover core tests using very small amounts of data, and with larger amounts of data can compute accurate predictions of the system dynamics.

1 Introduction

Representations of state in dynamical systems fall into three main categories. Methods like k-order Markov models attempt to identify state by remembering what has happened in the past. Methods such as partially observable Markov decision processes (POMDPs) identify state as a distribution over postulated base states. A more recently developed group of algorithms, known as *predictive representations*, identify state in dynamical systems by predicting what will happen in the future. Algorithms following this paradigm include observable operator models [1], predictive state representations [2, 3], TD-Nets [4] and TPSRs [5]. In this research we focus on predictive state representations (PSRs). PSRs are completely grounded in data obtained from the system, and they have been shown to be at least as general and as compact as other methods, like POMDPs [3].

Until recently, algorithms for discovery and learning of PSRs could be used only in special cases. They have required explicit control of the system using a reset action [6, 5], or have required the incoming data stream to be generated using an open-loop policy [7].

The algorithm presented in this paper does not require a reset action, nor does it make any assumptions about the policy used to generate the data stream. Furthermore, we focus on the *online* learning problem, *i.e.*, how can an estimate of the *current* state vector and parameters be maintained and improved during a single pass over a string of data. Like the myopic gradient descent algorithm [8], the algorithm we propose uses a gradient approach to move its predictions closer to its empirical observations; however, our algorithm also takes advantage of known constraints on valid test predictions. We show that this constrained gradient approach is capable of discovering a set of core tests quickly, and also of making online predictions that improve as more data is available.

2 Predictive State Representations

Predictive state representations (PSRs) were introduced by Littman *et al.* [2] as a method of modeling discrete-time, controlled dynamical systems. They possess several advantages over other popular models such as POMDPs and k-order Markov models, foremost being their ability to be learned entirely from sensorimotor data, requiring only a prior knowledge of the set of actions, $\mathcal{A}$, and observations, $\mathcal{O}$.

Notation.   An agent in a dynamical system experiences a sequence of action-observation pairs, or ao pairs. The sequence of ao pairs the agent has already experienced, beginning at the first time step, is known as a *history*. For instance, the history $h^n = a^1 o^1 a^2 o^2 \ldots a^n o^n$ of length n means that the agent chose action a^1 and perceived observation o^1 at the first time step, after which the agent chose a^2 and perceived o^2, and so on[1]. A *test* is a sequence of ao pairs that begins immediately after a history. A test is said to succeed if the observations in the sequence are observed in order, given that the actions in the sequence are chosen in order. For instance, the test $t = a_1 o_1 a_2 o_2$ succeeds if the agent observes o_1 followed by o_2, given that it performs actions a_1 followed by a_2. A test fails if the action sequence is taken but the observation sequence is not observed. A prediction about the outcome of a test t depends on the history h that preceded it, so we write predictions as $p(t|h)$, to represent the probability of t succeeding after history h. For test t of length n, we define a prediction $p(t|h)$ as $\prod_{i=1}^{n} \Pr(o_i|a_1 o_1 \ldots a_i)$. This definition is equivalent to the usual definition in the PSR literature, but makes it explicit that predictions are independent of the policy used to select actions. The special length zero test is called ε. If T is a set of tests and H is a set of histories, $p(t|h)$ is a single value, $p(T|h)$ is a row vector containing $p(t_i|h)$ for all tests $t_i \in T$, $p(t|H)$ is a column vector containing $p(t|h_j)$ for all histories $h_j \in H$, and $p(T|H)$ is a matrix containing $p(t_i|h_j)$ for all $t_i \in T$ and $h_j \in H$.

PSRS.   The fundamental principle underlying PSRs is that in most systems there exists a set of tests, Q, that at any history are a sufficient statistic for determining the probability of success for all possible tests. This means that for any test t there exists a function f_t such that $p(t|h) = f_t(p(Q|h))$. In this paper, we restrict our discussion of PSRs to *linear* PSRs, in which the function f_t is a linear function of the tests in Q. Thus, $p(t|h) = p(Q|h)m_t$, where m_t is a column vector of weights. The tests in Q are known as *core tests*, and determining which tests are core tests is known as the *discovery* problem. In addition to Q, it will be convenient to discuss the set of one-step extensions of Q. A one-step extension of a test t is a test aot, that prefixes the original test with a single ao pair. The set of all one-step extensions of $Q \cup \{\varepsilon\}$ will be called X.

The state vector of a PSR at time i is the set of predictions $p(Q|h^i)$. At each time step, the

---

[1]Much of the notation used in this paper is adopted from Wolfe *et al.* [7]. Here we use the notation that a superscript a^i or o^i indicates the time step of an action or observation, and a subscript a_i or o_i indicates that the action or observation is a particular element of the set $\mathcal{A}$ or $\mathcal{O}$.

state vector is updated by computing, for each $q_j \in Q$:

$$p(q_j|h^i) = \frac{p(a^i o^i q_j|h^{i-1})}{p(a^i o^i|h^{i-1})} = \frac{p(Q|h^{i-1})m_{a^i o^i q_j}}{p(Q|h^{i-1})m_{a^i o^i}}$$

Thus, in order to update the PSR at each time step, the vector m_t must be known for each test $t \in X$. This set of update vectors, that we will call m_X, are the parameters of the PSR, and estimation of these parameters is known as the *learning* problem.

3   Constrained Gradient Learning of PSRs

The goal of this paper is to develop an online algorithm for discovering and learning a PSR without the necessity of a reset action. To be online, the algorithm must always have an estimate of the current state vector, $p(Q|h^i)$, and estimates of the parameters m_X. In this section, we introduce our constrained gradient approach to solving this problem. A more complete explanation of this algorithm can be found in an expanded version of this work [9]. To begin, in Section 3.1, we will assume that the set of core tests Q is given to the algorithm; we describe how Q can be estimated online in Section 3.2.

3.1   Learning the PSR Parameters

The approach to learning taken by the constrained gradient algorithm is to approximate the matrix $p(T|H)$, for a selected set of tests T and histories H. We first discuss the proper selection of T and H, and then describe how this matrix can be constructed online. Finally, we show how the current PSR is extracted from the matrix.

Tests and Histories.   At a minimum, T must contain the union of Q and X, since Q is required to create the state vector and X is required to compute m_X. However, as will be explained in the next section, these tests are not sufficient to take full advantage of the structure in a prediction matrix. The constrained gradient algorithm requires the tests in T to satisfy two properties:

1. If $tao \in T$ then $t \in T$
2. If $tao_i \in T$ then $tao_j \in T$ $\forall o_j \in \mathcal{O}$

To build a valid set of tests, T is initialized to $Q \cup X$. Tests are iteratively added to T until it satisfies both of the above properties.

All histories in H are histories that have been experienced by the agent. The current history, h^i, must always be in H in order to make online predictions, and also to compute h^{i+1}. The only other requirement of H is that it contain sufficient histories to compute the linear functions m_t for the tests in T (see Section 3.1). Our strategy is impose a bound N on the size of H, and to restrict H to the N most recent histories encountered by the agent. When a new data point is seen and a new row is added to the matrix, the oldest row in the matrix is "forgotten." In addition to restricting the size of H, forgetting old rows has the side-effect that the rows estimated using the least amount of data are removed from the matrix, and no longer affect the computation of m_X.

Constructing the Prediction Matrix.   The approach used to build the matrix $p(T|H)$ is to estimate and append a new row, $p(T|h^i)$, after each new $a^i o^i$ pair is encountered. Once a row has been added, it is never changed. To initialize the algorithm, the first row of the matrix $p(T|h^0)$, is set to uniform probabilities.[2] The creation of the new row is performed in two stages: a row estimation stage, and a gradient descent stage.

---

[2] Each $p(t|h^0)$ is set to $1/|\mathcal{O}|^k$, where k is the length of test t.

Both stages take advantage of four constraints on the predictions $p(T|h)$ in order to be a valid row in the prediction matrix:

1. Range: $0 \leq p(t|h) \leq 1$
2. Null Test: $p(\varepsilon|h) = 1$
3. Internal Consistency: $p(t|h) = \sum_{o_j \in \mathcal{O}} p(tao_j|h) \quad \forall a \in \mathcal{A}$
4. Conditional Probability: $p(t|hao) = p(aot|h)/p(ao|h) \quad \forall a \in \mathcal{A}, o \in \mathcal{O}$

The range constraint restricts the entries in the matrix to be valid probabilities. The null test constraint defines the value of the null test. The internal consistency constraint ensures that the probabilities within a single row form valid probability distributions. The conditional probability constraint is required to maintain consistency between consecutive rows of the matrix.

Consider time $i - 1$ so that the last row of $p(T|H)$ is h^{i-1}. After action a^i is taken and observation o^i is seen, a new row for history $h^i = h^{i-1}a^io^i$ must be added to the matrix. First, as much of the new row as possible is computed using the conditional probability constraint, and the predictions for history h^{i-1}. For all tests $t \in T$ for which $a^io^it \in T$:

$$p(t|h^i) \leftarrow \frac{p(a^io^it|h^{i-1})}{p(a^io^i|h^{i-1})}$$

Because $X \subset T$, it is guaranteed that $p(Q|h^i)$ is estimated in this step.

The second phase of adding a new row is to compute predictions for the tests $t \in T$ for which $a^io^it \notin T$. An estimate of $p(t|h^i)$ can be found by computing $p(Q|h^i)m_t$ for an appropriate m_t, using the PSR assumption that any prediction is a linear combination of core test predictions. Regression is used to find a vector m_t that minimizes $||p(Q|H)m_t - p(t|H)||^2$. At this stage, the entire row for h^i has been estimated. The regression step can create probabilities that violate the range and normalization properties of a valid prediction. To enforce the range property, any predictions that are less than 0 are set to a small positive value[3]. Then, to ensure internal consistency within the row, the normalization property is enforced by setting predictions:

$$p(tao_j|h^i) \leftarrow \frac{p(t|h^i)p(tao_j|h^i)}{\sum_{o_i \in \mathcal{O}} p(tao_i|h^i)} \quad \forall o_j \in \mathcal{O}$$

This preserves the ratio among sibling predictions and creates a valid probability distribution from them. The normalization is performed by normalizing shorter tests first, which guarantees that a set of tests are not normalized to a value that will later change. The length one tests are normalized to sum to 1.

The gradient descent stage of estimating a new row moves the constraint-generated predictions in the direction of the gradient created by the new observation. Any prediction $p(tao|h^i)$ whose test tao is successfully executed over the next several time steps is updated using $p(tao|h^i) \leftarrow (1-\alpha)p(tao|h^i) + \alpha(p(t|h^i))$, for some learning rate $0 \leq \alpha \leq 1$. Note that this learning rule is a temporal difference update; prediction values are adjusted toward the value of their parent.[4] The update is accomplished by adding an appropriate positive value to $p(tao|h^i)$ and then running the normalization procedure on the row. The value is computed such that after normalization, $p(tao|h^i)$ contains the desired value. Tests

---

[3] Setting values to zero can cause division by zero errors, if the prediction probability was not actually supposed to be zero.

[4] When the algorithm is used online, looking forward into the stream is impossible. In this case, we maintain a buffer of ao pairs between the current time step and the histories that are added to the prediction matrix. The length of the buffer is the length of the longest test in T. To compute the predictions for the current time step, we iteratively update the PSR using the buffered data.

that are unsuccessfully executed (*i.e.* their action sequence is executed but their observation sequence is not observed) will have their probability reduced due to this re-normalization step. The learning parameter, α, is decayed throughout the learning process.

Extracting the PSR. Once a new row for h^i is estimated, the current PSR state vector is $p(Q|h^i)$. The parameters m_X can be found by using the output of the regression from the second phase, above. Thus, at every time step, the current best estimated PSR of the system is available.

3.2 Discovery of Core Tests

In the previous section, we assumed that the set of core tests was given to the algorithm. In general, though, Q is not known. A rudimentary, but effective, method of finding core tests is to choose tests whose corresponding columns of the matrix $p(T|H)$ are most linearly unrelated to the set of core tests already selected. Call the set of selected core tests $\widehat{Q}$. The condition number of the matrix $p(\{\widehat{Q}, t\}|H)$ is an indication of the linear relatedness of test t; if it is well-conditioned, the test is likely to be linearly independent. To choose core tests, we find the test t in X whose matrix $p(\{\widehat{Q}, t\}|H)$ is most well-conditioned. If the condition number of that test is below a threshold parameter, it is chosen as a new core test. The process can be repeated until no test can be added to $\widehat{Q}$ without surpassing the threshold. Because candidate tests are selected from X, the discovered set $\widehat{Q}$ will be a regular form PSR [10].

The set $\widehat{Q}$ is initialized to $\{\varepsilon\}$. The above core test selection procedure runs after every N data points are seen, where N is the maximum number of histories kept in H. After each new core test is selected, T is augmented with the one-step extensions of the new test, as well as any other tests needed to satisfy the rules in Section 3.1.

4 Experiments and Results

The goal of the constrained gradient algorithm is to choose a correct set of core tests and to make accurate, online predictions. In this section, we show empirical results that the algorithm is capable of these goals. We also show offline results, in order to compare our results with the suffix-history algorithm [7]. A more thorough suite of experiments can be found in an expanded version of this work [9].

We tested our algorithm on the same set of problems from Cassandra's POMDP page [11] used as the test domain in other PSR trials [8, 6, 7]. For each problem, 10 trials were run, with different training sequences and test sequences used for each trial. The sequences were generated using a uniform random policy over actions. The error for each history h^i was computed using the error measure $\frac{1}{|O|} \sum_{o_j \in O} (p(a^{i+1}o_j|h^i) - \hat{p}(a^{i+1}o_j|h^i))^2$ [7]. This measures the mean error in the one-step tests involving the action that was actually taken at step $i + 1$.

The same parameterization of the algorithm was used for all domains. The size bound on H was set to 1000, and the condition threshold for adding new tests was 10. The learning parameter α was initialized to 1 and halved every 100,000 time steps. The core test discovery procedure was run every 1000 data points.

4.1 Discovery Results

In this section, we examine the success of the constrained gradient algorithm at discovering core tests. Table 1 shows, for each test domain, the true number of core tests for the

Table 1: The number of core tests found by the constrained gradient algorithm. Data for the suffix-history algorithm [7] is repeated here for comparison. See text for explanation.

| Domain | | Constrained Gradient | | | Suffix-History | |
Name	$\|Q\|$	$\|\widehat{Q}\|$	Correct	# Data	$\|\widehat{Q}\|$/Correct	# Data
Float Reset	5	6.1	4.5	4000	-	-
Tiger	2	4.0	2.0	1000	2	4000
Paint	2	2.6	2.0	4000	2	4000
Shuttle	7	8.7	7.0	2000	7	1024000
4x3 Maze	10	10.4	8.6	2000	9	1024000
Cheese Maze	11	12.1	9.6	1000	9	32000
Bridge Repair	5	7.2	5.0	1000	5	1024000
Network	7	4.7	4.5	2000	3	2048000

dynamical system ($|Q|$), the number of core tests selected by the constrained gradient algorithm ($|\widehat{Q}|$), and how many of the selected core tests were *actually* core tests (*Correct*). The results are averaged over 10 trials. Table 1 also shows the time step at which the last core test was chosen (*# Data*). In all domains, the algorithm found a majority of the core tests after only several thousand data points; in several cases, the core tests were found after only a single run of the core test selection procedure.

Table 1 also shows discovery results published for the suffix-history algorithm [7]. All of the core tests found by the suffix-history algorithm were true core tests. In all cases except the 4x3 Maze, the constrained gradient algorithm was able to find at least as many core tests as the suffix-history method, and required significantly less data. To be fair, the suffix-history algorithm uses a conservative approach of selecting core tests, and therefore requires more data. The constrained gradient algorithm chooses tests that give an early indication of being linearly independent. Therefore, the constrained gradient finds most, or all, core tests extremely quickly, but can also choose tests that are not linearly independent.

4.2   Online and Offline Results

Figure 1 shows the performance of the constrained gradient approach, in online and offline settings. The question answered by the online experiments is: *How accurately can the constrained gradient algorithm predict the outcome of the next time step?* At each time i, we measured the error in the algorithm's predictions of $p(a^{i+1}o_j|h^i)$ for each $o_j \in O$. The 'Online' plot in Figure 1 shows the mean online error from the previous 1000 time steps.

The question posed for the offline experiments was: *What is the long-term performance of the PSRs learned by the constrained gradient algorithm?* To test this, we stopped the learning process at different points in the training sequence and computed the current PSR. The initial state vector for the offline tests was set to the column means of $p(\widehat{Q}|H)$, which approximates the state vector of the system's stationary distribution. In Figure 1, the 'Offline' plot shows the mean error of this PSR on a test sequence of length 10,000. The offline and online performances of the algorithm are very similar. This indicates that, after a given amount of data, the immediate error on the next observation and the long-term error of the generated PSR are approximately the same. This result is encouraging because it implies that the PSR remains stable in its predictions, even in the long term.

Previously published [7] performance results for the suffix-history algorithm are also shown in Figure 1. A direct comparison between the performance of the two algorithms is somewhat inappropriate, because the suffix-history algorithm solves the 'batch' problem and is able to make multiple passes over the data stream. However, the comparison does show that

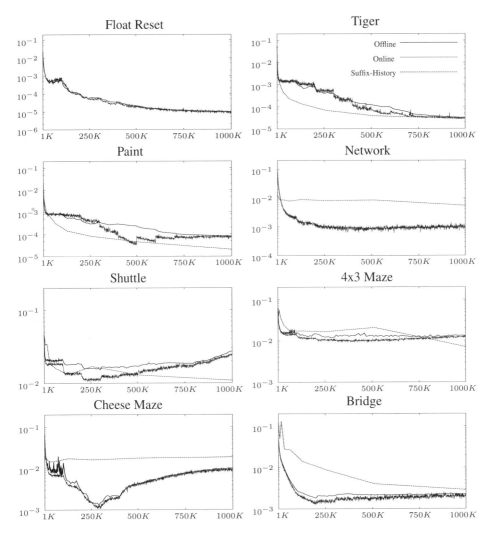

Figure 1: The PSR error on the test domains. The x-axis is the length of the sequence used for training, which ranges from 1,000 to 1,000,000. The y-axis shows the mean error on the one-step predictions (Online) or on a test sequence (Offline and Suffix-History). The results for Suffix-History are repeated from previous work [7]. See text for explanations.

the constrained gradient approach is competitive with current PSR learning algorithms.

The performance plateau in the 4x3 Maze and Network domains is unsurprising, because in these domains only a subset of the correct core tests were found (see Table 1). The plateau in the Bridge domain is more concerning, because in this domains all of the correct core tests were found. We suspect this may be due to a local minimum in the error space; more tests need to be performed to investigate this phenomenon.

5   Future Work and Conclusion

We have demonstrated that the constrained gradient algorithm can do online learning and discovery of predictive state representations from an arbitrary stream of experience. We

881

have also shown that it is competitive with the alternative batch methods. There are still a number of interesting directions for future improvement.

In the current method of core test selection, the condition of the core test matrix $p(\widehat{Q}|H)$ is important. If the matrix becomes ill-conditioned, it prevents new core tests from becoming selected. This can happen if the true core test matrix $p(Q|H)$ is poorly conditioned (because some core tests are similar), or if incorrect core tests are added to $\widehat{Q}$. To prevent this problem, there needs to be a mechanism for removing chosen core tests if they turn out to be linearly dependent. Also, the condition threshold should be gradually increased during learning, to allow more obscure core tests to be selected.

Another interesting modification to the algorithm is to replace the current multi-step estimation of new rows with a single optimization. We want to simultaneously minimize the regression error and next observation error subject to the constraints on valid predictions. This optimization could be solved with quadratic programming.

To date, the constrained gradient algorithm is the only PSR algorithm that takes advantage of the sequential nature of the data stream experienced by the agent, and the constraints such a sequence imposes on the system. It handles the lack of a reset action without partitioning histories. Also, at the end of learning the algorithm has an estimate of the current state, instead of a prediction of the initial distribution or a stationary distribution over states. Empirical results show that, while there is room for improvement, the constrained gradient algorithm is competitive in both discovery and learning of PSRs.

References

[1] Herbert Jaeger. Observable operator models for discrete stochastic time series. *Neural Computation*, 12(6):1371–1398, 2000.

[2] Michael Littman, Richard Sutton, and Satinder Singh. Predictive representations of state. In *Advances in Neural Information Processing Systems 14 (NIPS)*, pages 1555–1561, 2002.

[3] Satinder Singh, Michael R. James, and Matthew R. Rudary. Predictive state representations: A new theory for modeling dynamical systems. In *Uncertainty in Artificial Intelligence: Proceedings of the Twentieth Conference (UAI)*, pages 512–519, 2004.

[4] Richard Sutton and Brian Tanner. Temporal-difference networks. In *Advances in Neural Information Processing Systems 17*, pages 1377–1384, 2005.

[5] Matthew Rosencrantz, Geoff Gordon, and Sebastian Thrun. Learning low dimensional predictive representations. In *Twenty-First International Conference on Machine Learning (ICML)*, 2004.

[6] Michael R. James and Satinder Singh. Learning and discovery of predictive state representations in dynamical systems with reset. In *Twenty-First International Conference on Machine Learning (ICML)*, 2004.

[7] Britton Wolfe, Michael R. James, and Satinder Singh. Learning predictive state representations in dynamical systems without reset. In *Twenty-Second International Conference on Machine Learning (ICML)*, 2005.

[8] Satinder Singh, Michael Littman, Nicholas Jong, David Pardoe, and Peter Stone. Learning predictive state representations. In *Twentieth International Conference on Machine Learning (ICML)*, pages 712–719, 2003.

[9] Peter McCracken. An online algorithm for discovery and learning of prediction state representations. Master's thesis, University of Alberta, 2005.

[10] Eric Wiewiora. Learning predictive representations from a history. In *Twenty-Second International Conference on Machine Learning (ICML)*, 2005.

[11] Anthony Cassandra. Tony's POMDP file repository page. http://www.cs.brown.edu/-research/ai/pomdp/examples/index.html, 1999.

An Alternative Infinite Mixture Of Gaussian Process Experts

Edward Meeds and Simon Osindero
Department of Computer Science
University of Toronto
Toronto, M5S 3G4
{ewm,osindero}@cs.toronto.edu

Abstract

We present an infinite mixture model in which each component comprises a multivariate Gaussian distribution over an input space, and a Gaussian Process model over an output space. Our model is neatly able to deal with non-stationary covariance functions, discontinuities, multi-modality and overlapping output signals. The work is similar to that by Rasmussen and Ghahramani [1]; however, we use a full generative model over input and output space rather than just a conditional model. This allows us to deal with incomplete data, to perform inference over inverse functional mappings as well as for regression, and also leads to a more powerful and consistent Bayesian specification of the effective 'gating network' for the different experts.

1 Introduction

Gaussian process (GP) models are powerful tools for regression, function approximation, and predictive density estimation. However, despite their power and flexibility, they suffer from several limitations. The computational requirements scale cubically with the number of data points, thereby necessitating a range of approximations for large datasets. Another problem is that it can be difficult to specify priors and perform learning in GP models if we require non-stationary covariance functions, multi-modal output, or discontinuities.

There have been several attempts to circumvent some of these lacunae, for example [2, 1]. In particular the Infinite Mixture of Gaussian Process Experts (IMoGPE) model proposed by Rasmussen and Ghahramani [1] neatly addresses the aforementioned key issues. In a single GP model, an n by n matrix must be inverted during inference. However, if we use a model composed of multiple GP's, each responsible only for a subset of the data, then the computational complexity of inverting an n by n matrix is replaced by several inversions of smaller matrices — for large datasets this can result in a substantial speed-up and may allow one to consider large-scale problems that would otherwise be unwieldy. Furthermore, by combining multiple stationary GP experts, we can easily accommodate non-stationary covariance and noise levels, as well as distinctly multi-modal outputs. Finally, by placing a Dirichlet process prior over the experts we can allow the data and our prior beliefs (which may be rather vague) to automatically determine the number of components to use.

In this work we present an alternative infinite model that is strongly inspired by the work in [1], but which uses a different formulation for the mixture of experts that is in the style presented in, for example [3, 4]. This alternative approach effectively uses posterior re-

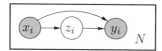 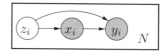

Figure 1: **Left:** Graphical model for the standard MoE model [6]. The expert indicators $\{z_{(i)}\}$ are specified by a gating network applied to the inputs $\{\mathbf{x}_{(i)}\}$. **Right:** An alternative view of MoE model using a full generative model [4]. The distribution of input locations is now given by a mixture model, with components for each expert. Conditioned on the input locations, the posterior responsibilities for each mixture component behave like a gating network.

sponsibilities from a mixture distribution as the gating network. Even if the task at hand is simply output density estimation or regression, we suggest a full generative model over inputs and outputs might be preferable to a purely conditional model. The generative approach retains all the strengths of [1] and also has a number of potential advantages, such as being able to deal with partially specified data (e.g. missing input co-ordinates) and being able to infer inverse functional mappings (i.e. the input space given an output value). The generative approach also affords us a richer and more consistent way of specifying our prior beliefs about how the covariance structure of the outputs might vary as we move within input space.

An example of the type of generative model which we propose is shown in figure 2. We use a Dirichlet process prior over a countably infinite number of experts and each expert comprises two parts: a density over input space describing the distribution of input points associated with that expert, and a Gaussian Process model over the outputs associated with that expert. In this preliminary exposition, we restrict our attention to experts whose input space densities are given a single full covariance Gaussian. Even this simple approach demonstrates interesting performance and capabilities. However, in a more elaborate setup the input density associated with each expert might itself be an infinite mixture of simpler distributions (for instance, an infinite mixture of Gaussians [5]) to allow for the most flexible partitioning of input space amongst the experts.

The structure of the paper is as follows. We begin in section 2 with a brief overview of two ways of thinking about Mixtures of Experts. Then, in section 3, we give the complete specification and graphical depiction of our generative model, and in section 4 we outline the steps required to perform Monte Carlo inference and prediction. In section 5 we present the results of several simple simulations that highlight some of the salient features of our proposal, and finally in section 6, we discuss our work and place it in relation to similar techniques.

2 Mixtures of Experts

In the standard mixture of experts (MoE) model [6], a gating network probabilistically mixes regression components. One subtlety in using GP's in a mixture of experts model is that IID assumptions on the data no longer hold and we must specify joint distributions for each possible assignment of experts to data. Let $\{\mathbf{x}_{(i)}\}$ be the set of d-dimensional input vectors, $\{y_{(i)}\}$ be the set of scalar outputs, and $\{z_{(i)}\}$ be the set of expert indicators which assign data points to experts.

The likelihood of the outputs, given the inputs, is specified in equation 1, where θ_r^{GP} represents the GP parameters of the rth expert, θ^g represents the parameters of the gating network, and the summation is over all possible configurations of indicator variables.

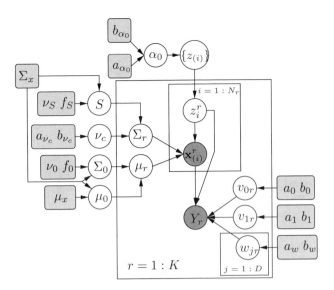

Figure 2: The graphical model representation of the alternative infinite mixture of GP experts (AiMoGPE) model proposed in this paper. We have used $\mathbf{x}^r_{(i)}$ to represent the ith data point in the set of input data whose expert label is r, and Y_r to represent the set of all output data whose expert label is r. In other words, input data are IID given their expert label, whereas the *sets* of output data are IID given their corresponding *sets* of input data. The lightly shaded boxes with rounded corners represent hyper-hyper parameters that are fixed (Ω in the text). The DP concentration parameter α_0, the expert indicators variables, $\{z_{(i)}\}$, the gate hyperparameters, $\phi^{\mathbf{x}} = \{\mu_0, \Sigma_0, \nu_c, S\}$, the gate component parameters, $\psi^{\mathbf{x}}_r = \{\mu_r, \Sigma_r\}$, and the GP expert parameters, $\theta^{\mathrm{GP}}_r = \{v_{0r}, v_{1r}, w_{jr}\}$, are all updated for all r and j.

$$P(\{y_{(i)}\}|\{\mathbf{x}_{(i)}\},\theta)=\sum_{\mathcal{Z}}P(\{z_{(i)}\}|\{\mathbf{x}_{(i)}\},\theta^g)\prod_r P(\{y_{(i)}: z_{(i)} = r\}|\{\mathbf{x}_{(i)}: z_{(i)} = r\},\theta^{\mathrm{GP}}_r)$$
(1)

There is an alternative view of the MoE model in which the experts also generate the inputs, rather than simply being conditioned on them [3, 4] (see figure 1). This alternative view employs a joint mixture model over input and output space, even though the objective is still primarily that of estimating conditional densities i.e. outputs given inputs. The gating network effectively gets specified by the posterior responsibilities of each of the different components in the mixture. An advantage of this perspective is that it can easily accommodate partially observed inputs and it also allows 'reverse-conditioning', should we wish to estimate where in input space a given output value is likely to have originated. For a mixture model using Gaussian Processes experts, the likelihood is given by

$$P(\{\mathbf{x}_{(i)}\},\{y_{(i)}\}|\theta) = \sum_{\mathcal{Z}} P(\{z_{(i)}\}|\theta^g)\times$$

$$\prod_r P(\{y_{(i)}: z_{(i)} = r\}|\{\mathbf{x}_{(i)}: z_{(i)} = r\}, \theta^{\mathrm{GP}}_r)P(\{\mathbf{x}_{(i)}: z_{(i)} = r\}|\theta^g) \quad (2)$$

where the description of the density over input space is encapsulated in θ^g.

3 Infinite Mixture of Gaussian Processes: A Joint Generative Model

The graphical structure for our full generative model is shown in figure 2. Our generative process does not produce IID data points and is therefore most simply formulated either as

885

a joint distribution over a dataset of a given size, or as a set of conditionals in which we incrementally add data points.To construct a complete set of N sample points from the prior (specified by top-level hyper-parameters Ω) we would perform the following operations:

1. Sample Dirichlet process concentration variable α_0 given the top-level hyper-parameters.
2. Construct a partition of N objects into at most N groups using a Dirichlet process. This assignment of objects is denoted by using a set the indicator variables $\{z_{(i)}\}_{i=1}^{N}$.
3. Sample the gate hyperparameters $\phi^{\mathbf{x}}$ given the top-level hyperparameters.
4. For each grouping of indicators $\{z_{(i)} : z_{(i)} = r\}$, sample the input space parameters $\psi_r^{\mathbf{x}}$ conditioned on $\phi^{\mathbf{x}}$. $\psi_r^{\mathbf{x}}$ defines the density in input space, in our case a full-covariance Gaussian.
5. Given the parameters $\psi_r^{\mathbf{x}}$ for each group, sample the locations of the input points $X_r \equiv \{\mathbf{x}_{(i)} : z_{(i)} = r\}$.
6. For each group, sample the hyper-parameters for the GP expert associated with that group, θ_r^{GP}.
7. Using the input locations X_r and hyper-parameters θ_r^{GP} for the individual groups, formulate the GP output covariance matrix and sample the set of output values, $Y_r \equiv \{y_{(i)} : z_{(i)} = r\}$ from this joint Gaussian distribution.

We write the full joint distribution of our model as follows.

$$P(\{\mathbf{x}_{(i)}, y_{(i)}\}_{i=1}^{N}, \{z_{(i)}\}_{i=1}^{N}, \{\psi_r^{\mathbf{x}}\}_{r=1}^{N}, \{\theta_r^{\mathrm{GP}}\}_{r=1}^{N}, \alpha_0, \phi^{\mathbf{x}} | N, \Omega) =$$

$$\prod_{r=1}^{N} \left[H_r^N P(\psi_r^{\mathbf{x}}|\phi^{\mathbf{x}}) P(X_r|\psi_r^{\mathbf{x}}) P(\theta_r^{\mathrm{GP}}|\Omega) P(Y_r|X_r, \theta_r^{\mathrm{GP}}) + (1 - H_r^N) D_0(\psi_r^{\mathbf{x}}, \theta_r^{\mathrm{GP}}) \right]$$

$$\times P(\{z_{(i)}\}_{i=1}^{N}|N, \alpha_0) P(\alpha_0|\Omega) P(\phi^{\mathbf{x}}|\Omega) \tag{3}$$

Where we have used the supplementary notation: $H_r^N = 0$ if $\{\{z_{(i)}\} : z_{(i)} = r\}$ is the empty set and $H_r^N = 1$ otherwise; and $D_0(\psi_r^{\mathbf{x}}, \theta_r^{\mathrm{GP}})$ is a delta function on an (irrelevant) dummy set of parameters to ensure proper normalisation.

For the GP components, we use a standard, stationary covariance function of the form

$$Q(\mathbf{x}_{(i)}, \mathbf{x}_{(h)}) = v_0 \exp\left(-\frac{1}{2}\sum_{j=1}^{D}\left(x_{(i)j} - x_{(h)j}\right)^2 / w_j^2\right) + \delta(i, h)v_1 \tag{4}$$

The individual distributions in equation 3 are defined as follows[1]:

$$P(\alpha_0|\Omega) = \mathcal{G}(\alpha_0; a_{\alpha_0}, b_{\alpha_0}) \tag{5}$$

$$P(\{z_{(i)}\}_{i=1}^{N}|N, \Omega) = \mathcal{PU}(\alpha_0, N) \tag{6}$$

$$P(\phi^{\mathbf{x}}|\Omega) = \mathcal{N}(\mu_0; \mu_x, \Sigma_x/f_0)\mathcal{W}(\Sigma_0^{-1}; \nu_0, f_0\Sigma_x^{-1}/\nu_0)$$

$$\mathcal{G}(\nu_c; a_{\nu_c}, b_{\nu_c})\mathcal{W}(S^{-1}; \nu_S, f_S\Sigma_x/\nu_S) \tag{7}$$

$$P(\psi_r^{\mathbf{x}}|\Omega) = \mathcal{N}(\mu_r; \mu_0, \Sigma_0)\mathcal{W}(\Sigma_r^{-1}; \nu_c, S/\nu_c) \tag{8}$$

$$P(X_r|\psi_r^{\mathbf{x}}) = \mathcal{N}(X_r; \mu_r, \Sigma_r) \tag{9}$$

$$P(\theta_r^{\mathrm{GP}}|\Omega) = \mathcal{G}(v_{0r}; a_0, b_0)\mathcal{G}(v_{1r}; a_1, b_1)\prod_{j=1}^{D}\mathcal{LN}(w_{jr}; a_w, b_w) \tag{10}$$

$$P(Y_r|X_r, \theta_r^{\mathrm{GP}}) = \mathcal{N}(Y_r; \mu_{Q_r}, \sigma_{Q_r}^2) \tag{11}$$

---

[1] We use the notation $\mathcal{N}$, $\mathcal{W}$, $\mathcal{G}$, and $\mathcal{LN}$ to represent the normal, the Wishart, the gamma, and the log-normal distributions, respectively; we use the parameterizations found in [7] (Appendix A). The notation $\mathcal{PU}$ refers to the Polya urn distribution [8].

In an approach similar to Rasmussen [5], we use the input data mean μ_x and covariance Σ_x to provide an automatic normalisation of our dataset. We also incorporate additional hyperparameters f_0 and f_S, which allow prior beliefs about the variation in location of μ_r and size of Σ_r, relative to the data covariance.

4 Monte Carlo Updates

Almost all the integrals and summations required for inference and learning operations within our model are analytically intractable, and therefore necessitate Monte Carlo approximations. Fortunately, all the necessary updates are relatively straightforward to carry out using a Markov Chain Monte Carlo (MCMC) scheme employing Gibbs sampling and Hybrid Monte Carlo. We also note that in our model the predictive density depends on the entire set of test locations (in input space). This transductive behaviour follows from the non-IID nature of the model and the influence that test locations have on the posterior distribution over mixture parameters. Consequently, the marginal predictive distribution at a given location can depend on the other locations for which we are making simultaneous predictions. This may or may not be desired. In some situations the ability to incorporate the additional information about the input density at test time may be beneficial. However, it is also straightforward to effectively 'ignore' this new information and simply compute a set of independent single location predictions.

Given a set of test locations $\{\mathbf{x}^*_{(t)}\}$, along with training data pairs $\{\mathbf{x}_{(i)}, y_{(i)}\}$ and top-level hyper-parameters Ω, we iterate through the following conditional updates to produce our predictive distribution for unknown outputs $\{y^*_{(t)}\}$. The parameter updates are all conjugate with the prior distributions, except where noted:

1. Update indicators $\{z_{(i)}\}$ by cycling through the data and sampling one indicator variable at a time. We use algorithm 8 from [9] with $m = 1$ to explore new experts.
2. Update input space parameters.
3. Update GP hyper-params using Hybrid Monte Carlo [10].
4. Update gate hyperparameters. Note that ν_c is updated using slice sampling [11].
5. Update DP hyperparameter α_0 using the data augmentation technique of Escobar and West [12].
6. Resample missing output values by cycling through the experts, and jointly sampling the missing outputs associated with that GP.

We perform some preliminary runs to estimate the longest auto-covariance time, τ_{max} for our posterior estimates, and then use a burn-in period that is about 10 times this timescale before taking samples every τ_{max} iterations.[2] For our simulations the auto-covariance time was typically 40 complete update cycles, so we use a burn-in period of 500 iterations and collect samples every 50.

5 Experiments

5.1 Samples From The Prior

In figure 3 (A) we give an example of data drawn from our model which is multi-modal and non-stationary. We also use this artificial dataset to confirm that our MCMC algorithm performs well and is able recover sensible posterior distributions. Posterior histograms for some of the inferred parameters are shown in figure 3 (B) and we see that they are well clustered around the 'true' values.

---

[2]This is primarily for convenience. It would also be valid to use all the samples after the burn-in period, and although they could not be considered independent, they could be used to obtain a more accurate estimator.

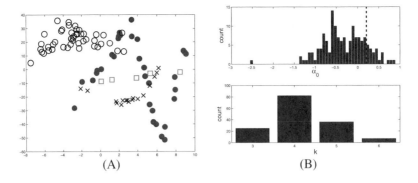

(A)   (B)

Figure 3: (A) A set of samples from our model prior. The different marker styles are used to indicate the sets of points from different experts. (B) The posterior distribution of $\log \alpha_0$ with its true value indicated by the dashed line (top) and the distribution of occupied experts (bottom). We note that the posterior mass is located in the vicinity of the true values.

5.2   Inference On Toy Data

To illustrate some of the features of our model we constructed a toy dataset consisting of 4 continuous functions, to which we added different levels of noise. The functions used were:

$$f_1(a_1) = 0.25a_1^2 - 40 \qquad\qquad a_1 \in (0\ldots15) \qquad \text{Noise SD: } 7 \quad (12)$$

$$f_2(a_2) = -0.0625(a_2 - 18)^2 + .5a_2 + 20 \qquad a_2 \in (35\ldots60) \qquad \text{Noise SD: } 7 \quad (13)$$

$$f_3(a_3) = 0.008(a_3 - 60)^3 - 70 \qquad\qquad a_3 \in (45\ldots80) \qquad \text{Noise SD: } 4 \quad (14)$$

$$f_4(a_4) = -\sin(0.25a_4) - 6 \qquad\qquad a_4 \in (80\ldots100) \qquad \text{Noise SD: } 2 \quad (15)$$

The resulting data has non-stationary noise levels, non-stationary covariance, discontinuities and significant multi-modality. Figure 4 shows our results on this dataset along with those from a single GP for comparison.

We see that in order to account for the entire data set with a single GP, we are forced to infer an unnecessarily high level of noise in the function. Also, a single GP is unable to capture the multi-modality or non-stationarity of the data distribution. In contrast, our model seems much more able to deal with these challenges.

Since we have a full generative model over both input and output space, we are also able to use our model to infer likely input locations given a particular output value. There are a number of applications for which this might be relevant, for example if one wanted to sample candidate locations at which to evaluate a function we are trying to optimise. We provide a simple illustration of this in figure 4 (B). We choose three output levels and conditioned on the output having these values, we sample for the input location. The inference seems plausible and our model is able to suggest locations in input space for a maximal output value ($+40$) that was not seen in the training data.

5.3   Regression on a simple "real-world" dataset

We also apply our model and algorithm to the motorcycle dataset of [13]. This is a commonly used dataset in the GP community and therefore serves as a useful basis for comparison. In particular, it also makes it easy to see how our model compares with standard GP's and with the work of [1]. Figure 5 compares the performance of our model with that of a single GP. In particular, we note that although the median of our model closely resembles the mean of the single GP, our model is able to more accurately model the low noise level

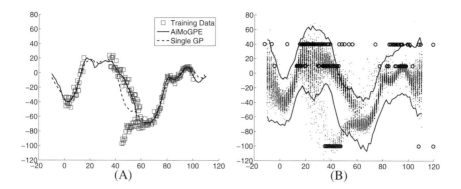

Figure 4: Results on a toy dataset. (A) The training data is shown along with the predictive mean of a stationary covariance GP and the median of the predictive distribution of our model. (B) The small dots are samples from the model (160 samples per location) evaluated at 80 equally spaced locations across the range (but plotted with a small amount of jitter to aid visualisation). These illustrate the predictive density from our model. The solid the lines show the $\pm$ 2 SD interval from a regular GP. The circular markers at ordinates of 40, 10 and -100 show samples from 'reverse-conditioning' where we sample likely abscissa locations given the test ordinate and the set of training data.

on the left side of the dataset. For the remainder of the dataset, the noise level modeled by our model and a single GP are very similar, although our model is better able to capture the behaviour of the data at around 30 ms. It is difficult to make an exact comparison to [1], however we can speculate that our model is more realistically modeling the noise at the beginning of the dataset by not inferring an overly "flat" GP expert at that location. We can also report that our expert adjacency matrix closely resembles that of [1].

6   Discussion

We have presented an alternative framework for an infinite mixture of GP experts. We feel that our proposed model carries over the strengths of [1] and augments these with the several desirable additional features. The pseudo-likelihood objective function used to adapt the gating network defined in [1] is not guaranteed to lead to a self-consistent distribution and therefore the results may depend on the order in which the updates are performed; our model incorporates a consistent Bayesian density formulation for both input and output spaces by definition. Furthermore, in our most general framework we are more naturally able to specify priors over the partitioning of space between different expert components. Also, since we have a full joint model we can infer inverse functional mappings.

There should be considerable gains to be made by allowing the input density models be more powerful. This would make it easier for arbitrary regions of space to share the same covariance structures; at present the areas 'controlled' by a particular expert tend to be local. Consequently, a potentially undesirable aspect of the current model is that strong clustering in input space can lead us to infer several expert components even if a single GP would do a good job of modelling the data. An elegant way of extending the model in this way might be to use a separate infinite mixture distribution for the input density of *each* expert, perhaps incorporating a hierarchical DP prior across the infinite set of experts to allow information to be shared.

With regard to applications, it might be interesting to further explore our model's capability to infer inverse functional mappings; perhaps this could be useful in an optimisation or active learning context. Finally, we note that although we have focused on rather small examples so far, it seems that the inference techniques should scale well to larger problems

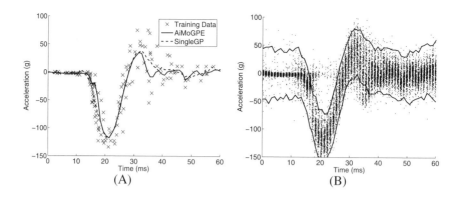

Figure 5: (A) Motorcycle impact data together with the median of our model's point-wise predictive distribution and the predictive mean of a stationary covariance GP model. (B) The small dots are samples from our model (160 samples per location) evaluated at 80 equally spaced locations across the range (but plotted with a small amount of jitter to aid visualisation). The solid lines show the ± 2 SD interval from a regular GP.

and more practical tasks.

Acknowledgments

Thanks to Ben Marlin for sharing slice sampling code and to Carl Rasmussen for making `minimize.m` available.

References

[1] C.E. Rasmussen and Z. Ghahramani. Infinite mixtures of Gaussian process experts. In *Advances in Neural Information Processing Systems 14*, pages 881–888. MIT Press, 2002.

[2] V. Tresp. Mixture of Gaussian processes. In *Advances in Neural Information Processing Systems*, volume 13. MIT Press, 2001.

[3] Z. Ghahramani and M. I. Jordan. Supervised learning from incomplete data via an EM approach. In *Advances in Neural Information Processing Systems 6*, pages 120–127. Morgan-Kaufmann, 1995.

[4] L. Xu, M. I. Jordan, and G. E. Hinton. An alternative model for mixtures of experts. In *Advances in Neural Information Processing Systems 7*, pages 633–640. MIT Press, 1995.

[5] C. E. Rasmussen. The infinite Gaussian mixture model. In *Advances in Neural Information Processing Systems*, volume 12, pages 554–560. MIT Press, 2000.

[6] R.A. Jacobs, M.I. Jordan, and G.E. Hinton. Adaptive mixture of local experts. *Neural Computation*, 3, 1991.

[7] A. Gelman, J. B. Carlin, H. S. Stern, and D. B. Rubin. *Bayesian Data Analysis*. Chapman and Hall, 2nd edition, 2004.

[8] D. Blackwell and J. B. MacQueen. Ferguson distributions via Polya urn schemes. *The Annals of Statistics*, 1(2):353–355, 1973.

[9] R. M. Neal. Markov chain sampling methods for Dirichlet process mixture models. *Journal of Computational and Graphical Statistics*, 9:249–265, 2000.

[10] R. M. Neal. Probabilistic inference using Markov chain Monte Carlo methods. Technical Report CRG-TR-93-1, University of Toronto, 1993.

[11] R. M. Neal. Slice sampling (with discussion). *Annals of Statistics*, 31:705–767, 2003.

[12] M. Escobar and M. West. Computing Bayesian nonparametric hierarchical models. In *Practical Nonparametric and Semiparametric Bayesian Statistics*, number 133 in Lecture Notes in Statistics. Springer-Verlag, 1998.

[13] B. W. Silverman. Some aspects of the spline smoothing approach to non-parametric regression curve fitting. *J. Royal Stayt Society. Ser. B*, 47:1–52, 1985.

Unbiased Estimator of Shape Parameter for Spiking Irregularities under Changing Environments

Keiji Miura
Kyoto University
JST PRESTO

Masato Okada
University of Tokyo
JST PRESTO
RIKEN BSI

Shun-ichi Amari
RIKEN BSI

Abstract

We considered a gamma distribution of interspike intervals as a statistical model for neuronal spike generation. The model parameters consist of a time-dependent firing rate and a shape parameter that characterizes spiking irregularities of individual neurons. Because the environment changes with time, observed data are generated from the time-dependent firing rate, which is an unknown function. A statistical model with an unknown function is called a semiparametric model, which is one of the unsolved problem in statistics and is generally very difficult to solve. We used a novel method of estimating functions in information geometry to estimate the shape parameter without estimating the unknown function. We analytically obtained an optimal estimating function for the shape parameter independent of the functional form of the firing rate. This estimation is efficient without Fisher information loss and better than maximum likelihood estimation.

1 Introduction

The firing patterns of cortical neurons look very noisy [1]. Consequently, probabilistic models are necessary to describe these patterns [2, 3, 4]. For example, Baker and Lemon showed that the firing patterns recorded from motor areas can be explained using a continuous-time rate-modulated gamma process [5]. Their model had a rate parameter, ξ, and a shape parameter, κ, that was related to spiking irregularity. ξ was assumed to be a function of time because it depended largely on the behavior of the monkey. κ was assumed to be unique to individual neurons and constant over time.

The assumption that κ is unique to individual neurons is also supported by other studies [6, 7, 8]. However, these indirect supports are not conclusive. Therefore, we need to accurately estimate κ to make the assumption more reliable. If the assumption is correct, neurons may be identified by κ estimated from the spiking patterns, and κ may provide useful information about the function of a neuron. In other words, it may be possible to classify neurons according to functional firing patterns rather than static anatomical properties. Thus, it is very important to accurately estimate κ in the field of neuroscience.

In reality, however, it is very difficult to estimate all the parameters in the model from the observed spike data. The reason for this is that the unknown function for the time-dependent firing rate, $\xi(t)$, has infinite degrees of freedom. This kind of estimation problem is called the semiparametric model [9] and is one of the unsolved problems in statistics. Are there any ingenious methods of estimating κ accurately to overcome this difficulty?

Ikeda pointed out that the problem we need to consider is the semiparametric model [10]. However, the problem remains unsolved. There is a method called estimating functions [11, 12] for semiparametric problems, and a general theory has been developed [13, 14, 15] from the viewpoint of information geometry [16, 17, 18]. However, the method of estimating functions cannot be applied to our problem in its original form.

In this paper, we consider the semiparametric model suggested by Ikeda instead of the continuous-time rate-modulated gamma process. In this discrete-time rate-modulated model, the firing rate varies for each interspike interval. This model is a mixture model and can represent various types of interspike interval distributions by adjusting its weight function. The model can be analyzed by using the method of estimating functions for semiparametric models.

Various attempts have been made to solve semiparametric models. Neyman and Scott pointed out that the maximum likelihood method does not generally provide a consistent estimator when the number of parameters and observations are the same [19]. In fact, we show that maximum likelihood estimation for our problem is biased. Ritov and Bickel considered asymptotic attainability of information bound purely mathematically [20, 21]. However, their results were not practical for application to our problem. Amari and Kawanabe showed a practical method of estimating finite parameters of interest without estimating an unknown function [15]. This is the method of estimating functions. If this method can be applied, κ can be estimated consistently independent of the functional form of a firing rate.

In this paper, we show that the model we consider here is the "exponential form" defined by Amari and Kawanabe [15]. However, an asymptotically unbiased estimating function does not exist unless multiple observations are given for each firing rate, ξ. We show that if multiple observations are given, the method of estimating functions can be applied. In that case, the estimating function of κ can be analytically obtained, and κ can be estimated consistently independent of the functional form of a firing rate. In general, estimation using estimating functions is not efficient. However, for our problem, this method yielded an optimal estimator in the sense of Fisher information [15]. That is, we obtained an efficient estimator.

2 Simple case

We considered the following statistical model of inter spike intervals proposed by Ikeda [10]. Interspike intervals are generated by a gamma distribution whose mean firing rate changes over time. The mean firing rate ξ at each observation is determined randomly according to an unknown probability distribution, $k(\xi)$. The model is described as

$$p(T; \kappa, k(\xi)) = \int q(T; \xi, \kappa) k(\xi) d\xi, \tag{1}$$

where

$$
\begin{aligned}
q(T; \xi, \kappa) &= \frac{(\xi\kappa)^\kappa}{\Gamma(\kappa)} T^{\kappa-1} e^{-\xi\kappa T} \\
&= e^{\xi(-\kappa T)+(\kappa-1)\log(T)-(-\kappa\log(\xi\kappa)+\log\Gamma(\kappa))} \\
&\equiv e^{\xi s(T,\kappa)+r(T,\kappa)-\psi(\kappa,\xi)}. \tag{2}
\end{aligned}
$$

Here, T denotes an interspike interval. We defined s, r, and ψ as

$$s(T, \kappa) = -\kappa T, \tag{3}$$

$$r(T, \kappa) = (\kappa - 1)\log(T), \text{ and} \tag{4}$$

$$\psi(\kappa, \xi) = -\kappa\log(\xi\kappa) + \log\Gamma(\kappa) \tag{5}$$

to demonstrate that the model is the exponential form defined by Amari and Kawanabe [15]. Note that this type of model is called a semiparametric model because it has both unknown finite parameters, κ, and function, $k(\xi)$.

In this mixture model, $\{\xi^{(1)}, \xi^{(2)}, \ldots\}$ is an unknown sequence where ξ is independently and identically distributed according to a probability density function $k(\xi)$. Then, l-th observation $T^{(l)}$ is distributed according to $q(T^{(l)}; \xi^{(l)}, \kappa)$. In effect, T is independently and identically distributed according to $p(T; \kappa, k(\xi))$.

An estimating function is a function of κ whose zero-crossing provides an estimate of κ, analogous to the derivative with respect to κ of the log-likelihood function. Note that the zero-crossings of the derivatives of the log-likelihood function with respect to parameters provide an maximum likelihood estimator.

Let us calculate the estimating function following Amari and Kawanabe [15] to estimate κ without estimating $k(\xi)$. They showed that for the exponential form of mixture distributions, the estimating function, u^I, is given by the projection of the score function, $u = \partial_\kappa \log p$, as

$$\begin{aligned} u^I(T, \kappa) &= u - E[u|s] \\ &= (\partial_\kappa s - E[\partial_\kappa s|s]) \cdot E_\xi[\xi|s] + \partial_\kappa r - E[\partial_\kappa r|s] \\ &= \partial_\kappa r - E[\partial_\kappa r|s], \end{aligned} \tag{6}$$

where

$$E_\xi[\xi|s] = \frac{\int \xi k(\xi)\exp(\xi \cdot s - \psi)d\xi}{\int k(\xi)\exp(\xi \cdot s - \psi)d\xi}. \tag{7}$$

The relation,

$$E[\partial_\kappa s|s] = \frac{s}{\kappa} = -T = \partial_\kappa s, \tag{8}$$

holds because the number of random variables, T, and s are the same. For the same reason,

$$E[\partial_\kappa r|s] = \log(T) = \partial_\kappa r. \tag{9}$$

Then,

$$u^I = 0. \tag{10}$$

This means that the set of estimating functions is an empty set. Therefore, we proved that no asymptotically unbiased estimating function of κ exists for the model.

Two or more random variables may be needed. Let us consider the multivariate model described as

$$p(T_1, \ldots, T_n; \kappa, k(\xi_1, \ldots, \xi_n)) = \int \prod_{i=1}^{n} q(T_i; \xi_i, \kappa)k(\xi_1, \ldots, \xi_n)d\xi. \tag{11}$$

Here, the number of random variables and s are also the same, and u^I becomes an empty set.

This result can be understood intuitively as follows. When the mean, μ, and variance, σ, of a normal distribution are estimated from a single observation, x, they are estimated as $\mu = x$ and $\sigma = 0$. Similarly, ξ and κ of a gamma distribution, $q(T; \xi, \kappa)$, are estimated from a single observation, T, as $\xi = \frac{1}{T}$ and $\kappa = \infty$ corresponding to 0 variance. Two or more observations are required to estimate κ. For the semiparametric model considered in this section, only one observation is given for each ξ. Two or more observations are needed for each ξ.

3 Cases with multiple observations for each ξ

Next we consider the case where m observations are given for each $\xi^{(l)}$, which may be distributed according to $k(\xi)$. Here, a consistent estimator of κ exists. Let $\{T\} = \{T_1, \ldots, T_m\}$ be the m observations, which are generated from the same distribution specified by ξ and κ. We have N such observations $\{T^{(l)}\}$, $l = 1, \ldots, N$, with a common κ and different $\xi^{(l)}$. Thus, $\{T_1^{(l)}, \ldots, T_m^{(l)}\}$ are generated from the same firing rate $\xi^{(l)}$. Let us take one $\{T\}$. The probability model can be written as

$$p(\{T\}; \kappa, k(\xi)) = \int \prod_{i=1}^{m} q(T_i; \xi, \kappa) k(\xi) d\xi, \tag{12}$$

where

$$
\begin{aligned}
\prod_{i=1}^{m} q(T_i; \xi, \kappa) &= \prod_{i=1}^{m} \frac{(\xi\kappa)^\kappa}{\Gamma(\kappa)} T_i^{\kappa-1} e^{-\xi\kappa T_i} \\
&= e^{\xi(-\kappa \sum_{i=1}^{m} T_i) + (\kappa-1)\sum_{i=1}^{m} \log(T_i) - (-m\kappa \log(\xi\kappa) + m \log \Gamma(\kappa))} \\
&\equiv e^{(\xi \cdot s(\{T\}, \kappa) + r(\{T\}, \kappa) - \psi(\kappa, \xi))}.
\end{aligned}
\tag{13}
$$

We defined s, r, and ψ as

$$s(\{T\}, \kappa) = -\kappa \sum_{i=1}^{m} T_i, \tag{14}$$

$$r(\{T\}, \kappa) = (\kappa - 1) \sum_{i=1}^{m} \log(T_i), \quad \text{and} \tag{15}$$

$$\psi(\kappa, \xi) = -m\kappa \log(\xi\kappa) + m \log \Gamma(\kappa). \tag{16}$$

Then, the estimating function is given by

$$
\begin{aligned}
u^I(\{T\}, \kappa) &= u - E[u|s] \\
&= (\partial_\kappa s - E[\partial_\kappa s|s]) \cdot E_\xi[\xi|s] + \partial_\kappa r - E[\partial_\kappa r|s] \\
&= \partial_\kappa r - E[\partial_\kappa r|s] \\
&= \sum_{i=1}^{m} \log(T_i) - m E[\log(T_1)|s],
\end{aligned}
\tag{17}
$$

where we used

$$E[\partial_\kappa s|s] = \frac{s}{\kappa} = \partial_\kappa s. \tag{18}$$

To calculate the conditional expectation of $\log T_1$, let us use Bayes's Theorem:

$$p(T|s) = \frac{p(T, s)}{p(s)}. \tag{19}$$

By transforming random variables, $(T_1, T_2, T_3, \ldots, T_m)$, into $(s, T_2, T_3, \ldots, T_m)$, we have

$$
\begin{aligned}
p(s) &= \int \prod_i q(T_i; \xi, \kappa) \delta(s + \kappa \sum_{i=1}^{m} T_i) k(\xi) d\xi dT \\
&= \prod_{i=1}^{m-1} B(i\kappa, \kappa) \frac{(-s)^{m\kappa-1}}{\Gamma(\kappa)^m} \int \xi^{m\kappa} e^{s\xi} k(\xi) d\xi.
\end{aligned}
\tag{20}
$$

894

where the beta function is defined as

$$B(x,y) = \frac{\Gamma(x)\Gamma(y)}{\Gamma(x+y)} = \frac{(x-1)!(y-1)!}{(x+y-1)!}. \tag{21}$$

Similarly, we have

$$
\begin{aligned}
E[\log(T_1)|s] &= \int \log(T_1) \prod_{i=1}^{m} q(T_i)\delta(s + \kappa \sum_{i=1}^{m} T_i)k(\xi)d\xi dT \frac{1}{p(s)} \\
&= \log(-\frac{s}{\kappa}) - \phi(m\kappa) + \phi(\kappa),
\end{aligned} \tag{22}
$$

where the digamma function is defined as

$$\phi(\kappa) = \frac{\Gamma'(\kappa)}{\Gamma(\kappa)}. \tag{23}$$

Note that $E[\log(T_1)|s]$ does not depend on the unknown function, $k(\xi)$. Thus, we have

$$u^I(\{T\}, \kappa) = \sum_{i=1}^{m} \log(T_i) - m\log(\sum_{i=1}^{m} T_i) + m\phi(m\kappa) - m\phi(\kappa). \tag{24}$$

The form of u^I can be understood as follows. If we scale T as $t = \xi T$, we have $E[t] = 1$. Then, we can show that u^I does not depend on ξ, because

$$\log(T) - E[\log T|s] = \log(t) - E[\log t|s]. \tag{25}$$

This implies that we can estimate κ without estimating ξ. The method of estimating function only works for gamma distributions. It crucially depends on the fact that the estimating function is invariant under scaling of T.

κ can be estimated consistently from N independent observations, $\{T^{(l)}\} = \{T_1^{(l)}, \ldots, T_m^{(l)}\}, l = 1, \ldots, N$, as the value of κ that solves

$$\sum_{l=1}^{N} u^I(\{T^{(l)}\}, \hat{\kappa}) = 0. \tag{26}$$

In fact, the expectation of u^I is 0 independent of $k(\xi)$:

$$
\begin{aligned}
E[u^I] &= \int (\int \prod_{i=1}^{m} q(T_i; \xi, \kappa)u^I dT)k(\xi)d\xi \\
&= \int E_q[u^I|s]p(s)ds \cdot \int k(\xi)d\xi \\
&= \int E_q[\log t - E[\log t|s]|s]p(s)ds \\
&= 0,
\end{aligned} \tag{27}
$$

where E_q denotes the expectation for $\prod_{i=1}^{m} q(t_i; 1, \kappa)$.

u^I yields an efficient estimating function [15, 21]. An efficient estimator is one whose variance attains the Cramer-Rao lower bound asymptotically. Thus, there is no estimator of κ whose mean-square estimation error is smaller than that given by u^I. As u^I does not depend on $k(\xi)$, it is the optimal estimating function whatever $k(\xi)$ is, or whatever the sequence $\xi^{(1)}, \ldots, \xi^{(N)}$ is.

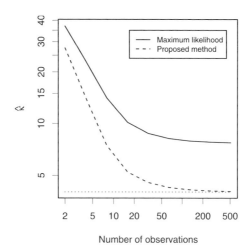

Figure 1: Biases of $\hat{\kappa}$ for maximum likelihood estimation and proposed method for $m = 2$. The dotted line represents the true value, $\kappa = 4$. The maximum likelihood estimation is biased even when an infinite number of observations are given while the estimating function is asymptotically unbiased.

The maximum likelihood estimation for this problem is given by

$$u^{MLE} = \sum_{i=1}^{m} \log(T_i) + m \log(\hat{\xi}) + m \log \kappa - m\phi(\kappa), \tag{28}$$

where

$$\frac{1}{\hat{\xi}} = \frac{1}{m} \sum_{i=1}^{m} T_i. \tag{29}$$

u^{MLE} is similar to u^I but different in terms of constant. As a result, the maximum likelihood estimator $\hat{\kappa}$ is biased (Figure 1).

So far, we have assumed that the firing rates for m observations are the same. Instead, let us consider a case where the firing rates have some relation. For example, consider the case where $E_q[t_1] = 2E_q[t_2]$. The model can be written as

$$p(t_1, t_2; \kappa, k(\xi)) = \int q(t_1; \xi, \kappa) q(t_2; 2\xi, \kappa) k(\xi) d\xi. \tag{30}$$

This model can be derived from Eq. (12) by rescaling as $T_1 = t_1$ and $T_2 = 2t_2$. Note that $q(2T; \xi, \kappa) = q(T; 2\xi, \kappa)$ because T always appears as ξT in $q(T; \xi, \kappa)$. Thus, Eq. (12) includes various kinds of models.

4   General case

Let us consider a general case where the firing rate changes stepwise. That is, $\{\xi_1, \ldots, \xi_n\}$ is distributed according to $k(\{\xi\}) = k(\xi_1, \ldots, \xi_n)$ and m_a observations are given for each ξ_a. The model can be written as

$$p(\{T\}; \kappa, k(\{\xi\}))$$
$$= \int \prod_{i_1=1}^{m_1} q(T_{i_1}^{(1)}; \xi_1, \kappa) \prod_{i_2=1}^{m_2} q(T_{i_2}^{(2)}; \xi_2, \kappa) \ldots \prod_{i_n=1}^{m_n} q(T_{i_n}^{(n)}; \xi_n, \kappa) k(\{\xi\}) d\xi_1 d\xi_2 \ldots d\xi_n,$$

where

$$(31)$$

$$
\prod_{i_1=1}^{m_1} q(T_{i_1}^{(1)}; \xi_1, \kappa) \prod_{i_2=1}^{m_2} q(T_{i_2}^{(2)}; \xi_2, \kappa) \dots \prod_{i_n=1}^{m_n} q(T_{i_n}^{(n)}; \xi_n, \kappa)
$$

$$
= \exp(\xi_1(-\kappa \sum_{i_1=1}^{m_1} T_{i_1}^{(1)}) + \xi_2(-\kappa \sum_{i_2=1}^{m_2} T_{i_2}^{(2)}) + \dots + \xi_n(-\kappa \sum_{i_n=1}^{m_n} T_{i_n}^{(n)})
$$

$$
+ (\kappa - 1)(\sum_{i_1=1}^{m_1} \log T_{i_1}^{(1)} + \sum_{i_2=1}^{m_2} \log T_{i_2}^{(2)} + \dots + \sum_{i_n=1}^{m_n} \log T_{i_n}^{(n)})
$$

$$
+ \sum_{a=1}^{n} m_a \kappa \log(\xi_a) + \sum_{a=1}^{n} m_a \kappa \log(\kappa) - \sum_{a=1}^{n} m_a \log \Gamma(\kappa)). \tag{32}
$$

We defined s_a, r, and ψ as

$$
s_a(\{T^{(a)}\}, \kappa) = -\kappa \sum_{i_a=1}^{m_a} T_{i_a}^{(a)}, \tag{33}
$$

$$
r(\{T\}, \kappa) = (\kappa - 1) \sum_{a=1}^{n} (\sum_{i_a=1}^{m_a} \log T_{i_a}^{(a)}), \tag{34}
$$

$$
\psi(\kappa, \{\xi\}) = -\sum_{a=1}^{n} m_a \kappa \log(\xi_a) - \sum_{a=1}^{n} m_a \kappa \log(\kappa) + \sum_{a=1}^{n} m_a \log \Gamma(\kappa). \tag{35}
$$

Then,

$$
\begin{aligned}
u^I(\{T\}, \kappa) &= u - E[u|s] \\
&= (\partial_\kappa s - E[\partial_\kappa s|s]) \cdot E[\xi|s] + \partial_\kappa r - E[\partial_\kappa r|s] \\
&= \partial_\kappa r - E[\partial_\kappa r|s] \\
&= \sum_{a=1}^{n} \{ \sum_{i_a=1}^{m_a} \log T_{i_a}^{(a)} - m_a \log(\sum_{i_a=1}^{m_a} T_{i_a}^{(a)}) + m_a \phi(m_a \kappa) - m_a \phi(\kappa) \}.
\end{aligned} \tag{36}
$$

Thus, κ is estimated with equal weight for every observation. Note that the conditional expectations can be calculated independently for each set of random variables. u^I yields an efficient estimating function. As this does not depend on $k(\{\xi\})$, u^I is the optimal estimating function at any $k(\{\xi\})$. There is no information loss. Note that $k(\{\xi\})$ can include correlations among ξ_a's. Nevertheless, the result is very similar to that of the previous section.

5   Summary and discussion

We estimated the shape parameter, κ, of the semiparametric model suggested by Ikeda without estimating the firing rate, ξ. The maximum likelihood estimator is not consistent for this problem because the number of nuisance parameters, ξ, increases with increasing observations, T. We showed that Ikeda's model is the exponential form defined by Amari and Kawanabe [15] and can be analyzed by a method of estimating functions for semiparametric models. We found that an estimating function does not exist unless multiple observations are given for each firing rate, ξ. If multiple observations are given, a method of estimating functions can be applied. In that case, the estimating function of κ can be analytically obtained, and κ can be estimated consistently independent of the functional form of the firing rate, $k(\xi)$. In general, the estimating function is not efficient. However, this method provided an optimal estimator in the sense of Fisher information for our problem. That is, we obtained an efficient estimator.

Acknowledgments

We are grateful to K. Ikeda for his helpful discussions. This work was supported in part by grants from the Japan Society for the Promotion of Science (Nos. 14084212 and 16500093).

References

[1] G. R. Holt, W. R. Softky, C. Koch, and R. J. Douglas, Comparison of discharge variability in vitro and in vivo in cat visual cortex neurons, J. Neurophysiol., Vol. 75, pp. 1806-14, 1996.

[2] H. C. Tuckwell, Introduction to theoretical neurobiology: volume 2, nonlinear and stochastic theories, Cambridge University Press, Cambridge, 1988.

[3] Y. Sakai, S. Funahashi, and S. Shinomoto, Temporally correlated inputs to leaky integrate-and-fire models can reproduce spiking statistics of cortical neurons, Neural Netw., Vol. 12, pp. 1181-1190, 1999.

[4] D. R. Cox and P. A. W. Lewis, The statistical analysis of series of events, Methuen, London, 1966.

[5] S. N. Baker and R. N. Lemon, Precise spatiotemporal repeating patterns in monkey primary and supplementary motor areas occur at chance levels, J. Neurophysiol., Vol. 84, pp. 1770-80, 2000.

[6] S. Shinomoto, K. Shima, and J. Tanji, Differences in spiking patterns among cortical neurons, Neural Comput.,Vol. 15, pp. 2823-42, 2003.

[7] S. Shinomoto, Y. Miyazaki, H. Tamura, and I. Fujita, Regional and laminar differences in in vivo firing patterns of primate cortical neurons, J. Neurophysiol., in press.

[8] S. Shinomoto, K. Miura, and S. Koyama, A measure of local variation of inter-spike intervals, Biosystems, Vol. 79, pp. 67-72, 2005.

[9] J. Pfanzagl, Estimation in semiparametric models, Springer-Verlag, Berlin, 1990.

[10] K. Ikeda, Information geometry of interspike intervals in spiking neurons, Neural Comput., in press.

[11] V. P. Godambe, An optimum property of regular maximum likelihood estimation, Ann. Math. Statist., Vol. 31, pp. 1208-1211, 1960.

[12] V. P. Godambe (ed.), Estimating functions, Oxford University Press, New York, 1991.

[13] S. Amari, Dual connections on the Hilbert bundles of statistical models, In C. T. J. Dodson (ed.), Geometrization of statistical theory, pp. 123-152, University of Lancaster Department of Mathematics, Lancaster, 1987.

[14] S. Amari and M. Kumon, Estimation in the presence of infinitely many nuisance parameters - geometry of estimating functions, Ann. Statist., Vol. 16, pp. 1044-1068, 1988.

[15] S. Amari and M. Kawanabe, Information geometry of estimating functions in semi-parametric statistical models, Bernoulli, Vol. 3, pp. 29-54, 1997.

[16] H. Nagaoka and S. Amari, Differential geometry of smooth families of probability distributions, Technical Report 82-7, University of Tokyo, 1982.

[17] S. Amari and H. Nagaoka, Methods of information geometry, American Mathematical Society, Providence, RI, 2001.

[18] S. Amari, Information geometry on hierarchy of probability distributions, IEEE Transactions on Information Theory, Vol. 47, pp. 1701-1711, 2001.

[19] J. Neyman and E. L. Scott, Consistent estimates based on partially consistent observations, Econometrica, Vol. 32, pp. 1-32, 1948.

[20] Y. Ritov and P. J. Bickel, Achieving information bounds in non and semiparametric models, Ann. Statist., Vol. 18, pp. 925-938, 1990.

[21] P. J. Bickel, C. A. J. Klaassen, Y. Ritov, and J. A. Wellner, Efficient and adaptive estimation for semiparametric models, Johns Hopkins University Press, Baltimore, MD, 1993.

Consensus Propagation

Ciamac C. Moallemi
Stanford University
Stanford, CA 95014 USA
ciamac@stanford.edu

Benjamin Van Roy
Stanford University
Stanford, CA 95014 USA
bvr@stanford.edu

Abstract

We propose *consensus propagation*, an asynchronous distributed protocol for averaging numbers across a network. We establish convergence, characterize the convergence rate for regular graphs, and demonstrate that the protocol exhibits better scaling properties than *pairwise averaging*, an alternative that has received much recent attention. Consensus propagation can be viewed as a special case of belief propagation, and our results contribute to the belief propagation literature. In particular, beyond singly-connected graphs, there are very few classes of relevant problems for which belief propagation is known to converge.

1 Introduction

Consider a network of n nodes in which the ith node observes a number $y_i \in [0, 1]$ and aims to compute the average $\sum_{i=1}^{n} y_i / n$. The design of scalable distributed protocols for this purpose has received much recent attention and is motivated by a variety of potential needs. In both wireless sensor and peer-to-peer networks, for example, there is interest in simple protocols for computing aggregate statistics (see, for example, the references in [1]), and averaging enables computation of several important ones. Further, averaging serves as a primitive in the design of more sophisticated distributed information processing algorithms. For example, a maximum likelihood estimate can be produced by an averaging protocol if each node's observations are linear in variables of interest and noise is Gaussian [2]. As another example, averaging protocols are central to policy-gradient-based methods for distributed optimization of network performance [3].

In this paper we propose and analyze a new protocol – **consensus propagation** – for asynchronous distributed averaging. As a baseline for comparison, we will also discuss another asychronous distributed protocol – **pairwise averaging** – which has received much recent attention. In pairwise averaging, each node maintains its current estimate of the average, and each time a pair of nodes communicate, they revise their estimates to both take on the mean of their previous estimates. Convergence of this protocol in a very general model of asynchronous computation and communication was established in [4]. Recent work [5, 6] has studied the convergence rate and its dependence on network topology and how pairs of nodes are sampled. Here, sampling is governed by a certain doubly stochastic matrix, and the convergence rate is characterized by its second-largest eigenvalue.

Consensus propagation is a simple algorithm with an intuitive interpretation. It can also be viewed as an asynchronous distributed version of belief propagation as applied to approximation of conditional distributions in a Gaussian Markov random field. When the network of interest is singly-connected, prior results about belief propagation imply convergence of consensus propagation. However, in most cases of interest, the network is not singly-connected and prior results have little to say about convergence. In particular, Gaussian belief propagation on a graph with cycles is not guaranteed to converge, as demonstrated by examples in [7].

In fact, there are very few relevant cases where belief propagation on a graph with cycles is known to converge. Some fairly general sufficient conditions have been established [8, 9, 10], but these conditions are abstract and it is difficult to identify interesting classes of problems that meet them. One simple case where belief propagation is guaranteed to converge is when the graph has only a single cycle [11, 12, 13]. Recent work proposes the use of belief propagation to solve maximum-weight matching problems and proves convergence in that context [14]. [15] proves convergence in the application of belief propogation to a classification problem. In the Gaussian case, [7, 16] provide sufficient conditions for convergence, but these conditions are difficult to interpret and do not capture situations that correspond to consensus propagation.

With this background, let us discuss the primary contributions of this paper: (1) we propose consensus propagation, a new asynchronous distributed protocol for averaging; (2) we prove that consensus propagation converges even when executed asynchronously. Since there are so few classes of relevant problems for which belief propagation is known to converge, even with *synchronous execution*, this is surprising; (3) We characterize the convergence time in regular graphs of the synchronous version of consensus propagation in terms of the the mixing time of a certain Markov chain over edges of the graph; (4) we explain why the convergence time of consensus propagation scales more gracefully with the number of nodes than does that of pairwise averaging, and for certain classes of graphs, we quantify the improvement.

2 Algorithm

Consider a connected undirected graph (V, E) with $|V| = n$ nodes. For each node $i \in V$, let $N(i) = \{j : (i,j) \in E\}$ be the set of neighbors of i. Each node $i \in V$ is assigned a number $y_i \in [0,1]$. The goal is for each node to obtain an estimate of $\bar{y} = \sum_{i \in V} y_i / n$ through an asynchronous distributed protocol in which each node carries out simple computations and communicates parsimonious messages to its neighbors.

We propose consensus propagation as an approach to the aforementioned problem. In this protocol, if a node i communicates to a neighbor j at time t, it transmits a message consisting of two numerical values. Let $\mu_{ij}^t \in \mathbb{R}$ and $K_{ij}^t \in \mathbb{R}_+$ denote the values associated with the most recently transmitted message from i to j at or before time t. At each time t, node j has stored in memory the most recent message from each neighbor: $\{\mu_{ij}^t, K_{ij}^t | i \in N(j)\}$. The initial values in memory before receiving any messages are arbitrary.

Consensus propagation is parameterized by a scalar $\beta > 0$ and a non-negative matrix $Q \in \mathbb{R}_+^{n \times n}$ with $Q_{ij} > 0$ if and only if $i \neq j$ and $(i,j) \in E$. Let $\vec{E} \subseteq V \times V$ be a set consisting of two directed edges (i,j) and (j,i) per undirected edge $(i,j) \in E$. For each $(i,j) \in \vec{E}$, it is useful to define the following three functions:

$$\mathcal{F}_{ij}(K) = \frac{1 + \sum_{u \in N(i) \setminus j} K_{ui}}{1 + \frac{1}{\beta Q_{ij}} \left(1 + \sum_{u \in N(i) \setminus j} K_{ui}\right)}, \tag{1}$$

$$\mathcal{G}_{ij}(\mu, K) = \frac{y_i + \sum_{u \in N(i) \setminus j} K_{ui} \mu_{ui}}{1 + \sum_{u \in N(i) \setminus j} K_{ui}}, \qquad \mathcal{X}_i(\mu, K) = \frac{y_i + \sum_{u \in N(i)} K_{ui} \mu_{ui}}{1 + \sum_{u \in N(i)} K_{ui}}. \tag{2}$$

For each t, denote by $U_t \subseteq \vec{E}$ the set of directed edges along which messages are transmitted at time t. Consensus propagation is presented below as Algorithm 1.

Algorithm 1 Consensus propagation.

1: **for** time $t = 1$ to ∞ **do**
2:     **for all** $(i,j) \in U_t$ **do**
3:         $K_{ij}^t \leftarrow \mathcal{F}_{ij}(K^{t-1})$
4:         $\mu_{ij}^t \leftarrow \mathcal{G}_{ij}(\mu^{t-1}, K^{t-1})$
5:     **end for**
6:     **for all** $(i,j) \notin U_t$ **do**
7:         $K_{ij}^t \leftarrow K_{ij}^{t-1}$
8:         $\mu_{ij}^t \leftarrow \mu_{ij}^{t-1}$
9:     **end for**
10:    $x^t \leftarrow \mathcal{X}(\mu^t, K^t)$
11: **end for**

Consensus propagation is a *distributed protocol* because computations at each node require only information that is locally available. In particular, the messages $\mathcal{F}_{ij}(K^{t-1})$ and $\mathcal{G}_{ij}(K^{t-1})$ transmitted from node i to node j depend only on $\{\mu_{ui}^{t-1}, K_{ui}^{t-1} | u \in N(i)\}$, which node i has stored in memory. Similarly, x_i^t, which serves as an estimate of $\bar{y}$, depends only on $\{\mu_{ui}^t, K_{ui}^t | u \in N(i)\}$.

Consensus propagation is an *asynchronous protocol* because only a subset of the potential messages are transmitted at each time. Our convergence analysis can also be extended to accommodate more general models of asynchronism that involve communication delays, as those presented in [17].

In our study of convergence *time*, we will focus on the *synchronous* version of consensus propagation. This is where $U_t = \vec{E}$ for all t. Note that synchronous consensus propagation is defined by:

$$K^t = \mathcal{F}(K^{t-1}), \quad \mu^t = \mathcal{G}(\mu^{t-1}, K^{t-1}), \quad x^t = \mathcal{X}(\mu^{t-1}, K^{t-1}). \tag{3}$$

2.1 Intuitive Interpretation

Consider the special case of a singly connected graph. For any $(i,j) \in \vec{E}$, there is a set $S_{ij} \subset V$ of nodes that can transmit information to $S_{ji} = V \setminus S_{ij}$ only through (i,j). In order for nodes in S_{ji} to compute $\bar{y}$, they must at least be provided with the average μ_{ij}^* among observations at nodes in S_{ij} and the cardinality $K_{ij}^* = |S_{ij}|$. The messages μ_{ij}^t and K_{ij}^t can be viewed as estimates. In fact, when $\beta = \infty$, μ_{ij}^t and K_{ij}^t converge to μ_{ij}^* and K_{ij}^*, as we will now explain.

Suppose the graph is singly connected, $\beta = \infty$, and transmissions are synchronous. Then,

$$K_{ij}^t = 1 + \sum_{u \in N(i) \setminus j} K_{ui}^{t-1}, \tag{4}$$

for all $(i,j) \in \vec{E}$. This is a recursive characterization of $|S_{ij}|$, and it is easy to see that it converges in a number of iterations equal to the diameter of the graph. Now consider the iteration

$$\mu_{ij}^t = \frac{y_i + \sum_{u \in N(i) \setminus j} K_{ui}^{t-1} \mu_{ui}^{t-1}}{1 + \sum_{u \in N(i) \setminus j} K_{ui}^{t-1}},$$

for all $(i,j) \in \vec{E}$. A simple inductive argument shows that at each time t, μ_{ij}^t is an average among observations at K_{ij}^t nodes in S_{ij}, and after a number of iterations equal to the diameter of the graph, $\mu^t = \mu^*$. Further, for any $i \in V$,

$$\overline{y} = \frac{y_i + \sum_{u \in N(i)} K_{ui}\mu_{ui}}{1 + \sum_{u \in N(i)} K_{ui}},$$

so x_i^t converges to $\overline{y}$. This interpretation can be extended to the asynchronous case where it elucidates the fact that μ^t and K^t become μ^* and K^* after every pair of nodes in the graph has established bilateral communication through some sequence of transmissions among adjacent nodes.

Suppose now that the graph has cycles. If $\beta = \infty$, for any $(i, j) \in \vec{E}$ that is part of a cycle, $K_{ij}^t \to \infty$ whether transmissions are synchronous or asynchronous, so long as messages are transmitted along each edge of the cycle an infinite number of times. A heuristic fix might be to compose the iteration (4) with one that attenuates: $\tilde{K}_{ij}^t \leftarrow 1 + \sum_{u \in N(i) \setminus j} K_{ui}^{t-1}$, and $K_{ij}^t \leftarrow \tilde{K}_{ij}^t / (1 + \epsilon_{ij} \tilde{K}_{ij}^t)$. Here, $\epsilon_{ij} > 0$ is a small constant. The message is essentially unaffected when $\epsilon_{ij} \tilde{K}_{ij}^t$ is small but becomes increasingly attenuated as $\tilde{K}_{ij}^t$ grows. This is exactly the kind of attenuation carried out by consensus propagation when $\beta Q_{ij} = 1/\epsilon_{ij} < \infty$. Understanding why this kind of attenuation leads to desirable results is a subject of our analysis.

2.2 Relation to Belief Propagation

Consensus propagation can also be viewed as a special case of belief propagation. In this context, belief propagation is used to approximate the marginal distributions of a vector $x \in \mathbb{R}^n$ conditioned on the observations $y \in \mathbb{R}^n$. The mode of each of the marginal distributions approximates $\overline{y}$.

Take the prior distribution over (x, y) to be the normalized product of potential functions $\{\psi_i(\cdot) | i \in V\}$ and compatibility functions $\{\psi_{ij}^\beta(\cdot) | (i, j) \in E\}$, given by $\psi_i(x_i) = \exp(-(x_i - y_i)^2)$, and $\psi_{ij}^\beta(x_i, x_j) = \exp(-\beta Q_{ij}(x_i - x_j)^2)$, where Q_{ij}, for each $(i, j) \in \vec{E}$, and β are positive constants. Note that β can be viewed as an inverse temperature parameter; as β increases, components of x associated with adjacent nodes become increasingly correlated.

Let Γ be a positive semidefinite symmetric matrix such that $x^T \Gamma x = \sum_{(i,j) \in E} Q_{ij}(x_i - x_j)^2$. Note that when $Q_{ij} = 1$ for all $(i, j) \in E$, Γ is the graph Laplacian. Given the vector y of observations, the conditional density of x is

$$p^\beta(x) \propto \prod_{i \in V} \psi_i(x_i) \prod_{(i,j) \in E} \psi_{ij}^\beta(x_i, x_j) = \exp\left(-\|x - y\|_2^2 - \beta x^T \Gamma x\right).$$

Let x^β denote the mode of $p^\beta(\cdot)$. Since the distribution is Gaussian, each component x_i^β is also the mode of the corresponding marginal distribution. Note that x^β it is the unique solution to the positive definite quadratic program

$$\underset{x}{\text{minimize}} \quad \|x - y\|_2^2 + \beta x^T \Gamma x. \tag{5}$$

The following theorem, whose proof can be found in [1], suggests that if β is sufficiently large each component x_i^β can be used as an estimate of the mean value $\overline{y}$.

Theorem 1. $\sum_i x_i^\beta / n = \overline{y}$ and $\lim_{\beta \uparrow \infty} x_i^\beta = \overline{y}$, for all $i \in V$.

In belief propagation, messages are passed along edges of a Markov random field. In our case, because of the structure of the distribution $p^\beta(\cdot)$, the relevant Markov random field has the same topology as the graph (V, E). The message $M_{ij}(\cdot)$ passed from node i to node j is a distribution on the variable x_j. Node i computes this message using incoming messages from other nodes as defined by the update equation

$$M_{ij}^t(x_j) = \kappa \int \psi_{ij}(x_i', x_j)\psi_i(x_i') \prod_{u \in N(i)\backslash j} M_{ui}^{t-1}(x_i') \, dx_i'. \tag{6}$$

Here, κ is a normalizing constant. Since our underlying distribution $p^\beta(\cdot)$ is Gaussian, it is natural to consider messages which are Gaussian distributions. In particular, let $(\mu_{ij}^t, K_{ij}^t) \in \mathbb{R} \times \mathbb{R}_+$ parameterize Gaussian message $M_{ij}^t(\cdot)$ according to $M_{ij}^t(x_j) \propto \exp\left(-K_{ij}^t(x_j - \mu_{ij}^t)^2\right)$. Then, (6) is equivalent to synchronous consensus propagation iterations for K^t and μ^t.

The sequence of densities

$$p_j^t(x_j) \propto \psi_j(x_j) \prod_{i \in N(j)} M_{ij}^t(x_j) = \exp\left(-(x_j - y_j)^2 - \sum_{i \in N(j)} K_{ij}^t(x_j - \mu_{ij}^t)^2\right),$$

is meant to converge to an approximation of the marginal conditional distribution of x_j. As such, an approximation to x_j^β is given by maximizing $p_j^t(\cdot)$. It is easy to show that, the maximum is attained by $x_j^t = \mathcal{X}_j(\mu^t, K^t)$. With this and aforementioned correspondences, we have shown that consensus propagation is a special case of belief propagation. Readers familiar with belief propagation will notice that in the derivation above we have used the sum product form of the algorithm. In this case, since the underlying distribution is Gaussian, the max product form yields equivalent iterations.

3 Convergence

The following theorem is our main convergence result.

Theorem 2. (i) *There are unique vectors (μ^β, K^β) such that $K^\beta = \mathcal{F}(K^\beta)$, and $\mu^\beta = \mathcal{G}(\mu^\beta, K^\beta)$.*

(ii) *Assume that each edge $(i, j) \in \vec{E}$ appears infinitely often in the sequence of communication sets $\{U_t\}$. Then, independent of the initial condition (μ^0, K^0), $\lim_{t\to\infty} K^t = K^\beta$, and $\lim_{t\to\infty} \mu^t = \mu^\beta$.*

(iii) *Given (μ^β, K^β), if $x^\beta = \mathcal{X}(\mu^\beta, K^\beta)$, then x^β is the mode of the distribution $p^\beta(\cdot)$.*

The proof of this theorem can be found in [1], but it rests on two ideas. First, notice that, according to the update equation (1), K^t evolves independently of μ^t. Hence, we analyze K^t first. Following the work of [7], we prove that the functions $\{\mathcal{F}_{ij}(\cdot)\}$ are monotonic. This property is used to establish convergence to a unique fixed point. Next, we analyze μ^t assuming that K^t has already converged. Given fixed K, the update equations for μ^t are linear, and we establish that they induce a contraction with respect to the maximum norm. This allows us to establish existence of a fixed point and asynchronous convergence.

4 Convergence Time for Regular Graphs

In this section, we will study the convergence time of synchronous consensus propagation. For $\epsilon > 0$, we will say that an estimate $\tilde{x}$ of $\bar{y}$ is ϵ-accurate if $\|\tilde{x} - \bar{y}\mathbf{1}\|_{2,n} \leq \epsilon$. Here, for integer m, $\|\cdot\|_{2,m}$ is the norm on $\mathbb{R}^m$ defined by $\|x\|_{2,m} = \|x\|_2/\sqrt{m}$. We are interested in the number of iterations required to obtain an ϵ-accurate estimate of the mean $\bar{y}$.

4.1 The Case of Regular Graphs

We will restrict our analysis of convergence time to cases where (V, E) is a d-regular graph, for $d \geq 2$. Extension of our analysis to broader classes of graphs remains an open issue. We will also make simplifying assumptions that $Q_{ij} = 1$, $\mu_{ij}^0 = y_i$, and $K^0 = [k_0]_{ij}$ for some scalar $k_0 \geq 0$.

In this restricted setting, the subspace of constant K vectors is invariant under $\mathcal{F}$. This implies that there is some scalar $k^\beta > 0$ so that $K^\beta = [k^\beta]_{ij}$. This k^β is the unique solution to the fixed point equation $k^\beta = (1 + (d-1)k^\beta) / ((1 + (1 + (d-1)k^\beta) / \beta)$. Given a uniform initial condition $K^0 = [k_0]_{ij}$, we can study the sequence of iterates $\{K^t\}$ by examining the scalar sequence $\{k_t\}$, defined by $k_t = (1 + (d-1)k_{t-1})(1 + (1 + (d-1)k_{t-1}) / \beta)$. In particular, we have $K^t = [k_t]_{ij}$, for all $t \geq 0$.

Similarly, in this setting, the equations for the evolution of μ^t take the special form

$$\mu_{ij}^t = \frac{y_i}{1 + (d-1)k_{t-1}} + \left(1 - \frac{1}{1 + (d-1)k_{t-1}}\right) \sum_{u \in N(i) \backslash j} \frac{\mu_{ui}^{t-1}}{d-1}.$$

Defining $\gamma_t = 1 / (1 + (d-1)k_t)$, we have, in vector form,

$$\mu^t = \gamma_{t-1} \hat{y} + (1 - \gamma_{t-1}) \hat{P} \mu^{t-1}, \tag{7}$$

where $\hat{y} \in \mathbb{R}^{nd}$ is a vector with $\hat{y}_{ij} = y_i$ and $\hat{P} \in \mathbb{R}_+^{nd \times nd}$ is a doubly stochastic matrix. The matrix $\hat{P}$ corresponds to a Markov chain on the set of directed edges $\vec{E}$. In this chain, an edge (i, j) transitions to an edge (u, i) with $u \in N(i) \backslash j$, with equal probability assigned to each such edge. As in (3), we associate each μ^t with an estimate x^t of x^β according to $x^t = y / (1 + dk^\beta) + dk^\beta A \mu^t / (1 + dk^\beta)$, where $A \in \mathbb{R}_+^{n \times nd}$ is a matrix defined by $(A\mu)_j = \sum_{i \in N(j)} \mu_{ij} / d$.

The update equation (7) suggests that the convergence of μ^t is intimately tied to a notion of mixing time associated with $\hat{P}$. Let $\hat{P}^\star$ be the Cesàro limit $\hat{P}^\star = \lim_{t \to \infty} \sum_{\tau=0}^{t-1} \hat{P}^\tau / t$. Define the *Cesàro mixing time* $\tau^\star$ by $\tau^\star = \sup_{t \geq 0} \| \sum_{\tau=0}^{t} (\hat{P}^\tau - \hat{P}^\star) \|_{2, nd}$. Here, $\| \cdot \|_{2, nd}$ is the matrix norm induced by the corresponding vector norm $\| \cdot \|_{2, nd}$. Since $\hat{P}$ is a stochastic matrix, $\hat{P}^\star$ is well-defined and $\tau^\star < \infty$. Note that, in the case where $\hat{P}$ is aperiodic, irreducible, and symmetric, $\tau^\star$ corresponds to the traditional definition of mixing time: the inverse of the spectral gap of $\hat{P}$.

A time t^* is said to be an ϵ-*convergence time* if estimates x^t are ϵ-accurate for all $t \geq t^*$. The following theorem, whose proof can be found in [1], establishes a bound on the ϵ-convergence time of synchronous consensus propagation given appropriately chosen β, as a function of ϵ and $\tau^\star$.

Theorem 3. *Suppose $k_0 \leq k^\beta$. If $d = 2$ there exists a $\beta = \Theta((\tau^\star / \epsilon)^2)$ and if $d > 2$ there exists a $\beta = \Theta(\tau^\star / \epsilon)$ such that some $t^* = O((\tau^\star / \epsilon) \log(\tau^\star / \epsilon))$ is an ϵ-convergence time. Alternatively, suppose $k_0 = k^\beta$. If $d = 2$ there exists a $\beta = \Theta((\tau^\star / \epsilon)^2)$ and if $d > 2$ there exists a $\beta = \Theta(\tau^\star / \epsilon)$ such that some $t^* = O((\tau^\star / \epsilon) \log(1/\epsilon))$ is an ϵ-convergence time.*

In the first part of the above theorem, k_0 is initialized arbitrarily so long as $k_0 \leq k^\beta$. Typically, one might set $k_0 = 0$ to guarantee this. The second case of interest is when $k_0 = k^\beta$, so that $k_t = k^\beta$ for all $t \geq 0$ Theorem 3 suggests that initializing with $k_0 = k^\beta$ leads to an improvement in convergence time. However, in our computational experience, we have found that an initial condition of $k_0 = 0$ consistently results in *faster* convergence than $k_0 = k^\beta$. Hence, we suspect that a convergence time bound of $O((\tau^\star / \epsilon) \log(1/\epsilon))$ also holds for the case of $k_0 = 0$. Proving this remains an open issue. Theorems 3 posits choices of β that require knowledge of $\tau^\star$, which may be both difficult to compute and also requires knowledge of the graph topology. This is not a major restriction, however. It is not difficult to imagine variations of Algorithm 1 which use a doubling sequence of guesses for the Cesáro mixing time $\tau^\star$. Each guess leads to a choice of β and a number of iterations t^* to run with that choice of β. Such a modified algorithm would still have an ϵ-convergence time of $O((\tau^\star/\epsilon)\log(\tau^\star/\epsilon))$.

5   Comparison with Pairwise Averaging

Using the results of Section 4, we can compare the performance of consensus propagation to that of pairwise averaging. Pairwise averaging is usually defined in an asynchronous setting, but there is a synchronous counterpart which works as follows. Consider a doubly stochastic symmetric matrix $P \in \mathbb{R}^{n \times n}$ such that $P_{ij} = 0$ if $(i,j) \notin E$. Evolve estimates according to $x^t = Px^{t-1}$, initialized with $x^0 = y$. Clearly $x^t = P^t y \to \bar{y}\mathbf{1}$ as $t \uparrow \infty$.

In the case of a singly-connected graph, synchronous consensus propagation converges exactly in a number of iterations equal to the diameter of the graph. Moreover, when $\beta = \infty$, this convergence is to the exact mean, as discussed in Section 2.1. This is the best one can hope for under any algorithm, since the diameter is the minimum amount of time required for a message to travel between the two most distant nodes. On the other hand, for a fixed accuracy ϵ, the worst-case number of iterations required by synchronous pairwise averaging on a singly-connected graph scales at least quadratically in the diameter [18].

The rate of convergence of synchronous pairwise averaging is governed by the relation $\|x^t - \bar{y}\mathbf{1}\|_{2,n} \leq \lambda_2^t$, where λ_2 is the second largest eigenvalue of P. Let $\tau_2 = 1/\log(1/\lambda_2)$, and call it the *mixing time* of P. In order to guarantee ϵ-accuracy (independent of y), $t > \tau_2 \log(1/\epsilon)$ suffices and $t = \Omega(\tau_2 \log(1/\epsilon))$ is required [6].

Consider d-regular graphs and fix a desired error tolerance ϵ. The number of iterations required by consensus propagation is $\Theta(\tau^\star \log \tau^\star)$, whereas that required by pairwise averaging is $\Theta(\tau_2)$. Both mixing times depend on the size and topology of the graph. τ_2 is the mixing time of a process on nodes that transitions along edges whereas $\tau^\star$ is the mixing time of a process on directed edges that transitions towards nodes. An important distinction is that the former process is allowed to "backtrack" where as the latter is not. By this we mean that a sequence of states $\{i,j,i\}$ can be observed in the vertex process, but the sequence $\{(i,j),(j,i)\}$ cannot be observed in the edge process. As we will now illustrate through an example, it is this difference that makes τ_2 larger than $\tau^\star$ and, therefore, pairwise averaging less efficient than consensus propagation.

In the case of a cycle ($d = 2$) with an even number of nodes n, minimizing the mixing time over P results in $\tau_2 = \Theta(n^2)$ [19]. For comparison, as demonstrated in the following theorem (whose proof can be found in [1]), $\tau^\star$ is linear in n.

Theorem 4. *For the cycle with n nodes, $\tau^\star \leq n/\sqrt{2}$.*

Intuitively, the improvement in mixing time arises from the fact that the edge process moves around the cycle in a single direction and therefore explores the entire graph within n iterations. The vertex process, on the other hand, randomly transitions back and forth among adjacent nodes, relying on chance to eventually explore the entire cycle.

The cycle example demonstrates a $\Theta(n/\log n)$ advantage offered by consensus propagation. Comparisons of mixing times associated with other graph topologies remains an issue for future analysis. But let us close by speculating on a uniform grid of n nodes over the m-dimensional unit torus. Here, $n^{1/m}$ is an integer, and each vertex has $2m$ neighbors, each a distance $n^{-1/m}$ away. With P optimized, it can be shown that $\tau_2 = \Theta(n^{2/m})$ [20]. We put forth a conjecture on $\tau^\star$.

Conjecture 1. *For the m-dimensional torus with n nodes, $\tau^\star = \Theta(n^{(2m-1)/m^2})$.*

Acknowledgments

The authors wish to thank Balaji Prabhakar and Ashish Goel for their insights and comments. The first author was supported by a Benchmark Stanford Graduate Fellowship. This research was supported in part by the National Science Foundation through grant IIS-0428868 and a supplement to grant ECS-9985229 provided by the Management of Knowledge Intensive Dynamic Systems Program (MKIDS).

References

[1] C. C. Moallemi and B. Van Roy. Consensus propagation. Technical report, Management Science & Engineering Deptartment, Stanford University, 2005. URL: `http://www.moallemi.com/ciamac/papers/cp-2005.pdf`.

[2] L. Xiao, S. Boyd, and S. Lall. A scheme for robust distributed sensor fusion based on average consensus. To appear in the proceedings of IPSN, 2005.

[3] C. C. Moallemi and B. Van Roy. Distributed optimization in adaptive networks. In *Advances in Neural Information Processing Systems 16*, 2004.

[4] J. N. Tsitsiklis. *Problems in Decentralized Decision-Making and Computation*. PhD thesis, Massachusetts Institute of Technology, Cambridge, MA, 1984.

[5] D. Kempe, A. Dobra, and J. Gehrke. Gossip-based computation of aggregate information. In *ACM Symposium on Theory of Computing*, 2004.

[6] S. Boyd, A. Ghosh, B. Prabhakar, and D. Shah. Gossip algorithms: Design, analysis and applications. To appear in the proceedings of INFOCOM, 2005.

[7] P. Rusmevichientong and B. Van Roy. An analysis of belief propagation on the turbo decoding graph with Gaussian densities. *IEEE Transactions on Information Theory*, 47(2):745–765, 2001.

[8] S. Tatikonda and M. I. Jordan. Loopy belief propagation and Gibbs measures. In *Proceedings of the 18th Conference on Uncertainty in Artificial Intelligence*, 2002.

[9] T. Heskes. On the uniqueness of loopy belief propagation fixed points. *Neural Computation*, 16(11):2379–2413, 2004.

[10] A. T. Ihler, J. W. Fisher III, and A. S. Willsky. Message errors in belief propagation. In *Advances in Neural Information Processing Systems*, 2005.

[11] G. Forney, F. Kschischang, and B. Marcus. Iterative decoding of tail-biting trelisses. In *Proceedings of the 1998 Information Theory Workshop*, 1998.

[12] S. M. Aji, G. B. Horn, and R. J. McEliece. On the convergence of iterative decoding on graphs with a single cycle. In *Proceedings of CISS*, 1998.

[13] Y. Weiss and W. T. Freeman. Correctness of local probability propagation in graphical models with loops. *Neural Computation*, 12:1–41, 2000.

[14] M. Bayati, D. Shah, and M. Sharma. Maximum weight matching via max-product belief propagation. preprint, 2005.

[15] V. Saligrama, M. Alanyali, and O. Savas. Asynchronous distributed detection in sensor networks. preprint, 2005.

[16] Y. Weiss and W. T. Freeman. Correctness of belief propagation in Gaussian graphical models of arbitrary topology. *Neural Computation*, 13:2173–2200, 2001.

[17] D. P. Bertsekas and J. N. Tsitsiklis. *Parallel and Distributed Computation: Numerical Methods*. Athena Scientific, Belmont, MA, 1997.

[18] S. Boyd, P. Diaconis, J. Sun, and L. Xiao. Fastest mixing Markov chain on a path. submitted to *The American Mathematical Monthly*, 2003.

[19] S. Boyd, A. Ghosh, B. Prabhakar, and D. Shah. Mixing times for random walks on geometric random graphs. To appear in the proceedings of SIAM ANALCO, 2005.

[20] S. Roch. Bounded fastest mixing. preprint, 2004.

Context as Filtering

Daichi Mochihashi
ATR, Spoken Language Communication
Research Laboratories
Hikaridai 2-2-2, Keihanna Science City
Kyoto, Japan
daichi.mochihashi@atr.jp

Yuji Matsumoto
Graduate School of Information Science
Nara Institute of Science and Technology
Takayama 8916-5, Ikoma City
Nara, Japan
matsu@is.naist.jp

Abstract

Long-distance language modeling is important not only in speech recognition and machine translation, but also in high-dimensional discrete sequence modeling in general. However, the problem of context length has almost been neglected so far and a naïve bag-of-words history has been employed in natural language processing. In contrast, in this paper we view topic shifts within a text as a latent stochastic process to give an explicit probabilistic generative model that has partial exchangeability. We propose an online inference algorithm using particle filters to recognize topic shifts to employ the most appropriate length of context automatically. Experiments on the BNC corpus showed consistent improvement over previous methods involving no chronological order.

1 Introduction

Contextual effect plays an essential role in the linguistic behavior of humans. We infer the context in which we are involved to make an adaptive linguistic response by selecting an appropriate model from that information. In natural language processing research, such models are called long-distance language models that incorporate distant effects of previous words over the short-term dependencies between a few words, which are called n-gram models. Besides apparent application in speech recognition and machine translation, we note that many problems of discrete data processing reduce to language modeling, such as information retrieval [1], Web navigation [2], human-machine interaction or collaborative filtering and recommendation [3].

From the viewpoint of signal processing or control theory, context modeling is clearly a filtering problem that estimates the states of a system sequentially along time to predict the outputs according to them. However, for the problem of long-distance language modeling, natural language processing has so far only provided simple averaging using a set of whole words from the beginning of a text, totally dropping chronological order and implicitly assuming that the text comes from a stationary information source [4, 5].

The inherent difficulties that have prevented filtering approaches to language modeling are its discreteness and high dimensionality, which precludes Kalman filters and their extensions that are all designed for vector spaces and distributions like Gaussians. As we note in the following, ordinary discrete HMMs are not powerful enough for this purpose because their true state is restricted to a single hidden component [6].

In contrast, this paper proposes to solve the *high-dimensional discrete filtering problem* directly using a Particle Filter. By combining a multinomial Particle Filter recently proposed in statistics for DNA sequence modeling [7] with Bayesian text models LDA and DM, we introduce two models that can track multinomial stochastic processes of natural language or similar high-dimensional discrete data domains that we often encounter.

2 Mean Shift Model of Context

2.1 HMM for Multinomial Distributions

The long-distance language models mentioned in Section 1 assume a hidden multinomial distribution, such as a unigram distribution or a mixture distribution over the latent topics, to predict the next word by updating its estimate according to the observations. Therefore, to track context shifts, we need a model that describes changes of multinomial distributions.

One model for this purpose is a multinomial extension to the Mean shift model (MSM) recently proposed in the field of statistics [7]. This is a kind of HMM, but note that it is different from traditional discrete HMMs. In discrete HMMs, the true state is one of M components and we estimate it stochastically as a multinomial over the M components. On the other hand, since the true state here is itself a multinomial over the components, we estimate it stochastically as (possibly a mixture of) a Dirichlet distribution, a distribution of multinomial distributions on the $(M-1)$-simplex. This HMM has some similarity to the Factorial HMM [6] in that it has a combinatorial representational power through a distributed state representation. However, because the true state here is a multinomial over the latent variables, there are dependencies between the states that are assumed independent in the FHMM. Below, we briefly introduce a multinomial Mean shift model following [7] and an associated solution using a Particle Filter.

2.2 Multinomial Mean Shift Model

The MSM is a generative model that describes the intermittent changes of hidden states and outputs according to them. Although there is a corresponding counterpart using Normal distribution that was first introduced [8, 9], here we concentrate on a multinomial extension of MSM, following [7] for DNA sequence modeling.

In a multinomial MSM, we assume time-dependent true multinomials $\boldsymbol{\theta}_t$ that may change occasionally and the following generative model for the discrete outputs $\mathbf{y}_t = y_1 y_2 \ldots y_t$ ($y_t \in \Sigma$; Σ is a set of symbols) according to $\boldsymbol{\theta}_1 \boldsymbol{\theta}_2 \ldots \boldsymbol{\theta}_t$:

$$\begin{cases} \boldsymbol{\theta}_t \sim \mathrm{Dir}(\boldsymbol{\alpha}) & \text{with probability } \rho \\ \quad = \boldsymbol{\theta}_{t-1} & \text{with probability } (1-\rho), \\ y_t \sim \mathrm{Mult}(\boldsymbol{\theta}_t) \end{cases} \tag{1}$$

where $\mathrm{Dir}(\boldsymbol{\alpha})$ and $\mathrm{Mult}(\boldsymbol{\theta})$ are a Dirichlet and multinomial distribution with parameters $\boldsymbol{\alpha}$ and $\boldsymbol{\theta}$, respectively. Here we assume that the hyperparameter $\boldsymbol{\alpha}$ is known and fixed, an assumption we will relax in Section 3.

This model first draws a multinomial $\boldsymbol{\theta}$ from $\mathrm{Dir}(\boldsymbol{\alpha})$ and samples output y according to $\boldsymbol{\theta}$ for a certain interval. When a change point occurs with probability ρ, a new $\boldsymbol{\theta}$ is sampled again from $\mathrm{Dir}(\boldsymbol{\alpha})$ and subsequent y is sampled from the new $\boldsymbol{\theta}$. This process continues recursively throughout which neither $\boldsymbol{\theta}_t$ nor the change points are known to us; all we know is the output sequence $\mathbf{y}_t$.

However, if we know that the change has occurred at time c, y can be predicted exactly. Let I_t be a binary variable that represents whether a change occurred at time t: that is, $I_t = 1$ means there was a change at t ($\boldsymbol{\theta}_t \neq \boldsymbol{\theta}_{t-1}$), and $I_t = 0$ means there was no change ($\boldsymbol{\theta}_t = \boldsymbol{\theta}_{t-1}$). When the last change occurred at time c,

1. For particles $i = 1 \ldots N$,
    (a) Calculate $f(t)$ and $g(t)$ according to (6).
    (b) Sample $I_t^{(i)} \sim \text{Bernoulli}\,(f(t)/(f(t)+g(t)))$, and update $\mathbf{I}_{t-1}^{(i)}$ to $\mathbf{I}_t^{(i)}$.
    (c) Update weight $w_t^{(i)} = w_{t-1}^{(i)} \cdot (f(t)+g(t))$.
2. Find a predictive distribution using $w_t^{(1)} \ldots w_t^{(N)}$ and $\mathbf{I}_t^{(1)} \ldots \mathbf{I}_t^{(N)}$:
$$p(y_{t+1}|\mathbf{y}_t) = \sum_{i=1}^{N} w_t^{(i)} p(y_{t+1}|\mathbf{y}_t, \mathbf{I}_t^{(i)}) \tag{4}$$
where $p(y_{t+1}|\mathbf{y}_t, \mathbf{I}_t^{(i)})$ is given by (3).

Figure 1: Algorithm of the Multinomial Particle Filter.

$$p(y_{t+1}=y \mid \mathbf{y}_t, I_c=1, I_{c+1}=\cdots=I_t=0) = \int p(y|\boldsymbol{\theta})p(\boldsymbol{\theta}|y_c \cdots y_t)d\boldsymbol{\theta} \tag{2}$$
$$= \frac{\alpha_y + n_y}{\sum_y (\alpha_y + n_y)}, \tag{3}$$

where α_y is the y'th element of $\boldsymbol{\alpha}$ and n_y is the number of occurrences of y in $y_c \cdots y_t$. Therefore, the essence of this problem lies in how to detect a change point given the data up to time t, a change point problem in discrete space. Actually, this problem can be solved by an efficient Particle Filter algorithm [10] shown below.

2.3 Multinomial Particle Filter

The prediction problem above can be solved by the efficient Particle Filter algorithm shown in Figure 1, graphically displayed in Figure 2 (excluding prior updates). The main intricacy involved is as follows. Let us denote $\mathbf{I}_t = \{I_1 \ldots I_t\}$. By Bayes' theorem,

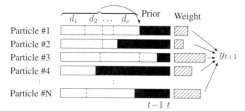

Figure 2: Multinomial Particle Filter in work.

$$p(I_t|\mathbf{I}_{t-1}, \mathbf{y}_t) \propto p(I_t, y_t|\mathbf{I}_{t-1}, \mathbf{y}_{t-1}) = p(y_t|\mathbf{y}_{t-1}, \mathbf{I}_{t-1}, I_t)p(I_t|\mathbf{I}_{t-1}) \tag{5}$$
$$= \begin{cases} p(y_t|\mathbf{y}_{t-1}, \mathbf{I}_{t-1}, I_t=1)p(I_t=1|\mathbf{I}_{t-1}) &=: f(t) \\ p(y_t|\mathbf{y}_{t-1}, \mathbf{I}_{t-1}, I_t=0)p(I_t=0|\mathbf{I}_{t-1}) &=: g(t) \end{cases} \tag{6}$$

leading
$$\begin{cases} p(I_t=1|\mathbf{I}_{t-1}, \mathbf{y}_t) = f(t)/(f(t)+g(t)) \\ p(I_t=0|\mathbf{I}_{t-1}, \mathbf{y}_t) = g(t)/(f(t)+g(t))\,. \end{cases} \tag{7}$$

In Expression (5), the first term is a likelihood of observation y_t when $\mathbf{I}_t$ has been fixed, which can be obtained through (3). The second term is a prior probability of change, which can be set tentatively by a constant ρ. However, when we endow ρ with a prior Beta distribution $\text{Be}(\alpha, \beta)$, posterior estimate of ρ_t given the binary change point history $\mathbf{I}_{t-1}$ can be obtained using the number of 1's in $\mathbf{I}_{t-1}$, $n_{t-1}(1)$, following a standard Bayesian method:
$$E[\rho_t|\mathbf{I}_{t-1}] = \frac{\alpha + n_{t-1}(1)}{\alpha + \beta + t - 1}\,. \tag{8}$$

This means that we can estimate a "rate of topic shifts" as time proceeds in a Bayesian fashion. Throughout the following experiments, we used this online estimate of ρ_t.

The above algorithm runs for each observation y_t ($t = 1 \ldots T$). If we observe a "strange" word that is more predictable from the prior than the contextual distribution, (6) makes $f(t)$ larger than $g(t)$, which leads to a higher probability that $I_t=1$ will be sampled in the Bernoulli trial of Algorithm 1(b).

3   Mean Shift Model of Natural Language

Chen and Lai [7] recently proposed the above algorithm to analyze DNA sequences. However, when extending this approach to natural language, i.e. word sequences, we meet two serious problems.

The first problem is that in a natural language the number of words is extremely large. As opposed to DNA, which has only four letters of A/T/G/C, a natural language usually contains a minimum of some tens of thousands of words and there are strong correlations between them. For example, if "nurse" follows "hospital"we believe that there has been no context shift; however, if "university" follows "hospital," the context probably has been shifted to a "medical school" subtopic, even though the two words are equally distinct from "hospital." Of course, this is due to the semantic relationship we can assume between these words. However, the original multinomial MSM cannot capture this relationship because it treats the words independently. To incorporate this relationship, we require an extensive prior knowledge of words as a probabilistic model.

The second problem is that in model equation (1), the hyperparameter α of prior Dirichlet distribution of the latent multinomials is assumed to be known. In the case of natural language, this means we know beforehand what words or topics will be spoken for all the texts. Apparently, this is not a natural assumption: we need an online estimation of α as well when we want to extend MSM to natural languages.

To solve these problems, we extended a multinomial MSM using two probabilistic text models, LDA and DM. Below we introduce MSM-LDA and MSM-DM, in this order.

3.1   MSM-LDA

Latent Dirichlet Allocation (LDA) [3] is a probabilistic text model that assumes a hidden multinomial topic distribution θ over the M topics on a document d to estimate it stochastically as a Dirichlet distribution $p(\theta|d)$. Context modeling using LDA [5] regards a history $\mathbf{h} = w_1 \ldots w_h$ as a pseudo document and estimates a variational approximation $q(\theta|\mathbf{h})$ of a topic distribution $p(\theta|\mathbf{h})$ through a variational Bayes EM algorithm on a document [3]. After obtaining topic distribution $q(\theta|\mathbf{h})$, we can predict the next word as follows.

$$p(y|\mathbf{h}) = \int p(y|\theta)q(\theta|\mathbf{h})d\theta = \sum_{i=1}^{M} p(y|\theta_i)\langle\theta_i\rangle_{q(\theta|\mathbf{h})} \tag{9}$$

When we use this prediction with an associated VB-EM algorithm in place of the naïve Dirichlet model (3) of MSM, we get an MSM-LDA that tracks a latent topic distribution θ instead of a word distribution. Since each particle computes a Dirichlet posterior of topic distribution, the final topic distribution of MSM-LDA is a mixture of Dirichlet distributions for predicting the next word through (4) and (9) as shown in Figure 3(a). Note that MSM-LDA has an implicit generative model corresponding to (1) in topic space. However, here we use a conditional model where LDA parameters are already known in order to estimate the context online.

In MSM-LDA, we can also update the hyperparameter α sequentially from the history. As seen in Figure 2, each particle has a history that has been segmented into pseudo "documents" $d_1 \ldots d_c$ by the change points sampled so far. Since each pseudo "document" has a Dirichlet posterior $q(\theta|d_i)$ $(i = 1 \ldots c)$, a common Dirichlet prior can be inferred by a linear-time Newton-Raphson algorithm [3]. Note that this computation needs only be run when a change point has been sampled. For this purpose, only the sufficient statistics $q(\theta|d_i)$ must be stored for each particle to render itself an online algorithm.

Note in passing that MSM-LDA is a model that only tracks a mixing distribution of a mixture model. Therefore, in principle this model is also applicable to other mixture models, e.g. Gaussian mixtures, where mixing distribution is not static but evolves according to (1).

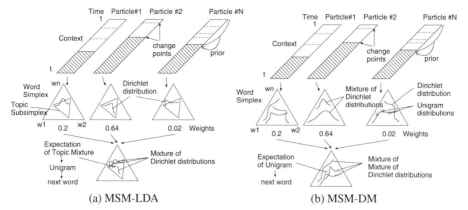

(a) MSM-LDA   (b) MSM-DM

Figure 3: MSM-LDA and MSM-DM in work.

However, in terms of multinomial estimation, this generality has a drawback because it uses a lower-dimensional topic representation to predict the next word, which may cause a loss of information. In contrast, MSM-DM is a model that works directly on the word space to predict the next word with no loss of information.

3.2 MSM-DM

Dirichlet Mixtures (DM) [11] is a novel Bayesian text model that has the lowest perplexity reported so far in context modeling. DM uses no intermediate "topic" variables, but places a *mixture of* Dirichlet distributions directly on the word simplex to model word correlations. Specifically, DM assumes the following generative model for a document $\mathbf{w} = w_1 \dots w_N$:[1]

1. Draw $m \sim \text{Mult}(\boldsymbol{\lambda})$.
2. Draw $\boldsymbol{p} \sim \text{Dir}(\boldsymbol{\alpha}_m)$.
3. For $n = 1 \dots N$,
   a. Draw $w_n \sim \text{Mult}(\boldsymbol{p})$.

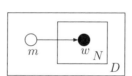

(a) Unigram Mixture (UM)   (b) Dirichlet Mixtures (DM)

Figure 4: Graphical models of UM and DM.

where $\boldsymbol{p}$ is a V-dimensional unigram distribution over words, $\boldsymbol{\alpha}_1 \dots \boldsymbol{\alpha}_M = \boldsymbol{\alpha}_1^M$ are parameters of Dirichlet prior distributions of $\boldsymbol{p}$, and $\boldsymbol{\lambda}$ is a M-dimensional prior mixing distribution of them. This model is considered a Bayesian extension of the Unigram Mixture [12] and has a graphical model shown in Figure 4. Given a set of documents $\mathcal{D} = \{\mathbf{w}_1, \mathbf{w}_2, \dots, \mathbf{w}_D\}$, parameters $\boldsymbol{\lambda}$ and $\boldsymbol{\alpha}_1^M$ can be iteratively estimated by a combination of EM algorithm and the modified Newton-Raphson method shown in Figure 5, which is a straight extension to the estimation of a Polya mixture [13]. [2]

Under DM, a predictive probability $p(y|\mathbf{h})$ is (omitting dependencies on $\boldsymbol{\lambda}$ and $\boldsymbol{\alpha}_1^M$):

$$p(y|\mathbf{h}) = \sum_{m=1}^{M} p(y|m,\mathbf{h})p(m|\mathbf{h}) = \sum_{m=1}^{M} \left(\int p(y|\boldsymbol{p})p(\boldsymbol{p}|\boldsymbol{\alpha}_m,\mathbf{h})d\boldsymbol{p} \right) \cdot p(m|\mathbf{h})$$

$$= \sum_{m=1}^{M} C_m \frac{\alpha_{my}+n_y}{\sum_y (\alpha_{my}+n_y)}, \tag{10}$$

---

[1]Step 1 of the generative model in fact can be replaced by a Dirichlet process prior. Full Bayesian treatment of DM through Dirichlet processes is now under our development.

[2]DM is an extension to the model for amino acids [14] to natural language with a huge number of parameters, which precludes the ordinary Newton-Raphson algorithm originally proposed in [14].

E step: $p(m|\mathbf{w}_i) \propto \lambda_m \dfrac{\Gamma(\sum_v \alpha_{mv})}{\Gamma(\sum_v \alpha_{mv} + \sum_v n_{iv})} \displaystyle\prod_{v=1}^{V} \dfrac{\Gamma(\alpha_{mv} + n_{iv})}{\Gamma(\alpha_{mv})}$ (13)

M step: $\lambda_m \propto \sum_{i=1}^{D} p(m|\mathbf{w}_i)\,,$ (14)

$$\alpha'_{mv} = \alpha_{mv} \cdot \frac{\sum_i p(m|\mathbf{w}_i)\, n_{iv}/(\alpha_{mv} + n_{iv} - 1)}{\sum_i p(m|\mathbf{w}_i)\, \sum_v n_{iv}/(\sum_v \alpha_{mv} + \sum_v n_{iv} - 1)}$$ (15)

Figure 5: EM-Newton algorithm of Dirichlet Mixtures.

where

$$C_m \propto \lambda_m \frac{\Gamma(\sum_v \alpha_{mv})}{\Gamma(\sum_v \alpha_{mv} + h)} \prod_{v=1}^{V} \frac{\Gamma(\alpha_{mv} + n_v)}{\Gamma(\alpha_{mv})}$$ (11)

and n_v is the number of occurrences of v in $\mathbf{h}$. This prediction can also be considered an extension to Dirichlet smoothing [15] with multiple hyperparameters $\boldsymbol{\alpha}_m$ to weigh them accordingly by C_m.[3]

When we replace a naïve Dirichlet model (3) by a DM prediction (10), we get a flexible MSM-DM dynamic model that works on word simplex directly. Since the original multinomial MSM places a Dirichlet prior in the model (1), MSM-DM is considered a natural extension to MSM by placing a mixture of Dirichlet priors rather than a single Dirichlet prior for multinomial unigram distribution. Because each particle calculates a mixture of Dirichlet posteriors for the current context, the final MSM-DM estimate is a mixture of them, again a mixture of Dirichlet distributions as shown in Figure 3(b).

In this case, we can also update the mixture prior $\boldsymbol{\lambda}$ sequentially. Because each particle has "pseudo documents" $\mathbf{w}_1 \ldots \mathbf{w}_c$ segmented by change points individually, posterior λ_m can be obtained similarly as (14),

$$\lambda_m \propto \sum_{i=1}^{c} p(m|\mathbf{w}_i)$$ (12)

where $p(m|\mathbf{w}_i)$ is obtained from (13). Also in this case, only the sufficient statistics $p(m|\mathbf{w}_i)$ ($i = 1 .. c$) must be stored to make MSM-DM a filtering algorithm.

4 Experiments

We conducted experiments using a standard British National Corpus (BNC). We randomly selected 100 files of BNC written texts as an evaluation set, and the remaining 2,943 files as a training set for parameter estimation of LDA and DM in advance.

4.1 Training and evaluation data

Since LDA and DM did not converge on the long texts like BNC, we divided training texts into pseudo documents with a minimum of ten sentences for parameter estimation. Due to the huge size of BNC, we randomly selected a maximum of 20 pseudo documents from each of the 2,943 files to produce a final corpus of 56,939 pseudo documents comprising 11,032,233 words. We used a lexicon of 52,846 words with a frequency ≥ 5. Note that this segmentation is optional and has an only indirect influence on the experiments. It only affects the clustering of LDA and DM: in fact, we could use another corpus, e.g. newspaper corpus, to estimate the parameters without any preprocessing.

Since the proposed method is an algorithm that simultaneously captures topic shifts and their rate in a text to predict the next word, we need evaluation texts that have different rates of topic shifts. For this purpose, we prepared four different text sets by sampling

---

[3]Therefore, MSM-DM is considered an ingenious dynamic Dirichlet smoothing as well as a context modeling.

Text	MSM-DM	DM	MSM-LDA	LDA
Raw	**870.06** (-6.02%)	925.83	**1028.04**	1037.42
Slow	**893.06** (-8.31%)	974.04	**1047.08**	1060.56
Fast	**898.34** (-9.10%)	988.26	**1044.56**	1061.01
VFast	**960.26** (-7.57%)	1038.89	1065.15	1050.83

Table 2: Contextual Unigram Perplexities for Evaluation Texts.

from the long BNC texts. Specifically, we conducted sentence-based random sampling as follows.

(1) Select a first sentence randomly for each text.
(2) Sample contiguous X sentences from that sentence.
(3) Skip Y sentences.
(4) Continue steps (2) and (3) until a desired length of text is obtained.

In the procedure above, X and Y are random variables that have uniform distributions given in Table 1. We sampled 100 sentences from each of the 100 files by this procedure to create the four evaluation text sets listed in the table.

4.2 Parameter settings

The number of latent classes in LDA and DM are set to 200 and 50, respectively.[4] The number of particles is set to $N = 20$, a relatively small number because each particle executes an exact Bayesian prediction once previous

Name	Property
Raw	$X = 100, Y = 0$
Slow	$1 \leq X \leq 10, 1 \leq Y \leq 3$
Fast	$1 \leq X \leq 10, 1 \leq Y \leq 10$
VeryFast	$X = 1, 1 \leq Y \leq 10$

Table 1: Types of Evaluation Texts.

change points have been sampled. Beta prior distribution of context change can be initialized as a uniform distribution, $(\alpha, \beta) = (1, 1)$. However, based on a preliminary experiment we set it to $(\alpha, \beta) = (1, 50)$: this means we initially assume a context change rate of once every 50 words in average, which will be updated adaptively.

4.3 Experimental results

Table 2 shows the unigram perplexity of contextual prediction for each type of evaluation set. Perplexity is a reciprocal of the geometric average of contextual predictions, thus better predictions yield lower perplexity. While MSM-LDA slightly improves LDA due to the topic space compression explained in Section 3.1, MSM-DM yields a consistently better prediction, and its performance is more significant for texts whose subtopics change faster.

Figure 6 shows a plot of the actual improvements relative to DM, $\text{PPL}_{\text{MSM}} - \text{PPL}_{\text{DM}}$. We can see that prediction improves for most documents by automatically selecting appropriate contexts. The maximum improvement was -365 in PPL for one of the evaluation texts. Finally, we show in Figure 7 a sequential plot of context change probabilities $p^{(i)}(I_t = 1)$ $(i = 1..N, t = 1..T)$ calculated by each particle for the first 1,000 words of one of the evaluation texts.

5 Conclusion and Future Work

In this paper, we extended the multinomial Particle Filter of a small number of symbols to natural language with an extremely large number of symbols. By combining original filter with Bayesian text models LDA and DM, we get two models, MSM-LDA and MSM-DM, that can incorporate semantic relationship between words and can update their hyperparam-

---

[4]We deliberately chose a smaller number of mixtures in DM because it is reported to have a better performance in small mixtures since it is essentially a unitopic model, in contrast to LDA.

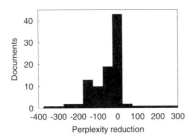

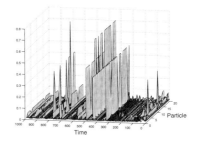

Figure 6: Perplexity reductions of MSM relative to DM.

Figure 7: Context change probabilities for 1,000 words text, sampled by the particles.

eter sequentially. According to this model, prediction is made using a mixture of different context lengths sampled by each Monte Carlo particle.

Although the proposed method is still in its fundamental stage, we are planning to extend it to larger units of change points beyond words, and to use a forward-backward MCMC or Expectation Propagation to model a semantic structure of text more precisely.

References

[1] Jay M. Ponte and W. Bruce Croft. A Language Modeling Approach to Information Retrieval. In *Proc. of SIGIR '98*, pages 275–281, 1998.

[2] David Cohn and Thomas Hofmann. The Missing Link: a probabilistic model of document content and hypertext connectivity. In *NIPS 2001*, 2001.

[3] David M. Blei, Andrew Y. Ng, and Michael I. Jordan. Latent Dirichlet Allocation. *Journal of Machine Learning Research*, 3:993–1022, 2003.

[4] Daniel Gildea and Thomas Hofmann. Topic-based Language Models Using EM. In *Proc. of EUROSPEECH '99*, pages 2167–2170, 1999.

[5] Takuya Mishina and Mikio Yamamoto. Context adaptation using variational Bayesian learning for ngram models based on probabilistic LSA. *IEICE Trans. on Inf. and Sys.*, J87-D-II(7):1409–1417, 2004.

[6] Zoubin Ghahramani and Michael I. Jordan. Factorial Hidden Markov Models. In *Advances in Neural Information Processing Systems (NIPS)*, volume 8, pages 472–478. MIT Press, 1995.

[7] Yuguo Chen and Tze Leung Lai. Sequential Monte Carlo Methods for Filtering and Smoothing in Hidden Markov Models. Discussion Paper 03-19, Institute of Statistics and Decision Sciences, Duke University, 2003.

[8] H. Chernoff and S. Zacks. Estimating the Current Mean of a Normal Distribution Which is Subject to Changes in Time. *Annals of Mathematical Statistics*, 35:999–1018, 1964.

[9] Yi-Chin Yao. Estimation of a noisy discrete-time step function: Bayes and empirical Bayes approaches. *Annals of Statistics*, 12:1434–1447, 1984.

[10] Arnaud Doucet, Nando de Freitas, and Neil Gordon. *Sequential Monte Carlo Methods in Practice*. Statistics for Engineering and Information Science. Springer-Verlag, 2001.

[11] Mikio Yamamoto and Kugatsu Sadamitsu. Dirichlet Mixtures in Text Modeling. CS Technical Report CS-TR-05-1, University of Tsukuba, 2005. http://www.mibel.cs.tsukuba.ac.jp/˜myama/pdf/dm.pdf.

[12] Kamal Nigam, Andrew K. McCallum, Sebastian Thrun, and Tom M. Mitchell. Text Classification from Labeled and Unlabeled Documents using EM. *Machine Learning*, 39(2/3):103–134, 2000.

[13] Thomas P. Minka. Estimating a Dirichlet distribution, 2000. http://research.microsoft.com/˜minka/papers/dirichlet/.

[14] K. Sjölander, K. Karplus, M.P. Brown, R. Hughey, R. Krogh, I.S. Mian, and D. Haussler. Dirichlet Mixtures: A Method for Improved Detection of Weak but Significant Protein Sequence Homology. *Computing Applications in the Biosciences*, 12(4):327–245, 1996.

[15] D. J. C. MacKay and L. Peto. A Hierarchical Dirichlet Language Model. *Natural Language Engineering*, 1(3):1–19, 1994.

Spectral Bounds for Sparse PCA: Exact and Greedy Algorithms

Baback Moghaddam
MERL
Cambridge MA, USA
baback@merl.com

Yair Weiss
Hebrew University
Jerusalem, Israel
yweiss@cs.huji.ac.il

Shai Avidan
MERL
Cambridge MA, USA
avidan@merl.com

Abstract

Sparse PCA seeks *approximate* sparse "eigenvectors" whose projections capture the maximal variance of data. As a cardinality-constrained and *non-convex* optimization problem, it is NP-hard and is encountered in a wide range of applied fields, from bio-informatics to finance. Recent progress has focused mainly on continuous approximation and convex relaxation of the hard cardinality constraint. In contrast, we consider an alternative *discrete* spectral formulation based on variational eigenvalue bounds and provide an effective greedy strategy as well as provably *optimal* solutions using branch-and-bound search. Moreover, the exact methodology used reveals a simple renormalization step that improves approximate solutions obtained by *any* continuous method. The resulting performance gain of discrete algorithms is demonstrated on real-world benchmark data and in extensive Monte Carlo evaluation trials.

1 Introduction

PCA is indispensable as a basic tool for factor analysis and modeling of data. But despite its power and popularity, one key drawback is its lack of sparseness (*i.e.,* factor loadings are linear combinations of *all* the input variables). Yet sparse representations are generally desirable since they aid human understanding (*e.g.,* with gene expression data), reduce computational costs and promote better generalization in learning algorithms. In machine learning, input sparseness is closely related to feature selection and automatic relevance determination, problems of enduring interest to the learning community.

The earliest attempts at "sparsifying" PCA in the statistics literature consisted of simple axis rotations and component thresholding [1] with the underlying goal being essentially that of subset selection, often based on the identification of *principal variables* [8]. The first true computational technique, called SCoTLASS by Jolliffe & Uddin [6], provided a proper optimization framework using Lasso [12] but it proved to be computationally impractical. Recently, Zou *et al.* [14] proposed an elegant algorithm (SPCA) using their "Elastic Net" framework for L_1-penalized regression on regular PCs, solved very efficiently using *least angle regression* (LARS). Subsequently, d'Aspremont *et al.* [3] relaxed the "hard" cardinality constraint and solved for a *convex* approximation using semi-definite programming (SDP). Their "direct" formulation for sparse PCA (called DSCPA) has yielded promising results that are comparable to (if not better than) Zou *et al.*'s Lasso-based method, as demonstrated on the standard "Pit Props" benchmark dataset, known in the statistics community for its lack of sparseness and subsequent difficulty of interpretation.

We pursued an alternative approach using a spectral formulation based on the variational principle of the Courant-Fischer "Min-Max" theorem for solving maximal eigenvalue problems in dimensionality-constrained subspaces. By its very nature, the discrete view leads to a simple post-processing (renormalization) step that improves *any* approximate solution (*e.g.,* those given in [6, 14, 3]), and also provides bounds on (sub)optimality. More importantly, it points the way towards *exact* and provably *optimal* solutions using branch-and-bound search [9]. Our exact computational strategy parallels that of Ko *et al.* [7] who solved a different optimization problem (maximizing entropy with bounds on *determinants*). In the experiments we demonstrate the power of greedy and exact algorithms by first solving for the optimal sparse factors of the real-world "Pit Props" data, a *de facto* benchmark used by [6, 14, 3], and then present summary findings from a large comparative study using extensive Monte Carlo evaluation of the leading algorithms.

2 Sparse PCA Formulation

Sparse PCA can be cast as a cardinality-constrained quadratic program (QP): given a symmetric positive-definite (covariance) matrix $A \in \mathcal{S}_+^n$, maximize the quadratic form $x'Ax$ (variance) with a *sparse* vector $x \in \mathcal{R}^n$ having no more than k non-zero elements:

$$\max \quad x'A\,x \tag{1}$$
$$\text{subject to} \quad x'x = 1$$
$$\text{card}(x) \leq k$$

where $\text{card}(x)$ denotes the L_0 norm. This optimization problem is non-convex, NP-hard and therefore *intractable*. Assuming we can solve for the optimal vector $\hat{x}$, subsequent sparse factors can be obtained using recursive *deflation* of A, as in standard numerical routines. The sparseness is controlled by the value(s) of k (in different factors) and can be viewed as a design parameter or as an unknown quantity itself (known only to the oracle). Alas, there are currently no guidelines for setting k, especially with multiple factors (*e.g.,* orthogonality is often relaxed) and unlike ordinary PCA some decompositions may not be unique.[1] Indeed, one of the contributions of this paper is in providing a sound theoretical basis for selecting k, thus clarifying the "art" of crafting sparse PCA factors.

Note that without the cardinality constraint, the quadratic form in Eq.(1) is a Rayleigh-Ritz quotient obeying the analytic bounds $\lambda_{\min}(A) \leq x'Ax/x'x \leq \lambda_{\max}(A)$ with corresponding unique eigenvector solutions. Therefore, the optimal objective value (variance) is simply the maximum eigenvalue $\lambda_n(A)$ of the principal eigenvector $\hat{x} = u_n$ — **Note:** throughout the paper the rank of all (λ_i, u_i) is in *increasing* order of magnitude, hence $\lambda_{\min} = \lambda_1$ and $\lambda_{\max} = \lambda_n$. With the (nonlinear) cardinality constraint however, the optimal objective value is strictly less than $\lambda_{\max}(A)$ for $k < n$ and the principal eigenvectors are no longer instrumental in the solution. Nevertheless, we will show that the *eigenvalues* of A continue to play a key role in the analysis and design of exact algorithms.

2.1 Optimality Conditions

First, let us consider what conditions *must* be true if the oracle revealed the optimal solution to us: a unit-norm vector $\hat{x}$ with cardinality k yielding the *maximum* objective value v^*. This would necessarily imply that $\hat{x}'A\,\hat{x} = z'A_k z$ where $z \in \mathcal{R}^k$ contains the same k non-zero elements in $\hat{x}$ and A_k is the $k \times k$ principal submatrix of A obtained by deleting the rows and columns corresponding to the zero indices of $\hat{x}$ (or equivalently, by extracting the rows and columns of non-zero indices). Like $\hat{x}$, the k-vector z will be unit norm and $z'A_k z$ is then equivalent to a standard *unconstrained* Rayleigh-Ritz quotient. Since this subproblem's maximum variance is $\lambda_{\max}(A_k)$, then this *must* be the optimal objective v^*. We will now summarize this important observation with the following proposition.

---

[1] We should note that the *multi-factor* version of Eq.(1) is *ill-posed* without additional constraints on basis orthogonality, cardinality, variable redundancy, ordinal rank and allocation of variance.

Proposition 1. *The optimal value v^* of the sparse PCA optimization problem in Eq.(1) is equal to $\lambda_{\max}(A_k^*)$, where A_k^* is the $k \times k$ principal submatrix of A with the largest maximal eigenvalue. In particular, the non-zero elements of the optimal sparse factor $\hat{x}$ are exactly equal to the elements of u_k^*, the principal eigenvector of A_k^*.*

This underscores the inherent combinatorial nature of sparse PCA and the equivalent class of cardinality-constrained optimization problems. However, despite providing an exact formulation and revealing necessary conditions for optimality (and in such simple matrix terms), this proposition does not suggest an efficient method for actually *finding* the principal submatrix A_k^* — short of an enumerative exhaustive search, which is impractical for $n > 30$ due to the exponential growth of possible submatrices. Still, exhaustive search is a viable method for small n which guarantees optimality for "toy problems" and small real-world datasets, thus calibrating the *quality* of approximations (via the optimality gap).

2.2   Variational Renormalization

Proposition 1 immediately suggests a rather simple but (as it turns out) quite effective computational "fix" for *improving* candidate sparse PC factors obtained by *any* continuous algorithm (*e.g.,* the various solutions found in [6, 14, 3]).

Proposition 2. *Let $\tilde{x}$ be a unit-norm candidate factor with cardinality k as found by any (approximation) technique. Let $\tilde{z}$ be the non-zero subvector of $\tilde{x}$ and u_k be the principal (maximum) eigenvector of the submatrix A_k defined by the same non-zero indices of $\tilde{x}$. If $\tilde{z} \neq u_k(A_k)$, then $\tilde{x}$ is not the optimal solution. Nevertheless, by replacing $\tilde{x}$'s nonzero elements with those of u_k we guarantee an increase in the variance, from $\tilde{v}$ to $\lambda_k(A_k)$.*

This variational renormalization suggests (somewhat ironically) that given a continuous (approximate) solution, it is almost certainly better to *discard* the loadings and keep only the sparsity pattern with which to solve the smaller *unconstrained* subproblem for the indicated submatrix A_k. This simple procedure (or "fix" as referred to herein) can *never* decrease the variance and will surely improve any continuous algorithm's performance.

In particular, the rather expedient but *ad-hoc* technique of "simple thresholding" (ST) [1] — *i.e.,* setting the $n - k$ *smallest* absolute value loadings of $u_n(A)$ to zero and then normalizing to unit-norm — is therefore *not* recommended for sparse PCA. In Section 3, we illustrate how this "straw-man" algorithm can be enhanced with proper renormalization. Consequently, past performance benchmarks using this simple technique may need revision — *e.g.,* previous results on the "Pit Props" dataset (Section 3). Indeed, most of the sparse PCA factors published in the literature can be readily improved (almost by inspection) with the proper renormalization, and at the mere cost of a single k-by-k eigen-decomposition.

2.3   Eigenvalue Bounds

Recall that the objective value v^* in Eq.(1) is bounded by the spectral radius $\lambda_{\max}(A)$ (by the Rayleigh-Ritz theorem). Furthermore, the spectrum of A's principal submatrices was shown to play a key role in *defining* the optimal solution. Not surprisingly, the two eigenvalue spectra are related by an inequality known as the *Inclusion Principle*.

Theorem 1 Inclusion Principle. *Let A be a symmetric $n \times n$ matrix with spectrum $\lambda_i(A)$ and let A_k be any $k \times k$ principal submatrix of A for $1 \leq k \leq n$ with eigenvalues $\lambda_i(A_k)$. For each integer i such that $1 \leq i \leq k$*

$$\lambda_i(A) \;\leq\; \lambda_i(A_k) \;\leq\; \lambda_{i+n-k}(A) \qquad (2)$$

Proof. The proof, which we omit, is a rather straightforward consequence of imposing a sparsity pattern of cardinality k as an additional orthogonality constraint in the variational inequality of the Courant-Fischer "Min-Max" theorem (see [13] for example).

In other words, the eigenvalues of a symmetric matrix form upper and lower bounds for the eigenvalues of all its principal submatrices. A special case of Eq.(2) with $k = n - 1$ leads to the well-known eigenvalue *interlacing property* of symmetric matrices:

$$\lambda_1(A_n) \leq \lambda_1(A_{n-1}) \leq \lambda_2(A_n) \leq \ldots \leq \lambda_{n-1}(A_n) \leq \lambda_{n-1}(A_{n-1}) \leq \lambda_n(A_n) \quad (3)$$

Hence, the spectra of A_n and A_{n-1} interleave or *interlace* each other, with the eigenvalues of the larger matrix "bracketing" those of the smaller one. Note that for *positive-definite* symmetric matrices (covariances), augmenting A_m to A_{m+1} (adding a new variable) will always *expand* the spectral range: reducing $\lambda_{\min}$ and increasing $\lambda_{\max}$. Thus for eigenvalue maximization, the inequality constraint $\operatorname{card}(x) \leq k$ in Eq.(1) is a tight *equality* at the optimum. Therefore, the maximum variance is achieved at the preset upper limit k of cardinality. Moreover, the function $v^*(k)$, the optimal variance for a given cardinality, is monotone *increasing* with range $[\sigma_{\max}^2(A), \lambda_{\max}(A)]$, where $\sigma_{\max}^2$ is the largest diagonal element (variance) in A. Hence, a concise and informative way to quantify the performance of an algorithm is to plot its variance curve $\tilde{v}(k)$ and compare it with the optimal $v^*(k)$.

Since we seek to *maximize* variance, the relevant inclusion bound is obtained by setting $i = k$ in Eq.(2), which yields lower and upper bounds for $\lambda_k(A_k) = \lambda_{\max}(A_k)$,

$$\lambda_k(A) \ \leq \ \lambda_{\max}(A_k) \ \leq \ \lambda_{\max}(A) \quad (4)$$

This shows that the k-th *smallest* eigenvalue of A is a *lower bound* for the maximum variance possible with cardinality k. The utility of this lower bound is in doing away with the "guesswork" (and the oracle) in setting k. Interestingly, we now see that the spectrum of A which has traditionally guided the selection of eigenvectors for dimensionality reduction (*e.g.,* in classical PCA), can also be consulted in sparse PCA to help pick the cardinality required to capture the desired (minimum) variance. The lower bound $\lambda_k(A)$ is also useful for speeding up branch-and-bound search (see next Section). Note that if $\lambda_k(A)$ is close to $\lambda_{max}(A)$ then practically any principal submatrix A_k can yield a near-optimal solution.

The right-hand inequality in Eq.(4) is a fixed (loose) upper bound $\lambda_{\max}(A)$ for *all* k. But in branch-and-bound search, any *intermediate* subproblem A_m, with $k \leq m \leq n$, yields a new and *tighter* bound $\lambda_{\max}(A_m)$ for the objective $v^*(k)$. Therefore, all bound computations are efficient and relatively inexpensive (*e.g.,* using the *power method*).

The inclusion principle also leads to some interesting constraints on *nested* submatrices. For example, among all m possible $(m-1)$-by-$(m-1)$ principal submatrices of A_m, obtained by deleting the j-th row and column, there is at least one submatrix $A_{m-1} = A_{\backslash j}$ whose maximal eigenvalue is a major fraction of its parent (*e.g.,* see p. 189 in [4])

$$\exists \ j : \ \lambda_{m-1}(A_{\backslash j}) \ \geq \ \frac{m-1}{m} \lambda_m(A_m) \quad (5)$$

The implication of this inequality for search algorithms is that it is simply not possible for the spectral radius of *every* submatrix $A_{\backslash j}$ to be arbitrarily small, especially for large m. Hence, with large matrices (or large cardinality) nearly all the variance $\lambda_n(A)$ is captured.

2.4 Combinatorial Optimization

Given Propositions 1 and 2, the inclusion principle, the interlacing property and especially the monotonic nature of the variance curves $v(k)$, a general class of (binary) *integer programming* (IP) optimization techniques [9] seem ideally suited for sparse PCA. Indeed, a greedy technique like *backward elimination* is already suggested by the bound in Eq.(5): start with the full index set $I = \{1, 2, \ldots, n\}$ and sequentially delete the variable j which yields the maximum $\lambda_{\max}(A_{\backslash j})$ until only k elements remain. However, for *small* cardinalities $k << n$, the computational cost of backward search can grow to near maximum complexity $\approx O(n^4)$. Hence its counterpart *forward selection* is preferred: start with the null index set $I = \{\}$ and sequentially add the variable j which yields the maximum $\lambda_{\max}(A_{+j})$ until k elements are selected. Forward greedy search has *worst-case* complexity $< O(n^3)$. The best overall strategy for this problem was empirically found to be a *bi-directional* greedy search: run a forward pass (from 1 to n) plus a second (independent) backward pass (from n to 1) and pick the better solution at each k. This proved to be remarkably effective under extensive Monte Carlo evaluation and with real-world datasets. We refer to this discrete algorithm as *greedy* sparse PCA or **GSPCA**.

Despite the expediency of near-optimal greedy search, it is nevertheless worthwhile to invest in optimal solution strategies, especially if the sparse PCA problem is in the application domain of finance or engineering, where even a small optimality gap can accrue substantial losses over time. As with Ko *et al.* [7], our branch-and-bound relies on computationally efficient bounds — in our case, the upper bound in Eq.(4), used on all active *sub*problems in a (FIFO) queue for *depth-first* search. The *lower* bound in Eq.(4) can be used to sort the queue for a more efficient *best-first* search [9]. This *exact* algorithm (referred to as **ESPCA**) is *guaranteed* to terminate with the optimal solution. Naturally, the search time depends on the quality (variance) of initial candidates. The solutions found by dual-pass greedy search (**GSPCA**) were found to be ideal for initializing **ESPCA**, as their quality was typically quite high. Note however, that even with good initializations, branch-and-bound search can take a *long* time (*e.g.* 1.5 hours for $n = 40$, $k = 20$). In practice, early termination with set thresholds based on eigenvalue bounds can be used.

In general, a cost-effective strategy that we can recommend is to first run GSPCA (or at least the forward pass) and then either settle for its (near-optimal) variance or else use it to initialize ESPCA for finding the optimal solution. A full GSPCA run has the added benefit of giving near-optimal solutions for *all* cardinalities at once, with run-times that are typically $O(10^2)$ faster than a *single* approximation with a continuous method.

3 Experiments

We evaluated the performance of GSPCA (and validated ESPCA) on various synthetic covariance matrices with $10 \leq n \leq 40$ as well as real-world datasets from the UCI ML repository with excellent results. We present few typical examples in order to illustrate the advantages and power of discrete algorithms. In particular, we compared our performance against 3 continuous techniques: simple thresholding (ST) [1], SPCA using an "Elastic Net" L_1-regression [14] and DSPCA using semidefinite programming [3].

We first revisited the "Pit Props" dataset [5] which has become a standard benchmark and a classic example of the difficulty of interpreting fully loaded factors with standard PCA. The first 6 ordinary PCs capture 87% of the total variance, so following the methodology in [3], we compared the explanatory power of our exact method (ESPCA) using 6 *sparse* PCs. Table 1 shows the first 3 PCs and their loadings. SPCA captures 75.8% of the variance with a cardinality pattern of 744111 (the k's for the 6 PCs) thus totaling 18 non-zero loadings [14] whereas DSPCA captures 77.3% with a sparser cardinality pattern 623111 totaling 14 non-zero loadings [3]. We aimed for an even sparser 522111 pattern (with only 12 non-zero loadings) yet captured nearly the same variance: 75.9% — *i.e.,* more than SPCA with 18 loadings and slightly less than DSPCA with 14 loadings.

Using the evaluation protocol in [3], we compared the cumulative variance and cumulative cardinality with the published results of SPCA and DSPCA in Figure 1. Our goal was to match the explained variance but do so with a sparser representation. The ESPCA loadings in Table 1 are optimal under the definition given in Section 2. The run-time of ESPCA, *including* initialization with a bi-directional pass of GSPCA, was negligible for this dataset ($n = 13$). Computing each factor took less than 50 msec in Matlab 7.0 on a 3GHz P4.

	x_1	x_2	x_3	x_4	x_5	x_6	x_7	x_8	x_9	x_{10}	x_{11}	x_{12}	x_{13}
SPCA : PC1	-.477	-.476	0	0	.177	0	-.250	-.344	-.416	-.400	-	0	0
PC2	0	0	.785	.620	0	0	0	-.021	0	0	0	.013	0
PC3	0	0	0	0	.640	.589	.492	0	0	0	0	0	-.015
DSPCA : PC1	-.560	-.583	0	0	0	0	-.263	-.099	-.371	-.362	0	0	0
PC2	0	0	.707	.707	0	0	0	0	0	0	0	0	0
PC3	0	0	0	0	0	-.793	-.610	0	0	0	0	0	.012
ESPCA : PC1	-.480	-.491	0	0	0	0	-.405	0	-.423	-.431	0	0	0
PC2	0	0	.707	.707	0	0	0	0	0	0	0	0	0
PC3	0	0	0	0	0	-.814	-.581	0	0	0	0	0	0

Table 1: Loadings for first 3 sparse PCs of the Pit Props data. See Figure 1(a) for plots of the corresponding cumulative variances. Original SPCA and DSPCA loadings taken from [14, 3].

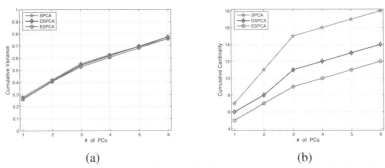

(a)   (b)

Figure 1: Pit Props: **(a)** cumulative variance and **(b)** cumulative cardinality for first 6 sparse PCs. Sparsity patterns (cardinality k_i for PC_i, with $i = 1, 2, \ldots, 6$) are 744111 for SPCA (magenta $\star$), 623111 for DSPCA (green $\diamond$) and an optimal 522111 for ESPCA (red $\circ$). The factor loadings for the first 3 sparse PCs are shown in Table 1. Original SPCA and DSPCA results taken from [14, 3].

To specifically demonstrate the benefits of the variational renormalization of Section 2.2, consider SPCA's first sparse factor in Table 1 (the 1st row of SPCA block) found by iterative (L_1-penalized) optimization and unit-norm scaling. It captures 28% of the total data variance, but after the variational renormalization the variance *increases* to 29%. Similarly, the first sparse factor of DSPCA in Table 1 (1st row of DSPCA block) captures 26.6% of the total variance, whereas after variational renormalization it captures 29% — a gain of 2.4% for the mere additional cost of a 7-by-7 eigen-decomposition. Given that variational renormalization results in the maximum variance possible for the indicated sparsity pattern, omitting such a simple post-processing step is counter-productive, since otherwise the approximations would be, in a sense, *doubly* sub-optimal: both globally and "locally" in the subspace (subset) of the sparsity pattern found.

We now give a representative summary of our extensive Monte Carlo (MC) evaluation of GSPCA and the 3 continuous algorithms. To show the most typical or average-case performance, we present results with random covariance matrices from synthetic stochastic Brownian processes of various degrees of smoothness, ranging from sub-Gaussian to super-Gaussian. Every MC run consisted of 50,000 covariance matrices and the (normalized) variance curves $\tilde{v}(k)$. For each matrix, **ESPCA** was used to find the *optimal* solution as "ground truth" for subsequent calibration, analysis and performance evaluation.

For SPCA we used the LARS-based "Elastic Net" SPCA Matlab toolbox of Sjöstrand [10] which is equivalent to Zou *et al.*'s SPCA source code, which is also freely available in R. For DSPCA we used the authors' own Matlab source code [2] which uses the SDP toolbox SeDuMi1.0x [11]. The main DSPCA routine *PrimalDec*(A, k) was called with $k-1$ instead of k, for all $k > 2$, as per the recommended calibration (see documentation in [3, 2]).

In our MC evaluations, all continuous methods (ST, SPCA and DSPCA) had variational renormalization post-processing (applied to their the "declared" solution). Note that comparing GSPCA with the *raw* output of these algorithms would be rather pointless, since

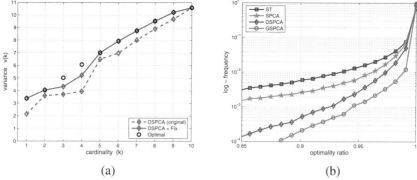

(a)   (b)

Figure 2: **(a)** Typical variance curve $v(k)$ for a continuous algorithm *without* post-processing (original: dash green) and *with* variational renormalization (+ Fix: solid green). Optimal variance (black ○) by **ESPCA**. At $k = 4$ optimality ratio *increases* from 0.65 to 0.86 (a 21% gain). **(b)** Monte Carlo study: log-likelihood of optimality ratio at max-complexity ($k = 8$, $n = 16$) for ST (blue []), DSPCA (green ◇), SPCA (magenta ⋆) and GSPCA (red ○). Continuous methods were "fixed" in (b).

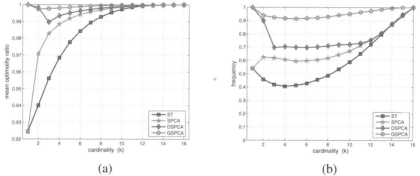

(a)   (b)

Figure 3: Monte Carlo summary statistics: **(a)** means of the distributions of optimality ratio (in Figure 2(b)) for all k and **(b)** estimated probability of finding the *optimal* solution for each cardinality.

without the "fix" their variance curves are markedly diminished, as in Figure 2(a).

Figure 2(b) shows the histogram of the optimality ratio — *i.e.,* ratio of the captured to optimal variance — shown here at "half-sparsity" ($k = 8, n = 16$) from a typical MC run of 50,000 different covariances matrices. In order to view the (one-sided) tails of the distributions we have plotted the *log* of the histogram values. Figure 3(a) shows the corresponding mean values of the optimality ratio for all k. Among continuous algorithms, the SDP-based DSPCA was generally more effective (almost comparable to GSPCA). For the smaller matrices ($n < 10$), LARS-based SPCA matched DSPCA for all k. In terms of complexity and speed however, SPCA was about 40 times faster than DSPCA. But GSPCA was 30 times faster than SPCA. Finally, we note that even simple thresholding (ST), once enhanced with the variational renormalization, performs quite adequately despite its simplicity, as it captures at least 92% of the optimal variance, as seen in Figure 3(a).

Figure 3(b) shows an alternative but more revealing performance summary: the fraction of the (50,000) trials in which the optimal solution was actually found (essentially, the likelihood of "success"). This *all-or-nothing* performance measure elicits important differences between the algorithms. In practical terms, only GSPCA is capable of finding the optimal factor more than 90% of the time (*vs.* 70% for DSPCA). Naturally, *without* the variational "fix" (not shown) continuous algorithms rarely ever found the optimal solution.

4 Discussion

The contributions of this paper can be summarized as: (1) an *exact* variational formulation of sparse PCA, (2) requisite eigenvalue bounds, (3) a principled choice of k, (4) a simple renormalization "fix" for *any* continuous method, (5) fast and effective greedy search (GSPCA) and (6) a less efficient but *optimal* method (ESPCA). Surprisingly, simple thresholding of the principal eigenvector (ST) was shown to be rather effective, especially given the perceived "straw-man" it was considered to be. Naturally, its performance will vary with the effective rank (or "eigen-gap") of the covariance matrix. In fact, it is not hard to show that if A is *exactly* rank-1, then ST is indeed an optimal strategy for all k. However, beyond such special cases, continuous methods can not ultimately be competitive with discrete algorithms without the variational renormalization "fix" in Section 2.2.

We should note that the somewhat remarkable effectiveness of GSPCA is not entirely unexpected and is supported by empirical observations in the combinatorial optimization literature: that greedy search with (sub)modular cost functions having the monotonicity property (*e.g.*, the variance curves $\tilde{v}(k)$) is known to produce good results [9]. In terms of quality of solutions, GSPCA consistently out-performed continuous algorithms, with run-times that were typically $O(10^2)$ faster than LARS-based SPCA and roughly $O(10^3)$ faster than SDP-based DSPCA (Matlab CPU times averaged over all k).

Nevertheless, we view discrete algorithms as complementary tools, especially since the leading continuous algorithms have distinct advantages. For example, with *very* high-dimensional datasets (*e.g.*, $n = 10,000$), Zou *et al.*'s LARS-based method is currently the only viable option, since it does not rely on computing or storing a *huge* covariance matrix. Although d'Aspremont *et al.* mention the possibility of solving "larger" systems much faster (using Nesterov's 1st-order method [3]), this would require a full matrix in memory (same as discrete algorithms). Still, their SDP formulation has an elegant *robustness* interpretation and can also be applied to *non-square* matrices (*i.e.*, for a sparse SVD).

Acknowledgments

The authors would like to thank Karl Sjöstrand (DTU) for his customized code and helpful advice in using the LARS-SPCA toolbox [10] and Gert Lanckriet (Berkeley) for providing the Pit Props data.

References

[1] J. Cadima and I. Jolliffe. Loadings and correlations in the interpretation of principal components. *Applied Statistics*, 22:203–214, 1995.

[2] A. d'Aspremont. DSPCA Toolbox. http://www.princeton.edu/~aspremon/DSPCA.htm.

[3] A. d'Aspremont, L. El Ghaoui, M. I. Jordan, and G. R. G. Lanckriet. A Direct Formulation for Sparse PCA using Semidefinite Programming. In *Advances in Neural Information Processing Systems (NIPS)*. Vancouver, BC, December 2004.

[4] R. A. Horn and C. R. Johnson. *Matrix Analysis*. Cambridge Press, Cambridge, England, 1985.

[5] J. Jeffers. Two cases studies in the application of principal components. *Applied Statistics*, 16:225–236, 1967.

[6] I. T. Jolliffe and M. Uddin. A Modified Principal Component Technique based on the Lasso. *Journal of Computational and Graphical Statistics*, 12:531–547, 2003.

[7] C. Ko, J. Lee, and M. Queyranne. An Exact Algorithm for Maximum Entropy Sampling. *Operations Research*, 43(4):684–691, July-August 1995.

[8] G. McCabe. Principal variables. *Technometrics*, 26:137–144, 1984.

[9] G. L. Nemhauser and L. A. Wolsey. *Integer and Combinatorial Optimization*. John Wiley, New York, 1988.

[10] K. Sjöstrand. Matlab implementation of LASSO, LARS, the Elastic Net and SPCA. Informatics and Mathematical Modelling, Technical University of Denmark (DTU), 2005.

[11] J. F. Sturm. SeDuMi1.0x, a MATLAB Toolbox for Optimization over Symmetric Cones. *Optimization Methods and Software*, 11:625–653, 1999.

[12] R. Tibshirani. Regression shrinkage and selection via Lasso. *Journal of the Royal Statistical Society B*, 58:267–288, 1995.

[13] J. H. Wilkinson. *The Algebraic Eigenvalue Problem*. Clarendon Press, Oxford, England, 1965.

[14] H. Zou, T. Hastie, and R. Tibshirani. Sparse Principal Component Analysis. Technical Report, Statistics Department, Stanford University, 2004.

Top-Down Control of Visual Attention: A Rational Account

Michael C. Mozer
Dept. of Comp. Science &
Institute of Cog. Science
University of Colorado
Boulder, CO 80309 USA

Michael Shettel
Dept. of Comp. Science &
Institute of Cog. Science
University of Colorado
Boulder, CO 80309 USA

Shaun Vecera
Dept. of Psychology
University of Iowa
Iowa City, IA 52242 USA

Abstract

Theories of visual attention commonly posit that early parallel processes extract conspicuous features such as color contrast and motion from the visual field. These features are then combined into a saliency map, and attention is directed to the most salient regions first. Top-down attentional control is achieved by modulating the contribution of different feature types to the saliency map. A key source of data concerning attentional control comes from behavioral studies in which the effect of recent experience is examined as individuals repeatedly perform a perceptual discrimination task (e.g., "what shape is the odd-colored object?"). The robust finding is that repetition of features of recent trials (e.g., target color) facilitates performance. We view this facilitation as an adaptation to the statistical structure of the environment. We propose a probabilistic model of the environment that is updated after each trial. Under the assumption that attentional control operates so as to make performance more efficient for more likely environmental states, we obtain parsimonious explanations for data from four different experiments. Further, our model provides a rational explanation for why the influence of past experience on attentional control is short lived.

1 INTRODUCTION

The brain does not have the computational capacity to fully process the massive quantity of information provided by the eyes. Selective attention operates to filter the spatiotemporal stream to a manageable quantity. Key to understanding the nature of attention is discovering the algorithm governing selection, i.e., understanding what information will be selected and what will be suppressed. Selection is influenced by attributes of the spatiotemporal stream, often referred to as *bottom-up* contributions to attention. For example, attention is drawn to abrupt onsets, motion, and regions of high contrast in brightness and color. Most theories of attention posit that some visual information processing is performed preattentively and in parallel across the visual field. This processing extracts *primitive* visual features such as color and motion, which provide the bottom-up cues for attentional guidance. However, attention is not driven willy nilly by these cues. The deployment of attention can be modulated by task instructions, current goals, and domain knowledge, collectively referred to as *top-down* contributions to attention.

How do bottom-up and top-down contributions to attention interact? Most psychologically and neurobiologically motivated models propose a very similar architecture in which information from bottom-up and top-down sources combines in a *saliency* (or *activation*) map (e.g., Itti et al., 1998; Koch & Ullman, 1985; Mozer, 1991; Wolfe, 1994). The saliency map indicates, for each location in the visual field, the relative importance of that location. Attention is drawn to the most salient locations first.

Figure 1 sketches the basic architecture that incorporates bottom-up and top-down contributions to the saliency map. The visual image is analyzed to extract maps of primitive features such as color and orientation. Associated with each location in a map is a scalar

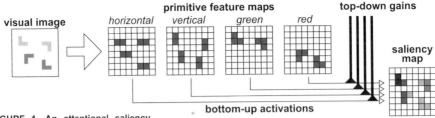

FIGURE 1. An attentional saliency map constructed from bottom-up and top-down information

FIGURE 2. Sample display from Experiment 1 of Maljkovic and Nakayama (1994)

response or *activation* indicating the presence of a particular feature. Most models assume that responses are stronger at locations with high local feature contrast, consistent with neurophysiological data, e.g., the response of a red feature detector to a red object is stronger if the object is surrounded by green objects. The saliency map is obtained by taking a sum of bottom-up activations from the feature maps. The bottom-up activations are modulated by a top-down *gain* that specifies the contribution of a particular map to saliency in the current task and environment. Wolfe (1994) describes a heuristic algorithm for determining appropriate gains in a *visual search* task, where the goal is to detect a *target* object among *distractor* objects. Wolfe proposes that maps encoding features that discriminate between target and distractors have higher gains, and to be consistent with the data, he proposes limits on the magnitude of gain modulation and the number of gains that can be modulated. More recently, Wolfe et al. (2003) have been explicit in proposing optimization as a principle for setting gains given the task definition and stimulus environment.

One aspect of optimizing attentional control involves configuring the attentional system to perform a given task; for example, in a visual search task for a red vertical target among green vertical and red horizontal distractors, the task definition should result in a higher gain for red and vertical feature maps than for other feature maps. However, there is a more subtle form of gain modulation, which depends on the statistics of display environments. For example, if green vertical distractors predominate, then red is a better discriminative cue than vertical; and if red horizontal distractors predominate, then vertical is a better discriminative cue than red.

In this paper, we propose a model that encodes statistics of the environment in order to allow for optimization of attentional control to the structure of the environment. Our model is designed to address a key set of behavioral data, which we describe next.

1.1 Attentional priming phenomena

Psychological studies involve a sequence of experimental *trials* that begin with a stimulus presentation and end with a response from the human participant. Typically, trial order is randomized, and the context preceding a trial is ignored. However, in *sequential studies*, performance is examined on one trial contingent on the past history of trials. These sequential studies explore how experience influences future performance. Consider a the sequential attentional task of Maljkovic and Nakayama (1994). On each trial, the stimulus display (Figure 2) consists of three notched diamonds, one a singleton in color—either green among red or red among green. The task is to report whether the singleton diamond, referred to as the *target*, is notched on the left or the right. The task is easy because the singleton *pops out*, i.e., the time to locate the singleton does not depend on the number of diamonds in the display. Nonetheless, the response time significantly depends on the sequence of trials leading up to the current trial: If the target is the same color on the current trial as on the previous trial, response time is roughly 100 ms faster than if the target is a different color on the current trial. Considering that response times are on the order of 700 ms, this effect, which we term *attentional priming*, is gigantic in the scheme of psychological phenomena.

2 ATTENTIONAL CONTROL AS ADAPTATION TO THE STATISTICS OF THE ENVIRONMENT

We interpret the phenomenon of attentional priming via a particular perspective on attentional control, which can be summarized in two bullets.

- The perceptual system dynamically constructs a probabilistic model of the environment based on its past experience.
- Control parameters of the attentional system are tuned so as to optimize performance under the current environmental model.

The primary focus of this paper is the environmental model, but we first discuss the nature of performance optimization.

The role of attention is to make processing of some stimuli more efficient, and consequently, the processing of other stimuli less efficient. For example, if the gain on the red feature map is turned up, processing will be efficient for red items, but competition from red items will reduce the efficiency for green items. Thus, optimal control should tune the system for the most likely states of the world by minimizing an objective function such as:

$$J(g) = \sum_e P(e)RT_g(e) \tag{1}$$

where g is a vector of top-down gains, e is an index over environmental states, $P(.)$ is the probability of an environmental state, and $RT_g(.)$ is the expected response time—assuming a constant error rate—to the environmental state under gains g. Determining the optimal gains is a challenge because every gain setting will result in facilitation of responses to some environmental states but hindrance of responses to other states.

The optimal control problem could be solved via direct reinforcement learning, but the rapidity of human learning makes this possibility unlikely: In a variety of experimental tasks, evidence suggests that adaptation to a new task or environment can occur in just one or two trials (e.g., Rogers & Monsell, 1996). Model-based reinforcement learning is an attractive alternative, because given a model, optimization can occur without further experience in the real world. Although the number of real-world trials necessary to achieve a given level of performance is comparable for direct and model-based reinforcement learning in stationary environments (Kearns & Singh, 1999), naturalistic environments can be viewed as highly nonstationary. In such a situation, the framework we suggest is well motivated: After each experience, the environment model is updated. The updated environmental model is then used to retune the attentional system.

In this paper, we propose a particular model of the environment suitable for visual search tasks. Rather than explicitly modeling the optimization of attentional control by setting gains, we assume that the optimization process will serve to minimize Equation 1. Because any gain adjustment will facilitate performance in some environmental states and hinder performance in others, an optimized control system should obtain faster reaction times for more probable environmental states. This assumption allows us to explain experimental results in a minimal, parsimonious framework.

3 MODELING THE ENVIRONMENT

Focusing on the domain of visual search, we characterize the environment in terms of a probability distribution over configurations of target and distractor features. We distinguish three classes of features: *defining, reported,* and *irrelevant.* To explain these terms, consider the task of searching a display of size varying, colored, notched diamonds (Figure 2), with the task of detecting the singleton in color and judging the notch location. Color is the defining feature, notch location is the reported feature, and size is an irrelevant feature. To simplify the exposition, we treat all features as having discrete values, an assumption which is true of the experimental tasks we model. We begin by considering displays containing a single target and a single distractor, and shortly generalize to multidistractor displays.

We use the framework of Bayesian networks to characterize the environment. Each feature of the target and distractor is a discrete random variable, e.g., T_{color} for target color and D_{notch} for the location of the notch on the distractor. The Bayes net encodes the probability distribution over environmental states; in our working example, this distribution is

$$\mathbf{P}(T_{color}, T_{size}, T_{notch}, D_{color}, D_{size}, D_{notch}).$$

The structure of the Bayes net specifies the relationships among the features. The simplest model one could consider would be to treat the features as independent, illustrated in Figure 3a for singleton-color search task. The opposite extreme would be the full joint distribution, which could be represented by a look up table indexed by the six features, or by the cascading Bayes net architecture in Figure 3b. The architecture we propose, which we'll refer to as the *dominance model* (Figure 3c), has an intermediate dependency structure, and expresses the joint distribution as:

$$\mathbf{P}(T_{color})\mathbf{P}(D_{color}|T_{color})\mathbf{P}(T_{size}|T_{color})\mathbf{P}(T_{notch}|T_{color})\mathbf{P}(D_{size}|D_{color})\mathbf{P}(D_{notch}|T_{color}).$$

The structured model is constructed based on three rules.

1. The defining feature of the target is at the root of the tree.

2. The defining feature of the distractor is conditionally dependent on the defining feature of the target. We refer to this rule as *dominance* of the target over the distractor.

3. The reported and irrelevant features of target (distractor) are conditionally dependent on the defining feature of the target (distractor). We refer to this rule as *dominance* of the defining feature over nondefining features.

As we will demonstrate, the dominance model produces a parsimonious account of a wide range of experimental data.

3.1 Updating the environment model

The model's parameters are the conditional distributions embodied in the links. In the example of Figure 3c with binary random variables, the model has 11 parameters. However, these parameters are determined by the environment: To be adaptive in nonstationary environments, the model must be updated following each experienced state. We propose a simple exponentially weighted averaging approach. For two variables V and W with observed values v and w on trial t, a conditional distribution, $P_t(V = u | W = w) = \delta_{uv}$, is

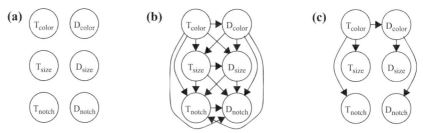

FIGURE 3. Three models of a visual-search environment with colored, notched, size-varying diamonds. (a) feature-independence model; (b) full-joint model; (c) dominance model.

defined, where δ is the Kronecker delta. The distribution representing the environment following trial t, denoted P_t^E, is then updated as follows:

$$P_t^E(V = u | W = w) = \alpha P_{t-1}^E(V = u | W = w) + (1 - \alpha) P_t(V = u | W = w) \quad (2)$$

for all u, where α is a memory constant. Note that no update is performed for values of W other than w. An analogous update is performed for unconditional distributions.

How the model is initialized—i.e., specifying P_0^E—is irrelevant, because all experimental tasks that we model, participants begin the experiment with many dozens of practice trials. Data is not collected during practice trials. Consequently, any transient effects of P_0^E do not impact the results. In our simulations, we begin with a uniform distribution for P_0^E, and include practice trials as in the human studies.

Thus far, we've assumed a single target and a single distractor. The experiments that we model involve multiple distractors. The simple extension we require to handle multiple distractors is to define a frequentist probability for each distractor feature V, $P_t(V = v | W = w) = C_{vw} / C_w$, where C_{vw} is the count of co-occurrences of feature values v and w among the distractors, and C_w is the count of w.

Our model is extremely simple. Given a description of the visual search task and environment, the model has only a single degree of freedom, α. In all simulations, we fix $\alpha = 0.75$; however, the choice of α does not qualitatively impact any result.

4 SIMULATIONS

In this section, we show that the model can explain a range of data from four different experiments examining attentional priming. All experiments measure response times of participants. On each trial, the model can be used to obtain a probability of the display configuration (the environmental state) on that trial, given the history of trials to that point. Our critical assumption—as motivated earlier—is that response times monotonically decrease with increasing probability, indicating that visual information processing is better configured for more likely environmental states. The particular relationship we assume is that response times are linear in log probability. This assumption yields long response time tails, as are observed in all human studies.

4.1 Maljkovic and Nakayama (1994, Experiment 5)

In this experiment, participants were asked to search for a singleton in color in a display of three red or green diamonds. Each diamond was notched on either the left or right side, and the task was to report the side of the notch on the color singleton. The well-practiced participants made very few errors. Reaction time (RT) was examined as a function of whether the target on a given trial is the same or different color as the target on trial n steps back or ahead. Figure 4 shows the results, with the human RTs in the left panel and the simulation log probabilities in the right panel. The horizontal axis represents n. Both graphs show the same outcome: repetition of target color facilitates performance. This influence lasts only for a half dozen trials, with an exponentially decreasing influence further into the past. In the model, this decreasing influence is due to the exponential decay of recent history (Equation 2). Figure 4 also shows that—as expected—the future has no influence on the current trial.

4.2 Maljkovic and Nakayama (1994, Experiment 8)

In the previous experiment, it is impossible to determine whether facilitation is due to repetition of the target's color or the distractor's color, because the display contains only two colors, and therefore repetition of target color implies repetition of distractor color. To unconfound these two potential factors, an experiment like the previous one was conducted using four distinct colors, allowing one to examine the effect of repeating the target color while varying the distractor color, and vice versa. The sequence of trials was composed of subsequences of up-to-six consecutive trials with either the target or distractor color held constant while the other color was varied trial to trial. Following each subsequence, both target and distractors were changed. Figure 5 shows that for both humans and the simulation, performance improves toward an asymptote as the number of target and distractor repetitions increases; in the model, the asymptote is due to the probability of the repeated color in the environment model approaching 1.0. The performance improvement is greater for target than distractor repetition; in the model, this difference is due to the dominance of the defining feature of the target over the defining feature of the distractor.

4.3 Huang, Holcombe, and Pashler (2004, Experiment 1)

Huang et al. (2004) and Hillstrom (2000) conducted studies to determine whether repetitions of one feature facilitate performance independently of repetitions of another feature. In the Huang et al. study, participants searched for a singleton in size in a display consisting of lines that were short and long, slanted left or right, and colored white or black. The reported feature was target slant. Slant, size, and color were uncorrelated. Huang et al. discovered that repeating an irrelevant feature (color or orientation) facilitated performance, but only when the defining feature (size) was repeated. As shown in Figure 6, the model replicates human performance, due to the dominance of the defining feature over the reported and irrelevant features.

4.4 Wolfe, Butcher, Lee, and Hyde (2003, Experiment 1)

In an empirical tour-de-force, Wolfe et al. (2003) explored singleton search over a range of environments. The task is to detect the presence or absence of a singleton in displays con-

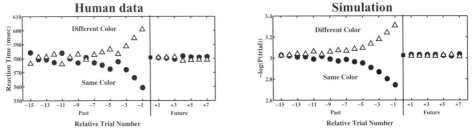

FIGURE 4. Experiment 5 of Maljkovic and Nakayama (1994): performance on a given trial conditional on the color of the target on a previous or subsequent trial. Human data is from subject KN.

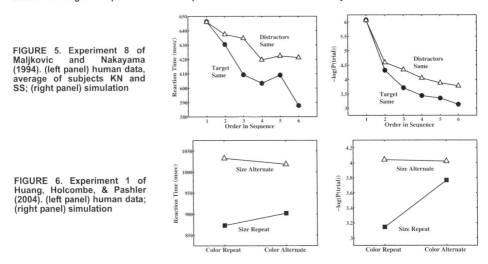

FIGURE 5. Experiment 8 of Maljkovic and Nakayama (1994). (left panel) human data, average of subjects KN and SS; (right panel) simulation

FIGURE 6. Experiment 1 of Huang, Holcombe, & Pashler (2004). (left panel) human data; (right panel) simulation

928

sisting of colored (red or green), oriented (horizontal or vertical) lines. Target-absent trials were used primarily to ensure participants were searching the display. The experiment examined seven experimental conditions, which varied in the amount of uncertainty as to the target identity. The essential conditions, from least to most uncertainty, are: *blocked* (e.g., target always red vertical among green horizontals), *mixed feature* (e.g., target always a color singleton), *mixed dimension* (e.g., target either red or vertical), and *fully mixed* (target could be red, green, vertical, or horizontal). With this design, one can ascertain how uncertainty in the environment and in the target definition influence task difficulty. Because the defining feature in this experiment could be either color or orientation, we modeled the environment with two Bayes nets—one color dominant and one orientation dominant—and performed model averaging. A comparison of Figures 7a and 7b show a correspondence between human RTs and model predictions. Less uncertainty in the environment leads to more efficient performance. One interesting result from the model is its prediction that the mixed-feature condition is easier than the fully-mixed condition; that is, search is more efficient when the *dimension* (i.e., color vs. orientation) of the singleton is known, even though the model has no abstract representation of feature dimensions, only feature values.

4.5 Optimal adaptation constant

In all simulations so far, we fixed the memory constant. From the human data, it is clear that memory for recent experience is relatively short lived, on the order of a half dozen trials (e.g., left panel of Figure 4). In this section we provide a rational argument for the short duration of memory in attentional control.

Figure 7c shows mean negative log probability in each condition of the Wolfe et al. (2003) experiment, as a function of α. To assess these probabilities, for each experimental condition, the model was initialized so that all of the conditional distributions were uniform, and then a block of trials was run. Log probability for all trials in the block was averaged. The negative log probability (y axis of the Figure) is a measure of the model's *misprediction* of the next trial in the sequence.

For complex environments, such as the fully-mixed condition, a small memory constant is detrimental: With rapid memory decay, the effective history of trials is a high-variance sample of the distribution of environmental states. For simple environments, a large memory constant is detrimental: With slow memory decay, the model does not transition quickly from the initial environmental model to one that reflects the statistics of a new environment. Thus, the memory constant is constrained by being large enough that the environment model can hold on to sufficient history to represent complex environments, and by being small enough that the model adapts quickly to novel environments. If the conditions in Wolfe et al. give some indication of the range of naturalistic environments an agent encounters, we have a rational account of why attentional priming is so short lived. Whether priming lasts 2 trials or 20, the surprising empirical result is that it does not last 200 or 2000 trials. Our rational argument provides a rough insight into this finding.

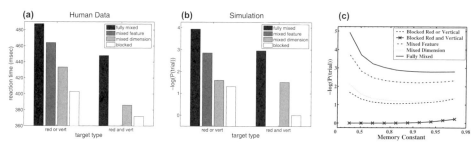

FIGURE 7. (a) Human data for Wolfe et al. (2003), Experiment 1; (b) simulation; (c) *misprediction* of model (i.e., lower y value = better) as a function of α for five experimental condition

5 DISCUSSION

The psychological literature contains two opposing accounts of attentional priming and its relation to attentional control. Huang et al. (2004) and Hillstrom (2000) propose an *episodic* account in which a distinct memory trace—representing the complete configuration of features in the display—is laid down for each trial, and priming depends on configural similarity of the current trial to previous trials. Alternatively, Maljkovic and Nakayama (1994) and Wolfe et al. (2003) propose a *feature-strengthening* account in which detection of a feature on one trial increases its ability to attract attention on subsequent trials, and priming is proportional to the number of overlapping features from one trial to the next. The episodic account corresponds roughly to the full joint model (Figure 3b), and the feature-strengthening account corresponds roughly to the independence model (Figure 3a). Neither account is adequate to explain the range of data we presented. However, an intermediate account, the dominance model (Figure 3c), is not only sufficient, but it offers a parsimonious, rational explanation. Beyond the model's basic assumptions, it has only one free parameter, and can explain results from diverse experimental paradigms.

The model makes a further theoretical contribution. Wolfe et al. distinguish the environments in their experiment in terms of the amount of top-down control available, implying that different mechanisms might be operating in different environments. However, in our account, top-down control is not some substance distributed in different amounts depending on the nature of the environment. Our account treats all environments uniformly, relying on attentional control to adapt to the environment at hand.

We conclude with two limitations of the present work. First, our account presumes a particular network architecture, instead of a more elegant Bayesian approach that specifies priors over architectures, and performs automatic model selection via the sequence of trials. We did explore such a Bayesian approach, but it was unable to explain the data. Second, at least one finding in the literature is problematic for the model. Hillstrom (2000) occasionally finds that RTs slow when an irrelevant target feature is repeated but the defining target feature is not. However, because this effect is observed only in some experiments, it is likely that *any* model would require elaboration to explain the variability.

ACKNOWLEDGEMENTS

We thank Jeremy Wolfe for providing the raw data from his experiment for reanalysis. This research was funded by NSF BCS Award 0339103.

REFERENCES

Huang, L, Holcombe, A. O., & Pashler, H. (2004). Repetition priming in visual search: Episodic retrieval, not feature priming. *Memory & Cognition, 32*, 12–20.

Hillstrom, A. P. (2000). Repetition effects in visual search. *Perception & Psychophysics*, **62**, 800-817.

Itti, L., Koch, C., & Niebur, E. (1998). A model of saliency-based visual attention for rapid scene analysis. *IEEE Trans. Pattern Analysis & Machine Intelligence*, **20**, 1254–1259.

Kearns, M., & Singh, S. (1999). Finite-sample convergence rates for Q-learning and indirect algorithms. In *Advances in Neural Information Processing Systems 11* (pp. 996–1002). Cambridge, MA: MIT Press.

Koch, C. and Ullman, S. (1985). Shifts in selective visual attention: towards the underlying neural circuitry. *Human Neurobiology*, 4, 219–227.

Maljkovic, V., & Nakayama, K. (1994). Priming of pop-out: I. Role of features. *Mem. & Cognition*, **22**, 657-672.

Mozer, M. C. (1991). The perception of multiple objects: A connectionist approach. Cambridge, MA: MIT Press.

Rogers, R. D., & Monsell, S. (1995). The cost of a predictable switch between simple cognitive tasks. *Journal of Experimental Psychology: General, 124*, 207–231.

Wolfe, J.M. (1994). Guided Search 2.0: A Revised Model of Visual Search. *Psych. Bull. & Rev.*, **1**, 202–238.

Wolfe, J. S., Butcher, S. J., Lee, C., & Hyde, M. (2003). Changing your mind: on the contributions of top-down and bottom-up guidance in visual search for feature singletons. *Journal of Exptl. Psychology: Human Perception & Performance*, *29*, 483-502.

Rate Distortion Codes in Sensor Networks: A System-level Analysis

Tatsuto Murayama and Peter Davis
NTT Communication Science Laboratories
Nippon Telegraph and Telephone Corporation
"Keihanna Science City", Kyoto 619-0237, Japan
{murayama,davis}@cslab.kecl.ntt.co.jp

Abstract

This paper provides a system-level analysis of a scalable distributed sensing model for networked sensors. In our system model, a data center acquires data from a bunch of L sensors which each independently encode their noisy observations of an original binary sequence, and transmit their encoded data sequences to the data center at a combined rate R, which is limited. Supposing that the sensors use independent LDGM rate distortion codes, we show that the system performance can be evaluated for any given finite R when the number of sensors L goes to infinity. The analysis shows how the optimal strategy for the distributed sensing problem changes at critical values of the data rate R or the noise level.

1 Introduction

Device and sensor networks are shaping many activities in our society. These networks are being deployed in a growing number of applications as diverse as agricultural management, industrial controls, crime watch, and military applications. Indeed, sensor networks can be considered as a promising technology with a wide range of potential future markets [1]. Still, for all the promise, it is often difficult to integrate the individual components of a sensor network in a smart way. Although we see many breakthroughs in component devices, advanced software, and power managements, system-level understanding of the emerging technology is still weak. It requires a shift in our notion of "what to look for". It requires a study of collective behavior and resulting trade-offs. This is the issue that we address in this article. We demonstrate the usefulness of adopting new approaches by considering the following scenario.

Consider that a data center is interested in the data sequence, $\{X(t)\}_{t=1}^{\infty}$, which cannot be observed directly. Therefore, the data center deploys a bunch of L sensors which each independently encodes its noisy observation of the sequence, $\{Y_i(t)\}_{t=1}^{\infty}$, without sharing any information, i.e., the sensors are not permitted to communicate and decide what to send to the data center beforehand. The data center collects separate samples from all the L sensors and uses them to recover the original sequence. However, since $\{X(t)\}_{t=1}^{\infty}$ is not the only pressing matter which the data center must consider, the combined data rate R at which the sensors can communicate with it is strictly limited. A formulation of decentralized communication with estimation task, the "CEO problem", was first proposed by Berger and Zhang [2], providing a new theoretical framework for large scale sensing systems. In this outstanding work, some interesting properties of such systems have been revealed. If the sensors were permitted to communicate on the basis of their pooled observations, then they would be able to smooth out their independent observation noises entirely as L goes to infinity. Therefore, the data center can achieve an arbitrary fidelity $D(R)$, where $D(\cdot)$ denotes the distortion rate function of $\{X(t)\}$. In particular, the data center recovers almost complete information if R exceeds the entropy rate of $\{X(t)\}$. However, if the sensors are not allowed to communicate with each other, there does not exist a finite value of R for which even infinitely many sensors can make D arbitrarily small [2].

In this paper, we introduce a new analytical model for a massive sensing system with a finite data rate R. More specifically, we assume that the sensors use LDGM codes for rate distortion coding, while the data center recovers the original sequence by using optimal "majority vote" estimation [3]. We consider the distributed sensing problem of deciding the optimal number of sensors L given the combined data rate R. Our asymptotic analysis successfully provides the performance of the whole sensing system when L goes to infinity, where the data rate for an individual sensor information vanishes. Here, we exploit statistical methods which have recently been developed in the field of disordered statistical systems, in particular, the spin glass theory. The paper is organized as follows. In Section 2, we introduce a system model for the sensor network. Section 3 summarizes the results of our approach, where the following section provides the outline of our analysis. Conclusions are given in the last section.

2 System Model

Let $P(x)$ be a probability distribution common to $\{X(t)\} \in \mathcal{X}$, and $W(y|x)$ be a stochastic matrix defined on $\mathcal{X} \times \mathcal{Y}$, with $\mathcal{Y}$ denotes the common alphabet of $\{Y_i(t)\}$, where $i = 1, \cdots, L$ and $t \geq 1$. In the general setup, we assume that the instantaneous joint probability distribution in the form

$$\Pr[x, y_1, \cdots, y_L] = P(x) \prod_{i=1}^{L} W(y_i|x)$$

for the temporally memoryless source $\{X(t)\}_{t=1}^{\infty}$. Here, the random variables $Y_i(t)$ are conditionally independent when $X(t)$ is given, and the conditional probabilities $W[y_i(t)|x(t)]$ are identical for all i and t. In this paper, we impose the binary assumptions to the problem, i.e., the data sequence $\{X(t)\}$ and its noisy observations $\{Y_i(t)\}$ are all assumed to be binary sequences. Therefore, the stochastic matrix can be parameterized as

$$W(y|x) = \begin{cases} 1 - p, & \text{if } y = x \\ p, & \text{otherwise} \end{cases},$$

where $p \in [0, 1]$ represents the observation noise. Note also that the alphabets have been selected as $\mathcal{X} = \mathcal{Y}$. Furthermore, for simplicity, we also assume that $P(x) = 1/2$ always holds, implying that a purely random source is observed.

At the encoding stage, a sensor i encodes a block $\boldsymbol{y}_i = [y_i(1), \cdots, y_i(n)]^T$ of length n from the noisy observation $\{y_i(t)\}_{t=1}^{\infty}$, into a block $\boldsymbol{z}_i = [z_i(1), \cdots, z_i(m)]^T$ of length m defined on $\mathcal{Z}$. Hereafter, we take the Boolean representation of the binary alphabet $\mathcal{X} = \{0, 1\}$, therefore $\mathcal{Y} = \mathcal{Z} = \{0, 1\}$ as well. Let $\hat{\boldsymbol{y}}_i$ be a reproduction sequence for the block, and we have a known integer $m < n$. Then, making use of a Boolean matrix A_i of dimensionality $n \times m$, we are to find an m bit codeword sequence $\boldsymbol{z}_i = [z_i(1), \cdots, z_i(m)]^T$ which satisfies

$$\hat{\boldsymbol{y}}_i = A_i \boldsymbol{z}_i \pmod{2}, \tag{1}$$

where the fidelity criterion

$$D = \frac{1}{n} d_\mathrm{H}(\boldsymbol{y}_i, \hat{\boldsymbol{y}}_i) \tag{2}$$

holds [4]. Here the Hamming distance $d_\mathrm{H}(\cdot, \cdot)$ is used for the distortion measure. Note that we have applied modulo-2 arithmetic for the additive operation in (1). Let A_i be characterized by K ones per row and C per column. The finite, and usually small, numbers K and C define a particular LDGM code family. The data center then collects the L codeword sequences, $\boldsymbol{z}_1, \cdots, \boldsymbol{z}_L$. Since all the L codewords are of the same length m, the combined data rate will be $R = L \times m/n$. Therefore, in our scenario, the data center deploys exchangeable sensors with fixed quality reproductions, $\hat{\boldsymbol{y}}_1, \cdots, \hat{\boldsymbol{y}}_L$. Lastly, the tth symbol of the estimate, $\hat{\boldsymbol{x}} = [\hat{x}(1), \cdots, \hat{x}(n)]^T$, is to be calculated by majority vote [3],

$$\hat{x}(t) = \begin{cases} 0, & \text{if } \hat{y}_1(t) + \cdots + \hat{y}_L(t) \leq L/2 \\ 1, & \text{otherwise} \end{cases}. \tag{3}$$

Therefore, overall performance of the system can be measured by the expected bit error frequency for decisions by the majority vote (3), $P_\mathrm{e} = \Pr[x \neq \hat{x}]$.

In this paper, we consider two limit cases of decentralization levels; (1) The extreme situation of $L \to \infty$, and (2) the case of $L = R$. The former case means that the data rate for an individual sensor information vanishes, while the latter case results in the transmission without coding techniques. In general, it is difficult to determine which level is optimal for the estimation, i.e., which scenario results in the smaller value of P_e. Indeed, by using the rate distortion codes, the data center could use as many sensors as possible for a given R. However, the quality of the individual reproduction would be less informative. The best choice seems to depend largely on R, as well as p.

3   Main Results

For simplicity, we consider the following two solvable cases; $K = 2$ for $C \geq K$ and the optimal case of $K \to \infty$. Let p be a given observation noise level, and R the finite real value of a given combined data rate. Letting $L \to \infty$, we find the expected bit error frequency to be

$$P_\mathrm{e}(p, R) = \int_{-\infty}^{-(1-2p)c_g\sqrt{R}} dr\, \mathrm{N}(0, 1) \tag{4}$$

with the constant value

$$c_g = \begin{cases} \frac{1}{\sqrt{2}} \left[\frac{\sqrt{\alpha}}{2} + \frac{2\ln 2}{\sqrt{\alpha}} - \left(\frac{\sqrt{\alpha}}{2} - \frac{\sigma^2}{\sqrt{\alpha}} \right) \langle \tanh^2 x \rangle_{\pi(x)} \right] & (K = 2) \\ \sqrt{2\ln 2} & (K \to \infty) \end{cases} \tag{5}$$

where the rescaled variance $\sigma^2 = \alpha \langle \hat{x}^2 \rangle_{\hat{\pi}(\hat{x})}$ and the *first step RSB* enforcement

$$-\frac{1}{2} + \frac{2}{\alpha}\ln 2 + \left(\frac{1}{2} - \frac{\sigma^2}{\alpha} \right) \langle \tanh^2 x\, (1 + 2x\,\mathrm{csch}\, x\,\mathrm{sech}\, x) \rangle_{\pi(x)} = 0$$

holds. Here $\mathrm{N}(X, Y)$ denotes the normal distribution with the mean X and the variance Y. The rescaled variance σ^2 and the scale invariant parameter α is determined numerically, where we use the following notations.

$$\langle \cdot \rangle_{\pi(x)} = \int_{-\infty}^{\infty} \frac{dx}{\sqrt{2\pi\sigma^2}} \exp\left[-\frac{x^2}{2\sigma^2} \right] (\cdot)\,,$$

$$\langle \cdot \rangle_{\hat{\pi}(\hat{x})} = \int_{-1}^{+1} \frac{d\hat{x}}{\sqrt{2\pi\sigma^2}} (1 - \hat{x}^2)^{-1} \exp\left[-\frac{(\tanh^{-1}\hat{x})^2}{2\sigma^2} \right] (\cdot)\,.$$

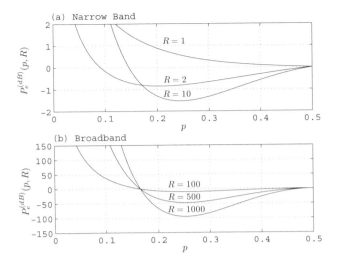

Figure 1: $P_e^{(\mathrm{dB})}(p, R)$ for $K = 2$. (a) Narrow band (b) Broadband

Therefore, it is straightforward to evaluate (4) with (5) for given parameters, p and R.

For a given *finite* value of R, we see what happens to the quality of the estimate when the noise level p varies. Fig. 1 and Fig. 2 shows the typical behavior of the bit error frequency, $P_e(p, R)$, in decibel (dB), where the reference level is chosen as

$$
P_e^{(0)}(p, R) = \begin{cases} \sum_{l=0}^{(R-1)/2} \binom{R}{l}(1-p)^l p^{R-l}, & (R \text{ is odd}) \\ \sum_{l=0}^{R/2-1} \binom{R}{l}(1-p)^l p^{R-l} + \frac{1}{2}\binom{R}{R/2}(1-p)^{R/2}p^{R/2} & (R \text{ is even}) \end{cases} \tag{6}
$$

for a given integer R. The reference (6) denotes P_e for the case of $L = R$, i.e., the case when the sensors are not allowed to compress their observations. Here, in decibel, we have

$$
P_e^{(\mathrm{dB})}(p, R) = 10 \log \frac{P_e(p, R)}{P_e^{(0)}(p, R)},
$$

where the log is to base 10. Note that the zero level in decibel occurs when the measured error frequency $P_e(p, R)$ is equal to the reference level. Therefore, it is also possible to have negative levels, which would mean an expected bit error frequency much smaller than the reference level. In the case of small combined data rate R, the narrow band case, the numerical results in Fig. 1 (a) and Fig. 2 (a) show that the quality of the estimate is sensitive to the parity of the integer R. In particular, the $R = 2$ case has the lowest threshold level, $p_c = 0.0921$ for Fig. 1 (a) and $p_c = 0.082$ for Fig. 2 (a) respectively, beyond which the $L \to \infty$ scenario outperforms the $L = R$ scenario, while the $R = 1$ case does not have such a threshold. In contrast, if the bandwidth is wide enough, the difference of the expected bit error probabilities in decibel, $P_e^{(\mathrm{dB})}(p, R)$, is proved to have similar qualitative characteristics as shown in Fig. 1 (b) and Fig. 2 (b). Moreover, our preliminary experiments for larger systems also indicate that the threshold p_c seems to converge to the value, 0.165 and 0.146 respectively, as L goes to infinity; we are currently working on the theoretical derivation.

4   Outline of Derivation

Since the predetermined matrices $A_1, \cdots, A_L$ are selected randomly, it is quite natural to say that the instantaneous series, defined by $\hat{\boldsymbol{y}}(t) = [\hat{y}_1(t), \cdots, \hat{y}_L(t)]^T$, can be modeled

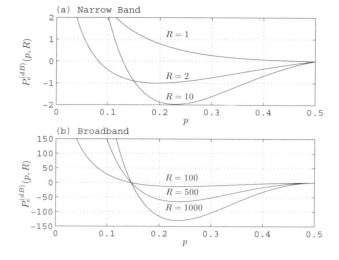

Figure 2: $P_{\mathrm{e}}^{(\mathrm{dB})}(p, R)$ for $K \to \infty$. (a) Narrow band (b) Broadband

using the Bernoulli trials. Here, the reproduction problem reduces to a channel model, where the stochastic matrix is defined as

$$W(\hat{y}|x) = \begin{cases} q, & \text{if } \hat{y} = x \\ 1 - q, & \text{otherwise} \end{cases}, \tag{7}$$

where q denotes the quality of the reproductions, i.e., $\Pr[x \neq \hat{y}_i] = 1 - q$ for $i = 1, \cdots, L$. Letting the channel model (7) for the reproduction problem be valid, the expected bit error frequency can be well captured by using the cumulative probability distributions

$$P_{\mathrm{e}} = \Pr[x \neq \hat{x}] = \begin{cases} B(\frac{L-1}{2} : L, q), & \text{if } L \text{ is odd} \\ B(\frac{L}{2} - 1 : L, q) + \frac{1}{2}b(\frac{L}{2} : L, q) & \text{otherwise} \end{cases} \tag{8}$$

with

$$B(L' : L, q) = \sum_{l=0}^{L'} b(l : L, q), \quad b(l : L, q) = \binom{L}{l} q^l (1 - q)^{L-l},$$

where an integer l be the total number of non-flipped elements in $\hat{y}(t)$, and the second term $(1/2)b(L/2 : L, q)$ represents random guessing with $l = L/2$. Note that the reproduction quality q can be easily obtained by the simple algebra $q = pD + (1 - p)(1 - D)$, where D is the distortion with respect to coding.

Since the error probability (8) is given by a function of q, we firstly derive an analytical solution for the quality q in the limit $L \to \infty$, keeping R finite. In this approach, we apply the method of statistical mechanics to evaluate the *typical* performance of the codes [4]. As a first step, we translate the Boolean alphabets $\mathcal{Z} = \{0, 1\}$ to the "Ising" ones, $\mathcal{S} = \{+1, -1\}$. Consequently, we need to translate the additive operations, such as, $z_i(s) + z_i(s') \pmod{2}$ into their multiplicative representations, $\sigma_i(s) \times \sigma_i(s') \in \mathcal{S}$ for $s, s' = 1, \cdots, m$. Similarly, we translate the Boolean $y_i(t)$s into the Ising $J_i(t)$s. For simplicity, we omit the subscript i, which labels the L agents, in the rest of this section. Following the prescription of Sourlas [5], we examine the *Gibbs-Boltzmann distribution*

$$\Pr[\boldsymbol{\sigma}] = \frac{\exp\left[-\beta H(\boldsymbol{\sigma}|\boldsymbol{J})\right]}{Z(\boldsymbol{J})} \quad \text{with} \quad Z(\boldsymbol{J}) = \sum_{\sigma} e^{-\beta H(\boldsymbol{\sigma}|\boldsymbol{J})}, \tag{9}$$

935

where the *Hamiltonian* of the Ising system is defined as

$$H(\boldsymbol{\sigma}|\boldsymbol{J}) = - \sum_{s_1 < \cdots < s_K} \mathcal{A}_{s_1 \ldots s_K} J_i[t(s_1, \ldots, s_K)]\sigma(s_1) \ldots \sigma(s_K) \,. \tag{10}$$

The observation index $t(s_1, \ldots, s_K)$ specifies the proper value of t given the set $s_1, \ldots, s_K$, so that it corresponds to the parity check equation (1). Here the elements of the symmetric tensor $\mathcal{A}_{s_1 \ldots s_K}$, representing dilution, is either zero or one depending on the set of indices $(s_1, \ldots, s_K)$. Since there are C non-zero elements randomly chosen for any given index s, we find $\sum_{s_2, \ldots, s_K} \mathcal{A}_{ss_2 \ldots s_K} = C$. The code rate is $R/L = K/C$ because a reproduction sequence has C bits per index s and carries K bits of the codeword. It is easy to see that the Hamiltonian (10) is counting the reproduction errors, $[1 - J_{t(s_1, \ldots, s_K)} \cdot \sigma(s_1) \ldots \sigma(s_K)]/2$.

Moreover, according to the statistical mechanics, we can easily derive the "observable" quantities using the *free energy* defined as

$$f = -\frac{1}{\beta} \langle \ln Z(\boldsymbol{J}) \rangle_{\mathcal{A}, \boldsymbol{J}}$$

which carries all information about the statistics of the system. Here, β denotes an "inverse temperature" for the Gibbs-Boltzmann distribution (9), and $\langle \cdot \rangle_{\mathcal{A}, \boldsymbol{J}}$ represents the configurational average. Therefore, we have to average the logarithm of the partition function $Z(\boldsymbol{J})$ over the given distribution $\langle \cdot \rangle_{\mathcal{A}, \boldsymbol{J}}$ after the calculation of the partition function. Finally, to perform such a program, the *replica trick* is used [6]. The theory of *replica symmetry breaking* can provide the free energy resulting in the expression

$$f = -\frac{1}{\beta n} \left[\ln \cosh \beta - K \left\langle \ln \left[1 + \tanh(\beta x) \tanh(\beta \hat{x}) \right] \right\rangle_{\pi(x), \hat{\pi}(\hat{x})} \right.$$

$$+ \frac{1}{2} \left\langle \sum_{J = \pm 1} \ln \left[1 + \tanh(\beta J) \prod_{l=1}^{K} \tanh(\beta x_l) \right] \right\rangle_{\pi(x)}$$

$$+ \left. \frac{C}{K} \left\langle \ln \sum_{\sigma = \pm 1} \prod_{l=1}^{C} [1 + \sigma \tanh(\beta \hat{x}_l)] \right\rangle_{\hat{\pi}(\hat{x})} \right], \tag{11}$$

where $\langle \cdot \rangle_{\pi(x)}$ denotes the averaging over $p(x_l)$s and so on. The variation of (11) by $\pi(x)$ and $\hat{\pi}(\hat{x})$ under the condition of normalization gives the saddle point condition

$$\pi(x) = \left\langle \delta \left[x - \sum_{l=1}^{C-1} \hat{x}_l \right] \right\rangle_{\hat{\pi}(\hat{x})} \quad , \quad \hat{\pi}(\hat{x}) = \left\langle \frac{1}{2} \sum_{J = \pm 1} \delta \left[\hat{x} - \mu(x_1, \ldots, x_{K-1}; J) \right] \right\rangle_{\pi(x)} \,,$$

where

$$\mu(x_1, \ldots, x_{K-1}; J) = \frac{1}{\beta} \tanh^{-1} \left[\tanh(\beta J) \prod_{l=1}^{K-1} \tanh(\beta x_l) \right] \,.$$

We now investigate the case of $K = 2$. Applying the central limit theorem to $\pi(x)$ [7], we get

$$\pi(x) = \frac{1}{\sqrt{2\pi C \sigma^2}} e^{-\frac{x^2}{2C\sigma^2}} \,, \tag{12}$$

where σ^2 is the variance of $\hat{\pi}(\hat{x})$. Here the resulting distribution (12) is a even function. The leading contribution to μ is then given by $\mu(x; J) \sim J \cdot \tanh(\beta x)$ as β goes to zero;

The expression is valid in the asymptotic region $L \gg 1$ for a fixed R. Then, the formula for the delta function yields [8]

$$
\begin{aligned}
\hat{\pi}(\hat{x}) &= \left\langle \delta\left[x - \frac{1}{\beta}\tanh^{-1}\hat{x}\right] \left|\rho'\left(\frac{1}{\beta}\tanh^{-1}\hat{x}; \hat{x}\right)\right|^{-1}\right\rangle_{\pi(x)} \\
&= \frac{(1-\hat{x}^2)^{-1}}{\sqrt{2\pi\beta^2 C\sigma^2}}\exp\left[-\frac{(\tanh^{-1}\hat{x})^2}{2\beta^2 C\sigma^2}\right],
\end{aligned} \tag{13}
$$

where we have used $\rho(x; \hat{x}) = \hat{x} - \tanh(\beta x)$. Therefore, we have

$$
\sigma^2 = \langle\hat{x}^2\rangle_{\hat{\pi}(\hat{x})} = \int_{-1}^{+1}\frac{d\hat{x}}{\sqrt{2\pi\beta^2 C\sigma^2}}\frac{\hat{x}^2}{1-\hat{x}^2}\exp\left[-\frac{(\tanh^{-1}\hat{x})^2}{2\beta^2 C\sigma^2}\right]
$$

for given $\beta^2 C$. Inserting (12), (13) into (11), we get

$$
f = -\frac{\beta}{2} - \frac{R}{\beta}\ln 2 + \frac{1-2\sigma^2}{2}\beta\langle\tanh^2\tilde{x}\rangle_{\tilde{\pi}(\tilde{x})} \quad \text{with} \quad \tilde{\pi}(\tilde{x}) = \frac{1}{\sqrt{2\pi\beta^2 C\sigma^2}}e^{-\frac{\tilde{x}^2}{2\beta^2 C\sigma^2}},
$$

where we rewrite $\tilde{x} = \beta x$. The theory of *replica symmetry breaking* tells us that relevant value of β should not be smaller than the "freezing point" β_g, which implies the vanishing entropy condition:

$$
\frac{\partial f}{\partial\beta} = -\frac{1}{2} + \frac{2}{\beta_g^2 C}\ln 2 + \frac{1-2\sigma^2}{2}\langle\tanh^2\tilde{x}\,(1 + 2\tilde{x}\operatorname{csch}\tilde{x}\operatorname{sech}\tilde{x})\rangle_{\tilde{\pi}(\tilde{x})} = 0.
$$

Accordingly, it is convenient for us to define a scaling invariant parameter $\alpha = \beta_g^2 C$, and to rewrite the variance $\tilde{\sigma}^2 = \alpha\sigma^2$ for simplicity. Introducing these newly defined parameters, the above results could be summarized as follows. Given R and L, we find

$$
f = \sqrt{\frac{R}{L}}\left[-\frac{1}{2}\sqrt{\frac{\alpha}{2}} - \ln 2\sqrt{\frac{2}{\alpha}} + \sqrt{\frac{\alpha}{2}}\left(\frac{1}{2} - \frac{\tilde{\sigma}^2}{\alpha}\right)\langle\tanh^2\tilde{x}\rangle_{\tilde{\pi}(\tilde{x})}\right]
$$

with $\tilde{\sigma}^2 = \alpha\langle\hat{x}^2\rangle_{\hat{\pi}(\hat{x})}$, where the condition

$$
-\frac{1}{2} + \frac{2}{\alpha}\ln 2 + \left(\frac{1}{2} - \frac{\tilde{\sigma}^2}{\alpha}\right)\langle\tanh^2\tilde{x}\,(1 + 2\tilde{x}\operatorname{csch}\tilde{x}\operatorname{sech}\tilde{x})\rangle_{\tilde{\pi}(\tilde{x})} = 0 \tag{14}
$$

holds. Here we denote

$$
\langle\,\cdot\,\rangle_{\tilde{\pi}(\tilde{x})} = \int_{-\infty}^{\infty}\frac{d\tilde{x}}{\sqrt{2\pi\tilde{\sigma}^2}}\exp\left[-\frac{\tilde{x}^2}{2\tilde{\sigma}^2}\right](\,\cdot\,),
$$

$$
\langle\,\cdot\,\rangle_{\hat{\pi}(\hat{x})} = \int_{-1}^{+1}\frac{d\hat{x}}{\sqrt{2\pi\tilde{\sigma}^2}}(1-\hat{x}^2)^{-1}\exp\left[-\frac{(\tanh^{-1}\hat{x})^2}{2\tilde{\sigma}^2}\right](\,\cdot\,).
$$

Lastly, by using the cumulative probability distribution, we get

$$
P_{\mathrm{e}} = \sum_{l=0}^{L/2}\binom{L}{l}q^l(1-q)^{L-l} \sim \int_0^{L/2}dr\,\mathrm{N}(Lq, Lq(1-q)). \tag{15}
$$

It is easy to see that (15) can be converted to a standard normal distribution by changing variables to $\tilde{r} = (r - Lq)/\sqrt{Lq(1-q)}$ [7], so $d\tilde{r} = dr/\sqrt{Lq(1-q)}$, yielding

$$
P_{\mathrm{e}} \sim \int_{-\sqrt{L}}^{\tilde{r}_g}d\tilde{r}\,\mathrm{N}(0, 1)
$$

937

with

$$\tilde{r}_g = 2\sqrt{L}(1-2p)\left(D - \frac{1}{2}\right)$$

$$= \sqrt{\frac{R}{2}}(1-2p)\left[-\frac{1}{2}\sqrt{\alpha} - \frac{2\ln 2}{\sqrt{\alpha}} + \sqrt{\alpha}\left(\frac{1}{2} - \frac{\tilde{\sigma}^2}{\alpha}\right)\langle\tanh^2 \tilde{x}\rangle_{\tilde{\pi}(\tilde{x})}\right].$$

Note that the relation $D = (1+f)/2$ holds at the vanishing entropy condition (14) [4]. Finally, we obtain the main result (4) in Section 3 in the limit $L \to \infty$, when we use proper notations for the variables and the name of the function.

We can investigate the asymptotic case of $K \to \infty$ in a similar way. Since the leading contribution to $\hat{\pi}(\hat{x})$ comes from the value of x in the vicinity of $\sqrt{C\sigma^2}$, we find the expression $\hat{\pi}(\hat{x}) \approx \left\langle\delta\left[\hat{x} - y\beta^K(C\sigma^2)^{\frac{K}{2}}\right]\right\rangle$ by using the power counting. Therefore, within the Parisi RSB scheme, one obtain a set of equations

$$\sqrt{L}f = -\frac{\sqrt{\alpha_c}}{2} - \frac{R}{\sqrt{\alpha_c}}\ln 2 , \quad -\frac{1}{2} + \frac{R}{\alpha_c}\ln 2 = 0$$

with the scale-invariant $\alpha_c = \beta^2 L$. This results in $c_g = \sqrt{2\ln 2}$, as is mentioned before.

5 Conclusion

This paper provides a system-level perspective for massive sensor networks. The decentralized sensing problem argued in this paper was first addressed by Berger and his collaborators. However, this paper is the first work that gives a scheme to analyze practically tractable codes in the given finite data rate, and shows the existence of threshold level of noise of which the optimal levels of decentralization changes. Future work includes the theoretical derivation of the threshold level p_c where R goes to infinity, as well as the implementation problem.

Acknowledgments

The authors thank Jun Muramatsu and Naonori Ueda for useful discussions. This work was supported by the Ministry of Education, Science, Sports and Culture (MEXT) of Japan, under the Grant-in-Aid for Young Scientists (B), 15760288.

References

[1] (2005) Intel@Mote. [Online]. Available: http://www.intel.com/research/exploratory/motes.htm

[2] T. Berger, Z. Zhang, and H. Viswanathan, "The CEO problem," *IEEE Trans. Inform. Theory*, vol. 42, pp. 887–902, May 1996.

[3] D. J. C. MacKay, *Information Theory, Inference and Learning Algorithms*. Cambridge, UK: Cambridge University Press, 2003.

[4] T. Murayama and M. Okada, "Rate distortion function in the spin glass state: a toy model," in *Advances in Neural Information Processing Systems 15 (NIPS'02)*, Denver, USA, Dec. 2002, pp. 423–430.

[5] N. Sourlas, "Spin-glass models as error-correcting codes," *Nature*, vol. 339, pp. 693–695, June 1989.

[6] V. Dotsenko, *Introduction to the Replica Theory of Disordered Statistical Systems*. Cambridge, UK: Cambridge University Press, 2001.

[7] W. Hays, *Statistics (5th Edition)*. Belmont, CA: Wadsworth Publishing, 1994.

[8] C. W. Wong, *Introduction to Mathematical Physics: Methods and Concepts*. Oxford, UK: Oxford University Press, 1991.

Gaussian Processes for Multiuser Detection in CDMA receivers

Juan José Murillo-Fuentes, Sebastian Caro
Dept. Signal Theory and Communications
University of Seville
{murillo,scaro}@us.es

Fernando Pérez-Cruz
Gatsby Computational Neuroscience
University College London
fernando@gatsby.ucl.ac.uk

Abstract

In this paper we propose a new receiver for digital communications. We focus on the application of Gaussian Processes (GPs) to the multiuser detection (MUD) in code division multiple access (CDMA) systems to solve the near-far problem. Hence, we aim to reduce the interference from other users sharing the same frequency band. While usual approaches minimize the mean square error (MMSE) to linearly retrieve the user of interest, we exploit the same criteria but in the design of a nonlinear MUD. Since the optimal solution is known to be nonlinear, the performance of this novel method clearly improves that of the MMSE detectors. Furthermore, the GP based MUD achieves excellent interference suppression even for short training sequences. We also include some experiments to illustrate that other nonlinear detectors such as those based on Support Vector Machines (SVMs) exhibit a worse performance.

1   Introduction

One of the major issues in present wireless communications is how users share the resources. And particularly, how they access to a common frequency band. Code division multiple access (CDMA) is one of the techniques exploited in third generation communications systems and is to be employed in the next generation. In CDMA each user uses direct sequence spread spectrum (DS-SS) to modulate its bits with an assigned code, spreading them over the entire frequency band. While typical receivers deal only with interferences and noise intrinsic to the channel (i.e. Inter-Symbolic Interference, intermodulation products, spurious frequencies, and thermal noise), in CDMA we also have interference produced by other users accessing the channel at the same time. Interference limitation due to the simultaneous access of multiple users systems has been the stimulus to the development of a powerful family of Signal Processing techniques, namely Multiuser Detection (MUD). These techniques have been extensively applied to CDMA systems. Thus, most of last generation digital communication systems such as Global Positioning System (GPS), wireless 802.11b, Universal Mobile Telecommunication System (UMTS), etc, may take advantage of any improvement on this topic.

In CDMA, we face the retrieval of a given user, the user of interest (UOI), with the knowledge of its associated code or even the whole set of users codes. Hence, we face the suppression of interference due to others users. If all users transmit with the same power,

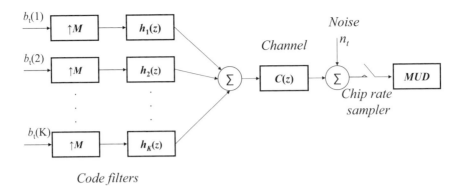

Figure 1: Synchronous CDMA system

but the UOI is far from the receiver, most users reach the receiver with a larger amplitude, making it more difficult to detect the bits of the UOI. This is well-known as the near-far problem. Simple detectors can be designed by minimizing the mean square error (MMSE) to linearly retrieve the user of interest [5]. However, these detectors need large sequences of training data. Besides, the optimal solution is known to be nonlinear.

There has been several attempts to solve the problem using nonlinear techniques. There are solutions based on Neural Networks such as multilayer perceptron or radial basis functions [1, 3], but training times are long and unpredictable. Recently, support vector machines (SVM) have been also applied to CDMA MUD [4]. This solution need very long training sequences (a few hundreds bits) and they are only tested in toy examples with very few users and short spreading sequences (the code for each user). In this paper, we will present a multiuser detector based on Gaussian Processes [7]. The MUD detector is inspired by the linear MMSE criteria, which can be interpreted as a Bayesian linear regressor. In this sense, we can extend the linear MMSE criteria to nonlinear decision functions using the same ideas developed in [6] to present Gaussian Processes for regression.

The rest of the paper is organised as follows. In Section 2, we present the multiuser detection problem in CDMA communication systems and the widely used minimum mean square error receiver. We propose a nonlinear receiver based on Gaussian Processes in Section 3. Section 4 is devoted to show, through computer experiments, the advantages of the GP-MUD receiver with short training sequences. We compare it to the linear MMSE and the nonlinear SVM MUD. We conclude the paper in Section 5 presenting some remarks and future work.

2 CDMA Communication System Model and MUD

Consider a synchronous CDMA digital communication system [5] as depicted in Figure 1. Its main goal is to share the channel between different users, discriminating between them by different assigned codes. Each transmitted bit is upsampled and multiplied by the users' spreading codes and then the chips for each bit are transmitted into the channel (each element of the spreading code is either +1 or −1 and they are known as chips). The channel is assumed to be linear and noisy, therefore the chips from different users are added together, plus Gaussian noise. Hence, the MUD has to recover from these chips the bits corresponding to each user. At each time step t, the signal in the receiver can be represented in matrix notation as:

$$\boldsymbol{x}_t = \boldsymbol{H}\boldsymbol{A}\boldsymbol{b}_t + \boldsymbol{n}_t \tag{1}$$

where $\boldsymbol{b}_t$ is a column vector that contains the bits ($+1$ or -1) for the K users at time k. The $K \times K$ diagonal matrix $\boldsymbol{A}$ contains the amplitude of each user, which represents the attenuation that each user's transmission suffers through the channel (this attenuation depends on the distance between the user and the receiver). $\boldsymbol{H}$ is an $L \times K$ matrix which contains in each column the L-dimensional spreading code for each of the K users. The spreading codes are designed to present a low cross-correlation between them and between any shifted version of the codes, to guarantee that the bits from each user can be readily recovered. The codes are known as spreading sequences, because they augment the occupied bandwidth of the transmitted signal by L. Finally, $\boldsymbol{x}_t$ represents the L received chips to which Gaussian noise has been added, which is denoted by $\boldsymbol{n}_t$.

At reception, we aim to estimate the original transmitted symbols of any user i, $\boldsymbol{b}_t(i)$, hereafter the user of interest. Linear MUDs estimate these bits as

$$\hat{\boldsymbol{b}}_t(i) = sgn\{\boldsymbol{w}_i^\top \boldsymbol{x}_t\} \tag{2}$$

The matched filter (MF) $\boldsymbol{w}_i = \boldsymbol{h}_i$, a simple correlation between $\boldsymbol{x}_t$ and the ith spreading code, is the optimal receiver if there were no additional users in the system, i.e. the received signal is only corrupted by Gaussian noise. The near-far problem arises when remaining users, apart from the UOI, are received with significantly higher amplitude. While the optimal solution is known to be nonlinear [5], some linear receivers such as the minimum mean square error (MMSE) present good performances and are used in practice. The MMSE receiver for the ith user solves:

$$\mathbf{w}_i^* = \arg\min_{\mathbf{w}_i} E\left[(\boldsymbol{b}_t(i) - \mathbf{w}_i^\top \boldsymbol{x}_t)^2\right] = \arg\min_{\mathbf{w}_i} E\left[(\boldsymbol{b}_t(i) - \mathbf{w}_i^\top(\boldsymbol{H}\boldsymbol{A}\boldsymbol{b}_t + \boldsymbol{\nu}_k))^2\right] \tag{3}$$

where $\mathbf{w}_i$ represents the decision function of the linear classifier. We can derive the MMSE receiver by taking derivatives with respect to $\mathbf{w}_i$ and equating to zero, obtaining:

$$\mathbf{w}_i^{MMSE_{de}} = \boldsymbol{R}_{xx}^{-1}\boldsymbol{h}_i \tag{4}$$

where $R_{xx} = \mathrm{E}[\boldsymbol{x}_t \boldsymbol{x}_t^\top]$ is the correlation between the received vectors and $\boldsymbol{h}_i$ represents the spreading sequence of the UOI. This receiver is known as the decentralized MMSE receiver as it can be implemented without knowing the spreading sequences of the remaining users. Its main limitation is its performance, which is very low even for high signal to noise ratio, and it needs many examples (thousands) before it can recover the received symbols.

If the spreading codes of all the users are available, as in the base station, this information can be used to improve the performance of the MMSE detector. We can define $\boldsymbol{z}_k = \boldsymbol{H}^\top \boldsymbol{x}_t$, which is a vector of sufficient statistics for this problem [5]. The vector $\boldsymbol{z}_k$ is the matched-filter output for each user and it reduces the dimensionality of our problem from the number of chips L to the number of users K, which is significantly lower in most applications. In this case the receiver is known as the centralized detector and it is defined as:

$$\mathbf{w}_i^{MMSE_{cent}} = \boldsymbol{H}\boldsymbol{R}_{zz}^{-1}\boldsymbol{H}^\top \boldsymbol{h}_i \tag{5}$$

where $R_{zz} = \mathrm{E}[\boldsymbol{z}_t \boldsymbol{z}_t^\top]$ is the correlation matrix of the received chips after the MFs.

These MUDs have good convergence properties and do not need a training sequence to decode the received bits, but they need large training sequences before their probability of error is low. Therefore the initially received bits will present a very high probability of error that will make impossible to send any information on them. Some improvements can be achieved by using higher order statistics [2], but still the training sequences are not short enough for most applications.

941

3 Gaussian Processes for Multiuser Detection

The MMSE detector minimizes the functional in (3), which gives the best linear classifier. As we know, the optimal classifier is nonlinear [5], and the MMSE criteria can be readily extended to provide nonlinear models by mapping the received chips to a higher dimensional space. In this case we will need to solve:

$$\mathbf{w}_i^* = \arg\min_{\mathbf{w}_i} \left\{ \sum_{k=1}^{N} \left(\boldsymbol{b}_t(i) - \mathbf{w}_i^\top \boldsymbol{\phi}(\boldsymbol{x}_t) \right)^2 + \lambda \|\mathbf{w}_i\|^2 \right\} \tag{6}$$

in which we have changed the expectation by the empirical mean over a training set and we have incorporated a regularizer to avoid overfitting. $\boldsymbol{\phi}(\cdot)$ represents the nonlinear mapping of the received chips. The $\mathbf{w}_i$ that minimizes (6) can be interpreted as the mode of the parameters in a Bayesian linear regressor, as noted in [6], and since the likelihood and the prior are both Gaussians, so it will be the posterior. For any received symbol $\boldsymbol{x}_*$, we know that it will be distributed as a Gaussian with mean:

$$\mu(\boldsymbol{x}_*) = \frac{1}{\lambda} \boldsymbol{\phi}^\top(\boldsymbol{x}_*) \mathbf{A}^{-1} \boldsymbol{\Phi}^\top \mathbf{b} \tag{7}$$

and variance

$$\sigma^2(\boldsymbol{x}_*) = \boldsymbol{\phi}^\top(\boldsymbol{x}_*) \mathbf{A}^{-1} \boldsymbol{\phi}(\boldsymbol{x}_*) \tag{8}$$

where $\boldsymbol{\Phi} = [\boldsymbol{\phi}(\boldsymbol{x}_1), \boldsymbol{\phi}(\boldsymbol{x}_2), \ldots, \boldsymbol{\phi}(\boldsymbol{x}_N)]^\top$, $\mathbf{b} = [\boldsymbol{b}_1(i), \boldsymbol{b}_2(i), \ldots, \boldsymbol{b}_N(i)]^\top$ and $\mathbf{A} = \boldsymbol{\Phi}^\top\boldsymbol{\Phi} + \frac{1}{\lambda}\mathbf{I}$.

In the case the nonlinear mapping is unknown, we can still obtain the mean and variance for each received sample using the kernel of the transformation, being the mean:

$$\mu(\boldsymbol{x}_*) = \mathbf{k}^\top \mathbf{P}^{-1} \mathbf{b} \tag{9}$$

and variance

$$\sigma^2(\boldsymbol{x}_*) = k(\boldsymbol{x}_*, \boldsymbol{x}_*) + \mathbf{k}^\top \mathbf{P}^{-1} \mathbf{k} \tag{10}$$

where $k(\cdot, \cdot) = \boldsymbol{\phi}^\top(\cdot)\boldsymbol{\phi}(\cdot)$ is the kernel of the nonlinear transformation, $\mathbf{k} = [k(\boldsymbol{x}_*, \boldsymbol{x}_1), k(\boldsymbol{x}_*, \boldsymbol{x}_2), \ldots, k(\boldsymbol{x}_*, \boldsymbol{x}_N)]$, and

$$\mathbf{P} = \boldsymbol{\Phi}\boldsymbol{\Phi}^\top + \lambda\mathbf{I} = \mathbf{K} + \lambda\mathbf{I} \tag{11}$$

where $(\mathbf{K})_{k\ell} = k(\boldsymbol{x}_t, \boldsymbol{x}_\ell)$. The kernel that we will use in our experiments are:

$$k(\boldsymbol{x}_t, \boldsymbol{x}_\ell) = e^{\theta[1]} \exp(-e^{\theta[4]} \|\boldsymbol{x}_t - \boldsymbol{x}_\ell\|^2) + e^{\theta[3]} \boldsymbol{x}_t^\top \boldsymbol{x}_\ell + e^{\theta[2]} \delta_{r,\ell} \tag{12}$$

The covariance function in (12) is a good kernel for solving the GP-MUD, because it contains a linear and a nonlinear part. The optimal decision surface for MUD is nonlinear, unless the spreading codes are orthogonal to each other, and its deviation from the linear solution depends on how strong the correlations between codes are. In most cases, a linear detector is very close to the optimal decision surface, as spreading codes are almost orthogonal, and only a minor correction is needed to achieve the optimal decision boundary. In this sense the proposed GP covariance function is ideal for the problem. The linear part can mimic the best linear decision boundary and the nonlinear part modifies it, where the linear explanation is not optimal. Also using a radial basis kernel for the nonlinear part is a good choice to achieve nonlinear decisions. Because, the received chips form a constellation of 2^K clouds of points with Gaussian spread around its centres.

Picturing the receiver as a Gaussian Process for regression, instead of a Regularised Least Square functional, allows us to either obtain the hyperparameters by maximizing the likelihood or marginalised them out using Monte Carlo techniques, as explained in [6]. For the

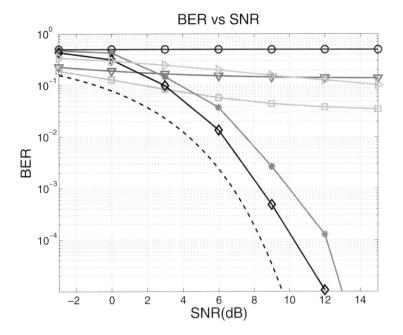

Figure 2: Bit Error Rate versus Signal to Noise ratio for the MF (∇), MMSE-Centralized ($\square$), MMSE-Decentralized ($\circ$), SVM-centralized ($\triangleright$), GP-Centralized ($\diamond$) and GP-Decentralized ($*$) with $k = 8$ users and $n = 30$ training samples. The powers of the interfering users is distributed homogeneously between 0 and 30 dB above that of the UOI.

problem at hand speed is a must and we will be using the maximum likelihood hyperparameters.

We have just shown above how we can make predictions in the nonlinear case (9) using the received symbols from the channel. In an analogy with the MMSE receiver, this will correspond to the decentralized GP-MUD detector as we will not need to know the other users' codes to detect the bits sent to us. It is also relevant to notice that we do not need our spreading code for detection, as the decentralized MMSE detector did. We can also obtain a centralized GP-MUD detector using as input vectors $z_t = H^\top x_t$.

4   Experiments

In this section we include the typical evaluation of the performance in a digital communications system, i.e., Bit Error Rate (BER). The test environment is a synchronous CDMA system in which the users are spread using Gold sequences with spreading factor $L = 31$ and $K = 8$ users, which are typical values in CDMA based mobile communication systems. We consider the same amplitude matrix in all experiments. These amplitudes are random values to achieve an interferer to signal ratio of 30 dB. Hence, the interferers are 30 dB over the UOI. We study the worse scenario and hence we will detect the user which arrives to the receiver with the lowest amplitude.

We compare the performance of the GP centralized and decentralized MUDs to the performance of the MMSE detectors, the Matched Filter detector and the (centralized) SVM-MUD in [4]. The SVM-MUD detector uses a Gaussian kernel and its width is adapted incorporating knowledge of the noise variance in the channel. We found that this setting

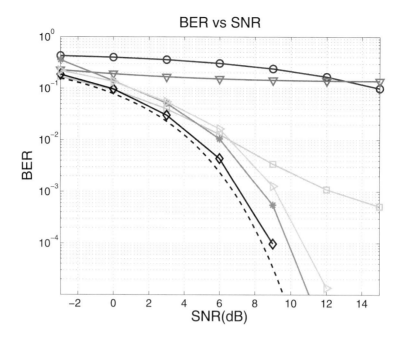

Figure 3: Bit Error Rate versus Signal to Noise ratio for the MF ($\triangledown$), MMSE-Centralized ($\square$), MMSE-Decentralized ($\circ$), SVM-centralized ($\triangleright$), GP-Centralized ($\diamond$) and GP-Decentralized ($*$) with $k = 8$ users and $n = 80$ training samples. The powers of the interfering users is distributed homogeneously between 0 and 30 dB above that of the UOI.

usually does not perform well for this experimental specification and we have set them using validation. We believe this might be due to either the reduced number of users in their experiments (2 or 3) or because they used the same amplitude for all the users, so they did not encounter the near-far problem.

We have included three experiments in which we have defined the number of training experiments equal to 30, 80 and 160. For each training set we have computed the BER for 10^6 bits. The reported results are mean curves for 50 different trials.

The results in Figure 2 show that the detectors based on GPs are able to reduce the probability of error as the signal to noise ratio in the channel decreases with only 30 samples in the training sequence. The GP centralized MUD is only 1.5-2dB worse than the best achievable probability of error, which is obtained in absence of interference (indicated by the dashed line). The GP decentralized MUD reduces the probability of error as the signal to noise increases, but it remains between 3-4dB from the optimal performance. The other detectors are not able to decrease the BER even for a very high signal to noise ratio in the channel. These figures show that the GP based MUD can outperform the other MUD when very short training sequences are available.

Figure 3 highlights that the SVM-MUD (centralized) and the MSSE centralized detectors are able to reduce the BER as the SNR increases, but they are still far from the performance of the GP-MUD. The centralized GP-MUD basically provides optimal performance as it is less than 0.3db from the possible achieved BER when there is no interference in the channel. The decentralized GP-MUD outperforms the other two centralized detectors (SVM and MMSE) since it is able to provide lower BER without needing to know the code of the remaining users.

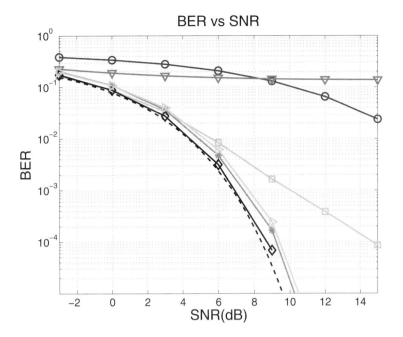

Figure 4: Bit Error Rate versus Signal to Noise ratio for the MF ($\triangledown$), MMSE-Centralized ($\square$), MMSE-Decentralized ($\circ$), SVM-centralized ($\triangleright$), GP-Centralized ($\diamond$) and GP-Decentralized ($*$) with $k = 8$ users and $n = 160$ training samples. The powers of the interfering users is distributed homogeneously between 0 and 30 dB above that of the UOI.

Finally, in Figure 4 we include the results for 160 training samples. In this case, the centralized GP-MUD lies above the optimal BER curve and the decentralized GP-MUD performs as the SVM-MUD detector. The centralized MMSE detector still presents very high probability of error for high signal to noise ratios and we need over 500 samples to obtain a performance similar to the centralized GP with 80 samples. For 160 samples the MMSE decentralized is already able to slightly reduce the bit error rate for very high signal to noise ratios. But to achieve the performance showed by the decentralized GP-MUD it needs several thousands samples.

5   Conclusions and Further Work

We propose a novel approach based on Gaussian Processes for regression to solve the near-far problem in CDMA receivers. Since the optimal solution is known to be nonlinear the Gaussian Processes are able to obtain this nonlinear decision surface with very few training examples. This is the main advantage of this method as it only requires a few tens training examples instead of the few hundreds needed by other nonlinear techniques as SVMs. This will allow its application in real communication systems, as training sequence of 26 samples are typically used in the GSM standard for mobile Telecommunications.

The most relevant result of this paper is the performance shown by the decentralized GP-MUD receiver, since it can be directly used over any CDMA system. The decentralized GP-MUD receiver does not need to know the codes from the other users and does not require the users to be aligned, as the other methods do. While the other receiver will degrade its performance if the users are not aligned, the decentralized GP-MUD receiver will not, providing a more robust solution to the near far problem.

We have presented some preliminary work, which shows that GPs for regression are suitable for the near-far problem in MUD. We have left for further work a more extensive set of experiments changing other parameters of the system such as: the number of users, the length of the spreading code, and the interferences with other users. But still, we believe the reported results are significant since we obtain low bit error rates for training sequences as short as 30 bits.

Acknowledgements

Fernando Pérez-Cruz is Supported by the Spanish Ministry of Education Postdoctoral Fellowships EX2004-0698. This work has been partially funded by research grants TIC2003-02602 and TIC2003-03781 by the Spanish Ministry of Education.

References

[1] G. C. Orsak B. Aazhang, B. P. Paris. Neural networks for multiuser detection in code-division multiple-access communications. *IEEE Transactions on Communications*, 40:1212–1222, 1992.

[2] Antonio Caamaño-Fernandez, Rafael Boloix-Tortosa, Javier Ramos, and Juan J. Murillo-Fuentes. High order statistics in multiuser detection. *IEEE Trans. on Man and Cybernetics C. Accepted for publication*, 2004.

[3] U. Mitra and H. V. Poor. Neural network techniques for adaptive multiuser demodulation. *IEEE Journal Selected Areas on Communications*, 12:14601470, 1994.

[4] L. Hanzo S. Chen, A. K. Samingan. Support vector machine multiuser receiver for DS-CDMA signals in multipath channels. *IEEE Transactions on Neural Network*, 12(3):604–611, December 2001.

[5] S. Verdú. *Multiuser Detection*. Cambridge University Press, 1998.

[6] C. Williams. Prediction with gaussian processes: From linear regression to linear prediction and beyond.

[7] Christopher K. I. Williams and Carl Edward Rasmussen. Gaussian processes for regression. In David S. Touretzky, Michael C. Mozer, and Michael E. Hasselmo, editors, *Proc. Conf. Advances in Neural Information Processing Systems, NIPS*, volume 8. MIT Press, 1995.

Nested sampling for Potts models

Iain Murray
Gatsby Computational Neuroscience Unit
University College London
i.murray@gatsby.ucl.ac.uk

David J.C. MacKay
Cavendish Laboratory
University of Cambridge
mackay@mrao.cam.ac.uk

Zoubin Ghahramani
Gatsby Computational Neuroscience Unit
University College London
zoubin@gatsby.ucl.ac.uk

John Skilling
Maximum Entropy
Data Consultants Ltd.
skilling@eircom.net

Abstract

Nested sampling is a new Monte Carlo method by Skilling [1] intended for general Bayesian computation. Nested sampling provides a robust alternative to annealing-based methods for computing normalizing constants. It can also generate estimates of other quantities such as posterior expectations. The key technical requirement is an ability to draw samples uniformly from the prior subject to a constraint on the likelihood. We provide a demonstration with the Potts model, an undirected graphical model.

1 Introduction

The computation of normalizing constants plays an important role in statistical inference. For example, Bayesian model comparison needs the evidence, or marginal likelihood of a model $\mathcal{M}$

$$\mathcal{Z} = p(\mathcal{D}|\mathcal{M}) = \int p(\mathcal{D}|\theta, \mathcal{M})p(\theta|\mathcal{M})\,\mathrm{d}\theta \equiv \int L(\theta)\pi(\theta)\,\mathrm{d}\theta, \tag{1}$$

where the model has prior π and likelihood L over parameters θ after observing data $\mathcal{D}$. This integral is usually intractable for models of interest. However, given its importance in Bayesian model comparison, many approaches—both sampling-based and deterministic—have been proposed for estimating it.

Often the evidence cannot be obtained using samples drawn from either the prior π, or the posterior $p(\theta|\mathcal{D}, \mathcal{M}) \propto L(\theta)\pi(\theta)$. Practical Monte Carlo methods need to sample from a sequence of distributions, possibly at different "temperatures" $p(\theta|\beta) \propto L(\theta)^\beta \pi(\theta)$ (see Gelman and Meng [2] for a review). These methods are sometimes cited as a gold standard for comparison with other approximate techniques, e.g. Beal and Ghahramani [3]. However, care is required in choosing intermediate distributions; appropriate temperature-based distributions may be difficult or impossible to find. Nested sampling provides an alternate standard, which makes no use of temperature and does not require tuning of intermediate distributions or other large sets of parameters.

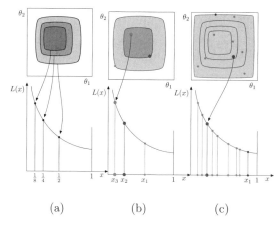

Figure 1: (a) Elements of parameter space (top) are sorted by likelihood and arranged on the x-axis. An eighth of the prior mass is inside the innermost likelihood contour in this figure. (b) Point x_i is drawn from the prior inside the likelihood contour defined by x_{i-1}. L_i is identified and $p(\{x_i\})$ is known, but exact values of x_i are not known. (c) With N particles, the least likely one sets the likelihood contour and is replaced by a new point inside the contour ($\{L_i\}$ and $p(\{x_i\})$ are still known).

(a) (b) (c)

Nested sampling uses a natural definition of $\mathcal{Z}$, a sum over prior mass. The weighted sum over likelihood elements is expressed as the area under a monotonic one-dimensional curve "L vs x" (figure 1(a)), where:

$$\mathcal{Z} = \int L(\theta)\pi(\theta) \ \mathrm{d}\theta = \int_0^1 L(\theta(x)) \ \mathrm{d}x. \tag{2}$$

This is a change of variables $\mathrm{d}x(\theta) = \pi(\theta)\mathrm{d}\theta$, where each volume element of the prior in the original θ-vector space is mapped onto a scalar element on the one-dimensional x-axis. The ordering of the elements on the x-axis is chosen to sort the prior mass in decreasing order of likelihood values ($x_1 < x_2 \Rightarrow L(\theta(x_1)) > L(\theta(x_2))$). See appendix A for dealing with elements with identical likelihoods.

Given some points $\{(x_i, L_i)\}_{i=1}^I$ ordered such that $x_i > x_{i+1}$, the area under the curve (2) is easily approximated. We denote by $\hat{\mathcal{Z}}$ estimates obtained using a trapezoidal rule. Rectangle rules upper and lower bound the error $\hat{\mathcal{Z}} - \mathcal{Z}$.

Points with known x-coordinates are unavailable in general. Instead we generate points, $\{\theta_i\}$, such that the *distribution* $p(\mathbf{x})$ is known (where $\mathbf{x} \equiv \{x_i\}$), and find their associated $\{L_i\}$. A simple algorithm to draw I points is algorithm 1, see also figure 1(b).

Algorithm 1	**Algorithm 2**
Initial point: draw $\theta_1 \sim \pi(\theta)$.	**Initialize:** draw N points $\theta^{(n)} \sim \pi(\theta)$
for i = 2 to I: draw $\theta_i \sim \breve{\pi}(\theta\|L(\theta_{i-1}))$,	**for i = 2 to I:**
where	

$$\breve{\pi}(\theta|L(\theta_{i-1})) \propto \begin{cases} \pi(\theta) & L(\theta) > L(\theta_{i-1}) \\ 0 & \text{otherwise.} \end{cases} \tag{3}$$

- $m = \mathrm{argmin}_n L(\theta^{(n)})$
- $\theta_{i-1} = \theta^{(m)}$
- draw $\theta_m \sim \breve{\pi}(\theta|L(\theta_{i-1}))$, given by equation (3)

We know $p(x_1) = \mathrm{Uniform}(0, 1)$, because x is a cumulative sum of prior mass. Similarly $p(x_i|x_{i-1}) = \mathrm{Uniform}(0, x_{i-1})$, as every point is drawn from the prior subject to $L(\theta_i) > L(\theta_{i-1}) \Rightarrow x_i < x_{i-1}$. This recursive relation allows us to compute $p(\mathbf{x})$.

A simple generalization, algorithm 2, uses multiple θ particles; at each step the least likely is replaced with a draw from a constrained prior (figure 1(c)). Now $p(x_1|N) = Nx_1^{N-1}$ and subsequent points have $p(x_i/x_{i-1}|x_{i-1}, N) = N(x_i/x_{i-1})^{N-1}$. This

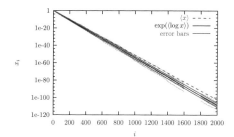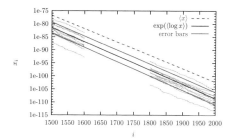

Figure 2: The arithmetic and geometric means of x_i against iteration number, i, for algorithm 2 with $N = 8$. Error bars on the geometric mean show $\exp(-i/N \pm \sqrt{i}/N)$. Samples of $p(\mathbf{x}|N)$ are superimposed ($i = 1600 \ldots 1800$ omitted for clarity).

distribution over $\mathbf{x}$ combined with observations $\{L_i\}$ gives a distribution over $\hat{\mathcal{Z}}$:

$$p(\hat{\mathcal{Z}}|\{L_i\}, N) \approx \int \delta(\hat{\mathcal{Z}}(\mathbf{x}) - \hat{\mathcal{Z}})p(\mathbf{x}|N)\,\mathrm{d}\mathbf{x}. \qquad (4)$$

Samples from the posterior over θ are also available, see Skilling [1] for details.

Nested sampling was introduced by Skilling [1]. The key idea is that samples from the prior, subject to a nested sequence of constraints (3), give a probabilistic realization of the curve, figure 1(a). Related work can be found in McDonald and Singer [4]. Explanatory notes and some code are available online[1]. In this paper we present some new discussion of important issues regarding the practical implementation of nested sampling and provide the first application to a challenging problem. This leads to the first cluster-based method for Potts models with first-order phase transitions of which we are aware.

2 Implementation issues

2.1 MCMC approximations

The nested sampling algorithm assumes obtaining samples from $\breve{\pi}(\theta|L(\theta_{i-1}))$, equation (3), is possible. Rejection sampling using π would slow down exponentially with iteration number i. We explore approximate sampling from $\breve{\pi}$ using Markov chain Monte Carlo (MCMC) methods.

In high-dimensional problems it is likely that the majority of $\breve{\pi}$'s mass is typically in a thin shell at the contour surface [5, p37]. This suggests finding efficient chains that sample at constant likelihood, a *microcanonical* distribution. In order to complete an ergodic MCMC method, we also need transition operators that can alter the likelihood (within the constraint). A simple Metropolis method may suffice.

We must initialize the Markov chain for each new sample somewhere. One possibility is to start at the position of the deleted point, θ_{i-1}, on the contour constraint, which is independent of the other points and not far from the bulk of the required uniform distribution. However, if the Markov chain mixes slowly amongst modes, the new point starting at θ_{i-1} may be trapped in an insignificant mode. In this case it would be better to start at one of the other $N-1$ existing points inside the contour constraint. They are all draws from the correct distribution, $\breve{\pi}(\theta|L(\theta_{i-1}))$, so represent modes fairly. However, this method may also require many Markov chain steps, this time to make the new point effectively independent of the point it cloned.

---

[1]http://www.inference.phy.cam.ac.uk/bayesys/

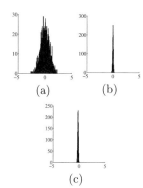

(a)   (b)

(c)

Figure 3: Histograms of errors in the point estimate $\log(\tilde{\mathcal{Z}})$ over 1000 random experiments for different approximations. The test system was a 40-dimensional hypercube of length 100 with uniform prior centered on the origin. The log-likelihood was $L = -\theta^\top\theta/2$. Nested sampling used $N = 10$, $I = 2000$. (a) Monte Carlo estimation (equation (5)) using $S = 12$ sampled trajectories (b) $S = 1200$ sampled trajectories. (c) Deterministic approximation using the geometric mean trajectory. In this example perfect integration over $p(\mathbf{x}|N)$ gives a distribution of width ≈ 3 over $\log(\hat{\mathcal{Z}})$. Therefore, improvements over (c) for approximating equation (5) are unwarranted.

2.2 Integrating out x

To estimate quantities of interest, we average over $p(\mathbf{x}|N)$, as in equation (4). The mean of a distribution over $\log(\hat{\mathcal{Z}})$ can be found by simple Monte Carlo estimation:

$$\log(\mathcal{Z}) \approx \int \log(\hat{\mathcal{Z}}(\mathbf{x}))p(\mathbf{x}|N)\,\mathrm{d}\mathbf{x} \approx \frac{1}{S}\sum_{s=1}^{S}\log(\hat{\mathcal{Z}}(\mathbf{x}^{(s)})) \qquad \mathbf{x}^{(s)} \sim p(\mathbf{x}|N). \quad (5)$$

This scheme is easily implemented for any expectation under $p(\mathbf{x}|N)$, including error bars from the variance of $\log(\hat{\mathcal{Z}})$. To reduce noise in comparisons between runs it is advisable to reuse the same samples from $p(\mathbf{x}|N)$ (e.g. clamp the seed used to generate them).

A simple deterministic approximation is useful for understanding, and also provides fast to compute, low variance estimators. Figure 2 shows sampled trajectories of x_i as the algorithm progresses. The geometric mean path, $x_i \approx \exp(\int p(x_i|N)\log x_i\,\mathrm{d}x_i) = e^{-i/N}$, follows the path of typical settings of $\mathbf{x}$. Using this single $\mathbf{x}$ setting is a reasonable and very cheap alternative to averaging over settings (equation 5); see figure 3.

Typically the trapezoidal estimate of the integral, $\hat{\mathcal{Z}}$, is dominated by a small number of trapezoids, around iteration i^* say. Considering uncertainty on just $\log x_{i^*} = -i^*/N \pm \sqrt{i^*}/N$ provides reasonable and convenient error bars.

3   Potts Models

The Potts model, an undirected graphical model, defines a probability distribution over discrete variables $\mathbf{s} = (s_1, \ldots, s_n)$, each taking on one of q distinct "colors":

$$P(\mathbf{s}|J,q) = \frac{1}{\mathcal{Z}_\mathrm{P}(J,q)}\exp\left(\sum_{(ij)\in\mathcal{E}}J(\delta_{s_i s_j} - 1)\right). \quad (6)$$

The variables exist as nodes on a graph where $(ij) \in \mathcal{E}$ means that nodes i and j are linked by an edge. The Kronecker delta, $\delta_{s_i s_j}$ is one when s_i and s_j are the same color and zero otherwise. Neighboring nodes pay an "energy penalty" of J when they are different colors. Here we assume identical positive couplings $J > 0$ on each edge (section 4 discusses the extension to different J_{ij}). The Ising model and Boltzmann machine are both special cases of the Potts model with $q=2$.

Our goal is to compute the normalization constant $\mathcal{Z}_\mathrm{P}(J,q)$, where the discrete variables $\mathbf{s}$ are the θ variables that need to be integrated (i.e. summed) over.

3.1 Swendsen–Wang sampling

We will take advantage of the "Fortuin-Kasteleyn-Swendsen-Wang" (FKSW) joint distribution identified explicitly in Edwards and Sokal [6] over color variables $\mathbf{s}$ and a bond variable for each edge in $\mathcal{E}$, $d_{ij} \in \{0, 1\}$:

$$P(\mathbf{s}, \mathbf{d}) = \frac{1}{\mathcal{Z}_P(J, q)} \prod_{(ij) \in \mathcal{E}} \left[(1 - p)\delta_{d_{ij}, 0} + p\delta_{d_{ij}, 1}\delta_{s_i, s_j} \right], \qquad p \equiv (1 - e^{-J}). \quad (7)$$

The marginal distribution over $\mathbf{s}$ in the FKSW model is the Potts distribution, equation (6). The marginal distribution over the bonds is the random cluster model of Fortuin and Kasteleyn [7]:

$$P(\mathbf{d}) = \frac{1}{\mathcal{Z}_P(J, q)} p^D (1 - p)^{|\mathcal{E}| - D} q^{C(\mathbf{d})} = \frac{1}{\mathcal{Z}_P(J, q)} \exp(D \log(e^J - 1)) e^{-J|\mathcal{E}|} q^{C(\mathbf{d})}, \quad (8)$$

where $C(\mathbf{d})$ is the number of connected components in a graph with edges wherever $d_{ij} = 1$, and $D = \sum_{(ij) \in \mathcal{E}} d_{ij}$. As the partition functions of equations 6, 7 and 8 are identical, we should consider using any of these distributions to compute $\mathcal{Z}_P(J, q)$. The algorithm of Swendsen and Wang [8] performs block Gibbs sampling on the joint model by alternately sampling from $P(d_{ij}|\mathbf{s})$ and $P(\mathbf{s}|d_{ij})$. This can convert a sample from any of the three distributions into a sample from one of the others.

3.2 Nested Sampling

A simple approximate nested sampler uses a fixed number of Gibbs sampling updates of $\breve{\pi}$. Cluster-based updates are also desirable in these models. Focusing on the random cluster model, we rewrite equation (8):

$$P(\mathbf{d}) = \frac{1}{\mathcal{Z}_N} L(\mathbf{d}) \pi(\mathbf{d}) \quad \text{where} \quad (9)$$

$$\mathcal{Z}_N = \frac{\mathcal{Z}_P(J, q)}{\mathcal{Z}_\pi} \exp(J|\mathcal{E}|), \quad L(\mathbf{d}) = \exp(D \log(e^J - 1)), \quad \pi(\mathbf{d}) = \frac{1}{\mathcal{Z}_\pi} q^{C(\mathbf{d})}.$$

Likelihood thresholds are thresholds on the total number of bonds D. Many states have identical D, which requires careful treatment, see appendix A. Nested sampling on this system will give the ratio of $\mathcal{Z}_P/\mathcal{Z}_\pi$. The prior normalization, $\mathcal{Z}_\pi$, can be found from the partition function of a Potts system at $J = \log(2)$.

The following steps give two MCMC operators to change the bonds $\mathbf{d} \to \mathbf{d}'$:

1. Create a random coloring, $\mathbf{s}$, uniformly from the $q^{C(\mathbf{d})}$ colorings satisfying the bond constraints $\mathbf{d}$, as in the Swendsen–Wang algorithm.
2. Count sites that allow bonds, $E = \sum_{(ij) \in \mathcal{E}} \delta_{s_i, s_j}$.
3. Either, operator 1: record the number of bonds $D' = \sum_{(ij) \in \mathcal{E}} d_{ij}$
   Or, operator 2: draw D' from $Q(D'|E(\mathbf{s})) \propto \binom{E(\mathbf{s})}{D'}$.
4. Throw away the old bonds, $\mathbf{d}$, and pick uniformly from one of the $\binom{E(\mathbf{s})}{D'}$ ways of setting D' bonds in the E available sites.

The probability of proposing a particular coloring and new setting of the bonds is

$$Q(\mathbf{s}, \mathbf{d}'|\mathbf{d}) = Q(\mathbf{d}'|\mathbf{s}, D') Q(D'|E(\mathbf{s})) Q(\mathbf{s}|\mathbf{d}) = \frac{1}{\binom{E(\mathbf{s})}{D'}} Q(D'|E(\mathbf{s})) \frac{1}{q^{C(\mathbf{d})}}. \quad (10)$$

Summing over colorings, the correct Metropolis-Hastings acceptance ratio is:

$$a = \frac{\pi(\mathbf{d}')}{\pi(\mathbf{d})} \cdot \frac{\sum_{\mathbf{s}} Q(\mathbf{s}, \mathbf{d}|\mathbf{d}')}{\sum_{\mathbf{s}} Q(\mathbf{s}, \mathbf{d}'|\mathbf{d})} = \frac{q^{C(\mathbf{d}')}}{q^{C(\mathbf{d})}} \cdot \frac{q^{C(\mathbf{d})}}{q^{C(\mathbf{d}')}} \frac{\sum_{\mathbf{s}} Q(D|\mathbf{s})/\binom{E(\mathbf{s})}{D}}{\sum_{\mathbf{s}} Q(D'|\mathbf{s})/\binom{E(\mathbf{s})}{D'}} = 1, \quad (11)$$

Table 1: Partition function results for 16×16 Potts systems (see text for details).

Method	$q = 2$ (Ising), $J = 1$	$q = 10$, $J = 1.477$
Gibbs AIS	7.1 ± 1.1	(1.5)
Swendsen–Wang AIS	7.4 ± 0.1	(1.2)
Gibbs nested sampling	7.1 ± 1.0	12.2 ± 2.4
Random-cluster nested sampling	7.1 ± 0.7	14.1 ± 1.8
Acceptance ratio	7.3	11.2

regardless of the choice in step 3. The simple first choice solves the difficult problem of navigating at constant D. The second choice defines an ergodic chain[2].

4 Results

Table 1 shows results on two example systems: an Ising model, $q = 1$, and a $q = 10$ Potts model in an difficult parameter regime. We tested nested samplers using Gibbs sampling and the cluster-based algorithm, annealed importance sampling (AIS) [9] using both Gibbs sampling and Swendsen–Wang cluster updates. We also developed an acceptance ratio method [10] based on our representation in equation (9), which we ran extensively and should give nearly correct results.

Annealed importance sampling (AIS) was run 100 times, with a geometric spacing of 10^4 settings of J as the annealing schedule. Nested sampling used $N = 100$ particles and 100 full-system MCMC updates to approximate each draw from $\check{\pi}$. Each Markov chain was initialized at one of the $N{-}1$ particles satisfying the current constraint. In trials using the other alternative (section 2.1) the Gibbs nested sampler could get stuck permanently in a local maximum of the likelihood, while the cluster method gave erroneous answers for the Ising system.

AIS performed very well on the Ising system. We took advantage of its performance in easy parameter regimes to compute $\mathcal{Z}_\pi$ for use in the cluster-based nested sampler. However, with a "temperature-based" annealing schedule, AIS was unable to give useful answers for the $q = 10$ system. While nested sampling appears to be correct within its error bars.

It is known that even the efficient Swendsen–Wang algorithm mixes slowly for Potts models with $q > 4$ near critical values of J [11], see figure 4. Typical Potts model states are either entirely disordered or ordered; disordered states contain a jumble of small regions with different colors (e.g. figure 4(b)), in ordered states the system is predominantly one color (e.g. figure 4(d)). Moving between these two phases is difficult; defining a valid MCMC method that moves between distinct phases requires knowledge of the relative probability of the whole collections of states in those phases.

Temperature-based annealing algorithms explore the model for a range of settings of J and fail to capture the correct behavior near the transition. Despite using closely related Markov chains to those used in AIS, nested sampling can work in all parameter regimes. Figure 4(e) shows how nested sampling can explore a mixture of ordered and disordered phases. By moving steadily through these states, nested sampling is able to estimate the prior mass associated with each likelihood value.

---

[2]Proof: with finite probability all s_i are given the same color, then any allowable D' is possible, in turn all allowable $\mathbf{d}'$ have finite probability.

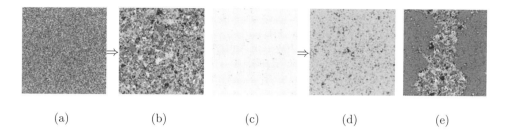

| (a) | (b) | (c) | (d) | (e) |

Figure 4: Two 256×256, $q = 10$ Potts models with starting states (a) and (c) were simulated with 5×10^6 full-system Swendsen–Wang updates with $J = 1.42577$. The corresponding results, (b) and (d) are typical of all the intermediate samples: Swendsen–Wang is unable to take (a) into an ordered phase, or (c) into a disordered phase, although both phases are typical at this J. (e) in contrast shows an intermediate state of nested sampling, which succeeds in bridging the phases.

This behaviour is not possible in algorithms that use J as a control parameter.

The potentials on every edge of the Potts model in this paper were the same. Much of the formalism above generalizes to allow different edge weights J_{ij} on each edge, and non-zero biases on each variable. Indeed Edwards and Sokal [6] gave a general procedure for constructing such auxiliary-variable joint distributions. This generalization would make the model more relevant to MRFs used in other fields (e.g. computer vision). The challenge for nested sampling remains the invention of effective sampling schemes that keep a system at or near constant energy. Generalizing step 4 in section 3.2 would be the difficult step.

Other temperatureless Monte Carlo methods exist, e.g. Berg and Neuhaus [12] study the Potts model using the *multicanonical ensemble*. Nested sampling has some unique properties compared to the established method. Formally it has only one free parameter, N the number of particles. Unless problems with multiple modes demand otherwise, $N = 1$ often reveals useful information, and if the error bars on $\mathcal{Z}$ are too large further runs with larger N may be performed.

5   Conclusions

We have applied nested sampling to compute the normalizing constant of a system that is challenging for many Monte Carlo methods.

- Nested sampling's key technical requirement, an ability to draw samples uniformly from a constrained prior, is largely solved by efficient MCMC methods.

- No complex schedules are required; steady progress towards compact regions of large likelihood is controlled by a single free parameter, N, the number of particles.

- Multiple particles, a built-in feature of this algorithm, are often necessary to obtain accurate results.

- Nested sampling has no special difficulties on systems with first order phase-transitions, whereas all temperature-based methods fail.

We believe that nested sampling's unique properties will be found useful in a variety of statistical applications.

A Degenerate likelihoods

The description in section 1 assumed that the likelihood function provides a total ordering of elements of the parameter space. However, distinct elements dx and dx' could have the same likelihood, either because the parameters are discrete, or because the likelihood is degenerate.

One way to break degeneracies is through a joint model with variables of interest θ and an independent variable $m \in [0, 1]$:

$$P(\theta, m) = P(\theta) \cdot P(m) = \frac{1}{\mathcal{Z}} L(\theta)\pi(\theta) \cdot \frac{1}{\mathcal{Z}_m} L(m)\pi(m) \tag{12}$$

where $L(m) = 1 + \epsilon(m - 0.5)$, $\pi(m) = 1$ and $\mathcal{Z}_m = 1$. We choose ϵ such that $\log(\epsilon)$ is smaller than the smallest difference in $\log(L(\theta))$ allowed by machine precision. Standard nested sampling is now possible. Assuming we have a likelihood constraint L_i, we need to be able to draw from

$$P(\theta', m' | \theta, m, L_i) \propto \begin{cases} \pi(\theta')\pi(m') & L(\theta')L(m') > L_i, \\ 0 & \text{otherwise.} \end{cases} \tag{13}$$

The additional variable can be ignored except for $L(\theta') = L(\theta_i)$, then only $m' > m$ are possible. Therefore, the probability of states with likelihood $L(\theta_i)$ are weighted by $(1 - m')$.

References

[1] John Skilling. Nested sampling. In R. Fischer, R. Preuss, and U. von Toussaint, editors, *Bayesian inference and maximum entropy methods in science and engineering*, AIP Conference Proceedings 735, pages 395–405, 2004.

[2] Andrew Gelman and Xiao-Li Meng. Simulating normalizing constants: from importance sampling to bridge sampling to path sampling. *Statist. Sci.*, 13(2):163–185, 1998.

[3] Matthew J. Beal and Zoubin Ghahramani. The variational Bayesian EM algorithm for incomplete data: with application to scoring graphical model structures. *Bayesian Statistics*, 7:453–464, 2003.

[4] I. R. McDonald and K. Singer. Machine calculation of thermodynamic properties of a simple fluid at supercritical temperatures. *J. Chem. Phys.*, 47(11):4766–4772, 1967.

[5] David J.C. MacKay. *Information Theory, Inference, and Learning Algorithms*. CUP, 2003. www.inference.phy.cam.ac.uk/mackay/itila/.

[6] Robert G. Edwards and Alan D. Sokal. Generalization of the Fortuin-Kasteleyn-Swendsen-Wang representation and Monte Carlo algorithm. *Phys.Rev. D*, 38(6), 1988.

[7] C. M. Fortuin and P. W. Kasteleyn. On the random-cluster model. I. Introduction and relation to other models. *Physica*, 57:536–564, 1972.

[8] R. H. Swendsen and J. S. Wang. Nonuniversal critical dynamics in Monte Carlo simulations. *Phys. Rev. Lett.*, 58(2):86–88, January 1987.

[9] Radford M. Neal. Annealed importance sampling. *Statistics and Computing*, 11: 125–139, 2001.

[10] Charles H. Bennett. Efficient estimation of free energy differences from Monte Carlo data. *Journal of Computational Physics*, 22(2):245–268, October 1976.

[11] Vivek K. Gore and Mark R. Jerrum. The Swendsen-Wang process does not always mix rapidly. In *29th ACM Symposium on Theory of Computing*, pages 674–681, 1997.

[12] Bernd A. Berg and Thomas Neuhaus. Multicanonical ensemble: A new approach to simulate first-order phase transitions. *Phys. Rev. Lett.*, 68(1):9–12, January 1992.

Diffusion Maps, Spectral Clustering and Eigenfunctions of Fokker-Planck Operators

Boaz Nadler*   **Stéphane Lafon**   **Ronald R. Coifman**
Department of Mathematics, Yale University, New Haven, CT 06520.
{boaz.nadler,stephane.lafon,ronald.coifman}@yale.edu

Ioannis G. Kevrekidis
Department of Chemical Engineering and Program in Applied Mathematics
Princeton University, Princeton, NJ 08544
yannis@princeton.edu

Abstract

This paper presents a diffusion based probabilistic interpretation of spectral clustering and dimensionality reduction algorithms that use the eigenvectors of the normalized graph Laplacian. Given the pairwise adjacency matrix of all points, we define a diffusion distance between any two data points and show that the low dimensional representation of the data by the first few eigenvectors of the corresponding Markov matrix is optimal under a certain mean squared error criterion. Furthermore, assuming that data points are random samples from a density $p(\boldsymbol{x}) = e^{-U(\boldsymbol{x})}$ we identify these eigenvectors as discrete approximations of eigenfunctions of a Fokker-Planck operator in a potential $2U(\boldsymbol{x})$ with reflecting boundary conditions. Finally, applying known results regarding the eigenvalues and eigenfunctions of the continuous Fokker-Planck operator, we provide a mathematical justification for the success of spectral clustering and dimensional reduction algorithms based on these first few eigenvectors. This analysis elucidates, in terms of the characteristics of diffusion processes, many empirical findings regarding spectral clustering algorithms.

Keywords: Algorithms and architectures, learning theory.

1 Introduction

Clustering and low dimensional representation of high dimensional data are important problems in many diverse fields. In recent years various spectral methods to perform these tasks, based on the eigenvectors of adjacency matrices of graphs on the data have been developed, see for example [1]-[10] and references therein. In the simplest version, known as the normalized graph Laplacian, given n data points $\{\boldsymbol{x}_i\}_{i=1}^n$ where each $\boldsymbol{x}_i \in \mathbb{R}^p$, we define a pairwise similarity matrix between points, for example using a Gaussian kernel

---

*Corresponding author. Currently at Weizmann Institute of Science, Rehovot, Israel.
http://www.wisdom.weizmann.ac.il/~nadler

with width ε,

$$L_{i,j} = k(\boldsymbol{x}_i, \boldsymbol{x}_j) = \exp\left(-\frac{\|\boldsymbol{x}_i - \boldsymbol{x}_j\|^2}{2\varepsilon}\right) \tag{1}$$

and a diagonal normalization matrix $D_{i,i} = \sum_j L_{i,j}$. Many works propose to use the first few eigenvectors of the normalized eigenvalue problem $L\phi = \lambda D\phi$, or equivalently of the matrix $M = D^{-1}L$, either as a low dimensional representation of data or as good coordinates for clustering purposes. Although eq. (1) is based on a Gaussian kernel, other kernels are possible. While for actual datasets the choice of a kernel $k(\boldsymbol{x}_i, \boldsymbol{x}_j)$ is crucial, it does not qualitatively change our asymptotic analysis [11].

The use of the first few eigenvectors of M as good coordinates is typically justified with heuristic arguments or as a relaxation of a discrete clustering problem [3]. In [4, 5] Belkin and Niyogi showed that when data is uniformly sampled from a low dimensional manifold of $\mathbb{R}^p$ the first few eigenvectors of M are discrete approximations of the eigenfunctions of the Laplace-Beltrami operator on the manifold, thus providing a mathematical justification for their use in this case. A different theoretical analysis of the eigenvectors of the matrix M, based on the fact that M is a stochastic matrix representing a random walk on the graph was described by Meilă and Shi [12], who considered the case of piecewise constant eigenvectors for specific lumpable matrix structures. Additional notable works that considered the random walk aspects of spectral clustering are [8, 13], where the authors suggest clustering based on the average commute time between points, and [14] which considered the relaxation process of this random walk.

In this paper we provide a unified probabilistic framework which combines these results and extends them in two different directions. First, in section 2 we define a distance function between any two points based on the random walk on the graph, which we naturally denote the *diffusion distance*. We then show that the low dimensional description of the data by the first few eigenvectors, denoted as the *diffusion map*, is optimal under a mean squared error criterion based on this distance. In section 3 we consider a statistical model, in which data points are iid random samples from a probability density $p(\boldsymbol{x})$ in a smooth bounded domain $\Omega \subset \mathbb{R}^p$ and analyze the asymptotics of the eigenvectors as the number of data points tends to infinity. This analysis shows that the eigenvectors of the finite matrix M are discrete approximations of the eigenfunctions of a Fokker-Planck (FP) operator with reflecting boundary conditions. This observation, coupled with known results regarding the eigenvalues and eigenfunctions of the FP operator provide new insights into the properties of these eigenvectors and on the performance of spectral clustering algorithms, as described in section 4.

2 Diffusion Distances and Diffusion Maps

The starting point of our analysis, as also noted in other works, is the observation that the matrix M is adjoint to a symmetric matrix

$$M_s = D^{1/2}MD^{-1/2}. \tag{2}$$

Thus, M and M_s share the same eigenvalues. Moreover, since M_s is symmetric it is diagonalizable and has a set of n real eigenvalues $\{\lambda_j\}_{j=0}^{n-1}$ whose corresponding eigenvectors $\{\boldsymbol{v}_j\}$ form an orthonormal basis of $\mathbb{R}^n$. The left and right eigenvectors of M, denoted ϕ_j and ψ_j are related to those of M_s according to

$$\phi_j = \boldsymbol{v}_j D^{1/2}, \qquad \psi_j = \boldsymbol{v}_j D^{-1/2} \tag{3}$$

Since the eigenvectors $\boldsymbol{v}_j$ are orthonormal under the standard dot product in $\mathbb{R}^n$, it follows that the vectors ϕ_j and ψ_k are bi-orthonormal

$$\langle \phi_i, \psi_j \rangle = \delta_{i,j} \tag{4}$$

where $\langle \boldsymbol{u}, \boldsymbol{v} \rangle$ is the standard dot product between two vectors in $\mathbb{R}^n$. We now utilize the fact that by construction M is a stochastic matrix with all row sums equal to one, and can thus be interpreted as defining a random walk on the graph. Under this view, $M_{i,j}$ denotes the transition probability from the point $\boldsymbol{x}_i$ to the point $\boldsymbol{x}_j$ in one time step. Furthermore, based on the similarity of the Gaussian kernel (1) to the fundamental solution of the heat equation, we define our time step as $\Delta t = \varepsilon$. Therefore,

$$\Pr\{\boldsymbol{x}(t + \varepsilon) = \boldsymbol{x}_j \,|\, \boldsymbol{x}(t) = \boldsymbol{x}_i\} = M_{i,j} \tag{5}$$

Note that ε has therefore a *dual* interpretation in this framework. The first is that ε is the (squared) radius of the neighborhood used to infer local geometric and density information for the construction of the adjacency matrix, while the second is that ε is the discrete time step at which the random walk jumps from point to point.

We denote by $p(t, \boldsymbol{y}|\boldsymbol{x})$ the probability distribution of a random walk landing at location $\boldsymbol{y}$ at time t, given a starting location $\boldsymbol{x}$ at time $t = 0$. For $t = k\,\varepsilon$, $p(t, \boldsymbol{y}|\boldsymbol{x}_i) = \boldsymbol{e}_i M^k$, where $\boldsymbol{e}_i$ is a row vector of zeros with a single one at the i-th coordinate. For ε large enough, all points in the graph are connected so that M has a unique eigenvalue equal to 1. The other eigenvalues form a non-increasing sequence of non-negative numbers: $\lambda_0 = 1 > \lambda_1 \geq \lambda_2 \geq \ldots \geq \lambda_{n-1} \geq 0$. Then, regardless of the initial starting point $\boldsymbol{x}$,

$$\lim_{t \to \infty} p(t, \boldsymbol{y}|\boldsymbol{x}) = \phi_0(\boldsymbol{y}) \tag{6}$$

where ϕ_0 is the left eigenvector of M with eigenvalue $\lambda_0 = 1$, explicitly given by

$$\phi_0(\boldsymbol{x}_i) = \frac{D_{i,i}}{\sum_j D_{j,j}} \tag{7}$$

This eigenvector also has a dual interpretation. The first is that ϕ_0 is the stationary probability distribution on the graph, while the second is that $\phi_0(\boldsymbol{x})$ is a density estimate at the point $\boldsymbol{x}$. Note that for a general shift invariant kernel $K(\boldsymbol{x} - \boldsymbol{y})$ and for the Gaussian kernel in particular, ϕ_0 is simply the well known Parzen window density estimator.

For any finite time t, we decompose the probability distribution in the eigenbasis $\{\phi_j\}$

$$p(t, \boldsymbol{y}|\boldsymbol{x}) = \phi_0(\boldsymbol{y}) + \sum_{j \geq 1} a_j(\boldsymbol{x}) \lambda_j^t \phi_j(\boldsymbol{y}) \tag{8}$$

where the coefficients a_j depend on the initial location $\boldsymbol{x}$. Using the bi-orthonormality condition (4) gives $a_j(\boldsymbol{x}) = \psi_j(\boldsymbol{x})$, with $a_0(\boldsymbol{x}) = \psi_0(\boldsymbol{x}) = 1$ already implicit in (8).

Given the definition of the random walk on the graph it is only natural to quantify the similarity between any two points according to the evolution of their probability distributions. Specifically, we consider the following distance measure at time t,

$$
\begin{aligned}
D_t^2(\boldsymbol{x}_0, \boldsymbol{x}_1) &= \|p(t, \boldsymbol{y}|\boldsymbol{x}_0) - p(t, \boldsymbol{y}|\boldsymbol{x}_1)\|_w^2 \\
&= \sum_{\boldsymbol{y}} (p(t, \boldsymbol{y}|\boldsymbol{x}_0) - p(t, \boldsymbol{y}|\boldsymbol{x}_1))^2 w(\boldsymbol{y})
\end{aligned}
\tag{9}
$$

with the specific choice $w(\boldsymbol{y}) = 1/\phi_0(\boldsymbol{y})$ for the weight function, which takes into account the (empirical) local density of the points.

Since this distance depends on the random walk on the graph, we quite naturally denote it as the *diffusion distance* at time t. We also denote the mapping between the original space and the first k eigenvectors as the *diffusion map*

$$\Psi_t(\boldsymbol{x}) = \left(\lambda_1^t \psi_1(\boldsymbol{x}), \lambda_2^t \psi_2(\boldsymbol{x}), \ldots, \lambda_k^t \psi_k(\boldsymbol{x})\right) \tag{10}$$

The following theorem relates the diffusion distance and the diffusion map.

Theorem: The diffusion distance (9) is equal to Euclidean distance in the diffusion map space with all $(n-1)$ eigenvectors.

$$D_t^2(\boldsymbol{x}_0, \boldsymbol{x}_1) = \sum_{j \geq 1} \lambda_j^{2t} \left(\psi_j(\boldsymbol{x}_0) - \psi_j(\boldsymbol{x}_1) \right)^2 = \| \Psi_t(\boldsymbol{x}_0) - \Psi_t(\boldsymbol{x}_1) \|^2 \qquad (11)$$

Proof: Combining (8) and (9) gives

$$D_t^2(\boldsymbol{x}_0, \boldsymbol{x}_1) = \sum_{\boldsymbol{y}} \left(\sum_j \lambda_j^t (\psi_j(\boldsymbol{x}_0) - \psi_j(\boldsymbol{x}_1)) \phi_j(\boldsymbol{y}) \right)^2 1/\phi_0(\boldsymbol{y}) \qquad (12)$$

Expanding the brackets, exchanging the order of summation and using relations (3) and (4) between ϕ_j and ψ_j yields the required result. Note that the weight factor $1/\phi_0$ is essential for the theorem to hold. $\qquad \square$.

This theorem provides a justification for using Euclidean distance in the diffusion map space for spectral clustering purposes. Therefore, geometry in diffusion space is meaningful and can be interpreted in terms of the Markov chain. In particular, as shown in [18], quantizing this diffusion space is equivalent to lumping the random walk. Moreover, since in many practical applications the spectrum of the matrix M has a *spectral gap* with only a few eigenvalues close to one and all additional eigenvalues much smaller than one, the diffusion distance at a large enough time t can be well approximated by only the first few k eigenvectors $\psi_1(\boldsymbol{x}), \ldots, \psi_k(\boldsymbol{x})$, with a negligible error of the order of $O((\lambda_{k+1}/\lambda_k)^t)$. This observation provides a theoretical justification for dimensional reduction with these eigenvectors. In addition, the following theorem shows that this k-dimensional approximation is *optimal* under a certain mean squared error criterion.

Theorem: Out of all k-dimensional approximations of the form

$$\hat{p}(t, \boldsymbol{y}|\boldsymbol{x}) = \phi_0(\boldsymbol{y}) + \sum_{j=1}^{k} a_j(t, \boldsymbol{x}) \boldsymbol{w}_j(\boldsymbol{y})$$

for the probability distribution at time t, the one that minimizes the mean squared error

$$\mathbb{E}_{\boldsymbol{x}} \{ \| p(t, \boldsymbol{y}|\boldsymbol{x}) - \hat{p}(t, \boldsymbol{y}|\boldsymbol{x}) \|_w^2 \}$$

where averaging over initial points $\boldsymbol{x}$ is with respect to the stationary density $\phi_0(\boldsymbol{x})$, is given by $\boldsymbol{w}_j(\boldsymbol{y}) = \phi_j(\boldsymbol{y})$ and $a_j(t, \boldsymbol{x}) = \lambda_j^t \psi_j(\boldsymbol{x})$. Therefore, the optimal k-dimensional approximation is given by the truncated sum

$$\hat{p}(\boldsymbol{y}, t|\boldsymbol{x}) = \phi_0(\boldsymbol{y}) + \sum_{j=1}^{k} \lambda_j^t \psi_j(\boldsymbol{x}) \phi_j(\boldsymbol{y}) \qquad (13)$$

Proof: The proof is a consequence of a weighted principal component analysis applied to the matrix M, taking into account the biorthogonality of the left and right eigenvectors.

We note that the first few eigenvectors are also optimal under other criteria, for example for data sampled from a manifold as in [4], or for multiclass spectral clustering [15].

3   The Asymptotics of the Diffusion Map

The analysis of the previous section provides a mathematical explanation for the success of the diffusion maps for dimensionality reduction and spectral clustering. However, it does not provide any information regarding the structure of the computed eigenvectors.

To this end, and similar to the framework of [16], we introduce a statistical model and assume that the data points $\{\boldsymbol{x}_i\}$ are i.i.d. random samples from a probability density $p(\boldsymbol{x})$

confined to a compact connected subset $\Omega \subset \mathbb{R}^p$ with smooth boundary $\partial\Omega$. Following the statistical physics notation, we write the density in Boltzmann form, $p(\boldsymbol{x}) = e^{-U(\boldsymbol{x})}$, where $U(\boldsymbol{x})$ is the (dimensionless) potential or energy of the configuration $\boldsymbol{x}$.

As shown in [11], in the limit $n \to \infty$ the random walk on the discrete graph converges to a random walk on the continuous space Ω. Then, it is possible to define forward and backward operators T_f and T_b as follows,

$$T_f[\phi](\boldsymbol{x}) = \int_\Omega M(\boldsymbol{x}|\boldsymbol{y})\phi(\boldsymbol{y})p(\boldsymbol{y})d\boldsymbol{y}, \quad T_b[\psi](\boldsymbol{x}) = \int_\Omega M(\boldsymbol{y}|\boldsymbol{x})\psi(\boldsymbol{y})p(\boldsymbol{y})d\boldsymbol{y} \quad (14)$$

where $M(\boldsymbol{x}|\boldsymbol{y}) = \exp(-\|\boldsymbol{x} - \boldsymbol{y}\|^2/2\varepsilon)/D(\boldsymbol{y})$ is the transition probability from $\boldsymbol{y}$ to $\boldsymbol{x}$ in time ε, and $D(\boldsymbol{y}) = \int \exp(-\|\boldsymbol{x} - \boldsymbol{y}\|^2/2\varepsilon)p(\boldsymbol{x})d\boldsymbol{x}$.

The two operators T_f and T_b have probabilistic interpretations. If $\phi(\boldsymbol{x})$ is a probability distribution on the graph at time $t = 0$, then $T_f[\phi]$ is the probability distribution at time $t = \varepsilon$. Similarly, $T_b[\psi](\boldsymbol{x})$ is the mean of the function ψ at time $t = \varepsilon$, for a random walk that started at location $\boldsymbol{x}$ at time $t = 0$. The operators T_f and T_b are thus the continuous analogues of the left and right multiplication by the finite matrix M.

We now take this analysis one step further and consider the limit $\varepsilon \to 0$. This is possible, since when $n = \infty$ each data point contains an infinite number of nearby neighbors. In this limit, since ε also has the interpretation of a time step, the random walk converges to a diffusion process, whose probability density evolves continuously in time, according to

$$\frac{\partial p(x,t)}{\partial t} = \lim_{\varepsilon\to 0} \frac{p(x, t + \varepsilon) - p(x, t)}{\varepsilon} = \lim_{\varepsilon\to 0} \frac{T_f - I}{\varepsilon}p(x,t) \quad (15)$$

in which case it is customary to study the infinitesimal generators (propagators)

$$\mathcal{H}_f = \lim_{\varepsilon\to 0} \frac{T_f - I}{\varepsilon}, \qquad \mathcal{H}_b = \lim_{\varepsilon\to 0} \frac{T_b - I}{\varepsilon} \quad (16)$$

Clearly, the eigenfunctions of T_f and T_b converge to those of $\mathcal{H}_f$ and $\mathcal{H}_b$, respectively.

As shown in [11], the backward generator is given by the following Fokker-Planck operator

$$\mathcal{H}_b\psi = \Delta\psi - 2\nabla\psi \cdot \nabla U \quad (17)$$

which corresponds to a diffusion process in a potential field of $2U(\boldsymbol{x})$

$$\dot{\boldsymbol{x}}(t) = -\nabla(2U) + \sqrt{2D}\dot{\boldsymbol{w}}(t) \quad (18)$$

where $\boldsymbol{w}(t)$ is standard Brownian motion in p dimensions and D is the diffusion coefficient, equal to one in equation (17). The Langevin equation (18) is a common model to describe stochastic dynamical systems in physics, chemistry and biology [19, 20]. As such, its characteristics as well as those of the corresponding FP equation have been extensively studied, see [19]-[22] and many others. The term $\nabla\psi \cdot \nabla U$ in (17) is interpreted as a *drift* term towards low energy (high-density) regions, and as discussed in the next section, may play a crucial part in the definition of clusters.

Note that when data is uniformly sampled from Ω, $\nabla U = 0$ so the drift term vanishes and we recover the Laplace-Beltrami operator on Ω. The connection between the discrete matrix M and the (weighted) Laplace-Beltrami or Fokker-Planck operator, as well as rigorous convergence proofs of the eigenvalues and eigenvectors of M to those of the integral operator T_b or infinitesimal generator $\mathcal{H}_b$ were considered in many recent works [4, 23, 17, 9, 24]. However, it seems that the important issue of boundary conditions was not considered.

Since (17) is defined in the bounded domain Ω, the eigenvalues and eigenfunctions of $\mathcal{H}_b$ depend on the boundary conditions imposed on $\partial\Omega$. As shown in [9], in the limit $\varepsilon \to 0$, the random walk satisfies reflecting boundary conditions on $\partial\Omega$, which translate into

$$\left.\frac{\partial\psi(\boldsymbol{x})}{\partial\boldsymbol{n}}\right|_{\partial\Omega} = 0 \quad (19)$$

Table 1: Random Walks and Diffusion Processes

Case	Operator	Stochastic Process
$\varepsilon > 0$ $n < \infty$	finite $n \times n$ matrix M	R.W. discrete in space discrete in time
$\varepsilon > 0$ $n \to \infty$	operators T_f, T_b	R.W. in continuous space discrete in time
$\varepsilon \to 0$ $n = \infty$	infinitesimal generator $\mathcal{H}_f$	diffusion process continuous in time & space

where $\boldsymbol{n}$ is a unit normal vector at the point $\boldsymbol{x} \in \partial\Omega$.

To conclude, the left and right eigenvectors of the finite matrix M can be viewed as discrete approximations to those of the operators T_f and T_b, which in turn can be viewed as approximations to those of $\mathcal{H}_f$ and $\mathcal{H}_b$. Therefore, if there are enough data points for accurate statistical sampling, the structure and characteristics of the eigenvalues and eigenfunctions of $\mathcal{H}_b$ are similar to the corresponding eigenvalues and discrete eigenvectors of M. For convenience, the three different stochastic processes are shown in table 1.

4 Fokker-Planck eigenfunctions and spectral clustering

According to (16), if λ_ε is an eigenvalue of the matrix M or of the integral operator T_b based on a kernel with parameter ε, then the corresponding eigenvalue of $\mathcal{H}_b$ is $\mu \approx (\lambda_\varepsilon - 1)/\varepsilon$. Therefore the largest eigenvalues of M correspond to the smallest eigenvalues of $\mathcal{H}_b$. These eigenvalues and their corresponding eigenfunctions have been extensively studied in the literature under various settings. In general, the eigenvalues and eigenfunctions depend both on the geometry of the domain Ω and on the profile of the potential $U(\boldsymbol{x})$. For clarity and due to lack of space we briefly analyze here two extreme cases. In the first case $\Omega = \mathbb{R}^p$ so geometry plays no role, while in the second $U(\boldsymbol{x}) = const$ so density plays no role. Yet we show that in both cases there can still be well defined clusters, with the unifying probabilistic concept being that the mean exit time from one cluster to another is much larger than the characteristic equilibration time inside each cluster.

Case I: Consider diffusion in a smooth potential $U(\boldsymbol{x})$ in $\Omega = \mathbb{R}^p$, where U has a few local minima, and $U(\boldsymbol{x}) \to \infty$ as $\|\boldsymbol{x}\| \to \infty$ fast enough so that $\int e^{-U} d\boldsymbol{x} = 1 < \infty$. Each such local minimum thus defines a metastable state, with transitions between metastable states being relatively rare events, depending on the barrier heights separating them. As shown in [21, 22] (and in many other works) there is an intimate connection between the smallest eigenvalues of $\mathcal{H}_b$ and mean exit times out of these metastable states. Specifically, in the asymptotic limit of small noise $D \ll 1$, exit times are exponentially distributed and the first non-trivial eigenvalue (after $\mu_0 = 0$) is given by $\mu_1 = 1/\bar{\tau}$ where $\bar{\tau}$ is the mean exit time to overcome the highest potential barrier on the way to the deepest potential well. For the case of two potential wells, for example, the corresponding eigenfunction is roughly constant in each well with a sharp transition near the saddle point between the wells. In general, in the case of k local minima there are asymptotically only k eigenvalues very close to zero. Apart from $\mu_0 = 0$, each of the other $k - 1$ eigenvalues corresponds to the mean exit time from one of the wells into the deepest one, with the corresponding eigenfunctions being almost constant in each well. Therefore, for a finite dataset the presence of only k eigenvalues close to 1 with a *spectral gap*, e.g. a large difference between λ_k and λ_{k+1} is indicative of k well defined *global* clusters. In figure 1 (left) an example of this case is shown, where $p(\boldsymbol{x})$ is the sum of two well separated Gaussian clouds leading to a double well potential. Indeed there are only two eigenvalues close or equal to 1 with a distinct spectral gap and the first eigenfunction being almost piecewise constant in each well.

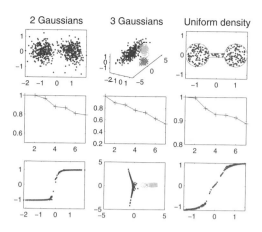

Figure 1: Diffusion map results on different datasets. Top - the datasets. Middle - the eigenvalues. Bottom - the first eigenvector vs. x_1 or the first and second eigenvectors for the case of three Gaussians.

In stochastic dynamical systems a spectral gap corresponds to a separation of time scales between long transition times from one well or metastable state to another as compared to short equilibration times inside each well. Therefore, clustering and identification of metastable states are very similar tasks, and not surprisingly algorithms similar to the normalized graph Laplacian have been independently developed in the literature [25].

The above mentioned results are asymptotic in the small noise limit. In practical datasets, there can be clusters of different scales, where a global analysis with a single ε is not suitable. As an example consider the second dataset in figure 1, with three clusters. While the first eigenvector distinguishes between the large cluster and the two smaller ones, the second eigenvector captures the equilibration inside the large cluster instead of further distinguishing the two small clusters. While a theoretical explanation is beyond the scope of this paper, a possible solution is to choose a location dependent ε, as proposed in [26].

Case II: Consider a uniform density in a region $\Omega \subset \mathbb{R}^3$ composed of two large containers connected by a narrow circular tube, as in the top right frame in figure 1. In this case $U(\boldsymbol{x}) = const$, so the second term in (17) vanishes. As shown in [27], the second eigenvalue of the FP operator is extremely small, of the order of a/V where a is the radius of the connecting tube and V is the volume of the containers, thus showing an interesting connection to the Cheeger constant on graphs. The corresponding eigenfunction is almost piecewise constant in each container with a sharp transition in the connecting tube. Even though in this case the density is uniform, there still is a spectral gap with two well defined clusters (the two containers), defined entirely by the geometry of Ω. An example of such a case and the results of the diffusion map are shown in figure 1 (right).

In summary the eigenfunctions and eigenvalues of the FP operator, and thus of the corresponding finite Markov matrix, depend on both geometry and density. The diffusion distance and its close relation to mean exit times between different clusters is the quantity that incorporates these two features. This provides novel insight into spectral clustering algorithms, as well as a theoretical justification for the algorithm in [13], which defines clusters according to mean travel times between points on the graph. A similar analysis could also be applied to semi-supervised learning based on spectral methods [28]. Finally, these eigenvectors may be used to design better search and data collection protocols [29].

Acknowledgments: The authors thank Mikhail Belkin and Partha Niyogi for interesting discussions. This work was partially supported by DARPA through AFOSR.

References

[1] B. Schölkopf, A. Smola and K.R. Müller. Nonlinear component analysis as a kernel eigenvalue problem, *Neural Computation* 10, 1998.

[2] Y. Weiss. Segmentation using eigenvectors: a unifying view. *ICCV* 1999.

[3] J. Shi and J. Malik. Normalized cuts and image segmentation, *PAMI*, Vol. 22, 2000.

[4] M. Belkin and P. Niyogi. Laplacian eigenmaps and spectral techniques for embedding and clustering, NIPS Vol. 14, 2002.

[5] M. Belkin and P. Niyogi. Laplacian eigenmaps for dimensionality reduction and data representation, *Neural Computation* 15:1373-1396, 2003.

[6] A.Y. Ng, M. Jordan and Y. Weiss. On spectral clustering, analysis and an algorithm, NIPS Vol. 14, 2002.

[7] X. Zhu, Z. Ghahramani, J. Lafferty, Semi-supervised learning using Gaussian fields and harmonic functions, Proceedings of the 20th international conference on machine learning, 2003.

[8] M. Saerens, F. Fouss, L. Yen and P. Dupont, The principal component analysis of a graph and its relationships to spectral clustering. ECML 2004.

[9] R.R. Coifman, S. Lafon, Diffusion Maps, to appear in Appl. Comp. Harm. Anal.

[10] R.R. Coifman & *al.*, Geometric diffusion as a tool for harmonic analysis and structure definition of data, parts I and II, *Proc. Nat. Acad. Sci.*, 102(21):7426-37 (2005).

[11] B. Nadler, S. Lafon, R.R. Coifman, I. G. Kevrekidis, Diffusion maps, spectral clustering, and the reaction coordinates of dynamical systems, to appear in Appl. Comp. Harm. Anal., available at http://arxiv.org/abs/math.NA/0503445.

[12] M. Meila, J. Shi. A random walks view of spectral segmentation, *AI and Statistics*, 2001.

[13] L. Yen L., Vanvyve D., Wouters F., Fouss F., Verleysen M. and Saerens M. , Clustering using a random-walk based distance measure. ESANN 2005, pp 317-324.

[14] N. Tishby, N. Slonim, Data Clustering by Markovian Relaxation and the information bottleneck method, NIPS, 2000.

[15] S. Yu and J. Shi. Multiclass spectral clustering. ICCV 2003.

[16] Y. Bengio et. al, Learning eigenfunctions links spectral embedding and kernel PCA, *Neural Computation*, 16:2197-2219 (2004).

[17] U. von Luxburg, O. Bousquet, M. Belkin, On the convergence of spectral clustering on random samples: the normalized case, NIPS, 2004.

[18] S. Lafon, A.B. Lee, Diffusion maps: A unified framework for dimension reduction, data partitioning and graph subsampling, submitted.

[19] C.W. Gardiner, *Handbook of stochastic methods*, third edition, Springer NY, 2004.

[20] H. Risken, *The Fokker Planck equation*, 2nd edition, Springer NY, 1999.

[21] B.J. Matkowsky and Z. Schuss, Eigenvalues of the Fokker-Planck operator and the approach to equilibrium for diffusions in potential fields, *SIAM J. App. Math.* 40(2):242-254 (1981).

[22] M. Eckhoff, Precise asymptotics of small eigenvalues of reversible diffusions in the metastable regime, *Annals of Prob.* 33:244-299, 2005.

[23] M. Belkin and P. Niyogi, Towards a theoeretical foundation for Laplacian-based manifold methods, COLT 2005 (to appear).

[24] M. Hein, J. Audibert, U. von Luxburg, From graphs to manifolds - weak and strong pointwise consistency of graph Laplacians, COLT 2005 (to appear).

[25] W. Huisinga, C. Best, R. Roitzsch, C. Schütte, F. Cordes, From simulation data to conformational ensembles, structure and dynamics based methods, *J. Comp. Chem.* 20:1760-74, 1999.

[26] L. Zelnik-Manor, P. Perona, Self-Tuning spectral clustering, NIPS, 2004.

[27] A. Singer, Z. Schuss, D. Holcman and R.S. Eisenberg, narrow escape, part I, submitted.

[28] D. Zhou & *al.*, Learning with local and global consistency, NIPS Vol. 16, 2004.

[29] I.G. Kevrekidis, C.W. Gear, G. Hummer, Equation-free: The computer-aided analysis of complex multiscale systems, *Aiche J.* 50:1346-1355, 2004.

Stimulus Evoked Independent Factor Analysis of MEG Data with Large Background Activity

S.S. Nagarajan
Biomagnetic Imaging Laboratory
Department of Radiology
University of California, San Francisco
San Francisco, CA 94122
sri@radiology.ucsf.edu

H.T. Attias
Golden Metallic, Inc.
P.O. Box 475608
San Francisco, CA 94147
htattias@goldenmetallic.com

K.E. Hild
Biomagnetic Imaging Laboratory
Department of Radiology
University of California, San Francisco
San Francisco, CA 94122
hild@mrsc.ucsf.edu

K. Sekihara
Dept. of Systems Design and Engineering
Tokyo Metropolitan University
Asahigaoka 6-6, Hino, Tokyo 191-0065
ksekiha@cc.tmit.ac.jp

Abstract

This paper presents a novel technique for analyzing electromagnetic imaging data obtained using the stimulus evoked experimental paradigm. The technique is based on a probabilistic graphical model, which describes the data in terms of underlying evoked and interference sources, and explicitly models the stimulus evoked paradigm. A variational Bayesian EM algorithm infers the model from data, suppresses interference sources, and reconstructs the activity of separated individual brain sources. The new algorithm outperforms existing techniques on two real datasets, as well as on simulated data.

1 Introduction

Electromagnetic source imaging, the reconstruction of the spatiotemporal activation of brain sources from MEG and EEG data, is currently being used in numerous studies of human cognition, both in normal and in various clinical populations [1]. A major advantage of MEG/EEG over other noninvasive functional brain imaging techniques, such as fMRI, is the ability to obtain valuable information about neural dynamics with high temporal resolution on the order of milliseconds. An experimental paradigm that is very popular in imaging studies is the stimulus evoked paradigm. In this paradigm, a stimulus, e.g., a tone at a particular frequency and duration, is presented to the subject at a series of equally spaced time points. Each presentation (or trial) produces activity in a set of brain sources, which generates an electromagnetic field captured by the sensor array. These data constitute the stimulus evoked response, and analyzing them can help to gain insights into the mechanism used by the brain to process the stimulus and similar sensory inputs. This paper presents a new technique for analyzing stimulus evoked electromagnetic imaging data.

963

An important problem in analyzing such data is that MEG/EEG signals, which are captured by sensors located outside the brain, contain not only signals generated by brain sources evoked by the stimulus, but also interference signals, generated by other sources such as spontaneous brain activity, eye blinks and other biological and non-biological sources of artifacts. Interference signals overlap spatially and temporally with the stimulus evoked signals, making it difficult to obtain accurate reconstructions of evoked brain sources. A related problem is that signals from different evoked sources themselves overlap with each other, making it difficult to localize individual sources and reconstruct their separate responses.

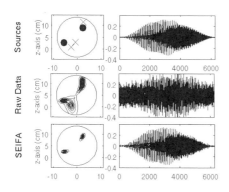

Figure 1: Simulation example (see text)

Many approaches have been taken to the problem of suppressing interference signals. One method is averaging over multiple trials, which reduces the contributions from interference sources, assuming that they are uncorrelated with the stimulus and that their autocorrelation time scale is shorter than the trial length. However, a successful application of this method requires a large number of trials, effectively limiting the number of stimulus conditions per experiment. It usually also requires manual rejection of trials containing conspicuous artifacts. A set of methods termed subspace techniques computes a projection of the sensor data onto the signal subspace, which corresponds to brain sources of interest. However, these methods rely on thresholding to determine the noise level, and tend to discard information below threshold. Consequently, those methods perform well only when the interference level is low.

Independent component analysis (ICA) techniques [4-8], introduced more recently, attempt to decompose the sensor data into a set of signals that are mutually statistically independent. Artifacts such as eye blinks are independent of brain source activity and ICA has been able in many cases to successfully separate the two types of signals into distinct groups of output variables. However, ICA techniques have several shortcomings. First, they require pre-processing the sensor data to reduce dimensionality from, which causes loss of information on brain sources with relatively low amplitude. This is because, for K sensors, ICA must learn a square $K \times K$ unmixing matrix from N data points; typical values such as $K = 275, N = 700$ can lead to poor performance due to local maxima, overfitting, and slow convergence. Second, ICA assumes $L + M = K'$, where L, M are the number of evoked and interference sources and $K' < K$ is the *reduced* input dimensionality. However, many cases have $L + M > K'$, which leads to suboptimal and sometime failed separation. Third, ICA requires post-processing of its output signals, usually via manual examination by experts (though sometime by thresholding), to determine which signals correspond evoked brain sources of interest.

The fourth drawback of ICA techniques is that, by design, they cannot exploit the advantage offered by the evoked stimulus paradigm. Whereas interference sources are continuously active, evoked sources become active at each trial only near the time of stimulus presentation, termed stimulus onset time. Hence, knowledge of the onset times can help separate the evoked sources. However, the onset times, which are determined by the experimental design and available during data analysis, are ignored by ICA.

In this paper we present a novel technique for suppressing interference signals and separating signals from individual evoked sources. The technique is based on a new probabilistic graphical model termed *stimulus evoked independent factor analysis* (SEIFA). This model, an extension of [2], describes the observed sensor data in terms of two sets of independent variables, termed factors, which are not directly observable. The factors in the first set represent evoked sources, and the factors in the second set represent interference sources. The sensor data are generated by linearly combining the factors in the two sets using two mixing matrices, followed by adding sensor noise. The mixing matrices and the precision matrix of the sensor noise constitute the SEIFA model parameters, and are inferred from data using a variational Bayesian EM algorithm [3], which computes their posterior distribution. Separation of the evoked sources is achieved in the course of processing by the algorithm.

The SEIFA model is free from the above four shortcomings. It can be applied directly to the sensor data without dimensionality reduction, therefore no information is lost. Rather than learning a square $K \times K$ unmixing matrix, it learns a $K \times (L + M)$ mixing matrix, where the number of interference factors M is minimized using automatic Bayesian model selection which is part of the algorithm. In addition, SEIFA is designed to explicitly model the stimulus evoked paradigm, hence it optimally exploits the knowledge of stimulus onset times. Consequently, evoked sources are automatically identified and no post-processing is required.

2 SEIFA
Probabilistic Graphical Model

This section presents the SEIFA probabilistic graphical model, which is the focus of this paper. The SEIFA model describes observed MEG sensor data in terms of three types of underlying, unobserved signals: (1) signals arising from stimulus evoked sources, (2) signals arising from interference sources, and (2) sensor noise signals. The model is inferred from data by an algorithm presented in the next section. Following inference, the model is used to separate the evoked source signals from those of the interference sources and from sensor noise, thus providing a clean version of the evoked response. The model further separates the evoked response into statistically inde-

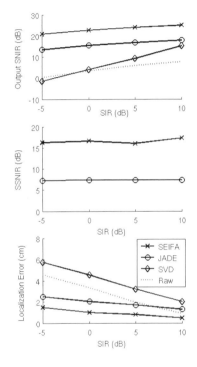

Figure 2: Performance on simulated data (see text)

pendent factors. In addition, it produces a regularized correlation matrix of the clean evoked response and of each independent factors, which facilitates localization.

Let y_{in} denote the signal recorded by sensor $i = 1 : K$ at time $n = 1 : N$. We assume that these signals arise from L evoked factors and M interference factors that are combined linearly. Let x_{jn} denote the signal of evoked factor $j = 1 : L$, and let u_{jn} denote the signal of interference factor $j = 1 : M$, both at time n. We use the term factor rather than source for a reason explained below. Let A_{ij} denote the evoked mixing matrix, and let B_{ij} denote the interference mixing matrix. Those matrices contain the coefficients of the linear combination of the factors that produces the data. They are analogous to the factor loading matrix in the factor analysis model. Let v_{in} denote the noise signal on sensor i.

We use an evoked stimulus paradigm, where a stimulus is presented at a specific time, termed the stimulus onset time, and is absent beforehand. The stimulus onset time is defined as $n = N_0 + 1$. The period preceding the onset $n = 1 : N_0$ is termed pre-stimulus period, and the period following the onset $n = N_0 + 1 : N$ is termed post-stimulus period. We assume the evoked factors are active only post stimulus and satisfy $x_{jn} = 0$ before its onset. Hence

$$
y_n = \begin{cases} Bu_n + v_n, & n = 1 : N_0 \\ Ax_n + Bu_n + v_n, & n = N_0 + 1 : N \end{cases} \tag{1}
$$

To turn (1) into a probabilistic model, each signal must be modelled by a probability distribution. Here, each evoked factor is modelled by a mixture of Gaussian (MOG) distributions. For factor j we have a MOG model with S_j components, also termed states,

$$
p(x_n) = \prod_{j=1}^{L} p(x_{jn}) , \qquad p(x_{jn}) = \sum_{s_j=1}^{S_j} \mathcal{N}(x_{jn} \mid \mu_{j,s_j}, \nu_{j,s_j}) \pi_{j,s_j} \tag{2}
$$

State s_j is a Gaussian with mean μ_{j,s_j} and precision ν_{j,s_j}, and its probability is π_{j,s_j}. We model the factors as mutually statistically independent.

There are three reasons for using MOG distributions, rather than Gaussians, to describe the evoked factors. First, evoked brain sources are often characterized by spikes or by modulated harmonic functions, leading to non-Gaussian distributions. Second, previous work on ICA has shown that independent Gaussian sources that are linearly mixed cannot be separated. Since we aim to separate the evoked response into contributions from individual factors, we must therefore use independent non-Gaussian factor distributions. Third, as is well known, a MOG model with a suitably chosen number of states can describe arbitrary distributions at the desired level of accuracy.

For interference signals and sensor noise we employ a Gaussian model. Each interference factor is modelled by an independent, zero-mean Gaussian distribution with unit precision,

$$
p(u_n) = \prod_{j=1}^{M} \mathcal{N}(u_{jn} \mid 0, 1) = \mathcal{N}(u_n \mid 0, I) \tag{3}
$$

The Gaussian model implies that we exploit only second order statistics of the interference signals. This contrasts with the evoked signals, whose MOG model facilitates exploiting higher order statistics, leading to more accurate reconstruction and to separation.

The sensor noise is modelled by a zero-mean Gaussian distribution with a diagonal precision matrix λ, $p(v_n) = \mathcal{N}(v_n \mid 0, \lambda)$. From (1) we obtain $p(y_n \mid x_n, u_n) = p(v_n)$ where we substitute $v_n = y_n - Ax_n - Bu_n$ with $x_n = 0$ for $n = 1 : N_0$. Hence, we obtain the distribution of the sensor signals conditioned on the evoked and interference factors,

$$
p(y_n \mid x_n, u_n, A, B) = \begin{cases} \mathcal{N}(y_n \mid Bu_n, \lambda), & n = 1 : N_0 \\ \mathcal{N}(y_n \mid Ax_n + Bu_n, \lambda), & n = N_0 + 1 : N \end{cases} \tag{4}
$$

SEIFA also makes an i.i.d. assumption, meaning the signals at different time points are independent. Hence $p(y, x, u \mid A, B) = \prod_n p(y_n \mid x_n, u_n, A, B)p(x_n)p(u_n)$. where y, x, u denote collectively the signals y_n, x_n, u_n at all time points. The i.i.d. assumption is made for simplicity, and implies that the algorithm presented below can exploit the spatial statistics of the data but not their temporal statistics.

To complete the definition of SEIFA, we must specify prior distributions over the model parameters. For the noise precision matrix λ we choose a flat prior, $p(\lambda) = const$. For the mixing matrices A, B we choose to use a conjugate prior

$$
p(A) = \prod_{ij} \mathcal{N}(A_{ij} \mid 0, \lambda_i \alpha_j) , \qquad p(B) = \prod_{ij} \mathcal{N}(B_{ij} \mid 0, \lambda_i \beta_j) \tag{5}
$$

where all matrix elements are independent zero-mean Gaussians and the precision of the ijth matrix element is proportional to the noise precision λ_i on sensor i. It is the λ dependence which makes this prior conjugate. The proportionality constants α_j and β_j constitute the parameters of the prior, a.k.a. hyperparameters. Eqs. (2,3,4,5) fully define the SEIFA model.

3 Inferring the SEIFA Model from Data: A VB-EM Algorithm

This section presents an algorithm that infers the SEIFA model from data. SEIFA is a probabilistic model with hidden variables, since the evoked and interference factors are not directly observable, hence it must be treated in the EM framework. We use variational Bayesian EM (VB-EM), which has two relevant advantages over standard EM. First, it is more robust to overfitting, which can be a significant problem when working with high-dimensional but relatively short time series (here we analyze $N < 1000$ point long, $K = 275$ dimensional data sequences). To achieve this robustness, VB-EM computes (using a variational approximation) a full posterior distribution over model parameters, rather than a single MAP estimate. This means that VB-EM considers all possible parameters values, and computes the probability of each value conditioned on the observed data. It also performs automatic model order selection by optimizing the hyperparameters, and consequently uses the minimum number of parameters needed to explain the data. Second, VB-EM produces automatically regularized estimators for the evoked response correlation matrices (required for source localization), where standard EM produces poorly conditioned ones. This is also a result of computing a parameter posterior.

VB-EM is an iterative algorithm, where each iteration consists of an E- and an M-step.

E-step. For the pre-stimulus period $n = 1 : N_0$ we compute the posterior over the interference factors u_n only. It is a Gaussian distribution with posterior mean $\bar{u}_n$ and covariance Φ given by

$$\bar{u}_n = \Phi \bar{B}^T \lambda y_n \, , \quad \Phi = \left(\bar{B}^T \lambda \bar{B} + I + K \Psi_{BB} \right)^{-1} \tag{6}$$

where $\bar{B}$ are Ψ_{BB} are the posterior mean and covariance of the interference mixing matrix B computed in the M-step below (more precisely, the posterior covariance of the ith row of B is Ψ_{BB}/λ_i).

For the post-stimulus period $n = N_0 + 1 : N$ we compute the posterior over the evoked and interference factors x_n, u_n, and the collective state s_n of the evoked factors. The latter is defined by the L-dimensional vector $s_n = (s_{1n}, s_{2n}, ..., s_{Ln})$, where $s_{jn} = 1 : S_j$ is the state of evoked factor j at time n. The total number of collective states is $S = \prod_j S_j$.

To simplify the notation, we combine the evoked and interference factors into a single $L' \times 1$ vector $x'_n = (x_n, u_n)$, where $L' = L + M$, and their mixing matrices into a single $K \times L'$ matrix $A' = (A, B)$. Now, at time n, let r run over all the S collective states. For each r, the posterior over the factors conditioned on $s_n = r$ is Gaussian, with posterior mean $\bar{x}_{rn}, \bar{u}_{rn}$ and covariance Γ_r given by

$$\bar{x}'_{rn} = \Gamma_r \left(\bar{A}'^T \lambda y_n + \nu'_r \mu'_r \right) \, , \quad \Gamma_r = \left(\bar{A}'^T \lambda \bar{A}' + \nu'_r + K \Psi \right)^{-1} \tag{7}$$

We have defined $\bar{x}'_{rn} = (\bar{x}_{rn}, \bar{u}_{rn})$ and $\bar{A}' = (\bar{A}, \bar{B})$. The $L \times 1$ vector μ'_r and the diagonal $L \times L$ matrix ν'_r contain the means and precisions of the individual states (see (2)) composing r. The posterior mean and covariance $\bar{A}', \Psi$ are computed in the M-step. Next, compute the posterior probability that $s_n = r$ by

$$\bar{\pi}_{rn} = \frac{1}{z_n} \pi_r \sqrt{|\nu_r||\Gamma_r|} \exp \left(-\frac{1}{2} y_n^T \lambda y_n + \frac{1}{2} \mu_r^T \nu_r \mu_r - \frac{1}{2} \bar{x}'_{rn} \Gamma_r^{-1} \bar{x}'_{rn} \right) \tag{8}$$

where z_n is a normalization constant and μ_r, ν_r, π_r are the MOG parameters of (2).

M-step. We divide the model parameters into two sets. The first set includes the mixing matrices A, B, for which we compute full posterior distributions. The second set includes the noise precision λ and the diagonal hyperparameters matrices α, β, for which we compute MAP estimates. The posterior over A, B is Gaussian factorized over their rows, where the mean is

$$\begin{aligned} \bar{A} &= R_{yx}\Psi \\ \bar{B} &= R_{yu}\Psi \end{aligned}, \qquad \Psi = \begin{pmatrix} R_{xx} + \alpha & R_{xu} \\ R_{xu}^T & R_{uu} + \beta \end{pmatrix}^{-1} \qquad (9)$$

and where the ith row of $A' = (A, B)$ has covariance Ψ/λ_i. The hyperparameters α_j, β_j are diagonal entries of diagonal matrices α, β. $R_{yx}, R_{yu}, R_{xx}, R_{xu}, R_{uu}$ are posterior correlations between the factors and the data and among the factors themselves, e.g., $R_{yx} = \sum_n \langle y_n x_n \rangle, R_{xx} = \sum_n \langle x_n x_n \rangle$, where $\langle \cdot \rangle$ denotes posterior averaging. They are easily computed in terms of the E-step quantities $\bar{u}_n, \bar{x}'_{rn}, \Phi, \Gamma_r, \bar{\pi}_{rn}$ and are omitted.

Next, the hyperparameter matrices α, β are updated by

$$\alpha^{-1} = \mathrm{diag}\left(\bar{A}^T \lambda \bar{A}/K + \Psi_{AA}\right), \qquad \beta^{-1} = \mathrm{diag}\left(\bar{B}^T \lambda \bar{B}/K + \Psi_{BB}\right) \qquad (10)$$

and the noise precision matrix by $\lambda^{-1} = \mathrm{diag}(R_{yy} - \bar{A}R_{yx}^T - \bar{B}R_{yu}^T)/N$. Ψ_{AA} and Ψ_{BB} are the appropriate blocks of Ψ in (9). The interference mixing matrix and the noise precision are initialized from pre-stimulus data. We used MOG parameters corresponding to peaky (super-Gaussian) distributions.

Estimating and Localizing Clean Evoked Responses. Let $z_{in}^j = \langle A_{ij} x_{jn} \rangle$ denote the inferred individual contribution from evoked factor j to sensor signal i. It is given via posterior averaging by

$$\bar{z}_{in}^j = \bar{A}_{ij} \bar{x}_{jn} \qquad (11)$$

where $\bar{x}_n = \sum_r \bar{\pi}_r \bar{x}_{rn}$. Computing this estimate amounts to obtaining a clean version of the individual contribution from each factor and of their combined contribution, and removing contributions from interference factors and sensor noise.

The localization of individual evoked factors using sensor signals z_n^j can be achieved by many algorithms. In this paper, we use adaptive spatial filters that take data correlation matrices as inputs for localization, because these methods have been shown to have superior spatial resolution and non-zero localization bias [6]. Let $C^j = \sum_n \langle z_n^j (z_n^j)^T \rangle$ denote the inferred sensor data correlation matrix corresponding to the individual contribution from evoked factor j. Then,

$$C^j = \left[\bar{A}^j (\bar{A}^j)^T + \lambda^{-1} (\Psi_{AA})_{jj}\right] (R_{xx})_{jj} \qquad (12)$$

where $\bar{A}^j$ is a $K \times 1$ vector denoting the jth column of $\bar{A}$. Notice that the VB-EM approach has produced a correlation matrix that is automatically regularized (due to the Ψ_{AA} term) and can be used for localization in its current form. In contrast, computing it from the signal estimates obtained by other methods, such as PCA or ICA, yields a poorly conditioned matrix that requires post-processing.

4 Experiments on Real and Simulated Data

Simulations. Fig. 1 shows a simulation with two evoked sources and three interference sources with $N = 10000$, signal-to-interference (SIR) of 0 dB and signal-to-sensor-noise (SNR) of 5dB. The true locations of the evoked sources, each of which is denoted by •, and the true locations of the background sources, each of which is denoted by × are shown in the top left panel. The right column in the top row shows the time courses of the evoked sources as they appear at the sensors. The time courses of the actual sensor signals, which also include the effects of background sources and sensor noise, are shown in the middle row (right column). The bottom row shows the localization and time-course of cleaned

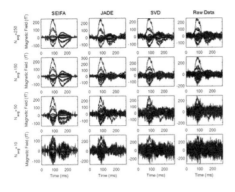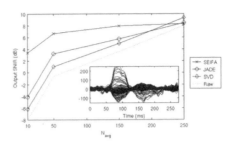

Figure 3: Estimating auditory-evoked responses from small trial averages (see text)

evoked sources estimated using SEIFA, which agrees with the true location and time-course. Fig. 2 shows the mean performance as a function of SIR, across 50 Monte Carlo trials for $N = 1000$ and SNR of 10 dB, for different locations of evoked and interference sources. Denoising performance is quantified by the output signal-to-(noise+interference) ratio (SNIR) and shown in the top panel. SEIFA outperforms both our benchmark methods, providing a 5-10 dB improvement over JADE [7] and SVD. Separation performance of individual evoked factors is quantified by (separated-signal)-to-(noise+interference) ratio (SSNIR) (definition omitted) and is shown in the middle panel. SEIFA far outperforms JADE for this set of examples. JADE is able to separate the background sources from the evoked sources (hence gives good denoising performance), but it is not always able to separate the evoked sources from each other. The Infomax algorithm [4] (results not shown) exhibited poor separation performance similar to JADE. Finally, localization performance is quantified by the mean distance in cm between the true evoked source locations and the estimated locations, as shown in the bottom panel. Here too, SEIFA far outperforms all other methods, especially for low SIR. Notably, SEIFA performance appears to be quite robust to the i.i.d. assumption of the evoked and background sources, because in these simulations evoked sources were assumed to be damped sinusoids and interference sources were sinusoids.

4.1 Real Data

Denoising averages from small number of trials. Auditory evoked responses from a particular subject obtained by averaging different number of trials are shown in figure 3 (left panel). SEIFA is able to clearly recover responses even from small trial averages. To quantify the performance of the different methods, a filtered version of the raw data for $N_{avg} = 250$ was assumed as "ground-truth", and is shown in the inset of the right panel. The output SNIR as a function of N_{avg} is also shown in figure 3 (right panel). SEIFA exhibits the best performance especially for small trial averages.

Separation of evoked sources. To highlight SEIFA's ability to separately localize evoked sources, we conducted an experiment involving simultaneous presentation of auditory and somatosensory stimuli. We expected the activation of contralateral auditory and somatosensory cortices to overlap in time. A pure tone (400ms duration, 1kHz, 5 ms ramp up/down) was presented binaurally with a delay of 50 ms following a pneumatic tap on the left index finger. Averaging is performed over $N_{avg} = 100$ trials triggered on the onset of the tap. Results from SEIFA for this experiment are shown in Figure 4. In these figures, one panel shows a contour map that shows the polarity and magnitude of the denoised and raw sensor signals in sensor space. The contour plot of the magnetic field on the sensor array, corresponding to the mapping of three-dimensional sensor surface array to points within a circle, shows the magnetic field profile at a particular instant of time relative to the stimulus presentation. Other panels show localization of a particular evoked factor overlaid on the subjects' MRI. Three orthogonal projections - axial, sagittal and coronal MRI slices, that highlight all voxels having activity that is $> 80\%$ of maximum are shown. Results are based on the right hemisphere channels above contralateral somatosensory and auditory cortices. Localization of time-course of the first two factors estimated by SEIFA are shown in left and middle panels of figure 4. The first two factors localize to primary somatosensory cortex (SI), however with differential latencies. The first factor shows a peak response at a latency of 50 ms, whereas the second factor shows the response at a later latency. Interestingly, the third factor localizes to auditory cortex and the extracted time-course corresponds well to an auditory evoked response that is well-separated from the somatosensory response (figure 3 right panels).

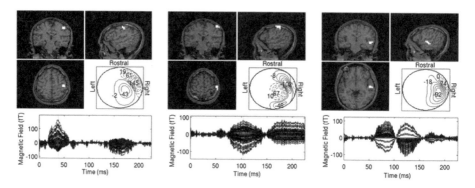

Figure 4: Estimated SEIFA factors for auditory-somatosensory experiment

5 Extensions

Whereas this paper uses fixed values for the number of evoked and interference sources L, M (though the effective number of interference sources was determined via optimizing the hyperparameter β), VB-EM facilitates inferring them from data, and we plan to investigate the effectiveness of this procedure. We also plan to infer the distribution of evoked sources (MOG parameters) from data rather than using a fixed distribution. Another extension that could enhance performance is exploiting temporal correlation in the data. We plan to do it by incorporating temporal (e.g., autoregressive) models into the source distributions and infer their parameters from data.

References

[1] S. Baillet, J. C. Mosher, and R. M. Leahy. Electromagnetic brain mapping.*Signal Processing Magazine*, 18:14-30, 2001.

[2] H. Attias (1999). Independent Factor Analysis. *Neur. Comp. 11*, 803-851.

[3] H. Attias (2000). A variational Bayes framework for graphical models. *Adv. Neur. Info. Proc. Sys. 12*, 209-215.

[4] T.-P. Jung, S. Makeig, M. Westerfield, J. Townsend, E. Courchesne, T.J. Sejnowski (2000). Removal of eye artifacts from visual event related potentials in normal and clinical subjects. *J. Clin. Neurophys. 40*, 516-520.

[5] S. Makeig, S. Debener, J. Onton, A. Delorme (2004). Mining event related brain dynamics. *Trends Cog. Sci. 8*, 204-210.

[6] K. Sekihara, S. Nagarajan, D. Poeppel, A. Marantz, Y. Miyashita (2001). Reconstructing spatio-temporal activities of neural sources using a MEG vector beamformer technique. *IEEE Trans. Biomed. Eng. 48*, 760-771.

[7] J.F.Cardoso (1999) High-order contrasts for independent component analysis, *Neural Computation*, 11(1):157–192.

[8] R. Vigario, J. Sarela, V. Jousmaki, M. Hamalainen, E. Oja (2000). Independent component approach to the analysis of EEG and MEG recordings. *IEEE Trans. Biomed. Eng. 47*, 589-593.

An Analog Visual Pre-Processing Processor Employing Cyclic Line Access in Only-Nearest-Neighbor-Interconnects Architecture

Yusuke Nakashita
Department of Frontier Informatics
School of Frontier Sciences
The University of Tokyo
5-1-5 Kashiwanoha, Kashiwa-shi, Chiba
277-8561, Japan
yusuke@else.k.u-tokyo.ac.jp

Yoshio Mita
Department of Electrical Engineering
School of Engineering
The University of Tokyo
7-3-1 Hongo, Bunkyo-ku,Tokyo
113-8656, Japan.
mita@ee.t.u-tokyo.ac.jp

Tadashi Shibata
Department of Frontier Informatics
School of Frontier Sciences
The University of Tokyo
5-1-5 Kashiwanoha, Kashiwa-shi, Chiba
277-8561, Japan
shibata@ee.t.u-tokyo.ac.jp

Abstract

An analog focal-plane processor having a 128×128 photodiode array has been developed for directional edge filtering. It can perform 4×4-pixel kernel convolution for entire pixels only with 256 steps of simple analog processing. Newly developed cyclic line access and row-parallel processing scheme in conjunction with the "only-nearest-neighbor interconnects" architecture has enabled a very simple implementation. A proof-of-concept chip was fabricated in a 0.35-μm 2-poly 3-metal CMOS technology and the edge filtering at a rate of 200 frames/sec. has been experimentally demonstrated.

1 Introduction

Directional edge detection in an input image is the most essential operation in early visual processing [1, 2]. Such spatial filtering operations are carried out by taking the convolution between a block of pixels and a weight matrix, requiring a number of multiply-and-accumulate operations. Since the convolution operation must be repeated pixel-by-pixel to scan the entire image, the computation is very expensive and software solutions are not compatible to real-time applications. Therefore, the hardware implementation of focal-plane parallel processing is highly demanded. However, there exists a hard problem which we call the *interconnects explosion* as illustrated in Fig. 1.

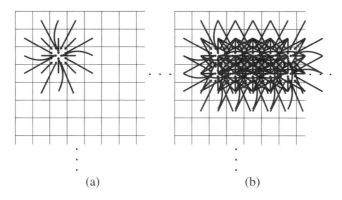

Figure 1: (a) Interconnects from nearest neighbor (N.N.) and second N.N. pixels to a single pixel at the center. (b) N.N. and second N.N. interconnects for pixels in the two rows, an illustrative example of *interconnecs explosion.*

In carrying out a filtering operation for one pixel, the luminance data must be gathered from the nearest-neighbor and second nearest-neighbor pixels. The interconnects necessary for this is illustrated in Fig. 1(a). If such wiring is formed for two rows of pixels, excessively high density overlapping interconnects are required. If we extend this to an entire chip, it is impossible to form the wiring even with the most advanced VLSI interconnects technology. Biology has solved the problem by real *3D-interconnects* structures. Since only two dimensional layouts are allowed with a limited number of stacks in VLSI technology, the *missing one dimension* is crucial. We must overcome the difficulty by introducing new architectures.

In order to achieve real-time performance in image filtering, a number of VLSI chips have been developed in both digital [3, 4] and analog [5, 6, 7] technologies. A flash-convolution processor [4] allows a single 5×5-pixel convolution operation in a single clock cycle by introducing a subtle memory access scheme. However, for an $N \times M$-pixel image, it takes $N \times M$ clock cycles to complete the processing. In the line-parallel processing scheme employed in [7], both row-parallel and column-parallel processing scan the target image several times and the entire filtering finishes in $O(N+M)$ steps. (A single step includes several clock cycles to control the analog processing.)

The purpose of this work is to present an analog focal-plane CMOS image sensor chip which carries out the directional edge filtering convolution for an $N \times M$-pixel image only in M (or N) steps. In order to achieve an efficient processing, two key technologies have been introduced: "only-nearest-neighbor interconnects" architecture and "cyclic line access and row-parallel processing". The former was first developed in [8], and has enabled the convolution including second-nearest-neighbor luminance data only using nearest neighbor interconnects, thus greatly reducing the interconnect complexity. However, the fill factor was sacrificed due to the pixel parallel organization. The problem has been resolved in the present work by "cyclic line access and row-parallel processing." Namely, the processing elements are separated from the array of photo diodes and the "only-nearest-neighbor interconnects" architecture was realized as a separate module of row-parallel processing elements. The cyclic line access scheme first introduced in the present work has eliminated the redundant data readout operations from the photodiode array and has established a very efficient processing. As a result, it has become possible to complete the edge filtering for a 128×128 pixel image only in 128×2 steps. A proof-of-concept chip was fabricated in a 0.35-μm 2-poly 3-metal CMOS technology, and the edge detection at a rate of 200 frames/sec. has been experimentally demonstrated.

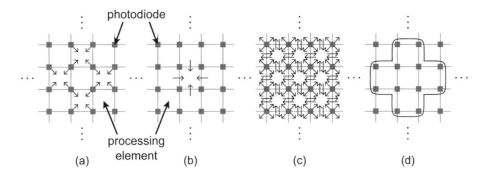

Figure 2: Edge filtering in the "only-nearest-neighbor interconnects" architecture: (a) first step; (b) second step; (c) all interconnects necessary for pixel parallel processing; (d) PD's involved in the convolution.

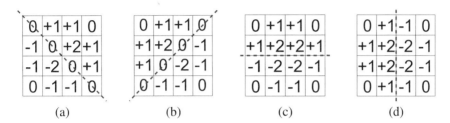

Figure 3: Edge filtering kernels realized in "only-nearest-neighbor interconnects" architecture: (a) $+45$ degree; (b) -45 degree; (c) horizontal; (d) vertical.

2 System Organization

The two key technologies employed in the present work are explained in the following.

2.1 "Only-Nearest-Neighbor Interconnects" Architecture

This architecture was first proposed in [8], and experimentally verified with small-scale test circuits (7×7 processing elements without photodiodes). The key feature of the architecture is that photodiodes (PD's) are placed at four corners of each processing element (PE), and that the luminance data of each PD are shared by four PE's as shown in Fig. 2.

The edge filtering is carried out as explained below. First, as shown in Fig. 2 (a), pre-processing is carried out in each PE using the luminance data taken from four PD's located at its corners. Then, the result is transferred to the center PE as shown in Fig. 2 (b) and necessary computation is carried out. This accomplishes the filtering processing for one half of the entire pixels. Then the roles of pre-processing PE's and center PE's are interchanged and the same procedure follows to complete the processing for the rest of the pixels. The interconnects necessary for the entire parallel processing is shown in Fig. 2(c). In this manner, every PE can gather all data necessary for the processing from its nearest-neighbor and second nearest-neighbor pixels without complicated crossover interconnects. The kernels illustrated in Fig. 3 have been all realized in this architecture. The luminance data from 12 PD's enclosed in Fig. 2 (d) are utilized to detect the edge information at the center location.

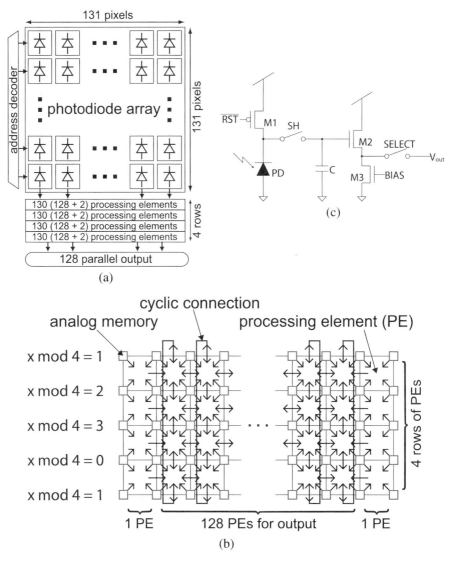

Figure 4: Block diagram of the chip (a), and organization of row-parallel processing module (b). x in (b) represents the row number $1 \sim 131$. (c) shows read out circuit of photodiode.

2.2 Cyclic Line Access and Row-Parallel Processing

A block diagram of the analog edge-filtering processor is given in Fig. 4 (a). It consists of an array of 131×131 photodiodes (PD's) and a module for row-parallel processing placed at the bottom of the PD array. Figure 4(b) illustrates the organization of the row processing module, which is composed of four rows of 130 PE's and five rows of 131 analog memory cells that temporarily store the luminance data read out from the PD array. It should be noted that only three rows of PE's and four rows of PD's are sufficient to carry out a single-row processing as explained in reference to Fig. 2(d). However, one extra row of PE's and one extra row of analog memories for PD data storage were included in the row-parallel processing module. This is essential to carry out a seamless data read out from the PD array and computation without analog data shift within the processing module. The chip yields

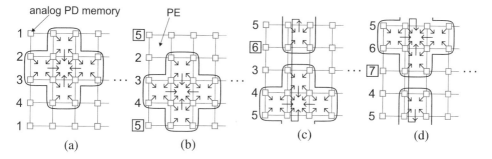

Figure 5: "Cyclic-line access and row-parallel processing" scheme.

the kernel convolution results for one of the rows in the PD array as 128 parallel outputs.

Now, the operation of the row-parallel processing module is explained with reference to Fig. 4 (b) and Fig. 5. In order to carry out the convolution for the data in Row 1~4, the PD data are temporarily stored in the analog memory array as shown in Fig. 5 (a). Imporatant to note is that the data from Row 1 are duplicated at the bottom. The convolution operation proceeds using the upper four rows of data as explained in Fig. 5 (a). In the next step, the data from Row 5 are overwritten to the sites of Row 1 data as shown in Fig. 5 (b). The operation proceeds using the lower four rows of data and the second set of outputs is produced. In the third step, the data from Row 6 is overwritten to the sites of Row 2 data (Fig. 5 (c)), and the convolution is taken using the data in the enclosure. Although a part of the data (top two rows) are separated from the rest, the topology of the hardware computation is identical to that explained in Fig. 5 (a). This is because the same set of data is stored in both top and bottom PD memories and the top and bottom PE's are connected by "cyclic connection" as illustrated in Fig. 4 (b). By introducing such one extra row of PD memories and one extra row of PE's with cyclic interconnections, row-parallel processing can be seamlessly performed with only a single-row PD data set download at each step.

3 Circuit Configurations

In this architecture, we need only two arithmetic operations, i.e., the sum of four inputs and the subtraction.

Figure 6(a) shows the adder circuit using the multiple-input floating-gate source follower [9]. The substrate of $M1$ is connected to the source to avoid the body effect. The transistor $M2$ operates as a current source for fast output voltage stabilization as well as to achieve good linearity. Due to the charge redistribution in the floating gate, the average of the four input voltages appears at the output as

$$V_{\text{out}} = \frac{V_1 + V_2 + V_3 + V_4}{4} + |V_{\text{th}}|,$$

where V_{th} represents the threshold voltage of $M1$. Here, the four coupling capacitors connected to the floating gate of $M1$ are identical and the capacitance coupling between the floating gate and the ground was assumed to be 0 for simplicity. The electrical charge in the floating gate is initialized periodically using the reset switch ($M3$). The coupling capacitors themselves are also utilized as temporary memories for the PD data read out from the PD array.

Figure 6(b) shows the subtraction circuit, where the same source follower was used. When SW1 and SW2 are turned on, and SW3 is turned off, the following voltage difference is

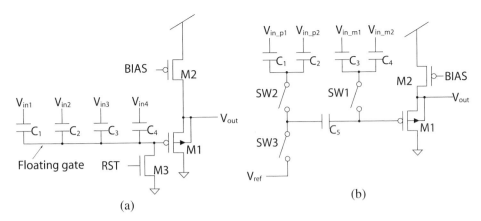

Figure 6: Adder circuit (a) and subtraction circuit (b) using floating-gate MOS technology.

developed across the capacitor C_5:

$$\frac{(V_{\text{in\_p1}} + V_{\text{in\_p2}}) - (V_{\text{in\_m1}} + V_{\text{in\_m2}})}{4}.$$

Then, SW1 and SW2 are turned off, and SW3 is turned on. As a result, the output voltage V_{out} becomes

$$V_{\text{out}} = \frac{(V_{\text{in\_p1}} + V_{\text{in\_p2}}) - (V_{\text{in\_m1}} + V_{\text{in\_m2}})}{4} + V_{\text{ref}} + |V_{\text{th}}|,$$

where V_{th} represents the threshold voltage of $M1$.

4   Experimental Results

A proof-of-concept chip was designed and fabricated in a 0.35-μm 2-poly 3-metal CMOS technology. Figure 7 shows the photomicrograph of the chip, and the chip specifications are given in Table 1. Since the pitch of a single PE unit is larger than the pitch of the PD array, 130 PE units are laid out as two separate L-shaped blocks at the periphery of the PD array as seen in the chip photomicrograph. Successful operation of the chip was experimentally verified.

An example is shown in Fig. 8, where the experimental results for -45-degree edge filtering are demonstrated. Since the thresholding circuitry was not implemented in the present chip, only the convolution results are shown. 128 parallel outputs from the test chip were multiplexed for observation using the external multiplexers mounted on a milled printed circuit board. The vertical stripes observed in the result are due to the resistance variation in the external interconnects poorly produced on the milled printed circuit board.

It was experimentally confirmed the chip operates at 1000 frames/sec. However, the operation is limited by the integration time of PD's and typical motion images are processed at about 200 frames/sec. The power dissipation in the PE's was 25 mW and that in the PD array was 40mW.

5   Conclusions

An analog edge-filtering processor has been developed based on the two key technologies: "only-nearest-neighbor interconnects" architecture and "cyclic line access and row-parallel

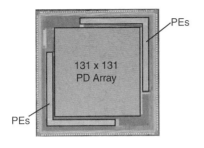

Figure 7: Chip photomicrograph.

Table 1: Chip Specifications.

Process Technology	0.35 μm CMOS, 2-Poly, 3-Metal
Die Size	9.8 mm x 9.8 mm
Voltage Supply	3.3 V
Operating Frequency	50M Hz
Power Dissipation	25 mW (PE Array)
PE Operation	1000 Frames/secl
Typical Frame Ratel	200 Frames / sec (limited by PD integration time)

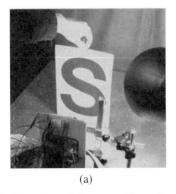
(a)

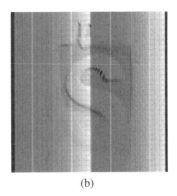
(b)

Figure 8: Experimental set up (a), and measurement results of -45 degree edge filtering convolution (b).

processing". As a result, the convolution operation involving second nearest-neighbor pixel data for an $N \times N$-pixel image can be performed only in $2N$ steps. The edge filtering operation for 128×128-pixel images at 200 frames/sec. has been experimentally demonstrated. The chip meets the requirement of low-power and real-time-response applications.

6 Acknowledgments

The VLSI chip in this study was fabricated in the chip fabrication program of VLSI Design and Education Center (VDEC), the University of Tokyo in collaboration with Rohm Corporation and Toppan Printing Corporation. The work is partially supported by the Ministry of Education, Science, Sports, and Culture under Grant-in-Aid for Scientific Research (No. 14205043).

References

[1] D. H. Hubel and T. N. Wiesel, "Receptive fields of single neurons in the cat's striate cortex," *Journal of Physiology*, vol. 148, pp. 574-591, 1959.

[2] M. Yagi and T. Shibata, "An image representation algorithm compatible with neural-associative-processor-based hardware recognition systems," *IEEE Trans. Neural Networks*, vol. 14(5), pp. 1144-1161, 2003.

[3] J. C. Gealow and C. G. Sodini, "A pixel parallel-processor using logic pitch-matched to dynamic memory," *IEEE J. Solid-State Circuits*, vol. 34, pp. 831-839, 1999.

[4] K. Ito, M. Ogawa and T. Shibata, "A variable-kernel flash-convolution image filtering processor," *Dig. Tech. Papers of Int. Solid-State Circuits Conf.*, pp. 470-471, 2003.

[5] L. D. McIlrath, "A CCD/CMOS focal plane array edge detection processor implementing the multiscale veto algorithm," *IEEE J. Solid-State Circuits*, vol. 31(9), pp. 1239-1247, 1996.

[6] R. Etiene-Cummings, Z. K. Kalayjian and D. Cai, "A programmable focal plane MIMD image processor chip," *IEEE J. Solid-State Circuits*, vol. 36(1), pp. 64-73, 2001.

[7] T. Taguchi, M. Ogawa and T. Shibata, "An Analog Image Processing LSI Employing Scanning Line Parallel Processing," *Proc. 29th European Solid-Sate Circuits Conference (ESSCIRC 2003)*, pp. 65-68, 2003.

[8] Y. Nakashita, Y. Mita and T. Shibata, "An Analog Edge-Filtering Processor Employing Only-Nearest-Neighbor Interconnects," *Ext. Abstracts of the International Conference on Solid State Devices and Materials (SSDM '04)*, pp. 356-357, 2004.

[9] T. Shibata and T. Ohmi, "A Functional MOS Transistor Featuring Gate-Level Weighted Sum and Threshold Operations," *IEEE Trans. Electron Devices*, vol. 39(6), pp. 1444-1455, 1992.

Q-Clustering

Mukund Narasimhan[†]   **Nebojsa Jojic**[‡]   **Jeff Bilmes**[†]

[†]Dept of Electrical Engineering, University of Washington, Seattle WA

[‡]Microsoft Research, Microsoft Corporation, Redmond WA

{mukundn,bilmes}@ee.washington.edu and jojic@microsoft.com

Abstract

We show that Queyranne's algorithm for minimizing symmetric submodular functions can be used for clustering with a variety of different objective functions. Two specific criteria that we consider in this paper are the single linkage and the minimum description length criteria. The first criterion tries to maximize the minimum distance between elements of different clusters, and is inherently "discriminative". It is known that optimal clusterings into k clusters for any given k in polynomial time for this criterion can be computed. The second criterion seeks to minimize the description length of the clusters given a probabilistic generative model. We show that the optimal partitioning into 2 clusters, and approximate partitioning (guaranteed to be within a factor of 2 of the the optimal) for more clusters can be computed. To the best of our knowledge, this is the first time that a tractable algorithm for finding the optimal clustering with respect to the MDL criterion for 2 clusters has been given. Besides the optimality result for the MDL criterion, the chief contribution of this paper is to show that the *same algorithm* can be used to optimize a broad class of criteria, and hence can be used for many application specific criterion for which efficient algorithm are not known.

1 Introduction

The clustering of data is a problem found in many pattern recognition tasks, often in the guises of unsupervised learning, vector quantization, dimensionality reduction, etc. Formally, the clustering problem can be described as follows. Given a finite set S, and a criterion function J_k defined on all partitions of S into k parts, find a partition of S into k parts $\{S_1, S_2, \ldots, S_k\}$ so that $J_k(\{S_1, S_2, \ldots, S_k\})$ is maximized. The number of k-clusters for a size $n > k$ data set is roughly $k^n/k!$ [5] so exhaustive search is not an efficient solution. The problem, in fact, is NP-complete for most desirable measures. Broadly speaking there are two classes of criteria for clustering. There are distance based criteria, for which a distance measure is specified between each pair of elements, and the criterion somehow combines either intercluster or intracluster distances into an objective function. The other class of criteria are model based, and for these, a probabilistic (generative) model is specified. There is no universally accepted criterion for clustering. The appropriate criterion is typically application dependent, and therefore, we do not claim that the two criteria considered in this paper are inherently better or more generally applicable than other criteria. However, we can show that for the single-linkage criterion, we can compute the optimal clustering into k parts (for any k), and for the MDL criterion, we can compute the optimal clustering into 2 parts using Queyranne's algorithm. More generally, any criterion from a broad class of criterion can be solved by the *same algorithm*, and this class of criteria is closed under linear combinations. In addition to the theoretical elegance of a single algorithm solving a number of very different criterion, this means that we can optimize (for example) for the sum of single-linkage and MDL criterions (or positively scaled versions thereof). The two criterion we consider are quite different. The first, "discriminative", criterion we consider is the single-linkage criterion. In this case, we are given distances $d(s_1, s_2)$ between all elements $s_1, s_2 \in S$, and we try and find clusters that maximize the minimum distance between elements of different clusters (i.e., maximize the separation of the clusters). This criterion has several advantages. Since we are only comparing distances, the distance measure can be chosen from any ordered set (addition/squaring/multiplication of distances need not be defined as is required for K-means, spectral clustering etc.). Further, this criterion only depends on the rank ordering of the distances, and so is completely insensitive to any monotone transformation of the distances. This gives a lot of flexibility in constructing a distance measure appropriate for an application. For example, it is a very natural candidate when the distance measure is derived from user studies (since users are more likely to be able to provide rankings than exact distances). On the other hand, this criterion is sensitive to outliers and may not be appropriate when there are a large number of outliers in the data set. The kernel based criterion considered in [3] is similar in spirit to this one. However, their algorithm only provides approximate solutions, and the extension to more than 2 clusters is not given. However, since they optimize the distance of the clusters to a hyperplane, it is more appropriate if the clusters are to be classified using a SVM.

The second criterion we consider is "generative" in nature and is based on the Minimum Description Length principle. In this case we are given a (generative) probability model for the elements, and we attempt to find clusters so that describing or encoding the clusters (separately) can be done using as few bits as possible. This is also a very natural criterion - grouping together data items that can be highly compressed translates to grouping elements that share common characteristics. This criterion has also been widely used in the past, though the algorithms given do not guarantee optimal solutions (even for 2 clusters).

Since these criteria seem quite different in nature, it is surprising that the same algorithm can be used to find the *optimal* partitions into two clusters in both cases. The key principle here is the notion of submodularity (and its variants) [1, 2]. We will show that the problem of finding the optimal clusterings minimizing the description length is equivalent to the problem of minimizing a symmetric submodular function, and the problem of maximizing the cluster separation is equivalent to minimizing a symmetric function which, while not submodular, is closely related, and can be minimized by the same algorithm.

2 Background and Notation

A *clustering* of a finite set S is a partition $\{S_1, S_2, \ldots, S_k\}$ of S. We will call the individual elements of the partition the clusters of the partition. If there are k clusters in the partition, then we say that the partition is a k-clustering. Let $\mathcal{C}_k(S)$ be the set of all k-clusterings for $1 \leq k \leq |S|$. For the first criterion, we assume we are given a function $d : S \times S \rightarrow \mathbb{R}$ that represents the "distance" between objects. Intuitively, we expect that $d(s, t)$ is large when the objects are dissimilar. We will assume that $d(\cdot, \cdot)$ is symmetric, but make no further assumptions. In particular we do not assume that $d(\cdot, \cdot)$ is a metric (Later on in this paper, we will not even assume that $d(s, t)$ is a (real) number, but instead will allow the range of d to be a ordered set). The distance between sets T and R is often defined to be the smallest distance between elements from these different clusters: $D(R, T) = \min_{r \in R, t \in T} d(r, t)$. The single-linkage criterion tries to maximize this distance, and hence an optimal 2-clustering is in $\arg\max_{\{S_1, S_2\} \in \mathcal{C}_2(S)} D(S_1, S_2)$. We let $\mathcal{O}_k(S)$ be the set of all optimal k-clusterings for $1 \leq k \leq |S|$ with respect to $D(\cdot, \cdot)$. It is known that an algorithm based on the Minimum Spanning Tree can be used to find optimal clusterings for the single-linkage criterion[8].

For the second criterion, we assume S is a collection of random variables, and for any subset $T = \{s_1, s_2, \ldots, s_m\}$ of S, we let $H(T)$ be the entropy of the set of random variables $\{s_1, s_2, \ldots, s_m\}$. Now, the (expected) total cost of encoding or describing the set T is $H(T)$. So a partition $\{S_1, S_2\}$ of S that minimizes the description length (DL) is in

$$\underset{\{S_1, S_2\} \in \mathcal{C}_2(S)}{\arg\min} \quad DL(S_1, S_2) = \underset{\{S_1, S_2\} \in \mathcal{C}_2(S)}{\arg\min} \quad H(S_1) + H(S_2)$$

We will denote by 2^S the set of all subsets of S. A set function $f : 2^S \to \mathbb{R}$ assigns a (real) number to every subset of S. We say that f is *submodular* if $f(A) + f(B) \geq f(A \cup B) + f(A \cap B)$ for every $A, B \subseteq S$. f is symmetric if $f(A) = f(S \setminus A)$. In [1], Queyranne gives a polynomial time algorithm that finds a set $A \in 2^S \setminus \{S, \phi\}$ that minimizes any symmetric submodular set function (specified in the form of an oracle). That is, Queyranne's algorithm finds a non-trivial partition $\{S_1, S \setminus S_1\}$ of S so that $f(S_1) \, (= f(S \setminus S_1))$ minimizes f over all non-trivial subsets of S. The problem of finding non-trivial minimizers of a symmetric submodular function can be thought of a a generalization of the graph-cut problem. For a symmetric set function f, we can think of $f(S_1)$ as $f(S_1, S \setminus S_1)$, and if we can extend f to be defined on all pairs of disjoint subsets of S, then Rizzi showed in [2] that Queyranne's algorithm works even when f is not submodular, as long as f is monotone and consistent, where f is *monotone* if for $R, T, T' \subseteq S$ with $T' \subseteq T$ and $R \cap T = \phi$ we have $f(R, T') \leq f(R, T)$ and f is *consistent* if $f(A, W \cup B) \geq f(B, A \cup W)$ whenever $A, B, W \subseteq S$ are disjoint sets satisfying $f(A, W) \geq f(B, W)$.

The rest of this paper is organized as follows. In Section 3, we show that Queyranne's algorithm can be used to find the optimal k-clustering (for any k) in polynomial time for the single-linkage criterion. In Section 4, we give an algorithm for finding the optimal clustering into 2 parts that minimizes the description length. In Section 5, we present some experimental results.

3 Single-Linkage: Maximizing the separation between clusters

In this section, we show that Queyranne's algorithm can be used for finding k-clusters (for any given k) that maximize the separation between elements of different clusters. We do this in two steps. First in Subsection 3.1, we show that Queyranne's algorithm can partition the set S into two parts to maximize the distance between these parts in polynomial time. Then in Subsection 3.2, we show how this subroutine can be used to find *optimal* k clusters, also in polynomial time.

3.1 Optimal 2-clusterings

In this section, we will show that the function $-D(\cdot, \cdot)$ is monotone and consistent. Therefore, by Rizzi's result, it follows that we can find a 2-clustering $\{S_1, S_2\} = \{S_1, S \setminus S_1\}$ that minimizes $-D(S_1, S_2)$, and hence maximizes $D(S_1, S_2)$.

Lemma 1. *If $R \subseteq T$, then $D(U, T) \leq D(U, R)$ (and hence $-D(U, R) \leq -D(U, T)$).*

This would imply that $-D$ is monotone. To see this, observe that

$$D(U, T) = \min_{u \in U, t \in T} d(u, t) = \min \left(\min_{u \in U, r \in R} d(u, r), \min_{u \in U, t \in T \setminus R} d(u, t) \right) \leq D(U, R)$$

Lemma 2. *Suppose that A, B, W are disjoint subsets of S and $D(A, W) \leq D(B, W)$. Then $D(A, W \cup B) \leq D(B, A \cup W)$.*

To see this first observe that $D(A, B \cup W) = \min(D(A, B), D(A, W))$ because

$$D(A, W \cup B) = \min_{a \in A, x \in W \cup B} D(a, x) = \min \left(\min_{a \in A, w \in W} D(a, w), \min_{a \in A, b \in B} D(A, b) \right)$$

It follows that $D(A, B \cup W) = \min(D(A, B), D(A, W)) \leq \min(D(A, B), D(B, W))$ $= \min(D(B, A), D(B, W)) = D(B, A \cup W)$. Therefore, if $-D(A, W) \geq -D(B, W)$, then $-D(A, W \cup B) \geq -D(B, A \cup W)$. Hence $-D(\cdot, \cdot)$ is consistent.

Therefore, $-D(\cdot, \cdot)$ is symmetric, monotone and consistent. Hence it can be minimized using Queyranne's algorithm [2]. Therefore, we have a procedure to compute optimal 2-clusterings. We now extend this to compute optimal k-clusterings.

3.2 Optimal k-clusterings

We start off by extending our objective function for k-clusterings in the obvious way. The function $D(R, T)$ can be thought of as defining the *separation* or *margin* between the clusters R and T. We can generalize this notion to more than two clusters as follows. Let

$$\mathsf{seperation}(\{S_1, S_2, \ldots, S_k\}) = \min_{i \neq j} D(S_i, S_j) = \min_{\substack{S_i \neq S_j \\ s_i \in S_i, s_j \in S_j}} d(s_i, s_j)$$

Note that $\mathsf{seperation}(\{R, T\}) = D(R, T)$ for a 2-clustering. The function $\mathsf{seperation} :$ $\cup_{k=1}^{|S|} \mathcal{C}_k(S) \to \mathbb{R}$ takes a single clustering as its argument. However, $D(\cdot, \cdot)$ takes two disjoint subsets of S as its arguments the union of which need not be S in general. The margin is the distance between the closest elements of different clusters, and hence we will be interested in finding k-clusters that maximize the margin. Therefore, we seek an element in $\mathcal{O}_k(S) = \arg\max_{\{S_1, S_2, \ldots, S_k\} \in \mathcal{C}_k(S)} \mathsf{seperation}(\{S_1, S_2, \ldots, S_k\})$. Let $v_k(S)$ be the margin of an element in $\mathcal{O}_k(S)$. Therefore, $v_k(S)$ is the best possible margin of any k-clustering of S. An obvious approach to generating optimal k-clusterings given a method of generating optimal 2-clusterings is the following. Start off with an optimal 2-clustering $\{S_1, S_2\}$. Then apply the procedure to find 2-clusterings of S_1 and S_2, and stop when you have enough clusters. There are two potential problems with this approach. First, it is not clear that an optimal k-clustering can be a refinement of an optimal 2-clustering. That is, we need to be sure that there is an optimal k-clustering in which S_1 is the union of some of the clusters, and S_2 is the union of the remaining. Second, we need to figure out how many of the clusters S_1 is the union of and how many S_2 is the union of. In this section, we will show that for any $k \geq 3$, there is always an optimal k-clustering that is a refinement of any given optimal 2-clustering. A simple dynamic programming algorithm takes care of the second potential problem.

We begin by establishing some relationships between the separation of clusterings of different sizes. To compare the separation of clusterings with different number of clusters, we can try and merge two of the clusters from the clustering with more clusters. Say that $\mathcal{S} = \{S_1, S_2, \ldots, S_k\} \in \mathcal{C}_k(S)$ is any k-clustering of S, and $\mathcal{S}'$ is a $(k-1)$-clustering of S obtained by merging two of the clusters (say S_1 and S_2). Then $\mathcal{S}' = \{S_1 \cup S_2, S_3, \ldots, S_k\} \in \mathcal{C}_{k-1}(S)$.

Lemma 3. *Suppose that* $\mathcal{S} = \{S_1, S_2, \ldots, S_k\} \in \mathcal{C}_k(S)$ *and* $\mathcal{S}' = \{S_1 \cup S_2, S_3, \ldots, S_k\} \in \mathcal{C}_{k-1}(S)$. *Then* $\mathsf{seperation}(\mathcal{S}) \leq \mathsf{seperation}(\mathcal{S}')$. *In other words, refining a partition can only reduce the margin.*

Therefore, refining a clustering (i.e., splitting a cluster) can only reduce the separation. An immediate corollary is the following.

Corollary 4. *If* $\mathcal{T}_l \in \mathcal{C}_l(S)$ *is a refinement of* $\mathcal{T}_k \in \mathcal{C}_k(S)$ *(for* $k < l$*) then* $\mathsf{seperation}(\mathcal{T}_l) \leq \mathsf{seperation}(\mathcal{T}_k)$. *It follows that* $v_k(S) \geq v_l(S)$ *if* $1 \leq k < l \leq n$.

Proof. It suffices to prove the result for $k = l - 1$. The first assertion follows immediately from Lemma 3. Let $\mathcal{S} \in \mathcal{O}_l(S)$ be an optimal l-clustering. Merge any two clusters to get $\mathcal{S}' \in \mathcal{C}_k(S)$. By Lemma 3, $v_k(S) \geq \mathsf{seperation}(\mathcal{S}') \geq \mathsf{seperation}(\mathcal{S}) = v_l(S)$. $\qquad\square$

Next, we consider the question of constructing larger partitions (i.e., partitions with more clusters) from smaller partitions. Given two clusterings $S = \{S_1, S_2, \ldots, S_k\} \in \mathcal{C}_k(S)$ and $\mathcal{T} = \{T_1, T_2, \ldots, T_l\} \in \mathcal{C}_l(S)$ of S, we can create a new clustering $\mathcal{U} = \{U_1, U_2, \ldots, U_m\} \in \mathcal{C}_m(S)$ to be their common refinement. That is, the clusters of $\mathcal{U}$ consist of those elements that are in the same clusters of both S and $\mathcal{T}$. Formally,

$$\mathcal{U} = \{ S_i \cap T_j : 1 \le i \le k, \, 1 \le j \le l \}$$

Lemma 5. *Let $S = \{S_1, S_2, \ldots, S_k\} \in \mathcal{C}_k(S)$ and $\mathcal{T} = \{T_1, T_2, \ldots, T_l\} \in \mathcal{C}_l(S)$ be any two partitions. Let $\mathcal{U} = \{U_1, U_2, \ldots, U_m\} \in \mathcal{C}_m(S)$ be their common refinement. Then* $\operatorname{seperation}(\mathcal{U}) = \min\left(\operatorname{seperation}(S), \operatorname{seperation}(\mathcal{T})\right)$.

Proof. It is clear that $\operatorname{seperation}(\mathcal{U}) \le \min\left(\operatorname{seperation}(S), \operatorname{seperation}(\mathcal{T})\right)$. To show equality, note that if a, b are in different clusters of $\mathcal{U}$, then a, b must have been in different clusters of either S or $\mathcal{T}$. $\qquad\square$

This result can be thought of as expressing a relationship between seperation and the lattice of partitions of S which will be important to our later robustness extension

Lemma 6. *Suppose that $S = \{S_1, S_2\} \in \mathcal{O}_2(S)$ is an optimal 2-clustering. Then there is always an optimal k-clustering that is a refinement of S.*

Proof. Suppose that this is not the case. If $\mathcal{T} = \{T_1, T_2, \ldots, T_k\} \in \mathcal{O}_k(S)$ is an optimal k-clustering, let r be the number of clusters of $\mathcal{T}$ that "do not respect" the partition $\{S_1, S_2\}$. That is, r is the number of clusters of $\mathcal{T}$ that intersect both S_1 and S_2 : $r = |\{1 \le i \le k : T_i \cap S_1 \ne \phi \text{ and } T_i \cap S_2 \ne \phi\}|$. Pick $\mathcal{T} \in \mathcal{O}_k(S)$ to have the smallest r. If $r = 0$, then $\mathcal{T}$ is a refinement of S and there is nothing to show. Otherwise, $r \ge 1$. Assume WLOG that $T_1^{(1)} = T_1 \cap S_1 \ne \phi$ and $T_1^{(2)} = T_1 \cap S_2 \ne \phi$. Then $\mathcal{T}' = \left\{ T_1^{(1)}, T_1^{(2)}, T_2, T_3, \ldots, T_k \right\} \in \mathcal{C}_{k+1}(S)$ is a refinement of $\mathcal{T}$ and satisfies $\operatorname{seperation}(\mathcal{T}') = \operatorname{seperation}(\mathcal{T})$. This follows from Lemma 3 along with the fact that **(1)** $D(T_i, T_j) \ge \operatorname{seperation}(\mathcal{T})$ for any $2 \le i < j \le k$, **(2)** $D(T_1^{(i)}, T_j) \ge \operatorname{seperation}(\mathcal{T})$ for any $i \in \{1, 2\}$ and $2 \le j \le k$, **(3)** $D(T_1^{(1)}, T_1^{(2)}) \ge \operatorname{seperation}(\{S_1, S_2\}) = v_2(S) \ge v_k(S) = \operatorname{seperation}(\mathcal{T})$.

Now, pick two clusters of $\mathcal{T}'$ that are either both contained in the same cluster of S or both "do not respect" S. Clearly this can always be done. Merge these clusters together to get an element $\mathcal{T}'' \in \mathcal{C}_k(S)$. By Lemma 3 merging clusters cannot decrease the margin. Therefore, $\operatorname{seperation}(\mathcal{T}'') = \operatorname{seperation}(\mathcal{T}') = \operatorname{seperation}(\mathcal{T})$. However, $\mathcal{T}''$ has fewer clusters that do not respect S hand $\mathcal{T}$ has, and hence we have a contradiction. $\qquad\square$

This lemma implies that Queyranne's algorithm, along with a simple dynamic programming algorithm can be used to find the best k clustering with time complexity $O(k|S|^3)$. Observe that in fact this problem can be solved in time $O(|S|^2)$ ([8]). Even though using Queyranne's algorithm is not the fastest algorithm for this problem, the fact that it optimizes this criterion implies that it can be used to optimize conic combinations of submodular criteria and the single-linkage criterion.

3.3 Generating robust clusterings

One possible issue with the metric we defined is that it is very sensitive to outliers and noise. To see this, note that if we have two very well separated clusters, then adding a few points "between" the clusters could dramatically decrease the separation. To increase the robustness of the algorithm, we can try to maximize the n smallest distances instead of maximizing just the smallest distance between clusters. If we give the nth smallest distance more importance than the smallest distance, this increases the noise tolerance by ignoring the effects of a few outliers. We will take $n \in \mathbb{N}$ to be some fixed positive integer specified by the user. This will represent the desired degree of noise tolerance (larger gives more noise tolerance). Let $\mathcal{R}_n$ be the set of decreasing n-tuples of elements in $\mathbb{R} \cup \{\infty\}$. Given disjoint sets $R, T \subseteq S$, let $D(R, T)$ be the element of $\mathcal{R}_n$ obtained as follows. Let $L(R, T) = \langle d_1, d_2, \ldots, d_{|R| \cdot |T|} \rangle$ be an ordered list of distances between elements of R and T arranged in decreasing order. So for example, if $R = \{1, 2\}$ and $T = \{3, 4\}$, with $d(r, t) = r \cdot t$, then $L(R, T) = \langle 8, 6, 4, 3 \rangle$. We define $D(R, T)$ as follows. If $|R| \cdot |T| \geq n$, then $D(R, T)$ is the last (and thus least) n elements of $L(R, T)$. Otherwise, if $|R| \cdot |T| < n$, then the first $n - |R| \cdot |T|$ elements of $D(R, T)$ are ∞, while the remaining elements are the elements of $L(R, T)$. So for example, if $n = 2$, then $D(R, T)$ in the above example would be $\langle 4, 3 \rangle$, if $n = 3$ then $D(R, T) = \langle 6, 4, 3 \rangle$ and if $n = 6$, then $D(R, T) = \langle \infty, \infty, 8, 6, 4, 3 \rangle$.

We define an operation $\oplus$ on $\mathcal{R}_n$ as follows. To get $\langle l_1, l_2, \ldots, l_n \rangle \oplus \langle r_1, r_2, \ldots, r_n \rangle$, order the elements of $\langle l_1, l_2, \ldots, l_n, r_1, r_2, \ldots, r_n \rangle$ in decreasing order, and let $\langle s_1, s_2, \ldots, s_n \rangle$ be the last n elements. For example, $\langle \infty, 3, 2 \rangle \oplus \langle \infty, 6, 5 \rangle = \langle 5, 3, 2 \rangle$ and $\langle 4, 3, 1 \rangle \oplus \langle 5, 4, 3 \rangle = \langle 3, 3, 1 \rangle$. So, the $\oplus$ operation picks off the n smallest elements. It is clear that this operation is commutative (symmetric), associative and that $\langle \infty, \infty, \ldots, \infty \rangle$ acts as an identity. Therefore, $\mathcal{R}_n$ forms a commutative semigroup. In fact, we can describe $D(R, T)$ as follows. For any pair of distinct elements $r, t \in S$, let $d'(r, t) = \langle \infty, \infty, \ldots, d(r, t) \rangle$. Then $D(R, T) = \bigoplus_{r \in R, t \in T} d'(r, t)$. Notice the similarity to $D(R, T) = \min_{r \in R, t \in T} d(r, t)$. In fact, if we take $n = 1$, then the $\oplus$ operation reduces to the minimum operation and we get back our original definitions. We can order $\mathcal{R}_n$ lexicographically. Therefore, $\mathcal{R}_n$ becomes an ordered semigroup. It is entirely straightforward to check that if $R \subseteq T$, then $D(U, T) \prec D(U, R)$, and that if A, B, W are disjoint sets with $D(A, W) \prec D(B, W)$, then $D(A, W \cup B) \prec D(B, A \cup W)$. It is also straightforward to extend Rizzi's proof to see that Queyranne's algorithm (with the obvious modifications) will generate a 2-clustering that minimizes this metric. It can also be verified that the results of Section 3.2 can be extended to this framework (also with the obvious modifications).

In our experiments, we observed that selecting the parameter n is quite tricky. Now, Queyranne's algorithm actually produces a (Gomory-Hu tree [1]) whose edges represent the cost of separating elements. In practice we noticed that restricting our search to only edges whose deletion results in clusters of at least certain sizes produces very good results. Other heuristics such as running the algorithm a number of times to eliminate outliers are also reasonable approaches. Modifying the algorithm to yield good results while retaining the theoretical guarantees is an open question.

4 MDL Clustering

We assume that S is a collection of random variables for which we have a (generative) probability model. Since we have the joint probabilities of all subsets of the random variables, the entropy of any collection of the variables is well defined. The expected coding (or description) length of any collection T of random variables using an optimal coding scheme (or a random coding scheme) is known to be $H(T)$. The partition $\{S_1, S_2\}$ of S that minimizes the coding length is therefore $\arg\min_{\{S_1, S_2\} \in \mathcal{C}_2(S)} H(S_1) + H(S_2)$. Now,

$$\arg\min_{\{S_1, S_2\} \in \mathcal{C}_2(S)} H(S_1) + H(S_2) = \arg\min_{\{S_1, S_2\} \in \mathcal{C}_2(S)} H(S_1) + H(S_2) - H(S)$$

$$= \arg\min_{\{S_1, S_2\} \in \mathcal{C}_2(S)} I(S_1; S_2)$$

where $I(S_1; S_2)$ is the mutual information between S_1 and S_2 because $S_1 \cup S_2 = S$ for all $\{S_1, S_2\} \in \mathcal{C}_2(S)$, Therefore, the problem of partitioning S into two parts to minimize the description length is equivalent to partitioning S into two parts to minimize the mutual information between the parts. It is shown in [9] that the function $f : 2^S \rightarrow \mathbb{R}$

defined by $f(T) = I(T; S \setminus T)$ is symmetric and submodular. Clearly the minima of this function correspond to partitions that minimize the mutual information between the parts. Therefore, the problem of partitioning in order to minimize the mutual information between the parts can be reduced to a symmetric submodular minimization problem, which can be solved using Queyranne's algorithm in time $O(|S|^3)$ assuming oracle queries to a mutual information oracle. While implementing such a mutual information oracle is not trivial, for many realistic applications (including one we consider in this paper), the cost of computing a mutual information query is bounded above by the size of the data set, and so the entire algorithm is polynomial in the size of the data set. Symmetric submodular functions generalize notions like graph-cuts, and indeed, Queyranne's algorithm generalizes an algorithm for computing graph-cuts. Since graph-cut based techniques are extensively used in many engineering applications, it might be possible to develop criteria that are more appropriate for these specific applications, while still retaining producing optimal partitions of size 2.

It should be noted that, in general, we cannot use the dynamic programming algorithm to produce optimal clusterings with $k > 2$ clusters for the MDL criterion (or for general symmetric submodular functions). The key reason is that we cannot prove the equivalent of Lemma 6 for the MDL criterion. However, such an algorithm seems reasonable, and it does produce reasonable results. Another approach (which is computationally cheaper) is to compute k clusters by deleting $k - 1$ edges of the Gomory-Hu tree produced by Queyranne's algorithm. It can be shown [9] that this will yield a factor 2 approximation to the optimal k-clustering. More generally, if we have an arbitrary increasing submodular function (such as entropy) $f : 2^S \to \mathbb{R}$, and we seek a clustering $\{S_1, S_2, \ldots, S_k\}$ to minimize the sum $\sum_{i=1}^{k} f(S_i)$, then we have an exact algorithm for 2-clusterings and a factor 2 approximation guarantee. Therefore, this generalizes approximation guarantees for graph k-cuts because for any graph $G = (V, E)$, the function $f : 2^V \to \mathbb{R}$ where $f(A)$ is the number of edges adjacent to the vertex set A is a submodular function. The finding a clustering to minimize $\sum_{i=1}^{k} f(S_i)$ is equivalent to finding a partition of the vertex set of size k to minimize the number of edges disconnected (i.e., to the graph k-cut problem). Another criterion which we can define similarly can be applied to clustering genomic sequences. Intuitively, two genomes are more closely related if they share more common subsequences. Therefore, a natural clustering criterion for sequences is to partition the sequences into clusters so that the sequences from different clusters share as few subsequences as possible. This problem too can be solved using this generic framework.

5   Results

Table 1 compares Q-Clustering with various other algorithms. The left part of the table shows the error rates (in percentages) of the (robust) single-linkage criterion and some other techniques on the same data set as is reported in [3]. The data sets are images (of digits and faces), and the distance function we used was the Euclidean distance between the vector of the pixels in the images. The right part of the table compares the Q-Clustering using MDL criterion with other state of the art algorithms for haplotype tagging of SNPs (single nucleotide polymorphisms) in the ACE gene on the data set reported in [4]. In this problem, the goal is to identify a set of SNPs that can accurately predict at least 90% of the SNPs in ACE gene. Typically the SNPs are highly correlated, and so it is necessary to cluster SNPs to identify the correlated SNPs. Note it is very important to identify as few SNPs as possible because the number of clinical trials required grows exponentially with the number of SNPs. As can be seen Q-Clustering does very well on this data set.

6   Conclusions

The maximum-separation (single-linkage) metric is a very natural "discriminative" criterion, and it has several advantages, including insensitivity to any monotone transformation of the distances. However, it is quite sensitive to outliers. The robust version does help

	Error rate on Digits	Error rate on Faces
Q-Clustering	1.4	0
Max-Margin[†]	3	0
Spectral Clust.[†]	6	16.7
K-means[†]	7	24.4

	#SNPs required
Q-Clustering	3
EigenSNP[‡]	5
Sliding Window[‡]	15
htStep (up)[‡]	7
htStep (down)[‡]	7

Table 1: Comparing (robust) max-separation and MDL Q-Clustering with other techniques. Results marked by [†] and [‡] are from [3] and [4] respectively.

a little, but it does require some additional knowledge (about the approximate number of outliers) and considerable tuning. It is possible that we could develop additional heuristics to automatically determine the parameters of the robust version. The MDL criterion is also a very natural one, and the results on haplotype tagging are quite promising. The MDL criterion can be seen as a generalization of graph cuts, and so it seems like Q-clustering can also be applied to optimize other criteria arising in problems like image segmentation, especially when there is a generative model. Another natural criterion for clustering strings is to partition the strings/sequences to minimize the number of common subsequences. This could have interesting applications in genomics. The key novelty of this paper is the guarantees of optimality produced by the algorithm, and the generaly framework into which a number of natural criterion fall.

7 Acknowledgments

The authors acknowledge the assistance of Linli Xu in obtaining the data to test the algorithm and for providing the code used in [3]. Gilles Blanchard pointed out that the MST algorithm finds the optimal solution for the single-linkage criterion. The first and third authors were supported by NSF grant IIS-0093430 and an Intel Corporation Grant.

References

[1] M. Queyranne. "Minimizing symmetric submodular functions", *Math. Programming*, 82, pages 3–12. 1998.

[2] R. Rizzi, "On Minimizing symmetric set functions", Combinatorica 20(3), pages 445–450, 2000.

[3] L. Xu, J. Neufeld, B. Larson and D. Schuurmans. "Maximum Margin Clustering", in Advances in Neural Information Processing Systems 17, pages 1537-1544, 2005.

[4] Z. Lin and R. B. Altman. "Finding Haplotype Tagging SNPs by Use of Principal Components Analysis", Am. J. Hum. Genet. 75, pages 850-861, 2004.

[5] Jain, A.K. and R.C. Dubes, "Algorithms for Clustering Data." Englewood Cliffs, N.J.: Prentice Hall, 1988.

[6] P. Brucker, "On the complexity of clustering problems," in R. Henn, B. Korte, and W. Oletti (eds.), Optimization and Operations Research, Lecture Notes in Economics and Mathematical Systems, Springer, Berlin 157.

[7] P. Kontkanen, P. Myllymäki, W. Buntine, J. Rissanen and H. Tirri. "An MDL framework for data clustering", HIIT Technical Report 2004.

[8] M. Delattre and P. Hansen. "Bicriterion Cluster Analysis", IEEE Transactions on Pattern Analysis and Machine Intelligence, Vol-2, No. 4, 1980

[9] M. Narasimhan, N. Jojic and J. Bilmes. "Q-Clustering", Technical Report, Dept. of Electrical Engg., University of Washington, UWEETR-2006-0001, 2005

Optimal cue selection strategy

Vidhya Navalpakkam
Department of Computer Science
USC, Los Angeles
navalpak@usc.edu

Laurent Itti
Department of Computer Science
USC, Los Angeles
itti@usc.edu

Abstract

Survival in the natural world demands the selection of relevant visual cues to rapidly and reliably guide attention towards prey and predators in cluttered environments. We investigate whether our visual system selects cues that guide search in an optimal manner. We formally obtain the optimal cue selection strategy by maximizing the signal to noise ratio ($\mathcal{SNR}$) between a search target and surrounding distractors. This optimal strategy successfully accounts for several phenomena in visual search behavior, including the effect of target-distractor discriminability, uncertainty in target's features, distractor heterogeneity, and linear separability. Furthermore, the theory generates a new prediction, which we verify through psychophysical experiments with human subjects. Our results provide direct experimental evidence that humans select visual cues so as to maximize SNR between the targets and surrounding clutter.

1 Introduction

Detecting a yellow tiger among distracting foliage in different shades of yellow and brown requires efficient top-down strategies that select relevant visual cues to enable rapid and reliable detection of the target among several distractors. For simple scenarios such as searching for a red target, the Guided Search theory [17] predicts that search efficiency can be improved by boosting the red feature in a top-down manner. But for more complex and natural scenarios such as detecting a tiger in the jungle or looking for a face in a crowd, finding the optimum amount of top-down enhancement to be applied to each low-level feature dimension encoded by the early visual system is non-trivial. It must not only consider features present in the target, but also those present in the distractors. In this paper, we formally obtain the optimal cue selection strategy and investigate whether our visual system has evolved to deploy it. In section 2, we formulate cue selection as an optimization problem where the relevant goal is to maximize the signal to noise ratio ($\mathcal{SNR}$) of the saliency map, so that the target becomes most salient and quickly draws attention, thereby minimizing search time. Next, we show through simulations that this optimal top-down guided search theory successfully accounts for several observed phenomena in visual search behavior, such as the effect of target-distractor discriminability, uncertainty in target's features, distractor heterogeneity, linear separability, and more. In section 4, we describe the design and analysis of psychophysics experiments to test new, counter-intuitive predictions of the theory. The results of our study suggest that humans deploy optimal cue selection strategies to detect targets in cluttered and distracting environments.

2 Formalizing visual search as an optimization problem

To quickly find a target among distractors, we wish to maximize the salience of the target relative to the distractors. Thus we can define the signal to noise ratio ($\mathcal{SNR}$) as the ratio of salience of the target to the distractors. Assuming that visual cues or features are encoded by populations of neurons in early visual areas, we define the optimal cue selection strategy as the best choice of neural response gain that maximizes the signal to noise ratio ($\mathcal{SNR}$). In the rest of this section, we formally obtain the optimal choice of gain in neural responses that will maximize $\mathcal{SNR}$.

$\mathcal{SNR}$ **in a visual search paradigm:** In a typical visual search paradigm, the salience of the target and distractors is a random variable that depends on their location in the search array, their features, the spatial configuration of target and distractors, and that varies between identical repeated trials due to internal noise in neural response to the visual input. Hence, we express $\mathcal{SNR}$ as the ratio of expected salience of the target over expected salience of the distractors, with the expectation taken over all possible target and distractor locations, their features and spatial configurations, and over several repeated trials.

$$\mathcal{SNR} = \frac{\text{Mean salience of the Target}}{\text{Mean salience of the distractor}}$$

Search array and its stimuli: Let search array A be a two-dimensional display that consists of one target T and several distractors D_j ($j = 1...N^2$-1). Let the display be divided into an invisible $N \times N$ grid, with one item occuring at each cell (x, y) in the grid. Let the color, contrast, orientation and other target parameters θ_T be chosen from a distribution $P(\theta|T)$. Similarly, for each distractor D_j, let its parameters θ_{D_j} be sampled independently from a distribution $P(\theta|D)$. Thus, search array A has a fixed choice of target and distractor parameters. Next, the spatial configuration C is decided by a random permutation of some assignment of the target and distractors to the N^2 cells in A (such that there is exactly one item in each cell). Thus, for a given search array A, the spatial configuration as well as stimulus parameters are fixed. Finally, given a choice of parameter θ and its spatial location (x, y), we generate an image pattern $R(\theta)$ (a set of pixels and their values) and embed it at location (x, y) in search array A. Thus, we generate search array A.

Saliency computation: Let the input search array A be processed by a population of neurons with gaussian tuning curves tuned to different stimulus parameters such as $\mu_1, \mu_2, ... \mu_n$. The output of this early visual processing stage is used to compute saliency maps $s_i(x, y, A)$ of search array A, that consist of the visual salience at every location (x, y) for feature-values $\mu_i(i = 1...n)$. Let $s_i(x, y, A)$ be combined linearly to form $S(x, y, A)$, the overall salience at location (x, y). Further, assuming a multiplicative gain g_i on the ith saliency map, we obtain:

$$S(x, y, A) \quad = \quad \sum_i g_i s_i(x, y, A) \tag{1}$$

Salience of the target and distractors: Let $S_T(A)$ be a random variable representing the salience of the target T in search array A. To factor out the variability due to internal noise η, we consider $E_\eta[S_T(A)]$, which is the mean salience of the target over repeated identical presentations of A. Further, let $E_C[S_T(A)]$ be the mean salience of the target averaged over all spatial configurations of a given set of target and distractor parameters. Similarly, $E_{\theta|T}[S_T(A)]$ is the mean salience of the target over all target parameters. The mean salience of the target combined over several repeated presentations of the search array A (to factor out internal noise η), over all spatial configurations C, and over all choices of target parameters $\theta|T$ is given below. Further, since η, C and θ are independent random variables, we can rewrite the joint expectation as follows:

$$E[S_T(A)] \quad = \quad E_{\theta|T}[E_C[E_\eta[S_T(A)]]] \tag{2}$$

Let $S_D(A)$ represent the mean salience of distractors D_j $(j = 1...N^2\text{-}1)$ in search array A. Similar to computing the mean salience of the target, we find the mean salience of distractors over all η, C and $\theta|D$.

$$S_D(A) \quad = \quad E_{D_j}[s_{iD_j}(A)] \tag{3}$$

$$E[S_D(A)] \quad = \quad E_{\theta|D}[E_C[E_\eta[S_D(A)]]] \tag{4}$$

$\mathcal{SNR}$ **and its optimization:** The additive salience and multiplicative gain hypothesis in eqn. 1 yields the following:

$$E[S_T(A)] \quad = \quad \sum_{i=1}^{n} g_i E_{\Theta|T}[E_C[E_\eta[s_{iT}(A)]]] \tag{5}$$

$$E[S_D(A)] \quad = \quad \sum_{i=1}^{n} g_i E_{\Theta|T}[E_C[E_\eta[s_{iT}(A)]]] \text{ (similarly)} \tag{6}$$

$\mathcal{SNR}$ can be expressed in terms of salience as:

$$\mathcal{SNR} \quad = \quad \frac{\sum_{i=1}^{n} g_i E_{\Theta|T}[E_C[E_\eta[s_{iT}(A)]]]}{\sum_{i=1}^{n} g_i E_{\Theta|D}[E_C[E_\eta[s_{iD}(A)]]]} \tag{7}$$

We wish to find the optimal choice of g_i that maximises $\mathcal{SNR}$. Hence, we differentiate $\mathcal{SNR}$ wrt g_i to get the following:

$$\frac{\partial}{\partial g_i}\mathcal{SNR} \quad = \quad \frac{\frac{E_{\Theta|T}[E_C[E_\eta[s_{iT}(A)]]]}{E_{\Theta|D}[E_C[E_\eta[s_{iD}(A)]]]} - \frac{\sum_{j=1}^{n} g_j E_{\Theta|T}[E_C[E_\eta[s_{jT}(A)]]]}{\sum_{j=1}^{n} g_j E_{\Theta|D}[E_C[E_\eta[s_{jD}(A)]]]}}{\frac{\sum_{j=1}^{n} g_j E_{\Theta|D}[E_C[E_\eta[s_{jD}(A)]]]}{E_{\Theta|D}[E_C[E_\eta[s_{iD}(A)]]]}} \tag{8}$$

$$= \quad \frac{\frac{\mathcal{SNR}_i}{\mathcal{SNR}} - 1}{\alpha_i} \tag{9}$$

where α_i is a normalization term and $\mathcal{SNR}_i$ is the signal-to-noise ratio of the ith saliency map.

$$\mathcal{SNR}_i = E_{\Theta|T}[E_C[E_\eta[s_{iT}(A)]]]/E_{\Theta|D}[E_C[E_\eta[s_{iD}(A)]]] \tag{10}$$

The sign of the derivative, $\left(\frac{d}{dg_i}\mathcal{SNR}\right)_{g_i=1}$ tells us whether g_i should be increased, decreased or maintained at the baseline activation 1 in order to maximize $\mathcal{SNR}$.

$$\frac{\mathcal{SNR}_i}{\mathcal{SNR}} \quad < \quad 1 \Rightarrow \frac{d}{dg_i}\mathcal{SNR} < 0 \Rightarrow \mathcal{SNR} \text{ increases as } g_i \text{ decreases} \Rightarrow g_i < 1 \tag{11}$$

$$= \quad 1 \Rightarrow \frac{d}{dg_i}\mathcal{SNR} = 0 \Rightarrow \mathcal{SNR} \text{ does not change with } g_i \Rightarrow g_i = 1 \tag{12}$$

$$> \quad 1 \Rightarrow \frac{d}{dg_i}\mathcal{SNR} > 0 \Rightarrow \mathcal{SNR} \text{ increases as } g_i \text{ increases} \Rightarrow g_i > 1 \tag{13}$$

Thus, we obtain an intuitive result that g_i increases as $\frac{\mathcal{SNR}_i}{\mathcal{SNR}}$ increases. We simplify this monotonic relationship assuming proportionality. Further, if we impose a restriction that the gains cannot be increased indiscriminately, but must sum to some constant, say the total number of saliency maps (n), we have the following:

$$\text{let } g_i \propto \frac{\mathcal{SNR}_i}{\mathcal{SNR}} \tag{14}$$

$$\text{if } \sum_i g_i = n \quad \Rightarrow \quad g_i = \frac{\mathcal{SNR}_i}{\frac{\sum_i \mathcal{SNR}_i}{n}} \tag{15}$$

Thus the gain of a saliency map tuned to a band of feature-values depends on the strength of the signal-to-noise ratio in that band compared to the mean signal-to-noise ratio in all bands in that feature dimension.

3 Predictions of the optimal cue selection strategy

To understand the implications of biasing features according to the optimal cue selection strategy, we simulate a simple model of early visual cortex. We assume that each feature dimension is encoded by a population of neurons with overlapping gaussian tuning curves that are broadly tuned to different features in that dimension. Let $f_i(\theta)$ represent the tuning curve of the ith neuron in a population of broadly tuned neurons with overlapping tuning curves. Let the tuning width σ and amplitude a be equal for all neurons, and μ_i represent the preferred stimulus parameter (or feature) of the ith neuron.

$$f_i(\theta) = \frac{a}{\sigma} \exp\left(-\frac{(\theta - \mu_i)^2}{2\sigma^2}\right) \qquad (16)$$

Let $\vec{r}(\Theta(x, y, A)) = \{r_1(\Theta(x, y, A))...r_n(\Theta(x, y, A))\}$ be the population response to a stimulus parameter $\Theta(x, y, A)$ at a location (x, y) in search array A, where r_i refers to the response of the ith neuron and n is the total number of neurons in the population. Let the neural response $r_i(\Theta(x, y, A))$ be a Poisson random variable.

$$P(r_i(\Theta(x, y, A)) = z) \quad = \quad P_{f_i(\Theta(x,y,A))}(z) \qquad (17)$$

For simplicity, let's assume that the local neural response $r_i(\Theta(x, y, A))$ is a measure of salience $s_i(x, y, A)$. Using eqns. 2, 4, 10, 16, 17, we can derive the mean salience of the target and distractor, and use it to compute $\mathcal{SNR}_i$.

$$s_i(x, y, A) \quad = \quad r_i(\Theta(x, y, A)) \qquad (18)$$
$$E[s_{iT}(A)] \quad = \quad E_{\theta|T}[f_i(\theta)] \qquad (19)$$
$$E[s_{iD}(A)] \quad = \quad E_{\theta|D}[f_i(\theta)] \qquad (20)$$
$$\mathcal{SNR}_i \quad = \quad \frac{E_{\theta|T}[f_i(\theta)]}{E_{\theta|D}[f_i(\theta)]} \qquad (21)$$

Finally, the gains g_i on each saliency map can be found using eqn. 15. Thus, for a given distribution of stimulus parameters for the target $P(\theta|T)$ and distractors $P(\theta|D)$, we simulate the above model of early visual cortex, compute salience of target and distractors, compute $\mathcal{SNR}_i$ and obtain g_i. In the rest of this section, we plot the distribution of optimal choice of gains g_i for an exhaustive list of conditions where knowledge of the target and distractors varies from complete certainty to uncertainty.

Unknown target and distractors: In the trivial case where there is no knowledge of the target and distractors, all cues are equally relevant and the optimal choice of gains is the same as baseline activation (unity). $\mathcal{SNR}$ is minimum leading to a slow search. This prediction is consistent with visual search experiments that observe slow search when the target and distractors are unknown due to reversal between trials [1, 2].

Search for a known target: During search for a known target, the optimal strategy predicts that $\mathcal{SNR}$ can be maximised by boosting neurons according to how strongly they respond to the target feature (as shown in figure 1, predicted $\mathcal{SNR}$ is 12.2 dB). Thus, a neuron that is optimally tuned to the target feature receives maximal gain. This prediction is consistent with single unit recordings on feature-based attention which show that the gain in neural response depends on the similarity between the neuron's preferred feature and the target feature [3, 4].

Role of uncertainty in target features: When there's uncertainty in the target's features, i.e., when the target's parameter assumes multiple values according to some probability distribution $P(\theta|T)$, the optimal strategy predicts that $\mathcal{SNR}$ decreases, leading to a slower search (as shown in figure 1, $\mathcal{SNR}$ decreases from 12.2 dB to 9 dB). This result is consistent with psychophysics experiments which suggest that better knowledge of the target leads to faster search [5, 6].

Distractor heterogeneity: While searching for an unknown target among known distractors, the optimal strategy predicts that $\mathcal{SNR}$ can be maximised by suppressing the neurons tuned to the distractors (see figure 1). But as we increase distractor heterogeneity or the number of distractor types, it predicts a decrease in $\mathcal{SNR}$ (from 36 dB to 17 dB, figure 1). This result is consistent with experimental data [10].

Discriminability between target and distractors: Several experiments and theories have studied the effect of target-distractor discriminability [10]-[17]. The optimal cue selection strategy also shows that if the target and distractors are very different or highly discriminable, $\mathcal{SNR}$ is high and the search is efficient ($\mathcal{SNR} = 51.4$ dB, see figure 1). Otherwise, if they are similar and not well separated in feature space, $\mathcal{SNR}$ is low and the search is hard ($\mathcal{SNR} = 16.3$ dB, see figure 1). Moreover, during search for a less discriminable target from distractors, the optimal strategy predicts that the neuron optimally tuned to the target may not be boosted maximally. Instead, a neuron that is sub-optimally tuned to the target and farther away from the distractors receives maximal gain. This new and counter-intuitive prediction is tested by visual search experiments described in the next section.

Linear separability effect: The optimal strategy also predicts the linear separability effect [18, 19] which suggests that when the target and distractors are less discriminable, search is easier if the target and distractors can be separated by a line in feature space (see figure 1). This effect has been demonstrated in size (e.g., search for the smallest or largest item is faster than search for a medium-sized item in the display)[20], chromaticity and luminance [21, 19], and orientation [22, 23].

4 Testing new predictions of the optimal cue selection strategy

In this section, we describe the design and analysis of psychophysics experiments to verify the counter-intuitive prediction mentioned in the previous section, i.e., during searching for a target that is less discriminable from the distractors, a neuron that is sub-optimally tuned to the target's feature will be boosted more than a neuron that is optimally tuned to the target's feature.

4.1 Design of psychophysics experiments

Our experiments are designed in two phases: phase 1 to set up the top-down bias and phase 2 to measure the bias.

Phase 1 - Setup the top-down bias: Subjects perform the primary task T1 which is a visual search for the target among distractors. This task sets the top-down bias on cues so that the target becomes the most salient item in the display, thus accelerating target detection. Subjects are trained on T1 trials until their performance stabilises with at least 80% accuracy. They are instructed to find the target ($55°$ tilt) among several distractors ($50°$ tilt). The target and distractors are the same for all T1 trials. To avoid false reports (which may occur due to boredom or lack of attention) and to verify that subjects indeed find the target, we introduce a novel *no cheat* scheme as follows: After finding the target among distractors, subjects press any key. Following the key press, we flash a grid of fineprint random numbers briefly (120ms) and ask subjects to report the number at the target's location. Online feedback on accuracy of report is provided. Thus, the top-down bias is set up by performing T1 trials.

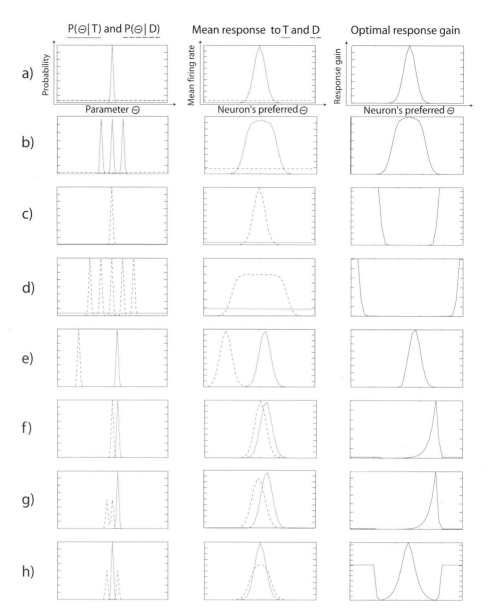

Figure 1: a) Search for a known target – left: Prior knowledge $P(\theta|T)$ has a peak at the known target feature and $P(\theta|D)$ is flat as the distractor is unknown, middle: The expected responses of a population of neurons to the target is highest for neurons tuned around the target's θ while the expected response to the distractors is flat, right: The optimal response gain in this situation is to boost the gain of the neurons that are tuned around the target's θ; b) Search for an uncertain target; c) Unknown target among a known distractor; d) Presence of heterogeneous distractors; e) High discriminability between target and distractors; f) Low discriminability; g) Search for an extreme feature (linearly separable) among others; h) Search for a mid feature (nonlinearly separable) among others.

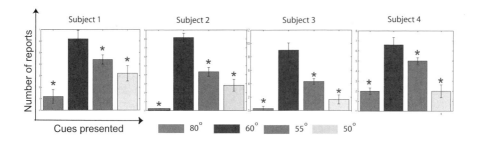

Figure 2: The results of the T2 trials described in section 4.1 (phase 2) are shown here. For each of the four subjects, the number of reports on the steepest ($80°$), relevant ($60°$), target ($55°$) and distractor ($50°$) cues are shown in these bar plots. As predicted by the theory, a paired t-test reveals that the number of reports on the relevant cue is significantly higher ($p < 0.05$) than the number of reports on the target, distractor and steepest cues, as indicated by the blue star.

Phase 2 - Measure the top-down bias: To measure the top-down bias generated by the above task, we randomly insert T2 trials in between T1 trials. Our theory predicts that during search for the target ($55°$) among distractors ($50°$), the most relevant cue will be around $60°$ and not $55°$. To test this, we briefly (200ms) flash four cues - steepest (S, $80°$), relevant as predicted by our theory (R, $60°$), target (T, $55°$) and distractor (D, $50°$). A cue that is biased more appears more salient, attracts a saccade, and gets reported. In other words, the greater the top-down bias on a cue, the higher the number of its reports. According to our theory, there should be higher number of reports on R than T.

Experimental details: We ran 4 naïve subjects. All were aged 22-30, had normal or corrected vision, volunteered or participated for course credit. As mentioned earlier, each subject received training on T1 trials for a few days until the performance (search speed) stabilised with atleast 80% accuracy. To become familiar with the secondary task, they were trained on 50 T2 trials. Finally, each subject performed 10 blocks of 50 trials each, with T2 trials randomly inserted in between T1 trials.

4.2 Results

For each of the four subjects, we extracted the number reports on the steepest (N_S), relevant (N_R), target (N_T) and distractor (N_D) cues, for each block. We used a paired t test to check for statistically significant differences between N_R and N_T, N_D, N_S. Results are shown in figure 2. As predicted by the theory, we found a significantly higher number of reports on the relevant cue than the target cue.

5 Discussion

In this paper, we have investigated whether our visual system has evolved to use optimal top-down strategies to select relevant cues that quickly and reliably detect the target among distracting environments. We formally obtained the optimal cue selection strategy where cues are chosen such that the signal-to-noise ratio ($\mathcal{SNR}$) of the saliency map is maximized, thus maximizing the target's salience relative to the distractors. The resulting optimal strategy is to boost a cue or feature if it provides higher signal-to-noise ratio than average. Through simulations, we confirmed the predictions of the optimal strategy with existing experimental data on visual search behavior, including the effect of distractor heterogeneity [10], uncertainty in target's features [5, 6], target-distractor discriminability [10], linear separabilty effect [18, 19]. Our study complements the recent work on optimal eye movement strategies [24]. While we focus on an early stage of visual processing - optimal cue selection in order to create a saliency map with maximum $\mathcal{SNR}$, their study focuses on a later stage of visual processing - optimal saccade generation such that for a given saliency map, the probability of subsequent target detection is maximized. Thus, both optimal cue selection and saccade generation are necessary for optimal visual search.

Acknowledgements

This work was supported by the National Science Foundation, National Eye Institute, National Imagery and Mapping Agency, Zumberge Innovation Fund, and Charles Lee Powell Foundation.

References

[1] V Maljkovic and K Nakayama. *Mem Cognit*, 22(6):657–672, Nov 1994.

[2] J. M. Wolfe, S. J. Butcher, and M. Hyle. *J Exp Psychol Hum Percept Perform*, 29(2):483–502, 2003.

[3] S Treue and J C Martinez Trujillo. *Nature*, 399(6736):575–579, Jun 1999.

[4] J. C. Martinez-Trujillo and S. Treue. *Curr Biol*, 14(9):744–751, May 2004.

[5] J. M. Wolfe, T. S. Horowitz, N. Kenner, M. Hyle, and N. Vasan. *Vision Res*, 44(12):1411–1426, Jun 2004.

[6] Timothy J Vickery, Li-Wei King, and Yuhong Jiang. *J Vis*, 5(1):81–92, Feb 2005.

[7] A. Triesman and J. Souther. *Journal of Experimental Psychology: Human Perception and Performance*, 14:107–141, 1986.

[8] A. Treisman and S. Gormican. *Psychological Review 95*, 1:15–48, 1988.

[9] R. Rosenholtz. *Percept Psychophys*, 63(3):476–489, Apr 2001.

[10] J Duncan and G W Humphreys. *Psychological Rev*, 96:433–458, 1989.

[11] A. L. Nagy and R. R. Sanchez. *Journal of the Optical Society of America A 7*, 7:1209–1217, 1990.

[12] H. Pashler. *Percept Psychophys*, 41(4):385–392, Apr 1987.

[13] K. Rayner and D. L. Fisher. *Percept Psychophys*, 42(1):87–100, Jul 1987.

[14] A. Treisman. *J Exp Psychol Hum Percept Perform*, 17(3):652–676, Aug 1991.

[15] J. Palmer, P. Verghese, and M. Pavel. *Vision Res*, 40(10-12):1227–1268, 2000.

[16] J. M. Wolfe, K. R. Cave, and S. L. Franzel. *J. Exper. Psychol.*, 15:419–433, 1989.

[17] J. M. Wolfe. *Psyonomic Bulletin and Review*, 1(2):202–238, 1994.

[18] M. D'Zmura. *Vision Research 31*, 6:951–966, 1991.

[19] B. Bauer, P. Jolicoeur, and W. B. Cowan. *Vision Research 36*, 10:1439–1465, 1996.

[20] A. Treisman and G. Gelade. *Cognitive Psychology*, 12:97–136, 1980.

[21] B. Bauer, P. Jolicoeur, and W. B. Cowan. *Vision Res*, 36(10):1439–1465, May 1996.

[22] J. M. Wolfe, S. R. Friedman-Hill, M. I. Stewart, and K. M. O' Connell. *J Exp Psychol Hum Percept Perform*, 18(1):34–49, Feb 1992.

[23] W. F. Alkhateeb, R. J. Morris, and K. H. Ruddock. *Spat Vis*, 5(2):129–141, 1990.

[24] J. Najemnik, W. S. Geisler. *Nature*, 434(7031):387–391, Mar 2005.

Nearest Neighbor Based Feature Selection for Regression and its Application to Neural Activity

Amir Navot[12] **Lavi Shpigelman**[12] **Naftali Tishby**[12] **Eilon Vaadia**[23]
[1]School of computer Science and Engineering
[2]Interdisciplinary Center for Neural Computation
[3]Dept. of Physiology, Hadassah Medical School
The Hebrew University Jerusalem, 91904, Israel
Email for correspondence: {anavot,shpigi}@cs.huji.ac.il

Abstract

We present a non-linear, simple, yet effective, feature subset selection method for regression and use it in analyzing cortical neural activity. Our algorithm involves a *feature-weighted* version of the k-nearest-neighbor algorithm. It is able to capture complex dependency of the target function on its input and makes use of the leave-one-out error as a natural regularization. We explain the characteristics of our algorithm on synthetic problems and use it in the context of predicting hand velocity from spikes recorded in motor cortex of a behaving monkey. By applying feature selection we are able to improve prediction quality and suggest a novel way of exploring neural data.

1 Introduction

In many supervised learning tasks the input is represented by a very large number of features, many of which are not needed for predicting the labels. Feature selection is the task of choosing a small subset of features that is sufficient to predict the target labels well. Feature selection reduces the computational complexity of learning and prediction algorithms and saves on the cost of measuring non selected features. In many situations, feature selection can also enhance the prediction accuracy by improving the signal to noise ratio. Another benefit of feature selection is that the identity of the selected features can provide insights into the nature of the problem at hand. Therefore *feature selection* is an important step in efficient learning of large multi-featured data sets.

Feature selection (variously known as *subset selection*, *attribute selection* or *variable selection*) has been studied extensively both in statistics and by the machine learning community over the last few decades. In the most common selection paradigm an evaluation function is used to assign scores to subsets of features and a search algorithm is used to search for a subset with a high score. The evaluation function can be based on the performance of a specific predictor (*wrapper* model, [1]) or on some general (typically cheaper to compute) relevance measure of the features to the prediction (*filter* model). In any case, an exhaustive search over all feature sets is generally intractable due to the exponentially large number of possible sets. Therefore, search methods are employed which apply a variety of heuristics, such as hill climbing and genetic algorithms. Other methods simply rank individual features, assigning a score to each feature independently. These methods are usually very fast, but inevitably fail in situations where only a combined set of features is predictive of the target function. See [2] for a comprehensive overview of feature selection and [3] which discusses selection methods for *linear* regression.

A possible choice of evaluation function is the leave-one-out (LOO) mean square error (MSE) of the *k-Nearest-Neighbor* (kNN) estimator ([4, 5]). This evaluation function has the advantage that it both gives a good approximation of the expected generalization error and can be computed quickly. [6] used this criterion on small synthetic problems (up to 12 features). They searched for good subsets using *forward selection*, *backward elimination* and an algorithm (called *schemata*) that *races* feature sets against each other (eliminating poor sets, keeping the fittest) in order to find a subset with a good score. All these algorithms perform a local search by flipping one or more features at a time. Since the space is discrete the direction of improvement is found by trial and error, which slows the search and makes it impractical for large scale real world problems involving many features.

In this paper we develop a novel selection algorithm. We extend the LOO-kNN-MSE evaluation function to assign scores to *weight vectors* over the features, instead of just to feature subsets. This results in a smooth ("almost everywhere") function over a continuous domain, which allows us to compute the gradient analytically and to employ a stochastic gradient ascent to find a locally optimal weight vector. The resulting weights provide a ranking of the features, which we can then threshold in order to produce a subset. In this way we can apply an easy-to-compute, gradient directed search, without relearning of a regression model at each step but while employing a strong non-linear function estimate (kNN) that can capture complex dependency of the function on its features[1].

Our motivation for developing this method is to address a major computational neuroscience question: which features of the neural code are relevant to the observed behavior. This is an important element of enabling interpretability of neural activity. Feature selection is a promising tool for this task. Here, we apply our feature selection method to the task of reconstructing hand movements from neural activity, which is one of the main challenges in implementing brain computer interfaces [8]. We look at neural population spike counts, recorded in motor cortex of a monkey while it performed hand movements and locate the most informative subset of neural features. We show that it is possible to improve prediction results by wisely selecting a subset of cortical units and their time lags, relative to the movement. Our algorithm, which considers feature subsets, outperforms methods that consider features on an individual basis, suggesting that complex dependency on a set of features exists in the code.

The remainder of the paper is organized as follows: we describe the problem setting in section 2. Our method is presented in section 3. Next, we demonstrate its ability to cope with a complicated dependency of the target function on groups of features using synthetic data (section 4). The results of applying our method to the hand movement reconstruction problem is presented in section 5.

2 Problem Setting

First, let us introduce some notation. Vectors in R^n are denoted by boldface small letters (e.g. $\mathbf{x}$, $\mathbf{w}$). Scalars are denoted by small letters (e.g. x, y). The i'th element of a vector $\mathbf{x}$ is denoted by x_i. Let $f(\mathbf{x})$, $f : R^n \longrightarrow R$ be a function that we wish to estimate. Given a set $S \subset R^n$, the empiric *mean square error* (MSE) of an estimator $\hat{f}$ for f is defined as

$$MSE_S(\hat{f}) = \frac{1}{|S|} \sum_{\mathbf{x} \in S} \left(f(\mathbf{x}) - \hat{f}(\mathbf{x}) \right)^2.$$

---

[1]The design of this algorithm was inspired by work done by Gilad-Bachrach et al. ([7]) which used a large margin based evaluation function to derive feature selection algorithms for classification.

kNN Regression *k-Nearest-Neighbor* (kNN) is a simple, intuitive and efficient way to estimate the value of an unknown function in a given point using its values in other (training) points. Let $S = \{\mathbf{x}_1, \ldots, \mathbf{x}_m\}$ be a set of training points. The kNN estimator is defined as the mean function value of the nearest neighbors: $\hat{f}(\mathbf{x}) = \frac{1}{k} \sum_{\mathbf{x}' \in N(\mathbf{x})} f(x')$ where $N(\mathbf{x}) \subset S$ is the set of k nearest points to $\mathbf{x}$ in S and k is a parameter([4, 5]). A softer version takes a *weighted* average, where the weight of each neighbor is proportional to its proximity. One specific way of doing this is

$$\hat{f}(\mathbf{x}) = \frac{1}{Z} \sum_{\mathbf{x}' \in N(\mathbf{x})} f(\mathbf{x}') e^{-d(\mathbf{x},\mathbf{x}')/\beta} \tag{1}$$

where $d(\mathbf{x}, \mathbf{x}') = \|\mathbf{x} - \mathbf{x}'\|_2^2$ is the ℓ_2 norm, $Z = \sum_{\mathbf{x}' \in N(\mathbf{x})} e^{-d(\mathbf{x},\mathbf{x}')/\beta}$ is a normalization factor and β is a parameter. The soft kNN version will be used in the remainder of this paper. This regression method is a special form of *locally weighted regression* (See [5] for an overview of the literature on this subject.) It has the desirable property that no learning (other than storage of the training set) is required for the regression. Also note that the Gaussian Radial Basis Function has the form of a *kernel* ([9]) and can be replaced with any operator on two data points that decays as a function of the difference between them (e.g. kernel induced distances). As will be seen in the next section, we use the MSE of a modified kNN regressor to guide the search for a set of features $F \subset \{1, \ldots n\}$ that achieves a low MSE. However, the MSE and the Gaussian kernel can be replaced by other loss measures and kernels (respectively) as long as they are differentiable almost everywhere.

3   The Feature Selection Algorithm

In this section we present our selection algorithm called *RGS* (Regression, Gradient guided, feature Selection). It can be seen as a filter method for general regression algorithms or as a wrapper for estimation by the kNN algorithm.

Our goal is to find subsets of features that induce a small estimation error. As in most supervised learning problems, we wish to find subsets that induce a small generalization error, but since it is not known, we use an *evaluation function* on the training set. This evaluation function is defined not only for subsets but for any weight vector over the features. This is more general because a feature subset can be represented by a binary weight vector that assigns a value of one to features in the set and zero to the rest of the features.

For a given weights vector over the features $\mathbf{w} \in R^n$, we consider the weighted squared ℓ_2 norm induced by $\mathbf{w}$, defined as $\|z\|_{\mathbf{w}}^2 = \sum_i z_i^2 w_i^2$. Given a training set S, we denote by $\hat{f}_{\mathbf{w}}(\mathbf{x})$ the value assigned to $\mathbf{x}$ by a weighted kNN estimator, defined in equation 1, using the weighted squared ℓ_2-norm as the distances $d(\mathbf{x}, \mathbf{x}')$ and the nearest neighbors are found among the points of S excluding $\mathbf{x}$. The evaluation function is defined as the negative (halved) square error of the weighted kNN estimator:

$$e(\mathbf{w}) = -\frac{1}{2} \sum_{\mathbf{x} \in S} \left(f(\mathbf{x}) - \hat{f}_w(\mathbf{x}) \right)^2. \tag{2}$$

This evaluation function scores weight vectors ($\mathbf{w}$). A change of weights will cause a change in the distances and, possibly, the identity of each point's nearest neighbors, which will change the function estimates. A weight vector that induces a distance measure in which neighbors have similar labels would receive a high score. The mean, $1/|S|$ is replaced with a $1/2$ to ease later differentiation. Note that there is no explicit regularization term in $e(\mathbf{w})$. This is justified by the fact that for each point, the estimate of its function value does not include that point as part of the training set. Thus, equation 2 is a leave-one-out cross validation error. Clearly, it is impossible to go over all the weight vectors (or even over all the feature subsets), and therefore some search technique is required.

Algorithm 1 $RGS(S, k, \beta, T)$

1. initialize $\mathbf{w} = (1, 1, \ldots, 1)$
2. for $t = 1 \ldots T$

    (a) pick randomly an instance $\mathbf{x}$ from S

    (b) calculate the gradient of $e(\mathbf{w})$:

$$\nabla e(\mathbf{w}) = -\sum_{\mathbf{x} \in S} \left(f(\mathbf{x}) - \hat{f}_w(\mathbf{x}) \right) \nabla_{\mathbf{w}} \hat{f}_{\mathbf{w}}(\mathbf{x})$$

$$\nabla_{\mathbf{w}} \hat{f}_{\mathbf{w}}(\mathbf{x}) = \frac{-\frac{4}{\beta} \sum_{\mathbf{x}'', \mathbf{x}' \in N(\mathbf{x})} f(x'') a(x', x'') \mathbf{u}(x', x'')}{\sum_{\mathbf{x}'', \mathbf{x}' \in N(\mathbf{x})} a(x', x'')}$$

    where $a(x', x'') = e^{-\left(||x - x'||_{\mathbf{w}}^2 + ||x - x''||_{\mathbf{w}}^2\right)/\beta}$

    and $\mathbf{u}(x', x'') \in R^n$ is a vector with $u_i = w_i \left[(x_i - x_i')^2 + (x_i - x_i'')^2 \right]$.

    (c) $\mathbf{w} = \mathbf{w} + \eta_t \nabla e(\mathbf{w}) = \mathbf{w} \left(1 + \eta_t \nabla_{\mathbf{w}} \hat{f}_{\mathbf{w}}(\mathbf{x}) \right)$ where η_t is a decay factor.

Our method finds a weight vector $\mathbf{w}$ that locally maximizes $e(\mathbf{w})$ as defined in (2) and then uses a threshold in order to obtain a feature subset. The threshold can be set either by cross validation or by finding a natural cutoff in the weight values. However, we later show that using the distance measure induced by $\mathbf{w}$ in the regression stage compensates for taking too many features. Since $e(\mathbf{w})$ is defined over a continuous domain and is smooth almost everywhere we can use gradient ascent in order to maximize it. *RGS* (algorithm 1) is a stochastic gradient ascent over $e(\mathbf{w})$. In each step the gradient is evaluated using one sample point and is added to the current weight vector. *RGS* considers the weights of all the features at the same time and thus it can handle dependency on a group of features. This is demonstrated in section 4. In this respect, it is superior to selection algorithms that scores each feature independently. It is also faster than methods that try to find a good subset directly by trial and error. Note, however, that convergence to global optima is not guaranteed and standard techniques to avoid local optima can be used.

The parameters of the algorithm are k (number of neighbors), β (Gaussian decay factor), T (number of iterations) and $\{\eta_t\}_{t=1}^T$ (step size decay scheme). The value of k can be tuned by cross validation, however a proper choice of β can compensate for a k that is too large. It makes sense to tune β to a value that places most neighbors in an active zone of the Gaussian. In our experiments, we set β to half of the mean distance between points and their k neighbors. It usually makes sense to use η_t that decays over time to ensure convergence, however, on our data, convergence was also achieved with $\eta_t = 1$.

The computational complexity of *RGS* is $\Theta(TNm)$ where T is the number of iterations, N is the number of features and m is the size of the training set S. This is correct for a naive implementation which finds the nearest neighbors and their distances from scratch at each step by measuring the distances between the current point to all the other points. RGS is basically an on line method which can be used in batch mode by running it in epochs on the training set. When it is run for only one epoch, $T = m$ and the complexity is $\Theta\left(m^2 N\right)$. Matlab code for this algorithm (and those that we compare with) is available at http://www.cs.huji.ac.il/labs/learning/code/fsr/

4 Testing on synthetic data

The use of synthetic data, where we can control the importance of each feature, allows us to illustrate the properties of our algorithm. We compare our algorithm with other common

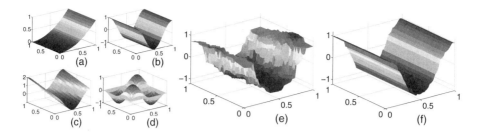

Figure 1: (a)-(d): Illustration of the four synthetic target functions. The plots shows the functions value as function of the first two features. (e),(f): demonstration of the effect of feature selection on estimating the second function using kNN regression ($k = 5$, $\beta = 0.05$). (e) using both features ($mse = 0.03$), (f) using the relevant feature only ($mse = 0.004$)

selection methods: *infoGain* [10], correlation coefficients (*corrcoef*) and *forward selection* (see [2]) . *infoGain* and *corrcoef* simply rank features according to the mutual information[2] or the correlation coefficient (respectively) between each feature and the labels (i.e. the target function value). Forward selection (*fwdSel*) is a greedy method in which features are iteratively added into a growing subset. In each step, the feature showing the greatest improvement (given the previously selected subset) is added. This is a search method that can be applied to any evaluation function and we use our criterion (equation 2 on feature subsets). This well known method has the advantages of considering feature subsets and that it can be used with non linear predictors. Another algorithm we compare with scores each feature independently using our evaluation function (2). This helps us in analyzing *RGS*, as it may help single out the respective contributions to performance of the properties of the evaluation function and the search method. We refer to this algorithm as *SKS* (Single feature, kNN regression, feature Selection).

We look at four different target functions over R^{50}. The training sets include 20 to 100 points that were chosen randomly from the $[-1, 1]^{50}$ cube. The target functions are given in the top row of figure 2 and are illustrated in figure 1(a-d). A random Gaussian noise with zero mean and a variance of $1/7$ was added to the function value of the training points. Clearly, only the first feature is relevant for the first two target functions, and only the first two features are relevant for the last two target functions. Note also that the last function is a smoothed version of parity function learning and is considered hard for many feature selection algorithms [2].

First, to illustrate the importance of feature selection on regression quality we use kNN to estimate the second target function. Figure 1(e-f) shows the regression results for target (b), using either only the relevant feature or both the relevant and an irrelevant feature. The addition of one irrelevant feature degrades the MSE ten fold. Next, to demonstrate the capabilities of the various algorithms, we run them on each of the above problems with varying training set size. We measure their success by counting the number of times that the relevant features were assigned the highest rank (repeating the experiment 250 times by re-sampling the training set). Figure 2 presents success rate as function of training set size. We can see that all the algorithms succeeded on the first function which is monotonic and depends on one feature alone. *infoGain* and *corrcoef* fail on the second, non-monotonic function. The three kNN based algorithms succeed because they only depend on local properties of the target function. We see, however, that RGS needs a larger training set to achieve a high success rate. The third target function depends on two features but the dependency is simple as each of them alone is highly correlated with the function value. The fourth, XOR-like function exhibits a complicated dependency that requires consideration of the two relevant features simultaneously. *SKS* which considers features separately sees the effect of all other features as noise and, therefore, has only marginal success on the third

---

[2]Feature and function values were "binarized" by comparing them to the median value.

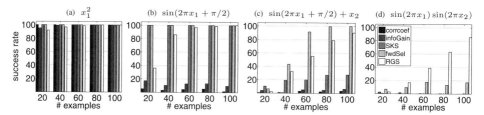

Figure 2: Success rate of the different algorithms on 4 synthetic regression tasks (averaged over 250 repetitions) as a function of the number of training examples. Success is measured by the percent of the repetitions in which the relevant feature(s) received first place(s).

function and fails on the fourth altogether. *RGS* and *fwdSel* apply different search methods. *fwdSel* considers subsets but can evaluate only one additional feature in each step, giving it some advantage over *RGS* on the third function but causing it to fail on the fourth. *RGS* takes a step in all features simultaneously. Only such an approach can succeed on the fourth function.

5 Hand Movements Reconstruction from Neural Activity

To suggest an interpretation of neural coding we apply *RGS* and compare it with the alternatives presented in the previous section[3] on the hand movement reconstruction task. The data sets were collected while a monkey performed a planar center-out reaching task with one or both hands [11]. 16 electrodes, inserted daily into novel positions in primary motor cortex were used to detect and sort spikes in up to 64 channels (4 per electrode). Most of the channels detected isolated neuronal spikes by template matching. Some, however, had templates that were not tuned, producing spikes during only a fraction of the session. Others (about 25%) contained unused templates (resulting in a constant zero producing channel or, possibly, a few random spikes). The rest of the channels (one per electrode) produced spikes by threshold passing. We construct a labeled regression data set as follows. Each example corresponds to one time point in a trial. It consists of the spike counts that occurred in the 10 previous consecutive $100ms$ long time bins from all 64 channels ($64 \times 10 = 640$ features) and the label is the X or Y component of the instantaneous hand velocity. We analyze data collected over 8 days. Each data set has an average of 5050 examples collected during the movement periods of the successful trials.

In order to evaluate the different feature selection methods we separate the data into training and test sets. Each selection method is used to produce a ranking of the features. We then apply kNN (based on the training set) using different size groups of top ranking features to the test set. We use the resulting MSE (or correlation coefficient between true and estimated movement) as our measure of quality. To test the significance of the results we apply 5-fold cross validation and repeat the process 5 times on different permutations of the trial ordering. Figure 3 shows the average (over permutations, folds and velocity components) MSE as a function of the number of selected features on four of the different data sets (results on the rest are similar and omitted due to lack of space)[4]. It is clear that *RGS* achieves better results than the other methods throughout the range of feature numbers.

To test whether the performance of *RGS* was consistently better than the other methods we counted winning percentages (the percent of the times in which *RGS* achieved lower MSE than another algorithm) in all folds of all data sets and as a function of the number of

---

[3]*fwdSel* was not applied due to its intractably high run time complexity. Note that its run time is at least r times that of *RGS* where r is the size of the optimal set and is longer in practice.

[4]We use $k = 50$ (approximately 1% of the data points). β is set automatically as described in section 3. These parameters were manually tuned for good kNN results and were not optimized for any of the feature selection algorithms. The number of epochs for *RGS* was set to 1 (i.e. $T = m$).

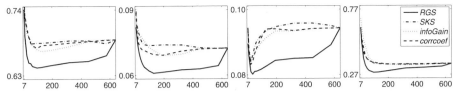

Figure 3: MSE results for the different feature selection methods on the neural activity data sets. Each sub figure is a different recording day. MSEs are presented as a function of the number of features used. Each point is a mean over all 5 cross validation folds, 5 permutations on the data and the two velocity component targets. Note that some of the data sets are harder than others.

features used. Figure 4 shows the winning percentages of *RGS* versus the other methods. For a very low number of features, while the error is still high, *RGS* winning scores are only slightly better than chance but once there are enough features for good predictions the winning percentages are higher than 90%. In figure 3 we see that the MSE achieved when using only approximately 100 features selected by *RGS* is better than when using all the features. This difference is indeed statistically significant (win score of 92%). If the MSE is replaced by correlation coefficient as the measure of quality, the average results (not shown due to lack of space) are qualitatively unchanged.

RGS not only ranks the features but also gives them weights that achieve locally optimal results when using kNN regression. It therefore makes sense not only to select the features but to weigh them accordingly. Figure 5 shows the winning percentages of *RGS* using the weighted features versus *RGS* using uniformly weighted features. The corresponding MSEs (with and without weights) on the first data set are also displayed. It is clear that using the weights improves the results in a manner that becomes increasingly significant as the number of features grows, especially when the number of features is greater than the optimal number. Thus, using weighted features can compensate for choosing too many by diminishing the effect of the surplus features.

To take a closer look at what features are selected, figure 6 shows the 100 highest ranking features for all algorithms on one data set. Similar selection results were obtained in the rest of the folds. One would expect to find that well isolated cells (template matching) are more informative than threshold based spikes. Indeed, all the algorithms select isolated cells more frequently within the top 100 features (*RGS* does so in 95% of the time and the rest in 70%-80%). A human selection of channels, based only on looking at raster plots and selecting channels with stable firing rates was also available to us. This selection was independent of the template/threshold categorisation. Once again, the algorithms selected the humanly preferred channels more frequently than the other channels. Another and more interesting observation that can also be seen in the figure is that while *corrcoef*, *SKS* and *infoGain* tend to select all time lags of a channel, *RGS*'s selections are more scattered (more channels and only a few time bins per channel). Since *RGS* achieves best results, we

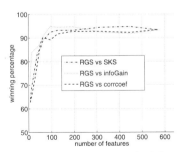

Figure 4: Winning percentages of *RGS* over the other algorithms. *RGS* achieves better MSEs consistently.

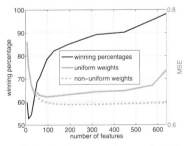

Figure 5: Winning percentages of *RGS* with and without weighting of features (black). Gray lines are corresponding MSEs of these methods on the first data set.

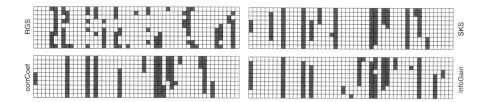

Figure 6: 100 highest ranking features (grayed out) selected by the algorithms. Results are for one fold of one data set. In each sub figure the bottom row is the ($100ms$) time bin with least delay and the higher rows correspond to longer delays. Each column is a channel (silent channels omitted).

conclude that this selection pattern is useful. Apparently *RGS* found these patterns thanks to its ability to evaluate complex dependency on feature subsets. This suggests that such dependency of the behavior on the neural activity does exist.

6 Summary

In this paper we present a new method of selecting features for function estimation and use it to analyze neural activity during a motor control task . We use the leave-one-out mean squared error of the kNN estimator and minimize it using a gradient ascent on an "almost" smooth function. This yields a selection method which can handle a complicated dependency of the target function on groups of features yet can be applied to large scale problems. This is valuable since many common selection methods lack one of these properties. By comparing the result of our method to other selection methods on the motor control task, we show that consideration of complex dependency helps to achieve better performance. These results suggest that this is an important property of the code.

Our future work is aimed at a better understanding of neural activity through the use of feature selection. One possibility is to perform feature selection on other kinds of neural data such as local field potentials or retinal activity. Another promising option is to explore the temporally changing properties of neural activity. Motor control is a dynamic process in which the input output relation has a temporally varying structure. *RGS* can be used in on line (rather than batch) mode to identify these structures in the code.

References

[1] R. Kohavi and G.H. John. Wrapper for feature subset selection. *Artificial Intelligence*, 97(1-2):273–324, 1997.

[2] I. Guyon and A. Elisseeff. An introduction to variable and feature selection. *JMLR*, 2003.

[3] A.J. Miller. *Subset Selection in Regression*. Chapman and Hall, 1990.

[4] L. Devroye. The uniform convergence of nearest neighbor regression function estimators and their application in optimization. *IEEE transactions in information theory*, 24(2), 1978.

[5] C. Atkeson, A. Moore, and S. Schaal. Locally weighted learning. *AI Review*, 11.

[6] O. Maron and A. Moore. The racing algorithm: Model selection for lazy learners. In *Artificial Intelligence Review*, volume 11, pages 193–225, April 1997.

[7] R. Gilad-Bachrach, A. Navot, and N. Tishby. Margin based feature selection - theory and algorithms. In *Proc. 21st (ICML)*, pages 337–344, 2004.

[8] D. M. Taylor, S. I. Tillery, and A. B. Schwartz. Direct cortical control of 3d neuroprosthetic devices. *Science*, 296(7):1829–1832, 2002.

[9] V. Vapnik. *The Nature Of Statistical Learning Theory*. Springer-Verlag, 1995.

[10] J. R. Quinlan. Induction of decision trees. In Jude W. Shavlik and Thomas G. Dietterich, editors, *Readings in Machine Learning*. Morgan Kaufmann, 1990. Originally published in *Machine Learning* 1:81–106, 1986.

[11] R. Paz, T. Boraud, C. Natan, H. Bergman, and E. Vaadia. Preparatory activity in motor cortex reflects learning of local visuomotor skills. *Nature Neuroscience*, 6(8):882–890, August 2003.

A Bayesian Spatial Scan Statistic

Daniel B. Neill   Andrew W. Moore
School of Computer Science
Carnegie Mellon University
Pittsburgh, PA 15213
{neill,awm}@cs.cmu.edu

Gregory F. Cooper
Center for Biomedical Informatics
University of Pittsburgh
Pittsburgh, PA 15213
gfc@cbmi.pitt.edu

Abstract

We propose a new Bayesian method for spatial cluster detection, the "Bayesian spatial scan statistic," and compare this method to the standard (frequentist) scan statistic approach. We demonstrate that the Bayesian statistic has several advantages over the frequentist approach, including increased power to detect clusters and (since randomization testing is unnecessary) much faster runtime. We evaluate the Bayesian and frequentist methods on the task of prospective disease surveillance: detecting spatial clusters of disease cases resulting from emerging disease outbreaks. We demonstrate that our Bayesian methods are successful in rapidly detecting outbreaks while keeping number of false positives low.

1 Introduction

Here we focus on the task of *spatial cluster detection*: finding spatial regions where some quantity is significantly higher than expected. For example, our goal may be to detect clusters of disease cases, which may be indicative of a naturally occurring epidemic (e.g. influenza), a bioterrorist attack (e.g. anthrax release), or an environmental hazard (e.g. radiation leak). [1] discusses many other applications of cluster detection, including mining astronomical data, medical imaging, and military surveillance. In all of these applications, we have two main goals: to identify the locations, shapes, and sizes of potential clusters, and to determine whether each potential cluster is more likely to be a "true" cluster or simply a chance occurrence. Thus we compare the null hypothesis H_0 of no clusters against some set of alternative hypotheses $H_1(S)$, each representing a cluster in some region or regions S. In the standard frequentist setting, we do this by significance testing, computing the p-values of potential clusters by randomization; here we propose a Bayesian framework, in which we compute posterior probabilities of each potential cluster.

Our primary motivating application is *prospective disease surveillance*: detecting spatial clusters of disease cases resulting from a disease outbreak. In this application, we perform surveillance on a daily basis, with the goal of finding emerging epidemics as quickly as possible. For this task, we are given the number of cases of some given syndrome type (e.g. respiratory) in each spatial location (e.g. zip code) on each day. More precisely, we typically cannot measure the actual number of cases, and instead rely on related observable quantities such as the number of Emergency Department visits or over-the-counter drug sales. We must then detect those increases which are indicative of emerging outbreaks, as close to the start of the outbreak as possible, while keeping the number of false positives low. In biosurveillance of disease, every hour of earlier detection can translate into thousands of lives saved by more timely administration of antibiotics, and this has led to widespread interest in systems for the rapid and automatic detection of outbreaks.

In this spatial surveillance setting, each day we have data collected for a set of discrete spatial locations s_i. For each location s_i, we have a *count* c_i (e.g. number of disease cases), and an underlying *baseline* b_i. The baseline may correspond to the underlying *population* at risk, or may be an estimate of the expected value of the count (e.g. derived from the time series of previous count data). Our goal, then, is to find if there is any spatial region S (set of locations s_i) for which the counts are significantly higher than expected, given the baselines. For simplicity, we assume here (as in [2]) that the locations s_i are aggregated to a uniform, two-dimensional, $N \times N$ grid G, and we search over the set of rectangular regions $S \subseteq G$. This allows us to search both compact and elongated regions, allowing detection of elongated disease clusters resulting from dispersal of pathogens by wind or water.

1.1 The frequentist scan statistic

One of the most important statistical tools for cluster detection is Kulldorff's *spatial scan statistic* [3-4]. This method searches over a given set of spatial regions, finding those regions which maximize a likelihood ratio statistic and thus are most likely to be generated under the alternative hypothesis of clustering rather than the null hypothesis of no clustering. Randomization testing is used to compute the *p*-value of each detected region, correctly adjusting for multiple hypothesis testing, and thus we can both identify potential clusters and determine whether they are significant. Kulldorff's framework assumes that counts c_i are Poisson distributed with $c_i \sim \mathrm{Po}(qb_i)$, where b_i represents the (known) census population of cell s_i and q is the (unknown) underlying disease rate. Then the goal of the scan statistic is to find regions where the disease rate is higher inside the region than outside. The statistic used for this is the likelihood ratio $F(S) = \frac{P(Data \mid H_1(S))}{P(Data \mid H_0)}$, where the null hypothesis H_0 assumes a uniform disease rate $q = q_{all}$. Under $H_1(S)$, we assume that $q = q_{in}$ for all $s_i \in S$, and $q = q_{out}$ for all $s_i \in G - S$, for some constants $q_{in} > q_{out}$. From this, we can derive an expression for $F(S)$ using maximum likelihood estimates of q_{in}, q_{out}, and q_{all}: $F(S) = \left(\frac{C_{in}}{B_{in}}\right)^{C_{in}} \left(\frac{C_{out}}{B_{out}}\right)^{C_{out}} \left(\frac{C_{all}}{B_{all}}\right)^{-C_{all}}$, if $\frac{C_{in}}{B_{in}} > \frac{C_{out}}{B_{out}}$, and $F(S) = 1$ otherwise. In this expression, we have $C_{in} = \sum_S c_i$, $C_{out} = \sum_{G-S} c_i$, $C_{all} = \sum_G c_i$, and similarly for the baselines $B_{in} = \sum_S b_i$, $B_{out} = \sum_{G-S} b_i$, and $B_{all} = \sum_G b_i$.

Once we have found the highest scoring region $S^* = \arg\max_S F(S)$ of grid G, and its score $F^* = F(S^*)$, we must still determine the statistical significance of this region by randomization testing. To do so, we randomly create a large number R of replica grids by sampling under the null hypothesis $c_i \sim \mathrm{Po}(q_{all}b_i)$, and find the highest scoring region and its score for each replica grid. Then the *p*-value of S^* is $\frac{R_{beat}+1}{R+1}$, where R_{beat} is the number of replicas G' with F^* higher than the original grid. If this *p*-value is less than some threshold (e.g. 0.05), we can conclude that the discovered region is unlikely to have occurred by chance, and is thus a significant spatial cluster; otherwise, no significant clusters exist.

The frequentist scan statistic is a useful tool for cluster detection, and is commonly used in the public health community for detection of disease outbreaks. However, there are three main disadvantages to this approach. First, it is difficult to make use of any prior information that we may have, for example, our prior beliefs about the size of a potential outbreak and its impact on disease rate. Second, the accuracy of this technique is highly dependent on the correctness of our maximum likelihood parameter estimates. As a result, the model is prone to parameter overfitting, and may lose detection power in practice because of model misspecification. Finally, the frequentist scan statistic is very time consuming, and may be computationally infeasible for large datasets. A naive approach requires searching over all rectangular regions, both for the original grid and for each replica grid. Since there are $O(N^4)$ rectangles to search for an $N \times N$ grid, the total computation time is $O(RN^4)$, where $R = 1000$ is a typical number of replications. In past work [5, 2, 6], we have shown how to reduce this computation time by a factor of 20-2000x through use of the "fast spatial scan" algorithm; nevertheless, we must still perform this faster search both for the original grid and for each replica.

We propose to remedy these problems through the use of a Bayesian spatial scan statistic. First, our Bayesian model makes use of prior information about the likelihood, size, and impact of an outbreak. If these priors are chosen well, we should achieve better detection power than the frequentist approach. Second, the Bayesian method uses a *marginal likelihood* approach, averaging over possible values of the model parameters q_{in}, q_{out}, and q_{all}, rather than relying on maximum likelihood estimates of these parameters. This makes the model more flexible and less prone to overfitting, and reduces the potential impact of model misspecification. Finally, under the Bayesian model there is no need for randomization testing, and (since we need only to search the original grid) even a naive search can be performed relatively quickly. We now present the Bayesian spatial scan statistic, and then compare it to the frequentist approach on the task of detecting simulated disease epidemics.

2 The Bayesian scan statistic

Here we consider the natural Bayesian extension of Kulldorff's scan statistic, moving from a Poisson to a conjugate Gamma-Poisson model. Bayesian Gamma-Poisson models are a common representation for count data in epidemiology, and have been used in disease mapping by Clayton and Kaldor [7], Mollié [8], and others. In disease mapping, the effect of the Gamma prior is to produce a spatially smoothed map of disease rates; here we instead focus on computing the posterior probabilities, allowing us to determine the likelihood that an outbreak has occurred, and to estimate the location and size of potential outbreaks.

For the Bayesian spatial scan, as in the frequentist approach, we wish to compare the null hypothesis H_0 of no clusters to the set of alternative hypotheses $H_1(S)$, each representing a cluster in some region S. As before, we assume Poisson likelihoods, $c_i \sim \mathrm{Po}(qb_i)$. The difference is that we assume a hierarchical Bayesian model where the disease rates q_{in}, q_{out}, and q_{all} are themselves drawn from Gamma distributions. Thus, under the null hypothesis H_0, we have $q = q_{all}$ for all $s_i \in G$, where $q_{all} \sim \mathrm{Ga}(\alpha_{all}, \beta_{all})$. Under the alternative hypothesis $H_1(S)$, we have $q = q_{in}$ for all $s_i \in S$ and $q = q_{out}$ for all $s_i \in G - S$, where we independently draw $q_{in} \sim \mathrm{Ga}(\alpha_{in}, \beta_{in})$ and $q_{out} \sim \mathrm{Ga}(\alpha_{out}, \beta_{out})$. We discuss how the α and β priors are chosen below. From this model, we can compute the posterior probabilities $P(H_1(S)|D)$ of an outbreak in each region S, and the probability $P(H_0|D)$ that no outbreak has occurred, given dataset D: $P(H_0|D) = \frac{P(D|H_0)P(H_0)}{P(D)}$ and $P(H_1(S)|D) = \frac{P(D|H_1(S))P(H_1(S))}{P(D)}$, where $P(D) = P(D|H_0)P(H_0) + \sum_S P(D|H_1(S))P(H_1(S))$. We discuss the choice of prior probabilities $P(H_0)$ and $P(H_1(S))$ below. To compute the marginal likelihood of the data given each hypothesis, we must integrate over all possible values of the parameters (q_{in}, q_{out}, q_{all}) weighted by their respective probabilities. Since we have chosen a conjugate prior, we can easily obtain a closed-form solution for these likelihoods:

$$P(D|H_0) = \int P(q_{all} \sim \mathrm{Ga}(\alpha_{all}, \beta_{all})) \prod_{s_i \in G} P(c_i \sim \mathrm{Po}(q_{all} b_i)) \, dq_{all}$$

$$P(D|H_1(S)) = \int P(q_{in} \sim \mathrm{Ga}(\alpha_{in}, \beta_{in})) \prod_{s_i \in S} P(c_i \sim \mathrm{Po}(q_{in} b_i)) \, dq_{in}$$

$$\times \int P(q_{out} \sim \mathrm{Ga}(\alpha_{out}, \beta_{out})) \prod_{s_i \in G - S} P(c_i \sim \mathrm{Po}(q_{out} b_i)) \, dq_{out}$$

Now, computing the integral, and letting $C = \sum c_i$ and $B = \sum b_i$, we obtain:

$$\int P(q \sim \mathrm{Ga}(\alpha, \beta)) \prod_{s_i} P(c_i \sim \mathrm{Po}(qb_i)) \, dq = \int \frac{\beta^\alpha}{\Gamma(\alpha)} q^{\alpha-1} e^{-\beta q} \prod_{s_i} \frac{(qb_i)^{c_i} e^{-qb_i}}{(c_i)!} \, dq \propto$$

$$\frac{\beta^\alpha}{\Gamma(\alpha)} \int q^{\alpha-1} e^{-\beta q} q^{\sum c_i} e^{-q \sum b_i} \, dq = \frac{\beta^\alpha}{\Gamma(\alpha)} \int q^{\alpha+C-1} e^{-(\beta+B)q} \, dq = \frac{\beta^\alpha \Gamma(\alpha+C)}{(\beta+B)^{\alpha+C} \Gamma(\alpha)}$$

Thus we have the following expressions for the marginal likelihoods: $P(D|H_0) \propto \frac{(\beta_{all})^{\alpha_{all}} \Gamma(\alpha_{all}+C_{all})}{(\beta_{all}+B_{all})^{\alpha_{all}+C_{all}} \Gamma(\alpha_{all})}$, and $P(D|H_1(S)) \propto \frac{(\beta_{in})^{\alpha_{in}} \Gamma(\alpha_{in}+C_{in})}{(\beta_{in}+B_{in})^{\alpha_{in}+C_{in}} \Gamma(\alpha_{in})} \times \frac{(\beta_{out})^{\alpha_{out}} \Gamma(\alpha_{out}+C_{out})}{(\beta_{out}+B_{out})^{\alpha_{out}+C_{out}} \Gamma(\alpha_{out})}$.

The Bayesian spatial scan statistic can be computed simply by first calculating the score $P(D \mid H_1(S))P(H_1(S))$ for each spatial region S, maintaining a list of regions ordered by score. We then calculate $P(D \mid H_0)P(H_0)$, and add this to the sum of all region scores, obtaining the probability of the data $P(D)$. Finally, we can compute the posterior probability $P(H_1(S) \mid D) = \frac{P(D \mid H_1(S))P(H_1(S))}{P(D)}$ for each region, as well as $P(H_0 \mid D) = \frac{P(D \mid H_0)P(H_0)}{P(D)}$. Then we can return all regions with non-negligible posterior probabilities, the posterior probability of each, and the overall probability of an outbreak. Note that no randomization testing is necessary, and thus overall complexity is proportional to number of regions searched, e.g. $O(N^4)$ for searching over axis-aligned rectangles in an $N \times N$ grid.

2.1 Choosing priors

One of the most challenging tasks in any Bayesian analysis is the choice of priors. For any region S that we examine, we must have values of the parameter priors $\alpha_{in}(S)$, $\beta_{in}(S)$, $\alpha_{out}(S)$, and $\beta_{out}(S)$, as well as the region prior probability $P(H_1(S))$. We must also choose the global parameter priors α_{all} and β_{all}, as well as the "no outbreak" prior $P(H_0)$.

Here we consider the simple case of a uniform region prior, with a known prior probability of an outbreak P_1. In other words, if there is an outbreak, it is assumed to be equally likely to occur in any spatial region. Thus we have $P(H_0) = 1 - P_1$, and $P(H_1(S)) = \frac{P_1}{N_{reg}}$, where N_{reg} is the total number of regions searched. The parameter P_1 can be obtained from historical data, estimated by human experts, or can simply be used to tune the sensitivity and specificity of the algorithm. The model can also be easily adapted to a non-uniform region prior, taking into account our prior beliefs about the size and shape of outbreaks.

For the parameter priors, we assume that we have access to a large number of days of past data, during which no outbreaks are known to have occurred. We can then obtain estimated values of the parameter priors under the null hypothesis by matching the moments of each Gamma distribution to their historical values. In other words, we set the expectation and variance of the Gamma distribution $Ga(\alpha_{all}, \beta_{all})$ to the sample expectation and variance of $\frac{C_{all}}{B_{all}}$ observed in past data: $\frac{\alpha_{all}}{\beta_{all}} = E_{sample}\left[\frac{C_{all}}{B_{all}}\right]$, and $\frac{\alpha_{all}}{\beta_{all}^2} = Var_{sample}\left[\frac{C_{all}}{B_{all}}\right]$. Solving for α_{all} and β_{all}, we obtain $\alpha_{all} = \frac{\left(E_{sample}\left[\frac{C_{all}}{B_{all}}\right]\right)^2}{Var_{sample}\left[\frac{C_{all}}{B_{all}}\right]}$ and $\beta_{all} = \frac{E_{sample}\left[\frac{C_{all}}{B_{all}}\right]}{Var_{sample}\left[\frac{C_{all}}{B_{all}}\right]}$.

The calculation of priors $\alpha_{in}(S)$, $\beta_{in}(S)$, $\alpha_{out}(S)$, and $\beta_{out}(S)$ is identical except for two differences: first, we must condition on the region S, and second, we must assume the alternative hypothesis $H_1(S)$ rather than the null hypothesis H_0. Repeating the above derivation for the "out" parameters, we obtain $\alpha_{out}(S) = \frac{\left(E_{sample}\left[\frac{C_{out}(S)}{B_{out}(S)}\right]\right)^2}{Var_{sample}\left[\frac{C_{out}(S)}{B_{out}(S)}\right]}$ and $\beta_{out}(S) = \frac{E_{sample}\left[\frac{C_{out}(S)}{B_{out}(S)}\right]}{Var_{sample}\left[\frac{C_{out}(S)}{B_{out}(S)}\right]}$, where $C_{out}(S)$ and $B_{out}(S)$ are respectively the total count $\sum_{G-S} c_i$ and total baseline $\sum_{G-S} b_i$ outside the region. Note that an outbreak in some region S does not affect the disease rate outside region S. Thus we can use the same values of $\alpha_{out}(S)$ and $\beta_{out}(S)$ whether we are assuming the null hypothesis H_0 or the alternative hypothesis $H_1(S)$.

On the other hand, the effect of an outbreak inside region S must be taken into account when computing $\alpha_{in}(S)$ and $\beta_{in}(S)$; since we assume that no outbreak has occurred in the past data, we cannot just use the sample mean and variance, but must consider what we expect these quantities to be in the event of an outbreak. We assume that the outbreak will increase q_{in} by a multiplicative factor m, thus multiplying the mean and variance of $\frac{C_{in}}{B_{in}}$ by m. To account for this in the Gamma distribution $Ga(\alpha_{in}, \beta_{in})$, we multiply α_{in} by m while leaving β_{in} unchanged. Thus we have $\alpha_{in}(S) = m\frac{\left(E_{sample}\left[\frac{C_{in}(S)}{B_{in}(S)}\right]\right)^2}{Var_{sample}\left[\frac{C_{in}(S)}{B_{in}(S)}\right]}$ and $\beta_{in}(S) = \frac{E_{sample}\left[\frac{C_{in}(S)}{B_{in}(S)}\right]}{Var_{sample}\left[\frac{C_{in}(S)}{B_{in}(S)}\right]}$, where $C_{in}(S) = \sum_S c_i$ and $B_{in}(S) = \sum_S b_i$. Since we typically do not know the exact value of m, here we use a discretized uniform distribution for m, ranging from $m = 1 \ldots 3$ at intervals of 0.2. Then scores can be calculated by averaging likelihoods over the distribution of m.

Finally, we consider how to deal with the case where the past values of the counts and baselines are not given. In this "blind Bayesian" (BBayes) case, we assume that counts are randomly generated under the null hypothesis $c_i \sim \text{Po}(q_0 b_i)$, where q_0 is the expected ratio of count to baseline under the null (for example, $q_0 = 1$ if baselines are obtained by estimating the expected value of the count). Under this simple assumption, we can easily compute the expectation and variance of the ratio of count to baseline under the null hypothesis: $\text{E}\left[\frac{C}{B}\right] = \frac{\text{E}[\text{Po}(q_0 B)]}{B} = \frac{q_0 B}{B} = q_0$, and $\text{Var}\left[\frac{C}{B}\right] = \frac{\text{Var}[\text{Po}(q_0 B)]}{B^2} = \frac{q_0 B}{B^2} = \frac{q_0}{B}$. Thus we have $\alpha = q_0 B$ and $\beta = B$ under the null hypothesis. This gives us $\alpha_{all} = q_0 B_{all}$, $\beta_{all} = B_{all}$, $\alpha_{out}(S) = q_0 B_{out}(S)$, $\beta_{out}(S) = B_{out}(S)$, $\alpha_{in}(S) = m q_0 B_{in}(S)$, and $\beta_{in}(S) = B_{in}(S)$. We can use a uniform distribution for m as before. In our empirical evaluation below, we consider both the Bayes and BBayes methods of generating parameter priors.

3   Results: detection power

We evaluated the Bayesian and frequentist methods on two types of simulated respiratory outbreaks, injected into real Emergency Department and over-the-counter drug sales data for Allegheny County, Pennsylvania. All data were aggregated to the zip code level to ensure anonymity, giving the daily counts of respiratory ED cases and sales of OTC cough and cold medication in each of 88 zip codes for one year. The baseline (expected count) for each zip code was estimated using the mean count of the previous 28 days. Zip code centroids were mapped to a 16×16 grid, and all rectangles up to 8×8 were examined. We first considered simulated aerosol releases of inhalational anthrax (e.g. from a bioterrorist attack), generated by the Bayesian Aerosol Release Detector, or BARD [9]. The BARD simulator uses a Bayesian network model to determine the number of spores inhaled by individuals in affected areas, the resulting number and severity of anthrax cases, and the resulting number of respiratory ED cases on each day of the outbreak in each affected zip code. Our second type of outbreak was a simulated "Fictional Linear Onset Outbreak" (or "FLOO"), as in [10]. A FLOO(Δ, T) outbreak is a simple simulated outbreak with duration T, which generates $t\Delta$ cases in each affected zip code on day t of the outbreak ($0 < t \leq T/2$), then generates $T\Delta/2$ cases per day for the remainder of the outbreak. Thus we have an outbreak where the number of cases ramps up linearly and then levels off. While this is clearly a less realistic outbreak than the BARD-simulated anthrax attack, it does have several advantages: most importantly, it allows us to precisely control the slope of the outbreak curve and examine how this affects our methods' detection ability.

To test detection power, a semi-synthetic testing framework similar to [10] was used: we first run our spatial scan statistic for each day of the last nine months of the year (the first three months are used only to estimate baselines and priors), and obtain the score F^* for each day. Then for each outbreak we wish to test, we inject that outbreak into the data, and obtain the score $F^*(t)$ for each day t of the outbreak. By finding the proportion of baseline days with scores higher than $F^*(t)$, we can determine the proportion of false positives we would have to accept to detect the outbreak on day t. This allows us to compute, for any given level of false positives, what proportion of outbreaks can be detected, and the mean number of days to detection. We compare three methods of computing the score F^*: the frequentist method (F^* is the maximum likelihood ratio $F(S)$ over all regions S), the Bayesian maximum method (F^* is the maximum posterior probability $P(H_1(S)\,|\,D)$ over all regions S), and the Bayesian total method (F^* is the sum of posterior probabilities $P(H_1(S)\,|\,D)$ over all regions S, i.e. total posterior probability of an outbreak). For the two Bayesian methods, we consider both Bayes and BBayes methods for calculating priors, thus giving us a total of five methods to compare (frequentist, Bayes_max, BBayes_max, Bayes_tot, BBayes_tot). In Table 1, we compare these methods with respect to proportion of outbreaks detected and

Table 1: Days to detect and proportion of outbreaks detected, 1 false positive/month

method	FLOO_ED (4,14)	FLOO_ED (2,20)	FLOO_ED (1,20)	BARD_ED (.125)	BARD_ED (.016)	FLOO_OTC (40,14)	FLOO_OTC (25,20)
frequentist	1.859 (100%)	3.324 (100%)	6.122 (96%)	1.733 (100%)	3.925 (88%)	3.582 (100%)	5.393 (100%)
Bayes_max	1.740 (100%)	2.875 (100%)	5.043 (100%)	**1.600** **(100%)**	3.755 (88%)	5.455 (63%)	7.588 (79%)
BBayes_max	**1.683** **(100%)**	**2.848** **(100%)**	**4.984** **(100%)**	**1.600** **(100%)**	**3.698** **(88%)**	5.164 (65%)	7.035 (77%)
Bayes_tot	1.882 (100%)	3.195 (100%)	5.777 (100%)	1.633 (100%)	3.811 (88%)	**3.475** **(100%)**	**5.195** **(100%)**
BBayes_tot	1.840 (100%)	3.180 (100%)	5.672 (100%)	1.617 (100%)	3.792 (88%)	4.380 (100%)	6.929 (99%)

mean number of days to detect, at a false positive rate of 1/month. Methods were evaluated on seven types of simulated outbreaks: three FLOO outbreaks on ED data, two FLOO outbreaks on OTC data, and two BARD outbreaks (with different amounts of anthrax release) on ED data. For each outbreak type, each method's performance was averaged over 100 or 250 simulated outbreaks for BARD or FLOO respectively.

In Table 1, we observe very different results for the ED and OTC datasets. For the five runs on ED data, all four Bayesian methods consistently detected outbreaks faster than the frequentist method. This difference was most evident for the more slowly growing (harder to detect) outbreaks, especially FLOO(1,20). Across all ED outbreaks, the Bayesian methods showed an average improvement of between 0.13 days (Bayes_tot) and 0.43 days (BBayes_max) as compared to the frequentist approach; "max" methods performed substantially better than "tot" methods, and "BBayes" methods performed slightly better than "Bayes" methods. For the two runs on OTC data, on the other hand, most of the Bayesian methods performed much worse (over 1 day slower) than the frequentist method. The exception was the Bayes_tot method, which again outperformed the frequentist method by an average of 0.15 days. We believe that the main reason for these differing results is that the OTC data is much noisier than the ED data, and exhibits much stronger seasonal trends. As a result, our baseline estimates (using mean of the previous 28 days) are reasonably accurate for ED, but for OTC the baseline estimates will lag behind the seasonal trends (and thus, underestimate the expected counts for increasing trends and overestimate for decreasing trends). The BBayes methods, which assume $E[C/B] = 1$ and thus rely heavily on the accuracy of baseline estimates, are not reasonable for OTC. On the other hand, the Bayes methods (which instead learn the priors from previous counts and baselines) can adjust for consistent misestimation of baselines and thus more accurately account for these seasonal trends. The "max" methods perform badly on the OTC data because a large number of baseline days have posterior probabilities close to 1; in this case, the maximum region posterior varies wildly from day to day, depending on how much of the total probability is assigned to a single region, and is not a reliable measure of whether an outbreak has occurred. The total posterior probability of an outbreak, on the other hand, will still be higher for outbreak than non-outbreak days, so the "tot" methods can perform well on OTC as well as ED data. Thus, our main result is that the Bayes_tot method, which infers baselines from past counts and uses total posterior probability of an outbreak to decide when to sound the alarm, consistently outperforms the frequentist method for both ED and OTC datasets.

4 Results: computation time

As noted above, the Bayesian spatial scan must search over all rectangular regions for the original grid only, while the frequentist scan (in order to calculate statistical significance by randomization) must also search over all rectangular regions for a large number (typically $R = 1000$) of replica grids. Thus, as long as the search time per region is comparable for the Bayesian and frequentist methods, we expect the Bayesian approach to be approximately 1000x faster. In Table 2, we compare the run times of the Bayes, BBayes, and frequen-

Table 2: Comparison of run times for varying grid size N

method	$N = 16$	$N = 32$	$N = 64$	$N = 128$	$N = 256$
Bayes (naive)	0.7 sec	10.8 sec	2.8 min	44 min	12 hrs
BBayes (naive)	0.6 sec	9.3 sec	2.4 min	37 min	10 hrs
frequentist (naive)	12 min	2.9 hrs	49 hrs	$\sim$31 days	$\sim$500 days
frequentist (fast)	20 sec	1.8 min	10.7 min	77 min	10 hrs

tist methods for searching a single grid and calculating significance (p-values or posterior probabilities for the frequentist and Bayesian methods respectively), as a function of the grid size N. All rectangles up to size $N/2$ were searched, and for the frequentist method $R = 1000$ replications were performed. The results confirm our intuition: the Bayesian methods are 900-1200x faster than the frequentist approach, for all values of N tested. However, the frequentist approach can be accelerated dramatically using our "fast spatial scan" algorithm [2], a multiresolution search method which can find the highest scoring region of a grid while searching only a small subset of regions. Comparing the fast spatial scan to the Bayesian approach, we see that the fast spatial scan is slower than the Bayesian method for grid sizes up to $N = 128$, but slightly faster for $N = 256$. Thus we now have two options for making the spatial scan statistic computationally feasible for large grid sizes: to use the fast spatial scan to speed up the frequentist scan statistic, or to use the Bayesian scan statistics framework (in which case the naive algorithm is typically fast enough). For even larger grid sizes, it may be possible to extend the fast spatial scan to the Bayesian approach: this would give us the best of both worlds, searching only one grid, and using a fast algorithm to do so. We are currently investigating this potentially useful synthesis.

5   Discussion

We have presented a Bayesian spatial scan statistic, and demonstrated several ways in which this method is preferable to the standard (frequentist) scan statistics approach. In Section 3, we demonstrated that the Bayesian method, with a relatively non-informative prior distribution, consistently outperforms the frequentist method with respect to detection power. Since the Bayesian framework allows us to easily incorporate prior information about size, shape, and impact of an outbreak, it is likely that we can achieve even better detection performance using more informative priors, e.g. obtained from experts in the domain. In Section 4, we demonstrated that the Bayesian spatial scan can be computed in much less time than the frequentist method, since randomization testing is unnecessary. This allows us to search large grid sizes using a naive search algorithm, and even larger grids might be searched by extending the fast spatial scan to the Bayesian framework.

We now consider three other arguments for use of the Bayesian spatial scan. First, the Bayesian method has easily interpretable results: it outputs the posterior probability that an outbreak has occurred, and the distribution of this probability over possible outbreak regions. This makes it easy for a user (e.g. public health official) to decide whether to investigate each potential outbreak based on the costs of false positives and false negatives; this type of decision analysis cannot be done easily in the frequentist framework. Another useful result of the Bayesian method is that we can compute a "map" of the posterior probabilities of an outbreak in each grid cell, by summing the posterior probabilities $P(H_1(S) \mid D)$ of all regions containing that cell. This technique allows us to deal with the case where the posterior probability mass is spread among many regions, by observing cells which are common to most or all of these regions. We give an example of such a map below:

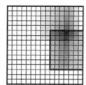

Figure 1: Output of Bayesian spatial scan on baseline OTC data, 1/30/05. Cell shading is based on posterior probability of an outbreak in that cell, ranging from white (0%) to black (100%). The bold rectangle represents the most likely region (posterior probability 12.27%) and the darkest cell is the most likely cell (total posterior probability 86.57%). Total posterior probability of an outbreak is 86.61%.

Second, calibration of the Bayesian statistic is easier than calibration of the frequentist statistic. As noted above, it is simple to adjust the sensitivity and specificity of the Bayesian method by setting the prior probability of an outbreak P_1, and then we can "sound the alarm" whenever posterior probability of an outbreak exceeds some threshold. In the frequentist method, on the other hand, many regions in the baseline data have sufficiently high likelihood ratios that no replicas beat the original grid; thus we cannot distinguish the p-values of outbreak and non-outbreak days. While one alternative is to "sound the alarm" when the likelihood ratio is above some threshold (rather than when p-value is below some threshold), this is technically incorrect: because the baselines for each day of data are different, the distribution of region scores under the null hypothesis will also differ from day to day, and thus days with higher likelihood ratios do not necessarily have lower p-values. Third, we argue that it is easier to combine evidence from multiple detectors within the Bayesian framework, i.e. by modeling the joint probability distribution. We are in the process of examining Bayesian detectors which look simultaneously at the day's Emergency Department records and over-the-counter drug sales in order to detect emerging clusters, and we believe that combination of detectors is an important area for future research.

In conclusion, we note that, though both Bayesian modeling [7-8] and (frequentist) spatial scanning [3-4] are common in the spatial statistics literature, this is (to the best of our knowledge) the first model which combines the two techniques into a single framework. In fact, very little work exists on Bayesian methods for spatial cluster detection. One notable exception is the literature on spatial cluster modeling [11-12], which attempts to infer the location of cluster centers by inferring parameters of a Bayesian process model. Our work differs from these methods both in its computational tractability (their models typically have no closed form solution, so computationally expensive MCMC approximations are used) and its easy interpretability (their models give no indication as to statistical significance or posterior probability of clusters found). Thus we believe that this is the first Bayesian spatial cluster detection method which is powerful and useful, yet computationally tractable. We are currently running the Bayesian and frequentist scan statistics on daily OTC sales data from over 10000 stores, searching for emerging disease outbreaks on a daily basis nationwide. Additionally, we are working to extend the Bayesian statistic to fMRI data, with the goal of discovering regions of brain activity corresponding to given cognitive tasks [13, 6]. We believe that the Bayesian approach has the potential to improve both speed and detection power of the spatial scan in this domain as well.

References

[1] M. Kulldorff. 1999. Spatial scan statistics: models, calculations, and applications. In J. Glaz and M. Balakrishnan, eds., *Scan Statistics and Applications*, Birkhauser, 303-322.

[2] D. B. Neill and A. W. Moore. 2004. Rapid detection of significant spatial clusters. In *Proc. 10th ACM SIGKDD Intl. Conf. on Knowledge Discovery and Data Mining*, 256-265.

[3] M. Kulldorff and N. Nagarwalla. 1995. Spatial disease clusters: detection and inference. *Statistics in Medicine* **14**, 799-810.

[4] M. Kulldorff. 1997. A spatial scan statistic. *Communications in Statistics: Theory and Methods* **26**(6), 1481-1496.

[5] D. B. Neill and A. W. Moore. 2004. A fast multi-resolution method for detection of significant spatial disease clusters. In *Advances in Neural Information Processing Systems* **16**, 651-658.

[6] D. B. Neill, A. W. Moore, F. Pereira, and T. Mitchell. 2005. Detecting significant multidimensional spatial clusters. In *Advances in Neural Information Processing Systems* **17**, 969-976.

[7] D. G. Clayton and J. Kaldor. 1987. Empirical Bayes estimates of age-standardized relative risks for use in disease mapping. *Biometrics* **43**, 671-681.

[8] A. Mollié. 1999. Bayesian and empirical Bayes approaches to disease mapping. In A. B. Lawson, et al., eds. *Disease Mapping and Risk Assessment for Public Health*. Wiley, Chichester.

[9] W. Hogan, G. Cooper, M. Wagner, and G. Wallstrom. 2004. A Bayesian anthrax aerosol release detector. Technical Report, RODS Laboratory, University of Pittsburgh.

[10] D. B. Neill, A. W. Moore, M. Sabhnani, and K. Daniel. 2005. Detection of emerging space-time clusters. In *Proc. 11th ACM SIGKDD Intl. Conf. on Knowledge Discovery and Data Mining*.

[11] R. E. Gangnon and M. K. Clayton. 2000. Bayesian detection and modeling of spatial disease clustering. *Biometrics* **56**, 922-935.

[12] A. B. Lawson and D. G. T. Denison, eds. 2002. *Spatial Cluster Modelling*. Chapman & Hall/CRC, Boca Raton, FL.

[13] X. Wang, R. Hutchinson, and T. Mitchell. 2004. Training fMRI classifiers to detect cognitive states across multiple human subjects. In *Advances in Neural Information Processing Systems* **16**, 709-716.

Divergences, surrogate loss functions and experimental design

XuanLong Nguyen
University of California
Berkeley, CA 94720
xuanlong@cs.berkeley.edu

Martin J. Wainwright
University of California
Berkeley, CA 94720
wainwrig@eecs.berkeley.edu

Michael I. Jordan
University of California
Berkeley, CA 94720
jordan@cs.berkeley.edu

Abstract

In this paper, we provide a general theorem that establishes a correspondence between surrogate loss functions in classification and the family of f-divergences. Moreover, we provide constructive procedures for determining the f-divergence induced by a given surrogate loss, and conversely for finding all surrogate loss functions that realize a given f-divergence. Next we introduce the notion of universal equivalence among loss functions and corresponding f-divergences, and provide necessary and sufficient conditions for universal equivalence to hold. These ideas have applications to classification problems that also involve a component of experiment design; in particular, we leverage our results to prove consistency of a procedure for learning a classifier under decentralization requirements.

1 Introduction

A unifying theme in the recent literature on classification is the notion of a *surrogate loss function*—a convex upper bound on the 0-1 loss. Many practical classification algorithms can be formulated in terms of the minimization of surrogate loss functions; well-known examples include the support vector machine (hinge loss) and Adaboost (exponential loss). Significant progress has been made on the theoretical front by analyzing the general statistical consequences of using surrogate loss functions [e.g., 2, 10, 13].

These recent developments have an interesting historical antecedent. Working in the context of experimental design, researchers in the 1960's recast the (intractable) problem of minimizing the probability of classification error in terms of the maximization of various surrogate functions [e.g., 5, 8]. Examples of experimental design include the choice of a quantizer as a preprocessor for a classifier [12], or the choice of a "signal set" for a radar system [5]. The surrogate functions that were used included the Hellinger distance and various forms of KL divergence; maximization of these functions was proposed as a criterion for the choice of a design. Theoretical support for this approach was provided by a classical theorem on the comparison of experiments due to Blackwell [3]. An important outcome of this line of work was the definition of a general family of "f-divergences" (also known as "Ali-Silvey distances"), which includes Hellinger distance and KL divergence as special cases [1, 4].

In broad terms, the goal of the current paper is to bring together these two literatures, in particular by establishing a correspondence between the family of surrogate loss functions and the family of f-divergences. Several specific goals motivate us in this regard: (1) different f-divergences are related by various well-known inequalities [11], so that a correspondence between loss functions and f-divergences would allow these inequalities to be harnessed in analyzing surrogate loss functions; (2) a correspondence could allow the definition of interesting equivalence classes of losses or divergences; and (3) the problem of experimental design, which motivated the classical research on f-divergences, provides new venues for applying the loss function framework from machine learning. In particular, one natural extension—and one which we explore towards the end of this paper—is in requiring consistency not only in the choice of an optimal discriminant function but also in the choice of an optimal experiment design.

The main technical contribution of this paper is to state and prove a general theorem relating surrogate loss functions and f-divergences. [1] We show that the correspondence is quite strong: any surrogate loss induces a corresponding f-divergence, and any f-divergence satisfying certain conditions corresponds to a family of surrogate loss functions. Moreover, exploiting tools from convex analysis, we provide a constructive procedure for finding loss functions from f-divergences. We also introduce and analyze a notion of *universal equivalence* among loss functions (and corresponding f-divergences). Finally, we present an application of these ideas to the problem of proving consistency of classification algorithms with an additional decentralization requirement.

2 Background and elementary results

Consider a covariate $X \in \mathcal{X}$, where $\mathcal{X}$ is a compact topological space, and a random variable $Y \in \mathcal{Y} := \{-1, +1\}$. The space $(X \times Y)$ is assumed to be endowed with a Borel regular probability measure P. In this paper, we consider a variant of the standard classification problem, in which the decision-maker, rather than having direct access to X, only observes some variable $Z \in \mathcal{Z}$ that is obtained via conditional probability $Q(Z|X)$. The stochastic map Q is referred to as an *experiment* in statistics; in the signal processing literature, where $\mathcal{Z}$ is generally taken to be discrete, it is referred to as a *quantizer*. We let $\mathcal{Q}$ denote the space of all stochastic Q and let $\mathcal{Q}_0$ denote its deterministic subset.

Given a fixed experiment Q, we can formulate a standard binary classification problem as one of finding a measurable function $\gamma \in \Gamma := \{\mathcal{Z} \to \mathbb{R}\}$ that minimizes the *Bayes risk* $P(Y \neq \text{sign}(\gamma(Z)))$. Our focus is the broader question of determining both the classifier $\gamma \in \Gamma$, as well as the experiment choice $Q \in \mathcal{Q}$ so as to minimize the Bayes risk.

The Bayes risk corresponds to the expectation of the 0-1 loss. Given the non-convexity of this loss function, it is natural to consider a surrogate loss function ϕ that we optimize in place of the 0-1 loss. We refer to the quantity $R_\phi(\gamma, Q) := \mathbb{E}\phi(Y\gamma(Z))$ as the *ϕ-risk*. For each fixed quantization rule Q, the optimal ϕ risk (as a function of Q) is defined as follows:

$$R_\phi(Q) := \inf_{\gamma \in \Gamma} R_\phi(\gamma, Q). \qquad (1)$$

Given priors $q = P(Y = -1)$ and $p = P(Y = 1)$, define nonnegative measures μ and π:

$$\mu(z) \quad = \quad P(Y = 1, Z = z) = p \int_x Q(z|x) dP(x|Y = 1)$$

$$\pi(z) \quad = \quad P(Y = -1, Z = z) = q \int_x Q(z|x) dP(x|Y = -1).$$

---

[1]Proofs are omitted from this manuscript for lack of space; see the long version of the paper [7] for proofs of all of our results.

As a consequence of Lyapunov's theorem, the space of $\{(\mu, \pi)\}$ obtained by varying $Q \in \mathcal{Q}$ (or $\mathcal{Q}_0$) is both compact and convex (see [12] for details). For simplicity, we assume that the space $\mathcal{Q}$ of Q is restricted such that both μ and π are strictly positive measures.

One approach to choosing Q is to define an f-divergence between μ and π; indeed this is the classical approach referred to earlier [e.g., 8]. Rather than following this route, however, we take an alternative path, setting up the problem in terms of ϕ-risk and optimizing out the discriminant function γ. Note in particular that the ϕ-risk can be represented in terms of the measures μ and π as follows:

$$R_\phi(\gamma, Q) \quad = \quad \sum_z \phi(\gamma(z))\mu(z) + \phi(-\gamma(z))\pi(z). \tag{2}$$

This representation allows us to compute the optimal value for $\gamma(z)$ for all $z \in \mathcal{Z}$, as well as the optimal ϕ risk for a fixed Q. We illustrate this calculation with several examples:

0-1 loss. If ϕ is 0-1 loss, then $\gamma(z) = \text{sign}(\mu(z) - \pi(z))$. Thus the optimal Bayes risk given a fixed Q takes the form: $R_{bayes}(Q) = \sum_{z \in \mathcal{Z}} \min\{\mu(z), \pi(z)\} = \frac{1}{2} - \frac{1}{2}\sum_{z \in \mathcal{Z}} |\mu(z) - \pi(z)| =: \frac{1}{2}(1 - V(\mu, \pi))$, where $V(\mu, \pi)$ denotes the variational distance between two measures μ and π.

Hinge loss. Let $\phi_{hinge}(y\gamma(z)) = (1 - y\gamma(z))_+$. In this case $\gamma(z) = \text{sign}(\mu(z) - \pi(z))$ and the optimal risk takes the form: $R_{hinge}(Q) = \sum_{z \in \mathcal{Z}} 2\min\{\mu(z), \pi(z)\} = 1 - \sum_{z \in \mathcal{Z}} |\mu(z) - \pi(z)| = 1 - V(\mu, \pi) = 2R_{bayes}(Q)$.

Least squares loss. Letting $\phi_{sqr}(y\gamma(z)) = (1 - y\gamma(z))^2$, we have $\gamma(z) = \frac{\mu(z) - \pi(z)}{\mu(z) + \pi(z)}$. The optimal risk takes the form: $R_{sqr}(Q) = \sum_{z \in \mathcal{Z}} \frac{4\mu(z)\pi(z)}{\mu(z) + \pi(z)} = 1 - \sum_{z \in \mathcal{Z}} \frac{(\mu(z) - \pi(z))^2}{\mu(z) + \pi(z)} =: 1 - \Delta(\mu, \pi)$, where $\Delta(\mu, \pi)$ denotes the *triangular discrimination* distance.

Logistic loss. Letting $\phi_{log}(y\gamma(z)) := \log\left(1 + \exp^{-y\gamma(z)}\right)$, we have $\gamma(z) = \log\frac{\mu(z)}{\pi(z)}$. The optimal risk for logistic loss takes the form: $R_{log}(Q) = \sum_{z \in \mathcal{Z}} \mu(z)\log\frac{\mu(z) + \pi(z)}{\mu(z)} + \pi(z)\log\frac{\mu(z) + \pi(z)}{\pi(z)} = \log 2 - KL(\mu||\frac{\mu + \pi}{2}) - KL(\pi||\frac{\mu + \pi}{2}) =: \log 2 - C(\mu, \pi)$, where $C(U, V)$ denotes the *capacitory discrimination* distance.

Exponential loss. Letting $\phi_{exp}(y\gamma(z)) = \exp(-y\gamma(z))$, we have $\gamma(z) = \frac{1}{2}\log\frac{\mu(z)}{\pi(z)}$. The optimal risk for exponential loss takes the form: $R_{exp}(Q) = \sum_{z \in \mathcal{Z}} 2\sqrt{\mu(z)\pi(z)} = 1 - \sum_{z \in \mathcal{Z}}(\sqrt{\mu(z)} - \sqrt{\pi(z)})^2 = 1 - 2h^2(\mu, \pi)$, where $h(\mu, \pi)$ denotes the Hellinger distance between measures μ and π.

All of the distances given above (e.g., variational, Hellinger) are all particular instances of f-divergences. This fact points to an interesting correspondence between optimized ϕ-risks and f-divergences. How general is this correspondence?

3 The correspondence between loss functions and f-divergences

In order to resolve this question, we begin with precise definitions of f-divergences, and surrogate loss functions. A f-*divergence functional* is defined as follows [1, 4]:

Definition 1. *Given any continuous convex function* $f : [0, +\infty) \rightarrow \mathbb{R} \cup \{+\infty\}$, *the f-divergence between measures μ and π is given by* $I_f(\mu, \pi) := \sum_z \pi(z)f\left(\frac{\mu(z)}{\pi(z)}\right)$.

For instance, the variational distance is given by $f(u) = |u - 1|$, KL divergence by $f(u) = u\log u$, triangular discrimination by $f(u) = (u - 1)^2/(u + 1)$, and Hellinger distance by $f(u) = \frac{1}{2}(\sqrt{u} - 1)^2$.

Surrogate loss ϕ. First, we require that any *surrogate* loss function ϕ is continuous and convex. Second, the function ϕ must be *classification-calibrated* [2], meaning that for any $a, b \geq 0$ and $a \neq b$, $\inf_{\alpha:\alpha(a-b)<0} \phi(\alpha)a + \phi(-\alpha)b > \inf_{\alpha\in\mathbb{R}} \phi(\alpha)a + \phi(-\alpha)b$. It can be shown [2] that in the convex case ϕ is classification-calibrated if and only if it is differentiable at 0 and $\phi'(0) < 0$. Lastly, let $\alpha^* = \inf_\alpha\{\phi(\alpha) = \inf \phi\}$. If $\alpha^* < +\infty$, then for any $\delta > 0$, we require that $\phi(\alpha^* - \delta) \geq \phi(\alpha^* + \delta)$. The interpretation of the last assumption is that one should penalize deviations away from α^* in the negative direction at least as strongly as deviations in the positive direction; this requirement is intuitively reasonable given the margin-based interpretation of α.

From ϕ-risk to f-divergence. We begin with a simple result that formalizes how any ϕ-risk induces a corresponding f-divergence. More precisely, the following lemma proves that the optimal ϕ risk for a fixed Q can be written as the negative of an f divergence.

Lemma 2. *For each fixed Q, let γ_Q denote the optimal decision rule. The ϕ risk for (Q, γ_Q) is an f-divergence between μ and π for some convex function f:*

$$R_\phi(Q) = -I_f(\mu, \pi). \tag{3}$$

Proof. The optimal ϕ risk takes the form:

$$R_\phi(Q) = \sum_{z\in\mathcal{Z}} \inf_\alpha (\phi(\alpha)\mu(z) + \phi(-\alpha)\pi(z)) = \sum_z \pi(z)\inf_\alpha\left(\phi(-\alpha) + \phi(\alpha)\frac{\mu(z)}{\pi(z)}\right).$$

For each z let $u = \frac{\mu(z)}{\pi(z)}$, then $\inf_\alpha(\phi(-\alpha) + \phi(\alpha)u)$ is a concave function of u (since minimization over a set of linear function is a concave function). Thus, the claim follows by defining (for $u \in \mathbb{R}$)

$$f(u) := -\inf_\alpha(\phi(-\alpha) + \phi(\alpha)u). \tag{4}$$

From f-divergence to ϕ-risk. In the remainder of this section, we explore the converse of Lemma 2. Given a divergence $I_f(\mu, \pi)$ for some convex function f, does there exist a loss function ϕ for which $R_\phi(Q) = -I_f(\mu, \pi)$? In the following, we provide a precise characterization of the set of f-divergences that can be realized in this way, as well as a constructive procedure for determining all ϕ that realize a given f-divergence.

Our method requires the introduction of several intermediate functions. First, let us define, for each β, the inverse mapping $\phi^{-1}(\beta) := \inf\{\alpha : \phi(\alpha) \leq \beta\}$, where $\inf \emptyset := +\infty$. Using the function ϕ^{-1}, we then define a new function $\Psi : \mathbb{R} \to \bar{\mathbb{R}}$ by

$$\Psi(\beta) := \begin{cases} \phi(-\phi^{-1}(\beta)) & \text{if } \phi^{-1}(\beta) \in \mathbb{R}, \\ +\infty & \text{otherwise.} \end{cases} \tag{5}$$

Note that the domain of Ψ is $\text{Dom}(\Psi) = \{\beta \in \mathbb{R} : \phi^{-1}(\beta) \in \mathbb{R}\}$. Define

$$\beta_1 := \inf\{\beta : \Psi(\beta) < +\infty\} \text{ and } \beta_2 := \inf\{\beta : \Psi(\beta) = \inf \Psi\}. \tag{6}$$

It is simple to check that $\inf \phi = \inf \Psi = \phi(\alpha^*)$, and $\beta_1 = \phi(\alpha^*)$, $\beta_2 = \phi(-\alpha^*)$. Furthermore, $\Psi(\beta_2) = \phi(\alpha^*) = \beta_1$, $\Psi(\beta_1) = \phi(-\alpha^*) = \beta_2$. With this set-up, the following lemma captures several important properties of Ψ:

Lemma 3.   (a) Ψ *is strictly decreasing in (β_1, β_2). If ϕ is decreasing, then Ψ is also decreasing in $(-\infty, +\infty)$. In addition, $\Psi(\beta) = +\infty$ for $\beta < \beta_1$.*

(b) Ψ *is convex in $(-\infty, \beta_2]$. If ϕ is decreasing, then Ψ is convex in $(-\infty, +\infty)$.*

(c) Ψ *is lower semi-continuous, and continuous in its domain.*

(d) *There exists $u^* \in (\beta_1, \beta_2)$ such that $\Psi(u^*) = u^*$.*

(e) There holds $\Psi(\Psi(\beta)) = \beta$ for all $\beta \in (\beta_1, \beta_2)$.

The connection between Ψ and an f-divergence arises from the following fact. Given the definition (5) of Ψ, it is possible to show that

$$f(u) = \sup_{\beta \in \mathbb{R}}(-\beta u - \Psi(\beta)) = \Psi^*(-u), \tag{7}$$

where Ψ^* denotes the conjugate dual of the function Ψ. Hence, if Ψ is a lower semicontinuous convex function, it is possible to recover Ψ from f by means of convex duality [9]: $\Psi(\beta) = f^*(-\beta)$. Thus, equation (5) provides means for recovering a loss function ϕ from Ψ. Indeed, the following theorem provides a constructive procedure for finding all such ϕ when Ψ satisfies necessary conditions specified in Lemma 3:

Theorem 4. *(a) Given a lower semicontinuous convex function $f : \mathbb{R} \to \overline{\mathbb{R}}$, define:*

$$\Psi(\beta) = f^*(-\beta). \tag{8}$$

If Ψ is a decreasing function satisfying the properties specified in parts (c), (d) and (e) of Lemma 3, then there exist convex continuous loss function ϕ for which (3) and (4) hold.

(b) More precisely, all such functions ϕ are of the form: For any $\alpha \geq 0$,

$$\phi(\alpha) = \Psi(g(\alpha + u^*)), \quad \text{and} \quad \phi(-\alpha) = g(\alpha + u^*), \tag{9}$$

where u^* satisfies $\Psi(u^*) = u^*$ for some $u^* \in (\beta_1, \beta_2)$ and $g : [u^*, +\infty) \to \overline{\mathbb{R}}$ is any increasing continuous convex function such that $g(u^*) = u^*$. Moreover, g is differentiable at u^*+ and $g'(u^*+) > 0$.

One interesting consequence of Theorem 4 that any realizable f-divergence can in fact be obtained from a fairly large set of ϕ loss functions. More precisely, examining the statement of Theorem 4(b) reveals that for $\alpha \leq 0$, we are free to choose a function g that must satisfy only mild conditions; given a choice of g, then ϕ is specified for $\alpha > 0$ accordingly by equation (9). We describe below how the Hellinger distance, for instance, is realized not only by the exponential loss (as described earlier), but also by many other surrogate loss functions. Additional examples can be found in [7].

Illustrative examples. Consider Hellinger distance, which is an f-divergence[2] with $f(u) = -2\sqrt{u}$. Augment the domain of f with $f(u) = +\infty$ for $u < 0$. Following the prescription of Theorem 4(a), we first recover Ψ from f:

$$\Psi(\beta) = f^*(-\beta) = \sup_{u \in \mathbb{R}}(-\beta u - f(u)) = \begin{cases} 1/\beta & \text{when } \beta > 0 \\ +\infty & \text{otherwise.} \end{cases}$$

Clearly, $u^* = 1$. Now if we choose $g(u) = e^{u-1}$, then we obtain the exponential loss $\phi(\alpha) = \exp(-\alpha)$. However, making the alternative choice $g(u) = u$, we obtain the function $\phi(\alpha) = 1/(\alpha+1)$ and $\phi(-\alpha) = \alpha+1$, which also realizes the Hellinger distance.

Recall that we have shown previously that the 0-1 loss induces the variational distance, which can be expressed as an f-divergence with $f_{\text{var}}(u) = -2\min(u, 1)$ for $u \geq 0$. It is thus of particular interest to determine other loss functions that also lead to variational distance. If we augment the function f_{var} by defining $f_{\text{var}}(u) = +\infty$ for $u < 0$, then we can recover Ψ from f_{var} as follows:

$$\Psi(\beta) = f^*_{\text{var}}(-\beta) = \sup_{u \in \mathbb{R}}(-\beta u - f_{\text{var}}(u)) = \begin{cases} (2 - \beta)_+ & \text{when } \beta \geq 0 \\ +\infty & \text{when } \beta < 0. \end{cases}$$

---

[2]We consider f-divergences for two convex functions f_1 and f_2 to be equivalent if f_1 and f_2 are related by a linear term, i.e., $f_1 = cf_2 + au + b$ for some constants $c > 0, a, b$, because then I_{f_1} and I_{f_2} are different by a constant.

Clearly $u^* = 1$. Choosing $g(u) = u$ leads to the hinge loss $\phi(\alpha) = (1 - \alpha)_+$, which is consistent with our earlier findings. Making the alternative choice $g(u) = e^{u-1}$ leads to a rather different loss—namely, $\phi(\alpha) = (2 - e^{\alpha})_+$ for $\alpha \geq 0$ and $\phi(\alpha) = e^{-\alpha}$ for $\alpha < 0$— that also realizes the variational distance.

Using Theorem 4 it can be shown that an f-divergence is realizable by a margin-based surrogate loss if and only if it is symmetric [7]. Hence, the list of non-realizable f-divergences includes the KL divergence $KL(\mu||\pi)$ (as well as $KL(\pi||\mu)$). The *symmetric* KL divergence $KL(\mu||\pi) + KL(\pi||\mu)$ is a realizable f-divergence. Theorem 4 allows us to construct all ϕ losses that realize it. One of them turns out to have the simple closed-form $\phi(\alpha) = e^{-\alpha} - \alpha$, but obtaining it requires some non-trivial calculations [7].

4 On comparison of loss functions and quantization schemes

The previous section was devoted to study of the correspondence between f-divergences and the optimal ϕ-risk $R_\phi(Q)$ for a fixed experiment Q. Our ultimate goal, however, is that of choosing an optimal Q, a problem known as experimental design in the statistics literature [3]. One concrete application is the design of quantizers for performing decentralized detection [12, 6] in a sensor network.

In this section, we address the experiment design problem via the joint optimization of ϕ-risk (or more precisely, its empirical version) over both the decision γ and the choice of experiment Q (hereafter referred to as a quantizer). This procedure raises the natural theoretical question: for what loss functions ϕ does such joint optimization lead to minimum Bayes risk? Note that the minimum here is taken over both the decision rule γ and the space of experiments Q, so that this question is not covered by standard consistency results [13, 10, 2]. Here we describe how the results of the previous section can be leveraged to resolve this issue of consistency.

4.1 Universal equivalence

The connection between f-divergences and 0-1 loss can be traced back to seminal work on the comparison of experiments [3]. Formally, we say that the quantization scheme Q_1 *dominates* than Q_2 if $R_{bayes}(Q_1) \leq R_{bayes}(Q_2)$ for any prior probabilities $q \in (0, 1)$. We have the following theorem [3] (see also [7] for a short proof):

Theorem 5. Q_1 *dominates* Q_2 iff $I_f(\mu^{Q_1}, \pi^{Q_1}) \geq I_f(\mu^{Q_2}, \pi^{Q_2})$, *for all convex functions* f. *The superscripts denote the dependence of* μ *and* π *on the quantizer rules* Q_1, Q_2.

Using Lemma 2, we can establish the following:

Corollary 6. Q_1 *dominates* Q_2 iff $R_\phi(Q_1) \leq R_\phi(Q_2)$ *for any surrogate loss* ϕ.

One implication of Corollary 6 is that if $R_\phi(Q_1) \leq R_\phi(Q_2)$ for some loss function ϕ, then $R_{bayes}(Q_1) \leq R_{bayes}(Q_2)$ for some set of prior probabilities on the labels Y. This fact justifies the use of a surrogate ϕ-loss as a proxy for the 0-1 loss, at least for a certain subset of prior probabilities. Typically, however, the goal is to select the optimal experiment Q for a pre-specified set of priors, in which context this implication is of limited use. We are thus motivated to consider a different method of determining which loss functions (or equivalently, f-divergences) lead to the same optimal experimental design as the 0-1 loss (respectively the variational distance). More generally, we are interested in comparing two arbitrary loss function ϕ_1 and ϕ_2, with corresponding divergences induced by f_1 and f_2 respectively:

Definition 7. *The surrogate loss functions* ϕ_1 *and* ϕ_2 *are* universally equivalent, *denoted by* $\phi_1 \overset{u}{\approx} \phi_2$ *(and* $f_1 \overset{u}{\approx} f_2$*), if for any* $P(X, Y)$ *and quantization rules* Q_1, Q_2*, there holds:*

$$R_{\phi_1}(Q_1) \leq R_{\phi_1}(Q_2) \Leftrightarrow R_{\phi_2}(Q_1) \leq R_{\phi_2}(Q_2). \tag{10}$$

The following result provides necessary and sufficient conditions for universal equivalence:

Theorem 8. *Suppose that f_1 and f_2 are differentiable a.e., convex functions that map $[0, +\infty)$ to $\mathbb{R}$. Then $f_1 \overset{u}{\approx} f_2$ if and only if $f_1(u) = cf_2(u) + au + b$ for some constants $a, b \in \mathbb{R}$ and $c > 0$.*

If we restrict our attention to convex and differentiable a.e. functions f, then it follows that all f-divergences univerally equivalent to the variational distance must have the form

$$f(u) = -c\min(u, 1) + au + b \qquad \text{with } c > 0. \tag{11}$$

As a consequence, the only ϕ-loss functions universally equivalent to 0-1 loss are those that induce an f-divergence of this form (11). One well-known example of such a function is the hinge loss; more generally, Theorem 4 allows us to construct all such ϕ.

4.2 Consistency in experimental design

The notion of universal equivalence might appear quite restrictive because condition (10) must hold for *any* underlying probability measure $P(X, Y)$. However, this is precisely what we need when $P(X, Y)$ is unknown. Assume that the knowledge about $P(X, Y)$ comes from an empirical data sample $(x_i, y_i)_{i=1}^n$.

Consider any algorithm (such as that proposed by Nguyen et al. [6]) that involves choosing a classifier-quantizer pair $(\gamma, Q) \in \Gamma \times \mathcal{Q}$ by minimizing an empirical version of ϕ-risk:

$$\hat{R}_\phi(\gamma, Q) := \frac{1}{n} \sum_{i=1}^n \sum_z \phi(y_i\gamma(z))Q(z|x_i).$$

More formally, suppose that $(\mathcal{C}_n, \mathcal{D}_n)$ is a sequence of increasing compact function classes such that $\mathcal{C}_1 \subseteq \mathcal{C}_2 \subseteq \ldots \subseteq \Gamma$ and $\mathcal{D}_1 \subseteq \mathcal{D}_2 \subseteq \ldots \subseteq \mathcal{Q}$. Let (γ_n^*, Q_n^*) be an optimal solution to the minimization problem $\min_{(\gamma, Q) \in (\mathcal{C}_n, \mathcal{D}_n)} \hat{R}_\phi(\gamma, Q)$, and let R_{bayes}^* denote the minimum Bayes risk achieved over the space of decision rules $(\gamma, Q) \in (\Gamma, \mathcal{Q})$. We call $R_{bayes}(\gamma_n^*, Q_n^*) - R_{bayes}^*$ the *Bayes error* of our estimation procedure. We say that such a procedure is *universally consistent* if the Bayes error tends to 0 as $n \to \infty$, i.e., for any (unknown) Borel probability measure P on $X \times Y$,

$$\lim_{n \to \infty} R_{bayes}(\gamma_n^*, Q_n^*) - R_{bayes}^* = 0 \quad \text{in probability.}$$

When the surrogate loss ϕ is universally equivalent to 0-1 loss, we can prove that suitable learning procedures are indeed universally consistent. Our approach is based on the framework developed by various authors [13, 10, 2] for the case of ordinary classification, and using the strategy of decomposing the Bayes error into a combination of (a) *approximation error* introduced by the bias of the function classes $\mathcal{C}_n \subseteq \Gamma$: $\mathcal{E}_0(\mathcal{C}_n, \mathcal{D}_n) = \inf_{(\gamma, Q) \in (\mathcal{C}_n, \mathcal{D}_n)} R_\phi(\gamma, Q) - R_\phi^*$, where $R_\phi^* := \inf_{(\gamma, Q) \in (\Gamma, \mathcal{Q})} R_\phi(\gamma, Q)$; and (b) *estimation error* introduced by the variance of using finite sample size n, $\mathcal{E}_1(\mathcal{C}_n, \mathcal{D}_n) = \mathbb{E} \sup_{(\gamma, Q) \in (\mathcal{C}_n, \mathcal{D}_n)} |\hat{R}_\phi(\gamma, Q) - R_\phi(\gamma, Q)|$, where the expectation is taken with respect to the (unknown) probability measure $P(X, Y)$.

Assumptions. Assume that the loss function ϕ is universally equivalent to the 0-1 loss. From Theorem 8, the corresponding f-divergence must be of the form $f(u) = -c\min(u, 1) + au + b$, for $a, b \in \mathbb{R}$ and $c > 0$. Finally, we also assume that $(a - b)(p - q) \geq 0$ and $\phi(0) \geq 0$.[3] In addition, for each $n = 1, 2, \ldots$, suppose that $M_n := \sup_{y,z} \sup_{(\gamma, Q) \in (\mathcal{C}_n, \mathcal{D}_n)} |\phi(y\gamma(z))| < +\infty$.

---

[3]These technical conditions are needed so that the approximation error due to varying Q dominates the approximation error due to varying γ. Setting $a = b$ is sufficient.

The following lemma plays a key role in our proof: it links the excess ϕ-risk to the Bayes error when performing joint minimization:

Lemma 9. *For any* (γ, Q), *we have* $\frac{c}{2}(R_{bayes}(\gamma, Q) - R^*_{bayes}) \leq R_\phi(\gamma, Q) - R^*_\phi$.

Finally, we can relate the Bayes error to the approximation error and estimation error, and provide general conditions for universal consistency:

Theorem 10. *(a) For any Borel probability measure P, with probability at least $1 - \delta$, there holds:* $R_{bayes}(\gamma^*_n, Q^*_n) - R^*_{bayes} \leq \frac{2}{c}(2\mathcal{E}_1(\mathcal{C}_n, \mathcal{D}_n) + \mathcal{E}_0(\mathcal{C}_n, \mathcal{D}_n) + 2M_n\sqrt{2\ln(2/\delta)/n})$.
(b) (Universal Consistency) If $\cup_{n=1}^\infty \mathcal{D}_n$ is dense in $\mathcal{Q}$ and if $\cup_{n=1}^\infty \mathcal{C}_n$ is dense in Γ so that $\lim_{n\to\infty} \mathcal{E}_0(\mathcal{C}_n, \mathcal{D}_n) = 0$, and if the sequence of function classes $(\mathcal{C}_n, \mathcal{D}_n)$ grows sufficiently slowly enough so that $\lim_{n\to\infty} \mathcal{E}_1(\mathcal{C}_n, \mathcal{D}_n) = \lim_{n\to\infty} M_n\sqrt{\ln n/n} = 0$, there holds $\lim_{n\to\infty} R_{bayes}(\gamma^*_n, Q^*_n) - R^*_{bayes} = 0$ in probability.

5 Conclusions

We have presented a general theoretical connection between surrogate loss functions and f-divergences. As illustrated by our application to decentralized detection, this connection can provide new domains of application for statistical learning theory. We also expect that this connection will provide new applications for f-divergences within learning theory; note in particular that bounds among f-divergences (of which many are known; see, e.g., [11]) induce corresponding bounds among loss functions.

References

[1] S. M. Ali and S. D. Silvey. A general class of coefficients of divergence of one distribution from another. *J. Royal Stat. Soc. Series B*, 28:131–142, 1966.

[2] P. Bartlett, M. I. Jordan, and J. D. McAuliffe. Convexity, classification and risk bounds. *Journal of the American Statistical Association*, 2005. To appear.

[3] D. Blackwell. Equivalent comparisons of experiments. *Annals of Statistics*, 24(2):265–272, 1953.

[4] I. Csiszár. Information-type measures of difference of probability distributions and indirect observation. *Studia Sci. Math. Hungar*, 2:299–318, 1967.

[5] T. Kailath. The divergence and Bhattacharyya distance measures in signal selection. *IEEE Trans. on Communication Technology*, 15(1):52–60, 1967.

[6] X. Nguyen, M. J. Wainwright, and M. I. Jordan. Nonparametric decentralized detection using kernel methods. *IEEE Transactions on Signal Processing*, 53(11):4053–4066, 2005.

[7] X. Nguyen, M. J. Wainwright, and M. I. Jordan. On divergences, surrogate loss functions and decentralized detection. Technical Report 695, Department of Statistics, University of California at Berkeley, September 2005.

[8] H. V. Poor and J. B. Thomas. Applications of Ali-Silvey distance measures in the design of generalized quantizers for binary decision systems. *IEEE Trans. on Communications*, 25:893–900, 1977.

[9] G. Rockafellar. *Convex Analysis*. Princeton University Press, Princeton, 1970.

[10] I. Steinwart. Consistency of support vector machines and other regularized kernel machines. *IEEE Trans. Info. Theory*, 51:128–142, 2005.

[11] F. Topsoe. Some inequalities for information divergence and related measures of discrimination. *IEEE Transactions on Information Theory*, 46:1602–1609, 2000.

[12] J. Tsitsiklis. Extremal properties of likelihood-ratio quantizers. *IEEE Trans. on Communication*, 41(4):550–558, 1993.

[13] T. Zhang. Statistical behavior and consistency of classification methods based on convex risk minimization. *Annal of Statistics*, 53:56–134, 2004.

How fast to work: Response vigor, motivation and tonic dopamine

Yael Niv[1,2]   Nathaniel D. Daw[2]   Peter Dayan[2]
[1]ICNC, Hebrew University, Jerusalem   [2]Gatsby Computational Neuroscience Unit, UCL
yaelniv@alice.nc.huji.ac.il   {daw,dayan}@gatsby.ucl.ac.uk

Abstract

Reinforcement learning models have long promised to unify computational, psychological and neural accounts of appetitively conditioned behavior. However, the bulk of data on animal conditioning comes from free-operant experiments measuring how fast animals will work for reinforcement. Existing reinforcement learning (RL) models are silent about these tasks, because they lack any notion of *vigor*. They thus fail to address the simple observation that hungrier animals will work harder for food, as well as stranger facts such as their sometimes greater productivity even when working for irrelevant outcomes such as water. Here, we develop an RL framework for free-operant behavior, suggesting that subjects choose how vigorously to perform selected actions by optimally balancing the costs and benefits of quick responding. Motivational states such as hunger shift these factors, skewing the tradeoff. This accounts normatively for the effects of motivation on response rates, as well as many other classic findings. Finally, we suggest that tonic levels of dopamine may be involved in the computation linking motivational state to optimal responding, thereby explaining the complex vigor-related effects of pharmacological manipulation of dopamine.

1   Introduction

A banal, but nonetheless valid, behaviorist observation is that hungry animals work harder to get food [1]. However, associated with this observation are two stranger experimental facts and a large theoretical failing. The first weird fact is that hungry animals will in some circumstances work more vigorously even for motivationally irrelevant outcomes such as water [2, 3], which seems highly counterintuitive. Second, contrary to the emphasis theoretical accounts have placed on the effects of dopamine (DA) on learning to choose between actions, the most overt behavioral effects of DA interventions are similar swings in undirected vigor [4], at least part of which appear immediately, without learning [5]. Finally, computational theories fail to deliver on the close link they trumpet between DA, behavior, and reinforcement learning (RL; *eg* [6]), as they do not address the whole experimental paradigm of *free-operant* tasks [7], whence hail those and many other results.

Rather than the standard RL problem of discrete choices between alternatives at prespecified timesteps [8], free-operant experiments investigate tasks in which subjects pace their own responding (typically on a lever or other manipulandum). The primary choice in these tasks is of how rapidly/vigorously to behave, rather than what behavior to choose (as typically only one relevant action is available). RL models are silent about these aspects, and thus fail to offer a principled understanding of the policies selected by the animals.

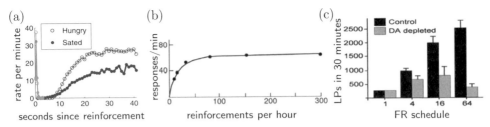

Figure 1: (a) Leverpress (blue, right) and consummatory nose poke (red, left) response rates of rats leverpressing for food on a modified RI30 schedule. Hungry rats (open circles) clearly press the lever at a higher rate than sated rats (filled circles). Data from [11], averaged over 19 rats in each group. (b) The relationship between rate of responding and rate of reinforcement (reciprocal of the interval) on an RI schedule, is hyperbolic (of the form $y = B \cdot x/(x + x_0)$). This is an instantiation of Herrnstein's matching law for one response (adapted from [9]). (c) Total number of leverpresses per session averaged over five 30 minute sessions by rats pressing for food on different FR schedules. Rats with nucleus accumbens 6-OHDA dopamine lesions (gray) press significantly less than control rats (black), with the difference larger for higher ratio requirements. Adapted from [12].

Here, we address these issues by constructing an RL account of behavior rates in free-operant settings (Sections 2,3). We consider optimal control in a continuous-time Markov Decision Process (MDP), in which agents must choose *both* an action and the latency with which to emit it (*ie* how vigorously, or at what instantaneous rate to perform it). Our model treats response vigor as being determined normatively, as the outcome of a battle between the cost of behaving more expeditiously and the benefit of achieving desirable outcomes more quickly. We show that this simple, normative framework captures many classic features of animal behavior that are obscure in our and others' earlier treatments (Section 4). These include the characteristic time-dependent profiles of response rates on tasks with different payoff scheduling [7], the hyperbolic relationship between response rate and payoff [9], and the difference in response rates between tasks in which reinforcements are allocated based on the number of responses emitted and those allocating reinforcements based on the passage of time [10].

A key feature of this model is that response rates are strongly dependent on the expected *average reward rate*, because this determines the opportunity cost of sloth. By influencing the value of reinforcers — and through this, the average reward rate — motivational states such as hunger influence the output response latencies (and not only response choice). Thus, in our model, hungry animals should *optimally* also work harder for water, since in typical circumstances, this should allow them to return more quickly to working for food. Further, we identify *tonic levels of dopamine* with the representation of average reward rate, and thereby suggest an account of a wealth of experiments showing that DA influences response vigor [4, 5], thus complementing existing ideas about the role of phasic DA signals in learned action selection (Section 5).

2 Free-operant behavior

We consider the free-operant scenario common in experimental psychology, in which an animal is placed in an experimental chamber, and can choose freely which actions to emit and when. Most actions have no programmed consequences; however, one action (*eg* leverpressing; LP) is rewarded with food (which falls into a food magazine) according to an experimenter-determined *schedule* of reinforcement. Food delivery makes a characteristic sound, signalling its availability for harvesting via a nose poke (NP) into the magazine.

The schedule of reinforcement defines the (possibly stochastic) relationship between the delivery of a reward and one or both of (a) the *number* of LPs, and (b) the *time* since the last reward was delivered. In common use are fixed-ratio (FR) schedules, in which a fixed number of LPs is required to obtain a reinforcer; random-ratio (RR) schedules, in which each LP has a constant probability of being reinforced; and random interval (RI) schedules, in which the first LP after an (exponentially distributed) interval of time has elapsed, is reinforced. Schedules are often labelled by their type and a parameter, so RI30 is a random interval schedule with the exponential waiting time having a mean of 30 seconds [7].

Different schedules induce different patterns of responding [7]. Fig 1a shows response metrics from rats leverpressing on an RI30 schedule. Leverpressing builds up to a relatively constant rate following a rather long pause after gaining each reward, during which the food is consumed. Hungry rats leverpress more vigorously than sated ones. A similar overall pattern is also characteristic of responding on RR schedules. Figure 1b shows the total number of LP responses in a 30 minute session for different interval schedules. The hyperbolic relationship between the reward rate (the inverse of the interval) and the response rate is a classic hallmark of free operant behavior [9].

3   The model

We model a free-operant task as a continuous MDP. Based on its state, the agent chooses both an action (a), and a latency (τ) at which to emit it. After time τ has elapsed, the action is completed, the agent receives rewards and incurs costs associated with its choice, and then selects a new (a, τ) pair based on its new state. We define three possible actions $a \in \{\texttt{LP}, \texttt{NP}, \texttt{other}\}$, where we take $a = \texttt{other}$ to include the various miscellaneous behaviors such as grooming, rearing, and sniffing which animals typically perform during the experiment. For simplicity we consider unit actions, with the latency τ related to the vigor with which this unit is performed. To account for consumption time (which is non-negligible [11, 13]), if the agent nose-pokes and food is available, a predefined time t_{eat} passes before the next decision point (and the next state) is reached.

Crucially, performing actions incurs costs as well as potentially gains rewards. Following Staddon [14], we assume one part of the cost of an action to be *proportional to the vigor* of its execution, *ie* inversely proportional to τ. The constant of proportionality K_v depends on both the previous and the current action, since switching between different action types can require travel between different parts of the experimental chamber (say, the magazine to the lever), and can thus be more costly. Each action also incurs a fixed 'internal' reward or cost of $\rho(a)$ per unit, typically with $\texttt{other}$ being rewarding. The reinforcement schedule defines the probability of reward delivery for each state-action-latency triplet. An available reward can be harvested by $a = \texttt{NP}$ into the magazine, and we assume that the thereby obtained subjective utility $U(r)$ of the food reward is *motivation-dependent*, such that food is worth more to a hungry animal than to a sated one.

We consider the simplified case of a state space comprised of all the parameters relevant to the task. Specifically, the state space includes the identity of the previous action, an indicator as to whether a reward is available in the food magazine, and, as necessary, the number of LPs since the previous reinforcement (for FR) or the elapsed time since the previous LP (for RI). The transitions between the states $P(S'|S, a, \tau)$ and the reward function $P_r(S, a, \tau)$ are defined by the dynamics of the schedule of reinforcement, and all rewards and costs are harvested at state transitions and considered as point events. In the following we treat the problem of optimising a policy (which action to take and with what latency, given the state) in order to maximize the average rate of return (rewards minus costs per time). An exponentially discounted model gives the same qualitative results.

In the average reward case [15, 16], the Bellman equation for the long-term differential (or

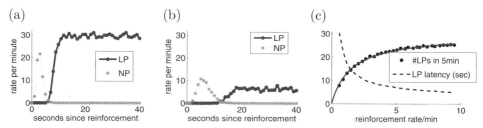

Figure 2: Data generated by the model captures the essence of the behavioral data: Lever-press (solid blue; circles) and nose poke (dashed red; stars) response rates on (a) an RR10 schedule and (b) a matched (yoked) RI schedule show constant LP rates which are higher for the ratio schedule. (c) The relationship between the total number of responses (circles) and rate of reinforcement is hyperbolic (solid line: hyperbolic curve fit). The mean latency to leverpress (dashed line) decreases as the rate of reinforcement increases.

average-adjusted) value of state S is:

$$V^*(S) = \max_{a,\tau} \left\{ \rho(a) - \frac{K_v(a_{prev}, a)}{\tau} + U(r)P_r(S, a, \tau) - \tau \cdot \bar{r} + \int dS' P(S'|S, a, \tau)V^*(S') \right\} \quad (1)$$

where $\bar{r}$ is the long term average reward rate (whose subtraction from the value quantifies the opportunity cost of delay). Building on ideas from [16], we suggest that the average reward rate is reported by tonic (baseline) levels of dopamine (and *not* serotonin [16]) in basal ganglia structures relevant for action selection, and that changes in tonic DA (*eg* as a result of pharmacological interventions) would thus alter the assumed average reward rate.

In this paper, we eschew learning, and examine the steady state behavior that arises when actions are chosen stochastically (via the so-called softmax or Boltzmann distribution) from the *optimal* one-step look-ahead model-based $Q(S, a, \tau)$ state-action-latency values. For ratio schedules, the simple transition structure of the task allows the Bellman equation to be solved analytically to determine the Q values. For interval schedules, we use average-reward value iteration [15] with time discretized at a resolution of 100ms. For simulations (*eg* of dopaminergic manipulations) where $\bar{r}$ was assumed to change independent of any change in the task contingencies, we used value iteration to find values approximately satisfying the Bellman equation (which is no longer exactly solvable). Our overriding aim is to replicate basic aspects of free operant behavior qualitatively, in order to understand the normative foundations of response vigor. We do not fit the parameters of the model to experimental data in a quantitative way, and the results we describe below are general, robust, characteristics of the model.

4   Results

Fig 2a depicts the behavior of our model on an RR10 schedule. In rough accordance with the behavior displayed by animals (which is similar to that shown in Fig 1a), the LP rate is constant over time, bar a pause for consumption. Fig 2b depicts the model's behavior in a *yoked* random interval schedule, in which the intervals between rewards were set to match exactly the intervals obtained by the agent trained on the ratio schedule in Fig 2a. The response rate is again constant over time, but it is also considerably *lower* than that in the corresponding RR schedule, although the external reward density is similar. This phenomenon has also been observed experimentally, and although the apparent anomaly has been much discussed in the associative learning literature, its explanation is not fully resolved [10]. Our model suggests that it is the result of an optimal cost/benefit tradeoff.

We can analyse this difference by considering the Q values for leverpressing at different latencies in random schedules

$$Q(S_{nr}, \text{LP}, \tau) = \rho(\text{LP}) - \frac{K_v(\text{LP}, \text{LP})}{\tau} - \tau \cdot \bar{r} + P(S_r|\tau)V^*(S_r) + [1 - P(S_r|\tau)]V^*(S_{nr}) \qquad (2)$$

where we are looking at consecutive leverpresses in the absence of available reward, and S_r and S_{nr} designate the states in which a reward is or is not available in the magazine, respectively. In ratio schedules, since $P(S_r|\tau)$ is independent of τ, the optimizing latency is $\tau_{\text{LP}}^* = \sqrt{K_v(\text{LP}, \text{LP})/\bar{r}}$, its inverse defining the optimal rate of leverpressing. In interval schedules, however, $P(S_r|\tau) = 1 - exp\{-\tau/T\}$ where T is the schedule interval. Taking the derivative of eq. (2) we find that the optimal latency to leverpress τ_{LP}^* satisfies $K_v(\text{LP}, \text{LP})/\tau_{\text{LP}}^{*2} - \bar{r} + (1/T)[V^*(S_r) - V^*(S_{nr})] \cdot exp\{-\tau_{\text{LP}}^*/T\} = 0$. Although no longer analytically solvable, it is easily seen that this latency will always be longer than that found above for ratio schedules. Intuitively, since longer inter-response intervals increase the probability of reward per press in interval schedules but not in ratio schedules, the optimal leverpressing rate is lower in the former than in the latter.

Fig 2c shows the average number of LPs in a 5 minute session for different interval schedules. This 'molar' measure of rate shows the well documented hyperbolic relationship (*cf* Fig 1b). On the 'molecular' level of single action choices, the mean latency $\langle \tau_{\text{LP}} \rangle$ between consecutive LPs decreases as the probability of reinforcement increases. This measure of response vigor is actually more accurate than the overall response measure, as it is not contaminated by competition with other actions, or confounded with the number of reinforcers per session for different schedules (and the time forgone when consuming them). For this reason, although we (correctly; see [13]) predict that inter-response latency should slow for higher ratio requirements, raw LP counts can actually increase, as in Fig. 1c, probably due to fewer rewards and less time spent eating [13].

5 Drive and dopamine

Having provided a qualitative account of the basic patterns of free operant rates of behavior, we turn to the main theoretical conundrum — the effects of drive and DA manipulations on response vigor. The key to understanding these is the role that the average reward $\bar{r}$ plays in the tradeoffs determining optimal response vigor. In effect, the average expected reward per unit time quantifies the opportunity cost for doing nothing (and receiving no reward) for that time; its increase thus produces general pressure for faster work. A direct consequence of making the agent hungrier is that the subjective utility of food is enhanced. This will have interrelated effects on the optimal average reward $\bar{r}$, the optimal values V^*, and the resultant optimal action choices and vigors. Notably, so long as the policy obtains food, its average reward rate will *increase*.

Consider a fixed or random ratio schedule. The increase in $\bar{r}$ will increase the optimal LP rate $1/\tau_{\text{LP}}^* = \sqrt{\bar{r}/K_v(\text{LP}, \text{LP})}$, as the higher reward utility offsets higher procurement costs. Importantly, because the optimal τ^* has a similar dependence on $\bar{r}$ even for actions irrelevant to obtaining food, they also become more vigorous. The explanation of this effect is presented graphically in Fig 3e. The higher $\bar{r}$ increases the cost of sloth, since every τ time without reward forgoes an expected $(\tau \cdot \bar{r})$ mean reward. Higher average rewards penalize late actions more than they do early ones, thus tilting action selection toward faster behavior, for *all* pre-potent actions. Essentially, hunger encourages the agent to complete irrelevant actions faster, in order to be able to resume leverpressing more quickly.

For other schedules, the same effects generally hold (although the analytical reasoning is complicated by the fact that the optimal latencies may in these cases depend not only on the new average reward but also on the new values V^*). Fig 3a shows simulated responding on an RI25 schedule in which the internal reward for the food-irrelevant action other has been set high enough to warrant non-negligible base responding. Fig 3b shows that when

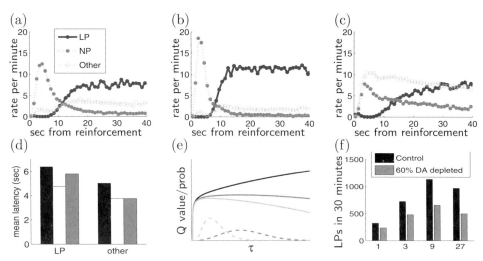

Figure 3: The effects of drive on response rates. (a) Responding on a RI25 schedule, with high internal rewards (0.35) for $a = \texttt{other}$ (open circles). (b) The effects of hunger: $U(r)$ was changed from 10 to 15. (c) The effect of an irrelevant drive (hungry animals lever-pressing for water rewards): $\bar{r}$ was increased by 4% compared to (a). (d) Mean latencies to responding $\langle \tau \rangle$ for LP and $\texttt{other}$ in baseline (a; black), increased hunger (b; white) and irrelevant drive (c; gray). (e) Q values for leverpressing at different latencies τ. In black (top) are the unadjusted Q values, before subtracting $(\tau \cdot \bar{r})$. In red (middle, solid) and green (bottom, solid) are the values adjusted for two different average reward rates. The higher reward rate penalizes late actions more, thereby causing *faster* responding, as shown by the corresponding softmaxed action probability curves (dashed). (f) Simulation of DA depletion: overall leverpress count over 30 minute sessions (each bar averaging 15 sessions), for different FR requirements (bottom). In black is the control condition, and in gray is simulated DA depletion, attained by lowering $\bar{r}$ by 60%. The effects of the depletion seem more pronounced in higher schedules (compare to Fig 1c), but this actually results from the interaction with the number of rewards attained (see text).

the utility of food is increased by 50%, the agent chooses to leverpress more, at the expense of $\texttt{other}$ actions. This illustrates the 'directing' effect of motivation, by which the agent is directed more forcefully toward the motivationally relevant action [17]. Furthermore, the second, 'driving' effect, by which motivation increases vigor globally [17], is illustrated in Fig 3d which shows that, in fact, the latency to both actions has *decreased*. Thus, although selected less often, when $\texttt{other}$ is selected, it is performed more vigorously than it was when the agent was sated.

This general drive effect can be better isolated if we examine hungry agents leverpressing for water (rather than food), without competition from actions for food. We can view our leverpressing MDP as a portion of a larger one, which also includes (for instance) occasional opportunities for visits to a home cage where food is available. Without explicitly specifying all this extra structure, a good approximation is to take hunger as again causing an increase in the global rate of reinforcement $\bar{r}$, reflecting the increase in the utility of food received elsewhere. Fig 3c shows the effects on responding on an interval schedule, of estimating the average reward rate to be 4% higher than in Fig 3a, and deriving new Q values from the previous V^* with this new $\bar{r}$ as illustrated in Fig 3e. As above, the adjusted vigors of all behaviors are faster (Fig 3d, gray bars), as a result of the higher 'drive'.

How do these drive effects relate to dopamine? Pharmacological and lesion studies show that enhancing DA levels (through agonists such as amphetamine) increases general activity

[5, 18, 19], while depleting or antagonising DA causes a general slowing of responding (*eg* [4]). Fig. 1c is representative of a host of results from the lab of Salamone [4, 12] which show that lower levels of DA in the nucleus accumbens (a structure in the basal ganglia implicated in action selection) result in lower response rates. This effect seems more pronounced in higher fixed-ratio schedules, those requiring more work per reinforcer. As a result of this apparent dependence on the response requirement, Salamone and his colleagues have hypothesized that DA enables animals to overcome higher work demands.

We suggest that tonic levels of DA represent the average reward rate (a role tentatively proposed for *serotonin* in [16]). Thus a higher tonic level of DA represents a situation akin to higher drive, in which behavior is more vigorous, and lower tonic levels of DA cause a general slowing of behavior. Fig. 3f shows the simulated response counts for different FR schedules in two conditions. The control condition is the standard model described above; DA depletion was modeled by decreasing tonic DA levels (and therefore $\bar{r}$) to 40% of their original levels. The results match the data in Fig. 1c. Here, the apparently small effect on the number of LPs for low ratio schedules actually arises because of the large amount of time spent eating. Thus, according to the model DA is not really allowing animals to cope with higher work requirements, but rather is important for optimal choice of vigor at any work requirement, with the slowing effect of DA depletion more prominent (in the crude measure of LPs per session) when more time is spent leverpressing.

6 Discussion

The present model brings the computational machinery and neural grounding of RL models fully into contact with the vast reservoir of data from free-operant tasks. Classic quantitative accounts of operant behavior (such as Herrnstein's matching law [9], and variations such as melioration) lack RL's normative grounding in sound control theory, and tend instead toward descriptive curve-fitting. Most of these theories do not address that fine scale (molecular) structure of behavior, and instead concentrate on fairly crude molar measures such as total number of leverpresses over long durations. In addition to the normative starting point it offers for investigations of response vigor, our theory provides a relatively fine scalpel for dissecting the temporal details of behavior, such as the distributions of inter-response intervals at particular state transitions. There is thus great scope for revealing re-analyses of many existing data sets. In particular, the effects of generalized drive have proved mixed and complex [17]. Our theory suggests that studies of inter-response intervals (*eg* Fig 3d) may reveal more robust changes in vigor, uncontaminated by shifts in overall action propensity.

Response vigor and dopamine's role in controlling it have appeared in previous RL models of behavior [20, 21], but only as fairly ad-hoc bolt-ons — for instance, using repeated choices between doing nothing versus something to capture response latency. Here, these aspects are wholly integrated into the explanatory framework: optimizing response vigor is treated as itself an RL problem, with a natural dopaminergic substrate. To account for immediate (unlearned) effects of motivational or dopaminergic manipulations, the main assumption we make is that tonic levels of DA can be sensitive to predicted changes in the average reward occasioned by changes in the motivational state, and that behavioral policies are in turn immediately affected. This sensitivity would be easy to embed in a temporal-difference RL system, producing flexible adaptation of response vigor. By contrast, due to the way they cache outcome values, the action choices of such RL systems are characteristically *insensitive* to the 'directing' effects of motivational manipulations [22]. In animal behavior, 'habitual actions' (the ones associated with the DA system) are indeed motivationally insensitive for action choice, but show a direct effect of drive on vigor [23].

Our model is easy to accommodate within a framework of temporal difference (TD) learning. Thus, it naturally preserves the link between phasic DA signals and online learning of optimal values [24]. We further elaborate this link by suggesting an additional role for tonic levels of DA in online vigor selection. A major question remains as to whether phasic responses (which are known to correlate with response latency [25]) play an additional role in determining response vigor. Further, it is pressing to reconcile the present account with our previous suggestion (based on microdialysis findings) [16] that tonic levels of DA might track average *punishment*.

The most critical avenues to develop this work will be an account of learning, and neurally and psychologically more plausible state and temporal representations. On-line value learning should be a straightforward adaptation of existing TD models of phasic DA based on the continuous-time semi-Markov setting [26]. The representation of state is more challenging — the assumption of a fully observable state space automatically appropriate for the schedule of reinforcement is not realistic. Indeed, apparently sub-optimal actions emitted by animals, *eg* engaging in excessive nose-poking even when a reward has not audibly dropped into the food magazine [11], may provide clues to this issue. Finally, it will be crucial to consider the fact that animals' decisions about vigor may translate only noisily into response times, due, for instance, to the variability of internal timing [27].

Acknowledgments

This work was funded by the Gatsby Charitable Foundation, a Dan David fellowship (YN), the Royal Society (ND) and the EU BIBA project (ND and PD). We are grateful to Jonathan Williams for discussions on free operant behavior.

References

[1] Dickinson A. and Balleine B.W. The role of learning in the operation of motivational systems. Steven's Handbook of Experimental Psychology Volume 3, pages 497–533. John Wiley & Sons, New York, 2002.

[2] Hull C.L. *Principles of behavior: An introduction to behavior theory*. Appleton-Century-Crofts, New York, 1943.

[3] Bélanger D. and Tétreau B. L'influence d'une motivation inappropriate sur le comportement du rat et sa fréquence cardiaque. *Can. J. of Psych.*, 15:6–14, 1961.

[4] Salamone J.D. and Correa M. Motivational views of reinforcement: implications for understanding the behavioral functions of nucleus accumbens dopamine. *Behavioural Brain Research*, 137:3–25, 2002.

[5] Ikemoto S. and Panksepp J. The role of nucleus accumbens dopamine in motivated behavior: a unifying interpretation with special reference to reward-seeking. *Brain Res. Rev.*, 31:6–41, 1999.

[6] Schultz W. Predictive reward signal of dopamine neurons. *J. Neurophys.*, 80:1–27, 1998.

[7] Domjan M. *The principles of learning and behavior*. Brooks/Cole, Pacific Grove, California, 3rd edition, 1993.

[8] R. S. Sutton and A. G. Barto. *Reinforcement learning: An introduction*. MIT Press, 1998.

[9] Herrnstein R.J. On the law of effect. *J. of the Exp. Anal. of Behav.*, 13(2):243–266, 1970.

[10] Dawson G.R. and Dickinson A. Performance on ratio and interval schedules with matched reinforcement rates. *Q. J. of Exp. Psych. B*, 42:225–239, 1990.

[11] Niv Y., Daw N.D., Joel D., and Dayan P. Motivational effects on behavior: Towards a reinforcement learning model of rates of responding. In *CoSyNe*, Salt Lake City, Utah, 2005.

[12] Aberman J.E. and Salamone J.D. Nucleus accumbens dopamine depletions make rats more sensitive to high ratio requirements but do not impair primary food reinforcement. *Neuroscience*, 92(2):545–552, 1999.

[13] Foster T.M., Blackman K.A., and Temple W. Open versus closed economies: performance of domestic hens under fixed-ratio schedules. *J. of the Exp. Anal. of Behav.*, 67:67–89, 1997.

[14] Staddon J.E.R. *Adaptive dynamics*. MIT Press, Cambridge, Mass., 2001.

[15] Mahadevan S. Average reward reinforcement learning: Foundations, algorithms and empirical results. *Machine Learning*, 22:1–38, 1996.

[16] Daw N.D., Kakade S., and Dayan P. Opponent interactions between serotonin and dopamine. *Neural Networks*, 15(4-6):603–616, 2002.

[17] Bolles R.C. *Theory of Motivation*. Harper & Row, 1967.

[18] Carr G.D. and White N.M. Effects of systemic and intracranial amphetamine injections on behavior in the open field: a detailed analysis. *Pharmacol. Biochem. Behav.*, 27:113–122, 1987.

[19] Jackson D.M., Anden N., and Dahlstrom A. A functional effect of dopamine in the nucleus accumbens and in some other dopamine-rich parts of the rat brain. *Psychopharmacologia*, 45:139–149, 1975.

[20] Dayan P. and Balleine B.W. Reward, motivation and reinforcement learning. *Neuron*, 36:285–298, 2002.

[21] McClure S.M., Daw N.D., and Montague P.R. A computational substrate for incentive salience. *Trends in Neurosc.*, 26(8):423–428, 2003.

[22] Daw N.D., Niv Y., and Dayan P. Uncertainty based competition between prefrontal and dorsolateral striatal systems for behavioral control. *Nature Neuroscience*, 8(12):1704–1711, 2005.

[23] Dickinson A., Balleine B., Watt A., Gonzalez F., and Boakes R.A. Motivational control after extended instrumental training. *Anim. Learn. and Behav.*, 23(2):197–206, 1995.

[24] Montague P.R., Dayan P., and Sejnowski T.J. A framework for mesencephalic dopamine systems based on predictive hebbian learning. *J. of Neurosci.*, 16(5):1936–1947, 1996.

[25] Satoh T., Nakai S., Sato T., and Kimura M. Correlated coding of motivation and outcome of decision by dopamine neurons. *J. of Neurosci.*, 23(30):9913–9923, 2003.

[26] Daw N.D., Courville A.C., and Touretzky D.S. Timing and partial observability in the dopamine system. In T.G. Dietterich, S. Becker, and Z. Ghahramani, editors, *NIPS*, volume 14, Cambridge, MA, 2002. MIT Press.

[27] Gallistel C.R. and Gibbon J. Time, rate and conditioning. *Psych. Rev.*, 107:289–344, 2000.

Analyzing Coupled Brain Sources: Distinguishing True from Spurious Interaction

Guido Nolte[1], Andreas Ziehe[3], Frank Meinecke[1] and Klaus-Robert Müller[1,2]

[1] Fraunhofer FIRST.IDA, Kekuléstr. 7, 12489 Berlin, Germany
[2] Dept. of CS, University of Potsdam, August-Bebel-Strasse 89, 14482 Potsdam, Germany
[3] TU Berlin, Inst. for Software Engineering, Franklinstr. 28/29, 10587 Berlin, Germany
{nolte,ziehe,meinecke,klaus}@first.fhg.de

Abstract

When trying to understand the brain, it is of fundamental importance to analyse (e.g. from EEG/MEG measurements) what parts of the cortex interact with each other in order to infer more accurate models of brain activity. Common techniques like Blind Source Separation (BSS) can estimate brain sources and single out artifacts by using the underlying assumption of source signal independence. However, physiologically interesting brain sources typically interact, so BSS will—by construction—fail to characterize them properly. Noting that there are truly interacting sources and signals that only seemingly interact due to effects of volume conduction, this work aims to contribute by *distinguishing* these effects. For this a new BSS technique is proposed that uses anti-symmetrized cross-correlation matrices and subsequent diagonalization. The resulting decomposition consists of the truly interacting brain sources and suppresses any spurious interaction stemming from volume conduction. Our new concept of interacting source analysis (ISA) is successfully demonstrated on MEG data.

1 Introduction

Interaction between brain sources, phase synchrony or coherent states of brain activity are believed to be fundamental for neural information processing (e.g. [2, 6, 5]). So it is an important topic to devise new methods that can more reliably characterize interacting sources in the brain. The macroscopic nature and the high temporal resolution of electroencephalography (EEG) and magnetoencephalography (MEG) in the millisecond range makes these measurement technologies ideal candidates to study brain interactions. However, interpreting data from EEG/MEG channels in terms of connections between brain sources is largely hampered by artifacts of volume conduction, i.e. the fact that activities of single sources are observable as superposition in all channels (with varying amplitude). So ideally one would like to discard all—due to volume conduction—seemingly interacting signals and retain only truly linked brain source activity.

So far neither existing source separation methods nor typical phase synchronization analysis (e.g. [1, 5] and references therein) can adequately handle signals when the sources are both superimposed and interacting i.e. non-independent (cf. discussions in [3, 4]). It is here where we contribute in this paper by proposing a new algorithm to distinguish true from spurious interaction. A prerequisite to achieve this goal was recently established by [4]: as a consequence of instantaneous and linear volume conduction, the cross-spectra of independent sources are real-valued, regardless of the specifics of the volume conductor, number of sources or source configuration. Hence, a non-vanishing imaginary part of the cross-spectra must necessarily reflect a true interaction. Drawbacks of Nolte's method are: (a) cross-spectra for all frequencies in multi-channel systems contain a huge amount of information and it can be tedious to find the interesting structures, (b) it is very much possible that the interacting brain consists of several subsystems which are independent of each other but are not separated by that method, and (c) the method is well suited for rhythmic interactions while wide-band interactions are not well represented.

A recent different approach by [3] uses BSS as preprocessing step before phase synchronization is measured. The drawback of this method is the assumption that there are not more sources than sensors, which is often heavily violated because, e.g., channel noise trivially consists of as many sources as channels, and, furthermore, brain noise can be very well modelled by assuming thousands of randomly distributed and independent dipoles.

To avoid the drawbacks of either method we will formulate an algorithm called interacting source analysis (ISA) which is technically based on BSS using second order statistics but is only sensitive to interacting sources and, thus, can be applied to systems with *arbitrary* noise structure. In the next section, after giving a short introduction to BSS as used for this paper, we will derive some fundamental properties of our new method. In section 3 we will show in simulated data and real MEG examples that the ISA procedure finds the interacting components and separates interacting subsystems which are independent of each other.

2   Theory

The fundamental assumption of ICA is that a data matrix X, without loss of generality assumed to be zero mean, originates from a superposition of independent sources S such that

$$X = AS \tag{1}$$

where A is called the mixing matrix which is assumed to be invertible. The task is to find A and hence S (apart from meaningless ordering and scale transformations of the columns of A and the rows of S) by merely exploiting statistical independence of the sources. Since independence implies that the sources are uncorrelated we may choose W, the estimated inverse mixing matrix, such that the covariance matrix of

$$\hat{S} \equiv WX \tag{2}$$

is equal to the identity matrix. This, however, does not uniquely determine W because for any such W also UW, where U is an arbitrary orthogonal matrix, leads to a unit covariance matrix of $\hat{S}$. Uniqueness can be restored if we require that W not only diagonalizes the covariance matrix but also cross-correlation matrices for various delays τ, i.e. we require that

$$WC^X(\tau)W^\dagger = diag \tag{3}$$

with

$$C^X(\tau) \equiv \langle \mathbf{x}(t)\mathbf{x}^\dagger(t+\tau)\rangle \tag{4}$$

where $\mathbf{x}(t)$ is the $t.th$ column of X and $\langle . \rangle$ means expectation value which is estimated by the average over t. Although at this stage all expressions are real-valued we introduce a complex formulation for later use.

Note, that since under the ICA assumption the cross-correlation matrices $C^S(\tau)$ of the source signals are diagonal

$$C_{ij}^S(\tau) = \langle s_i(t) s_i(t + \tau) \rangle \delta_{ij} = C_{ji}^S, \tag{5}$$

the cross-correlation matrices of the mixtures are symmetric:

$$C^X(\tau) = AC^S(\tau)A^\dagger = \left(AC^S(\tau)A^\dagger\right)^\dagger = C^{X\dagger}(\tau) \tag{6}$$

Hence, the antisymmetric part of $C^X(\tau)$ can only arise due to meaningless fluctuations and can be ignored. In fact, the above TDSEP algorithm uses symmetrized versions of $C^X(\tau)$ [8].

Now, the key and new point of our method is that we will turn the above argument upside down. Since non-interacting sources do not contribute (systematically) to the anti-symmetrized correlation matrices

$$D(\tau) \equiv C^X(\tau) - C^{X\dagger}(\tau) \tag{7}$$

any (significant) non-vanishing elements in $D(\tau)$ must arise from interacting sources, and hence the analysis of $D(\tau)$ is ideally suited to study the interacting brain. In doing so we exploit that neuronal interactions necessarily take some time which is well above the typical time resolution of EEG/MEG measurements.

It is now our goal to identify one or many interacting systems from a suitable spatial transformation which corresponds to a demixing of the systems rather than individual sources. Although we concentrate on those components which explicitly violate the independence assumption we will use the technique of simultaneous diagonalization to achieve this goal. We first note that a diagonalization of $D(\tau)$ using a real-valued W is meaningless since with $D(\tau)$ also $WD(\tau)W^\dagger$ is anti-symmetric and always has vanishing diagonal elements. Hence $D(\tau)$ can only be diagonalized with a complex-valued W with subsequent interpretation of it in terms of a real-valued transformation.

We will here discuss the case where all interacting systems consist of pairs of neuronal sources. Properties of systems with more than two interacting systems will be discussed below. Furthermore, for simplicity we assume an even number of channels. Then a real-valued spatial transformation W_1 exists such that the set of $D(\tau)$ becomes decomposed into $K = N/2$ blocks of size 2×2

$$W_1 D(\tau) W_1^\dagger = \begin{pmatrix} \alpha_1(\tau) \begin{pmatrix} 0 & 1 \\ -1 & 0 \end{pmatrix} & 0 & 0 \\ 0 & \ddots & 0 \\ 0 & 0 & \alpha_K(\tau) \begin{pmatrix} 0 & 1 \\ -1 & 0 \end{pmatrix} \end{pmatrix} \tag{8}$$

Each block can be diagonalized e.g. with

$$\tilde{W}_2 = \begin{pmatrix} 1 & -i \\ 1 & i \end{pmatrix} \tag{9}$$

and with

$$W_2 = id_{K \times K} \otimes \tilde{W}_2 \tag{10}$$

we get

$$W_2 W_1 D(\tau) W_1^\dagger W_2^\dagger = diag \tag{11}$$

From a simultaneous diagonalization of $D(\tau)$ we obtain an estimate of the demixing matrix $\hat{W}$ of the true demixing matrix $W = W_2 W_1$. We are interested in the columns of W_1^{-1} which correspond to the spatial patterns of the interacting sources. Let us denote the $N \times 2$

submatrix of a matrix B consisting of the $(2k-1).th$ and the $2k.th$ column as $(B)_k$. Then we can write

$$(W_1^{-1})_k \sim (W^{-1})_k \tilde{W}_2 \tag{12}$$

and hence the desired spatial patterns of the $k.th$ system are a complex linear superposition of the $(2k-1).th$ and the $2k.th$ column of W. The subspace spanned in channel-space by the two interacting sources, denoted as $span((A)_k)$, can now be found by separating real and imaginary part of W^{-1}

$$span((A)_k) = span\left(\left(\Re((W^{-1})_k), \Im((W^{-1})_k)\right)\right) \tag{13}$$

According to (13) we can calculate from W just the 2D-subspaces spanned by the interacting systems but not the patterns of the sources themselves. The latter would indeed be impossible because all we analyze are anti-symmetric matrices which are, for each system, constructed as anti-symmetric outer products of the two respective field patterns. These anti-symmetric matrices are, apart from an irrelevant global scale, invariant with respect to a linear and real-valued mixing of the sources within each system.

The general procedure can now be outlined as follows.

1. From the data construct anti-symmetric cross-correlation matrices as defined in Eq.(7) for reasonable set of delays τ.

2. Find a complex matrix W such that $WD(\tau)W^\dagger$ is approximately diagonal for all τ.

3. If the system consists of subsystems of paired interactions (and indeed, according to our own experience, very much in practice) the diagonal elements in $WD(\tau)W^\dagger$ come in pairs in the form $\pm i\lambda$. Each pair constitutes one interacting system. The corresponding two columns in W^{-1}, with separated real and imaginary parts, form an $N \times 4$ matrix V with rank 2. The span of V coincides with the space spanned by the respective system. In practice, V will have two singular values which are just very small rather than exactly zero. The corresponding singular vectors should then be discarded. Instead of analyzing V in the above way it is also possible to simply take the real and imaginary part of either one of the two columns.

4. Similar to the spatial analysis, it is not possible to separate the time-courses of two interacting sources within one subsystem. In general, two *estimated* time-courses, say $\hat{s}_1(t)$ and $\hat{s}_2(t)$, are an unknown linear combination of the true source activations $s_1(t)$ and $s_2(t)$. To understand the type of interaction it is still recommended to look at the power and autocorrelation functions. Invariant with respect to linear mixing with one subsystem is the anti-symmetrized cross-correlation between $\hat{s}_1(t)$ and $\hat{s}_2(t)$ and, equivalently, the imaginary part of the cross-spectral density. For the $k.th$ system, these quantities are given by the $k.th$ diagonal $\lambda_k(\tau)$ and their respective Fourier transforms.

While (approximate) simultaneous diagonalization of $D(\tau)$ using complex demixing matrices is always possible with pairwise interactions we can expect only block-diagonal structure if a larger number of sources are interacting within one or more subsystems. We will show below for simulated data that the algorithm still finds these blocks although the actual goal, i.e. diagonal $WD(\tau)W^\dagger$, is not reachable.

3 Results

3.1 Simulated data

Matrices were approximately simultaneously diagonalized with the DOMUNG-algorithm [7], which was generalized to the complex domain. Here, an initial guess for the demixing matrix W is successively optimized using a natural gradient approach combined with line search according to the requirement that the off-diagonals are minimal under the constraint $det(W) = 1$. Special care has to be taken in the choice of the initial guess. Due to the complex-conjugation symmetry of our problem (i.e., W^* diagonalizes as well as W) the initial guess may not be set to a real-valued matrix because then the component of the gradient in imaginary direction will be zero and W will converge to a real-valued saddle point.

We simulated two random interacting subsystems of dimensions N_A and N_B which were assumed to be mutually independent. The two subsystems were mapped into $N = N_A + N_B$ channels with a random mixture matrix. The anti-symmetrized cross-correlation matrices read

$$D(\tau) = A \begin{pmatrix} D_A(\tau) & 0 \\ 0 & D_B(\tau) \end{pmatrix} A^\dagger \tag{14}$$

where A is a random real-valued $N \times N$ matrix, and $D_A(\tau)$ ($D_B(\tau)$), with $\tau = 1...20$, are a set of random anti-symmetric $N_A \times N_A$ ($N_B \times N_B$) matrices. Note, that in this context, τ has no physical meaning.

As expected, we have found that if one of the subsystems is two-dimensional the respective block can always be diagonalized exactly for any number of τs. We have also seen, that the diagonalization procedure always perfectly separates the two subsystems even if a diagonalization within a subsystem is not possible. A typical result for $N_A = 2$ and $N_B = 3$ is presented in Fig.1. In the left panel we show the average of the absolute value of correlation matrices before spatial mixing. In the middle panel we show the respective result after random spatial mixture and subsequent demixing, and in the right panel we show $W_1 A$ where W_1 is the estimated real version of the demixing matrix as explained in the preceding section. We note again, that also for the two-dimensional block, which can always be diagonalized exactly, one can only recover the corresponding two-dimensional subspace and not the source components themselves.

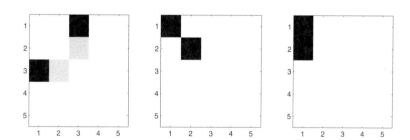

Figure 1: Left: average of the absolute values of correlation matrices before spatial mixing; middle: same after random spatial mixture and subsequent demixing; right: product of the estimated demixing matrix and the true mixing matrix ($W_1 A$). White indicates zero and black the maximum value for each matrix.

3.2 Real MEG data

We applied our method to real data gathered in 93 MEG channels during triggered finger movements of the right or left hand. We recall that for each interacting component we get two results: a) the 2D subspace spanned by the two components and b) the diagonals of the demixed system, say $\pm i\lambda_k(\tau)$. To visualize the 2D subspace in a unique way we construct from the two patterns of the $k.th$ system, say $\mathbf{x}_1$ and $\mathbf{x}_2$, the anti-symmetric outer product

$$D_k \equiv \mathbf{x}_1\mathbf{x}_2^T - \mathbf{x}_2\mathbf{x}_1^T \tag{15}$$

Indeed, the $k.th$ subsystem contributes this matrix to the anti-symmetrized cross-correlations $D(\tau)$ with varying amplitude for all τ.

The matrix D_k is now visualized as shown in Figs.3. The $i.th$ row of D_k corresponds to the interaction of the $i.th$ channel to all others and this interaction is represented by the contour-plot within the $i.th$ circle located at the respective channel location. In this example, the observed structure clearly corresponds to the interaction between eye-blinks and visual cortex since occipital channels interact with channels close to the eyes and vice versa.

In the upper panels of Fig.2 we show the corresponding temporal and spectral structures of this interaction, represented by $\lambda_k(\tau)$, and its Fourier transform, respectively. We observe in the temporal domain a peak at a delay around 120 ms (indicated by the arrow) which corresponds well to the response time of the primary visual cortex to visual input.

In the lower panels of Fig.2 we show the temporal and spectral pattern of another interacting component with a clear peak in the alpha range (10 Hz). The corresponding spatial pattern (Fig.4) clearly indicates an interacting system in occipital-parietal areas.

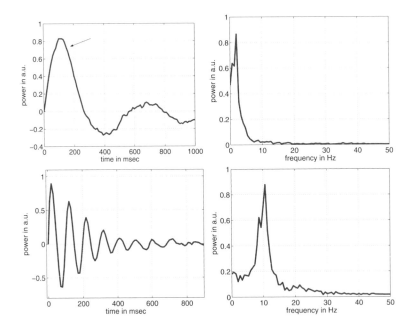

Figure 2: Diagonals of demixed antisymmetric correlation matrices as a function of delay τ (left panels) and, after Fourier transformation, as a function of frequency (right panels). Top: interaction of eye-blinks and visual cortex; bottom: interaction of alpha generators.

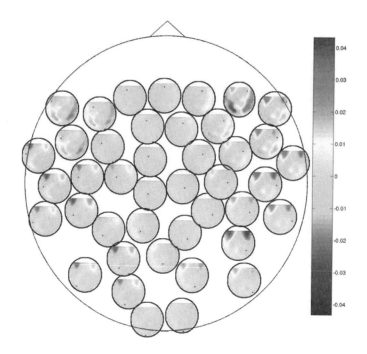

Figure 3: Spatial pattern corresponding to the interaction between eye-blinks and visual cortex.

4 Conclusion

When analyzing interaction between brain sources from macroscopic measurements like EEG/MEG it is important to distinguish physiologically reasonable patterns of interaction and spurious ones. In particular, volume conduction effects make large parts of the cortex seemingly interact although in reality such contributions are purely artifactual. Existing BSS methods that have been used with success for artifact removal and for estimation of brain sources will by construction fail when attempting to separate interacting i.e. non-independent brain sources. In this work we have proposed a new BSS algorithm that uses anti-symmetrized cross-correlation matrices and subsequent diagonalization and can thus reliably extract meaningful interaction while ignoring all spurious effects. Experiments using our interacting source analysis (ISA) reveal interesting relationships that are found *blindly*, e.g. inferring a component that links both eyes with visual cortex activity in a self-paced finger movement experiment. A more detailed look at the spectrum exhibits a peak at the typing frequency, and, in fact going back to the original MEG traces, eye-blinks were strongly coupled with the typing speed. This simple finding exemplifies that ISA is a powerful new technique for analyzing dynamical correlations in macroscopic brain measurements.

Future studies will therefore apply ISA to other neurophysiological paradigms in order to gain insights into the coherence and synchronicity patterns of cortical dynamics. It is especially of high interest to explore the possibilities of using true brain interactions as revealed by the imaginary part of cross-spectra as complementing information to improve the performance of brain computer interfaces.

Acknowledgements. We thank G. Curio for valuable discussions. This work was supported in part by the IST Programme of the European Community, under PASCAL Network

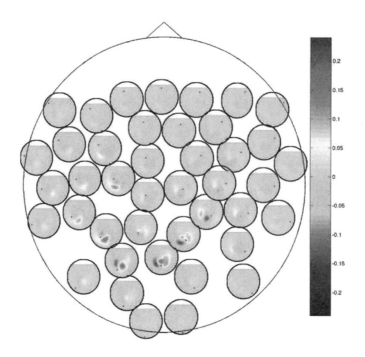

Figure 4: Spatial pattern corresponding to the interaction between alpha generators.

of Excellence, IST-2002-506778 and the BMBF in the BCI III project (grant 01BE01A). This publication only reflects the author's views.

References

[1] A. Hyvarinen, J. Karhunen, and E. Oja. *Independent Component Analysis.* Wiley, 2001.

[2] V.K. Jirsa. Connectivity and dynamics of neural information processing. *Neuroinformatics*, (2):183–204, 2004.

[3] Frank Meinecke, Andreas Ziehe, Jürgen Kurths, and Klaus-Robert Müller. Measuring Phase Synchronization of Superimposed Signals. *Physical Review Letters*, 94(8), 2005.

[4] G. Nolte, O. Bai, L. Wheaton, Z. Mari, S. Vorbach, and M. Hallet. Identifying true brain interaction from eeg data using the imaginary part of coherency. *Clinical Neurophysiology*, 115:2292–2307, 2004.

[5] A. Pikovsky, M. Rosenblum, and J. Kurths. *Synchronization – A Universal Concept in Nonlinear Sciences.* Cambridge University Press, 2001.

[6] W. Singer. Striving for coherence. *Nature*, 397(6718):391–393, Feb 1999.

[7] A. Yeredor, A. Ziehe, and K.-R. Müller. Approximate joint diagonalization using a natural-gradient approach. In Carlos G. Puntonet and Alberto Prieto, editors, *Lecture Notes in Computer Science*, volume 3195, pages 89–96, Granada, 2004. Springer-Verlag. Proc. ICA 2004.

[8] A. Ziehe and K.-R. Müller. TDSEP – an efficient algorithm for blind separation using time structure. In L. Niklasson, M. Bodén, and T. Ziemke, editors, *Proceedings of the 8th International Conference on Artificial Neural Networks, ICANN'98*, Perspectives in Neural Computing, pages 675 – 680, Berlin, 1998. Springer Verlag.

An Approximate Inference Approach for the PCA Reconstruction Error

Manfred Opper
Electronics and Computer Science
University of Southampton
Southampton, SO17 1BJ
mo@ecs.soton.ac.uk

Abstract

The problem of computing a resample estimate for the reconstruction error in PCA is reformulated as an inference problem with the help of the replica method. Using the expectation consistent (EC) approximation, the intractable inference problem can be solved efficiently using only two variational parameters. A perturbative correction to the result is computed and an alternative simplified derivation is also presented.

1 Introduction

This paper was motivated by recent joint work with Ole Winther on approximate inference techniques (the expectation consistent (EC) approximation [1] related to Tom Minka's EP [2] approach) which allows us to tackle high–dimensional sums and integrals required for Bayesian probabilistic inference.

I was looking for a nice model on which I could test this approximation. It had to be simple enough so that I would not be bogged down by large numerical simulations. But it had to be nontrivial enough to be of at least modest interest to Machine Learning. With the somewhat unorthodox application of approximate inference to resampling in PCA I hope to be able to stress the following points:

- Approximate efficient inference techniques can be useful in areas of Machine Learning where one would not necessarily assume that they are applicable. This can happen when the underlying probabilistic model is not immediately visible but shows only up as a result a of mathematical transformation.

- Approximate inference methods can be highly robust allowing for analytic continuations of model parameters to the complex plane or even noninteger dimensions.

- It is not always necessary to use a large number of variational parameters in order to get reasonable accuracy.

- Inference methods could be systematically improved using perturbative corrections.

The work was also stimulated by previous joint work with Dörthe Malzahn [3] on resampling estimates for generalization errors of Gaussian process models and Supportvector–Machines.

2 Resampling estimators for PCA

Principal Component Analysis (PCA) is a well known and widely applied tool for data analysis. The goal is to project data vectors $\mathbf{y}$ from a typically high (d-) dimensional space into an optimally chosen lower (q-) dimensional linear space with $q << d$, thereby minimizing the expected projection error $\varepsilon = E||\mathbf{y} - P_q[\mathbf{y}]||^2$, where $P_q[\mathbf{y}]$ denotes the projection. E stands for an expectation over the distribution of the data. In practice where the distribution is not available, one has to work with a data sample D_0 consisting of N vectors $\mathbf{y}_k = (y_k(1), y_k(2), \ldots, y_k(d))^T$, $k = 1, \ldots, N$. We arrange these vectors into a $(d \times N)$ data matrix $\mathbf{Y} = (\mathbf{y}_1, \mathbf{y}_2, \ldots, \mathbf{y}_N)$. Assuming centered data, the optimal subspace is spanned by the eigenvectors $\mathbf{u}_l$ of the $d \times d$ *data covariance matrix* $\mathbf{C} = \frac{1}{N}\mathbf{Y}\mathbf{Y}^T$ corresponding to the q largest eigenvalues λ_k. We will assume that these correspond to all eigenvectors $\lambda_k > \lambda$ above some threshold value λ.

After computing the PCA projection, one would be interested in finding out if the computed subspace represents the data well by estimating the average projection error on *novel data* $\mathbf{y}$ (ie not contained in D_0) which are drawn from the same distribution.

Fixing the projection P_q, the error can be rewritten as

$$\mathcal{E} = \sum_{\lambda_l < \lambda} E \operatorname{Tr} \left[\mathbf{y}\mathbf{y}^T \mathbf{u}_l \mathbf{u}_l^T \right] \tag{1}$$

where the expectation is only over $\mathbf{y}$ and the training data are fixed. The *training error* $\mathcal{E}_t = \sum_{\lambda_l < \lambda} \lambda_l^2$ can be obtained without knowledge of the distribution but will usually only give an optimistically biased estimate for $\mathcal{E}$.

2.1 A resampling estimate for the error

New artificial data samples D of arbitrary size can be created by resampling a number of data points from D_0 with or without replacement. A simple choice would be to choose all data independently with the same probability $1/N$, but other possibilities can also be implemented within our formalism. Thus, some $\mathbf{y}_i$ in D_0 may appear multiple times in D and others not at all. The idea of performing PCA on resampled data sets D and testing on the remaining data $D_0 \backslash D$, motivates the following definition of a *resample averaged reconstruction error*

$$\mathcal{E}_r = \frac{1}{N_0} E_D \left[\sum_{\mathbf{y}_i \notin D; \lambda_l < \lambda} \operatorname{Tr} \left(\mathbf{y}_i \mathbf{y}_i^T \mathbf{u}_l \mathbf{u}_l^T \right) \right] \tag{2}$$

as a proxy for $\mathcal{E}$. E_D is the expectation over the resampling process. This is an estimator of the *bootstrap* type [3,4]. N_0 is the expected number of data in D_0 which are not contained in the random set D. The rest of the paper will discuss a method for efficiently approximating (2).

2.2 Basic formalism

We introduce "occupation numbers" s_i which count how many times $\mathbf{y}_i$ is containd in D. We also introduce two matrices $\mathbf{D}$ and $\mathbf{C}$. $\mathbf{D}$ is a *diagonal random matrix*

$$\mathbf{D}_{ii} = D_i = \frac{1}{\mu \Gamma}(s_i + \epsilon \delta_{s_i,0}) \qquad \mathbf{C}(\epsilon) = \frac{\Gamma}{N}\mathbf{Y}\mathbf{D}\mathbf{Y}^T \,. \tag{3}$$

$\mathbf{C}(0)$ is proportional to the covariance matrix of the *resampled* data. μ is the sampling rate, i.e. $\mu N = E_D[\sum_i s_i]$ is the expected number of data in D (counting multiplicities). The role of Γ will be explained later. Using ϵ, we can generate expressions that can be used in (2) to sum over the data which are not contained in the set D

$$\mathbf{C}'(0) = \frac{1}{\mu N} \sum_j \delta_{s_j,0} \mathbf{y}_j \mathbf{y}_j^T .$$ (4)

In the following λ_k and $\mathbf{u}_k$ will always denote eigenvalues and eigenvectors of the data dependent (i.e. random) covariance matrix $\mathbf{C}(0)$.

The desired averages can be constructed from the $d \times d$ matrix *Green's function*

$$\mathbf{G}(\Gamma) = (\mathbf{C}(0) + \Gamma \mathbf{I})^{-1} = \sum_k \frac{\mathbf{u}_k \mathbf{u}_k^T}{\lambda_k + \Gamma}$$ (5)

Using the well known representation of the *Dirac* δ distribution given by $\delta(x) = \lim_{\eta \to 0^+} \Im \frac{1}{\pi(x - i\eta)}$ where $i = \sqrt{-1}$ and $\Im$ denotes the imaginary part, we get

$$\lim_{\eta \to 0^+} \frac{1}{\pi} \Im \, \mathbf{G}(\Gamma - i\eta) = \sum_k \mathbf{u}_k \mathbf{u}_k^T \delta(\lambda_k + \Gamma) .$$ (6)

Hence, we have

$$\mathcal{E}_r = \mathcal{E}_r^0 + \int_{0^+}^{\lambda} d\lambda' \, \varepsilon_r(\lambda')$$ (7)

where

$$\varepsilon_r(\lambda) = \frac{1}{\pi} \lim_{\eta \to 0^+} \Im \frac{1}{N_0} E_D \left[\sum_j \delta_{s_j,0} \mathrm{Tr} \left(\mathbf{y}_j \mathbf{y}_j^T \mathbf{G}(-\lambda - i\eta) \right) \right]$$ (8)

defines the *error density* from all eigenvalues > 0 and $\mathcal{E}_r^0$ is the contribution from the eigenspace with $\lambda_k = 0$. The latter can also be easily expressed from $\mathbf{G}$ as

$$\mathcal{E}_r^0 = \lim_{\Gamma \to 0} \frac{1}{N_0} E_D \left[\sum_j \delta_{s_j,0} \mathrm{Tr} \left(\mathbf{y}_j \mathbf{y}_j^T \Gamma \mathbf{G}(\Gamma) \right) \right]$$ (9)

We can also compute the resample averaged density of eigenvalues using

$$\rho(\lambda) = \frac{1}{\pi \mu N} \lim_{\eta \to 0^+} \Im \, E_D \left[\mathrm{Tr} \, \mathbf{G}(-\lambda - i\eta) \right]$$ (10)

3 A Gaussian probabilistic model

The matrix Green's function for $\Gamma > 0$ can be generated from a Gaussian partition function Z. This is a well known construction in statistical physics, and has also been used within the NIPS community to study the distribution of eigenvalues for an average case analysis of PCA [5]. Its use for computing the expected reconstruction error is to my knowledge new.

With the $(N \times N)$ *kernel matrix* $\mathbf{K} = \frac{1}{N} \mathbf{Y}^T \mathbf{Y}$ we define the Gaussian partition function

$$Z = \int d\mathbf{x} \, \exp \left[-\frac{1}{2} \mathbf{x}^T \left(\mathbf{K}^{-1} + \mathbf{D} \right) \mathbf{x} \right]$$ (11)

$$= |\mathbf{K}|^{\frac{1}{2}} \Gamma^{d/2} (2\pi)^{(N-d)/2} \int d^d \mathbf{z} \, \exp \left[-\frac{1}{2} \mathbf{z}^T \left(\mathbf{C}(\epsilon) + \Gamma \mathbf{I} \right) \mathbf{z} \right] .$$ (12)

x is an N dimensional integration variable. The equality can be easily shown by expressing the integrals as determinants. [1] The first representation (11) is useful for computing the resampling average and the second one connects directly to the definition of the matrix Green's function $\mathbf{G}$. Note, that by its dependence on the kernel matrix $\mathbf{K}$, a generalization to $d = \infty$ dimensional feature spaces and *kernel PCA* is straightforward. The partition function can then be understood as a certain Gaussian process expectation. We will not discuss this point further.

The *free energy* $F = -\ln Z$ enables us to generate the following quantities

$$-2\frac{\partial \ln Z}{\partial \epsilon}\bigg|_{\epsilon=0} = \frac{1}{\mu N}\sum_{j=1}^{N}\delta_{s_j,0}\operatorname{Tr}\mathbf{y}_j\mathbf{y}_j^T\mathbf{G}(\Gamma) \tag{13}$$

$$-2\frac{\partial \ln Z}{\partial \Gamma} = \frac{d}{\Gamma} + \operatorname{Tr}\mathbf{G}(\Gamma) \tag{14}$$

where we have used (4) for (13). (13) will be used for the computation of (8) and (14) applies to the density of eigenvalues. Note that the definition of the partition function Z requires that $\Gamma > 0$, whereas the application to the reconstruction error (7) needs negative values $\Gamma = -\lambda < 0$. Hence, an analytic continuation of end results must be performed.

4 Resampling average and replicas

(13) and (14) show that we can compute the desired resampling averages from the expected free energy $-E_D[\ln Z]$. This can be expressed using the "replica trick" of statistical physics (see e.g. [6]) using

$$E_D[\ln Z] = \lim_{n\to 0}\frac{1}{n}\ln E_D[Z^n]\,, \tag{15}$$

where one attempts an approximate computation of $E_D[Z^n]$ for *integer* n and uses a continuation to real numbers at the end. The n times replicated and averaged partition function (11) can be written in the form

$$Z^{(n)} \doteq E_D[Z^n] = \int dx\ \psi_1(x)\ \psi_2(x) \tag{16}$$

where we set $x \doteq (\mathbf{x}_1,\ldots,\mathbf{x}_n)$ and

$$\psi_1(x) = E_D\left[\exp\left\{-\frac{1}{2}\sum_{a=1}^{n}\mathbf{x}_a^T\mathbf{D}\mathbf{x}_a\right\}\right] \qquad \psi_2(x) = \exp\left[-\frac{1}{2}\sum_{a=1}^{n}\mathbf{x}_a^T\mathbf{K}^{-1}\mathbf{x}_a\right] \tag{17}$$

The *unaveraged* partition function Z (11) is Gaussian, but the *averaged* $Z^{(n)}$ is not and usually intractable.

5 Approximate inference

To approximate $Z^{(n)}$, we will use the EC approximation recently introduced by Opper & Winther [1]. For this method we need two auxiliary distributions

$$p_1(x) = \frac{1}{Z_1}\psi_1(x)e^{-\Lambda_1 x^T x} \qquad p_0(x) = \frac{1}{Z_0}e^{-\frac{1}{2}\Lambda_0 x^T x}\,, \tag{18}$$

where Λ_1 and Λ_0 are "variational" parameters to be optimized. p_1 tries to mimic the intractable $p(x) \propto \psi_1(x)\ \psi_2(x)$, replacing the multivariate Gaussian ψ_2 by a simpler, i.e.

---

[1] If $\mathbf{K}$ has zero eigenvalues, a division of Z by $|\mathbf{K}|^{\frac{1}{2}}$ is necessary. This additive renormalization of the free energy $-\ln Z$ will not influence the subsequent computations.

tractable diagonal one. One may think of using a general diagonal matrix Λ_1, but we will restrict ourselves in the present case to the simplest case of a spherical Gaussian with a *single parameter* Λ_1.

The strategy is to split $Z^{(n)}$ into a product of Z_1 and a term that has to be further approximated:

$$Z^{(n)} = Z_1 \int dx\ p_1(x)\ \psi_2(x)\ e^{\Lambda_1 x^T x} \tag{19}$$

$$\approx Z_1 \int dx\ p_0(x)\ \psi_2(x)\ e^{\Lambda_1 x^T x} \equiv Z_{EC}^{(n)}(\Lambda_1, \Lambda_0)\ .$$

The approximation replaces the intractable average over p_1 by a tractable one over p_0. To optimize Λ_1 and Λ_0 we argue as follows: We try to make p_0 as close as possible to p_1 by matching the moments $\langle x^T x \rangle_1 = \langle x^T x \rangle_0$. The index denotes the distribution which is used for averaging. By this step, Λ_0 becomes a function of Λ_1. Second, since the true partition function $Z^{(n)}$ is *independent* of Λ_1, we expect that a good approximation to $Z^{(n)}$ should be stationary with respect to variations of Λ_1. Both conditions can be expressed by the requirement that $\ln Z_{EC}^{(n)}(\Lambda_1, \Lambda_0)$ must be stationary with respect to variations of Λ_1 and Λ_0.

Within this EC approximation we can carry out the replica limit $E_D[\ln Z] \approx \ln Z_{EC} = \lim_{n\to 0} \frac{1}{n} \ln Z_{EC}^{(n)}$ and get after some calculations

$$-\ln Z_{EC} = -E_D \left[\ln \int dx\ e^{-\frac{1}{2} x^T (D + (\Lambda_0 - \Lambda) I) x} \right] - \tag{20}$$

$$-\ln \int dx\ e^{-\frac{1}{2} x^T (K^{-1} + \Lambda I) x} + \ln \int dx\ e^{-\frac{1}{2} \Lambda_0 x^T x}$$

where we have set $\Lambda = \Lambda_0 - \Lambda_1$. Since the first Gaussian integral factorises, we can now perform the resampling average in (20) relatively easy for the case when all s_j's in (3) are independent. Assuming e.g. *Poisson* probabilities $p(s) = e^{-\mu} \frac{\mu^s}{s!}$ gives a good approximation for the case of resampling μN points with replacement.

The variational equations which make (20) stationary are

$$E_D \left(\frac{1}{\Lambda_0 - \Lambda + D_i} \right) = \frac{1}{\Lambda_0} \qquad \frac{1}{N} \sum_k \frac{\omega_i}{1 + \omega_k \Lambda} = \frac{1}{\Lambda_0} \tag{21}$$

where ω_k are the eigenvalues of the matrix K. The variational equations have to be solved in the region $\Gamma = -\lambda < 0$ where the original partition function does not exist. The resulting parameters Λ_0 and Λ will usually come out as *complex* numbers.

6 Experiments

By eliminating the parameter Λ_0 from (21) it is possible to reduce the numerical computations to solving a nonlinear equation for a single *complex* parameter Λ which can be solved easily and fast by a Newton method. While the analytical results are based on *Poisson* statistics, the simulations of random resampling was performed by choosing a *fixed* number (equal to the expected number of the Poisson distribution) of data at random with replacement.

The first experiment was for a set of data generated at random from a spherical Gaussian. To show that resampling maybe useful, we give on on the left hand side of Figure 1 the reconstruction error as a function of the value of λ below which eigenvalues are dicarded.

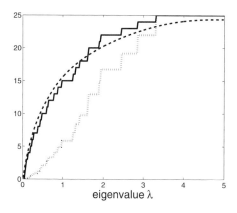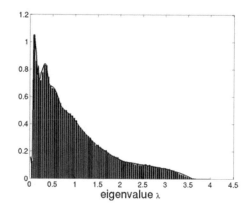

Figure 1: *Left:* Errors for PCA on $N = 32$ spherically Gaussian data with $d = 25$ and $\mu = 3$. Smooth curve: approximate resampled error estimate, upper step function: true error. Lower step function: Training error. *Right:* Comparison of EC approximation (line) and simulation (histogramme) of the resampled density of eigenvalues for $N = 50$ spherically Gaussian data of dimensionality $d = 25$. The sampling rate was $\mu = 3$.

The smooth function is the approximate resampling error (3× oversampled to leave not many data out of the samples) from our method. The upper step function gives the true reconstruction error (easy to calculate for spherical data) from (1). The lower step function is the training error. The right panel demonstrates the *accuracy* of the approximation on a similar set of data. We compare the analytically approximated density of states with the results of a true resampling experiment, where eigenvalues for many samples are counted into small bins. The theoretical curve follows closely the experiment.

Since the good accuracy might be attributed to the high symmetry of the toy data, we have also performed experiments on a set of $N = 100$ handwritten digits with $d = 784$. The results in Figure 2 are promising. Although the density of eigenvalues is more accurate than the resampling error, the latter comes still out reasonable.

7 Corrections

I will show next that the EC approximation can be augmented by a perturbation expansion. Going back to (19), we can write

$$\frac{Z^{(n)}}{Z_1} = \int dx\, p_1(x)\, \psi_2(x)\, e^{\Lambda_1 x^T x} = \int dx\, \psi_2(x)\, e^{\frac{1}{2}\Lambda x^T x} \left\{ \int \frac{dk}{(2\pi)^{Nn}} e^{-ik^T x} \chi(k) \right\}$$

where $\chi(k) \doteq \int dx\, p_1(x) e^{ik^T x}$ is the *characteristic function* of the density p_1 (18). $\ln \chi(k)$ is the *cumulant generating function*. Using the symmetries of the density p_1, we can perform a power series expansion of $\ln \chi(k)$, which starts with a quadratic term (second cumulant)

$$\ln \chi(k) = -\frac{M_2}{2} k^T k + R(k) , \tag{22}$$

where $M_2 = \langle x_a^T x_a \rangle_1$. It can be shown that if we neglect $R(k)$ (containing the higher order cumulants) and carry out the integral over k, we end up replacing p_1 by a simpler Gaussian p_0 with matching moments M_2, i.e. the EC approximation. Higher order corrections to the free energy $-E_D[\ln Z] = -\ln Z_{EC} + \Delta F_1 + \ldots$ can be obtained perturbatively by writing $\chi(k) = e^{-\frac{M_2}{2} k^T k}(1 + R(k) + \ldots)$. This expansion is similar in spirit to *Edgeworth*

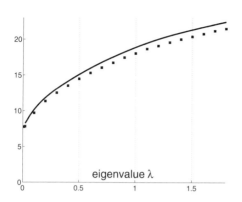
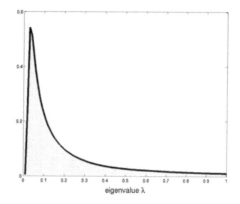

Figure 2: *Left:* Resampling error ($\mu = 1$) for PCA on a set of 100 handwritten digits ("5") with $d = 784$. The approximation (line) for $\mu = 1$ is compared with simulations of the random resampling. *Right:* Resampled density of eigenvalues for the same data set. Only the nonzero eigenvalues are shown.

expansions in statistics. The present case is more complicated by the extra dimensions introduced by the *replicating* of variables and the limit $n \to 0$. After a lengthy calculation one finds for the lowest order correction (containing the monomials in k of order 4) to the free energy:

$$\Delta F_1 = -\frac{1}{4} E_D \left(\frac{\Lambda_0}{\Lambda_0 - \Lambda + D_i} - 1 \right)^2 \times \sum_i \left(\Lambda_0 \left(\mathbf{K}^{-1} + \Lambda \mathbf{I} \right)_{ii}^{-1} - 1 \right)^2 \quad (23)$$

I illustrate the effect of ΔF_1 on a correction to the reconstruction error in the "zero–subspace" using (9) and (13) for the digit data as a function of μ. Resampling used the Poisson approximation. The left panel of Figure 3 demonstrates that the true correction is fairly small. The right panel shows that the lowest order term ΔF_1 accounts for a major part of the true correction when $\mu < 3$. The strong underestimation for larger μ needs further investigation.

8 The calculation without replicas

Knowing with hindsight how the final EC result (20) looks like, we can rederive it using another method which does not rely on the "replica trick". We first write down an exact expression for $-\ln Z$ *before* averaging. Expressing Gaussian integrals by determinants yields

$$-\ln Z = -\ln \int d\mathbf{x} \, e^{-\frac{1}{2}\mathbf{x}^T (\mathbf{D} + (\Lambda_0 - \Lambda)\mathbf{I})\mathbf{x}} - \ln \int d\mathbf{x} \, e^{-\frac{1}{2}\mathbf{x}^T (\mathbf{K}^{-1} + \Lambda \mathbf{I})\mathbf{x}} + \quad (24)$$

$$+ \ln \int d\mathbf{x} \, e^{-\frac{1}{2}\Lambda_0 \mathbf{x}^T \mathbf{x}} + \frac{1}{2} \ln \det(\mathbf{I} + \mathbf{r})$$

where the matrix $\mathbf{r}$ has elements $\mathbf{r}_{ij} = \left(1 - \frac{\Lambda_0}{\Lambda_0 - \Lambda + D_i} \right) \left(\Lambda_0 \left(\mathbf{K}^{-1} + \Lambda \mathbf{I} \right)^{-1} - \mathbf{I} \right)_{ij}$. The EC approximation is obtained by simply neglecting $\mathbf{r}$. Corrections to this are found by expanding

$$\ln \det \left(\mathbf{I} + \mathbf{r} \right) = \operatorname{Tr} \ln \left(\mathbf{I} + \mathbf{r} \right) = \sum_{k=1}^{\infty} \frac{(-1)^{k+1}}{k} \operatorname{Tr} \left(\mathbf{r}^k \right) \quad (25)$$

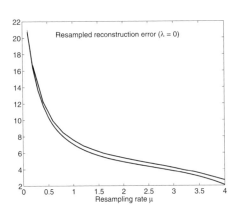
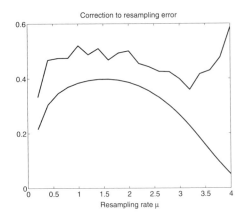

Figure 3: *Left:* Resampling error $\mathcal{E}_r^0$ from the $\lambda = 0$ subspace as a function of resampling rate for the digits data. The approximation (lower line) is compared with simulations of the random resampling (upper line). *Right:* The difference between approximation and simulations (upper curve) and its estimate (lower curve) from the perturbative correction (23).

The first order term in the expansion (25) vanishes after averaging (see (21)) and the second order term gives exactly the correction of the cumulant method (23).

9 Outlook

It will be interesting to extend the perturbative framework for the computation of corrections to inference approximations to other, more complex models. However, our results indicate that the use and convergence of such perturbation expansion needs to be critically investigated and that the lowest order may not always give a clear indication of the accuracy of the approximation. The alternative derivation for our simple model could present an interesting ground for testing these ideas.

Acknowledgments

I would like to thank Ole Winther for the great collaboration on the EC approximation.

References

[1] Manfred Opper and Ole Winther. Expectation consistent free energies for approximate inference. In *NIPS 17*, 2005.

[2] T. P. Minka. Expectation propagation for approximate Bayesian inference. In *UAI 2001*, pages 362–369, 2001.

[3] D. Malzahn and M. Opper. An approximate analytical approach to resampling averages. *Journal of Machine Learning Research*, pages 1151–1173, 2003.

[4] B. Efron, R. J. Tibshirani. *An Introduction to the Bootstrap*. Monographs on Statistics and Applied Probability 57, Chapman & Hall, 1993.

[5] D. C. Hoyle and M. Rattray Limiting form of the sample covariance matrix eigenspectrum in PCA and kernel PCA. In *NIPS 16*, 2003.

[6] A. Engel and C. Van den Broeck, *Statistical Mechanics of Learning* (Cambridge University Press, 2001).

Bayesian model learning in
human visual perception

Gergő Orbán
Collegium Budapest
Institute for Advanced Study
2 Szentháromság utca, Budapest,
1014 Hungary
ogergo@colbud.hu

József Fiser
Department of Psychology and
Volen Center for Complex Systems
Brandeis University
Waltham, Massachusetts 02454, USA
fiser@brandeis.edu

Richard N. Aslin
Department of Brain and Cognitive
Sciences, Center for Visual Science
University of Rochester
Rochester, New York 14627, USA
aslin@cvs.rochester.edu

Máté Lengyel
Gatsby Computational Neuroscience Unit
University College London
17 Queen Square, London WC1N 3AR
United Kingdom
lmate@gatsby.ucl.ac.uk

Abstract

Humans make optimal perceptual decisions in noisy and ambiguous conditions. Computations underlying such optimal behavior have been shown to rely on probabilistic inference according to generative models whose structure is usually taken to be known a priori. We argue that Bayesian model selection is ideal for inferring similar and even more complex model structures from experience. We find in experiments that humans learn subtle statistical properties of visual scenes in a completely unsupervised manner. We show that these findings are well captured by Bayesian model learning within a class of models that seek to explain observed variables by independent hidden causes.

1 Introduction

There is a growing number of studies supporting the classical view of perception as probabilistic inference [1, 2]. These studies demonstrated that human observers parse sensory scenes by performing optimal estimation of the parameters of the objects involved [3, 4, 5]. Even single neurons in primary sensory cortices have receptive field properties that seem to support such a computation [6]. A core element of this Bayesian probabilistic framework is an internal model of the world, the generative model, that serves as a basis for inference. In principle, inference can be performed on several levels: the generative model can be used for inferring the values of hidden variables from observed information, but also the model itself may be inferred from previous experience [7].

Most previous studies testing the Bayesian framework in human psychophysical experiments used highly restricted generative models of perception, usually consisting of a few observed and latent variables, of which only a limited number of parameters needed to be adjusted by experience. More importantly, the generative models considered in these studies were tailor-made to the specific pscychophysical task presented in the experiment. Thus, it remains to be shown whether more flexible, 'open-ended' generative models are used and learned by humans during perception.

Here, we use an unsupervised visual learning task to show that a general class of generative models, sigmoid belief networks (SBNs), perform similarly to humans (also reproducing paradoxical aspects of human behavior), when not only the parameters of these models but also their structure is subject to learning. Crucially, the applied Bayesian model learning embodies the Automatic Occam's Razor (AOR) effect that selects the models that are 'as simple as possible, but no simpler'. This process leads to the extraction of independent causes that efficiently and sufficiently account for sensory experience, without a pre-specification of the number or complexity of potential causes.

In section 2, we describe the experimental protocol we used in detail. Next, the mathematical framework is presented that is used to study model learning in SBNs (Section 3). In Section 4, experimental results on human performance are compared to the prediction of our Bayes-optimal model learning in the SBN framework. All the presented human experimental results were reproduced and had identical roots in our simulations: the modal model developed latent variables corresponding to the unknown underlying causes that generated the training scenes.

In Section 5, we discuss the implications of our findings. Although structure and parameter learning are not fundamentally different computations in Bayesian inference, we argue that the natural integration of these two kinds of learning lead to a behavior that accounts for human data which cannot be reproduced in some simpler alternative learning models with parameter but without structure learning. Given the recent surge of biologically plausible neural network models performing inference in belief networks we also point out challenges that our findings present for future models of probabilistic neural computations.

2 Experimental paradigm

Human adult subjects were trained and then tested in an unsupervised learning paradigm with a set of complex visual scenes consisting of 6 of 12 abstract unfamiliar black *shapes* arranged on a 3x3 (Exp 1) or 5x5 (Exps 2-4) white grid (Fig. 1, left panel). Unbeknownst to subjects, various subsets of the shapes were arranged into fixed spatial combinations *(combos)* (doublets, triplets, quadruplets, depending on the experiment). Whenever a combo appeared on a training scene, its constituent shapes were presented in an invariant spatial arrangement, and in no scenes elements of a combo could appear without all the other elements of the same combo also appearing. Subjects were presented with 100–200 training scenes, each scene was presented for 2 seconds with a 1-second pause between scenes. No specific instructions were given to subjects prior to training, they were only asked to pay attention to the continuous sequence of scenes.

The test phase consisted of 2AFC trials, in which two arrangements of shapes were shown sequentially in the same grid that was used in the training, and subjects were asked which of the two scenes was more familiar based on the training. One of the presented scenes was either a combo that was actually used for constructing the training set *(true combo)*, or a part of it *(embedded combo)* (e.g., a pair of adjacent shapes from a triplet or quadruplet combo). The other scene consisted of the same number of shapes as the first scene in an arrangement that might or might not have occurred during training, but was in fact a mixture of shapes from different true combos *(mixture combo)*.

Here four experiments are considered that assess various aspects of human observational

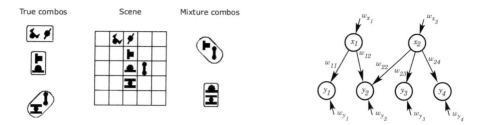

Figure 1: Experimental design (*left panel*) and explanation of graphical model parameters (*right panel*).

learning, the full set of experiments are presented elsewhere [8, 9]. Each experiment was run with 20 naïve subjects.

1. Our first goal was to establish that humans are sensitive to the statistical structure of visual experience, and use this experience for judging familiarity. In the baseline experiment 6 doublet combos were defined, three of which were presented simultaneously in any given training scene, allowing 144 possible scenes [8]. Because the doublets were not marked in any way, subjects saw only a group of random shapes arranged on a grid. The occurrence frequency of doublets and individual elements was equal across the set of scenes, allowing no obvious bias to remember any element more than others. In the test phase a true and a mixture doublet were presented sequentially in each 2AFC trial. The mixture combo was presented in a spatial position that had never appeared before.

2. In the previous experiment the elements of mixture doublets occurred together fewer times than elements of real doublets, thus a simple strategy based on tracking co-occurrence frequencies of shape-pairs would be sufficient to distinguish between them. The second, frequency-balanced experiment tested whether humans are sensitive to higher-order statistics (at least cross-correlations, which are co-occurence frequencies normalized by respective invidual occurence frequencies).

   The structure of Experiment 1 was changed so that while the 6 doublet combo architecture remained, their appearance frequency became non-uniform introducing *frequent* and *rare combos*. Frequent doublets were presented twice as often as rare ones, so that certain mixture doublets consisting of shapes from frequent doublets appeared just as often as rare doublets. Note, that the frequency of the constituent shapes of these mixture doublets was higher than that of rare doublets. The training session consisted of 212 scenes, each scene being presented twice. In the test phase, the familiarity of both single shapes and doublet combos was tested. In the doublet trials, rare combos with low appearance frequency but high correlations between elements were compared to mixed combos with higher element and equal pair appearance frequency, but lower correlations between elements.

3. The third experiment tested whether human performance in this paradigm can be fully accounted for by learning cross-correlations. Here, four triplet combos were formed and presented with equal occurrence frequencies. 112 scenes were presented twice to subjects. In the test phase two types of tests were performed. In the first type, the familiarity of a true triplet and a mixture triplet was compared, while in the second type doublets consisting of adjacent shapes embedded in a triplet combo (*embedded doublet*) were tested against mixture doublets.

4. The fourth experiment compared directly how humans treat embedded and independent (non-embedded) combos of the same spatial dimensions. Here two

quadruplet combos and two doublet combos were defined and presented with equal frequency. Each training scene consisted of six shapes, one quadruplet and one doublet. 120 such scenes were constructed. In the test phase three types of tests were performed. First, true quadruplets were compared to mixture quadruplets; next, embedded doublets were compared to mixture doublets, finally true doublets were compared to mixture doublets.

3   Modeling framework

The goal of Bayesian learning is to 'reverse-engineer' the generative model that could have generated the training data. Because of inherent ambiguity and stochasticity assumed by the generative model itself, the objective is to establish a *probability distribution* over possible models. Importantly, because models with parameter spaces of different dimensionality are compared, the likelihood term (Eq. 3) will prefer the simplest model (in our case, the one with fewest parameters) that can effectively account for (generate) the training data due to the AOR effect in Bayesian model comparison [7].

Sigmoid belief networks   The class of generative models we consider is that of two-layer sigmoid belief networks (SBNs, Fig. 1). The same modelling framework has been successfully aplied to animal learning in classical conditioning [10, 11]. The SBN architecture assumes that the state of observed binary variables (y_j, in our case: shapes being present or absent in a training scene) depends through a sigmoidal activation function on the state of a set of hidden binary variables ($\mathbf{x}$), which are not directly observable:

$$P\left(y_j = 1 | \mathbf{x}, \mathbf{w}_m, m\right) = \left(1 + \exp\left(-\sum_i w_{ij} x_i - w_{y_j}\right)\right)^{-1} \quad (1)$$

where w_{ij} describes the (real-valued) influence of hidden variable x_i on observed variable y_j, w_{y_j} determines the spontaneous activation bias of y_j, and m indicates the model structure, including the number of latent variables and identity of the observeds they can influence (the w_{ij} weights that are allowed to have non-zero value).

Observed variables are independent conditioned on the latents (i.e. any correlation between them is assumed to be due to shared causes), and latent variables are marginally independent and have Bernoulli distributions parametrised by $\mathbf{w}_x$:

$$P\left(\mathbf{y} | \mathbf{x}, \mathbf{w}_m, m\right) = \prod_j P\left(y_j | \mathbf{x}, \mathbf{w}_m, m\right), \ P\left(\mathbf{x} | \mathbf{w}_m, m\right) = \prod_i \left(1 + \exp\left(-1^{x_i} w_{x_i}\right)\right)^{-1}$$

$$(2)$$

Finally, scenes ($\mathbf{y}^{(t)}$) are assumed to be iid samples from the same generative distribution, and so the probability of the training data ($\mathcal{D}$) given a specific model is:

$$P\left(\mathcal{D} | \mathbf{w}_m, m\right) = \prod_t P\left(\mathbf{y}^{(t)} | \mathbf{w}_m, m\right) = \prod_t \sum_{\mathbf{x}} \prod_j P\left(y_j^{(t)}, \mathbf{x} | \mathbf{w}_m, m\right) \quad (3)$$

The 'true' generative model that was actually used for generating training data in the experiments (Section 2) is closely related to this model, with the combos corresponding to latent variables. The main difference is that here we ignore the spatial aspects of the task, i.e. only the occurrence of a shape matters but not *where* it appears on the grid. Although in general, space is certainly not a negligible factor in vision, human behavior in the present experiments depended on the fact of shape-appearances sufficiently strongly so that this simplification did not cause major confounds in our results.

A second difference between the model and the human experiments was that in the experiments, combos were not presented completely randomly, because the number of combos per scene was fixed (and not binomially distributed as implied by the model, Eq. 2). Nevertheless, our goal was to demonstrate the use of a general-purpose class of generative models, and although truly independent causes are rare in natural circumstances, always a fixed number of them being present is even more so. Clearly, humans are able to capture dependences between latent variables, and these should be modeled as well ([12]). Similarly, for simplicity we also ignored that subsequent scenes are rarely independent (Eq. 3) in natural vision.

Training Establishing the posterior probability of any given model is straightforward using Bayes' rule:

$$P(\mathbf{w}_m, m | \mathcal{D}) \propto P(\mathcal{D} | \mathbf{w}_m, m) \ P(\mathbf{w}_m, m) \tag{4}$$

where the first term is the likelihood of the model (Eq. 3), and the second term is the prior distribution of models. Prior distributions for the weights were: $P(w_{ij}) = \text{Laplace}(12, 2)$, $P(w_{x_i}) = \text{Laplace}(0, 2)$, $P(w_{x_j}) = \delta(-6)$. The prior over model structure preferred simple models and was such that the distributions of the number of latents and of the number of links conditioned on the number of latents were both $\text{Geometric}(0.1)$. The effect of this preference is 'washed out' with increasing training length as the likelihood term (Eq. 3) sharpens.

Testing When asked to compare the familiarity of two scenes ($\mathbf{y}^A$ and $\mathbf{y}^B$) in the testing phase, the optimal strategy for subjects would be to compute the posterior probability of both scenes based on the training data

$$P(\mathbf{y}^Z | \mathcal{D}) = \sum_m \int d\mathbf{w}_m \sum_{\mathbf{x}} P(\mathbf{y}^Z, \mathbf{x} | \mathbf{w}_m, m) \ P(\mathbf{w}_m, m | \mathcal{D}) \tag{5}$$

and always (ie, with probability one) choose the one with the higher probability. However, as a phenomenological model of all kinds of possible sources of noise (sensory noise, model noise, etc) we chose a soft threshold function for computing choice probability:

$$P(\text{choose A}) = \left(1 + \exp\left(-\beta \log \frac{P(\mathbf{y}^A | \mathcal{D})}{P(\mathbf{y}^B | \mathcal{D})}\right)\right)^{-1} \tag{6}$$

and used $\beta = 1$ ($\beta = \infty$ corresponds to the optimal strategy).

Note that when computing the probability of a test scene, we seek the probability that exactly the given scene was generated by the learned model. This means that we require not only that all the shapes that are present in the test scene are present in the generated data, but also that all the shapes that are absent from the test scene are absent from the generated data. A different scheme, in which only the presence but not the absence of the shapes need to be matched (i.e. absent observeds are marginalized out just as latents are in Eq. 5) could also be pursued, but the results of the embedding experiments (Exp. 3 and 4, see below) discourage it.

The model posterior in Eq. 4 is analytically intractable, therefore an exchange reversible-jump Markov chain Monte Carlo sampling method [10, 13, 14] was applied, that ensured fair sampling from a model space containing subspaces of differring dimensionality, and integration over this posterior in Eq. 5 was approximated by a sum over samples.

4 Results

Pilot studies were performed with reduced training datasets in order to test the performance of the model learning framework. First, we trained the model on data consisting of 8 observed variables ('shapes'). The 8 'shapes' were partitioned into three 'combos' of different

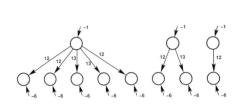 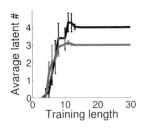

Figure 2: Bayesian learning in sigmoid belief networks. *Left panel:* MAP model of a 30-trial-long training with 8 observed variables and 3 combos. Latent variables of the MAP model reflect the relationships defined by the combos. *Right panel:* Increasing model complexity with increasing training experience. Average number of latent variables ($\pm$SD) in the model posterior distribution as a function of the length of training data was obtained by marginalizing Eq. 4 over weights $\mathbf{w}$.

sizes (5, 2, 1), two of which were presented simultaneously in each training trial. The AOR effect in Bayesian model learning should select the model structure that is of just the right complexity for describing the data. Accordingly, after 30 trials, the *maximum a posteriori* (MAP) model had three latents corresponding to the underlying 'combos' (Fig. 2, left panel). Early on in training simpler model structures dominated because of the prior preference for low latent and link numbers, but due to the simple structure of the training data the likelihood term won over in as few as 10 trials, and the model posterior converged to the true generative model (Fig. 2, right panel, gray line). Importantly, presenting more data with the same statistics did not encourage the fitting of over-complicated model structures. On the other hand, if data was generated by using more 'combos' (4 'doublets'), model learning converged to a model with a correspondingly higher number of latents (Fig. 2, right panel, black line).

In the baseline experiment (Experiment 1) human subjects were trained with six equal-sized doublet combos and were shown to recognize true doublets over mixture doublets (Fig. 3, first column). When the same training data was used to compute the choice probability in 2AFC tests with model learning, true doublets were reliably preferred over mixture doublets. Also, the MAP model showed that the discovered latent variables corresponded to the combos generating the training data (data not shown).

In Experiment 2, we sought to answer the question whether the statistical learning demonstrated in Experiment 1 was solely relying on co-occurrence frequencies, or was using something more sophisticated, such as at least cross-correlations between shapes. Bayesian model learning, as well as humans, could distinguish between rare doublet combos and mixtures from frequent doublets (Fig. 3, second column) despite their balanced co-occurrence frequencies. Furthermore, although in this comparison rare doublet combos were preferred, both humans and the model learned about the frequencies of their constituent shapes and preferred constituent single shapes of frequent doublets over those of rare doublets. Nevertheless, it should be noted that while humans showed greater preference for frequent singlets than for rare doublets our simulations predicted an opposite trend[1].

We were interested whether the performance of humans could be fully accounted for by the learning of cross-correlations, or they demonstrated more sophisticated computations.

---

[1]This discrepancy between theory and experiments may be explained by Gestalt effects in human vision that would strongly prefer the independent processing of constituent shapes due to their clear spatial separation in the training scenes. The reconciliation of such Gestalt effects with pure statistical learning is the target of further investigations.

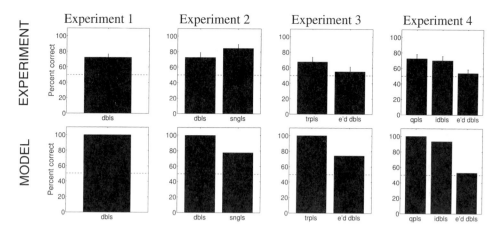

Figure 3: Comparison of human and model performance in four experiments. Bars show percent 'correct' values (choosing a true or embedded combo over a mixture combo, or a frequent singlet over a rare singlet) for human experiments (average over subjects ±SEM), and 'correct' choice probabilities (Eq. 6) for computer simulations. *Sngls:* Single shapes; *dbls*: Doublet combos; *trpls:* triplet combos; *e'd dbls:* embedded doublet combos; *qpls:* quadruple combos; *idbls:* independent doublet combos.

In Experiment 3, training data was composed of triplet combos, and beside testing true triplets against mixture triplets, we also tested embedded doublets (pairs of shapes from the same triplet) against mixture doublets (pairs of shapes from different triplets). If learning only depends on cross-correlations, we expect to see similar performance on these two types of tests. In contrast, human performace was significantly different for triplets (true triplets were preferred) and doublets (embedded and mixture doublets were not distinguished) (Fig. 3, third column). This may be seen as Gestalt effects being at work: once the 'whole' triplet is learned, its constituent parts (the embedded doublets) loose their significance. Our model reproduced this behavior and provided a straightforward explanation: latent-to-observed weights (w_{ij}) in the MAP model were so strong that whenever a latent was switched on it could almost only produce triplets, therefore doublets were created by spontaneous independent activation of observeds which thus produced embedded and mixture doublets with equal chance. In other words, doublets were seen as mere noise under the MAP model.

The fourth experiment tested explicitly whether embedded combos and equal-sized independent real combos are distinguished and not only size effects prevented the recognition of embedded small structures in the previous experiment. Both human experiments and Bayesian model selection demonstrated that quadruple combos as well as stand-alone doublets were reliably recognized (Fig. 3, fourth column), while embedded doublets were not.

5 Discussion

We demonstrated that humans flexibly yet automatically learn complex generative models in visual perception. Bayesian model learning has been implicated in several domains of high level human cognition, from causal reasoning [15] to concept learning [16]. Here we showed it being at work already at a pre-verbal stage.

We emphasized the importance of learning the *structure* of the generative model, not only its parameters, even though it is quite clear that the two cannot be formally distinguished. Nevertheless we have two good reasons to believe that structure learning is indeed important in our case. (1) Sigmoid belief networks identical to ours but without structure learning have been shown to perform poorly on a task closely related to ours [17], Földiák's bar test [18]. More complicated models will of course be able to produce identical results, but we think our model framework has the advantage of being intuitively simple: it seeks to find the simplest possible explanation for the data assuming that it was generated by independent causes. (2) Structure learning allows Occam's automatic razor to come to play. This is computationally expensive, but together with the generative model class we use provides a neat and highly efficient way to discover 'independent components' in the data. We experienced difficulties with other models [17] developed for similar purposes when trying to reproduce our experimental findings.

Our approach is very much in the tradition that sees the finding of independent causes behind sensory data as one of the major goals of perception [2]. Although neural network models that can produce such computations exist [6, 19], none of these does model selection. Very recently, several models have been proposed for doing inference in belief networks [20, 21] but parameter learning let alone structure learning proved to be non-trivial in them. Our results highlight the importance of considering model structure learning in neural models of Bayesian inference.

Acknowledgements

We were greatly motivated by the earlier work of Aaron Courville and Nathaniel Daw [10, 11], and hugely benefited from several useful discussions with them. We would also like to thank the insightful comments of Peter Dayan, Maneesh Sahani, Sam Roweis, and Zoltán Szatmáry on an earlier version of this work. This work was supported by IST-FET-1940 program (GO), NIH research grant HD-37082 (RNA, JF), and the Gatsby Charitable Foundation (ML).

References

[1] Helmholtz HLF. Treatise on Physiological Optics. New York: Dover, 1962.
[2] Barlow HB. Vision Res 30:1561, 1990.
[3] Ernst MO, Banks MS. Nature 415:429, 2002.
[4] Körding KP, Wolpert DM. Nature 427:244, 2004.
[5] Kersten D, et al. Annu Rev Psychol 55, 2004.
[6] Olshausen BA, Field DJ. Nature 381:607, 1996.
[7] MacKay DJC. Network: Comput Neural Syst 6:469, 1995.
[8] Fiser J, Aslin RN. Psych Sci 12:499, 2001.
[9] Fiser J, Aslin RN. J Exp Psychol Gen , in press.
[10] Courville AC, et al. In NIPS 16 , Cambridge, MA, 2004. MIT Press.
[11] Courville AC, et al. In NIPS 17 , Cambridge, MA, 2005. MIT Press.
[12] Hinton GE, et al. In Artificial Intelligence and Statistics , Barbados, 2005.
[13] Green PJ. Biometrika 82:711, 1995.
[14] Iba Y. Int J Mod Phys C 12:623, 2001.
[15] Tenenbaum JB, Griffiths TL. In NIPS 15 , 35, Cambridge, MA, 2003. MIT Press.
[16] Tenenbaum JB. In NIPS 11 , 59, Cambridge, MA, 1999. MIT Press.
[17] Dayan P, Zemel R. Neural Comput 7:565, 1995.
[18] Földiak P. Biol Cybern 64:165, 1990.
[19] Dayan P, et al. Neural Comput 7:1022, 1995.
[20] Rao RP. Neural Comput 16:1, 2004.
[21] Deneve S. In NIPS 17 , Cambridge, MA, 2005. MIT Press.

Spiking Inputs to a Winner-take-all Network

Matthias Oster and Shih-Chii Liu
Institute of Neuroinformatics
University of Zurich and ETH Zurich
Winterthurerstrasse 190
CH-8057 Zurich, Switzerland
{mao,shih}@ini.phys.ethz.ch

Abstract

Recurrent networks that perform a winner-take-all computation have been studied extensively. Although some of these studies include spiking networks, they consider only analog input rates. We present results of this winner-take-all computation on a network of integrate-and-fire neurons which receives spike trains as inputs. We show how we can configure the connectivity in the network so that the winner is selected after a pre-determined number of input spikes. We discuss spiking inputs with both regular frequencies and Poisson-distributed rates. The robustness of the computation was tested by implementing the winner-take-all network on an analog VLSI array of 64 integrate-and-fire neurons which have an innate variance in their operating parameters.

1 Introduction

Recurrent networks that perform a winner-take-all computation are of great interest because of the computational power they offer. They have been used in modelling attention and recognition processes in cortex [Itti et al., 1998, Lee et al., 1999] and are thought to be a basic building block of the cortical microcircuit [Douglas and Martin, 2004]. Descriptions of theoretical spike-based models [Jin and Seung, 2002] and analog VLSI (aVLSI) implementations of both spike and non-spike models [Lazzaro et al., 1989, Indiveri, 2000, Hahnloser et al., 2000] can be found in the literature. Although the competition mechanism in these models uses spike signals, they usually consider the external input to the network to be either an analog input current or an analog value that represents the spike rate.

We describe the operation and connectivity of a winner-take-all network that receives input spikes. We consider the case of the hard winner-take-all mode, where only the winning neuron is active and all other neurons are suppressed. We discuss a scheme for setting the excitatory and inhibitory weights of the network so that the winner which receives input with the shortest inter-spike interval is selected after a pre-determined number of input spikes. The winner can be selected with as few as two input spikes, making the selection process fast [Jin and Seung, 2002].

We tested this computation on an aVLSI chip with 64 integrate-and-fire neurons and various dynamic excitatory and inhibitory synapses. The distribution of mismatch (or variance) in the operating parameters of the neurons and synapses has been reduced using a spike coding

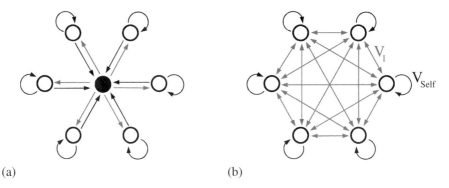

(a)   (b)

Figure 1: Connectivity of the winner-take-all network: (a) in biological networks, inhibition is mediated by populations of global inhibitory interneurons (filled circle). To perform a winner-take-all operation, they are driven by excitatory neurons (unfilled circles) and in return, they inhibit all excitatory neurons (black arrows: excitatory connections; dark arrows: inhibitory). (b) Network model in which the global inhibitory interneuron is replaced by full inhibitory connectivity of efficacy V_I. Self excitation of synaptic efficacy V_{self} stabilizes the selection of the winning neuron.

mismatch compensation procedure described in [Oster and Liu, 2004]. The results shown in Section 3 of this paper were obtained with a network that has been calibrated so that the neurons have about 10% variance in their firing rates in response to a common input current.

1.1 Connectivity

We assume a network of integrate-and-fire neurons that receive external excitatory or inhibitory spiking input. In biological networks, inhibition between these array neurons is mediated by populations of global inhibitory interneurons (Fig. 1a). They are driven by the excitatory neurons and inhibit them in return. In our model, we assume the forward connections between the excitatory and the inhibitory neurons to be strong, so that each spike of an excitatory neuron triggers a spike in the global inhibitory neurons. The strength of the total inhibition between the array neurons is adjusted by tuning the backward connections from the global inhibitory neurons to the array neurons. This configuration allows the fastest spreading of inhibition through the network and is consistent with findings that inhibitory interneurons tend to fire at high frequencies.

With this configuration, we can simplify the network by replacing the global inhibitory interneurons with full inhibitory connectivity between the array neurons (Fig. 1b). In addition, each neuron has a self-excitatory connection that facilitates the selection of this neuron as winner for repeated input.

2 Network Connectivity Constraints for a Winner-Take-All Mode

We first discuss the conditions for the connectivity under which the network operates in a hard winner-take-all mode. For this analysis, we assume that the neurons receive spike trains of regular frequency. We also assume the neurons to be non-leaky.

The membrane potentials V_i, $i = 1 \ldots N$ then satisfy the equation of a non-leaky integrate-

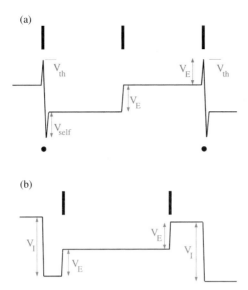

Figure 2: Membrane potential of the winning neuron k (a) and another neuron in the array (b). Black bars show the times of input spikes. Traces show the changes in the membrane membrane potential caused by the various synaptic inputs. Black dots show the times of output spikes of neuron k.

and-fire neuron model with non-conductance-based synapses:

$$\frac{dV_i}{dt} = V_E \sum_n \delta(t - t_i^{(n)}) - V_I \sum_{\substack{j=1 \\ j \neq i}}^{N} \sum_m \delta(t - s_j^{(m)}) \tag{1}$$

The membrane resting potential is set to 0. Each neuron receives external excitatory input and inhibitory connections from all other neurons. All inputs to a neuron are spikes and its output is also transmitted as spikes to other neurons. We neglect the dynamics of the synaptic currents and the delay in the transmission of the spikes. Each input spike causes a fixed discontinuous jump in the membrane potential (V_E for the excitatory synapse and V_I for the inhibitory). Each neuron i spikes when $V_i \geq V_{th}$ and is reset to $V_i = 0$. Immediately afterwards, it receives a self-excitation of weight V_{self}. All potentials satisfy $0 \leq V_i \leq V_{th}$, that is, an inhibitory spike can not drive the membrane potential below ground. All neurons $i \in 1 \dots N, i \neq k$ receive excitatory input spike trains of constant frequency r_i. Neuron k receives the highest input frequency ($r_k > r_i \ \forall \ i \neq k$).

As soon as neuron k spikes once, it has won the computation. Depending on the initial conditions, other neurons can at most have transient spikes before the first spike of neuron k. For this hard winner-take-all mode, the network has to fulfill the following constraints (Fig. 2):

(a) Neuron k (the winning neuron) spikes after receiving $n_k = n$ input spikes that cause its membrane potential to exceed threshold. After every spike, the neuron is reset to V_{self}:

$$V_{self} + n_k V_E \geq V_{th} \tag{2}$$

(b) As soon as neuron k spikes once, no other neuron $i \neq k$ can spike because it receives an inhibitory spike from neuron k. Another neuron can receive up to n spikes even if its input spike frequency is lower than that of neuron k because the neuron is reset to V_{self}

after a spike, as illustrated in Figure 2. The resulting membrane voltage has to be smaller than before:

$$n_i \cdot V_E \leq n_k \cdot V_E \leq V_I \tag{3}$$

(c) If a neuron j other than neuron k spikes in the beginning, there will be some time in the future when neuron k spikes and becomes the winning neuron. From then on, the conditions (a) and (b) hold, so a neuron $j \neq k$ can at most have a few transient spikes.

Let us assume that neurons j and k spike with almost the same frequency (but $r_k > r_j$). For the inter-spike intervals $\Delta_i = 1/r_i$ this means $\Delta_j > \Delta_k$. Since the spike trains are not synchronized, an input spike to neuron k has a changing phase offset ϕ from an input spike of neuron j. At every output spike of neuron j, this phase decreases by $\Delta\phi = n_k(\Delta_j - \Delta_k)$ until $\phi < n_k(\Delta_j - \Delta_k)$. When this happens, neuron k receives $(n_k + 1)$ input spikes before neuron j spikes again and crosses threshold:

$$(n_k + 1) \cdot V_E \geq V_{th} \tag{4}$$

We can choose $V_{self} = V_E$ and $V_I = V_{th}$ to fulfill the inequalities (2)-(4). V_E is adjusted to achieve the desired n_k.

Case (c) happens only under certain initial conditions, for example when $V_k \ll V_j$ or when neuron j initially received a spike train of higher frequency than neuron k. A leaky integrate-and-fire model will ensure that all membrane potentials are discharged ($V_i = 0$) at the onset of a stimulus. The network will then select the winning neuron after receiving a pre-determined number of input spikes and this winner will have the first output spike.

2.1 Poisson-Distributed Inputs

In the case of Poisson-distributed spiking inputs, there is a probability associated with the correct winner being selected. This probability depends on the Poisson rate ν and the number of spikes needed for the neuron to reach threshold n. The probability that m input spikes arrive at a neuron in the period T is given by the Poisson distribution

$$P(m, \nu T) = e^{-\nu T} \frac{(\nu T)^m}{m!} \tag{5}$$

We assume that all neurons i receive an input rate ν_i, except the winning neuron which receives a higher rate ν_k. All neurons are completely discharged at $t = 0$.

The network will make a correct decision at time T, if the winner crosses threshold exactly then with its nth input spike, while all other neuron received less than n spikes until then.

The winner receives the nth input spike at T, if it received $n-1$ input spikes in $[0; T[$ and one at time T. This results in the probability density function

$$p_k(T) = \nu_k P(n-1, \nu_k T) \tag{6}$$

The probability that the other $N-1$ neurons receive less or equal than $n-1$ spikes in $[0; T[$ is

$$P_0(T) = \prod_{\substack{i=1 \\ i \neq k}}^{N} \left(\sum_{j=0}^{n-1} P(j, \nu_i T) \right) \tag{7}$$

For a correct decision, the output spike of the winner can happen at any time $T > 0$, so we integrate over all times T:

$$P = \int_0^\infty p_k(T) \cdot P_0(T) \, dT = \int_0^\infty \nu_k P(n-1, \nu_k T) \cdot \prod_{\substack{j=1 \\ i \neq k}}^{N} \left(\sum_{i=0}^{n-1} P(j, \nu_i T) \right) dT \tag{8}$$

We did not find a closed solution for this integral, but we can discuss its properties n is varied by changing the synaptic efficacies. For $n = 1$ every input spike elicits an output spike. The probability of a having an output spike from neuron k is then directly dependent on the input rates, since no computation in the network takes place. For $n \to \infty$, the integration times to determine the rates of the Poisson-distributed input spike trains are large, and the neurons perform a good estimation of the input rate. The network can then discriminate small changes in the input frequencies. This gain in precision leads a slow response time of the network, since a large number of input spike is integrated before an output spike of the network.

The winner-take-all architecture can also be used with a latency spike code. In this case, the delay of the input spikes after a global reset determines the strength of the signal. The winner is selected after the first input spike to the network ($n_k = 1$). If all neurons are discharged at the onset of the stimulus, the network does not require the global reset. In general, the computation is finished at a time $n_k \cdot \Delta_k$ after the stimulus onset.

3 Results

We implemented this architecture on a chip with 64 integrate-and-fire neurons implemented in analog VLSI technology. These neurons follow the model equation 1, except that they also show a small linear leakage. Spikes from the neurons are communicated off-chip using an asynchronous event representation transmission protocol (AER). When a neuron spikes, the chip outputs the address of this neuron (or spike) onto a common digital bus (see Figure 3). An external spike interface module (consisting of a custom computer board that can be programmed through the PCI bus) receives the incoming spikes from the chip, and retransmits spikes back to the chip using information stored in a routing table. This module can also monitor spike trains from the chip and send spikes from a stored list. Through this module and the AER protocol, we implement the connectivity needed for the winner-take-all network in Figure 1. All components have been used and described in previous work [Boahen, 2000, Liu et al., 2001].

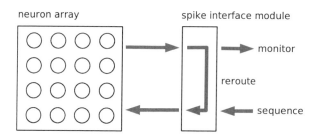

Figure 3: The connections are implemented by transmitting spikes over a common bus (grey arrows). Spikes from aVLSI neurons in the network are recorded by the digital interface and can be monitored and rerouted to any neuron in the array. Additionally, externally generated spike trains can be transmitted to the array through the sequencer.

We configure this network according to the constraints which are described above. Figure 4 illustrates the network behaviour with a spike raster plot. At time $t = 0$, the neurons receive inputs with the same regular firing frequency of 100Hz except for one neuron which received a higher input frequency of 120Hz. The synaptic efficacies were tuned so that threshold is reached with 6 input spikes, after which the network does select the neuron with the strongest input as the winner.

We characterized the discrimination capability of the winner-take-all implementation by

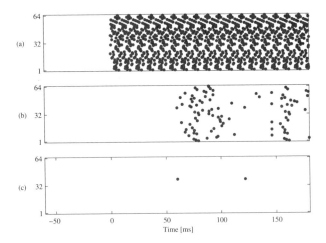

Figure 4: Example raster plot of the spike trains to and from the neurons: (a) Input: starting from 0 ms, the neurons are stimulated with spike trains of a regular frequency of 100Hz, but randomized phase. Neuron number 42 receives an input spike train with an increased frequency of 120Hz. (b) Output without WTA connectivity: after an adjustable number of input spikes, the neurons start to fire with a regular output frequency. The output frequencies of the neurons are slightly different due to mismatch in the synaptic efficacies. Neuron 42 has the highest output frequency since it receives the strongest input. (c) Output with WTA connectivity: only neuron 42 with the strongest input fires, all other neurons are suppressed.

measuring to which minimal frequency, compared to the other input, the input rate to this neuron has to be raised to select it as the winner. The neuron being tested receives an input of regular frequency of $f \cdot 100$Hz, while all other neuron receive 100Hz. The histogram of the minimum factors f for all neurons is shown in Figure 5. On average, the network can discriminate a difference in the input frequency of 10%. This value is identical with the variation in the synaptic efficacies of the neurons, which had been compensated to a mismatch of 10%. We can therefore conclude that the implemented winner-take-all network functions according to the above discussion of the constraints. Since only the timing information of the spike trains is used, the results can be extended to a wide range of input frequencies different from 100Hz.

To test the performance of the network with Poisson inputs, we stimulated all neurons with Poisson-distibuted spike rates of rate ν, except neuron k which received the rate $\nu_k = f\nu$. Eqn. 8 then simplifies to

$$P = \int_0^\infty f\nu\, \mathrm{P}(n-1, f\nu\, T) \cdot \left(\sum_{i=0}^{n-1} P(i, \nu T) \right)^{N-1} \mathrm{d}T \qquad (9)$$

We show measured data and theoretical predictions for a winner-take-all network of 2 and 8 neurons (Fig. 6). Obviously, the discrimation performance of the network is substantially limited by the Poisson nature of the spike trains compared to spike trains of regular frequency.

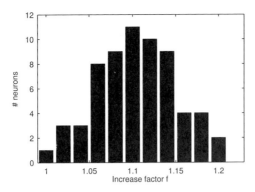

Figure 5: Discrimination capability of the winner-take-all network: X-axis: factor f to which the input frequency of a neuron has to be increased, compared to the input rate of the other neurons, in order for that neuron to be selected as the winner. Y-axis: histogram of all 64 neurons.

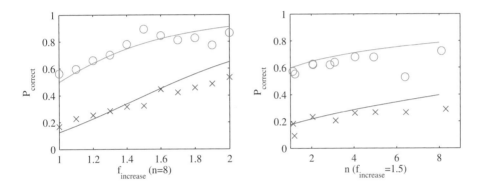

Figure 6: Probability of a correct decision of the winner-take-all network, versus difference in frequencies (left), and number of input spikes n for a neuron to reach threshold (right). The measured data (crosses/circles) is shown with the prediction of the model (continuous lines), for a winner-take-all network of 2 neurons (red,circles) and 8 neurons (blue, crosses).

4 Conclusion

We analysed the performance and behavior of a winner-take-all spiking network that receives input spike trains. The neuron that receives spikes with the highest rate is selected as the winner after a pre-determined number of input spikes. Assuming a non-leaky integrate-and-fire model neuron with constant synaptic weights, we derived constraints for the strength of the inhibitory connections and the self-excitatory connection of the neuron. A large inhibitory synaptic weight is in agreement with previous analysis for analog inputs [Jin and Seung, 2002]. The ability of a single spike from the inhibitory neuron to inhibit all neurons removes constraints on the matching of the time constants and efficacy of the connections from the excitatory neurons to the inhibitory neuron and vice versa. This feature makes the computation tolerant to variance in the synaptic parameters as demonstrated by the results of our experiment.

We also studied whether the network is able to select the winner in the case of input spike trains which have a Poisson distribution. Because of the Poisson distributed inputs, the network does not always chose the right winner (that is, the neuron with the highest input frequency) but there is a certain probability that the network does select the right winner. Results from the network show that the measured probabilities match that of the theoretical results. We are currently extending our analysis to a leaky integrate-and-fire neuron model and conductance-based synapses, which results in a more complex description of the network.

Acknowledgments

This work was supported in part by the IST grant IST-2001-34124. We acknowledge Sebastian Seung for discussions on the winner-take-all mechanism.

References

[Boahen, 2000] Boahen, K. A. (2000). Point-to-point connectivity between neuromorphic chips using address-events. *IEEE Transactions on Circuits & Systems II*, 47(5):416–434.

[Douglas and Martin, 2004] Douglas, R. and Martin, K. (2004). Cortical microcircuits. *Annual Review of Neuroscience*, 27(1f).

[Hahnloser et al., 2000] Hahnloser, R., Sarpeshkar, R., Mahowald, M. A., Douglas, R. J., and Seung, S. (2000). Digital selection and analogue amplification coexist in a cortex-inspired silicon circuit. *Nature*, 405:947–951.

[Indiveri, 2000] Indiveri, G. (2000). Modeling selective attention using a neuromorphic analog VLSI device. *Neural Computation*, 12(12):2857–2880.

[Itti et al., 1998] Itti, C., Niebur, E., and Koch, C. (1998). A model of saliency-based fast visual attention for rapid scene analysis. *IEEE Transactions on Pattern Analysis and Machine Intelligence*, 20(11):1254–1259.

[Jin and Seung, 2002] Jin, D. Z. and Seung, H. S. (2002). Fast computation with spikes in a recurrent neural network. *Physical Review E*, 65:051922.

[Lazzaro et al., 1989] Lazzaro, J., Ryckebusch, S., Mahowald, M. A., and Mead, C. A. (1989). Winner-take-all networks of O(n) complexity. In Touretzky, D., editor, *Advances in Neural Information Processing Systems*, volume 1, pages 703–711. Morgan Kaufmann, San Mateo, CA.

[Lee et al., 1999] Lee, D., Itti, C., Koch, C., and Braun, J. (1999). Attention activates winner-take-all competition among visual filters. *Nature Neuroscience*, 2:375–381.

[Liu et al., 2001] Liu, S.-C., Kramer, J., Indiveri, G., Delbrück, T., Burg, T., and Douglas, R. (2001). Orientation-selective aVLSI spiking neurons. *Neural Networks: Special Issue on Spiking Neurons in Neuroscience and Technology*, 14(6/7):629–643.

[Oster and Liu, 2004] Oster, M. and Liu, S.-C. (2004). A winner-take-all spiking network with spiking inputs. In *11th IEEE International Conference on Electronics, Circuits and Systems*. ICECS '04: Tel Aviv, Israel, 13–15 December.

Variational EM Algorithms for
Non-Gaussian Latent Variable Models

J. A. Palmer, D. P. Wipf, K. Kreutz-Delgado, and B. D. Rao
Department of Electrical and Computer Engineering
University of California San Diego, La Jolla, CA 92093
{japalmer,dwipf,kreutz,brao}@ece.ucsd.edu

Abstract

We consider criteria for variational representations of non-Gaussian latent variables, and derive variational EM algorithms in general form. We establish a general equivalence among convex bounding methods, evidence based methods, and ensemble learning/Variational Bayes methods, which has previously been demonstrated only for particular cases.

1 Introduction

Probabilistic methods have become well-established in the analysis of learning algorithms over the past decade, drawing largely on classical Gaussian statistical theory [21, 2, 28]. More recently, variational Bayes and ensemble learning methods [22, 13] have been proposed. In addition to the evidence and VB methods, variational methods based on convex bounding have been proposed for dealing with non-gaussian latent variables [18, 14]. We concentrate here on the theory of the linear model, with direct application to ICA [14], factor analysis [2], mixture models [13], kernel regression [30, 11, 32], and linearization approaches to nonlinear models [15]. The methods can likely be applied in other contexts.

In Mackay's evidence framework, "hierarchical priors" are employed on the latent variables, using Gamma priors on the inverse variances, which has the effect of making the marginal distribution of the latent variable prior the non-Gaussian Student's t [30]. Based on Mackay's framework, Tipping proposed the Relevance Vector Machine (RVM) [30] for estimation of sparse solutions in the kernel regression problem. A relationship between the evidence framework and ensemble/VB methods has been noted in [22, 6] for the particular case of the RVM with t hyperprior. Figueiredo [11] proposed EM algorithms based on hyperprior representations of the Laplacian and Jeffrey's priors. In [14], Girolami employed the convex variational framework of [16] to derive a different type of variational EM algorithm using a convex variational representation of the Laplacian prior. Wipf et al. [32] demonstrated the equivalence between the variational approach of [16, 14] and the evidence based RVM for the case of t priors, and thus via [6], the equivalence of the convex variational method and the ensemble/VB methods for the particular case of the t prior.

In this paper we consider these methods from a unifying viewpoint, deriving algorithms in more general form and establishing a more general relationship among the methods than has previously been shown. In §2, we define the model and estimation problems we shall be concerned with, and in §3 we discuss criteria for variational representations. In §4 we consider the relationships among these methods.

2 The Bayesian linear model

Throughout we shall consider the following model,

$$\mathbf{y} = \mathbf{A}\mathbf{x} + \nu, \tag{1}$$

where $\mathbf{A} \in \mathbb{R}^{m \times n}$, $\mathbf{x} \sim p(\mathbf{x}) = \prod_i p(x_i)$, and $\nu \sim \mathcal{N}(\mathbf{0}, \Sigma_\nu)$, with $\mathbf{x}$ and ν independent. The important thing to note for our purposes is that the x_i are non-Gaussian.

We consider two types of variational representation of the non-Gaussian priors $p(x_i)$, which we shall call *convex type* and *integral type*. In the convex type of variational representation, the density is represented as a supremum over Gaussian functions of varying scale,

$$p(x) = \sup_{\xi > 0} \mathcal{N}(x; 0, \xi^{-1}) \, \varphi(\xi). \tag{2}$$

The essential property of "concavity in x^2" leading to this representation was used in [29, 17, 16, 18, 6] to represent the Logistic link function. A convex type representation of the Laplace density was applied to learning overcomplete representations in [14].

In the integral type of representation, the density $p(x)$ is represented as an integral over the scale parameter of the density, with respect to some positive measure μ,

$$p(x) = \int_0^\infty \mathcal{N}(x; 0, \xi^{-1}) \, d\mu(\xi). \tag{3}$$

Such representations with a general kernel are referred to as scale mixtures [19]. Gaussian scale mixtures were discussed in the examples of Dempster, Laird, and Rubin's original EM paper [9], and treated more extensively in [10]. The integral representation has been used, sometimes implicitly, for kernel-based estimation [30, 11] and ICA [20]. The distinction between MAP estimation of components and estimation of hyperparameters has been discussed in [23] and [30] for the case of Gamma distributed inverse variance.

We shall be interested in variational EM algorithms for solving two basic problems, corresponding essentially to the two methods of handling hyperparameters discussed in [23]: the MAP estimate of the latent variables

$$\hat{\mathbf{x}} = \arg \max_{\mathbf{x}} p(\mathbf{x}|\mathbf{y}) \tag{4}$$

and the MAP estimate of the hyperparameters,

$$\hat{\xi} = \arg \max_{\xi} p(\xi|\mathbf{y}). \tag{5}$$

The following section discusses the criteria for and relationship between the two types of variational representation. In §4, we discuss algorithms for each problem based on the two types of variational representations, and determine when these are equivalent. We also discuss the approximation of the likelihood $p(\mathbf{y}; \mathbf{A})$ using the ensemble learning or VB method, which approximates the posterior $p(\mathbf{x}, \xi|\mathbf{y})$ by a factorial density $q(\mathbf{x}|\mathbf{y})q(\xi|\mathbf{y})$. We show that the ensemble method is equivalent to the hyperparameter MAP method.

3 Variational representations of super-Gaussian densities

In this section we discuss the criteria for the convex and integral type representations.

3.1 Convex variational bounds

We wish to determine when a symmetric, unimodal density $p(x)$ can be represented in the form (2) for some function $\varphi(\xi)$. Equivalently, when,

$$-\log p(x) = -\sup_{\xi > 0} \log \mathcal{N}(x; 0, \xi^{-1}) \varphi(\xi) = \inf_{\xi > 0} \tfrac{1}{2} x^2 \xi - \log \xi^{\frac{1}{2}} \varphi(\xi)$$

for all $x > 0$. The last formula says that $-\log p(\sqrt{x})$ is the concave conjugate of (the closure of the convex hull of) the function, $\log \xi^{\frac{1}{2}} \varphi(\xi)$ [27, §12]. This is possible if and only if $-\log p(\sqrt{x})$ is closed, increasing and concave on $(0, \infty)$. Thus we have the following.

Theorem 1. *A symmetric probability density* $p(x) \equiv \exp(-g(x^2))$ *can be represented in the convex variational form,*

$$p(x) = \sup_{\xi > 0} \mathcal{N}(x; 0, \xi^{-1}) \, \varphi(\xi)$$

if and only if $g(x) \equiv -\log p(\sqrt{x})$ *is increasing and concave on* $(0, \infty)$. *In this case we can use the function,*

$$\varphi(\xi) = \sqrt{2\pi/\xi} \, \exp\big(g^*(\xi/2)\big) \,,$$

where g^* *is the concave conjugate of* g.

Examples of densities satisfying this criterion include: (i) Generalized Gaussian $\propto \exp(-|x|^\beta)$, $0 < \beta \leq 2$, (ii) Logistic $\propto 1/\cosh^2(x/2)$, (iii) Student's $t \propto (1 + x^2/\nu)^{-(\nu+1)/2}$, $\nu > 0$, and (iv) symmetric α-stable densities (having characteristic function $\exp(-|\omega|^\alpha)$, $0 < \alpha \leq 2$).

The convex variational representation motivates the following definition.

Definition 1. *A symmetric probability density* $p(x)$ *is* **strongly super-gaussian** *if* $p(\sqrt{x})$ *is log-convex on* $(0, \infty)$, *and* **strongly sub-gaussian** *if* $p(\sqrt{x})$ *is log-concave on* $(0, \infty)$.

An equivalent definition is given in [5, pp. 60-61], which defines $p(x) = \exp(-f(x))$ to be sub-gaussian (super-gaussian) if $f'(x)/x$ is increasing (decreasing) on $(0, \infty)$. This condition is equivalent to $f(x) = g(x^2)$ with g concave, i.e. g' decreasing. The property of being strongly sub- or super-gaussian is independent of scale.

3.2   Scale mixtures

We now wish to determine when a probability density $p(x)$ can be represented in the form (3) for some $\mu(\xi)$ non-decreasing on $(0, \infty)$. A fundamental result dealing with integral representations was given by Bernstein and Widder (see [31]). It uses the following definition.

Definition 1. *A function* $f(x)$ *is* **completely monotonic** *on* (a, b) *if,*

$$(-1)^n f^{(n)}(x) \geq 0 \,, \quad n = 0, 1, \ldots$$

for every $x \in (a, b)$.

That is, $f(x)$ is completely monotonic if it is positive, decreasing, convex, and so on. Bernstein's theorem [31, Thm. 12b] states:

Theorem 2. *A necessary and sufficient condition that* $p(x)$ *should be completely monotonic on* $(0, \infty)$ *is that,*

$$p(x) = \int_0^\infty e^{-tx} d\alpha(t) \,,$$

where $\alpha(t)$ *is non-decreasing on* $(0, \infty)$.

Thus for $p(x)$ to be a Gaussian scale mixture,

$$p(x) = e^{-f(x)} = e^{-g(x^2)} = \int_0^\infty e^{-\frac{1}{2}tx^2} d\alpha(t) \,,$$

a necessary and sufficient condition is that $p(\sqrt{x}) = e^{-g(x)}$ be completely monotonic for $0 < x < \infty$, and we have the following (see also [19, 1]),

Theorem 3. *A function* $p(x)$ *can be represented as a Gaussian scale mixture if and only if* $p(\sqrt{x})$ *is completely monotonic on* $(0, \infty)$.

3.3 Relationship between convex and integral type representations

We now consider the relationship between the convex and integral types of variational representation. Let $p(x) = \exp(-g(x^2))$. We have seen that $p(x)$ can be represented in the form (2) if and only if $g(x)$ is symmetric and concave on $(0, \infty)$. And we have seen that $p(x)$ can be represented in the form (3) if and only if $p(\sqrt{x}) = \exp(-g(x))$ is completely monotonic. We shall consider now whether or not complete monotonicity of $p(\sqrt{x})$ implies the concavity of $g(x) = -\log p(\sqrt{x})$, that is whether representability in the integral form implies representability in the convex form.

Complete monotonicity of a function $q(x)$ implies that $q \geq 0$, $q' \leq 0$, $q'' \geq 0$, etc. For example, if $p(\sqrt{x})$ is completely monotonic, then,

$$\frac{d^2}{dx^2} p(\sqrt{x}) = \frac{d^2}{dx^2} e^{-g(x)} = e^{-g(x)} \left(g'(x)^2 - g''(x) \right) \geq 0.$$

Thus if $g'' \leq 0$, then $p(\sqrt{x})$ is convex, but the converse does not necessarily hold. That is, concavity of g does not follow from convexity of $p(\sqrt{x})$, as the latter only requires that $g'' \leq g'^2$.

Concavity of g does follow however from the complete monotonicity of $p(\sqrt{x})$. For example, we can use the following result [8, §3.5.2].

Theorem 4. *If the functions $f_t(x)$, $t \in \mathcal{D}$, are convex, then $\int_{\mathcal{D}} e^{f_t(x)} dt$ is convex.*

Thus completely monotonic functions, being scale mixtures of the log convex function e^{-x} by Theorem 2, are also log convex. We thus see that *any function representable in the integral variational form* (3) *is also representable in the convex variational form* (2).

In fact, a stronger result holds. The following theorem [7, Thm. 4.1.5] establishes the equivalence between $q(x)$ and $g'(x) = d/dx - \log q(x)$ in terms of complete monotonicity.

Theorem 5. *If $g(x) > 0$, then $e^{-ug(x)}$ is completely monotonic for every $u > 0$, if and only if $g'(x)$ is completely monotonic.*

In particular, it holds that $q(x) \equiv p(\sqrt{x}) = \exp(-g(x))$ is convex only if $g''(x) \leq 0$.

To summarize, let $p(x) = e^{-g(x^2)}$. If g is increasing and concave for $x > 0$, then $p(x)$ admits the convex type of variational representation (2). If, in addition, the higher derivatives satisfy $g^{(3)}(x) \geq 0$, $g^{(4)}(x) \leq 0$, $g^{(5)}(x) \geq 0$, etc., then $p(x)$ also admits the Gaussian scale mixture representation (3).

4 General equivalences among Variational methods

4.1 MAP estimation of components

Consider first the MAP estimate of the latent variables (4).

4.1.1 Component MAP – Integral case

Following [10][1], consider an EM algorithm to estimate $\mathbf{x}$ when the $p(x_i)$ are independent Gaussian scale mixtures as in (3). Differentiating inside the integral gives,

$$p'(x) = \frac{d}{dx} \int_0^\infty p(x|\xi)p(\xi)d\xi = -\int_0^\infty \xi x p(x, \xi) \, d\xi$$

$$= -x p(x) \int_0^\infty \xi p(\xi|x) \, d\xi.$$

---

[1]In [10], the x_i in (1) are actually estimated as non-random parameters, with the noise ν being non-gaussian, but the underlying theory is essentially the same.

Thus, with $p(x) \equiv \exp(-f(x))$, we see that,

$$E(\xi_i | x_i) = \int_0^\infty \xi_i p(\xi_i | x_i) \, d\xi_i = -\frac{p'(x_i)}{x_i p(x_i)} = \frac{f'(x_i)}{x_i} \,. \tag{6}$$

The EM algorithm alternates setting $\hat{\xi}_i$ to the posterior mean, $E(\xi_i | x_i) = f'(x_i)/x_i$, and setting $\mathbf{x}$ to minimize,

$$-\log p(\mathbf{y}|\mathbf{x})p(\mathbf{x}|\hat{\xi}) = \tfrac{1}{2}\mathbf{x}^T\mathbf{A}^T\boldsymbol{\Sigma}_\nu^{-1}\mathbf{A}\mathbf{x} - \mathbf{y}^T\boldsymbol{\Sigma}_\nu^{-1}\mathbf{A}\mathbf{x} + \tfrac{1}{2}\mathbf{x}^T\boldsymbol{\Lambda}\mathbf{x} + \text{const.}, \tag{7}$$

where $\boldsymbol{\Lambda} = \text{diag}(\hat{\xi})^{-1}$. At iteration k, we put $\xi_i^k = f'(x_i^k)/x_i^k$, and $\boldsymbol{\Lambda}^k = \text{diag}(\xi^k)^{-1}$, and

$$\mathbf{x}^{k+1} = \boldsymbol{\Lambda}^k\mathbf{A}^T(\mathbf{A}\boldsymbol{\Lambda}^k\mathbf{A}^T + \boldsymbol{\Sigma}_\nu)^{-1}\mathbf{y} \,.$$

4.1.2 Component MAP – Convex case

Again consider the MAP estimate of $\mathbf{x}$. For strongly super-gaussian priors, $p(x_i)$, we have,

$$\arg\max_{\mathbf{x}} p(\mathbf{x}|\mathbf{y}) = \arg\max_{\mathbf{x}} p(\mathbf{y}|\mathbf{x})p(\mathbf{x}) = \arg\max_{\mathbf{x}} \max_{\xi} p(\mathbf{y}|\mathbf{x})p(\mathbf{x};\xi)\varphi(\xi)$$

Now since,

$$-\log p(\mathbf{y}|\mathbf{x})p(\mathbf{x};\xi)\varphi(\xi) = \tfrac{1}{2}\mathbf{x}^T\mathbf{A}^T\boldsymbol{\Sigma}_\nu^{-1}\mathbf{A}\mathbf{x} - \mathbf{y}^T\boldsymbol{\Sigma}_\nu^{-1}\mathbf{A}\mathbf{x} + \sum_{i=1}^n \tfrac{1}{2}x_i^2\xi_i - g^*(\xi_i/2) \,,$$

the MAP estimate can be improved iteratively by alternately maximizing $\mathbf{x}$ and ξ,

$$\xi_i^k = 2\,g^{*\prime-1}(x_i^{k\,2}) = 2\,g'(x_i^{k\,2}) = \frac{f'(x_i^k)}{x_i^k} \,, \tag{8}$$

with $\mathbf{x}$ updated as in §4.1.1. We thus see that this algorithm is equivalent to the MAP algorithm derived in §4.1.1 for Gaussian scale mixtures. That is, for direct MAP estimation of latent variable $\mathbf{x}$, the EM Gaussian scale mixture method and the variational bounding method yield the same algorithm.

This algorithm has also been derived in the image restoration literature [12] as the "half-quadratic" algorithm, and it is the basis for the FOCUSS algorithms derived in [26, 25]. The regression algorithm given in [11] for the particular cases of Laplacian and Jeffrey's priors is based on the theory in §4.1.1, and is in fact equivalent to the FOCUSS algorithm derived in [26].

4.2 MAP estimate of variational parameters

Now consider MAP estimation of the (random) variational hyperparameters ξ.

4.2.1 Hyperparameter MAP – Integral case

Consider an EM algorithm to find the MAP estimate of the hyperparameters ξ in the integral representation (Gaussian scale mixture) case, where the latent variables $\mathbf{x}$ are hidden. For the complete likelihood, we have,

$$p(\xi, \mathbf{x}|\mathbf{y}) \propto p(\mathbf{y}|\mathbf{x},\xi)p(\mathbf{x}|\xi)p(\xi) = p(\mathbf{y}|\mathbf{x})p(\mathbf{x}|\xi)p(\xi) \,.$$

The function to be minimized over ξ is then,

$$\left\langle -\log p(\mathbf{x}|\xi)p(\xi) \right\rangle_{\mathbf{x}} = \sum_i \tfrac{1}{2}\langle x_i^2 \rangle \xi_i - \log\sqrt{\xi_i}\,p(\xi_i) + \text{const.} \tag{9}$$

If we define $h(\xi) \equiv \log\sqrt{\xi_i}\,p(\xi_i)$, and assume that this function is concave, then the optimal value of ξ is given by,

$$\xi_i = h^{*\prime}\big(\tfrac{1}{2}\langle x_i^2 \rangle\big) \,.$$

This algorithm converges to a local maximum of $p(\xi|\mathbf{y})$, $\hat{\xi}$, which then yields an estimate of $\mathbf{x}$ by taking $\hat{\mathbf{x}} = E(\mathbf{x}|\mathbf{y},\hat{\xi})$. Alternative algorithms result from using this method to find the MAP estimate of different functions of the scale random variable ξ.

4.2.2 Hyperparameter MAP – Convex case

In the convex representation, the ξ parameters do not actually represent a probabilistic quantity, but rather arise as parameters in a variational inequality. Specifically, we write,

$$
\begin{aligned}
p(\mathbf{y}) &= \int p(\mathbf{y}, \mathbf{x}) \, d\mathbf{x} = \int \max_{\xi} p(\mathbf{y}|\mathbf{x}) \, p(\mathbf{x}|\xi) \, \varphi(\xi) \, d\mathbf{x} \\
&\geq \max_{\xi} \int p(\mathbf{y}|\mathbf{x}) \, p(\mathbf{x}|\xi) \, \varphi(\xi) \, d\mathbf{x} \\
&= \max_{\xi} \mathcal{N}\left(\mathbf{y}; \mathbf{0}, \mathbf{A}\mathbf{\Lambda}\mathbf{A}^{T} + \mathbf{\Sigma}_{\nu}\right) \varphi(\xi) .
\end{aligned}
$$

Now we define the function,

$$
\tilde{p}(\mathbf{y}; \xi) \equiv \mathcal{N}\left(\mathbf{y}; \mathbf{0}, \mathbf{A}\mathbf{\Lambda}\mathbf{A}^{T} + \mathbf{\Sigma}_{\nu}\right) \varphi(\xi)
$$

and try to find $\hat{\xi} = \arg\max \tilde{p}(\mathbf{y}; \xi)$. We maximize $\tilde{p}$ by EM, marginalizing over $\mathbf{x}$,

$$
\tilde{p}(\mathbf{y}; \xi) = \int p(\mathbf{y}|\mathbf{x}) \, p(\mathbf{x}|\xi) \, \varphi(\xi) \, d\mathbf{x} .
$$

The algorithm is then equivalent to that in §4.1.2 except that the expectation is taken of x^2 as the E step, and the diagonal weighting matrix becomes,

$$
\xi_i = \frac{f'(\sigma_i)}{\sigma_i} ,
$$

where $\sigma_i = \sqrt{E\left(x_i^2 | \mathbf{y}; \xi_i\right)}$. Although $\tilde{p}$ is not a true probability density function, the proof of convergence for EM does not assume unit normalization. This theory is the basis for the algorithm presented in [14] for the particular case of a Laplacian prior (where in addition $\mathbf{A}$ in the model (1) is updated according to the standard EM update.)

4.3 Ensemble learning

In the ensemble learning approach (also Variational Bayes [4, 3, 6]) the idea is to find the approximate separable posterior that minimizes the KL divergence from the true posterior, using the following decomposition of the log likelihood,

$$
\begin{aligned}
\log p(\mathbf{y}) &= \int q(\mathbf{z}|\mathbf{y}) \log \frac{p(\mathbf{z}, \mathbf{y})}{q(\mathbf{z}|\mathbf{y})} \, d\mathbf{z} + D\big(q(\mathbf{z}|\mathbf{y}) \| p(\mathbf{z}|\mathbf{y})\big) \\
&\equiv -F(q) + D(q\|p) .
\end{aligned}
$$

The term $F(q)$ is commonly called the *variational free energy* [29, 24]. Minimizing the F over q is equivalent to minimizing D over q. The posterior approximating distribution is taken to be factorial,

$$
q(\mathbf{z}|\mathbf{y}) = q(\mathbf{x}, \xi|\mathbf{y}) = q(\mathbf{x}|\mathbf{y}) q(\xi|\mathbf{y}) .
$$

For fixed $q(\xi|\mathbf{y})$, the free energy F is given by,

$$
-\iint q(\mathbf{x}|\mathbf{y}) q(\xi|\mathbf{y}) \log \frac{p(\mathbf{x}, \xi|\mathbf{y})}{q(\mathbf{x}|\mathbf{y}) q(\xi|\mathbf{y})} \, d\xi \, d\mathbf{x} = D\left(q(\mathbf{x}|\mathbf{y}) \| e^{\langle \log p(\mathbf{x}, \xi|\mathbf{y})\rangle_\xi}\right) + \text{const.},
\tag{10}
$$

where $\langle \cdot \rangle_\xi$ denotes expectation with respect to $q(\xi|\mathbf{y})$, and the constant is the entropy, $H\big(q(\xi|\mathbf{y})\big)$. The minimum of the KL divergence in (10) is attained if and only if

$$
q(\mathbf{x}|\mathbf{y}) \propto \exp\left\langle \log p(\mathbf{x}, \xi|\mathbf{y})\right\rangle_\xi \propto p(\mathbf{y}|\mathbf{x}) \exp\left\langle \log p(\mathbf{x}|\xi)\right\rangle_\xi
$$

almost surely. An identical derivation yields the optimal

$$
q(\xi|\mathbf{y}) \propto \exp\left\langle \log p(\mathbf{x}, \xi|\mathbf{y})\right\rangle_\mathbf{x} \propto p(\xi) \exp\left\langle \log p(\mathbf{x}|\xi)\right\rangle_\mathbf{x}
$$

when $q(\mathbf{x}|\mathbf{y})$ is fixed. The ensemble (or VB) algorithm consists of alternately updating the parameters of these approximating marginal distributions.

In the linear model with Gaussian scale mixture latent variables, the complete likelihood is again,

$$p(\mathbf{y}, \mathbf{x}, \xi) \;=\; p(\mathbf{y}|\mathbf{x})p(\mathbf{x}|\xi)p(\xi)\,.$$

The optimal approximate posteriors are given by,

$$q(\mathbf{x}|\mathbf{y}) \;=\; \mathcal{N}(\mathbf{x}; \mu_{\mathbf{x}|\mathbf{y}}, \Sigma_{\mathbf{x}|\mathbf{y}})\,, \qquad q(\xi_i|\mathbf{y}) \;=\; p\left(\xi_i \mid x_i = \langle x_i^2\rangle^{1/2}\right),$$

where, letting $\Lambda = \mathrm{diag}((\langle\xi\rangle))^{-1}$, the posterior moments are given by,

$$\mu_{\mathbf{x}|\mathbf{y}} \;\equiv\; \Lambda\mathbf{A}^T(\mathbf{A}\Lambda\mathbf{A}^T + \Sigma_\nu)^{-1}\mathbf{y}$$

$$\Sigma_{\mathbf{x}|\mathbf{y}} \;\equiv\; (\mathbf{A}^T\Sigma_\nu^{-1}\mathbf{A} + \Lambda^{-1})^{-1} \;=\; \Lambda - \Lambda\mathbf{A}^T(\mathbf{A}\Lambda\mathbf{A}^T + \Sigma_\nu)^{-1}\mathbf{A}\Lambda\,.$$

The only relevant fact about $q(\xi|\mathbf{y})$ that we need is $\langle\xi\rangle$, for which we have, using (6),

$$\langle\xi_i\rangle \;=\; \int \xi_i q(\xi_i|\mathbf{y})\,d\xi_i \;=\; \int \xi_i p\left(\xi_i \mid x_i = \langle x_i^2\rangle^{1/2}\right)d\xi_i \;=\; \frac{f'(\sigma_i)}{\sigma_i}\,,$$

where $\sigma_i = \sqrt{E\left(x_i^2|\mathbf{y};\xi_i\right)}$. We thus see that the ensemble learning algorithm is equivalent to the approximate hyperparameter MAP algorithm of §4.2.2. Note also that this shows that the VB methods can be applied to any Gaussian scale mixture density, using only the form of the latent variable prior $p(x)$, without needing the marginal hyperprior $p(\xi)$ in closed form. This is particularly important in the case of the Generalized Gaussian and Logistic densities, whose scale parameter densities are α-Stable and Kolmogorov [1] respectively.

5 Conclusion

In this paper, we have discussed criteria for variational representations of non-Gaussian latent variables, and derived general variational EM algorithms based on these representations. We have shown a general equivalence between the two representations in MAP estimation taking hyperparameters as hidden, and we have shown the general equivalence between the variational convex approximate MAP estimate of hyperparameters and the ensemble learning or VB method.

References

[1] D. F. Andrews and C. L. Mallows. Scale mixtures of normal distributions. *J. Roy. Statist. Soc. Ser. B*, 36:99–102, 1974.

[2] H. Attias. Independent factor analysis. *Neural Computation*, 11:803–851, 1999.

[3] H. Attias. A variational Bayesian framework for graphical models. In *Advances in Neural Information Processing Systems 12*. MIT Press, 2000.

[4] M. J. Beal and Z. Ghahrramani. The variational Bayesian EM algorithm for incomplete data: with application to scoring graphical model structures. In *Bayesian Statistics 7*, pages 453–464. University of Oxford Press, 2002.

[5] A. Benveniste, M. Métivier, and P. Priouret. *Adaptive algorithms and stochastic approximations*. Springer-Verlag, 1990.

[6] C. M. Bishop and M. E. Tipping. Variational relevance vector machines. In C. Boutilier and M. Goldszmidt, editors, *Proceedings of the 16th Conference on Uncertainty in Artificial Intelligence*, pages 46–53. Morgan Kaufmann, 2000.

[7] S. Bochner. *Harmonic analysis and the theory of probability*. University of California Press, Berkeley and Los Angeles, 1960.

[8] S. Boyd and L. Vandenberghe. *Convex Optimization.* Cambridge University Press, 2004.

[9] A. P. Dempster, N. M. Laird, and D. B. Rubin. Maximum likelihood from incomplete data via the EM algorithm. *Journal of the Royal Statistical Society, Series B*, 39:1–38, 1977.

[10] A. P. Dempster, N. M. Laird, and D. B. Rubin. Iteratively reweighted least squares for linear regression when errors are Normal/Independent distributed. In P. R. Krishnaiah, editor, *Multivariate Analysis V*, pages 35–57. North Holland Publishing Company, 1980.

[11] M. Figueiredo. Adaptive sparseness using Jeffreys prior. In T. G. Dietterich, S. Becker, and Z. Ghahramani, editors, *Advances in Neural Information Processing Systems 14*, Cambridge, MA, 2002. MIT Press.

[12] D. Geman and G. Reynolds. Constrained restoration and the recovery of discontinuities. *IEEE Trans. Pattern Analysis and Machine Intelligence*, 14(3):367–383, 1992.

[13] Z. Ghahramani and M. J. Beal. Variational inference for Bayesian mixtures of factor analysers. In *Advances in Neural Information Processing Systems 12*. MIT Press, 2000.

[14] M. Girolami. A variational method for learning sparse and overcomplete representations. *Neural Computation*, 13:2517–2532, 2001.

[15] A. Honkela and H. Valpola. Unsupervised variational Bayesian learning of nonlinear models. In *Advances in Neural Information Processing Systems 17*. MIT Press, 2005.

[16] T. S. Jaakkola. *Variational Methods for Inference and Estimation in Graphical Models.* PhD thesis, Massachusetts Institute of Technology, 1997.

[17] T. S. Jaakkola and M. I. Jordan. A variational approach to Bayesian logistic regression models and their extensions. In *Proceedings of the 1997 Conference on Artificial Intelligence and Statistics*, 1997.

[18] M. I. Jordan, Z. Ghahramani, T. S. Jaakkola, and L. K. Saul. An introduction to variational methods for graphical models. In M. I. Jordan, editor, *Learning in Graphical Models.* Kluwer Academic Publishers, 1998.

[19] J. Keilson and F. W. Steutel. Mixtures of distributions, moment inequalities, and measures of exponentiality and Normality. *The Annals of Probability*, 2:112–130, 1974.

[20] H. Lappalainen. Ensemble learning for independent component analysis. In *Proceedings of the First International Workshop on Independent Component Analysis*, 1999.

[21] D. J. C. MacKay. Bayesian interpolation. *Neural Computation*, 4(3):415–447, 1992.

[22] D. J. C. MacKay. Ensemble learning and evidence maximization. Unpublished manuscript, 1995.

[23] D. J. C. Mackay. Comparison of approximate methods for handling hyperparameters. *Neural Computation*, 11(5):1035–1068, 1999.

[24] R. M. Neal and G. E. Hinton. A view of the EM algorithm that justifies incremental, sparse, and other variants. In M. I. Jordan, editor, *Learning in Graphical Models*, pages 355–368. Kluwer, 1998.

[25] B. D. Rao, K. Engan, S. F. Cotter, J. Palmer, and K. Kreutz-Delgado. Subset selection in noise based on diversity measure minimization. *IEEE Trans. Signal Processing*, 51(3), 2003.

[26] B. D. Rao and I. F. Gorodnitsky. Sparse signal reconstruction from limited data using FOCUSS: a re-weighted minimum norm algorithm. *IEEE Trans. Signal Processing*, 45:600–616, 1997.

[27] R. T. Rockafellar. *Convex Analysis.* Princeton, 1970.

[28] Sam Roweis and Zoubin Ghahramani. A unifying review of linear gaussian models. *Neural Computation*, 11(5):305–345, 1999.

[29] L. K. Saul, T. S. Jaakkola, and M. I. Jordan. Mean field theory for sigmoid belief networks. *Journal of Artificial Intelligence Research*, 4:61–76, 1996.

[30] M. E. Tipping. Sparse Bayesian learning and the Relevance Vector Machine. *Journal of Machine Learning Research*, 1:211–244, 2001.

[31] D. V. Widder. *The Laplace Transform.* Princeton University Press, 1946.

[32] D. Wipf, J. Palmer, and B. Rao. Perspectives on sparse bayesian learning. In S. Thrun, L. Saul, and B. Schölkopf, editors, *Advances in Neural Information Processing Systems 16*, Cambridge, MA, 2003. MIT Press.

Nonparametric inference of prior probabilities from Bayes-optimal behavior

Liam Paninski[*]
Department of Statistics, Columbia University
liam@stat.columbia.edu; http://www.stat.columbia.edu/~liam

Abstract

We discuss a method for obtaining a subject's *a priori* beliefs from his/her behavior in a psychophysics context, under the assumption that the behavior is (nearly) optimal from a Bayesian perspective. The method is nonparametric in the sense that we do not assume that the prior belongs to any fixed class of distributions (e.g., Gaussian). Despite this increased generality, the method is relatively simple to implement, being based in the simplest case on a linear programming algorithm, and more generally on a straightforward maximum likelihood or maximum *a posteriori* formulation, which turns out to be a convex optimization problem (with no non-global local maxima) in many important cases. In addition, we develop methods for analyzing the uncertainty of these estimates. We demonstrate the accuracy of the method in a simple simulated coin-flipping setting; in particular, the method is able to precisely track the evolution of the subject's posterior distribution as more and more data are observed. We close by briefly discussing an interesting connection to recent models of neural population coding.

Introduction

Bayesian methods have become quite popular in psychophysics and neuroscience (*1–5*); in particular, a recent trend has been to interpret observed biases in perception and/or behavior as optimal, in a Bayesian (average) sense, under ecologically-determined prior distributions on the stimuli or behavioral contexts under study. For example, (*2*) interpret visual motion illusions in terms of a prior weighted towards slow, smooth movements of objects in space.

In an experimental context, it is clearly desirable to empirically obtain estimates of the prior the subject is operating under; the idea would be to then compare these experimental estimates of the subject's prior with the ecological prior he or she "should" have been using. Conversely, such an approach would have the potential to establish that the subject is not behaving Bayes-optimally under any prior, but rather is in fact using a different, non-Bayesian strategy. Such tools would also be quite useful in the context of studies of learning and generalization, in which we would like to track the time course of a subject's adaptation to an experimentally-chosen prior distribution (*5*). Such estimates of the subject's prior have in the past been rather qualitative, and/or limited to simple parametric families (e.g.,

---

[*]We thank N. Daw, P. Hoyer, S. Inati, K. Koerding, I. Nemenman, E. Simoncelli, A. Stocker, and D. Wolpert for helpful suggestions, and in particular P. Dayan for pointing out the connection to neural population coding models. This work was supported by funding from the Howard Hughes Medical Institute, Gatsby Charitable Trust, and by a Royal Society International Fellowship.

the width of a Gaussian may be fit to the experimental data, but the actual Gaussian identity of the prior is not examined systematically).

We present a more quantitative method here. We first discuss the method in the general case of an arbitrarily-chosen loss function (the "cost" which we assume the subject is attempting to minimize, on average), then examine a few special important cases (e.g., mean-square and mean-absolute error) in which the technique may be simplified somewhat. The algorithms for determining the subject's prior distributions turn out to be surprisingly quick and easy to code: the basic idea is that each observed stimulus-response pair provides a set of constraints on what the actual prior could be. In the simplest case, these constraints are linear, and the resulting algorithm is simply a version of linear programming, for which very efficient algorithms exist. More generally, the constraints are probabilistic, and we discuss likelihood-based methods for combining these noisy constraints (and in particular when the resulting maximum likelihood, or maximum *a posteriori*, problem can be solved efficiently via ascent methods, without fear of getting trapped in non-global local maxima). Finally, we discuss Bayesian methods for representing the uncertainty in our estimates.

We should point out that related problems have appeared in the statistics literature, particularly under the subject of elicitation of expert opinion (*6–8*); in the machine learning literature, most recently in the area of "inverse reinforcement learning" (*9*); and in the economics/ game theory literature on utility learning (*10*). The experimental economics literature in particular is quite vast (where the relevance to gambling, price setting, etc. is discussed at length, particularly in settings in which "rational" — expected utility-maximizing — behavior seems to break down); see, e.g. Wakker's recent bibliography (www1.fee.uva.nl/creed/wakker/refs/rfrncs.htm) for further references. Finally, it is worth noting that the question of determining a subject's (or more precisely, an opponent's) priors in a gambling context — in particular, in the binary case of whether or not an opponent will accept a bet, given a fixed table of outcomes vs. payoffs — has received attention going back to the foundations of decision theory, most prominently in the discussions of de Finetti and Savage. Nevertheless, we are unaware of any previous application of similar techniques (both for estimating a subject's true prior and for analyzing the uncertainty associated with these estimates) in the psychophysical or neuroscience literature.

General case

Our technique for determining the subject's prior is based on several assumptions (some of which will be relaxed below). To begin, we assume that the subject is behaving optimally in a Bayesian sense. To be precise, we have four ingredients: a prior distribution on some hidden parameter θ; observed input (stimulus) data, dependent in some probabilistic way on θ; the subject's corresponding output estimates of the underlying θ, given the input data; and finally a loss function $D(.,.)$ that penalizes bad estimates for θ. The fundamental assumption is that, on each trial i, the subject is choosing the estimate $\hat{\theta}_i$ of the underlying parameter, given data x_i, to minimize the posterior average error

$$\int p(\theta|x_i)D(\hat{\theta}_i,\theta)d\theta \sim \int p(\theta)p(x_i|\theta)D(\hat{\theta}_i,\theta)d\theta, \tag{1}$$

where $p(\theta)$ is the prior on hidden parameters (the unknown object the experimenter is trying to estimate), and $p(x_i|\theta)$ is the likelihood of data x_i given θ. For example, in the visual motion example, θ could be the true underlying velocity of an object moving through space, the observed data x_i could be a short, noise-contaminated movie of the object's motion, and the subject would be asked to estimate the true motion θ given the data x_i and any prior conceptions, $p(\theta)$, of how one expects objects to move. Note that we have also implicitly assumed, in this simplest case, that both the loss $D(.,.)$ and likelihood functions $p(x_i|\theta)$ are known, both to the subject and to the experimenter (perhaps from a preceding set of "learning" trials).

So how can the experimenter actually estimate $p(\theta)$, given the likelihoods $p(x|\theta)$, the loss function $D(.,.)$, and some set of data $\{x_i\}$ with corresponding estimates $\{\hat{\theta}_i\}$ minimizing the posterior expected loss (1)? This turns out to be a linear programming problem (*11*), for which very efficient algorithms exist (e.g., "linprog.m" in Matlab). To see why, first note that the right hand side of expression (1) is linear in the prior $p(\theta)$. Second, we have a large collection of linear constraints on $p(\theta)$: we know that

$$p(\theta) \geq 0 \quad \forall \theta \tag{2}$$

$$\int p(\theta) d\theta = 1 \tag{3}$$

$$\int p(\theta) p(x_i|\theta) \Big[D(\hat{\theta}_i, \theta) - D(z, \theta) \Big] d\theta \leq 0 \quad \forall z \tag{4}$$

where (2-3) are satisfied by any proper prior distribution and (4) is the maximizer condition (1) expressed in slightly different language. (See also (*10*), who noted the same linear programming structure in an application to cost function estimation, rather than the prior estimation examined here.)

The solution to the linear programming problem defined by (2-4) isn't necessarily unique; it corresponds to an intersection of half-spaces, which is convex in general. To come up with a unique solution, we could maximimize a concave "regularizing" function on this convex set; possible such functions include, e.g., the entropy of $p(\theta)$, or its negative mean-square derivative (this function is strictly concave on the space of all functions whose integral is held fixed, as is the case here given constraint (3)); more generally, if we have some prior information on the form of the priors the subject might be using, and this information can be expressed in the "energy" form

$$P[p(\theta)] \sim e^{q[p(\theta)]},$$

for a concave functional $q[.]$, we could use the log of this "prior on priors" P. An alternative solution would be to modify constraint (4) to

$$\int p(\theta) p(x_i|\theta) \Big[D(\hat{\theta}_i, \theta) - D(z, \theta) \Big] \leq -\epsilon \quad \forall z,$$

where we can then adjust the slack variable ϵ until the contraint set shrinks to a single point. This leads directly to another linear programming problem (where we want to make the linear function ϵ as large as possible, under the above constraints). Note that for this last approach to work — for the linear programming problem to have a solution — we need to ensure that the set defined by the constraints (2-4) is compact; this basically means that the constraint set (4) needs to be sufficiently rich, which, in turn, means that sufficient data (or sufficiently strong prior constraints) are required. We will return to this point below.

Finally, what if our primary assumption is not met? That is, what if subjects are not quite behaving optimally with respect to $p(\theta)$? It is possible to detect this situation in the above framework, for example if the slack variable ϵ above is found to be negative. However, a different, more probabilistic viewpoint can be taken. Assume the value of the choice $\hat{\theta}_i$ is optimal under some "comparison" noise, that is,

$$\int p(\theta) p(x_i|\theta) \Big[D(\hat{\theta}_i, \theta) - D(z, \theta) \Big] \leq \sigma \eta_i(z) \quad \forall z,$$

with $\eta_i(z)$ a random variable of scale $\sigma > 0$ (assume η to be i.i.d. for now, although this may be generalized). If we assume this decision noise η has a log-concave density (i.e., the log of the density is a concave function; e.g., Gaussian, or exponential), then so does its integral (*12*), and the resulting maximum likelihood problem has no non-global local maxima and is therefore solvable by ascent methods. To see this, write the log-likelihood of (p, σ) given data $\{x_i, \hat{\theta}_i\}$ as

$$L_{\{x_i, \hat{\theta}_i\}}(p, \sigma) = \sum \log \int_{-\infty}^{u_i(z)} dp(\eta),$$

with the sum over the set of all the constraints in (4) and

$$u_i(z) \equiv \frac{1}{\sigma} \int p(\theta) p(x_i | \theta) \left[D(\hat{\theta}_i, \theta) - D(z, \theta) \right].$$

L is the sum of concave functions in u_i, and hence is concave itself, and has no non-global local maxima in these variables; since σ and p are linearly related through u_i (and (p, σ) live in a convex set), L has no non-global local maxima in (p, σ), either. Once again, this maximum likelihood problem may be regularized by prior information[1], maximizing the *a posteriori* likelihood $L(p) - q[p]$ instead of $L(p)$; this problem is similarly tractable by ascent methods, by the concavity of $-q[.]$ (note that this "soft-constraint" problem reduces exactly to the "hard" constraint problem (4) as the noise $\sigma \to 0$)[2].

Note that the estimated value of the noise scale σ plays a similar role to that of the slack variable ϵ, above, with the difference that ϵ can be much more sensitive to the worst trial (that is, the trial on which the subject behaves most suboptimally); we can use either of these slack variables to go back and ask about how close to optimally the subjects were actually performing — large values of σ, for example, imply sub-optimal performance. An additional interesting idea is to use the computed value of η as a kind of outlier test; η large implies the trial was particularly suboptimal.

Special cases

Maximum *a posteriori* estimation: The maximum *a posteriori* (MAP) estimator corresponds to the Hamming distance loss function,

$$D(i, j) = 1(i \neq j);$$

this implies that the constraints (4) have the simple form

$$p(\hat{\theta}_i) - p(z) L(\hat{\theta}_i, z) \geq 0,$$

with $L(\hat{\theta}_i, z)$ defined as the largest observed likelihood ratio for $\hat{\theta}_i$ and z, that is,

$$L(\hat{\theta}_i, z) \equiv \max_{x_i} \frac{p(x_i | z)}{p(x_i | \hat{\theta}_i)},$$

---

[1]Overfitting here is a symptom of the fact that in some cases — particularly when few data samples have been observed — many priors (even highly implausible priors) can explain the observed data fairly well; in this case, it is often quite useful to penalize these "implausible" priors, thus effectively regularizing our estimates. Similar observations have appeared in the context of medical applications of Markov random field methods (*13*).

[2]Another possible application of this regularization idea is as follows. We may incorporate improper priors — that is, priors which may not integrate to unity (such priors frequently arise in the analysis of reparameterization-invariant decision procedures, for example) — without any major conceptual modification in our analysis, simply by removing the normalization contraint (3). However, a problem arises: the zero measure, $p(\theta) \equiv 0$, will always trivially satisfy the remaining constraints (2) and (4). This problem could potentially be ameliorated by introducing a convex regularizing term (or equivalently, a log-concave prior) on the total mass $\int p(\theta) d\theta$.

with the maximum taken over all x_i which led to the estimate $\hat{\theta}_i$. This setup is perhaps most appropriate for a two-alternative forced choice situation, where the problem is one of classification or discrimination, not estimation.

Mean-square and absolute-error regression: Our discussion assumes an even simpler form when the loss function $D(.,.)$ is taken to be squared error, $D(x, y) = (x - y)^2$, or absolute error, $D(x, y) = |x - y|$. In this case it is convenient to work with a slightly different noise model than the classification noise discussed above; instead, we may model the subject's responses as optimal plus estimation noise. For squared-error, the optimal $\hat{\theta}_i$ is known to be uniquely defined as the conditional mean of θ given x_i. Thus we may replace the collection of linear inequality constraints (4) with a much smaller set of linear *equalities* (a single equality per trial, instead of a single inequality per trial per z):

$$\int \left(p(x_i|\theta)(\theta - \hat{\theta}_i) \right) p(\theta) d\theta = \sigma \eta_i; \tag{5}$$

the corresponding likelihood, again, has no non-global local maxima if η has a log-concave density. In the simplest case of Gaussian η, the maximum likelihood problem may be solved by standard nonnegative least-squares (e.g., "lsqnonneg" or "quadprog" in Matlab).

In the absolute error case, the optimal $\hat{\theta}_i$ is given by the conditional median of θ given x_i (although recall that the median is not necessarily unique here); thus, the inequality constraints (4) may again be replaced by equalities which are linear in $p(\theta)$:

$$\int_{-\infty}^{\hat{\theta}_i} p(\theta)p(x_i|\theta) - \int_{\hat{\theta}_i}^{\infty} p(\theta)p(x_i|\theta) = \sigma \eta_i;$$

again, for Gaussian η this may be solved via standard nonnegative regression, albeit with a different constraint matrix. In each case, η_i retains its utility as an outlier score.

A worked example: learning the fairness of a coin

In this section we will work through a concrete example, to show how to put the ideas discussed above into practice. We take perhaps the simplest possible example, for clarity: the subject observes some number N of independent, identically distributed coin flips, and on each trial i tells us his/her probability of observing tails on the next trial, given that $t = t(i)$ tails were observed in the first i trials[3]. Here the likelihood functions $p(x_i|\theta)$ take the standard binomial form $p(t(i)|p_{tails}) = \binom{i}{t} p_{tails}^t (1 - p_{tails})^{i-t}$ (note that it is reasonable to assume that these likelihoods are known to the subject, at least approximately, due to the ubiquity of binomial data).

Under our assumptions, the subject's estimates $\hat{p}_{tails,i}$ are given as the posterior mean of p_{tails} given the number of tails observed up to trial i. This puts us directly in the mean-square framework discussed in equation (5); we assume Gaussian estimation noise η, construct a regression matrix A of N rows, with the i-th row given by $p(t(i)|p_{tails})(p_{tails} - \hat{p}_{tails,i})$. To regularize our estimates, we add a small square-difference penalty of the form $q[p(\theta)] = \int |dp(\theta)/d\theta|^2 d\theta$. Finally, we estimate

$$\hat{p}(\theta) = \arg \min_{p \geq 0; \int_0^1 p(\theta)d\theta = 1} ||Ap||_2^2 + \epsilon q[p],$$

for $\epsilon \approx 10^{-7}$; this estimate is equivalent to MAP estimation under a (weak) Gaussian prior on the function $p(\theta)$ (truncated so that $p(\theta) \geq 0$), and is computed using quadprog.m.

---

[3]We note in passing that this simple binomial paradigm has potential applications to ideal-observer analysis of classical neuroscientific tasks (e.g., synaptic release detection, or photon counting in retina) in addition to potential applications in psychophysics.

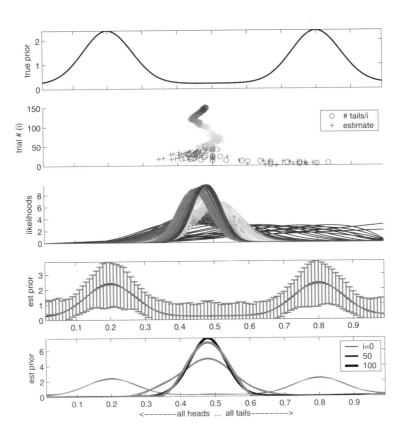

Figure 1: Learning the fairness of a coin (numerical simulation). **Top panel**: True prior distribution on coin fairness. The bimodal nature of this prior indicates that the subject expects coins to be unfair (skewed towards heads, $p_{tails} < .5$, or tails, $p_{tails} > .5$) more often than fair ($p_{tails} = .5$). **Second**: Observed data. Open circles indicate the fraction of observed tails $t = t(i)$ as a function of trial number i (the maximum likelihood estimate, MLE, of the fairness and a minimal sufficient statistic for this problem); $+$ symbols indicate the subject's estimate of the coin's fairness, assumed to correspond to the posterior mean of the fairness under the subject's prior. Note the systematic deviations of the subject's estimate from the MLE; these deviations shrink as i increases and the strength of the prior relative to the likelihood term decreases. **Third**: Binomial likelihood terms $\binom{i}{t} p_{tails}^{t} (1 - p_{tails})^{i-t}$. Color of trace correponds to trial number i, as indicated in previous panel (traces are normalized for clarity). **Fourth**: Estimate of prior given 150 trials. Black trace indicates true prior (as in top panel); red indicates estimate ± 1 posterior standard error (computed via importance sampling). **Bottom**: Tracking the evolution of the posterior. Black traces indicate the subject's true posterior after observing 0 (thin trace), 50 (medium trace), and 100 (thick trace) sample coin flips; as more data are observed, the subject becomes more and more confident about the true fairness of the coin ($p = .5$), and the posteriors match the likelihood terms (c.f. third panel) more closely. Red traces indicate the estimated posterior given the full 150 or just the last 100 or 50 trials, respectively (errorbars omitted for visibility). Note that the procedure tracks the evolution of the subject's posterior quite accurately, given relatively few trials.

To place Bayesian confidence intervals around our estimate, we sample from the corresponding (truncated) Gaussian posterior distribution on $p(\theta)$ (via importance sampling with a suitably shifted, rescaled truncated Gaussian proposal density; similar methods are applicable more generally in the non-Gaussian case via the usual posterior approximation techniques, e.g. Laplace approximation). Figs. 1-2 demonstrate the accuracy of the estimated $\hat{p}(\theta)$; in particular, the bottom panels show that the method accurately tracks the evolution of the model subjects' posteriors as an increasing amount of data are observed.

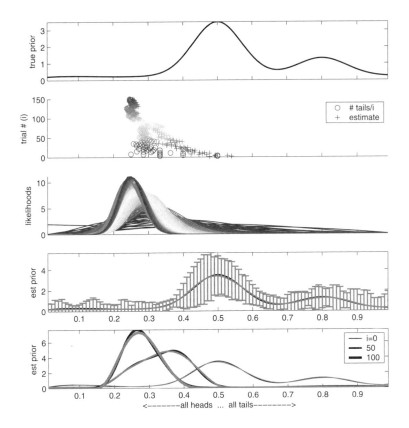

Figure 2: Learning an unfair coin ($p_{tails} = .25$). Conventions as in Fig. 1.

Connection to neural population coding

It is interesting to note a connection to the neural population coding model studied in (*14*) (with more recent work reviewed in (*15*)). The basic idea is that neural populations encode not just stimuli, but probability distributions over stimuli (where the distribution describes the uncertainty in the state of the encoded object). Here the experimentally observed data are neural firing rates, which provide constraints on the underlying encoded "prior" distribution in terms of the individual tuning function of each cell in the observed population.

The simplest model is as follows: the observed spikes n_i from the i-th cell are Poisson-distributed, with rate a nonlinear function of a linear functional of some prior distribution,

$$n_i \sim \text{Poiss}\left(g\left(\int p(\theta) f(x_i, \theta) \right) \right),$$

where the kernel f is considered as the cell's "tuning function"; the log-concavity of the likelihood of p is preserved for any nonlinearity g that is convex and log-concave, a class including the linear rectifiers, exponentials, and power-laws (and studied more extensively in (*16*)). Alternately, a simplified model is often used, e.g.:

$$n_i \sim q\left(\frac{n_i - \int p(\theta) f(x_i, \theta)}{\sigma} \right),$$

with q a log-concave density (typically Gaussian) to preserve the concavity of the log-likelihood; in this case, the scale σ of the noise does not vary with the mean firing rate, as it does in the Poisson model. In both cases, the observed firing rates act as constraints oriented linearly with respect to p; in the latter case, the noise scale σ sets the strength, or confidence, of each such constraint ($2, 3$). Thus, under this framework, given the simultaneously recorded activity of many cells $\{n_i\}$ and some model for the tuning functions $f(x_i, \theta)$, we can infer $p(\theta)$ (and represent the uncertainty in these estimates) using methods quite similar to those developed above.

Directions

The obvious open avenue for future research (aside from application to experimental data) is to relax the assumptions: that the likelihood and cost function are both known, and that the data are observed directly (without any noise). It seems fair to conjecture that the subject can learn the likelihood and cost functions given enough data, but one would like to test this directly, e.g. by estimating $D(., .)$ and p together, perhaps under restrictions on the form of $D(., .)$. As emphasized above, the utility estimation problem has received a great deal of attention, and it is plausible to expect that the methods proposed here for estimation of the prior might be combined with previously-studied methods for utility elicitation and estimation. It is also interesting to consider these elicitation methods in the context of experimental design ($8, 17, 18$), in which we might actively seek stimuli x_i to maximally constrain the possible form of the prior and/or cost function.

References

1. D. Knill, W. Richards, eds., *Perception as Bayesian Inference* (Cambridge University Press, 1996).

2. Y. Weiss, E. Simoncelli, E. Adelson, *Nature Neuroscience* **5**, 598 (2002).

3. Y. Weiss, D. Fleet, *Statistical Theories of the Cortex* (MIT Press, 2002), chap. Velocity likelihoods in biological and machine vision, pp. 77–96.

4. D. Kersten, P. Mamassian, A. Yuille, *Annual Review of Psychology* **55**, 271 (2004).

5. K. Koerding, D. Wolpert, *Nature* **427**, 244 (2004).

6. R. Hogarth, *Journal of the American Statistical Association* **70**, 271 (1975).

7. J. Oakley, A. O'Hagan, *Biometrika* **under review** (2003).

8. P. Garthwaite, J. Kadane, A. O'Hagan, *Handbook of Statistics* (2004), chap. Elicitation.

9. A. Ng, S. Russell, *ICML-17* (2000).

10. J. Blythe, *AAAI02* (2002).

11. G. Strang, *Linear algebra and its applications* (Harcourt Brace, New York, 1988).

12. Y. Rinott, *Annals of Probability* **4**, 1020 (1976).

13. M. Henrion, *et al.*, Why is diagnosis using belief networks insensitive to imprecision in probabilities?, *Tech. Rep. SMI-96-0637*, Stanford (1996).

14. R. Zemel, P. Dayan, A. Pouget, *Neural Computation* **10**, 403 (1998).

15. A. Pouget, P. Dayan, R. Zemel, *Annual Reviews of Neuroscience* **26**, 381 (2003).

16. L. Paninski, *Network: Computation in Neural Systems* **15**, 243 (2004).

17. K. Chaloner, I. Verdinelli, *Statistical Science* **10**, 273 (1995).

18. L. Paninski, *Advances in Neural Information Processing Systems* **16** (2003).

Neuronal Fiber Delineation in Area of Edema from Diffusion Weighted MRI

Ofer Pasternak[*]
School of Computer Science
Tel-Aviv University
Tel-Aviv, ISRAEL 69978
oferpas@post.tau.ac.il

Nir Sochen
Department of Applied Mathematics
Tel-Aviv University
sochen@post.tau.ac.il

Nathan Intrator
School of Computer Science
Tel-Aviv University
nin@post.tau.ac.il

Yaniv Assaf
Department of Neurobiochemistry
Faculty of Life Science
Tel-Aviv University
assafyan@post.tau.ac.il

Abstract

Diffusion Tensor Magnetic Resonance Imaging (DT-MRI) is a non invasive method for brain neuronal fibers delineation. Here we show a modification for DT-MRI that allows delineation of neuronal fibers which are infiltrated by edema. We use the Muliple Tensor Variational (MTV) framework which replaces the diffusion model of DT-MRI with a multiple component model and fits it to the signal attenuation with a variational regularization mechanism. In order to reduce free water contamination we estimate the free water compartment volume fraction in each voxel, remove it, and then calculate the anisotropy of the remaining compartment. The variational framework was applied on data collected with conventional clinical parameters, containing only six diffusion directions. By using the variational framework we were able to overcome the highly ill posed fitting. The results show that we were able to find fibers that were not found by DT-MRI.

1 Introduction

Diffusion weighted Magnetic Resonance Imaging (DT-MRI) enables the measurement of the apparent water self-diffusion along a specified direction [1]. Using a series of Diffusion Weighted Images (DWIs) DT-MRI can extract quantitative measures of water molecule diffusion anisotropy which characterize tissue microstructure [2]. Such measures are in particular useful for the segmentation of neuronal fibers from other brain tissue which then allows a noninvasive delineation and visualization of major brain neuronal fiber bundles in vivo [3]. Based on the assumptions that each voxel can be represented by a single diffusion compartment and that the diffusion within this compartment has a Gaussian distribution

---

[*]http://www.cs.tau.ac.il/~oferpas

DT-MRI states the relation between the signal attenuation, E, and the diffusion tensor, D, as follows [4, 5, 6]:

$$E(q_k) = \frac{A(q_k)}{A(0)} = \exp(-bq_k^T D q_k) \,, \tag{1}$$

where $A(q_k)$ is the DWI for the k'th applied diffusion gradient direction q_k. The notation $A(0)$ is for the non weighted image and b is a constant reflecting the experimental diffusion weighting [2]. D is a second order tensor, *i.e.*, a 3×3 positive semidefinite matrix, that requires at least 6 DWIs from different non-collinear applied gradient directions to uniquely determine it. The symmetric diffusion tensor has a spectral decomposition for three eigenvectors U^a and three positive eigenvalues λ^a. The relation between the eigenvalues determines the diffusion anisotropy using measures such as Fractional Anisotropy (FA) [5]:

$$FA = \sqrt{\frac{3((\lambda_1 - \langle D \rangle)^2 + (\lambda_2 - \langle D \rangle)^2 + (\lambda_3 - \langle D \rangle)^2)}{2(\lambda_1^2 + \lambda_2^2 + \lambda_3^2)}} \,, \tag{2}$$

where $\langle D \rangle = (\lambda_1 + \lambda_2 + \lambda_3)/3$. FA is relatively high in neuronal fiber bundles (white matter), where the cylindrical geometry of fibers causes the diffusion perpendicular to the fibers be much smaller than parallel to them. Other brain tissues, such as gray matter and Cerebro-Spinal Fluid (CSF), are less confined with diffusion direction and exhibit isotropic diffusion. In cases of partial volume where neuronal fibers reside other tissue type in the same voxel, or present complex architecture, the diffusion has no longer a single pronounced orientation and therefore the FA value of the fitted tensor is decreased. The decreased FA values causes errors in segmentation and in any proceeding fiber analysis.

In this paper we focus on the case where partial volume occurs when fiber bundles are infiltrated with edema. Edema might occur in response to brain trauma, or surrounding a tumor. The brain tissue accumulate water which creates pressure and might change the fiber architecture, or infiltrate it. Since the edema consists mostly of relatively free diffusing water molecules, the diffusion attenuation increases and the anisotropy decreases. We chose to reduce the effect of edema by changing the diffusion model to a dual compartment model, assuming an isotropic compartment added to a tensor compartment.

2 Theory

The method we offer is based on the dual compartment model which was already demonstrated as able to reduce CSF contamination [7], where it required a large number of diffusion measurement with different diffusion times. Here we require the conventional DT-MRI data of only six diffusion measurement, and apply it on the edema case.

2.1 The Dual Compartment Model

The dual compartment model is described as follows:

$$E(q_k) = f \exp(-bq_k^T D_1 q_k) + (1 - f) \exp(-bD_2) \,. \tag{3}$$

The diffusion tensor for the tensor compartment is denoted by D_1, and the diffusion coefficient of the isotropic water compartment is denoted by D_2. The compartments have relative volume of f and $1 - f$. Finding the best fitting parameters D_1, D_2 and f is highly ill-posed, especially in the case of six measurement, where for any arbitrarily chosen isotropic compartment there could be found a tensor compartment which exactly fits the data.

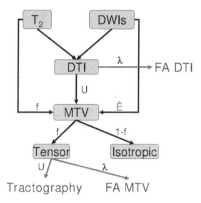

Figure 1: The initialization scheme. In addition to the DWI data, MTV uses the T_2 image to initialize f. The initial orientation for the tensor compartment are those that DT-MRI calculated.

2.2 The Variational Framework

In order to stabilize the fitting process we chose to use the Multiple Tensor Variational (MTV) framework [8] which was previously used to resolve partial volume caused by complex fiber architecture [9], and to reduce CSF contamination in cases of hydrocephalus [10]. We note that the dual compartment model is a special case of the more general multiple tensor model, where the number of the compartments is restricted to 2 and one of the compartments is restricted to equal eigenvalues (isotropy). Therefore the MTV framework adapted for separation of fiber compartments from edema is composed of the following functional, whose minima should provide the wanted diffusion parameters:

$$S(f, D_1, D_2) = \int_\Omega \left[\alpha \sum_{k=1}^{d} (E(q_k) - \hat{E}(q_k))^2 + \phi(|\nabla U_i^1|) \right] d\Omega . \tag{4}$$

The notation $\hat{E}$ is for the observed diffusion signal attenuation and E is calculated using (3) for d different acquisition directions. Ω is the image domain with $3D$ axis (x, y, z), $|\nabla I| = \sqrt{(\frac{\partial I}{\partial x})^2 + (\frac{\partial I}{\partial y})^2 + (\frac{\partial I}{\partial z})^2}$ is defined as the vector gradient norm. The notation U_i^1 stands for the principal eigenvector of the i'th diffusion tensor. The fixed parameters α is set to keep the solution closer to the observed diffusion signal. The function ϕ is a diffusion flow function, which controls the regularization behavior. Here we chose to use $\phi_i(s) = \sqrt{1 + \frac{s^2}{K_i^2}}$ which lead to anisotropic diffusion-like flow while preserving discontinuities [11]. The regularized fitting allows the identification of smoothed fiber compartments and reduces noise. The minimum of (4) solves the Euler-Lagrange equations, and can be found by the gradient descent scheme.

2.3 Initialization Scheme

Since the functional space is highly irregular (not enough measurements), the minimization process requires initial guess (figure 1), which is as close as possible to the global minimum. In order to apriori estimate the relative volume of the isotropic compartment we used a normalized diffusion non-weighted image, where high contrast correlates to larger fluid volume. In order to apriori estimate the parameters of D_1 we used the result of conventional DT-MRI fitting on the original data. The DT-MRI results were spectrally decomposed and the eigenvectors were used as initial guess for the eigenvectors of D_1. The initial guess for the eigenvalues of D_1 were set to $\lambda_1 = 1.5$, $\lambda_2 = \lambda_3 = 0.4$.

3 Methods

We demonstrate how partial volume of neuronal fiber and edema can be reduced by applying the modified MTV framework on a brain slice taken from a patient with sever edema surrounding a brain tumor. MRI was performed on a $1.5T$ MRI scanner (GE, Milwaukee). DT-MRI experiments were performed using a diffusion-weighted spin-echo echo-planar-imaging (DWI-EPI) pulse sequence. The experimental parameters were as follows: $TR/TE = 10000/98ms$, $\Delta/\delta = 31/25ms$, $b = 1000s/mm2$ with six diffusion gradient directions. 48 slices with thickness of $3mm$ and no gap were acquired covering the whole brain with FOV of $240mm2$ and matrix of $128x128$. Number of averages was 4, and the total experimental time was about 6 minutes. Head movement and image distortions were corrected using a mutual information based registration algorithm [12]. The corrected DWIs were fitted to the dual compartment model via the modified MTV framework, then the isotropic compartment was omitted. FA was calculated for the remaining tensor for which FA higher than 0.25 was considered as white matter. We compared these results to single component DT-MRI with no regularization, which was also used for initialization of the MTV fitting.

4 Results and Discussion

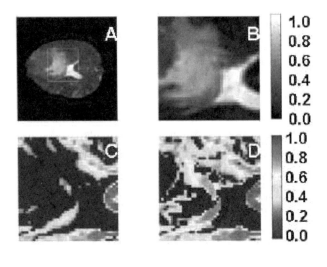

Figure 2: A single slice of a patient with edema. (A) a non diffusion weighted image with ROI marked. Showing the tumor in black surrounded by sever edema which appear bright. (B) Normalized T_2 of the ROI, used for f initialization. (C) FA map from DT-MRI (threshold of FA> 0.25). Large parts of the corpus callosum are obscured. (D) FA map of D_1 from MTV (thresholds f> 0.35, FA> 0.25). A much larger part of the corpus callosum is revealed

Figure (2) shows the Edema case, where DTI was unable to delineate large parts of the corpus callosum. Since the corpus callosum is one of the largest fiber bundles in the brain it was highly unlikely that the fibers were disconnected or disappeared. The expected FA should have been on the same order as on the opposite side of the brain, where the corpus callosum shows high FA values. Applying the MTV on the slice and mapping the FA value of the tensor compartment reveals considerably much more pixels of higher FA in the area of the corpus callosum. In general the FA values of most pixels were increased, which was predicted, since by removing any size of a sphere (isotropic compartment) we should be left with a shape which is less spherical, and therefore with increased FA. The benefit of using the MTV framework over an overall reduce of FA threshold in recognizing neuronal fiber voxels is that the amount of FA increase is not uniform in all tissue types. In areas where the partial volume was not big due to the edema, the increase was much lower than in areas contaminated with edema. This keeps the nice contrast reflected by FA values between neuronal fibers and other tissue types. Reducing the FA threshold on original DT-MRI results would cause a less clear separation between the fiber bundles and other tissue types. This tool could be used for fiber tracking in the vicinity of brain tumors, or with stroke, where edema contaminates the fibers and prevents fiber delineation with the conventional DT-MRI.

5 Conclusions

We show that by modifying the MTV framework to fit the dual compartment model we can reduce the contamination of edema, and delineate much larger fiber bundle areas. By using the MTV framework we stabilize the fitting process, and also include some biological constraints, such as the piece-wise smoothness nature of neuronal fibers in the brain. There is no doubt that using a much larger number of diffusion measurements should increase the stabilization of the process, and will increase its accuracy. However, more measurement require much more scan time, which might not be available in some cases. The variational framework is a powerful tool for the modeling and regularization of various mappings. It is applied, with great success, to scalar and vector fields in image processing and computer vision. Recently it has been generalized to deal with tensor fields which are of great interest to brain research via the analysis of DWIs and DT-MRI. We show that the more realistic model of multi-compartment voxels conjugated with the variational framework provides much improved results.

Acknowledgments

We acknowledge the support of the Edersheim - Levi - Gitter Institute for Functional Human Brain Mapping of Tel-Aviv Sourasky Medical Center and Tel-Aviv University, the Adams super-center for brain research of Tel-Aviv University, the Israel Academy of Sciences, Israel Ministry of Science, and the Tel-Aviv University research fund.

References

[1] E Stejskal and JE Tanner. Spin diffusion measurements: Spin echoes in the presence of a time-dependant field gradient. *J. Chem. Phys.*, 42:288–292, 1965.

[2] D. Le-Bihan, J.-F. Mangin, C. Poupon, C.A. Clark, S. Pappata, N. Molko, and H. Chabriat. Diffusion tensor imaging: concepts and applications. *Journal of Magnetic Resonance Imaging*, 13:534–546, 2001.

[3] S. Mori and P.C. van Zijl. Fiber tracking: principles and strategies - a technical review. *NMR Biomed.*, 15:468–480, 2002.

[4] P.J. Basser, J. Mattiello, and D. Le-Bihan. MR diffusion tensor spectroscopy and imaging. *Biophysical Journal*, 66:259–267, 1994.

[5] P.J. Basser and C. Pierpaoli. Microstructural and physiological features of tissues elucidated by quantitative-diffusion-tensor MRI. *Journal of Magnetic Resonance*, 111(3):209–219, June 1996.

[6] C. Pierpaoli, P. Jezzard, P.J. Basser, A. Barnett, and G. Di-Chiro. Diffusion tensor MR imaging of human brain. *Radiology*, 201:637–648, 1996.

[7] C. Pierpaoli and D. K. Jones. Removing CSF contamination in brain DT-MRIs by using a two-compartment tensor model. In *Proc. International Society for Magnetic Resonance in Medicine 12th Scientific meeting ISMRM04*, page 1215, Kyoto, Japan, 2004.

[8] O. Pasternak, N. Sochen, and Y. Assaf. Variational regularization of multiple diffusion tensor fields. In J. Weickert and H. Hagen, editors, *Visualization and Processing of Tensor Fields*. Springer, Berlin, 2005.

[9] O. Pasternak, N. Sochen, and Y. Assaf. Separation of white matter fascicles from diffusion MRI using ϕ-functional regularization. In *Proceedings of 12th Annual Meeting of the ISMRM*, page 1227, 2004.

[10] O. Pasternak, N. Sochen, and Y. Assaf. CSF partial volume reduction in hydrocephalus using a variational framework. In *Proceedings of 13th Annual Meeting of the ISMRM*, page 1100, 2005.

[11] G. Aubert and P. Kornprobst. *Mathematical Problems in Image Processing: Partial Differential Equations and the Calculus of Variations*, volume 147 of *Applied Mathematical Sciences*. Springer-Verlag, 2002.

[12] G.K. Rohde, A.S. Barnett, P.J. Basser, S. Marenco, and C. Pierpaoli. Comprehensive approach for correction of motion and distortion in diffusion-weighted MRI. *Magnetic Resonance in Medicine*, 51:103–114, 2004.

Beyond Pair-Based STDP: a Phenomenogical Rule for Spike Triplet and Frequency Effects

Jean-Pascal Pfister and Wulfram Gerstner
School of Computer and Communication Sciences
and Brain-Mind Institute,
Ecole Polytechnique Fédérale de Lausanne (EPFL), CH-1015 Lausanne
{jean-pascal.pfister, wulfram.gerstner}@epfl.ch

Abstract

While classical experiments on spike-timing dependent plasticity analyzed synaptic changes as a function of the timing of *pairs* of pre- and postsynaptic spikes, more recent experiments also point to the effect of spike *triplets*. Here we develop a mathematical framework that allows us to characterize timing based learning rules. Moreover, we identify a candidate learning rule with five variables (and 5 free parameters) that captures a variety of experimental data, including the dependence of potentiation and depression upon pre- and postsynaptic firing frequencies. The relation to the Bienenstock-Cooper-Munro rule as well as to some timing-based rules is discussed.

1 Introduction

Most experimental studies of Spike-Timing Dependent Plasticity (STDP) have focused on the timing of spike pairs [1, 2, 3] and so do many theoretical models. The spike-pair based models can be divided into two classes: either all pairs of spikes contribute in a homogeneous fashion [4, 5, 6, 7, 8, 9, 10] (called 'all-to-all' interaction in the following) or only pairs of 'neighboring' spikes [11, 12, 13] (called 'nearest-spike' interaction in the following); cf. [14, 15]. Apart from these phenomenological models, there are also models that are somewhat closer to the biophysics of synaptic changes [16, 17, 18, 19].

Recent experiments have furthered our understanding of timing effects in plasticity and added at least two different aspects: firstly, it has been shown that the mechanism of potentiation in STDP is different from that of depression [20] and secondly, it became clear that not only the timing of pairs, but also of triplets of spikes contributes to the outcome of plasticity experiments [21, 22].

In this paper, we introduce a learning rule that takes these two aspects partially into account in a simple way. Depression is triggered by *pairs* of spikes with *post-before-pre* timing, whereas potentiation is triggered by *triplets* of spikes consisting of 1 pre- and 2 postsynaptic spikes. Moreover, in our model the pair-based depression includes an explicit dependence upon the mean postsynaptic firing rate. We show that such a learning rule accounts for two important stimulation paradigms:

P1 (Relative Spike Timing): *Both the pre- and postsynaptic spike trains consist of a burst* *of N spikes at regular intervals T, but the two spike trains are shifted by a time* $\Delta t = t^{\text{post}} - t^{\text{pre}}$.

The total weight change is a function of the relative timing Δt (this gives the standard STDP function), but also a function of the firing frequency $\rho = 1/T$ during the burst; cf. Fig. 1A (data from L5 pyramidal neurons in visual cortex).

P2 (Poisson Firing): *The pre- and postsynaptic spike trains are generated by two independent Poisson processes with rates* ρ_x *and* ρ_y *respectively.*

Protocol P2 has less experimental support but it helps to establish a relation to the Bienenstock-Cooper-Munro (BCM) model [23]. To see that relation, it is useful to plot the weight change as a function of the postsynaptic firing rate, i.e., $\Delta w \propto \phi(\rho_y)$ (cf. Fig 1B). Note that the function ϕ has only been measured indirectly in experiments [24, 25].

We emphasize that in the BCM model,

$$\Delta w = \rho_x \phi(\rho_y, \bar{\rho}_y) \tag{1}$$

the function ϕ depends not only on the current firing rate ρ_y, but also on the *mean* firing rate $\bar{\rho}_y$ averaged over the recent past which has the effect that the threshold between depression and potentiation is not fixed but dynamic. More precisely, this threshold θ depends non-linearly on the mean firing rate $\bar{\rho}_y$:

$$\theta = \alpha \bar{\rho}_y^p, \quad p > 1 \tag{2}$$

with parameters α and p. Previous models of STDP have already discussed the relation of STDP to the BCM rule [16, 12, 17, 26], but none of these seems to be completely satisfactory as discussed in Section 4. We will also compare our results to the rule of [21] which was together with the work of [16] amongst the first triplet rules to be proposed.

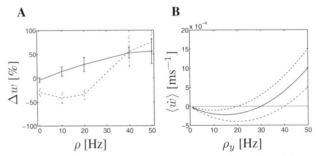

Figure 1: **A**. Weight change in an experiment on cortical synapses using pairing protocol (P1) (solid line: $\Delta t = 10$ ms, dot-dashed line $\Delta t = -10$ ms) as a function of the frequency ρ. Figure redrawn from [11]. **B**. Weight change in protocol P2 according to the BCM rule for $\theta = 20, 30, 40$ Hz.

2   A Framework for STDP

Several learning rules in the modeling literature can be classified according to the two criteria introduced above: (i) all-to-all interaction vs. nearest spike interaction; (ii) pair-based vs. triplet based rules. Point (ii) can be elaborated further in the context of an expansion (pairs, triplets, quadruplets, ... of spikes) that we introduce now.

2.1   Volterra Expansion ('all-to-all')

For the sake of simplicity, we assume that weight changes occur at the moment of presynaptic spike arrival or at the moment of postsynaptic firing. The direction and amplitude of the weight change depends on the configuration of spikes in the presynaptic spike train $X(t) = \sum_k \delta(t - t_x^k)$ and the postsynaptic spike train $Y(t) = \sum_k \delta(t - t_y^k)$. With some arbitrary functionals $F[X, Y]$ and $G[X, Y]$, we write (see also [8])

$$\dot{w}(t) = X(t)F[X, Y] + Y(t)G[X, Y] \tag{3}$$

Clearly, there can be other neuronal variables that influence the synaptic dynamics. For example, the weight change can depend on the current weight value w [8, 15, 10], the Ca^{2+} concentration [17, 19], the depolarization [25, 27, 28], the mean postsynaptic firing rate $\bar{\rho}_y(t)$ [23],.... Here, we will consider only the dependence upon the history of the pre- and postsynaptic firing times and the mean postsynaptic firing rate $\bar{\rho}_y$. Note that even if $\bar{\rho}_y$ depends via a low-pass filter $\tau_\rho \dot{\bar{\rho}}_y = -\bar{\rho}_y + Y(t)$ on the past spike train Y of the postsynaptic neuron, the description of the problem will turn out to be simpler if the mean firing rate is considered as a separate variable. Therefore, let us write the instantaneous weight change as

$$\dot{w}(t) = X(t)F([X, Y], \bar{\rho}_y(t)) + Y(t)G([X, Y], \bar{\rho}_y(t)) \tag{4}$$

The goal is now to determine the simplest functionals F and G that would be consistent with the experimental protocols $P1$ and $P2$ introduced above. Since the functionals are unknown, we perform a Volterra expansion of F and G in the hope that a small number of low-order terms are sufficient to explain a large body of experimental data. The Volterra expansion [29] of the functional G can be written as[1]

$$
\begin{aligned}
G([X, Y]) &= G_1^y + \int_0^\infty G_2^{xy}(s)X(t - s)ds + \int_0^\infty G_2^{yy}(s)Y(t - s)ds \\
&+ \int_0^\infty \int_0^\infty G_3^{xxy}(s, s')X(t - s)X(t - s')ds'ds \\
&+ \int_0^\infty \int_0^\infty \mathbf{G}_3^{xyy}(s, s')X(t - s)Y(t - s')ds'ds \\
&+ \int_0^\infty \int_0^\infty G_3^{yyy}(s, s')Y(t - s)Y(t - s')ds'ds + \dots
\end{aligned} \tag{5}
$$

Similarly, the expansion of F yields

$$F([X, Y]) = F_1^x + \int_0^\infty F_2^{xx}(s)X(t - s)ds + \int_0^\infty \mathbf{F}_2^{xy}(s)Y(t - s)ds + \dots \tag{6}$$

Note that the upper index in functions represents the type of interaction. For example, G_3^{xyy} (in bold face above) refers to a triplet interaction consisting of 1 pre- and 2 postsynaptic spikes. Note that the G_3^{xyy} term could correspond to a *pre-post-post* sequence as well as a *post-pre-post* sequence. Similarly the term F_2^{xy} picks up the changes caused by arrival of a presynaptic spike after postsynaptic spike firing. Several learning rules with all-to-all interaction can be classified in this framework, e.g. [5, 6, 7, 8, 9, 10].

2.2 Our Model

Not all term in the expansion need to be non-zero. In fact, in the results section we will show that a learning rule with $G_3^{xyy}(s, s') \geq 0$ for all $s, s' > 0$ and $F_2^{xy}(s) \leq 0$ for $s > 0$ and all other terms set to zero is sufficient to explain the results from protocols P1 and P2. Thus, in our learning rule an isolated pair of spikes in configuration *post-before-pre* will lead to depression. An isolated spike pair *pre-before-post*, on the other hand, would not be sufficient to trigger potentiation, whereas a triplet *pre-post-post* or *post-pre-post* will do so (see Fig. 2).

---

[1]For the sake of clarity we have omitted the dependence on $\bar{\rho}_y$.

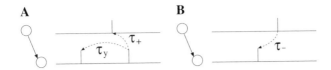

Figure 2: **A**. Triplet interaction for LTP **B**. Pair interaction for LTD.

To be specific, we consider

$$F_2^{xy}(s) = -A_-(\bar{\rho}_y)e^{-\frac{s}{\tau_-}} \quad \text{and} \quad G_3^{xyy}(s, s') = A_+ e^{-\frac{s}{\tau_+}} e^{-\frac{s'}{\tau_y}}. \tag{7}$$

Such an exponential model can be implemented by a mechanistic update involving three variables (the dot denotes a temporal derivative)

$$\dot{a} = -\frac{a}{\tau_+}; \quad \text{if } t = t_x^k \text{ then } a \to a+1$$

$$\dot{b} = -\frac{b}{\tau_-}; \quad \text{if } t = t_y^k \text{ then } b \to b+1 \tag{8}$$

$$\dot{c} = -\frac{c}{\tau_y}; \quad \text{if } t = t_y^k \text{ then } c \to c+1$$

The weight update is then

$$\dot{w}(t) = -A_-(\bar{\rho}_y)X(t)b(t) + A_+Y(t)a(t)c(t). \tag{9}$$

2.3 Nearest Spike Expansion (truncated model)

Following ideas of [11, 12, 13], the expansion can also be restricted to neighboring spikes only. Let us denote by $f_y(t)$ the firing time of the last postsynaptic spike before time t. Similarly, $f_x(t')$ denotes the timing of the last presynaptic spike preceding t'. With this notation the Volterra expansion of the preceding section can be repeated in a form that only nearest spikes play a role. A classification of the models [11, 12, 13] is hence possible.

We focus immediately on the truncated version of our model

$$\dot{w}(t) = X(t)F_2^{xy}(t - f_y(t), \bar{\rho}_y(t)) + Y(t)G_3^{xyy}(t - f_x(t), t - f_y(t)) \tag{10}$$

The mechanistic model that generates the truncated version of the model is similar to Eq. (8) except that under the appropriate update condition, the variable goes to one, i.e. $a \to 1, b \to 1$ and $c \to 1$. The weight update is identical to that of the all-to-all model, Eq. (9).

3 Results

One advantage of our formulation is that we can derive explicit formulas for the total weight changes induced by protocols P1 and P2.

3.1 All-to-all Interaction

If we use protocol P1 with a total of N pre- and postsynaptic spikes at frequency ρ shifted by a time Δt, then the total weight change Δw is for our model with all-to-all interaction

$$\begin{aligned}
\Delta w = {} & A_+ \sum_{k=0}^{N-1} \sum_{k'=1}^{N-1} (N - \max(k, k')) \exp\left(-\frac{k/\rho + \Delta t}{\tau_+}\right) \exp\left(-\frac{k'}{\tau_y \rho}\right) \lambda_k(-\Delta t) \\
& - A_-(\bar{\rho}_y) \sum_{k=0}^{N-1} (N-k) \exp\left(-\frac{k/\rho - \Delta t}{\tau_-}\right) \lambda_k(\Delta t)
\end{aligned} \tag{11}$$

where $\lambda_k(\Delta t) = 1 - \delta_{k0}\Theta(\Delta t)$ with Θ the Heaviside step function. The results are plotted in Fig. 3 top-left for $N = 60$ spikes.

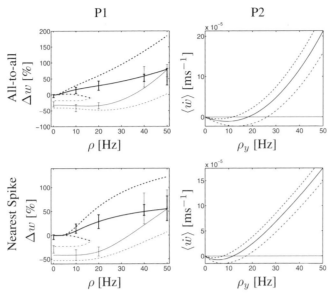

Figure 3: Triplet learning rule. Summary of all results of protocol $P1$ (left) and $P2$ (right) for an all-to-all (top) and nearest-spike (bottom) interaction scheme. For the left column, the upper thick lines correspond to positive timing ($\Delta t > 0$) while the lower thin lines to negative timing. Dashed line: $\Delta t = \pm 2$ ms, solid line: $\Delta t = \pm 10$ ms and dot-dashed line $\Delta t = \pm 30$ ms. The error bars indicate the experimental data points of Fig. 1A. Right column: dashed-line $\bar{\rho}_y = 8$ Hz, solid line $\bar{\rho}_y = 10$ Hz and dot-dashed line $\bar{\rho}_y = 12$ Hz. Top: $\tau_y = 200$ ms, bottom: $\tau_y = 40$ ms.

The mean firing rate $\bar{\rho}_y$ reflects the firing activity during the recent past (i.e. *before* the start of the experiment) and is assumed as fixed during the experiment. The exact value does not matter. Overall, the frequency dependence of changes Δw is very similar to that observed in experiments. If X and Y are independent Poisson process, the protocol P2 gives a total weight change that can be calculated using standard arguments [8]

$$\langle \dot{w} \rangle = -A_-(\bar{\rho}_y)\rho_x\rho_y\tau_- + A_+\rho_x\rho_y^2\tau_+\tau_y \tag{12}$$

As before, the mean firing rate $\bar{\rho}_y$ reflects the firing activity during the recent past and is assumed as fixed during the experiment. In order to implement a sliding threshold as in the BCM rule, we take $A_-(\bar{\rho}_y) = \beta_-\bar{\rho}_y^2/\rho_0^2$ where we set $\rho_0 = 10$ Hz. This yields a frequency dependent threshold $\theta(\bar{\rho}_y) = \beta_-\tau_-\bar{\rho}_y^2/(A_+\tau_+\tau_y\rho_0^2)$. As can be seen in Fig. 3 top-right our model exhibits all essential features of a BCM rule.

3.2 Nearest Spike Interaction

We now apply protocols P1 and P2 to our truncated rule, i.e. restricted to the *nearest-spike* interaction; cf. Eq. (10) where the expression of F_2^{xy} and G_3^{xyy} are taken from Eq. (7). The weight change Δw for the protocol $P1$ can be calculated explicitly and is plotted in Fig. 3 bottom-left. For protocol $P2$ (see Fig. 3 bottom-right) we find

$$\langle \dot{w} \rangle = \rho_x \left(-\frac{A_-(\bar{\rho}_y)\rho_y}{\rho_y + \alpha_-} + \frac{A_+}{\rho_x + \alpha_+}\frac{\rho_y^2}{\rho_y + \alpha_y} \right) \tag{13}$$

where $\alpha_y = \tau_y^{-1}$. If we assume that $\rho_x \ll \alpha_x$, Eq. (13) is a BCM learning rule.

In summary, both versions of our learning rule (all-to-all or nearest-spike) yield a frequency dependence that is consistent with experimental results under protocol P1 and with the BCM rule tested under protocol P2. We note that our learning rule contains only two terms, i.e., a triplet term (1 pre and 2 post) for potentiation and a *post-pre* pair term for depression. The dynamics is formulated using five variables $(a, b, c, \bar{\rho}_y, w)$ and five parameters $(\tau_+, \tau_-, \tau_y, A_+, \beta_-)$. $\tau_+ = 16.8$ ms and $\tau_- = 33.7$ ms are taken from [14]. A_+ and β_- are chosen such that the weight changes for $\Delta t = \pm 10$ ms and $\rho = 20$ Hz fit the experimental data [11].

4 Discussion - Comparison with Other Rules

While we started out developing a general framework, we focused in the end on a simple model with only five parameters - why, then, this model and not some other combination of terms? To answer this question we apply our approach to a couple of other models, i.e., pair-based models (all-to-all or nearest spike), triplet-based models, and others.

4.1 STDP Models Based on Spike Pairs

Pair-based models with all-to-all interaction [4, 5, 6, 7, 8, 9, 10] yield under Poisson stimulation (protocol P2) a total weight change that is linear in presynaptic and postsynaptic frequencies. Thus, as a function of postsynaptic frequency we always find a straight line with a slope that depends on the integral of the STDP function [5, 7]. Thus pair-based models with all-to-all interaction need to be excluded in view of BCM features of plasticity [25, 24].

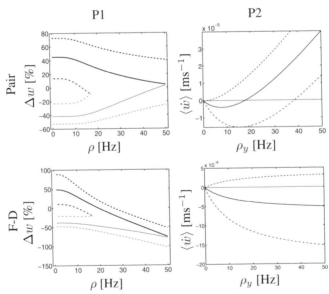

Figure 4: Pair learning rule in a nearest spike interaction scheme (top) and Froemke-Dan rule (bottom). For the left column, the higher thick lines correspond to positive timing ($\Delta t > 0$) while the lower thin lines to negative timing. Dashed line: $\Delta t = \pm 2$ ms, solid line: $\Delta t = \pm 10$ ms and dot-dashed line $\Delta t = \pm 30$ ms. Right column: dashed-line $\bar{\rho}_y = 8$ Hz, solid line $\bar{\rho}_y = 10$ Hz and dot-dashed line $\bar{\rho}_y = 12$ Hz. The parameters of the F-D model are taken from [21]. The dependence upon $\bar{\rho}_y$ has been added to the original F-D rule ($A_- \rightarrow \beta_- \bar{\rho}_y^2 / \rho_0^2$).

A pair-based model with nearest-spike interaction, however, can give a non-linear dependence upon the postsynaptic frequency under protocol P2 with fixed threshold between depression and potentation [12]. We can go beyond the results of [12] by adding a suitable dependence of the parameter A_- upon $\bar{\rho}_y$ which yields a sliding threshold; cf. Fig. 4 top right.

But even a pair rule restricted to nearest-spike interaction is unable to account for the results of protocol P1. An important feature of the experimental results with protocol P1 is that potentiation only occurs above a minimal firing frequency of the postsynaptic neuron (cf. Fig. 1A) whereas pair-based rules *always* exhibit potentiation with pre-before-post timing even in the limit of low frequencies; cf. Fig. 4 top left. The intuitive reason is that at low frequency the total weight change is proportional to the number of *pre-post* pairings and this argument can be directly transformed into a mathematical proof (details omitted). Thus, pair-based rules of potentiation (all-to-all or nearest spike) cannot account for results of protocol P1 and must be excluded.

4.2 Comparison with Triplet-Based Learning Rules

The model of Senn et al. [16] can well account of the results under protocol P1. A classification of this rule within our framework reveals that the update algorithm generates pair terms of the form *pre-post* and *post-pre*, as well as triplet terms of the form *pre-post-post* and *post-pre-pre*. As explained in the previous paragraph, a pair term *pre-post* generated potentiation even at very low frequencies which is not realistic. In order to avoid this effect in their model, Senn et al. included additional threshold values which increased the number of parameters in their model to 9 [16] while the number of variables is 5 as in our model. Moreover, the mapping of the model of Senn et al. to the BCM rule is not ideal, since the sliding threshold is different for each individual synapse [16].

An explicit triplet rule has been proposed by Froemke and Dan [21]. In our framework, the rule can be classified as a combination of triplet terms for potentiation and depression. Following the same line or argument as in the preceding sections we can calculate the total weight change for protocols P1 and P2. The result is shown in Fig. 4 bottom. We can clearly see that the pairing experiment $P1$ yields a behavior opposite to the one found experimentally and the BCM behavior is not at all reproduced in protocol P2.

4.3 Summary

We consider our model as a minimal model to account for results of protocol P1 and P2, but, of course, several factors are not captured by the model. First, our model has no dependence upon the current weight value, but, in principle, this could be included along the lines of [10]. Second, the model has no explicit dependence upon the membrane potential or calcium concentration, but the postsynaptic neuron enters only via its firing activity. Third, and most importantly, there are other experimental paradigms that have to be taken care of.

In a recent series of experiments Bi and colleagues [22] have systematically studied the effect of symmetric spike triplets (*pre-post-pre* or *post-pre-post*) and spike quadruplets (e.g., *pre-post-post-pre*) in hippocampal cultures. While the model presented in this paper is intended to model the synaptic dynamic for L5 pyramidal neurons in the visual cortex [11], it is possible to consider a similar model for the hippocampus containing two extra terms (a pair term for potentiation and and triplet term for depression).

References

[1] Markram, H., Lübke, J., Frotscher, M., and Sakmann, B. *Science* **275**, 213–215 (1997).

[2] Zhang, L., Tao, H., Holt, C., W.A.Harris, and Poo, M.-M. *Nature* **395**, 37–44 (1998).

[3] Bi, G. and Poo, M. *Ann. Rev. Neurosci.* **24**, 139–166 (2001).

[4] Gerstner, W., Kempter, R., van Hemmen, J. L., and Wagner, H. *Nature* **383**, 76–78 (1996).

[5] Kempter, R., Gerstner, W., and van Hemmen, J. L. *Phys. Rev. E* **59**, 4498–4514 (1999).

[6] Roberts, P. *J. Computational Neuroscience* **7**, 235–246 (1999).

[7] Song, S., Miller, K., and Abbott, L. *Nature Neuroscience* **3**, 919–926 (2000).

[8] Kistler, W. M. and van Hemmen, J. L. *Neural Comput.* **12**, 385–405 (2000).

[9] Rubin, J., Lee, D. D., and Sompolinsky, H. *Physical Review Letters* **86**, 364–367 (2001).

[10] Gütig, R., Aharonov, R., Rotter, S., and Sompolinsky, H. *J. Neuroscience* **23**, 3697–3714 (2003).

[11] Sjöström, P., Turrigiano, G., and Nelson, S. *Neuron* **32**, 1149–1164 (2001).

[12] Izhikevich, E. and Desai, N. *Neural Computation* **15**, 1511–1523 (2003).

[13] Burkitt, A. N., Meffin, M. H., and Grayden, D. *Neural Computation* **16**, 885–940 (2004).

[14] Bi, G.-Q. *Biological Cybernetics* **319-332** (2002).

[15] van Rossum, M. C. W., Bi, G. Q., and Turrigiano, G. G. *J. Neuroscience* **20**, 8812–8821 (2000).

[16] Senn, W., Tsodyks, M., and Markram, H. *Neural Computation* **13**, 35–67 (2001).

[17] Shouval, H. Z., Bear, M. F., and Cooper, L. N. *Proc. Natl. Acad. Sci. USA* **99**, 10831–10836 (2002).

[18] Abarbanel, H., Huerta, R., and Rabinovich, M. *Proc. Natl. Academy of Sci. USA* **59**, 10137–10143 (2002).

[19] Karmarkar, U., Najarian, M., and Buonomano, D. *Biol. Cybernetics* **87**, 373–382 (2002).

[20] Sjöström, P., Turrigiano, G., and Nelson, S. *Neuron* **39**, 641–654 (2003).

[21] Froemke, R. and Dan, Y. *Nature* **416**, 433–438 (2002).

[22] Wang, H. X., Gerkin, R. C., Nauen, D. W., and Bi, G. Q. *Nature Neuroscience* **8**, 187–193 (2005).

[23] Bienenstock, E., Cooper, L., and Munro, P. *Journal of Neuroscience* **2**, 32–48 (1982). reprinted in Anderson and Rosenfeld, 1990.

[24] Kirkwood, A., Rioult, M. G., and Bear, M. F. *Nature* **381**, 526–528 (1996).

[25] Artola, A. and Singer, W. *Trends Neurosci.* **16**(11), 480–487 (1993).

[26] Toyoizumi, T., Pfister, J.-P., Aihara, K., and Gerstner, W. In *Advances in Neural Information Processing Systems 17*, Saul, L. K., Weiss, Y., and Bottou, L., editors, 1409–1416. MIT Press, Cambridge, MA (2005).

[27] Fusi, S., Annunziato, M., Badoni, D., Salamon, A., and D.J.Amit. *Neural Computation* **12**, 2227–2258 (2000).

[28] Toyoizumi, T., Pfister, J.-P., Aihara, K., and Gerstner, W. *Proc. National Academy Sciences (USA)* **102**, 5239–5244 (2005).

[29] Volterra, V. *Theory of Functionals and of Integral and Integro-Differential Equations.* Dover, New York, (1930).

Scaling Laws in Natural Scenes and the Inference of 3D Shape

Brian Potetz
Department of Computer Science
Center for the Neural Basis of Cognition
Carnegie Mellon University
Pittsburgh, PA 15213
bpotetz@cs.cmu.edu

Tai Sing Lee
Department of Computer Science
Center for the Neural Basis of Cognition
Carnegie Mellon University
Pittsburgh, PA 15213
tai@cnbc.cmu.edu

Abstract

This paper explores the statistical relationship between natural images and their underlying range (depth) images. We look at how this relationship changes over scale, and how this information can be used to enhance low resolution range data using a full resolution intensity image. Based on our findings, we propose an extension to an existing technique known as shape recipes [3], and the success of the two methods are compared using images and laser scans of real scenes. Our extension is shown to provide a two-fold improvement over the current method. Furthermore, we demonstrate that ideal linear shape-from-shading filters, when learned from natural scenes, may derive even more strength from shadow cues than from the traditional linear-Lambertian shading cues.

1   Introduction

The inference of depth information from single images is typically performed by devising models of image formation based on the physics of light interaction and then inverting these models to solve for depth. Once inverted, these models are highly underconstrained, requiring many assumptions such as Lambertian surface reflectance, smoothness of surfaces, uniform albedo, or lack of cast shadows. Little is known about the relative merits of these assumptions in real scenes. A statistical understanding of the joint distribution of real images and their underlying 3D structure would allow us to replace these assumptions and simplifications with probabilistic priors based on real scenes. Furthermore, statistical studies may uncover entirely new sources of information that are not obvious from physical models. Real scenes are affected by many regularities in the environment, such as the natural geometry of objects, the arrangements of objects in space, natural distributions of light, and regularities in the position of the observer. Few current shape inference algorithms make use of these trends. Despite the potential usefulness of statistical models and the growing success of statistical methods in vision, few studies have been made into the statistical relationship between images and range (depth) images. Those studies that have examined this relationship in nature have uncovered meaningful and exploitable statistical trends in real scenes which may be useful for designing new algorithms in surface inference, and also for understanding how humans perceive depth in real scenes [6, 4, 8].

In this paper, we explore some of the properties of the statistical relationship between images and their underlying range (depth) images in real scenes, using images acquired by laser scanner in natural environments. Specifically, we will examine the cross-covariance between images and range images, and how this structure changes over scale. We then illustrate how our statistical findings can be applied to inference problems by analyzing and extending the shape recipe depth inference algorithm.

2   Shape recipes

We will motivate our statistical study with an application. Often, we may have a high-resolution color image of a scene, but only a low spatial resolution range image (range images record the 3D distance between the scene and the camera for each pixel). This often happens if our range image was acquired by applying a stereo depth inference algorithm. Stereo algorithms rely on smoothness constraints, either explicitly or implicitly, and so the high-frequency components of the resulting range image are not reliable [1, 7]. Low-resolution range data may also be the output of a laser range scanner, if the range scanner is inexpensive, or if the scan must be acquired quickly (range scanners typically acquire each pixel sequentially, taking up to several minutes for a high-resolution scan).

It should be possible to improve our estimate of the high spatial frequencies of the range image by using monocular cues from the high-resolution intensity (or color) image. Shape recipes [3, 9] provide one way of doing this. The basic principle of shape recipes is that a relationship between shape and light intensity could be *learned* from the low resolution image pair, and then *extrapolated* and applied to the high resolution intensity image to infer the high spatial frequencies of the range image. One advantage of this approach is that hidden variables important to inference from monocular cues, such as illumination direction and material reflectance properties, might be implicitly learned from the low-resolution range and intensity images. However, for this approach to work, we require some model of how the relationship between shape and intensity changes over scale, which we discuss below.

For shape recipes, both the high resolution intensity image and the low resolution range image are decomposed into steerable wavelet filter pyramids, linearly breaking the image down according to scale and orientation [2]. Linear regression is then used between the highest frequency band of the available low-resolution range image and the corresponding band of the intensity image, to learn a linear filter that best predicts the range band from the image band. The hypothesis of the model is that this filter can then be used to predict high frequency range bands from the high frequency image bands. We describe the implementation in more detail below.

Let $i_{m,\phi}$ and $z_{m,\phi}$ be steerable filter pyramid subbands of the intensity and range image respectively, at spatial resolution m and orientation ϕ (both are integers). Number the band levels so that $m=0$ is the highest frequency subband of the intensity image, and $m=n$ is the highest available frequency subband of the low-resolution range image. Thus, higher level numbers correspond to lower spatial frequencies. Shape recipes work by learning a linear filter $k_{n,\phi}$ at level n by minimizing sum-squared error $\sum(z_{n,\phi} - k_{n,\phi} \star i_{n,\phi})^2$, where $\star$ denotes convolution. Higher resolution subbands of the range image are inferred by:

$$\hat{z}_{m,\phi} = \frac{1}{c^{n-m}}(k_{n,\phi} \star i_{m,\phi}) \tag{1}$$

where $c = 2$. The choice of $c = 2$ in the shape recipe model is motivated by the linear Lambertian shading model [9]. We will discuss this choice of constant in section 3.

The underlying assumption of shape recipes is that the convolution kernel $k_{m,\phi}$ should be roughly constant over the four highest resolution bands of the steerable filter pyramid. This is based on the idea that shape recipe kernels should vary slowly over scale. In this section, we show mathematically that this model is internally inconsistent. To do this, we first re-express the shape recipe process in the Fourier domain. The operations of shape recipes (pyramid decomposition, convolution, and image reconstruction) are all linear operations, and so they can be combined into a single linear convolution. In other words, we can think of shape recipes as inferring the high resolution range data z_{high} via a single convolution

$$Z_{high}(u, v) = I(u, v) \cdot K_{recipe}(u, v) \qquad (2)$$

where I is the Fourier transform of the intensity image i. (In general, we will use capital letters to denote functions in the Fourier domain). K_{recipe} is a filter in the Fourier domain, of the same size as the image, whose construction is discussed below. Note that K_{recipe} is zero in the low frequency bands where Z_{low} is available. Once z_{high} (the inverse Fourier transform of Z_{high}) is estimated, it can be combined with the known low-resolution range data simply by adding them together: $z_{recipe}(x, y) = z_{low}(x, y) + z_{high}(x, y)$.

For shorthand, we will write $I(u, v)I^*(u, v)$ as $II(u, v)$ and $Z(u, v)I^*(u, v)$ as $ZI(u, v)$. II is also known as the power spectrum, and it is the Fourier transform of the autocorrelation of the intensity image. ZI is the Fourier transform of the cross-correlation between the intensity and range images, and it has both real and imaginary parts. Let $K = ZI/II$. Observe that $I \cdot K$ is a perfect reconstruction of the original high resolution range image (as long as $II(u, v) \neq 0$). Because we do not have the full-resolution range image, we can only compute the low spatial frequencies of $ZI(u, v)$. Let $K_{low} = ZI_{low}/II$, where ZI_{low} is the Fourier transform of the cross-correlation between the low-resolution range image, and a low-resolution version of the intensity image. K_{low} is zero in the high frequency bands. We can then think of K_{recipe} as an approximation of $K = ZI/II$ formed by *extrapolating* K_{low} into the higher spatial frequencies.

In the appendix, we show that shape recipes implicitly perform this extrapolation by learning the highest available frequency octave of K_{low}, and duplicating this octave into all successive octaves of K_{recipe}, multiplied by a scale factor. However, there is a problem with this approach. First, there is no reason to expect that features in the range/intensity relationship should repeat once every octave. Figure 1a shows a plot of ZI from a scene in our database of ground-truth range data (to be described in section 3). The fine structures in real$[K]$ do not duplicate themselves every octave. Second and more importantly, octave duplication violates Freeman and Torralba's assumption that shape recipe kernels should change slowly over scale, which we take to mean over *all* scales, not just over successive octaves. Even if octave 2 of K is made identical to octave 1, it is mathematically impossible for fractional octaves of K like 1.5 to also be identical unless ZI/II is completely smooth and devoid of fine structure. The fine structures in K therefore cannot possibly generalize over *all* scales.

In the next section, we use laser scans of real scenes to study the joint statistics of range and intensity images in greater detail, and use our results to form a statistically-motivated model of ZI. We believe that a greater understanding of the joint distribution of natural images and their underlying 3D structure will have a broad impact on the development of robust depth inference algorithms, and also on understanding human depth perception. More immediately, our statistical observations lead to a more accurate way to extrapolate K_{low}, which in turn results in a more accurate shape recipe method.

3   Scaling laws in natural scene statistics

To study the correlational structures between depth and intensity in natural scenes, we have collected a database of coregistered intensity and high-resolution range images (corresponding pixels of the two images correspond to the same point in space). Scans were collected using the Riegl LMS-Z360 laser range scanner with integrated color photosensor.

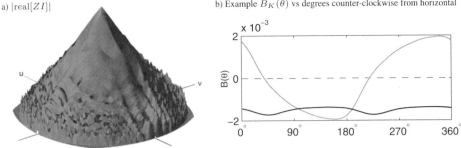

Figure 1: **a)** A log-log polar plot of $|real[ZI]|$ from a scene in our database. ZI contains extensive fine structures that do not repeat at each octave. However, along all orientations, the general form of $|real[ZI]|$ is a power-law. $|imag[ZI]|$ similarly obeys a power-law. **b)** A plot of $B_K(\theta)$ for the scene in figure 2. $real[B_K(\theta)]$ is drawn in black and $imag[B_K(\theta)]$ in grey. This plot is typical of most scenes in our database. As predicted by equation 4, $imag[B_K(\theta)]$ reaches its minima at the illumination direction (in this case, to the extreme left, almost $180°$). Also typical is that $real[B_K(\theta)]$ is uniformly negative, most likely caused by cast shadows in object concavities [6].

Scans were taken of a variety of rural and urban scenes. All images were taken outdoors, under sunny conditions, while the scanner was level with ground. The shape recipe model was intended for scenes with homogenous albedo and surface material. To test this algorithm in real scenes of this type, we selected 28 single-texture image sections from our database. These textures include statue surfaces and faceted building exteriors, such as archways and church facades (12 scenes), rocky terrain and rock piles (8), and leafy foliage (8). No logarithm or other transformation was applied to the intensity or range data (measured in meters), as this would interfere with the Lambertian model that motivates the shape recipe technique. Average size of these textures was 172,669 pixels per image.

We show a log-log polar plot of $|real[ZI(r, \theta)]|$ from one image in our database in figure 1a. As can be seen in the figure, this structure appears to closely follow a power law. We claim that ZI can be reasonably modeled by $B(\theta)/r^\alpha$, where r is spatial frequency in polar coordinates, and $B(\theta)$ is a parameter of the model (with both real and imaginary parts) that depends only on polar angle θ. We test this claim by dividing the Fourier plane into four $45°$ octants (vertical, forward diagonal, horizontal, and backward diagonal), and measuring the drop-off rate in each octant separately. For each octant, we average over the octant's included orientations and fit the result to a power-law. The resulting values of α (averaged over all 28 images) are listed in the table below:

orientation	II	$real[ZI]$	$imag[ZI]$	ZZ
horizontal	2.47 ± 0.10	3.61 ± 0.18	3.84 ± 0.19	2.84 ± 0.11
forward diagonal	2.61 ± 0.11	3.67 ± 0.17	3.95 ± 0.17	2.92 ± 0.11
vertical	2.76 ± 0.11	3.62 ± 0.15	3.61 ± 0.24	2.89 ± 0.11
backward diagonal	2.56 ± 0.09	3.69 ± 0.17	3.84 ± 0.23	2.86 ± 0.10
mean	2.60 ± 0.10	3.65 ± 0.14	3.87 ± 0.16	2.88 ± 0.10

For each octant, the correlation coefficient between the power-law fit and the actual spectrum ranged from 0.91 to 0.99, demonstrating that each octant is well-fit by a power-law (Note that averaging over orientation smooths out some fine structures in each spectrum). Furthermore, α varies little across orientations, showing that our model fits ZI closely.

The above findings predict that $K = ZI/II$ also obeys a power-law. Subtracting α_{II} from $\alpha_{real[ZI]}$ and $\alpha_{imag[ZI]}$, we find that $real[K]$ drops off at $1/r^{1.1}$ and $imag[K]$ drops off at $1/r^{1.2}$. Thus, we have that $K(r, \theta) \approx B_K(\theta)/r$.

Now that we know that K can be fit (roughly) by a $1/r$ power-law, we can offer some insight into why K tends to approximate this general form. The $1/r$ drop-off in the imaginary part of K can be explained by the linear Lambertian model of shading, with oblique lighting conditions. This argument was used by Freeman and Torralba [9] in their theoretical motivation for choosing $c = 2$. The linear Lambertian model is obtained by taking only the linear terms of the Taylor series of the Lambertian equation. Under this model, if constant albedo is assumed, and no occlusion is present, then with lighting from above, $i(x, y) = a\, \partial z/\partial y$, where a is some constant. In the Fourier domain, $I(u, v) = a2\pi jv Z(u, v)$, where $j = \sqrt{-1}$. Thus, we have that

$$ZI(r, \theta) = -\frac{j}{a2\pi\, r\sin(\theta)} II(r, \theta) \tag{3}$$

$$K(r, \theta) = -j\frac{1}{r}\frac{1}{a2\pi\sin(\theta)} \tag{4}$$

In other words, under this model, K obeys a $1/r$ power-law. This means that each octave of K is half of the octave before it. Our empirical finding that the imaginary part of K obeys a $1/r$ power-law confirms Freeman and Torralba's reasoning behind choosing $c = 2$ for shape recipes.

However, the linear Lambertian shading model predicts that only the imaginary part of ZI should obey a power-law. In fact, according to equation 3, this model predicts that the real part of ZI should be zero. Yet, in our database, the real part of ZI was typically stronger than the imaginary part. The real part of ZI is the Fourier transform of the even-symmetric part of the cross-correlation function, and it includes the direct correlation $\mathrm{cov}[i, z]$. In a previous study of the statistics of natural range images [6], we have found that darker pixels in the image tend to be farther away, resulting in significantly negative $\mathrm{cov}[i, z]$. We attributed this phenomenon to cast shadows in complex scenes: object interiors and concavities are farther away than object exteriors, and these regions are the most likely to be in shadow. This effect can be observed wherever shadows are found, such as the crevices of figure 2a. However, the effect appears strongest in complex objects with many shadows and concavities, like folds of cloth, or foliage. We found that the real part of ZI is especially likely to be strongly negative in images of foliage. Such correlation between depth and darkness has been predicted theoretically for diffuse lighting conditions, such as cloudy days, when viewed from directly above [5]. The fact that all of our images were taken under cloudless, sunny conditions and with oblique lighting from above suggests that this cue may be more important than at first realized. Psychophysical experiments have demonstrated that in the absence of all other cues, darker image regions appear farther, suggesting that the human visual system makes use of this cue for depth inference (see [6] for a review, also [10]). We believe that the $1/r$ drop-off rate observed in $\mathrm{real}[K]$ is due to the fact that concavities with smaller apertures but equal depths tend to be darker. In other words, for a given level of darkness, a smaller aperture corresponds to a more shallow hole.

4 Inference using power-law models

Armed with a better understanding of the statistics of real scenes, we are better prepared to develop successful depth inference algorithms. We now know that fine details in ZI/II do not generalize across scales, but that its coarse structure roughly follows a $1/r$ power-law. We can exploit this statistical trend directly. We can simply fit our $B_K(\theta)/r$ power law to ZI_{low}/II, and then use this estimate of K to reconstruct the high frequency range data.

Specifically, from the low-resolution range and intensity image, we compute low resolution spectra of ZI and II. From the highest frequency octave of the low-resolution images, we estimate $B_{II}(\theta)$ and $B_{ZI}(\theta)$. Any standard interpolation method will work to estimate these functions. We chose a $cos^3(\theta + \pi\phi/4)$ basis function based on steerable filters [2].

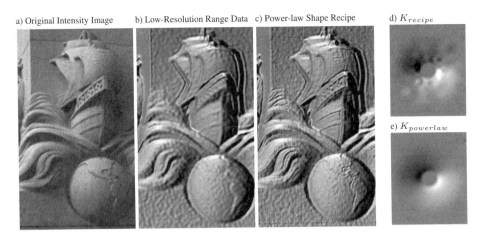

a) Original Intensity Image   b) Low-Resolution Range Data   c) Power-law Shape Recipe   d) K_{recipe}

e) $K_{powerlaw}$

Figure 2: **a)** An example intensity image from our database. **b)** A Lambertian rendering of the corresponding low resolution range image. **c)** Power-law method output. Shape recipe reconstructions show a similar amount of texture, but tests show that texture generated by the power-law method is more highly correlated with the true texture. **d)** The imaginary parts of K_{recipe} and **e)** $K_{powerlaw}$ for the same scene. Dark regions are negative, light regions are positive. The grey center region in each estimate of K corresponds to the low spatial frequencies, where range data is not inferred because it is already known. Notice that K_{recipe} oscillates over scale.

We now can estimate the high spatial frequencies of the range image, z. Define

$$K_{powerlaw}(r, \theta) = F_{high}(r) \cdot (B_{ZI}(\theta)/B_{II}(\theta))/r \tag{5}$$

$$Z_{powerlaw} = Z_{low} + I \cdot K_{powerlaw} \tag{6}$$

where F_{high} is the high-pass filter associated with the two highest resolution bands of the steerable filter pyramid of the full-resolution image.

5   Empirical evaluation

In this section, we compare the performance of shape recipes with our new approach, using our ground-truth database of high-resolution range and intensity image pairs described in section 3. For each range image in our database, a low-resolution (but still full-sized) range image, z_{low}, was generated by setting to zero the top two steerable filter pyramid layers. Both algorithms accepted as input the low-resolution range image and high-resolution intensity image, and the output was compared with the original high-resolution range image. The high resolution output corresponds to a 4-fold increase in spatial resolution (or a 16-fold increase in total size).

Although encouraging enhancements of stereo output were given by the authors, shape recipes has not been evaluated with real, ground-truth high resolution range data. To maximize its performance, we implemented shape recipes using ridge regression, with the ridge coefficient obtained using cross-validation. Linear kernels were learned (and the output evaluated) over a region of the image at least 21 pixels from the image border.

For each high-resolution output, we measured the sum squared error between the reconstruction (z_{recipe} or $z_{powerlaw}$) and the original range image (z). We compared this with the sum-squared error of the low-resolution range image z_{low} to get the percent reduction in sum-squared error: $error\_reduction_{recipe} = \frac{err_{low} - err_{recipe}}{err_{low}}$. This measure of error reflects the performance of the method independently of the variance or absolute depth of the range image. On average, shape recipe reconstructions had 1.3% less mean-squared error than z_{low}. Shape recipes improved 21 of the 28 images. Our new approach had 2.2% less mean-squared error than z_{low}, and improved 26 of the 28 images.

We cannot expect the error reduction values to be very high, partly because our images are highly complex natural scenes, and also because some noise was present in both the range and intensity images. Therefore, it is difficult to assess how much of the remaining error could be recovered by a superior algorithm, and how much is simply due to sensor noise. As a comparison, we generated an optimal linear reconstruction, z_{optlin}, by learning 11×11 shape recipe kernels for the two high resolution pyramid bands directly from the ground-truth high resolution range image. This reconstruction provides a loose upper bound on the degree of improvement possible by linear shape methods. We then measured the percentage of linearly achievable improvement for each image: $improvement_{recipe} = \frac{err_{low} - err_{recipe}}{err_{low} - err_{optlin}}$ Shape recipes yielded an average improvement of 23%. Our approach achieved an improvement of 44%, nearly a two-fold enhancement over shape recipes.

6   The relative strengths of shading and shadow cues

Earlier we showed that Lambertian shading alone predicts that the real part of ZI in natural scenes is empty of useful correlations between images and range images. Yet in our database, the real part of ZI, which we believe is related to shadow cues, was often *stronger* than the imaginary component. Our depth-inference algorithm offers an opportunity to compare the performance of shading cues versus shadow cues. We ran our algorithm again, except that we set the real part of $K_{powerlaw}$ to zero. This yielded only a 12% improvement. However, when we ran the algorithm after setting $\mathrm{imag}[K]$ to zero, 32% improvement was achieved. Thus, 72% of the algorithm's total improvement was due to shadow cues. When the database is broken down into categories, the real part of ZI is responsible for 96% of total improvement in foliage scenes, 76% in rocky terrain scenes, and 35% in urban scenes (statue surfaces and building facades). As expected, the algorithm relies more heavily on the real part of ZI in environments rich in cast shadows. These results show that shadow cues are far more useful than was previously expected, and also that they can be exploited more easily than was previously thought possible, using only simple linear relationships that might easily be incorporated into linear shape-from-shading techniques. We feel that these insights into natural scene statistics are the most important contributions of this paper.

7   Discussion

The power-law extension to shape recipes not only offers a substantial improvement in performance, but it also greatly reduces the number of parameters that must be learned. The original shape recipes required one 11×11 kernel, or 121 parameters, for each orientation of the steerable filters. The new algorithm requires only two parameters for each orientation (the real and the imaginary parts of $B_K(\theta)$). This suggests that the new approach has captured only those components of K that generalize across scales, disregarding all others.

While it is encouraging that the power-law algorithm is highly parsimonious, it also means that fewer scene properties are encoded in the shape recipe kernels than was previously hoped [3]. For example, complex properties of the material and surface reflectance cannot be encoded. We believe that the $B(\theta)$ parameter of the power-law model can be determined almost entirely by the direction of illumination and the prominence of cast shadows (see figure 1b). This suggests that the power-law algorithm of this paper would work equally well for scenes with multiple materials. To capture more complex material properties, nonlinear methods and probabilistic methods may achieve greater success. However, when designing these more sophisticated methods, care must be taken to avoid the same pitfall encountered by shape recipes: not all properties of a scene can be scale-invariant simultaneously.

8 Appendix

Shape recipes infer each high resolution band of the range using equation 1. Let $\sigma = 2^{n-m}$. If we take the Fourier transform of equation 1, we get

$$Z_{high} \cdot F_{m,\phi} = \frac{1}{c^{n-m}} K_{n,\phi} \left(\frac{u}{\sigma}, \frac{v}{\sigma} \right) \cdot (I \cdot F_{m,\phi}) \tag{7}$$

where $F_{m,\phi}$ is the Fourier transform of the steerable filter at level m and orientation ϕ, and Z_{high} is the inferred high spatial frequency components of the range image. If we take the steerable pyramid decomposition of Z_{high} and then transform it back, we get Z_{high} again, and so:

$$I \cdot K_{recipe} = Z_{high} = \sum_{m,\phi}^{m<n} Z_{high} F_{m,\phi} F_{m,\phi}^* \tag{8}$$

$$= I \sum_{m,\phi}^{m<n} \frac{1}{c^{n-m}} K_{n,\phi} \left(\frac{u}{\sigma}, \frac{v}{\sigma} \right) \cdot F_{m,\phi} \cdot F_{m,\phi}^* \tag{9}$$

The steerable filters at each level are simply a dilation of the steerable filters of preceding levels: $F_{m,\phi}(u,v) = F_{n,\phi} \left(\frac{u}{\sigma}, \frac{v}{\sigma} \right)$. Thus, recalling that $\sigma = 2^{n-m}$, we have

$$K_{recipe} = \sum_{m,\phi}^{m<n} \frac{1}{c^{n-m}} K_{n,\phi}(\frac{u}{\sigma}, \frac{v}{\sigma}) \cdot F_{n,\phi}(\frac{u}{\sigma}, \frac{v}{\sigma}) \cdot F_{n,\phi}^*(\frac{u}{\sigma}, \frac{v}{\sigma}) \tag{10}$$

The steerable filters $F_{n,\phi}$ are band-pass filters, and they are essentially zero outside of octave n. Thus, each octave of K_{recipe} is identical to the octave before it, except reduced by a constant scale factor c. In other words, shape recipes extrapolate K_{low} by copying the highest available octave of K_{low} (or some estimation of it) into each successive octave. An example of K_{recipe} can be seen in figure 2d.

This research was funded in part by NSF IIS-0413211, Penn Dept of Health-MPC 05-06-2. Brian Potetz is supported by an NSF Graduate Research Fellowship.

References

[1] J. E. Cryer, P. S. Tsai and M. Shah, "Integration of shape from shading and stereo," Pattern Recognition, 28(7):1033–1043, 1995.

[2] W. T. Freeman, E. H. Adelson, "The design and use of steerable filters," IEEE Transactions on Pattern Analysis and Machine Intelligence, **13**, 891–906 1991.

[3] W. T. Freeman and A. Torralba, "Shape Recipes: Scene representations that refer to the image," Advances in Neural Information Processing Systems 15 (NIPS), MIT Press, 2003.

[4] C. Q. Howe and D. Purves, "Range image statistics can explain the anomalous perception of length," Proc. Nat. Acad. Sci. U.S.A. **99** 13184–13188 2002.

[5] M. S. Langer and S. W. Zucker, "Shape-from-shading on a cloudy day," J. Opt. Soc. Am. A **11**, 467–478 (1994).

[6] B. Potetz, T. S. Lee, "Statistical correlations between two-dimensional images and three-dimensional structures in natural scenes," J. Opt. Soc. Amer. A, **20**, 1292–1303 2003.

[7] D. Scharstein and R. Szeliski, "A taxonomy and evaluation of dense two-frame stereo correspondence algorithms," IJCV 47(1/2/3):7–42, April-June 2002.

[8] A. Torralba, A. Oliva, "Depth estimation from image structure," IEEE Transactions on Pattern Analysis and Machine Intelligence. 24(9): 1226–1238 2002.

[9] A. Torralba and W. T. Freeman, "Properties and applications of shape recipes," IEEE Computer Society Conference on Computer Vision and Pattern Recognition, 2003.

[10] C. W. Tyler, "Diffuse illumination as a default assumption for shape-from-shading in the absence of shadows," J. Imaging Sci. Technol. **42**, 319–325 1998.

Off-policy Learning with Options and Recognizers

Doina Precup
McGill University
Montreal, QC, Canada

Richard S. Sutton
University of Alberta
Edmonton, AB, Canada

Cosmin Paduraru
University of Alberta
Edmonton, AB, Canada

Anna Koop
University of Alberta
Edmonton, AB, Canada

Satinder Singh
University of Michigan
Ann Arbor, MI, USA

Abstract

We introduce a new algorithm for off-policy temporal-difference learning with function approximation that has lower variance and requires less knowledge of the behavior policy than prior methods. We develop the notion of a *recognizer*, a filter on actions that distorts the behavior policy to produce a related target policy with low-variance importance-sampling corrections. We also consider target policies that are deviations from the state distribution of the behavior policy, such as potential temporally abstract options, which further reduces variance. This paper introduces recognizers and their potential advantages, then develops a full algorithm for linear function approximation and proves that its updates are in the same direction as on-policy TD updates, which implies asymptotic convergence. Even though our algorithm is based on importance sampling, we prove that it requires absolutely no knowledge of the behavior policy for the case of state-aggregation function approximators.

Off-policy learning is learning about one way of behaving while actually behaving in another way. For example, Q-learning is an off-policy learning method because it learns about the optimal policy while taking actions in a more exploratory fashion, e.g., according to an ε-greedy policy. Off-policy learning is of interest because only one way of selecting actions can be used at any time, but we would like to learn about many different ways of behaving from the single resultant stream of experience. For example, the options framework for temporal abstraction involves considering a variety of different ways of selecting actions. For each such option one would like to learn a model of its possible outcomes suitable for planning and other uses. Such option models have been proposed as fundamental building blocks of grounded world knowledge (Sutton, Precup & Singh, 1999; Sutton, Rafols & Koop, 2005). Using off-policy learning, one would be able to learn predictive models for many options at the same time from a single stream of experience.

Unfortunately, off-policy learning using temporal-difference methods has proven problematic when used in conjunction with function approximation. Function approximation is essential in order to handle the large state spaces that are inherent in many problem domains. Q-learning, for example, has been proven to converge to an optimal policy in the tabular case, but is unsound and may diverge in the case of linear function approximation (Baird, 1996). Precup, Sutton, and Dasgupta (2001) introduced and proved convergence for the first off-policy learning algorithm with linear function approximation. They addressed the problem of learning the expected value of a target policy based on experience generated using a different behavior policy. They used importance sampling techniques to reduce the off-policy case to the on-policy case, where existing convergence theorems apply (Tsitsiklis & Van Roy, 1997; Tadic, 2001). There are two important difficulties with that approach. First, the behavior policy needs to be stationary and known, because it is needed to compute the importance sampling corrections. Second, the importance sampling weights are often ill-conditioned. In the worst case, the variance could be infinite and convergence would not occur. The conditions required to prevent this were somewhat awkward and, even when they applied and asymptotic convergence was assured, the variance could still be high and convergence could be slow.

In this paper we address both of these problems in the context of off-policy learning for options. We introduce the notion of a *recognizer*. Rather than specifying an explicit target policy (for instance, the policy of an option), about which we want to make predictions, a recognizer specifies a condition on the actions that are selected. For example, a recognizer for the temporally extended action of picking up a cup would not specify which hand is to be used, or what the motion should be at all different positions of the cup. The recognizer would recognize a whole variety of directions of motion and poses as part of picking the cup. The advantage of this strategy is not that one might prefer a multitude of different behaviors, but that the behavior may be based on a variety of different strategies, all of which are relevant, and we would like to learn from any of them. In general, a recognizer is a function that recognizes or accepts a space of different ways of behaving and thus, can learn from a wider range of data.

Recognizers have two advantages over direct specification of a target policy: 1) they are a natural and easy way to specify a target policy for which importance sampling will be well conditioned, and 2) they do not require the behavior policy to be known. The latter is important because in many cases we may have little knowledge of the behavior policy, or a stationary behavior policy may not even exist. We show that for the case of state aggregation, even if the behavior policy is unknown, convergence to a good model is achieved.

1 Non-sequential example

The benefits of using recognizers in off-policy learning can be most easily seen in a non-sequential context with a single continuous action. Suppose you are given a sequence of sample actions $a_i \in [0, 1]$, selected i.i.d. according to probability density $b : [0, 1] \mapsto \Re^+$ (the behavior density). For example, suppose the behavior density is of the oscillatory form shown as a red line in Figure 1. For each each action, a_i, we observe a corresponding outcome, $z_i \in \Re$, a random variable whose distribution depends only on a_i. Thus the behavior density induces an outcome density. The on-policy problem is to estimate the mean m^b of the outcome density. This problem can be solved simply by averaging the sample outcomes: $\hat{m}^b = (1/n) \sum_{i=1}^{n} z_i$. The off-policy problem is to use this same data to learn what the mean would be if actions were selected in some way other than b, for example, if the actions were restricted to a designated range, such as between 0.7 and 0.9.

There are two natural ways to pose this off-policy problem. The most straightforward way is to be equally interested in all actions within the designated region. One professes to be interested in actions selected according to a target density $\pi : [0, 1] \mapsto \Re^+$, which in the example would be 5.0 between 0.7 and 0.9, and zero elsewhere, as in the dashed line in

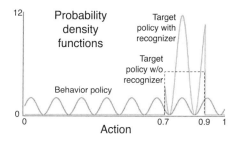

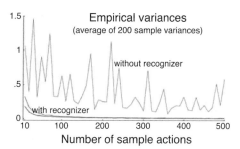

Figure 1: The left panel shows the behavior policy and the target policies for the formulations of the problem with and without recognizers. The right panel shows empirical estimates of the variances for the two formulations as a function of the number sample actions. The lowest line is for the formulation using empirically-estimated recognition probabilities.

Figure 1 (left). The importance- sampling estimate of the mean outcome is

$$\hat{m}^\pi = \frac{1}{n} \sum_{i=1}^{n} \frac{\pi(a_i)}{b(a_i)} z_i. \tag{1}$$

This approach is problematic if there are parts of the region of interest where the behavior density is zero or very nearly so, such as near 0.72 and 0.85 in the example. Here the importance sampling ratios are exceedingly large and the estimate is poorly conditioned (large variance). The upper curve in Figure 1 (right) shows the empirical variance of this estimate as a function of the number of samples. The spikes and uncertain decline of the empirical variance indicate that the distribution is very skewed and that the estimates are very poorly conditioned.

The second way to pose the problem uses recognizers. One professes to be interested in actions to the extent that they are both selected by b and within the designated region. This leads to the target policy shown in blue in the left panel of Figure 1 (it is taller because it still must sum to 1). For this problem, the variance of (1) is much smaller, as shown in the lower two lines of Figure 1 (right). To make this way of posing the problem clear, we introduce the notion of a recognizer function $c : \mathcal{A} \mapsto \mathfrak{R}^+$. The action space in the example is $\mathcal{A} = [0,1]$ and the recognizer is $c(a) = 1$ for a between 0.7 and 0.9 and is zero elsewhere. The target policy is defined in general by

$$\pi(a) = \frac{c(a)b(a)}{\sum_x c(x)b(x)} = \frac{c(a)b(a)}{\mu}. \tag{2}$$

where $\mu = \sum_x c(x)b(x)$ is a constant, equal to the probability of recognizing an action from the behavior policy. Given π, $\hat{m}^\pi$ from (1) can be rewritten in terms of the recognizer as

$$\hat{m}^\pi = \frac{1}{n} \sum_{i=1}^{n} z_i \frac{\pi(a_i)}{b(a_i)} = \frac{1}{n} \sum_{i=1}^{n} z_i \frac{c(a_i)b(a_i)}{\mu} \frac{1}{b(a_i)} = \frac{1}{n} \sum_{i=1}^{n} z_i \frac{c(a_i)}{\mu} \tag{3}$$

Note that the target density does not appear at all in the last expression and that the behavior distribution appears only in μ, which is independent of the sample action. If this constant is known, then this estimator can be computed with no knowledge of π or b. The constant μ can easily be estimated as the fraction of recognized actions in the sample. The lowest line in Figure 1 (right) shows the variance of the estimator using this fraction in place of the recognition probability. Its variance is low, no worse than that of the exact algorithm, and apparently slightly lower. Because this algorithm does not use the behavior density, it can be applied when the behavior density is unknown or does not even exist. For example, suppose actions were selected in some deterministic, systematic way that in the long run produced an empirical distribution like b. This would be problematic for the other algorithms but would require no modification of the recognition-fraction algorithm.

2 Recognizers improve conditioning of off-policy learning

The main use of recognizers is in formulating a target density π about which we can successfully learn predictions, based on the current behavior being followed. Here we formalize this intuition.

Theorem 1 *Let $A = \{a_1, \ldots a_k\} \subseteq \mathcal{A}$ be a subset of all the possible actions. Consider a fixed behavior policy b and let π_A be the class of policies that only choose actions from A, i.e., if $\pi(a) > 0$ then $a \in A$. Then the policy induced by b and the binary recognizer c_A is the policy with minimum-variance one-step importance sampling corrections, among those in π_A:*

$$\pi \text{ as given by (2)} = \arg\min_{\pi \in \pi_A} E_b \left[\left(\frac{\pi(a_i)}{b(a_i)} \right)^2 \right] \tag{4}$$

Proof: Denote $\pi(a_i) = \pi_i$, $b(a_i) = b_i$. Then the expected variance of the one-step importance sampling corrections is:

$$E_b \left[\left(\frac{\pi_i}{b_i} \right)^2 \right] - E_b^2 \left[\left(\frac{\pi_i}{b_i} \right) \right] = \sum_i b_i \left(\frac{\pi_i}{b_i} \right)^2 - 1 = \sum_i \frac{\pi_i^2}{b_i} - 1,$$

where the summation (here and everywhere below) is such that the action $a_i \in A$. We want to find π_i that minimizes this expression, subject to the constraint that $\sum_i \pi_i = 1$. This is a constrained optimization problem. To solve it, we write down the corresponding Lagrangian:

$$L(\pi_i, \beta) = \sum_i \frac{\pi_i^2}{b_i} - 1 + \beta(\sum_i \pi_i - 1)$$

We take the partial derivatives wrt π_i and β and set them to 0:

$$\frac{\partial L}{\partial \pi_i} = \pi_i \frac{2}{b_i} + \beta = 0 \Rightarrow \pi_i = -\frac{\beta b_i}{2} \tag{5}$$

$$\frac{\partial L}{\partial \beta} = \sum_i \pi_i - 1 = 0 \tag{6}$$

By taking (5) and plugging into (6), we get the following expression for β:

$$-\frac{\beta}{2} \sum_i b_i = 1 \Rightarrow \beta = -\frac{2}{\sum_i b_i}$$

By substituting β into (5) we obtain:

$$\pi_i = \frac{b_i}{\sum_i b_i}$$

This is exactly the policy induced by the recognizer defined by $c(a_i) = 1$ iff $a_i \in A$. $\diamond$

We also note that it is advantageous, from the point of view of minimizing the variance of the updates, to have recognizers that accept a broad range of actions:

Theorem 2 *Consider two binary recognizers c_1 and c_2, such that $\mu_1 > \mu_2$. Then the importance sampling corrections for c_1 have lower variance than the importance sampling corrections for c_2.*

Proof: From the previous theorem, we have the variance of a recognizer c_A:

$$Var = \sum_i \frac{\pi_i^2}{b_i} - 1 = \sum_i \left(\frac{b_i}{\sum_{j \in A} b_j} \right)^2 \frac{1}{b_i} - 1 = \frac{1}{\sum_{j \in A} b_j} - 1 = \frac{1}{\mu} - 1 \qquad \diamond$$

3   Formal framework for sequential problems

We turn now to the full case of learning about sequential decision processes with function approximation. We use the standard framework in which an agent interacts with a stochastic environment. At each time step t, the agent receives a state s_t and chooses an action a_t. We assume for the moment that actions are selected according to a fixed behavior policy, $b : S \times \mathcal{A} \to [0,1]$ where $b(s,a)$ is the probability of selecting action a in state s. The behavior policy is used to generate a sequence of experience (observations, actions and rewards). The goal is to learn, from this data, predictions about different ways of behaving. In this paper we focus on learning predictions about expected returns, but other predictions can be tackled as well (for instance, predictions of transition models for options (Sutton, Precup & Singh, 1999), or predictions specified by a TD-network (Sutton & Tanner, 2005; Sutton, Rafols & Koop, 2006)). We assume that the state space is large or continuous, and function approximation must be used to compute any values of interest. In particular, we assume a space of feature vectors Φ and a mapping $\phi : S \to \Phi$. We denote by ϕ_s the feature vector associated with s.

An option is defined as a triple $o = \langle I, \pi, \beta \rangle$ where $I \subseteq S$ is the set of states in which the option can be initiated, π is the internal policy of the option and $\beta : S \to [0,1]$ is a stochastic termination condition. In the option work (Sutton, Precup & Singh, 1999), each of these elements has to be explicitly specified and fixed in order for an option to be well defined. Here, we will instead define options implicitly, using the notion of a recognizer.

A recognizer is defined as a function $c : S \times \mathcal{A} \to [0,1]$, where $c(s,a)$ indicates to what extent the recognizer allows action a in state s. An important special case, which we treat in this paper, is that of binary recognizers. In this case, c is an indicator function, specifying a subset of actions that are allowed, or recognized, given a particular state. Note that recognizers do not specify policies; instead, they merely give restrictions on the policies that are allowed or recognized.

A recognizer c together with a behavior policy b generates a *target policy* π, where:

$$\pi(s,a) = \frac{b(s,a)c(s,a)}{\sum_x b(s,x)c(s,x)} = \frac{b(s,a)c(s,a)}{\mu(s)} \tag{7}$$

The denominator of this fraction, $\mu(s) = \sum_x b(s,x)c(s,x)$, is the *recognition probability* at s, i.e., the probability that an action will be accepted at s when behavior is generated according to b. The policy π is only defined at states for which $\mu(s) > 0$. The numerator gives the probability that action a is produced by the behavior and recognized in s. Note that if the recognizer accepts all state-action pairs, i.e. $c(s,a) = 1, \forall s,a$, then π is the same as b.

Since a recognizer and a behavior policy can specify together a target policy, we can use recognizers as a way to specify policies for options, using (7). An option can only be initiated at a state for which at least one action is recognized, so $\mu(s) > 0, \forall s \in I$. Similarly, the termination condition of such an option, β, is defined as $\beta(s) = 1$ if $\mu(s) = 0$. In other words, the option must terminate if no actions are recognized at a given state. At all other states, β can be defined between 0 and 1 as desired.

We will focus on computing the reward model of an option o, which represents the expected total return. The expected values of different features at the end of the option can be estimated similarly. The quantity that we want to compute is

$$E_o\{R(s)\} = E\{r_1 + r_2 + \ldots + r_T \mid s_0 = s, \pi, \beta\}$$

where $s \in I$, experience is generated according to the policy of the option, π, and T denotes the random variable representing the time step at which the option terminates according to β. We assume that linear function approximation is used to represent these values, i.e.

$$E_o\{R(s)\} \approx \theta^T \phi_s$$

where θ is a vector of parameters.

4 Off-policy learning algorithm

In this section we present an adaptation of the off-policy learning algorithm of Precup, Sutton & Dasgupta (2001) to the case of learning about options. Suppose that an option's policy π was used to generate behavior. In this case, learning the reward model of the option is a special case of temporal-difference learning of value functions. The forward view of this algorithm is as follows. Let $\bar{R}_t^{(n)}$ denote the truncated n-step return starting at time step t and let y_t denote the 0-step truncated return, $\bar{R}_t^{(0)}$. By the definition of the n-step truncated return, we have:

$$\bar{R}_t^{(n)} = r_{t+1} + (1 - \beta_{t+1})\bar{R}_{t+1}^{(n-1)}.$$

This is similar to the case of value functions, but it accounts for the possibility of terminating the option at time step $t+1$. The λ-return is defined in the usual way:

$$\bar{R}_t^\lambda = (1 - \lambda) \sum_{n=1}^\infty \lambda^{n-1} \bar{R}_t^{(n)}.$$

The parameters of the linear function approximator are updated on every time step proportionally to:

$$\Delta\bar{\theta}_t = \left[\bar{R}_t^\lambda - y_t\right] \nabla_\theta y_t (1 - \beta_1) \cdots (1 - \beta_t).$$

In our case, however, trajectories are generated according to the behavior policy b. The main idea of the algorithm is to use importance sampling corrections in order to account for the difference in the state distribution of the two policies.

Let $\rho_t = \frac{\pi(s_t, a_t)}{b(s_t, a_t)}$ be the importance sampling ratio at time step t. The truncated n-step return, $R_t^{(n)}$, satisfies:

$$R_t^{(n)} = \rho_t [r_{t+1} + (1 - \beta_{t+1})R_{t+1}^{(n-1)}].$$

The update to the parameter vector is proportional to:

$$\Delta\theta_t = \left[R_t^\lambda - y_t\right] \nabla_\theta y_t \rho_0 (1 - \beta_1) \cdots \rho_{t-1}(1 - \beta_t).$$

The following result shows that the expected updates of the on-policy and off-policy algorithms are the same.

Theorem 3 *For every time step $t \geq 0$ and any initial state s,*

$$E_b[\Delta\theta_t|s] = E_\pi[\Delta\bar{\theta}_t|s].$$

Proof: First we will show by induction that $E_b\{R_t^{(n)}|s\} = E_\pi\{\bar{R}_t^{(n)}|s\}, \forall n$ (which implies that $E_b\{R_t^\lambda|s\} = E_\pi(\bar{R}_t^\lambda|s\})$. For $n = 0$, the statement is trivial. Assuming that it is true for $n-1$, we have

$$
\begin{aligned}
E_b\left\{R_t^{(n)}|s\right\} &= \sum_a b(s,a) \sum_{s'} P_{ss'}^a \rho(s,a) \left[r_{ss'}^a + (1 - \beta(s'))E_b\left\{R_{t+1}^{(n-1)}|s'\right\}\right] \\
&= \sum_a \sum_{s'} P_{ss'}^a b(s,a) \frac{\pi(s,a)}{b(s,a)} \left[r_{ss'}^a + (1 - \beta(s'))E_\pi\left\{\bar{R}_{t+1}^{(n-1)}|s'\right\}\right] \\
&= \sum_a \pi(s,a) \sum_{s'} P_{ss'}^a \left[r_{ss'}^a + (1 - \beta(s'))E_\pi\left\{\bar{R}_{t+1}^{(n-1)}|s'\right\}\right] = E_\pi\left\{\bar{R}_t^{(n)}|s\right\}.
\end{aligned}
$$

Now we are ready to prove the theorem's main statement. Defining Ω_t to be the set of all trajectory components up to state s_t, we have:

$$E_b\{\Delta\theta_t|s\} = \sum_{\omega \in \Omega_t} P_b(\omega|s)E_b\left\{(R_t^\lambda - y_t)\nabla_\theta y_t|\omega\right\} \prod_{i=0}^{t-1} \rho_i(1 - \beta_{i+1})$$

$$= \sum_{\omega \in \Omega_t} \left(\prod_{i=0}^{t-1} b_i P_{s_i s_{i+1}}^{a_i} \right) \left[E_b \left\{ R_t^{\lambda} | s_t \right\} - y_t \right] \nabla_{\theta} y_t \prod_{i=0}^{t-1} \frac{\pi_i}{b_i} (1 - \beta_{i+1})$$

$$= \sum_{\omega \in \Omega_t} \left(\prod_{i=0}^{t-1} \pi_i P_{s_i s_{i+1}}^{a_i} \right) \left[E_{\pi} \left\{ \bar{R}_t^{\lambda} | s_t \right\} - y_t \right] \nabla_{\theta} y_t (1 - \beta_1) \ldots (1 - \beta_t)$$

$$= \sum_{\omega \in \Omega_t} P_{\pi}(\omega | s) E_{\pi} \left\{ (\bar{R}_t^{\lambda} - y_t) \nabla_{\theta} y_t | \omega \right\} (1 - \beta_1) \ldots (1 - \beta_t) = E_{\pi} \left\{ \Delta \bar{\theta}_t | s \right\}.$$

Note that we are able to use s_t and ω interchangeably because of the Markov property. $\diamond$

Since we have shown that $E_b[\Delta \theta_t | s] = E_{\pi}[\Delta \bar{\theta}_t | s]$ for any state s, it follows that the expected updates will also be equal for any distribution of the initial state s. When learning the model of options with data generated from the behavior policy b, the starting state distribution with respect to which the learning is performed, I_0 is determined by the stationary distribution of the behavior policy, as well as the initiation set of the option I. We note also that the importance sampling corrections only have to be performed for the trajectory since the initiation of the updates for the option. No corrections are required for the experience prior to this point. This should generate updates that have significantly lower variance than in the case of learning values of policies (Precup, Sutton & Dasgupta, 2001).

Because of the termination condition of the option, β, $\Delta\theta$ can quickly decay to zero. To avoid this problem, we can use a *restart function* $g : S \rightarrow [0,1]$, such that $g(s_t)$ specifies the extent to which the updating episode is considered to start at time t. Adding restarts generates a new forward update:

$$\Delta\theta_t = (R_t^{\lambda} - y_t) \nabla_{\theta} y_t \sum_{i=0}^{t} g_i \rho_i \ldots \rho_{t-1} (1 - \beta_{i+1}) \ldots (1 - \beta_t), \qquad (8)$$

where R_t^{λ} is the same as above. With an adaptation of the proof in Precup, Sutton & Dasgupta (2001), we can show that we get the same expected value of updates by applying this algorithm from the original starting distribution as we would by applying the algorithm without restarts from a starting distribution defined by I_0 and g. We can turn this forward algorithm into an incremental, backward view algorithm in the following way:

- Initialize $k_0 = g_0, e_0 = k_0 \nabla_{\theta} y_0$
- At every time step t:

$$\delta_t = \rho_t (r_{t+1} + (1 - \beta_{t+1}) y_{t+1}) - y_t$$
$$\theta_{t+1} = \theta_t + \alpha \delta_t e_t$$
$$k_{t+1} = \rho_t k_t (1 - \beta_{t+1}) + g_{t+1}$$
$$e_{t+1} = \lambda \rho_t (1 - \beta_{t+1}) e_t + k_{t+1} \nabla_{\theta} y_{t+1}$$

Using a similar technique to that of Precup, Sutton & Dasgupta (2001) and Sutton & Barto (1998), we can prove that the forward and backward algorithm are equivalent (omitted due to lack of space). This algorithm is guaranteed to converge if the variance of the updates is finite (Precup, Sutton & Dasgupta, 2001). In the case of options, the termination condition β can be used to ensure that this is the case.

5   Learning when the behavior policy is unknown

In this section, we consider the case in which the behavior policy is unknown. This case is generally problematic for importance sampling algorithms, but the use of recognizers will allow us to define importance sampling corrections, as well as a convergent algorithm. Recall that when using a recognizer, the target policy of the option is defined as:

$$\pi(s,a) = \frac{c(s,a) b(s,a)}{\mu(s)}$$

and the recognition probability becomes:

$$\rho(s,a) = \frac{\pi(s,a)}{b(s,a)} = \frac{c(s,a)}{\mu(s)}$$

Of course, $\mu(s)$ depends on b. If b is unknown, instead of $\mu(s)$, we will use a maximum likelihood estimate $\hat{\mu} : S \to [0,1]$. The structure used to compute $\hat{\mu}$ will have to be compatible with the feature space used to represent the reward model. We will make this more precise below. Likewise, the recognizer $c(s,a)$ will have to be defined in terms of the features used to represent the model. We will then define the importance sampling corrections as:

$$\hat{\rho}(s,a) = \frac{c(s,a)}{\hat{\mu}(s)}$$

We consider the case in which the function approximator used to model the option is actually a state aggregator. In this case, we will define recognizers which behave consistently in each partition, i.e., $c(s,a) = c(p,a), \forall s \in p$. This means that an action is either recognized or not recognized in all states of the partition. The recognition probability $\hat{\mu}$ will have one entry for every partition p of the state space. Its value will be:

$$\hat{\mu}(p) = \frac{N(p, c = 1)}{N(p)}$$

where $N(p)$ is the number of times partition p was visited, and $N(p, c = 1)$ is the number of times the action taken in p was recognized. In the limit, w.p.1, $\hat{\mu}$ converges to $\sum_s d^b(s|p) \sum_a c(p,a) b(s,a)$ where $d^b(s|p)$ is the probability of visiting state s from partition p under the stationary distribution of b. At this limit, $\hat{\pi}(s,a) = \hat{\rho}(s,a) b(s,a)$ will be a well-defined policy (i.e., $\sum_a \hat{\pi}(s,a) = 1$). Using Theorem 3, off-policy updates using importance sampling corrections $\hat{\rho}$ will have the same expected value as on-policy updates using $\hat{\pi}$. Note though that the learning algorithm never uses $\hat{\pi}$; the only quantities needed are $\hat{\rho}$, which are learned incrementally from data.

For the case of general linear function approximation, we conjecture that a similar idea can be used, where the recognition probability is learned using logistic regression. The development of this part is left for future work.

Acknowledgements

The authors gratefully acknowledge the ideas and encouragement they have received in this work from Eddie Rafols, Mark Ring, Lihong Li and other members of the rlai.net group. We thank Csaba Szepesvari and the reviewers of the paper for constructive comments. This research was supported in part by iCore, NSERC, Alberta Ingenuity, and CFI.

References

Baird, L. C. (1995). Residual algorithms: Reinforcement learning with function approximation. In *Proceedings of ICML*.

Precup, D., Sutton, R. S. and Dasgupta, S. (2001). Off-policy temporal-difference learning with function approximation. In *Proceedings of ICML*.

Sutton, R.S., Precup D. and Singh, S (1999). Between MDPs and semi-MDPs: A framework for temporal abstraction in reinforcement learning. *Artificial Intelligence*, vol . 112, pp. 181–211.

Sutton,, R.S. and Tanner, B. (2005). Temporal-difference networks. In *Proceedings of NIPS-17*.

Sutton R.S., Raffols E. and Koop, A. (2006). Temporal abstraction in temporal-difference networks". In *Proceedings of NIPS-18*.

Tadic, V. (2001). On the convergence of temporal-difference learning with linear function approximation. In *Machine learning* vol. 42, pp. 241-267.

Tsitsiklis, J. N., and Van Roy, B. (1997). An analysis of temporal-difference learning with function approximation. *IEEE Transactions on Automatic Control* 42:674–690.

Estimation of Intrinsic Dimensionality Using High-Rate Vector Quantization

Maxim Raginsky and Svetlana Lazebnik
Beckman Institute, University of Illinois
405 N Mathews Ave, Urbana, IL 61801
{maxim,slazebni}@uiuc.edu

Abstract

We introduce a technique for dimensionality estimation based on the notion of *quantization dimension*, which connects the asymptotic optimal quantization error for a probability distribution on a manifold to its intrinsic dimension. The definition of quantization dimension yields a family of estimation algorithms, whose limiting case is equivalent to a recent method based on packing numbers. Using the formalism of high-rate vector quantization, we address issues of statistical consistency and analyze the behavior of our scheme in the presence of noise.

1. Introduction

The goal of *nonlinear dimensionality reduction* (NLDR) [1, 2, 3] is to find low-dimensional manifold descriptions of high-dimensional data. Most NLDR schemes require a good estimate of the intrinsic dimensionality of the data to be available in advance. A number of existing methods for estimating the intrinsic dimension (e.g., [3, 4, 5]) rely on the fact that, for data uniformly distributed on a d-dimensional compact smooth submanifold of $\mathbb{R}^D$, the probability of a small ball of radius ϵ around any point on the manifold is $\Theta(\epsilon^d)$. In this paper, we connect this argument with the notion of *quantization dimension* [6, 7], which relates the intrinsic dimension of a manifold (a *topological* property) to the asymptotic optimal quantization error for distributions on the manifold (an *operational* property). Quantization dimension was originally introduced as a theoretical tool for studying "nonstandard" signals, such as singular distributions [6] or fractals [7]. However, to the best of our knowledge, it has not been previously used for dimension estimation in manifold learning. The definition of quantization dimension leads to a family of dimensionality estimation algorithms, parametrized by the *distortion exponent* $r \in [1, \infty)$, yielding in the limit of $r = \infty$ a scheme equivalent to Kégl's recent technique based on packing numbers [4].

To date, many theoretical aspects of intrinsic dimensionality estimation remain poorly understood. For instance, while the estimator bias and variance are assessed either heuristically [4] or exactly [5], scant attention is paid to robustness of each particular scheme against noise. Moreover, existing schemes do not fully utilize the potential for statistical consistency afforded by ergodicity of i.i.d. data: they compute the dimensionality estimate from a fixed training sequence (typically, the entire dataset of interest), whereas we show that an independent *test sequence* is necessary to avoid overfitting. In addition, using the framework of high-rate vector quantization allows us to analyze the performance of our scheme in the presence of noise.

2. Quantization-based estimation of intrinsic dimension

Let us begin by introducing the definitions and notation used in the rest of the paper. A *D-dimensional k-point vector quantizer* [6] is a measurable map $Q_k : \mathbb{R}^D \to \mathcal{C}$, where $\mathcal{C} = \{y_1, \ldots, y_k\} \subset \mathbb{R}^D$ is called the *codebook* and the y_i's are called the *codevectors*. The number $\log_2 k$ is called the *rate* of the quantizer, in bits per vector. The sets $R_i \triangleq \{x \in \mathbb{R}^D : Q_k(x) = y_i\}, 1 \leq i \leq k$, are called the *quantizer cells* (or *partition regions*). The quantizer performance on a random vector X distributed according to a probability distribution μ (denoted $X \sim \mu$) is measured by the *average rth-power distortion* $\delta_r(Q_k|\mu) \triangleq \mathbb{E}_\mu \|X - Q_k(X)\|^r$, $r \in [1, \infty)$, where $\|\cdot\|$ is the Euclidean norm on $\mathbb{R}^D$. In the sequel, we will often find it more convenient to work with the *quantizer error* $e_r(Q_k|\mu) \triangleq \delta_r(Q_k|\mu)^{1/r}$. Let $\mathcal{Q}_k$ denote the set of all D-dimensional k-point quantizers. Then the performance achieved by an *optimal k-point quantizer* on X is $\delta_r^*(k|\mu) \triangleq \inf_{Q_k \in \mathcal{Q}_k} \delta_r(Q_k|\mu)$ or equivalently, $e_r^*(k|\mu) \triangleq \delta_r^*(k|\mu)^{1/r}$.

2.1. Quantization dimension

The dimensionality estimation method presented in this paper exploits the connection between the intrinsic dimension d of a smooth compact manifold $M \subset \mathbb{R}^D$ (from now on, simply referred to as "manifold") and the asymptotic optimal quantization error for a regular probability distribution[1] on M. When the quantizer rate is high, the partition cells can be well approximated by D-dimensional balls around the codevectors. Then the regularity of μ ensures that the probability of such a ball of radius ϵ is $\Theta(\epsilon^d)$, and it can be shown [7, 6] that $e_r^*(k|\mu) = \Theta(k^{-1/d})$. This is referred to as the *high-rate* (or *high-resolution*) *approximation*, and motivates the definition of *quantization dimension* of order r:

$$d_r(\mu) \triangleq -\lim_{k \to \infty} \frac{\log k}{\log e_r^*(k|\mu)}.$$

The theory of high-rate quantization confirms that, for a regular μ supported on the manifold M, $d_r(\mu)$ exists for all $1 \leq r \leq \infty$ and equals the intrinsic dimension of M [7, 6]. (The $r = \infty$ limit will be treated in Sec. 2.2.)

This definition immediately suggests an empirical procedure for estimating the intrinsic dimension of a manifold from a set of samples. Let $X^n = (X_1, \ldots, X_n)$ be n i.i.d. samples from an unknown regular distribution μ on the manifold. We also fix some $r \in [1, \infty)$. Briefly, we select a range $k_1 \leq k \leq k_2$ of codebook sizes for which the high-rate approximation holds (see Sec. 3 for implementation details), and design a sequence of quantizers $\{\hat{Q}_k\}_{k=k_1}^{k_2}$ that give us good approximations $\hat{e}_r(k|\mu)$ to the optimal error $e_r^*(k|\mu)$ over the chosen range of k. Then an estimate of the intrinsic dimension is obtained by plotting $\log k$ vs. $-\log \hat{e}_r(k|\mu)$ and measuring the slope of the plot over the chosen range of k (because the high-rate approximation holds, the plot is linear).

This method hinges on estimating reliably the optimal errors $e_r^*(k|\mu)$. Let us explain how this can be achieved. The ideal quantizer for each k should minimize the *training error*

$$e_r(Q_k|\mu_{\text{train}}) = \left(\frac{1}{n} \sum_{i=1}^n \|X_i - Q_k(X_i)\|^r \right)^{1/r},$$

---

[1] A probability distribution μ on $\mathbb{R}^D$ is *regular of dimension d* [6] if it has compact support and if there exist constants $c, \epsilon_0 > 0$, such that $c^{-1}\epsilon^d \leq \mu(B(a, \epsilon)) \leq c\epsilon^d$ for all $a \in \text{supp}(\mu)$ and all $\epsilon \in (0, \epsilon_0)$, where $B(a, \epsilon)$ is the open ball of radius ϵ centered at a. If $M \subset \mathbb{R}^D$ is a d-dimensional smooth compact manifold, then any μ with $M = \text{supp}(\mu)$ that possesses a smooth, strictly positive density w.r.t. the normalized surface measure on M is regular of dimension d.

where μ_{train} is the corresponding empirical distribution. However, finding this *empirically optimal* quantizer is, in general, an intractable problem, so in practice we merely strive to produce a quantizer $\hat{Q}_k$ whose error $e_r(\hat{Q}_k|\mu_{\text{train}})$ is a good approximation to the *minimal empirical error* $e_r^*(k|\mu_{\text{train}}) \triangleq \inf_{Q_k \in \mathcal{Q}_k} e_r(Q_k|\mu_{\text{train}})$ (the issue of quantizer design is discussed in Sec. 3). However, while minimizing the training error is necessary for obtaining a statistically consistent approximation to an optimal quantizer for μ, the training error itself is an optimistically biased estimate of $e_r^*(k|\mu)$ [8]: intuitively, this is due to the fact that an empirically designed quantizer overfits the training set. A less biased estimate is given by the performance of $\hat{Q}_k$ on a *test sequence* independent from the training set. Let $Z^m = (Z_1, \ldots, Z_m)$ be m i.i.d. samples from μ, independent from X^n. Provided m is sufficiently large, the law of large numbers guarantees that the empirical average

$$e_r(\hat{Q}_k|\mu_{\text{test}}) = \left(\frac{1}{m} \sum_{i=1}^m \|Z_i - \hat{Q}_k(Z_i)\|^r \right)^{1/r}$$

will be a good estimate of the *test error* $e_r(\hat{Q}_k|\mu)$. Using learning-theoretic formalism [8], one can show that the test error of an empirically optimal quantizer is a *strongly consistent* estimate of $e_r^*(k|\mu)$, i.e., it converges almost surely to $e_r^*(k|\mu)$ as $n \to \infty$. Thus, we take $\hat{e}_r(k|\mu) = e_r(\hat{Q}_k|\mu_{\text{test}})$. In practice, therefore, the proposed scheme is statistically consistent to the extent that $\hat{Q}_k$ is close to the optimum.

2.2. The $r = \infty$ limit and packing numbers

If the support of μ is compact (which is the case with all probability distributions considered in this paper), then the limit $e_\infty(Q_k|\mu) = \lim_{r \to \infty} e_r(Q_k|\mu)$ exists and gives the "worst-case" quantization error of X by Q_k:

$$e_\infty(Q_k|\mu) = \max_{x \in \text{supp}(\mu)} \|x - Q_k(x)\|.$$

The optimum $e_\infty^*(k|\mu) = \inf_{Q_k \in \mathcal{Q}_k} e_\infty(Q_k|\mu)$ has an interesting interpretation as the smallest covering radius of the most parsimonious covering of $\text{supp}(\mu)$ by k or fewer balls of equal radii [6]. Let us describe how the $r = \infty$ case is equivalent to dimensionality estimation using packing numbers [4]. The *covering number* $N_M(\epsilon)$ of a manifold $M \subset \mathbb{R}^D$ is defined as the size of the smallest covering of M by balls of radius $\epsilon > 0$, while the *packing number* $P_M(\epsilon)$ is the cardinality of the maximal set $S \subset M$ with $\|x - y\| \geq \epsilon$ for all distinct $x, y \in S$. If d is the dimension of M, then $N_M(\epsilon) = \Theta(\epsilon^{-d})$ for small enough ϵ, leading to the definition of the *capacity dimension*: $d_{\text{cap}}(M) \triangleq -\lim_{\epsilon \to 0} \frac{\log N_M(\epsilon)}{\log \epsilon}$. If this limit exists, then it equals the intrinsic dimension of M. Alternatively, Kégl [4] suggests using the easily proved inequality $N_M(\epsilon) \leq P_M(\epsilon) \leq N_M(\epsilon/2)$ to express the capacity dimension in terms of packing numbers as $d_{\text{cap}}(M) = -\lim_{\epsilon \to 0} \frac{\log P_M(\epsilon)}{\log \epsilon}$.

Now, a simple geometric argument shows that, for any μ supported on M, $P_M(e_\infty^*(k|\mu)) > k$ [6]. On the other hand, $N_M(e_\infty^*(k|\mu)) \leq k$, which implies that $P_M(2e_\infty^*(k|\mu)) \leq k$. Let $\{\epsilon_k\}$ be a sequence of positive reals converging to zero, such that $\epsilon_k = e_\infty^*(k|\mu)$. Let k_0 be such that $\log \epsilon_k < 0$ for all $k \geq k_0$. Then it is not hard to show that

$$-\frac{\log P_M(2\epsilon_k)}{\log 2\epsilon_k - 1} \leq -\frac{\log k}{\log e_\infty^*(k|\mu)} < -\frac{\log P_M(\epsilon_k)}{\log \epsilon_k}, \qquad k \geq k_0.$$

In other words, there exists a decreasing sequence $\{\epsilon_k\}$, such that for sufficiently large values of k (i.e., in the high-rate regime) the ratio $-\log k / \log e_\infty^*(k|\mu)$ can be approximated increasingly finely both from below and from above by quantities involving the packing numbers $P_M(\epsilon_k)$ and $P_M(2\epsilon_k)$ and converging to the common value $d_{\text{cap}}(M)$.

This demonstrates that the $r = \infty$ case of our scheme is numerically equivalent to Kégl's method based on packing numbers.

For a finite training set, the $r = \infty$ case requires us to find an empirically optimal k-point quantizer w.r.t. the worst-case ℓ_2 error — a task that is much more computationally complex than for the $r = 2$ case (see Sec. 3 for details). In addition to computational efficiency, other important practical considerations include sensitivity to sampling density and noise. In theory, this worst-case quantizer is completely insensitive to variations in sampling density, since the optimal error $e_\infty^*(k|\mu)$ is the same for all μ with the same support. However, this advantage is offset in practice by the increased sensitivity of the $r = \infty$ scheme to noise, as explained next.

2.3. Estimation with noisy data

Random noise transforms "clean" data distributed according to μ into "noisy" data distributed according to some other distribution ν. This will cause the empirically designed quantizer to be matched to the noisy distribution ν, whereas our aim is to estimate optimal quantizer performance on the original clean data. To do this, we make use of the rth-order *Wasserstein distance* [6] between μ and ν, defined as $\bar{\rho}_r(\mu, \nu) \overset{\triangle}{=} \inf_{X \sim \mu, Y \sim \nu}(\mathrm{E}\,\|X - Y\|^r)^{1/r}$, $r \in [1, \infty)$, where the infimum is taken over all pairs (X, Y) of jointly distributed random variables with the respective marginals μ and ν. It is a natural measure of *quantizer mismatch*, i.e., the difference in performance that results from using a quantizer matched to ν on data distributed according to μ [9]. Let ν_n denote the empirical distribution of n i.i.d. samples of ν. It is possible to show (details omitted for lack of space) that for an empirically optimal k-point quantizer $Q_{k,r}^*$ trained on n samples of ν, $|e_r(Q_{k,r}^*|\nu) - e_r^*(k|\mu)| \leq 2\bar{\rho}_r(\nu_n, \nu) + \bar{\rho}_r(\mu, \nu)$. Moreover, ν_n converges to ν in the Wasserstein sense [6]: $\lim_{n \to \infty} \bar{\rho}_r(\nu_n, \nu) = 0$. Thus, provided the training set is sufficiently large, the distortion estimation error is controlled by $\bar{\rho}_r(\mu, \nu)$.

Consider the case of isotropic additive Gaussian noise. Let W be a D-dimensional zero-mean Gaussian with covariance matrix $K = \sigma^2 I_D$, where I_D is the $D \times D$ identity matrix. The noisy data are described by the random variable $X + W = Y \sim \nu$, and

$$\bar{\rho}_r(\mu, \nu) \leq \sqrt{2}\sigma \left[\frac{\Gamma((r + D)/2)}{\Gamma(D/2)} \right]^{1/r},$$

where Γ is the gamma function. In particular, $\bar{\rho}_2(\mu, \nu) \leq \sigma\sqrt{D}$. The magnitude of the bound, and hence the worst-case sensitivity of the estimation procedure to noise, is controlled by the noise variance, by the extrinsic dimension, and by the distortion exponent. The factor involving the gamma functions grows without bound both as $D \to \infty$ and as $r \to \infty$, which suggests that the susceptibility of our algorithm to noise increases with the extrinsic dimension of the data and with the distortion exponent.

3. Experimental results

We have evaluated our quantization-based scheme for two choices of the distortion exponent, $r = 2$ and $r = \infty$. For $r = 2$, we used the k-means algorithm to design the quantizers. For $r = \infty$, we have implemented a Lloyd-type algorithm, which alternates two steps: (1) the *minimum-distortion encoder*, where each sample X_i is mapped to its nearest neighbor in the current codebook, and (2) the *centroid decoder*, where the center of each region is recomputed as the center of the minimum enclosing ball of the samples assigned to that region. It is clear that the decoder step locally minimizes the worst-case error (the largest distance of any sample from the center). Using a simple randomized algorithm, the minimum enclosing ball can be found in $O((D + 1)!(D + 1)N)$ time, where N is the number of samples in the region [10]. Because of this dependence on D, the running time of the Lloyd algorithm becomes prohibitive in high dimensions, and even for $D < 10$ it is an

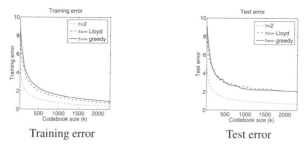

Training error   Test error

Figure 1: Training and test error vs. codebook size on the swiss roll (Figure 2 (a)). Dashed line: $r = 2$ (k-means), dash-dot: $r = \infty$ (Lloyd-type), solid: $r = \infty$ (greedy).

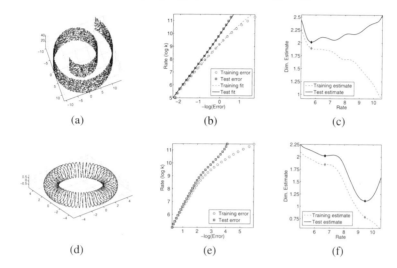

Figure 2: (a) The swiss roll (20,000 samples). (b) Plot of rate vs. negative log of the quantizer error (log-log curves), together with parametric curves fitted using linear least squares (see text). (c) Slope (dimension) estimates: 1.88 (training) and 2.04 (test). (d) Toroidal spiral (20,000 samples). (e) Log-log curves, exhibiting two distinct linear parts. (f) Dimension estimates: 1.04 (training), 2.02 (test) in the low-rate region, 0.79 (training), 1.11 (test) in the high-rate region.

order of magnitude slower than k-means. Thus, we were compelled to also implement a greedy algorithm reminiscent of Kégl's algorithm for estimating the packing number [4]: supposing that $k-1$ codevectors have already been selected, the kth one is chosen to be the sample point with the largest distance from the nearest codevector. Because this is the point that gives the worst-case error for codebook size $k-1$, adding it to the codebook lowers the error. We generate several codebooks, initialized with different random samples, and then choose the one with the smallest error. For the experiment shown in Figure 3, the training error curves produced by this greedy algorithm were on average 21% higher than those of the Lloyd algorithm, but the test curves were only 8% higher. In many cases, the two test curves are visually almost coincident (Figure 1). Therefore, in the sequel, we report only the results for the greedy algorithm for the $r = \infty$ case.

Our first synthetic dataset (Fig. 2 (a)) is the 2D "swiss roll" embedded in $\mathbb{R}^3$ [2]. We split the samples into 4 equal parts and use each part in turn for training and the rest for testing. This cross-validation setup produces four sets of error curves, which we average to obtain an improved estimate. We sample quantizer rates in increments of 0.1 bits. The lowest rate is 5 bits, and the highest rate is chosen as $\log(n/2)$, where n is the size of the training set.

The high-rate approximation suggests the asymptotic form $\Theta(k^{-1/d})$ for the quantizer error as a function of codebook size k. To validate this approximation, we use linear least squares to fit curves of the form $a + b\,k^{-1/2}$ to the $r = 2$ training and test distortion curves for the the swiss roll. The fitting procedure yields estimates of $-0.22 + 29.70k^{-1/2}$ and $0.10 + 28.41k^{-1/2}$ for the training and test curves, respectively. These estimates fit the observed data well, as shown in Fig. 2(b), a plot of rate vs. the negative logarithm of the training and test error ("log-log curves" in the following). Note that the additive constant for the training error is negative, reflecting the fact that the training error of the empirical quantizer is identically zero when $n = k$ (each sample becomes a codevector). On the other hand, the test error has a positive additive constant as a consequence of quantizer suboptimality. Significantly, the fit deteriorates as $n/k \to 1$, as the average number of training samples per quantizer cell becomes too small to sustain the exponentially slow decay required for the high-rate approximation.

Fig. 2(c) shows the slopes of the training and test log-log curves, obtained by fitting a line to each successive set of 10 points. These slopes are, in effect, rate-dependent dimensionality estimates for the dataset. Note that the training slope is always below the test slope; this is a consequence of the "optimism" of the training error and the "pessimism" of the test error (as reflected in the additive constants of the parametric fits). The shapes of the two slope curves are typical of many "well-behaved" datasets. At low rates, both the training and the test slopes are close to the extrinsic dimension, reflecting the global geometry of the dataset. As rate increases, the local manifold structure is revealed, and the slope yields its intrinsic dimension. However, as $n/k \to 1$, the quantizer begins to "see" isolated samples instead of the manifold structure. Thus, the training slope begins to fall to zero, and the test slope rises, reflecting the failure of the quantizer to generalize to the test set. For most datasets in our experiments, a good intrinsic dimensionality estimate is given by the first minimum of the test slope where the line-fitting residual is sufficiently low (marked by a diamond in Fig. 2(c)). For completeness, we also report the slope of the training curve at the same rate (note that the training curve may not have local minima because of its tendency to fall as the rate increases). Interestingly, some datasets yield several well-defined dimensionality estimates at different rates. Fig. 2(d) shows a toroidal spiral embedded in $\mathbb{R}^3$, which at larger scales "looks" like a torus, while at smaller scales the 1D curve structure becomes more apparent. Accordingly, the log-log plot of the test error (Fig. 2(e)) has two distinct linear parts, yielding dimension estimates of 2.02 and 1.11, respectively (Fig. 2(f)).

Recall from Sec. 2.1 that the high-rate approximation for regular probability distributions is based on the assumption that the intersection of each quantizer cell with the manifold is a d-dimensional neighborhood of that manifold. Because we compute our dimensionality estimate at a rate for which this approximation is valid, we know that the empirically optimal quantizer at this rate partitions the data into clusters that are locally d-dimensional. Thus, our dimensionality estimation procedure is also useful for finding a clustering of the data that respects the intrinsic neighborhood structure of the manifold from which it is sampled. As an expample, for the toroidal spiral of Fig. 2(c), we obtain two distinct dimensionality estimates of 2 and 1 at rates 6.6 and 9.4, respectively (Fig. 2(f)). Accordingly, quantizing the spiral at the lower (resp. higher) rate yields clusters that are locally two-dimensional (resp. one-dimensional).

To ascertain the effect of noise and extrinsic dimension on our method, we have embedded the swiss roll in dimensions 4 to 8 by zero-padding the coordinates and applying a random orthogonal matrix, and added isotropic zero-mean Gaussian noise in the high-dimensional space, with $\sigma = 0.2, 0.4, \dots, 1$. First, we have verified that the $r = 2$ estimator behaves in agreement with the Wasserstein bound from Sec. 2.3. The top part of Fig. 3(a) shows the maximum differences between the noisy and the noiseless test error curves for each combination of D and σ, and the bottom part shows the corresponding values of the Wasserstein bound $\sigma\sqrt{D}$ for comparison. For each value of σ, the test error of the empirically designed quantizer differs from the noiseless case by $O(\sqrt{D})$, while, for a fixed D, the difference

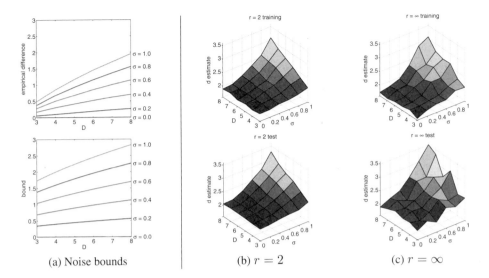

| (a) Noise bounds | (b) $r = 2$ | (c) $r = \infty$ |

Figure 3: (a) Top: empirically observed differences between noisy and noiseless test curves; bottom: theoretically derived bound $\left(\sigma\sqrt{D}\right)$. (b) Height plot of dimension estimates for the $r = 2$ algorithm as a function of D and σ. Top: training estimates, bottom: test estimates. (c) Dimension estimates for $r = \infty$. Top: training, bottom: test. Note that the training estimates are consistently lower than the test estimates: the average difference is 0.17 (resp. 0.28) for the $r = 2$ (resp. $r = \infty$) case.

of the noisy and noiseless test errors grows as $O(\sigma)$. As predicted by the bound, the additive constant in the parametric form of the test error increases with σ, resulting in larger slopes of the log-log curve and therefore higher dimension estimates. This is reflected in Figs. 3(b) and (c), which show training and test dimensionality estimates for $r = 2$ and $r = \infty$, respectively. The $r = \infty$ estimates are much less stable than those for $r = 2$ because the $r = \infty$ (worst-case) error is controlled by outliers and often stays constant over a range of rates. The piecewise-constant shape of the test error curves (see Fig. 1) results in log-log plots with unstable slopes.

Table 1 shows a comparative evaluation on the MNIST handwritten digits database[2] and a face video.[3] The MNIST database contains 70,000 images at resolution 28×28 $(D = 784)$, and the face video has 1965 frames at resolution 28×20 $(D = 560)$. For each of the resulting 11 datasets (taking each digit separately), we used half the samples for training and half for testing. The first row of the table shows dimension estimates obtained using a baseline regression method [3]: for each sample point, a local estimate is given by the first local minimum of the curve $\frac{\mathrm{d} \log \ell}{\mathrm{d} \log \epsilon(\ell)}$, where $\epsilon(\ell)$ is the distance from the point to its ℓth nearest neighbor, and a global estimate is then obtained by averaging the local estimates. The rest of the table shows the estimates obtained from the training and test curves of the $r = 2$ quantizer and the (greedy) $r = \infty$ quantizer. Comparative examination of the results shows that the $r = \infty$ estimates tend to be fairly low, which is consistent with the experimental findings of Kégl [4]. By contrast, the $r = 2$ estimates seem to be most resistant to negative bias. The relatively high values of the dimension estimates reflect the many degrees of freedom found in handwritten digits, including different scale, slant and thickness of the strokes, as well as the presence of topological features (i.e., loops in 2's or extra horizontal bars in 7's). The lowest dimensionality is found for 1's, while the highest is found for 8's, reflecting the relative complexities of different digits. For the face dataset, the different dimensionality estimates range from 4.25 to 8.30. This dataset certainly contains enough degrees of freedom to justify such high estimates, including changes in pose

---

[2]http://yann.lecun.com/exdb/mnist/
[3]http://www.cs.toronto.edu/~roweis/data.html, B. Frey and S. Roweis.

Table 1: Performance on the MNIST dataset and on the Frey faces dataset.

	Handwritten digits (MNIST data set)										Faces
	0	1	2	3	4	5	6	7	8	9	
# samples	6903	7877	6990	7141	6824	6313	6876	7293	6825	6958	1965
Regression	11.14	7.86	12.79	13.39	11.98	13.05	11.19	10.42	13.79	11.26	5.63
$r = 2$ train	12.39	6.51	16.04	15.38	13.22	14.63	12.05	12.32	19.80	13.44	5.70
$r = 2$ test	15.47	7.11	20.89	19.78	16.79	19.80	16.02	16.02	20.07	17.46	8.30
$r = \infty$ train	10.33	8.19	10.15	12.63	9.87	8.49	9.85	8.10	10.88	7.40	4.25
$r = \infty$ test	9.02	6.61	13.98	12.21	7.26	10.46	9.08	9.92	14.03	9.59	6.39

and facial expression, as well as camera jitter.[4] Finally, for both the digits and the faces, significant noise in the dataset additionally inflated the estimates.

4. Discussion

We have demonstrated an approach to intrinsic dimensionality estimation based on high-rate vector quantization. A crucial distinguishing feature of our method is the use of an independent test sequence to ensure statistical consistency and avoid underestimating the dimension. Many existing methods are well-known to exhibit a negative bias in high dimensions [4, 5]. This can have serious implications in practice, as it may result in low-dimensional representations that lose essential features of the data. Our results raise the possibility that this negative bias may be indicative of overfitting. In the future we plan to integrate our proposed method into a unified package of quantization-based algorithms for estimating the intrinsic dimension of the data, obtaining its dimension-reduced manifold representation, and compressing the low-dimensional data [11].

Acknowledgments

Maxim Raginsky was supported by the Beckman Institute Postdoctoral Fellowship. Svetlana Lazebnik was partially supported by the National Science Foundation grants IIS-0308087 and IIS-0535152.

References

[1] S.T. Roweis and L.K. Saul. Nonlinear dimensionality reduction by locally linear embedding. *Science*, 290:2323–2326, December 2000.

[2] J.B. Tenenbaum, V. de Silva, and J.C. Langford. A global geometric framework for nonlinear dimensionality reduction. *Science*, 290:2319–2323, December 2000.

[3] M. Brand. Charting a manifold. In *NIPS 15*, pages 977–984, Cambridge, MA, 2003. MIT Press.

[4] B. Kégl. Intrinsic dimension estimation using packing numbers. In *NIPS 15*, volume 15, Cambridge, MA, 2003. MIT Press.

[5] E. Levina and P.J. Bickel. Maximum likelihood estimation of intrinsic dimension. In *NIPS 17*, Cambridge, MA, 2005. MIT Press.

[6] S. Graf and H. Luschgy. *Foundations of Quantization for Probability Distributions*. Springer-Verlag, Berlin, 2000.

[7] P.L. Zador. Asymptotic quantization error of continuous signals and the quantization dimension. *IEEE Trans. Inform. Theory*, IT-28:139–149, March 1982.

[8] T. Linder. Learning-theoretic methods in vector quantization. In L. Györfi, editor, *Principles of Nonparametric Learning*. Springer-Verlag, New York, 2001.

[9] R.M. Gray and L.D. Davisson. Quantizer mismatch. *IEEE Trans. Commun.*, 23:439–443, 1975.

[10] E. Welzl. Smallest enclosing disks (balls and ellipsoids). In *New Results and New Trends in Computer Science*, volume 555 of *LNCS*, pages 359–370. Springer, 1991.

[11] M. Raginsky. A complexity-regularized quantization approach to nonlinear dimensionality reduction. *Proc. 2005 IEEE Int. Symp. Inform. Theory*, pages 352–356.

---

[4] Interestingly, Brand [3] reports an intrinsic dimension estimate of 3 for this data set. However, he used only a 500-frame subsequence and introduced additional mirror symmetry.

Preconditioner Approximations for Probabilistic Graphical Models

Pradeep Ravikumar   John Lafferty
School of Computer Science
Carnegie Mellon University

Abstract

We present a family of approximation techniques for probabilistic graphical models, based on the use of graphical preconditioners developed in the scientific computing literature. Our framework yields rigorous upper and lower bounds on event probabilities and the log partition function of undirected graphical models, using non-iterative procedures that have low time complexity. As in mean field approaches, the approximations are built upon tractable subgraphs; however, we recast the problem of optimizing the tractable distribution parameters and approximate inference in terms of the well-studied linear systems problem of obtaining a good matrix preconditioner. Experiments are presented that compare the new approximation schemes to variational methods.

1 Introduction

Approximate inference techniques are enabling sophisticated new probabilistic models to be developed and applied to a range of practical problems. One of the primary uses of approximate inference is to estimate the partition function and event probabilities for undirected graphical models, which are natural tools in many domains, from image processing to social network modeling. A central challenge is to improve the accuracy of existing approximation methods, and to derive rigorous rather than heuristic bounds on probabilities in such graphical models. In this paper, we present a simple new approach to the approximate inference problem, based upon non-iterative procedures that have low time complexity. We follow the variational mean field intuition of focusing on tractable subgraphs, however we recast the problem of optimizing the tractable distribution parameters as a generalized linear system problem. In this way, the task of deriving a tractable distribution conveniently reduces to the well-studied problem of obtaining a good *preconditioner* for a matrix (Boman and Hendrickson, 2003). This framework has the added advantage that tighter bounds can be obtained by reducing the sparsity of the preconditioners, at the expense of increasing the time complexity for computing the approximation.

In the following section we establish some notation and background. In Section 3, we outline the basic idea of our proposed framework, and explain how to use preconditioners for deriving tractable approximate distributions. In Sections 3.1 and 4, we then describe the underlying theory, which we call the generalized support theory for graphical models. In Section 5 we present experiments that compare the new approximation schemes to some of the standard variational and optimization based methods.

2 Notation and Background

Consider a graph $G = (V, E)$, where V denotes the set of nodes and E denotes the set of edges. Let X_i be a random variable associated with node i, for $i \in V$, yielding a random vector $X = \{X_1, \ldots, X_n\}$. Let $\phi = \{\phi_\alpha, \alpha \in I\}$ denote the set of *potential functions* or *sufficient statistics*, for a set I of cliques in G. Associated with ϕ is a vector of parameters $\theta = \{\theta_\alpha, \alpha \in I\}$. With this notation, the exponential family of distributions of X, associated with ϕ and G, is given by

$$p(x; \theta) = \exp\left(\sum_\alpha \theta_\alpha \phi_\alpha - \Psi(\theta) \right). \tag{1}$$

For traditional reasons through connections with statistical physics, $Z = \exp \Psi(\theta)$ is called the *partition function*. As discussed in (Yedidia et al., 2001), at the expense in increasing the state space one can assume without loss of generality that the graphical model is a pairwise Markov random field, *i.e.*, the set of cliques I is the set of edges $\{(s, t) \in E\}$. We shall assume a pairwise random field, and thus can express the potential function and parameter vectors in more compact form as matrices:

$$\Theta := \begin{pmatrix} \theta_{11} & \cdots & \theta_{1n} \\ \vdots & \vdots & \vdots \\ \theta_{n1} & \cdots & \theta_{nn} \end{pmatrix} \quad \Phi(x) := \begin{pmatrix} \phi_{11}(x_1, x_1) & \cdots & \phi_{1n}(x_1, x_n) \\ \vdots & \vdots & \vdots \\ \phi_{n1}(x_n, x_1) & \cdots & \phi_{nn}(x_n, x_n) \end{pmatrix} \tag{2}$$

In the following we will denote the trace of the product of two matrices A and B by the inner product $\langle\langle A, B \rangle\rangle$. Assuming that each X_i is finite-valued, the partition function $Z(\Theta)$ is then given by $Z(\Theta) = \sum_{x \in \chi} \exp \langle\langle \Theta, \Phi(x) \rangle\rangle$. The computation of $Z(\Theta)$ has a complexity exponential in the tree-width of the graph G and hence is intractable for large graphs. Our goal is to obtain rigorous upper and lower bounds for this partition function, which can then be used to obtain rigorous upper and lower bounds for general event probabilities; this is discussed further in (Ravikumar and Lafferty, 2004).

2.1 Preconditioners in Linear Systems

Consider a linear system, $Ax = c$, where the variable x is n dimensional, and A is an $n \times n$ matrix with m non-zero entries. Solving for x via direct methods such as Gaussian elimination has a computational complexity $O(n^3)$, which is impractical for large values of n. Multiplying both sides of the linear system by the inverse of an invertible matrix B, we get an equivalent "preconditioned" system, $B^{-1}Ax = B^{-1}c$. If B is similar to A, $B^{-1}A$ is in turn similar to I, the identity matrix, making the preconditioned system easier to solve. Such an approximating matrix B is called a preconditioner.

The computational complexity of preconditioned conjugate gradient is given by

$$T(A) = \sqrt{\kappa(A, B)} \, (m + T(B)) \log\left(\frac{1}{\epsilon}\right) \tag{3}$$

where $T(A)$ is the time required for an ϵ-approximate solution; $\kappa(A, B)$ is the *condition number* of A and B which intuitively corresponds to the quality of the approximation B, and $T(B)$ is the time required to solve $By = c$.

Recent developments in the theory of preconditioners are in part based on *support graph theory*, where the linear system matrix is viewed as the Laplacian of a graph, and graph-based techniques can be used to obtain good approximations. While these methods require diagonally dominant matrices ($A_{ii} \geq \sum_{j \neq i} |A_{ij}|$), they yield "ultra-sparse" (tree plus a constant number of edges) preconditioners with a low condition number. In our experiments, we use two elementary tree-based preconditioners in this family, Vaidya's Spanning Tree preconditioner Vaidya (1990), and Gremban-Miller's Support Tree preconditioner Gremban (1996).

3 Graphical Model Preconditioners

Our proposed framework follows the generalized mean field intuition of looking at sparse graph approximations of the original graph, but solving a different optimization problem. We begin by outlining the basic idea, and then develop the underlying theory.

Consider the graphical model with graph G, potential-function matrix $\Phi(x)$, and parameter matrix Θ. For purposes of intuition, think of the graphical model "energy" $\langle\!\langle \Theta, \Phi(x) \rangle\!\rangle$ as the matrix norm $x^\top \Theta x$. We would like to obtain a sparse approximation B for Θ. If B approximates Θ well, then the condition number κ is small:

$$\kappa(\Theta, B) \;=\; \max_x \frac{x^\top \Theta x}{x^\top B x} \;\bigg/\; \min_x \frac{x^\top \Theta x}{x^\top B x} \;=\; \lambda_{max}(\Theta, B) \,/\, \lambda_{min}(\Theta, B) \qquad (4)$$

This suggests the following procedure for approximate inference. First, choose a matrix B that minimizes the condition number with Θ (rather than KL divergence as in mean-field). Then, scale B appropriately, as detailed in the following sections. Finally, use the scaled matrix B as the parameter matrix for approximate inference. Note that if B corresponds to a tree, approximate inference has linear time complexity.

3.1 Generalized Eigenvalue Bounds

Given a graphical model with graph G, potential-function matrix $\Phi(x)$, and parameter matrix Θ, our goal is to obtain parameter matrices Θ_U and Θ_L, corresponding to sparse graph approximations of G, such that

$$Z(\Theta_L) \;\leq\; Z(\Theta) \;\leq\; Z(\Theta_U). \qquad (5)$$

That is, the partition functions of the sparse graph parameter matrices Θ_U and Θ_L are upper and lower bounds, respectively, of the partition function of the original graph. However, we will instead focus on a seemingly much *stronger* condition; in particular, we will look for Θ_L and Θ_U that satisfy

$$\langle\!\langle \Theta_L, \Phi(x) \rangle\!\rangle \;\leq\; \langle\!\langle \Theta, \Phi(x) \rangle\!\rangle \;\leq\; \langle\!\langle \Theta_U, \Phi(x) \rangle\!\rangle \qquad (6)$$

for all x. By monotonicity of $\exp$, this stronger condition implies condition (5) on the partition function, by summing over the values of X. However, this stronger condition will give us greater flexibility, and rigorous bounds for general event probabilities since then

$$\frac{\exp \langle\!\langle \Theta_L, \Phi(x) \rangle\!\rangle}{Z(\Theta_U)} \;\leq\; p(x; \Theta) \;\leq\; \frac{\exp \langle\!\langle \Theta_U, \Phi(x) \rangle\!\rangle}{Z(\Theta_L)}. \qquad (7)$$

In contrast, while variational methods give bounds on the log partition function, the derived bounds on general event probabilities via the variational parameters are only heuristic.

Let $\mathcal{S}$ be a set of sparse graphs; for example, $\mathcal{S}$ may be the set of all trees. Focusing on the upper bound, we for now would like to obtain a graph $G' \in \mathcal{S}$ with parameter matrix B, which approximates G, and whose partition function upper bounds the partition function of the original graph. Following (6), we require,

$$\langle\!\langle \Theta, \Phi(x) \rangle\!\rangle \;\leq\; \langle\!\langle B, \Phi(x) \rangle\!\rangle, \text{ such that } G(B) \in \mathcal{S} \qquad (8)$$

where $G(B)$ denotes the graph corresponding to the parameter matrix B. Now, we would like the distribution corresponding to B to be as close as possible to the distribution corresponding to Θ; that is, $\langle\!\langle B, \Phi(x) \rangle\!\rangle$ should not only upper bound $\langle\!\langle \Theta, \Phi(x) \rangle\!\rangle$ but should be close to it. The distance measure we use for this is the minimax distance. In other words, while the upper bound requires that

$$\frac{\langle\!\langle \Theta, \Phi(x) \rangle\!\rangle}{\langle\!\langle B, \Phi(x) \rangle\!\rangle} \leq 1, \tag{9}$$

we would like

$$\min_x \frac{\langle\!\langle \Theta, \Phi(x) \rangle\!\rangle}{\langle\!\langle B, \Phi(x) \rangle\!\rangle} \tag{10}$$

to be as high as possible. Expressing these desiderata in the form of an optimization problem, we have

$$B^\star = \underset{B:\, G(B) \in \mathcal{S}}{\arg\max} \ \min_x \ \frac{\langle\!\langle \Theta, \Phi(x) \rangle\!\rangle}{\langle\!\langle B, \Phi(x) \rangle\!\rangle}, \quad \text{such that} \quad \frac{\langle\!\langle \Theta, \Phi(x) \rangle\!\rangle}{\langle\!\langle B, \Phi(x) \rangle\!\rangle} \leq 1.$$

Before solving this problem, we first make some definitions, which are generalized versions of standard concepts in linear systems theory.

Definition 3.1. *For a pairwise Markov random field with potential function matrix $\Phi(x)$, the generalized eigenvalues of a pair of parameter matrices (A, B) are defined as*

$$\lambda^{\Phi}_{max}(A, B) = \max_{x:\, \langle\!\langle B, \Phi(x) \rangle\!\rangle \neq 0} \frac{\langle\!\langle A, \Phi(x) \rangle\!\rangle}{\langle\!\langle B, \Phi(x) \rangle\!\rangle} \tag{11}$$

$$\lambda^{\Phi}_{min}(A, B) = \min_{x:\, \langle\!\langle B, \Phi(x) \rangle\!\rangle \neq 0} \frac{\langle\!\langle A, \Phi(x) \rangle\!\rangle}{\langle\!\langle B, \Phi(x) \rangle\!\rangle}. \tag{12}$$

Note that

$$\lambda^{\Phi}_{max}(A, \alpha B) = \max_{x:\, \langle\!\langle \alpha B, \Phi(x) \rangle\!\rangle \neq 0} \frac{\langle\!\langle A, \Phi(x) \rangle\!\rangle}{\langle\!\langle \alpha B, \Phi(x) \rangle\!\rangle} \tag{13}$$

$$= \frac{1}{\alpha} \max_{x:\, \langle\!\langle B, \Phi(x) \rangle\!\rangle \neq 0} \frac{\langle\!\langle A, \Phi(x) \rangle\!\rangle}{\langle\!\langle B, \Phi(x) \rangle\!\rangle} = \alpha^{-1} \lambda^{\Phi}_{max}(A, B). \tag{14}$$

We state the basic properties of the generalized eigenvalues in the following lemma.

Lemma 3.2 *The generalized eigenvalues satisfy*

$$\lambda^{\Phi}_{min}(A, B) \leq \frac{\langle\!\langle A, \Phi(x) \rangle\!\rangle}{\langle\!\langle B, \Phi(x) \rangle\!\rangle} \leq \lambda^{\Phi}_{max}(A, B) \tag{15}$$

$$\lambda^{\Phi}_{max}(A, \alpha B) = \alpha^{-1} \lambda^{\Phi}_{max}(A, B) \tag{16}$$

$$\lambda^{\Phi}_{min}(A, \alpha B) = \alpha^{-1} \lambda^{\Phi}_{min}(A, B) \tag{17}$$

$$\lambda^{\Phi}_{min}(A, B) = \frac{1}{\lambda^{\Phi}_{max}(B, A)}. \tag{18}$$

In the following, we will use A to generically denote the parameter matrix Θ of the model. We can now rewrite the optimization problem for the upper bound in equation (11) as

$$(\text{Problem } \Lambda_1) \qquad \max_{B:\, G(B) \in \mathcal{S}} \ \lambda^{\Phi}_{min}(A, B), \quad \text{such that} \quad \lambda^{\Phi}_{max}(A, B) \leq 1 \tag{19}$$

We shall express the optimal solution of Problem Λ_1 in terms of the optimal solution of a companion problem. Towards that end, consider the optimization problem

$$(\text{Problem } \Lambda_2) \qquad \min_{C:\, G(C) \in \mathcal{S}} \ \frac{\lambda^{\Phi}_{max}(A, C)}{\lambda^{\Phi}_{min}(A, C)}. \tag{20}$$

The following proposition shows the sense in which these problems are equivalent.

Proposition 3.3. *If $\widehat{C}$ attains the optimum in Problem Λ_2, then $\widetilde{C} = \lambda^{\Phi}_{max}(A, \widehat{C})\,\widehat{C}$ attains the optimum of Problem Λ_1.*

Proof. For any feasible solution B of Problem Λ_1, we have

$$\lambda^{\Phi}_{\min}(A, B) \;\leq\; \frac{\lambda^{\Phi}_{\min}(A, B)}{\lambda^{\Phi}_{\max}(A, B)} \quad (\text{since } \lambda^{\Phi}_{\max}(A, B) \leq 1) \tag{21}$$

$$\leq\; \frac{\lambda^{\Phi}_{\min}(A, \widehat{C})}{\lambda^{\Phi}_{\max}(A, \widehat{C})} \quad (\text{since } \widehat{C} \text{ is the optimum of Problem } \Lambda_2) \tag{22}$$

$$=\; \lambda^{\Phi}_{\min}\left(A, \lambda^{\Phi}_{\max}(A, \widehat{C})\widehat{C}\right) \quad (\text{from Lemma 3.2}) \tag{23}$$

$$=\; \lambda^{\Phi}_{\min}(A, \widetilde{C}). \tag{24}$$

Thus, $\widetilde{C}$ upper bounds all feasible solutions in Problem Λ_1. However, it itself is a feasible solution, since

$$\lambda^{\Phi}_{\max}(A, \widetilde{C}) \;=\; \lambda^{\Phi}_{\max}\left(A, \lambda^{\Phi}_{\max}(A, \widehat{C})\widehat{C}\right) \;=\; \frac{1}{\lambda^{\Phi}_{\max}(A, \widehat{C})}\lambda^{\Phi}_{\max}(A, \widehat{C}) \;=\; 1 \tag{25}$$

from Lemma 3.2. Thus, $\widetilde{C}$ attains the maximum in the upper bound Problem Λ_1. $\square$

The analysis for obtaining an upper bound parameter matrix B for a given parameter matrix A carries over for the lower bound; we need to replace a maximin problem with a minimax problem. For the lower bound, we want a matrix B such that

$$B_\star \;=\; \min_{B:\, G(B)\in\mathcal{S}}\; \max_{\{x:\,\langle\langle B, \Phi(x)\rangle\rangle\neq 0\}}\; \frac{\langle\langle A, \Phi(x)\rangle\rangle}{\langle\langle B, \Phi(x)\rangle\rangle}, \quad \text{such that}\quad \frac{\langle\langle A, \Phi(x)\rangle\rangle}{\langle\langle B, \Phi(x)\rangle\rangle} \geq 1 \tag{26}$$

This leads to the following lower bound optimization problem.

$$(\text{Problem } \Lambda_3)\qquad \min_{B:\, G(B)\in\mathcal{S}}\; \lambda^{\Phi}_{\max}(A, B), \quad \text{such that}\quad \lambda^{\Phi}_{\min}(A, B) \geq 1. \tag{27}$$

The proof of the following statement closely parallels the proof of Proposition 3.3.

Proposition 3.4. *If $\widehat{C}$ attains the optimum in Problem Λ_2, then $\underline{C} = \lambda^{\Phi}_{min}(A, \widehat{C})\widehat{C}$ attains the optimum of the lower bound Problem Λ_3.*

Finally, we state the following basic lemma, whose proof is easily verified.

Lemma 3.5. *For any pair of parameter-matrices (A, B), we have*

$$\langle\langle \lambda^{\Phi}_{min}(A, B)B, \Phi(x)\rangle\rangle \;\leq\; \langle\langle A, \Phi(x)\rangle\rangle \;\leq\; \langle\langle \lambda^{\Phi}_{max}(A, B)B, \Phi(x)\rangle\rangle. \tag{28}$$

3.2 Main Procedure

We now have in place the machinery necessary to describe the procedure for solving the main problem in equation (6), to obtain upper and lower bound matrices for a graphical model. Lemma 3.5 shows how to obtain upper and lower bound parameter matrices with respect to any matrix B, given a parameter matrix A, by solving a generalized eigenvalue problem. Propositions 3.3 and 3.4 tell us, in principle, how to obtain the optimal such upper and lower bound matrices. We thus have the following procedure. First, obtain a parameter matrix C such that $G(C) \in \mathcal{S}$, which minimizes $\lambda^{\Phi}_{\max}(\Theta, C)/\lambda^{\Phi}_{\min}(\Theta, C)$. Then $\lambda^{\Phi}_{\max}(\Theta, C)\,C$ gives the optimal upper bound parameter matrix and $\lambda^{\Phi}_{\min}(\Theta, C)\,C$ gives the optimal lower bound parameter matrix. However, as things stand, this recipe appears to be even more challenging to work with than the generalized mean field procedures. The difficulty lies in obtaining the matrix C. In the following section we offer a series of relaxations that help to simplify this task.

4   Generalized Support Theory for Graphical Models

In what follows, we begin by assuming that the potential function matrix is positive semi-definite, $\Phi(x) \succeq 0$, and later extend our results to general Φ.

Definition 4.1. *For a pairwise MRF with potential function matrix $\Phi(x) \succeq 0$, the generalized support number of a pair of parameter matrices (A, B), where $B \succeq 0$, is*

$$\sigma^\Phi(A, B) = \min \{\tau \in \mathbf{R} \mid \langle\langle \tau B, \Phi(x) \rangle\rangle \geq \langle\langle A, \Phi(x) \rangle\rangle \text{ for all } x\} \quad (29)$$

The generalized support number can be thought of as the "number of copies" τ of B required to "support" A so that $\langle\langle \tau B - A, \Phi(x) \rangle\rangle \geq 0$. The usefulness of this definition is demonstrated by the following result.

Proposition 4.2. *If $B \succeq 0$ then $\lambda^\Phi_{max}(A, B) \leq \sigma^\Phi(A, B)$.*

Proof. From the definition of the generalized support number for a graphical model, we have that $\langle\langle \sigma^\Phi(A, B)B - A, \Phi(x) \rangle\rangle \geq 0$. Now, since we assume that $\Phi(x) \succeq 0$, if also $B \succeq 0$ then $\langle\langle B, \Phi(x) \rangle\rangle \geq 0$. Therefore, it follows that $\frac{\langle\langle A, \Phi(x) \rangle\rangle}{\langle\langle B, \Phi(x) \rangle\rangle} \leq \sigma^\Phi(A, B)$, and thus

$$\lambda^\Phi_{max}(A, B) = \max_x \frac{\langle\langle A, \Phi(x) \rangle\rangle}{\langle\langle B, \Phi(x) \rangle\rangle} \leq \sigma^\Phi(A, B) \quad (30)$$

giving the statement of the proposition. $\square$

This leads to our first relaxation of the generalized eigenvalue bound for a model. From Lemma 3.2 and Proposition 4.2 we see that

$$\frac{\lambda^\Phi_{max}(A, B)}{\lambda^\Phi_{min}(A, B)} = \lambda^\Phi_{max}(A, B)\lambda^\Phi_{max}(B, A) \leq \sigma^\Phi(A, B)\sigma^\Phi(B, A) \quad (31)$$

Thus, this result suggests that to approximate the graphical model (Θ, Φ) we can search for a parameter matrix $B^\star$, with corresponding simple graph $G(B^\star) \in \mathcal{S}$, such that

$$B^\star = \arg\min_B \sigma^\Phi(\Theta, B)\sigma^\Phi(B, \Theta) \quad (32)$$

While this relaxation may lead to effective bounds, we will now go further, to derive an additional relaxation that relates our generalized graphical model support number to the "classical" support number.

Proposition 4.3. *For a potential function matrix $\Phi(x) \succeq 0$, $\sigma^\Phi(A, B) \leq \sigma(A, B)$, where $\sigma(A, B) = \min\{\tau \mid (\tau B - A) \succeq 0\}$.*

Proof. Since $\sigma(A, B)B - A \succeq 0$ by definition and $\Phi(x) \succeq 0$ by assumption, we have that $\langle\langle \sigma(A, B)B - A, \Phi(x) \rangle\rangle \geq 0$. Therefore, $\sigma^\Phi(A, B) \leq \sigma(A, B)$ from the definition of generalized support number. $\square$

The above result reduces the problem of approximating a graphical model to the problem of minimizing classical support numbers, the latter problem being well-studied in the scientific computing literature (Boman and Hendrickson, 2003; Bern et al., 2001), where the expression $\sigma(A, C)\sigma(C, A)$ is called the *condition number*, and a matrix that minimizes it within a simple family of graphs is called a *preconditioner*. We can thus plug in any algorithm for finding a sparse preconditioner for Θ, carrying out the optimization

$$B^\star = \arg\min_B \sigma(\Theta, B)\,\sigma(B, \Theta) \quad (33)$$

and then use that matrix B^* in our basic procedure.

One example is Vaidya's preconditioner Vaidya (1990), which is essentially the maximum spanning tree of the graph. Another is the support tree of Gremban (1996), which introduces Steiner nodes, in this case auxiliary nodes introduced via a recursive partitioning of the graph. We present experiments with these basic preconditioners in the following section.

Before turning to the experiments, we comment that our generalized support number analysis assumed that the potential function matrix $\Phi(x)$ was positive semi-definite. The case when it is not can be handled as follows. We first add a large positive diagonal matrix D so that $\Phi'(x) = \Phi(x) + D \succeq 0$. Then, for a given parameter matrix Θ, we use the above machinery to get an upper bound parameter matrix B such that

$$\langle\langle A, \Phi(x) + D \rangle\rangle \leq \langle\langle B, \Phi(x) + D \rangle\rangle \;\Rightarrow\; \langle\langle A, \Phi(x) \rangle\rangle \leq \langle\langle B, \Phi(x) \rangle\rangle + \langle\langle B - A, D \rangle\rangle.$$
(34)

Exponentiating and summing both sides over x, we then get the required upper bound for the parameter matrix A; the same can be done for the lower bound.

5 Experiments

As the previous sections detailed, the preconditioner based bounds are in principle quite easy to compute—we compute a sparse preconditioner for the parameter matrix (typically $O(n)$ to $O(n^3)$) and use the preconditioner as the parameter matrix for the bound computation (which is linear if the preconditioner matrix corresponds to a tree). This yields a simple, non-iterative deterministic procedure as compared to the more complex propagation-based or iterative update procedures. In this section we evaluate these bounds on small graphical models for which exact answers can be readily computed, and compare the bounds to variational approximations.

We show simulation results averaged over a randomly generated set of graphical models. The graphs used were 2D grid graphs, and the edge potentials were selected according to a uniform distribution Uniform$(-2d_{coup}, 0)$ for various coupling strengths d_{coup}. We report the relative error, (bound − log-partition-function)/log-partition-function.

As a baseline, we use the mean field and structured mean field methods for the lower bound, and the Wainwright et al. (2003) tree-reweighted belief propagation approximation for the upper bound. For the preconditioner based bounds, we use two very simple preconditioners, (a) Vaidya's maximum spanning tree preconditioner (Vaidya, 1990), which assumes the input parameter matrix to be a Laplacian, and (b) Gremban (1996)'s support tree preconditioner, which also gives a sparse parameter matrix corresponding to a tree, with Steiner (auxiliary) nodes. To compute bounds over these larger graphs with Steiner nodes we average an internal node over its children; this is the technique used with such preconditioners for solving linear systems. We note that these preconditioners are quite basic, and the use of better preconditioners (yielding a better condition number) has the potential to achieve much better bounds, as shown in Propositions 3.3 and 3.4. We also reiterate that while our approach can be used to derive bounds on event probabilities, the variational methods yield bounds only for the partition function, and only apply heuristically to estimating simple event probabilities such as marginals.

As the plots in Figure 1 show, even for the simple preconditioners used, the new bounds are quite close to the actual values, outperforming the mean field method and giving comparable results to the tree-reweighted belief propagation method. The spanning tree preconditioner provides a good lower bound, while the support tree preconditioner provides a good upper bound, however not as tight as the bound obtained using tree-reweighted belief propagation. Although we cannot compute the exact solution for large graphs, we can

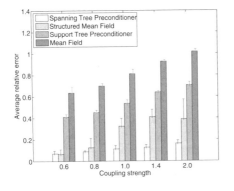

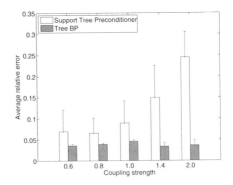

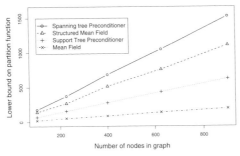

Figure 1: Comparison of lower bounds (top left), and upper bounds (top right) for small grid graphs, and lower bounds for grid graphs of increasing size (left).

compare bounds. The bottom plot of Figure 1 compares lower bounds for graphs with up to 900 nodes; a larger bound is necessarily tighter, and the preconditioner bounds are seen to outperform mean field.

Acknowledgments

We thank Gary Miller for helpful discussions. Research supported in part by NSF grants IIS-0312814 and IIS-0427206.

References

M. Bern, J. R. Gilbert, B. Hendrickson, N. Nguyen, and S. Toledo. Support-graph preconditioners. Submitted to *SIAM J. Matrix Anal. Appl.*, 2001.

E. G. Boman and B. Hendrickson. Support theory for preconditioning. *SIAM Journal on Matrix Analysis and Applications*, 25, 2003.

K. Gremban. Combinatorial preconditioners for sparse, symmetric, diagonally dominant linear systems. *Ph.D. Thesis, Carnegie Mellon University, 1996*, 1996.

P. Ravikumar and J. Lafferty. Variational Chernoff bounds for graphical models. *Proceedings of Uncertainty in Artificial Intelligence (UAI)*, 2004.

P. M. Vaidya. Solving linear equations with symmetric diagonally dominant matrices by constructing good preconditioners. 1990. Unpublished manuscript, UIUC.

M. J. Wainwright, T. Jaakkola, and A. S. Willsky. Tree-reweighted belief propagation and approximate ML estimation by pseudo-moment matching. *9th Workshop on Artificial Intelligence and Statistics*, 2003.

J. S. Yedidia, W. T. Freeman, and Y. Weiss. Understanding belief propagation and its generalizations. *IJCAI 2001 Distinguished Lecture track*, 2001.

Cue Integration for Figure/Ground Labeling

Xiaofeng Ren, Charless C. Fowlkes and Jitendra Malik
Computer Science Division, University of California, Berkeley, CA 94720
`{xren,fowlkes,malik}@cs.berkeley.edu`

Abstract

We present a model of edge and region grouping using a conditional random field built over a scale-invariant representation of images to integrate multiple cues. Our model includes potentials that capture low-level similarity, mid-level curvilinear continuity and high-level object shape. Maximum likelihood parameters for the model are learned from human labeled groundtruth on a large collection of horse images using belief propagation. Using held out test data, we quantify the information gained by incorporating generic mid-level cues and high-level shape.

1 Introduction

Figure/ground organization, the binding of contours to surfaces, is a classical problem in vision. In the 1920s, Edgar Rubin pointed to several generic properties, such as closure, which governed the perception of figure/ground. However, it is clear that in the context of natural scenes, such processing must be closely intertwined with many low- and mid-level grouping cues as well as a priori object knowledge [10].

In this paper, we study a simplified task of figure/ground labeling in which the goal is to label every pixel as belonging to either a figural object or background. Our goal is to understand the role of different cues in this process, including low-level cues, such as edge contrast and texture similarity; mid-level cues, such as curvilinear continuity; and high-level cues, such as characteristic shape or texture of the object. We develop a conditional random field model [7] over edges, regions and objects to integrate these cues. We train the model from human-marked groundtruth labels and quantify the relative contributions of each cue on a large collection of horse images[2].

In computer vision, the work of Geman and Geman [3] inspired a whole subfield of work on Markov Random Fields in relation to segmentation and denoising. More recently, *Conditional Random Fields* (CRF) have been applied to low-level segmentation [6, 12, 4] and have shown performance superior to traditional MRFs. However, most of the existing MRF/CRF models focus on pixel-level labeling, requiring inferences over millions of pixels. Being tied to the pixel resolution, they are also unable to deal with scale change or explicitly capture mid-level cues such as junctions. Our approach overcomes these difficulties by utilizing a scale-invariant representation of image contours and regions where each variable in our model can correspond to hundreds of pixels. It is also quite straightforward to design potentials which capture complicated relationships between these mid-level tokens in a transparent way.

Interest in combining object knowledge with segmentation has grown quickly over the

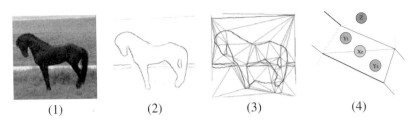

(1)   (2)   (3)   (4)

Figure 1: A scale-invariant representation of images: Given the input (1), we estimate the local probability of boundary Pb based on gradients (2). We then build a piecewise linear approximation of the edge map and complete it with *Constrained Delaunay Triangulation* (CDT). The black edges in (3) are gradient edges detected in (2); the green edges are potential completions generated by CDT. (4) We perform inference in a probabilistic model built on top of this representation and extract marginal distributions on edges X, triangular regions Y and object pose Z.

last few years [2, 16, 14]. Our probabilistic approach is similar in spirit to [14] however we focus on learning parameters of a discriminative model and quantify our performance on test data. Compared to previous techniques which rely heavily on top-down template matching [2, 5], our approach has three major advantages: (1) We are able to use mid-level grouping cues including junctions and continuity. Our results show these cues make quantitatively significant contributions. (2) We combine cues in a probabilistic framework where the relative weighting of cues is learned from training data resulting in weights that are easy to interpret. (3) The role of different cues can be easily studied by "surgically removing" them refitting the remaining parameters.

2   A conditional random field for figure/ground labeling

Figure 1 provides an overview of our technique for building a discrete, scale-independent representation of image boundaries from a low-level detector. First we compute an edge map using the boundary detector of [9] which utilizes both brightness and texture contrast to estimate the probability of boundary, Pb at each pixel. Next we use Canny's hysteresis thresholding to trace the Pb boundaries and then recursively split the boundaries using angles, a scale-invariant measure, until each segment is approximately linear. Finally we utilize the *Constrained Delaunay Triangulation* [13] to complete the piecewise linear approximations. CDT often completes gaps in object boundaries where local gradient information is absent. More details about this construction can be found in [11].

Let G be the resulting CDT graph. The edges and triangles in G are natural entities for figure/ground labeling. We introduce the following random variables:

- Edges: X_e is 1 if edge e in the CDT is a true boundary and 0 otherwise.

- Regions: Y_t is 1 if triangle t corresponds to figure and 0 otherwise.

- Pose: Z encodes the figural object's pose in the scene. We use a very simple Z which considers a discrete configuration space given by a grid of 25 possible image locations. Z is easily augmented to include an indicator of object category or aspect as well as location.

We now describe a conditional random field model on $\{X, Y, Z\}$ used to integrate multiple grouping cues. The model takes the form of a log-linear combination of features which are functions of variables and image measurements. We consider Z a latent variable which is marginalized out by assuming a uniform distribution over aspects and locations.

$$P(X, Y | Z, I, \Theta) = \frac{1}{\mathcal{Z}(I, \Theta)} e^{-E(X, Y | Z, I, \Theta)}$$

where the energy E of a configuration is linear in the parameters $\Theta = \{\alpha, \vec{\beta}, \vec{\delta}, \gamma, \vec{\eta}, \kappa, \vec{\nu}\}$ and given by

$$E = -\alpha \sum_e L_1(X_e | I) - \vec{\beta} \cdot \sum_{\langle s, t \rangle} \vec{L}_2(Y_s, Y_t | I) - \vec{\delta} \cdot \sum_V \vec{M}_1(X_V | I)$$

$$-\gamma \sum_{\langle s, t \rangle} M_2(Y_s, Y_t, X_e) - \vec{\eta} \cdot \sum_t \vec{H}_1(Y_t | I) - \kappa \sum_t H_2(Y_t | Z, I) - \vec{\nu} \cdot \sum_e \vec{H}_3(X_e | Z, I)$$

The table below gives a summary of each potential. The next section fills in details.

Similarity	Edge energy along e	$L_1(X_e	I)$
	Brightness/Texture similarity between s and t	$L_2(Y_s, Y_t	I)$
Continuity	Collinearity and junction frequency at vertex V	$M_1(X_V	I)$
Closure	Consistency of edge and adjoining regions	$M_2(Y_s, Y_t, X_e)$
	Similarity of region t to exemplar texture	$H_1(Y_t	I)$
Familiarity	Compatibility of region shape with pose	$H_2(Y_t	Z, I)$
	Compatibility of local edge shape with pose	$H_3(X_e	Z, I)$

3 Cues for figure/ground labeling

3.1 Low-level Cues: Similarity of Brightness and Texture

To capture the locally measured edge contrast, we assign a singleton edge potential whose energy is

$$L_1(X_e | I) = \log(Pb_e) X_e$$

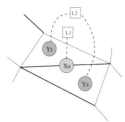

where Pb_e is the average Pb recorded over the pixels corresponding to edge e.

Since the triangular regions have larger support than the local edge detector, we also include a pairwise, region-based similarity cue, computed as

$$\vec{\beta} \cdot \vec{L}_2(Y_s, Y_t | I) = (\beta_B \log(f(|I_s - I_t|)) + \beta_T \log(g(\chi^2(h_s, h_t)))) \mathbf{1}_{\{Y_s = Y_t\}}$$

where f predicts the likelihood of s and t belonging to the same group given the difference of average image brightness and g makes a similar prediction based on the χ^2 difference between histograms of vector quantized filter responses (referred to as textons [8]) which describe the texture in the two regions.

3.2 Mid-level Cues: Curvilinear Continuity and Closure

There are two types of edges in the CDT graph, gradient-edges (detected by Pb) and completed-edges (filled in by the triangulation). Since true boundaries are more commonly marked by a gradient, we keep track of these two types of edges separately when modeling junctions. To capture continuity and the frequency of different junction types, we assign energy:

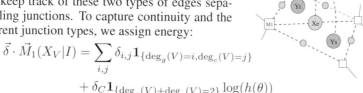

$$\vec{\delta} \cdot \vec{M}_1(X_V | I) = \sum_{i,j} \delta_{i,j} \mathbf{1}_{\{\deg_g(V) = i, \deg_c(V) = j\}}$$

$$+ \delta_C \mathbf{1}_{\{\deg_g(V) + \deg_c(V) = 2\}} \log(h(\theta))$$

where $X_V = \{X_{e_1}, X_{e_2}, \ldots\}$ is the set of edge variables incident on V, $\deg_g(V)$ is the number of gradient-edges at vertex V for which $X_e = 1$. Similarly $\deg_c(V)$ is the number of completed-edges that are "turned on". When the total degree of a vertex is 2, δ_C weights the continuity of the two edges. h is the output of a logistic function fit to $|\theta|$ and the probability of continuation. It is smooth and symmetric around $\theta = 0$ and falls of as $\theta \to \pi$. If the angle between the two edges is close to 0, they form a good continuation, $f(\theta)$ is large, and they are more likely to both be turned on.

In order to assert the duality between segments and boundaries, we use a compatibility term

$$M_2(Y_s, Y_t, X_e) = \mathbf{1}_{\{Y_s = Y_t, X_e = 0\}} + \mathbf{1}_{\{Y_s \neq Y_t, X_e = 1\}}$$

which simply counts when the label of s and t is consistent with that of e.

3.3 High-level Cues: Familiarity of Shape and Texture

We are interested in encoding high-level knowledge about object categories. In this paper we experiment with a single object category, horses, but we believe our high-level cues will scale to multiple objects in a natural way.

We compute texton histograms h_t for each triangular region (as in L_1). From the set of training images, we use k-medoids to find 10 representative histograms $\{h_1^F, \ldots, h_{10}^F\}$ for the collection of segments labeled as figure and 10 histograms $\{h_1^G, \ldots, h_{10}^G\}$ for the set of background segments. Each segment in a test image is compared to the set of exemplar histograms using the χ^2 histogram difference. We use the energy term

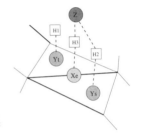

$$H_1(Y_t|I) = \log \left(\frac{\min_i \chi^2(h_t, h_i^F)}{\min_i \chi^2(h_t, h_i^G)} \right) Y_t$$

to capture the cue of texture familiarity.

We describe the global shape of the object using a template $T(x, y)$ generated by averaging the groundtruth object segmentation masks. This yields a silhouette with quite fuzzy boundaries due to articulations and scale variation. Figure 3.3(a) shows the template extracted from our training data. Let $O(Z, t)$ be the normalized overlap between template centered at $Z = (x_0, y_0)$ with the triangular region corresponding to Y_t. This is computed as the integral of $T(x, y)$ over the triangle t divided by the area of t. We then use energy

$$\vec{\eta} \cdot \vec{H}_2(Y_t|Z) = \eta_F \log(O(Z, t)) Y_t + \eta_G \log(1 - O(Z, t))(1 - Y_t)$$

In the case of multiple objects or aspects of a single object, we use multiple templates and augment Z with an indicator of the aspect $Z = (x, y, a)$. In our experiments on the dataset considered here, we found that the variability is too small (all horses facing left) to see a significant impact on performance from adding multiple aspects.

Lastly, we would like to capture the spatial layout of articulated structures such as the horses legs and head. To describe characteristic configuration of edges, we utilize the *geometric blur*[1] descriptor applied to the output of the Pb boundary detector. The *geometric blur* centered at location x, $GB_x(y)$, is a linear operator applied to $Pb(x, y)$ whose value is another image given by the "convolution" of $Pb(x, y)$ with a spatially varying Gaussian. Geometric blur is motivated by the search for a linear operator which will respond strongly to a particular object feature and is invariant to some set of transformations of the image.

We use the geometric blur computed at the set of image edges ($Pb > 0.05$) to build a library of 64 prototypical "shapemes" from the training data by vector quantization. For each edge X_e which expresses a particular shapeme we would like to know whether X_e should be

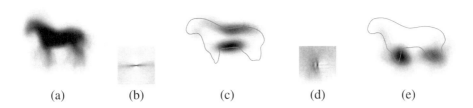

(a)   (b)   (c)   (d)   (e)

Figure 2: Using a priori shape knowledge: (a) average horse template. (b) one shapeme, capturing long horizontal curves. Shown here is the average shape in this shapeme cluster. (c) on a horse, this shapeme occurs at horse back and stomach. Shown here is the density of the shapeme M^{ON} overlayed with a contour plot of the average mask. (d) another shapeme, capturing parallel vertical lines. (e) on a horse, this shapeme occurs at legs.

"turned on". This is estimated from training data by building spatial maps $M_i^{ON}(x, y)$ and $M_i^{OFF}(x, y)$ for each shapeme relative to the object center which record the frequency of a true/false boundary expressing shapeme i. Figure 3.3(b-e) shows two example shapemes and their corresponding M^{ON} map. Let $S_{e,i}(x, y)$ be the indicator of the set of pixels on edge e which express shapeme i. For an object in pose $Z = (x_0, y_0)$ we use the energy

$$\vec{\nu} \cdot \sum_e \vec{H}_3(X_e | Z, I) = \sum_e \frac{1}{|e|} (\nu_{ON} \sum_{i,x,y} \log(M_i^{ON}(x - x_0, y - y_0)) S_{e,i}(x, y) X_e +$$

$$\nu_{OFF} \sum_{i,x,y} \log(M_i^{OFF}(x - x_0, y - y_0)) S_{e,i}(x, y) (1 - X_e))$$

4 Learning cue integration

We carry out approximate inference using loopy belief propagation [15] which appears to converge quickly to a reasonable solution for the graphs and potentials in question.

To fit parameters of the model, we maximize the joint likelihood over X, Y, Z taking each image as an iid sample. Since our model is log-linear in the parameters Θ, partial derivatives always yield the difference between the empirical expectation of a feature given by the training data and the expected value given the model parameters. For example, the derivative with respect to the continuation parameter δ_0 for a single training image/ground truth labeling, (I, X, Y, Z) is:

$$\frac{\partial}{\partial \delta_0} - \log P(X, Y | Z, I, \Theta)$$

$$= \frac{\partial}{\partial \delta_0} \log \mathcal{Z}(I_n, \Theta) - \sum_V \frac{\partial}{\partial \delta_0} \{\delta_0 \mathbf{1}_{\{\deg_g(V) + \deg_c(V) = 2\}} log(f(\theta))\}$$

$$= \left\langle \sum_V \mathbf{1}_{\{deg_g(V) + \deg_c(V) = 2\}} log(f(\theta)) \right\rangle - \sum_V \mathbf{1}_{\{\deg_g(V) + \deg_c(V) = 2\}} log(f(\theta))$$

where the expectation is taken with respect to $P(X, Y | Z, I, \Theta)$.

Given this estimate, we optimize the parameters by gradient descent. We have also used the difference of the energy and the Bethe free energy given by the beliefs as an estimate of the log likelihood in order to support line-search in conjugate gradient or quasi-newton routines. For our model, we find that gradient descent with momentum is efficient enough.

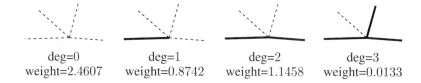

| deg=0 | deg=1 | deg=2 | deg=3 |
| weight=2.4607 | weight=0.8742 | weight=1.1458 | weight=0.0133 |

Figure 3: Learning about junctions: (a) deg=0, no boundary detected; the most common case. (b) line endings. (c) continuations of contours, more common than line endings. (d) T-junctions, very rare for the horse dataset. Compare with hand set potentials of Geman and Geman [3].

5   Experiments

In our experiments we use 344 grayscale images of the horse dataset of Borenstein et al [2]. Half of the images are used for training and half for testing. Human-marked segmentations are used[1] for both training and evaluation.

Training: loopy belief propagation on a typical CDT graph converges in about 1 second. The gradient descent learning described above converges within 1000 iterations. To understand the weights given by the learning procedure, Figure 3 shows some of the junction types in M_1 and their associated weights δ.

Testing: we evaluate the performance of our model on both edge and region labels. We present the results using a *precision-recall curve* which shows the trade-off between false positives and missed detections. For each edge e, we assign the marginal probability $E[X_e]$ to all pixels (x, y) belonging to e. Then for each threshold r, pixels above r are matched to human-marked boundaries H. The precision $P = P(H(x, y) = 1 | P_E(x, y) > r)$ and recall $R = P(P_E(x, y) > r | H(x, y) = 1)$ are recorded. Similarly, each pixel in a triangle t is assigned the marginal probability $E[Y_t]$ and the precision and recall of the ground-truth figural pixels computed.

The evaluations are shown in Figure 4 for various combinations of cues. Figure 5 shows our results on some of the test images.

6   Conclusion

We have introduced a conditional random field model on a triangulated representation of images for figure/ground labeling. We have measured the contributions of mid- and high-level cues by quantitative evaluations on held out test data. Our findings suggest that mid-level cues provide useful information, even in the presence of high-level shape cues. In future work we plan to extend this model to multiple object categories.

References

[1] A. Berg and J. Malik. Geometric blur for template matching. In *CVPR*, 2001.

[2] E. Borenstein and S. Ullman. Class-specific, top-down segmentation. In *Proc. 7th Europ. Conf. Comput. Vision*, volume 2, pages 109–124, 2002.

[3] S. Geman and D. Geman. Stochastic relaxation, gibbs distribution, and the bayesian retoration of images. *IEEE Trans. Pattern Analysis and Machine Intelligence*, 6:721–41, Nov. 1984.

---

[1]From the human segmentations on pixel-grid, we use two simple techniques to establish groundtruth labels on the CDT edges X_e and triangles Y_t. For X_e, we run a maximum-cardinality bipartite matching between the human marked boundaries and the CDT edges. We label $X_e = 1$ if 75% of the pixels lying under the edge e are matched to human boundaries. For Y_t, we label $Y_t = 1$ if at least half of the pixels within the triangle are figural pixels in the human segmentation.

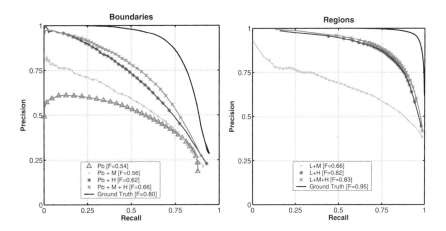

Figure 4: Performance evaluation: (a) precision-recall curves for horse boundaries, models with low-level cues only (Pb), low- plus mid-level cues ($Pb+M$), low- plus high-level cues ($Pb+H$), and all three classes of cues combined ($Pb+M+H$). The *F-measure* recorded in the legend is the maximal harmonic mean of precision and recall and provides an overall ranking. Using high-level cues greatly improves the boundary detection performance. Mid-level continuity cues are useful with or without high-level cues. (b) precision-recall for regions. The poor performance of the baseline $L+M$ model indicates the ambiguity of figure/ground labeling at low-level despite successful boundary detection. High-level shape knowledge is the key, consistent with evidence from psychophysics [10]. In both boundary and region cases, the groundtruth labels on CDTs are nearly perfect, indicating that the CDT graphs preserve most of the image structure.

[4] X. He, R. Zemel, and M. Carreira-Perpinan. Multiscale conditional random fields for image labelling. In *IEEE Conference on Computer Vision and Pattern Recognition*, 2004.

[5] M. P. Kumar, P. H. S. Torr, and A. Zisserman. OBJ CUT. In *CVPR*, 2005.

[6] S. Kumar and M. Hebert. Discriminative random fields: A discriminative framework for contextual interaction in classification. In *ICCV*, 2003.

[7] John Lafferty, Andrew McCallum, and Fernando Pereira. Conditional random fields: Probabilistic models for segmenting and labeling sequence data. In *Proc. 18th International Conf. on Machine Learning*, 2001.

[8] J. Malik, S. Belongie, J. Shi, and T. Leung. Textons, contours and regions: Cue integration in image segmentation. In *Proc. 7th Int'l. Conf. Computer Vision*, pages 918–925, 1999.

[9] D. Martin, C. Fowlkes, and J. Malik. Learning to detect natural image boundaries using brightness and texture. In *Advances in Neural Information Processing Systems 15*, 2002.

[10] M. A. Peterson and B. S. Gibson. Object recognition contributions to figure-ground organization. *Perception and Psychophysics*, 56:551–564, 1994.

[11] X. Ren, C. Fowlkes, and J. Malik. Mid-level cues improve boundary detection. Technical Report UCB//CSD-05-1382, UC Berkeley, January 2005.

[12] N. Shental, A. Zomet, T. Hertz, and Y. Weiss. Pairwise clustering and graphical models. In *NIPS 2003*, 2003.

[13] J. Shewchuk. Triangle: Engineering a 2d quality mesh generator and delaunay triangulator. In *First Workshop on Applied Computational Geometry*, pages 124–133, 1996.

[14] Z.W. Tu, X.R. Chen, A.L Yuille, and S.C. Zhu. Image parsing: segmentation, detection, and recognition. In *ICCV*, 2003.

[15] Y. Weiss. Correctness of local probability propagation in graphical models with loops. *Neural Computation*, 2000.

[16] S. Yu, R. Gross, and J. Shi. Concurrent object segmentation and recognition with graph partitioning. In *Advances in Neural Information Processing Systems 15*, 2002.

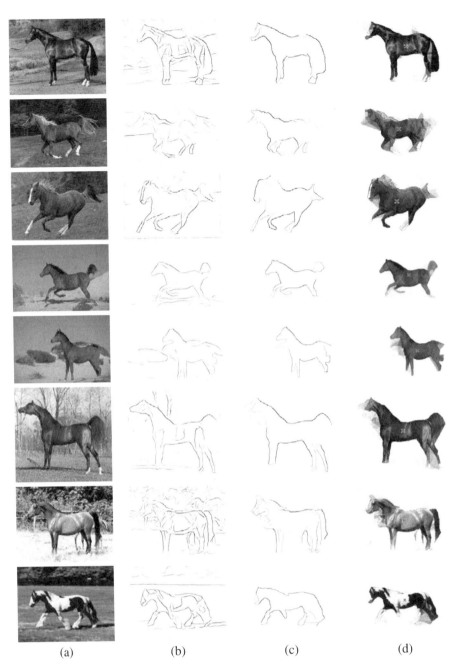

| (a) | (b) | (c) | (d) |

Figure 5: Sample results. (a) the input grayscale images. (b) the low-level boundary map output by Pb. (c) the edge marginals under our full model and (d) the image masked by the output region marginals. A red cross in (d) indicates the most probably object center. By combining relatively simple low-/mid-/high-level cues in a learning framework, We are able to find and segment horses under varying conditions with only a simple object mode. The boundary maps show the model is capable of suppressing strong gradients in the scene background while boosting low-contrast edges between figure and ground. (Row 3) shows an example of an unusual pose. In (Row 5) we predict a correct off-center object location and (Row 8) demonstrates grouping together figure with non-homogeneous appearance.

Generalization to Unseen Cases

Teemu Roos
Helsinki Institute for Information Technology
P.O.Box 68, 00014 Univ. of Helsinki, Finland
teemu.roos@cs.helsinki.fi

Peter Grünwald
CWI, P.O.Box 94079, 1090 GB,
Amsterdam, The Netherlands
pdg@cwi.nl

Petri Myllymäki
Helsinki Institute for Information Technology
P.O.Box 68, 00014 Univ of Helsinki, Finland
petri.myllymaki@cs.helsinki.fi

Henry Tirri
Nokia Research Center
P.O.Box 407 Nokia Group, Finland
henry.tirri@nokia.com

Abstract

We analyze classification error on unseen cases, i.e. cases that are different from those in the training set. Unlike standard generalization error, this *off-training-set error* may differ significantly from the empirical error with high probability even with large sample sizes. We derive a data-dependent bound on the difference between off-training-set and standard generalization error. Our result is based on a new bound on the missing mass, which for small samples is stronger than existing bounds based on Good-Turing estimators. As we demonstrate on UCI data-sets, our bound gives nontrivial generalization guarantees in many practical cases. In light of these results, we show that certain claims made in the No Free Lunch literature are overly pessimistic.

1 Introduction

A large part of learning theory deals with methods that bound the generalization error of hypotheses in terms of their empirical errors. The standard definition of generalization error allows overlap between the training sample and test cases. When such overlap is not allowed, i.e., when considering *off-training-set error* [1]–[5] defined in terms of only previously unseen cases, usual generalization bounds do not apply. The off-training-set error and the empirical error sometimes differ significantly with high probability even for large sample sizes. In this paper, we show that in many practical cases, one can nevertheless bound this difference. In particular, we show that with high probability, in the realistic situation where the number of *repeated* cases, or duplicates, relative to the total sample size is small, the difference between the off-training-set error and the standard generalization error is also small. In this case *any* standard generalization error bound, no matter how it is arrived at, transforms into a similar bound on the off-training-set error.

Our Contribution   We show that with probability at least $1-\delta$, if there are r repetitions in the training sample, then the difference between the off-training-set error and the standard generalization error is at most of order $O\left(\sqrt{\frac{1}{n}\left(\log\frac{4}{\delta}+r\log n\right)}\right)$ (Thm. 2). Our main result (Corollary 1 of Thm. 1) gives a stronger non-asymptotic bound that can be evaluated numerically. The proof of Thms. 1 and 2 is based on Lemma 2, which is of independent interest, giving a new lower bound on the so-called *missing mass*, the total probability of as yet unseen cases. For small samples and few repetitions, this bound is significantly stronger than existing bounds based on Good-Turing estimators [6]–[8].

Properties of Our Bounds Our bounds hold (1) *uniformly*, are (2) *distribution-free* and (3) *data-dependent*, yet (4) *relevant for data-sets encountered in practice*. Let us consider these properties in turn. Our bounds hold uniformly in that they hold for *all* hypotheses (functions from features to labels) at the same time. Thus, unlike many bounds on standard generalization error, our bounds do not depend in any way on the richness of the hypothesis class under consideration measured in terms of, for instance, its VC dimension, or the margin of the selected hypothesis on the training sample, or any other property of the mechanism with which the hypothesis is chosen. Our bounds are distribution-free in that they hold no matter what the (unknown) data-generating distribution is. Our bounds depend on the *data*: they are useful only if the number of repetitions in the training set is very small compared to the training set size. However, in machine learning practice this is often the case as demonstrated in Sec. 3 with several UCI data-sets.

Relevance Why are our results interesting? There are at least three reasons, the first two of which we discuss extensively in Sec. 4: (1) The use of off-training-set error is an essential ingredient of the No Free Lunch (NFL) theorems [1]–[5]. Our results counter-balance some of the overly pessimistic conclusions of this work. This is all the more relevant since the NFL theorems have been quite influential in shaping the thinking of both theoretical and practical machine learning researchers (see, e.g., Sec. 9.2 of the well-known textbook [5]). (2) The off-training-set error is an intuitive measure of generalization performance. Yet in practice it differs from standard generalization error (even with continuous feature spaces). Thus, we feel, it is worth studying. (3) Technically, we establish a surprising connection between off-training-set error (a concept from classification) and missing mass (a concept mostly applied in language modeling), and give a new lower bound on the missing mass.

The paper is organized as follows: In Sec. 2 we fix notation, including the various error functionals considered, and state some preliminary results. In Sec. 3 we state our bounds, and we demonstrate their use on data-sets from the UCI machine learning repository. We discuss the implications of our results in Sec. 4. Postponed proofs are in Appendix A.

2 Preliminaries and Notation

Let $\mathcal{X}$ be an arbitrary space of inputs, and let $\mathcal{Y}$ be a discrete space of labels. A learner observes a random *training sample*, D, of size n, consisting of the values of a sequence of input–label pairs $((X_1, Y_1), ..., (X_n, Y_n))$, where $(X_i, Y_i) \in \mathcal{X} \times \mathcal{Y}$. Based on the sample, the learner outputs a hypothesis $h : \mathcal{X} \to \mathcal{Y}$ that gives, for each possible input value, a prediction of the corresponding label. The learner is successful if the produced hypothesis has high probability of making a correct prediction when applied to a test case. (X_{n+1}, Y_{n+1}). Both the training sample and the test case are independently drawn from a common *generating distribution* P^*. We use the following error functionals:

Definition 1 (errors). *Given a training sample D of size n, the* i.i.d., off-training-set, *and* empirical error *of a hypothesis h are given by*

$$
\begin{aligned}
\mathcal{E}_{\mathrm{iid}}(h) &:= \Pr[Y \neq h(X)] & \textit{i.i.d. error,} \\
\mathcal{E}_{\mathrm{ots}}(h, D) &:= \Pr[Y \neq h(X) \mid X \notin \mathcal{X}_D] & \textit{off-training-set error,} \\
\mathcal{E}_{\mathrm{emp}}(h, D) &:= \tfrac{1}{n} \sum_{i=1}^{n} \mathbb{I}_{\{h(X_i) \neq Y_i\}} & \textit{empirical error,}
\end{aligned}
$$

where $\mathcal{X}_D$ is the set of X-values occurring in sample D, and the indicator function $\mathbb{I}_{\{\cdot\}}$ takes value one if its argument is true and zero otherwise.

The first one of these is just the standard generalization error of learning theory. Following [2], we call it i.i.d. error. For general input spaces and generating distributions $\mathcal{E}_{\text{ots}}(h, D)$ may be undefined for some D. In either case, this is not a problem. First, if $\mathcal{X}_D$ has measure one, the off-training-set error is undefined and we need not concern ourselves with it; the relevant error measure is $\mathcal{E}_{\text{iid}}(h)$ and standard results apply[1]. If, on the other hand, $\mathcal{X}_D$ has measure zero, the off-training-set error and the i.i.d. error are equivalent and our results (in Sec. 3 below) hold trivially. Thus, *if* off-training-set error is relevant, our results hold.

Definition 2. *Given a training sample D, the* sample coverage $p(\mathcal{X}_D)$ *is the probability that a new X-value appears in D: $p(\mathcal{X}_D) := \Pr[X \in \mathcal{X}_D]$, where $\mathcal{X}_D$ is as in Def. 1. The remaining probability, $1 - p(\mathcal{X}_D)$, is called the* missing mass.

Lemma 1. *For any training set D such that $\mathcal{E}_{\text{ots}}(h, D)$ is defined, we have*

$$a) \quad |\mathcal{E}_{\text{ots}}(h, D) - \mathcal{E}_{\text{iid}}(h)| \leq p(\mathcal{X}_D) \ ,$$

$$b) \quad \mathcal{E}_{\text{ots}}(h, D) - \mathcal{E}_{\text{iid}}(h) \leq \frac{p(\mathcal{X}_D)}{1 - p(\mathcal{X}_D)} \mathcal{E}_{\text{iid}}(h) \ .$$

Proof. Both bounds follow essentially from the following inequalities[2]:

$$
\begin{aligned}
\mathcal{E}_{\text{ots}}(h, D) &= \frac{\Pr[Y \neq h(X), X \notin \mathcal{X}_D]}{\Pr[X \notin \mathcal{X}_D]} \leq \frac{\Pr[Y \neq h(X)]}{\Pr[X \notin \mathcal{X}_D]} \wedge 1 = \frac{\mathcal{E}_{\text{iid}}(h)}{1 - p(\mathcal{X}_D)} \wedge 1 \\
&= \left(\frac{\mathcal{E}_{\text{iid}}(h)}{1 - p(\mathcal{X}_D)} \wedge 1 \right)(1 - p(\mathcal{X}_D)) + \left(\frac{\mathcal{E}_{\text{iid}}(h)}{1 - p(\mathcal{X}_D)} \wedge 1 \right) p(\mathcal{X}_D) \\
&\leq \mathcal{E}_{\text{iid}}(h) + p(\mathcal{X}_D) \ ,
\end{aligned}
$$

where $\wedge$ denotes the minimum. This gives one direction of Lemma 1.a (an *upper* bound on $\mathcal{E}_{\text{ots}}(h, D)$); the other direction is obtained by using analogous inequalities for the quantity $1 - \mathcal{E}_{\text{ots}}(h, D)$, with $Y \neq h(X)$ replaced by $Y = h(X)$, which gives the upper bound $1 - \mathcal{E}_{\text{ots}}(h, D) \leq 1 - \mathcal{E}_{\text{iid}}(h) + p(\mathcal{X}_D)$. Lemma 1.b follows from the first line by ignoring the upper bound 1, and subtracting $\mathcal{E}_{\text{iid}}(h)$ from both sides. $\square$

Given the value of (or an upper bound on) $\mathcal{E}_{\text{iid}}(h)$, the upper bound of Lemma 1.b may be significantly stronger than that of Lemma 1.a. However, in this work we only use Lemma 1.a for simplicity since it depends on $p(\mathcal{X}_D)$ alone. The lemma would be of little use without a good enough upper bound on the sample coverage $p(\mathcal{X}_D)$, or equivalently, a lower bound on the missing mass. In the next section we obtain such a bound.

3 An Off-training-set Error Bound

Good-Turing estimators [6], named after Irving J. Good, and Alan Turing, are widely used in language modeling to estimate the missing mass. The known small bias of such estimators, together with a rate of convergence, can be used to obtain lower and upper bound for the missing mass [7, 8]. Unfortunately, for the sample sizes we are interested in, the lower bounds are not quite tight enough (see Fig. 1 below). In this section we state a new lower bound, not based on Good-Turing estimators, that is practically useful in our context. We compare this bound to the existing ones after Thm. 2.

Let $\bar{\mathcal{X}}_n \subset \mathcal{X}$ be the set consisting of the n most probable individual values of X. In case there are several such subsets any one of them will do. In case $\mathcal{X}$ has less than n elements, $\bar{\mathcal{X}}_n := \mathcal{X}$. Denote for short $\bar{p}_n := \Pr[X \in \bar{\mathcal{X}}_n]$. No assumptions are made regarding the value of $\bar{p}_n$, it may or may not be zero. The reason for us being interested in $\bar{p}_n$ is that

---

[1]Note however, that a continuous feature space does not necessarily imply this, see Sec. 4.
[2]This neat proof is due to Gilles Blanchard (personal communication).

it gives us an upper bound $p(\mathcal{X}_D) \leq \bar{p}_n$ on the sample coverage that holds for all D. We prove that when $\bar{p}_n$ is large it is likely that a sample of size n will have several repeated X-values so that the number of distinct X-values is less than n. This implies that if a sample with a small number of repeated X-values is observed, it is safe to assume that $\bar{p}_n$ is small and therefore, the sample coverage $p(\mathcal{X}_D)$ must also be small.

Lemma 2. *The probability of obtaining a sample of size $n \geq 1$ with at most $0 \leq r < n$ repeated X-values is upper-bounded by* $\Pr[\text{"at most } r \text{ repetitions"}] \leq \Delta(n, r, \bar{p}_n)$ *, where*

$$\Delta(n, r, \bar{p}_n) := \sum_{k=0}^{n} \binom{n}{k} \bar{p}_n^k (1 - \bar{p}_n)^{n-k} f(n, r, k) \tag{1}$$

and $f(n, r, k)$ *is given by* $f(n, r, k) := \begin{cases} 1 & \text{if } k < r \\ \min\left(\binom{k}{r} \frac{n!}{(n-k+r)!} n^{-(k-r)}, 1\right) & \text{if } k \geq r. \end{cases}$

$\Delta(n, r, \bar{p}_n)$ *is a non-increasing function of* $\bar{p}_n$.

For a proof, see Appendix A. Given a fixed confidence level $1 - \delta$ we can now define a data-dependent upper bound on the sample coverage

$$\mathcal{B}(\delta, D) := \arg \min_p \{p \ : \ \Delta(n, r, p) \leq \delta\} \ , \tag{2}$$

where r is the number of repeated X-values in D, and $\Delta(n, r, p)$ is given by Eq. (1).

Theorem 1. *For any $0 \leq \delta \leq 1$, the upper bound $\mathcal{B}(\delta, D)$ on the sample coverage given by Eq. (2) holds with at least probability $1 - \delta$:*

$$\Pr[p(\mathcal{X}_D) \leq \mathcal{B}(\delta, D)] \geq 1 - \delta \ .$$

Proof. Consider fixed values of the confidence level $1 - \delta$, sample size n, and probability $\bar{p}_n$. Let R be the largest integer for which $\Delta(n, R, \bar{p}_n) \leq \delta$. By Lemma 2 the probability of obtaining at most R repetitions is upper-bounded by δ. Thus, it is sufficient that the bound holds whenever the number of repetitions is greater than R. For any such $r > R$, we have $\Delta(n, r, \bar{p}_n) > \delta$. By Lemma 2 the function $\Delta(n, r, \bar{p}_n)$ is non-increasing in $\bar{p}_n$, and hence it must be that $\bar{p}_n < \arg \min_p \{p \ : \ \Delta(n, r, p) \leq \delta\} = \mathcal{B}(\delta, D)$. Since $p(\mathcal{X}_D) \leq \bar{p}_n$, the bound then holds for all $r > R$. $\square$

Rather than the sample coverage $p(\mathcal{X}_D)$, the real interest is often in off-training-set error. Using the relation between the two quantities, one gets the following corollary that follows directly from Lemma 1.a and Thm. 1.

Corollary 1 (main result: off-training-set error bound). *For any $0 \leq \delta \leq 1$, the difference between the i.i.d. error and the off-training-set error is bounded by*

$$\Pr[\forall h \ |\mathcal{E}_{\text{ots}}(h, D) - \mathcal{E}_{\text{iid}}(h)| \leq \mathcal{B}(\delta, D)] \geq 1 - \delta \ .$$

Corollary 1 implies that the off-training-set error and the i.i.d. error are entangled, thus transforming all distribution-free bounds on the i.i.d. error to similar bounds on the off-training-set error. Since the probabilistic part of the result (Lemma 1) does not involve a specific hypothesis, Corollary 1 holds for all hypotheses at the same time, and does not depend on the richness of the hypothesis class in terms of, for instance, its VC dimension.

Figure 1 illustrates the behavior of the bound (2) as the sample size grows. It can be seen that for a small number of repetitions the bound is nontrivial already at moderate sample sizes. Moreover, the effect of repetitions is tolerable, and it diminishes as the number of repetitions grows. Table 1 lists values of the bound for a number of data-sets from the UCI machine learning repository [9]. In many cases the bound is about 0.10–0.20 or less.

Theorem 2 gives an upper bound on the rate with which the bound decreases as n grows.

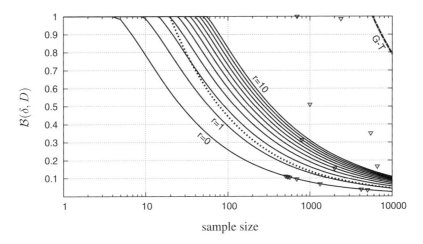

Figure 1: Upper bound $\mathcal{B}(\delta, D)$ given by Eq. (2) for samples with zero ($r = 0$) to ten ($r = 10$) repeated X-values on the 95 % confidence level ($\delta = 0.05$). The dotted curve is an asymptotic version for $r = 0$ given by Thm. 2. The curve labeled 'G-T' (for $r = 0$) is based on Good-Turing estimators (Thm. 3 in [7]). Asymptotically, it exceeds our $r = 0$ bound by a factor $O(\log n)$. Bound for the UCI data-sets in Table 1 are marked with small triangles ($\triangledown$). Note the log-scale for sample size.

Theorem 2 (a weaker bound in closed-form). *For all n and all $\bar{p}_n$, all $r < n$, the function $\mathcal{B}(\delta, D)$ has the upper bound $\mathcal{B}(\delta, D) \leq 3\sqrt{\frac{1}{2n}\left(\log \frac{4}{\delta} + 2r \log n\right)}$.*

For a proof, see Appendix A. Let us compare Thm. 2 to the existing bounds on $\mathcal{B}(\delta, D)$ based on Good-Turing estimators [7, 8]. For fixed δ, Thm. 3 in [7] gives an upper bound of $O\left(r/n + \log n/\sqrt{n}\right)$. The exact bound is drawn as the G-T curve in Fig. 1. In contrast, our bound gives $O\left(\sqrt{C + r \log n}/\sqrt{n}\right)$, for a known constant $C > 0$. For fixed r and increasing n, this gives an improvement over the G-T bound of order $O(\log n)$ if $r = 0$, and $O(\sqrt{\log n})$ if $r > 0$. For r growing faster than $O(\sqrt{\log n})$, asymptotically our bound becomes uncompetitive[3]. The real advantage of our bound is that, in contrast to G-T, it gives nontrivial bounds for sample sizes and number of repetitions that typically occur in classification problems. For practical applications in language modeling (large samples, many repetitions), the existing G-T bound of [7] is probably preferable.

The developments in [8] are also relevant, albeit in a more indirect manner. In Thm. 10 of that paper, it is shown that the probability that the missing mass is larger than its expected value by an amount ϵ is bounded by $e^{-(e/2)n\epsilon^2}$. In [7], Sec. 4, some techniques are developed to bound the expected missing mass in terms of the number of repetitions in the sample. One might conjecture that, combined with Thm. 10 of [8], these techniques can be extended to yield an upper bound on $\mathcal{B}(\delta, D)$ of order $O(r/n + 1/\sqrt{n})$ that would be asymptotically stronger than the current bound. We plan to investigate this and other potential ways to improve the bounds in future work. Any advance in this direction makes the implications of our bounds even more compelling.

---

[3]If data are i.i.d. according to a fixed P^*, then, as follows from the strong law of large numbers, r, considered as a function of n, will either remain zero for ever or will be larger than cn for some $c > 0$, for all n larger than some n_0. In practice, our bound is still relevant because typical data-sets often have r very small compared to n (see Table 1). This is possible because apparently $n \ll n_0$.

Table 1: Bounds on the difference between the i.i.d. error and the off-training-set error given by Eq. (2) on confidence level 95% ($\delta = 0.05$). A dash (-) indicates no repetitions. Bounds greater than 0.5 are in parentheses.

DATA	SAMPLE SIZE	REPETITIONS	BOUND
Abalone	4177	-	0.0383
Adult	32562	25	0.0959
Annealing	798	8	0.3149
Artificial Characters	1000	34	(0.5112)
Breast Cancer (Diagnostic)	569	-	0.1057
Breast Cancer (Original)	699	236	(1.0)
Credit Approval	690	-	0.0958
Cylinder Bands	542	-	0.1084
Housing	506	-	0.1123
Internet Advertisement	2385	441	(0.9865)
Isolated Letter Speech Recogn.	1332	-	0.0685
Letter Recognition	20000	1332	(0.6503)
Multiple Features	2000	4	0.1563
Musk	6598	17	0.1671
Page Blocks	5473	80	0.3509
Water Treatment Plant	527	-	0.1099
Waveform	5000	-	0.0350

4 Discussion – Implications of Our Results

The use of off-training-set error is an essential ingredient of the influential No Free Lunch theorems [1]–[5]. Our results imply that, while the NFL theorems themselves are valid, some of the conclusions drawn from them are overly pessimistic, and should be reconsidered. For instance, it has been suggested that the tools of conventional learning theory (dealing with standard generalization error) are "ill-suited for investigating off-training-set error" [3]. With the help of the little add-on we provide in this paper (Corollary 1), *any* bound on standard generalization error can be converted to a bound on off-training-set error. Our empirical results on UCI data-sets show that the resulting bound is often not essentially weaker than the original one. Thus, the conventional tools turn out not to be so 'ill-suited' after all. Secondly, contrary to what is sometimes suggested[4], we show that one *can* relate performance on the training sample to performance on as yet unseen cases.

On the other side of the debate, it has sometimes been claimed that the off-training-set error is irrelevant to much of modern learning theory where often the feature space is continuous. This may seem to imply that off-training-set error coincides with standard generalization error (see remark after Def. 1). However, this is true only if the associated *distribution* is continuous: *then* the probability of observing the same X-value twice is zero. However, in practice even when the feature space has continuous components, data-sets sometimes contain repetitions (e.g., Adult, see Table 1), if only for the reason that continuous features may be discretized or truncated. In practice repetitions occur in many data-sets, implying that off-training-set error can be different from the standard i.i.d. error. Thus, off-training-set error is *relevant*. Also, it measures a quantity that is in some ways close to the meaning of 'inductive generalization' – in dictionaries the words 'induction' and 'generalization' frequently refer to 'unseen instances'. Thus, off-training-set error is not just relevant but also *intuitive*. This makes it all the more interesting that standard generalization bounds transfer to off-training-set error – and that is the central implication of this paper.

---

[4]For instance, "if we are interested in the error for [unseen cases], the NFL theorems tell us that (in the absence of prior assumptions) [empirical error] is meaningless" [2].

Acknowledgments

We thank Gilles Blanchard for useful discussions. Part of this work was carried out while the first author was visiting CWI. This work was supported in part by the Academy of Finland (Minos, Prima), Nuffic, and IST Programme of the European Community, under the PASCAL Network, IST-2002-506778. This publication only reflects the authors' views.

References

[1] Wolpert, D.H.: On the connection between in-sample testing and generalization error. Complex Systems **6** (1992) 47–94

[2] Wolpert, D.H.: The lack of *a priori* distinctions between learning algorithms. Neural Computation **8** (1996) 1341–1390

[3] Wolpert, D.H.: The supervised learning no-free-lunch theorems. In: Proc. 6th Online World Conf. on Soft Computing in Industrial Applications (2001).

[4] Schaffer, C.: A conservation law for generalization performance. In: Proc. 11th Int. Conf. on Machine Learning (1994) 259–265

[5] Duda, R.O., Hart, P.E., Stork, D.G.: *Pattern Classification*, 2nd Edition. Wiley, 2001.

[6] Good, I.J.: The population frequencies of species and the estimation of population parameters. Biometrika **40** (1953) 237–264

[7] McAllester, D.A., Schapire, R.E.: On the convergence rate of Good-Turing estimators. In: Proc. 13th Ann. Conf. on Computational Learning Theory (2000) 1–6

[8] McAllester, D.A., Ortiz L.: Concentration inequalities for the missing mass and for histogram rule error. Journal of Machine Learning Research **4** (2003) 895–911.

[9] Blake, C., and Merz, C.: UCI repository of machine learning databases. Univ. of California, Dept. of Information and Computer Science (1998)

A   Postponed Proofs

We first state two propositions that are useful in the proof of Lemma 2.

Proposition 1. *Let $\mathcal{X}_m$ be a domain of size m, and let $P^*_{\mathcal{X}_m}$ be an associated probability distribution. The probability of getting no repetitions when sampling $1 \leq k \leq m$ items with replacement from distribution $P^*_{\mathcal{X}_m}$ is upper-bounded by*

$$\Pr[\text{``no repetitions''} \mid k] \leq \frac{m!}{(m-k)!m^k} \ .$$

Proof Sketch of Proposition 1. By way of contradiction it is possible to show that the probability of obtaining no repetitions is maximized when $P^*_{\mathcal{X}_m}$ is uniform. After this, it is easily seen that the maximal probability equals the right-hand side of the inequality. $\square$

Proposition 2. *Let $\mathcal{X}_m$ be a domain of size m, and let $P^*_{\mathcal{X}_m}$ be an associated probability distribution. The probability of getting at most $r \geq 0$ repeated values when sampling $1 \leq k \leq m$ items with replacement from distribution $P^*_{\mathcal{X}_m}$ is upper-bounded by*

$$\Pr[\text{``at most } r \text{ repetitions''} \mid k] \leq \begin{cases} 1 & \text{if } k < r \\ \min\left(\binom{k}{r}\frac{m!}{(m-k+r)!}m^{-(k-r)}, 1\right) & \text{if } k \geq r. \end{cases}$$

Proof of Proposition 2. The case $k < r$ is trivial. For $k \geq r$, the event "at most r repetitions in k draws" is equivalent to the event that there is at least one subset of size $k - r$ of the X-variables $\{X_1, \ldots, X_k\}$ such that all variables in the subset take distinct values. For a subset of size $k - r$, Proposition 1 implies that the probability that all values are distinct is at most $\frac{m!}{(m-k+r)!}m^{-(k-r)}$. Since there are $\binom{k}{r}$ subsets of the X-variables of size $k - r$, the union bound implies that multiplying this by $\binom{k}{r}$ gives the required result. $\square$

Proof of Lemma 2. The probability of getting at most r repeated X-values can be upper bounded by considering repetitions in the maximally probable set $\bar{\mathcal{X}}_n$ only. The probability of no repetitions in $\bar{\mathcal{X}}_n$ can be broken into $n+1$ mutually exclusive cases depending on how many X-values fall into the set $\bar{\mathcal{X}}_n$. Thus we get

$$\Pr[\text{"at most } r \text{ repetitions in } \bar{\mathcal{X}}_n\text{"}] = \sum_{k=0}^{n} \Pr[\text{"at most } r \text{ repetitions in } \bar{\mathcal{X}}_n\text{"} \mid k]\Pr[k] \ ,$$

where $\Pr[\cdot \mid k]$ denotes probability under the condition that k of the n cases fall into $\bar{\mathcal{X}}_n$, and $\Pr[k]$ denotes the probability of the latter occurring. Proposition 2 gives an upper bound on the conditional probability. The probability $\Pr[k]$ is given by the binomial distribution with parameter $\bar{p}_n$: $\Pr[k] = \text{Bin}(k \ ; \ n, \bar{p}_n) = \binom{n}{k}\bar{p}_n^k(1-\bar{p}_n)^{n-k}$. Combining these gives the formula for $\Delta(n, r, \bar{p}_n)$. Showing that $\Delta(n, r, \bar{p}_n)$ is non-increasing in $\bar{p}_n$ is tedious but uninteresting and we only sketch the proof: It can be checked that the conditional probability given by Proposition 2 is non-increasing in k (the min operator is essential for this). From this the claim follows since for increasing $\bar{p}_n$ the binomial distribution puts more weight to terms with large k, thus not increasing the sum. □

Proof of Thm. 2. The first three factors in the definition (1) of $\Delta(n, r, \bar{p}_n)$ are equal to a binomial probability $\text{Bin}(k \ ; \ n, \bar{p}_n)$, and the expectation of k is thus $n\bar{p}_n$. By the Hoeffding bound, for all $\epsilon > 0$, the probability of $k < n(\bar{p}_n - \epsilon)$ is bounded by $\exp(-2n\epsilon^2)$. Applying this bound with $\epsilon = \bar{p}_n/3$ we get that the probability of $k < \frac{2}{3}\bar{p}_n$ is bounded by $\exp(-\frac{2}{9}n\bar{p}_n^2)$. Combined with (1) this gives the following upper bound on $\Delta(n, r, \bar{p}_n)$:

$$\exp\left(-\frac{2}{9}n\bar{p}_n^2\right) \max_{k<n\frac{2}{3}\bar{p}_n} f(n, r, k) + \max_{k\geq n\frac{2}{3}\bar{p}_n} f(n, r, k) \leq \exp\left(-\frac{2}{9}n\bar{p}_n^2\right) + \max_{k\geq n\frac{2}{3}\bar{p}_n} f(n, r, k) \tag{3}$$

where the maxima are taken over integer-valued k. In the last inequality we used the fact that for all n, r, k, it holds that $f(n, r, k) \leq 1$. Now note that for $k \geq r$, we can bound

$$f(n, r, k) \leq \binom{k}{r} \prod_{j=0}^{k-r-1} \frac{n-j}{n} \leq \binom{n}{r} \prod_{j=0}^{k} \frac{n-j}{n} \prod_{j=k-r}^{k} \frac{n}{n-j} \leq$$

$$\binom{n}{r} \prod_{j=1}^{k} \frac{n-j}{n} \left(\frac{n}{n-k}\right)^{r+1} \leq n^{2r} \frac{n}{n-k} \prod_{j=1}^{k} \frac{n-j}{n} \ . \tag{4}$$

If $k < r$, $f(n, r, k) = 1$ so that (4) holds in fact for all k with $1 \leq k \leq n$. We bound the last factor $\prod_{j=1}^{k} \frac{n-j}{n}$ further as follows. The average of the k factors of this product is less than or equal to $\frac{n-k/2}{n} = 1 - \frac{k}{2n}$. Since a product of k factors is always less than or equal to the average of the factors to the power of k, we get the upper bound $\left(1 - \frac{k}{2n}\right)^k \leq \exp\left(-\frac{k \cdot k}{2n}\right) \leq \exp\left(-\frac{k^2}{2n}\right)$, where the first inequality follows from $1 - x \leq \exp(-x)$ for $x < 1$. Plugging this into (4) gives $f(n, r, k) \leq n^{2r} \frac{n}{n-k} \exp\left(-\frac{k^2}{2n}\right)$. Plugging this back into (3) gives $\Delta(n, r, \bar{p}_n) \leq \exp(-\frac{2}{9}n\bar{p}_n^2) + \max_{k\geq n\frac{2}{3}\bar{p}_n} 3n^{2r} \exp\left(-\frac{k^2}{2n}\right) \leq \exp(-\frac{2}{9}n\bar{p}_n^2) + 3n^{2r}\exp(-\frac{2}{9}n\bar{p}_n^2) \leq 4n^{2r}\exp(-\frac{2}{9}n\bar{p}_n^2)$.

Recall that $\mathcal{B}(\delta, D) := \arg\min_p \{p \ : \ \Delta(n, r, p) \leq \delta\}$. Replacing $\Delta(n, r, p)$ by the above upper bound, makes the set of p satisfying the inequality smaller. Thus, the minimal member of the reduced set is greater than or equal to the minimal member of the set with $\Delta(n, r, p) \leq \delta$, giving the following bound on $\mathcal{B}(\delta, D)$:

$$\mathcal{B}(\delta, D) \leq \arg\min_p \left\{p \ : \ 4n^{2r}\exp\left(-\frac{2}{9}np^2\right) \leq \delta\right\} = 3\sqrt{\frac{1}{2n}\left(\log\frac{4}{\delta} + 2r\log n\right)} \ . \quad □$$

Visual Encoding with Jittering Eyes

Michele Rucci[*]
Department of Cognitive and Neural Systems
Boston University
Boston, MA 02215
rucci@cns.bu.edu

Abstract

Under natural viewing conditions, small movements of the eye and body prevent the maintenance of a steady direction of gaze. It is known that stimuli tend to fade when they are stabilized on the retina for several seconds. However, it is unclear whether the physiological self-motion of the retinal image serves a visual purpose during the brief periods of natural visual fixation. This study examines the impact of fixational instability on the statistics of visual input to the retina and on the structure of neural activity in the early visual system. Fixational instability introduces fluctuations in the retinal input signals that, in the presence of natural images, lack spatial correlations. These input fluctuations strongly influence neural activity in a model of the LGN. They decorrelate cell responses, even if the contrast sensitivity functions of simulated cells are not perfectly tuned to counter-balance the power-law spectrum of natural images. A decorrelation of neural activity has been proposed to be beneficial for discarding statistical redundancies in the input signals. Fixational instability might, therefore, contribute to establishing efficient representations of natural stimuli.

1 Introduction

Models of the visual system often examine steady-state levels of neural activity during presentations of visual stimuli. It is difficult, however, to envision how such steady-states could occur under natural viewing conditions, given that the projection of the visual scene on the retina is never stationary. Indeed, the physiological instability of visual fixation keeps the retinal image in permanent motion even during the brief periods in between saccades.

Several sources cause this constant jittering of the eye. Fixational eye movements, of which we are not aware, alternate small saccades with periods of drifts, even when subjects are instructed to maintain steady fixation [8]. Following macroscopic redirection of gaze, other small eye movements, such as corrective saccades and post-saccadic drifts, are likely to occur. Furthermore, outside of the controlled conditions of a laboratory, when the head is not constrained by a bite bar, movements of the body, as well as imperfections in the vestibulo-ocular reflex, significantly amplify the motion of the retinal image. In the light of

---

[*]Webpage: www.cns.bu.edu/~rucci

this constant jitter, it is remarkable that the brain is capable of constructing a stable percept, as fixational instability moves the stimulus by an amount that should be clearly visible (see, for example, [7]).

Little is known about the purposes of fixational instability. It is often claimed that small saccades are necessary to refresh neuronal responses and prevent the disappearance of a stationary scene, a claim that has remained controversial given the brief durations of natural visual fixation (reviewed in [16]). Yet, recent theoretical proposals [1, 11] have claimed that fixational instability plays a more central role in the acquisition and neural encoding of visual information than that of simply refreshing neural activity. Consistent with the ideas of these proposals, neurophysiological investigations have shown that fixational eye movements strongly influence the activity of neurons in several areas of the monkey's brain [5, 14, 6]. Furthermore, modeling studies that simulated neural responses during free-viewing suggest that fixational instability profoundly affects the statistics of thalamic [13] and thalamocortical activity [10].

This paper summarizes an alternative theory for the existence of fixational instability. Instead of regarding the jitter of visual fixation as necessary for *refreshing* neuronal responses, it is argued that the self-motion of the retinal image is essential for properly *structuring* neural activity in the early visual system into a format that is suitable for processing at later stages. It is proposed that fixational instability is part of a strategy of acquisition of visual information that enables compact visual representations in the presence of natural visual input.

2 Neural decorrelation and fixational instability

It is a long-standing proposal that an important function of early visual processing is the removal of part of the redundancy that characterizes natural visual input [3]. Less redundant signals enable more compact representations, in which the same amount of information can be represented by smaller neuronal ensembles. While several methods exist for eliminating input redundancies, a possible approach is the removal of pairwise correlations between the intensity values of nearby pixels [2]. Elimination of these spatial correlations allows efficient representations in which neuronal responses tend to be less statistically dependent.

According to the theory described in this paper, fixational instability contributes to decorrelating the responses of cells in the retina and the LGN during viewing of natural scenes. This theory is based on two factors, which are described separately in the following sections. The first component, analyzed in Section 2.1, is the spatially uncorrelated input signal that occurs when natural scenes are scanned by jittering eyes. The second factor is an amplification of this spatially uncorrelated input, which is mediated by cell response characteristics. Section 2.2 examines the interaction between the dynamics of fixational instability and the temporal characteristics of neurons in the Lateral Geniculate Nucleus (LGN), the main relay of visual information to the cortex.

2.1 Influence of fixational instability on visual input

To analyze the effect of fixational instability on the statistics of geniculate activity, it is useful to approximate the input image in a neighborhood of a fixation point $\mathbf{x}_0$ by means of its Taylor series:

$$I(\mathbf{x}) \approx I(\mathbf{x}_0) + \nabla I(\mathbf{x}_0) \cdot (\mathbf{x} - \mathbf{x}_0)^T + \mathbf{o}(|\mathbf{x} - \mathbf{x}_0|^2) \tag{1}$$

If the jittering produced by fixational instability is sufficiently small, high-order derivatives can be neglected, and the input to a location $\mathbf{x}$ on the retina during visual fixation can be approximated by its first-order expansion:

$$S(\mathbf{x}, t) \approx I(\mathbf{x}) + \boldsymbol{\xi}^T(t) \cdot \nabla I(\mathbf{x}) = I(\mathbf{x}) + \tilde{I}(\mathbf{x}, t) \tag{2}$$

where $\boldsymbol{\xi}(t) = [\xi_x(t), \xi_y(t)]$ is the trajectory of the center of gaze during the period of fixation, t is the time elapsed from fixation onset, $I(\mathbf{x})$ is the visual input at $t = 0$, and $\tilde{I}(\mathbf{x}, t) = \frac{\partial I(\mathbf{x})}{\partial x}\xi_x(t) + \frac{\partial I(\mathbf{x})}{\partial y}\xi_y(t)$ is the dynamic fluctuation in the visual input produced by fixational instability.

Eq. 2 allows an analytical estimation of the power spectrum of the signal entering the eye during the self-motion of the retinal image. Since, according to Eq. 2, the retinal input $S(\mathbf{x}, t)$ can be approximated by the sum of two contributions, I and $\tilde{I}$, its power spectrum R_{SS} consists of three terms:

$$R_{SS}(\mathbf{u}, w) \approx R_{II} + R_{\tilde{I}\tilde{I}} + 2R_{I\tilde{I}}$$

where $\mathbf{u}$ and w represent, respectively, spatial and temporal frequency.

Fixational instability can be modeled as an ergodic process with zero mean and uncorrelated components along the two axes, $i.e.$, $\langle \boldsymbol{\xi} \rangle_T = \mathbf{0}$ and $R_{\xi_x \xi_y}(t) = 0$. Although not necessary for the proposed theory, these assumptions simplify our statistical analysis, as $R_{I\tilde{I}}$ is zero, and the power spectrum of the visual input is given by:

$$R_{SS} \approx R_{II} + R_{\tilde{I}\tilde{I}} \qquad (3)$$

where R_{II} is the power spectrum of the stimulus, and $R_{\tilde{I}\tilde{I}}$ depends on both the stimulus and fixational instability.

To determine $R_{\tilde{I}\tilde{I}}(\mathbf{u}, w)$, from Eq. 2 follows that

$$\tilde{I}(\mathbf{u}, w) = iu_x I(\mathbf{u})\xi_x(w) + iu_y I(\mathbf{u})\xi_y(w)$$

and under the assumption of uncorrelated motion components, approximating the power spectrum via finite Fourier Transform yields:

$$R_{\tilde{I}\tilde{I}}(\mathbf{u}, w) = \lim_{T \to \infty} < \frac{1}{T}|\tilde{I}_T(\mathbf{u}, w)|^2 >_{\xi, \mathcal{I}} = R_{\xi\xi}(w)R_{II}(\mathbf{u})|\mathbf{u}|^2 \qquad (4)$$

where $\tilde{I}_T$ is the Fourier Transform of a signal of duration T, and we have assumed identical second-order statistics of retinal image motion along the two Cartesian axes. As shown in Fig. 1 is clear that the presence of the term $\mathbf{u}^2$ in Eq. 4 compensates for the scaling invariance of natural images. That is, since for natural images $R_{II}(\mathbf{u}) \propto \mathbf{u}^{-2}$, the product $R_{II}(\mathbf{u})|\mathbf{u}|^2$ whitens R_{II} by producing a power spectrum $R_{\tilde{I}\tilde{I}}$ that remains virtually constant at all spatial frequencies.

2.2 Influence of fixational instability on neural activity

This section analyzes the structure of correlated activity during fixational instability in a model of the LGN. To delineate the important elements of the theory, we consider linear approximations of geniculate responses provided by space-time separable kernels. This assumption greatly simplifies the analysis of levels of correlation. Results are, however, general, and the outcomes of simulations with space-time inseparable kernels and different levels of rectification (the most prominent nonlinear behavior of parvocellular geniculate neurons) can be found in [13, 10].

Mean instantaneous firing rates were estimated on the basis of the convolution between the input I and the cell spatiotemporal kernel h_α:

$$\alpha(t) = h_\alpha(\mathbf{x}, t) \star I(\mathbf{x}, t) = \int_0^t \int_{-\infty}^\infty \int_{-\infty}^\infty h_\alpha(x', y', t')I(x - x', y - y', t - t')\,dx'\,dy'\,dt'$$

where $h_\alpha(\mathbf{x}, t) = g_\alpha(t)f_\alpha(\mathbf{x})$. Kernels were designed on the basis of data from neurophysiological recordings to replicate the responses of parvocellular ON-center cells in the LGN

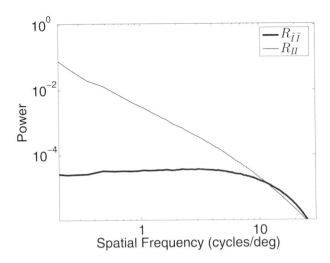

Figure 1: Fixational instability introduces a spatially uncorrelated component in the visual input to the retina during viewing of natural scenes. The graph compares the power spectrum of natural images (R_{II}) to the dynamic power spectrum introduced by fixational instability ($R_{\bar{I}\bar{I}}$). The two curves represent radial averages evaluated over 15 pictures of natural scenes.

of the macaque. The spatial component $f_\alpha(\mathbf{x})$ was modeled by a standard difference of Gaussian [15]. The temporal kernel $g_\alpha(t)$ possessed a biphasic profile with positive peak at 50 ms, negative peak at 75 ms, and overall duration of less than 200 ms [4].

In this section, levels of correlation in the activity of pairs of geniculate neurons are summarized by the correlation pattern $\hat{c}_{\alpha\alpha}(\mathbf{x})$:

$$\hat{c}_{\alpha\alpha}(\mathbf{x}) = \langle \alpha_{\mathbf{y}}(t)\alpha_{\mathbf{z}}(t)\rangle \Big|_{T,\mathcal{I}} \tag{5}$$

where $\alpha_{\mathbf{y}}(t)$ and $\alpha_{\mathbf{z}}(t)$ are the responses of cells with receptive fields centered at $\mathbf{y}$ and $\mathbf{z}$, and $\mathbf{x} = \mathbf{y} - \mathbf{z}$ is the separation between receptive field centers. The average is evaluated over time T and over a set of stimuli $\mathcal{I}$.

With linear models, $\hat{c}_{\alpha\alpha}(\mathbf{x})$ can be estimated on the basis of the input power spectrum $R_{SS}(\mathbf{u}, w)$:

$$\hat{c}_{\alpha\alpha}(\mathbf{x}) = c_{\alpha\alpha}(\mathbf{x}, t)\Big|_{t=0} \quad \text{and} \quad c_{\alpha\alpha}(\mathbf{x}, t) = \mathcal{F}^{-1}\{R_{\alpha\alpha}\} \tag{6}$$

where $R_{\alpha\alpha} = |H_\alpha|^2 R_{SS}(\mathbf{u}, w)$ is the power spectrum of LGN activity ($H_\alpha(\mathbf{u}, w)$ is the spatiotemporal Fourier transform of the kernel $h_\alpha(\mathbf{x}, t)$), and $\mathcal{F}^{-1}$ represents the inverse Fourier transform operator.

To evaluate $R_{\alpha\alpha}$, substitution of R_{SS} from Eq. 3 and separation of spatial and temporal elements yield:

$$R_{\alpha\alpha} \approx |G_\alpha|^2|F_\alpha|^2 R_{II} + |G_\alpha|^2|F_\alpha|^2 R_{\bar{I}\bar{I}} = R_{\alpha\alpha}^S + R_{\alpha\alpha}^D \tag{7}$$

where $F_\alpha(\mathbf{u})$ and $G_\alpha(w)$ represent the Fourier Transforms of the spatial and temporal kernels. Eq. 7 shows that, similar to the retinal input, also the power spectrum of geniculate activity can be approximated by the sum of two separate elements. Only $R_{\alpha\alpha}^D$ depends on fixational instability. The first term, $R_{\alpha\alpha}^S$, is determined by the power spectrum of the stimulus and the characteristics of geniculate cells but does not depend on the motion of the eye during the acquisition of visual information.

By substituting in Eq. 6 the expression of $R_{\alpha\alpha}$ from Eq. 7, we obtain

$$c_{\alpha\alpha}(\mathbf{x}, t) \approx c_{\alpha\alpha}^S(\mathbf{x}, t) + c_{\alpha\alpha}^D(\mathbf{x}, t) \tag{8}$$

where

$$c_{\alpha\alpha}^S(\mathbf{x}, t) = \mathcal{F}^{-1}\{R_{\alpha\alpha}^S(\mathbf{u}, w)\} \text{ and } c_{\alpha\alpha}^D(\mathbf{x}, t) = \mathcal{F}^{-1}\{R_{\alpha\alpha}^D(\mathbf{u}, w)\}$$

Eq. 8 shows that fixational instability adds the term $c_{\alpha\alpha}^D$ to the pattern of correlated activity $c_{\alpha\alpha}^S$ that would obtained with presentation of the same set of stimuli without the self-motion of the eye.

With presentation of pictures of natural scenes, $R_{II}(w) = 2\pi\delta(w)$, and the two input signals $R_{\alpha\alpha}^S$ and $R_{\alpha\alpha}^D$ provide, respectively, a static and a dynamic contribution to the spatiotemporal correlation of geniculate activity. The first term in Eq. 8 gives a correlation pattern:

$$\hat{c}_{\alpha\alpha}^S(\mathbf{x}) = k_S \mathcal{F}_S^{-1}\{|F_\alpha|^2 R_{II}^S(\mathbf{u})\} \tag{9}$$

where $k_S = |G(0)|^2$.

By substituting $R_{\tilde{I}\tilde{I}}$ from Eq. 4, the second term in Eq. 8 gives a correlation pattern:

$$\hat{c}_{\alpha\alpha}^D(\mathbf{x}) = k_D \mathcal{F}_S^{-1}\{|F_\alpha|^2 R_{II}^S(\mathbf{u})|\mathbf{u}|^2\} \tag{10}$$

where $k_D = \mathcal{F}_T^{-1}\{|G_\alpha(w)|^2 R_{\xi\xi}(w)\}\Big|_{t=0}$ is a constant given by the temporal dynamics of cell response and fixational instability. $\mathcal{F}_T^{-1}$ and $\mathcal{F}_S^{-1}$ indicate the operations of inverse Fourier Transform in time and space.

To summarize, during the physiological instability of visual fixation, the structure of correlated activity in a linear model of the LGN is given by the superposition of two spatial terms, each of them weighted by a coefficient (k_S and k_D) that depends on dynamics:

$$\hat{c}_{\alpha\alpha}(\mathbf{x}) = k_S \mathcal{F}_S^{-1}\{(|F_\alpha|^2 R_{II}^S(\mathbf{u})\} + k_D \mathcal{F}_S^{-1}\{|F_\alpha|^2 R_{II}^S(\mathbf{u})|\mathbf{u}|^2\} \tag{11}$$

Whereas the stimulus contributes to the structure of correlated activity by means of the power spectrum R_{II}^S, the contribution introduced by fixational instability depends on $R_{\tilde{I}\tilde{I}}^S$, a signal that discards the broad correlation of natural images. Since in natural images, most power is concentrated at low spatial frequencies, the uncorrelated fluctuations in the input signals generated by fixational instability have small amplitudes. That is, R_{II}^D provides less power than R_{II}^S. However, geniculate cells tend to respond more strongly to changing stimuli than stationary ones, and k_D is larger than k_S. Therefore, the small input modulations introduced by fixational instability are amplified by the dynamics of geniculate cells.

Fig. 2 shows the structure of correlated activity in the model when images of natural scenes are examined in the presence of fixational instability. In this example, fixational instability was assumed to possess Gaussian temporal correlation, $R_{\xi\xi}(w)$, with standard deviation $\sigma_T = 22$ ms and amplitude $\sigma_S = 12$ arcmin. In addition to the total pattern of correlation given by Eq. 11, Fig. 2 also shows the patterns of correlation produced by the two components $\hat{c}_{\alpha\alpha}^S$ and $\hat{c}_{\alpha\alpha}^D$. Whereas $\hat{c}_{\alpha\alpha}^S$ was strongly influenced by the broad spatial correlations of natural images, $\hat{c}_{\alpha\alpha}^D$, due to its dependence on the whitened power spectrum $R_{\tilde{I}\tilde{I}}$, was determined exclusively by cell receptive fields. Due to the amplification factor k_D, $\hat{c}_{\alpha\alpha}^D$ provided a stronger contribution than $\hat{c}_{\alpha\alpha}^S$ and heavily influenced the global structure of correlated activity.

To examine the relative influence of the two terms $\hat{c}_{\alpha\alpha}^S$ and $\hat{c}_{\alpha\alpha}^D$ on the structure of correlated activity, Fig. 3 shows their ratio at separation zero, $\rho_{DS} = \hat{c}_{\alpha\alpha}^D(0)/\hat{c}_{\alpha\alpha}^S(0)$, with

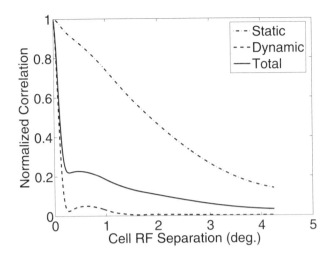

Figure 2: Patterns of correlation obtained from Eq. 11 when natural images are examined in the presence of fixational instability. The three curves represent the total level of correlation (Total), the correlation $\hat{c}^S_{\alpha\alpha}(\mathbf{x})$ that would be present if the same images were examined in the absence of fixational instability (Static), and the contribution $\hat{c}^D_{\alpha\alpha}(\mathbf{x})$ of fixational instability (Dynamic). Data are radial averages evaluated over pairs of cells with the same separation $\|\mathbf{x}\|$ between their receptive fields.

presentation of natural images and for various parameters of fixational instability. Fig. 3 (a) shows the effect of varying the spatial amplitude of the retinal jitter. In order to remain within the range of validity of the Taylor approximation in Eq. 2, only small amplitude values are considered. As shown by Fig. 3 (a), the larger the instability of visual fixation, the larger the contribution of the dynamic term $\hat{c}^D_{\alpha\alpha}$ with respect to $\hat{c}^S_{\alpha\alpha}$. Except for very small values of σ_S, ρ_{DS} is larger than one, indicating that $\hat{c}^D_{\alpha\alpha}$ influences the structure of correlated activity more strongly than $\hat{c}^S_{\alpha\alpha}$. Fig. 3 (b) shows the impact of varying σ_T, which defines the temporal window over which fixational jitter is correlated. Note that ρ_{DS} is a non-monotonic function of σ_T. For a range of σ_T corresponding to intervals shorter than the typical duration of visual fixation, $\hat{c}^D_{\alpha\alpha}$ is significantly larger than $\hat{c}^S_{\alpha\alpha}$. Thus, fixational instability strongly influences correlated activity in the model when it moves the direction of gaze within a range of a few arcmin and is correlated over a fraction of the duration of visual fixation. This range of parameters is consistent with the instability of fixation observed in primates.

3   Conclusions

It has been proposed that neurons in the early visual system decorrelate their responses to natural stimuli, an operation that is believed to be beneficial for the encoding of visual information [2]. The original claim, which was based on psychophysical measurements of human contrast sensitivity, relies on an inverse proportionality between the spatial response characteristics of retinal and geniculate neurons and the structure of natural images. However, data from neurophysiological recordings have clearly shown that neurons in the retina and the LGN respond significantly to low spatial frequencies, in a way that is not compatible with the requirements of Atick and Redlich's proposal. During natural viewing, input signals to the retina depend not only on the stimulus, but also on the physiological instability of visual fixation. The results of this study show that when natural scenes are examined

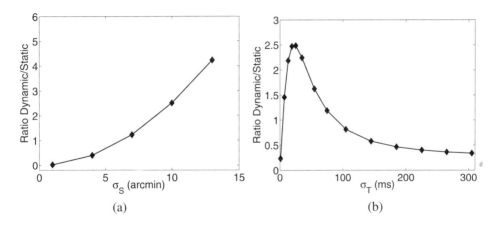

Figure 3: Influence of the characteristics of fixational instability on the patterns of correlated activity during presentation of natural images. The two graphs show the ratio ρ_{DS} between the peaks of the two terms $\hat{c}^D_{\alpha\alpha}$ and $\hat{c}^S_{\alpha\alpha}$ in Eq. 8. Fixational instability was assumed to possess a Gaussian correlation with standard deviation σ_T and amplitude σ_S. (a) Effect of varying σ_S ($\sigma_T = 22$ ms). (b) Effect of varying σ_T ($\sigma_S = 12$ arcmin).

with jittering eyes, as occurs under natural viewing conditions, fixational instability tends to decorrelate cell responses even if the contrast sensitivity functions of individual neurons do not counterbalance the power spectrum of visual input.

The theory described in this paper relies of two main elements. The first component is the presence of a spatially uncorrelated input signal during presentation of natural visual stimuli ($R_{\tilde{I}\tilde{I}}$ in Eq. 3). This input signal is a direct consequence of the scale invariance of natural images. It is a property of natural images that, although the intensity values of nearby pixels tend to be correlated, changes in intensity around pairs of pixels are uncorrelated. This property is not satisfied by an arbitrary image. In a spatial grating, for example, intensity changes at any two locations are highly correlated. During the instability of visual fixation, neurons receive input from the small regions of the visual field covered by the jittering of their receptive fields. In the presence of natural images, although the inputs to cells with nearby receptive fields are on average correlated, the fluctuations in these input signals produced by fixational instability are not correlated. Fixational instability appears to be tuned to the statistics of natural images, as it introduces a spatially uncorrelated signal only in the presence of visual input with a power spectrum that declines as u^{-2} with spatial frequency.

The second element of the theory is the neuronal amplification of the spatially uncorrelated input signal introduced by the self-motion of the retinal image. This amplification originates from the interaction between the dynamics of fixational instability and the temporal sensitivity of geniculate units. Since $R_{\tilde{I}\tilde{I}}$ attenuates the low spatial frequencies of the stimulus, it tends to possess less power than R_{II}. However, in Eq. 11, the contributions of the two input signals are modulated by the multiplicative terms k_S and k_D, which depend on the temporal characteristics of cell responses (both k_S and k_D) and fixational instability (k_D only). Since geniculate neurons respond more strongly to changing stimuli than to stationary ones, k_D tends to be higher than k_S. Correspondingly, in a linear model of the LGN, units are highly sensitive to the uncorrelated fluctuations in the input signals produced by fixational instability.

The theory summarized in this study is consistent with the strong modulations of neural responses observed during fixational eye movements [5, 14, 6], as well as with the results of recent psychophysical experiments aimed at investigating perceptual influences of fixational instability [12, 9]. It should be observed that, since patterns of correlations were evaluated via Fourier analysis, this study implicitly assumed a steady-state condition of visual fixation. Further work is needed to extend the proposed theory in order to take into account time-varying natural stimuli and the nonstationary regime produced by the occurrence of saccades.

Acknowledgments

The author thanks Antonino Casile and Gaelle Desbordes for many helpful discussions. This material is based upon work supported by the National Institute of Health under Grant EY15732-01 and the National Science Foundation under Grant CCF-0432104.

References

[1] E. Ahissar and A. Arieli. Figuring space by time. *Neuron*, 32(2):185–201, 2001.

[2] J. J. Atick and A. Redlich. What does the retina know about natural scenes? *Neural Comp.*, 4:449–572, 1992.

[3] H. B. Barlow. The coding of sensory messages. In W. H. Thorpe and O. L. Zangwill, editors, *Current Problems in Animal Behaviour*, pages 331–360. Cambridge University Press, Cambridge, 1961.

[4] E. A. Benardete and E. Kaplan. Dynamics of primate P retinal ganglion cells: Responses to chromatic and achromatic stimuli. *J. Physiol.*, 519(3):775–790, 1999.

[5] D. A. Leopold and N. K. Logothetis. Microsaccades differentially modulate neural activity in the striate and extrastriate visual cortex. *Exp. Brain. Res.*, 123:341–345, 1998.

[6] S. Martinez-Conde, S. L. Macknik, and D. H. Hubel. The function of bursts of spikes during visual fixation in the awake primate lateral geniculate nucleus and primary visual cortex. *Proc. Natl. Acad. Sci. USA*, 99(21):13920–13925, 2002.

[7] I. Murakami and P. Cavanagh. A jitter after-effect reveals motion-based stabilization of vision. *Nature*, 395(6704):798–801, 1998.

[8] F. Ratliff and L. A. Riggs. Involuntary motions of the eye during monocular fixation. *J. Exp. Psychol.*, 40:687–701, 1950.

[9] M. Rucci and J. Beck. Effects of ISI and flash duration on the identification of briefly flashed stimuli. *Spatial Vision*, 18(2):259–274, 2005.

[10] M. Rucci and A. Casile. Decorrelation of neural activity during fixational instability: Possible implications for the refinement of V1 receptive fields. *Visual Neurosci.*, 21:725–738, 2004.

[11] M. Rucci and A. Casile. Fixational instability and natural image statistics: Implications for early visual representations. *Network: Computation in Neural Systems*, 16(2-3):121–138, 2005.

[12] M. Rucci and G. Desbordes. Contributions of fixational eye movements to the discrimination of briefly presented stimuli. *J. Vision*, 3(11):852–64, 2003.

[13] M. Rucci, G. M. Edelman, and J. Wray. Modeling LGN responses during free-viewing: A possible role of microscopic eye movements in the refinement of cortical orientation selectivity. *J. Neurosci*, 20(12):4708–4720, 2000.

[14] D. M. Snodderly, I. Kagan, and M. Gur. Selective activation of visual cortex neurons by fixational eye movements: Implications for neural coding. *Vis. Neurosci.*, 18:259–277, 2001.

[15] P. D. Spear, R. J. Moore, C. B. Y. Kim, J. T. Xue, and N. Tumosa. Effects of aging on the primate visual system: spatial and temporal processing by lateral geniculate neurons in young adult and old rhesus monkeys. *J. Neurophysiol.*, 72:402–420, 1994.

[16] R.M. Steinman and J.Z. Levinson. The role of eye movements in the detection of contrast and spatial detail. In E. Kowler, editor, *Eye Movements and their Role in Visual and Cognitive Processes*, pages 115–212. Elsevier Science, 1990.

Dynamic Social Network Analysis using Latent Space Models

Purnamrita Sarkar, Andrew W. Moore
Center for Automated Learning and Discovery
Carnegie Mellon University
Pittsburgh, PA 15213
(psarkar,awm)@cs.cmu.edu

Abstract

This paper explores two aspects of social network modeling. First, we generalize a successful static model of relationships into a dynamic model that accounts for friendships drifting over time. Second, we show how to make it tractable to learn such models from data, even as the number of entities n gets large. The generalized model associates each entity with a point in p-dimensional Euclidian latent space. The points can move as time progresses but large moves in latent space are improbable. Observed links between entities are more likely if the entities are close in latent space. We show how to make such a model tractable (sub-quadratic in the number of entities) by the use of appropriate kernel functions for similarity in latent space; the use of low dimensional kd-trees; a new efficient dynamic adaptation of multidimensional scaling for a first pass of approximate projection of entities into latent space; and an efficient conjugate gradient update rule for non-linear local optimization in which amortized time per entity during an update is $O(\log n)$. We use both synthetic and real-world data on upto 11,000 entities which indicate linear scaling in computation time and improved performance over four alternative approaches. We also illustrate the system operating on twelve years of NIPS co-publication data. We present a detailed version of this work in [1].

1   Introduction

Social network analysis is becoming increasingly important in many fields besides sociology including intelligence analysis [2], marketing [3] and recommender systems [4]. Here we consider learning in systems in which relationships drift over time.

Consider a friendship graph in which the nodes are entities and two entities are linked if and only if they have been observed to collaborate in some way. In 2002, Raftery et al [5]introduced a model similar to Multidimensional Scaling in which entities are associated with locations in p-dimensional space, and links are more likely if the entities are close in latent space. In this paper we suppose that each observed link is associated with a discrete timestep, so each timestep produces its own graph of observed links, and information is preserved between timesteps by two assumptions. First we assume entities can move in latent space between timesteps, but large moves are improbable. Second, we make a standard Markov assumption that latent locations at time $t + 1$ are conditionally independent of all previous locations given the latent locations at time t and that the observed graph at time t is conditionally independent of all other positions and graphs, given the locations at time t (see Figure 1).

Let G_t be the graph of observed pairwise links at time t. Assuming n entities, and a p-dimensional latent space, let X_t be an $n \times p$ matrix in which the ith row, called x_i, corresponds to the latent position of entity i at time t. Our conditional independence structure, familiar in HMMs and Kalman filters, is shown in Figure 1. For most of this paper we treat the problem as a tracking problem in which we estimate X_t at each timestep as a function of the current observed graph G_t and the previously estimated positions X_{t-1}. We want

$$X_t = \arg\max_X P(X|G_t, X_{t-1}) = \arg\max_X P(G_t|X)P(X|X_{t-1}) \tag{1}$$

In Section 2 we design models of $P(G_t|X_t)$ and $P(X_t|X_{t-1})$ that meet our modeling needs *and* which have learning times that are tractable as n gets large. In Sections 3 and 4 we introduce a two-stage procedure for locally optimizing equation (1). The first stage generalizes linear multidimensional scaling algorithms to the dynamic case while carefully maintaining the ability to computationally exploit sparsity in the graph. This gives an approximate estimate of X_t. The second stage refines this estimate using an augmented conjugate gradient approach in which gradient updates can use kd-trees over latent space to allow $O(n \log n)$ computation per step.

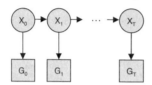

Figure 1: Model through time

2 The DSNL (Dynamic Social Network in Latent space) Model

Let $d_{ij} = |x_i - x_j|$ be the Euclidian distance between entities i and j in latent space at time t. For clarity we will not use a t subscript on these variables except where it is needed. We denote linkage at time t by $i \sim j$, and absence of a link by $i \nsim j$. $p(i \sim j)$ denotes the probability of observing the link. We use $p(i \sim j)$ and p_{ij} interchangeably.

2.1 Observation Model

The likelihood score function $P(G_t|X_t)$ intuitively measures how well the model explains pairs of entities which are actually connected in the training graph as well as those that are not. Thus it is simply

$$P(G_t|X_t) = \prod_{i \sim j} p_{ij} \prod_{i \nsim j} (1 - p_{ij}) \tag{2}$$

Following [5] the link probability is a logistic function of d_{ij} and is denoted as p_{ij}^L, i.e.

$$p_{ij}^L = \frac{1}{1 + e^{(d_{ij} - \alpha)}} \tag{3}$$

where α is a constant whose significance is explained shortly. So far this model is similar to [5]. To extend this model to the dynamic case, we now make two important alterations.

First, we allow entities to vary their sociability. Some entities participate in many links while others are in few. We give each entity a *radius*, which will be used as a sphere of interaction within latent space. We denote entity i's radius as r_i. We introduce the term r_{ij} to replace α in equation (3). r_{ij} is the maximum of the radii of i and j. Intuitively, an entity with higher degree will have a larger radius. Thus we define the radius of entity i with degree δ_i as, $c(\delta_i + 1)$, so that r_{ij} is $c \times (max(\delta_i, \delta_j) + 1)$, and c will be estimated from the data. In practice, we estimate the constant c by a simple line-search on the score function. The constant 1 ensures a nonzero radius.

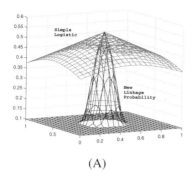
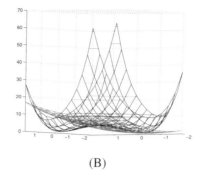

|(A)|(B)|

Figure 2: A. The actual logistic function, and our kernelized version with $\rho = 0.1$. B.The actual (flat, with one minimum), and the modified (steep with two minima) constraint functions, for two dimensions, with X_t varying over a 2-d grid, from $(-2, -2)$ to $(2, 2)$, and $X_{t-1} = (1, 1)$

The second alteration is to weigh the link probabilities by a kernel function. We alter the simple logistic link probability p_{ij}^L, such that two entities have high probability of linkage only if their latent coordinates are within distance r_{ij} of one another. Beyond this range there is a constant noise probability ρ of linkage. Later we will need the kernelized function to be continuous and differentiable at r_{ij}. Thus we pick the biquadratic kernel.

$$K(d_{ij}) = (1 - (d_{ij}/r_{ij})^2)^2, \qquad\qquad \text{when } d_{ij} \leq r_{ij}$$
$$= 0, \qquad\qquad \text{otherwise} \qquad (4)$$

Using this function we redefine our link probability p_{ij} as $p_{ij}^L K(d_{ij}) + \rho(1 - K(d_{ij}))$. This is equivalent to having,

$$p_{ij} = \frac{1}{1 + e^{(d_{ij} - r_{ij})}} K(d_{ij}) + \rho(1 - K(d_{ij})) \qquad\qquad \text{when } d_{ij} \leq r_{ij}$$
$$= \rho \qquad\qquad \text{otherwise} \qquad (5)$$

We plot this function in Figure 2A.

2.2 Transition Model

The second part of the score penalizes large displacements from the previous time step. We use the most obvious Gaussian model: each coordinate of each latent position is independently subjected to a Gaussian perturbation with mean 0 and variance σ^2. Thus

$$\log P(X_t | X_{t-1}) = -\sum_{i=1}^{n} |X_{i,t} - X_{i,t-1}|^2 / 2\sigma^2 + const \qquad (6)$$

3   Learning Stage One: Linear Approximation

We generalize classical multidimensional scaling (MDS) [6] to get an initial estimate of the positions in the latent space. We begin by recapping what MDS does. It takes as input an $n \times n$ matrix of non-negative distances D where $D_{i,j}$ denotes the target distance between entity i and entity j. It produces an $n \times p$ matrix X where the ith row is the position of entity i in p-dimensional latent space. MDS finds $\arg\min_X |\tilde{D} - XX^T|_F$ where $|\cdot|_F$ denotes the Frobenius norm [7]. $\tilde{D}$ is the similarity matrix obtained from D, using standard linear algebra operations. Let Γ be the matrix of the eigenvectors of $\tilde{D}$, and Λ be a diagonal matrix with the corresponding eigenvalues. Denote the matrix of the p positive eigenvalues by Λ_p and the corresponding columns of Γ by Γ_p. From this follows the expression of classical MDS, i.e. $X = \Gamma_p \Lambda_p^{\frac{1}{2}}$.

Two questions remain. Firstly, what should be our target distance matrix D? Secondly, how should this be extended to account for time? The first answer follows from [5] and defines D_{ij} as length of the shortest path from i to j in graph G. We restrict this length to a maximum of three hops in order to avoid the full n^2 computation of all-shortest paths. D thus has a dense mostly constant structure.

When accounting for time, we do not want the positions of entities to change drastically from one time step to another. Hence we try to minimize $|X_t - X_{t-1}|_F$ along with the main objective of MDS. Let $\tilde{D}_t$ denote the $\tilde{D}$ matrix derived from G_t. We formulate the above problem as minimization of $|\tilde{D}_t - X_t X_t^T|_F + \lambda |X_t - X_{t-1}|_F$, where λ is a parameter which controls the importance of the two parts of the objective function. The above does not have a closed form solution. However, by constraining the objective function further, we can obtain a closed form solution for a closely related problem. The idea is to work with the distances and not the positions themselves. Since we are learning the positions from distances, we change our constraint (during this linear stage of learning) to encourage the pairwise distance between all pairs of entities to change little between each time step, instead of encouraging the individual coordinates to change little. Hence we try to minimize

$$|\tilde{D}_t - X_t X_t^T|_F + \lambda |X_t X_t^T - X_{t-1} X_{t-1}^T|_F \qquad (7)$$

which is equivalent to minimizing the trace of $(\tilde{D}_t - X_t X_t^T)^T (\tilde{D}_t - X_t X_t^T) + \lambda (X_t X_t^T - X_{t-1} X_{t-1}^T)^T (X_t X_t^T - X_{t-1} X_{t-1}^T)$. The above expression has an analytical solution: an affine combination of the current information from the graph and the coordinates at the last timestep. Namely, the new solution satisfies,

$$X_t X_t^T = \frac{1}{1+\lambda} \tilde{D}_t + \frac{\lambda}{1+\lambda} X_{t-1} X_{t-1}^T \qquad (8)$$

We plot the two constraint functions in Figure 2B. When λ is zero, $X_t X_t^T$ equals $\tilde{D}_t$, and when $\lambda \to \infty$, it is equal to $X_{t-1} X_{t-1}^T$. As in MDS, eigendecomposition of the right hand side of equation 8 yields the solution X_t which minimizes the objective function in equation 7.

We now have a method which finds latent coordinates for time t that are consistent with G_t and have similar pairwise distances as X_{t-1}. But although all pairwise distances may be similar, the coordinates may be very different. Indeed, even if λ is very large and we only care about preserving distances, the resulting X may be any reflection, rotation or translation of the original X_{t-1}. We solve this by applying the *Procrustes* transform to the solution X_t of equation 8. This transform finds the linear area-preserving transformation of X_t that brings it closest to the previous configuration X_{t-1}. The solution is unique if $X_t^T X_{t-1}$ is nonsingular [8], and for zero centered X_t and X_{t-1}, is given by $X_t^* = X_t U V^T$, where $X_t^T X_{t-1} = U S V^T$ using Singular Value Decomposition (SVD).

Before moving on to stage two's nonlinear optimization we must address the scalability of stage one. The naive implementation (SVD of the matrix from equation 8) has a cost of $O(n^3)$, for n nodes, since both $\tilde{D}_t$, and $X_t X_t^T$, are dense $n \times n$ matrices. However in [1] we show how we use the power method [9] to exploit the dense mostly constant structure of D_t and the fact that $X_t X_t^T$ is just an outer product of two thin $n \times p$ matrices. The power method is an iterative eigendecomposition technique which only involves multiplying a matrix by a vector. Its net cost can be shown to be $O(n^2 f + n + pn)$ per iteration, where f is the fraction of non-constant entries in D_t.

4 Stage Two: Nonlinear Search

Stage One places entities in reasonably consistent locations which fit our intuition, but it is not tied to the probabilistic model from Section 2. Stage two uses these locations as initializations for applying nonlinear optimization directly to the model in equation 1. We use conjugate gradient (CG) which was the most effective of several alternatives attempted. The most important practical question is how to make these gradient computations tractable, especially when the model likelihood involves a double sum over all entities. We must compute the partial derivatives of $logP(G_t|X_t) + logP(X_t|X_{t-1})$ with respect to all values $x_{i,k,t}$ for $i \in 1...n$ and $k \in 1..p$. First consider the $P(G_t|X_t)$ term:

$$\frac{\partial \log P(G_t|X_t)}{\partial X_{i,k,t}} = \sum_{j,i \sim j} \frac{\partial \log p_{ij}}{\partial X_{i,k,t}} + \sum_{j,i \nsim j} \frac{\partial log(1-p_{ij})}{\partial X_{i,k,t}} = \sum_{j,i \sim j} \frac{\partial p_{ij}/\partial X_{i,k,t}}{p_{ij}} - \sum_{j,i \nsim j} \frac{\partial p_{ij}/\partial X_{i,k,t}}{1 - p_{ij}}$$
(9)

$$\partial p_{ij}/\partial X_{i,k,t} = \frac{\partial(p_{ij}^L K + \rho(1-K))}{\partial X_{i,k,t}} = K \frac{\partial p_{ij}^L}{\partial X_{i,k,t}} + p_{ij}^L \frac{\partial K}{\partial X_{i,k,t}} - \rho \frac{\partial K}{\partial X_{i,k,t}} = \psi_{i,j,k,t}$$
(10)

However K, the biquadratic kernel introduced in equation 4, evaluates to zero and has a zero derivative when $d_{ij} > r_{ij}$. Plugging this information in (10), we have,

$$\partial p_{ij}/\partial X_{i,k,t} = \begin{cases} \psi_{i,j,k,t} & \text{when } d_{ij} \leq r_{ij}, \\ 0 & \text{otherwise.} \end{cases}$$
(11)

Equation (9) now becomes

$$\frac{\partial \log P(G_t|X_t)}{\partial X_{i,k,t}} = \sum_{\substack{j,i \sim j \\ d_{ij} \leq r_{ij}}} \frac{\psi_{i,j,k,t}}{p_{ij}} - \sum_{\substack{j,i \nsim j \\ d_{ij} \leq r_{ij}}} \frac{\psi_{i,j,k,t}}{1 - p_{ij}}$$
(12)

when $d_{ij} \leq r_{ij}$ and zero otherwise. This simplification is very important because we can now use a spatial data structure such as a kd-tree in the low dimensional latent space to retrieve all pairs of entities that lie within each other's radius in time $O(rn + n \log n)$ where r is the average number of in-radius neighbors of an entity [10, 11]. The computation of the gradient involves only those pairs. A slightly more sophisticated trick, omitted for space reasons, lets us compute $\log P(G_t|X_t)$, in $O(rn + n \log n)$ time. From equation(6), we have

$$\frac{\partial \log P(X_t|X_{t-1})}{\partial X_{i,k,t}} = -\frac{X_{i,k,t} - X_{i,k,t-1}}{\sigma^2}$$
(13)

In the early stages of Conjugate Gradient, there is a danger of a plateau in our score function in which our first derivative is insensitive to two entities that are connected, but are not within each other's radius. To aid the early steps of CG, we add an additional term to the score function, which penalizes all pairs of connected entities according to the square of their separation in latent space, i.e. $\sum_{i \sim j} d_{ij}^2$. Weighting this by a constant $pConst$, our final CG gradient becomes

$$\frac{\partial Score_t}{\partial X_{i,k,t}} = \frac{\partial \log P(G_t|X_t)}{\partial X_{i,k,t}} + \frac{\partial \log P(X_t|X_{t-1})}{\partial X_{i,k,t}} - pConst \times 2 \sum_{\substack{j \\ i \sim j}} (X_{i,k,t} - X_{j,k,t})$$

5   Results

We report experiments on synthetic data generated by a model described below and the NIPS co-publication data [1]. We investigate three things: ability of the algorithm to reconstruct the latent space based only on link observations, anecdotal evaluation of what happens to the NIPS data, and scalability results on large datasets from Citeseer.

5.1   Comparing with ground truth

We generate synthetic data for six consecutive timesteps. At each timestep the next set of two-dimensional latent coordinates are generated with the former positions as mean, and a gaussian noise of standard deviation $\sigma = 0.01$. Each entity is assigned a random radius. At each step , each entity is linked with a relatively higher probability to the ones falling within its radius, or containing it within their radii. There is a noise probability of 0.1, by

---

[1] See http://www.cs.toronto.edu/~roweis/data.html

which any two entities i and j outside the maximum pairwise radii r_{ij} are connected. We generate graphs of sizes 20 to 1280, doubling the size every time. Accuracy is measured by drawing a test set from the same model, and determining the ROC curve for predicting whether a pair of entities will be linked in the test set. We experiment with six approaches:

A. The True model that was used to generate the data (this is an upper bound on the performance of any learning algotihm).
B. The DSNL model learned using the above algorithms.
C. A random model, guessing link probabilities randomly (this should have an AUC of 0.5).
D. The *Simple Counting* model (Control Experiment). This ranks the likelihood of being linked in the testset according to the frequency of linkage in the training set. It can be considered as the equivalent of the 1-nearest-neighbor method in classification: it does not generalize, but merely duplicates the training set.
E. Time-varying MDS: The model that results from running stage one only.
F. MDS with no time: The model that results from ignoring time information and running independent MDS on each timestep.

Figure 3 shows the ROC curves for the third timestep on a test set of size 160. Table 1 shows the AUC scores of our approach and the five alternatives for 3 different sizes of the dataset over the first, third, and last time steps.

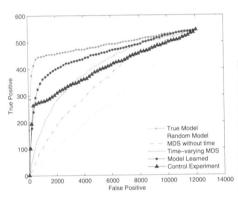

Figure 3: ROC curves of the six different models described earlier for test set of size 160 at timestep 3, in simulated data.

Table 1. AUC score on graphs of size n for six different models (A) True (B) Model learned by DSNL,(C) Random Model,(D) Simple Counting model(Control), (E) MDS with time, and (F) MDS without time.

Time	A	B	C	D	E	F
			n=80			
1	0.94	0.85	0.48	0.76	0.77	0.67
3	0.93	0.88	0.48	0.81	0.77	0.65
6	0.93	0.82	0.50	0.76	0.77	0.67
			n=320			
1	0.86	0.83	0.50	0.70	0.72	0.65
3	0.86	0.79	0.51	0.70	0.72	0.62
6	0.86	0.81	0.50	0.71	0.74	0.64
			n=1280			
1	0.81	0.79	0.50	0.68	0.61	0.70
3	0.80	0.79	0.50	0.69	0.74	0.71
6	0.81	0.78	0.50	0.68	0.70	0.70

In all the cases we see that the true model has the highest AUC score, followed by the model learned by DSNL. The simple counting model rightly guesses some of the links in the test graph from the training graph. However it also predicts the noise as links, and ends up being beaten by the model we learn. The results show that it is not sufficient to only perform Stage One. When the number of links is small, MDS without time does poorly compared to our temporal version. However as the number of links grows quadratically with the number of entities, regular MDS does almost as well as the temporal version: this is not a surprise because the generalization benefit from the previous timestep becomes unnecessary with sufficient data on the current timestep. Further experiments we conducted [1] show that the experiments initialized with time-variant MDS converges almost twice as fast as those with random initialization, and also converges to a better log-likelihood.

5.2 Visualizing the NIPS coauthorship data over time

For clarity we present a subset of the NIPS dataset, obtained by choosing a well-connected author, and including all authors and links within a few hops. We dropped authors who appeared only once and we merged the timesteps into three groups: 1987-1990 (Figure 4A), 1991-1994(Figure 4B), and 1995-1998(Figure 4C). In each picture we have the links for that timestep, a few well connected people highlighted, with their radii. These radii are learnt from the model. Remember that the distance between two people is related to the radii. Two people with very small radii, are considered far apart in the model even if they are physically close. To give some intuition of the movement of the rest of the points, we divided the area in the first timestep in 4 parts, and colored and shaped the points in each differently. This coloring and shaping is preserved throughout all the timesteps.

In this paper we limit ourselves to anecdotal examination of the latent positions. For example, with $Burges_C$ and $Vapnik_V$ we see that they had very small radii in the first four years, and were further apart from one another, since there was no co-publication. However in the second timestep they move closer, though there are no direct links. This is because of the fact that they both had co-published with neighbors of one another. On the third time step they make a connection, and are assigned almost identical coordinates, since they have a very overlapping set of neighbors.

We end the discussion with entities $Hinton_G$, $Ghahramani_Z$, and $Jordan_M$. In the first timestep they did not coauthor with one another, and were placed outside one-another's radii. In the second timestep $Ghahramani_Z$, and $Hinton_G$ coauthor with $Jordan_M$. However since $Hinton_G$ had a large radius and more links than the former, it is harder for him to meet all the constraints, and he doesn't move very close to $Jordan_M$. In the next timestep however $Ghahramani_Z$ has a link with both of the others, and they move substantially closer to one another.

5.3 Performance Issues

Figure 4D shows the performance against the number of entities. When kd-trees are used and the graphs are sparse scaling is clearly sub-quadratic and nearly linear in the number of entities, meeting our expectation of $O(n \log n)$ performance. We successfully applied our algorithms to networks of sizes up to 11,000 [1]. The results show subquadratic time-complexity along with satisfactory link prediction on test sets.

6 Conclusions and Future Work

This paper has described a method for modeling relationships that change over time. We believe it is useful both for understanding relationships in a mass of historical data and also as a tool for predicting future interactions, and we plan to explore both directions further. In [1] we develop a forward-backward algorithm, optimizing the global likelihood instead of treating the model as a tracking model. We also plan to extend this to find the posterior distributions of the coordinates following the approach used by [5].

Acknowledgments

We are very grateful to Anna Goldenberg for her valuable insights. We also thank Paul Komarek and Sajid Siddiqi for some very helpful discussions and useful comments. This work was partially funded by DARPA EELD grant F30602-01-2-0569.

References

[1] P. Sarkar and A. Moore. Dynamic social network analysis using latent space models. *SIGKDD Explorations: Special Issue on Link Mining*, 2005.

[2] J. Schroeder, J. J. Xu, and H. Chen. Crimelink explorer: Using domain knowledge to facilitate automated crime association analysis. In *ISI*, pages 168–180, 2003.

[3] J. J. Carrasco, D. C. Fain, K. J. Lang, and L. Zhukov. Clustering of bipartite advertiser-keyword graph. In *ICDM*, 2003.

[4] J. Palau, M. Montaner, and B. López. Collaboration analysis in recommender systems using social networks. In *Eighth Intl. Workshop on Cooperative Info. Agents (CIA'04)*, 2004.

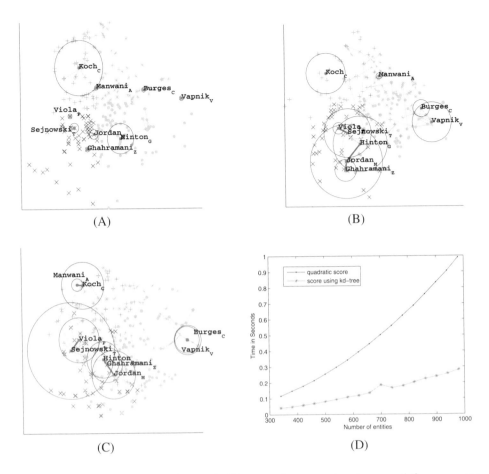

Figure 4: NIPS coauthorship data at **A**. Timestep 1: green stars in upper-left corner, magenta pluses in top right, cyan spots in lower right, and blue crosses in the bottom-left. **B**. Timestep 2. **C**. Timestep 3. **D**. Time taken for score calculation vs number of entities.

[5] A. E. Raftery, M. S. Handcock, and P. D. Hoff. Latent space approaches to social network analysis. *J. Amer. Stat. Assoc.*, 15:460, 2002.

[6] R. L. Breiger, S. A. Boorman, and P. Arabie. An algorithm for clustering relational data with applications to social network analysis and comparison with multidimensional scaling. *J. of Math. Psych.*, 12:328–383, 1975.

[7] I. Borg and P. Groenen. *Modern Multidimensional Scaling*. Springer-Verlag, 1997.

[8] R. Sibson. Studies in the robustness of multidimensional scaling : Perturbational analysis of classical scaling. *J. Royal Stat. Soc. B, Methodological*, 41:217–229, 1979.

[9] David S. Watkins. *Fundamentals of Matrix Computations*. John Wiley & Sons, 1991.

[10] F. Preparata and M. Shamos. *Computational Geometry: An Introduction*. Springer, 1985.

[11] A. G. Gray and A. W. Moore. N-body problems in statistical learning. In *NIPS*, 2001.

Logic and MRF Circuitry for Labeling Occluding and Thinline Visual Contours

Eric Saund
Palo Alto Research Center
3333 Coyote Hill Rd.
Palo Alto, CA 94304
saund@parc.com

Abstract

This paper presents representation and logic for labeling contrast edges and ridges in visual scenes in terms of both surface occlusion (border ownership) and thinline objects. In natural scenes, thinline objects include sticks and wires, while in human graphical communication thinlines include connectors, dividers, and other abstract devices. Our analysis is directed at both natural and graphical domains. The basic problem is to formulate the logic of the interactions among local image events, specifically contrast edges, ridges, junctions, and alignment relations, such as to encode the natural constraints among these events in visual scenes. In a sparse heterogeneous Markov Random Field framework, we define a set of interpretation nodes and energy/potential functions among them. The minimum energy configuration found by Loopy Belief Propagation is shown to correspond to preferred human interpretation across a wide range of prototypical examples including important illusory contour figures such as the Kanizsa Triangle, as well as more difficult examples. In practical terms, the approach delivers correct interpretations of inherently ambiguous hand-drawn box-and-connector diagrams at low computational cost.

1   Introduction

A great deal of attention has been paid to the curious phenomenon of illusory contours in visual scenes [5]. The most famous example is the Kanizsa Triangle (Figure 1). Although a number of explanations have been proposed, computational accounts have converged on the understanding that illusory contours are an outcome of the more general problem of labeling scene contours in terms of causal events such as surface overlap. Illusory contours are the visual system's way of expressing belief in an occlusion relation between two surfaces having the same lightness and therefore lacking a visible contrast edge. The phenomena are interesting in their revelation of interactions among multiple factors comprising the visual system's prior assumptions about what constitutes likely interpretations of ambiguous input.

Several computational models for this process have generated interpretations of Kanizsa-like figures corresponding to human perception. Williams[9] formulated an integer-linear

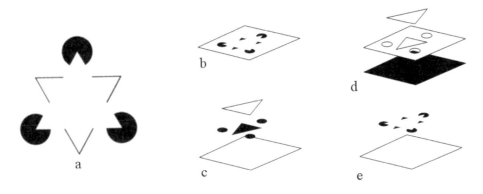

Figure 1: a. Original Kanizsa Triangle. b. Solid surface version. c. Human preferred interpretation. d, e. Other valid interpretations.

optimization problem with hard constrains originating from the topology of contours and junctions, and soft constraints representing figural biases for non-accidental interpretations and figural closure. Heitger and von der Heydt[2] implemented a series of nonlinear filtering operations that enacted interactions among line terminations and junctions to infer modal completions corresponding to illusory contours. Geiger[1] used a dense Markov Random Field to represent surface depths explicitly and propagated local evidence through a diffusion process. Saund[6] enumerated possible generic and non-generic interpretations of T- and L-junctions to set up an optimization problem solved by deterministic annealing. Liu and Wang[4] set up a network of contours traversing the boundaries of segmented regions, which interact to propagate local information through an iterative updating scheme.

This paper expands this body of previous work in the following ways:

- The computational model is expressed in terms of a sparse heterogeneous Markov Random Field whose solution is accessible to fast techniques such as Loopy Belief Propagation.

- We introduce interpretations of thinlines in addition to solid surfaces, adding a significant layer of richness and complexity.

- The model infers occlusion relations of surfaces depicted by line drawings of their borders, as well as solid graphics depictions.

- We devise MRF energy functions that implement circuitry for sophisticated logical constraints of the domain.

The result is a formulation that is both fast and effective at correctly interpreting a greater range of psychophysical and near-practical contour configuration examples than has heretofore been demonstrated. The model exposes aspects of fundamental ambiguity to be resolved by the incorporation of additional constraints and domain-specific knowledge.

2 Interpretation Nodes and Relations

2.1 Visible Contours and Contour Ends

Early vision studies commonly distinguish several models for visible contour creation and measurement, including contrast edges, lines or ridges, ramps, color and texture edges, etc. Let us idealize to consider only contrast edges and ridges (also known as "bars"), measured at a single scale. We include in our domain of interest human-generated graphical

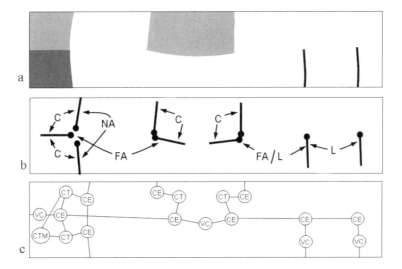

Figure 2: a. Sample image region. b. Spatial relation categories characterizing links in the MRF among Contour End nodes: Corner, Near Alignment, Far Alignment, Lateral. c. Resulting MRF including nodes of type Visible Contour, Contour End, Corner Tie, and Corner Tie Mediator.

figures. Contrast edges arise from distinct regions or surfaces, while ridges may represent either a boundary between regions or else a "thinline", i.e. a physical or graphical object whose shape is essentially defined by a one-dimensional path at our scale of measurement. Examples of thinlines in photographic imagery include twigs, sidewalk cracks, and telephone wires, while in graphical images thinlines include separators, connectors, and arrow shafts. Figure 7e shows a hand-drawn sketch in which some lines (measured as ridges) are intended to define boxes and therefore represent region boundaries, while others are connectors between boxes. We take the contour interpretation problem to include the analysis of this type of scene in addition to classical illusory contour figures.

For any input data, we may construct a Markov Random Field consisting of four types of nodes derived from measured contrast edge and ridge contours. An interpretation is an assignment of states to nodes. Local potentials and the potential matrices associated with pairwise links between nodes encode constraints and biases among interpretation states based on the spatial relations among the visible contours. Figure 2 illustrates MRF nodes types and links for a simple example input image, as explained below.

Let us assume that contours defining region boundaries are assigned an occlusion direction, equivalent to relative surface depth and hence boundary ownership. Figure 3 shows the possible mappings between visible image contours measured as contrast edges or ridges, and their interpretation in terms of direction of surface overlap or else thinline object. Contrast edges always correspond to surface occlusion, while ridges may represent either a surface boundary or a thinline object. Correspondingly, the simplest MRF node type is the Visible Contour node which has state dimension 3 corresponding to two possible overlap directions and one thinline interpretation.

Most of the interesting evidence and interaction occurs at terminations and junctions of visible contours. Contour End nodes are given the job of explaining why a smooth visible edge or ridge contour has terminated visibility, and hence they will encode the bulk of the modal (illusory) and amodal (occluded) completion information of a computed interpretation. Smooth visible contours may terminate in four ways:

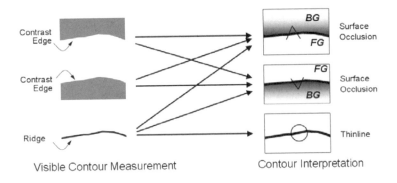

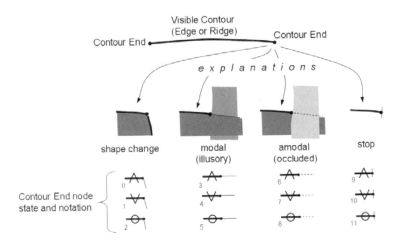

Figure 3: Permissible mappings between visible edge and ridge contours and interpretations. Wedges indicate direction of surface overlap: white (FG) surface occludes shaded (BG) surface.

1. The surface boundary contour or thinline object changes direction (turns a corner)

2. The contour becomes modal because the background surface lacks a visible edge with the foreground surface.

3. The contour becomes amodal because it becomes occluded by another surface.

4. The contour simply terminates when an surface overlap meets the end of a fold, or when a thin object or graphic stops.

Contour Ends therefore have 3x4 = 12 interpretation states as shown in Figure 4.

Figure 4: Contour End nodes have state dimension 12 indicating contour overlap type/direction (overlap or thinline) and one of four explanations for termination of the visible contour.

Every Visible Contour node is linked to its two corresponding Contour End nodes through energy matrices (or equivalently, potential matrices, using Potential $\psi = \exp^{-E}$) representing simple compatibility among overlap direction/thinline interpretation states. Additional links in the network are created based on spatial relations among Contour Ends as described next.

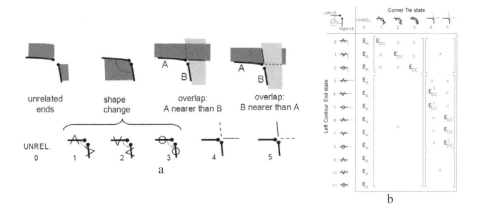

Figure 5: a. Corner Tie nodes have state dimension 6 indicating the causal relationship between the Contour End nodes they link. b. Energy matrix linking the Left Contour End of a pair of corner-relation Contour Ends to their Corner Tie. X indicates high energy prohibiting the state combination. E_A refers to a low penalty for Accidental Coincidence of the Contour Ends. E_{DC} refers to a (typically low) penalty of two Contour Ends failing to meet the ideal geometrical constraints of meeting at a corner. The subscripts refer to necessary Near-Alignment Relations on the Contour Ends. The energy matrix linking the Right End Contour to the Corner Tie swaps the 5th and 6th columns.

2.2 Contour Ends Relation Links

Let us consider five classes of pairwise geometric relations among observed contour ends: Corner, Near-Alignment, Far-Alignment, Lateral, and Unrelated. Mathematical expressions forming the bases for these relations may be engineered as measures of distance and smooth continuation such as used by Saund [6]. The Corner relation depends only on proximity; Near-Alignment depends on proximity and alignment; Far-Alignment omits the proximity requirement.

Within this framework a further refinement distinguishes ridge Contour Ends from those arising from contrast edges. Namely, ridge ends are permitted to form Lateral relation links which correspond to potential modal contours. Contrast edge Contour Ends are excluded from this link type because they terminate at junctions which distribute modal and amodal completion roles to their participating Contour Ends. Contour End nodes from ridge contours may participate in Far-Alignment links but their local energies are set to preclude them from taking states representing modal completions.

In this way the present model fixes the topology of related ends in the process of setting up the Markov Graph. An important problem for future research is to formulate the Markov Graph to include *all* plausible Contour End pairings and have the actual pairings sort themselves out at solution time.

Biases about preferred and less-preferred interpretations are represented through the terms in the energy matrices linking related Contour Ends. In accordance with prior work, we bias energy terms associated with curved Visible Contours and junctions of Contour Ends in favor of convex object interpretations. Space limitations preclude presenting the energy matrices in detail, but we discuss the main novel and significant considerations.

The simplest case is pairs of Contour Ends sharing a Near-Alignment or Far-Alignment relation. These energy matrices are constructed to trade off priors regarding accidental alignment versus amodal or modal invisible contour completion interpretations. For Con-

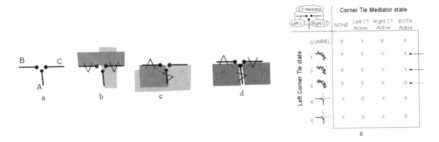

Figure 6: The Corner Tie Mediator node restricts border ownership of occluding contours to physically consistent interpretations. The energy matrix shown in e links the Corner Tie Mediator to the Left Corner Tie of a pair sharing a Contour End. X indicates high energy. The energy matrix for the link to the Right Corner Tie swaps the second and third columns.

tour End pairs that are relatively near and well aligned, energy terms corresponding to causally unrelated interpretations (CE states 0,1,2) are large, while terms corresponding to amodal completion with compatible overlap/thinline property (CE states 6,7,8) are small. Actual energy values for the matrices are assigned by straightforward formulas derived from the Proximity and Smooth Continuation terms mentioned above. Per Kanizsa, modal completion interpretations (CE states 3,4,5) are somewhat more expensive than amodal interpretations, by a constant factor. Energy terms shift their relative weights in favor of causally unrelated interpretations (CE corner states 0,1,2) as the Contour Ends become more distant and less aligned.

Contour Ends sharing a Corner relation can be related in one of three ways: they can be causally unrelated and unordered in depth; they can represent a turning of a surface boundary or thinline object; they can represent overlap of one contour above the other. In order to exploit the geometry of Contour Ends as local evidence, these alternatives must be articulated and entered into the MRF node graph. To do this we therefore introduce a third type of node, the Corner Tie node, possessing six states as illustrated in Figure 5a.

The energy matrix relating Contour End nodes and Corner Tie nodes is shown in Figure 5b. It contains low energy terms representing the Corner Tie's belief that the Contour End termination is due to direction change (turning a corner). It also contains low energy terms representing the conditions of one Contour End's owning surface overlapping the other contour, i.e. the relative depth relation between these contours in the scene.

2.3   Constraints on Overlaps and Thinlines at Junctions

Physical considerations impose hard constraints on the interpretations of End Pairs meeting at a junction. Consider the T-junction in Figure 6a. One preferred interpretation for a T-junction is occlusion (6b). A less-preferred but possible interpretation is a change of direction (corner) by one surface, with accidental alignment by another contour (6c). What is *impossible* is for a surface boundary to bifurcate and "belong" to both sides of the T (6d).

This type of constraint cannot be enforced by the purely pairwise Corner Tie node. We therefore introduce a fourth node type, the Corner Tie Mediator. This node governs the number of Corner Ties that any Contour End can claim to form a direction change (corner turn) relation with. The energy matrix for the Corner Tie Mediator node is shown in Figure 6e: multiple Corner-Ties in the overlap direction-turn states (CT states 1 & 2) are excluded (solid arrows). But note that the matrix contains a low energy term (dashed arrow) for the formation of multiple direction-turn Corner-Ties provided they are in the Thinline state (CT state 3); branching of thinline objects *is* physically permissible.

3 Experiments and Conclusion

Loopy Belief Propagation under the Max-Product algorithm seeks the MAP configuration which is equivalent to the minimum-energy assignment of states [8]. We have not encountered a failure of LBP to converge, and it is quite rare to encounter a lower-energy assignment of states than the algorithm delivers starting from an initial uniform distribution over states. However, multiple stable fixed points can exist. For some ambiguous figures such as Figure 7e in which qualitatively different interpretations have similar energies, one may clamp one or more nodes to alternative states, leading to LBP solutions which persist once the clamping is removed. This invites the exploration of N-best configuration solution techniques [10].

Figure 7 demonstrates MAP assignments corresponding to preferred human interpretations of the classic Kanizsa illusory contour figure and others containing both aligning L-junction and ridge termination evidence for modal contours, amodal completions, and thinline objects. Note that the MRF correctly predicts that outline drawings of surface boundaries do not induce illusory contours.

Figure 7g borrows from experiments by Szummer and Cowans[7] toward a practical application in line drawing interpretation, in which closed boxes define regions while connectors remain interpreted as thinline objects. For this scene containing 369 nodes and 417 links, the entire process of forming the MRF and performing 100 iterations of LBP takes less than a second. The major pressures operating in these situations are a figural bias toward interpreting closed paths as convex regions, and a preference to interpret ridge contours participating in T- and X- junctions as thinline objects.

We have shown how explicit consideration of ridge features and thinline interpretations brings new complexity to the logic of sorting out depth relations in visual scenes. This investigation suggests that a sparse heterogeneous Markov Random Field approach may provide a suitable basis for such models.

References

[1] Geiger, D., Kumaran, K, & Parida, L. (1996) Visual organization for figure/ground separation. in *Proc. IEEE CVPR* pp. 155-160.

[2] Heitger, F., & von der Heydt, R. (1993) A Computational Model of Neural Contour Processing: Figure-Ground Segregation and Illusory Contours. *Proc. ICCV '93*.

[3] Kanizsa, G. (1979) *Organization in Vision,* Praeger, New York.

[4] Liu, X., Wang, D. (2000) Perceptual Organization Based on Temporal Dynamics. in S.A. Solla, T.K. Leen, K.-R. Muller (eds.), *Advances in Neural Information Processing Systems 12*, pp. 38-44. MIT Press.

[5] Petry, S., & Meyer, G. (eds.) (1987) *The Perception of Illusory Contours,* Springer-Verlag, New York.

[6] Saund, E. (1999) Perceptual Organization of Occluding Contours of Opaque Surfaces, *CVIU* V. 76, No. 1, pp. 70-82.

[7] Szummer, M., & Cowans, P. (2004) Incorporating Context and User Feedback in Pen-Based Interfaces. *AAAI TR FS-04-06* (Papers from the 2004 AAAI Fall Symposium.)

[8] Weiss, Y., and Freeman, W.T. (2001) On the optimality of solutions of the max-product belief propagation algorithm in arbitrary graphs, *IEEE Trans. Inf. Theory* 47:2, pp. 723-735.

[9] Williams, L. (1990) Perceptual Organization of Occluding Contours. *Proc. ICCV '90*. pp. 639-649.

[10] Yanover, C. and Weiss, Y. (2003) Finding the M Most Probable Configurations Using Loopy Belief Propagation. in S. Thrun, L. Saul and B. Schölkpf, eds., *Advances in Neural Information Processing Systems 16*, MIT Press.

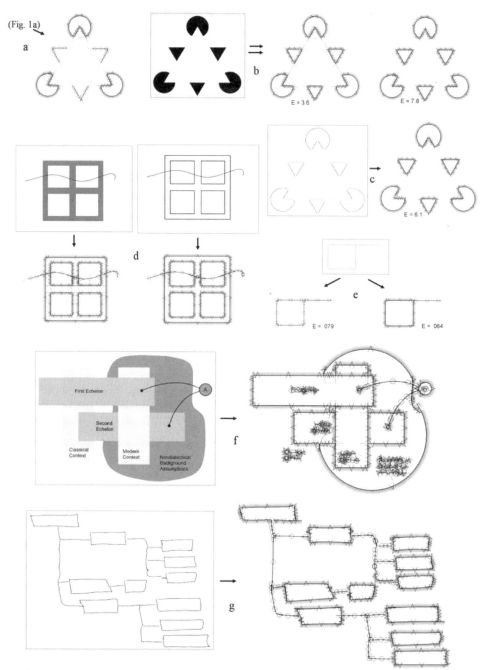

Figure 7: Experimental results. Arrow leads from input image to MRF interpretations. Curved contours are approximated by circular arcs. a. Original Kanizsa Triangle. b. Energies for preferred and "pac-man" interpretations. c. No illusory contour interpretations arise from outline drawing. d. Similar interpretations of solid and outline graphical windows overlain by a line. e. Similar energies obtain for an inherently ambiguous thinline/region figure. f. Graphical figure. g. Hand-drawn figure from [7] interpreted as closed regions and connectors.

1160

Learning Depth from Single Monocular Images

Ashutosh Saxena, Sung H. Chung, and Andrew Y. Ng
Computer Science Department
Stanford University
Stanford, CA 94305
asaxena@stanford.edu,
{codedeft,ang}@cs.stanford.edu

Abstract

We consider the task of depth estimation from a single monocular image. We take a supervised learning approach to this problem, in which we begin by collecting a training set of monocular images (of unstructured outdoor environments which include forests, trees, buildings, etc.) and their corresponding ground-truth depthmaps. Then, we apply supervised learning to predict the depthmap as a function of the image. Depth estimation is a challenging problem, since local features alone are insufficient to estimate depth at a point, and one needs to consider the global context of the image. Our model uses a discriminatively-trained Markov Random Field (MRF) that incorporates multiscale local- and global-image features, and models both depths at individual points as well as the relation between depths at different points. We show that, even on unstructured scenes, our algorithm is frequently able to recover fairly accurate depthmaps.

1 Introduction

Recovering 3-D depth from images is a basic problem in computer vision, and has important applications in robotics, scene understanding and 3-D reconstruction. Most work on visual 3-D reconstruction has focused on binocular vision (stereopsis) [1] and on other algorithms that require multiple images, such as structure from motion [2] and depth from defocus [3]. Depth estimation from a *single* monocular image is a difficult task, and requires that we take into account the global structure of the image, as well as use prior knowledge about the scene. In this paper, we apply supervised learning to the problem of estimating depth from single monocular images of unstructured outdoor environments, ones that contain forests, trees, buildings, people, buses, bushes, etc.

In related work, Michels, Saxena & Ng [4] used supervised learning to estimate 1-D distances to obstacles, for the application of autonomously driving a remote control car. Nagai et al. [5] performed surface reconstruction from single images for known, fixed, objects such as hands and faces. Gini & Marchi [6] used single-camera vision to drive an indoor robot, but relied heavily on known ground colors and textures. Shape from shading [7] offers another method for monocular depth reconstruction, but is difficult to apply to scenes that do not have fairly uniform color and texture. In work done independently of ours, Hoiem, Efros and Herbert (personal communication) also considered monocular 3-D reconstruction, but focused on generating 3-D graphical images rather than accurate metric depthmaps. In this paper, we address the task of learning full depthmaps from single images of unconstrained environments.

Markov Random Fields (MRFs) and their variants are a workhorse of machine learning, and have been successfully applied to numerous problems in which local features were insufficient and more contextual information had to be used. Examples include text segmentation [8], object classification [9], and image labeling [10]. To model spatial dependencies in images, Kumar and Hebert's Discriminative Random Fields algorithm [11] uses logistic regression to identify man-made structures in natural images. Because MRF learning is intractable in general, most of these model are trained using pseudo-likelihood.

Our approach is based on capturing depths and relationships between depths using an MRF. We began by using a 3-D distance scanner to collect training data, which comprised a large set of images and their corresponding ground-truth depthmaps. Using this training set, the MRF is discriminatively trained to predict depth; thus, rather than modeling the joint distribution of image features and depths, we model only the posterior distribution of the depths given the image features. Our basic model uses L_2 (Gaussian) terms in the MRF interaction potentials, and captures depths and interactions between depths at multiple spatial scales. We also present a second model that uses L_1 (Laplacian) interaction potentials. Learning in this model is approximate, but exact MAP posterior inference is tractable (similar to Gaussian MRFs) via linear programming, and it gives significantly better depthmaps than the simple Gaussian model.

2 Monocular Cues

Humans appear to be extremely good at judging depth from single monocular images. [12] This is done using monocular cues such as texture variations, texture gradients, occlusion, known object sizes, haze, defocus, etc. [4, 13, 14] For example, many objects' texture will look different at different distances from the viewer. Texture gradients, which capture the distribution of the direction of edges, also help to indicate depth.[1] Haze is another depth cue, and is caused by atmospheric light scattering.

Most of these monocular cues are "contextual information," in the sense that they are global properties of an image and cannot be inferred from small image patches. For example, occlusion cannot be determined if we look at just a small portion of an occluded object. Although local information such as the texture and color of a patch can give some information about its depth, this is usually insufficient to accurately determine its absolute depth. For another example, if we take a patch of a clear blue sky, it is difficult to tell if this patch is infinitely far away (sky), or if it is part of a blue object. Due to ambiguities like these, one needs to look at the *overall* organization of the image to determine depths.

3 Feature Vector

In our approach, we divide the image into small patches, and estimate a single depth value for each patch. We use two types of features: *absolute* depth features—used to estimate the absolute depth at a particular patch—and *relative* features, which we use to estimate relative depths (magnitude of the difference in depth between two patches). We chose features that capture three types of local cues: texture variations, texture gradients, and haze.

Texture information is mostly contained within the image intensity channel,[2] so we apply Laws' masks [15, 4] to this channel to compute the texture energy (Fig. 1). Haze is reflected in the low frequency information in the color channels, and we capture this by applying a local averaging filter (the first Laws mask) to the color channels. Lastly, to compute an

---

[1]For example, a tiled floor with parallel lines will appear to have tilted lines in an image. The distant patches will have larger variations in the line orientations, and nearby patches will have smaller variations in line orientations. Similarly, a grass field when viewed at different distances will have different texture gradient distributions.

[2]We represent each image in YCbCr color space, where Y is the intensity channel, and Cb and Cr are the color channels.

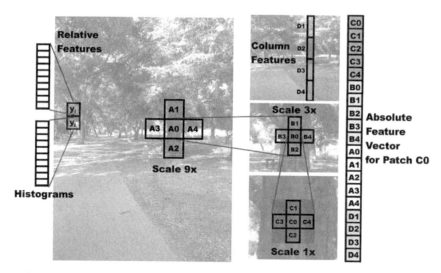

Figure 1: The convolutional filters used for texture energies and gradients. The first nine are 3x3 Laws' masks. The last six are the oriented edge detectors spaced at 30^0 intervals. The nine Law's masks are used to perform local averaging, edge detection and spot detection.

Figure 2: The absolute depth feature vector for a patch, which includes features from its immediate neighbors and its more distant neighbors (at larger scales). The relative depth features for each patch use histograms of the filter outputs.

estimate of texture gradient that is robust to noise, we convolve the intensity channel with six oriented edge filters (shown in Fig. 1).

3.1 Features for absolute depth

Given some patch i in the image $I(x, y)$, we compute summary statistics for it as follows. We use the output of each of the 17 (9 Laws' masks, 2 color channels and 6 texture gradients) filters $F_n(x, y)$, $n = 1, ..., 17$ as: $E_i(n) = \sum_{(x,y)\in\text{patch}(i)} |I(x, y) * F_n(x, y)|^k$, where $k = \{1, 2\}$ give the sum absolute energy and sum squared energy respectively. This gives us an initial feature vector of dimension 34.

To estimate the absolute depth at a patch, local image features centered on the patch are insufficient, and one has to use more global properties of the image. We attempt to capture this information by using image features extracted at multiple scales (image resolutions). (See Fig. 2.) Objects at different depths exhibit very different behaviors at different resolutions, and using multiscale features allows us to capture these variations [16].[3] In addition to capturing more global information, computing features at multiple spatial scales also help accounts for different relative sizes of objects. A closer object appears larger in the image, and hence will be captured in the larger scale features. The same object when far away will be small and hence be captured in the small scale features. Such features may be strong indicators of depth.

To capture additional global features (e.g. occlusion relationships), the features used to predict the depth of a particular patch are computed from that patch as well as the four neighboring patches. This is repeated at each of the three scales, so that the feature vector

---

[3]For example, blue sky may appear similar at different scales; but textured grass would not.

at a patch includes features of its immediate neighbors, and its far neighbors (at a larger scale), and its very far neighbors (at the largest scale), as shown in Fig. 2. Lastly, many structures (such as trees and buildings) found in outdoor scenes show vertical structure, in the sense that they are vertically connected to themselves (things cannot hang in empty air). Thus, we also add to the features of a patch additional summary features of the column it lies in.

For each patch, after including features from itself and its 4 neighbors at 3 scales, and summary features for its 4 column patches, our vector of features for estimating depth at a particular patch is $19 * 34 = 646$ dimensional.

3.2 Features for relative depth

We use a different feature vector to learn the dependencies between two neighboring patches. Specifically, we compute a histogram (with 10 bins) of each of the 17 filter outputs $|I(x, y) * F_n(x, y)|$, giving us a total of 170 features y_i for each patch i. These features are used to estimate how the depths at two different locations are related. We believe that learning these estimates requires less global information than predicting absolute depth,[4] but more detail from the individual patches. Hence, we use as our relative depth features the differences between the histograms computed from two neighboring patches $y_{ij} = y_i - y_j$.

4 The Probabilistic Model

The depth of a particular patch depends on the features of the patch, but is also related to the depths of other parts of the image. For example, the depths of two adjacent patches lying in the same building will be highly correlated. We will use an MRF to model the relation between the depth of a patch and the depths of its neighboring patches. In addition to the interactions with the immediately neighboring patches, there are sometimes also strong interactions between the depths of patches which are not immediate neighbors. For example, consider the depths of patches that lie on a large building. All of these patches will be at similar depths, even if there are small discontinuities (such as a window on the wall of a building). However, when viewed at the smallest scale, some adjacent patches are difficult to recognize as parts of the same object. Thus, we will also model interactions between depths at multiple spatial scales.

Our first model will be a jointly Gaussian MRF. To capture the multiscale depth relations, let us define $d_i(s)$ as follows. For each of three scales $s = 1, 2, 3$, define $d_i(s + 1) = (1/5) \sum_{j \in N_s(i) \cup \{i\}} d_j(s)$. Here, $N_s(i)$ are the 4 neighbors of patch i at scale s. I.e., the depth at a higher scale is constrained to be the average of the depths at lower scales. Our model over depths is as follows:

$$P(d|X; \theta, \sigma) = \frac{1}{Z} \exp\left(-\sum_{i=1}^{M} \frac{(d_i(1) - x_i^T \theta_r)^2}{2\sigma_{1r}^2} - \sum_{s=1}^{3} \sum_{i=1}^{M} \sum_{j \in N_s(i)} \frac{(d_i(s) - d_j(s))^2}{2\sigma_{2rs}^2}\right)$$

(1)

Here, M is the total number of patches in the image (at the lowest scale); x_i is the absolute depth feature vector for patch i; and θ and σ are parameters of the model. In detail, we use different parameters $(\theta_r, \sigma_{1r}, \sigma_{2r})$ for each row in the image, because the images we consider are taken from a horizontally mounted camera, and thus different rows of the image have different statistical properties.[5] Z is the normalization constant for the model.

---

[4]For example, given two adjacent patches of a distinctive, unique, color and texture, we may be able to safely conclude that they are part of the same object, and thus that their depths are close, even without more global features.

[5]For example, a blue patch might represent sky if it is in upper part of image, and might be more likely to be water if in the lower part of the image.

We estimate the parameters θ_r in Eq. 1 by maximizing the conditional likelihood $p(d|X;\theta_r)$ of the training data. Since the model is a multivariate Gaussian, the maximum likelihood estimate of parameters θ_r is obtained by solving a linear least squares problem.

The first term in the exponent above models depth as a function of multiscale features of a single patch i. The second term in the exponent places a soft "constraint" on the depths to be smooth. If the variance term σ_{2rs}^2 is a fixed constant, the effect of this term is that it tends to smooth depth estimates across nearby patches. However, in practice the dependencies between patches are not the same everywhere, and our expected value for $(d_i - d_j)^2$ may depend on the features of the local patches.

Therefore, to improve accuracy we extend the model to capture the "variance" term σ_{2rs}^2 in the denominator of the second term as a linear function of the patches i and j's relative depth features y_{ijs} (discussed in Section 3.2). We use $\sigma_{2rs}^2 = u_{rs}^T |y_{ijs}|$. This helps determine which neighboring patches are likely to have similar depths. E.g., the "smoothing" effect is much stronger if neighboring patches are similar. This idea is applied at multiple scales, so that we learn different σ_{2rs}^2 for the different scales s (and rows r of the image). The parameters u_{rs} are chosen to fit σ_{2rs}^2 to the expected value of $(d_i(s) - d_j(s))^2$, with a constraint that $u_{rs} \geq 0$ (to keep the estimated σ_{2rs}^2 non-negative).

Similar to our discussion on σ_{2rs}^2, we also learn the variance parameter $\sigma_{1r}^2 = v_r^T x_i$ as a linear function of the features. The parameters v_r are chosen to fit σ_{1r}^2 to the expected value of $(d_i(r) - \theta_r^T x_i)^2$, subject to $v_r \geq 0$.[6] This σ_{1r}^2 term gives a measure of the uncertainty in the first term, and depends on the features. This is motivated by the observation that in some cases, depth cannot be reliably estimated from the local features. In this case, one has to rely more on neighboring patches' depths to infer a patch's depth (as modeled by the second term in the exponent).

After learning the parameters, given a new test-set image we can find the MAP estimate of the depths by maximizing Eq. 1 in terms of d. Since Eq. 1 is Gaussian, $\log P(d|X;\theta,\sigma)$ is quadratic in d, and thus its maximum is easily found in closed form (taking at most 2-3 seconds per image, including feature computation time).

4.1 Laplacian model

We now present a second model that uses Laplacians instead of Gaussians to model the posterior distribution of the depths. Our motivation for doing so is three-fold. First, a histogram of the relative depths $(d_i - d_j)$ empirically appears Laplacian, which strongly suggests that it is better modeled as one. Second, the Laplacian distribution has heavier tails, and is therefore more robust to outliers in the image features and error in the training-set depthmaps (collected with a laser scanner; see Section 5.1). Third, the Gaussian model was generally unable to give depthmaps with sharp edges; in contrast, Laplacians tend to model sharp transitions/outliers better. Our model is as follows:

$$P(d|X;\theta,\lambda) = \frac{1}{Z} \exp\left(-\sum_{i=1}^{M} \frac{|d_i(1) - x_i^T \theta_r|}{\lambda_{1r}} - \sum_{s=1}^{3}\sum_{i=1}^{M}\sum_{j\in N_s(i)} \frac{|d_i(s) - d_j(s)|}{\lambda_{2rs}}\right) \quad (2)$$

Here, the parameters are the same as Eq. 1, except for the variance terms. Here, λ_{1r} and λ_{2rs} are the *Laplacian spread* parameters. Maximum-likelihood parameter estimation for the Laplacian model is not tractable (since the partition function depends on θ_r). But by analogy to the Gaussian case, we approximate this by solving a linear system of equations $X_r\theta_r \approx d_r$ to minimize L_1 (instead of L_2) error. Here X_r is the matrix of absolute-depth features. Following the Gaussian model, we also learn the Laplacian spread parameters in the denominator in the same way, except that the instead of estimating the expected value of $(d_i - d_j)^2$, we estimate the expected value of $|d_i - d_j|$. Even though maximum

---

[6]The absolute depth features x_{ir} are non-negative; thus, the estimated σ_{1r}^2 is also non-negative.

likelihood parameter estimation for θ_r is intractable in the Laplacian model, given a new test-set image, MAP inference for the depths d is tractable. Specifically, $P(d|X; \theta, \lambda)$ is easily maximized in terms of d using linear programming.

Remark. We can also extend these models to combine Gaussian and Laplacian terms in the exponent, for example by using a L_2 norm term for absolute depth, and a L_1 norm term for the interaction terms. MAP inference remains tractable in this setting, and can be solved using convex optimization as a QP (quadratic program).

5 Experiments

5.1 Data collection

We used a 3-D laser scanner to collect images and their corresponding depthmaps. The scanner uses a SICK 1-D laser range finder mounted on a motor to get 2D scans. We collected a total of 425 image+depthmap pairs, with an image resolution of 1704x2272 and a depthmap resolution of 86x107. In the experimental results reported here, 75% of the images/depthmaps were used for training, and the remaining 25% for hold-out testing. Due to noise in the motor system, the depthmaps were not perfectly aligned with the images, and had an alignment error of about 2 depth patches. Also, the depthmaps had a maximum range of 81m (the maximum range of the laser scanner), and had minor additional errors due to reflections and missing laser scans. Prior to running our learning algorithms, we transformed all the depths to a log scale so as to emphasize multiplicative rather than additive errors in training. In our earlier experiments (not reported here), learning using linear depth values directly gave poor results.

5.2 Results

We tested our model on real-world test-set images of forests (containing trees, bushes, etc.), campus areas (buildings, people, and trees), and indoor places (such as corridors). The algorithm was trained on a training set comprising images from *all* of these environments. Table 1 shows the test-set results when using different feature combinations. We see that using multiscale and column features significantly improves the algorithm's performance.

Including the interaction terms further improved its performance, and the Laplacian model performs better than the Gaussian one. Empirically, we also observed that the Laplacian model does indeed give depthmaps with significantly sharper boundaries (as in our discussion in Section 4.1; also see Fig. 3). Table 1 shows the errors obtained by our algorithm on a variety of forest, campus, and indoor images. The results on the test set show that the algorithm estimates the depthmaps with a average error of 0.132 orders of magnitude. It works well even in the varied set of environments as shown in Fig. 3 (last column). It also appears to be very robust towards variations caused by shadows.

Informally, our algorithm appears to predict the relative depths of objects quite well (i.e., their relative distances to the camera), but seems to make more errors in absolute depths. Some of the errors can be attributed to errors or limitations of the training set. For example, the training set images and depthmaps are slightly misaligned, and therefore the edges in the learned depthmap are not very sharp. Further, the maximum value of the depths in the training set is 81m; therefore, far-away objects are all mapped to the one distance of 81m.

Our algorithm appears to incur the largest errors on images which contain very irregular trees, in which most of the 3-D structure in the image is dominated by the shapes of the leaves and branches. However, arguably even human-level performance would be poor on these images.

6 Conclusions

We have presented a discriminatively trained MRF model for depth estimation from single monocular images. Our model uses monocular cues at multiple spatial scales, and also

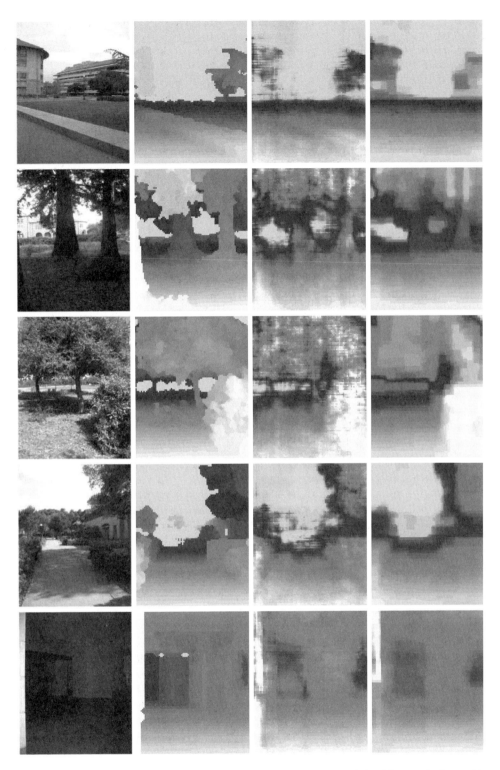

Figure 3: Results for a varied set of environments, showing original image (column 1), ground truth depthmap (column 2), predicted depthmap by Gaussian model (column 3), predicted depthmap by Laplacian model (column 4). (**Best viewed in color**)

Table 1: Effect of multiscale and column features on accuracy. The average absolute errors (RMS errors gave similar results) are on a log scale (base 10). H_1 and H_2 represent summary statistics for $k = 1, 2$. S_1, S_2 and S_3 represent the 3 scales. C represents the column features. Baseline is trained with only the bias term (no features).

FEATURE	ALL	FOREST	CAMPUS	INDOOR
BASELINE	.295	.283	.343	.228
GAUSSIAN ($S_1, S_2, S_3, H_1, H_2, no\ neighbors$)	.162	.159	.166	.165
GAUSSIAN (S_1, H_1, H_2)	.171	.164	.189	.173
GAUSSIAN (S_1, S_2, H_1, H_2)	.155	.151	.164	.157
GAUSSIAN (S_1, S_2, S_3, H_1, H_2)	.144	.144	.143	.144
GAUSSIAN (S_1, S_2, S_3, C, H_1)	.139	.140	.141	.122
GAUSSIAN ($S_1, S_2, S_3, C, H_1, H_2$)	.133	.135	.132	.124
LAPLACIAN	.132	.133	.142	.084

incorporates interaction terms that model relative depths, again at different scales. In addition to a Gaussian MRF model, we also presented a Laplacian MRF model in which MAP inference can be done efficiently using linear programming. We demonstrated that our algorithm gives good 3-D depth estimation performance on a variety of images.

Acknowledgments

We give warm thanks to Jamie Schulte, who designed the 3-D scanner, for help in collecting the data used in this work. We also thank Larry Jackel for helpful discussions. This work was supported by the DARPA LAGR program under contract number FA8650-04-C-7134.

References

[1] D. Scharstein and R. Szeliski. A taxonomy and evaluation of dense two-frame stereo correspondence algorithms. *Int'l Journal of Computer Vision*, 47:7–42, 2002.

[2] David A. Forsyth and Jean Ponce. *Computer Vision : A Modern Approach*. Prentice Hall, 2003.

[3] S. Das and N. Ahuja. Performance analysis of stereo, vergence, and focus as depth cues for active vision. *IEEE Trans Pattern Analysis & Machine Intelligence*, 17:1213–1219, 1995.

[4] J. Michels, A. Saxena, and A.Y. Ng. High speed obstacle avoidance using monocular vision and reinforcement learning. In *ICML*, 2005.

[5] T. Nagai, T. Naruse, M. Ikehara, and A. Kurematsu. Hmm-based surface reconstruction from single images. In *Proc IEEE Int'l Conf Image Processing*, volume 2, 2002.

[6] G. Gini and A. Marchi. Indoor robot navigation with single camera vision. In *PRIS*, 2002.

[7] M. Shao, T. Simchony, and R. Chellappa. New algorithms from reconstruction of a 3-d depth map from one or more images. In *Proc IEEE CVPR*, 1988.

[8] J. Lafferty, A. McCallum, and F. Pereira. Discriminative fields for modeling spatial dependencies in natural images. In *ICML*, 2001.

[9] K. Murphy, A. Torralba, and W.T. Freeman. Using the forest to see the trees: A graphical model relating features, objects, and scenes. In *NIPS 16*, 2003.

[10] Xuming He, Richard S. Zemel, and Miguel A. Carreira-Perpinan. Multiscale conditional random fields for image labeling. In *proc. CVPR*, 2004.

[11] S. Kumar and M. Hebert. Discriminative fields for modeling spatial dependencies in natural images. In *NIPS 16*, 2003.

[12] J.M. Loomis. Looking down is looking up. *Nature News and Views*, 414:155–156, 2001.

[13] B. Wu, T.L. Ooi, and Z.J. He. Perceiving distance accurately by a directional process of integrating ground information. *Letters to Nature*, 428:73–77, 2004.

[14] P. Sinha I. Blthoff, H. Blthoff. Top-down influences on stereoscopic depth-perception. *Nature Neuroscience*, 1:254–257, 1998.

[15] E.R. Davies. Laws' texture energy in TEXTURE. In *Machine Vision: Theory, Algorithms, Practicalities 2nd Edition*. Academic Press, San Diego, 1997.

[16] A.S. Willsky. Multiresolution markov models for signal and image processing. *IEEE*, 2002.

Identifying Distributed Object Representations in Human Extrastriate Visual Cortex

Rory Sayres

Department of Neuroscience
Stanford University
Stanford, CA 94305
sayres@stanford.edu

David Ress

Department of Neuroscience
Brown University
Providence, RI 02912
ress@brown.edu

Kalanit Grill-Spector

Departments of Neuroscience and Psychology
Stanford University
Stanford, CA 94305
kalanit@psych.stanford.edu

Abstract

The category of visual stimuli has been reliably decoded from patterns of neural activity in extrastriate visual cortex [1]. It has yet to be seen whether object identity can be inferred from this activity. We present fMRI data measuring responses in human extrastriate cortex to a set of 12 distinct object images. We use a simple winner-take-all classifier, using half the data from each recording session as a training set, to evaluate encoding of object identity across fMRI voxels. Since this approach is sensitive to the inclusion of noisy voxels, we describe two methods for identifying subsets of voxels in the data which optimally distinguish object identity. One method characterizes the reliability of each voxel within subsets of the data, while another estimates the mutual information of each voxel with the stimulus set. We find that both metrics can identify subsets of the data which reliably encode object identity, even when noisy measurements are artificially added to the data. The mutual information metric is less efficient at this task, likely due to constraints in fMRI data.

1   Introduction

Humans and other primates can perform fast and efficient object recognition. This ability is mediated within a large extent of occipital and temporal cortex, sometimes referred to as the ventral processing stream [10]. This cortex has been examined using electrophysiological recordings, optical imaging techniques, and a variety of neuroimaging techniques including functional magnetic resonance imaging (fMRI) [refs]. With fMRI, these regions can be reliably identified by their strong preferential response to intact objects over other visual stimuli [9,10].

The functional organization of object-selective cortex is unclear. A number of regions have been identified within this cortex, which preferentially respond to particular categories of images [refs]; it has been proposed that these regions are specialized for processing visual information about those categories [refs]. A recent study by Haxby and colleagues [1] found that the category identity of different stimuli could be decoded from fMRI response patterns, using a simple classifier in which half of each data set was used as a training set and half as a test set. These results were interpreted as evidence for a distributed representation of objects across ventral cortex, in which both positive and negative responses contribute information about object identity. It is not clear, however, to what extent information about objects is processed at the category level, and to what extent it reflects individual object identity, or features within objects [1,8].

The study in [1] is one of a growing number of recent attempts to decode stimulus identity by examining fMRI response patterns across cortex [1-4]. fMRI data has particular advantages and disadvantages for this approach. Among its advantages are the ability to make many measurements across a large extent of cortex in awake, behaving humans. Its disadvantages include temporal and spatial resolution constraints, which limit the number of trials that may be collected; the ability to examine trial-by-trial variation; and potentially limit the localization of small neuronal populations. A further potential disadvantage arises from the little-understood functional organization of object-selective cortical regions. Because it is not clear which parts of this cortex are involved in representing different objects and which aren't, analyses may include fMRI image locations (voxels) which are not involved in object representation.

The present study addresses a number of these questions by examining the response patterns across object-selective cortex to a set of 12 individual object images, using high-resolution fMRI. We sought to address the following experimental questions: (1) Can individual object identity be decoded from fMRI responses in object-selective cortex? (2) How can one identify those subsets of fMRI voxels which reliably encode identity about a stimulus, among a large set of potentially unrelated voxels? We adopt a similar approach to that described in [1], subdividing each data set into training and test subsets, and evaluate the efficiency of a set of voxels in discriminating object identity among the 12 possible images with a simple winner-take-all classifier. We then describe two metrics from which to identify sets of voxels which reliably discriminate different objects. The first metric estimates the replicability of voxels to each stimulus between the training and the test data. The second metric estimates the mutual information each voxel has with the stimulus set.

2 Experimental design and data collection

Our experimental design is summarized in Figure 1. We chose a stimulus set of 12 line drawings of different object stimuli, shown in Figure 1a. These objects can be readily categorized as faces, animals, or vehicles; these categories have been previously identified as producing distinct patterns of blood-oxygenation-level-dependent (BOLD) response in object-selective cortex [10]. This allows us to compare category and object identity as potential explanatory factors for BOLD response patterns. Further, the use of black-and-white line drawings reduces the number of stimulus features which differentiate the stimuli, such as spatial frequency bands.

A typical trial is illustrated in Figure 1b. We presented one of the 12 object images to the subject within the foveal 5 degrees of visual field for 2 sec, then masked the image with a scrambled version of a random image for 10 sec. These scrambled images are known to produce minimal response in our regions of interest [11], and serve as a baseline condition for these experiments. Each scan contained one trial per image, presented in a randomized order. We ran 10-15 event-related scans for each scanning session. This allowed us to collect full hemodynamic responses to each image, which in BOLD signal lags several seconds after stimulus onset. In this way we were able to analyze trial-by-trial variations in response to different images, without the analytic and design restrictions involved in analyzing fMRI data with more closely-spaced trials [5]. This feature was essential for computing the mutual information of a voxel with the stimulus set.

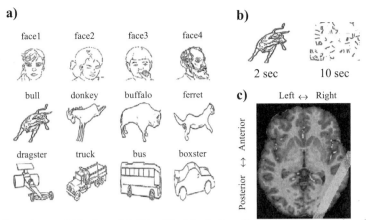

Figure 1: Experimental Design. **(a)** The 12 object stimuli used. **(b)** Example of a typical trial. **(c)** Depiction of imaged region during one session. The image is an axial slice from a T1-weighted anatomical image for one subject. The blue region shows the region imaged at high resolution. The white outlines show gray matter within the imaged area.

We obtained high-resolution fMRI images at 3 Tesla using a spiral-out protocol. We used a custom-built receive-only surface coil. This coil was small and flexible, with a 7.5 cm diameter, and could be placed on a subject's skull directly over the region to be imaged. Because of the restricted field of view of this coil, we imaged only right hemisphere cortex for these experiments. We imaged 4 subjects (1 female), each of whom participated in multiple recording sessions. For each recording session, we imaged 12 oblique slices, with voxel dimensions of 1 x 1 x 1 mm and a frame period of 2 seconds. (More typical fMRI resolutions are around 3 x 3 x 3 mm–3x3x6 mm, at least 27 times lower in resolution.) A typical imaging prescription, superimposed over a high-resolution T1-weighted anatomical image, is shown in Figure 1c.

Functional data from these experiments are illustrated in Figure 2. Within each session, we identified object-selective voxels by applying a general linear model to the time series data, estimating the amplitude of BOLD response to different images [5]. We then computed contrast maps representing T tests of response of different images against the baseline scrambled condition. An example of voxels localized in this way is illustrated in Figure 2a, superimposed over mean T1-weighted anatomical images for two slices. Our criterion for defining object-selective voxels was that a voxel needed to respond to at least one of the 12 stimulus images relative to baseline with a significance level of $p \leq 0.001$. Each data set contained between 600 and 2500 object-selective voxels.

The design of our surface coil, combined with its proximity to the imaged cortex, allowed us to observe significant event-related responses within single voxels. Figure 2b shows peri-stimulus time courses to each image from four sample voxels. These responses are summarized by subtracting the mean BOLD response after stimulus onset with the response during the baseline period, as illustrated in Figure 2c. In this way we can summarize a data set as a matrix $\mathbf{A}$ of response amplitudes to different voxels, where $\mathbf{A}_{i,j}$ represents the response to the ith image of the jth voxel. These responses are statistically significant (T test, $p < 0.001$) for many stimuli, yet the voxels are heterogeneous in their responses—different voxels respond to different stimuli. This response diversity prompts the questions of deciding which sets of responses, if any, are informative of image identity.

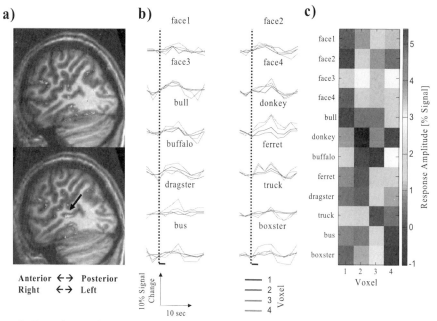

Figure 2: Experimental Data. **(a)** T1-weighted anatomical images from a sample session, with object-selective voxels indicated in orange. **(b)** Mean peristimulus time courses from 4 object-selective voxels in the lower slice of **(a)** (locations indicated by arrow), for each image. Dotted lines indicate trial onset; dark bars at bottom indicate stimulus presentation duration. Scale bars indicate 10 seconds duration and 10 percent BOLD signal change relative to baseline. **(c)** Mean response amplitudes from the voxels depicted in **(b)**, represented as a set of column vectors for each voxel. Color indicates mean amplitude during post-stimulus period relative to pre-stimulus period.

3   Winner-take-all classifier

Given a set of response amplitudes across object-selective voxels, how can we characterize the discriminabilty of responses to different stimuli? This question can be answered by constructing a classifier, which takes a set of responses to an unknown stimulus, and compares it to a training set of responses to known stimuli. This general approach has been successfully applied to fMRI responses in early visual cortex [3-4], object-selective cortex [1], and across multiple cortical regions [2].

For our classifier, we adopt the approach used in [1], with a few refinements. As in the previous study, we subdivide each data set into a training set and a test set, with the training set representing odd-numbered runs and the test set representing even-numbered runs. (Since each run contains one trial per image, this is equivalent to using odd- and even-numbered trials). We construct a training matrix, $A_{training}$, in which each row represents the response across voxels to a different image in the training data set. We construct a second matrix, A_{test}, which contains the responses to different images during the test set. These matrices are illustrated for one data set in Figure 3a. Each row of A_{test} is considered to be the response to an unknown stimulus, and is compared to each of the rows in $A_{training}$. The overall performance of the classifier is evaluated by its success rate at classifying test responses based on the correlation to training responses.

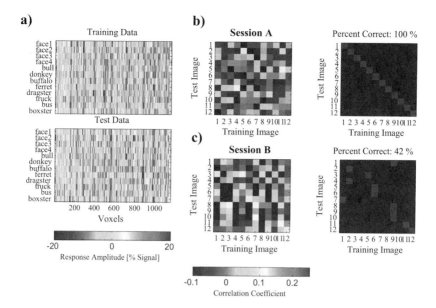

Figure 3: Illustration of winner-take-all classifier for two sample sessions. **(a)** Response amplitudes for all object-selective voxels for the training *(top)* and test *(bottom)* data sets, for one recording session. **(b)** Classifier results for the same session as in **(a)**. *Left:* Correlation matrix between the training and test sets. *Right:* Results of the winner-take-all algorithm. The red square in each row represents the image from the test set that produced the highest correlation with the training set, and is the "guess" of the classifier. The percent correct is evaluated as the number of guesses that lie along the diagonal (the same image in the training and test sets produces the highest correlation). **(c)** Results for a second session, in the same format as **(b)**.

We evaluate classifier performance with a winner-take-all criterion, which is more conservative than the criterion in [1]. First, a correlation matrix $\mathbf{R}$ is constructed containing correlation coefficients for each pairwise comparison of rows in $\mathbf{A}_{\text{training}}$ and $\mathbf{A}_{\text{test}}$ (shown on the left in Figure 3b and 3c for two data sets). The element $\mathbf{R}_{i,j}$ represents the correlation coefficient between row i of $\mathbf{A}_{\text{test}}$ and row j of $\mathbf{A}_{\text{training}}$. Then, for each row in the correlation matrix, the classifier "guesses" the identity of the test stimulus by selecting the element with the highest coefficient (shown on the right in Figure 3b and 3c). Correct guesses lie along the diagonal of this matrix, $\mathbf{R}_{i,i}$.

The previously-used method evaluated classifier performance by successively pairing off the correct stimulus with incorrect stimuli from the training set [1]. With this criterion, responses from the test set which do not correlate maximally with the same stimulus in the training set might still lead to high classifier performance. For instance, if an element $\mathbf{R}_{i,i}$ is larger than all but one coefficient in row i, pairwise comparisons would reveal correct guesses for 10 out of 11 comparisons, or 91% correct, while the winner-take-all criterion would consider this 0%. This conservative criterion reduces chance performance from 1/2 to 1/12, and ensures that high classifier performance reflects a high level of discriminability between different stimuli, providing a stringent test for decoding.

4 Identifying voxels which distinguish objects

When we examined response patterns across all object-selective voxels, we observed high levels of classifier performance from some recording sessions, as shown in Session A in Figure 3. Many sessions, however, were more similar to Session B: limited success at decoding object identity when using all voxels.

For both cases, a relevant question is the extent to which information is contained within a subset of the selected voxel. The distributed representation implied in Session A may be driven by only a few informative voxels; conversely, excessively noisy or unrelated activity from other voxels may be affected classifier performance on Session B. This is of particular concern given that the functional organization of this cortex is not well understood. In addition to using such classifiers to test a hypothesis that a pre-defined region of interest can discriminate stimuli, it would be highly useful to use the classifier to identify cortical regions which represent a stimulus.

To identify subsets of the data which reliably represent different stimuli, we search among the set of object-selective voxels using two metrics to rank voxels: (1) The reliability of each voxel between the training and test data subsets; and (2) The mutual information of each voxel with the stimulus set.

4.1 Voxel reliability metric

The voxel reliability metric is computed for each voxel by taking the vectors of 12 response amplitudes to each stimulus in the training and test sets, and calculating their correlation coefficient. Voxels with high reliability will have high values for the diagonal elements in the **R** correlation matrix, but this does not place constraints on correlations for the off-diagonal comparisons. For instance, persistently active and nonspecific voxels (such as might be expected from draining veins or sinuses) would have high voxel reliability, but also high correlation for all pairwise comparisons between stimuli in test and training sets, so as not to guarantee high classifier performance.

4.2 Mutual information metric

The mutual information for a voxel is computed as the difference between the overall entropy of the voxel and the "noise entropy", the sum over all stimuli of the entropy of the voxel given each stimulus [6]:

$$I_m = H - H_{noise} = -\sum_r P(r)\log_2 P(r) + \sum_{s,r} P(s)P(r|s)\log_2 P(r|s) \quad (1)$$

In this formula, P(r) represents the probability of observing a response level r and P(r|s) represents the probability of observing response r given stimulus s. Computing these probabilities presents a difficulty for fMRI data, since an accurate estimate requires many trials. Given the hemodynamic lag of 9-16 sec inherent to measuring BOLD signal, and the limitations of keeping a human observer in an MRI scanner before motion artifacts or attentional drifts confound the signals, it is difficult to obtain many trials over which to evaluate different response probabilities. There are two possible solutions to this: find ways of obtaining large number of trials, e. g. through co-registering data across many sessions; and reduce the number of possible response bins for the data. While the first option is an area of active pursuit for us, we will focus here on the second approach.

Given the low number of trials per image, we reduce the number of possible response levels to only two bins, 0 and 1. This allows for a wider range of possible values for P(r) and P(r|s) at the expense of ignoring potential information contained in varying response levels. Given these two bins, the next question is deciding how to threshold responses to decide if a given voxel responded significantly (r=1) or not (r=0) on a given trial. Since we do not have an *a priori* hypothesis about the value of this threshold, we choose it separately for each voxel, such that it maximizes the mutual information of that voxel. This approach has been used previously to reduce free parameters while developing artificial recognition models[7].

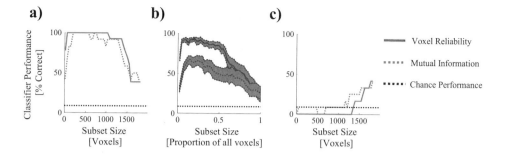

Figure 4: Comparison of metrics for identifying reliable subsets of voxels in data sets. **(a)** Performance on winner-take-all classifier of different-sized subsets of one data set ("Session B" in Figure 3), sorted by voxel reliability *(gray, solid)* and mutual information *(red, dashed)* metrics. **(b)** Performance of the two metrics across 12 data sets. Each curve represents the mean (thick line) ± standard error of the mean across data sets. **(c)** Performance on data set from **(a)** when reverse-sorting voxels by each metric. Dotted black line indicates chance performance.

After ranking each voxel with the two metrics, we evaluated how well these voxels found reliable object representations. To do this, we sorted the voxels in descending order according to each metric; selected progressively larger subsets of voxels, starting with the 10 highest-ranked voxels and proceeding to the full set of voxels; and evaluated performance on the classifier for each subset. Results of these analyses are summarized in Figure 4. Figure 4a shows performance curves for the two sortings on data from the "Session B" data set illustrated in Figure 3. As can be seen, while performance using all voxels is at 42% correct, by removing voxels, performance quickly reaches 100% using the reliability criterion. The mutual information metric also converges to 100%, albeit slightly more slowly. Also note that for very small subset sizes, performance decreases again: correct discrimination requires information distributed across a set of voxels.

Finally, we repeated our analyses across 12 data sets collected from 4 subjects. Figure 4c shows the mean performance across sessions for the two metrics. These curves are normalized by the proportion of total available voxels for each data set. Overall, the voxel reliability metric was significantly better at identifying subsets of voxels which could discriminate object identity, although both metrics performed significantly better than the 1/12 chance performance at the classifier task, and both produced pronounced improvements in performance for smaller subsets compared to using the entire data sets. Note that simply removing voxels does not guarantee the better performance on the classifier. If the voxels are sorted in reverse order, starting with e. g. the lowest values of voxel reliability or mutual information, subsets containing half the voxels are consistently at or below chance performance (Figure 4c).

5 Summary and conclusions

Developing and training classifiers to identify cognitive states based on fMRI data is a growing and promising approach for neuroscience [1-4]. One drawback to these methods, however, is that they often require prior knowledge of which voxels are involved in specifying a cognitive state, and which aren't. Given the poorly-understood functional organization of the majority of cortex, an important goal is to develop methods to search across cortex for regions which represent such states. The results described here represent one step in this direction.

Our voxel-ranking metrics successfully identified subsets of object-selective voxels which discriminate object identity. This demonstrates the feasibility of adapting classifier methods to search across cortical regions. However, these methods can be refined considerably. The most important improvement is providing a larger set of trials from which to compute response probabilities. This is currently being pursued by combining data sets from multiple recording sessions in a reference volume. Given more extensive data, the set of possible response bins can be increased from the current binary set, which should improve performance of our mutual information metric.

Our results also have several implications for object recognition. We found a high ability to discriminate between individual images in our data sets. Moreover, this discrimination could be performed with sets of voxels of widely varying sizes. For some sessions, perfect discrimination could be achieved using all object-selective voxels, which number in the thousands (Figure 3a, 3b); for many others, perfect discrimination was possible using subsets as small as a few dozen voxels. This has implications for the distributed nature of object representation in extrastriate cortex. However, it raises the question of identifying redundant information within these representations. The distributed representations may reflect functionally distinct areas which are processing different aspects of each stimulus, as in earlier visual cortex. Mutual information approaches have succeeded at identifying redundant coding of information in other sensory areas [10], and can be tested on the known functional subdivisions in early visual cortex. In this way, we can use intuitions generated by ideal observers of the data, such as the classifier described here, and apply them to understanding how the brain processes this information.

Acknowledgments

We would like to thank Gal Chechik and Brian Wandell for input on analysis techniques. This work was supported by NEI National Research Service Award 5F31EY015937-02 to RAS, and a research grant 2005-05-111-RES from the Whitehall Foundation to KGS.

References

[1] Haxby JV, Gobbini MI, Furey ML, Ishai A, Schouten JL, and Pietrini P. (2001) Distributed and overlapping representations of faces and objects in ventral temporal cortex. *Science* 293:2425-30.

[2] Wang X, Hutchinson R, and Mitchell TM (2004) Training fMRI classifiers to distinguish cognitive states across multiple subjects. In S. Thrun, L. Saul and B. Scholköpf (eds.), Advances in Neural Information Processing Systems 16. Cambridge, MA: MIT Press.

[3] Kamitani Y and Tong F. (2005) Decoding the visual and subjective contents of the human brain. *Nat Neurosci.* 8:679-85.

[4] Haynes JD and Rees G. (2005) Predicting the orientation of invisible stimuli from activity in human primary visual cortex. *Nat Neurosci.* 8:686-691.

[5] Burock MA and Dale AM. (2000) Estimation and Detection of Event-Related fMRI Signals with temporally correlated noise: a statistically efficient and unbiased approach. *Human Brain Mapping* 11:249-260.

[6] Abbott L and Dayan P (2001) Theoretical Neuroscience. Cambridge, MA: MIT Press.

[7] Ullman S, Vidal-Naquet M, and Sali E. Visual features of intermediate complexity and their use in classification. *Nat Neurosci.* 5(7):682-7.

[8] Tsunoda K, Yamane Y, Nishizaki M, and Tanifuji M. (2001) Complex objects are represented in macaque inferotemporal cortex by the combination of feature columns. *Nat Neurosci.* 4:832-8.

[9] Grill-Spector K, Kushnir T, Hendler T, and Malach R. (2000) The dynamics of object-selective activation correlate with recognition performance in humans. *Nat Neurosci.* 3:837-43.

[10] Malach R, Reppas JB, Benson RR, Kwong KK, Jiang H, Kennedy WA, Ledden PJ, Brady TJ, Rosen BR, and Tootell RB. (1995) Object-related activity revealed by functional magnetic resonance imaging in human occipital cortex. *Proc Natl Acad Sci U S A* 92:8135-8139.

[11] Chechik G, Globerson A, Anderson MJ, Young ED, Nelken I, and Tishby N. (2001) Groups redundancy measures reveal redundancy reduction along the auditory pathway. Advances in Neural Information Processing Systems 14. Cambridge, MA: MIT Press.

On the Accuracy of Bounded Rationality: How Far from Optimal Is Fast and Frugal?

Michael Schmitt
Ludwig-Marum-Gymnasium
Schlossgartenstraße 11
76327 Pfinztal, Germany
mschmittm@googlemail.com

Laura Martignon
Institut für Mathematik und Informatik
Pädagogische Hochschule Ludwigsburg
Reuteallee 46, 71634 Ludwigsburg, Germany
martignon@ph-ludwigsburg.de

Abstract

Fast and frugal heuristics are well studied models of bounded rationality. Psychological research has proposed the take-the-best heuristic as a successful strategy in decision making with limited resources. Take-the-best searches for a sufficiently good ordering of cues (features) in a task where objects are to be compared lexicographically. We investigate the complexity of the problem of approximating optimal cue permutations for lexicographic strategies. We show that no efficient algorithm can approximate the optimum to within any constant factor, if $P \neq NP$. We further consider a greedy approach for building lexicographic strategies and derive tight bounds for the performance ratio of a new and simple algorithm. This algorithm is proven to perform better than take-the-best.

1 Introduction

In many circumstances the human mind has to make decisions when time and knowledge are limited. Cognitive psychology categorizes human judgments made under such constraints as being boundedly rational if they are "satisficing" (Simon, 1982) or, more generally, if they do not fall too far behind the rational standards. A class of models for human reasoning studied in the context of bounded rationality consists of simple algorithms termed "fast and frugal heuristics". These were the topic of major psychological research (Gigerenzer and Goldstein, 1996; Gigerenzer et al., 1999). Great efforts have been put into testing these heuristics by empirical means in experiments with human subjects (Bröder, 2000; Bröder and Schiffer, 2003; Lee and Cummins, 2004; Newell and Shanks, 2003; Newell et al., 2003; Slegers et al., 2000) or in simulations on computers (Bröder, 2002; Hogarth and Karelaia, 2003; Nellen, 2003; Todd and Dieckmann, 2005). (See also the discussion and controversies documented in the open peer commentaries on Todd and Gigerenzer, 2000.)

Among the fast and frugal heuristics there is an algorithm called "take-the-best" (TTB) that is considered a process model for human judgments based on one-reason decision making. Which of the two cities has a larger population: (a) Düsseldorf (b) Hamburg? This is the task originally studied by Gigerenzer and Goldstein (1996) where German cities with a population of more than 100,000 inhabitants had to be compared. The available information on each city consists of the values of nine binary cues, or attributes, indicating

	Soccer Team	State Capital	License Plate
Hamburg	1	1	0
Essen	0	0	1
Düsseldorf	0	1	1
Validity	1	1/2	0

Table 1: Part of the German cities task of Gigerenzer and Goldstein (1996). Shown are profiles and validities of three cues for three cities. Cue validities are computed from the data as given here. The original data has different validities but the same cue ranking.

presence or absence of a feature. The cues being used are, for instance, whether the city is a state capital, whether it is indicated on car license plates by a single letter, or whether it has a soccer team in the national league. The judgment which city is larger is made on the basis of the two binary vectors, or cue profiles, representing the two cities. TTB performs a lexicographic strategy, comparing the cues one after the other and using the first cue that discriminates as the one reason to yield the final decision. For instance, if one city has a university and the other does not, TTB would infer that the first city is larger than the second. If the cue values of both cities are equal, the algorithm passes on to the next cue.

TTB examines the cues in a certain order. Gigerenzer and Goldstein (1996) introduced ecological validity as a numerical measure for ranking the cues. The validity of a cue is a real number in the interval $[0, 1]$ that is computed in terms of the known outcomes of paired comparisons. It is defined as the number of pairs the cue discriminates correctly (i.e., where it makes a correct inference) divided by the number of pairs it discriminates (i.e., where it makes an inference, be it right or wrong). TTB always chooses a cue with the highest validity, that is, it "takes the best" among those cues not yet considered. Table 1 shows cue profiles and validities for three cities. The ordering defined by the size of their population is given by

$$\{\langle \text{ Düsseldorf}, \text{Essen }\rangle, \langle \text{ Düsseldorf}, \text{Hamburg }\rangle, \langle \text{ Essen}, \text{Hamburg }\rangle\},$$

where a pair $\langle a, b\rangle$ indicates that a has less inhabitants than b. As an example for calculating the validity, the state-capital cue distinguishes the first and the third pair but is correct only on the latter. Hence, its validity has value $1/2$.

The order in which the cues are ranked is crucial for success or failure of TTB. In the example of Düsseldorf and Hamburg, the car-license-plate cue would yield that Düsseldorf (D) is larger than Hamburg (HH), whereas the soccer-team cue would correctly favor Hamburg. Thus, how successful a lexicographic strategy is in a comparison task consisting of a partial ordering of cue profiles depends on how well the cue ranking minimizes the number of incorrect comparisons. Specifically, the accuracy of TTB relies on the degree of optimality achieved by the ranking according to decreasing cue validities. For TTB and the German cities task, computer simulations have shown that TTB discriminates at least as accurate as other models (Gigerenzer and Goldstein, 1996; Gigerenzer et al., 1999; Todd and Dieckmann, 2005). TTB made as many correct inferences as standard algorithms proposed by cognitive psychology and even outperformed some of them.

Partial results concerning the accuracy of TTB compared to the accuracy of other strategies have been obtained analytically by Martignon and Hoffrage (2002). Here we subject the problem of finding optimal cue orderings to a rigorous theoretical analysis employing methods from the theory of computational complexity (Ausiello et al., 1999). Obviously, TTB runs in polynomial time. Given a list of ordered pairs, it computes all cue validities in polynomially many computing steps in terms of the size of the list. We define the optimization problem MINIMUM INCORRECT LEXICOGRAPHIC STRATEGY as the task of minimizing the number of incorrect inferences for the lexicographic strategy on a given list of pairs. We show that, unless P = NP, there is no polynomial-time approximation algorithm that computes solutions for MINIMUM INCORRECT LEXICOGRAPHIC STRATEGY that are only a constant factor worse than the optimum, unless $P = NP$. This means that the approximating factor, or performance ratio, must grow with the size of the problem.

As an extension of TTB we consider an algorithm for finding cue orderings that was called "TTB by Conditional Validity" in the context of bounded rationality. It is based on the greedy method, a principle widely used in algorithm design. This greedy algorithm runs in polynomial time and we derive tight bounds for it, showing that it approximates the optimum with a performance ratio proportional to the number of cues. An important consequence of this result is a guarantee that for those instances that have a solution that discriminates all pairs correctly, the greedy algorithm always finds a permutation attaining this minimum. We are not aware that this quality has been established for any of the previously studied heuristics for paired comparison. In addition, we show that TTB does not have this property, concluding that the greedy method of constructing cue permutations performs provably better than TTB. For a more detailed account and further results we refer to the complete version of this work (Schmitt and Martignon, 2006).

2 Lexicographic Strategies

A *lexicographic strategy* is a method for comparing elements of a set $B \subseteq \{0,1\}^n$. Each component $1, \ldots, n$ of these vectors is referred to as a *cue*. Given $a, b \in B$, where $a = (a_1, \ldots, a_n)$ and $b = (b_1, \ldots, b_n)$, the lexicographic strategy searches for the smallest cue index $i \in \{1, \ldots, n\}$ such that a_i and b_i are different. The strategy then outputs one of " $<$ " or " $>$ " according to whether $a_i < b_i$ or $a_i > b_i$ assuming the usual order $0 < 1$ of the truth values. If no such cue exists, the strategy returns " $=$ ". Formally, let diff : $B \times B \to \{1, \ldots, n+1\}$ be the function where $\mathrm{diff}(a,b)$ is the smallest cue index on which a and b are different, or $n + 1$ if they are equal, that is,

$$\mathrm{diff}(a, b) \;=\; \min\{\{i : a_i \neq b_i\} \cup \{n+1\}\}.$$

Then, the function $S : B \times B \to \{\text{" } < \text{ "}, \text{" } = \text{ "}, \text{" } > \text{ "}\}$ computed by the lexicographic strategy is

$$S(a,b) \;=\; \begin{cases} \text{" } < \text{ "} & \text{if } \mathrm{diff}(a,b) \leq n \text{ and } a_{\mathrm{diff}(a,b)} < b_{\mathrm{diff}(a,b)}, \\ \text{" } > \text{ "} & \text{if } \mathrm{diff}(a,b) \leq n \text{ and } a_{\mathrm{diff}(a,b)} > b_{\mathrm{diff}(a,b)}, \\ \text{" } = \text{ "} & \text{otherwise.} \end{cases}$$

Lexicographic strategies may take into account that the cues come in an order that is different from $1, \ldots, n$. Let $\pi : \{1, \ldots, n\} \to \{1, \ldots, n\}$ be a permutation of the cues. It gives rise to a mapping $\overline{\pi} : \{0,1\}^n \to \{0,1\}^n$ that permutes the components of Boolean vectors by $\overline{\pi}(a_1, \ldots, a_n) = (a_{\pi(1)}, \ldots, a_{\pi(n)})$. As $\overline{\pi}$ is uniquely defined given π, we simplify the notation and write also π for $\overline{\pi}$. The *lexicographic strategy under cue permutation* π passes through the cues in the order $\pi(1), \ldots, \pi(n)$, that is, it computes the function $S_\pi : B \times B \to \{\text{" } < \text{ "}, \text{" } = \text{ "}, \text{" } > \text{ "}\}$ defined as

$$S_\pi(a, b) \;=\; S(\pi(a), \pi(b)).$$

The problem we study is that of finding a cue permutation that minimizes the number of incorrect comparisons in a given list of element pairs using the lexicographic strategy. An instance of this problem consists of a set B of elements and a set of pairs $L \subseteq B \times B$. Each pair $\langle a, b \rangle \in L$ represents an inequality $a \leq b$. Given a cue permutation π, we say that the lexicographic strategy under π *infers* the pair $\langle a, b \rangle$ correctly if $S_\pi(a, b) \in \{\text{" } < \text{ "}, \text{" } = \text{ "}\}$, otherwise the inference is incorrect. The task is to find a permutation π such that the number of incorrect inferences in L using S_π is minimal, that is, a permutation π that minimizes

$$\mathrm{INCORRECT}(\pi, L) \;=\; |\{\langle a, b \rangle \in L : S_\pi(a, b) = \text{" } > \text{ "}\}|.$$

1179

3 Approximability of Optimal Cue Permutations

A large class of optimization problems, denoted APX, can be solved efficiently if the solution is required to be only a constant factor worse than the optimum (see, e.g., Ausiello et al., 1999). Here, we prove that, if $P \neq NP$, there is no polynomial-time algorithm whose solutions yield a number of incorrect comparisons that is by at most a constant factor larger than the minimal number possible. It follows that the problem of approximating the optimal cue permutation is even harder than any problem in APX. The optimization problem is formally stated as follows.

> MINIMUM INCORRECT LEXICOGRAPHIC STRATEGY
> Instance: A set $B \subseteq \{0,1\}^n$ and a set $L \subseteq B \times B$.
> Solution: A permutation π of the cues of B.
> Measure: The number of incorrect inferences in L for the lexicographic strategy under cue permutation π, that is, INCORRECT(π, L).

Given a real number $r > 0$, an algorithm is said to approximate MINIMUM INCORRECT LEXICOGRAPHIC STRATEGY to within a factor of r if for every instance (B, L) the algorithm returns a permutation π such that

$$\text{INCORRECT}(\pi, L) \leq r \cdot \text{opt}(L),$$

where opt(L) is the minimal number of incorrect comparisons achievable on L by any permutation. The factor r is also known as the performance ratio of the algorithm. The following optimization problem plays a crucial role in the derivation of the lower bound for the approximability of MINIMUM INCORRECT LEXICOGRAPHIC STRATEGY.

> MINIMUM HITTING SET
> Instance: A collection C of subsets of a finite set U.
> Solution: A hitting set for C, that is, a subset $U' \subseteq U$ such that U' contains at least one element from each subset in C.
> Measure: The cardinality of the hitting set, that is, $|U'|$.

MINIMUM HITTING SET is equivalent to MINIMUM SET COVER. Bellare et al. (1993) have shown that MINIMUM SET COVER cannot be approximated in polynomial time to within any constant factor, unless $P = NP$. Thus, if $P \neq NP$, MINIMUM HITTING SET cannot be approximated in polynomial time to within any constant factor as well.

Theorem 1. *For every r, there is no polynomial-time algorithm that approximates* MINIMUM INCORRECT LEXICOGRAPHIC STRATEGY *to within a factor of r, unless* $P = NP$.

Proof. We show that the existence of a polynomial-time algorithm that approximates MINIMUM INCORRECT LEXICOGRAPHIC STRATEGY to within some constant factor implies the existence of a polynomial-time algorithm that approximates MINIMUM HITTING SET to within the same factor. Then the statement follows from the equivalence of MINIMUM HITTING SET with MINIMUM SET COVER and the nonapproximability of the latter (Bellare et al., 1993). The main part of the proof consists in establishing a specific approximation preserving reduction, or AP-reduction, from MINIMUM HITTING SET to MINIMUM INCORRECT LEXICOGRAPHIC STRATEGY. (See Ausiello et al., 1999, for a definition of the AP-reduction.).

We first define a function f that is computable in polynomial time and maps each instance of MINIMUM HITTING SET to an instance of MINIMUM INCORRECT LEXICOGRAPHIC STRATEGY. Let $\mathbf{1}$ denote the n-bit vector with a 1 everywhere and $\mathbf{1}_{i_1,\dots,i_\ell}$ the vector with 0 in positions $i_1, \dots, i_\ell$ and 1 elsewhere. Given the collection C of subsets of the set $U = \{u_1, \dots, u_n\}$, the function f maps C to (B, L), where $B \subseteq \{0,1\}^{n+1}$ is defined as follows:

1. Let $(\mathbf{1}, 0) \in B$.
2. For $i = 1, \ldots, n$, let $(\mathbf{1}_i, 1) \in B$.
3. For every $\{u_{i_1}, \ldots, u_{i_\ell}\} \in C$, let $(\mathbf{1}_{i_1, \ldots, i_\ell}, 1) \in B$.

Further, the set L is constructed as

$$L = \{\langle (\mathbf{1}, 0), (\mathbf{1}_i, 1) \rangle : i = 1, \ldots, n\} \cup \{\langle (\mathbf{1}_{i_1, \ldots, i_\ell}, 1), (\mathbf{1}, 0) \rangle : \{u_{i_1}, \ldots, u_{i_\ell}\} \in C\}. \quad (1)$$

In the following, a pair from the first and second set on the right-hand side of equation (1) is referred to as an element pair and a subset pair, respectively. Obviously, the function f is computable in polynomial time. It has the following property.

Claim 1. *Let $f(C) = (B, L)$. If C has a hitting set of cardinality k or less then $f(C)$ has a cue permutation π where $\mathrm{INCORRECT}(\pi, L) \leq k$.*

To prove this, assume without loss of generality that C has a hitting set U' of cardinality exactly k, say $U' = \{u_{j_1}, \ldots, u_{j_k}\}$, and let $U \setminus U' = \{u_{j_{k+1}}, \ldots, u_{j_n}\}$. Then the cue permutation

$$j_1, \ldots, j_k, n+1, j_{k+1}, \ldots, j_n.$$

results in no more than k incorrect inferences in L. Indeed, consider an arbitrary subset pair $\langle (\mathbf{1}_{i_1, \ldots, i_\ell}, 1), (\mathbf{1}, 0) \rangle$. To not be an error, one of $i_1, \ldots, i_\ell$ must occur in the hitting set $j_1, \ldots, j_k$. Hence, the first cue that distinguishes this pair has value 0 in $(\mathbf{1}_{i_1, \ldots, i_\ell}, 1)$ and value 1 in $(\mathbf{1}, 0)$, resulting in a correct comparison. Further, let $\langle (\mathbf{1}, 0), (\mathbf{1}_i, 1) \rangle$ be an element pair with $u_i \notin U'$. This pair is distinguished correctly by cue $n + 1$. Finally, each element pair $\langle (\mathbf{1}, 0), (\mathbf{1}_i, 1) \rangle$ with $u_i \in U'$ is distinguished by cue i with a result that disagrees with the ordering given by L. Thus, only element pairs with $u_i \in U'$ yield incorrect comparisons and no subset pair. Hence, the number of incorrect inferences is not larger than $|U'|$.

Next, we define a polynomial-time computable function g that maps each collection C of subsets of a finite set U and each cue permutation π for $f(C)$ to a subset of U. Given that $f(C) = (B, L)$, the set $g(C, \pi) \subseteq U$ is defined as follows:

1. For every element pair $\langle (\mathbf{1}, 0), (\mathbf{1}_i, 1) \rangle \in L$ that is compared incorrectly by π, let $u_i \in g(C, \pi)$.

2. For every subset pair $\langle (\mathbf{1}_{i_1, \ldots, i_\ell}, 1), (\mathbf{1}, 0) \rangle \in L$ that is compared incorrectly by π, let one of the elements $u_{i_1}, \ldots, u_{i_\ell} \in g(C, \pi)$.

Clearly, the function g is computable in polynomial time. It satisfies the following condition.

Claim 2. *Let $f(C) = (B, L)$. If $\mathrm{INCORRECT}(\pi, L) \leq k$ then $g(C, \pi)$ is a hitting set of cardinality k or less for C.*

Obviously, if $\mathrm{INCORRECT}(\pi, L) \leq k$ then $g(C, \pi)$ has cardinality at most k. To show that it is a hitting set, assume the subset $\{u_{i_1}, \ldots, u_{i_\ell}\} \in C$ is not hit by $g(C, \pi)$. Then neither of $u_{i_1}, \ldots, u_{i_\ell}$ is in $g(C, \pi)$. Hence, we have correct comparisons for the element pairs corresponding to $u_{i_1}, \ldots, u_{i_\ell}$ and for the subset pair corresponding to $\{u_{i_1}, \ldots, u_{i_\ell}\}$. As the subset pair is distinguished correctly, one of the cues $i_1, \ldots, i_\ell$ must be ranked before cue $n + 1$. But then at least one of the element pairs for $u_{i_1}, \ldots, u_{i_\ell}$ yields an incorrect comparison. This contradicts the assertion that the comparisons for these element pairs are all correct. Thus, $g(C, \pi)$ is a hitting set and the claim is established.

Assume now that there exists a polynomial-time algorithm A that approximates MINIMUM INCORRECT LEXICOGRAPHIC STRATEGY to within a factor of r. Consider the algorithm that, for a given instance C of MINIMUM HITTING SET as input, calls algorithm A with input $(B, L) = f(C)$, and returns $g(C, \pi)$ where π is the output provided by A. Clearly, this new algorithm runs in polynomial time. We show that it approximates MINIMUM

Algorithm 1 GREEDY CUE PERMUTATION

Input: a set $B \subseteq \{0,1\}^n$ and a set $L \subseteq B \times B$
Output: a cue permutation π for n cues
$\quad I := \{1, \ldots, n\};$
$\quad$**for** $i = 1, \ldots, n$ **do**
$\quad\quad$ let $j \in I$ be a cue where $\text{INCORRECT}(j, L) = \min_{j' \in I} \text{INCORRECT}(j', L);$
$\quad\quad \pi(i) := j;$
$\quad\quad I := I \setminus \{j\};$
$\quad\quad L := L \setminus \{\langle a, b \rangle : a_j \neq b_j\}$
$\quad$**end for**.

HITTING SET to within a factor of r. By the assumed approximation property of algorithm A, we have

$$\text{INCORRECT}(\pi, L) \leq r \cdot \text{opt}(L).$$

Together with Claim 2, this implies that $g(\pi, C)$ is a hitting set for C satisfying

$$|g(C, \pi)| \leq r \cdot \text{opt}(L).$$

From Claim 1 we obtain $\text{opt}(L) \leq \text{opt}(C)$ and, thus,

$$|g(C, \pi)| \leq r \cdot \text{opt}(C).$$

Thus, the proposed algorithm for MINIMUM HITTING SET violates the approximation lower bound that holds for this problem under the assumption $P \neq NP$. This proves the statement of the theorem. $\qquad\square$

4 Greedy Approximation of Optimal Cue Permutations

The so-called greedy approach to the solution of an approximation problem is helpful when it is not known which algorithm performs best. It is a simple heuristic that in practice often provides satisfactory solutions in many situations. The algorithm GREEDY CUE PERMU-TATION that we introduce here is based on the greedy method. The idea is to select the first cue according to which single cue makes a minimum number of incorrect inferences (choosing one arbitrarily if there are two or more). After that the algorithm removes those pairs that are distinguished by the selected cue, which is reasonable as the distinctions drawn by this cue cannot be undone by later cues. This procedure is then repeated on the set of pairs left. The description of GREEDY CUE PERMUTATION is given as Algorithm 1. It employs an extension of the function INCORRECT applicable to single cues, such that for a cue i we have

$$\text{INCORRECT}(i, L) = |\{\langle a, b \rangle \in L : a_i > b_i\}|.$$

It is evident that Algorithm 1 runs in polynomial time, but how good is it? The least one should demand from a good heuristic is that, whenever a minimum of zero is attainable, it finds such a solution. This is indeed the case with GREEDY CUE PERMUTATION as we show in the following result. Moreover, it asserts a general performance ratio for the approximation of the optimum.

Theorem 2. *The algorithm* GREEDY CUE PERMUTATION *approximates* MINIMUM IN-CORRECT LEXICOGRAPHIC STRATEGY *to within a factor of* n, *where* n *is the number of cues. In particular, it always finds a cue permutation with no incorrect inferences if one exists.*

Proof. We show by induction on n that the permutation returned by the algorithm makes a number of incorrect inferences no larger than $n \cdot \text{opt}(L)$. If $n = 1$, the optimal cue

$$\langle\, 001\, ,\, 010\, \rangle$$
$$\langle\, 010\, ,\, 100\, \rangle$$
$$\langle\, 010\, ,\, 101\, \rangle$$
$$\langle\, 100\, ,\, 111\, \rangle$$

Figure 1: A set of lexicographically ordered pairs with nondecreasing cue validities $(1, 1/2,$ and $2/3)$. The cue ordering of TTB $(1, 3, 2)$ causes an incorrect inference on the first pair. By Theorem 2, GREEDY CUE PERMUTATION finds the lexicographic ordering.

permutation is definitely found. Let $n > 1$. Clearly, as the incorrect inferences of a cue cannot be reversed by other cues, there is a cue j with

$$\text{INCORRECT}(j, L) \le \text{opt}(L).$$

The algorithm selects such a cue in the first round of the loop. During the rest of the rounds, a permutation of $n - 1$ cues is constructed for the set of remaining pairs. Let j be the cue that is chosen in the first round, $I' = \{1, \ldots, j - 1, j + 1, \ldots, n\}$, and $L' = L \setminus \{\langle a, b \rangle : a_j \ne b_j\}$. Further, let $\text{opt}_{I'}(L')$ denote the minimum number of incorrect inferences taken over the permutations of I' on the set L'. Then, we observe that

$$\text{opt}(L) \ge \text{opt}(L') = \text{opt}_{I'}(L').$$

The inequality is valid because of $L \supseteq L'$. (Note that $\text{opt}(L')$ refers to the minimum taken over the permutations of all cues.) The equality holds as cue j does not distinguish any pair in L'. By the induction hypothesis, rounds 2 to n of the loop determine a cue permutation π' with $\text{INCORRECT}(\pi', L') \le (n-1) \cdot \text{opt}_{I'}(L')$. Thus, the number of incorrect inferences made by the permutation π finally returned by the algorithm satisfies

$$\text{INCORRECT}(\pi, L) \quad \le \quad \text{INCORRECT}(j, L) + (n-1) \cdot \text{opt}_{I'}(L'),$$

which is, by the inequalities derived above, not larger than $\text{opt}(L) + (n-1) \cdot \text{opt}(L)$ as stated. □

Corollary 3. *On inputs that have a cue ordering without incorrect comparisons under the lexicographic strategy,* GREEDY CUE PERMUTATION *can be better than TTB.*

Proof. Figure 1 shows a set of four lexicographically ordered pairs. According to Theorem 2, GREEDY CUE PERMUTATION comes up with the given permutation of the cues. The validities are $1, 1/2$, and $2/3$. Thus, TTB ranks the cues as $1, 3, 2$ whereupon the first pair is inferred incorrectly. □

Finally, we consider lower bounds on the performance ratio of GREEDY CUE PERMUTATION. The proof of this claim is omitted here.

Theorem 4. *The performance ratio of* GREEDY CUE PERMUTATION *is at least* $\max\{n/2, |L|/2\}$.

5 Conclusions

The result that the optimization problem MINIMUM INCORRECT LEXICOGRAPHIC STRATEGY cannot be approximated in polynomial time to within any constant factor answers a long-standing question of psychological research into models of bounded rationality: How accurate are fast and frugal heuristics? It follows that no fast, that is, polynomial-time, algorithm can approximate the optimum well, under the widely accepted assumption that $P \ne NP$. A further question is concerned with a specific fast and frugal heuristic: How accurate is TTB? The new algorithm GREEDY CUE PERMUTATION has been shown to perform provably better than TTB. In detail, it always finds accurate solutions when they exist, in contrast to TTB. With this contribution we pose a challenge to cognitive psychology: to study the relevance of the greedy method as a model for bounded rationality.

Acknowledgment. The first author has been supported in part by the Deutsche Forschungsgemeinschaft (DFG).

References

Ausiello, G., Crescenzi, P., Gambosi, G., Kann, V., Marchetti-Spaccamela, A., and Protasi, M. (1999). *Complexity and Approximation: Combinatorial Problems and Their Approximability Properties*. Springer-Verlag, Berlin.

Bellare, M., Goldwasser, S., Lund, C., and Russell, A. (1993). Efficient probabilistically checkable proofs and applications to approximation. In *Proceedings of the 25th Annual ACM Symposium on Theory of Computing*, pages 294–304. ACM Press, New York, NY.

Bröder, A. (2000). Assessing the empirical validity of the "take-the-best" heuristic as a model of human probabilistic inference. *Journal of Experimental Psychology: Learning, Memory, and Cognition*, 26:1332–1346.

Bröder, A. (2002). Take the best, Dawes' rule, and compensatory decision strategies: A regression-based classification method. *Quality & Quantity*, 36:219–238.

Bröder, A. and Schiffer, S. (2003). Take the best versus simultaneous feature matching: Probabilistic inferences from memory and effects of representation format. *Journal of Experimental Psychology: General*, 132:277–293.

Gigerenzer, G. and Goldstein, D. G. (1996). Reasoning the fast and frugal way: Models of bounded rationality. *Psychological Review*, 103:650–669.

Gigerenzer, G., Todd, P. M., and the ABC Research Group (1999). *Simple Heuristics That Make Us Smart*. Oxford University Press, New York, NY.

Hogarth, R. M. and Karelaia, N. (2003). "Take-the-best" and other simple strategies: Why and when they work "well" in binary choice. DEE Working Paper 709, Universitat Pompeu Fabra, Barcelona.

Lee, M. D. and Cummins, T. D. R. (2004). Evidence accumulation in decision making: Unifying the "take the best" and the "rational" models. *Psychonomic Bulletin & Review*, 11:343–352.

Martignon, L. and Hoffrage, U. (2002). Fast, frugal, and fit: Simple heuristics for paired comparison. *Theory and Decision*, 52:29–71.

Nellen, S. (2003). The use of the "take the best" heuristic under different conditions, modeled with ACT-R. In Detje, F., Dörner, D., and Schaub, H., editors, *Proceedings of the Fifth International Conference on Cognitive Modeling*, pages 171–176, Universitätsverlag Bamberg, Bamberg.

Newell, B. R. and Shanks, D. R. (2003). Take the best or look at the rest? Factors influencing "One-Reason" decision making. *Journal of Experimental Psychology: Learning, Memory, and Cognition*, 29:53–65.

Newell, B. R., Weston, N. J., and Shanks, D. R. (2003). Empirical tests of a fast-and-frugal heuristic: Not everyone "takes-the-best". *Organizational Behavior and Human Decision Processes*, 91:82–96.

Schmitt, M. and Martignon, L. (2006). On the complexity of learning lexicographic strategies. *Journal of Machine Learning Research*, 7(Jan):55–83.

Simon, H. A. (1982). *Models of Bounded Rationality, Volume 2*. MIT Press, Cambridge, MA.

Slegers, D. W., Brake, G. L., and Doherty, M. E. (2000). Probabilistic mental models with continuous predictors. *Organizational Behavior and Human Decision Processes*, 81:98–114.

Todd, P. M. and Dieckmann, A. (2005). Heuristics for ordering cue search in decision making. In Saul, L. K., Weiss, Y., and Bottou, L., editors, *Advances in Neural Information Processing Systems 17*, pages 1393–1400. MIT Press, Cambridge, MA.

Todd, P. M. and Gigerenzer, G. (2000). Précis of "Simple Heuristics That Make Us Smart". *Behavioral and Brain Sciences*, 23:727–741.

Fast Online Policy Gradient Learning with SMD Gain Vector Adaptation

Nicol N. Schraudolph   Jin Yu   Douglas Aberdeen
Statistical Machine Learning, National ICT Australia, Canberra
{nic.schraudolph,douglas.aberdeen}@nicta.com.au

Abstract

Reinforcement learning by direct policy gradient estimation is attractive in theory but in practice leads to notoriously ill-behaved optimization problems. We improve its robustness and speed of convergence with stochastic meta-descent, a gain vector adaptation method that employs fast Hessian-vector products. In our experiments the resulting algorithms outperform previously employed online stochastic, offline conjugate, and natural policy gradient methods.

1   Introduction

Policy gradient reinforcement learning (RL) methods train controllers by estimating the gradient of a long-term reward measure with respect to the parameters of the controller [1]. The advantage of policy gradient methods, compared to value-based RL, is that we avoid the often redundant step of accurately estimating a large number of values. Policy gradient methods are particularly appealing when large state spaces make representing the exact value function infeasible, or when partial observability is introduced. However, in practice policy gradient methods have shown slow convergence [2], not least due to the stochastic nature of the gradients being estimated.

The *stochastic meta-descent* (SMD) gain adaptation algorithm [3, 4] can considerably accelerate the convergence of stochastic gradient descent. In contrast to other gain adaptation methods, SMD copes well not only with stochasticity, but also with non-i.i.d. sampling of observations, which necessarily occurs in RL. In this paper we derive SMD in the context of policy gradient RL, and obtain over an order of magnitude improvement in convergence rate compared to previously employed policy gradient algorithms.

2   Stochastic Meta-Descent

2.1   Gradient-based gain vector adaptation

Let R be a scalar objective function we wish to maximize with respect to its adaptive parameter vector $\theta \in \mathbb{R}^n$, given a sequence of observations $x_t \in \mathcal{X}$ at time $t = 1, 2, \ldots$ Where R is not available or expensive to compute, we use the *stochastic approximation* $R_t : \mathbb{R}^n \times \mathcal{X} \to \mathbb{R}$ of R instead, and maximize the expectation $\mathbb{E}_t[R_t(\theta_t, x_t)]$. Assuming that R_t is twice differentiable wrt. θ, with gradient and Hessian given by

$$g_t = \tfrac{\partial}{\partial \theta} R_t(\theta, x_t)|_{\theta=\theta_t} \quad \text{and} \quad H_t = \tfrac{\partial^2}{\partial \theta\, \partial \theta^\top} R_t(\theta, x_t)|_{\theta=\theta_t}, \tag{1}$$

1185

respectively, we maximize $\mathbb{E}_t[R_t(\boldsymbol{\theta})]$ by the stochastic gradient ascent

$$\boldsymbol{\theta}_{t+1} = \boldsymbol{\theta}_t + \boldsymbol{\gamma}_t \cdot \boldsymbol{g}_t , \tag{2}$$

where $\cdot$ denotes element-wise (Hadamard) multiplication. The gain vector $\boldsymbol{\gamma}_t \in (\mathbb{R}^+)^n$ serves as a diagonal conditioner, providing each element of $\boldsymbol{\theta}$ with its own positive gradient step size. We adapt $\boldsymbol{\gamma}$ by a simultaneous meta-level gradient ascent in the objective R_t. A straightforward implementation of this idea is the *delta-delta* algorithm [5], which would update $\boldsymbol{\gamma}$ via

$$\boldsymbol{\gamma}_{t+1} = \boldsymbol{\gamma}_t + \mu \frac{\partial R_{t+1}(\boldsymbol{\theta}_{t+1})}{\partial \boldsymbol{\gamma}_t} = \boldsymbol{\gamma}_t + \mu \frac{\partial R_{t+1}(\boldsymbol{\theta}_{t+1})}{\partial \boldsymbol{\theta}_{t+1}} \cdot \frac{\partial \boldsymbol{\theta}_{t+1}}{\partial \boldsymbol{\gamma}_t} = \boldsymbol{\gamma}_t + \mu \boldsymbol{g}_{t+1} \cdot \boldsymbol{g}_t , \tag{3}$$

where $\mu \in \mathbb{R}$ is a scalar meta-step size. In a nutshell, gains are decreased where a negative autocorrelation of the gradient indicates oscillation about a local minimum, and increased otherwise. Unfortunately such a simplistic approach has several problems: Firstly, (3) allows gains to become negative. This can be avoided by updating $\boldsymbol{\gamma}$ multiplicatively, *e.g.* via the *exponentiated gradient* algorithm [6].

Secondly, delta-delta's cure is worse than the disease: individual gains are meant to address ill-conditioning, but (3) actually squares the condition number. The autocorrelation of the gradient must therefore be normalized before it can be used. A popular (if extreme) form of normalization is to consider only the sign of the autocorrelation. Such sign-based methods [5, 7–9], however, do not cope well with stochastic approximation of the gradient since the non-linear sign function does not commute with the expectation operator [10]. More recent algorithms [3, 4, 10] therefore use multiplicative (hence linear) normalization factors to condition the meta-level update.

Finally, (3) fails to take into account that gain changes affect not only the current, but also future parameter updates. In recognition of this shortcoming, $\boldsymbol{g}_t$ in (3) is often replaced with a running average of past gradients. Though such ad-hoc smoothing does improve performance, it does not properly capture long-term dependences, the average still being one of immediate, single-step effects. By contrast, Sutton [11] modeled the long-term effect of gains on future parameter values in a linear system by carrying the relevant partials forward in time, and found that the resulting gain adaptation can outperform a less than perfectly matched Kalman filter. Stochastic meta-descent (SMD) extends this approach to arbitrary twice-differentiable nonlinear systems, takes into account the full Hessian instead of just the diagonal, and applies a decay to the partials being carried forward.

2.2 The SMD Algorithm

SMD employs two modifications to address the problems described above: it adjusts gains in log-space, and optimizes over an exponentially decaying trace of gradients. Thus $\ln \boldsymbol{\gamma}$ is updated as follows:

$$\ln \boldsymbol{\gamma}_{t+1} = \ln \boldsymbol{\gamma}_t + \mu \sum_{i=0}^{t} \lambda^i \frac{\partial R(\boldsymbol{\theta}_{t+1})}{\partial \ln \boldsymbol{\gamma}_{t-i}}$$

$$= \ln \boldsymbol{\gamma}_t + \mu \frac{\partial R(\boldsymbol{\theta}_{t+1})}{\partial \boldsymbol{\theta}_{t+1}} \cdot \sum_{i=0}^{t} \lambda^i \frac{\partial \boldsymbol{\theta}_{t+1}}{\partial \ln \boldsymbol{\gamma}_{t-i}} =: \ln \boldsymbol{\gamma}_t + \mu \boldsymbol{g}_{t+1} \cdot \boldsymbol{v}_{t+1}, \tag{4}$$

where the vector $\boldsymbol{v} \in \mathbb{R}^n$ characterizes the long-term dependence of the system parameters on their gain history over a time scale governed by the decay factor $0 \le \lambda \le 1$. Element-wise exponentiation of (4) yields the desired multiplicative update

$$\boldsymbol{\gamma}_{t+1} = \boldsymbol{\gamma}_t \cdot \exp(\mu \boldsymbol{g}_{t+1} \cdot \boldsymbol{v}_{t+1}) \approx \boldsymbol{\gamma}_t \cdot \max(\tfrac{1}{2}, 1 + \mu \boldsymbol{g}_{t+1} \cdot \boldsymbol{v}_{t+1}). \tag{5}$$

The linearization $e^u \approx \max(\tfrac{1}{2}, 1+u)$ eliminates an expensive exponentiation for each gain update, improves its robustness by reducing the effect of outliers ($|u| \gg 0$), and ensures that γ remains positive. To compute the gradient trace v efficiently, we expand θ_{t+1} in terms of its recursive definition (2):

$$v_{t+1} = \sum_{i=0}^{t} \lambda^i \frac{\partial \theta_{t+1}}{\partial \ln \gamma_{t-i}} = \sum_{i=0}^{t} \lambda^i \frac{\partial \theta_t}{\partial \ln \gamma_{t-i}} + \sum_{i=0}^{t} \lambda^i \frac{\partial (\gamma_t \cdot g_t)}{\partial \ln \gamma_{t-i}} \tag{6}$$

$$\approx \lambda v_t + \gamma_t \cdot g_t + \gamma_t \cdot \left[\frac{\partial g_t}{\partial \theta_t} \sum_{i=0}^{t} \lambda^i \frac{\partial \theta_t}{\partial \ln \gamma_{t-i}} \right]$$

Noting that $\frac{\partial g_t}{\partial \theta_t}$ is the Hessian H_t of $R_t(\theta_t)$, we arrive at the simple iterative update

$$v_{t+1} = \lambda v_t + \gamma_t \cdot (g_t + \lambda H_t v_t); \quad v_0 = 0. \tag{7}$$

Although the Hessian of a system with n parameters has $O(n^2)$ entries, efficient indirect methods from algorithmic differentiation are available to compute its product with an arbitrary vector in the same time as 2–3 gradient evaluations [12, 13]. To improve stability, SMD employs an extended Gauss-Newton approximation of H_t for which a similar (even faster) technique is available [4]. An iteration of SMD—comprising (5), (2), and (7)—thus requires less than 3 times the floating-point operations of simple gradient ascent. The extra computation is typically more than compensated for by the faster convergence of SMD. Fast convergence minimizes the number of expensive world interactions required, which in RL is typically of greater concern than computational cost.

3 Policy Gradient Reinforcement Learning

A Markov decision process (MDP) consists of a finite[1] set of states $s \in \mathcal{S}$ of the world, actions $a \in \mathcal{A}$ available to the agent in each state, and a (possibly stochastic) reward function $r(s)$ for each state s. In a partially observable MDP (POMDP), the controller sees only an observation $x \in \mathcal{X}$ of the current state, sampled stochastically from an unknown distribution $\mathbb{P}(x|s)$. Each action a determines a stochastic matrix $P(a) = [\mathbb{P}(s'|s,a)]$ of transition probabilities from state s to state s' given action a. The methods discussed in this paper do not assume explicit knowledge of $P(a)$ or of the observation process. All policies are stochastic, with a probability of choosing action a given state s, and parameters $\theta \in \mathbb{R}^n$ of $\mathbb{P}(a|\theta, s)$. The evolution of the state s is Markovian, governed by an $|\mathcal{S}| \times |\mathcal{S}|$ transition probability matrix $P(\theta) = [\mathbb{P}(s'|\theta, s)]$ with entries given by

$$\mathbb{P}(s'|\theta, s) = \sum_{a \in \mathcal{A}} \mathbb{P}(a|\theta, s)\, \mathbb{P}(s'|s, a). \tag{8}$$

3.1 GPOMDP Monte Carlo estimates of gradient and hessian

GPOMDP is an infinite-horizon policy gradient method [1] to compute the gradient of the *long-term average reward*

$$R(\theta) := \lim_{T \to \infty} \frac{1}{T} \mathbb{E}_\theta \left[\sum_{t=1}^{T} r(s_t) \right], \tag{9}$$

with respect the policy parameters θ. The expectation $\mathbb{E}_\theta$ is over the distribution of state trajectories $\{s_0, s_1, \dots\}$ induced by $P(\theta)$.

Theorem 1 (1) *Let I be the identity matrix, and u a column vector of ones. The gradient of the long-term average reward wrt. a policy parameter θ_i is*

$$\nabla_{\theta_i} R(\theta) = \pi(\theta)^\top \nabla_{\theta_i} P(\theta)[I - P(\theta) + u\pi(\theta)^\top]^{-1} r, \tag{10}$$

where $\pi(\theta)$ is the stationary distribution of states induced by θ.

---

[1]For uncountably infinite state spaces, the derivation becomes more complex without substantially altering the resulting algorithms.

Note that (10) requires knowledge of the underlying transition probabilities $P(\boldsymbol{\theta})$, and the inversion of a potentially large matrix. The GPOMDP algorithm instead computes a Monte-Carlo approximation of (10): the agent interacts with the environment, producing an observation, action, reward sequence $\{\boldsymbol{x}_1, a_1, r_1, \boldsymbol{x}_2, \ldots, \boldsymbol{x}_T, a_T, r_T\}$.[2] Under mild technical assumptions, including ergodicity and bounding all the terms involved, Baxter and Bartlett [1] obtain

$$\widehat{\nabla}_{\boldsymbol{\theta}} R = \frac{1}{T} \sum_{t=0}^{T-1} \nabla_{\boldsymbol{\theta}} \ln \mathbb{P}(a_t | \boldsymbol{\theta}, s_t) \sum_{\tau=t+1}^{T} \beta^{\tau-t-1} r(s_\tau) , \tag{11}$$

where a discount factor $\beta \in [0, 1)$ implicitly assumes that rewards are exponentially more likely to be due to recent actions. Without it, rewards would be assigned over a potentially infinite horizon, resulting in gradient estimates with infinite variance. As β decreases, so does the variance, but the bias of the gradient estimate increases [1]. In practice, (11) is implemented efficiently via the discounted *eligibility trace*

$$e_t = \beta e_{t-1} + \boldsymbol{\delta}_t , \quad \text{where} \quad \boldsymbol{\delta}_t := \nabla_{\boldsymbol{\theta}} \mathbb{P}(a_t | \boldsymbol{\theta}, s_t) / \mathbb{P}(a_t | \boldsymbol{\theta}, s_t) . \tag{12}$$

Now $g_t = r_t e_t$ is the gradient of $R(\boldsymbol{\theta})$ arising from assigning the instantaneous reward to all log action gradients, where β gives exponentially more credit to recent actions. Likewise, Baxter and Bartlett [1] give the Monte Carlo estimate of the Hessian as $\boldsymbol{H}_t = r_t(\boldsymbol{E}_t + e_t e_t^\top)$, using an eligibility trace *matrix*

$$\boldsymbol{E}_t = \beta \boldsymbol{E}_{t-1} + \boldsymbol{G}_t - \boldsymbol{\delta}_t \boldsymbol{\delta}_t^\top , \quad \text{where} \quad \boldsymbol{G}_t := \nabla_{\boldsymbol{\theta}}^2 \mathbb{P}(a_t | \boldsymbol{\theta}, s_t) / \mathbb{P}(a_t | \boldsymbol{\theta}, s_t) . \tag{13}$$

Maintaining $\boldsymbol{E}$ would be $O(n^2)$, thus computationally expensive for large policy parameter spaces. Noting that SMD only requires the product of $\boldsymbol{H}_t$ with a vector v, we instead use

$$\boldsymbol{H}_t v = r_t [d_t + e_t (e_t^\top v)] , \quad \text{where} \quad d_t = \beta d_{t-1} + \boldsymbol{G}_t v - \boldsymbol{\delta}_t (\boldsymbol{\delta}_t^\top v) \tag{14}$$

is an eligibility trace vector that can be maintained in $O(n)$. We describe the efficient computation of $\boldsymbol{G}_t v$ in (14) for a specific action selection method in Section 3.3 below.

3.2 GPOMDP-Based optimization algorithms

Baxter et al. [2] proposed two optimization algorithms using GPOMDP's policy gradient estimates g_t: OLPOMDP is a simple online stochastic gradient descent (2) with scalar gain γ_t. Alternatively, CONJPOMDP performs Polak-Ribière conjugation of search directions, using a noise-tolerant line search to find the approximately best scalar step size in a given search direction. Since conjugate gradient methods are very sensitive to noise [14], CONJPOMDP must average g_t over many steps to obtain a reliable gradient measurement; this makes the algorithm inherently inefficient (*cf.* Section 4).

OLPOMDP, on the other hand, is robust to noise but converges only very slowly. We can, however, employ SMD's gain vector adaptation to greatly accelerate it while retaining the benefits of high noise tolerance and online learning. Experiments (Section 4) show that the resulting SMDPOMDP algorithm can greatly outperform OLPOMDP and CONJPOMDP.

Kakade [15] has applied natural gradient [16] to GPOMDP, premultiplying the policy gradient by the inverse of the online estimate

$$\boldsymbol{F}_t = (1 - \tfrac{1}{t}) \boldsymbol{F}_{t-1} + \tfrac{1}{t} (\boldsymbol{\delta}_t \boldsymbol{\delta}_t^\top + \epsilon \boldsymbol{I}) \tag{15}$$

of the Fisher information matrix for the parameter update: $\boldsymbol{\theta}_{t+1} = \boldsymbol{\theta}_t + \gamma_0 \cdot r_t \boldsymbol{F}_t^{-1} e_t$. This approach can yield very fast convergence on small problems, but in our experience does not scale well at all to larger, more realistic tasks; see our experiments in Section 4.

---

[2] We use r_t as shorthand for $r(s_t)$, making it clear that only the reward value is known, not the underlying state s_t.

3.3 Softmax action selection

For discrete action spaces, a vector of action probabilities $z_t := \mathbb{P}(a_t|y_t)$ can be generated from the output $y_t := f(\theta_t, x_t)$ of a parameterised function $f : \mathbb{R}^n \times \mathcal{X} \to \mathbb{R}^{|\mathcal{A}|}$ (such as a neural network) via the *softmax* function:

$$z_t := \text{softmax}(y_t) = \frac{e^{y_t}}{\sum_{m=1}^{|\mathcal{A}|}[e^{y_t}]_m}. \tag{16}$$

Given action $a_t \sim z_t$, GPOMDP's instantaneous log-action gradient wrt. y is then

$$\tilde{g}_t := \nabla_y[z_t]_{a_t}/[z_t]_{a_t} = u_{a_t} - z_t, \tag{17}$$

where u_i is the unity vector in direction i. The action gradient wrt. θ is obtained by backpropagating $\tilde{g}_t$ through f's *adjoint* system [13], performing an efficient multiplication by the transposed Jacobian of f. The resulting gradient $\delta_t := J_f^\top \tilde{g}_t$ is then accumulated in the eligibility trace (12). GPOMDP's instantaneous Hessian for softmax action selection is

$$\tilde{H}_t := \nabla_y^2[z_t]_{a_t}/[z_t]_{a_t} = (u_{a_t} - z_t)(u_{a_t} - z_t)^\top + z_t z_t^\top - \text{diag}(z_t). \tag{18}$$

It is indefinite but reasonably well-behaved: the Gerschgorin circle theorem can be employed to show that its eigenvalues must all lie in the interval $[-\frac{1}{4}, 2]$. Furthermore, its expectation over possible actions is zero:

$$\mathbb{E}_{z_t}(\tilde{H}_t) = [\text{diag}(z_t) - 2z_t z_t^\top + z_t z_t^\top] + z_t z_t^\top - \text{diag}(z_t) = 0. \tag{19}$$

The extended Gauss-Newton matrix-vector product [4] employed by SMD is then given by

$$G_t v_t := J_f^\top \tilde{H}_t J_f v_t, \tag{20}$$

where the multiplication by the Jacobian of f (resp. its transpose) is implemented efficiently by propagating v_t through f's *tangent linear* (resp. adjoint) system [13].

Algorithm 1 SMDPOMDP with softmax action selection

---

1. Given (a) an ergodic POMDP with observations $x_t \in \mathcal{X}$, actions $a_t \in \mathcal{A}$, bounded rewards $r_t \in \mathbb{R}$, and softmax action selection

    (b) a differentiable parametric map $f : \mathbb{R}^n \times \mathcal{X} \to \mathbb{R}^{|\mathcal{A}|}$ (neural network)

    (c) f's adjoint ($u \to J_f^\top u$) and tangent linear ($v \to J_f v$) maps

    (d) free parameters: $\mu \in \mathbb{R}_+$; $\beta, \lambda \in [0,1]$; $\gamma_0 \in \mathbb{R}_+^n$; $\theta_1 \in \mathbb{R}^n$

2. Initialize in $\mathbb{R}^n$: $e_0 = d_0 = v_0 = 0$

3. For $t = 1$ to ∞: (a) interact with POMDP:

    i. observe feature vector x_t

    ii. compute $z_t := \text{softmax}(f(\theta_t, x_t))$

    iii. perform action $a_t \sim z_t$

    iv. observe reward r_t

    (b) maintain eligibility traces:

    i. $\delta_t := J_f^\top(u_{a_t} - z_t)$

    ii. $p_t := J_f v_t$

    iii. $q_t := (u_{a_t} - z_t)(\delta_t^\top v_t) + z_t(z_t^\top p_t) - z_t \cdot p_t$

    iv. $e_t = \beta e_{t-1} + \delta_t$

    v. $d_t = \beta d_{t-1} + J_f^\top q_t - \delta_t(\delta_t^\top v_t)$

    (c) update SMD parameters:

    i. $\gamma_t = \gamma_{t-1} \cdot \max(\frac{1}{2}, 1 + \mu\, r_t e_t \cdot v_t)$

    ii. $\theta_{t+1} = \theta_t + r_t \gamma_t \cdot e_t$

    iii. $v_{t+1} = \lambda v_t + r_t \gamma_t \cdot [(1 + \lambda e_t^\top v_t)e_t + \lambda d_t]$

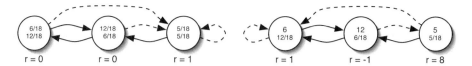

Fig. 1: Left: Baxter et al.'s simple 3-state POMDP. States are labelled with their observable features and instantaneous reward r; arrows indicate the 80% likely transition for the first (solid) *resp.* second (dashed) action. Right: our modified, more difficult 3-state POMDP.

4 Experiments

4.1 Simple Three-State POMDP

Fig. 1 (left) depicts the simple 3-state POMDP used by Baxter et al. [2, Tables 1&2]. Of the two possible transitions from each state, the preferred one occurs with 80% probability, the other with 20%. The preferred transition is determined by the action of a simple probabilistic adaptive controller that receives two state-dependent feature values as input, and is trained to maximize the expected average reward by policy gradient methods.

Using the original code of Baxter et al. [2], we replicated their experimental results for the OLPOMDP and CONJPOMDP algorithms on this simple POMDP. We can accurately reproduce all essential features of their graphed results on this problem [2, Figures 7&8]. We then implemented SMDPOMDP (Algorithm 1), and ran a comparison of algorithms, using the best free parameter settings found by Baxter et al. [2] (in particular: $\beta = 0, \gamma_0 = 1$), and $\mu = \lambda = 1$ for SMDPOMDP. We always match random seeds across algorithms.

Baxter et al. [2] collect and plot results for CONJPOMDP in terms of its T parameter, which specifies the number of Markov chain iterations *per gradient evaluation*. For a fair comparison of convergence speed we added code to record the *total* number of Markov chain iterations consumed by CONJPOMDP, and plot performance for all three algorithms in those terms, with error bars along both axes for CONJPOMDP.

The results are shown in Fig. 2 (left), averaged over 500 runs. While early on CONJPOMDP *on average* reaches a given level of performance about three times faster than OLPOMDP, it does so at the price of far higher variance. Moreover, CONJPOMDP is the only algorithm that fails to asymptotically approach optimal performance ($R = 0.8$; Fig. 2 left, inset). Once its step size adaptation gets going, SMDPOMDP converges asymptotically to the op-

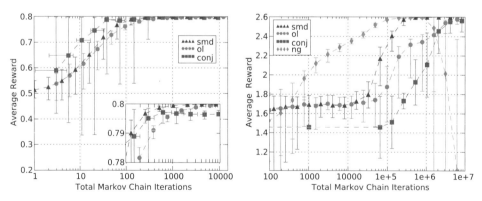

Fig. 2: Left: The POMDP of Fig. 1 (left) is easy to learn. CONJPOMDP converges faster but to asymptotically inferior solutions (see inset) than the two online algorithms. Right: SMDPOMDP outperforms OLPOMDP and CONJPOMDP on the difficult POMDP of Fig. 1 (right). Natural policy gradient has rapid early convergence but diverges asymptotically.

timal policy about three times faster than OLPOMDP in terms of Markov chain iterations, making the two algorithms roughly equal in terms of computational expense.

CONJPOMDP on average performs *less than two iterations* of conjugate gradient in each run. While this is perfectly understandable — the controller only has two trainable parameters — it bears keeping in mind that the performance of CONJPOMDP here is almost entirely governed by the line search rather than the conjugation of search directions.

4.2 Modified Three-State POMDP

The three-state POMDP employed by Baxter et al. [2] has the property that greedy maximization of instantaneous reward leads to the optimal policy. Non-trivial temporal credit assignment — the hallmark of reinforcement learning — is not needed. The best results are obtained with the eligibility trace turned off ($\beta = 0$). To create a more challenging problem, we rearranged the POMDP's state transitions and reward structure so that the instantaneous reward becomes deceptive (Fig. 1, right). We also multiplied one state feature by 18 to create an ill-conditioned input to the controller, while leaving the actions and relative transition probabilities (80% resp. 20%) unchanged. In our modified POMDP, the high-reward state can only be reached through an intermediate state with negative reward.

Fig. 2 (right) shows our experimental results for this harder POMDP, averaged over 100 runs. Free parameters were tuned to $\theta_1 \in [-0.1, 0.1]$, $\beta = 0.6$, $\gamma_0 = 0.001$; $T = 10^5$ for CONJPOMDP; $\mu = 0.002$, $\lambda = 1$ for SMDPOMDP. CONJPOMDP now performs the worst, which is expected because conjugation of directions is known to collapse in the presence of noise [14]. SMDPOMDP converges about 20 times faster than OLPOMDP because its adjustable gains compensate for the ill-conditioned input. Kakade's natural gradient (using $\epsilon = 0.01$) performs extremely well early on, taking 2–3 times fewer iterations than SMD-POMDP to reach optimal performance ($R = 2.6$). It does, however, diverge asymptotically.

4.3 Puck World

We also implemented the Puck World benchmark of Baxter et al. [2], with the free parameters settings $\theta_1 \in [-0.1, 0.1]$, $\beta = 0.95$ $\gamma_0 = 2 \cdot 10^{-6}$; $T = 10^6$ for CONJPOMDP; $\mu = 100$, $\lambda = 0.999$ for SMDPOMDP; $\epsilon = 0.01$ for natural policy gradient. To improve its stability, we modified SMD here to track instantaneous log-action gradients δ_t instead of noisy $r_t e_t$ estimates of $\nabla_\theta R$. CONJPOMDP used a quadratic weight penalty of initially 0.5, with the adaptive reduction schedule described by Baxter et al. [2, page 369]; the online algorithms did not require a weight penalty.

Fig. 3 shows our results averaged over 100 runs, except for natural policy gradient where only a single typical run is shown. This is because its $O(n^3)$ time complexity per iteration[3]

---

[3]The Sherman-Morrison formula cannot be used here because of the diagonal term in (15).

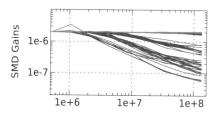

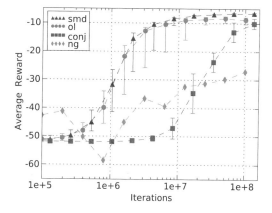

Fig. 3: The action-gradient version of SMDPOMDP yields better asymptotic results on PuckWorld than OL-POMDP; CONJPOMDP is inefficient; natural policy gradient even more so.

makes natural policy gradient intolerably slow for this task, where $n = 88$. Moreover, its convergence is quite poor here in terms of the number of iterations required as well.

CONJPOMDP is again inferior to the best online algorithms by over an order of magnitude. Early on, SMDPOMDP matches OLPOMDP, but then reaches superior solutions with small variance. SMDPOMDP-trained controllers achieve a long-term average reward of -6.5, significantly above the optimum of -8 hypothesized by Baxter et al. [2, page 369] based on their experiments with CONJPOMDP.

5 Conclusion

On several non-trivial RL problems we find that our SMDPOMDP consistently outperforms OLPOMDP, which in turn outperforms CONJPOMDP. Natural policy gradient can converge rapidly, but is too unstable and computationally expensive for all but very small controllers.

Acknowledgements

We are indebted to John Baxter for his code and helpful comments. National ICT Australia is funded by the Australian Government's Backing Australia's Ability initiative, in part through the Australian Research Council. This work is also supported by the IST Program of the European Community, under the Pascal Network of Excellence, IST-2002-506778.

References

[1] J. Baxter and P. L. Bartlett. Infinite-horizon policy-gradient estimation. *Journal of Artificial Intelligence Research*, 15:319–350, 2001.

[2] J. Baxter, P. L. Bartlett, and L. Weaver. Experiments with infinite-horizon, policy-gradient estimation. *Journal of Artificial Intelligence Research*, 15:351–381, 2001.

[3] N. N. Schraudolph. Local gain adaptation in stochastic gradient descent. In *Proc. Intl. Conf. Artificial Neural Networks*, pages 569–574, Edinburgh, Scotland, 1999. IEE, London.

[4] N. N. Schraudolph. Fast curvature matrix-vector products for second-order gradient descent. *Neural Computation*, 14(7):1723–1738, 2002.

[5] R. Jacobs. Increased rates of convergence through learning rate adaptation. *Neural Networks*, 1:295–307, 1988.

[6] J. Kivinen and M. K. Warmuth. Additive versus exponentiated gradient updates for linear prediction. In *Proc. 27th Annual ACM Symposium on Theory of Computing*, pages 209–218. ACM Press, New York, NY, 1995.

[7] T. Tollenaere. SuperSAB: Fast adaptive back propagation with good scaling properties. *Neural Networks*, 3:561–573, 1990.

[8] F. M. Silva and L. B. Almeida. Acceleration techniques for the backpropagation algorithm. In L. B. Almeida and C. J. Wellekens, editors, *Neural Networks: Proc. EURASIP Workshop*, volume 412 of *Lecture Notes in Computer Science*, pages 110–119. Springer Verlag, 1990.

[9] M. Riedmiller and H. Braun. A direct adaptive method for faster backpropagation learning: The RPROP algorithm. In *Proc. Intl. Conf. Neural Networks*, pages 586–591. IEEE, 1993.

[10] L. B. Almeida, T. Langlois, J. D. Amaral, and A. Plakhov. Parameter adaptation in stochastic optimization. In D. Saad, editor, *On-Line Learning in Neural Networks*, Publications of the Newton Institute, chapter 6, pages 111–134. Cambridge University Press, 1999.

[11] R. S. Sutton. Gain adaptation beats least squares? In *Proceedings of the 7th Yale Workshop on Adaptive and Learning Systems*, pages 161–166, 1992.

[12] B. A. Pearlmutter. Fast exact multiplication by the Hessian. *Neural Comput.*, 6(1):147–60, 1994.

[13] A. Griewank. *Evaluating Derivatives: Principles and Techniques of Algorithmic Differentiation*. Frontiers in Applied Mathematics. SIAM, Philadelphia, 2000.

[14] N. N. Schraudolph and T. Graepel. Combining conjugate direction methods with stochastic approximation of gradients. In C. M. Bishop and B. J. Frey, editors, *Proc. 9th Intl. Workshop Artificial Intelligence and Statistics*, pages 7–13, Key West, Florida, 2003.

[15] S. Kakade. A natural policy gradient. In T. G. Dietterich, S. Becker, and Z. Ghahramani, editors, *Advances in Neural Information Processing Systems 14*, pages 1531–1538. MIT Press, 2002.

[16] S. Amari. Natural gradient works efficiently in learning. *Neural Comput.*, 10(2):251–276, 1998.

The Information-Form Data Association Filter

Brad Schumitsch, Sebastian Thrun, Gary Bradski, and Kunle Olukotun

Stanford AI Lab
Stanford University, Stanford, CA 94305

Abstract

This paper presents a new filter for online data association problems in high-dimensional spaces. The key innovation is a representation of the data association posterior in information form, in which the "proximity" of objects and tracks are expressed by numerical links. Updating these links requires linear time, compared to exponential time required for computing the exact posterior probabilities. The paper derives the algorithm formally and provides comparative results using data obtained by a real-world camera array and by a large-scale sensor network simulation.

1 Introduction

This paper addresses the problem of data association in online object tracking [6]. The data association problem arises in a large number of application domains, including computer vision, robotics, and sensor networks.

Our setup assumes an online tracking system that receives two types of data: *sensor data*, conveying information about the identity or type of objects that are being tracked; and *transition data*, characterizing the uncertainty introduced through the tracker's inability to reliably track individual objects over time. The setup is motivated by a camera network which we recently deployed in our lab. Here sensor data relates to the color of clothing of individual people, which enables us to identify them. Tracks are lost when people walk too closely together, or when they occlude each other.

We show that the standard probabilistic solution to the discrete data association problem requires exponential update time and exponential memory. This is because each data association hypothesis is expressed by a permutation matrix that assigns computer-internal tracks to objects in the physical world. An optimal filter would therefore need to maintain a probability distribution over the space of all permutation matrices, which grows exponentially with N, the number of objects in the world. The common remedy involves the selection of a small number K of likely hypotheses. This is the core of numerous widely-used multi-hypothesis tracking algorithms [9, 1]. More recent solutions involve particle filters [3], which maintain stochastic samples of hypotheses. Both of these techniques are very effective for small N, but the number of hypothesis they require grows exponentially with N.

This paper provides a filter algorithm that scales to much larger problems. This filter maintains an information matrix Ω of size $N \times N$, which relates tracks to physical objects in the world. The rows of Ω correspond to object identities, the columns to the tracks of the tracker. Ω is a matrix in *information form*, that is, it can be thought of as a non-normalized log-probability.

Fig. 1a shows an example. The highlighted first column corresponds to track 1 in the tracker. The numerical values in this column suggest that this track is most strongly

(a) Example: Information matrix

$$\Omega = \begin{pmatrix} \mathbf{2} & 12 & 4 & 4 \\ 1 & 2 & 11 & 0 \\ \mathbf{10} & 4 & 4 & 15 \\ 5 & 2 & 1 & 2 \end{pmatrix}$$

(b) Most likely data association

$$\hat{A} = \underset{A}{\operatorname{argmax}} \operatorname{tr} A^T \Omega = \begin{pmatrix} 0 & 1 & 0 & 0 \\ 0 & 0 & 1 & 0 \\ 0 & 0 & 0 & 1 \\ 1 & 0 & 0 & 0 \end{pmatrix}$$

(c) Update: Associating track 2 with object 4

$$\begin{pmatrix} 2 & 12 & 4 & 4 \\ 1 & 2 & 11 & 0 \\ 10 & 4 & 4 & 15 \\ 5 & \boxed{2} & 1 & 2 \end{pmatrix} \longrightarrow \begin{pmatrix} 2 & 12 & 4 & 4 \\ 1 & 2 & 11 & 0 \\ 10 & 4 & 4 & 15 \\ 5 & \boxed{3} & 1 & 2 \end{pmatrix}$$

(d) Update: Tracks 2 and 3 merge

$$\begin{pmatrix} 2 & \boxed{12} & \boxed{4} & 4 \\ 1 & \boxed{2} & \boxed{11} & 0 \\ 10 & \boxed{4} & \boxed{4} & 15 \\ 5 & \boxed{3} & \boxed{1} & 2 \end{pmatrix} \longrightarrow \begin{pmatrix} 2 & \boxed{11.31} & \boxed{11.31} & 4 \\ 1 & \boxed{10.31} & \boxed{10.31} & 0 \\ 10 & \boxed{4} & \boxed{4} & 15 \\ 5 & \boxed{2.43} & \boxed{2.43} & 2 \end{pmatrix}$$

(e) Graphical network interpretation of the information form

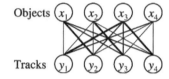

Objects x_1 x_2 x_3 x_4

Tracks y_1 y_2 y_3 y_4

Figure 1: Illustration of the information form filter for data association in object tracking

associated with object 3, since the value 10 dominates all other values in this column. Thus, looking at column 1 of Ω in isolation would have us conclude that the most likely association of track 1 is object 3. However, the most likely permutation matrix is shown in Fig. 1b; from all possible data association assignments, this matrix receives the highest score. Its score is $\operatorname{tr} \hat{A}^T \Omega = 5 + 12 + 11 + 15 = 43$ (here "tr" denotes the trace of a matrix). This permutation matrix associates object 3 with track 4, while associating track 1 with object 4.

The key question now pertains to the construction of Ω. As we shall see, the update operations for Ω are simple and parallelizable. Suppose we receive a measurement that associates track 2 with object 4 (e.g., track 2's hair color appears to be the same as person 4's hair color in our camera array). As a result, our approach adds a value to the element in Ω that links object 4 and track 2, as illustrated in Fig. 1c (the exact magnitude of this value will be discussed below). Similarly, suppose our tracker is unable to distinguish between objects 2 and 3, perhaps because these objects are so close together in a camera image that they cannot be tracked individually. Such a situation leads to a new information matrix, in which both columns assume the same values, as illustrated in Fig. 1d. The exact values in this new information matrix are the result of an exponentiated averaging explained below. All of these updates are easily parallelized, and hence are applicable to a decentralized network of cameras. The exact update and inference rules are based on a probabilistic model that is also discussed below.

Given the importance of data association, it comes as no surprise that our algorithm is related to a rich body of prior work. The data association problem has been studied as an *offline* problem, in which all data is memorized and inference takes place after data collection. There exists a wealth of powerful methods, such as RANSAC [4] and MCMC [6, 2], but those are inherently offline and their memory requirements increase over time. The dominant online, or filter, paradigm involves the selection of K representative samples of the data association matrix, but such algorithms tend to work only for small N [11]. Relatively little work has focused on the development of compact sufficient statistics for data association. One alternative $O(N^2)$ technique to the one proposed here was explored in [8]. This technique uses doubly stochastic matrices, which are computationally hard to maintain. The first mention of information filters is in [8], but the update rules there were computationally less efficient (in $O(N^4)$) and required central optimization.

The work in this paper does not address the continuous-valued aspects of object tracking. Those are very well understood, and information representations have been successfully applied [5, 10].

Information representations are popular in the field of graphical networks. Our approach can be viewed as a learning algorithm for a Markov network [7] of a special topology, where any track and any object are connected by an edge. Such a network is shown in Fig. 1e. The filter update equations manipulate the strength of the edges based on data.

2   Problem Setup and Bayes Filter Solution

We begin with a formal definition of the data association problem and derive the obvious but inefficient Bayes filter solution. Throughout this paper, we make the closed world assumption, that is, there are always the same N known objects in the world.

2.1   Data Association

We assume that we are given a tracking algorithm that maintains N internal tracks of the moving objects. Due to insufficient information, this assumed tracking algorithm does not always know the exact mapping of identities to internal tracks. Hence, the same internal track may correspond to different identities at different times.

The data association problem is the problem of assigning these N tracks to N objects. Each data association hypothesis is characterized by a permutation matrix of the type shown in Fig. 1b. The columns of this matrix correspond to the internal tracks, and the rows to the objects. We will denote the data association matrix by A (not to be confused with the information matrix Ω). In our closed world, A is always a permutation matrix; hence all elements are 0 or 1. There are exponentially many permutation matrices, which is a reason why data association is considered a hard problem.

2.2   Identity Measurement

The correct data association matrix A is unobservable. Instead, the sensors produce local information about the relation of individual tracks to individual objects. We will denote sensor measurements by z_j, where j is the index of the corresponding track. Each $z_j = \{z_{ij}\}$ specifies a local probability distribution in the corresponding object space:

$$p(x_i = y_j \mid z_j) \quad = \quad z_{ij} \quad \text{with} \quad \sum_i z_{ij} = 1 \tag{1}$$

Here x_i is the i-th object in the world, and y_j is the j-th track.

The measurement in our introductory example (see Fig. 1c) was of a special form, in that it elevated one specific correspondence over the others. This occurs when $z_{ij} = \alpha$ for some $\alpha \approx 1$, and $z_{kj} = \frac{1-\alpha}{N-1}$ for all $k \neq i$. Such a measurement arises when the tracker receives evidence that a specific track y_j corresponds with high likelihood to a specific object x_i. Specifically, the measurement likelihood of this correspondence is α, and the error probability is $1 - \alpha$.

2.3   State Transitions

As time passes by, our tracker may confuse tracks, which is a loss of information with respect to the data association. The tracker confusing two objects amounts to a random flip of two columns in the data association matrix A.

The model adopted in this paper generalizes this example to arbitrary distributions over permutations of the columns in A. Let $\{B_1, \ldots, B_M\}$ be a set of permutation matrices, and $\{\beta_1, \ldots, \beta_M\}$ with $\sum_m \beta_m = 1$ be a set of associated probabilities. The "true" permutation matrix undergoes a random transition from A to $A\,B_m$ with probability β_m:

$$A \quad \overset{\text{prob}=\beta_m}{\longrightarrow} \quad A\,B_m \tag{2}$$

The sets $\{B_1, \ldots, B_M\}$ and $\{\beta_1, \ldots, \beta_M\}$ are given to us by the tracker. For the example in Fig. 1d, in which tracks 2 and 3 merge, the following two permutation matrices will implement such a merge:

$$B_1 = \begin{pmatrix} 1 & 0 & 0 & 0 \\ 0 & 1 & 0 & 0 \\ 0 & 0 & 1 & 0 \\ 0 & 0 & 0 & 1 \end{pmatrix} ; \beta_1 = 0.5 \quad B_2 = \begin{pmatrix} 1 & 0 & 0 & 0 \\ 0 & 0 & 1 & 0 \\ 0 & 1 & 0 & 0 \\ 0 & 0 & 0 & 1 \end{pmatrix} ; \beta_2 = 0.5 \quad (3)$$

The first such matrix leaves the association unchanged, whereas the second swaps columns 2 and 3. Since $\beta_1 = \beta_2 = 0.5$, such a swap happens exactly with probability 0.5.

2.4 Inefficient Bayesian Solution

For small N, the data association problem now has an obvious Bayes filter solution. Specifically, let $\mathcal{A}$ be the space of all permutation matrices. The Bayesian filter solves the identity tracking problem by maintaining a probabilistic belief over the space of all permutation matrices $A \in \mathcal{A}$. For each A, it maintains a posterior probability denoted $p(A)$. This probability is updated in two different ways, reminiscent of the measurement and state transition updates in DBNs and EKFs.

The measurement step updates the belief in response to a measurement z_j. This update is an application of Bayes rule:

$$p(A) \longleftarrow \frac{1}{L} p(A) \sum_i a_{ij} z_{ij} \quad (4)$$

$$\text{with } L = \sum_{\bar{A}} p(\bar{A}) \sum_i \bar{a}_{ij} z_{ij} \quad (5)$$

Here a_{ij} denotes the ij-th element of the matrix A. Because A is a permutation matrix, only one element in the sum over i is non-zero (hence there is not really a summation here).

The state transition updates the belief in accordance with the permutation matrices B_m and associated probabilities β_m (see Eq. 2):

$$p(A) \longleftarrow \sum_m \beta_m \, p(A \, B_m^T) \quad (6)$$

We use here that the inverse of a permutation matrix is its transpose.

This Bayesian filter is an exact solution to our identity tracking problem. Its problem is complexity: there are $N!$ permutation matrices A, and we have to compute probabilities for all of them. Thus, the exact filter is only applicable to problems with small N. Even if we want to keep track of $K \ll N$ *likely* permutations—as attempted by filters like the multi-hypothesis EKF or the particle filter—the required number of tracks K will generally have to scale exponentially with N (albeit at a slower rate). This exponential scaling renders the Bayesian filter ultimately inapplicable to the identity tracking problem with large N.

3 The Information-Form Solution

Our data association filter represents the posterior in condensed form, using an $N \times N$ information matrix. As a result, it requires linear update time and quadratic memory, instead of the exponential time and memory requirements of the Bayes filter.

However, we give two caveats regarding our method: it is approximate, and it does not maintain probabilities. The approximation is the result of a Jensen approximation, which we will show is empirically accurate. The calculation of probabilities from an information matrix requires inference, and we will provide several options for performing this inference.

3.1 The Information Matrix

The information matrix, denoted Ω, is a matrix of size $N \times N$ whose elements are non-negative. Ω induces a probability distribution over the space of all data association matrices

$\mathcal{A}$, through the following definition:

$$p(A) = \frac{1}{Z} \exp \operatorname{tr} A \,\Omega \quad \text{with} \quad Z = \sum_A \exp \operatorname{tr} A \,\Omega \tag{7}$$

Here tr is the trace of a matrix, and Z is the partition function.

Computing the posterior probability $p(A)$ from Ω is hard, due to the difficulty of computing the partition function Z. However, as we shall see, maintaining Ω is surprisingly easy, and it is also computationally efficient.

3.2 Measurement Update in Information Form

In information form, the measurement update is a local addition of the form:

$$\Omega \;\longleftarrow\; \Omega + \begin{pmatrix} 0\cdots0 & \log z_{1j} & 0\cdots0 \\ \vdots\ddots\vdots & \vdots & \vdots\ddots\vdots \\ 0\cdots0 & \log z_{1N} & 0\cdots0 \end{pmatrix} \tag{8}$$

This follows directly from Eq. 4. The complexity of this update is $O(N)$.

Of particular interest is the case where one specific association was affirmed with probability $z_{ij} = \alpha$, while all others were true with the error probability $z_{kj} = \frac{1-\alpha}{N-1}$. Then the update is of the form

$$\Omega \;\longleftarrow\; \Omega + \begin{pmatrix} 0\cdots0 & c & 0\cdots0 \\ \vdots\ddots\vdots & \vdots & \vdots\ddots\vdots \\ 0\cdots0 & c & 0\cdots0 \\ \vdots\ddots\vdots & \log\alpha & \vdots\ddots\vdots \\ 0\cdots0 & c & 0\cdots0 \\ \vdots\ddots\vdots & \vdots & \vdots\ddots\vdots \\ 0\cdots0 & c & 0\cdots0 \end{pmatrix} \quad \text{with} \quad c = \log \frac{1-\alpha}{N-1} \tag{9}$$

However, since Ω is a non-normalized matrix (it is normalized via the partition function Z in Eq. 7), we can modify Ω as long as $\exp \operatorname{tr} A\,\Omega$ is changed by the same factor for any A. In particular, we can subtract c from an entire column in Ω; this will affect the result of $\exp \operatorname{tr} A\,\Omega$ by a factor of $\exp c$, which is independent of A and hence will be subsumed by the normalizer Z. This allows us to perform a more efficient update

$$\omega_{ij} \;\longleftarrow\; \omega_{ij} + \log\alpha - \log\frac{1-\alpha}{N-1} \tag{10}$$

where ω_{ij} is the ij-th element of Ω. This update is indeed of the form shown in Fig. 1c. It requires $O(1)$ time, is entirely local, and is an exact realization of Bayes rule in information form.

3.3 State Transition Update in Information Form

The state transition update is also simple, but it is approximate. We show that using a Jensen bound, we obtain the following update for the information matrix:

$$\Omega \;\longleftarrow\; \log \sum_m \beta_m B_m^T \exp\Omega \tag{11}$$

Here the expression "$\exp\Omega$" denotes a component-wise exponentiation of the matrix Ω; the result is also a matrix. This update implements a "dual" of a geometric mean; here the exponentiation is applied to the individual elements of this mean, and the logarithm is applied to the result. It is important to notice that this update only affects elements in Ω that might be affected by a permutation B_m; all others remain the same.

A numerical example of this update was given in Fig. 1d, assuming the permutation matrices in Eq. 3. The values there are the result of applying this update formula. For example, for the first row we get $\log\frac{1}{2}(\exp 12 + \exp 4) = 11.3072$.

1197

The derivation of this update formula is straightforward. We begin with Eq. 6, written in logarithmic form. The transformations rely heavily on the fact that A and B_m are permutation matrices. We use the symbol "tr*" for a multiplicative version of the matrix trace, in which all elements on the diagonal are multiplied.

$$
\begin{aligned}
\log p(A) \quad \longleftarrow \quad & \log \sum_m \beta_m \, p(A \, B_m^T) \\
= \quad & \text{const.} + \log \sum_m \beta_m \, \exp \text{tr} \, A \, B_m^T \, \Omega \\
= \quad & \text{const.} + \log \sum_m \beta_m \, \text{tr}^* \exp A \, B_m^T \, \Omega \\
= \quad & \text{const.} + \log \sum_m \beta_m \, \text{tr}^* \, A \, B_m^T \, \exp \Omega \\
\leq \quad & \text{const.} + \log \text{tr}^* \, A \, \sum_m \beta_m \, B_m^T \, \exp \Omega \\
= \quad & \text{const.} + \text{tr} \, A \left[\log \sum_m \beta_m \, B_m^T \, \exp \Omega \right]
\end{aligned}
\tag{12}
$$

The result is of the form of (the logarithm of) Eq. 7. The expression in brackets is equivalent to the right-hand side of the update Eq. 11. A benefit of this update rule is that it only affects columns in Ω that are affected by a permutation B_m; all other columns are unchanged.

We note that the approximation in this derivation is the result of applying a Jensen bound. As a result, we gain a compact closed-form solution to the update problem, but the state transition step may sacrifice information in doing so (as indicated by the "$\leq$" sign). In our experimental results section, however, we find that this approximation is extremely accurate in practice.

4   Computing the Data Association

The previous section formally derived our update rules, which are simple and local. We now address the problem of recovering actual data association hypotheses from the information matrix, along with the associated probabilities.

We consider three cases: the computation of the most likely data association matrix as illustrated in Fig. 1b; the computation of a relative probability of the form $p(A)/p(A')$; and the computation of an absolute probability or expectation.

To recover $\text{argmax}_A \, p(A)$, we need only solve a linear program.

Relative probabilities are also easy to recover. Consider, for example, the quotient of the probability $p(A)/p(A')$ for two identity matrices A and A'. When calculating this quotient from Eq. 7, the normalizer Z cancels out:

$$
\frac{p(A)}{p(A')} \quad = \quad \exp \text{tr}(A - A') \, \Omega
\tag{13}
$$

Absolute probabilities and expectations are generally the most difficult to compute. This is because of the partition function Z in Eq. 7, whose exact calculation requires considering $N!$ permutation matrices.

Our approximate method for recovering probabilities/expectations is based on the Metropolis algorithm. Specifically, consider the expectation of a function f:

$$
E[f(A)] \quad = \quad \sum_A f(A) \, p(A)
\tag{14}
$$

Our method approximates this expression through a finite sample of matrices $A^{[1]}, A^{[2]}, \ldots,$ using Metropolis and the proposal distribution defined in Eq. 13. This proposal generates excellent results for simple functions f (e.g., the marginal of a single identity). For more

(a) camera   **(b)** array of 16 ceiling-mounted cameras   **(c)** camera images   **(d)** 2 of the tracks

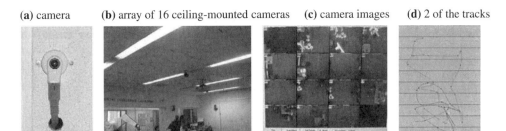

Figure 2: The camera array, part of the common area in the Stanford AI Lab. Panel (d) compares our esitmate with ground truth for two of the tracks. The data association is essentially correct at all times.

(a) Comparison K-hypothesis vs. information-theoretic tracker   **(b)** Comparison using a DARPA challenge data set produced by Northrop Grumman

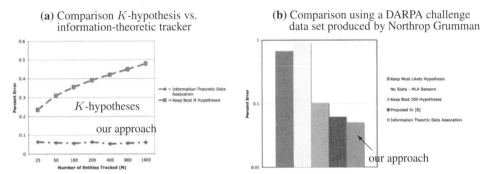

Figure 3: Results for our approach information-form filter the common multi-hypothesis approach for (a) synthetic data and (b) a DARPA challenge data set. The comparison (b) involves additional algorithms, including one published in [8].

complex functions f, we refer the reader to improved proposal distributions that have been found to be highly efficient in related problems [6, 2].

5   Experimental Results

To evaluate this algorithm, we deployed a network of ceiling-mounted cameras in our lab, shown in Fig. 2. We used 16 cameras to track individuals walking through the lab. The tracker uses background subtraction to find blobs and uses a color histogram to classify these blobs. Only when two or more people come very close to each other might the tracker lose track of individual people. We find that for $N = 5$ our method tracks people nearly perfectly, but so does the full-blown Bayesian solution, as well as the K-best multi-hypothesis method that is popular in the tracking literature.

To investigate scaling to larger N, we compared our approach on two data sets: a synthetic one with up to $N = 1,600$ objects, and a dataset using an sensor network simulation provided to us by Northrop Grumman through an ongoing DARPA program. The latter set is thought to be realistic. It was chosen because it involves a large number ($N = 200$) of moving objects, whose motion patterns come from a behavioral model. In all cases, we measured the number of objects mislabeled in the maximum likelihood hypothesis (as found by solving the LP). All results are averaged over 50 runs.

The comparison in Fig. 3a shows that our approach outperforms the traditional K-best hypothesis approach (with $K = N$) by a large margin. Furthermore, our approach seems to be unaffected by N, the number of entities in the environment, whereas the traditional approach deteriorates. This comes as no surprise, since the traditional approach requires increasing numbers of samples to cover the space of all data associations. The results in Fig. 3b compare (from left to right), the most likely hypothesis, the most recent sensor measurement, the K-best approach with $K = 200$, an approach proposed in [8], and our approach. Notice that this plot is in log-form.

No comparisons were attempted with offline techniques, such as the ones in [4, 6], because the data sets used here are quite large and our interest is online filtering.

6 Conclusion

We have provided an information form algorithm for the data association problem in object tracking. The key idea of this approach is to maintain a cumulative matrix of information associating computer-internal tracks with physical objects. Updating this matrix is easy; furthermore, efficient methods were proposed for extracting concrete data association hypotheses from this representation. Empirical work using physical networks of camera arrays illustrated that our approach outperforms alternative paradigms that are commonly used throughout all of science.

Despite these advances, the work possesses a number of limitations. Specifically, our closed world assumption is problematic, although we believe the extension to open worlds is relatively straightforward. Also missing is a tight integration of our discrete formulation into continuous-valued traditional tracking algorithms such as EKFs. Such extensions warrant further research.

We believe the key innovation here is best understood from a graphical model perspective. Sampling K good data associations *cannot* exploit conditional independence in the data association posterior, hence will always require that K is an exponential function of N. The information form and the equivalent graphical network in Fig. 1e exploits conditional independences. This subtle difference makes it possible to get away with $O(N^2)$ memory and $O(N)$ computation without a loss of accuracy when N increases, as shown in Fig. 3a. The information form discussed here—and the associated graphical networks— promise to overcome a key brittleness associated with the current state-of-the-art in online data association.

Acknowledgements

We gratefully thank Jaewon Shin and Leo Guibas for helpful discussions.

This research was sponsored by the Defense Advanced Research Projects Agency (DARPA) under the ACIP program and grant number NBCH104009.

References

[1] Y. Bar-Shalom and X.-R. Li. *Estimation and Tracking: Principles, Techniques, and Software.* YBS, Danvers, MA, 1998.

[2] F. Dellaert, S.M. Seitz, C. Thorpe, and S. Thrun. EM, MCMC, and chain flipping for structure from motion with unknown correspondence. *Machine Learning*, 50(1-2):45–71, 2003.

[3] A. Doucet, J.F.G. de Freitas, and N.J. Gordon, editors. *Sequential Monte Carlo Methods in Practice.* Springer, 2001.

[4] M. A. Fischler and R. C. Bolles. Random sample consensus: A paradigm for model fitting with applications to image analysis and automated cartography. *Communications of the ACM*, 24:381–395, 1981.

[5] P. Maybeck. *Stochastic Models, Estimation, and Control, Volume 1.* Academic Press, 1979.

[6] H. Pasula, S. Russell, M. Ostland, and Y. Ritov. Tracking many objects with many sensors. IJCAI-99.

[7] J. Pearl. *Probabilistic reasoning in intelligent systems: networks of plausible inference.* Morgan Kaufmann, 1988.

[8] J. Shin, N. Lee, S. Thrun, and L. Guibas. Lazy inference on object identities in wireless sensor networks. IPSN-05.

[9] D.B. Reid. An algorithm for tracking multiple targets. *IEEE Transactions on Aerospace and Electronic Systems*, AC-24:843–854, 1979.

[10] S. Thrun, Y. Liu, D. Koller, A.Y. Ng, Z. Ghahramani, and H. Durrant-Whyte. Simultaneous localization and mapping with sparse extended information filters. IJRR, 23(7/8), 2004.

[11] D. Fox, J. Hightower, L. Lioa, D. Schulz, and G. Borriello. Bayesian Filtering for Location Estimation. IEEE Pervasive Computing, 2003.

A Bayesian Framework for
Tilt Perception and Confidence

Odelia Schwartz
HHMI and Salk Institute
La Jolla, CA 92014
odelia@salk.edu

Terrence J. Sejnowski
HHMI and Salk Institute
La Jolla, CA 92014
terry@salk.edu

Peter Dayan
Gatsby, UCL
17 Queen Square, London
dayan@gatsby.ucl.ac.uk

Abstract

The misjudgement of tilt in images lies at the heart of entertaining visual illusions and rigorous perceptual psychophysics. A wealth of findings has attracted many mechanistic models, but few clear computational principles. We adopt a Bayesian approach to perceptual tilt estimation, showing how a smoothness prior offers a powerful way of addressing much confusing data. In particular, we faithfully model recent results showing that *confidence* in estimation can be systematically affected by the same aspects of images that affect bias. Confidence is central to Bayesian modeling approaches, and is applicable in many other perceptual domains.

Perceptual anomalies and illusions, such as the misjudgements of motion and tilt evident in so many psychophysical experiments, have intrigued researchers for decades.[1–3] A Bayesian view[4–8] has been particularly influential in models of motion processing, treating such anomalies as the normative product of prior information (often statistically codifying Gestalt laws) with likelihood information from the actual scenes presented. Here, we expand the range of statistically normative accounts to tilt estimation, for which there are classes of results (on estimation confidence) that are so far not available for motion.

The tilt illusion arises when the perceived tilt of a center target is misjudged (*ie bias*) in the presence of flankers. Another phenomenon, called Crowding, refers to a loss in the confidence (*ie sensitivity*) of perceived target tilt in the presence of flankers. Attempts have been made to formalize these phenomena quantitatively. Crowding has been modeled as compulsory feature pooling (*ie* averaging of orientations), ignoring spatial positions.[9, 10] The tilt illusion has been explained by lateral interactions[11, 12] in populations of orientation-tuned units; and by *calibration*.[13]

However, most models of this form cannot explain a number of crucial aspects of the data. First, the *geometry* of the positional arrangement of the stimuli affects attraction versus repulsion in bias, as emphasized by Kapadia *et al*[14] (figure 1A), and others.[15, 16] Second, Solomon et al. recently measured bias *and* sensitivity simultaneously.[11] The rich and surprising range of sensitivities, far from flat as a function of flanker angles (figure 1B), are outside the reach of standard models. Moreover, current explanations do not offer a computational account of tilt perception as the outcome of a normative inference process.

Here, we demonstrate that a Bayesian framework for orientation estimation, with a prior favoring smoothness, can naturally explain a range of seemingly puzzling tilt data. We explicitly consider both the geometry of the stimuli, and the issue of confidence in the esti-

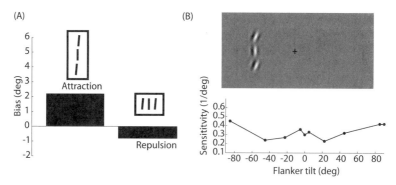

Figure 1: Tilt biases and sensitivities in visual perception. **(A)** Kapadia *et al* demonstrated the importance of geometry on tilt bias, with bar stimuli in the fovea (and similar results in the periphery). When 5 degrees clockwise flankers are arranged colinearly, the center target appears attracted in the direction of the flankers; when flankers are lateral, the target appears repulsed. Data are an average of 5 subjects.[14] **(B)** Solomon *et al* measured both biases and sensitivities for gratings in the visual periphery.[11] On the top are example stimuli, with flankers tilted 22.5 degrees clockwise. This constitutes the classic tilt illusion, with a repulsive bias percept. In addition, sensitivities vary as a function of flanker angles, in a systematic way (even in cases when there are no biases at all). Sensitivities are given in units of the inverse of standard deviation of the tilt estimate. More detailed data for both experiments are shown in the results section.

mation. Bayesian analyses have most frequently been applied to bias. Much less attention has been paid to the equally important phenomenon of sensitivity. This aspect of our model should be applicable to other perceptual domains.

In section 1 we formulate the Bayesian model. The prior is determined by the principle of creating a smooth contour between the target and flankers. We describe how to extract the bias and sensitivity. In section 2 we show experimental data of Kapadia *et al* and Solomon *et al*, alongside the model simulations, and demonstrate that the model can account for both geometry, and bias and sensitivity measurements in the data. Our results suggest a more unified, rational, approach to understanding tilt perception.

1   Bayesian model

Under our Bayesian model, inference is controlled by the posterior distribution over the tilt of the target element. This comes from the combination of a prior favoring smooth configurations of the flankers and target, and the likelihood associated with the actual scene. A complete distribution would consider all possible angles and relative spatial positions of the bars, and marginalize the posterior over all but the tilt of the central element. For simplicity, we make two benign approximations: conditionalizing over (*ie* clamping) the *angles* of the flankers, and exploring only a small neighborhood of their positions. We now describe the steps of inference.

Smoothness prior: Under these approximations, we consider a given *actual* configuration (see fig 2A) of flankers $f_1 = (\phi_1, x_1)$, $f_2 = (\phi_2, x_2)$ and center target $c = (\phi_c, x_c)$, arranged from top to bottom. We have to generate a prior over ϕ_c and $\delta_1 = x_1 - x_c$ and $\delta_2 = x_2 - x_c$ based on the principle of smoothness. As a less benign approximation, we do this in two stages: articulating a principle that determines a single optimal configuration; and generating a prior as a mixture of a Gaussian about this optimum and a uniform distribution, with the mixing proportion of the latter being determined by the smoothness of the optimum.

Smoothness has been extensively studied in the computer vision literature.[17–20] One widely

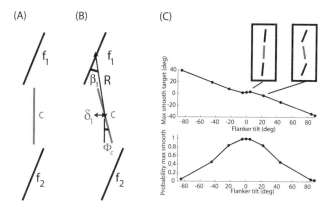

Figure 2: Geometry and smoothness for flankers, f_1 and f_2, and center target, c. **(A)** Example *actual* configuration of flankers and target, aligned along the y axis from top to bottom. **(B)** The elastica procedure can rotate the target angle (to Φ_c) and shift the relative flanker and target positions on the x axis (to δ_1 and δ_2) in its search for the maximally smooth solution. Small spatial shifts (up to $1/15$ the size of R) of positions are allowed, but positional shift is over-emphasized in the figure for visibility. **(C)** Top: center tilt that results in maximal smoothness, as a function of flanker tilt. Boxed cartoons show examples for given flanker tilts, of the optimally smooth configuration. Note attraction of target towards flankers for small flanker angles; here flankers and target are positioned in a nearly colinear arrangement. Note also repulsion of target away from flankers for intermediate flanker angles. Bottom: $P[c, f_1, f_2]$ for center tilt that yields maximal smoothness. The y axis is normalized between 0 and 1.

used principle, *elastica*, known even to Euler, has been applied to contour completion[21] and other computer vision applications.[17] The basic idea is to find the curve with minimum energy (*ie*, square of curvature). Sharon *et al*[19] showed that the elastica function can be well approximated by a number of simpler forms. We adopt a version that Leung and Malik[18] adopted from Sharon *et al*.[19] We assume that the probability for completing a smooth curve, can be factorized into two terms:

$$P[c, f_1, f_2] = G(c, f_1)G(c, f_2) \qquad (1)$$

with the term $G(c, f_1)$ (and similarly, $G(c, f_2)$) written as:

$$G(c, f_1) = \exp(-\frac{R}{\sigma_R} - \frac{D_\beta}{\sigma_\beta}) \qquad \text{where} \qquad D_\beta = \beta_1^2 + \beta_c^2 - \beta_1\beta_c \qquad (2)$$

and β_1 (and similarly, β_c) is the angle between the orientation at f_1, and the line joining f_1 and c. The distance between the centers of f_1 and c is given by R. The two constants, σ_β and σ_R, control the relative contribution to smoothness of the angle versus the spatial distance. Here, we set $\sigma_\beta = 1$, and $\sigma_R = 1.5$. Figure 2B illustrates an example geometry, in which ϕ_c, δ_1, and δ_2, have been shifted from the actual scene (of figure 2A).

We now estimate the smoothest solution for given configurations. Figure 2C shows for given flanker tilts, the center tilt that yields maximal smoothness, and the corresponding probability of smoothness. For near vertical flankers, the spatial lability leads to very weak attraction and high probability of smoothness. As the flanker angle deviates farther from vertical, there is a large repulsion, but also lower probability of smoothness. These observations are key to our model: the maximally smooth center tilt will influence attractive and repulsive interactions of tilt estimation; the probability of smoothness will influence the relative weighting of the prior versus the likelihood.

From the smoothness principle, we construct a two dimensional prior (figure 3A). One dimension represents tilt, the other dimension, the overall positional shift between target

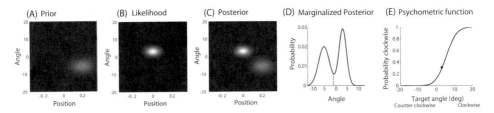

Figure 3: Bayes model for example flankers and target. **(A)** Prior 2D distribution for flankers set at 22.5 degrees (note repulsive preference for -5.5 degrees). **(B)** Likelihood 2D distribution for a target tilt of 3 degrees; **(C)** Posterior 2D distribution. All 2D distributions are drawn on the same grayscale range, and the presence of a larger baseline in the prior causes it to appear more dimmed. **(D)** Marginalized posterior, resulting in 1D distribution over tilt. Dashed line represents the mean, with slight preference for negative angle. **(E)** For this target tilt, we calculate probability clockwise, and obtain one point on psychometric curve.

and flankers (called 'position'). The prior is a 2D Gaussian distribution, sat upon a constant baseline.[22] The Gaussian is centered at the estimated smoothest target angle and relative position, and the baseline is determined by the probability of smoothness. The baseline, and its dependence on the flanker orientation, is a key difference from Weiss *et al*'s Gaussian prior for smooth, slow motion. It can be seen as a mechanism to allow segmentation (see Posterior description below). The standard deviation of the Gaussian is a free parameter.

Likelihood: The likelihood over tilt and position (figure 3B) is determined by a 2D Gaussian distribution with an added baseline.[22] The Gaussian is centered at the actual target tilt; and at a position taken as zero, since this is the actual position, to which the prior is compared. The standard deviation and baseline constant are free parameters.

Posterior and marginalization: The posterior comes from multiplying likelihood and prior (figure 3C) and then marginalizing over position to obtain a 1D distribution over tilt. Figure 3D shows an example in which this distribution is bimodal. Other likelihoods, with closer agreement between target and smooth prior, give unimodal distributions. Note that the bimodality is a direct consequence of having an added baseline to the prior and likelihood (if these were Gaussian without a baseline, the posterior would always be Gaussian). The viewer is effectively assessing whether the target is associated with the same object as the flankers, and this is reflected in the baseline, and consequently, in the bimodality, and confidence estimate. We define α as the mean angle of the 1D posterior distribution (*eg*, value of dashed line on the x axis), and β as the height of the probability distribution at that mean angle (*eg*, height of dashed line). The term β is an indication of confidence in the angle estimate, where for larger values we are more certain of the estimate.

Decision of probability clockwise: The probability of a clockwise tilt is estimated from the marginalized posterior:

$$P = \frac{1}{1 + \exp\left(\frac{-\alpha . *k}{-\log(\beta+\eta)}\right)} \tag{3}$$

where α and β are defined as above, k is a free parameter and η a small constant. Free parameters are set to a single constant value for all flanker and center configurations. Weiss *et al* use a similar compressive nonlinearity, but without the term β. We also tried a decision function that integrates the posterior, but the resulting curves were far from the sigmoidal nature of the data.

Bias and sensitivity: For one target tilt, we generate a single probability and therefore a single point on the psychometric function relating tilt to the probability of choosing clockwise. We generate the full psychometric curve from all target tilts and fit to it a cumulative

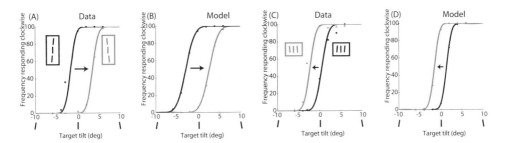

Figure 4: Kapadia *et al* data,[14] versus Bayesian model. Solid lines are fits to a cumulative Gaussian distribution. **(A)** Flankers are tilted 5 degrees clockwise (black curve) or anti-clockwise (gray) of vertical, and positioned spatially in a colinear arrangement. The center bar appears tilted in the direction of the flankers (attraction), as can be seen by the attractive shift of the psychometric curve. The boxed stimuli cartoon illustrates a vertical target amidst the flankers. **(B)** Model for colinear bars also produces attraction. **(C)** Data and **(D)** model for lateral flankers results in repulsion. All data are collected in the fovea for bars.

Gaussian distribution $N(\mu, \sigma)$ (figure 3E). The mean μ of the fit corresponds to the bias, and $\frac{1}{\sigma}$ to the sensitivity, or confidence in the bias. The fit to a cumulative Gaussian and extraction of these parameters exactly mimic psychophysical procedures.[11]

2 Results: data versus model

We first consider the geometry of the center and flanker configurations, modeling the full psychometric curve for colinear and parallel flanks (recall that figure 1A showed summary biases). Figure 4A;B demonstrates attraction in the data and model; that is, the psychometric curve is shifted towards the flanker, because of the nature of smooth completions for colinear flankers. Figure 4C;D shows repulsion in the data and model. In this case, the flankers are arranged laterally instead of colinearly. The smoothest solution in the model arises by shifting the target estimate away from the flankers. This shift is rather minor, because the configuration has a low probability of smoothness (similar to figure 2C), and thus the prior exerts only a weak effect.

The above results show examples of changes in the psychometric curve, but do not address both bias and, particularly, sensitivity, across a whole range of flanker configurations. Figure 5 depicts biases and sensitivity from Solomon *et al*, versus the Bayes model. The data are shown for a representative subject, but the qualitative behavior is consistent across all subjects tested. In figure 5A, bias is shown, for the condition that both flankers are tilted at the same angle. The data exhibit small attraction at near vertical flanker angles (this arrangement is close to colinear); large repulsion at intermediate flanker angles of 22.5 and 45 degrees from vertical; and minimal repulsion at large angles from vertical. This behavior is also exhibited in the Bayes model (Figure 5B). For intermediate flanker angles, the smoothest solution in the model is repulsive, and the effect of the prior is strong enough to induce a significant repulsion. For large angles, the prior exerts almost no effect.

Interestingly, sensitivity is far from flat in both data and model. In the data (Figure 5C), there is most loss in sensitivity at intermediate flanker angles of 22.5 and 45 degrees (*ie*, the subject is less certain); and sensitivity is higher for near vertical or near horizontal flankers. The model shows the same qualitative behavior (Figure 5D). In the model, there are two factors driving sensitivity: one is the probability of completing a smooth curvature for a given flanker configuration, as in Figure 2B; this determines the strength of the prior. The other factor is certainty in a particular center estimation; this is determined by β, derived from the posterior distribution, and incorporated into the decision stage of the model

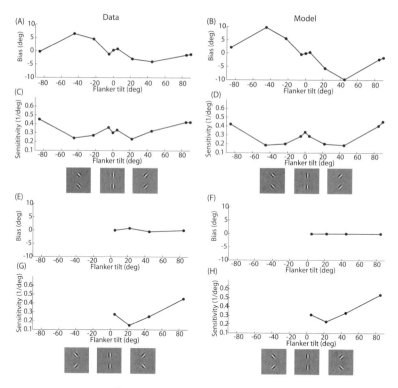

Figure 5: Solomon *et al* data[11] (subject FF), versus Bayesian model. **(A)** Data and **(B)** model biases with same-tilted flankers; **(C)** Data and **(D)** model sensitivities with same-tilted flankers; **(E;G)** data and **(F;H)** model as above, but for opposite-tilted flankers (note that opposite-tilted data was collected for less flanker angles). Each point in the figure is derived by fitting a cumulative Gaussian distribution $N(\mu, \sigma)$ to corresponding psychometric curve, and setting bias equal to μ and sensitivity to $\frac{1}{\sigma}$. In all experiments, flanker and target gratings are presented in the visual periphery. Both data and model stimuli are averages of two configurations, on the left hand side (9 O'clock position) and right hand side (3 O'clock position). The configurations are similar to Figure 1 (B), but slightly shifted according to an iso-eccentric circle, so that all stimuli are similarly visible in the periphery.

(equation 3). For flankers that are far from vertical, the prior has minimal effect because one cannot find a smooth solution (*eg*, the likelihood dominates), and thus sensitivity is higher. The low sensitivity at intermediate angles arises because the prior has considerable effect; and there is conflict between the prior (tilt, position), and likelihood (tilt, position). This leads to uncertainty in the target angle estimation . For flankers near vertical, the prior exerts a strong effect; but there is less conflict between the likelihood and prior estimates (tilt, position) for a vertical target. This leads to more confidence in the posterior estimate, and therefore, higher sensitivity. The only aspect that our model does not reproduce is the (more subtle) sensitivity difference between 0 and +/- 5 degree flankers.

Figure 5E-H depict data and model for opposite tilted flankers. The bias is now close to zero in the data (Figure 5E) and model (Figure 5F), as would be expected (since the maximally smooth angle is now always roughly vertical). Perhaps more surprisingly, the sensitivities continue to to be non-flat in the data (Figure 5G) and model (Figure 5H). This behavior arises in the model due to the strength of prior, and positional uncertainty. As before, there is most loss in sensitivity at intermediate angles.

Note that to fit Kapadia *et al*, simulations used a constant parameter of $k = 9$ in equation

3, whereas for the Solomon et al. simulations, $k = 2.5$. This indicates that, in our model, there was higher confidence in the foveal experiments than in the peripheral ones.

3 Discussion

We applied a Bayesian framework to the widely studied tilt illusion, and demonstrated the model on examples from two different data sets involving foveal and peripheral estimation. Our results support the appealing hypothesis that perceptual misjudgements are not a consequence of poor system design, but rather can be described as optimal inference.[4–8] Our model accounts correctly for both attraction and repulsion, determined by the smoothness prior and the geometry of the scene.

We emphasized the issue of estimation confidence. The dataset showing how confidence is affected by the same issues that affect bias,[11] was exactly appropriate for a Bayesian formulation; other models in the literature typically do not incorporate confidence in a thoroughly probabilistic manner. In fact, our model fits the confidence (and bias) data more proficiently than an account based on lateral interactions among a population of orientation-tuned cells.[11] Other Bayesian work, by Stocker *et al*,[6] utilized the full slope of the psychometric curve in fitting a prior and likelihood to motion data, but did not examine the issue of confidence. Estimation confidence plays a central role in Bayesian formulations as a whole. Understanding how priors affect confidence should have direct bearing on many other Bayesian calculations such as multimodal integration.[23]

Our model is obviously over-simplified in a number of ways. First, we described it in terms of tilts and spatial positions; a more complete version should work in the pixel/filtering domain.[18,19] We have also only considered two flanking elements; the model is extendible to a full-field surround, whereby smoothness operates along a range of geometric directions, and some directions are more (smoothly) dominant than others. Second, the prior is constructed by summarizing the maximal smoothness information; a more probabilistically correct version should capture the full probability of smoothness in its prior. Third, our model does not incorporate a formal noise representation; however, sensitivities could be influenced both by stimulus-driven noise and confidence. Fourth, our model does not address attraction in the so-called indirect tilt illusion, thought to be mediated by a different mechanism. Finally, we have yet to account for neurophysiological data within this framework, and incorporate constraints at the neural implementation level. However, versions of our computations are oft suggested for intra-areal and feedback cortical circuits; and smoothness principles form a key part of the association field connection scheme in Li's[24] dynamical model of contour integration in V1.

Our model is connected to a wealth of literature in computer vision and perception. Notably, occlusion and contour completion might be seen as the extreme example in which there is no likelihood information at all for the center target; a host of papers have shown that under these circumstances, smoothness principles such as *elastica* and variants explain many aspects of perception. The model is also associated with many studies on contour integration motivated by Gestalt principles;[25,26] and exploration of natural scene statistics and Gestalt,[27,28] including the relation to contour grouping within a Bayesian framework.[29,30] Indeed, our model could be modified to include a prior from natural scenes.

There are various directions for the experimental test and refinement of our model. Most pressing is to determine bias and sensitivity for different center and flanker contrasts. As in the case of motion, our model predicts that when there is more uncertainty in the center element, prior information is more dominant. Another interesting test would be to design a task such that the center element is actually part of a different figure and unrelated to the flankers; our framework predicts that there would be minimal bias, because of segmentation. Our model should also be applied to other tilt-based illusions such as the Fraser spiral and Zöllner. Finally, our model can be applied to other perceptual domains;[31] and given the apparent similarities between the tilt illusion and the tilt after-effect, we plan to extend the model to adaptation, by considering smoothness in time as well as space.

Acknowledgements This work was funded by the HHMI (OS, TJS) and the Gatsby Charitable Foundation (PD). We are very grateful to Serge Belongie, Leanne Chukoskie, Philip Meier and Joshua Solomon for helpful discussions.

References

[1] J J Gibson. Adaptation, after-effect, and contrast in the perception of tilted lines. *Journal of Experimental Psychology*, 20:553–569, 1937.

[2] C Blakemore, R H S Carpentar, and M A Georgeson. Lateral inhibition between orientation detectors in the human visual system. *Nature*, 228:37–39, 1970.

[3] J A Stuart and H M Burian. A study of separation difficulty: Its relationship to visual acuity in normal and amblyopic eyes. *American Journal of Ophthalmology*, 53:471–477, 1962.

[4] A Yuille and H H Bulthoff. Perception as bayesian inference. In Knill and Whitman, editors, *Bayesian decision theory and psychophysics*, pages 123–161. Cambridge University Press, 1996.

[5] Y Weiss, E P Simoncelli, and E H Adelson. Motion illusions as optimal percepts. *Nature Neuroscience*, 5:598–604, 2002.

[6] A Stocker and E P Simoncelli. Constraining a bayesian model of human visual speed perception. *Adv in Neural Info Processing Systems*, 17, 2004.

[7] D Kersten, P Mamassian, and A Yuille. Object perception as bayesian inference. *Annual Review of Psychology*, 55:271–304, 2004.

[8] K Kording and D Wolpert. Bayesian integration in sensorimotor learning. *Nature*, 427:244–247, 2004.

[9] L Parkes, J Lund, A Angelucci, J Solomon, and M Morgan. Compulsory averaging of crowded orientation signals in human vision. *Nature Neuroscience*, 4:739–744, 2001.

[10] D G Pelli, M Palomares, and N J Majaj. Crowding is unlike ordinary masking: Distinguishing feature integration from detection. *Journal of Vision*, 4:1136–1169, 2002.

[11] J Solomon, F M Felisberti, and M Morgan. Crowding and the tilt illusion: Toward a unified account. *Journal of Vision*, 4:500–508, 2004.

[12] J A Bednar and R Miikkulainen. Tilt aftereffects in a self-organizing model of the primary visual cortex. *Neural Computation*, 12:1721–1740, 2000.

[13] C W Clifford, P Wenderoth, and B Spehar. A functional angle on some after-effects in cortical vision. *Proc Biol Sci*, 1454:1705–1710, 2000.

[14] M K Kapadia, G Westheimer, and C D Gilbert. Spatial distribution of contextual interactions in primary visual cortex and in visual perception. *J Neurophysiology*, 4:2048–262, 2000.

[15] C C Chen and C W Tyler. Lateral modulation of contrast discrimination: Flanker orientation effects. *Journal of Vision*, 2:520–530, 2002.

[16] I Mareschal, M P Sceniak, and R M Shapley. Contextual influences on orientation discrimination: binding local and global cues. *Vision Research*, 41:1915–1930, 2001.

[17] D Mumford. Elastica and computer vision. In Chandrajit Bajaj, editor, *Algebraic geometry and its applications*. Springer Verlag, 1994.

[18] T K Leung and J Malik. Contour continuity in region based image segmentation. In *Proc. ECCV*, pages 544–559, 1998.

[19] E Sharon, A Brandt, and R Basri. Completion energies and scale. *IEEE Pat. Anal. Mach. Intell.*, 22(10), 1997.

[20] S W Zucker, C David, A Dobbins, and L Iverson. The organization of curve detection: coarse tangent fields. *Computer Graphics and Image Processing*, 9(3):213–234, 1988.

[21] S Ullman. Filling in the gaps: the shape of subjective contours and a model for their generation. *Biological Cybernetics*, 25:1–6, 1976.

[22] G E Hinton and A D Brown. Spiking boltzmann machines. *Adv in Neural Info Processing Systems*, 12, 1998.

[23] R A Jacobs. What determines visual cue reliability? *Trends in Cognitive Sciences*, 6:345–350, 2002.

[24] Z Li. A saliency map in primary visual cortex. *Trends in Cognitive Science*, 6:9–16, 2002.

[25] D J Field, A Hayes, and R F Hess. Contour integration by the human visual system: evidence for a local "association field". *Vision Research*, 33:173–193, 1993.

[26] J Beck, A Rosenfeld, and R Ivry. Line segregation. *Spatial Vision*, 4:75–101, 1989.

[27] M Sigman, G A Cecchi, C D Gilbert, and M O Magnasco. On a common circle: Natural scenes and gestalt rules. *PNAS*, 98(4):1935–1940, 2001.

[28] S Mahumad, L R Williams, K K Thornber, and K Xu. Segmentation of multiple salient closed contours from real images. *IEEE Pat. Anal. Mach. Intell.*, 25(4):433–444, 1997.

[29] W S Geisler, J S Perry, B J Super, and D P Gallogly. Edge co-occurence in natural images predicts contour grouping performance. *Vision Research*, 6:711–724, 2001.

[30] J H Elder and R M Goldberg. Ecological statistics of gestalt laws for the perceptual organization of contours. *Journal of Vision*, 4:324–353, 2002.

[31] S R Lehky and T J Sejnowski. Neural model of stereoacuity and depth interpolation based on a distributed representation of stereo disparity. *Journal of Neuroscience*, 10:2281–2299, 1990.

1208

Learning Minimum Volume Sets

Clayton Scott
Statistics Department
Rice University
Houston, TX 77005
cscott@rice.edu

Robert Nowak
Electrical and Computer Engineering
University of Wisconsin
Madison, WI 53706
nowak@engr.wisc.edu

Abstract

Given a probability measure P and a reference measure μ, one is often interested in the minimum μ-measure set with P-measure at least α. Minimum volume sets of this type summarize the regions of greatest probability mass of P, and are useful for detecting anomalies and constructing confidence regions. This paper addresses the problem of estimating minimum volume sets based on independent samples distributed according to P. Other than these samples, no other information is available regarding P, but the reference measure μ is assumed to be known. We introduce rules for estimating minimum volume sets that parallel the empirical risk minimization and structural risk minimization principles in classification. As in classification, we show that the performances of our estimators are controlled by the rate of uniform convergence of empirical to true probabilities over the class from which the estimator is drawn. Thus we obtain finite sample size performance bounds in terms of VC dimension and related quantities. We also demonstrate strong universal consistency and an oracle inequality. Estimators based on histograms and dyadic partitions illustrate the proposed rules.

1 Introduction

Given a probability measure P and a reference measure μ, the minimum volume set (MV-set) with mass at least $0 < \alpha < 1$ is

$$G_\alpha^* = \arg \min\{\mu(G) : P(G) \geq \alpha, G \text{ measurable}\}.$$

MV-sets summarize regions where the mass of P is most concentrated. For example, if P is a multivariate Gaussian distribution and μ is the Lebesgue measure, then the MV-sets are ellipsoids (see also Figure 1). Applications of minimum volume sets include outlier/anomaly detection, determining highest posterior density or multivariate confidence regions, tests for multimodality, and clustering. In comparison to the closely related problem of density level set estimation [1, 2], the minimum volume approach seems preferable in practice because the mass α is more easily specified than a level of a density. See [3, 4, 5] for further discussion of MV-sets.

This paper considers the problem of MV-set estimation using a training sample drawn from P, which in most practical settings is the only information one has

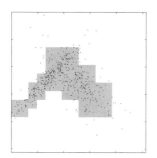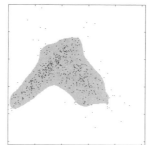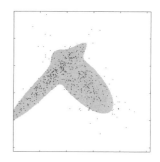

Figure 1: Gaussian mixture data, 500 samples, $\alpha = 0.9$. (Left and Middle) Minimum volume set estimates based on recursive dyadic partitions, discussed in Section 6. (Right) True MV set.

about P. The specifications to the estimation process are the significance level α, the reference measure μ, and a collection of candidate sets $\mathcal{G}$. All proofs, as well as additional results and discussion, may be found in [6] . To our knowledge, ours is the first work to establish finite sample bounds, an oracle inequality, and universal consistency for the MV-set estimation problem.

The methods proposed herein are primarily of theoretical interest, although they may be implemented efficiently for certain partition-based estimators as discussed later. As a more practical alternative, the MV-set problem may be reduced to Neyman-Pearson classification [7, 8] by simulating realizations from.

1.1 Notation

Let $(\mathcal{X}, \mathcal{B})$ be a measure space with $\mathcal{X} \subset \mathbb{R}^d$. Let X be a random variable taking values in $\mathcal{X}$ with distribution P. Let $S = (X_1, \ldots, X_n)$ be an independent and identically distributed (IID) sample drawn according to P. Let G denote a subset of $\mathcal{X}$, and let $\mathcal{G}$ be a collection of such subsets. Let $\widehat{P}$ denote the empirical measure based on S: $\widehat{P}(G) = (1/n) \sum_{i=1}^{n} I(X_i \in G)$. Here $I(\cdot)$ is the indicator function. Set

$$\mu_\alpha^* = \inf_G \{\mu(G) : P(G) \geq \alpha\}, \tag{1}$$

where the inf is over all measurable sets. A minimum volume set, G_α^*, is a minimizer of (1), when it exists. Let $\mathcal{G}$ be a class of sets. Given $\alpha \in (0, 1)$, denote $\mathcal{G}_\alpha = \{G \in \mathcal{G} : P(G) \geq \alpha\}$, the collection of all sets in $\mathcal{G}$ with mass at least alpha. Define $\mu_{\mathcal{G},\alpha} = \inf\{\mu(G) : G \in \mathcal{G}_\alpha\}$ and $G_{\mathcal{G},\alpha} = \arg\min\{\mu(G) : G \in \mathcal{G}_\alpha\}$ when it exists. Thus $G_{\mathcal{G},\alpha}$ is the best approximation to the MV-set G_α^* from $\mathcal{G}$. Existence and uniqueness of these and related quantities are discussed in [6] .

2 Minimum Volume Sets and Empirical Risk Minimization

In this section we introduce a procedure inspired by the empirical risk minimization (ERM) principle for classification. In classification, ERM selects a classifier from a fixed set of classifiers by minimizing the empirical error (risk) of a training sample. Vapnik and Chervonenkis established the basic theoretical properties of ERM (see [9, 10]), and we find similar properties in the minimum volume setting. In this and the next section we do not assume P has a density with respect to μ.

Let $\phi(G, S, \delta)$ be a function of $G \in \mathcal{G}$, the training sample S, and a confidence parameter $\delta \in (0, 1)$. Set $\widehat{\mathcal{G}}_\alpha = \{G \in \mathcal{G} : \widehat{P}(G) \geq \alpha - \phi(G, S, \delta)\}$ and

$$\widehat{G}_{\mathcal{G},\alpha} = \arg\min\{\mu(G) : G \in \widehat{\mathcal{G}}_\alpha\}. \tag{2}$$

We refer to the rule in (2) as MV-ERM because of the analogy with empirical risk minimization in classification. The quantity ϕ acts as a kind of "tolerance" by which the empirical mass estimate may deviate from the targeted value of α. Throughout this paper we assume that ϕ satisfies the following.

Definition 1. *We say ϕ is a (distribution free) complexity penalty for $\mathcal{G}$ if and only if for all distributions P and all $\delta \in (0, 1)$,*

$$P^n\left(\left\{S : \sup_{G \in \mathcal{G}}\left(\left|P(G) - \widehat{P}(G)\right| - \phi(G, S, \delta)\right) > 0\right\}\right) \leq \delta.$$

Thus, ϕ controls the rate of uniform convergence of $\widehat{P}(G)$ to $P(G)$ for $G \in \mathcal{G}$. It is well known that the performance of ERM (for binary classification) relative to the performance of the best classifier in the given class is controlled by the uniform convergence of true to empirical probabilities. A similar result holds for MV-ERM.

Theorem 1. *If ϕ is a complexity penalty for $\mathcal{G}$, then*

$$P^n\left(\left(P(\widehat{G}_{\mathcal{G},\alpha}) < \alpha - 2\phi(\widehat{G}_{\mathcal{G},\alpha}, S, \delta)\right) \text{ or } \left(\mu(\widehat{G}_{\mathcal{G},\alpha}) > \mu_{\mathcal{G},\alpha}\right)\right) \leq \delta.$$

Proof. Consider the sets

$$
\begin{aligned}
\Theta_P &= \{S : P(\widehat{G}_{\mathcal{G},\alpha}) < \alpha - 2\phi(\widehat{G}_{\mathcal{G},\alpha}, S, \delta)\}, \\
\Theta_\mu &= \{S : \mu(\widehat{G}_{\mathcal{G},\alpha}) > \mu(G_{\mathcal{G},\alpha})\}, \\
\Omega_P &= \left\{S : \sup_{G \in \mathcal{G}}\left(\left|P(G) - \widehat{P}(G)\right| - \phi(G, S, \delta)\right) > 0\right\}.
\end{aligned}
$$

The result follows easily from the following lemma.

Lemma 1. *With Θ_P, Θ_μ, and Ω_P defined as above and $\widehat{G}_{\mathcal{G},\alpha}$ as defined in (2) we have $\Theta_P \cup \Theta_\mu \subset \Omega_P$.*

The proof of this lemma (see [6]) follows closely the proof of Lemma 1 in [7]. This result may be understood by analogy with the result from classification that says $R(\widehat{f}) - \inf_{f \in \mathcal{F}} R(f) \leq 2\sup_{f \in \mathcal{F}}|R(f) - \widehat{R}(f)|$ (see [10], Ch. 8). Here R and $\widehat{R}$ are the true and empirical risks, $\widehat{f}$ is the empirical risk minimizer, and $\mathcal{F}$ is a set of classifiers. Just as this result relates uniform convergence bounds to empirical risk minimization in classification, so does Lemma 1 relate uniform convergence to the performance of MV-ERM. $\qquad\square$

The theorem above allows direct translation of uniform convergence results into performance guarantees for MV-ERM. Fortunately, many penalties (uniform convergence results) are known. We now give to important examples, although many others, such as the Rademacher penalty, are possible.

2.1 Example: VC Classes

Let $\mathcal{G}$ be a class of sets with VC dimension V, and define

$$\phi(G, S, \delta) = \sqrt{32\frac{V\log n + \log(8/\delta)}{n}}. \tag{3}$$

By a version of the VC inequality [10], we know that ϕ is a complexity penalty for $\mathcal{G}$, and therefore Theorem 1 applies. To view this result in perhaps a more recognizable way, let $\epsilon > 0$ and choose δ such that $2\phi(G, S, \delta) = \epsilon$. By inverting the relationship between δ and ϵ, we have the following.

Corollary 1. *With the notation defined above,*

$$P^n \left(\left(P(\widehat{G}_{\mathcal{G},\alpha}) < \alpha - \epsilon \right) \text{ or } \left(\mu(\widehat{G}_{\mathcal{G},\alpha}) > \mu_{\mathcal{G},\alpha} \right) \right) \leq 8n^V e^{-n\epsilon^2/128}.$$

Thus, for any fixed $\epsilon > 0$, the probability of being within ϵ of the target mass α and being less than the target volume $\mu_{\mathcal{G},\alpha}$ approaches one exponentially fast as the sample size increases. This result may also be used to calculate a distribution free upper bound on the sample size needed to be within a given tolerance ϵ of α and with a given confidence $1 - \delta$. In particular, the sample size will grow no faster than a polynomial in $1/\epsilon$ and $1/\delta$, paralleling results for classification.

2.2 Example: Countable Classes

Suppose $\mathcal{G}$ is a countable class of sets. Assume that to every $G \in \mathcal{G}$ a number $[\![G]\!]$ is assigned such that $\sum_{G \in \mathcal{G}} 2^{-[\![G]\!]} \leq 1$. In light of the Kraft inequality for prefix codes, $[\![G]\!]$ may be defined as the codelength of a codeword for G in a prefix code for $\mathcal{G}$. Let $\delta > 0$ and define

$$\phi(G, S, \delta) = \sqrt{\frac{[\![G]\!] \log 2 + \log(2/\delta)}{2n}}. \tag{4}$$

By Chernoff's bound together with the union bound, ϕ is a penalty for $\mathcal{G}$. Therefore Theorem 1 applies and we have obtained a result analogous to the Occam's Razor bound for classification.

As a special case, suppose $\mathcal{G}$ is finite and take $[\![G]\!] = \log_2 |\mathcal{G}|$. Setting $2\phi(G, S, \delta) = \epsilon$ and inverting the relationship between δ and ϵ, we have

Corollary 2. *For the MV-ERM estimate $\widehat{G}_{\mathcal{G},\alpha}$ from a finite class $\mathcal{G}$*

$$P^n \left(\left(P(\widehat{G}_{\mathcal{G},\alpha}) < \alpha - \epsilon \right) \text{ or } \left(\mu(\widehat{G}_{\mathcal{G},\alpha}) > \mu_{\mathcal{G},\alpha} \right) \right) \leq 2|\mathcal{G}|e^{-n\epsilon^2/2}.$$

3 Consistency

A minimum volume set estimator is consistent if its volume and mass tend to the optimal values μ_α^* and α as $n \to \infty$. Formally, define the error quantity

$$\mathcal{M}(G) := (\mu(G) - \mu_\alpha^*)_+ + (\alpha - P(G))_+,$$

where $(x)_+ = \max(x, 0)$. (Note that without the $(\cdot)_+$ operator, this would not be a meaningful error since one term could be negative and cause $\mathcal{M}$ to tend to zero, even if the other error term does not go to zero.) We are interested in MV-set estimators such that $\mathcal{M}(\widehat{G}_{\mathcal{G},\alpha})$ tends to zero as $n \to \infty$.

Definition 2. *A learning rule $\widehat{G}_{\mathcal{G},\alpha}$ is strongly consistent if $\lim_{n \to \infty} \mathcal{M}(\widehat{G}_{\mathcal{G},\alpha}) = 0$ with probability 1. If $\widehat{G}_{\mathcal{G},\alpha}$ is strongly consistent for every possible distribution of X, then $\widehat{G}_{\mathcal{G},\alpha}$ is strongly universally consistent.*

To see how consistency might result from MV-ERM, it helps to rewrite Theorem 1 as follows. Let $\mathcal{G}$ be fixed and let $\phi(G, S, \delta)$ be a penalty for $\mathcal{G}$. Then with probability at least $1 - \delta$, both

$$\mu(\widehat{G}_{\mathcal{G},\alpha}) - \mu_\alpha^* \leq \mu(G_{\mathcal{G},\alpha}) - \mu_\alpha^* \tag{5}$$

and
$$\alpha - P(\widehat{G}_{\mathcal{G},\alpha}) \leq 2\phi(\widehat{G}_{\mathcal{G},\alpha}, S, \delta) \qquad (6)$$

hold. We refer to the left-hand side of (5) as the *excess volume* of the class $\mathcal{G}$ and the left-hand side of (6) as the *missing mass* of $\widehat{G}_{\mathcal{G},\alpha}$. The upper bounds on the right-hand sides are an approximation error and a stochastic error, respectively. The idea is to let $\mathcal{G}$ grow with n so that both errors tend to zero as $n \to \infty$. If $\mathcal{G}$ does not change with n, universal consistency is impossible.

To have both stochastic and approximation errors tend to zero, we apply MV-ERM to a class $\mathcal{G}^k$ from a sequence of classes $\mathcal{G}^1, \mathcal{G}^2, \ldots$, where $k = k(n)$ grows with the sample size. Consider the estimator $\widehat{G}_{\mathcal{G}^k,\alpha}$.

Theorem 2. *Choose $k = k(n)$ and $\delta = \delta(n)$ such that $k(n) \to \infty$ as $n \to \infty$ and $\sum_{n=1}^{\infty} \delta(n) < \infty$. Assume the sequence of sets $\mathcal{G}^k$ and penalties ϕ_k satisfy*

$$\lim_{k \to \infty} \inf_{G \in \mathcal{G}^k_\alpha} \mu(G) = \mu^*_\alpha \qquad (7)$$

and

$$\lim_{n \to \infty} \sup_{G \in \mathcal{G}^k_\alpha} \phi_k(G, S, \delta(n)) = o(1). \qquad (8)$$

Then $\widehat{G}_{\mathcal{G}^k,\alpha}$ is strongly universally consistent.

The proof combines the Borel-Cantelli lemma and the distribution-free result of Theorem 1 with the stated assumptions. Examples satisfying the hypotheses of the theorem include families of VC classes with arbitrary approximating power (e.g., generalized linear discriminant rules with appropriately chosen basis functions and neural networks), and histogram rules. See [6] for further discussion.

4 Structural Risk Minimization and an Oracle Inequality

In the previous section the rate of convergence of the two errors to zero is determined by the choice of $k = k(n)$, which must be chosen a priori. Hence it is possible that the excess volume decays much more quickly than the missing mass, or vice versa. In this section we introduce a new rule called MV-SRM, inspired by the principle of structural risk minimization (SRM) from the theory of classification [11, 12], that automatically balances the two errors.

The result in this section is not distribution free. We assume

A1 P has a density f with respect to μ.

A2 G^*_α exists and $P(G^*_\alpha) = \alpha$.

Under these assumptions (see [6]) there exists $\gamma_\alpha > 0$ such that for any MV-set G^*_α, $\{x : f(x) > \gamma_\alpha\} \subset G^*_\alpha \subset \{x : f(x) \geq \gamma_\alpha\}$.

Let $\mathcal{G}$ be a class of sets. Conceptualize $\mathcal{G}$ as a collection of sets of varying capacities, such as a union of VC classes or a union of finite classes. Let $\phi(G, S, \delta)$ be a penalty for $\mathcal{G}$. The MV-SRM principle selects the set

$$\widehat{G}_{\mathcal{G},\alpha} = \arg\min_{G \in \mathcal{G}} \left\{ \mu(G) + \phi(G, S, \delta) : \widehat{P}(G) \geq \alpha - \phi(G, S, \delta) \right\}. \qquad (9)$$

Note that MV-SRM is different from MV-ERM because it minimizes a complexity penalized volume instead of simply the volume. We have the following.[1]

---

[1] Although the value of $1/\gamma_\alpha$ is in practice unknown, it can be bounded by $1/\gamma_\alpha \leq (1 - \mu^*_\alpha)/(1 - \alpha) \leq 1/(1 - \alpha)$. This follows from the bound $1 - \alpha \leq \gamma_\alpha \cdot (1 - \mu^*_\alpha)$ on the mass outside the minimum volume set.

Theorem 3. *Let $\widehat{G}_{\mathcal{G},\alpha}$ be the MV-set estimator in (9). With probability at least $1 - \delta$ over the training sample S,*

$$\mathcal{M}(\widehat{G}_{\mathcal{G},\alpha}) \leq \left(1 + \frac{1}{\gamma_\alpha}\right) \inf_{G \in \mathcal{G}_\alpha} \left\{ \mu(G) - \mu_\alpha^* + 2\phi(G, S, \delta) \right\}. \tag{10}$$

Sketch of proof: The proof is similar in some respects to oracle inequalities for classification. The key difference is in the form of the error term $\mathcal{M}(G) = (\mu(G) - \mu_\alpha^*)_+ + (\alpha - P(G))_+$. In classification both approximation and stochastic errors are positive, whereas with MV-sets the excess volume $\mu(G) - \mu_\alpha^*$ or missing mass $\alpha - P(G)$ could be negative. This necessitates the $(\cdot)_+$ operators, without which the error would not be meaningful as mentioned earlier. The proof considers three cases separately: (1) $\mu(\widehat{G}_{\mathcal{G},\alpha}) \geq \mu_\alpha^*$ and $P(\widehat{G}_{\mathcal{G},\alpha}) < \alpha$, (2) $\mu(\widehat{G}_{\mathcal{G},\alpha}) \geq \mu_\alpha^*$ and $P(\widehat{G}_{\mathcal{G},\alpha}) \geq \alpha$, and (3) $\mu(\widehat{G}_{\mathcal{G},\alpha}) < \mu_\alpha^*$ and $P(\widehat{G}_{\mathcal{G},\alpha}) < \alpha$. In the first case, both volume and mass errors are positive and the argument follows standard lines. The second case can be seen to follow easily from the first. The third case (which occurs most frequently in practice) is most involved and requires use of the fact that $\mu_\alpha^* - \mu_{\alpha-\epsilon}^* \leq \epsilon/\gamma_\alpha$ for $\epsilon > 0$, which can be deduced from basic properties of MV and density level sets. $\qquad\square$

The oracle inequality says that MV-SRM performs about as well as the set chosen by an oracle to optimize the tradeoff between the stochastic and approximation errors. To illustrate the power of the oracle inequality, in [6] we demonstrate that MV-SRM applied to recursive dyadic partition-based estimators adapts optimally to the number of relevant features (unknown a priori).

5 Damping the Penalty

In Theorem 1, the reader may have noticed that MV-ERM does not equitably balance the volume error with the mass error. Indeed, with high probability, $\mu(\widehat{G}_{\mathcal{G},\alpha})$ is *less* than $\mu(G_{\mathcal{G},\alpha})$, while $P(\widehat{G}_{\mathcal{G},\alpha})$ is only guaranteed to be within $\phi(\widehat{G}_{\mathcal{G},\alpha})$ of α. The net effect is that MV-ERM (and MV-SRM) underestimates the MV-set. Experimental comparisons have confirmed this to be the case [6].

A minor modification of MV-ERM and MV-SRM leads to a more equitable distribution of error between the volume and mass, instead of having all the error reside in the mass term. The idea is simple: scale the penalty in the constraint by a damping factor $\nu < 1$. In the case of MV-SRM, the penalty in the objective function also needs to be scaled by $1+\nu$. Moreover, the theoretical properties of these estimators stated above are retained (the statements, omitted here, are slightly more involved [6]). Notice that in the case $\nu = 1$ we recover the original estimators. Also note that the above theorem encompasses the generalized quantile estimate of [3], which corresponds to $\nu = 0$. Thus we have finite sample size guarantees for that estimator to match Polonik's asymptotic analysis.

6 Experiments: Histograms and Trees

To gain some insight into the basic properties of our estimators, we devised some simple numerical experiments. In the case of histograms, MV-SRM can be implemented in a two step process. First, compute the MV-ERM estimate (a very simple procedure) for each $\mathcal{G}^k$, $k = 1, \ldots, K$, where $1/k$ is the bin-width. Second, choose the final estimate by minimizing the penalized volume of the MV-ERM estimates.

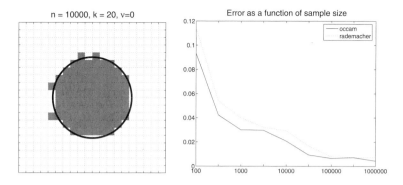

Figure 2: Results for histograms. (Left) A typical MV-ERM estimate with bin-width $1/20$, $\nu = 0$, and based on 10000 points. True MV-set indicated by solid line. (Right) The error of the MV-SRM estimate $\mathcal{M}(\widehat{G}_{\mathcal{G},\alpha})$ as a function of sample size when $\nu = 0$. The results indicated that the Occam's Razor bound is tighter and yields better performance than Rademacher.

We consider two penalties: one based on an Occam style bound, the other on the (conditional) Rademacher average. As a data set we consider $\mathcal{X} = [0,1]^2$, the unit square, and data generated by a two-dimensional truncated Gaussian distribution, centered at the point $(1/2, 1/2)$ and having spherical variance with parameter $\sigma = 0.15$. Other parameter settings are $\alpha = 0.8$, $K = 40$, and $\delta = 0.05$. All experiments were conducted at nine different sample sizes, logarithmically spaced from 100 to 1000000, and repeated 100 times. Results are summarized in Figure 2.

To illustrate the potential improvement offered by spatially adaptive partitioning methods, we consider a minimum volume set estimator based on recursive dyadic (quadsplit) partitions. We employ a penalty that is additive over the cells A of the partition. The precise form of the penalty $\phi(A)$ for each cell is given in [6], but loosely speaking it is proportional to the square-root of the ratio of the empirical mass of the cell to the sample size n. In this case, MV-SRM with $\nu = 0$ is

$$\min_{G \in \mathcal{G}^L} \sum_A [\mu(A)\ell(A) + \phi(A)] \quad \text{subject to} \quad \sum_A \widehat{P}(A)\ell(A) \geq \alpha \qquad (11)$$

where $\mathcal{G}^L$ is the collection of all partitions with dyadic cell sidelengths no smaller than 2^{-L} and $\ell(A) = 1$ if A belongs to the candidate set and $\ell(A) = 0$ otherwise (see [6] for further details). Although directly optimization appears formidable, an efficient alternative is to consider the Lagrangian and conduct a bisection search over the Lagrange multiplier until the mass constraint is nearly achieved with equality (10 iterations is sufficient in practice). For each iteration, minimization of the Lagrangian can be performed very rapidly using standard tree pruning techniques.

An experimental demonstration of the dyadic partition estimator is depicted in Figure 1. In the experiments we employed a dyadic quadtree structure with $L = 8$ (i.e., cell sidelengths no smaller than 2^{-8}) and pruned according to the theoretical penalty $\phi(A)$ formally defined in [6] weighted by a factor of $1/30$ (in practice the optimal weight could be found via cross-validation or other techniques). Figure 1 shows the results with data distributed according to a two-component Gaussian mixture distribution. This figure (middle image) additionally illustrates the improvement possible by "voting" over shifted partitions, which in principle is equivalent to constructing $2^L \times 2^L$ different trees, each based on a partition offset by an integer multiple of the base sidelength 2^{-L}, and taking a majority vote over all the resulting set estimates to form the final estimate. This strategy mitigates the "blocky" structure due to the underlying dyadic partitions, and can be computed almost as rapidly as a single tree estimate (within a factor of L) due to the large amount of redundancy among trees. The actual running time was one to two seconds.

7 Conclusions

In this paper we propose two rules, MV-ERM and MV-SRM, for estimation of minimum volume sets. Our theoretical analysis is made possible by relating the performance of these rules to the uniform convergence properties of the class of sets from which the estimate is taken. Ours are the first known results to feature finite sample bounds, an oracle inequality, and universal consistency.

Acknowledgements

The authors thank Ercan Yildiz and Rebecca Willett for their assistance with the experiments involving dyadic trees.

References

[1] I. Steinwart, D. Hush, and C. Scovel, "A classification framework for anomaly detection," *J. Machine Learning Research*, vol. 6, pp. 211–232, 2005.

[2] S. Ben-David and M. Lindenbaum, "Learning distributions by their density levels – a paradigm for learning without a teacher," *Journal of Computer and Systems Sciences*, vol. 55, no. 1, pp. 171–182, 1997.

[3] W. Polonik, "Minimum volume sets and generalized quantile processes," *Stochastic Processes and their Applications*, vol. 69, pp. 1–24, 1997.

[4] G. Walther, "Granulometric smoothing," *Ann. Stat.*, vol. 25, pp. 2273–2299, 1997.

[5] B. Schölkopf, J. Platt, J. Shawe-Taylor, A. Smola, and R. Williamson, "Estimating the support of a high-dimensional distribution," *Neural Computation*, vol. 13, no. 7, pp. 1443–1472, 2001.

[6] C. Scott and R. Nowak, "Learning minimum volume sets," UW-Madison, Tech. Rep. ECE-05-2, 2005. [Online]. Available: http://www.stat.rice.edu/~cscott

[7] A. Cannon, J. Howse, D. Hush, and C. Scovel, "Learning with the Neyman-Pearson and min-max criteria," Los Alamos National Laboratory, Tech. Rep. LA-UR 02-2951, 2002. [Online]. Available: http://www.c3.lanl.gov/~kelly/ml/pubs/2002_minmax/paper.pdf

[8] C. Scott and R. Nowak, "A Neyman-Pearson approach to statistical learning," *IEEE Trans. Inform. Theory*, 2005, (in press).

[9] V. Vapnik, *Statistical Learning Theory*. New York: Wiley, 1998.

[10] L. Devroye, L. Györfi, and G. Lugosi, *A Probabilistic Theory of Pattern Recognition*. New York: Springer, 1996.

[11] V. Vapnik, *Estimation of Dependencies Based on Empirical Data*. New York: Springer-Verlag, 1982.

[12] G. Lugosi and K. Zeger, "Concept learning using complexity regularization," *IEEE Trans. Inform. Theory*, vol. 42, no. 1, pp. 48–54, 1996.

AER Building Blocks for Multi-Layer Multi-Chip Neuromorphic Vision Systems

R. Serrano-Gotarredona[1], M. Oster[2], P. Lichtsteiner[2], A. Linares-Barranco[4], R. Paz-Vicente[4], F. Gómez-Rodríguez[4], H. Kolle Riis[3], T. Delbrück[2], S. C. Liu[2], S. Zahnd[2], A. M. Whatley[2], R. Douglas[2], P. Häfliger[3], G. Jimenez-Moreno[4], A. Civit[4], T. Serrano-Gotarredona[1], A. Acosta-Jiménez[1], B. Linares-Barranco[1]

[1]Instituto de Microelectrónica de Sevilla (IMSE-CNM-CSIC) Sevilla Spain, [2]Institute of Neuroinformatics (INI-ETHZ) Zurich Switzerland, [3]University of Oslo Norway (UIO), [4]University of Sevilla Spain (USE).

Abstract

A 5-layer neuromorphic vision processor whose components communicate spike events asynchronously using the address-event-representation (AER) is demonstrated. The system includes a retina chip, two convolution chips, a 2D winner-take-all chip, a delay line chip, a learning classifier chip, and a set of PCBs for computer interfacing and address space remappings. The components use a mixture of analog and digital computation and will learn to classify trajectories of a moving object. A complete experimental setup and measurements results are shown.

1 Introduction

The Address-Event-Representation (AER) is an event-driven asynchronous inter-chip communication technology for neuromorphic systems [1][2]. Senders (e.g. pixels or neurons) asynchronously generate events that are represented on the AER bus by the source addresses. AER systems can be easily expanded. The events can be merged with events from other senders and broadcast to multiple receivers [3]. Arbitrary connections, remappings and transformations can be easily performed on these digital addresses.

A potentially huge advantage of AER systems is that computation is event driven and thus can be very fast and efficient. Here we describe a set of AER building blocks and how we assembled them into a prototype vision system that learns to classify trajectories of a moving object. All modules communicate asynchronously using AER. The building blocks and demonstration system have been developed in the EU funded research project CAVIAR (Convolution AER VIsion Architecture for Real-time). The building blocks (Fig. 1) consist of: (1) a retina loosely modeled on the magnocellular pathway that responds to brightness changes, (2) a convolution chip with programmable convolution kernel of arbitrary shape and size, (3) a multi-neuron 2D competition chip, (4) a spatio-temporal pattern classification learning module, and (5) a set of FPGA-based PCBs for address remapping and computer interfaces.

Using these AER building blocks and tools we built the demonstration vision system shown schematically in Fig. 1, that detects a moving object and learns to classify its

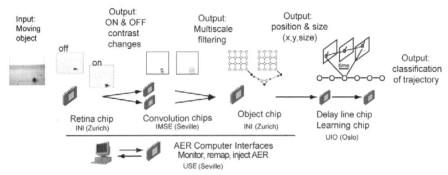

Fig. 1: Demonstration AER vision system

trajectories. It has a front end retina, followed by an array of convolution chips, each programmed to detect a specific feature with a given spatial scale. The competition or 'object' chip selects the most salient feature and scale. A spatio-temporal pattern classification module categorizes trajectories of the object chip outputs.

2 Retina

Biological vision uses asynchronous events (spikes) delivered from the retina. The stream of events encodes dynamic scene contrast. Retinas are optimized to deliver relevant information and to discard redundancy. CAVIAR's input is a dynamic visual scene. We developed an AER silicon retina chip 'TMPDIFF' that generates events corresponding to *relative changes in image intensity* [8]. These address-events are broadcast asynchronously on a shared digital bus to the convolution chips. Static scenes produce no output. The events generated by TMPDIFF represent relative changes in intensity that exceed a user-defined threshold and are ON or OFF type depending on the sign of the change since the last event. This silicon retina loosely models the magnocellular retinal pathway.

The front-end of the pixel core (see Fig. 2a) is an active unity-gain logarithmic photoreceptor that can be self-biased by the average photocurrent [7]. The active feedback speeds up the response compared to a passive log photoreceptor and greatly increases bandwidth at low illumination. The photoreceptor output is buffered to a voltage-mode capacitive-feedback amplifier with closed-loop gain set by a well-matched capacitor ratio. The amplifier is balanced after transmission of each event by the AER handshake. ON and OFF events are detected by the comparators that follow. Mismatch of the event threshold is determined by only 5 transistors and is effectively further reduced by the gain of the amplifier. Much higher contrast resolution than in previous work [6] is obtained by using the excellent matching between capacitors to form a self-clocked switched-capacitor change amplifier, allowing for operation with scene contrast down to about 20%. A chip photo is shown in Fig. 2b.

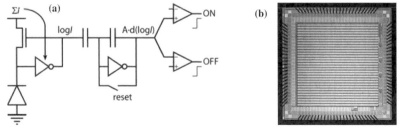

Fig. 2. Retina. a) core of pixel circuit, b) chip photograph.

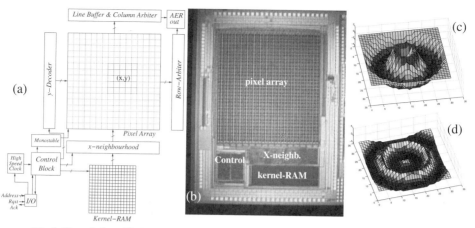

Fig. 3. Convolution chip (a) architecture of the convolution chip. (b) microphotograph of fabricated chip. (c) kernel for detecting circumferences of radius close to 4 pixels and (d) close to 9 pixels.

TMPDIFF has 64x64 pixels, each with 2 outputs (ON and OFF), which are communicated off-chip on a 16-bit AER bus. It is fabricated in a 0.35μm process. Each pixel is 40x40 μm^2 and has 28 transistors and 3 capacitors. The operating range is at least 5 decades and minimum scene illumination with f/1.4 lens is less than 10 lux.

3   Convolution Chip

The convolution chip is an AER transceiver with an array of event integrators. Foreach incoming event, integrators within a projection field around the addressed pixel compute a weighted event integration. The weight of this integration is defined by the convolution kernel [4]. This event-driven computation puts the kernel onto the integrators.

Fig. 3a shows the block diagram of the convolution chip. The main parts of the chip are: (1) An array of 32x32 pixels. Each pixel contains a binary weighted signed current source and an integrate-and-fire signed integrator [5]. The current source is controlled by the kernel weight read from the RAM and stored in a dynamic register. (2) A 32x32 kernel RAM. Each kernel weight value is stored with signed 4-bit resolution. (3) A digital controller handles all sequence of operations. (4) A monostable. For each incoming event, it generates a pulse of fixed duration that enables the integration simultaneously in all the pixels. (5) X-Neighborhood Block. This block performs a displacement of the kernel in the x direction. (6) Arbitration and decoding circuitry that generate the output address events. It uses Boahen's burst mode fully parallel AER [2].

The chip operation sequence is as follows: (1) Each time an input address event is received, the digital control block stores the (x,y) address and acknowledges reception of the event. (2) The control block computes the x-displacement that has to be applied to the kernel and the limits in the y addresses where the kernel has to be copied. (3) The Afterwards, the control block generates signals that control on a row-by-row basis the copy of the kernel to the corresponding rows in the pixel array. (4) Once the kernel copy is finished, the control block activates the generation of a monostable pulse. This way, in each pixel a current weighted by the corresponding kernel weight is integrated during a fixed time interval. Afterwards, kernel weights in the pixels are erased. (5) When the integrator voltage in a pixel reaches a threshold, that pixel asynchronously sends an event, which is arbitrated and decoded in the periphery of the array. The pixel voltage is reset upon reception of the acknowledge from the periphery.

A prototype convolution chip has been fabricated in a CMOS 0.35μm process. Both the size of the pixel array and the size of the kernel storage RAM are 32x32. The input address space can be up to 128x128. In the experimental setup of Section 7, the 64x64 retina output is fed to the convolution chip, whose pixel array addresses are centered on that of the retina. The pixel size is 92.5μm x 95μm. The total chip area is 5.4x4.2 mm². Fig. 3b shows the microphotograph of the fabricated chip. AER events can be fed-in up to a peak rate of 50 Mevent/s. Output event rate depends on kernel lines n_k. The measured output AER peak delay is $(40 + 20 \times n_k)$ ns/event.

4 Competition 'Object' Chip

This AER transceiver chip consists of a group of VLSI integrate-and-fire neurons with various types of synapses [9]. It reduces the dimensionality of the input space by preserving the strongest input and suppressing all other inputs. The strongest input is determined by configuring the architecture on the 'Object' chip as a spiking winner-take-all network. Each convolution chip convolves the output spikes of the retina with its preprogrammed feature kernel (in our example, this kernel consists of a ring filter of a particular resolution). The 'Object' chip receives the outputs of several convolution chips and computes the winner (strongest input) in two dimensions. First, it determines the strongest input in each feature map and in addition, it determines the strongest feature. The computation to determine the strongest input in each feature map is carried out using a two-dimensional winner-take-all circuit as shown in Fig. 4. The network is configured so that it implements a hard winner-take-all, that is, only one neuron is active at a time. The activity of the winner is proportional to the winner's input activity.

The winner-take-all circuit can reliably select the winner given a difference of input firing rate of only 10% assuming that it receives input spike trains having a regular firing rate [10]. Each excitatory input spike charges the membrane of the post-synaptic neuron until one neuron in the array--the winner--reaches threshold and is reset. All other neurons are then inhibited via a global inhibitory neuron which is driven by all the excitatory neurons. Self-excitation provides hysteresis for the winning neuron by facilitating the selection of this neuron as the next winner.

Because of the moving stimulus, the network has to determine the winner using an estimate of the instantaneous input firing rates. The number of spikes that the neuron must integrate before eliciting an output spike can be adjusted by varying the efficacies of the input synapses.

To determine the winning feature, we use the activity of the global inhibitory neuron (which reflects the activity of the strongest input within a feature map) of each feature map in a second layer of competition. By adding a second global inhibitory neuron to each feature map and by driving this neuron through the outputs of the first global inhibitory neurons of all feature maps, only the strongest feature map will survive. The output of the object chip will be spikes encoding the spatial location of the stimulus and the identity of the winning feature. (In the characterization shown in Section 7, the global competition was disabled, so both objects could be simultaneously localized by the object chip).

We integrated the winner-take-all circuits for four feature maps on a single chip with a total of 16x16 neurons; each feature uses an 8x8 array. The chip was fabricated in a 0.35 μm CMOS process with an area of 8.5 mm².

5 Learning Spatio-Temporal Pattern Classification

The last step of data reduction in the CAVIAR demonstrator is a subsystem that learns to classify the spatio-temporal patterns provided by the object chip. It consists of three

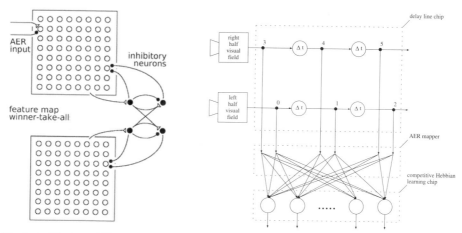

Fig. 4: Architecture of 'Object' chip configured for competition within two feature maps and competition across the two feature maps.

Fig. 5: System setup for learning direction of motion

components: a delay line chip, a competitive Hebbian learning chip [11], and an AER mapper that connects the two. The task of the delay line chip is to project the temporal dimension into a spatial dimension. The competitive Hebbian learning chip will then learn to classify the resulting patterns. The delay line chip consists of one cascade of 880 delay elements. 16 monostables in series form one delay element. The output of every delay element produces an output address event. A pulse can be inserted at every delay-element by an input address event. The cascade can be programmed to be interrupted or connected between any two subsequent delay-elements. The associative Hebbian learning chip consists of 32 neurons with 64 learning synapses each. Each synapse includes learning circuitry with a weak multi-level memory cell for spike-based learning [11].

A simple example of how this system may be configured is depicted in Fig. 5: the mapper between the object chip and the delay line chip is programmed to project all activity from the left half of the field of vision onto the input of one delay line, and from the right half of vision onto another. The mapper between the delay line chip and the competitive Hebbian learning chip taps these two delay lines at three different delays and maps these 6 outputs onto 6 synapses of each of the 32 neurons in the competitive Hebbian learning chip. This configuration lets the system learn the direction of motion.

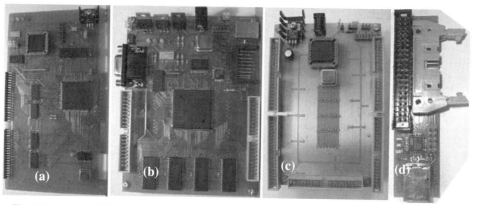

Fig. 6: Developed AER interfacing PCBs. (a) PCI-AER, (b) USB-AER, (c) AER-switch, (d) mini-USB

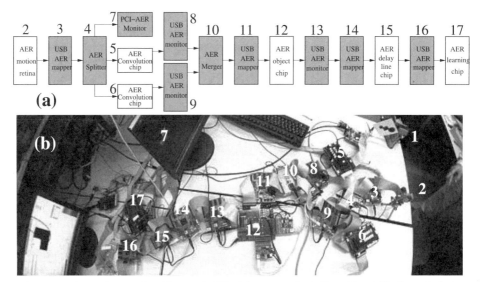

Fig. 7: Experimental setup of multi-layered AER vision system for ball tracking (white boxes include custom designed chips, blue boxes are interfacing PCBs). (a) block diagram, (b) photograph of setup.

6 Computer Interfaces

When developing and tuning complex hierarchical multi-chips AER systems it is crucial to have available proper computer interfaces for (a) reading AER traffic and visualizing it, and (b) for injecting synthesized or recorded AER traffic into AER buses. We developed several solutions. Fig. 6(a) shows a PCI-AER interfacing PCB capable of transmitting AER streams from within the computer or, vice versa, capturing them from an AER bus and into computer memory. It uses a Spartan-II FPGA, and can achieve a peak rate of 15 Mevent/s using PCI mastering. Fig. 5(b) shows a USB-AER board that does not require a PCI slot and can be controlled through a USB port. It uses a Spartan II 200 FPGA with a Silicon Labs C8051F320 microcontroller. Depending on the FPGA firmware, it can be used to perform five different functions: (a) transform sequence of frames into AER in real time [13], (b) histogram AER events into sequences of frames in real time, (c) do remappings of addresses based on look-up-tables, (d) capture timestamped events for off-line analysis, (e) reproduce time-stamped sequences of events in real time. This board can also work without a USB connection (stand-alone mode) by loading the firmware through MMC/SD cards, used in commercial digital cameras. This PCB can handle AER traffic of up to 25 Mevent/s. It also includes a VGA output for visualizing histogrammed frames. The third PCB, based on a simple CPLD, is shown in Fig. 6(c). It splits one AER bus into 2, 3 or 4 buses, and vice versa, merges 2, 3 or 4 buses into a single bus, with proper handling of handshaking signals. The last board in Fig. 6(d) is a lower performance but more compact single-chip bus-powered USB interface based on a C8051F320 microcontroller. It captures timestamped events to a computer at rates of up to 100 kevent/s and is particularly useful for demonstrations and field capture of retina output.

7 Demonstration Vision System

To test CAVIAR's capabilities, we built a demonstration system that could simultaneously track two objects of different size. A block diagram of the complete system is shown in Fig. 7(a), and a photograph of the complete experimental setup is given in Fig. 7(b). The

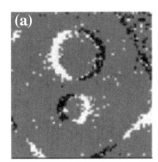
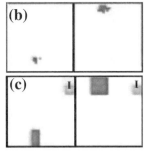

Fig. 8: Captured AER outputs at different stages of processing chain. (a) at the retina output, (b) at the output of the 2 convolution chips, (c) at the output of the object chip. 'I' labels the activity of the inhibitory neurons.

complete chain consisted of 17 pieces (chips and PCBs), all numbered in Fig. 7: (1) The rotating wheel stimulus. (2) The retina. The retina looked at a rotating disc with two solid circles on it of two different radii. (3) A USB-AER board as mapper to reassign addresses and eliminate the polarity of brightness change. (4) A 1-to-3 splitter (one output for the PCI-AER board (7) to visualize the retina output, as shown in Fig. 8(a), and two outputs for two convolution chips). (5-6) Two convolution chips programmed with the kernels in Fig. 3c-d, to detect circumferences of radius 4 pixels and 9 pixels, respectively. They see the complete 64x64 retina image (with rectified activity; polarity is ignored) but provide a 32x32 output for only the central part of the retina image. This eliminates convolution edge effects. The output of each convolution chip is fed to a USB-AER board working as a monitor (8-9) to visualize their outputs (Fig. 8b). The left half is for the 4-radius kernel and the right half for the 9-radius kernel. The outputs of the convolution chips provide the center of the circumferences only if they have radius close to 4 pixels or 9 pixels, respectively. As can be seen, each convolution chip detects correctly the center of its corresponding circumference, but not the other. Both chips are tuned for the same feature but with different spatial scale. Both convolution chips outputs are merged onto a single AER bus using a merger (10) and then fed to a mapper (11) to properly reassign the address and bit signs for the winner-take-all 'object' chip (12), which correctly decides the centers of the convolution chip outputs. The object chip output is fed to a monitor (13) for visualization purposes. This output is shown in Fig. 8(c). The output of this chip is transformed using a mapper (14) and fed to the delay line chip (15), the outputs of which are fed through a mapper (16) to the learning (17) chip. The system as characterized can simultaneously trach two objects of different shape; we have connected but not yet studied trajectory learning and classification.

8 Conclusions

In terms of the number of independent components, CAVIAR demonstrates the largest AER system yet assembled. It consists of 5 custom neuromorphic AER chips and at least 6 custom AER digital boards. Its functioning shows that AER can be used for assembling complex real time sensory processing systems and that relevant information about object size and location can be extracted and restored through a chain of feedforward stages. The CAVIAR system is a useful environment to develop reusable AER infrastructure and is capable of fast visual computation that is not limited by normal imager frame rate. Its continued development will result in insights about spike coding and representation.

Acknowledgements

This work was sponsored by EU grant IST-2001-34124 (CAVIAR), and Spanish grant TIC-2003-08164-C03 (SAMANTA). We thank K. Boahen for sharing AER interface technology and the EU project ALAVLSI for sharing chip development and other AER computer interfaces [14].

References

[1] M. Sivilotti, *Wiring Considerations in Analog VLSI Systems with Application to Field-Programmable Networks*, Ph.D. Thesis, California Institute of Technology, Pasadena CA, 1991.

[2] K. Boahen, "Point-to-Point Connectivity Between Neuromorphic Chips Using Address Events," *IEEE Trans. on Circuits and Systems Part-II*, vol. 47, No. 5, pp. 416-434, May 2000.

[3] J. P. Lazzaro and J. Wawrzynek, "A Multi-Sender Asynchronous Extension to the Address-Event Protocol," *16th Conference on Advanced Research in VLSI*, W. J. Dally, J. W. Poulton, and A. T. Ishii (Eds.), pp. 158-169, 1995.

[4] T. Serrano-Gotarredona, A. G. Andreou, and B. Linares-Barranco, "AER Image Filtering Architecture for Vision Processing Systems," *IEEE Trans. Circuits and Systems (Part II): Analog and Digital Signal Processing*, vol. 46, No. 9, pp. 1064-1071, September 1999.

[5] R. Serrano-Gotarredona, B. Linares-Barranco, and T. Serrano-Gotarredona, "A New Charge-Packet Driven Mismatch-Calibrated Integrate-and-Fire Neuron for Processing Positive and Negative Signals in AER-based Systems," In *Proc. of the IEEE Int. Symp. Circ. Syst.*, (ISCAS04), vol. 5, pp. 744-747 ,Vancouver, Canada, May 2004.

[6] P. Lichtsteiner, T. Delbrück, and J. Kramer, "Improved ON/OFF temporally differentiating address-event imager," in *11th IEEE International Conference on Electronics, Circuits and Systems* (ICECS2004), Tel Aviv, Israel, 2004, pp. 211-214.

[7] T. Delbrück and D. Oberhoff, "Self-biasing low-power adaptive photoreceptor," in *Proc. of the IEEE Int. Symp. Circ. Syst.* (ISCAS04), pp. IV-844-847, 2004.

[8] P. Lichtsteiner and T. Delbrück "64x64 AER Logarithmic Temporal Derivative Silicon Retina," *Research in Microelectronics and Electronics*, Vol. 2, pp. 202-205, July 2005.

[9] Liu, S.-C. and Kramer, J. and Indiveri, G. and Delbrück, T. and Burg, T. and Douglas, R. "Orientation-selective aVLSI spiking neurons", *Neural Networks*, 14:(6/7) 629-643, Jul, 2001

[10] Oster, M. and Liu, S.-C. "A Winner-take-all Spiking Network with Spiking Inputs", in *11th IEEE International Conference on Electronics, Circuits and Systems* (ICECS 2004), Tel Aviv, pp. 203-206, 2004

[11] H. Kolle Riis and P. Haefliger, "Spike based learning with weak multi-level static memory," In *Proc. of the IEEE Int. Symp. Circ. Syst.* (ISCAS04), vol. 5, pp. 393-395, Vancouver, Canada, May 2004.

[12] P. Häfliger and H. Kolle Riis, "A Multi-Level Static Memory Cell," In *Proc. of the IEEE Int. Symp. Circ. Syst.* (ISCAS04), vol. 1, pp. 22-25, Bangkok, Thailand, May 2003.

[13] A. Linares-Barranco, G. Jiménez-Moreno, B. Linares-Barranco, and A. Civit-Ballcels, "On Algorithmic Rate-Coded AER Generation," accepted for publication in *IEEE Trans. Neural Networks*, May 2006 (tentatively).

[14] V. Dante, P. Del Giudice, and A. M. Whatley, "PCI-AER Hardware and Software for Interfacing to Address-Event Based Neuromorphic Systems", *The Neuromorphic Engineer*, 2:(1) 5-6, 2005.

Fast Gaussian Process Regression using KD-Trees

Yirong Shen
Electrical Engineering Dept.
Stanford University
Stanford, CA 94305

Andrew Y. Ng
Computer Science Dept.
Stanford University
Stanford, CA 94305

Matthias Seeger
Computer Science Div.
UC Berkeley
Berkeley, CA 94720

Abstract

The computation required for Gaussian process regression with n training examples is about $O(n^3)$ during training and $O(n)$ for each prediction. This makes Gaussian process regression too slow for large datasets. In this paper, we present a fast approximation method, based on kd-trees, that significantly reduces both the prediction and the training times of Gaussian process regression.

1 Introduction

We consider (regression) estimation of a function $x \mapsto u(x)$ from noisy observations. If the data-generating process is not well understood, simple parametric learning algorithms, for example ones from the generalized linear model (GLM) family, may be hard to apply because of the difficulty of choosing good features. In contrast, the nonparametric *Gaussian process (GP)* model [19] offers a flexible and powerful alternative. However, a major drawback of GP models is that the computational cost of learning is about $O(n^3)$, and the cost of making a single prediction is $O(n)$, where n is the number of training examples. This high computational complexity severely limits its scalability to large problems, and we believe has proved a significant barrier to the wider adoption of the GP model.

In this paper, we address the scaling issue by recognizing that learning and predictions with a GP regression (GPR) model can be implemented using the matrix-vector multiplication (MVM) primitive $z \mapsto Kz$. Here, $K \in \mathbb{R}^{n,n}$ is the *kernel matrix*, and $z \in \mathbb{R}^n$ is an arbitrary vector. For the wide class of so-called *isotropic* kernels, MVM can be approximated efficiently by arranging the dataset in a tree-type multiresolution data structure such as *kd-trees* [13], *ball trees* [11], or *cover trees* [1]. This approximation can sometimes be made orders of magnitude faster than the direct computation, without sacrificing much in terms of accuracy.

Further, the storage requirements for the tree is $O(n)$, while a direct storage of the kernel matrix would require $O(n^2)$ spare. We demonstrate the efficiency of the tree approach on several large datasets.

In the sequel, for the sake of simplicity we will focus on kd-trees (even though it is known that kd-trees do not scale well to high dimensional data). However, it is also completely straightforward to apply the ideas in this paper to other tree-type data structures, for example ball trees and cover trees, which typically scale significantly better to high dimensional data.

2 The Gaussian Process Regression Model

Suppose that we observe some data $D = \{(x_i, y_i) \mid i = 1, \ldots, n\}$, $x_i \in \mathcal{X}$, $y_i \in \mathbb{R}$, sampled independently and identically distributed (i.i.d.) from some unknown distribution.

Our goal is to predict the response y_* on future test points $\boldsymbol{x}_*$ with small mean-squared error under the data distribution. Our model consists of a latent (unobserved) function $\boldsymbol{x} \mapsto u$ so that $y_i = u_i + \varepsilon_i$, where $u_i = u(\boldsymbol{x}_i)$, and the ε_i are independent Gaussian noise variables with zero mean and variance $\sigma^2 > 0$. Following the Bayesian paradigm, we place a prior distribution $P(u(\cdot))$ on the function $u(\cdot)$ and use the posterior distribution

$$P(u(\cdot)|D) \propto N(\boldsymbol{y}|\boldsymbol{u}, \sigma^2 \boldsymbol{I}) P(u(\cdot))$$

in order to predict y_* on new points $\boldsymbol{x}_*$. Here, $\boldsymbol{y} = [y_1, \ldots, y_n]^T$ and $\boldsymbol{u} = [u_1, \ldots, u_n]^T$ are vectors in $\mathbb{R}^n$, and $N(\cdot|\mu, \Sigma)$ is the density of a Gaussian with mean μ and covariance Σ. For a GPR model, the prior distribution is a (zero-mean) Gaussian process defined in terms of a positive definite kernel (or covariance) function $K : \mathcal{X}^2 \to \mathbb{R}$. For the purposes of this paper, a GP can be thought of as a mapping from arbitrary finite subsets $\{\tilde{\boldsymbol{x}}_i\} \subset \mathcal{X}$ of points, to corresponding zero-mean Gaussian distributions with covariance matrix $\tilde{\boldsymbol{K}} = (K(\tilde{\boldsymbol{x}}_i, \tilde{\boldsymbol{x}}_j))_{i,j}$. (This notation indicates that $\tilde{\boldsymbol{K}}$ is a matrix whose (i, j)-element is $K(\tilde{\boldsymbol{x}}_i, \tilde{\boldsymbol{x}}_j)$.) In this paper, we focus on the problem of speeding up GPR under the assumption that the kernel is monotonic isotropic. A kernel function $K(\boldsymbol{x}, \boldsymbol{x}')$ is called *isotropic* if it depends only on the Euclidean distance $r = \|\boldsymbol{x} - \boldsymbol{x}'\|_2$ between the points, and it is *monotonic isotropic* if it can be written as a monotonic function of r.

3   Fast GPR predictions

Since $u(\boldsymbol{x}_1), u(\boldsymbol{x}_2), \ldots, u(\boldsymbol{x}_n)$ and $u(\boldsymbol{x}_*)$ are jointly Gaussian, it is easy to see that the predictive (posterior) distribution $P(u_*|D)$, $u_* = u(\boldsymbol{x}_*)$ is given by

$$P(u_*|D) = N\left(u_* \mid \boldsymbol{k}_*^T \boldsymbol{M}^{-1} \boldsymbol{y}, \ K(\boldsymbol{x}_*, \boldsymbol{x}_*) - \boldsymbol{k}_*^T \boldsymbol{M}^{-1} \boldsymbol{k}_*\right), \tag{1}$$

where $\boldsymbol{k}_* = [K(\boldsymbol{x}_*, \boldsymbol{x}_1), \ldots, K(\boldsymbol{x}_*, \boldsymbol{x}_n)]^T \in \mathbb{R}^n$, and $\boldsymbol{M} = \boldsymbol{K} + \sigma^2 \boldsymbol{I}$, $\boldsymbol{K} = (K(\boldsymbol{x}_i, \boldsymbol{x}_j))_{i,j}$. Therefore, if $\boldsymbol{p} = \boldsymbol{M}^{-1} \boldsymbol{y}$, the optimal prediction under the model is $\hat{u}_* = \boldsymbol{k}_*^T \boldsymbol{p}$, and the predictive variance (of $P(u_*|D)$) can be used to quantify our uncertainty in the prediction. Details can be found in [19]. ([16] also provides a tutorial on GPs.)

Once $\boldsymbol{p}$ is determined, making a prediction now requires that we compute

$$\boldsymbol{k}_*^T \boldsymbol{p} = \sum_{i=1}^{n} K(\boldsymbol{x}_*, \boldsymbol{x}_i) p_i = \sum_{i=1}^{n} w_i p_i \tag{2}$$

which is $O(n)$ since it requires scanning through the entire training set and computing $K(\boldsymbol{x}_*, \boldsymbol{x}_i)$ for each $\boldsymbol{x}_i$ in the training set. When the training set is very large, this becomes prohibitively slow. In such situations, it is desirable to use a fast approximation instead of the exact direct implementation.

3.1   Weighted Sum Approximation

The computations in Equation 2 can be thought of as a weighted sum, where $w_i = K(\boldsymbol{x}_*, \boldsymbol{x}_i)$ is the weight on the i-th summand p_i. We observe that if the dataset is divided into groups where all data points in a group have similar weights, then it is possible to compute a fast approximation to the above weighted sum. For example, let G be a set of data points that all have weights near some value w. The contribution to the weighted sum by points in G is

$$\sum_{i:\boldsymbol{x}_i \in G} w_i p_i = \sum_{i:\boldsymbol{x}_i \in G} w p_i + \sum_{i:\boldsymbol{x}_i \in G} (w_i - w) p_i = w \sum_{i:\boldsymbol{x}_i \in G} p_i + \sum_{i:\boldsymbol{x}_i \in G} \epsilon_i p_i$$

Where $\epsilon_i = w_i - w$. Assuming that $\sum_{i:\boldsymbol{x}_i \in G} p_i$ is known in advance, $w \sum_{i:\boldsymbol{x}_i \in G} p_i$ can then be computed in constant time and used as an approximation to $\sum_{i:\boldsymbol{x}_i \in G} w_i p_i$ if $\sum_{i:\boldsymbol{x}_i \in G} \epsilon_i p_i$ is small.

We note that for a continuous isotropic kernel function, the weights $w_i = K(\boldsymbol{x}_*, \boldsymbol{x}_i)$ and $w_j = K(\boldsymbol{x}_*, \boldsymbol{x}_j)$ will be similar if $\boldsymbol{x}_i$ and $\boldsymbol{x}_j$ are close to each other. In addition, if the

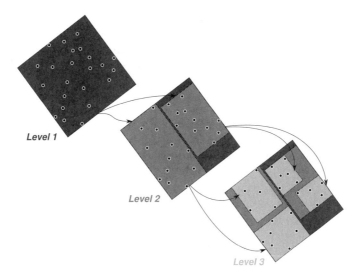

Level 1

Level 2

Level 3

Figure 1: Example of bounding rectangles for nodes in the first three levels of a kd-tree.

kernel function monotonically decreases to zero with increasing $\|\boldsymbol{x}_i - \boldsymbol{x}_j\|$, then points that are far away from the query point $\boldsymbol{x}_*$ will all have weights near zero.

Given a new query, we would like to automatically group points together that have similar weights. But the weights are dependent on the query point and hence the best grouping of the data will also be dependent on the query point. Thus, the problem we now face is, given query point, how to quickly divide the dataset into groups such that data points in the same group have similar weights. Our solution to this problem takes inspiration and ideas from [9], and uses an enhanced kd-tree data structure.

3.2 The kd-tree algorithm

A kd-tree [13] is a binary tree that recursively partitions a set of data points. Each node in the kd-tree contains a subset of the data, and records the bounding hyper-rectangle for this subset. The root node contains the entire dataset. Any node that contains more than 1 data point has two child nodes, and the data points contained by the parent node are split among the children by cutting the parent node's bounding hyper-rectangle in the middle of its widest dimension.[1] An example with inputs of dimension 2 is illustrated in Figure 1.

For our algorithm, we will enhance the kd-tree with additional cached information at each node. At a node $\mathbf{ND}$ whose set of data points is $\mathcal{X}_{\mathbf{ND}}$, in addition to the bounding box we also store

1. $N_{\mathbf{ND}} = |\mathcal{X}_{\mathbf{ND}}|$: the number of data points contained by $\mathbf{ND}$.

2. $S_{\mathbf{ND}}^{\text{Unweighted}} = \sum_{\boldsymbol{x}_i \in \mathcal{X}_{\mathbf{ND}}} p_i$: the unweighted sum corresponding to the data contained by $\mathbf{ND}$.

Now, let

$$S_{\mathbf{ND}}^{\text{Weighted}} = \sum_{i:\boldsymbol{x}_i \in \mathcal{X}_{\mathbf{ND}}} K(\boldsymbol{x}_*, \boldsymbol{x}_i) p_i \tag{3}$$

be the weighted sum corresponding to node $\mathbf{ND}$. One way to calculate $S_{\mathbf{ND}}^{\text{Weighted}}$ is to simply have the 2 children of $\mathbf{ND}$ recursively compute $S_{\text{Left}(\mathbf{ND})}^{\text{Weighted}}$ and $S_{\text{Right}(\mathbf{ND})}^{\text{Weighted}}$ (where

---

[1]There are numerous other possible kd-tree splitting criteria. Our criteria is the same as the one used in [9] and [5]

Left(**ND**) and Right(**ND**) are the 2 children of **ND**) and then sum the two results. This takes $O(n)$ time—same as the direct computation—since all $O(n)$ nodes need to be processed. However, if we only want an approximate result for the weighted sum, then we can cut off the recursion at nodes whose data points have nearly identical weights for the given query point.

Since each node maintains a bounding box of the data points that it owns, we can easily bound the maximum weight variation of the data points owned by a node (as in [9]). The nearest and farthest points in the bounding box to the query point can be computed in O(input dimension) operations, and since the kernel function is isotropic monotonic, these points give us the maximum and minimum possible weights $w_{\max}$ and $w_{\min}$ of any data point in the bounding box.

Now, whenever the difference between $w_{\max}$ and $w_{\min}$ is small, we can cutoff the recursion and approximate the weighted sum in Equation 3 by $w * S_{\mathbf{ND}}^{\text{Unweighted}}$ where $w = \frac{1}{2}(w_{\min} + w_{\max})$. The speed and accuracy of the approximation is highly dependent on the cutoff criteria. Moore et al. used the following cutoff rule in [9]:

$$w_{\max} - w_{\min} \leq 2\epsilon(W_{\text{SoFar}} + N_{\mathbf{ND}}w_{\min}).$$

Here, W_{SoFar} is the weight accumulated so far in the computation and $W_{\text{SoFar}} + N_{\mathbf{ND}}w_{\min}$ serves as a lower bound on the total sum of weights involved in the regression. In our experiments, we found that although the above cutoff rule ensures the error incurred at any particular data point in **ND** is small, the total error incurred by all the data points in **ND** can still be high if $N_{\mathbf{ND}}$ is very large. In our experiments (not reported here), their method gave poor performance on the GPR task, in many cases incurring significant errors in the predictions (or, alternatively running no faster than exact computation, if sufficiently small ϵ is chosen to prevent the large accumulation of errors). Hence, we chose instead the following cutoff rule:

$$N_{\mathbf{ND}}(w_{\max} - w_{\min}) \leq 2\epsilon(W_{\text{SoFar}} + N_{\mathbf{ND}}w_{\min}),$$

which also takes into account the total number of points contained in a node.

From the forumla above, we see that the decision of whether to cutoff computation at a node depends on the value of W_{SoFar} (the total weight of all the points that have been added to the summation so far). Thus it is desirable to quickly accumulate weights at the beginning of the computations, so that more of the later recursions can be cut off. This can be accomplished by going into the child node that's nearer to the query point first when we recurse into the children of a node that doesn't meet the cutoff criteria. (In contrast, [9] always visits the children in left-right order, which in our experiments also gave significantly worse performance than our version.) Our overall algorithm is summarized below:

WeightedSum$(x_*, \mathbf{ND}, W_{\text{SoFar}}, \epsilon)$

compute $w_{\max}$ and $w_{\min}$ for the given query point x_*
$S_{\mathbf{ND}}^{\text{Weighted}} = 0$
if $(w_{\max} - w_{\min}) \leq 2\epsilon(W_{\text{SoFar}} + N_{\mathbf{ND}}w_{\min})$
then
$\quad S_{\mathbf{ND}}^{\text{Weighted}} = \frac{1}{2}(w_{\min} + w_{\max})S_{\mathbf{ND}}^{\text{Unweighted}}$
$\quad W_{\text{SoFar}} = W_{\text{SoFar}} + w_{\min}N_{\mathbf{ND}}$
$\quad$**return** $S_{\mathbf{ND}}^{\text{Weighted}}$
else
$\quad$determine which child is nearer to the query point x_*
$\quad S_{\text{Nearer}}^{\text{Weighted}} = $ **WeightedSum**$(x_*, \text{Nearer child of ND}, W_{\text{SoFar}}, \epsilon)$
$\quad S_{\text{Farther}}^{\text{Weighted}} = $ **WeightedSum**$(x_*, \text{Farther child of ND}, W_{\text{SoFar}}, \epsilon)$
$\quad S_{\mathbf{ND}}^{\text{Weighted}} = S_{\text{Nearer}}^{\text{Weighted}} + S_{\text{Farther}}^{\text{Weighted}}$
$\quad$**return** $S_{\mathbf{ND}}^{\text{Weighted}}$

4 Fast Training

Training (or first-level inference) in the GPR model requires solving the positive definite linear system

$$Mp = y, \quad M = K + \sigma^2 I \tag{4}$$

for the vector p, which in the previous section we assumed had already been pre-computed. Directly calculating p by inverting the matrix M costs about $O(n^3)$ in general. However, in practice there are many ways to quickly obtain approximate solutions to linear systems. Since the system matrix is symmetric positive definite, the *conjugate gradient (CG)* algorithm can be applied. CG is an iterative method which searches for p by maximizing the quadratic function

$$q(z) = y^T z - \frac{1}{2} z^T M z.$$

Briefly, CG ensures that z after iteration k is a maximizer of q over a (Krylow) subspace of dimension k. For details about CG and many other approximate linear solvers, see [15]. Thus, z "converges" to p (the unconstrained maximizer of q) after n steps, but intermediate z can be used as approximate solutions. The speed of convergence depends on the eigenstructure of M. In our case, M typically has only a few large eigenvalues, and most of the spectrum is close to the lower bound σ^2; under these conditions CG is known to produce good approximations after only a few iterations. Crucially, the only operation on M performed in each iteration of CG is a matrix-vector multiplication (MVM) with M.

Since $M = K + \sigma^2 I$, speeding up MVM with M is critically dependent on our ability to perform fast MVM with the kernel matrix K. We can apply the algorithm from Section 3 to perform fast MVM.

Specifically, observe that the i-th row of K is given by $k_i = [K(x_i, x_1), \ldots, K(x_i, x_n)]^T$. Thus, k_i has the same form as that of the vector k_* used in the prediction step. Hence to compute the matrix-vector product Kv, we simply need to compute the inner products

$$k_i^T v = \sum_{j=1}^n K(x_i, x_j) v_j$$

for $i = 1, \ldots, n$. Following exactly the method presented in Section 3, we can do this efficiently using a kd-tree, where here v now plays the role of p in Equation 2.

Two additional optimizations are possible. First, in different iterations of conjugate gradient, we can use the same kd-tree structure to compute $k_i^T v$ for different i and different v. Indeed, given a dataset, we need only ever find a single kd-tree structure for it, and the same kd-tree structure can then be used to make multiple predictions or multiple MVM operations. Further, given fixed v, to compute $k_i^T v$ for different $i = 1, \ldots, n$ (to obtain the vector resulting from one MVM operation), we can also share the same pre-computed partial unweighted sums in the internal nodes of the tree. Only when v (or p) changes do we need to change the partial unweighted sums (discussed in Section 3.2) of v stored in the internal nodes (an $O(n)$ operation).

5 Performance Evaluation

We evaluate our kd-tree implementation of GPR and an implementation that uses direct computation for the inner products. Our experiments were performed on the nine regression datasets in Table 1. [2]

---

[2]Data for the Helicopter experiments come from an autonomous helicopter flight project, [10] and the three tasks were to model three subdynamics of the helicopter, namely its yaw rate, forward velocity, and lateral velocity one timestep later as a function of the helicopter's current state. The temperature and humidity experiments use data from a sensornet comprising a network of simple sensor motes, [2] and the goal here is to predict the conditions at a mote from the measurements

Data set name	Input dimension	Training set size	Test set size
Helicopter yaw rate	3	40000	4000
Helicopter x-velocity	2	40000	4000
Helicopter y-velocity	2	40000	4000
Mote 10 temperature	2	20000	5000
Mote 47 temperature	3	20000	5000
Mote 47 humidity	3	20000	5000
Housing income	2	18000	2000
Housing value	2	18000	2000
Housing age	2	18000	2000

Table 1: Datasets used in our experiments.

	Exact cost	Tree cost	Speedup	Exact error	Tree error
Helicopter yaw rate	14.95	0.31	47.8	0.336	0.336
Helicopter x-velocity	12.37	0.41	30.3	0.594	0.595
Helicopter y-velocity	11.25	0.41	27.3	0.612	0.614
Mote 10 temperature	4.54	0.69	6.6	0.278	0.258
Mote 47 temperature	4.34	1.11	3.9	0.385	0.433
Mote 47 humidity	3.87	0.82	4.7	1.189	1.273
Housing income	2.75	0.76	3.6	0.478	0.478
Housing value	4.47	0.51	8.8	0.496	0.496
Housing age	3.21	1.15	2.8	0.787	0.785

Table 2: Prediction performance on 9 regression problems. **Exact** uses exact computation of Equation 2. **Tree** is the kd-tree based implementation described in Section 3.2. Cost is the computation time measured in milliseconds per prediction. The error reported is the mean absolute prediction error.

For all experiments, we used the Gaussian RBF kernel

$$K(\boldsymbol{x}, \boldsymbol{x}') = \exp -\frac{\|\boldsymbol{x} - \boldsymbol{x}'\|^2}{2d^2},$$

which is monotonic isotropic, with d and σ chosen to be reasonable values for each problem (via cross validation). The ϵ parameter used in the cutoff rule was set to be 0.001 for all experiments.

5.1 Prediction performance

Our first set of experiments compare the prediction time of the kd-tree algorithm with exact computation, given a precomputed p. Our average prediction times are given in Table 2. These numbers include the cost of building the kd-tree (but remain small since the cost is then amortized over all the examples in the test set). As we see, our algorithm runs 2.8-47.8 times faster than exact computation. Further, it incurs only a very small amount of additional error compared to the exact algorithm.

5.2 Learning performance

Our second set of experiments examine the running times for learning (i.e., solving the system of Equations 4,) using our kd-tree algorithm for the MVM operation, compared to exact computation. For both approximate and exact MVM, conjugate gradient was used

---

of nearby motes. The housing experiments make use of data collected from the 1990 Census in California. [12] The median income of a block group is predicted from the median house value and average number of rooms per person; the median house value is predicted using median housing age and median income; the median housing age is predicted using median house value and average number of rooms per household.

	Exact cost	Tree cost	Speedup	Exact error	Tree error
Helicopter yaw rate	22885	279	82.0	0.336	0.336
Helicopter x-velocity	23412	619	37.9	0.594	0.595
Helicopter y-velocity	14341	443	32.4	0.612	0.614
Mote 10 temperature	2071	253	8.2	0.278	0.258
Mote 47 temperature	2531	487	5.2	0.385	0.433
Mote 47 humidity	2121	398	5.3	1.189	1.273
Housing income	1922	581	3.3	0.478	0.478
Housing value	997	138	7.2	0.496	0.496
Housing age	1496	338	4.4	0.787	0.785

Table 3: Training time on the 9 regression problems. Cost is the computation time measured in seconds.

(with the same number of iterations). Here, we see that our algorithm performs 3.3-82 times faster than exact computation.[3]

6 Discussion

6.1 Related Work

Multiresolution tree data structures have been used to speed up the computation of a wide variety of machine learning algorithms [9, 5, 7, 14]. GP regression was introduced to the machine learning community by Rasmussen and Williams [19]. The use of CG for efficient first-level inference is described by Gibbs and MacKay [6]. The stability of Krylov subspace iterative solvers (such as CG) with approximate matrix-vector multiplication is discussed in [4].

Sparse approximations to GP inference provide a different way of overcoming the $O(n^3)$ scaling [18, 3, 8], by selecting a representative subset of D of size $d \ll n$. Sparse methods can typically be trained in $O(n\,d^2)$ (including the active forward selection of the subset) and require $O(d)$ prediction time only. In contrast, in our work here we make use of all of the data for prediction, achieving better scaling by exploiting cluster structure in the data through a kd-tree representation.

More closely related to our work is [20], where the MVM primitive is also approximated using a special data structure for D. Their approach, called the improved fast Gauss transform (IFGT), partitions the space with a k-centers clustering of D and uses a Taylor expansion of the RBF kernel in order to cache repeated computations. The IFGT is limited to the RBF kernel, while our method can be used with all monotonic isotropic kernels. As a topic for future work, we believe it may be possible to apply IFGT's Taylor expansions at each node of the kd-tree's query-dependent multiresolution clustering, to obtain an algorithm that enjoys the best properties of both.

6.2 Isotropic Kernels

Recall that an isotropic kernel $K(\boldsymbol{x}, \boldsymbol{x}')$ can be written as a function of the Euclidean distance $r = \|\boldsymbol{x} - \boldsymbol{x}'\|$. While the RBF kernel of the form $\exp(-r^2)$ is the most frequently used isotropic kernel in machine learning, there are many other isotropic kernels to which our method here can be applied without many changes (since the kd-tree cutoff criteria depends on the pairwise Euclidean distances only). An interesting class of kernels is the *Matérn* model (see [17], Sect. 2.10) $K(r) \propto (\alpha r)^\nu K_\nu(\alpha r)$, $\alpha = 2\nu^{1/2}$, where K_ν is the modified Bessel function of the second kind. The parameter ν controls the roughness of functions sampled from the process, in that they are $\lfloor \nu \rfloor$ times mean-square differentiable.

---

[3]The errors reported in this table are identical to Table 2, since for the kd-tree results we always trained and made predictions both using the fast approximate method. This gives a more reasonable test of the "end-to-end" use of kd-trees.

For $\nu = 1/2$ we have the "random walk" Ornstein-Uhlenbeck kernel of the form $e^{-\alpha r}$, and the RBF kernel is obtained in the limit $\nu \to \infty$. The RBF kernel forces $u(\cdot)$ to be very smooth, which can lead to bad predictions for training data with partly rough behaviour, and its uncritical usage is therefore discouraged in Geostatistics (where the use of GP models was pioneered). Here, other Matérn kernels are sometimes preferred. We believe that our kd-trees approach holds rich promise for speeding up GPR with other isotropic kernels such the Matérn and Ornstein-Uhlenbeck kernels.

References

[1] Alina Beygelzimer, Sham Kakade, and John Langford. Cover trees for nearest neighbor. (Unpublished manuscript), 2005.

[2] Phil Buonadonna, David Gay, Joseph M. Hellerstein, Wei Hong, and Samuel Madden. Task: Sensor network in a box. In *Proceedings of European Workshop on Sensor Networks*, 2005.

[3] Lehel Csató and Manfred Opper. Sparse on-line Gaussian processes. *Neural Computation*, 14:641–668, 2002.

[4] Nando de Freitas, Yang Wang, Maryam Mahdaviani, and Dustin Lang. Fast krylov methods for n-body learning. In *Advances in NIPS 18*, 2006.

[5] Kan Deng and Andrew Moore. Multiresolution instance-based learning. In *Proceedings of the Twelfth International Joint Conference on Artificial Intelligence*, pages 1233–1239. Morgan Kaufmann, 1995.

[6] Mark N. Gibbs. *Bayesian Gaussian Processes for Regression and Classification*. PhD thesis, University of Cambridge, 1997.

[7] Alexander Gray and Andrew Moore. N-body problems in statistical learning. In *Advances in NIPS 13*, 2001.

[8] N. D. Lawrence, M. Seeger, and R. Herbrich. Fast sparse Gaussian process methods: The informative vector machine. In *Advances in NIPS 15*, pages 609–616, 2003.

[9] Andrew Moore, Jeff Schneider, and Kan Deng. Efficient locally weighted polynomial regression predictions. In *Proceedings of the Fourteenth International Conference on Machine Learning*, pages 236–244. Morgan Kaufmann, 1997.

[10] Andrew Y. Ng, Adam Coates, Mark Diel, Varun Ganapathi, Jamie Schulte, Ben Tse, Eric Berger, and Eric Liang. Inverted autonomous helicopter flight via reinforcement learning. In *International Symposium on Experimental Robotics*, 2004.

[11] Stephen M. Omohundro. Five balltree construction algorithms. Technical Report TR-89-063, International Computer Science Institute, 1989.

[12] R. Kelley Pace and Ronald Barry. Sparse spatial autoregressions. *Statistics and Probability Letters*, 33(3):291–297, May 5 1997.

[13] F.P. Preparata and M. Shamos. *Computational Geometry*. Springer-Verlag, 1985.

[14] Nathan Ratliff and J. Andrew Bagnell. Kernel conjugate gradient. Technical Report CMU-RI-TR-05-30, Robotics Institute, Carnegie Mellon University, June 2005.

[15] Y. Saad. *Iterative Methods for Sparse Linear Systems*. International Thomson Publishing, 1st edition, 1996.

[16] M. Seeger. Gaussian processes for machine learning. *International Journal of Neural Systems*, 14(2):69–106, 2004.

[17] M. Stein. *Interpolation of Spatial Data: Some Theory for Kriging*. Springer, 1999.

[18] Michael Tipping. Sparse Bayesian learning and the relevance vector machine. *Journal of Machine Learning Research*, 1:211–244, 2001.

[19] C. Williams and C. Rasmussen. Gaussian processes for regression. In *Advances in NIPS 8*, 1996.

[20] C. Yang, R. Duraiswami, and L. Davis. Efficient kernel machines using the improved fast Gauss transform. In *Advances in NIPS 17*, pages 1561–1568, 2005.

Learning Shared Latent Structure for Image Synthesis and Robotic Imitation

Aaron P. Shon †   **Keith Grochow** †   **Aaron Hertzmann** ‡   **Rajesh P. N. Rao** †
†Department of Computer Science and Engineering
University of Washington
Seattle, WA 98195 USA
‡Department of Computer Science
University of Toronto
Toronto, ON M5S 3G4 Canada
{*aaron,keithg,rao*}*@cs.washington.edu, hertzman@dgp.toronto.edu*

Abstract

We propose an algorithm that uses Gaussian process regression to learn common hidden structure shared between corresponding sets of heterogenous observations. The observation spaces are linked via a single, reduced-dimensionality latent variable space. We present results from two datasets demonstrating the algorithms's ability to synthesize novel data from learned correspondences. We first show that the method can learn the nonlinear mapping between corresponding views of objects, filling in missing data as needed to synthesize novel views. We then show that the method can learn a mapping between human degrees of freedom and robotic degrees of freedom for a humanoid robot, allowing robotic imitation of human poses from motion capture data.

1   Introduction

Finding common structure between two or more concepts lies at the heart of analogical reasoning. Structural commonalities can often be used to interpolate novel data in one space given observations in another space. For example, predicting a 3D object's appearance given corresponding poses of another, related object relies on learning a parameterization common to both objects. Another domain where finding common structure is crucial is imitation learning, also called "learning by watching" [11, 12, 6]. In imitation learning, one agent, such as a robot, learns to perform a task by observing another agent, for example, a human instructor. In this paper, we propose an efficient framework for discovering parameterizations shared between multiple observation spaces using Gaussian processes.

Gaussian processes (GPs) are powerful models for classification and regression that subsume numerous classes of function approximators, such as single hidden-layer neural networks and RBF networks [8, 15, 9]. Recently, Lawrence proposed the Gaussian process latent variable model (GPLVM) [4] as a new technique for nonlinear dimensionality reduction and data visualization [13, 10]. An extension of this model, the scaled GPLVM (SGPLVM), has been used successfully for dimensionality reduction on human motion capture data for motion synthesis and visualization [1].

In this paper, we propose a generalization of the GPLVM model that can handle multiple observation spaces, where each set of observations is parameterized by a different set of kernel parameters. Observations are linked via a single, reduced-dimensionality latent variable space. Our framework can be viewed as a nonlinear extension to canonical correlation analysis (CCA), a framework for learning correspondences between sets of observations. Our goal is to find correspondences on testing data, given a limited set of corresponding training data from two observation spaces. Such an algorithm can be used in a variety of applications, such as inferring a novel view of an object given a corresponding view of a different object and estimating the kinematic parameters for a humanoid robot given a human pose.

Several properties motivate our use of GPs. First, finding latent representations for correlated, high-dimensional sets of observations requires non-linear mappings, so linear CCA is not viable. Second, GPs reduce the number of free parameters in the regression model, such as number of basis units needed, relative to alternative regression models such as neural networks. Third, the probabilistic nature of GPs facilitates learning from multiple sources with potentially different variances. Fourth, probabilistic models provide an estimate of uncertainty in classification or interpolating between data; this is especially useful in applications such as robotic imitation where estimates of uncertainty can be used to decide whether a robot should attempt a particular pose or not. GPs can also generate samples of novel data, unlike many nonlinear dimensionality reduction methods [10, 13].

Fig. 1(a) shows the graphical model for learning shared structure using Gaussian processes. A latent space X maps to two (or more) observation spaces Y, Z using nonlinear kernels, and "inverse" Gaussian processes map back from observations to latent coordinates. Synthesis employs a map from latent coordinates to observations, while recognition employs an inverse mapping. We demonstrate our approach on two datasets. The first is an image dataset containing corresponding views of two different objects. The challenge is to predict corresponding views of the second object given novel views of the first based on a limited training set of corresponding object views. The second dataset consists of human poses derived from motion capture data and corresponding kinematic poses from a humanoid robot. The challenge is to estimate the kinematic parameters for robot pose, given a potentially novel pose from human motion capture, thereby allowing robotic imitation of human poses. Our results indicate that the model generalizes well when only limited training correspondences are available, and that the model remains robust when testing data is noisy.

2 Latent Structure Model

The goal of our model is to find a shared latent variable parameterization in a space X that relates corresponding pairs of observations from two (or more) different spaces Y, Z. The observation spaces might be very dissimilar, despite the observations sharing a common structure or parameterization. For example, a robot's joint space may have very different degrees of freedom than a human's joint space, although they may both be made to assume similar poses. The latent variable space then characterizes the common pose space.

Let $\mathbf{Y}, \mathbf{Z}$ be matrices of observations (training data) drawn from spaces of dimensionality D_Y, D_Z respectively. Each row represents one data point. These observations are drawn so that the first observation $\mathbf{y}_1$ corresponds to the observation $\mathbf{z}_1$, observation $\mathbf{y}_2$ corresponds to observation $\mathbf{z}_2$, etc. up to the number of observations N. Let X be a "latent space" of dimensionality $D_X \ll D_Y, D_Z$. We initialize a matrix of latent points $\mathbf{X}$ by averaging the top D_X principal components of $\mathbf{Y}, \mathbf{Z}$. As with the original GPLVM, we optimize over a limited subset of training points (the *active set*) to accelerate training, determined by the informative vector machine (IVM) [5]. The SGPLVM assumes that a diagonal "scaling matrix" $\mathbf{W}$ scales the variances of each dimension k of the $\mathbf{Y}$ matrix (a similar matrix $\mathbf{V}$ scales each dimension m of $\mathbf{Z}$). The scaling matrix helps in domains where different output dimensions (such as the degrees of freedom of a robot) can have vastly different variances.

We assume that each latent point $\mathbf{x}_i$ generates a pair of observations $\mathbf{y}_i, \mathbf{z}_i$ via a nonlinear function parameterized by a kernel matrix. GPs parameterize the functions $f_Y : X \mapsto Y$ and $f_Z : X \mapsto Z$. The SGPLVM model uses an exponential (RBF) kernel, defining the similarity between two data points $\mathbf{x}, \mathbf{x}'$ as:

$$k\left(\mathbf{x}, \mathbf{x}'\right) = \alpha_Y \exp\left(-\frac{\gamma_Y}{2}||\mathbf{x} - \mathbf{x}'||^2\right) + \delta_{\mathbf{x},\mathbf{x}'}\beta_Y^{-1} \tag{1}$$

given hyperparameters for the $\mathbf{Y}$ space $\theta_Y = \{\alpha_Y, \beta_Y, \gamma_Y\}$. δ represents the delta function. Following standard notation for GPs [8, 15, 9], the priors $P(\theta_Y), P(\theta_Z), P(\mathbf{X})$, the likelihoods $P(\mathbf{Y}), P(\mathbf{Z})$ for the $\mathbf{Y}, \mathbf{Z}$ observation spaces, and the joint likelihood $P_{GP}(\mathbf{X}, \mathbf{Y}, \mathbf{Z}, \theta_Y, \theta_Z)$ are given by:

$$P(\mathbf{Y}|\theta_Y, \mathbf{X}) = \frac{|\mathbf{W}|^N}{\sqrt{(2\pi)^{ND_Y}|\mathbf{K}|^{D_Y}}} \exp\left(-\frac{1}{2}\sum_{k=1}^{D_Y} w_k^2 \mathbf{Y}_k^{\mathrm{T}} \mathbf{K}_Y^{-1} \mathbf{Y}_k\right) \tag{2}$$

$$P(\mathbf{Z}|\theta_Z, \mathbf{X}) = \frac{|\mathbf{V}|^N}{\sqrt{(2\pi)^{ND_Z}|\mathbf{K}|^{D_Z}}} \exp\left(-\frac{1}{2}\sum_{m=1}^{D_Z} v_m^2 \mathbf{Z}_m^{\mathrm{T}} \mathbf{K}_Z^{-1} \mathbf{Z}_m\right) \tag{3}$$

$$P(\theta_Y) \propto \frac{1}{\alpha_Y \beta_Y \gamma_Y} \qquad P(\theta_Z) \propto \frac{1}{\alpha_Z \beta_Z \gamma_Z} \tag{4}$$

$$P(\mathbf{X}) = \frac{1}{\sqrt{2\pi}} \exp\left(-\frac{1}{2}\sum_i ||\mathbf{x}_i||^2\right) \tag{5}$$

$$P_{GP}(\mathbf{X}, \mathbf{Y}, \mathbf{Z}, \theta_Y, \theta_Z) = P(\mathbf{Y}|\theta_Y, \mathbf{X})P(\mathbf{Z}|\theta_Z, \mathbf{X})P(\theta_Y)P(\theta_Z)P(\mathbf{X}) \tag{6}$$

where $\alpha_Z, \beta_Z, \gamma_Z$ are hyperparameters for the Z space, and w_k, v_m respectively denote the diagonal entries for matrices $\mathbf{W}, \mathbf{V}$. Let $\overline{\mathbf{Y}}, \overline{\mathbf{K}}_Y^{-1}$ respectively denote the $\mathbf{Y}$ observations from the active set (with mean μ_Y subtracted out) and the kernel matrix for the active set. The joint negative log likelihood of a latent point $\mathbf{x}$ and observations $\mathbf{y}, \mathbf{z}$ is:

$$L_{\mathbf{y}|\mathbf{x}}(\mathbf{x}, \mathbf{y}) = \frac{||\mathbf{W}(\mathbf{y} - f_Y(\mathbf{x}))||^2}{2\sigma_Y^2(\mathbf{x})} + \frac{D_Y}{2}\ln\left(\sigma_Y^2(\mathbf{x})\right) \tag{7}$$

$$f_Y(\mathbf{x}) = \mu_Y + \overline{\mathbf{Y}}^{\mathrm{T}}\overline{\mathbf{K}}_Y^{-1}\mathbf{k}(\mathbf{x}) \tag{8}$$

$$\sigma_Y^2(\mathbf{x}) = k(\mathbf{x}, \mathbf{x}) - \mathbf{k}(\mathbf{x})^{\mathrm{T}}\overline{\mathbf{K}}_Y^{-1}\mathbf{k}(\mathbf{x}) \tag{9}$$

$$L_{\mathbf{z}|\mathbf{x}}(\mathbf{x}, \mathbf{z}) = \frac{||\mathbf{V}(\mathbf{z} - f_Z(\mathbf{x}))||^2}{2\sigma_Z^2(\mathbf{x})} + \frac{D_Z}{2}\ln\left(\sigma_Z^2(\mathbf{x})\right) \tag{10}$$

$$f_Z(\mathbf{x}) = \mu_Z + \overline{\mathbf{Z}}^{\mathrm{T}}\overline{\mathbf{K}}_Z^{-1}\mathbf{k}(\mathbf{x}) \tag{11}$$

$$\sigma_Z^2(\mathbf{x}) = k(\mathbf{x}, \mathbf{x}) - \mathbf{k}(\mathbf{x})^{\mathrm{T}}\overline{\mathbf{K}}_Z^{-1}\mathbf{k}(\mathbf{x}) \tag{12}$$

$$L_{\mathbf{x},\mathbf{y},\mathbf{z}} = L_{\mathbf{y}|\mathbf{x}} + L_{\mathbf{z}|\mathbf{x}} + \frac{1}{2}||\mathbf{x}||^2 \tag{13}$$

The model learns a separate kernel for each observation space, but a single set of common latent points. A conjugate gradient solver adjusts model parameters and latent coordinates to maximize Eq. 6.

Given a trained SGPLVM, we would like to infer the parameters in one observation space given parameters in the other (e.g., infer robot pose $\mathbf{z}$ given human pose $\mathbf{y}$). We solve this problem in two steps. First, we determine the most likely latent coordinate $\mathbf{x}$ given the observation $\mathbf{y}$ using $\mathrm{argmax}_{\mathbf{x}} L_X(\mathbf{x}, \mathbf{y})$. In principle, one could find $\mathbf{x}$ at $\frac{\partial L_X}{\partial \mathbf{x}} = 0$ using gradient descent. However, to speed up recognition, we instead learn a separate "inverse" Gaussian process $f_Y^{-1} : \mathbf{y} \mapsto \mathbf{x}$ that maps back from the space Y to the space X. Once the correct latent coordinate $\mathbf{x}$ has been inferred for a given $\mathbf{y}$, the model uses the trained SGPLVM to predict the corresponding observation $\mathbf{z}$.

3 Results

We first demonstrate how the our model can be used to synthesize new views of an object, character or scene from known views of another object, character or scene, given a common latent variable model. For ease of visualization, we used 2D latent spaces for all results shown here. The model was applied to image pairs depicting corresponding views of 3D objects. Different views show the objects[1] rotated at varying degrees out of the camera plane. We downsampled the images to 32×32 grayscale pixels. For fitting images, the scaling matrices $\mathbf{W}, \mathbf{V}$ are of minimal importance (since we expect all pixels should *a priori* have the same variance). We also found empirically that using $f_Y(\mathbf{x}) = \mathbf{Y}^{\mathrm{T}} \overline{\mathbf{K}}_Y^{-1} \mathbf{k}(\mathbf{x})$ instead of Eqn. 8 produced better renderings. We rescaled each f_Y to use the full range of pixel values $[0 \dots 255]$, creating the images shown in the figures.

Fig. 1(b) shows how the model extrapolates to novel datasets given a limited set of training correspondences. We trained the model using 72 corresponding views of two different objects, a coffee cup and a toy truck. Fixing the latent coordinates learned during training, we then selected 8 views of a third object (a toy car). We selected latent points corresponding to those views, and learned kernel parameters for the 8 images. Empirically, priors on kernel parameters are critical for acceptable performance, particularly when only limited data are available such as the 8 different poses for the toy car. In this case, we used the kernel parameters learned for the cup and toy truck (based on 72 different poses) to impose a Gaussian prior on the kernel parameters for the car (replacing $P(\theta)$ in Eqn. 4):

$$ -\log P(\theta_{\mathrm{car}}) = -\log P_{GP} + (\theta_{\mathrm{car}} - \theta_\mu)^{\mathrm{T}} \, \Gamma_\theta^{-1} \, (\theta_{\mathrm{car}} - \theta_\mu) \qquad (14) $$

where $\theta_{\mathrm{car}}, \theta_\mu, \Gamma_\theta^{-1}$ are respectively kernel parameters for the car, the mean kernel parameters for previously learned kernels (for the cup and truck), and inverse covariance matrix for learned kernel parameters. $\theta_\mu, \Gamma_\theta^{-1}$ in this case are derived from only two samples, but nonetheless successfully constrain the kernel parameters for the car so the model functions on the limited set of 8 example poses.

To test the model's robustness to noise and missing data, we randomly selected 10 latent coordinates corresponding to a subset of learned cup and truck image pairs. We then added varying displacements to the latent coordinates and synthesized the corresponding *novel* views for all 3 observation spaces. Displacements varied from 0 to 0.45 (all 72 latent coordinates lie on the interval [-0.70,-0.87] to [0.72,0.56]). The synthesized views are shown in Fig. 1(b), with images for the cup and truck in the first two rows. Latent coordinates in regions of low model likelihood generate images that appear blurry or noisy. More interestingly, despite the small number of images used for the car, the model correctly matches the orientation of the car to the synthesized images of the cup and truck. Thus, the model can synthesize reasonable correspondences (given a latent point) even if the number of training examples used to learn kernel parameters is small.

Fig. 2 illustrates the recognition performance of the "inverse" Gaussian process model as a function of the amount of noise added to the inputs. Using the latent space and kernel parameters learned for Fig. 1, we present 72 views of the coffee cup with varying amounts of additive, zero-mean white noise, and determine the fraction of the 72 poses correctly classified by the model. The model estimates the pose using 1-nearest-neighbor classification of the latent coordinates $\mathbf{x}$ learned during training:

$$ \underset{\mathbf{x}'}{\operatorname{argmax}} \, k\left(\mathbf{x}, \mathbf{x}'\right) \qquad (15) $$

The recognition performance degrades gracefully with increasing noise power. Fig. 2 also plots sample images from one pose of the cup at several different noise levels. For two of the noise levels, we show the "denoised" cup image selected using the nearest-neighbor

---

[1]http://www1.cs.columbia.edu/CAVE/research/softlib/coil-100.html

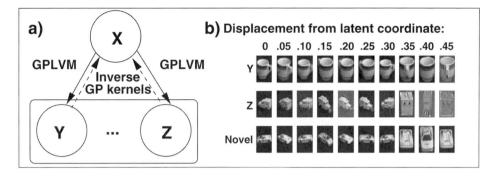

Figure 1: **Pose synthesis for multiple objects using shared structure:** (a) Graphical model for our shared structure latent variable model. The latent space X maps to two (or more) observation spaces Y, Z using a nonlinear kernel. "Inverse" Gaussian process kernels map back from observations to latent coordinates. (b) The model learns pose correspondences for images of the coffee cup and toy truck (**Y** and **Z**) by fitting kernel parameters and a 2-dimensional latent variable space. After learning the latent coordinates for the cup and truck, we fit kernel parameters for a novel object (the toy car). Unlike the cup and truck, where 72 pairs of views were used to fit kernel parameters and latent coordinates, only 8 views were used to fit kernel parameters for the car. The model is robust to noise in the latent coordinates; numbers above each column represent the amount of noise added to the latent coordinates used to synthesize the images. Even at points where the model is uncertain (indicated by the rightmost results in the **Y** and **Z** rows), the learned kernel extrapolates the correct view of the toy car (the "novel" row).

classification, and the corresponding reconstructed truck. This illustrates how even noisy observations in one space can predict corresponding observations in the companion space.

Fig. 3 illustrates the ability of the model to synthesize novel views of one object given a novel view of a different object. A limited set of corresponding poses (24 of 72 total) of a cat figurine and a mug were used to train the GP model. The remaining 48 poses of the mug were then used as testing data. For each snapshot of the mug, we inferred a latent point using the "inverse" Gaussian process model and used the learned model to synthesize what the cat figurine should look like in the same pose. A subset of these results is presented in the rows on the left in Fig. 3: the "Test" rows show novel images of the mug, the "Inferred" rows show the model's best estimate for the cat figurine, and the "Actual" rows show the ground truth. Although the images for some poses are blurry and the model fails to synthesize the correct image for pose 44, the model nevertheless manages to capture fine detail on most of the images.

The grayscale plot at upper right in Fig. 3 shows model certainty $1/\left[\sigma_Y^2(\mathbf{x}) + \sigma_Z^2(\mathbf{x})\right]$, with white where the model is highly certain and black where the model is highly uncertain. Arrows indicate the path in latent space formed by the training images. The dashed line indicates latent points inferred from testing images of the mug. Numbered latent coordinates correspond to the synthesized images at left. The latent space shows structure: latent points for similar poses are grouped together, and tend to move along a smooth curve in latent space, with coordinates for the final pose lying close to coordinates for the first pose (as desired for a cyclic image sequence). The bar graph at lower right compares model certainty for the numbered latent coordinates; higher bars indicate greater model certainty. The model appears particularly uncertain for blurry inferred images, such as 8, 14, and 26.

Fig. 4 shows an application of our framework to the problem of robotic imitation of human actions. We trained our model on a dataset containing human poses (acquired with a Vicon motion capture system) and corresponding poses of a Fujitsu HOAP-2 humanoid robot. Note that the robot has 25 degrees-of-freedom which differ significantly from the degrees-

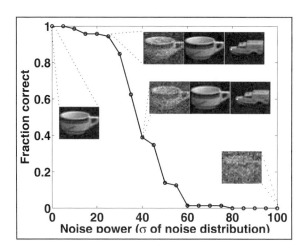

Figure 2: **Recognition using a Learned Latent Variable Space:** After learning from 72 paired correspondences between poses of a coffee cup and of a toy truck, the model is able to recognize different poses of the coffee cup in the presence of additive white noise. Fraction of images recognized are plotted on the Y axis and standard deviation of white noise is plotted on the X axis. One pose of the cup (of 72 total) is plotted for various noise levels (see text for details). "Denoised" images obtained from nearest-neighbor classification and the corresponding images for the Z space (the toy truck) are also shown.

of-freedom of the human skeleton used in motion capture. After training on 43 roughly matching poses (only linear time scaling applied to align training poses), we tested the model by presenting a set of 123 human motion capture poses (which includes the original training set). Because the recognition model $f_Y^{-1} : \mathbf{y} \mapsto \mathbf{x}$ is not trained from samples from the prior distribution of the data, $P(\mathbf{x}, \mathbf{y})$, we found it necessary to approximate $\mathbf{k}(\mathbf{x})$ for the recognition model by rescaling $\mathbf{k}(\mathbf{x})$ for the testing points to lie on the same interval as the $\mathbf{k}(\mathbf{x})$ values of the training points. We suspect that providing proper samples from the prior will improve recognition performance. As illustrated in Fig. 4 (inset panels, human and robot skeletons), the model was able to correctly infer appropriate robot kinematic parameters given a range of novel human poses. These inferred parameters were used in conjunction with a simple controller to instantiate the pose in the humanoid robot (see photos in the inset panels).

4 Discussion

Our Gaussian process model provides a novel method for learning nonlinear relationships between corresponding sets of data. Our results demonstrate the model's utility for diverse tasks such as image synthesis and robotic programming by demonstration. The GP model is closely related to other kernel methods for solving CCA [3] and similar problems [2].

The problems addressed by our model can also be framed as a type of nonlinear CCA. Our method differs from the latent variable method proposed in [14] by using Gaussian process regression. Disadvantages of our method with respect to [14] include lack of global optimality for the latent embedding; advantages include fewer independent parameters and the ability to easily impose priors on the latent variable space (since GPLVM regression uses conjugate gradient optimization instead of eigendecomposition). Empirically we found the flexiblity of the GPLVM approach desirable for modeling a diversity of data sources.

Our framework learns mappings between each observation space and a latent space, rather than mapping directly between the observation spaces. This makes visualization and interaction much easier. An intermediate mapping to a latent space is also more economical in

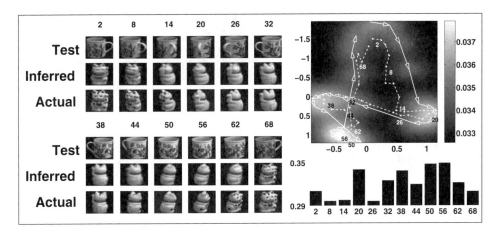

Figure 3: **Synthesis of novel views using a shared latent variable model:** After training on 24 paired images of a mug with a cat figurine (out of 72 total paired images), we ask the model to infer what the remaining 48 poses of the cat would look like given 48 novel views of the mug. The system uses an inverse Gaussian process model to infer a 2D latent point for each of the 48 novel mug views, then synthesizes a corresponding view of the cat figurine. At left we plot the novel testing mug images given to the system ("test"), the synthesized cat images ("inferred"), and the actual views of the cat figurine from the database ("actual"). At upper right we plot the model uncertainty in the latent space. The 24 latent coordinates from the training data are plotted as arrows, while the 48 novel latent points are plotted as crosses on a dashed line. At lower right we show model certainty for the cat figurine data $(1/\sigma_Z^2(\mathbf{x}))$ for each testing latent point $\mathbf{x}$. Note the low certainty for the blurry inferred images labeled 8, 14, and 26.

the limit of many correlated observation spaces. Rather than learning all pairwise relations between observation spaces (requiring a number of parameters quadratic in the number of observation spaces), our method learns one generative and one inverse mapping between each observation space and the latent space (so the number of parameters grows linearly).

From a cognitive science perspective, such an approach is similar to the Active Intermodal Mapping (AIM) hypothesis of imitation [6]. In AIM, an imitating agent maps its own actions and its perceptions of others' actions into a single, modality-independent space. This modality-independent space is analogous to the latent variable space in our model. Our model does not directly address the "correspondence problem" in imitation [7], where correspondences between an agent and a teacher are established through some form of un-supervised feature matching. However, it is reasonable to assume that imitation by a robot of human activity could involve some initial, explicit correspondence matching based on simultaneity. Turn-taking behavior is an integral part of human-human interaction. Thus, to bootstrap its database of corresponding data points, a robot could invite a human to take turns playing out motor sequences. Initially, the human would imitate the robot's actions and the robot could use this data to learn correspondences using our GP model; later, the robot could check and if necessary, refine its learned model by attempting to imitate the human's actions.

Acknowledgements: This work was supported by NSF AICS grant no. 130705 and an ONR YIP award/NSF Career award to RPNR. We thank the anonymous reviewers for their comments.

References

[1] K. Grochow, S. L. Martin, A. Hertzmann, and Z. Popović. Style-based inverse kinematics. In *Proc. SIGGRAPH*, 2004.

[2] J. Ham, D. Lee, and L. Saul. Semisupervised alignment of manifolds. In *AISTATS*, 2004.

[3] P. L. Lai and C. Fyfe. Kernel and nonlinear canonical correlation analysis. *Int. J. Neural Sys.*, 10(5):365–377, 2000.

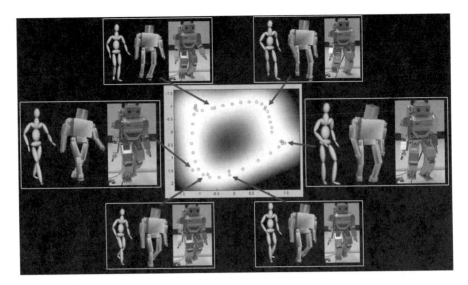

Figure 4: **Learning shared latent structure for robotic imitation of human actions:** The plot in the center shows the latent training points (red circles) and model precision $1/\sigma_Z^2$ for the robot model (grayscale plot), with examples of recovered latent points for testing data (blue diamonds). Model precision is qualitatively similar for the human model. Inset panels show the pose of the human motion capture skeleton, the simulated robot skeleton, and the humanoid robot for each example latent point. The model correctly infers robot poses from the human walking data (inset panels).

[4] N. D. Lawrence. Gaussian process models for visualization of high dimensional data. In S. Thrun, L. Saul, and B. Schölkopf, editors, *Advances in NIPS 16*.

[5] N. D. Lawrence, M. Seeger, and R. Herbrich. Fast sparse Gaussian process methods: the informative vector machine. In S. Becker, S. Thrun, and K. Obermayer, editors, *Advances in NIPS 15*, 2003.

[6] A. N. Meltzoff. Elements of a developmental theory of imitation. In A. N. Meltzoff and W. Prinz, editors, *The imitative mind: Development, evolution, and brain bases*, pages 19–41. Cambridge: Cambridge University Press, 2002.

[7] C. Nehaniv and K. Dautenhahn. The correspondence problem. In *Imitation in Animals and Artifacts*. MIT Press, 2002.

[8] A. O'Hagan. On curve fitting and optimal design for regression. *Journal of the Royal Statistical Society B*, 40:1–42, 1978.

[9] C. E. Rasmussen. *Evaluation of Gaussian Processes and other Methods for Non-Linear Regression*. PhD thesis, University of Toronto, 1996.

[10] S. Roweis and L. Saul. Nonlinear dimensionality reduction by locally linear embedding. *Science*, 290(5500):2323–2326, 2000.

[11] S. Schaal, A. Ijspeert, and A. Billard. Computational approaches to motor learning by imitation. *Phil. Trans. Royal Soc. London: Series B*, 358:537–547, 2003.

[12] A. P. Shon, D. B. Grimes, C. L. Baker, and R. P. N. Rao. A probabilistic framework for model-based imitation learning. In *Proc. 26th Ann. Mtg. Cog. Sci. Soc.*, 2004.

[13] J. B. Tenenbaum, V. de Silva, and J. C. Langford. A global geometric framework for nonlinear dimensionality reduction. *Science*, 290(5500):2319–2323, 2000.

[14] J. J. Verbeek, S. T. Roweis, and N. Vlassis. Non-linear CCA and PCA by alignment of local models. In *Advances in NIPS 16*, pages 297–304. 2003.

[15] C. K. I. Williams. Computing with infinite networks. In M. C. Mozer, M. I. Jordan, and T. Petsche, editors, *Advances in NIPS 9*. Cambridge, MA: MIT Press, 1996.

Selecting Landmark Points for Sparse Manifold Learning

J. G. Silva
ISEL/ISR
R. Conselheiro Emidio Navarro
1950.062 Lisbon, Portugal
jgs@isel.ipl.pt

J. S. Marques
IST/ISR
Av. Rovisco Pais
1949-001 Lisbon, Portugal
jsm@isr.ist.utl.pt

J. M. Lemos
INESC-ID/IST
R. Alves Redol, 9
1000-029 Lisbon, Portugal
jlml@inesc-id.pt

Abstract

There has been a surge of interest in learning non-linear manifold models to approximate high-dimensional data. Both for computational complexity reasons and for generalization capability, sparsity is a desired feature in such models. This usually means dimensionality reduction, which naturally implies estimating the intrinsic dimension, but it can also mean selecting a subset of the data to use as landmarks, which is especially important because many existing algorithms have quadratic complexity in the number of observations. This paper presents an algorithm for selecting landmarks, based on LASSO regression, which is well known to favor sparse approximations because it uses regularization with an l_1 norm. As an added benefit, a continuous manifold parameterization, based on the landmarks, is also found. Experimental results with synthetic and real data illustrate the algorithm.

1 Introduction

The recent interest in manifold learning algorithms is due, in part, to the multiplication of very large datasets of high-dimensional data from numerous disciplines of science, from signal processing to bioinformatics [6].

As an example, consider a video sequence such as the one in Figure 1. In the absence of features like contour points or wavelet coefficients, each image of size 71×71 pixels is a point in a space of dimension equal to the number of pixels, $71 \times 71 = 5041$. The observation space is, therefore, $\mathbb{R}^{5041}$. More generally, each observation is a vector $\mathbf{y} \in \mathbb{R}^m$ where m may be very large.

A reasonable assumption, when facing an observation space of possibly tens of thousands of dimensions, is that the data are not dense in such a space, because several of the mea-

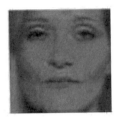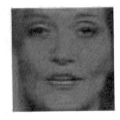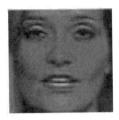

Figure 1: Example of a high-dimensional dataset: each image of size 71×71 pixels is a point in $\mathbb{R}^{5041}$.

sured variables must be dependent. In fact, in many problems of interest, there are only a few free parameters, which are embedded in the observed variables, frequently in a non-linear way. Assuming that the number of free parameters remains the same throughout the observations, and also assuming smooth variation of the parameters, one is in fact dealing with geometric restrictions which can be well modelled as a manifold.

Therefore, the data must lie on, or near (accounting for noise) a manifold embedded in observation, or ambient space. Learning this manifold is a natural approach to the problem of modelling the data, since, besides computational issues, sparse models tend to have better generalization capability. In order to achieve sparsity, considerable effort has been devoted to reducing the dimensionality of the data by some form of non-linear projection. Several algorithms ([10], [8], [3]) have emerged in recent years that follow this approach, which is closely related to the problem of feature extraction. In contrast, the problem of finding a relevant subset of the observations has received less attention.

It should be noted that the complexity of most existing algorithms is, in general, dependent not only on the dimensionality but also on the number of observations. An important example is the ISOMAP [10], where the computational cost is quadratic in the number of points, which has motivated the L-ISOMAP variant [3] which uses a randomly chosen subset of the points as *landmarks* (L is for Landmark).

The proposed algorithm uses, instead, a principled approach to select the landmarks, based on the solutions of a regression problem minimizing a regularized cost functional. When the regularization term is based on the l_1 norm, the solution tends to be sparse. This is the motivation for using the Least Absolute value Subset Selection Operator (LASSO) [5].

Finding the LASSO solutions used to require solving a quadratic programming problem, until the development of the Least Angle Regression (LARS[1]) procedure [4], which is much faster (the cost is equivalent to that of ordinary least squares) and not only gives the LASSO solutions but also provides an estimator of the risk as a function of the regularization tuning parameter. This means that the correct amount of regularization can be automatically found.

In the specific context of selecting landmarks for manifold learning, with some care in the LASSO problem formulation, one is able to avoid a difficult problem of sparse regression with Multiple Measurement Vectors (MMV), which has received considerable interest in its own right [2].

The idea is to use local information, found by local PCA as usual, and preserve the smooth variation of the tangent subspace over a larger scale, taking advantage of any known embedding. This is a natural extension of the Tangent Bundle Approximation (TBA) algorithm, proposed in [9], since the principal angles, which TBA computes anyway, are readily avail-

---

[1]The S in LARS stands for Stagewise and LASSO, an allusion to the relationship between the three algorithms.

able and appropriate for this purpose. Nevertheless, the method proposed here is independent of TBA and could, for instance, be plugged into a global procedure like L-ISOMAP.

The algorithm avoids costly global computations, that is, it doesn't attempt to preserve geodesic distances between faraway points, and yet, unlike most local algorithms, it is explicitly designed to be sparse while retaining generalization ability.

The remainder of this introduction formulates the problem and establishes the notation. The selection procedure itself is covered in section 2, while also providing a quick overview of the LASSO and LARS methods. Results are presented in section 3 and then discussed in section 4.

1.1 Problem formulation

The problem can be formulated as following: given N vectors $\mathbf{y} \in \mathbb{R}^m$, suppose that the $\mathbf{y}$ can be approximated by a differentiable n-manifold $\mathcal{M}$ embedded in $\mathbb{R}^m$. This means that $\mathcal{M}$ can be *charted* through one or more invertible and differentiable mappings of the type

$$g_i(\mathbf{y}) = \mathbf{x} \tag{1}$$

to vectors $\mathbf{x} \in \mathbb{R}^n$ so that open sets $\mathcal{P}_i \subset \mathcal{M}$, called *patches*, whose union covers $\mathcal{M}$, are diffeomorphically mapped onto other open sets $\mathcal{U}_i \subset \mathbb{R}^n$, called *parametric domains*. $\mathbb{R}^n$ is the lower dimensional parameter space and n is the intrinsic dimension of $\mathcal{M}$. The g_i are called *charts*, and manifolds with complex topology may require several g_i. Equivalently, since the charts are invertible, inverse mappings $h_i : \mathbb{R}^n \to \mathbb{R}^m$, called *parameterizations* can be also be found.

Arranging the original data in a matrix $\mathbf{Y} \in \mathbb{R}^{m \times N}$, with the $\mathbf{y}$ as column vectors and assuming, for now, only one mapping g, the charting process produces a matrix $\mathbf{X} \in \mathbb{R}^{n \times N}$:

$$\mathbf{Y} = \begin{bmatrix} y_{11} & \cdots & y_{1N} \\ \vdots & \ddots & \vdots \\ y_{m1} & \cdots & y_{mN} \end{bmatrix} \quad \mathbf{X} = \begin{bmatrix} x_{11} & \cdots & x_{1N} \\ \vdots & \ddots & \vdots \\ x_{n1} & \cdots & x_{nN} \end{bmatrix} \tag{2}$$

The n rows of $\mathbf{X}$ are sometimes called *features* or *latent variables*. It is often intended in manifold learning to estimate the correct intrinsic dimension, n, as well as the chart g or at least a column-to-column mapping from $\mathbf{Y}$ to $\mathbf{X}$. In the present case, this mapping will be assumed known, and so will n.

What is intended is to select a subset of the *columns* of $\mathbf{X}$ (or of $\mathbf{Y}$, since the mapping between them is known) to use as landmarks, while retaining enough information about g, resulting in a reduced $n \times N'$ matrix with $N' < N$. N' is the number of landmarks, and should also be automatically determined.

Preserving g is equivalent to preserving its inverse mapping, the parameterization h, which is more practical because it allows the following generative model:

$$\mathbf{y} = h(\mathbf{x}) + \boldsymbol{\eta} \tag{3}$$

in which $\boldsymbol{\eta}$ is zero mean Gaussian observation noise. How to find the fewest possible landmarks so that h can still be well approximated?

2 Landmark selection

2.1 Linear regression model

To solve the problem, it is proposed to start by converting the non-linear regression in (3) to a *linear* regression by offloading the non-linearity onto a kernel, as described in numerous works, such as [7]. Since there are N columns in $\mathbf{X}$ to start with, let $\mathbf{K}$ be a square, $N \times N$, symmetric semidefinite positive matrix such that

$$
\begin{aligned}
\mathbf{K} &= \{k_{ij}\} \\
k_{ij} &= K(\mathbf{x}_i, \mathbf{x}_j) \\
K(\mathbf{x}, \mathbf{x}_j) &= \exp(-\frac{\|\mathbf{x} - \mathbf{x}_j\|^2}{2\sigma_K^2}).
\end{aligned}
\tag{4}
$$

The function K can be readily recognized as a Gaussian kernel. This allows the reformulation, in matrix form, of (3) as

$$
\mathbf{Y}^T = \mathbf{K}\mathbf{B} + \mathbf{E}
\tag{5}
$$

,

where $\mathbf{B}, \mathbf{E} \in \mathbb{R}^{N \times m}$ and each line of $\mathbf{E}$ is a realization of η above. Still, it is difficult to proceed directly from (5), because neither the response, $\mathbf{Y}^T$, nor the regression parameters, $\mathbf{B}$, are column vectors. This leads to a Multiple Measurement Vectors (MMV) problem, and while there is nothing to prevent solving it separately for each column, this makes it harder to impose sparsity in all columns *simultaneously*. Two alternative approaches present themselves at this point:

- Solve a sparse regression problem for each column of $\mathbf{Y}^T$ (and the corresponding column of $\mathbf{B}$), find a way to force several *lines* of $\mathbf{B}$ to zero.
- Re-formulate (5) is a way that turns it to a single measurement value problem.

The second approach is better studied, and it will be the one followed here. Since the parameterization h is known and must be, at the very least, bijective and continuous, then it must preserve the smoothness of quantities like the geodesic distance and the principal angles. Therefore, it is proposed to re-formulate (5) as

$$
\boldsymbol{\theta} = \mathbf{K}\boldsymbol{\beta} + \boldsymbol{\epsilon}
\tag{6}
$$

where the new response, $\boldsymbol{\theta} \in \mathbb{R}^N$, as well as $\boldsymbol{\beta} \in \mathbb{R}^N$ and $\boldsymbol{\epsilon} \in \mathbb{R}^N$ are now column vectors, allowing the use of known subset selection procedures.

The elements of $\boldsymbol{\theta}$ can be, for example, the geodesic distances to the $\mathbf{y}_\mu = h(\mathbf{x}_\mu)$ observation corresponding to the mean, $\mathbf{x}_\mu$ of the columns of $\mathbf{X}$. This would be a possibility if an algorithm like ISOMAP were used to find the chart from $\mathbf{Y}$ to $\mathbf{X}$. However, since the whole point of using landmarks is to know them beforehand, so as to avoid having to compute $N \times N$ geodesic distances, this is not the most interesting alternative.

A better way is to use a computationally lighter quantity like the maximum principal angle between the tangent subspace at $\mathbf{y}_\mu$, $T_{\mathbf{y}_\mu}(\mathcal{M})$, and the tangent subspaces at all other $\mathbf{y}$.

Given a point $\mathbf{y}_0$ and its k nearest neighbors, finding the tangent subspace can be done by local PCA. The sample covariance matrix $\mathbf{S}$ can be decomposed as

$$\mathbf{S} = \frac{1}{k} \sum_{i=0}^{k} (\mathbf{y}_i - \mathbf{y}_0)(\mathbf{y}_i - \mathbf{y}_0)^T \tag{7}$$

$$\mathbf{S} = \mathbf{V}\mathbf{D}\mathbf{V}^T \tag{8}$$

where the columns of $\mathbf{V}$ are the eigenvectors $\mathbf{v}_i$ and $\mathbf{D}$ is a diagonal matrix containing the eigenvalues λ_i, in descending order. The eigenvectors form an orthonormal basis aligned with the principal directions of the data. They can be divided in two groups: tangent and normal vectors, spanning the tangent and normal subspaces, with dimensions n and $m - n$, respectively. Note that $m - n$ is the *codimension* of the manifold. The tangent subspaces are spanned from the n most important eigenvectors. The principal angles between two different tangent subspaces at different points $\mathbf{y}_0$ can be determined from the column spaces of the corresponding matrices $\mathbf{V}$.

An in-depth description of the principal angles, as well as efficient algorithms to compute them, can be found, for instance, in [1]. Note that, should the $T_\mathbf{y}(\mathcal{M})$ be already available from the eigenvectors found during some local PCA analysis, e. g., during estimation of the intrinsic dimension, there would be little extra computational burden. An example is [9], where the principal angles already are an integral part of the procedure - namely for partitioning the manifold into patches.

Thus, it is proposed to use θ_j equal to the maximum principal angle between $T_{\mathbf{y}_\mu}(\mathcal{M})$ and $T_{\mathbf{y}_j}(\mathcal{M})$, where $\mathbf{y}_j$ is the j-th column of $\mathbf{Y}$. It remains to be explained how to achieve a sparse solution to (6).

2.2 Sparsity with LASSO and LARS

The idea is to find an estimate $\hat{\boldsymbol{\beta}}$ that minimizes the functional

$$E = \|\boldsymbol{\theta} - \mathbf{K}\hat{\boldsymbol{\beta}}\|^2 + \gamma\|\hat{\boldsymbol{\beta}}\|_q^q. \tag{9}$$

Here, $\|\hat{\boldsymbol{\beta}}\|_q$ denotes the l_q norm of $\hat{\boldsymbol{\beta}}$, i. e. $\sqrt[q]{\sum_{i=1}^m |\hat{\beta}_i|^q}$, and γ is a tuning parameter that controls the amount of regularization. For the most sparseness, the ideal value of q would be zero. However, minimizing E with the l_0 norm is, in general, prohibitive in computational terms. A sub-optimal strategy is to use $q = 1$ instead. This is the usual formulation of a LASSO regression problem. While minimization of (9) can be done using quadratic programming, the recent development of the LARS method has made this unnecessary. For a detailed description of LARS and its relationship with the LASSO, *vide* [4].

Very briefly, LARS starts with $\hat{\boldsymbol{\beta}} = \mathbf{0}$ and adds covariates (the columns of $\mathbf{K}$) to the model according to their correlation with the prediction error vector, $\boldsymbol{\theta} - \mathbf{K}\hat{\boldsymbol{\beta}}$, setting the corresponding $\hat{\beta}_j$ to a value such that another covariate becomes equally correlated with the error and is, itself, added to the model - it becomes *active*. LARS then proceeds in a direction equiangular to all the active $\hat{\beta}_j$ and the process is repeated until all covariates have been added. There are a total of m steps, each of which adds a new $\hat{\beta}_j$, making it non-zero. With slight modifications, these steps correspond to a sampling of the tuning parameter γ in (9) under LASSO. Moreover, [4] shows that the risk, as a function of the number, p, of non-zero $\hat{\beta}_j$, can be estimated (under mild assumptions) as

$$R(\hat{\boldsymbol{\beta}}_p) = \|\boldsymbol{\theta} - \mathbf{K}\hat{\boldsymbol{\beta}}_p\|^2/\bar{\sigma}^2 - m + 2p \tag{10}$$

where $\bar{\sigma}^2$ can be found from the unconstrained least squares solution of (6). Computing $R(\hat{\boldsymbol{\beta}}_p)$ requires no more than the $\hat{\boldsymbol{\beta}}_p$ themselves, which are already provided by LARS anyway.

2.3 Landmarks and parameterization of the manifold

The landmarks are the columns $\mathbf{x}_j$ of $\mathbf{X}$ (or of $\mathbf{Y}$) with the same indexes j as the non-zero elements of $\boldsymbol{\beta}_p$, where

$$p = \arg\min_p R(\boldsymbol{\beta}_p). \tag{11}$$

There are $N' = p$ landmarks, because there are p non-zero elements in $\boldsymbol{\beta}_p$. This criterion ensures that the landmarks are the kernel centers that minimize the risk of the regression in (6).

As an interesting byproduct, regardless of whether h was a continuous or point-to-point mapping to begin with, it is now also possible to obtain a new, continuous parameterization $h_{\mathbf{B},\mathbf{X}'}$ by solving a reduced version of (5):

$$\mathbf{Y}^T = \mathbf{B}\mathbf{K}' + \mathbf{E} \tag{12}$$

where $\mathbf{K}'$ only has N' columns, with the same indexes as $\mathbf{X}'$. In fact, $\mathbf{K}' \in \mathbb{R}^{N \times N'}$ is no longer square. Also, now $\mathbf{B} \in \mathbb{R}^{N' \times m}$. The new, smaller regression (12) can be solved separately for each column of $\mathbf{Y}^T$ and $\mathbf{B}$ by *unconstrained* least squares. For a new feature vector, $\mathbf{x}$, in the parametric domain, a new vector $\mathbf{y} \in \mathcal{M}$ in observation space can be synthesized by

$$\begin{aligned} \mathbf{y} = h_{\mathbf{B},\mathbf{X}'}(\mathbf{x}) &= [y_1(\mathbf{x}) \dots y_m(\mathbf{x})]^T \\ y_j(\mathbf{x}) &= \sum_{\mathbf{x}_i \in \mathbf{X}'} b_{ij} K(\mathbf{x}_i, \mathbf{x}) \end{aligned} \tag{13}$$

where the $\{b_{ij}\}$ are the elements of $\mathbf{B}$.

3 Results

The algorithm has been tested in two synthetic datasets: the traditional synthetic "swiss roll" and a sphere, both with 1000 points embedded in $\mathbb{R}^{10}$, with a small amount of isotropic Gaussian noise ($\sigma_{\mathbf{y}} = 0.01$) added in all dimensions, as shown in Figure 2. These manifolds have intrinsic dimension $n = 2$. A global embedding for the swiss roll was found by ISOMAP, using $k = 8$. On the other hand, TBA was used for the sphere, resulting in multiple patches and charts - a necessity, because otherwise the sphere's topology would make ISOMAP fail. Therefore, in the sphere, each patch has its own landmark points, and the manifold require the union of all such points. All are shown in Figure 2, as selected by our procedure.

Additionally, a real dataset was used: images from the video sequence shown above in Figure 1. This example is known [9] to be reasonably well modelled by as few as 2 free parameters.

The sequence contains $N = 194$ frames with $m = 5041$ pixels. A first step was to perform global PCA in order to discard irrelevant dimensions. Since it obviously isn't possible

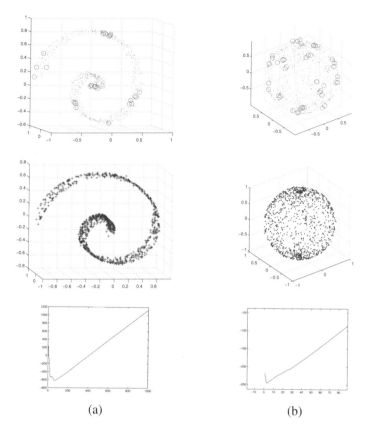

Figure 2: *Above*: landmarks; *Middle*: interpolated points using $h_{\mathbf{B},\mathbf{X}'}$; *Below*: risk estimates. For the sphere, the risk plot is for the largest patch. Total landmarks, $N' = 27$ for the swiss roll, 42 for the sphere.

to compute a covariance matrix of size 5000×5000 from 194 samples, the problem was transposed, leading to the computation of the eigenvectors of a $N \times N$ covariance, from which the first $N - 1$ eigenvectors of the non-transposed problem can easily be found [11]. This resulted in an estimated 15 globally significant principal directions, on which the data were projected.

After this pre-processing, the effective values of m and N were, respectively, 15 and 194. An embedding was found using TBA with 2 features (ISOMAP would have worked as well). The results obtained for this case are shown in Figure 3. Only 4 landmarks were needed, and they correspond to very distinct face expressions.

4   Discussion

A new approach for selecting landmarks in manifold learning, based on LASSO and LARS regression, has been presented. The proposed algorithm finds geometrically meaningful landmarks and successfully circumvents a difficult MMV problem, by using the intuition that, since the variation of the maximum principal angle is a measure of curvature, the points that are important in preserving it should also be important in preserving the overall manifold geometry. Also, a continuous manifold parameterization is given with very little

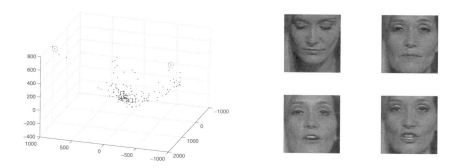

Figure 3: Landmarks for the video sequence: $N' = 4$, marked over a scatter plot of the first 3 eigen-coordinates. The corresponding pictures are also shown.

additional computational cost.

The entire procedure avoids expensive, quadratic programming computations - its complexity is dominated by the LARS step, which has the same cost as a least squares fit [4]. The proposed approach has been validated with experiments on synthetic and real datasets.

Acknowledgments

This work was partially supported by FCT POCTI, under project 37844.

References

[1] A. Bjorck and G. H. Golub. Numerical methods for computing angles between linear subspaces. *Mathematical Computation*, 27, 1973.

[2] J. Chen and X. Huo. Sparse representation for multiple measurement vectors (mmv) in an over-complete dictionary. *ICASSP*, 2005.

[3] V. de Silva and J. B. Tenenbaum. Global versus local methods in nonlinear dimensionality reduction. *NIPS*, 15, 2002.

[4] B. Efron, T. Hastie, I. Johnstone, and R. Tibshirani. Least angle regression. *Annals of Statistics*, 2003.

[5] T. Hastie, R. Tibshirani, and J. H. Friedman. *The Elements of Statistical Learning*. Springer, 2001.

[6] H. Lädesmäki, O. Yli-Harja, W. Zhang, and I. Shmulevich. Intrinsic dimensionality in gene expression analysis. *GENSIPS*, 2005.

[7] T. Poggio and S. Smale. The mathematics of learning: Dealing with data. *Notices of the American Mathematical Society*, 2003.

[8] S. T. Roweis and L. K. Saul. Nonlinear dimensionality reduction by locally linear embedding. *Science*, 290:2323–2326, 2000.

[9] J. Silva, J. Marques, and J. M. Lemos. Non-linear dimension reduction with tangent bundle approximation. *ICASSP*, 2005.

[10] J. B. Tenenbaum, V. de Silva, and J. C. Langford. A global geometric framework for nonlinear dimensionality reduction. *Science*, 290:2319–2323, 2000.

[11] M. Turk and A. Pentland. Eigenfaces for recognition. *Journal of Cognitive Neuroscience*, 3:71–86, 1991.

Conditional Visual Tracking in Kernel Space

Cristian Sminchisescu[1,2,3] **Atul Kanujia**[3] **Zhiguo Li**[3] **Dimitris Metaxas**[3]
[1]TTI-C, 1497 East 50th Street, Chicago, IL, 60637, USA
[2]University of Toronto, Department of Computer Science, Canada
[3]Rutgers University, Department of Computer Science, USA
`crismin@cs.toronto.edu`, {`kanaujia,zhli,dnm`}`@cs.rutgers.edu`

Abstract

We present a conditional temporal probabilistic framework for reconstructing 3D human motion in monocular video based on descriptors encoding image silhouette observations. For computational efficiency we restrict visual inference to low-dimensional kernel induced non-linear state spaces. Our methodology (kBME) combines kernel PCA-based non-linear dimensionality reduction (kPCA) and Conditional Bayesian Mixture of Experts (BME) in order to learn complex multivalued predictors between observations and model hidden states. This is necessary for accurate, inverse, visual perception inferences, where several probable, distant 3D solutions exist due to noise or the uncertainty of monocular perspective projection. Low-dimensional models are appropriate because many visual processes exhibit strong non-linear correlations in both the image observations and the target, hidden state variables. The learned predictors are temporally combined within a conditional graphical model in order to allow a principled propagation of uncertainty. We study several predictors and empirically show that the proposed algorithm positively compares with techniques based on regression, Kernel Dependency Estimation (KDE) or PCA alone, and gives results competitive to those of high-dimensional mixture predictors at a fraction of their computational cost. We show that the method successfully reconstructs the complex 3D motion of humans in real monocular video sequences.

1 Introduction and Related Work

We consider the problem of inferring 3D articulated human motion from monocular video. This research topic has applications for scene understanding including human-computer interfaces, markerless human motion capture, entertainment and surveillance. A monocular approach is relevant because in real-world settings the human body parts are rarely completely observed even when using multiple cameras. This is due to occlusions form other people or objects in the scene. A robust system has to necessarily deal with incomplete, ambiguous and uncertain measurements. Methods for 3D human motion reconstruction can be classified as *generative* and *discriminative*. They both require a state representation, namely a 3D human model with kinematics (joint angles) or shape (surfaces or joint positions) and they both use a set of image features as observations for state inference. The computational goal in both cases is the conditional distribution for the model state given image observations.

Generative model-based approaches [6, 16, 14, 13] have been demonstrated to flexibly reconstruct complex unknown human motions and to naturally handle problem constraints. However it is difficult to construct reliable observation likelihoods due to the complexity of modeling human appearance. This varies widely due to different clothing and deformation, body proportions or lighting conditions. Besides being somewhat indirect, the generative approach further imposes strict conditional independence assumptions on the temporal observations given the states in order to ensure computational tractability. Due to these factors inference is expensive and produces highly multimodal state distributions [6, 16, 13]. Generative inference algorithms require complex annealing schedules [6, 13] or systematic non-linear search for local optima [16] in order to ensure continuing tracking.

These difficulties motivate the advent of a complementary class of discriminative algorithms [10, 12, 18, 2], that approximate the state conditional directly, in order to simplify inference. However, inverse, observation-to-state multivalued mappings are difficult to learn (see *e.g.* fig. 1a) and a probabilistic temporal setting is necessary. In an earlier paper [15] we introduced a probabilistic discriminative framework for human motion reconstruction. Because the method operates in the originally selected state and observation spaces that can be task generic, therefore redundant and often high-dimensional, inference is more expensive and can be less robust. To summarize, reconstructing 3D human motion in a

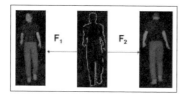 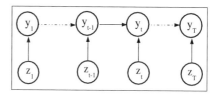

Figure 1: *(a, Left)* Example of 180° ambiguity in predicting 3D human poses from silhouette image features (center). It is essential that multiple plausible solutions (*e.g.* F_1 and F_2) are correctly represented and tracked over time. A single state predictor will either average the distant solutions or zig-zag between them, see also tables 1 and 2. *(b, Right)* A conditional chain model. The local distributions $p(\mathbf{y}_t|\mathbf{y}_{t-1}, \mathbf{z}_t)$ or $p(\mathbf{y}_t|\mathbf{z}_t)$ are learned as in fig. 2. For inference, the predicted local state conditional is recursively combined with the filtered prior *c.f.* (1).

conditional temporal framework poses the following difficulties: (*i*) The mapping between temporal observations and states is multivalued (*i.e.* the local conditional distributions to be learned are multimodal), therefore it cannot be accurately represented using global function approximations. (*ii*) Human models have multivariate, high-dimensional continuous states of 50 or more human joint angles. The temporal state conditionals are multimodal which makes efficient Kalman filtering algorithms inapplicable. General inference methods (particle filters, mixtures) have to be used instead, but these are expensive for high-dimensional models (*e.g.* when reconstructing the motion of several people that operate in a joint state space). (*iii*) The components of the human state and of the silhouette observation vector exhibit strong correlations, because many repetitive human activities like walking or running have low intrinsic dimensionality. It appears wasteful to work with high-dimensional states of 50+ joint angles. Even if the space were truly high-dimensional, predicting correlated state dimensions independently may still be suboptimal.

In this paper we present a conditional temporal estimation algorithm that restricts visual inference to low-dimensional, kernel induced state spaces. To exploit correlations among observations and among state variables, we model the local, temporal conditional distributions using ideas from Kernel PCA [11, 19] and conditional mixture modeling [7, 5], here adapted to produce multiple probabilistic predictions. The corresponding predictor is referred to as a *Conditional Bayesian Mixture of Low-dimensional Kernel-Induced Experts (kBME)*. By integrating it within a conditional graphical model framework (fig. 1b), we can exploit temporal constraints probabilistically. We demonstrate that this methodology is effective for reconstructing the 3D motion of multiple people in monocular video. Our contribution w.r.t. [15] is a probabilistic conditional inference framework that operates over a non-linear, kernel-induced low-dimensional state spaces, and a set of experiments (on both real and artificial image sequences) that show how the proposed framework positively compares with powerful predictors based on KDE, PCA, or with the high-dimensional models of [15] at a fraction of their cost.

2 Probabilistic Inference in a Kernel Induced State Space

We work with conditional graphical models with a chain structure [9], as shown in fig. 1b, These have continuous temporal states $\mathbf{y}_t$, $t = 1 \ldots T$, observations $\mathbf{z}_t$. For compactness, we denote joint states $\mathbf{Y}_t = (\mathbf{y}_1, \mathbf{y}_2, \ldots, \mathbf{y}_t)$ or joint observations $\mathbf{Z}_t = (\mathbf{z}_1, \ldots, \mathbf{z}_t)$. Learning and inference are based on local conditionals: $p(\mathbf{y}_t|\mathbf{z}_t)$ and $p(\mathbf{y}_t|\mathbf{y}_{t-1}, \mathbf{z}_t)$, with $\mathbf{y}_t$ and $\mathbf{z}_t$ being low-dimensional, kernel induced representations of some initial model having state $\mathbf{x}_t$ and observation $\mathbf{r}_t$. We obtain $\mathbf{z}_t, \mathbf{y}_t$ from $\mathbf{r}_t, \mathbf{x}_t$ using kernel PCA [11, 19]. *Inference is performed in a low-dimensional, non-linear, kernel induced latent state space* (see fig. 1b and fig. 2 and (1)). For display or error reporting, we compute the original conditional $p(\mathbf{x}|\mathbf{r})$, or a temporally filtered version $p(\mathbf{x}_t|\mathbf{R}_t)$, $\mathbf{R}_t = (\mathbf{r}_1, \mathbf{r}_2, \ldots, \mathbf{r}_t)$, using a learned pre-image state map [3].

2.1 Density Propagation for Continuous Conditional Chains

For online filtering, we compute the optimal distribution $p(\mathbf{y}_t|\mathbf{Z}_t)$ for the state $\mathbf{y}_t$, conditioned by observations $\mathbf{Z}_t$ up to time t. The filtered density can be recursively derived as:

$$p(\mathbf{y}_t|\mathbf{Z}_t) = \int_{\mathbf{y}_{t-1}} p(\mathbf{y}_t|\mathbf{y}_{t-1}, \mathbf{z}_t) p(\mathbf{y}_{t-1}|\mathbf{Z}_{t-1}) \tag{1}$$

We compute using a conditional mixture for $p(\mathbf{y}_t|\mathbf{y}_{t-1}, \mathbf{z}_t)$ (a Bayesian mixture of experts *c.f.* §2.2) and the prior $p(\mathbf{y}_{t-1}|\mathbf{Z}_{t-1})$, each having, say M components. We integrate M^2 pairwise products of Gaussians analytically. The means of the expanded posterior are clustered and the centers are used to initialize a reduced M-component Kullback-Leibler approximation that is refined using gradient descent [15]. The propagation rule (1) is similar to the one used for discrete state labels [9], but here we work with multivariate continuous state spaces and represent the local multimodal state conditionals using kBME (fig. 2), and not log-linear models [9] (these would require intractable normalization). This complex continuous model rules out inference based on Kalman filtering or dynamic programming [9].

2.2 Learning Bayesian Mixtures over Kernel Induced State Spaces (kBME)

In order to model conditional mappings between low-dimensional non-linear spaces we rely on kernel dimensionality reduction and conditional mixture predictors. The authors of KDE [19] propose a powerful structured unimodal predictor. This works by decorrelating the output using kernel PCA and learning a ridge regressor between the input and each decorrelated output dimension.

Our procedure is also based on kernel PCA but takes into account the structure of the studied visual problem where both inputs and outputs are likely to be low-dimensional and the mapping between them multivalued. The output variables $\mathbf{x}_i$ are projected onto the column vectors of the principal space in order to obtain their principal coordinates $\mathbf{y}_i$. A

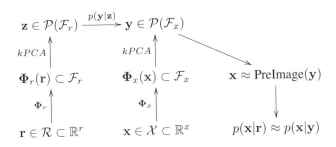

Figure 2: The learned low-dimensional predictor, kBME, for computing $p(\mathbf{x}|\mathbf{r}) \equiv p(\mathbf{x}_t|\mathbf{r}_t), \forall t$. (We similarly learn $p(\mathbf{x}_t|\mathbf{x}_{t-1}, \mathbf{r}_t)$, with input $(\mathbf{x}, \mathbf{r})$ instead of $\mathbf{r}$ – here we illustrate only $p(\mathbf{x}|\mathbf{r})$ for clarity.) The input $\mathbf{r}$ and the output $\mathbf{x}$ are decorrelated using Kernel PCA to obtain $\mathbf{z}$ and $\mathbf{y}$ respectively. The kernels used for the input and output are $\boldsymbol{\Phi}_r$ and $\boldsymbol{\Phi}_x$, with induced feature spaces $\mathcal{F}_r$ and $\mathcal{F}_x$, respectively. Their principal subspaces obtained by kernel PCA are denoted by $\mathcal{P}(\mathcal{F}_r)$ and $\mathcal{P}(\mathcal{F}_x)$, respectively. A conditional Bayesian mixture of experts $p(\mathbf{y}|\mathbf{z})$ is learned using the low-dimensional representation $(\mathbf{z}, \mathbf{y})$. Using learned local conditionals of the form $p(\mathbf{y}_t|\mathbf{z}_t)$ or $p(\mathbf{y}_t|\mathbf{y}_{t-1}, \mathbf{z}_t)$, temporal inference can be efficiently performed in a *low-dimensional kernel induced state space* (see *e.g.* (1) and fig. 1b). For visualization and error measurement, the filtered density, *e.g.* $p(\mathbf{y}_t|\mathbf{Z}_t)$, can be mapped back to $p(\mathbf{x}_t|\mathbf{R}_t)$ using the pre-image *c.f.* (3).

similar procedure is performed on the inputs $\mathbf{r}_i$ to obtain $\mathbf{z}_i$. In order to relate the reduced feature spaces of $\mathbf{z}$ and $\mathbf{y}$ ($\mathcal{P}(\mathcal{F}_r)$ and $\mathcal{P}(\mathcal{F}_x)$), we estimate a probability distribution over mappings from training pairs $(\mathbf{z}_i, \mathbf{y}_i)$. We use a conditional Bayesian mixture of experts (BME) [7, 5] in order to account for ambiguity when mapping similar, possibly identical reduced feature inputs to very different feature outputs, as common in our problem (fig. 1a). This gives a model that is a conditional mixture of low-dimensional kernel-induced experts (kBME):

$$p(\mathbf{y}|\mathbf{z}) = \sum_{j=1}^{M} g(\mathbf{z}|\boldsymbol{\delta}_j)\mathcal{N}(\mathbf{y}|\mathbf{W}_j\mathbf{z}, \boldsymbol{\Sigma}_j) \tag{2}$$

where $g(\mathbf{z}|\boldsymbol{\delta}_j)$ is a softmax function parameterized by $\boldsymbol{\delta}_j$ and $(\mathbf{W}_j, \boldsymbol{\Sigma}_j)$ are the parameters and the output covariance of expert j, here a linear regressor. As in many Bayesian settings [17, 5], the weights of the experts and of the gates, $\mathbf{W}_j$ and $\boldsymbol{\delta}_j$, are controlled by hierarchical priors, typically Gaussians with 0 mean, and having inverse variance hyperparameters controlled by a second level of Gamma distributions. We learn this model using a double-loop EM and employ ML-II type approximations [8, 17] with greedy (weight) subset selection [17, 15].

Finally, the kBME algorithm requires the computation of pre-images in order to recover the state distribution $\mathbf{x}$ from it's image $\mathbf{y} \in \mathcal{P}(\mathcal{F}_x)$. This is a closed form computation for polynomial kernels of odd degree. For more general kernels optimization or learning (regression based) methods are necessary [3]. Following [3, 19], we use a sparse Bayesian kernel regressor to learn the pre-image. This is based on training data $(\mathbf{x}_i, \mathbf{y}_i)$:

$$p(\mathbf{x}|\mathbf{y}) = \mathcal{N}(\mathbf{x}|\mathbf{A}\boldsymbol{\Phi}_y(\mathbf{y}), \boldsymbol{\Omega}) \tag{3}$$

with parameters and covariances $(\mathbf{A}, \boldsymbol{\Omega})$. Since temporal inference is performed in the low-dimensional kernel induced state space, the pre-image function needs to be calculated only for visualizing results or for the purpose of error reporting. Propagating the result from the reduced feature space $\mathcal{P}(\mathcal{F}_x)$ to the output space $\mathcal{X}$ produces a Gaussian mixture with M elements, having coefficients $g(\mathbf{z}|\boldsymbol{\delta}_j)$ and components $\mathcal{N}(\mathbf{x}|\mathbf{A}\boldsymbol{\Phi}_y(\mathbf{W}_j\mathbf{z}), \mathbf{A}\mathbf{J}_{\boldsymbol{\Phi}_y}\boldsymbol{\Sigma}_j\mathbf{J}_{\boldsymbol{\Phi}_y}^\top\mathbf{A}^\top + \boldsymbol{\Omega})$, where $\mathbf{J}_{\boldsymbol{\Phi}_y}$ is the Jacobian of the mapping $\boldsymbol{\Phi}_y$.

3 Experiments

We run experiments on both real image sequences (fig. 5 and fig. 6) and on sequences where silhouettes were artificially rendered. The prediction error is reported in degrees (for mixture of experts, this is w.r.t. the most probable one, but see also fig. 4a), and normalized per joint angle, per frame. The models are learned using standard cross-validation. Pre-images are learned using kernel regressors and have average error 1.7°.

Training Set and Model State Representation: For training we gather pairs of 3D human poses together with their image projections, here silhouettes, using the graphics package Maya. We use realistically rendered computer graphics human surface models which we animate using human motion capture [1]. Our original human representation ($\mathbf{x}$) is based on articulated skeletons with spherical joints and has 56 skeletal d.o.f. including global translation. The database consists of 8000 samples of human activities including walking, running, turns, jumps, gestures in conversations, quarreling and pantomime.

Image Descriptors: We work with image silhouettes obtained using statistical background subtraction (with foreground and background models). Silhouettes are informative for pose estimation although prone to ambiguities (*e.g.* the left / right limb assignment in side views) or occasional lack of observability of some of the d.o.f. (*e.g.* 180° ambiguities in the global azimuthal orientation for frontal views, *e.g.* fig. 1a). These are multiplied by intrinsic forward / backward monocular ambiguities [16]. As observations $\mathbf{r}$, we use shape contexts extracted on the silhouette [4] (5 radial, 12 angular bins, size range 1/8 to 3 on log scale).

The features are computed at different scales and sizes for points sampled on the silhouette. To work in a common coordinate system, we cluster all features in the training set into $K = 50$ clusters. To compute the representation of a new shape feature (a point on the silhouette), we 'project' onto the common basis by (inverse distance) weighted voting into the cluster centers. To obtain the representation ($\mathbf{r}$) for a new silhouette we regularly sample 200 points on it and add all their feature vectors into a feature histogram. Because the representation uses *overlapping features of the observation* the elements of the descriptor are not independent. However, a conditional temporal framework (fig. 1b) flexibly accommodates this.

For experiments, we use Gaussian kernels for the joint angle feature space and dot product kernels for the observation feature space. We learn state conditionals for $p(\mathbf{y}_t|\mathbf{z}_t)$ and $p(\mathbf{y}_t|\mathbf{y}_{t-1}, \mathbf{z}_t)$ using 6 dimensions for the joint angle kernel induced state space and 25 dimensions for the observation induced feature space, respectively. In fig. 3b) we show an evaluation of the efficacy of our kBME predictor for different dimensions in the joint angle kernel induced state space (the observation feature space dimension is here 50). On the analyzed dancing sequence, that involves complex motions of the arms and the legs, the non-linear model significantly outperforms alternative PCA methods and gives good predictions for compact, low-dimensional models.[1]

In tables 1 and 2, as well as fig. 4, we perform quantitative experiments on artificially rendered silhouettes. 3D ground truth joint angles are available and this allows a more

---

[1]**Running times:** On a Pentium 4 PC (3 GHz, 2 GB RAM), a full dimensional BME model with 5 experts takes 802s to train $p(\mathbf{x}_t|\mathbf{x}_{t-1}, \mathbf{r}_t)$, whereas a kBME (including the pre-image) takes 95s to train $p(\mathbf{y}_t|\mathbf{y}_{t-1}, \mathbf{z}_t)$. The prediction time is 13.7s for BME and 8.7s (including the pre-image cost 1.04s) for kBME. The integration in (1) takes 2.67s for BME and 0.31s for kBME. The speed-up for kBME is significant and likely to increase with original models having higher dimensionality.

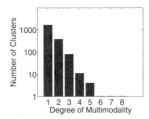 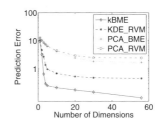

Figure 3: *(a, Left)* Analysis of 'multimodality' for a training set. The input $\mathbf{z}_t$ dimension is 25, the output $\mathbf{y}_t$ dimension is 6, both reduced using kPCA. We cluster independently in $(\mathbf{y}_{t-1}, \mathbf{z}_t)$ and $\mathbf{y}_t$ using many clusters (2100) to simulate small input perturbations and we histogram the $\mathbf{y}_t$ clusters falling within each cluster in $(\mathbf{y}_{t-1}, \mathbf{z}_t)$. This gives intuition on the degree of ambiguity in modeling $p(\mathbf{y}_t|\mathbf{y}_{t-1}, \mathbf{z}_t)$, for small perturbations in the input. *(b, Right)* Evaluation of dimensionality reduction methods for an artificial dancing sequence (models trained on 300 samples). The kBME is our model §2.2, whereas the KDE-RVM is a KDE model learned with a Relevance Vector Machine (RVM) [17] feature space map. PCA-BME and PCA-RVM are models where the mappings between feature spaces (obtained using PCA) is learned using a BME and a RVM. The non-linearity is significant. Kernel-based methods outperform PCA and give low prediction error for 5-6d models.

systematic evaluation. Notice that the kernelized low-dimensional models generally outperform the PCA ones. At the same time, they give results competitive to the ones of high-dimensional BME predictors, while being lower-dimensional and therefore significantly less expensive for inference, *e.g.* the integral in (1).

In fig. 5 and fig. 6 we show human motion reconstruction results for two real image sequences. Fig. 5 shows the good quality reconstruction of a person performing an agile jump. (Given the missing observations in a side view, 3D inference for the occluded body parts would not be possible without using prior knowledge!) For this sequence we do inference using conditionals having 5 modes and reduced 6d states. We initialize tracking using $p(\mathbf{y}_t|\mathbf{z}_t)$, whereas for inference we use $p(\mathbf{y}_t|\mathbf{y}_{t-1}, \mathbf{z}_t)$ within (1). In the second sequence in fig. 6, we simultaneously reconstruct the motion of two people mimicking domestic activities, namely washing a window and picking an object. Here we do inference over a product, 12-dimensional state space consisting of the joint 6d state of each person. We obtain good 3D reconstruction results, using only 5 hypotheses. Notice however, that the results are not perfect, there are small errors in the elbow and the bending of the knee for the subject at the l.h.s., and in the different wrist orientations for the subject at the r.h.s. This reflects the bias of our training set.

	KDE-RR	RVM	KDE-RVM	BME	kBME
Walk and turn	10.46	4.95	7.57	4.27	4.69
Conversation	7.95	4.96	6.31	4.15	4.79
Run and turn left	5.22	5.02	6.25	5.01	4.92

Table 1: Comparison of average joint angle prediction error for different models. All kPCA-based models use 6 output dimensions. Testing is done on 100 video frames for each sequence, the inputs are artificially generated silhouettes, not in the training set. 3D joint angle ground truth is used for evaluation. KDE-RR is a KDE model with ridge regression (RR) for the feature space mapping, KDE-RVM uses an RVM. BME uses a Bayesian mixture of experts with no dimensionality reduction. kBME is our proposed model. kPCA-based methods use kernel regressors to compute pre-images.

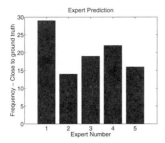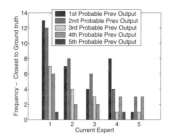

Figure 4: *(a, Left)* Histogram showing the accuracy of various expert predictors: how many times the expert ranked as the k-th most probable by the model (horizontal axis) is closest to the ground truth. The model is consistent (the most probable expert indeed is the most accurate most frequently), but occasionally less probable experts are better. *(b, Right)* Histograms show the dynamics of $p(\mathbf{y}_t|\mathbf{y}_{t-1}, \mathbf{z}_t)$, *i.e.* how the probability mass is redistributed among experts between two successive time steps, in a conversation sequence.

	KDE-RR	RVM	KDE-RVM	BME	kBME
Walk and turn back	7.59	6.9	7.15	3.6	3.72
Run and turn	17.7	16.8	16.08	8.2	8.01

Table 2: Joint angle prediction error computed for two complex sequences with walks, runs and turns, thus more ambiguity (100 frames). Models have 6 state dimensions. Unimodal predictors average competing solutions. kBME has significantly lower error.

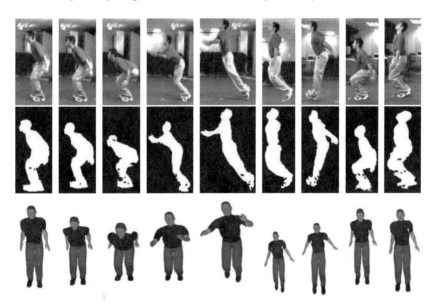

Figure 5: Reconstruction of a jump (selected frames). *Top:* original image sequence. *Middle:* extracted silhouettes. *Bottom:* 3D reconstruction seen from a synthetic viewpoint.

4 Conclusion

We have presented a probabilistic framework for conditional inference in latent kernel-induced low-dimensional state spaces. Our approach has the following properties: *(a)*

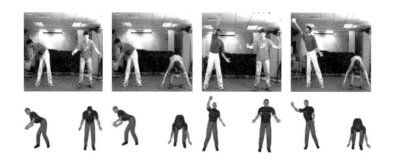

Figure 6: Reconstructing the activities of 2 people operating in an 12-d state space (each person has its own 6d state). *Top:* original image sequence. *Bottom:* 3D reconstruction seen from a synthetic viewpoint.

Accounts for non-linear correlations among input or output variables, by using kernel non-linear dimensionality reduction (kPCA); *(b)* Learns probability distributions over mappings between low-dimensional state spaces using conditional Bayesian mixture of experts, as required for accurate prediction. In the resulting low-dimensional kBME predictor ambiguities and multiple solutions common in visual, inverse perception problems are accurately represented. *(c)* Works in a continuous, conditional temporal probabilistic setting and offers a formal management of uncertainty. We show comparisons that demonstrate how the proposed approach outperforms regression, PCA or KDE alone for reconstructing the 3D human motion in monocular video. Future work we will investigate scaling aspects for large training sets and alternative structured prediction methods.

References

[1] CMU Human Motion DataBase. Online at http://mocap.cs.cmu.edu/search.html, 2003.
[2] A. Agarwal and B. Triggs. 3d human pose from silhouettes by Relevance Vector Regression. In *CVPR*, 2004.
[3] G. Bakir, J. Weston, and B. Scholkopf. Learning to find pre-images. In *NIPS*, 2004.
[4] S. Belongie, J. Malik, and J. Puzicha. Shape matching and object recognition using shape contexts. *PAMI*, 24, 2002.
[5] C. Bishop and M. Svensen. Bayesian mixtures of experts. In *UAI*, 2003.
[6] J. Deutscher, A. Blake, and I. Reid. Articulated Body Motion Capture by Annealed Particle Filtering. In *CVPR*, 2000.
[7] M. Jordan and R. Jacobs. Hierarchical mixtures of experts and the EM algorithm. *Neural Computation*, (6):181–214, 1994.
[8] D. Mackay. Bayesian interpolation. *Neural Computation*, 4(5):720–736, 1992.
[9] A. McCallum, D. Freitag, and F. Pereira. Maximum entropy Markov models for information extraction and segmentation. In *ICML*, 2000.
[10] R. Rosales and S. Sclaroff. Learning Body Pose Via Specialized Maps. In *NIPS*, 2002.
[11] B. Schölkopf, A. Smola, and K. Müller. Nonlinear component analysis as a kernel eigenvalue problem. *Neural Computation*, 10:1299–1319, 1998.
[12] G. Shakhnarovich, P. Viola, and T. Darrell. Fast Pose Estimation with Parameter Sensitive Hashing. In *ICCV*, 2003.
[13] L. Sigal, S. Bhatia, S. Roth, M. Black, and M. Isard. Tracking Loose-limbed People. In *CVPR*, 2004.
[14] C. Sminchisescu and A. Jepson. Generative Modeling for Continuous Non-Linearly Embedded Visual Inference. In *ICML*, pages 759–766, Banff, 2004.
[15] C. Sminchisescu, A. Kanaujia, Z. Li, and D. Metaxas. Discriminative Density Propagation for 3D Human Motion Estimation. In *CVPR*, 2005.
[16] C. Sminchisescu and B. Triggs. Kinematic Jump Processes for Monocular 3D Human Tracking. In *CVPR*, volume 1, pages 69–76, Madison, 2003.
[17] M. Tipping. Sparse Bayesian learning and the Relevance Vector Machine. *JMLR*, 2001.
[18] C. Tomasi, S. Petrov, and A. Sastry. 3d tracking = classification + interpolation. In *ICCV*, 2003.
[19] J. Weston, O. Chapelle, A. Elisseeff, B. Scholkopf, and V. Vapnik. Kernel dependency estimation. In *NIPS*, 2002.

Sparse Gaussian Processes using Pseudo-inputs

Edward Snelson   **Zoubin Ghahramani**

Gatsby Computational Neuroscience Unit
University College London
17 Queen Square, London WC1N 3AR, UK
{snelson,zoubin}@gatsby.ucl.ac.uk

Abstract

We present a new Gaussian process (GP) regression model whose covariance is parameterized by the the locations of M pseudo-input points,
which we learn by a gradient based optimization. We take $M \ll N$,
where N is the number of real data points, and hence obtain a sparse
regression method which has $\mathcal{O}(M^2 N)$ training cost and $\mathcal{O}(M^2)$ prediction cost per test case. We also find hyperparameters of the covariance function in the same joint optimization. The method can be viewed
as a Bayesian regression model with particular input dependent noise.
The method turns out to be closely related to several other sparse GP approaches, and we discuss the relation in detail. We finally demonstrate
its performance on some large data sets, and make a direct comparison to
other sparse GP methods. We show that our method can match full GP
performance with small M, i.e. very sparse solutions, and it significantly
outperforms other approaches in this regime.

1   Introduction

The Gaussian process (GP) is a popular and elegant method for Bayesian non-linear non-
parametric regression and classification. Unfortunately its non-parametric nature causes
computational problems for large data sets, due to an unfavourable N^3 scaling for training,
where N is the number of data points. In recent years there have been many attempts to
make sparse approximations to the full GP in order to bring this scaling down to $M^2 N$
where $M \ll N$ [1, 2, 3, 4, 5, 6, 7, 8, 9]. Most of these methods involve selecting a subset
of the training points of size M (active set) on which to base computation. A typical way of
choosing such a subset is through some sort of information criterion. For example, Seeger
et al. [7] employ a very fast approximate information gain criterion, which they use to
greedily select points into the active set.

A major common problem to these methods is that they lack a reliable way of learning
kernel hyperparameters, because the active set selection interferes with this learning procedure. Seeger et al. [7] construct an approximation to the full GP marginal likelihood, which
they try to maximize to find the hyperparameters. However, as the authors state, they have
persistent difficulty in practically doing this through gradient ascent. The reason for this
is that reselecting the active set causes non-smooth fluctuations in the marginal likelihood

and its gradients, meaning that they cannot get smooth convergence. Therefore the speed of active set selection is somewhat undermined by the difficulty of selecting hyperparameters. Inappropriately learned hyperparameters will adversely affect the quality of solution, especially if one is trying to use them for *automatic relevance determination* (ARD) [10].

In this paper we circumvent this problem by constructing a GP regression model that enables us to find active set point locations and hyperparameters in one smooth joint optimization. The covariance function of our GP is parameterized by the locations of pseudo-inputs — an active set not constrained to be a subset of the data, found by a continuous optimization. This is a further major advantage, since we can improve the quality of our fit by the fine tuning of their precise locations.

Our model is closely related to several sparse GP approximations, in particular Seeger's method of *projected latent variables* (PLV) [7, 8]. We discuss these relations in section 3. In principle we could also apply our technique of moving active set points off data points to approximations such as PLV. However we empirically demonstrate that a crucial difference between PLV and our method (SPGP) prevents this idea from working for PLV.

1.1 Gaussian processes for regression

We provide here a concise summary of GPs for regression, but see [11, 12, 13, 10] for more detailed reviews. We have a data set $\mathcal{D}$ consisting of N input vectors $\mathbf{X} = \{\mathbf{x}_n\}_{n=1}^{N}$ of dimension D and corresponding real valued targets $\mathbf{y} = \{y_n\}_{n=1}^{N}$. We place a zero mean Gaussian process prior on the underlying latent function $f(x)$ that we are trying to model. We therefore have a multivariate Gaussian distribution on any finite subset of latent variables; in particular, at $\mathbf{X}$: $p(\mathbf{f}|\mathbf{X}) = \mathcal{N}(\mathbf{f}|\mathbf{0}, \mathbf{K}_N)$, where $\mathcal{N}(\mathbf{f}|\mathbf{m}, \mathbf{V})$ is a Gaussian distribution with mean $\mathbf{m}$ and covariance $\mathbf{V}$. In a Gaussian process the covariance matrix is constructed from a covariance function, or kernel, K which expresses some prior notion of smoothness of the underlying function: $[\mathbf{K}_N]_{nn'} = K(\mathbf{x}_n, \mathbf{x}_{n'})$. Usually the covariance function depends on a small number of hyperparameters $\boldsymbol{\theta}$, which control these smoothness properties. For our experiments later on we will use the standard Gaussian covariance with ARD hyperparameters:

$$K(\mathbf{x}_n, \mathbf{x}_{n'}) = c \exp\left[-\tfrac{1}{2} \sum_{d=1}^{D} b_d\big(x_n^{(d)} - x_{n'}^{(d)}\big)^2\right], \qquad \boldsymbol{\theta} = \{c, \mathbf{b}\} . \tag{1}$$

In standard GP regression we also assume a Gaussian noise model or likelihood $p(\mathbf{y}|\mathbf{f}) = \mathcal{N}(\mathbf{y}|\mathbf{f}, \sigma^2\mathbf{I})$. Integrating out the latent function values we obtain the marginal likelihood:

$$p(\mathbf{y}|\mathbf{X}, \boldsymbol{\theta}) = \mathcal{N}(\mathbf{y}|\mathbf{0}, \mathbf{K}_N + \sigma^2\mathbf{I}) , \tag{2}$$

which is typically used to train the GP by finding a (local) maximum with respect to the hyperparameters $\boldsymbol{\theta}$ and σ^2.

Prediction is made by considering a new input point $\mathbf{x}$ and conditioning on the observed data and hyperparameters. The distribution of the target value at the new point is then:

$$p(y|\mathbf{x}, \mathcal{D}, \boldsymbol{\theta}) = \mathcal{N}\big(y|\mathbf{k}_\mathbf{x}^\top (\mathbf{K}_N + \sigma^2\mathbf{I})^{-1}\mathbf{y}, \; K_{\mathbf{xx}} - \mathbf{k}_\mathbf{x}^\top (\mathbf{K}_N + \sigma^2\mathbf{I})^{-1}\mathbf{k}_\mathbf{x} + \sigma^2\big) , \tag{3}$$

where $[\mathbf{k}_\mathbf{x}]_n = K(\mathbf{x}_n, \mathbf{x})$ and $K_{\mathbf{xx}} = K(\mathbf{x}, \mathbf{x})$. The GP is a non-parametric model, because the training data are explicitly required at test time in order to construct the predictive distribution, as is clear from the above expression.

GPs are prohibitive for large data sets because training requires $\mathcal{O}(N^3)$ time due to the inversion of the covariance matrix. Once the inversion is done, prediction is $\mathcal{O}(N)$ for the predictive mean and $\mathcal{O}(N^2)$ for the predictive variance per new test case.

2 Sparse Pseudo-input Gaussian processes (SPGPs)

In order to derive a sparse model that is computationally tractable for large data sets, which still preserves the desirable properties of the full GP, we examine in detail the GP predictive distribution (3). Consider the mean and variance of this distribution as functions of $\mathbf{x}$, the new input. Regarding the hyperparameters as known and fixed for now, these functions are effectively parameterized by the locations of the N training input and target pairs, $\mathbf{X}$ and $\mathbf{y}$. In this paper we consider a model with likelihood given by the GP predictive distribution, and parameterized by a *pseudo data set*. The sparsity in the model will arise because we will generally consider a pseudo data set $\bar{\mathcal{D}}$ of size $M < N$: pseudo-inputs $\bar{\mathbf{X}} = \{\bar{\mathbf{x}}_m\}_{m=1}^M$ and pseudo targets $\bar{\mathbf{f}} = \{\bar{f}_m\}_{m=1}^M$. We have denoted the pseudo targets $\bar{\mathbf{f}}$ instead of $\bar{\mathbf{y}}$ because as they are not real observations, it does not make much sense to include a noise variance for them. They are therefore equivalent to the latent function values $\mathbf{f}$. The actual observed target value will of course be assumed noisy as before. These assumptions therefore lead to the following single data point likelihood:

$$p(y|\mathbf{x}, \bar{\mathbf{X}}, \bar{\mathbf{f}}) = \mathcal{N}\left(y|\mathbf{k}_{\mathbf{x}}^\top \mathbf{K}_M^{-1}\bar{\mathbf{f}}, \ K_{\mathbf{xx}} - \mathbf{k}_{\mathbf{x}}^\top \mathbf{K}_M^{-1}\mathbf{k}_{\mathbf{x}} + \sigma^2\right), \tag{4}$$

where $[\mathbf{K}_M]_{mm'} = K(\bar{\mathbf{x}}_m, \bar{\mathbf{x}}_{m'})$ and $[\mathbf{k}_{\mathbf{x}}]_m = K(\bar{\mathbf{x}}_m, \mathbf{x})$, for $m = 1, \ldots, M$.

This can be viewed as a standard regression model with a particular form of parameterized mean function and input-dependent noise model. The target data are generated i.i.d. given the inputs, giving the complete data likelihood:

$$p(\mathbf{y}|\mathbf{X}, \bar{\mathbf{X}}, \bar{\mathbf{f}}) = \prod_{n=1}^N p(y_n|\mathbf{x}_n, \bar{\mathbf{X}}, \bar{\mathbf{f}}) = \mathcal{N}(\mathbf{y}|\mathbf{K}_{NM}\mathbf{K}_M^{-1}\bar{\mathbf{f}}, \ \mathbf{\Lambda} + \sigma^2\mathbf{I}), \tag{5}$$

where $\mathbf{\Lambda} = \mathrm{diag}(\boldsymbol{\lambda})$, $\lambda_n = K_{nn} - \mathbf{k}_n^\top \mathbf{K}_M^{-1}\mathbf{k}_n$, and $[\mathbf{K}_{NM}]_{nm} = K(\mathbf{x}_n, \bar{\mathbf{x}}_m)$.

Learning in the model involves finding a suitable setting of the parameters – an appropriate pseudo data set that explains the real data well. However rather than simply maximize the likelihood with respect to $\bar{\mathbf{X}}$ and $\bar{\mathbf{f}}$ it turns out that we can integrate out the pseudo targets $\bar{\mathbf{f}}$. We place a Gaussian prior on the pseudo targets:

$$p(\bar{\mathbf{f}}|\bar{\mathbf{X}}) = \mathcal{N}(\bar{\mathbf{f}}|\mathbf{0}, \mathbf{K}_M). \tag{6}$$

This is a very reasonable prior because we expect the pseudo data to be distributed in a very similar manner to the real data, if they are to model them well. It is not easy to place a prior on the pseudo-inputs and still remain with a tractable model, so we will find these by maximum likelihood (ML). For the moment though, consider the pseudo-inputs as known.

We find the posterior distribution over pseudo targets $\bar{\mathbf{f}}$ using Bayes rule on (5) and (6):

$$p(\bar{\mathbf{f}}|\mathcal{D}, \bar{\mathbf{X}}) = \mathcal{N}\left(\bar{\mathbf{f}}|\mathbf{K}_M\mathbf{Q}_M^{-1}\mathbf{K}_{MN}(\mathbf{\Lambda} + \sigma^2\mathbf{I})^{-1}\mathbf{y}, \ \mathbf{K}_M\mathbf{Q}_M^{-1}\mathbf{K}_M\right), \tag{7}$$

where $\mathbf{Q}_M = \mathbf{K}_M + \mathbf{K}_{MN}(\mathbf{\Lambda} + \sigma^2\mathbf{I})^{-1}\mathbf{K}_{NM}$.

Given a new input $\mathbf{x}_*$, the predictive distribution is then obtained by integrating the likelihood (4) with the posterior (7):

$$p(y_*|\mathbf{x}_*, \mathcal{D}, \bar{\mathbf{X}}) = \int d\bar{\mathbf{f}} \, p(y_*|\mathbf{x}_*, \bar{\mathbf{X}}, \bar{\mathbf{f}}) \, p(\bar{\mathbf{f}}|\mathcal{D}, \bar{\mathbf{X}}) = \mathcal{N}(y_*|\mu_*, \sigma_*^2), \tag{8}$$

where

$$\mu_* = \mathbf{k}_*^\top \mathbf{Q}_M^{-1}\mathbf{K}_{MN}(\mathbf{\Lambda} + \sigma^2\mathbf{I})^{-1}\mathbf{y}$$
$$\sigma_*^2 = K_{**} - \mathbf{k}_*^\top(\mathbf{K}_M^{-1} - \mathbf{Q}_M^{-1})\mathbf{k}_* + \sigma^2.$$

Note that inversion of the matrix $\mathbf{\Lambda} + \sigma^2\mathbf{I}$ is not a problem because it is diagonal. The computational cost is dominated by the matrix multiplication $\mathbf{K}_{MN}(\mathbf{\Lambda} + \sigma^2\mathbf{I})^{-1}\mathbf{K}_{NM}$ in the calculation of $\mathbf{Q}_M$ which is $\mathcal{O}(M^2N)$. After various precomputations, prediction can then be made in $\mathcal{O}(M)$ for the mean and $\mathcal{O}(M^2)$ for the variance per test case.

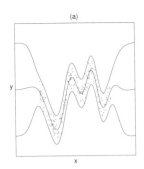 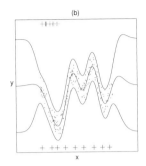 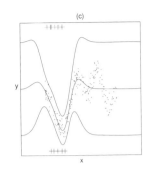

Figure 1: Predictive distributions (mean and two standard deviation lines) for: (a) full GP, (b) SPGP trained using gradient ascent on (9), (c) SPGP trained using gradient ascent on (10). Initial pseudo point positions are shown at the top as red crosses; final pseudo point positions are shown at the bottom as blue crosses (the y location on the plots of these crosses is *not* meaningful).

We are left with the problem of finding the pseudo-input locations $\bar{\mathbf{X}}$ and hyperparameters $\boldsymbol{\Theta} = \{\boldsymbol{\theta}, \sigma^2\}$. We can do this by computing the marginal likelihood from (5) and (6):

$$
\begin{aligned}
p(\mathbf{y}|\mathbf{X}, \bar{\mathbf{X}}, \boldsymbol{\Theta}) &= \int d\bar{\mathbf{f}}\; p(\mathbf{y}|\mathbf{X}, \bar{\mathbf{X}}, \bar{\mathbf{f}})\, p(\bar{\mathbf{f}}|\bar{\mathbf{X}}) \\
&= \mathcal{N}(\mathbf{y}|\mathbf{0},\; \mathbf{K}_{NM}\mathbf{K}_M^{-1}\mathbf{K}_{MN} + \boldsymbol{\Lambda} + \sigma^2\mathbf{I}) \;.
\end{aligned}
\tag{9}
$$

The marginal likelihood can then be maximized with respect to all these parameters $\{\bar{\mathbf{X}}, \boldsymbol{\Theta}\}$ by gradient ascent. The details of the gradient calculations are long and tedious and therefore omitted here for brevity. They closely follow the derivations of hyperparameter gradients of Seeger et al. [7] (see also section 3), and as there, can be most efficiently coded with Cholesky factorisations. Note that $\mathbf{K}_M$, $\mathbf{K}_{MN}$ and $\boldsymbol{\Lambda}$ are all functions of the M pseudo-inputs $\bar{\mathbf{X}}$ and $\boldsymbol{\theta}$. The exact form of the gradients will of course depend on the functional form of the covariance function chosen, but our method will apply to any covariance that is differentiable with respect to the input points. It is worth saying that the SPGP can be viewed as a standard GP with a particular non-stationary covariance function parameterized by the pseudo-inputs.

Since we now have $MD + |\boldsymbol{\Theta}|$ parameters to fit, instead of just $|\boldsymbol{\Theta}|$ for the full GP, one may be worried about overfitting. However, consider the case where we let $M = N$ and $\bar{\mathbf{X}} = \mathbf{X}$ – the pseudo-inputs coincide with the real inputs. At this point the marginal likelihood is equal to that of a full GP (2). This is because at this point $\mathbf{K}_{MN} = \mathbf{K}_M = \mathbf{K}_N$ and $\boldsymbol{\Lambda} = \mathbf{0}$. Moreover the predictive distribution (8) also collapses to the full GP predictive distribution (3). These are clearly desirable properties of the model, and they give confidence that a good solution will be found when $M < N$. However it is the case that hyperparameter learning complicates matters, and we discuss this further in section 4.

3 Relation to other methods

It turns out that Seeger's method of PLV [7, 8] uses a very similar marginal likelihood approximation and predictive distribution. If you remove $\boldsymbol{\Lambda}$ from all the SPGP equations you get precisely their expressions. In particular the marginal likelihood they use is:

$$
p(\mathbf{y}|\mathbf{X}, \bar{\mathbf{X}}, \boldsymbol{\Theta}) = \mathcal{N}(\mathbf{y}|\mathbf{0},\; \mathbf{K}_{NM}\mathbf{K}_M^{-1}\mathbf{K}_{MN} + \sigma^2\mathbf{I}) \;,
\tag{10}
$$

which has also been used elsewhere before [1, 4, 5]. They have derived this expression from a somewhat different route, as a direct approximation to the full GP marginal likelihood.

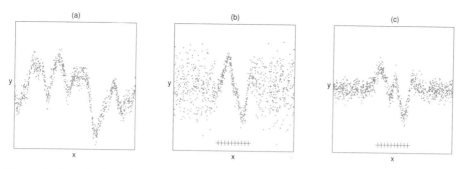

Figure 2: Sample data drawn from the marginal likelihood of: (a) a full GP, (b) SPGP, (c) PLV. For (b) and (c), the blue crosses show the location of the 10 pseudo-input points.

As discussed earlier, the major difference between our method and these other methods, is that they do not use this marginal likelihood to learn locations of active set input points – only the hyperparameters are learnt from (10). This begged the question of what would happen if we tried to use their marginal likelihood approximation (10) instead of (9) to try to learn pseudo-input locations by gradient ascent. We show that the Λ that appears in the SPGP marginal likelihood (9) is crucial for finding pseudo-input points by *gradients*.

Figure 1 shows what happens when we try to optimize these two likelihoods using gradient ascent with respect to the pseudo inputs, on a simple 1D data set. Plotted are the predictive distributions, initial and final locations of the pseudo inputs. Hyperparameters were fixed to their true values for this example. The initial pseudo-input locations were chosen adversarially: all towards the left of the input space (red crosses). Using the SPGP likelihood, the pseudo-inputs spread themselves along the extent of the training data, and the predictive distribution matches the full GP very closely (Figure 1(b)). Using the PLV likelihood, the points begin to spread, but very quickly become stuck as the gradient pushing the points towards the right becomes tiny (Figure 1(c)).

Figure 2 compares data sampled from the marginal likelihoods (9) and (10), given a particular setting of the hyperparameters and a small number of pseudo-input points. The major difference between the two is that the SPGP likelihood has a constant marginal variance of $K_{nn} + \sigma^2$, whereas the PLV decreases to σ^2 away from the pseudo-inputs. Alternatively, the *noise* component of the PLV likelihood is a constant σ^2, whereas the SPGP noise grows to $K_{nn} + \sigma^2$ away from the pseudo-inputs. If one is in the situation of Figure 1(c), under the SPGP likelihood, moving the rightmost pseudo-input slightly to the right will immediately start to reduce the noise in this region from $K_{nn} + \sigma^2$ towards σ^2. Hence there will be a strong gradient pulling it to the right. With the PLV likelihood, the noise is fixed at σ^2 everywhere, and moving the point to the right does not improve the quality of fit of the mean function enough locally to provide a significant gradient. Therefore the points become stuck, and we believe this effect accounts for the failure of the PLV likelihood in Figure 1(c).

It should be emphasised that the *global* optimum of the PLV likelihood (10) may well be a good solution, but it is going to be difficult to find with *gradients*. The SPGP likelihood (9) also suffers from local optima of course, but not so catastrophically. It may be interesting in the future to compare which performs better for hyperparameter optimization.

4   Experiments

In the previous section we showed our gradient method successfully learning the pseudo-inputs on a 1D example. There the initial pseudo input points were chosen adversarially, but on a real problem it is sensible to initialize by randomly placing them on real data points,

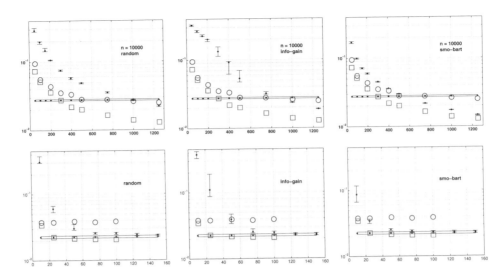

Figure 3: Our results have been added to plots reproduced with kind permission from [7]. The plots show mean square test error as a function of active/pseudo set size M. Top row – data set *kin-40k*, bottom row – *pumadyn-32nm*[1]. We have added circles which show SPGP with both hyperparameter and pseudo-input learning from random initialisation. For *kin-40k* the squares show SPGP with hyperparameters obtained from a full GP and fixed. For *pumadyn-32nm* the squares show hyperparameters *initialized* from a full GP. *random*, *info-gain* and *smo-bart* are explained in the text. The horizontal lines are a full GP trained on a subset of the data.

and this is what we do for all of our experiments. To compare our results to other methods we have run experiments on exactly the same data sets as in Seeger et al. [7], following precisely their preprocessing and testing methods. In Figure 3, we have reproduced their learning curves for two large data sets[1], superimposing our test error (mean squared).

Seeger et al. compare three methods: *random*, *info-gain* and *smo-bart*. *random* involves picking an active set of size M randomly from among training data. *info-gain* is their own greedy subset selection method, which is extremely cheap to train – barely more expensive than *random*. *smo-bart* is Smola and Bartlett's [1] more expensive greedy subset selection method. Also shown with horizontal lines is the test error for a full GP trained on a subset of the data of size 2000 for data set *kin-40k* and 1024 for *pumadyn-32nm*. For these learning curves, they do *not* actually learn hyperparameters by maximizing their approximation to the marginal likelihood (10). Instead they fix them to those obtained from the full GP[2].

For *kin-40k* we follow Seeger et al.'s procedure of setting the hyperparameters from the full GP on a subset. We then optimize the pseudo-input positions, and plot the results as red squares. We see the SPGP learning curve lying significantly below all three other methods in Figure 3. We rapidly approach the error of a full GP trained on 2000 points, using a pseudo set of only a few hundred points. We then try the harder task of also finding the hyperparameters at the same time as the pseudo-inputs. The results are plotted as blue circles. The method performs extremely well for small M, but we see some overfitting

---

[1]*kin-40k*: 10000 training, 30000 test, 9 attributes, see *www.igi.tugraz.at/aschwaig/data.html*. *pumadyn-32nm*: 7168 training, 1024 test, 33 attributes, see *www.cs.toronto/ delve*.

[2]Seeger et al. have a separate section testing their likelihood approximation (10) to learn hyperparameters, in conjunction with the active set selection methods. They show that it can be used to reliably learn hyperparameters with *info-gain* for active set sizes of 100 and above. They have more trouble reliably learning hyperparameters for very small active sets.

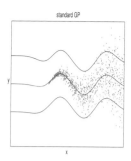
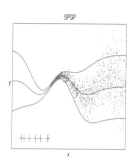

Figure 4: Regression on a data set with input dependent noise. Left: standard GP. Right: SPGP. Predictive mean and two standard deviation lines are shown. Crosses show final locations of pseudo-inputs for SPGP. Hyperparameters are also learnt.

behaviour for large M which seems to be caused by the noise hyperparameter being driven too small (the blue circles have higher likelihood than the red squares below them).

For data set *pumadyn-32nm*, we again try to jointly find hyperparameters and pseudo-inputs. Again Figure 3 shows SPGP with extremely low error for small pseudo set size – with just 10 pseudo-inputs we are already close to the error of a full GP trained on 1024 points. However, in this case increasing the pseudo set size does not decrease our error. In this problem there is a large number of irrelevant attributes, and the relevant ones need to be singled out by ARD. Although the hyperparameters learnt by our method are reasonable (2 out of the 4 relevant dimensions are found), they are not good enough to get down to the error of the full GP. However if we initialize our gradient algorithm with the hyperparameters of the full GP, we get the points plotted as squares (this time red likelihoods > blue likelihoods, so it is a problem of local optima not overfitting). Now with only a pseudo set of size 25 we reach the performance of the full GP, and significantly outperform the other methods (which also had their hyperparameters set from the full GP).

Another main difference between the methods lies in training time. Our method performs optimization over a potentially large parameter space, and hence is relatively expensive to train. On the face of it methods such as *info-gain* and *random* are extremely cheap. However all these methods must be combined with obtaining hyperparameters in some way – either by a full GP on a subset (generally expensive), or by gradient ascent on an approximation to the likelihood. When you consider this combined task, and that all methods involve some kind of gradient based procedure, then none of the methods are particularly cheap. We believe that the gain in accuracy achieved by our method can often be worth the extra training time associated with optimizing in a larger parameter space.

5 Conclusions, extensions and future work

Although GPs are very flexible regression models, they are still limited by the form of the covariance function. For example it is difficult to model non-stationary processes with a GP because it is hard to construct sensible non-stationary covariance functions. Although the SPGP is not specifically designed to model non-stationarity, the extra flexibility associated with moving pseudo inputs around can actually achieve this to a certain extent. Figure 4 shows the SPGP fit to some data with an input dependent noise variance. The SPGP achieves a much better fit to the data than the standard GP by moving almost all the pseudo-input points outside the region of data[3]. It will be interesting to test these capabilities further in the future. The extension to classification is also a natural avenue to explore.

We have demonstrated a significant decrease in test error over the other methods for a given small pseudo/active set size. Our method runs into problems when we consider much larger

---

[3]It should be said that there are local optima in this problem, and other solutions looked closer to the standard GP. We ran the method 5 times with random initialisations. All runs had higher likelihood than the GP; the one with the highest likelihood is plotted.

pseudo set size and/or high dimensional input spaces, because the space in which we are optimizing becomes impractically big. However we have currently only tried using an 'off the shelf' conjugate gradient minimizer, or L-BFGS, and there are certainly improvements that can be made in this area. For example we can try optimizing subsets of variables iteratively (chunking), or stochastic gradient ascent, or we could make a hybrid by picking some points randomly and optimizing others. In general though we consider our method most useful when one wants a very sparse (hence fast prediction) and accurate solution. One further way in which to deal with large D is to learn a low dimensional projection of the input space. This has been considered for GPs before [14], and could easily be applied to our model.

In conclusion, we have presented a new method for sparse GP regression, which shows a significant performance gain over other methods especially when searching for an extremely sparse solution. We have shown that the added flexibility of moving pseudo-input points which are not constrained to lie on the true data points leads to better solutions, and even some non-stationary effects can be modelled. Finally we have shown that hyperparameters can be jointly learned with pseudo-input points with reasonable success.

Acknowledgements

Thanks to the authors of [7] for agreeing to make their results and plots available for reproduction. Thanks to all at the Sheffield GP workshop for helping to clarify this work.

References

[1] A. J. Smola and P. Bartlett. Sparse greedy Gaussian process regression. In *Advances in Neural Information Processing Systems 13*. MIT Press, 2000.

[2] C. K. I. Williams and M. Seeger. Using the Nyström method to speed up kernel machines. In *Advances in Neural Information Processing Systems 13*. MIT Press, 2000.

[3] V. Tresp. A Bayesian committee machine. *Neural Computation*, 12:2719–2741, 2000.

[4] L. Csató. Sparse online Gaussian processes. *Neural Computation*, 14:641–668, 2002.

[5] L. Csató. *Gaussian Processes — Iterative Sparse Approximations*. PhD thesis, Aston University, UK, 2002.

[6] N. D. Lawrence, M. Seeger, and R. Herbrich. Fast sparse Gaussian process methods: the informative vector machine. In *Advances in Neural Information Processing Systems 15*. MIT Press, 2002.

[7] M. Seeger, C. K. I. Williams, and N. D. Lawrence. Fast forward selection to speed up sparse Gaussian process regression. In C. M. Bishop and B. J. Frey, editors, *Proceedings of the Ninth International Workshop on Artificial Intelligence and Statistics*, 2003.

[8] M. Seeger. *Bayesian Gaussian Process Models: PAC-Bayesian Generalisation Error Bounds and Sparse Approximations*. PhD thesis, University of Edinburgh, 2003.

[9] J. Quiñonero Candela. *Learning with Uncertainty — Gaussian Processes and Relevance Vector Machines*. PhD thesis, Technical University of Denmark, 2004.

[10] D. J. C. MacKay. Introduction to Gaussian processes. In C. M. Bishop, editor, *Neural Networks and Machine Learning*, NATO ASI Series, pages 133–166. Kluwer Academic Press, 1998.

[11] C. K. I. Williams and C. E. Rasmussen. Gaussian processes for regression. In *Advances in Neural Information Processing Systems 8*. MIT Press, 1996.

[12] C. E. Rasmussen. *Evaluation of Gaussian Processes and Other Methods for Non-Linear Regression*. PhD thesis, University of Toronto, 1996.

[13] M. N. Gibbs. *Bayesian Gaussian Processes for Regression and Classification*. PhD thesis, Cambridge University, 1997.

[14] F. Vivarelli and C. K. I. Williams. Discovering hidden features with Gaussian processes regression. In *Advances in Neural Information Processing Systems 11*. MIT Press, 1998.

Phase Synchrony Rate for the Recognition of Motor Imagery in Brain-Computer Interface

Le Song
Nation ICT Australia
School of Information Technologies
The University of Sydney
NSW 2006, Australia
lesong@it.usyd.edu.au

Evian Gordon
Brain Resource Company
Scientific Chair, Brain Dynamics Center
Westmead Hospitial
NSW 2006, Australia
eviang@brainresource.com

Elly Gysels
Swiss Center for Electronics and Microtechnology
Neuchâtel, CH-2007 Switzerland
elly.gysels@csem.ch

Abstract

Motor imagery attenuates EEG μ and β rhythms over sensorimotor cortices. These amplitude changes are most successfully captured by the method of Common Spatial Patterns (CSP) and widely used in brain-computer interfaces (BCI). BCI methods based on amplitude information, however, have not incoporated the rich phase dynamics in the EEG rhythm. This study reports on a BCI method based on phase synchrony rate (SR). SR, computed from binarized phase locking value, describes the number of discrete synchronization events within a window. Statistical nonparametric tests show that SRs contain significant differences between 2 types of motor imageries. Classifiers trained on SRs consistently demonstrate satisfactory results for all 5 subjects. It is further observed that, for 3 subjects, phase is more discriminative than amplitude in the first 1.5-2.0 s, which suggests that phase has the potential to boost the information transfer rate in BCIs.

1 Introduction

A brain-computer interface (BCI) is a communication system that relies on the brain rather than the body for control and feedback. Such an interface offers hope not only for those severely paralyzed to control wheelchairs but also to enhance normal performance. Current BCI research is still in its infancy. Most studies focus on finding useful brain signals and designing algorithms to interpret them [1, 2].

The most exploited signal in BCI is the scalp-recorded electroencephalogram (EEG). EEG is a noninvasive measurement of the brain's electrical activities and has a temporal resolution of milliseconds. It is well known that motor imagery attenuates EEG μ and β rhythm over sensorimotor cortices. Depending on the part of the body imagined moving, the amplitude of multichannel EEG recordings exhibits distinctive spatial patterns. Classification of these patterns is used to control computer applications. Currently, the most successful method for BCI is called Common Spatial Patterns (CSP). The CSP method constructs a few new time series whose variances contain the most discriminative information. For the problem of classifying 2 types of motor imageries, the CSP method is able to correctly recognize 90% of the single trials in many studies [3, 4]. Ongoing research on the CSP method mainly focuses on its extension to the multi-class problem [5] and its integration with other forms of EEG amplitude information [4].

EEG signals contain both amplitude and phase information. Phase, however, has been largely ignored in BCI studies. Literature from neuroscience suggests, instead, that phase can be more discriminative than amplitude [6, 7]. For example, compared to a stimuli in which no face is present, face perception induces significant changes in γ synchrony, but not in amplitude [6]. Phase synchrony has been proposed as a mechanism for dynamic integration of distributed neural networks in the brain. Decreased synchrony, on the other hand, is associated with active unbinding of the neural assemblies and preparation of the brain for the next mental state (see [7] for a review). Accumulating evidence from both micro-electrode recordings [8,9] and EEG measurements [6] provides support to the notion that phase dynamics subserve all mental processes, including motor planning and imagery.

In the BCI community, only a paucity of results has demonstrated the relevance of phase information [10–12]. Fewer studies still have ever compared the difference between amplitude and phase information for BCI. To address these deficits, this paper focuses on three issues:

- Does binarized phase locking value (PLV) contain relevant information for the classification of motor imageries?
- How does the performance of binarized PLV compare to that of non-binarized PLV?
- How does the performance of methods based on phase information compare to that of the CSP method?

In the remainder of the paper, the experimental paradigm will be described first. The details of the method based on binarized PLV are presented in Section 3. Comparison between PLV, binarized PLV and CSP are then made in Section 4. Finally, conclusions are provided in Section 5.

2   Recording paradigm

Data set IVa provided by the Berlin BCI group [5] is investigated in this paper (available from the BCI competition III web site). Five healthy subjects (labeled 'aa', 'al', 'av', 'aw' and 'ay' respectively) participated in the EEG recordings. Based on the visual cues, they were required to imagine for 3.5 s either right hand (type 1) or right foot movements (type 2). Each type of motor imagery was carried out 140 times, which results in 280 labeled trials for each subject. Furthermore, the down-sampled data (at 100 Hz) is used. For the convenience of explanation, the length of the data is also referred to as time points. Therefore, the window for the full length of a trial is [1, 350].

3   Feature from phase

3.1   Phase locking value

Two EEG signals $x_i(t)$ and $x_j(t)$ are said to be synchronized, if their instantaneous phase difference $\psi_{ij}(t)$ (complex-valued with unit modulus) stays constant for a period of time

Δ_ψ. Phase locking value (PLV) is commonly used to quantify the degree of synchrony, i.e.

$$PLV_{ij}(t) = \frac{1}{\Delta_\psi} \left| \sum_{t-\Delta_\psi}^{t} \psi_{ij}(t) \right| \in [0, 1], \tag{1}$$

where 1 represents perfect synchrony. The instantaneous phase difference $\psi_{ij}(t)$ can be computed using either wavelet analysis or Hilbert transformation. Studies show that these two approaches are equivalent for the analysis of EEG signals [13]. In this study, Hilbert transformation is employed in a similar manner to [10].

3.2 Synchrony rate

Neuroscientists usually threshold the phase locking value and focus on statistically significant periods of strong synchrony. Only recently, researchers begin to study the transition between high and low levels of synchrony [6, 14, 15]. Most notably, the researcher in [15] transformed PLV into discrete values called link rates and showed that link rates could be a sensitive measure to relevant changes in synchrony. To investigate the usefulness of discretization for BCIs, we binarize the time series of PLV and define synchrony rate based on them.

The threshold chosen to binarize PLV minimizes the quantization error. Suppose that the distribution of PLV is $p(x)$, then the threshold th_0 is determined by

$$th_0 = \arg\min_{th} \int_0^1 (x - g(x - th))^2 p(x)\mathrm{d}x, \tag{2}$$

where $g(\cdot)$ is the hard-limit transfer function which assumes 1 for non-negative numbers and 0 otherwise. In practice, $p(x)$ is computed at discrete locations and the integration is replaced by summation. For the data set investigated, th_0s are similar across 5 subjects ($\simeq$ 0.5) when EEG signals are filtered between 4 and 40Hz and Δ_ψ is 0.25 s (These parameters are used in the Result section for all 5 subjects). The thresholded sequences are binary and denoted by $b_{ij}(t)$.

The ones in $b_{ij}(t)$ can be viewed as discrete events of strong synchrony, while zeros are those of weak synchrony. The resemblance of $b_{ij}(t)$ to the spike trains of neurons prompts us to define synchrony rate (SR)—the number of discrete events of strong synchrony per second. Formally, given a window Δ_b, the synchrony rate $r_{ij}(t)$ at time t is:

$$r_{ij}(t) = \frac{1}{\Delta_b} \sum_{t-\Delta_b}^{t} b_{ij}(t). \tag{3}$$

SR describes the average level of synchrony between a pair of electrodes in a given window. The size of the window will affect the value of the SR. In the next section, we will detail the choice of the windows and the selection of features from SRs.

3.3 Feature extraction

Before computing synchrony rates, a circular Laplacian [16] is applied to boost the spatial resolution of the raw EEG. This method first interpolates the scalp EEG, and then re-references EEG using interpolated values on a circle around an electrode. Varying the radius of the circles achieves different spatial filtering effects, and the best radius is tuned for individual subject.

Spatially filtered EEG is split into 6 sliding windows of length 100, namely [1, 100], [51, 150], [101, 200], [151, 250], [201, 300] and [251, 350]. Each window is further divivded

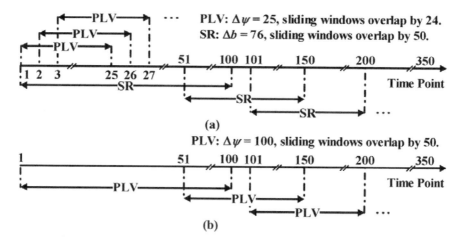

Figure 1: Overall scheme of window division for (a) the synchrony rate (SR) method and (b) the phase locking value (PLV) method. Δ_ψ for the SR method covers the length of a micro-window, while that for the PLV method corresponds to the length of a sliding window. Δ_b is equal to $100 - \Delta_\psi + 1$. (Note: time axis is NOT uniformly scaled.)

into 76 micro-windows (with size 25 and overlap by 24). PLVs are then computed and binarized for each micro-window (according to (1)). Averaging the 76 binarized PLVs results in the SR (according to (3)). As a whole, 6 SRs will be computed for each electrode pair in a trial. SRs from all electrode pairs will be passed to statistical tests and further used as features for classification. The overall scheme of this window division is illustrated in Fig 1(a). In order to compare PLV and SR, PLVs are also computed for the full length of each sliding window (Fig. 1(b)), which results in 6 PLVs for each electrode pair. These PLVs will go through the same statistical tests and classification stage.

3.4 Statistical test

A key observation is that both PLVs and SRs contain many statistically significant differences between the 2 types of motor imagery in almost every sliding window. Statistical nonparametric tests [17] are employed to locate these differences. For each electrode pair, a null hypothesis—H_0: The difference of the mean SR/PLV for the 2 types of motor imagery is zero—is formulated for each sliding window. Then the distribution of the difference is obtained by 1000 randomization. The hypothesis is rejected if the difference of the original data is larger than 99.5% or smaller than 0.5% of those from randomized data (equivalent to $p < 0.01$).

Fig. 2 illustrates the test results with data from subject 'av'. For simplicity, only those SRs with significant increase are displayed. Although the exact locations of these increases differ from window to window, some general patterns can be observed. Roughly speaking, window 2, 3 and 4 can be grouped as similar, while window 1, 5 and 6 are different from each other. Window 1 reflects changes in the early stage of a motor imagery, consisting increased couplings mainly within visual cortices and between visual and motor cortices. Then (window 2, 3 and 4) increased couplings occur between motor cortices of both hemispheres and between lateral and mesial areas of the motor cortices. During the last stage, these couplings first (window 5) shift to the left hemisphere and then (window 6) reduce to some sparse distant interactions. Similar patterns can also be discovered from the PLVs (not illustrated). Although the exact functional interpretation of these patterns awaits further investigation, they can be treated as potential features for classification.

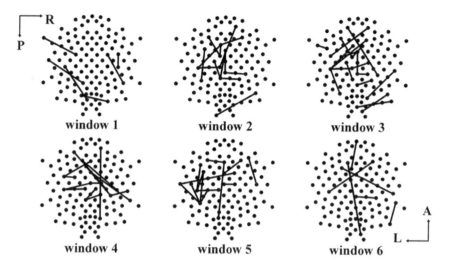

Figure 2: Significantly increased synchrony rates in right hand motor imagery. Data are from subject 'av'. (A: anterior; L: left; P: posterior; R: right.)

4 Classification strategy

To evaluate the usefulness of synchrony rate for the classification of motor imagery, 50×2-fold cross validation is employed to compute the generalization error. This scheme randomizes the order of the trials for 50 times. Each randomization further splits the trials into two equal halves (of 70 trials), each serving as training data once. There are four steps in each fold. Averaging the prediction errors from each fold results in the generalization error.

- Compute SRs for each trial (including both training and test data). As illustrated in Fig. 1(a), this results in a 6 dimensional (one for each window) feature vector for each electrode pair ($6903 = \frac{118 \times (118-1)}{2}$ pairs in total). Alternatively, it can be viewed as a 6903 dimensional feature vector for each window.

- Filter features using the Fisher ratio. The Fisher ratio (a variant, $\frac{|\mu_+ - \mu_-|}{\sigma_+ + \sigma_-}$, is used in the actual computation) measures the discriminability of individual feature for classification task. It is computed using training data only, and then compared to a threshold (0.3), below which a feature is discarded. The indices of the selected features are further used to filter the test data. The selected features are not necessarily all those located by the statistical tests. Generally, they are only a subset of the most significant SRs.

- Train a linear SVM for each window and use meta-training scheme to combine them. The evolving nature of the SRs (illustrated in Fig. 2) suggests that information in the 6 windows may be complementary to each other. Similar to [4], a second level of linear SVM is trained on the output of the SVMs for individual windows. This meta-training scheme allows us to exploit the inter-window relations. (Note that this step is carried out strictly on the training data.)

- Predict the label of the test data. Test data are fed into the two-level SVM, and the prediction error is measured as the proportion of the misclassified trials.

The above four steps are also used to compute the generalization errors for the PLV method. The only modification is in step one, where PLVs are computed instead of SRs (Fig. 1(b)). In the next section, we will present the generalization errors for both SR and PLV method, and compare them to those of the CSP method.

5 Result and comparison

5.1 Generalization error

Table 1 shows the generalization errors in percentage (with standard deviations) for both synchrony rate and PLV method. For comparison, we also computed the generalization errors of the CSP method [3] using linear SVM and 50×2-fold cross validation. The parameters of the CSP method (including filtering frequency, the number of channels used and the number of spatial patterns selected) are individually tuned for each subject according the competition winning entry of data set IVa [18]. Note that all errors in Table 1 are computed using the full length (3.5 s) of a trial.

Generally, the errors of the SR method is higher than those of the PLV method. This is because SR is an approximation of PLV by definition. Remember that during the computation of SRs, the PLVs in the micro-windows are first binarized with a threshold th_0. This threshold is so chosen that the approximation is as close to its original as possible. It works especially well for two of the subjects ('al' and 'ay'), with the difference between the two methods less than 1%. Although SR method produces higher errors, it may have some advantages in practice. Especially for hardware implemented BCI systems, smaller window for PLV computation means smaller buffer and binarized PLV makes further processing easier and faster.

The errors of the CSP method is lowest for most of the subjects. For subject 'aa' and 'aw', it is better than the other two methods by 10-20%, but the gaps are narrowed for subject 'al' and 'av' (less than 2.5%). Most notably, for subject 'ay', the SR method even outperforms the CSP method by about 5%. Remember that the CSP method is implemented using individually optimized parameters, while those for the SR and PLV method are the same across the 5 subjects. Fine tuning the parameters has the potential to further improve the performance of the latter two methods. The errors computed above, however, reveals only partial difference between the three methods. In the next subsection, a more thorough investigation will be carried out using information transfer rates.

5.2 Information transfer rate

Information transfer rate (ITR) [1] is the amount of information (measured in bits) generated by a BCI system within a second. It takes both the error and the length of a trial into account. If two BCI systems produce the same error, the one with a short trial will have higher information transfer rate. To investigate the performance of the three methods in this context, we shortened the trials into 5 different lengths, namely 1.0 s, 1.5 s, 2.0 s, 2.5 s and 3.0 s. The generalization errors are computed for these shortened trials and then converted into information transfer rates, as showed in Fig. 3.

Interesting results emerge from the curves in Fig. 3. Most subjects (except subject 'aw') achieve the highest information transfer rates within the first 1.5-2.0 s. Although longer trials usually decrease the errors, they do not necessarily result in increased information transfer rates. Furthermore, for subject 'al', 'av' and 'ay', the highest information transfer

Table 1: Generalization errors (%) of the synchrony rate (SR), PLV and CSP methods

Subject	aa	al	av	aw	ay
SR	29.34±3.97	4.05±1.28	32.67±3.41	22.96±4.39	5.93±1.75
PLV	23.05±3.39	3.59±1.28	29.91±3.23	18.65±3.48	5.41±1.53
CSP	12.58±2.56	2.65±1.35	30.30±3.02	3.16±1.32	11.43±2.34

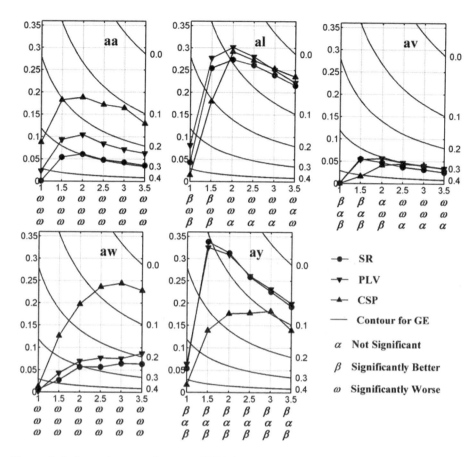

Figure 3: Information transfer rates (ITR) for synchrony rate (SR), PLV and CSP method. Horizontal axis is time T (in seconds). Vertical axis on the left measures information transfer rate (in bit/second) and that on the right shows the generalization error (GE) in decimals. The three lines of Greek characters under each subplot code the results of statistical comparisons (Student's t-test, significance level 0.01) of different methods. Line 1 is the comparison between SR and CSP methods; Line 2 is between SR and PLV method; and Line 3 between PLV and CSP method.

rates are achieved by methods based on phase. Especially for subject 'ay', phase generates about 0.2 bits more information per second. The qualitative similarity between SR and PLV method suggests that phase can be more discriminative than amplitude within the first 1.5-2.0 s. Common to the three methods, however, the near zero information transfer rates within the first second virtually pose a limit for BCIs. In the case where real-time application is of high priority, such as navigating wheelchairs, this problem is even more pronounced. Incorporating phase information and continuing the search for new features have the potential to overcome this limit.

6   Conclusion

EEG phase contains complex dynamics. Changes of phase synchrony provide complementary information to EEG amplitude. Our results show that within the first 1.5-2.0 s of a motor imagery, phase can be more useful for classification and can be exploited by our synchrony rate method. Although methods based on phase have achieved good results in some subjects, the subject-wise difference and the exact functional interpretation of the selected features need further investigation. Solving these problems have the potential to boost information transfer rates in BCIs.

Acknowledgments

The author would like to thank Ms. Yingxin Wu and Dr. Julien Epps from NICTA, and Dr. Michael Breakspear from Brain Dynamics Center for discussion.

References

[1] J.R. Wolpaw et al., "Brain-computer interface technology: a review of the first international meeting," *IEEE Trans. Rehab. Eng.*, vol. 8, pp. 164-173, 2000.

[2] T.M. Vaughan et al., "Brain-computer interface technonolgy: a review of the second international meeting," *IEEE Trans. Rehab. Eng.*, vol. 11, pp. 94-109, 2003.

[3] H. Ramoser, J. Müller-Gerking, and G. Pfurtscheller, "Optimal spatial filtering of single trial EEG during imagined hand movement," *IEEE Trans. Rehab. Eng.*, vol. 8, pp. 441-446, 2000.

[4] G. Dornhege, B. Blankertz, G. Curio, and K.R. Müller, "Combining features for BCI," *Advances in Neural Inf. Proc. Systems (NIPS 02)*, vol. 15, pp. 1115-1122, 2003.

[5] G. Dornhege, B. Blankertz, G. Curio, and K.R. Müller, "Boosting bit rates in non-invasive EEG single-trial classifications by feature combination and multi-class paradigms," *IEEE Trans. Biomed. Eng.*, vol. 51, pp. 993-1002, 2004.

[6] E. Rodriguez et al., "Perception's shadow: long distance synchronization of human brain activity," *Nature*, vol. 397, pp. 430-433, 1999.

[7] F. Varela, J.P. Lachaux, E. Rodriguez, and J. Martinerie, "The brainweb: phase synchronization and large-scale integration," *Nature Reviews Neuroscience*, vol. 2, pp. 229-239, 2001.

[8] W. Singer, and C.M. Gray, "Visual feature integration and the temporal correlation hypothesis," *Annu. Rev. Neurosci*, vol. 18, pp. 555-586, 1995.

[9] P.R. Roelfsema, A.K. Engel, P. König, and W. Singer, "Visuomotor integration is associated with zero time-lag synchronization among cortical areas," *Nature*, vol. 385, pp. 157-161, 1997.

[10] E. Gysels, and P. Celka, "Phase synchronization for the recognition of mental tasks in brain-computer interface," *IEEE Trans. Neural Syst. Rehab. Eng.*, vol. 12, pp. 406-415, 2004.

[11] C. Brunner, B. Graimann, J.E. Huggins, S.P Levine and G. Pfurtscheller, "Phase relationships between different subdural electrode recordings in man," *Neurosci. Lett.*, vol. 275, pp.69-74, 2005.

[12] L. Song, "Desynchronization network analysis for the recognition of imagined movement in BCIs,", *Proc. of 27th IEEE EMBS conference*, Shanghai, China, September 2005.

[13] M. Le Van Quyen et al., "Comparison of Hilbert transform and wavelet methods for the analysis of neuronal synchrony," *J. Neurosci. Methods*, vol. 111, pp. 83-98, 2001.

[14] M. Breakspear, L. Williams, and C.J. Stam, "A novel method for the topographic analysis of neural activity reveals formation and dissolution of 'dynmaic cell assemblies'," *J. Comput. Neurosci.*, vol. 16, pp. 49-68, 2004.

[15] M.J.A.M van Putten, "Proposed link rates in the human brain," *J. of Neurosci. Methods*, vol. 127, pp. 1-10, 2003.

[16] L. Song, and J. Epps, "Improving separability of EEG signals during motor imagery with an efficient circular Laplacian," in preparation.

[17] T.E. Nichols, and A.P. Holmes, "Nonparametric permutation tests for functional neuroimaging: a primer with examples," *Human Brain Mapping*, vol. 15, pp. 1-25, 2001.

[18] Y.J. Wang, X.R. Gao, Z.G. Zhang, B. Hong, and S.K. Gao, "BCI competition III—data set IVa: classifying single-trial EEG during motor imagery with a small training set," *IEEE Trans. Neural Syst. Rehab. Eng.*, submitted.

A General and *Efficient* Multiple Kernel Learning Algorithm

Sören Sonnenburg[*]
Fraunhofer FIRST
Kekuléstr. 7
12489 Berlin
Germany
sonne@first.fhg.de

Gunnar Rätsch
Friedrich Miescher Lab
Max Planck Society
Spemannstr. 39
Tübingen, Germany
raetsch@tue.mpg.de

Christin Schäfer
Fraunhofer FIRST
Kekuléstr. 7
12489 Berlin
Germany
christin@first.fhg.de

Abstract

While classical kernel-based learning algorithms are based on a single kernel, in practice it is often desirable to use multiple kernels. Lankriet et al. (2004) considered conic combinations of kernel matrices for classification, leading to a convex quadratically constraint quadratic program. We show that it can be rewritten as a semi-infinite linear program that can be efficiently solved by recycling the standard SVM implementations. Moreover, we generalize the formulation and our method to a larger class of problems, including regression and one-class classification. Experimental results show that the proposed algorithm helps for automatic model selection, improving the interpretability of the learning result and works for hundred thousands of examples or hundreds of kernels to be combined.

1 Introduction

Kernel based methods such as Support Vector Machines (SVMs) have proven to be powerful for a wide range of different data analysis problems. They employ a so-called kernel function $\mathbf{k}(\mathbf{x}_i, \mathbf{x}_j)$ which intuitively computes the similarity between two examples $\mathbf{x}_i$ and $\mathbf{x}_j$. The result of SVM learning is a α-weighted linear combination of kernel elements and the bias b:

$$f(\mathbf{x}) = \text{sign}\left(\sum_{i=1}^{N} \alpha_i y_i \mathbf{k}(\mathbf{x}_i, \mathbf{x}) + b\right), \tag{1}$$

where the $\mathbf{x}_i$'s are N labeled training examples ($y_i \in \{\pm 1\}$).

Recent developments in the literature on the SVM and other kernel methods have shown the need to consider multiple kernels. This provides flexibility, and also reflects the fact that typical learning problems often involve multiple, heterogeneous data sources. While this so-called "multiple kernel learning" (MKL) problem can in principle be solved via cross-validation, several recent papers have focused on more efficient methods for multiple kernel learning [4, 5, 1, 7, 3, 9, 2].

One of the problems with kernel methods compared to other techniques is that the resulting decision function (1) is hard to interpret and, hence, is difficult to use in order to extract rel-

---

[*]For more details, datasets and pseudocode see http://www.fml.tuebingen.mpg.de/raetsch/projects/mkl_silp.

evant knowledge about the problem at hand. One can approach this problem by considering convex combinations of K kernels, i.e.

$$\mathbf{k}(\mathbf{x}_i, \mathbf{x}_j) = \sum_{k=1}^{K} \beta_k \mathbf{k}_k(\mathbf{x}_i, \mathbf{x}_j) \tag{2}$$

with $\beta_k \geq 0$ and $\sum_k \beta_k = 1$, where each kernel $\mathbf{k}_k$ uses only a distinct set of features of each instance. For appropriately designed sub-kernels $\mathbf{k}_k$, the optimized combination coefficients can then be used to understand which features of the examples are of importance for discrimination: if one would be able to obtain an accurate classification by a *sparse* weighting β_k, then one can quite easily interpret the resulting decision function. We will illustrate that the considered MKL formulation provides useful insights and is at the same time is very efficient. This is an important property missing in current kernel based algorithms.

We consider the framework proposed by [7], which results in a convex optimization problem - a quadratically-constrained quadratic program (QCQP). This problem is more challenging than the standard SVM QP, but it can in principle be solved by general-purpose optimization toolboxes. Since the use of such algorithms will only be feasible for small problems with few data points and kernels, [1] suggested an algorithm based on sequential minimization optimization (SMO) [10]. While the kernel learning problem is convex, it is also non-smooth, making the direct application of simple local descent algorithms such as SMO infeasible. [1] therefore considered a smoothed version of the problem to which SMO can be applied.

In this work we follow a different direction: We reformulate the problem as a semi-infinite linear program (SILP), which can be efficiently solved using an off-the-shelf LP solver and a standard SVM implementation (cf. Section 2 for details). Using this approach we are able to solve problems with more than hundred thousand examples or with several hundred kernels quite efficiently. We have used it for the analysis of sequence analysis problems leading to a better understanding of the biological problem at hand [16, 13]. We extend our previous work and show that the transformation to a SILP works with a large class of convex loss functions (cf. Section 3). Our column-generation based algorithm for solving the SILP works by repeatedly using an algorithm that can efficiently solve the single kernel problem in order to solve the MKL problem. Hence, if there exists an algorithm that solves the simpler problem efficiently (like SVMs), then our new algorithm can efficiently solve the multiple kernel learning problem.

We conclude the paper by illustrating the usefulness of our algorithms in several examples relating to the interpretation of results and to automatic model selection.

2 Multiple Kernel Learning for Classification using SILP

In the Multiple Kernel Learning (MKL) problem for binary classification one is given N data points $(\mathbf{x}_i, y_i)$ $(y_i \in \{\pm 1\})$, where $\mathbf{x}_i$ is translated via a mapping $\Phi_k(\mathbf{x}) \mapsto \mathbb{R}^{D_k}$, $k = 1 \dots K$ from the input into K feature spaces $(\Phi_1(\mathbf{x}_i), \dots, \Phi_K(\mathbf{x}_i))$ where D_k denotes the dimensionality of the k-th feature space. Then one solves the following optimization problem [1], which is equivalent to the linear SVM for $K = 1$:[1]

$$\min_{\mathbf{w}_k \in \mathbb{R}^{D_k}, \boldsymbol{\xi} \in \mathbb{R}^N_+, \boldsymbol{\beta} \in \mathbb{R}^K_+, b \in \mathbb{R}} \quad \frac{1}{2}\left(\sum_{k=1}^{K} \beta_k \|\mathbf{w}_k\|_2\right)^2 + C \sum_{i=1}^{N} \xi_i \tag{3}$$

$$\text{s.t.} \quad y_i \left(\sum_{k=1}^{K} \beta_k \mathbf{w}_k^\top \Phi_k(\mathbf{x}_i) + b\right) \geq 1 - \xi_i \text{ and } \sum_{k=1}^{K} \beta_k = 1.$$

---

[1] [1] used a slightly different but equivalent (assuming $\operatorname{tr}(K_k) = 1$, $k = 1, \dots, K$) formulation without the β's, which we introduced for illustration.

Note that the ℓ_1-norm of $\boldsymbol{\beta}$ is constrained to one, while one is penalizing the ℓ_2-norm of $\mathbf{w}_k$ in each block k separately. The idea is that ℓ_1-norm constrained or penalized variables tend to have sparse optimal solutions, while ℓ_2-norm penalized variables do not [11]. Thus the above optimization problem offers the possibility to find sparse solutions on the block level with non-sparse solutions within the blocks.

Bach et al. [1] derived the dual for problem (3), which can be equivalently written as:

$$\min_{\gamma \in \mathbb{R}, 1C \geq \boldsymbol{\alpha} \in \mathbb{R}_+^N} \gamma \quad \text{s.t.} \quad \underbrace{\frac{1}{2} \sum_{i,j=1}^N \alpha_i \alpha_j y_i y_j \mathbf{k}_k(\mathbf{x}_i, \mathbf{x}_j) - \sum_{i=1}^N \alpha_i}_{=:S_k(\boldsymbol{\alpha})} \leq \gamma \quad \text{and} \quad \sum_{i=1}^N \alpha_i y_i = 0 \quad (4)$$

for $k = 1, \ldots, K$, where $\mathbf{k}_k(\mathbf{x}_i, \mathbf{x}_j) = (\Phi_k(\mathbf{x}_i), \Phi_k(\mathbf{x}_j))$. Note that we have one quadratic constraint per kernel ($S_k(\boldsymbol{\alpha}) \leq \gamma$). In the case of $K = 1$, the above problem reduces to the original SVM dual.

In order to solve (4), one may solve the following saddle point problem (Lagrangian):

$$\mathcal{L} := \gamma + \sum_{k=1}^K \beta_k (S_k(\boldsymbol{\alpha}) - \gamma) \tag{5}$$

minimized w.r.t. $\boldsymbol{\alpha} \in \mathbb{R}_+^N, \gamma \in \mathbb{R}$ (subject to $\boldsymbol{\alpha} \leq C\mathbf{1}$ and $\sum_i \alpha_i y_i = 0$) and maximized w.r.t. $\boldsymbol{\beta} \in \mathbb{R}_+^K$. Setting the derivative w.r.t. to γ to zero, one obtains the constraint $\sum_k \beta_k = 1$ and (5) simplifies to: $\mathcal{L} = S(\boldsymbol{\alpha}, \boldsymbol{\beta}) := \sum_{k=1}^K \beta_k S_k(\boldsymbol{\alpha})$ and leads to a min-max problem:

$$\max_{\boldsymbol{\beta} \in \mathbb{R}_+^K} \min_{1C \geq \boldsymbol{\alpha} \in \mathbb{R}_+^N} \sum_{k=1}^K \beta_k S_k(\boldsymbol{\alpha}) \quad \text{s.t.} \quad \sum_{i=1}^N \alpha_i y_i = 0 \quad \text{and} \quad \sum_{k=1}^K \beta_k = 1. \tag{6}$$

Assume $\boldsymbol{\alpha}^*$ would be the optimal solution, then $\theta^* := S(\boldsymbol{\alpha}^*, \boldsymbol{\beta})$ is minimal and, hence, $S(\boldsymbol{\alpha}, \boldsymbol{\beta}) \geq \theta^*$ for all $\boldsymbol{\alpha}$ (subject to the above constraints). Hence, finding a saddle-point of (5) is equivalent to solving the following semi-infinite linear program:

$$\max_{\theta \in \mathbb{R}, \boldsymbol{\beta} \in \mathbb{R}_+^M} \theta \quad \text{s.t.} \quad \sum_k \beta_k = 1 \quad \text{and} \quad \sum_{k=1}^K \beta_k S_k(\boldsymbol{\alpha}) \geq \theta \tag{7}$$

$$\text{for all } \boldsymbol{\alpha} \text{ with } 0 \leq \boldsymbol{\alpha} \leq C\mathbf{1} \text{ and } \sum_i y_i \alpha_i = 0$$

Note that this is a linear program, as θ and $\boldsymbol{\beta}$ are only linearly constrained. However there are infinitely many constraints: one for each $\boldsymbol{\alpha} \in \mathbb{R}^N$ satisfying $0 \leq \boldsymbol{\alpha} \leq C$ and $\sum_{i=1}^N \alpha_i y_i = 0$. Both problems (6) and (7) have the same solution. To illustrate that, consider $\boldsymbol{\beta}$ is fixed and we maximize $\boldsymbol{\alpha}$ in (6). Let $\boldsymbol{\alpha}^*$ be the solution that maximizes (6). Then we can decrease the value of θ in (7) as long as no $\boldsymbol{\alpha}$-constraint (7) is violated, i.e. down to $\theta = \sum_{k=1}^K \beta_k S_k(\boldsymbol{\alpha}^*)$. Similarly, as we increase θ for a fixed $\boldsymbol{\alpha}$ the maximizing $\boldsymbol{\beta}$ is found. We will discuss in Section 4 how to solve such semi infinite linear programs.

3 Multiple Kernel Learning with General Cost Functions

In this section we consider the more general class of MKL problems, where one is given an *arbitrary* strictly convex differentiable loss function, for which we derive its MKL SILP formulation. We will then investigate in this general MKL SILP using different loss functions, in particular the soft-margin loss, the ϵ-insensitive loss and the quadratic loss.

We define the MKL primal formulation for a strictly convex and differentiable loss function L as: (for simplicity we omit a bias term)

$$\min_{\mathbf{w}_k \in \mathbb{R}^{D_k}} \frac{1}{2} \left(\sum_{k=1}^K \|\mathbf{w}_k\| \right)^2 + \sum_{i=1}^N L(f(\mathbf{x}_i), y_i) \quad \text{s.t.} \quad f(\mathbf{x}_i) = \sum_{k=1}^K (\Phi_k(\mathbf{x}_i), \mathbf{w}_k) \tag{8}$$

1275

In analogy to [1] we treat problem (8) as a second order cone program (SOCP) leading to the following dual (see Supplementary Website or [17] for details):

$$\min_{\gamma \in \mathbb{R}, \boldsymbol{\alpha} \in \mathbb{R}^N} \quad \gamma - \sum_{i=1}^{N} L(L'^{-1}(\alpha_i, y_i), y_i) + \sum_{i=1}^{N} \alpha_i L'^{-1}(\alpha_i, y_i) \tag{9}$$

$$\text{s.t.} : \quad \frac{1}{2} \left\| \sum_{i=1}^{N} \alpha_i \Phi_k(\mathbf{x}_i) \right\|_2^2 \leq \gamma, \ \forall k = 1 \dots K$$

To derive the SILP formulation we follow the same recipe as in Section 2: deriving the Lagrangian leads to a max-min problem formulation to be eventually reformulated to a SILP:

$$\max_{\theta \in \mathbb{R}, \boldsymbol{\beta} \in \mathbb{R}^K} \ \theta \quad \text{s.t.} \quad \sum_{k=1}^{K} \beta_k = 1 \quad \text{and} \quad \sum_{k=1}^{K} \beta_k S_k(\boldsymbol{\alpha}) \geq \theta, \ \forall \boldsymbol{\alpha} \in \mathbb{R}^N,$$

where $S_k(\boldsymbol{\alpha}) = - \sum_{i=1}^{N} L(L'^{-1}(\alpha_i, y_i), y_i) + \sum_{i=1}^{N} \alpha_i L'^{-1}(\alpha_i, y_i) + \frac{1}{2} \left\| \sum_{i=1}^{N} \alpha_i \Phi_k(\mathbf{x}_i) \right\|_2^2.$

We assumed that $L(x, y)$ is strictly convex and differentiable in x. Unfortunately, the soft margin and ϵ-insensitive loss do not have these properties. We therefore consider them separately in the sequel.

Soft Margin Loss We use the following loss in order to approximate the soft margin loss: $L_\sigma(x, y) = \frac{C}{\sigma} \log(1 + \exp((1 - xy)\sigma))$. It is easy to verify that $\lim_{\sigma \to \infty} L_\sigma(x, y) = C(1 - xy)_+$. Moreover, L_σ is strictly convex and differentiable for $\sigma < \infty$. Using this loss and assuming $y_i \in \{\pm 1\}$, we obtain :

$$S_k(\boldsymbol{\alpha}) = - \sum_{i=1}^{N} \frac{C}{\sigma} \left(\log \left(\frac{C y_i}{\alpha_i + C y_i} \right) + \log \left(-\frac{\alpha_i}{\alpha_i + C y_i} \right) \right) + \sum_{i=1}^{N} \alpha_i y_i + \frac{1}{2} \left\| \sum_{i=1}^{N} \alpha_i \Phi_k(\mathbf{x}_i) \right\|_2^2.$$

If $\sigma \to \infty$, then the first two terms vanish provided that $-C \leq \alpha_i \leq 0$ if $y_i = 1$ and $0 \leq \alpha_i \leq C$ if $y_i = -1$. Substituting $\alpha = -\tilde{\alpha}_i y_i$, we then obtain $S_k(\tilde{\boldsymbol{\alpha}}) = - \sum_{i=1}^{N} \tilde{\alpha}_i + \frac{1}{2} \left\| \sum_{i=1}^{N} \tilde{\alpha}_i y_i \Phi_k(\mathbf{x}_i) \right\|_2^2$, with $0 \leq \tilde{\alpha}_i \leq C$ $(i = 1, \dots, N)$, which is very similar to (4): only the $\sum_i \alpha_i y_i = 0$ constraint is missing, since we omitted the bias.

One-Class Soft Margin Loss The one-class SVM soft margin (e.g. [15]) is very similar to the two class case and leads to $S_k(\boldsymbol{\alpha}) = \frac{1}{2} \left\| \sum_{i=1}^{N} \alpha_i \Phi_k(\mathbf{x}_i) \right\|_2^2$ subject to $\mathbf{0} \leq \boldsymbol{\alpha} \leq \frac{1}{\nu N} \mathbf{1}$ and $\sum_{i=1}^{N} \alpha_i = 1$.

ϵ-insensitive Loss Using the same technique for the epsilon insensitive loss $L(x, y) = C(1 - |x - y|)_+$, we obtain

$$S_k(\boldsymbol{\alpha}, \boldsymbol{\alpha}^*) = \frac{1}{2} \left\| \sum_{i=1}^{N} (\alpha_i - \alpha_i^*) \Phi_k(\mathbf{x}_i) \right\|_2^2 - \sum_{i=1}^{N} (\alpha_i + \alpha_i^*) \epsilon - \sum_{i=1}^{N} (\alpha_i - \alpha_i^*) y_i,$$

with $\mathbf{0} \leq \boldsymbol{\alpha}, \boldsymbol{\alpha}^* \leq C\mathbf{1}$. When including a bias term, we additionally have the constraint $\sum_{i=1}^{N} (\alpha_i - \alpha_i^*) y_i = 0$.

It is straightforward to derive the dual problem for other loss functions such as the quadratic loss. Note that the dual SILP's only differ in the definition of S_k and the domains of the $\boldsymbol{\alpha}$'s.

4 Algorithms to solve SILPs

The SILPs considered in this work all have the following form:

$$\max_{\theta \in \mathbb{R}, \boldsymbol{\beta} \in \mathbb{R}_+^M} \ \theta \quad \text{s.t.} \quad \sum_{k=1}^{K} \beta_k = 1 \quad \text{and} \quad \sum_{k=1}^{M} \beta_k S_k(\boldsymbol{\alpha}) \geq \theta \text{ for all } \boldsymbol{\alpha} \in \mathcal{C} \tag{10}$$

for some appropriate $S_k(\boldsymbol{\alpha})$ and the feasible set $\mathcal{C} \subseteq \mathbb{R}^N$ of $\boldsymbol{\alpha}$ depending on the choice of the cost function. Using Theorem 5 in [12] one can show that the above SILP has a solution if the corresponding primal is feasible and bounded. Moreover, there is no duality gap, if $\mathcal{M} = \mathrm{co}\{[S_1(\boldsymbol{\alpha}), \ldots, S_K(\boldsymbol{\alpha})]^\top \mid \boldsymbol{\alpha} \in \mathcal{C}\}$ is a closed set. For all loss functions considered in this paper this holds true. We propose to use a technique called Column Generation to solve (10). The basic idea is to compute the optimal $(\boldsymbol{\beta}, \theta)$ in (10) for a restricted subset of constraints. It is called the *restricted master problem*. Then a second algorithm generates a new constraint determined by $\boldsymbol{\alpha}$. In the best case the other algorithm finds the constraint that maximizes the constraint violation for the given intermediate solution $(\boldsymbol{\beta}, \theta)$, i.e.

$$\boldsymbol{\alpha_\beta} := \underset{\boldsymbol{\alpha} \in \mathcal{C}}{\mathrm{argmin}} \sum_k \beta_k S_k(\boldsymbol{\alpha}). \tag{11}$$

If $\boldsymbol{\alpha_\beta}$ satisfies the constraint $\sum_{k=1}^K \beta_k S_k(\boldsymbol{\alpha_\beta}) \geq \theta$, then the solution is optimal. Otherwise, the constraint is added to the set of constraints.

Algorithm 1 is a special case of the set of SILP algorithms known as **exchange methods**. These methods are known to converge (cf. Theorem 7.2 in [6]). However, no convergence rates for such algorithm are so far known.[2] Since it is often sufficient to obtain an approximate solution, we have to define a suitable convergence criterion. Note that the problem is solved when all constraints are satisfied. Hence, it is a natural choice to use the normalized maximal constraint violation as a convergence criterion, i.e. $\epsilon := \left| 1 - \frac{\sum_{k=1}^K \beta_k^t S_k(\boldsymbol{\alpha}^t)}{\theta^t} \right|$, where $(\boldsymbol{\beta}^t, \theta^t)$ is the optimal solution at iteration $t-1$ and $\boldsymbol{\alpha}^t$ corresponds to the newly found maximally violating constraint of the next iteration.

We need an algorithm to identify unsatisfied constraints, which, fortunately, turns out to be particularly simple. Note that (11) is for all considered cases exactly the dual optimization problem of the single kernel case for fixed $\boldsymbol{\beta}$. For instance for binary classification, (11) reduces to the standard SVM dual using the kernel $\mathbf{k}(\mathbf{x}_i, \mathbf{x}_j) = \sum_k \beta_k \mathbf{k}_k(\mathbf{x}_i, \mathbf{x}_j)$:

$$\min_{\boldsymbol{\alpha} \in \mathbb{R}^N} \sum_{i,j=1}^N \alpha_i \alpha_j y_i y_j \mathbf{k}(\mathbf{x}_i, \mathbf{x}_j) - \sum_{i=1}^N \alpha_i \quad \text{with} \quad \mathbf{0} \leq \boldsymbol{\alpha} \leq C\mathbf{1} \text{ and } \sum_{i=1}^N \alpha_i y_i = 0.$$

We can therefore use a standard SVM implementation in order to identify the most violated constraint. Since there exist a large number of efficient algorithms to solve the single kernel problems for all sorts of cost functions, we have therefore found an easy way to extend their applicability to the problem of Multiple Kernel Learning. In some cases it is possible to extend existing SMO based implementations to simultaneously optimize $\boldsymbol{\beta}$ and $\boldsymbol{\alpha}$. In [16] we have considered such an algorithm for the binary classification case that frequently recomputes the $\boldsymbol{\beta}$'s.[3] Empirically it is a few times faster than the column generation algorithm, but it is on the other hand much harder to implement.

5   Experiments

In this section we will discuss toy examples for binary classification and regression, demonstrating that MKL can recover information about the problem at hand, followed by a brief review on problems for which MKL has been successfully used.

5.1   Classifications

In Figure 1 we consider a binary classification problem, where we used MKL-SVMs with five RBF-kernels with different widths, to distinguish the dark star-like shape from the

---

[2]It has been shown that solving semi-infinite problems like (7), using a method related to boosting (e.g. [8]) one requires at most $T = \mathcal{O}(\log(M)/\hat{\epsilon}^2)$ iterations, where $\hat{\epsilon}$ is the remaining constraint violation and the constants may depend on the kernels and the number of examples N [11, 14]. At least for not too small values of $\hat{\epsilon}$ this technique produces reasonably fast good approximate solutions.

[3]Simplex based LP solvers often offer the possibility to efficient restart the computation when adding only a few constraints.

Algorithm 1 The column generation algorithm employs a linear programming solver to iteratively solve the semi-infinite linear optimization problem (10). The accuracy parameter ϵ is a parameter of the algorithm. $S_k(\boldsymbol{\alpha})$ and $\mathcal{C}$ are determined by the cost function.

$S^0 = 1, \theta^1 = -\infty, \beta_k^1 = \frac{1}{K}$ for $k = 1, \ldots, K$

for $t = 1, 2, \ldots$ **do**

Compute $\boldsymbol{\alpha}^t = \underset{\boldsymbol{\alpha} \in \mathcal{C}}{\operatorname{argmin}} \sum_{k=1}^{K} \beta_k^t S_k(\boldsymbol{\alpha})$ by single kernel algorithm with $K = \sum_{k=1}^{K} \beta_k^t K_k$

$S^t = \sum_{k=1}^{K} \beta_k^t S_k(\boldsymbol{\alpha}^t)$

if $|1 - \frac{S^t}{\theta^t}| \leq \epsilon$ **then break**

$(\boldsymbol{\beta}^{t+1}, \theta^{t+1}) = \operatorname{argmax} \theta$

w.r.t. $\boldsymbol{\beta} \in \mathbb{R}_+^K, \theta \in \mathbb{R}$ with $\sum_{k=1}^{K} \beta_k = 1$ and $\sum_{k=1}^{K} \beta_k S_k^r \geq \theta$ for $r = 1, \ldots, t$

end for

---

light star. (The distance between the stars increases from left to right.) Shown are the obtained kernel weightings for the five kernels and the test error which quickly drops to zero as the problem becomes separable. Note that the RBF kernel with largest width was not appropriate and thus never chosen. Also with increasing distance between the stars kernels with greater widths are used. This illustrates that MKL one can indeed recover such tendencies.

5.2 Regression

We applied the newly derived MKL support vector regression formulation, to the task of learning a sine function using three RBF-kernels with different widths. We then increased the frequency of the sine wave. As can be seen in Figure 2, MKL-SV regression abruptly switches to the width of the RBF-kernel fitting the regression problem best. In another regression experiment, we combined a linear function with two sine waves, one of lower frequency and one of high frequency, i.e. $f(x) = c \cdot x + \sin(ax) + \sin(bx)$. Using ten RBF-kernels of different width (see Figure 3) we trained a MKL-SVR and display the learned weights (a column in the figure). The largest selected width (100) models the linear component (since RBF with large widths are effectively linear) and the medium width (1) corresponds to the lower frequency sine. We varied the frequency of the high frequency sine wave from low to high (left to right in the figure). One observes that MKL determines

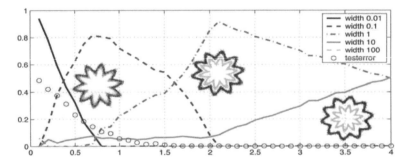

Figure 1: A 2-class toy problem where the dark grey star-like shape is to be distinguished from the light grey star inside of the dark grey star. For details see text.

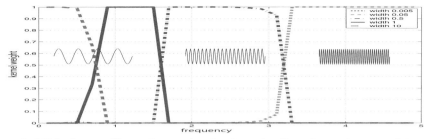

Figure 2: MKL-Support Vector Regression for the task of learning a sine wave (please see text for details).

an appropriate combination of kernels of low and high widths, while decreasing the RBF-kernel width with increased frequency. This shows that MKL can be more powerful than cross-validation: To achieve a similar result with cross-validation one has to use 3 nested loops to tune 3 RBF-kernel sigmas, e.g. train $10 \cdot 9 \cdot 8/6 = 120$ SVMs, which in preliminary experiments was much slower then using MKL (800 vs. 56 seconds).

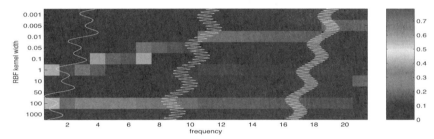

Figure 3: MKL support vector regression on a linear combination of three functions: $f(x) = c \cdot x + \sin(ax) + \sin(bx)$. MKL recovers that the original function is a combination of functions of low and high complexity. For more details see text.

5.3 Applications in the Real World

MKL has been successfully used on real-world datasets in the field of computational biology [7, 16]. It was shown to improve classification performance on the task of ribosomal and membrane protein prediction, where a weighting over different kernels each corresponding to a different feature set was learned. Random channels obtained low kernel weights. Moreover, on a splice site recognition task we used MKL as a tool for interpreting the SVM classifier [16], as is displayed in Figure 4. Using specifically optimized string kernels, we were able to solve the classification MKL SILP for $N = 1.000.000$ examples and $K = 20$ kernels, as well as for $N = 10.000$ examples and $K = 550$ kernels.

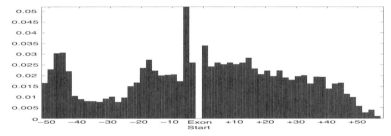

Figure 4: The figure shows an importance weighting for each position in a DNA sequence (around a so called splice site). MKL was used to learn these weights, each corresponding to a sub-kernel which uses information at that position to discriminate true splice sites from fake ones. Different peaks correspond to different biologically known signals (see [16] for details). We used 65.000 examples for training with 54 sub-kernels.

6 Conclusion

We have proposed a simple, yet efficient algorithm to solve the multiple kernel learning problem for a large class of loss functions. The proposed method is able to exploit the existing single kernel algorithms, whereby extending their applicability. In experiments we have illustrated that the MKL for classification and regression can be useful for automatic model selection and for obtaining comprehensible information about the learning problem at hand. It is future work to evaluate MKL algorithms for unsupervised learning such as Kernel PCA and one-class classification.

Acknowledgments

The authors gratefully acknowledge partial support from the PASCAL Network of Excellence (EU #506778), DFG grants JA 379 / 13-2 and MU 987/2-1. We thank Guido Dornhege, Olivier Chapelle, Olaf Weiss, Joaquin Quiñoñero Candela, Sebastian Mika and K.-R. Müller for great discussions.

References

[1] Francis R. Bach, Gert R. G. Lanckriet, and Michael I. Jordan. Multiple kernel learning, conic duality, and the SMO algorithm. In *Twenty-first international conference on Machine learning*. ACM Press, 2004.

[2] Kristin P. Bennett, Michinari Momma, and Mark J. Embrechts. Mark: a boosting algorithm for heterogeneous kernel models. *KDD*, pages 24–31, 2002.

[3] Jinbo Bi, Tong Zhang, and Kristin P. Bennett. Column-generation boosting methods for mixture of kernels. *KDD*, pages 521–526, 2004.

[4] O. Chapelle, V. Vapnik, O. Bousquet, and S. Mukherjee. Choosing multiple parameters for support vector machines. *Machine Learning*, 46(1-3):131–159, 2002.

[5] I. Grandvalet and S. Canu. Adaptive scaling for feature selection in SVMs. In *In Advances in Neural Information Processing Systems*, 2002.

[6] R. Hettich and K.O. Kortanek. Semi-infinite programming: Theory, methods and applications. *SIAM Review*, 3:380–429, September 1993.

[7] G.R.G. Lanckriet, T. De Bie, N. Cristianini, M.I. Jordan, and W.S. Noble. A statistical framework for genomic data fusion. *Bioinformatics*, 2004.

[8] R. Meir and G. Rätsch. An introduction to boosting and leveraging. In S. Mendelson and A. Smola, editors, *Proc. of the first Machine Learning Summer School in Canberra*, LNCS, pages 119–184. Springer, 2003. in press.

[9] C.S. Ong, A.J. Smola, and R.C. Williamson. Hyperkernels. In *In Advances in Neural Information Processing Systems*, volume 15, pages 495–502, 2003.

[10] J. Platt. Fast training of support vector machines using sequential minimal optimization. In B. Schölkopf, C.J.C. Burges, and A.J. Smola, editors, *Advances in Kernel Methods — Support Vector Learning*, pages 185–208, Cambridge, MA, 1999. MIT Press.

[11] G. Rätsch. *Robust Boosting via Convex Optimization*. PhD thesis, University of Potsdam, Computer Science Dept., August-Bebel-Str. 89, 14482 Potsdam, Germany, 2001.

[12] G. Rätsch, A. Demiriz, and K. Bennett. Sparse regression ensembles in infinite and finite hypothesis spaces. *Machine Learning*, 48(1-3):193–221, 2002. Special Issue on New Methods for Model Selection and Model Combination. Also NeuroCOLT2 Technical Report NC-TR-2000-085.

[13] G. Rätsch, S. Sonnenburg, and C. Schäfer. Learning interpretable svms for biological sequence classification. *BMC Bioinformatics, Special Issue from NIPS workshop on New Problems and Methods in Computational Biology Whistler, Canada, 18 December 2004*, 7(Suppl. 1:S9), February 2006.

[14] G. Rätsch and M.K. Warmuth. Marginal boosting. NeuroCOLT2 Technical Report 97, Royal Holloway College, London, July 2001.

[15] B. Schölkopf and A. J. Smola. *Learning with Kernels*. MIT Press, Cambridge, MA, 2002.

[16] S. Sonnenburg, G. Rätsch, and C. Schäfer. Learning interpretable SVMs for biological sequence classification. In *RECOMB 2005, LNBI 3500*, pages 389–407. Springer-Verlag Berlin Heidelberg, 2005.

[17] S. Sonnenburg, G. Rätsch, S. Schäfer, and B. Schölkopf. Large scale multiple kernel learning. *Journal of Machine Learning Research*, 2006. accepted.

Prediction and Change Detection

Mark Steyvers
msteyver@uci.edu
University of California, Irvine
Irvine, CA 92697

Scott Brown
scottb@uci.edu
University of California, Irvine
Irvine, CA 92697

Abstract

We measure the ability of human observers to predict the next datum in a sequence that is generated by a simple statistical process undergoing change at random points in time. Accurate performance in this task requires the identification of changepoints. We assess individual differences between observers both empirically, and using two kinds of models: a Bayesian approach for change detection and a family of cognitively plausible fast and frugal models. Some individuals detect too many changes and hence perform sub-optimally due to excess variability. Other individuals do not detect enough changes, and perform sub-optimally because they fail to notice short-term temporal trends.

1 Introduction

Decision-making often requires a rapid response to change. For example, stock analysts need to quickly detect changes in the market in order to adjust investment strategies. Coaches need to track changes in a player's performance in order to adjust strategy. When tracking changes, there are costs involved when either more or less changes are observed than actually occurred. For example, when using an overly conservative change detection criterion, a stock analyst might miss important short-term trends and interpret them as random fluctuations instead. On the other hand, a change may also be detected too readily. For example, in basketball, a player who makes a series of consecutive baskets is often identified as a "hot hand" player whose underlying ability is perceived to have suddenly increased [1,2]. This might lead to sub-optimal passing strategies, based on random fluctuations.

We are interested in explaining individual differences in a sequential prediction task. Observers are shown stimuli generated from a simple statistical process with the task of predicting the next datum in the sequence. The latent parameters of the statistical process change discretely at random points in time. Performance in this task depends on the accurate detection of those changepoints, as well as inference about future outcomes based on the outcomes that followed the most recent inferred changepoint. There is much prior research in statistics on the problem of identifying changepoints [3,4,5]. In this paper, we adopt a Bayesian approach to the changepoint identification problem and develop a simple inference procedure to predict the next datum in a sequence. The Bayesian model serves as an ideal observer model and is useful to characterize the ways in which individuals deviate from optimality.

The plan of the paper is as follows. We first introduce the sequential prediction task and discuss a Bayesian analysis of this prediction problem. We then discuss the results from a few individuals in this prediction task and show how the Bayesian approach can capture individual differences with a single "twitchiness" parameter that describes how readily changes are perceived in random sequences. We will show that some individuals are too twitchy: their performance is too variable because they base their predictions on too little of the recent data. Other individuals are not twitchy enough, and they fail to capture fast changes in the data. We also show how behavior can be explained with a set of *fast and frugal* models [6]. These are cognitively realistic models that operate under plausible computational constraints.

2 A prediction task with multiple changepoints

In the prediction task, stimuli are presented sequentially and the task is to predict the next stimulus in the sequence. After t trials, the observer has been presented with stimuli $y_1, y_2, \ldots, y_t$ and the task is to make a prediction about y_{t+1}. After the prediction is made, the actual outcome y_{t+1} is revealed and the next trial proceeds to the prediction of y_{t+2}. This procedure starts with y_1 and is repeated for T trials.

The observations y_t are D-dimensional vectors with elements sampled from binomial distributions. The parameters of those distributions change discretely at random points in time such that the mean increases or decreases after a change point. This generates a sequence of observation vectors, $y_1, y_2, \ldots, y_T$, where each $y_t = \{y_{t,1} \ldots y_{t,D}\}$. Each of the $y_{t,d}$ is sampled from a binomial distribution $\text{Bin}(\theta_{t,d}, K)$, so $0 \leq y_{t,d} \leq K$. The parameter vector $\theta_t = \{\theta_{t,1} \ldots \theta_{t,D}\}$ changes depending on the locations of the changepoints. At each time step, x_t is a binary indicator for the occurrence of a changepoint occurring at time $t+1$. The parameter α determines the probability of a change occurring in the sequence. The generative model is specified by the following algorithm:

1. For $d=1..D$ sample $\theta_{1,d}$ from a Uniform(0,1) distribution

2. For $t=2..T$,

   (a) Sample x_{t-1} from a Bernoulli(α) distribution

   (b) If $x_{t-1}=0$, then $\theta_t=\theta_{t-1}$, else

       for $d=1..D$ sample $\theta_{t,d}$ from a Uniform(0,1) distribution

   (c) for $d=1..D$, sample y_t from a $\text{Bin}(\theta_{t,d}, K)$ distribution

Table 1 shows some data generated from the changepoint model with $T=20$, $\alpha=.1$, and $D=1$. In the prediction task, y will be observed, but x and θ are not.

Table 1: Example data

t	1	2	3	4	5	6	7	8	9	10	11	12	13	14	15	16	17	18	19	20
x	0	0	0	1	0	0	1	0	0	0	0	0	1	0	1	0	0	0	0	0
θ	.68	.68	.68	.68	.48	.48	.48	.74	.74	.74	.74	.74	.74	.19	.19	.87	.87	.87	.87	.87
y	9	7	8	7	4	4	4	9	8	3	6	7	8	2	1	8	9	9	8	8

3   A Bayesian prediction model

In both our Bayesian and fast-and-frugal analyses, the prediction task is decomposed into two inference procedures. First, the changepoint locations are identified. This is followed by predictive inference for the next outcome based on the most recent changepoint locations. Several Bayesian approaches have been developed for changepoint problems involving single or multiple changepoints [3,5]. We apply a Markov Chain Monte Carlo (MCMC) analysis to approximate the joint posterior distribution over changepoint assignments x while integrating out θ. Gibbs sampling will be used to sample from this posterior marginal distribution. The samples can then be used to predict the next outcome in the sequence.

3.1   Inference for changepoint assignments.

To apply Gibbs sampling, we evaluate the conditional probability of assigning a changepoint at time i, given all other changepoint assignments and the current α value. By integrating out θ, the conditional probability is

$$P\left(x_i \mid x_{-i}, y, \alpha\right) = \int_\theta P\left(x_i, \theta, \alpha \mid x_{-i}, y\right) \tag{1}$$

where x_{-i} represents all switch point assignments except x_i. This can be simplified by considering the location of the most recent changepoint preceding and following time i and the outcomes occurring between these locations. Let n_i^L be the number of time steps from the last changepoint up to and including the current time step i such that $x_{i-n_i^L} = 1$ and $x_{i-n_i^L+j} = 0$ for $0 < j < n_i^L$. Similarly, let n_i^R be the number of time steps that follow time step i up to the next changepoint such that $x_{i+n_i^R} = 1$ and $x_{i+n_i^R-j} = 0$ for $0 < j < n_i^R$. Let $y_i^L = \sum_{i-n_i^L < k \leq i} y_k$ and $y_i^R = \sum_{k < k \leq i+n_i^R} y_k$. The update equation for the changepoint assignment can then be simplified to

$$
P\left(x_i = m \mid x_{-i}\right) \propto
$$
$$
\begin{cases}
(1-\alpha)\displaystyle\prod_{j=1}^{D} \frac{\Gamma\left(1+y_{i,j}^L+y_{i,j}^R\right)\Gamma\left(1+Kn_i^L+Kn_i^R-y_{i,j}^L-y_{i,j}^R\right)}{\Gamma\left(2+Kn_i^L+Kn_i^R\right)} & m=0 \\[3ex]
\alpha\displaystyle\prod_{j=1}^{D} \frac{\Gamma\left(1+y_{i,j}^L\right)\Gamma\left(1+Kn_i^L-y_{i,j}^L\right)\Gamma\left(1+y_{i,j}^R\right)\Gamma\left(1+Kn_i^R-y_{i,j}^R\right)}{\Gamma\left(2+Kn_i^L\right)\Gamma\left(2+Kn_i^R\right)} & m=1
\end{cases}
\tag{2}
$$

We initialize the Gibbs sampler by sampling each x_t from a Bernoulli(α) distribution. All changepoint assignments are then updated sequentially by the Gibbs sampling equation above. The sampler is run for M iterations after which one set of changepoint assignments is saved. The Gibbs sampler is then restarted multiple times until S samples have been collected.

Although we could have included an update equation for α, in this analysis we treat α as a known constant. This will be useful when characterizing the differences between human observers in terms of differences in α.

3.2 Predictive inference

The next latent parameter value θ_{t+1} and outcome y_{t+1} can be predicted on the basis of observed outcomes that occurred after the last inferred changepoint:

$$\theta_{t+1,j} = \sum_{i=t^*+1}^{t} y_{i,j} / K, \qquad y_{t+1,j} = \text{round}\left(\theta_{t+1,j} K\right) \tag{3}$$

where t^* is the location of the most recent change point. By considering multiple Gibbs samples, we get a distribution over outcomes y_{t+1}. We base the model predictions on the mean of this distribution.

3.3 Illustration of model performance

Figure 1 illustrates the performance of the model on a one dimensional sequence ($D=1$) generated from the changepoint model with $T=160$, $\alpha=0.05$, and $K=10$. The Gibbs sampler was run for $M=30$ iterations and S=200 samples were collected. The top panel shows the actual changepoints (triangles) and the distribution of changepoint assignments averaged over samples. The bottom panel shows the observed data y (thin lines) as well as the θ values in the generative model (rescaled between 0 and 10).

At locations with large changes between observations, the marginal changepoint probability is quite high. At other locations, the true change in the mean is very small, and the model is less likely to put in a changepoint. The lower right panel shows the distribution over predicted θ_{t+1} values.

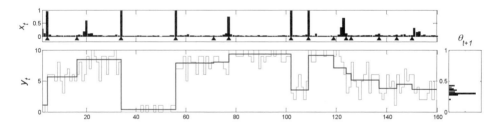

Figure 1. Results of model simulation.

4 Prediction experiment

We tested performance of 9 human observers in the prediction task. The observers included the authors, a visitor, and one student who were aware of the statistical nature of the task as well as naïve students. The observers were seated in front of an LCD touch screen displaying a two-dimensional grid of 11 x 11 buttons. The changepoint model was used to generate a sequence of $T=1500$ stimuli for two binomial variables y_1 and y_2 ($D=2$, $K=10$). The change probability α was set to 0.1. The two variables y_1 and y_2 specified the two-dimensional button location. The same sequence was used for all observers.

On each trial, the observer touched a button on the grid displayed on the touch screen. Following each button press, the button corresponding to the next $\{y_1, y_2\}$ outcome in the sequence was highlighted. Observers were instructed to press the button that best predicted the next location of the highlighted button. The 1500 trials were divided into three blocks of 500 trials. Breaks were allowed between blocks. The whole experiment lasted between 15 and 30 minutes. Figure 2 shows the first 50 trials from the third block of the experiment. The top and bottom panels show the actual outcomes for the y_1 and y_2 button grid coordinates as well as the predictions for two observers (SB and MY). The figure shows that at trial 15, the y_1 and y_2 coordinates show a large shift followed by an immediate shift in observer's MY predictions (on trial 16). Observer SB waits until trial 17 to make a shift.

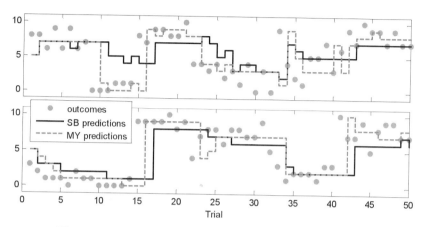

Figure 2. Trial by trial predictions from two observers.

4.1 Task error

We assessed prediction performance by comparing the prediction with the actual outcome in the sequence. Task error was measured by normalized city-block distance

$$\text{task error} = \frac{1}{(T-1)} \sum_{t=2}^{T} \left| y_{t,1} - y_{t,1}^O \right| + \left| y_{t,2} - y_{t,2}^O \right| \tag{4}$$

where y^O represents the observer's prediction. Note that the very first trial is excluded from this calculation. Even though more suitable probabilistic measures for prediction error could have been adopted, we wanted to allow comparison of observer's performance with both probabilistic and non-probabilistic models. Task error ranged from 2.8 (for participant MY) to 3.3 (for ML). We also assessed the performance of five models – their task errors ranged from 2.78 to 3.20. The Bayesian models (Section 3) had the lowest task errors, just below 2.8. This fits with our definition of the Bayesian models as "ideal observer" models – their task error is lower than any other model's and any human observer's task error. The fast and frugal models (Section 5) had task errors ranging from 2.85 to 3.20.

5 Modeling Results

We will refer to the models with the following letter codes: B=Bayesian Model, LB=limited Bayesian model, FF1..3=fast and frugal models 1..3. We assessed model fit by comparing the model's prediction against the human observers' predictions, again using a normalized city-block distance

$$\text{model error} = \frac{1}{(T-1)} \sum_{t=2}^{T} \left| y_{t,1}^{M} - y_{t,1}^{O} \right| + \left| y_{t,2}^{M} - y_{t,2}^{O} \right| \tag{5}$$

where y^M represents the model's prediction. The model error for each individual observer is shown in Figure 3. It is important to note that because each model is associated with a set of free parameters, the parameters optimized for task error and model error are different. For Figure 3, the parameters were optimized to minimize Equation (5) for each individual observer, showing the extent to which these models can capture the performance of individual observers, not necessarily providing the best task performance.

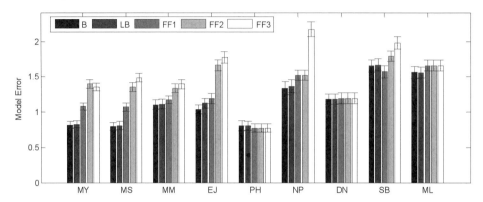

Figure 3. Model error for each individual observer.[1]

5.1 Bayesian prediction models

At each trial t, the model was provided with the sequence of all previous outcomes. The Gibbs sampling and inference procedures from Eq. (2) and (3) were applied with $M=30$ iterations and $S=200$ samples. The change probability α was a free parameter. In the full Bayesian model, the whole sequence of observations up to the current trial is available for prediction, leading to a memory requirement of up to $T=1500$ trials – a psychologically unreasonable assumption. We therefore also simulated a limited Bayesian model (LB) where the observed sequence was truncated to the last 10 outcomes. The LB model showed almost no decrement in task performance compared to the full Bayesian model. Figure 3 also shows that it fit human data quite well.

5.2 Individual Differences

The right-hand panel of Figure 4 plots each observer's task error as a function of the mean city-block distance between their subsequent button presses. This shows a clear U-shaped function. Observers with very variable predictions (e.g., ML and DN) had large average changes between successive button pushes, and also had large task error: These observers were too "twitchy". Observers with very small average button changes (e.g., SB and NP) were not twitchy enough, and also had large task error. Observers in the middle had the lowest task error (e.g., MS and MY). The left-hand panel of Figure 4 shows the same data, but with the x-axis based on the Bayesian model fits. Instead of using mean button change distance to index twitchiness (as in

---

[1] Error bars indicate bootstrapped 95% confidence intervals.

the right-hand panel), the left-hand panel uses the estimated α parameters from the Bayesian model. A similar U-shaped pattern is observed: individuals with too large or too small α estimates have large task errors.

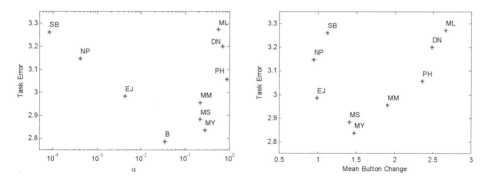

Figure 4. Task error vs. "twitchiness". Left-hand panel indexes twitchiness using estimated α parameters from Bayesian model fits. Right-hand panel uses mean distance between successive predictions.

5.3 Fast-and-Frugal (FF) prediction models

These models perform the prediction task using simple heuristics that are cognitively plausible. The FF models keep a short memory of previous stimulus values and make predictions using the same two-step process as the Bayesian model. First, a decision is made as to whether the latent parameter θ has changed. Second, remembered stimulus values that occurred after the most recently detected changepoint are used to generate the next prediction.

A simple heuristic is used to detect changepoints: If the distance between the most recent observation and prediction is greater than some threshold amount, a change is inferred. We defined the distance between a prediction (p) and an observation (y) as the difference between the log-likelihoods of y assuming $\theta = p$ and $\theta = y$. Thus, if $f_B(.|\theta, K)$ is the binomial density with parameters θ and K, the distance between observation y and prediction p is defined as $d(y,p)=\log(f_B(y|y,K))-\log(f_B(y|p,K))$. A changepoint on time step $t+1$ is inferred whenever $d(y_t, p_t) > C$. The parameter C governs the twitchiness of the model predictions. If C is large, only very dramatic changepoints will be detected, and the model will be too conservative. If C is small, the model will be too twitchy, and will detect changepoints on the basis of small random fluctuations.

Predictions are based on the most recent M observations, which are kept in memory, unless a changepoint has been detected in which case only those observations occurring after the changepoint are used for prediction. The prediction for time step $t+1$ is simply the mean of these observations, say p. Human observers were reticent to make predictions very close to the boundaries. This was modeled by allowing the FF model to change its prediction for the next time step, y_{t+1}, towards the mean prediction (0.5). This change reflects a two-way bet. If the probability of a change occurring is α, the best guess will be 0.5 if that change occurs, or the mean p if the change does not occur. Thus, the prediction made is actually $y_{t+1}=1/2\ \alpha+(1-\alpha)p$. Note that we do not allow perfect knowledge of the probability of a changepoint, α. Instead, an estimated value of α is used based on the number of changepoints detected in the data series up to time t.

The FF model nests two simpler FF models that are psychologically interesting. If the twitchiness threshold parameter C becomes arbitrarily large, the model *never* detects a change and instead becomes a continuous running average model. Predictions from this model are simply a boxcar smooth of the data. Alternatively, if we assume no memory the model must based each prediction on only the previous stimulus (i.e., $M=1$). Above, in Figure 3, we labeled the complete FF model as FF1, the boxcar model as FF2 and the memoryless model FF3.

Figure 3 showed that the complete FF model (FF1) fit the data from all observers significantly better than either the boxcar model (FF2) or the memoryless model (FF3). Exceptions were observers PH, DN and ML, for whom all three FF model fit equally well. This result suggests that our observers were (mostly) doing more than just keeping a running average of the data, or using only the most recent observation. The FF1 model fit the data about as well as the Bayesian models for all observers except MY and MS. Note that, in general, the FF1 and Bayesian model fits are very good: the average city block distance between the human data and the model prediction is around 0.75 (out of 10) buttons on both the x- and y-axes.

6 Conclusion

We used an online prediction task to study changepoint detection. Human observers had to predict the next observation in stochastic sequences containing random changepoints. We showed that some observers are too "twitchy": They perform poorly on the prediction task because they see changes where only random fluctuation exists. Other observers are not twitchy enough, and they perform poorly because they fail to see small changes. We developed a Bayesian changepoint detection model that performed the task optimally, and also provided a good fit to human data when sub-optimal parameter settings were used. Finally, we developed a fast-and-frugal model that showed how participants may be able to perform well at the task using minimal information and simple decision heuristics.

Acknowledgments

We thank Eric-Jan Wagenmakers and Mike Yi for useful discussions related to this work. This work was supported in part by a grant from the US Air Force Office of Scientific Research (AFOSR grant number FA9550-04-1-0317).

References

[1] Gilovich, T., Vallone, R. and Tversky, A. (1985). The hot hand in basketball: on the misperception of random sequences. *Cognitive Psychology17*, 295-314.

[2] Albright, S.C. (1993a). A statistical analysis of hitting streaks in baseball. *Journal of the American Statistical Association, 88*, 1175-1183.

[3] Stephens, D.A. (1994). Bayesian retrospective multiple changepoint identification. *Applied Statistics* **43**(1), 159-178.

[4] Carlin, B.P., Gelfand, A.E., & Smith, A.F.M. (1992). Hierarchical Bayesian analysis of changepoint problems. *Applied Statistics* **41**(2), 389-405.

[5] Green, P.J. (1995). Reversible jump Markov chain Monte Carlo computation and Bayesian model determination. *Biometrika* **82**(4), 711-732.

[6] Gigerenzer, G., & Goldstein, D.G. (1996). Reasoning the fast and frugal way: Models of bounded rationality. *Psychological Review, 103*, 650-669.

Sensory Adaptation within a Bayesian Framework for Perception

Alan A. Stocker[*] and **Eero P. Simoncelli**

Howard Hughes Medical Institute and
Center for Neural Science
New York University

Abstract

We extend a previously developed Bayesian framework for perception to account for sensory adaptation. We first note that the perceptual effects of adaptation seems inconsistent with an adjustment of the internally represented prior distribution. Instead, we postulate that adaptation increases the signal-to-noise ratio of the measurements by adapting the operational range of the measurement stage to the input range. We show that this changes the likelihood function in such a way that the Bayesian estimator model can account for reported perceptual behavior. In particular, we compare the model's predictions to human motion discrimination data and demonstrate that the model accounts for the commonly observed perceptual adaptation effects of repulsion and enhanced discriminability.

1 Motivation

A growing number of studies support the notion that humans are nearly optimal when performing perceptual estimation tasks that require the combination of sensory observations with *a priori* knowledge. The Bayesian formulation of these problems defines the optimal strategy, and provides a principled yet simple computational framework for perception that can account for a large number of known perceptual effects and illusions, as demonstrated in sensorimotor learning [1], cue combination [2], or visual motion perception [3], just to name a few of the many examples.

Adaptation is a fundamental phenomenon in sensory perception that seems to occur at all processing levels and modalities. A variety of computational principles have been suggested as explanations for adaptation. Many of these are based on the concept of maximizing the sensory information an observer can obtain about a stimulus despite limited sensory resources [4, 5, 6]. More mechanistically, adaptation can be interpreted as the attempt of the sensory system to adjusts its (limited) dynamic range such that it is maximally informative with respect to the statistics of the stimulus. A typical example is observed in the retina, which manages to encode light intensities that vary over nine orders of magnitude using ganglion cells whose dynamic range covers only two orders of magnitude. This is achieved by adapting to the local mean as well as higher order statistics of the visual input over short time-scales [7].

---

[*]corresponding author.

If a Bayesian framework is to provide a valid computational explanation of perceptual processes, then it needs to account for the behavior of a perceptual system, regardless of its adaptation state. In general, adaptation in a sensory estimation task seems to have two fundamental effects on subsequent perception:

- *Repulsion:* The estimate of parameters of subsequent stimuli are repelled by those of the adaptor stimulus, *i.e.* the perceived values for the stimulus variable that is subject to the estimation task are more distant from the adaptor value after adaptation. This repulsive effect has been reported for perception of visual speed (*e.g.* [8, 9]), direction-of-motion [10], and orientation [11].

- *Increased sensitivity:* Adaptation increases the observer's discrimination ability around the adaptor (*e.g.* for visual speed [12, 13]), however it also seems to decrease it further away from the adaptor as shown in the case of direction-of-motion discrimination [14].

In this paper, we show that these two perceptual effects can be explained within a Bayesian estimation framework of perception. Note that our description is at an abstract functional level - we do not attempt to provide a computational model for the underlying *mechanisms* responsible for adaptation, and this clearly separates this paper from other work which might seem at first glance similar [e.g., 15].

2 Adaptive Bayesian estimator framework

Suppose that an observer wants to estimate a property of a stimulus denoted by the variable θ, based on a measurement m. In general, the measurement can be vector-valued, and is corrupted by both internal and external noise. Hence, combining the noisy information gained by the measurement m with *a priori* knowledge about θ is advantageous. According to Bayes' rule

$$p(\theta|m) = \frac{1}{\alpha}p(m|\theta)p(\theta) \ . \tag{1}$$

That is, the probability of stimulus value θ given m (*posterior*) is the product of the *likelihood* $p(m|\theta)$ of the particular measurement and the *prior* $p(\theta)$. The normalization constant α serves to ensure that the posterior is a proper probability distribution. Under the assumption of a squared-error loss function, the optimal estimate $\hat{\theta}(m)$ is the mean of the posterior, thus

$$\hat{\theta}(m) = \int_0^\infty \theta \, p(\theta|m) \, d\theta \ . \tag{2}$$

Note that $\hat{\theta}(m)$ describes an estimate for a single measurement m. As discussed in [16], the measurement will vary stochastically over the course of many exposures to the same stimulus, and thus the estimator will also vary. We return to this issue in Section 3.2.

Figure 1a illustrates a Bayesian estimator, in which the shape of the (arbitrary) prior distribution leads on average to a shift of the estimate toward a lower value of θ than the true stimulus value θ_{stim}. The likelihood and the prior are the fundamental constituents of the Bayesian estimator model. Our goal is to describe how adaptation alters these constituents so as to account for the perceptual effects of repulsion and increased sensitivity.

Adaptation does not change the prior ...

An intuitively sensible hypothesis is that adaptation changes the prior distribution. Since the prior is meant to reflect the knowledge the observer has about the distribution of occurrences of the variable θ in the world, repeated viewing of stimuli with the same parameter

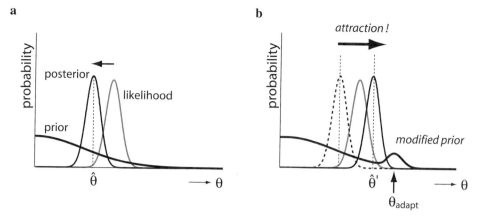

Figure 1: *Hypothetical model in which adaptation alters the prior distribution.* a) Unadapted Bayesian estimation configuration in which the prior leads to a shift of the estimate $\hat{\theta}$, relative to the stimulus parameter θ_{stim}. Both the likelihood function and the prior distribution contribute to the exact value of the estimate $\hat{\theta}$ (mean of the posterior). b) Adaptation acts by increasing the prior distribution around the value, θ_{adapt}, of the adapting stimulus parameter. Consequently, an subsequent estimate $\hat{\theta}'$ of the same stimulus parameter value θ_{stim} is *attracted* toward the adaptor. This is the opposite of observed perceptual effects, and we thus conclude that adjustments of the prior in a Bayesian model do not account for adaptation.

value θ_{adapt} should presumably increase the prior probability in the vicinity of θ_{adapt}. Figure 1b schematically illustrates the effect of such a change in the prior distribution. The estimated (perceived) value of the parameter under the adapted condition is *attracted* to the adapting parameter value. In order to account for observed perceptual repulsion effects, the prior would have to *decrease* at the location of the adapting parameter, a behavior that seems fundamentally inconsistent with the notion of a prior distribution.

... but increases the reliability of the measurements

Since a change in the prior distribution is not consistent with repulsion, we are led to the conclusion that adaptation must change the likelihood function. But why, and how should this occur?

In order to answer this question, we reconsider the functional purpose of adaptation. We assume that adaptation acts to allocate more resources to the representation of the parameter values in the vicinity of the adaptor [4], resulting in a local increase in the signal-to-noise ratio (SNR). This can be accomplished, for example, by dynamically adjusting the operational range to the statistics of the input. This kind of increased operational *gain* around the adaptor has been effectively demonstrated in the process of retinal adaptation [17]. In the context of our Bayesian estimator framework, and restricting to the simple case of a scalar-valued measurement, adaptation results in a narrower conditional probability density $p(m|\theta)$ in the immediate vicinity of the adaptor, thus an increase in the reliability of the measurement m. This is offset by a broadening of the conditional probability density $p(m|\theta)$ in the region beyond the adaptor vicinity (we assume that total resources are conserved, and thus an increase around the adaptor must necessarily lead to a decrease elsewhere).

Figure 2 illustrates the effect of this local increase in signal-to-noise ratio on the likeli-

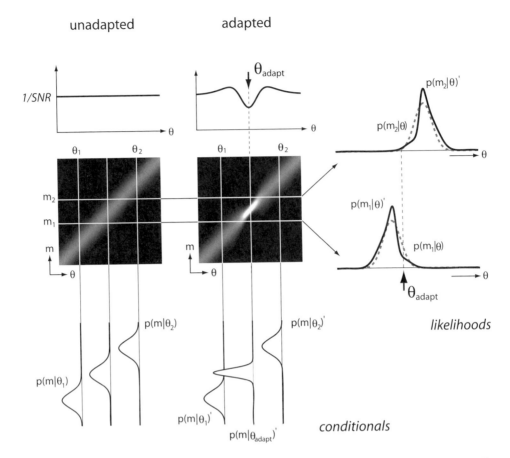

Figure 2: *Measurement noise, conditionals and likelihoods.* The two-dimensional conditional density, $p(m|\theta)$, is shown as a grayscale image for both the unadapted and adapted cases. We assume here that adaptation increases the reliability (SNR) of the measurement around the parameter value of the adaptor. This is balanced by a decrease in SNR of the measurement further away from the adaptor. Because the likelihood is a function of θ (horizontal slices, shown plotted at right), this results in an *asymmetric* change in the likelihood that is in agreement with a repulsive effect on the estimate.

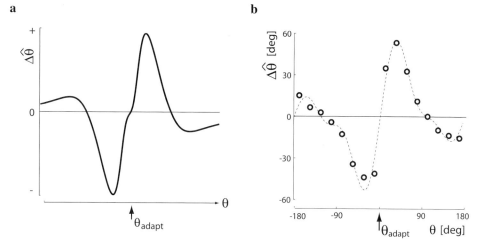

Figure 3: *Repulsion: Model predictions vs. human psychophysics.* a) Difference in perceived direction in the pre- and post-adaptation condition, as predicted by the model. Post-adaptive percepts of motion direction are repelled away from the direction of the adaptor. b) Typical human subject data show a qualitatively similar repulsive effect. Data (and fit) are replotted from [10].

hood function. The two gray-scale images represent the conditional probability densities, $p(m|\theta)$, in the unadapted and the adapted state. They are formed by assuming additive noise on the measurement m of constant variance (unadapted) or with a variance that decreases symmetrically in the vicinity of the adaptor parameter value θ_{adapt}, and grows slightly in the region beyond. In the unadapted state, the likelihood is convolutional and the shape and variance are equivalent to the distribution of measurement noise. However, in the adapted state, because the likelihood is a function of θ (horizontal slice through the conditional surface) it is no longer convolutional around the adaptor. As a result, the mean is pushed away from the adaptor, as illustrated in the two graphs on the right. Assuming that the prior distribution is fairly smooth, this repulsion effect is transferred to the posterior distribution, and thus to the estimate.

3 Simulation Results

We have qualitatively demonstrated that an increase in the measurement reliability around the adaptor is consistent with the repulsive effects commonly seen as a result of perceptual adaptation. In this section, we simulate an adapted Bayesian observer by assuming a simple model for the changes in signal-to-noise ratio due to adaptation. We address both repulsion and changes in discrimination threshold. In particular, we compare our model predictions with previously published data from psychophysical experiments examining human perception of motion direction.

3.1 Repulsion

In the unadapted state, we assume the measurement noise to be additive and normally distributed, and constant over the whole measurement space. Thus, assuming that m and θ live in the same space, the likelihood is a Gaussian of constant width. In the adapted state, we assume a simple functional description for the variance of the measurement noise around the adapter. Specifically, we use a constant plus a difference of two Gaussians,

a   **b**

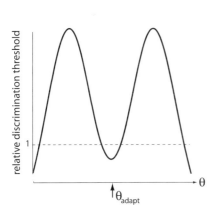
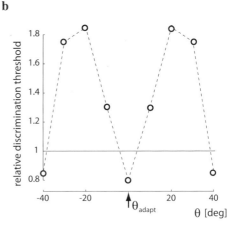

Figure 4: *Discrimination thresholds: Model predictions vs. human psychophysics.* a) The model predicts that thresholds for direction discrimination are reduced at the adaptor. It also predicts two side-lobes of increased threshold at further distance from the adaptor. b) Data of human psychophysics are in qualitative agreement with the model. Data are replotted from [14] (see also [11]).

each having equal area, with one twice as broad as the other (see Fig. 2). Finally, for simplicity, we assume a flat prior, but any reasonable smooth prior would lead to results that are qualitatively similar. Then, according to (2) we compute the predicted estimate of motion direction in both the unadapted and the adapted case.

Figure 3a shows the predicted difference between the pre- and post-adaptive average estimate of direction, as a function of the stimulus direction, θ_{stim}. The adaptor is indicated with an arrow. The repulsive effect is clearly visible. For comparison, Figure 3b shows human subject data replotted from [10]. The perceived motion direction of a grating was estimated, under both adapted and unadapted conditions, using a two-alternative-forced-choice experimental paradigm. The plot shows the change in perceived direction as a function of test stimulus direction relative to that of the adaptor. Comparison of the two panels of Figure 3 indicate that despite the highly simplified construction of the model, the prediction is quite good, and even includes the small but consistent repulsive effects observed 180 degrees from the adaptor.

3.2 Changes in discrimination threshold

Adaptation also changes the ability of human observers to discriminate between the direction of two different moving stimuli. In order to model discrimination thresholds, we need to consider a Bayesian framework that can account not only for the mean of the estimate but also its variability. We have recently developed such a framework, and used it to quantitatively constrain the likelihood and the prior from psychophysical data [16]. This framework accounts for the effect of the measurement noise on the variability of the estimate $\hat{\theta}$. Specifically, it provides a characterization of the *distribution* $p(\hat{\theta}|\theta_{\text{stim}})$ of the estimate for a given stimulus direction in terms of its expected value and its variance as a function of the measurement noise. As in [16] we write

$$\text{var}\langle\hat{\theta}|\theta_{\text{stim}}\rangle = \text{var}\langle m\rangle (\frac{\partial\hat{\theta}(m)}{\partial m})^2|_{m=\theta_{\text{stim}}} . \tag{3}$$

Assuming that discrimination threshold is proportional to the standard deviation,

$\sqrt{\text{var}\langle\hat{\theta}|\theta_{\text{stim}}\rangle}$, we can now predict how discrimination thresholds should change after adaptation. Figure 4a shows the predicted change in discrimination thresholds relative to the unadapted condition for the same model parameters as in the repulsion example (Figure 3a). Thresholds are slightly reduced at the adaptor, but increase symmetrically for directions further away from the adaptor. For comparison, Figure 4b shows the relative change in discrimination thresholds for a typical human subject [14]. Again, the behavior of the human observer is qualitatively well predicted.

4 Discussion

We have shown that adaptation can be incorporated into a Bayesian estimation framework for human sensory perception. Adaptation seems unlikely to manifest itself as a change in the internal representation of prior distributions, as this would lead to perceptual bias effects that are opposite to those observed in human subjects. Instead, we argue that adaptation leads to an increase in reliability of the measurement in the vicinity of the adapting stimulus parameter. We show that this change in the measurement reliability results in changes of the likelihood function, and that an estimator that utilizes this likelihood function will exhibit the commonly-observed adaptation effects of repulsion and changes in discrimination threshold. We further confirm our model by making quantitative predictions and comparing them with known psychophysical data in the case of human perception of motion direction.

Many open questions remain. The results demonstrated here indicate that a resource allocation explanation is consistent with the functional effects of adaptation, but it seems unlikely that theory alone can lead to a unique quantitative prediction of the detailed form of these effects. Specifically, the constraints imposed by biological implementation are likely to play a role in determining the changes in measurement noise as a function of adaptor parameter value, and it will be important to characterize and interpret neural response changes in the context of our framework. Also, although we have argued that changes in the prior seem inconsistent with adaptation effects, it may be that such changes do occur but are offset by the likelihood effect, or occur only on much longer timescales.

Last, if one considers sensory perception as the result of a cascade of successive processing stages (with both feedforward and feedback connections), it becomes necessary to expand the Bayesian description to describe this cascade [e.g., 18, 19]. For example, it may be possible to interpret this cascade as a sequence of Bayesian estimators, in which the measurement of each stage consists of the estimate computed at the previous stage. Adaptation could potentially occur in each of these processing stages, and it is of fundamental interest to understand how such a cascade can perform useful stable computations despite the fact that each of its elements is constantly readjusting its response properties.

References

[1] K. Körding and D. Wolpert. Bayesian integration in sensorimotor learning. *Nature*, 427(15):244–247, January 2004.

[2] D C Knill and W Richards, editors. *Perception as Bayesian Inference*. Cambridge University Press, 1996.

[3] Y. Weiss, E. Simoncelli, and E. Adelson. Motion illusions as optimal percept. *Nature Neuroscience*, 5(6):598–604, June 2002.

[4] H.B. Barlow. *Vision: Coding and Efficiency*, chapter A theory about the functional role and synaptic mechanism of visual after-effects, pages 363–375. Cambridge University Press., 1990.

[5] M.J. Wainwright. Visual adaptation as optimal information transmission. *Vision Research*, 39:3960–3974, 1999.

[6] N. Brenner, W. Bialek, and R. de Ruyter van Steveninck. Adaptive rescaling maximizes information transmission. *Neuron*, 26:695–702, June 2000.

[7] S.M. Smirnakis, M.J. Berry, D.K. Warland, W. Bialek, and M. Meister. Adaptation of retinal processing to image contrast and spatial scale. *Nature*, 386:69–73, March 1997.

[8] P. Thompson. Velocity after-effects: the effects of adaptation to moving stimuli on the perception of subsequently seen moving stimuli. *Vision Research*, 21:337–345, 1980.

[9] A.T. Smith. Velocity coding: evidence from perceived velocity shifts. *Vision Research*, 25(12):1969–1976, 1985.

[10] P. Schrater and E. Simoncelli. Local velocity representation: evidence from motion adaptation. *Vision Research*, 38:3899–3912, 1998.

[11] C.W. Clifford. Perceptual adaptation: motion parallels orientation. *Trends in Cognitive Sciences*, 6(3):136–143, March 2002.

[12] C. Clifford and P. Wenderoth. Adaptation to temporal modulaton can enhance differential speed sensitivity. *Vision Research*, 39:4324–4332, 1999.

[13] A. Kristjansson. Increased sensitivity to speed changes during adaptation to first-order, but not to second-order motion. *Vision Research*, 41:1825–1832, 2001.

[14] R.E. Phinney, C. Bowd, and R. Patterson. Direction-selective coding of stereoscopic (cyclopean) motion. *Vision Research*, 37(7):865–869, 1997.

[15] N.M. Grzywacz and R.M. Balboa. A Bayesian framework for sensory adaptation. *Neural Computation*, 14:543–559, 2002.

[16] A.A. Stocker and E.P. Simoncelli. Constraining a Bayesian model of human visual speed perception. In Lawrence K. Saul, Yair Weiss, and Léon Bottou, editors, *Advances in Neural Information Processing Systems NIPS 17*, pages 1361–1368, Cambridge, MA, 2005. MIT Press.

[17] D. Tranchina, J. Gordon, and R.M. Shapley. Retinal light adaptation – evidence for a feedback mechanism. *Nature*, 310:314–316, July 1984.

[18] S. Deneve. Bayesian inference in spiking neurons. In Lawrence K. Saul, Yair Weiss, and Léon Bottou, editors, *Adv. Neural Information Processing Systems (NIPS*04)*, vol 17, Cambridge, MA, 2005. MIT Press.

[19] R. Rao. Hierarchical Bayesian inference in networks of spiking neurons. In Lawrence K. Saul, Yair Weiss, and Léon Bottou, editors, *Adv. Neural Information Processing Systems (NIPS*04)*, vol 17, Cambridge, MA, 2005. MIT Press.

Describing Visual Scenes using Transformed Dirichlet Processes

Erik B. Sudderth, Antonio Torralba, William T. Freeman, and Alan S. Willsky
Department of Electrical Engineering and Computer Science
Massachusetts Institute of Technology
esuddert@mit.edu, torralba@csail.mit.edu, billf@mit.edu, willsky@mit.edu

Abstract

Motivated by the problem of learning to detect and recognize objects with minimal supervision, we develop a hierarchical probabilistic model for the spatial structure of visual scenes. In contrast with most existing models, our approach explicitly captures uncertainty in the *number* of object instances depicted in a given image. Our scene model is based on the transformed Dirichlet process (TDP), a novel extension of the hierarchical DP in which a set of stochastically transformed mixture components are shared between multiple groups of data. For visual scenes, mixture components describe the spatial structure of visual features in an object–centered coordinate frame, while transformations model the object positions in a particular image. Learning and inference in the TDP, which has many potential applications beyond computer vision, is based on an empirically effective Gibbs sampler. Applied to a dataset of partially labeled street scenes, we show that the TDP's inclusion of spatial structure improves detection performance, flexibly exploiting partially labeled training images.

1 Introduction

In this paper, we develop methods for analyzing the features composing a *visual scene*, thereby localizing and categorizing the objects in an image. We would like to design learning algorithms that exploit relationships among multiple, partially labeled object categories during training. Working towards this goal, we propose a hierarchical probabilistic model for the expected spatial locations of objects, and the appearance of visual features corresponding to each object. Given a new image, our model provides a globally coherent explanation for the observed scene, including estimates of the location and category of an *a priori* unknown number of objects.

This generative approach is motivated by the pragmatic need for learning algorithms which require little manual supervision and labeling. While discriminative models may produce accurate classifiers, they typically require very large training sets even for relatively simple categories [1]. In contrast, generative approaches can discover large, visually salient categories (such as foliage and buildings [2]) without supervision. Partial segmentations can then be used to learn semantically interesting categories (such as cars and pedestrians) which are less visually distinctive, or present in fewer training images. Moreover, generative models provide a natural framework for learning contextual relationships between objects, and transferring knowledge between related, but distinct, visual scenes.

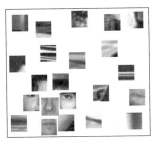 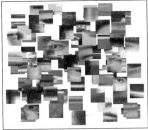 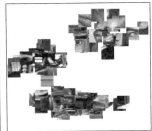

Constellation	LDA	Transformed DP

Figure 1: A scene with faces as described by three generative models. *Constellation:* Fixed parts of a single face in unlocalized clutter. *LDA:* Bag of unlocalized face and background features. *TDP:* Spatially localized clusters of background clutter, and one or more faces (in this case, the sample contains one face and two background clusters). *Note:* The LDA and TDP images are sampled from models learned from training images, while the Constellation image is a hand-constructed illustration.

The principal challenge in developing hierarchical models for scenes is specifying tractable, scalable methods for handling uncertainty in the number of objects. This issue is entirely ignored by most existing models. We address this problem using Dirichlet processes [3], a tool from nonparametric Bayesian analysis for learning mixture models whose number of components is not fixed, but instead estimated from data. In particular, we extend the recently proposed *hierarchical Dirichlet process* (HDP) [4, 5] framework to allow more flexible sharing of mixture components between images. The resulting *transformed Dirichlet process* (TDP) is naturally suited to our scene understanding application, as well as many other domains where "style and content" are combined to produce the observed data [6].

We begin in Sec. 2 by reviewing several related generative models for objects and scenes. Sec. 3 then introduces Dirichlet processes and develops the TDP model, including MCMC methods for learning and inference. We specialize the TDP to visual scenes in Sec. 4, and conclude in Sec. 5 by demonstrating object recognition and segmentation in street scenes.

2 Generative Models for Objects and Scenes

Constellation models [7] describe single objects via the appearance of a fixed, and typically small, set of spatially constrained parts (see Fig. 1). Although they can successfully recognize objects in cluttered backgrounds, they do not directly provide a mechanism for detecting multiple object instances. In addition, it seems difficult to generalize the fixed set of constellation parts to problems where the number of objects is uncertain.

Grammars, and related rule–based systems, were one of the earliest approaches to scene understanding [8]. More recently, distributions over hierarchical tree–structured partitions of image pixels have been used to segment simple scenes [9, 10]. In addition, an *image parsing* [11] framework has been proposed which explains an image using a set of regions generated by generic or object–specific processes. While this model allows uncertainty in the number of regions, and hence the number of objects, the high dimensionality of the model state space requires good, discriminatively trained bottom–up proposal distributions for acceptable MCMC performance. We also note that the BLOG language [12] provides a promising framework for reasoning about unknown objects. As of yet, however, the computational tools needed to apply BLOG to large–scale applications are unavailable.

Inspired by techniques from the text analysis literature, several recent papers analyze scenes using a spatially unstructured *bag of features* extracted from local image patches (see Fig. 1). In particular, *latent Dirichlet allocation* (LDA) [13] describes the features x_{ji} in image j using a K component mixture model with parameters θ_k. Each image reuses these same mixture parameters in different proportions π_j (see the graphical model of Fig. 2). By appropriately defining these shared mixtures, LDA may be used to discover object categories from images of single objects [2], categorize natural scenes [14], and (with a slight extension) parse presegmented captioned images [15].

While these LDA models are sometimes effective, their neglect of spatial structure ignores valuable information which is critical in challenging object detection tasks. We recently proposed a hierarchical extension of LDA which learns shared parts describing the internal structure of objects, and contextual relationships among known groups of objects [16]. The *transformed Dirichlet process* (TDP) addresses a key limitation of this model by allowing uncertainty in the number and identity of the objects depicted in each image. As detailed in Sec. 4 and illustrated in Fig. 1, the TDP effectively provides a *textural* model in which locally unstructured clumps of features are given global spatial structure by the inferred set of objects underlying each scene.

3 Hierarchical Modeling using Dirichlet Processes

In this section, we review Dirichlet process mixture models (Sec. 3.1) and previously proposed hierarchical extensions (Sec. 3.2). We then introduce the *transformed Dirichlet process* (TDP) (Sec. 3.3), and discuss Monte Carlo methods for learning TDPs (Sec. 3.4).

3.1 Dirichlet Process Mixture Models

Let θ denote a parameter taking values in some space Θ, and H be a measure on Θ. A *Dirichlet process* (DP), denoted by $\mathrm{DP}(\gamma, H)$, is then a distribution over measures on Θ, where the concentration parameter γ controls the similarity of samples $G \sim \mathrm{DP}(\gamma, H)$ to the base measure H. Samples from DPs are discrete with probability one, a property highlighted by the following *stick–breaking construction* [4]:

$$G(\theta) = \sum_{k=1}^{\infty} \beta_k \delta(\theta, \theta_k) \qquad \beta_k' \sim \mathrm{Beta}(1, \gamma) \qquad \beta_k = \beta_k' \prod_{\ell=1}^{k-1}(1 - \beta_\ell') \qquad (1)$$

Each parameter $\theta_k \sim H$ is independently sampled, while the weights $\boldsymbol{\beta} = (\beta_1, \beta_2, \dots)$ use Beta random variables to partition a unit–length "stick" of probability mass.

In nonparametric Bayesian statistics, DPs are commonly used as prior distributions for mixture models with an unknown number of components [3]. Let $F(\theta)$ denote a family of distributions parameterized by θ. Given $G \sim \mathrm{DP}(\gamma, H)$, each observation x_i from an exchangeable data set $\mathbf{x}$ is generated by first choosing a parameter $\bar{\theta}_i \sim G$, and then sampling $x_i \sim F(\bar{\theta}_i)$. Computationally, this process is conveniently described by a set $\mathbf{z}$ of independently sampled variables $z_i \sim \mathrm{Mult}(\boldsymbol{\beta})$ indicating the component of the mixture $G(\theta)$ (see eq. (1)) associated with each data point $x_i \sim F(\theta_{z_i})$.

Integrating over G, the indicator variables $\mathbf{z}$ demonstrate an important clustering property. Letting n_k denote the number of times component θ_k is chosen by the first $(i-1)$ samples,

$$p\left(z_i \mid z_1, \dots, z_{i-1}, \gamma\right) = \frac{1}{\gamma + i - 1}\left[\sum_k n_k \delta(z_i, k) + \gamma \delta(z_i, \bar{k})\right] \qquad (2)$$

Here, $\bar{k}$ indicates a previously unused mixture component (*a priori*, all unused components are equivalent). This process is sometimes described by analogy to a Chinese restaurant in which the (infinite collection of) tables correspond to the mixture components θ_k, and customers to observations x_i [4]. Customers are social, tending to sit at tables with many other customers (observations), and each table shares a single dish (parameter).

3.2 Hierarchical Dirichlet Processes

In many domains, there are several groups of data produced by related, but distinct, generative processes. For example, in this paper's applications each group is an image, and the data are visual features composing a scene. Given J groups of data, let $\mathbf{x}_j = (x_{j1}, \dots, x_{jn_j})$ denote the n_j exchangeable data points in group j.

Hierarchical Dirichlet processes (HDPs) [4, 5] describe grouped data with a coupled set of

1299

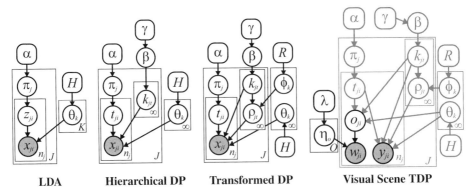

LDA	Hierarchical DP	Transformed DP	Visual Scene TDP

Figure 2: Graphical representations of the LDA, HDP, and TDP models for sharing mixture components θ_k, with proportions π_j, among J groups of exchangeable data $\mathbf{x}_j = (x_{j1}, \ldots, x_{jn_j})$. LDA directly assigns observations x_{ji} to clusters via indicators z_{ji}. HDP and TDP models use "table" indicators t_{ji} as an intermediary between observations and assignments k_{jt} to an infinite global mixture with weights β. TDPs augment each table t with a transformation ρ_{jt} sampled from a distribution parameterized by $\phi_{k_{jt}}$. Specializing the TDP to visual scenes (right), we model the position y_{ji} and appearance w_{ji} of features using distributions η_o indexed by unobserved object categories o_{ji}.

mixture models. To construct an HDP, a global probability measure $G_0 \sim \mathrm{DP}(\gamma, H)$ is first chosen to define a set of shared mixture components. A measure $G_j \sim \mathrm{DP}(\alpha, G_0)$ is then independently sampled for each group. Because G_0 is discrete (as in eq. (1)), groups G_j will reuse the same mixture components θ_k in different proportions:

$$G_j(\theta) = \sum_{k=1}^{\infty} \pi_{jk} \delta(\theta, \theta_k) \qquad \pi_j \sim \mathrm{DP}(\alpha, \beta) \qquad (3)$$

In this construction, shared components improve generalization when learning from few examples, while distinct mixture weights capture differences between groups.

The generative process underlying HDPs may be understood in terms of an extension of the DP analogy known as the *Chinese restaurant franchise* [4]. Each group defines a separate restaurant in which customers (observations) x_{ji} sit at tables t_{ji}. Each table shares a single dish (parameter) θ, which is ordered from a menu G_0 shared among restaurants (groups). Letting k_{jt} indicate the parameter $\theta_{k_{jt}}$ assigned to table t in group j, we may integrate over G_0 and G_j (as in eq. (2)) to find the conditional distributions of these indicator variables:

$$p\left(t_{ji} \mid t_{j1}, \ldots, t_{ji-1}, \alpha\right) \propto \sum_t n_{jt} \delta(t_{ji}, t) + \alpha \delta(t_{ji}, \bar{t}) \qquad (4)$$

$$p\left(k_{jt} \mid \mathbf{k}_1, \ldots, \mathbf{k}_{j-1}, k_{j1}, \ldots, k_{jt-1}, \gamma\right) \propto \sum_k m_k \delta(k_{jt}, k) + \gamma \delta(k_{jt}, \bar{k}) \qquad (5)$$

Here, m_k is the number of tables previously assigned to θ_k. As before, customers prefer tables t at which many customers n_{jt} are already seated (eq. (4)), but sometimes choose a new table $\bar{t}$. Each new table is assigned a dish $k_{j\bar{t}}$ according to eq. (5). Popular dishes are more likely to be ordered, but a new dish $\theta_{\bar{k}} \sim H$ may also be selected.

The HDP generative process is summarized in the graphical model of Fig. 2. Given the assignments $\mathbf{t}_j$ and $\mathbf{k}_j$ for group j, observations are sampled as $x_{ji} \sim F(\theta_{z_{ji}})$, where $z_{ji} = k_{jt_{ji}}$ indexes the shared parameters assigned to the table associated with x_{ji}.

3.3 Transformed Dirichlet Processes

In the HDP model of Fig. 2, the group distributions G_j are derived from the global distribution G_0 by resampling the mixture weights from a Dirichlet process (see eq. (3)), leaving the component parameters θ_k unchanged. In many applications, however, it is difficult to define θ so that parameters may be exactly reused between groups. Consider, for example, a Gaussian distribution describing the location at which object features are detected in an image. While the covariance of that distribution may stay relatively constant across object instances, the mean will change dramatically from image to image (group to group), depending on the objects' position relative to the camera.

Motivated by these difficulties, we propose the *Transformed Dirichlet Process* (TDP), an extension of the HDP in which global mixture components undergo a set of random transformations before being reused in each group. Let ρ denote a transformation of the parameter vector $\theta \in \Theta$, $\phi \in \Phi$ the parameters of a distribution Q over transformations, and R a measure on Φ. We begin by augmenting the DP stick–breaking construction of eq. (1) to create a global measure describing both parameters and transformations:

$$G_0(\theta, \rho) = \sum_{k=1}^{\infty} \beta_k \delta(\theta, \theta_k) q(\rho \mid \phi_k) \qquad \theta_k \sim H \qquad \phi_k \sim R \qquad (6)$$

As before, $\boldsymbol{\beta}$ is sampled from a stick–breaking process with parameter γ. For each group, we then sample a measure $G_j \sim \mathrm{DP}(\alpha, G_0)$. Marginalizing over transformations ρ, $G_j(\theta)$ reuses parameters from $G_0(\theta)$ exactly as in eq. (3). Because samples from DPs are discrete, the joint measure for group j then has the following form:

$$G_j(\theta, \rho) = \sum_{k=1}^{\infty} \pi_{jk} \delta(\theta, \theta_k) \left[\sum_{\ell=1}^{\infty} \omega_{jk\ell} \delta(\rho, \rho_{jk\ell}) \right] \qquad \sum_{\ell=1}^{\infty} \omega_{jk\ell} = 1 \qquad (7)$$

Note that within the jth group, each shared parameter vector θ_k may potentially be reused multiple times with different transformations $\rho_{jk\ell}$. Conditioning on θ_k, it can be shown that $G_j(\rho \mid \theta_k) \sim \mathrm{DP}(\alpha \beta_k, Q(\phi_k))$, so that the proportions $\boldsymbol{\omega}_{jk}$ of features associated with each transformation of θ_k follow a stick–breaking process with parameter $\alpha \beta_k$.

Each observation x_{ji} is now generated by sampling $(\bar{\theta}_{ji}, \bar{\rho}_{ji}) \sim G_j$, and then choosing $x_{ji} \sim F(\bar{\theta}_{ji}, \bar{\rho}_{ji})$ from a distribution which transforms $\bar{\theta}_{ji}$ by $\bar{\rho}_{ji}$. Although the global family of transformation distributions $Q(\phi)$ is typically non–atomic, the discreteness of G_j ensures that transformations are shared between observations within group j.

Computationally, the TDP is more conveniently described via an extension of the Chinese restaurant franchise analogy (see Fig. 2). As before, customers (observations) x_{ji} sit at tables t_{ji} according to the clustering bias of eq. (4), and new tables choose dishes according to their popularity across the franchise (eq. (5)). Now, however, the dish (parameter) $\theta_{k_{jt}}$ at table t is seasoned (transformed) according to $\rho_{jt} \sim q(\rho_{jt} \mid \phi_{k_{jt}})$. Each time a dish is ordered, the recipe is seasoned differently.

3.4 Learning via Gibbs Sampling

To learn the parameters of a TDP, we extend the HDP Gibbs sampler detailed in [4]. The simplest implementation samples table assignments $\mathbf{t}$, cluster assignments $\mathbf{k}$, transformations $\boldsymbol{\rho}$, and parameters $\boldsymbol{\theta}, \boldsymbol{\phi}$. Let $\mathbf{t}^{-ji}$ denote all table assignments excluding t_{ji}, and define $\mathbf{k}^{-jt}$, $\boldsymbol{\rho}^{-jt}$ similarly. Using the Markov properties of the TDP (see Fig. 2), we have

$$p\left(t_{ji} = t \mid \mathbf{t}^{-ji}, \mathbf{k}, \boldsymbol{\rho}, \boldsymbol{\theta}, \mathbf{x}\right) \propto p\left(t \mid \mathbf{t}^{-ji}\right) f\left(x_{ji} \mid \theta_{k_{jt}}, \rho_{jt}\right) \qquad (8)$$

The first term is given by eq. (4). For a fixed set of transformations $\boldsymbol{\rho}$, the second term is a simple likelihood evaluation for existing tables, while new tables may be evaluated by marginalizing over possible cluster assignments (eq. (5)).

Because cluster assignments k_{jt} and transformations ρ_{jt} are strongly coupled in the posterior, a blocked Gibbs sampler which jointly resamples them converges much more rapidly:

$$p\left(k_{jt} = k, \rho_{jt} \mid \mathbf{k}^{-jt}, \boldsymbol{\rho}^{-jt}, \mathbf{t}, \boldsymbol{\theta}, \boldsymbol{\phi}, \mathbf{x}\right) \propto p\left(k \mid \mathbf{k}^{-jt}\right) q\left(\rho_{jt} \mid \phi_k\right) \prod_{t_{ji}=t} f\left(x_{ji} \mid \theta_k, \rho_{jt}\right)$$

For the models considered in this paper, F is conjugate to Q for any fixed observation value. We may thus analytically integrate over ρ_{jt} and, combined with eq. (5), sample a

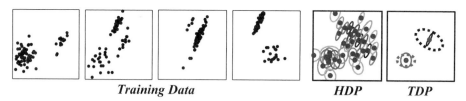

Figure 3: Comparison of hierarchical models learned via Gibbs sampling from synthetic 2D data. *Left:* Four of 50 "images" used for training. *Center:* Global distribution $G_0(\theta)$ for the HDP, where ellipses are covariance estimates and intensity is proportional to prior probability. *Right:* Global TDP distribution $G_0(\theta, \rho)$ over both clusters θ (solid) and translations ρ of those clusters (dashed).

new cluster assignment $\bar{k}_{jt}$. Conditioned on $\bar{k}_{jt}$, we again use conjugacy to sample $\bar{\rho}_{jt}$. We also choose the parameter priors H and R to be conjugate to Q and F, respectively, so that standard formulas may be used to resample θ, ϕ.

4 Transformed Dirichlet Processes for Visual Scenes

4.1 Context–Free Modeling of Multiple Object Categories

In this section, we adapt the TDP model of Sec. 3.3 to describe the spatial structure of visual scenes. Groups j now correspond to training, or test, images. For the moment, we assume that the observed data $x_{ji} = (o_{ji}, y_{ji})$, where y_{ji} is the position of a feature corresponding to object category o_{ji}, and the number of object categories O is known (see Fig. 2). We then choose cluster parameters $\theta_k = (\bar{o}_k, \mu_k, \Lambda_k)$ to describe the mean μ_k and covariance Λ_k of a Gaussian distribution over feature positions, as well as the *single* object category $\bar{o}_k$ assigned to *all* observations sampled from that cluster. Although this cluster parameterization does not capture contextual relationships between object categories, the results of Sec. 5 demonstrate that it nevertheless provides an effective model of the spatial variability of individual categories across many different scenes.

To model the variability in object location from image to image, transformation parameters ρ_{jt} are defined to *translate* feature position relative to that cluster's "canonical" mean μ_k:

$$p(o_{ji}, y_{ji} \mid t_{ji} = t, \mathbf{k}_j, \boldsymbol{\rho}_j, \boldsymbol{\theta}) = \delta(o_{ji}, \bar{o}_{k_{jt}}) \times \mathcal{N}(y_{ji}; \mu_{k_{jt}} + \rho_{jt}, \Lambda_{k_{jt}}) \quad (9)$$

We note that there is a different translation ρ_{jt} associated with each table t, allowing the same object cluster to be reused at multiple locations within a single image. This flexibility, which is not possible with HDPs, is critical to accurately modeling visual scenes. Density models for spatial transformations have been previously used to recognize isolated objects [17], and estimate layered decompositions of video sequences [18]. In contrast, the proposed TDP models the variability of object positions across scenes, and couples this with a nonparametric prior allowing uncertainty in the number of objects.

To ensure that the TDP scene model is identifiable, we define $p(\rho_{jt} \mid \mathbf{k}_j, \phi)$ to be a zero–mean Gaussian with covariance $\phi_{k_{jt}}$. The parameter prior R is uniform across object categories, while R and H both use inverse–Wishart position distributions, weakly biased towards moderate covariances. Fig. 3 shows a 2D synthetic example based on a single object category ($O = 1$). Following 100 Gibbs sampling iterations, the TDP correctly discovers that the data is composed of elongated "bars" in the upper right, and round "blobs" in the lower left. In contrast, the learned HDP uses a large set of global clusters to discretize the transformations underlying the data, and thus generalizes poorly to new translations.

4.2 Detecting Objects from Image Features

To apply the TDP model of Sec. 4.1 to images, we must learn the relationship between object categories and visual features. As in [2, 16], we obtain discrete features by vector quantizing SIFT descriptors [19] computed over locally adapted elliptical regions. To improve discriminative power, we divide these elliptical regions into three groups (roughly circular, and horizontally or vertically elongated) prior to quantizing SIFT values, producing a discrete vocabulary with 1800 appearance "words". Given the density of feature detection, these descriptors essentially provide a multiscale over–segmentation of the image.

We assume that the appearance w_{ji} of each detected feature is independently sampled conditioned on the underlying object category o_{ji} (see Fig. 2). Placing a symmetric Dirichlet prior, with parameter λ, on each category's multinomial appearance distribution η_o,

$$p\left(w_{ji} = b \mid o_{ji} = o, \mathbf{w}^{-ji}, \mathbf{t}, \mathbf{k}, \boldsymbol{\theta}\right) \propto c_{bo} + \lambda \qquad (10)$$

where c_{bo} is the number of times feature b is currently assigned to object o. Because a single object category is associated with each cluster, the Gibbs sampler of Sec. 3.4 may be easily adapted to this case by incorporating eq. (10) into the assignment likelihoods.

5 Analyzing Street Scenes

To demonstrate the potential of our TDP scene model, we consider a set of street scene images (250 training, 75 test) from the MIT-CSAIL database. These images contain three "objects": buildings, cars (side views), and roads. All categories were labeled in 112 images, while in the remainder only cars were segmented. Training from semi–supervised data is accomplished by restricting object category assignments for segmented features.

Fig. 4 shows the four global object clusters learned following 100 Gibbs sampling iterations. There is one elongated car cluster, one large building cluster, and two road clusters with differing shapes. Interestingly, the model has automatically determined that building features occur in large homogeneous patches, while road features are sparse and better described by many smaller transformed clusters. To segment test images, we run the Gibbs sampler for 50 iterations from each of 10 random initializations. Fig. 4 shows segmentations produced by averaging these samples, as well as transformed clusters from the final iteration. Qualitatively, results are typically good, although foliage is often mislabeled as road due to the textural similarities with features detected in shadows across roads.

For comparison, we also trained an LDA model based solely on feature appearance, allowing three topics per object category and again using object labels to restrict the Gibbs sampler's assignments [16]. As shown by the ROC curves of Fig. 4, our TDP model of spatial scene structure significantly improves segmentation performance. In addition, through the set of transformed car clusters generated by the Gibbs sampler, the TDP explicitly estimates the number of object *instances* underlying each image. These detections, which are not possible using LDA, are based on a single global parsing of the scene which automatically estimates object locations without a "sliding window" [1].

6 Discussion

We have developed the transformed Dirichlet process, a hierarchical model which shares a set of stochastically transformed clusters among groups of data. Applied to visual scenes, TDPs provide a model of spatial structure which allows the number of objects generating an image to be automatically inferred, and lead to improved detection performance. We are currently investigating extensions of the basic TDP scene model presented in this paper which describe the internal structure of objects, and also incorporate richer contextual cues.

Acknowledgments

Funding provided by the National Geospatial-Intelligence Agency NEGI-1582-04-0004, the National Science Foundation NSF-IIS-0413232, the ARDA VACE program, and a grant from BAE Systems.

References

[1] P. Viola and M. J. Jones. Robust real–time face detection. *IJCV*, 57(2):137–154, 2004.
[2] J. Sivic, B. C. Russell, A. A. Efros, A. Zisserman, and W. T. Freeman. Discovering objects and their location in images. In *ICCV*, 2005.

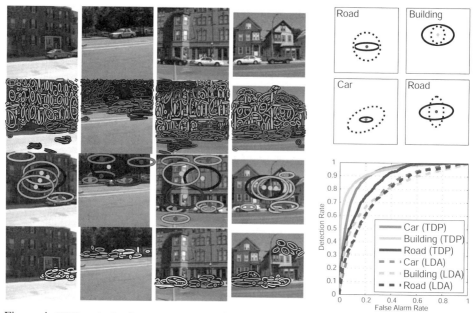

Figure 4: TDP analysis of street scenes containing cars (red), buildings (green), and roads (blue). *Top right:* Global model G_0 describing object shape (solid) and expected transformations (dashed). *Bottom right:* ROC curves comparing TDP feature segmentation performance to an LDA model of feature appearance. *Left:* Four test images (first row), estimated segmentations of features into object categories (second row), transformed global clusters associated with each image interpretation (third row), and features assigned to different instances of the transformed car cluster (fourth row).

[3] M. D. Escobar and M. West. Bayesian density estimation and inference using mixtures. *J. Amer. Stat. Assoc.*, 90(430):577–588, June 1995.

[4] Y. W. Teh, M. I. Jordan, M. J. Beal, and D. M. Blei. Hierarchical Dirichlet processes. Technical Report 653, U.C. Berkeley Statistics, October 2004.

[5] Y. W. Teh, M. I. Jordan, M. J. Beal, and D. M. Blei. Hierarchical Dirichlet processes. In *NIPS 17*, pages 1385–1392. MIT Press, 2005.

[6] J. B. Tenenbaum and W. T. Freeman. Separating style and content with bilinear models. *Neural Comp.*, 12:1247–1283, 2000.

[7] L. Fei-Fei, R. Fergus, and P. Perona. A Bayesian approach to unsupervised one-shot learning of object categories. In *ICCV*, volume 2, pages 1134–1141, 2003.

[8] J. M. Tenenbaum and H. G. Barrow. Experiments in interpretation-guided segmentation. *Artif. Intel.*, 8:241–274, 1977.

[9] A. J. Storkey and C. K. I. Williams. Image modeling with position-encoding dynamic trees. *IEEE Trans. PAMI*, 25(7):859–871, July 2003.

[10] J. M. Siskind et al. Spatial random tree grammars for modeling hierarchal structure in images. Submitted to IEEE Tran. PAMI, 2004.

[11] Z. Tu, X. Chen, A. L. Yuille, and S. C. Zhu. Image parsing: Unifying segmentation, detection, and recognition. In *ICCV*, volume 1, pages 18–25, 2003.

[12] B. Milch, B. Marthi, S. Russell, D. Sontag, D. L. Ong, and A. Kolobov. BLOG: Probabilistic models with unknown objects. In *IJCAI 19*, pages 1352–1359, 2005.

[13] D. M. Blei, A. Y. Ng, and M. I. Jordan. Latent Dirichlet allocation. *JMLR*, 3:993–1022, 2003.

[14] L. Fei-Fei and P. Perona. A Bayesian hierarchical model for learning natural scene categories. In *CVPR*, volume 2, pages 524–531, 2005.

[15] K. Barnard et al. Matching words and pictures. *JMLR*, 3:1107–1135, 2003.

[16] E. B. Sudderth, A. Torralba, W. T. Freeman, and A. S. Willsky. Learning hierarchical models of scenes, objects, and parts. In *ICCV*, 2005.

[17] E. G. Miller, N. E. Matsakis, and P. A. Viola. Learning from one example through shared densities on transforms. In *CVPR*, volume 1, pages 464–471, 2000.

[18] N. Jojic and B. J. Frey. Learning flexible sprites in video layers. In *CVPR*, volume 1, pages 199–206, 2001.

[19] D. G. Lowe. Distinctive image features from scale–invariant keypoints. *IJCV*, 60(2):91–110, 2004.

Active Learning for Misspecified Models

Masashi Sugiyama
Department of Computer Science, Tokyo Institute of Technology
2-12-1, O-okayama, Meguro-ku, Tokyo, 152-8552, Japan
sugi@cs.titech.ac.jp

Abstract

Active learning is the problem in supervised learning to design the locations of training input points so that the generalization error is minimized.
Existing active learning methods often assume that the model used for
learning is correctly specified, i.e., the learning target function can be expressed by the model at hand. In many practical situations, however, this
assumption may not be fulfilled. In this paper, we first show that the existing active learning method can be theoretically justified under slightly
weaker condition: the model does not have to be correctly specified, but
slightly misspecified models are also allowed. However, it turns out that
the weakened condition is still restrictive in practice. To cope with this
problem, we propose an alternative active learning method which can be
theoretically justified for a wider class of misspecified models. Thus,
the proposed method has a broader range of applications than the existing method. Numerical studies show that the proposed active learning
method is robust against the misspecification of models and is thus reliable.

1 Introduction and Problem Formulation

Let us discuss the regression problem of learning a real-valued function $f(\boldsymbol{x})$ defined on
$\mathbb{R}^d$ from training examples

$$\{(\boldsymbol{x}_i, y_i) \mid y_i = f(\boldsymbol{x}_i) + \epsilon_i\}_{i=1}^n,$$

where $\{\epsilon_i\}_{i=1}^n$ are i.i.d. noise with mean zero and unknown variance σ^2. We use the following linear regression model for learning.

$$\widehat{f}(\boldsymbol{x}) = \sum_{i=1}^p \alpha_i \varphi_i(\boldsymbol{x}),$$

where $\{\varphi_i(\boldsymbol{x})\}_{i=1}^p$ are fixed linearly independent functions and $\boldsymbol{\alpha} = (\alpha_1, \alpha_2, \ldots, \alpha_p)^\top$
are parameters to be learned.

We evaluate the goodness of the learned function $\widehat{f}(\boldsymbol{x})$ by the expected squared test error
over test input points and noise (i.e., the *generalization error*). When the test input points
are drawn independently from a distribution with density $p_t(\boldsymbol{x})$, the generalization error is
expressed as

$$G = \mathbb{E}_\epsilon \int \left(\widehat{f}(\boldsymbol{x}) - f(\boldsymbol{x})\right)^2 p_t(\boldsymbol{x}) d\boldsymbol{x},$$

where $\mathbb{E}_{\epsilon}$ denotes the expectation over the noise $\{\epsilon_i\}_{i=1}^n$. In the following, we suppose that $p_t(\boldsymbol{x})$ is known[1].

In a standard setting of regression, the training input points are provided from the environment, i.e., $\{\boldsymbol{x}_i\}_{i=1}^n$ independently follow the distribution with density $p_t(\boldsymbol{x})$. On the other hand, in some cases, the training input points can be designed by users. In such cases, it is expected that the accuracy of the learning result can be improved if the training input points are chosen appropriately, e.g., by densely locating training input points in the regions of high uncertainty.

Active learning—also referred to as *experimental design*—is the problem of optimizing the location of training input points so that the generalization error is minimized. In active learning research, it is often assumed that the regression model is correctly specified [2, 1, 3], i.e., the learning target function $f(\boldsymbol{x})$ can be expressed by the model. In practice, however, this assumption is often violated.

In this paper, we first show that the existing active learning method can still be theoretically justified when the model is approximately correct in a strong sense. Then we propose an alternative active learning method which can also be theoretically justified for approximately correct models, but the condition on the approximate correctness of the models is weaker than that for the existing method. Thus, the proposed method has a wider range of applications.

In the following, we suppose that the training input points $\{\boldsymbol{x}_i\}_{i=1}^n$ are independently drawn from a user-defined distribution with density $p_x(\boldsymbol{x})$, and discuss the problem of finding the optimal density function.

2   Existing Active Learning Method

The generalization error G defined by Eq.(1) can be decomposed as

$$G = B + V,$$

where B is the (squared) *bias* term and V is the *variance* term given by

$$B = \int \left(\mathbb{E}_{\epsilon}\widehat{f}(\boldsymbol{x}) - f(\boldsymbol{x})\right)^2 p_t(\boldsymbol{x})d\boldsymbol{x} \quad \text{and} \quad V = \mathbb{E}_{\epsilon} \int \left(\widehat{f}(\boldsymbol{x}) - \mathbb{E}_{\epsilon}\widehat{f}(\boldsymbol{x})\right)^2 p_t(\boldsymbol{x})d\boldsymbol{x}.$$

A standard way to learn the parameters in the regression model (1) is the *ordinary least-squares learning*, i.e., parameter vector $\boldsymbol{\alpha}$ is determined as follows.

$$\widehat{\boldsymbol{\alpha}}_{OLS} = \operatorname*{argmin}_{\boldsymbol{\alpha}} \left[\sum_{i=1}^n \left(\widehat{f}(\boldsymbol{x}_i) - y_i\right)^2 \right].$$

It is known that $\widehat{\boldsymbol{\alpha}}_{OLS}$ is given by

$$\widehat{\boldsymbol{\alpha}}_{OLS} = \boldsymbol{L}_{OLS}\boldsymbol{y},$$

where

$$\boldsymbol{L}_{OLS} = (\boldsymbol{X}^\top \boldsymbol{X})^{-1}\boldsymbol{X}^\top, \quad X_{i,j} = \varphi_j(\boldsymbol{x}_i), \quad \text{and} \quad \boldsymbol{y} = (y_1, y_2, \ldots, y_n)^\top.$$

Let G_{OLS}, B_{OLS} and V_{OLS} be G, B and V for the learned function obtained by the ordinary least-squares learning, respectively. Then the following proposition holds.

---

[1]In some application domains such as web page analysis or bioinformatics, a large number of *unlabeled samples*—input points without output values independently drawn from the distribution with density $p_t(\boldsymbol{x})$—are easily gathered. In such cases, a reasonably good estimate of $p_t(\boldsymbol{x})$ may be obtained by some standard density estimation method. Therefore, the assumption that $p_t(\boldsymbol{x})$ is known may not be so restrictive.

Proposition 1 ([2, 1, 3]) *Suppose that the model is correctly specified, i.e., the learning target function $f(x)$ is expressed as*

$$f(x) = \sum_{i=1}^{p} \alpha_i^* \varphi_i(x).$$

Then B_{OLS} and V_{OLS} are expressed as

$$B_{OLS} = 0 \quad and \quad V_{OLS} = \sigma^2 J_{OLS},$$

where

$$J_{OLS} = \mathrm{tr}(U L_{OLS} L_{OLS}^\top) \quad and \quad U_{i,j} = \int \varphi_i(x)\varphi_j(x)p_t(x)dx.$$

Therefore, for the correctly specified model (1), the generalization error G_{OLS} is expressed as

$$G_{OLS} = \sigma^2 J_{OLS}.$$

Based on this expression, the existing active learning method determines the location of training input points $\{x_i\}_{i=1}^n$ (or the training input density $p_x(x)$) so that J_{OLS} is minimized [2, 1, 3].

3   Analysis of Existing Method under Misspecification of Models

In this section, we investigate the validity of the existing active learning method for misspecified models.

Suppose the model does not exactly include the learning target function $f(x)$, but it *approximately* includes it, i.e., for a scalar δ such that $|\delta|$ is small, $f(x)$ is expressed as

$$f(x) = g(x) + \delta r(x),$$

where $g(x)$ is the orthogonal projection of $f(x)$ onto the span of $\{\varphi_i(x)\}_{i=1}^p$ and the residual $r(x)$ is orthogonal to $\{\varphi_i(x)\}_{i=1}^p$:

$$g(x) = \sum_{i=1}^{p} \alpha_i^* \varphi_i(x) \quad and \quad \int r(x)\varphi_i(x)p_t(x)dx = 0 \ \text{ for } i = 1, 2, \ldots, p.$$

In this case, the bias term B is expressed as

$$B = \int \left(\mathbb{E}_\epsilon \widehat{f}(x) - g(x) \right)^2 p_t(x)dx + C, \quad where \quad C = \int \left(g(x) - f(x) \right)^2 p_t(x)dx.$$

Since C is constant which does not depend on the training input density $p_x(x)$, we subtract C in the following discussion.

Then we have the following lemma[2].

Lemma 2 *For the approximately correct model (3), we have*

$$B_{OLS} - C = \delta^2 \langle U L_{OLS} z_r, L_{OLS} z_r \rangle = \mathcal{O}(\delta^2),$$
$$V_{OLS} = \sigma^2 J_{OLS} = \mathcal{O}_p(n^{-1}),$$

where

$$z_r = \left(r(x_1), r(x_2), \ldots, r(x_n) \right)^\top.$$

---

[2]Proofs of lemmas are provided in an extended version [6].

Note that the asymptotic order in Eq.(1) is in probability since V_{OLS} is a random variable that includes $\{x_i\}_{i=1}^n$. The above lemma implies that

$$G_{OLS} - C = \sigma^2 J_{OLS} + o_p(n^{-1}) \quad \text{if } \delta = o_p(n^{-\frac{1}{2}}).$$

Therefore, the existing active learning method of minimizing J_{OLS} is still justified if $\delta = o_p(n^{-\frac{1}{2}})$. However, when $\delta \neq o_p(n^{-\frac{1}{2}})$, the existing method may not work well because the bias term $B_{OLS} - C$ is not smaller than the variance term V_{OLS}, so it can not be neglected.

4 New Active Learning Method

In this section, we propose a new active learning method based on the weighted least-squares learning.

4.1 Weighted Least-Squares Learning

When the model is correctly specified, $\hat{\alpha}_{OLS}$ is an unbiased estimator of α^*. However, for misspecified models, $\hat{\alpha}_{OLS}$ is generally biased even asymptotically if $\delta = \mathcal{O}_p(1)$.

The bias of $\hat{\alpha}_{OLS}$ is actually caused by the *covariate shift* [5]—the training input density $p_x(x)$ is different from the test input density $p_t(x)$. For correctly specified models, influence of the covariate shift can be ignored, as the existing active learning method does. However, for misspecified models, we should explicitly cope with the covariate shift.

Under the covariate shift, it is known that the following *weighted least-squares learning* is asymptotically unbiased even if $\delta = \mathcal{O}_p(1)$ [5].

$$\hat{\alpha}_{WLS} = \operatorname*{argmin}_{\alpha} \left[\sum_{i=1}^n \frac{p_t(x_i)}{p_x(x_i)} \left(\hat{f}(x_i) - y_i \right)^2 \right].$$

Asymptotic unbiasedness of $\hat{\alpha}_{WLS}$ would be intuitively understood by the following identity, which is similar in spirit to *importance sampling*:

$$\int \left(\hat{f}(x) - f(x) \right)^2 p_t(x) dx = \int \left(\hat{f}(x) - f(x) \right)^2 \frac{p_t(x)}{p_x(x)} p_x(x) dx.$$

In the following, we assume that $p_x(x)$ is strictly positive for all x. Let D be the diagonal matrix with the i-th diagonal element

$$D_{i,i} = \frac{p_t(x_i)}{p_x(x_i)}.$$

Then it can be confirmed that $\hat{\alpha}_{WLS}$ is given by

$$\hat{\alpha}_{WLS} = L_{WLS} y, \quad \text{where} \quad L_{WLS} = (X^\top D X)^{-1} X^\top D.$$

4.2 Active Learning Based on Weighted Least-Squares Learning

Let G_{WLS}, B_{WLS} and V_{WLS} be G, B and V for the learned function obtained by the above weighted least-squares learning, respectively. Then we have the following lemma.

Lemma 3 *For the approximately correct model (3), we have*

$$B_{WLS} - C = \delta^2 \langle U L_{WLS} z_r, L_{WLS} z_r \rangle = \mathcal{O}_p(\delta^2 n^{-1}),$$
$$V_{WLS} = \sigma^2 J_{WLS} = \mathcal{O}_p(n^{-1}),$$

where

$$J_{WLS} = \operatorname{tr}(U L_{WLS} L_{WLS}^\top).$$

This lemma implies that

$$G_{WLS} - C = \sigma^2 J_{WLS} + o_p(n^{-1}) \quad \text{if } \delta = o_p(1).$$

Based on this expression, we propose determining the training input density $p_x(x)$ so that J_{WLS} is minimized.

The use of the proposed criterion J_{WLS} can be theoretically justified when $\delta = o_p(1)$, while the existing criterion J_{OLS} requires $\delta = o_p(n^{-\frac{1}{2}})$. Therefore, the proposed method has a wider range of applications. The effect of this extension is experimentally investigated in the next section.

5   Numerical Examples

We evaluate the usefulness of the proposed active learning method through experiments.

Toy Data Set: We first illustrate how the proposed method works under a controlled setting.

Let $d = 1$ and the learning target function $f(x)$ be $f(x) = 1 - x + x^2 + \delta x^3$. Let $n = 100$ and $\{\epsilon_i\}_{i=1}^{100}$ be i.i.d. Gaussian noise with mean zero and standard deviation 0.3. Let $p_t(x)$ be the Gaussian density with mean 0.2 and standard deviation 0.4, which is assumed to be known here. Let $p = 3$ and the basis functions be $\varphi_i(x) = x^{i-1}$ for $i = 1, 2, 3$. Let us consider the following three cases. $\delta = 0, 0.04, 0.5$, where each case corresponds to "*correctly specified*", "*approximately correct*", and "*misspecified*" (see Figure 1). We choose the training input density $p_x(x)$ from the Gaussian density with mean 0.2 and standard deviation $0.4c$, where

$$c = 0.8, 0.9, 1.0, \ldots, 2.5.$$

We compare the accuracy of the following three methods:

(A) Proposed active learning criterion + WLS learning : The training input density is determined so that J_{WLS} is minimized. Following the determined input density, training input points $\{x_i\}_{i=1}^{100}$ are created and corresponding output values $\{y_i\}_{i=1}^{100}$ are observed. Then WLS learning is used for estimating the parameters.

(B) Existing active learning criterion + OLS learning [2, 1, 3]: The training input density is determined so that J_{OLS} is minimized. OLS learning is used for estimating the parameters.

(C) Passive learning + OLS learning: The test input density $p_t(x)$ is used as the training input density. OLS learning is used for estimating the parameters.

First, we evaluate the accuracy of J_{WLS} and J_{OLS} as approximations of G_{WLS} and G_{OLS}. The means and standard deviations of G_{WLS}, J_{WLS}, G_{OLS}, and J_{OLS} over 100 runs are depicted as functions of c in Figure 2. These graphs show that when $\delta = 0$ ("*correctly specified*"), both J_{WLS} and J_{OLS} give accurate estimates of G_{WLS} and G_{OLS}. When $\delta = 0.04$ ("*approximately correct*"), J_{WLS} again works well, while J_{OLS} tends to be negatively biased for large c. This result is surprising since as illustrated in Figure 1, the learning target functions with $\delta = 0$ and $\delta = 0.04$ are visually quite similar. Therefore, it intuitively seems that the result of $\delta = 0.04$ is not much different from that of $\delta = 0$. However, the simulation result shows that this slight difference makes J_{OLS} unreliable. When $\delta = 0.5$ ("*misspecified*"), J_{WLS} is still reasonably accurate, while J_{OLS} is heavily biased.

These results show that as an approximation of the generalization error, J_{WLS} is more robust against the misspecification of models than J_{OLS}, which is in good agreement with the theoretical analyses given in Section 3 and Section 4.

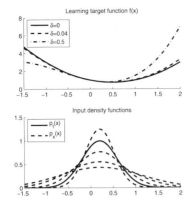

Figure 1: Learning target function and input density functions.

Table 1: The means and standard deviations of the generalization error for Toy data set. The best method and comparable ones by the t-test at the significance level 5% are described with boldface. The value of method (B) for $\delta = 0.5$ is extremely large but it is not a typo.

	$\delta = 0$	$\delta = 0.04$	$\delta = 0.5$
(A)	1.99 ± 0.07	$\mathbf{2.02 \pm 0.07}$	$\mathbf{5.94 \pm 0.80}$
(B)	$\mathbf{1.34 \pm 0.04}$	3.27 ± 1.23	303 ± 197
(C)	2.60 ± 0.44	2.62 ± 0.43	6.87 ± 1.15

All values in the table are multiplied by 10^3.

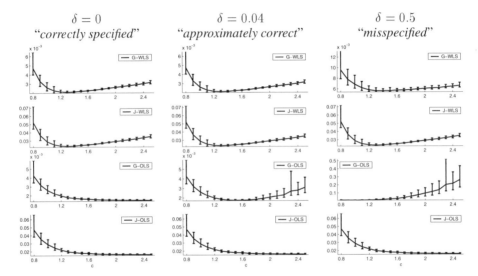

Figure 2: The means and error bars of G_{WLS}, J_{WLS}, G_{OLS}, and J_{OLS} over 100 runs as functions of c.

In Table 1, the mean and standard deviation of the generalization error obtained by each method is described. When $\delta = 0$, the existing method (B) works better than the proposed method (A). Actually, in this case, training input densities that approximately minimize G_{WLS} and G_{OLS} were found by J_{WLS} and J_{OLS}. Therefore, the difference of the errors is caused by the difference of WLS and OLS: WLS generally has larger variance than OLS. Since bias is zero for both WLS and OLS if $\delta = 0$, OLS would be more accurate than WLS. Although the proposed method (A) is outperformed by the existing method (B), it still works better than the passive learning scheme (C). When $\delta = 0.04$ and $\delta = 0.5$ the proposed method (A) gives significantly smaller errors than other methods.

Overall, we found that for all three cases, the proposed method (A) works reasonably well and outperforms the passive learning scheme (C). On the other hand, the existing method (B) works excellently in the correctly specified case, although it tends to perform poorly once the correctness of the model is violated. Therefore, the proposed method (A) is found to be robust against the misspecification of models and thus it is reliable.

Table 2: The means and standard deviations of the test error for DELVE data sets. All values in the table are multiplied by 10^3.

	Bank-8fm	Bank-8fh	Bank-8nm	Bank-8nh
(A)	$\mathbf{0.31 \pm 0.04}$	$\mathbf{2.10 \pm 0.05}$	$\mathbf{24.66 \pm 1.20}$	$\mathbf{37.98 \pm 1.11}$
(B)	0.44 ± 0.07	2.21 ± 0.09	27.67 ± 1.50	39.71 ± 1.38
(C)	0.35 ± 0.04	2.20 ± 0.06	26.34 ± 1.35	39.84 ± 1.35

	Kin-8fm	Kin-8fh	Kin-8nm	Kin-8nh
(A)	1.59 ± 0.07	5.90 ± 0.16	$\mathbf{0.72 \pm 0.04}$	3.68 ± 0.09
(B)	$\mathbf{1.49 \pm 0.06}$	$\mathbf{5.63 \pm 0.13}$	0.85 ± 0.06	$\mathbf{3.60 \pm 0.09}$
(C)	1.70 ± 0.08	6.27 ± 0.24	0.81 ± 0.06	3.89 ± 0.14

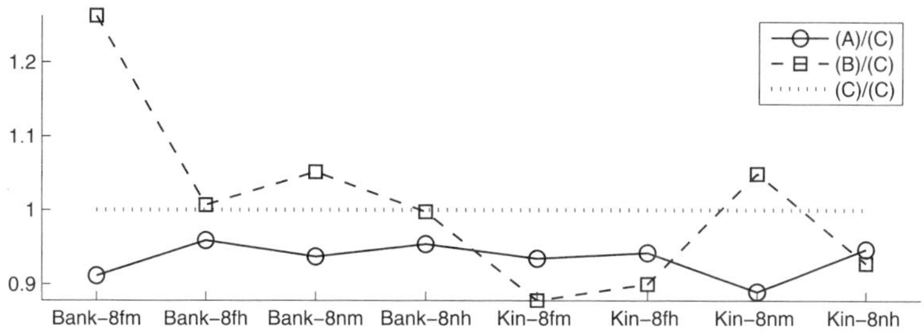

Figure 3: Mean relative performance of (A) and (B) compared with (C). For each run, the test errors of (A) and (B) are normalized by the test error of (C), and then the values are averaged over 100 runs. Note that the error bars were reasonably small so they were omitted.

Realistic Data Set: Here we use eight practical data sets provided by DELVE [4]: *Bank-8fm, Bank-8fh, Bank-8nm, Bank-8nh, Kin-8fm, Kin-8fh, Kin-8nm*, and *Kin-8nh*. Each data set includes 8192 samples, consisting of 8-dimensional input and 1-dimensional output values. For convenience, every attribute is normalized into $[0, 1]$.

Suppose we are given all 8192 *input* points (i.e., unlabeled samples). Note that output values are unknown. From the pool of unlabeled samples, we choose $n = 1000$ input points $\{x_i\}_{i=1}^{1000}$ for training and observe the corresponding output values $\{y_i\}_{i=1}^{1000}$. The task is to predict the output values of all unlabeled samples.

In this experiment, the test input density $p_t(x)$ is unknown. So we estimate it using the independent Gaussian density.

$$p_t(x) = (2\pi \widehat{\gamma}_{MLE}^2)^{-\frac{d}{2}} \exp\left(-\|x - \widehat{\mu}_{MLE}\|^2 / (2\widehat{\gamma}_{MLE}^2)\right),$$

where $\widehat{\mu}_{MLE}$ and $\widehat{\gamma}_{MLE}$ are the maximum likelihood estimates of the mean and standard deviation obtained from all unlabeled samples. Let $p = 50$ and the basis functions be

$$\varphi_i(x) = \exp\left(-\|x - t_i\|^2 / 2\right) \quad \text{for } i = 1, 2, \ldots, 50,$$

where $\{t_i\}_{i=1}^{50}$ are template points randomly chosen from the pool of unlabeled samples.

We select the training input density $p_x(x)$ from the independent Gaussian density with mean $\widehat{\mu}_{MLE}$ and standard deviation $c\widehat{\gamma}_{MLE}$, where

$$c = 0.7, 0.75, 0.8, \ldots, 2.4.$$

In this simulation, we can not create the training input points in an arbitrary location because we only have 8192 samples. Therefore, we first create temporary input points following the determined training input density, and then choose the input points from the pool of unlabeled samples that are closest to the temporary input points. For each data set, we repeat this simulation 100 times, by changing the template points $\{t_i\}_{i=1}^{50}$ in each run.

The means and standard deviations of the test error over 100 runs are described in Table 2. The proposed method (A) outperforms the existing method (B) for five data sets, while it is outperformed by (B) for the other three data sets. We conjecture that the model used for learning is almost correct in these three data sets. This result implies that the proposed method (A) is slightly better than the existing method (B).

Figure 3 depicts the relative performance of the proposed method (A) and the existing method (B) compared with the passive learning scheme (C). This shows that (A) outperforms (C) for all eight data sets, while (B) is comparable or is outperformed by (C) for five data sets. Therefore, the proposed method (A) is overall shown to work better than other schemes.

6 Conclusions

We argued that active learning is essentially the situation under the covariate shift—the training input density is different from the test input density. When the model used for learning is correctly specified, the covariate shift does not matter. However, for misspecified models, we have to explicitly cope with the covariate shift. In this paper, we proposed a new active learning method based on the weighted least-squares learning.

The numerical study showed that the existing method works better than the proposed method if model is correctly specified. However, the existing method tends to perform poorly once the correctness of the model is violated. On the other hand, the proposed method overall worked reasonably well and it consistently outperformed the passive learning scheme. Therefore, the proposed method would be robust against the misspecification of models and thus it is reliable.

The proposed method can be theoretically justified if the model is approximately correct in a weak sense. However, it is no longer valid for totally misspecified models. A natural future direction would be therefore to devise an active learning method which has theoretical guarantee with totally misspecified models. It is also important to notice that when the model is totally misspecified, even learning with optimal training input points would not be successful anyway. In such cases, it is of course important to carry out *model selection*. In active learning research—including the present paper, however, the location of training input points are designed for a *single* model at hand. That is, the model should have been chosen *before* performing active learning. Devising a method for simultaneously optimizing models and the location of training input points would be a more important and promising future direction.

Acknowledgments: The author would like to thank MEXT (Grant-in-Aid for Young Scientists 17700142) for partial financial support.

References

[1] D. A. Cohn, Z. Ghahramani, and M. I. Jordan. Active learning with statistical models. *Journal of Artificial Intelligence Research*, 4:129–145, 1996.

[2] V. V. Fedorov. *Theory of Optimal Experiments*. Academic Press, New York, 1972.

[3] K. Fukumizu. Statistical active learning in multilayer perceptrons. *IEEE Transactions on Neural Networks*, 11(1):17–26, 2000.

[4] C. E. Rasmussen, R. M. Neal, G. E. Hinton, D. van Camp, M. Revow, Z. Ghahramani, R. Kustra, and R. Tibshirani. The DELVE manual, 1996.

[5] H. Shimodaira. Improving predictive inference under covariate shift by weighting the log-likelihood function. *Journal of Statistical Planning and Inference*, 90(2):227–244, 2000.

[6] M. Sugiyama. Active learning for misspecified models. Technical report, Department of Computer Science, Tokyo Institute of Technology, 2005.

Temporal Abstraction
in Temporal-difference Networks

Richard S. Sutton, Eddie J. Rafols, Anna Koop
Department of Computing Science
University of Alberta
Edmonton, AB, Canada T6G 2E8
{sutton,erafols,anna}@cs.ualberta.ca

Abstract

We present a generalization of temporal-difference networks to include temporally abstract options on the links of the question network. Temporal-difference (TD) networks have been proposed as a way of representing and learning a wide variety of predictions about the interaction between an agent and its environment. These predictions are *compositional* in that their targets are defined in terms of other predictions, and *subjunctive* in that that they are about what would happen if an action or sequence of actions were taken. In conventional TD networks, the inter-related predictions are at successive time steps and contingent on a single action; here we generalize them to accommodate extended time intervals and contingency on whole ways of behaving. Our generalization is based on the options framework for temporal abstraction. The primary contribution of this paper is to introduce a new algorithm for intra-option learning in TD networks with function approximation and eligibility traces. We present empirical examples of our algorithm's effectiveness and of the greater representational expressiveness of temporally-abstract TD networks.

The primary distinguishing feature of temporal-difference (TD) networks (Sutton & Tanner, 2005) is that they permit a general compositional specification of the *goals* of learning. The goals of learning are thought of as predictive questions being asked by the agent in the learning problem, such as "What will I see if I step forward and look right?" or "If I open the fridge, will I see a bottle of beer?" Seeing a bottle of beer is of course a complicated perceptual act. It might be thought of as obtaining a set of predictions about what would happen if certain reaching and grasping actions were taken, about what would happen if the bottle were opened and turned upside down, and of what the bottle would look like if viewed from various angles. To predict seeing a bottle of beer is thus to make a prediction about a set of other predictions. The target for the overall prediction is a composition in the mathematical sense of the first prediction with each of the other predictions.

TD networks are the first framework for representing the goals of predictive learning in a compositional, machine-accessible form. Each node of a TD network represents an individual question—something to be predicted—and has associated with it a value representing an answer to the question—a prediction of that something. The questions are represented by a set of directed links between nodes. If node 1 is linked to node 2, then node 1 represents a question incorporating node 2's question; its value is a prediction about node 2's prediction. Higher-level predictions can be composed in several ways from lower ones, producing a powerful, structured representation language for the targets of learning. The compositional structure is not just in a human designer's head; it is expressed in the links and thus is accessible to the agent and its learning algorithm.

The network of these links is referred to as the *question network*. An entirely separate set of directed links between the nodes is used to compute the values (predictions, answers) associated with each node. These links collectively are referred to as the *answer network*. The computation in the answer network is compositional in a conventional way—node values are computed from other node values. The essential insight of TD networks is that the notion of compositionality should apply to questions as well as to answers.

A secondary distinguishing feature of TD networks is that the predictions (node values) at each moment in time can be used as a representation of the state of the world at that time. In this way they are an instance of the idea of *predictive state representations* (PSRs) introduced by Littman, Sutton and Singh (2002), Jaeger (2000), and Rivest and Schapire (1987). Representing a state by its predictions is a potentially powerful strategy for state abstraction (Rafols et al., 2005). We note that the questions used in all previous work with PSRs are defined in terms of concrete actions and observations, not other predictions. They are not compositional in the sense that TD-network questions are.

The questions we have discussed so far are *subjunctive*, meaning that they are conditional on a certain way of behaving. We predict what we would see *if we were* to step forward and look right, or *if we were* to open the fridge. The questions in conventional TD networks are subjunctive, but they are conditional only on primitive actions or open-loop sequences of primitive actions (as are conventional PSRs). It is natural to generalize this, as we have in the informal examples above, to questions that are conditional on closed-loop temporally extended ways of behaving. For example, opening the fridge is a complex, high-level action. The arm must be lifted to the door, the hand shaped for grasping the handle, etc. To ask questions like "if I were to go to the coffee room, would I see John?" would require substantial temporal abstraction in addition to state abstraction.

The options framework (Sutton, Precup & Singh, 1999) is a straightforward way of talking about temporally extended ways of behaving and about predictions of their outcomes. In this paper we extend the options framework so that it can be applied to TD networks. Significant extensions of the original options framework are needed. Novel features of our option-extended TD networks are that they 1) predict components of option outcomes rather than full outcome probability distributions, 2) learn according to the first intra-option method to use eligibility traces (see Sutton & Barto, 1998), and 3) include the possibility of options whose 'policies' are indifferent to which of several actions are selected.

1 The options framework

In this section we present the essential elements of the options framework (Sutton, Precup & Singh, 1999) that we will need for our extension of TD networks. In this framework, an agent and an environment interact at discrete time steps $t = 1, 2, 3....$ In each state $s_t \in \mathcal{S}$, the agent selects an action $a_t \in \mathcal{A}$, determining the next state s_{t+1}.[1] An action is a way of behaving for one time step; the options framework lets us talk about temporally extended ways of behaving. An individual option consists of three parts. The first is the *initiation set*, $\mathcal{I} \subset \mathcal{S}$, the subset of states in which the option can be started. The second component of an option is its *policy*, $\pi : \mathcal{S} \times \mathcal{A} \Rightarrow [0, 1]$, specifying how the agent behaves when

---

[1] Although the options framework includes rewards, we omit them here because we are concerned only with prediction, not control.

following the option. Finally, a termination function, $\beta : \mathcal{S} \times \mathcal{A} \Rightarrow [0,1]$, specifies how the option ends: $\beta(s)$ denotes the probability of terminating when in state s. The option is thus completely and formally defined by the 3-tuple $(\mathcal{I}, \pi, \beta)$.

2   Conventional TD networks

In this section we briefly present the details of the structure and the learning algorithm comprising TD networks as introduced by Sutton and Tanner (2005). TD networks address a prediction problem in which the agent may not have direct access to the state of the environment. Instead, at each time step the agent receives an *observation* $o_t \in \mathcal{O}$ dependent on the state. The experience stream thus consists of a sequence of alternating actions and observations, $o_1, a_1, o_2, a_2, o_3 \cdots$.

The TD network consists of a set of nodes, each representing a single scalar prediction, interlinked by the question and answer networks as suggested previously. For a network of n nodes, the vector of all predictions at time step t is denoted $\mathbf{y}_t = (y_t^1, \ldots, y_t^n)^T$. The predictions are estimates of the expected value of some scalar quantity, typically of a bit, in which case they can be interpreted as estimates of probabilities. The predictions are updated at each time step according to a vector-valued function $\mathbf{u}$ with modifiable parameter $\mathbf{W}$, which is often taken to be of a linear form:

$$\mathbf{y}_t = \mathbf{u}(\mathbf{y}_{t-1}, a_{t-1}, o_t, \mathbf{W}_t) = \boldsymbol{\sigma}(\mathbf{W}_t \mathbf{x}_t), \tag{1}$$

where $\mathbf{x}_t \in \Re^m$ is an m-vector of features created from $(\mathbf{y}_{t-1}, a_{t-1}, o_t)$, $\mathbf{W}_t$ is an $n \times m$ matrix (whose elements are sometimes referred to as weights), and $\boldsymbol{\sigma}$ is the n-vector form of either the identity function or the S-shaped logistic function $\sigma(s) = \frac{1}{1+e^{-s}}$. The feature vector is an arbitrary vector-valued function of $\mathbf{y}_{t-1}$, a_{t-1}, and o_t. For example, in the simplest case the feature vector is a unit basis vector with the location of the one communicating the current state. In a partially observable environment, the feature vector may be a combination of the agent's action, observations, and predictions from the previous time step. The overall update $\mathbf{u}$ defines the answer network.

The question network consists of a set of *target functions*, $z^i : \mathcal{O} \times \Re^n \to \Re$, and *condition functions*, $c^i : \mathcal{A} \times \Re^n \to [0,1]^n$. We define $z_t^i = z^i(o_{t+1}, \tilde{\mathbf{y}}_{t+1})$ as the target for prediction y_t^i.[2] Similarly, we define $c_t^i = c^i(a_t, \mathbf{y}_t)$ as the condition at time t. The learning algorithm for each component w_t^{ij} of $\mathbf{W}_t$ can then be written

$$w_{t+1}^{ij} = w_t^{ij} + \alpha \left(z_t^i - y_t^i \right) c_t^i \frac{\partial y_t^i}{\partial w_t^{ij}}, \tag{2}$$

where α is a positive step-size parameter. Note that the targets here are functions of the observation and predictions exactly one time step later, and that the conditions are functions of a single primitive action. This is what makes this algorithm suitable only for learning about one-step TD relationships. By chaining together multiple nodes, Sutton and Tanner (2005) used it to predict k steps ahead, for various particular values of k, and to predict the outcome of specific action sequences (as in PSRs, e.g., Littman et al., 2002; Singh et al., 2004). Now we consider the extension to temporally abstract actions.

3   Option-extended TD networks

In this section we present our intra-option learning algorithm for TD networks with options and eligibility traces. As suggested earlier, each node's outgoing link in the question

---

[2]The quantity $\tilde{\mathbf{y}}$ is almost the same as $\mathbf{y}$, and we encourage the reader to think of them as identical here. The difference is that $\tilde{\mathbf{y}}$ is calculated by weights that are one step out of date as compared to $\mathbf{y}$, i.e., $\tilde{\mathbf{y}}_t = \mathbf{u}(\mathbf{y}_{t-1}, a_{t-1}, o_t, \mathbf{W}_{t-1})$ (cf. equation 1).

network will now correspond to an option applying over possibly many steps. The policy of the ith node's option corresponds to the condition function c^i, which we think of as a *recognizer* for the option. It inspects each action taken to assess whether the option is being followed: $c_t^i = 1$ if the agent is acting consistently with the option policy and $c_t^i = 0$ otherwise (intermediate values are also possible). When an agent ceases to act consistently with the option policy, we say that the option has *diverged*. The possibility of recognizing more than one action as consistent with the option is a significant generalization of the original idea of options. If no actions are recognized as acceptable in a state, then the option cannot be followed and thus cannot be initiated. Here we take the set of states with at least one recognized action to be the initiation set of the option.

The option-termination function β generalizes naturally to TD networks. Each node i is given a corresponding termination function, $\beta^i : \mathcal{O} \times \Re^n \to [0, 1]$, where $\beta_t^i = \beta^i(o_{t+1}, \mathbf{y}_t)$ is the probability of terminating at time t.[3] $\beta_t^i = 1$ indicates that the option has terminated at time t; $\beta_t^i = 0$ indicates that it has not, and intermediate values of β correspond to soft or stochastic termination conditions. If an option terminates, then z_t^i acts as the target, but if the option is ongoing without termination, then the node's own next value, $\tilde{y}_{t+1}^i$, should be the target. The termination function specifies which of the two targets (or mixture of the two targets) is used to produce a form of TD error for each node i:

$$\delta_t^i = \beta_t^i z_t^i + (1 - \beta_t^i)\tilde{y}_{t+1}^i - y_t^i. \tag{3}$$

Our option-extended algorithm incorporates eligibility traces (see Sutton & Barto, 1998) as short-term memory variables organized in an $n \times m$ matrix $\mathbf{E}$, paralleling the weight matrix. The traces are a record of the effect that each weight could have had on each node's prediction during the time the agent has been acting consistently with the node's option. The components e^{ij} of the eligibility matrix are updated by

$$e_t^{ij} = c_t^i \left[\lambda e_{t-1}^{ij}(1 - \beta_t^i) + \frac{\partial y_t^i}{\partial w_t^{ij}} \right], \tag{4}$$

where $0 \leq \lambda \leq 1$ is the trace-decay parameter familiar from the TD(λ) learning algorithm. Because of the c_t^i factor, all of a node's traces will be immediately reset to zero whenever the agent deviates from the node's option's policy. If the agent follows the policy and the option does not terminate, then the trace decays by λ and increments by the gradient in the way typical of eligibility traces. If the policy is followed and the option does terminate, then the trace will be reset to zero on the immediately following time step, and a new trace will start building. Finally, our algorithm updates the weights on each time step by

$$w_{t+1}^{ij} = w_t^{ij} + \alpha \, \delta_t^i \, e_t^{ij}. \tag{5}$$

4 Fully observable experiment

This experiment was designed to test the correctness of the algorithm in a simple gridworld where the environmental state is observable. We applied an options-extended TD network to the problem of learning to predict observations from interaction with the gridworld environment shown on the left in Figure 1. Empty squares indicate spaces where the agent can move freely, and colored squares (shown shaded in the figure) indicate walls. The agent is egocentric. At each time step the agent receives from the environment six bits representing the color it is facing (red, green, blue, orange, yellow, or white). In this first experiment we also provided $6 \times 6 \times 4 = 144$ other bits directly indicating the complete state of the environment (square and orientation).

---

[3]The fact that the option depends only on the current predictions, action, and observation means that we are considering only *Markov* options.

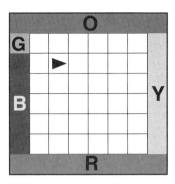
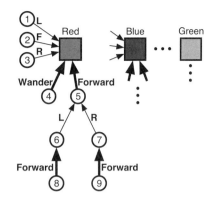

Figure 1: The test world (left) and the question network (right) used in the experiments. The triangle in the world indicates the location and orientation of the agent. The walls are labeled R, O, Y, G, and B representing the colors red, orange, yellow, green and blue. Note that the left wall is mostly blue but partly green. The right diagram shows in full the portion of the question network corresponding to the red bit. This structure is repeated, but not shown, for the other four (non-white) colors. L, R, and F are primitive actions, and Forward and Wander are options.

There are three possible actions: $\mathcal{A} = \{\text{F, R, L}\}$. Actions were selected according to a fixed stochastic policy independent of the state. The probability of the F, L, and R actions were 0.5, 0.25, and 0.25 respectively. L and R cause the agent to rotate 90 degrees to the left or right. F causes the agent to move ahead one square with probability $1 - p$ and to stay in the same square with probability p. The probability p is called the *slipping probability*. If the forward movement would cause the agent to move into a wall, then the agent does not move. In this experiment, we used $p = 0$, $p = 0.1$, and $p = 0.5$.

In addition to these primitive actions, we provided two temporally abstract options, Forward and Wander. The Forward option takes the action F in every state and terminates when the agent senses a wall (color) in front of it. The policy of the Wander option is the same as that actually followed by the agent. Wander terminates with probability 1 when a wall is sensed, and spontaneously with probability 0.5 otherwise.

We used the question network shown on the right in Figure 1. The predictions of nodes 1, 2, and 3 are estimates of the probability that the red bit would be observed if the corresponding primitive action were taken. Node 4 is a prediction of whether the agent will see the red bit upon termination of the Wander option if it were taken. Node 5 predicts the probability of observing the red bit given that the Forward option is followed until termination. Nodes 6 and 7 represent predictions of the outcome of a primitive action followed by the Forward option. Nodes 8 and 9 take this one step further: they represent predictions of the red bit if the Forward option were followed to termination, then a primitive action were taken, and then the Forward option were followed again to termination.

We applied our algorithm to learn the parameter $\mathbf{W}$ of the answer network for this question network. The step-size parameter α was 1.0, and the trace-decay parameter λ was 0.9. The initial $\mathbf{W}_0$, $\mathbf{E}_0$, and $\mathbf{y}_0$ were all 0. Each run began with the agent in the state indicated in Figure 1 (left). In this experiment $\boldsymbol{\sigma}(\cdot)$ was the identity function.

For each value of p, we ran 50 runs of 20,000 time steps. On each time step, the root-mean-squared (RMS) error in each node's prediction was computed and then averaged over all the nodes. The nodes corresponding to the Wander option were not included in the average because of the difficulty of calculating their correct predictions. This average was then

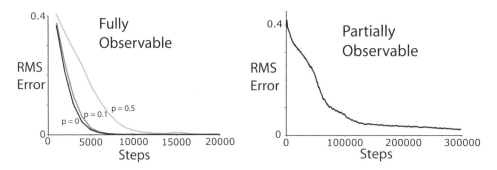

Figure 2: Learning curves in the fully-observable experiment for each slippage probability (left) and in the partially-observable experiment (right).

itself averaged over the 50 runs and bins of 1,000 time steps to produce the learning curves shown on the left in Figure 2.

For all slippage probabilities, the error in all predictions fell almost to zero. After approximately 12,000 trials, the agent made almost perfect predictions in all cases. Not surprisingly, learning was slower at the higher slippage probabilities. These results show that our augmented TD network is able to make a complete temporally-abstract model of this world.

5 Partially observable experiment

In our second experiment, only the six color observation bits were available to the agent. This experiment provides a more challenging test of our algorithm. To model the environment well, the TD network must construct a representation of state from very sparse information. In fact, completely accurate prediction is not possible in this problem with our question network.

In this experiment the input vector consisted of three groups of 46 components each, 138 in total. If the action was R, the first 46 components were set to the 40 node values and the six observation bits, and the other components were 0. If the action was L, the next group of 46 components was filled in in the same way, and the first and third groups were zero. If the action was F, the third group was filled. This technique enables the answer network as function approximator to represent a wider class of functions in a linear form than would otherwise be possible. In this experiment, $\sigma(\cdot)$ was the S-shaped logistic function. The slippage probability was $p = 0.1$.

As our performance measure we used the RMS error, as in the first experiment, except that the predictions for the primitive actions (nodes 1-3) were not included. These predictions can never become completely accurate because the agent can't tell in detail where it is located in the open space. As before, we averaged RMS error over 50 runs and 1,000 time step bins, to produce the learning curve shown on the right in Figure 2. As before, the RMS error approached zero.

Node 5 in Figure 1 holds the prediction of red if the agent were to march forward to the wall ahead of it. Corresponding nodes in the other subnetworks hold the predictions of the other colors upon Forward. To make these predictions accurately, the agent must keep track of which wall it is facing, even if it is many steps away from it. It has to learn a sort of compass that it can keep updated as it turns in the middle of the space. Figure 3 is a demonstration of the compass learned after a representative run of 200,000 time steps. At the end of the run, the agent was driven manually to the state shown in the first row (relative time index $t = 1$). On steps 1-25 the agent was spun clockwise in place. The third column shows the prediction for node 5 in each portion of the question network. That is, the predictions shown are for each color-observation bit at termination of the Forward option. At $t = 1$, the agent is facing the orange wall and it predicts that the Forward option would result in seeing the orange bit and none other. Over steps 2-5 we see that the predictions are maintained accurately as the agent spins despite the fact that its observation bits remain the same. Even after spinning for 25 steps the agent knows exactly which way it is facing. While spinning, the agent correctly never predicts seeing the green bit (after Forward), but if it is driven up and turned, as in the last row of the figure, the green bit is accurately predicted.

The fourth column shows the prediction for node 8 in each portion of the question network. Recall that these nodes correspond to the sequence Forward, L, Forward. At time $t = 1$, the agent accurately predicts that Forward will bring it to orange (third column) and also predicts that Forward, L, Forward will bring it to green. The predictions made for node 8 at each subsequent step of the sequence are also correct.

These results show that the agent is able to accurately maintain its long term predictions without directly encountering sensory verification. How much larger would the TD network have to be to handle a 100x100 gridworld? The answer is *not at all*. The same question network applies to any size problem. If the layout of the colored walls remain the same, then even the answer network transfers across worlds of widely varying sizes. In other experiments, training on successively larger problems, we have shown that the same TD network as used here can learn to make all the long-term predictions correctly on a 100x100 version of the 6x6 gridworld used here.

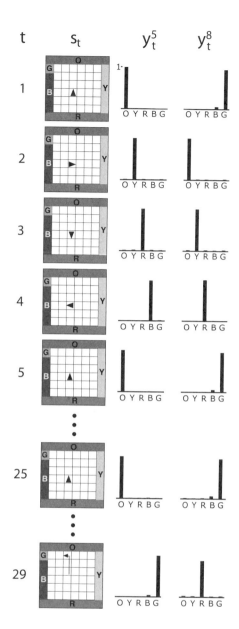

Figure 3: An illustration of part of what the agent learns in the partially observable environment. The second column is a sequence of states with (relative) time index as given by the first column. The sequence was generated by controlling the agent manually. On steps 1-25 the agent was spun clockwise in place, and the trajectory after that is shown by the line in the last state diagram. The third and fourth columns show the values of the nodes corresponding to 5 and 8 in Figure 1, one for each color-observation bit.

6 Conclusion

Our experiments show that option-extended TD networks can learn effectively. They can learn facts about their environments that are not representable in conventional TD networks or in any other method for learning models of the world. One concern is that our intra-option learning algorithm is an off-policy learning method incorporating function approximation and bootstrapping (learning from predictions). The combination of these three is known to produce convergence problems for some methods (see Sutton & Barto, 1998), and they may arise here. A sound solution may require modifications to incorporate importance sampling (see Precup, Sutton & Dasgupta, 2001). In this paper we have considered only intra-option eligibility traces—traces extending over the time span within an option but not persisting across options. Tanner and Sutton (2005) have proposed a method for *inter*-option traces that could perhaps be combined with our intra-option traces.

The primary contribution of this paper is the introduction of a new learning algorithm for TD networks that incorporates options and eligibility traces. Our experiments are small and do little more than exercise the learning algorithm, showing that it does not break immediately. More significant is the greater representational power of option-extended TD networks. Options are a general framework for temporal abstraction, predictive state representations are a promising strategy for state abstraction, and TD networks are able to represent compositional questions. The combination of these three is potentially very powerful and worthy of further study.

Acknowledgments

The authors gratefully acknowledge the ideas and encouragement they have received in this work from Mark Ring, Brian Tanner, Satinder Singh, Doina Precup, and all the members of the rlai.net group.

References

Jaeger, H. (2000). Observable operator models for discrete stochastic time series. *Neural Computation*, 12(6):1371-1398. MIT Press.

Littman, M., Sutton, R. S., & Singh, S. (2002). Predictive representations of state. In T. G. Dietterich, S. Becker and Z. Ghahramani (eds.), *Advances In Neural Information Processing Systems 14*, pp. 1555-1561. MIT Press.

Precup, D., Sutton, R. S., & Dasgupta, S. (2001). Off-policy temporal-difference learning with function approximation. In C. E. Brodley, A. P. Danyluk (eds.), *Proceedings of the Eighteenth International Conference on Machine Learning*, pp. 417-424. San Francisco, CA: Morgan Kaufmann.

Rafols, E. J., Ring, M., Sutton, R.S., & Tanner, B. (2005). Using predictive representations to improve generalization in reinforcement learning. To appear in *Proceedings of the Nineteenth International Joint Conference on Artificial Intelligence*.

Rivest, R. L., & Schapire, R. E. (1987). Diversity-based inference of finite automata. In *Proceedings of the Twenty Eighth Annual Symposium on Foundations of Computer Science*, (pp. 78–87). IEEE Computer Society.

Singh, S., James, M. R., & Rudary, M. R. (2004). Predictive state representations: A new theory for modeling dynamical systems. In *Uncertainty in Artificial Intelligence: Proceedings of the Twentieth Conference in Uncertainty in Artificial Intelligence*, (pp. 512–519). AUAI Press.

Sutton, R. S., & Barto, A. G. (1998). *Reinforcement learning: An introduction*. Cambridge, MA: MIT Press.

Sutton, R. S., Precup, D., Singh, S. (1999). Between MDPs and semi-MDPs: A framework for temporal abstraction in reinforcement learning. *Artificial Intelligence*, *112*, pp. 181-211.

Sutton, R. S., & Tanner, B. (2005). Temporal-difference networks. To appear in *Neural Information Processing Systems Conference 17*.

Tanner, B., Sutton, R. S. (2005) Temporal-difference networks with history. To appear in *Proceedings of the Nineteenth International Joint Conference on Artificial Intelligence*.

Sequence and Tree Kernels
with Statistical Feature Mining

Jun Suzuki and Hideki Isozaki
NTT Communication Science Laboratories, NTT Corp.
2-4 Hikaridai, Seika-cho, Soraku-gun, Kyoto,619-0237 Japan
{jun, isozaki}@cslab.kecl.ntt.co.jp

Abstract

This paper proposes a new approach to feature selection based on a statistical feature mining technique for sequence and tree kernels. Since natural language data take discrete structures, convolution kernels, such as sequence and tree kernels, are advantageous for both the concept and accuracy of many *natural language processing* tasks. However, experiments have shown that the best results can only be achieved when limited small sub-structures are dealt with by these kernels. This paper discusses this issue of convolution kernels and then proposes a statistical feature selection that enable us to use larger sub-structures effectively. The proposed method, in order to execute efficiently, can be embedded into an original kernel calculation process by using *sub-structure mining* algorithms. Experiments on real NLP tasks confirm the problem in the conventional method and compare the performance of a conventional method to that of the proposed method.

1 Introduction

Since natural language data take the form of sequences of words and are generally analyzed into discrete structures, such as trees (parsed trees), *discrete kernels*, such as sequence kernels [7, 1] and tree kernels [2, 5], have been shown to offer excellent results in the *natural language processing (NLP)* field. Conceptually, these proposed kernels are defined as instances of *convolution kernels* [3, 11], which provides the concept of kernels over discrete structures.

However, unfortunately, experiments have shown that in some cases there is a critical issue with convolution kernels in NLP tasks [2, 1, 10]. That is, since natural language data contain many types of symbols, NLP tasks usually deal with extremely high dimension and sparse feature space. As a result, the convolution kernel approach can never be trained effectively, and it behaves like a nearest neighbor rule. To avoid this issue, we generally eliminate large sub-structures from the set of features used. However, the main reason for using convolution kernels is that we aim to use structural features easily and efficiently. If their use is limited to only very small structures, this negates the advantages of using convolution kernels.

This paper discusses this issue of convolution kernels, in particular sequence and tree kernels, and proposes a new method based on statistical significant test. The proposed method deals only with those features that are statistically significant for solving the target task, and large significant sub-structures can be used without over-fitting. Moreover, by using *sub-structure mining* algorithms, the proposed method can be executed efficiently by embedding it in an original kernel calculation process, which is defined by the *dynamic-programming* (DP) based calculation.

2 Convolution Kernels for Sequences and Trees

Convolution kernels have been proposed as a concept of kernels for discrete structures, such as sequences, trees and graphs. This framework defines the kernel function between input objects as the convolution of "sub-kernels", i.e. the kernels for the decompositions (parts or sub-structures) of the objects. Let X and Y be discrete objects. Conceptually, convolution kernels $K(X, Y)$ enumerate all sub-structures occurring in X and Y and then calculate their inner product, which is simply written as: $K(X, Y) = \langle \phi(X), \phi(Y) \rangle = \sum_i \phi_i(X) \cdot \phi_i(Y)$. ϕ represents the feature mapping from the discrete object to the feature space; that is, $\phi(X) = (\phi_1(X), \ldots, \phi_i(X), \ldots)$. Therefore, with sequence kernels, input objects X and Y are sequences, and $\phi_i(X)$ is a sub-sequence; with tree kernels, X and Y are trees, and $\phi_i(X)$ is a sub-tree. Up to now, many kinds of sequence and tree kernels have been proposed for a variety of different tasks. To clarify the discussion, this paper basically follows the framework of [1], which proposed a *gapped word sequence kernel*, and [5], which introduced a *labeled ordered tree kernel*.

We can treat that sequence is one of the special form of trees if we say sequences are rooted by their last symbol and each node has one child each of a previous symbol. Thus, in this paper, the word 'tree' is always including sequence. Let $\mathcal{L}$ be a set of finite symbols. Then, let $\mathcal{L}^n$ be a set of symbols whose sizes are n and $P(\mathcal{L}^n)$ be a set of trees that are constructed by $\mathcal{L}^n$. The meaning of "size" in this paper is the the number of nodes in a tree. We denote a tree $u \in P(\mathcal{L}_1^n)$ whose size is n or less, where $\cup_{m=1}^n \mathcal{L}^m = \mathcal{L}_1^n$. Let T be a tree and $\mathrm{sub}(T)$ be a function that returns a set of all possible sub-trees in T. We define a function $C_u(t)$ that returns a constant, $\lambda(0 < \lambda \le 1)$, if the sub-tree t covers u with the same root symbol. For example, a sub-tree 'a-b-c-d', where 'a', 'b', 'c' and 'd' represent symbols and '-' represents an edge between symbols, covers sub-trees 'd', 'a-c-d' and 'b-d'. That is, $C_u(t) = \lambda$ if u matches t allowing the node skip, 0 otherwise. We also define a function $\gamma_u(t)$ that returns the difference of size of sub-trees t and u. For example, if $t = \text{a-b-c-d}$ and $u = \text{a-b}$, then $\gamma_u(t) = |4 - 2| = 2$.

Formally, sequence and tree kernels can be defined as the same form as

$$K^{\mathrm{SK,TK}}(T^1, T^2) = \sum_{u \in P(\mathcal{L}_1^n)} \sum_{t^1 \in \mathrm{sub}(T^1)} C_u(t^1)^{\gamma_u(t^1)} \sum_{t^2 \in \mathrm{sub}(T^2)} C_u(t^2)^{\gamma_u(t^2)}. \quad (1)$$

Note that this formula is also including the node skip framework that is generally introduced only in sequence kernels[7, 1]; λ is the decay factor that handles the gap present in sub-trees u and t.

Sequence and tree kernels are defined in recursive formula to calculate them efficiently instead of the explicit calculation of Equation (1). Moreover, when implemented, these kernels can calculated in $O(n|T^1||T^2|)$, where $|T|$ represents the number of nodes in T, by using the DP technique. Note, that if the kernel does not use size restriction, the calculation cost becomes $O(|T^1||T^2|)$.

3 Problem of Applying Convolution Kernels to Real tasks

 According to the original definition of convolution kernels, all of the sub-structures are enumerated and calculated for the kernels. The number of sub-structures in the input object usually becomes exponential against input object size. The number of symbols, $|\mathcal{L}|$, is generally very large number (i.e. more than 10,000) since words are treated as symbols. Moreover, the appearance of sub-structures (sub-sequences and sub-trees) are highly correlated with that of sub-structures of sub-structures themselves. As a result, the dimension of feature space becomes extremely high, and all kernel values $K(X,Y)$ are very small compared to the kernel value of the object itself, $K(X,X)$. In this situation, the convolution kernel approach can never be trained effectively, and it will behave like a nearest neighbor rule; we obtain a result that is very precise but with very low recall. The details of this issue were described in [2].

To avoid this, most conventional methods use an approach that involves smoothing the kernel values or eliminating features based on the sub-structure size. For sequence kernels, [1] use a feature elimination method based on the size of sub-sequence n. This means that the kernel calculation deals only with those sub-sequences whose length is n or less. As well as the sequence kernel, [2] proposed a method that restricts the features based on sub-tree depth for tree kernels. These methods seem to work well on the surface, however, good results can only be achieved when n is very small, i.e. $n = 2$ or 3. For example, $n = 3$ showed the best performance for parsing in the experimental results of [2], and $n = 2$ showed the best for the text classification task in [1]. The main reason for using these kernels is that they allow us to employ structural features simply and efficiently. When only small-sized sub-structures are used (i.e. $n = 2$ or 3), the full benefits of the kernels are missed.

Moreover, these results do not mean that no larger-sized sub-structures are useful. In some cases we already know that certain larger sub-structures can be significant features for solving the target problem. That is, significant larger sub-structures, which the conventional methods cannot deal with efficiently, should have the possibility of further improving the performance. The aim of the work described in this paper is to be able to use any significant sub-structure efficiently, regardless of its size, to better solve NLP tasks.

4 Statistical Feature Mining Method for Sequence and Tree Kernels

This section proposes a new approach to feature selection, which is based on statistical significant test, in contrast to the conventional methods, which use sub-structure size.

To simplify the discussion, we restrict ourselves to dealing hereafter with the two-class (positive and negative) supervised classification problem. In our approach, we test the statistical deviation of all sub-structures in the training samples between the appearance of positive samples and negative samples, and then, select only the sub-structures which are larger than a certain threshold τ as features. This allows us to select only the statistically significant sub-structures. In this paper, we explains our proposed method by using the chi-squared (χ^2) value as a statistical metric.

We note, however, we can use many types of statistical metrics in our proposed method.

Table 1: Contingency table and notation for the chi-squared value

	c	$\bar{c}$	$\sum$ row
u	O_{uc}	$O_{u\bar{c}}$	O_u
$\bar{u}$	$O_{\bar{u}c}$	$O_{\bar{u}\bar{c}}$	$O_{\bar{u}}$
$\sum$ column	O_c	$O_{\bar{c}}$	N

First, we briefly explain how to calculate the χ^2 value by referring to Table 1. c and $\bar{c}$ represent the names of classes, c for the positive class and $\bar{c}$ for the negative class. O_{ij}, where $i \in \{u, \bar{u}\}$ and $j \in \{c, \bar{c}\}$, represents the number of samples in each case. $O_{u\bar{c}}$, for instance, represents the number of u that appeared in $\bar{c}$. Let N be the total number of training samples. Since N and O_c are constant for training samples, χ^2 can be obtained as a function of O_u and O_{uc}. The χ^2 value expresses the normalized deviation of the observation from the expectation: $\text{chi}(O_u, O_{uc}) = \sum_{i \in \{u, \bar{u}\}, j \in \{c, \bar{c}\}} (O_{ij} - E_{ij})^2 / E_{ij}$, where $E_{ij} = n \cdot O_i / n \cdot O_j / n$, which represents the expectation. We simply represent $\text{chi}(O_u, O_{uc})$ as $\chi^2(u)$.

In the kernel calculation with the statistical feature selection, if $\chi^2(u) < \tau$ holds, that is, u is not statistically significant, then u is eliminated from the features, and the value of u is presumed to be 0 for the kernel value. Therefore, the sequence and tree kernel with feature selection (SK,TK+FS) can be defined as follows:

$$K^{\text{SK,TK+FS}}(T^1, T^2) = \sum_{u \in \{u | \tau \leq \chi^2(u), u \in P(\mathcal{L}_1^n)\}} \sum_{t^1 \in \text{sub}(T^1)} C_u(t^1)^{\gamma_u(t^1)} \sum_{t^2 \in \text{sub}(T^2)} C_u(t^2)^{\gamma_u(t^2)}.$$

(2)

The difference with their original kernels is simply the condition of the first summation, which is $\tau \leq \chi^2(u)$.

The basic idea of using a statistical metric to select features is quite natural, but it is not a very attractive approach. We note, however, it is not clear how to calculate that kernels efficiently with a statistical feature selection. It is computationally infeasible to calculate $\chi^2(u)$ for all possible u with a naive exhaustive method. In our approach, we take advantage of *sub-structure mining* algorithms in order to calculate $\chi^2(u)$ efficiently and to embed statistical feature selection to the kernel calculation. Formally, sub-structure mining is to find the complete set, but no-duplication, of all significant (generally frequent) sub-structures from dataset. Specifically, we apply combination of a sequential pattern mining technique, PrefixSpan [9], and a statistical metric pruning (SMP) method, Apriori SMP [8]. PrefixSpan can substantially reduce the search space of enumerating all significant sub-sequences. Briefly saying, it finds any sub-sequences uw whose size is n, by searching a single symbol w in the projected database of the sub-sequence (prefix) u of size $n - 1$. The projected database is a partial database which only contains all postfixes (pointers in the implementation) of appeared the prefix u in the database. It starts searching from $n = 1$, that is, it enumerates all the significant sub-sequences by the recursive calculation of *pattern-growth*, searching in the projected database of prefix u and adding a symbol w to u, and *prefix-projection*, making projected database of uw.

Before explaining the algorithm of the proposed kernels, we introduce the upper bound of the χ^2 value. The upper bound of the χ^2 value of a sequence uv, which is the concatenation of sequences u and v, can be calculated by the value of the contingency table of the prefix u [8]: $\chi^2(uv) \leq \hat{\chi}^2(u) = \max\left(\text{chi}(O_{uc}, O_{uc}), \text{chi}(O_u - O_{uc}, 0)\right)$. This upper bound indicates that if $\hat{\chi}^2(u) < \tau$ holds, no (super-)sequences uv, whose prefix is u, can be larger than threshold, $\tau \leq \chi^2(uv)$. In our context, we can eliminate all (super-)sequences uv from candidates of the feature without the explicit evaluation of uv.

Using this property in the PrefixSpan algorithm, we can eliminate to evaluate all the (super-)sequences uv by evaluating the upper bound of sequence u. After finding the number of individual symbol w appeared in projected database of u, we evaluate uw in the following three conditions: (1) $\tau \leq \chi^2(uw)$, (2) $\tau > \chi^2(uw)$, $\tau > \hat{\chi}^2(uw)$, and (3) $\tau > \chi^2(uw)$, $\tau \leq \hat{\chi}^2(uw)$. With condition (1), sub-sequence uw is selected as the feature. With condition (2), uw is pruned, that is, all uwv are also pruned from search space. With condition (3), uw is not a significant, however, uwv can be a significant; thus uw is not selected as features, however, mining is continue to uwv. Figure 1 shows an example of searching and pruning the sub-sequences to select significant features by the PrefixSpan with SMP algorithm.

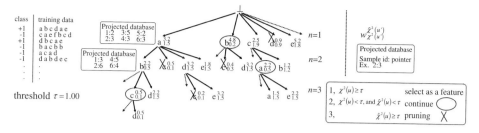

Figure 1: Example of searching and pruning the sub-sequences by PrefixSpan with SMP algorithm

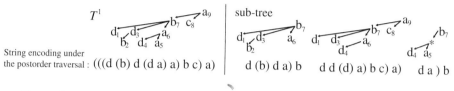

String encoding under the postorder traversal : $(((d \ (b) \ d \ (d \ a) \ a) \ b \ c) \ a)$ | $d \ (b) \ d \ a) \ b$ $d \ d \ (d) \ a) \ b \ c) \ a)$ $d \ a \ ) \ b$

Figure 2: Example of the string encoding for trees under the postorder traversal

The famous tree mining algorithm [12] cannot be simply applied as a feature selection method for the proposed tree kernels, because this tree mining executes preorder search of trees while tree kernels calculate the kernel in postorder. Thus, we take advantage of the *string (sequence) encoding* method for trees and treat them in sequence kernels. Figure 2 shows an example of the string encoding for trees under the postorder traversal. The brackets indicate the hierarchical relation between their left and right hand side nodes. We treat these brackets as a special symbol during the sequential pattern mining phase. Sub-trees are evaluated as the same if and only if the string encoded sub-sequences are exactly the same including brackets. For example, 'd) b) a' and 'd b) a' are different.

We previously said that sequence can be treated as one of trees. We also encode in the case of sequence; for example a sequence 'a b c d' is encoded in '((((a) b) c) d)'. That is, we can define sequence and tree kernels with our feature selection method in the same form.

Sequence and Tree Kernels with Statistical Feature Mining: Sequence and Tree kernels with our proposed feature selection method is defined in the following equations.

$$K^{\text{SK,TK+FS}}(T^1, T^2; \mathcal{D}) = \sum_{1 \leq i \leq |T^1|} \sum_{1 \leq j \leq |T^2|} \mathcal{H}_n(T_i^1, T_j^2; \mathcal{D}) \tag{3}$$

$\mathcal{D}$ represents the training data, and i and j represent indices of nods in postorder of T^1 and T^2, respectively. Let $\mathcal{H}_n(T_i^1, T_j^2; \mathcal{D})$ be a function that returns the sum value of all statistically significant common sub-sequences u if $t_i^1 = t_j^2$ and $|u| \leq n$.

$$\mathcal{H}_n(T_i^1, T_j^2; \mathcal{D}) = \sum_{u \in \Gamma_n(T_i^1, T_j^2; \mathcal{D})} \mathcal{J}_u(T_i^1, T_j^2; \mathcal{D}), \tag{4}$$

where $\Gamma_n(T_i^1, T_j^2; \mathcal{D})$ represents a set of sub-sequences, which is $|u| \leq n$, that satisfy the above condition 1. Then, let $\mathcal{J}_u(T_i^1, T_j^2; \mathcal{D})$, $\mathcal{J}_u'(T_i^1, T_j^2; \mathcal{D})$ and $\mathcal{J}_u''(T_i^1, T_j^2; \mathcal{D})$ be functions that calculate the value of the common sub-sequences between T_i^1 and T_j^2 recursively.

$$\mathcal{J}_{uw}(T_i^1, T_j^2) = \begin{cases} \mathcal{J}_u'(T_i^1, T_j^2; \mathcal{D}) \cdot \mathcal{I}_w(t_i^1, t_j^2) & \text{if } uw \in \widehat{\Gamma}_n(T_i^1, T_j^2; \mathcal{D}), \\ 0 & \text{otherwise,} \end{cases} \tag{5}$$

where $\mathcal{I}_w(t_i^1, t_j^2)$ is a function that returns 1 iff $t_i^1 = w$ and $t_j^2 = w$, and 0 otherwise. $\widehat{\Gamma}_n(T_i^1, T_j^2; \mathcal{D})$ is a set of sub-sequences, which is $|u| \leq n$, that satisfy condition (3). We introduce a special symbol Λ to represent an "empty sequence", and define $\Lambda w = w$ and $|\Lambda w| = 1$.

$$\mathcal{J}_u'(T_i^1, T_j^2; \mathcal{D}) = \begin{cases} 1 & \text{if } u = \Lambda, \\ 0 & \text{if } j = 0 \text{ and } u \neq \Lambda, \\ \lambda \mathcal{J}_u'(T_i^1, T_{j-1}^2; \mathcal{D}) + \mathcal{J}_u''(T_i^1, T_{j-1}^2, \mathcal{D}) & \text{otherwise,} \end{cases} \quad (6)$$

$$\mathcal{J}_u''(T_i^1, T_j^2; \mathcal{D}) = \begin{cases} 0 & \text{if } i = 0, \\ \lambda \mathcal{J}_u''(T_{i-1}^1, T_j^2; \mathcal{D}) + \mathcal{J}_u(T_{i-1}^1, T_j^2; \mathcal{D}) & \text{otherwise.} \end{cases} \quad (7)$$

The following equations are introduced to select a set of significant sub-sequences.

$$\Gamma_n(T_i^1, T_j^2; \mathcal{D}) = \{u \mid u \in \widehat{\Gamma}_n(T_i^1, T_j^2; \mathcal{D}), \tau \leq \chi^2(u), u_{|u|} \in \cap_{i=1}^{|u|-1} \mathrm{ans}(u_i)\} \quad (8)$$

$u_{|u|} \in \cap_{i=1}^{|u|-1} \mathrm{ans}(u_i)$ evaluates if a sub-sequence u is complete sub-tree, where $\mathrm{ans}(u_i)$ returns ancestor of the node u_i. For example, 'd) b a' is not a complete subtree, because the last node 'a' is not an ancestor of 'd' and 'b'.

$$\widehat{\Gamma}_n(T_i^1, T_j^2; \mathcal{D}) = \begin{cases} \Psi_n(\widehat{\Gamma}_n'(T_i^1, T_j^2; \mathcal{D}), t_i^1) \cup \{t_i^1\} & \text{if } t_i^1 = t_j^2, \\ \emptyset & \text{otherwise,} \end{cases} \quad (9)$$

where $\Psi_n(F, w) = \{uw \mid u \in F, \tau \leq \widehat{\chi}^2(uw), |uw| \leq n\}$, and F represents a set of sub-sequences. Note that $\Gamma_n(T_i^1, T_j^2; \mathcal{D})$ and $\widehat{\Gamma}_n(T_i^1, T_j^2; \mathcal{D})$ have only sub-sequences u that satisfy $\tau \leq \chi^2(uw)$ and $\tau \leq \widehat{\chi}^2(uw)$, respectively, iff $t_i^1 = t_j^2$ and $|uw| \leq n$; otherwise they become empty sets.

The following two equations are introduced for recursive the set operation to calculate $\Gamma_n(T_i^1, T_j^2; \mathcal{D})$ and $\widehat{\Gamma}_n(T_i^1, T_j^2; \mathcal{D})$.

$$\widehat{\Gamma}_n'(T_i^1, T_j^2; \mathcal{D}) = \begin{cases} \emptyset & \text{if } j = 0, \\ \widehat{\Gamma}_n'(T_i^1, T_{j-1}^2; \mathcal{D}) \cup \widehat{\Gamma}_n''(T_i^1, T_{j-1}^2; \mathcal{D}) & \text{otherwise,} \end{cases} \quad (10)$$

$$\widehat{\Gamma}_n''(T_i^1, T_j^2; \mathcal{D}) = \begin{cases} \emptyset & \text{if } i = 0, \\ \widehat{\Gamma}_n''(T_{i-1}^1, T_j^2; \mathcal{D}) \cup \widehat{\Gamma}_n(T_{i-1}^1, T_j^2; \mathcal{D}) & \text{otherwise.} \end{cases} \quad (11)$$

In the implementation, $\chi^2(uw)$ and $\widehat{\chi}^2(uw)$, where uw represents a concatenation of a sequence u and a symbol w, can be calculated by a set of pointers of u against data and the number of appearance of w in backside of the pointers. We note that the set of pointers of uw can be simply obtained from previous search of u. With condition (1), uw is stored in Γ_n and $\widehat{\Gamma}_n$. With condition (3), uw is only stored in $\widehat{\Gamma}_n$.

There are some technique in order to calculate kernel faster in the implementation. For example, since $\chi^2(u)$ and $\widehat{\chi}^2(u)$ are constant against the same data, we only have to calculate them once. We store the internal search results of PrefixSpan with SMP algorithm in a TRIE structure. After that, we look in that results in TRIE instead of explicitly calculate $\chi^2(u)$ again when the kernel finds the same sub-sequence. Moreover, when the projected database is exactly the same, these sub-sequences can be merged since the value of $\chi^2(uv)$ and $\widehat{\chi}^2(uv)$ for any postfix v are exactly the same. Moreover, we introduce a 'transposed index' for fast evaluation of $\chi^2(u)$ and $\widehat{\chi}^2(u)$. By using that, we only have to look up that index of w to evaluate whether or not any uw are significant features.

Equations (4) to (7) can be performed in the same as the original DP based kernel calculation. The recursive set operations of Equations (9) to (11) can be executed as well as

Table 2: Experimental Results

n	Question Classification					Subjectivity Detection					Polarity Identification				
	1	2	3	4	∞	1	2	3	4	∞	1	2	3	4	∞
SK+FS	-	.823	.827	.824	.822	-	.822	.839	.841	.842	-	.824	.838	.839	.839
SK	-	.808	.818	.808	.797	-	.823	.824	.809	.772	-	.835	.835	.833	.789
TK+FS	-	.812	.815	.812	.812	-	.834	.857	.854	.856	-	.830	.832	.835	.833
TK	-	.802	.802	.797	.783	-	.842	.850	.830	.755	-	.828	.827	.820	.745
BOW-K	.754	.792	.790	.778	-	.717	729	.715	.649	-	.740	.810	.822	.795	-

Equations (5) to (7). Moreover, calculating $\chi^2(u)$ and $\hat{\chi}^2(u)$ with sub-structure mining algorithms allow to calculate the same order of the DP based kernel calculation. As a result, statistical feature selection can be embedded in original kernel calculation based on the DP.

Essentially, the worst case time complexity of the proposed method will become exponential, since we enumerate individual sub-structures in sub-structure mining phase. However, actual calculation time in the most cases of our experiments is even faster than original kernel calculation, since search space pruning efficiently remove vain calculation and the implementation techniques briefly explained above provide practical calculation speed.

We note that if we set $\tau = 0$, which means all features are dealt with kernel calculation, we can get exactly the same kernel value as the original tree kernel.

5 Experiments and Results

We evaluated the performance of the proposed method in actual NLP tasks, namely *English question classification* (EQC), *subjectivity detection* (SD) and *polarity identification* (PI) tasks. These tasks are defined as a text categorization task: it maps a given sentence into one of the pre-defined classes. We used data provided by [6] for EQC, that contains about 5500 questions with 50 question types. SD data was created from Mainichi news articles, and the size was 2095 sentences consisting of 822 subjective sentences. PI data has 5564 sentences with 2671 positive opinion. By using these data, we compared the proposed method (SK+FS and TK+FS) with a conventional method (SK or TK), as discussed in Section 3, and with *bag-of-words* (BOW) Kernel (BOW-K)[4] as baseline methods. We used word sequences for input objects of sequence kernels and word dependency trees for tree kernels.

Support Vector Machine (SVM) was selected as the kernel-based classifier for training and classification with a soft margin parameter $C = 1000$. We used the *one-vs-rest* classifier of SVM as the multi-class classification method for EQC. We evaluated the performance with label accuracy by using ten-fold cross validation: eight for training, one for development and remaining one for test set. The parameter λ and τ was automatically selected from the value set of $\lambda = \{0.1, 0.3, 0.5, 0.7, 0.9\}$ and $\tau = \{3.84, 6.63\}$ by the development test. Note that these two values represent the 10% and 5% levels of significance in the χ^2 distribution with one degree of freedom, which used the χ^2 significant test.

Tables 2 shows our experimental results. where n in each table indicates the restriction of the sub-structure size, and $n = \infty$ means all possible sub-structures are used. As shown in this table, SK or TK achieve maximum performance when $n = 2$ or 3. The performance deteriorates considerably once n exceeds 4 or more. This implies that larger sub-structures degrade classification performance, which showed the same tendency as in the previous studies discussed in Section 3. This is evidence of over-fitting in learning. On the other hand, SK+FS and TK+FS provided consistently better performance than the conventional methods. Moreover, the experiments confirmed one important fact: in some cases, maximum performance was achieved with $n = \infty$. This indicates that certain sub-sequences created using very large structures can be extremely effective. If the performance is improved by using a larger n, this means that significant features do exist. Thus, we can improve the performance of some classification problems by dealing with larger substructures. Even if optimum performance was not achieved with $n = \infty$, the difference from the performance of a smaller n is quite small compared to that of SK and TK. This indicates that our method is very robust against sub-structure size.

6 Conclusions

This paper proposed a statistical feature selection method for sequence kernels and tree kernels. Our approach can select significant features automatically based on a statistical significance test. The proposed method can be embedded in the original DP based kernel calculation process by using sub-structure mining algorithms.

Our experiments demonstrated that our method is superior to conventional methods. Moreover, the results indicate that complex features exist and can be effective. Our method can employ them without over-fitting problems, which yields benefits in terms of concept and performance.

References

[1] N. Cancedda, E. Gaussier, C. Goutte, and J.-M. Renders. Word-Sequence Kernels. *Journal of Machine Learning Research*, 3:1059–1082, 2003.

[2] M. Collins and N. Duffy. Convolution kernels for natural language. In *Proc. of Neural Information Processing Systems (NIPS'2001)*, 2001.

[3] D. Haussler. Convolution kernels on discrete structures. In *Technical Report UCS-CRL-99-10*. UC Santa Cruz, 1999.

[4] T. Joachims. Text Categorization with Support Vector Machines: Learning with Many Relevant Features. In *Proc. of European Conference on Machine Learning (ECML '98)*, pages 137–142, 1998.

[5] H. Kashima and T. Koyanagi. Kernels for Semi-Structured Data. In *Proc. 19th International Conference on Machine Learning (ICML2002)*, pages 291–298, 2002.

[6] X. Li and D. Roth. Learning Question Classifiers. In *Proc. of the 19th International Conference on Computational Linguistics (COLING 2002)*, pages 556–562, 2002.

[7] H. Lodhi, C. Saunders, J. Shawe-Taylor, N. Cristianini, and C. Watkins. Text Classification Using String Kernel. *Journal of Machine Learning Research*, 2:419–444, 2002.

[8] S. Morishita and J. Sese. Traversing Itemset Lattices with Statistical Metric Pruning. In *Proc. of ACM SIGACT-SIGMOD-SIGART Symp. on Database Systems (PODS'00)*, pages 226–236, 2000.

[9] J. Pei, J. Han, B. Mortazavi-Asl, and H. Pinto. PrefixSpan: Mining Sequential Patterns Efficiently by Prefix-Projected Pattern Growth. In *Proc. of the 17th International Conference on Data Engineering (ICDE 2001)*, pages 215–224, 2001.

[10] J. Suzuki, Y. Sasaki, and E. Maeda. Kernels for Structured Natural Language Data. In *Proc. of the 17th Annual Conference on Neural Information Processing Systems (NIPS2003)*, 2003.

[11] C. Watkins. Dynamic alignment kernels. In *Technical Report CSD-TR-98-11*. Royal Holloway, University of London Computer Science Department, 1999.

[12] M. J. Zaki. Efficiently Mining Frequent Trees in a Forest. In *Proc. of the 8th International Conference on Knowledge Discovery and Data Mining (KDD'02)*, pages 71–80, 2002.

Silicon Growth Cones Map Silicon Retina

Brian Taba and Kwabena Boahen[*]
Department of Bioengineering
University of Pennsylvania
Philadelphia, PA 19104
{btaba,boahen}@seas.upenn.edu

Abstract

We demonstrate the first fully hardware implementation of retinotopic self-organization, from photon transduction to neural map formation. A silicon retina transduces patterned illumination into correlated spike trains that drive a population of silicon growth cones to automatically wire a topographic mapping by migrating toward sources of a diffusible guidance cue that is released by postsynaptic spikes. We varied the pattern of illumination to steer growth cones projected by different retinal ganglion cell types to self-organize segregated or coordinated retinotopic maps.

1 Introduction

Engineers have long admired the brain's ability to effortlessly adapt to novel situations without instruction, and sought to endow digital computers with a similar capacity for unsupervised self-organization. One prominent example is Kohonen's self-organizing map [1], which achieved popularity by distilling neurophysiological insights into a simple set of mathematical equations. Although these algorithms are readily simulated in software, previous hardware implementations have required high precision components that are expensive in chip area (e.g. [2, 3]). By contrast, neurobiological systems can self-organize components possessing remarkably heterogeneous properties. To pursue this biological robustness against component mismatch, we designed circuits that mimic neurophysiological function down to the subcellular level. In this paper, we demonstrate topographic refinement of connections between a silicon retina and the first neuromorphic self-organizing map chip, previously reported in [5], which is based on axon migration in the developing brain.

During development, neurons wire themselves into their mature circuits by extending axonal and dendritic precursors called *neurites*. Each neurite is tipped by a motile sensory structure called a *growth cone* that guides the elongating neurite based on local chemical cues. Growth cones move by continually sprouting and retracting finger-like extensions called *filopodia* whose dynamics can be biased by diffusible ligands in an activity-dependent manner [4]. Based on these observations, we designed and fabricated the Neurotrope1 chip to implement a population of silicon growth cones [5]. We interfaced Neu-

---

[*]www.neuroengineering.upenn.edu/boahen

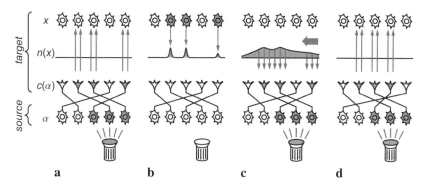

Figure 1: Neurotropic axon guidance. **a.** Active source cells (grey) relay spikes down their axons to their growth cones, which excite nearby target cells. **b.** Active target cell bodies secrete neurotropin. **c.** Neurotropin spreads laterally, establishing a spatial concentration gradient that is sampled by active growth cones. **d.** Active growth cones climb the local neurotropin gradient, translating temporal activity coincidence into spatial position coincidence. Growth cones move by displacing other growth cones.

rotrope1 directly to a spiking silicon retina to illustrate its applicability to larger neuromorphic systems.

This paper is organized as follows. In Section 2, we present an algorithm for axon migration under the guidance of a diffusible chemical whose release and uptake is gated by activity. In Section 3, we describe our hardware implementation of this algorithm. In Section 4, we examine the Neurotrope1 system's performance on a topographic refinement task when driven by spike trains generated by a silicon retina in response to several types of illumination stimuli.

2   Neurotropic axon guidance

We model the self-organization of connections between two layers of neurons (Fig. 1). Cells in the *source layer* innervate cells in the *target layer* with excitatory axons that are tipped by motile growth cones. Growth cones tow their axons within the target layer as directed by a diffusible guidance factor called *neurotropin* that they bind from the local extracellular environment. Neurotropin is released by postsynaptically active target cell bodies and bound by presynaptically active growth cones, so the retrograde transfer of neurotropin from a target cell to a source cell measures the temporal coincidence of their spike activities. Growth cones move to maximize their neurotropic uptake, a Hebbian-like learning rule that causes cells that fire at the same time to wire to the same place. To prevent the population of growth cones from attempting to trivially maximize their uptake by all exciting the same target cell, we impose a synaptic density constraint that requires a migrating growth cone to displace any other growth cone occupying its path.

To state the model more formally, source cell bodies occupy nodes of a regular two-dimensional (2D) lattice embedded in the source layer, while growth cones and target cell bodies occupy nodes on separate 2D lattices that are interleaved in the target layer. We index nodes by their positions in their respective layers, using Greek letters for source layer positions (e.g., $\alpha \in \mathbb{Z}^2$) and Roman letters for target layer positions (e.g., $x, c \in \mathbb{Z}^2$).

Each source cell α fires spikes at a rate $a_{\mathrm{SC}}(\alpha)$ and conveys this presynaptic activity down an axon that elaborates an excitatory arbor in the target layer centered on $c(\alpha)$. In principle, every branch of this arbor is tipped by its own motile growth cone, but to facilitate efficient

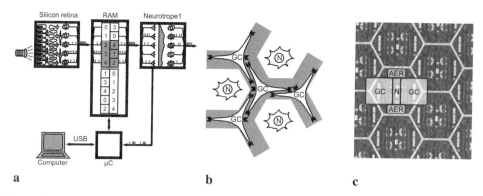

a   b   c

Figure 2: **a.** Neurotrope1 system. Spike communication is by address-events (AER). **b.** Neurotrope1 cell mosaic. The extracellular medium (grey) is laid out as a monolithic honeycomb lattice. Growth cones (GC) occupy nodes of this lattice and extend filopodia to the adjacent nodes. Neurotropin receptors (black) are located at the tip of each filopodium and at the growth cone body. Target cells (N) occupy nodes of an interleaved triangular lattice. **c.** Detail of chip layout.

hardware implementation, we abstract the collection of branch growth cones into a single central growth cone that tows the arbor's trunk around the target layer, dragging the rest of the arbor with it. The arbor overlaps nearby target cells with a branch density $A(x - c(\alpha))$ that diminishes with distance $\|x - c(\alpha)\|$ from the arbor center. The postsynaptic activity $a_{TC}(x)$ of target cell x is proportional to the linear sum of its excitation.

$$a_{TC}(x) = \sum_{\alpha} a_{SC}(\alpha) A(x - c(\alpha)) \tag{1}$$

Postsynaptically active target cell bodies release neurotropin, which spreads laterally until consumed by constitutive decay processes. The neurotropin $n(x')$ present at target site x' is assembled from contributions from all active release sites. The contribution of each target cell x is proportional to its postsynaptic activity and weighted by a spreading kernel $N(x - x')$ that is a decreasing function of its distance $\|x - x'\|$ from the measurement site x'.

$$n(x') = \sum_{x} a_{TC}(x) N(x - x') \tag{2}$$

A presynaptically active growth cone located at $c(\alpha)$ computes the direction of the local neurotropin gradient by identifying the adjacent lattice node $c'(\alpha) \in \mathcal{C}(c(\alpha))$ with the most neurotropin, where $\mathcal{C}(c(\alpha))$ includes $c(\alpha)$ and its nearest neighbors.

$$c'(\alpha) = \arg\max_{x' \in \mathcal{C}(c(\alpha))} n(x') \tag{3}$$

Once the growth cone has identified $c'(\alpha)$, it swaps positions with the growth cone already located at $c'(\alpha)$, increasing its own neurotropic uptake while preserving a constant synaptic density. Growth cones compute position updates independently, at a rate $\lambda(\alpha) \propto a_{SC}(\alpha) \max_{y \in \mathcal{C}(c(\alpha))} n(x')$. Updates are executed asynchronously, in order of their arrival.

Software simulation of a similar set of equations generates self-organized feature maps when driven by appropriately correlated source cell activity [6]. Here, we illustrate topographic map formation in hardware using correlated spike trains generated by a silicon retina.

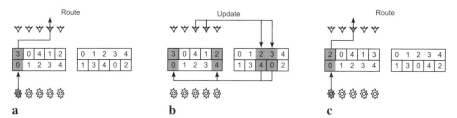

Figure 3: Virtual axon remapping. **a.** Cell bodies tag their spikes with their own source layer addresses, which the forward lookup table translates into target layer destinations. **b.** Axon updates are computed by growth cones, which decode their own target layer addresses through the reverse lookup table to obtain the source layer addresses of their cell bodies that identify their entries in the forward lookup table. **c.** Growth cones move by modifying their entries in the forward and reverse lookup tables to reroute their spikes to updated locations.

3 Neurotrope1 system

Our hardware implementation splits the model into three stages: the source layer, the target layer, and the intervening axons (Fig. 2a). Any population of spiking neurons can act as a source layer; in this paper we employ the silicon retina of [7]. The target layer is implemented by a full custom VLSI chip that interleaves a 48×20 array of growth cone circuits with a 24×20 array of target cell circuits. There is also a spreading network that represents the intervening medium for propagating neurotropin. The Neurotrope1 chip was fabricated by MOSIS using the TSMC 0.35μm process and has an area of 11.5 mm^2. Connections are specified as entries in a pair of lookup tables, stored in an off-chip RAM, that are updated by a Ubicom ip2022 microcontroller as instructed by the Neurotrope1 chip. The ip2022 also controls a USB link that allows a computer to write and read the contents of the RAM. Subsection 3.1 explains how updates are computed by the Neurotrope1 chip and Subsection 3.2 describes the procedure for executing these updates.

3.1 Axon updates

Axon updates are computed by the Neurotrope1 chip using the transistor circuits described in [5]. Here, we provide a brief description. The Neurotrope1 chip represents neurotropin as charge spreading through a monolithic transistor channel laid out as a honeycomb lattice. Each growth cone occupies one node of this lattice and extends filopodia to the three adjacent nodes, expressing neurotropin receptors at all four locations (Fig. 2b-c). When a growth cone receives a presynaptic spike, its receptor circuits tap charge from all four nodes onto separate capacitors. The first capacitor voltage to integrate to a threshold resets all of the growth cone's capacitors and transmits a request off-chip to update the growth cone's position by swapping locations with the growth cone currently occupying the winning node.

3.2 Address-event remapping

Chips in the Neurotrope1 system exchange spikes encoded in the address-event representation (AER) [8], an asynchronous communication protocol that merges spike trains from every cell on the same chip onto a single shared data link instead of requiring a dedicated wire for each connection. Each spike is tagged with the address of its originating cell for transmission off-chip. Between chips, spikes are routed through a *forward lookup table* that translates their original source layer addresses into their destined target layer addresses

1332

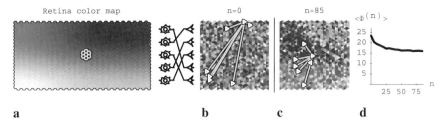

Figure 4: Retinotopic self-organization of ON-center RGCs. **a.** Silicon retina color map of ON-center RGC body positions. A representative RGC body is outlined in white, as are the RGC neighbors that participate in its topographic order parameter $\Phi^{(n)}$. **b.** Target layer color map of growth cone positions for sample $n = 0$, colored by the retinal positions of their cell bodies. Growth cones projected by the representative RGC and its nearest neighbors are outlined in white. Grey lines denote target layer distances used to compute $\Phi^{(n)}$. **c.** Target layer color map at $n = 85$. **d.** Order parameter evolution.

on the receiving chip (Fig. 3a). An axon entry in this forward lookup table is indexed by the source layer address of its cell body and contains the target layer address of its growth cone. The virtual axon moves by updating this entry.

Axon updates are computed by growth cone circuits on the Neurotrope1 chip, encoded as address-events, and sent to the ip2022 for processing. Each update identifies a pair of axon terminals to be swapped. These growth cone addresses are translated through a *reverse lookup table* into the source layer addresses that index the relevant forward lookup table entries (Fig. 3b). Modification of the affected entries in each lookup table completes the axon migration (Fig. 3c).

4 Retinotopic self-organization

We programmed the growth cone population to self-organize retinotopic maps by driving them with correlated spike trains generated by the silicon retina. The silicon retina translates patterned illumination in real-time into spike trains that are fed into the Neurotrope1 chip as presynaptic input from different retinal ganglion cell (RGC) types. An ON-center RGC is excited by a spot of light in the center of its receptive field and inhibited by light in the surrounding annulus, while an OFF-center RGC responds analogously to the absence of light. There is an ON-center and an OFF-center RGC located at every retinal coordinate.

To generate appropriately correlated RGC spike trains, we illuminated the silicon retina with various mixtures of light and dark spot stimuli. Each spot stimulus was presented against a uniformly grey background for 100 ms and covered a contiguous cluster of RGCs centered on a pseudorandomly selected position in the retinal plane, eliciting overlapping bursts of spikes whose coactivity established a spatially restricted presynaptic correlation kernel containing enough information to instruct topographic ordering [9]. Strongly driven RGCs could fire at nearly 1 kHz, which was the highest mean rate at which the silicon retina could still be tuned to roughly balance ON- and OFF-center RGC excitability. We tracked the evolution of the growth cone population by reading out the contents of the lookup table every five minutes, a sampling interval selected to include enough patch stimuli to allow each of the 48×20 possible patches to be activated on average at least once per sample.

We first induced retinotopic self-organization within a single RGC cell type by illuminating the silicon retina with a sequence of randomly centered spots of light presented against a grey background, selectively activating only ON-center RGCs. Each of the 960 growth

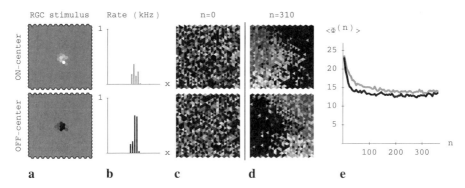

Figure 5: Segregation by cell type under separate light and dark spot stimulation. Top: ON-center; bottom: OFF-center. **a.** Silicon retina image of representative spot stimulus. Light or dark intensity denotes relative ON- or OFF-center RGC output rate. **b.** Spike rates for ON-center (grey) and OFF-center (black) RGCs in column x of a cross-section of a representative spot stimulus. **c.** Target layer color maps of RGC growth cones at sample $n = 0$. Black indicates the absence of a growth cone projected by an RGC of this cell type. Other colors as in Fig. 4. **d.** Target layer color maps at $n = 310$. **e.** Order parameter evolution for ON-center (grey) and OFF-center (black) RGCs.

cones was randomly assigned to a different ON-center RGC, creating a scrambled map from retina to target layer (Fig. 4a-b). The ON-center RGC growth cone population visibly refined the topography of the nonretinotopic initial state (Fig. 4c). We quantify this observation by introducing an *order parameter* $\Phi^{(n)}$ whose value measures the instantaneous retinotopy for an RGC at the nth sample. The definition of retinotopy is that adjacent RGCs innervate adjacent target cells, so we define $\Phi^{(n)}$ for a given RGC to be the average target layer distance separating its growth cone from the growth cones projected by the six adjacent RGCs of the same cell type. The population average $\langle \Phi^{(n)} \rangle$ converges to a value that represents the achievable performance on this task (Fig. 4d).

We next induced growth cones projected by each cell type to self-organize disjoint topographic maps by illuminating the silicon retina with a sequence of randomly centered light or dark spots presented against a grey background (Fig. 5a-b). Half the growth cones were assigned to ON-center RGCs and the other half were assigned to the corresponding OFF-center RGCs. We seeded the system with a random projection that evenly distributed growth cones of both cell types across the entire target layer (Fig. 5c). Since only RGCs of the same cell type were coactive, growth cones segregated into ON- and OFF-center clusters on opposite sides of the target layer (Fig. 5d). OFF-center RGCs were slightly more excitable on average than ON-center RGCs, so their growth cones refined their topography more quickly (Fig. 5e) and clustered in the right half of the target layer, which was also more excitable due to poor power distribution on the Neurotrope1 chip.

Finally, we induced growth cones of both cell types to self-organize coordinated retinotopic maps by illuminating the retina with center-surround stimuli that oscillate radially from light to dark or vice versa (Fig. 6). The light-dark oscillation injected enough coactivity between neighboring ON- and OFF-center RGCs to prevent their growth cones from segregating by cell type into disjoint clusters. Instead, both subpopulations developed and maintained coarse retinotopic maps that cover the entire target layer and are oriented in register with one another, properties sufficient to seed more interesting circuits such as oriented receptive fields [10].

Performance in this hardware implementation is limited mainly by variability in the behav-

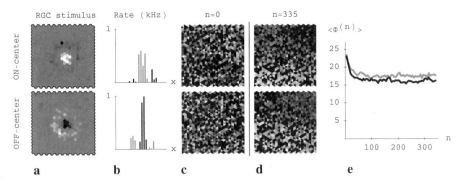

Figure 6: Coordinated retinotopy under center-surround stimulation. Top: ON-center; bottom: OFF-center. **a.** Silicon retina image of a representative center-surround stimulus. Light or dark intensity denotes relative ON- or OFF-center RGC output rate. **b.** Spike rates for ON-center (grey) and OFF-center (black) RGCs in column x of a cross-section of a representative center-surround stimulus. **c.** Target layer color maps of RGC growth cones for sample $n = 0$. Colors as in Fig. 5. **d.** Target layer color maps at $n = 335$. **e.** Order parameter evolution for ON-center (grey) and OFF-center (black) RGCs.

ior of nominally identical circuits on the Neurotrope1 chip and the silicon retina. In the silicon retina, the wide variance of the RGC output rates [7] limits both the convergence speed and the final topographic level achieved by the spot-driven growth cone population. Growth cones move faster when stimulated at higher rates, but elevating the mean output rate of the RGC population allows more excitable RGCs to fire spontaneously at a sustained rate, swamping growth cone-specific guidance signals with stimulus-independent postsynaptic activity that globally attracts all growth cones. The mean RGC output rate must remain low enough to suppress these spontaneous distractors, limiting convergence speed. Variance in the output rates of neighboring RGCs also distorts the shape of the spot stimulus, eroding the fidelity of the correlation-encoded instructions received by the growth cones.

Variability in the Neurotrope1 chip further limits topographic convergence. Migrating growth cones are directed by the local neurotropin landscape, which forms an image of recent presynaptic activity correlations as filtered through the postsynaptic activation of the target cell population. This image is distorted by variations between the properties of individual target cell and neurotropin circuits that are introduced during fabrication. In particular, poor power distribution on the Neurotrope1 chip creates a systematic gradient in target cell excitability that warps a growth cone's impression of the relative coactivity of its neighbors, attracting it preferentially toward the more excitable target cells on the right side of the array.

5   Conclusions

In this paper, we demonstrated a completely neuromorphic implementation of retinotopic self-organization. This is the first time every stage of the process has been implemented entirely in hardware, from photon transduction through neural map formation. The only comparable system was described in [11], which processed silicon retina data offline using a software model of neurotrophic guidance running on a workstation. Our system computes results in real time at low power, two prerequisites for autonomous mobile applications.

The novel infrastructure developed to implement virtual axon migration allows silicon growth cones to directly interface with an existing family of AER-compliant devices, enabling a host of multimodal neuromorphic self-organizing applications. In particular, the silicon retina's ability to translate arbitrary visual stimuli into growth cone-compatible spike trains in real-time opens the door to more ambitious experiments such as using natural video correlations to automatically wire more complicated visual feature maps.

Our faithful adherence to cellular level details yields an algorithm that is well suited to physical implementation. In contrast to all previous self-organizing map chips (e.g. [2, 3]), which implemented a global winner-take-all function to induce competition, our silicon growth cones compute their own updates using purely local information about the neurotropin gradient, a cellular approach that scales effortlessly to larger populations. Performance might be improved by supplementing our purely morphogenetic model with additional physiologically-inspired mechanisms to prune outliers and consolidate well-placed growth cones into permanent synapses.

Acknowledgments

We would like to thank J. Arthur for developing a USB system to facilitate data collection. This project was funded by the David and Lucille Packard Foundation and the NSF/BITS program (EIA0130822).

References

[1] T. Kohonen (1982), "Self-organized formation of topologically correct feature maps," *Biol. Cybernetics*, vol. 43, no. 1, pp. 59-69.

[2] W.-C. Fang, B.J. Sheu, O.T.-C. Chen, and J. Choi (1992), "A VLSI neural processor for image data compression using self-organization networks," *IEEE Trans. Neural Networks*, vol. 3, no. 3, pp. 506-518.

[3] S. Rovetta and R. Zunino (1999), "Efficient training of neural gas vector quantizers with analog circuit implementation," *IEEE Trans. Circ. & Sys. II*, vol. 46, no. 6, pp. 688-698.

[4] E.W. Dent and F.B. Gertler (2003), "Cytoskeletal dynamics and transport in growth cone mobility and axon guidance," *Neuron*, vol. 40, pp. 209-227.

[5] B. Taba and K. Boahen (2003), "Topographic map formation by silicon growth cones," in: *Advances in Neural Information Processing Systems 15* (MIT Press, Cambridge, eds. S. Becker, S. Thrun, and K. Obermayer), pp. 1163-1170.

[6] S.Y.M. Lam, B.E. Shi, and K.A. Boahen (2005), "Self-organized cortical map formation by guiding connections," *Proc. 2005 IEEE Int. Symp. Circ. & Sys.*, in press.

[7] K.A. Zaghloul and K. Boahen (2004), "Optic nerve signals in a neuromorphic chip I: Outer and inner retina models," *IEEE Trans. Bio-Med. Eng.*, vol. 51, no. 4, pp. 657-666.

[8] K. Boahen (2000), "Point-to-point connectivity between neuromorphic chips using address-events," *IEEE Trans. Circ. & Sys. II*, vol. 47, pp. 416-434.

[9] K. Miller (1994), "A model for the development of simple cell receptive fields and the ordered arrangement of orientation columns through activity-dependent competition between on- and off-center inputs," *J. Neurosci.*, vol. 14, no. 1, pp. 409-441.

[10] D. Ringach (2004), "Haphazard wiring of simple receptive fields and orientation columns in visual cortex," *J. Neurophys.*, vol. 92, no. 1, pp. 468-476.

[11] T. Elliott and J. Kramer (2002), "Coupling an aVLSI neuromorphic vision chip to a neurotrophic model of synaptic plasticity: the development of topography," *Neural Comp.*, vol. 14, no. 10, pp. 2353-2370.

Temporally changing synaptic plasticity

Minija Tamosiunaite[1,2]**, Bernd Porr**[3]**, and Florentin Wörgötter**[1,4]

[1] Department of Psychology, University of Stirling
Stirling FK9 4LA, Scotland
[2] Department of Informatics, Vytautas Magnus University
Kaunas, Lithuania
[3] Department of Electronics & Electrical Engineering, University of Glasgow
Glasgow, GT12 8LT, Scotland
[4] Bernstein Centre for Computational Neuroscience, University of Göttingen, Germany
{minija,worgott}@cn.stir.ac.uk; b.porr@elec.gla.ac.uk

Abstract

Recent experimental results suggest that dendritic and back-propagating spikes can influence synaptic plasticity in different ways [1]. In this study we investigate how these signals could temporally interact at dendrites leading to changing plasticity properties at local synapse clusters. Similar to a previous study [2], we employ a differential Hebbian plasticity rule to emulate spike-timing dependent plasticity. We use dendritic (D-) and back-propagating (BP-) spikes as post-synaptic signals in the learning rule and investigate how their interaction will influence plasticity. We will analyze a situation where synapse plasticity characteristics change in the course of time, depending on the type of post-synaptic activity momentarily elicited. Starting with weak synapses, which only elicit local D-spikes, a slow, unspecific growth process is induced. As soon as the soma begins to spike this process is replaced by fast synaptic changes as the consequence of the much stronger and sharper BP-spike, which now dominates the plasticity rule. This way a winner-take-all-mechanism emerges in a two-stage process, enhancing the best-correlated inputs. These results suggest that synaptic plasticity is a temporal changing process by which the computational properties of dendrites or complete neurons can be substantially augmented.

1 Introduction

The traditional view on Hebbian plasticity is that the correlation between pre- and postsynaptic events will drive learning. This view ignores the fact that synaptic plasticity is driven by a whole sequence of events and that some of these events are causally related. For example, usually through the synaptic activity at a cluster of synapses the postsynaptic spike will be triggered. This signal can then travel retrogradely into the dendrite (as a so-called back-propagating- or BP-spike, [3]), leading to a depolarization at this and other clusters of synapses by which their plasticity will be influenced. More locally, something similar can happen if a cluster of synapses is able to elicit a dendritic spike (D-spike, [4, 5]), which may not travel far, but which certainly leads to a local depolarization "under" these and adjacent synapses, triggering synaptic plasticity of one kind or another. Hence synaptic plasticity seems to be to some degree influenced by recurrent processes. In this study, we will use a differential Hebbian learning rule [2, 6] to emulate spike timing dependent plasticity (STDP, [7, 8]). With one specifically chosen example architecture we will investigate how the temporal relation between dendritic- and back propagating spikes could influence plasticity. Specifically we will report how learning could change *during* the course of network development, and how that could enrich the computational properties of the affected neuronal compartments.

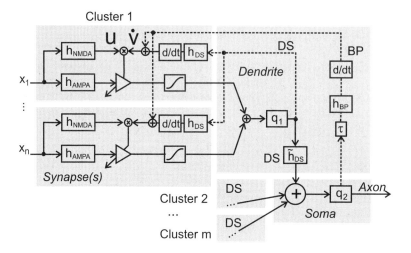

Figure 1: Basic learning scheme with $x_1, ..., x_n$ representing inputs to cluster 1, h_{AMPA}, h_{NMDA} - filters shaping AMPA and NMDA signals, h_{DS}, $\tilde{h}_{DS}$, h_{BP} - filters shaping D and BP-spikes, q_1, q_2 - differential thresholds, τ - a delay. Weight impact is saturated. Only the first of m clusters is shown explicitly; clusters $2, 3, ..., m$ would be employing the same BP spike (not shown). The symbol $\oplus$ represents a summation node and $\otimes$ multiplication.

2   The Model

A block diagram of the model is shown in Fig. 1. The model includes several clusters of synapses located on dendritic branches. Dendritic spikes are elicited following the summation of several AMPA signals passing threshold q_1. NMDA receptor influence on dendritic spike generation was not considered as the contribution of NMDA potentials to the total membrane potential is substantially smaller than that of AMPA channels at a mixed synapse.

Inputs to the model arrive in groups, but each input line gets only one pulse in a given group (Fig. 2 C). Each synaptic cluster is limited to generating one dendritic spike from one arriving pulse group. Cell firing is not explicitly modelled but said to be achieved when the summation of several dendritic spikes at the cell soma has passed threshold q_2. This leads to a BP-spike. Progression of signals along a dendrite is not modelled explicitly, but expressed by means of delays. Since we do not model biophysical processes, all signal *shapes* are obtained by appropriate filters h, where $u = x * h$ is the convolution of spike train x with filter h.

A differential Hebbian-type learning rule is used to drive synaptic plasticity [2, 6] with $\dot{\rho} = \mu u \dot{v}$, where ρ denotes synaptic weight, u stands for the synaptic input, v for the output, and μ for the learning rate. see e.g.; u and $\dot{v}$ annotations in Fig. 1, top left.

NMDA signals are used as the pre-synaptic signals, dendritic spikes, or dendritic spikes complemented by back-propagating spikes, define the post-synaptic signals for the learning rule. In addition, synaptic weights were sigmoidally saturated with limits zero and one. Filter shapes forming AMPA and NMDA channel responses, as well as back- propagating spikes and some forms of dendritic spikes used in this study were described by:

$$h(t) = \frac{e^{-2\pi t/\tau} - e^{-8\pi t/\tau}}{6\pi/\tau} \tag{1}$$

where τ determines the total duration of the pulse. The ratio between rise and fall time is $1 : 4$. We use for AMPA channels: $\tau = 6\ ms$, for NMDA channels: $\tau = 120\ ms$, for dendritic spikes: $\tau = 235\ ms$, and for BP-spikes: $\tau = 40\ ms$.

Note, we are approximating the NMDA characteristic by a non-voltage dependent filter function. In conjunction with STDP, this simplification is justified by Saudargiene et al [2, 9], showing that voltage dependency induces only a second-order effect on the shape of the STDP curve.

Individual input timings are drawn from a uniform distribution from within a pre-specified interval which can vary under different conditions. We distinguish three basic input groups: *strongly correlated* inputs (several inputs over an interval of up to 10 ms), *less correlated* (dispersed over an interval of 10-100 ms) and *uncorrelated* (dispersed over the interval of more than 100 ms).

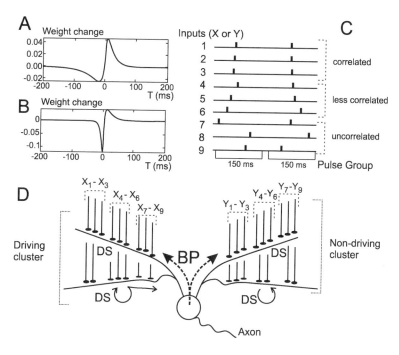

Figure 2: Example STDP curves (A,B), input pulse distribution (C), and model setup (D). A) STDP curve obtained with a D-spike using Eq. 1 with $\tau = 235\ ms$, B) from a BP spike with $\tau = 40\ ms$. C) Example input pulse distribution for two pulse groups. D) Model neuron with two dendritic branches (left and right), consisting of two sub-branches which get inputs X or Y, which are similar for either side. DS stands for D-spike, BP for a BP-spike.

3 Results

3.1 Experimental setup

Fig. 2 A,B shows two STDP curves, one obtained with a wide D-spike the other one with a much sharper BP-spike. The study investigates interactions of such post-synaptic signals in time. Though the signals interact linearly, the much stronger BP signal dominates learning when elicited. In the absence of a BP spike the D-spike dominates plasticity. This seems to correspond to new physiological observations concerning the relations between post-synaptic signals and the actually expressed form of plasticity [10]. We specifically investigate a two-phase processes, where plasticity is *first* dominated by the D- spike and *later* by a BP-spike.

Fig. 2 D shows a setup in which two-phase plasticity could arise. We assume that inputs to compact clusters of synapses are similar (e.g. all left branches in Fig. 2 D) but dissimilar over larger distances (between left and right branches). First, e.g. early in development, synapses may be weak and only the conjoint action of many synchronous inputs will lead to a local D-spike. Local plasticity from these few D-spikes (indicated by the circular arrow under the dendritic branches in Fig. 2) strengthens these synapses and at some point D-spikes are elicited more reliably at conjoint branches. This could finally also lead to spiking at the soma and, hence, to a BP-spike, changing plasticity of the individual synapses.

To emulate such a multi-cluster system we actually model only one left and one right branch. Plasticity in both branches is driven by D-spikes in the first part of the experiment. Assuming that at some point the cell will be driven into spiking, a BP-spike is added after several hundred pulse groups (second part of the experiment).

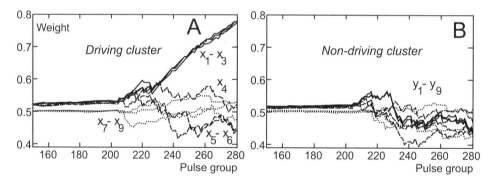

Figure 3: Temporal weight development for the setup shown in Fig 2 with one sub-branch for the driving cluster (A), and one for the non-driving cluster (B). Initially all weights grow gradually until the driving cluster leads to a BP-spike after 200 pulse groups. Thus only the weights of its group $x_1 - x_3$ will continue to grow, now at an increased rate.

3.2 An emerging winner-take-all mechanism

In Fig. 3 we have simulated two clusters each with nine synapses. For both clusters, we assume that the input activity for three synapses is closely correlated and that they occur in a temporal interval of 6 ms (group x, y: $1 - 3$). Three other inputs are wider dispersed (interval of 35 ms, group x, y: $4 - 6$) and the three remaining ones arrive uncorrelated in an interval of 150 ms (group x, y: $7 - 9$). The activity of the second cluster is determined by the same parameters. Pulse groups arriving at the second cluster, however, were randomly shifted by maximally ± 20 ms relative to the centre of the pulse group of the first cluster.

All synapses start with weights 0.5, which will not suffice to drive the soma of the cell into spiking. Hence initially plasticity can only take place by D-spikes, and we assume that D-spikes will not reach the other cluster. Hence, learning is local. The wide D-spike leads to a broad learning curve which has a span of about $\pm 17.5 ms$ around zero, covering the dispersion of input groups $1 - 3$ as well as $4 - 6$. Furthermore it has a slightly bigger area under the LTP part as compared to the LTD part. As a consequence, in both diagrams (Fig. 3 A,B) we see that *all* weights $1 - 6$ grow, only for the least correlated input $6 - 9$ the weights remain close their origin. The correlated group $1 - 3$, however, benefits most strongly, because it is more likely that a D-spike will be elicited by this group than by any other combination.

Conjoint growth at a whole cluster of such synapses would at some point drive the cell into somatic firing. Here we just assume that this happens for one cluster (Fig. 3 A) at a certain time point. This can, for example, be the case when the input properties of the two input groups are different leading to (slightly) less weight growth in the other cluster. As soon as this happens a BP-spike is triggered and the STDP curve takes a narrow shape similar to that in Fig. 2 B now strongly enhancing all causally driving synapses, hence group $x_1 - x_3$ (Fig. 3 A). This group grows at an increased rate while all other synapses shrink. Hence, in general this system exhibits two-phase plasticity. This result was reproduced in a model with 100 synapses in each input group (data not shown) and in the next sections we will show that a system with two growth phases is rather robust against parameter variations.

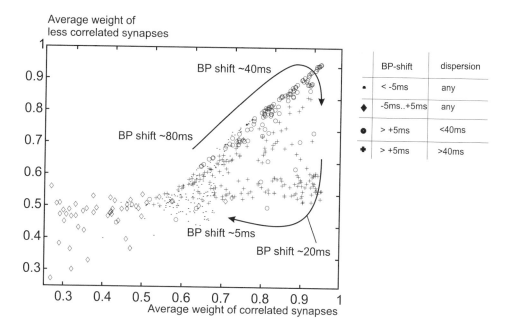

Figure 4: Robustness of the observed effects. Plotted are the average weights of the less correlated group (ordinate) against the correlated group (abscissa). Simulation with three correlated and three less correlated inputs, for AMPA: $\tau = 6\,ms$, for NMDA: $\tau = 117\,ms$, for D-spike: $\tau = 235\,ms$, for BP-spike: $\tau = 6 - 66\,ms$, $q_1 = 0.14$. D/BP spike amplitude relation from $1/1.5$ to $1/15$, depending on BP-spike width, and keeping the area under the BP-spike constant, $\mu = 0.2$. For further explanation see text.

3.3 Robustness

This system is not readily suited for analytical investigation like the simpler ones in [9]. However, a fairly exhaustive parameter analysis is performed. Fig. 4 shows a plot of 350 experiments with the same basic architecture, using only one synapse cluster and the same chain of events as before but with different parameter settings. Only "strong correlated" ($< 10 \ ms$) and "less correlated" ($10 - 100 \ ms$) inputs were used in this experiment. Each point represents one experiment consisting of 600 pulse groups. On the abscissa we plot the average weight of the three correlated synapses; on the ordinate the average weight of the three less correlated synapses after these 600 pulse groups. We assume, as in the last experiment, that a BP-spike is triggered as soon as q_2 is passed, which happens around pulse group 200 in all cases.

Four parameters were varied to obtain this plot. **(1)** The width of the BP-spike was varied between $5 \ ms$ and $50 \ ms$. **(2)** The interval width for the temporal distribution of the three correlated spikes was varied between $1 \ ms$ and $10 \ ms$. Hence $1 \ ms$ amounts to three synchronously elicited spikes. **(3)** The interval width for the temporal distribution of the three less correlated spikes was varied between $1 \ ms$ and $100 \ ms$. **(4)** The shift of the BP-spike with respect to the beginning of the D-spike was varied in an interval of $\pm 80 \ ms$.

Mainly parameters 3 and 4 have an effect on the results. The first parameter, BP spike width, shows some small interference with the spike shift for the widest spikes. The second parameter has almost no influence, due to the small parameter range ($10 \ ms$). Symbol coding is used in Fig. 4 to better depict the influence of parameters 3 and 4 in their different ranges. Symbols "dots", "diamonds" and "others" (circles and plusses) refer to a BP-spike shifts: of less than $-5 \ ms$ (dots), between $-5 \ ms$ and $+5 \ ms$ (diamonds) and larger than $+5 \ ms$ (circles and pluses). Circles in the latter region show cases with the less correlated dispersion interval below $40 \ ms$, and plusses the cases of the dispersion $40 \ ms$ or higher. The "dot" region ($-5 \ ms$) shows cases where correlated synapses will grow, while less correlated synapses can grow or shrink. This happens because the BP spike is too early to influence plasticity in the strongly correlated group, which will grow by the DS-mechanism only, but the BP-spike still falls in the dispersion range of the less correlated group, influencing its weights. At a shift of $-5 \ ms$ a fast transition in the weight development occurs. The reason for this transition is that the BP-spike, being very close to the D-spike, overrules the effect of the D-spike. The randomness whether the input falls into pre- or post-output zone in both, correlated and less correlated, groups is large enough, and leads to weights staying close to origin or to shrinkage. The circles and plusses encode the dispersion of the wide, less correlated spike distributions in the case when time shifts of the BP-spike are positive ($> 5 \ ms$, hence BP-spike after D-spike). Dispersions are getting wider essentially from top to bottom (circle to dot). Clearly this shows that there are many cases corresponding to the example depicted in Fig. 3 (horizontal tail of Fig. 4 A), but there are also many conventional situations, where both weight-groups just grow in a similar way (diagonal).

The data points show a certain regularity when the BP spike shift moves from big values towards the borderline of $+5 \ ms$, where the weights stop to grow. For big shifts, points cluster on the upper, diagonal tail in or near the dot region. With a smaller BP spike shift points move up this tail and then drop down to the horizontal tail, which occurs for shifts of about $20 \ ms$. This pattern is typical for the bigger dispersion in the range of $20 - 60 \ ms$ and data points essentially follow the circle drawn in the figure.

This happens because as soon as the BP-spike gets closer to the D-spike, it will start to exert its influence. But this will first only affect the less correlated group as there are almost always some inputs so late that they "collide" with the BP-spike. Time of collision, however, is random and sometimes these input are "pre" while sometimes they are "post" with respect to the BP-spike. Hence LTP and LTD will be essentially balanced in the less correlated group, leading on average to zero weight growth. This effect is most pronounced when the less correlated group has an intermediate dispersion (see the circles from the upper tail dropping to the lower tail in the range of dispersions $20 - 40\ ms$), while it does not occur if the dispersion of correlated and less correlated groups are similar ($1 - 20\ ms$).

Furthermore, the clear separation into the top- (circles, $1 - 40\ ms$) and bottom-tail (plusses, $61 - 100\ ms$) indicates that it is possible to let the parameters drift quite a bit without leaving the respective regions. Hence, while the moment-to-moment weight growth might change, the general pattern will stay the same.

4   Discussion

Just like with the famous Baron von Münchausen, who was able to pull himself out of a swamp by his own hair, the current study suggests that plasticity change as a consequence of itself might lead to specific functional properties. In order to arrive at this conclusion, we have used a simplified model of STDP and combined it with a custom designed and also simplified dendritic architecture. Hence, can the conclusions of this study be valid and where are the limitations? We believe that answer to the first question is affirmative because the degree of abstraction used in this model and the complexity of the results match. This model never attempted to address the difficult issues of the biophysics of synaptic plasticity (for a discussion see [2]) and it was also not our goal to investigate the mechanisms of signal propagation in a dendrite [11]. Both aspects had been reduced to a few basic descriptors and this way we were able to show for the first time that a useful synaptic selection process can develop over time. The system consisted of a first "pre-growth" phase (until the BP-spike sets in) followed by a second phase where only one group of synapses grows strongly, while the others shrink again. In general this example describes a scenario where groups of synapses first undergo less selective classical Hebbian-like growth, while later more pronounced STDP sets in, selecting only the main driving group. We believe that in the early development of a real brain such a two-phase system might be beneficial for the stable selection of those synapses that are better correlated. It is conceivable that at early developmental stages correlations are in general weaker, while the number of inputs to a cell is probably much higher than in the adult stage, where many have been pruned. Hence highly selective and strong STDP-like plasticity employed too early might lead to a noise-induced growth of "the wrong" synapses. This, however, might be prevented by just such a soft pre-selection mechanisms which would gradually drive clusters of synapses apart by a local dendritic process before the stronger influence of the back-propagating spike sets in. This is supported by recent results from Holthoff et al [1, 12], who have shown that D-spikes will lead to a different type of plasticity than BP-spikes in layer 5 pyramidal cells in mouse cortex. Many more complications exist, for example the assumed chain of events of D- and BP-spikes may be very different in different neurons and the interactions between these signals may be far more non-linear (but see [10]). This will require to re-address these issues in greater detail when dealing with a specific given neuron but the general conclusions about the self-influencing and local [2, 13] character of synaptic plasticity and their possible functional use should hopefully remain valid.

5   Acknowledgements

The authors acknowledge the support from SHEFC INCITE and IBRO. We are grateful to B. Graham, L. Smith and D. Sterratt for their helpful comments on this work. The authors wish to especially express their thanks to A. Saudargiene for her help at many stages in this project.

References

[1] K. Holthoff, Y. Kovalchuk, R. Yuste, and A. Konnerth. Single-shock plasticity induced by local dendritic spikes. In *Proc. Göttingen NWG Conference*, page 245B, 2005.

[2] A. Saudargiene, B. Porr, and F. Wörgötter. How the shape of pre- and postsynaptic signals can influence STDP: a biophysical model. *Neural Comp.*, 16:595–626, 2004.

[3] N.L. Golding, W. L. Kath, and N. Spruston. Dichotomy of action-potential backpropagation in ca1 pyramidal neuron dendrites. *J Neurophysiol.*, 86:2998–3010, 2001.

[4] M. E. Larkum, J. J. Zhu, and B. Sakmann. Dendritic mechanisms underlying the coupling of the dendritic with the axonal action potential initiation zone of adult rat layer 5 pyramidal neurons. *J. Physiol. (Lond.)*, 533:447–466, 2001.

[5] N. L. Golding, P. N. Staff, and N. Spurston. Dendritic spikes as a mechanism for cooperative long-term potentiation. *Nature*, 418:326–331, 2002.

[6] B. Porr and F. Wörgötter. Isotropic sequence order learning. *Neural Comp.*, 15:831–864, 2003.

[7] J. C. Magee and D. Johnston. A synaptically controlled, associative signal for Hebbian plasticity in hippocampal neurons. *Science*, 275:209–213, 1997.

[8] H. Markram, J. Lübke, M. Frotscher, and B. Sakmann. Regulation of synaptic efficacy by coincidence of postsynaptic APs and EPSPs. *Science*, 275:213–215, 1997.

[9] A. Saudargiene, B. Porr, and F. Wörgötter. Local learning rules: predicted influence of dendritic location on synaptic modification in spike-timing-dependent plasticity. *Biol. Cybern.*, 92:128–138, 2005.

[10] H.-X. Wang, Gerkin R. C., D. W. Nauen, and G.-Q. Bi. Coactivation and timing-dependent integration of synaptic potentiation and depression. *Nature Neurosci.*, 8:187–193, 2005.

[11] P. Vetter, A. Roth, and M. Häusser. Propagation of action potentials in dendrites depends on dendritic morphology. *J. Neurophsiol.*, 85:926–937, 2001.

[12] K. Holthoff, Y. Kovalchuk, R. Yuste, and A. Konnerth. Single-shock LTD by local dendritic spikes in pyramidal neurons of mouse visual cortex. *J. Physiol.*, 560.1:27–36, 2004.

[13] R. C. Froemke, M-m. Poo, and Y. Dan. Spike-timing-dependent synaptic plasticity depends on dendritic location. *Nature*, 434:221–225, 2005.

Structured Prediction via the Extragradient Method

Ben Taskar
Computer Science
UC Berkeley, Berkeley, CA 94720
taskar@cs.berkeley.edu

Simon Lacoste-Julien
Computer Science
UC Berkeley, Berkeley, CA 94720
slacoste@cs.berkeley.edu

Michael I. Jordan
Computer Science and Statistics
UC Berkeley, Berkeley, CA 94720
jordan@cs.berkeley.edu

Abstract

We present a simple and scalable algorithm for large-margin estimation of structured models, including an important class of Markov networks and combinatorial models. We formulate the estimation problem as a convex-concave saddle-point problem and apply the extragradient method, yielding an algorithm with linear convergence using simple gradient and projection calculations. The projection step can be solved using combinatorial algorithms for min-cost quadratic flow. This makes the approach an efficient alternative to formulations based on reductions to a quadratic program (QP). We present experiments on two very different structured prediction tasks: 3D image segmentation and word alignment, illustrating the favorable scaling properties of our algorithm.

1 Introduction

The scope of discriminative learning methods has been expanding to encompass prediction tasks with increasingly complex structure. Much of this recent development builds upon graphical models to capture sequential, spatial, recursive or relational structure, but as we will discuss in this paper, the structured prediction problem is broader still. For graphical models, two major approaches to discriminative estimation have been explored: (1) maximum conditional likelihood [13] and (2) maximum margin [6, 1, 20]. For the broader class of models that we consider here, the conditional likelihood approach is intractable, but the large margin formulation yields tractable convex problems.

We interpret the term *structured output model* very broadly, as a compact scoring scheme over a (possibly very large) set of combinatorial structures and a method for finding the highest scoring structure. In graphical models, the scoring scheme is embodied in a probability distribution over possible assignments of the prediction variables as a function of input variables. In models based on combinatorial problems, the scoring scheme is usually a simple sum of weights associated with vertices, edges, or other components of a structure; these weights are often represented as parametric functions of a set of features. Given training instances labeled by desired structured outputs (e.g., matchings) and a set of features that parameterize the scoring function, the learning problem is to find parameters such that the highest scoring outputs are as close as possible to the desired outputs.

Example of prediction tasks solved via combinatorial optimization problems include bipartite and non-bipartite matching in alignment of 2D shapes [5], word alignment in natural language translation [14] and disulfide connectivity prediction for proteins [3]. All of these problems can be formulated in terms of a tractable optimization problem. There are also interesting subfamilies of graphical models for which large-margin methods are tractable whereas likelihood-based methods are not; an example is the class of Markov random fields with restricted potentials used for object segmentation in vision [12, 2].

Tractability is not necessarily sufficient to obtain algorithms that work effectively in practice. In particular, although the problem of large margin estimation can be formulated as a quadratic program (QP) in several cases of interest [2, 19], and although this formulation exploits enough of the problem structure so as to achieve a polynomial representation in terms of the number of variables and constraints, off-the-shelf QP solvers scale poorly with problem and training sample size for these models. To solve large-scale machine learning problems, researchers often turn to simple gradient-based algorithms, in which each individual step is cheap in terms of computation and memory. Examples of this approach in the structured prediction setting include the Structured Sequential Minimal Optimization algorithm [20, 18] and the Structured Exponentiated Gradient algorithm [4]. These algorithms are first-order methods for solving QPs arising from low-treewidth Markov random fields and other decomposable models. They are able to scale to significantly larger problems than off-the-shelf QP solvers. However, they are limited in scope in that they rely on dynamic programming to compute essential quantities such as gradients. They do not extend to models in which dynamic programming is not applicable, for example, to problems such as matchings and min-cuts.

In this paper, we present an estimation methodology for structured prediction problems that does not require a general-purpose QP solver. We propose a saddle-point formulation which allows us to exploit simple gradient-based methods [11] with linear convergence guarantees. Moreover, we show that the key computational step in these methods—a certain projection operation—inherits the favorable computational complexity of the underlying optimization problem. This important result makes our approach viable computationally. In particular, for matchings and min-cuts, projection involves a min-cost quadratic flow computation, a problem for which efficient, highly-specialized algorithms are available. We illustrate the effectiveness of this approach on two very different large-scale structured prediction tasks: 3D image segmentation and word alignment in translation.

2 Structured models

We begin by discussing two special cases of the general framework that we subsequently present: (1) a class of Markov networks used for segmentation, and (2) a bipartite matching model for word alignment. Despite significant differences in the setup for these models, they share the property that in both cases the problem of finding the highest-scoring output can be formulated as a linear program (LP).

Markov networks. We consider a special class of Markov networks, common in vision applications, in which inference reduces to a tractable min-cut problem [7]. Focusing on binary variables, $\mathbf{y} = \{y_1, \ldots, y_N\}$, and pairwise potentials, we define a joint distribution over $\{0, 1\}^N$ via $P(\mathbf{y}) \propto \prod_{j \in \mathcal{V}} \phi_j(y_j) \prod_{jk \in \mathcal{E}} \phi_{jk}(y_j, y_k)$, where $(\mathcal{V}, \mathcal{E})$ is an undirected graph, and where $\{\phi_j(y_j); j \in \mathcal{V}\}$ are the node potentials and $\{\phi_{jk}(y_j, y_k), jk \in \mathcal{E}\}$ are the edge potentials.

In image segmentation (see Fig. 1(a)), the node potentials capture local evidence about the label of a pixel or laser scan point. Edges usually connect nearby pixels in an image, and serve to correlate their labels. Assuming that such correlations tend to be *positive*

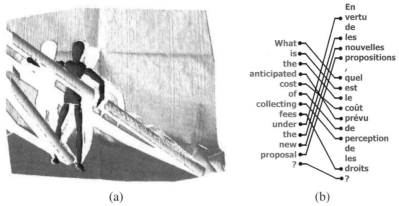

<table>
(a)   (b)
</table>

Figure 1: Examples of structured prediction applications: (a) articulated object segmentation and (b) word alignment in machine translation.

(connected nodes tend to have the same label), we restrict the form of edge potentials to be of the form $\phi_{jk}(y_j, y_k) = \exp\{-s_{jk} \mathbb{I}(y_j \neq y_k)\}$, where s_{jk} is a non-negative penalty for assigning y_j and y_k different labels. Expressing node potentials as $\phi_j(y_j) = \exp\{s_j y_j\}$, we have $P(\mathbf{y}) \propto \exp\left\{\sum_{j \in \mathcal{V}} s_j y_j - \sum_{jk \in \mathcal{E}} s_{jk} \mathbb{I}(y_j \neq y_k)\right\}$. Under this restriction of the potentials, it is known that the problem of computing the maximizing assignment, $\mathbf{y}^* = \arg\max P(\mathbf{y} \mid \mathbf{x})$, has a tractable formulation as a min-cut problem [7]. In particular, we obtain the following LP:

$$\max_{0 \leq \mathbf{z} \leq 1} \sum_{j \in \mathcal{V}} s_j z_j - \sum_{jk \in \mathcal{E}} s_{jk} z_{jk} \quad \text{s.t.} \quad z_j - z_k \leq z_{jk}, \ z_k - z_j \leq z_{jk}, \ \forall jk \in \mathcal{E}. \quad (1)$$

In this LP, a continuous variable z_j is a relaxation of the binary variable y_j. Note that the constraints are equivalent to $|z_j - z_k| \leq z_{jk}$. Because s_{jk} is positive, $z_{jk} = |z_k - z_j|$ at the maximum, which is equivalent to $\mathbb{I}(z_j \neq z_k)$ if the z_j, z_k variables are binary. An integral optimal solution always exists, as the constraint matrix is totally unimodular [17] (that is, the relaxation is not an approximation).

We can parametrize the node and edge weights s_j and s_{jk} in terms of user-provided features $\mathbf{x}_j$ and $\mathbf{x}_{jk}$ associated with the nodes and edges. In particular, in 3D range data, $\mathbf{x}_j$ might be spin image features or spatial occupancy histograms of a point j, while $\mathbf{x}_{jk}$ might include the distance between points j and k, the dot-product of their normals, etc. The simplest model of dependence is a linear combination of features: $s_j = \mathbf{w}_n^\top \mathbf{f}_n(\mathbf{x}_j)$ and $s_{jk} = \mathbf{w}_e^\top \mathbf{f}_e(\mathbf{x}_{jk})$, where $\mathbf{w}_n$ and $\mathbf{w}_e$ are node and edge parameters, and $\mathbf{f}_n$ and $\mathbf{f}_e$ are node and edge feature mappings, of dimension d_n and d_e, respectively. To ensure non-negativity of s_{jk}, we assume the edge features $\mathbf{f}_e$ to be non-negative and restrict $\mathbf{w}_e \geq 0$. This constraint is easily incorporated into the formulation we present below. We assume that the feature mappings $\mathbf{f}$ are provided by the user and our goal is to estimate parameters $\mathbf{w}$ from labeled data. We abbreviate the score assigned to a labeling $\mathbf{y}$ for an input $\mathbf{x}$ as $\mathbf{w}^\top \mathbf{f}(\mathbf{x}, \mathbf{y}) = \sum_j y_j \mathbf{w}_n^\top \mathbf{f}_n(\mathbf{x}_j) - \sum_{jk \in \mathcal{E}} y_{jk} \mathbf{w}_e^\top \mathbf{f}_e(\mathbf{x}_{jk})$, where $y_{jk} = \mathbb{I}(y_j \neq y_k)$.

Matchings. Consider modeling the task of word alignment of parallel bilingual sentences (see Fig. 1(b)) as a maximum weight bipartite matching problem, where the nodes $\mathcal{V} = \mathcal{V}^s \cup \mathcal{V}^t$ correspond to the words in the "source" sentence $(\mathcal{V}^s)$ and the "target" sentence $(\mathcal{V}^t)$ and the edges $\mathcal{E} = \{jk : j \in \mathcal{V}^s, k \in \mathcal{V}^t\}$ correspond to possible alignments between them. For simplicity, assume that each word aligns to one or zero words in the other sentence. The edge weight s_{jk} represents the degree to which word j in one sentence can translate into the word k in the other sentence. Our objective is to find an alignment that maximizes the sum of edge scores. We represent a matching using a set of binary variables

1347

y_{jk} that are set to 1 if word j is assigned to word k in the other sentence, and 0 otherwise. The score of an assignment is the sum of edge scores: $s(\mathbf{y}) = \sum_{jk \in \mathcal{E}} s_{jk} y_{jk}$. The maximum weight bipartite matching problem, $\arg \max_{\mathbf{y} \in \mathcal{Y}} s(\mathbf{y})$, can be found by solving the following LP:

$$\max_{0 \leq \mathbf{z} \leq 1} \sum_{jk \in \mathcal{E}} s_{jk} z_{jk} \text{ s.t. } \sum_{j \in \mathcal{V}^s} z_{jk} \leq 1, \forall k \in \mathcal{V}^t; \quad \sum_{k \in \mathcal{V}^t} z_{jk} \leq 1, \forall j \in \mathcal{V}^s, \quad (2)$$

where again the continuous variables z_{jk} correspond to the relaxation of the binary variables y_{jk}. As in the min-cut problem, this LP is guaranteed to have integral solutions for any scoring function $s(\mathbf{y})$ [17].

For word alignment, the scores s_{jk} can be defined in terms of the word pair jk and input features associated with $\mathbf{x}_{jk}$. We can include the identity of the two words, relative position in the respective sentences, part-of-speech tags, string similarity (for detecting cognates), etc. We let $s_{jk} = \mathbf{w}^\top \mathbf{f}(\mathbf{x}_{jk})$ for some user-provided feature mapping $\mathbf{f}$ and abbreviate $\mathbf{w}^\top \mathbf{f}(\mathbf{x}, \mathbf{y}) = \sum_{jk} y_{jk} \mathbf{w}^\top \mathbf{f}(\mathbf{x}_{jk})$.

General structure. More generally, we consider prediction problems in which the input $\mathbf{x} \in \mathcal{X}$ is an arbitrary structured object and the output is a vector of values $\mathbf{y} = (y_1, \ldots, y_{L_\mathbf{x}})$, for example, a matching or a cut in the graph. We assume that the length $L_\mathbf{x}$ and the structure of $\mathbf{y}$ depend deterministically on the input $\mathbf{x}$. In our word alignment example, the output space is defined by the length of the two sentences. Denote the output space for a given input $\mathbf{x}$ as $\mathcal{Y}(\mathbf{x})$ and the entire output space as $\mathcal{Y} = \bigcup_{\mathbf{x} \in \mathcal{X}} \mathcal{Y}(\mathbf{x})$.

Consider the class of structured prediction models $\mathcal{H}$ defined by the linear family: $h_\mathbf{w}(\mathbf{x}) = \arg \max_{\mathbf{y} \in \mathcal{Y}(\mathbf{x})} \mathbf{w}^\top \mathbf{f}(\mathbf{x}, \mathbf{y})$, where $\mathbf{f}(\mathbf{x}, \mathbf{y})$ is a vector of functions $\mathbf{f} : \mathcal{X} \times \mathcal{Y} \mapsto \mathbb{R}^n$. This formulation is very general. Indeed, it is too general for our purposes—for many $\mathbf{f}, \mathcal{Y}$ pairs, finding the optimal $\mathbf{y}$ is intractable. Below, we specialize to the class of models in which the $\arg \max$ problem can be solved in polynomial time using linear programming (and more generally, convex optimization); this is still a very large class of models.

3 Max-margin estimation

We assume a set of training instances $S = \{(\mathbf{x}_i, \mathbf{y}_i)\}_{i=1}^m$, where each instance consists of a structured object $\mathbf{x}_i$ (such as a graph) and a target solution $\mathbf{y}_i$ (such as a matching). Consider learning the parameters $\mathbf{w}$ in the conditional likelihood setting. We can define $P_\mathbf{w}(\mathbf{y} \mid \mathbf{x}) = \frac{1}{Z_\mathbf{w}(\mathbf{x})} \exp\{\mathbf{w}^\top \mathbf{f}(\mathbf{x}, \mathbf{y})\}$, where $Z_\mathbf{w}(\mathbf{x}) = \sum_{\mathbf{y}' \in \mathcal{Y}(\mathbf{x})} \exp\{\mathbf{w}^\top \mathbf{f}(\mathbf{x}, \mathbf{y}')\}$, and maximize the conditional log-likelihood $\sum_i \log P_\mathbf{w}(\mathbf{y}_i \mid \mathbf{x}_i)$, perhaps with additional regularization of the parameters $\mathbf{w}$. However, computing the partition function $Z_\mathbf{w}(\mathbf{x})$ is #P-complete [23, 10] for the two structured prediction problems we presented above, matchings and min-cuts. Instead, we adopt the max-margin formulation of [20], which directly seeks to find parameters $\mathbf{w}$ such that: $\mathbf{y}_i = \arg \max_{\mathbf{y}_i' \in \mathcal{Y}_i} \mathbf{w}^\top \mathbf{f}(\mathbf{x}_i, \mathbf{y}_i'), \quad \forall i$, where $\mathcal{Y}_i = \mathcal{Y}(\mathbf{x}_i)$ and $\mathbf{y}_i$ denotes the appropriate vector of variables for example i. The solution space $\mathcal{Y}_i$ depends on the structured object $\mathbf{x}_i$; for example, the space of possible matchings depends on the precise set of nodes and edges in the graph.

As in univariate prediction, we measure the error of prediction using a loss function $\ell(\mathbf{y}_i, \mathbf{y}_i')$. To obtain a convex formulation, we upper bound the loss $\ell(\mathbf{y}_i, h_\mathbf{w}(\mathbf{x}_i))$ using the hinge function: $\max_{\mathbf{y}_i' \in \mathcal{Y}_i} [\mathbf{w}^\top \mathbf{f}_i(\mathbf{y}_i') + \ell_i(\mathbf{y}_i')] - \mathbf{w}^\top \mathbf{f}_i(\mathbf{y}_i)$, where $\ell_i(\mathbf{y}_i') = \ell(\mathbf{y}_i, \mathbf{y}_i')$, and $\mathbf{f}_i(\mathbf{y}_i') = \mathbf{f}(\mathbf{x}_i, \mathbf{y}_i')$. Minimizing this upper bound will force the true structure $\mathbf{y}_i$ to be optimal with respect to $\mathbf{w}$ for each instance i. We add a standard L_2 weight penalty $\frac{\|\mathbf{w}\|^2}{2C}$:

$$\min_{\mathbf{w} \in \mathcal{W}} \frac{\|\mathbf{w}\|^2}{2C} + \sum_i \max_{\mathbf{y}_i' \in \mathcal{Y}_i} [\mathbf{w}^\top \mathbf{f}_i(\mathbf{y}_i') + \ell_i(\mathbf{y}_i')] - \mathbf{w}^\top \mathbf{f}_i(\mathbf{y}_i), \quad (3)$$

where C is a regularization parameter and $\mathcal{W}$ is the space of allowed weights (for example, $\mathcal{W} = \mathbb{R}^n$ or $\mathcal{W} = \mathbb{R}^n_+$). Note that this formulation is equivalent to the standard formulation using slack variables ξ and slack penalty C presented in [20, 19].

The key to solving Eq. (3) efficiently is the *loss-augmented inference problem*, $\max_{\mathbf{y}'_i \in \mathcal{Y}_i} [\mathbf{w}^\top \mathbf{f}_i(\mathbf{y}'_i) + \ell_i(\mathbf{y}'_i)]$. This optimization problem has precisely the same form as the prediction problem whose parameters we are trying to learn—$\max_{\mathbf{y}'_i \in \mathcal{Y}_i} \mathbf{w}^\top \mathbf{f}_i(\mathbf{y}'_i)$— but with an additional term corresponding to the loss function. Tractability of the loss-augmented inference thus depends not only on the tractability of $\max_{\mathbf{y}'_i \in \mathcal{Y}_i} \mathbf{w}^\top \mathbf{f}_i(\mathbf{y}'_i)$, but also on the form of the loss term $\ell_i(\mathbf{y}'_i)$. A natural choice in this regard is the Hamming distance, which simply counts the number of variables in which a candidate solution $\mathbf{y}'_i$ differs from the target output $\mathbf{y}_i$. In general, we need only assume that the loss function decomposes over the variables in $\mathbf{y}_i$.

For example, in the case of bipartite matchings the Hamming loss counts the number of different edges in the matchings $\mathbf{y}_i$ and $\mathbf{y}'_i$ and can be written as: $\ell_i^H(\mathbf{y}'_i) = \sum_{jk} y_{i,jk} + \sum_{jk}(1 - 2y'_{i,jk})y_{i,jk}$. Thus the loss-augmented matching problem for example i can be written as an LP similar to Eq. (2) (without the constant term $\sum_{jk} y_{i,jk}$):

$$\max_{0 \leq \mathbf{z} \leq 1} \quad \sum_{jk} z_{i,jk}[\mathbf{w}^\top \mathbf{f}(\mathbf{x}_{i,jk}) + 1 - 2y_{i,jk}] \quad \text{s.t.} \quad \sum_j z_{i,jk} \leq 1, \quad \sum_k z_{i,jk} \leq 1.$$

Generally, when we can express $\max_{\mathbf{y}'_i \in \mathcal{Y}_i} \mathbf{w}^\top \mathbf{f}_i(\mathbf{y}'_i)$ as an LP, $\max_{\mathbf{z}_i \in \mathcal{Z}_i} \mathbf{w}^\top \mathbf{F}_i \mathbf{z}_i$, where $\mathcal{Z}_i = \{\mathbf{z}_i : \mathbf{A}_i \mathbf{z}_i \leq \mathbf{b}_i, \ \mathbf{z}_i \geq 0\}$, for appropriately defined constraints $\mathbf{A}_i, \mathbf{b}_i$ and feature matrix $\mathbf{F}_i$, we have a similar LP for the loss-augmented inference for each example i: $d_i + \max_{\mathbf{z}_i \in \mathcal{Z}_i}(\mathbf{w}^\top \mathbf{F}_i + \mathbf{c}_i)^\top \mathbf{z}_i$ for appropriately defined $d_i, \mathbf{F}_i, \mathbf{c}_i, \mathbf{A}_i, \mathbf{b}_i$. Let $\mathbf{z} = \{\mathbf{z}_1, \ldots, \mathbf{z}_m\}$, $\mathcal{Z} = \mathcal{Z}_1 \times \ldots \times \mathcal{Z}_m$.

We could proceed by making use of Lagrangian duality, which yields a joint convex optimization problem; this is the approach described in [19]. Instead we take a different tack here, posing the problem in its natural saddle-point form:

$$\min_{\mathbf{w} \in \mathcal{W}} \max_{\mathbf{z} \in \mathcal{Z}} \quad \frac{\|\mathbf{w}\|^2}{2C} + \sum_i \left[\mathbf{w}^\top \mathbf{F}_i \mathbf{z}_i + \mathbf{c}_i^\top \mathbf{z}_i - \mathbf{w}^\top \mathbf{f}_i(\mathbf{y}_i) \right]. \tag{4}$$

As we discuss in the following section, this approach allows us to exploit the structure of $\mathcal{W}$ and $\mathcal{Z}$ *separately*, allowing for efficient solutions for a wider range of structure spaces.

4 Extragradient method

The key operations of the method we present below are gradient calculations and Euclidean projections. We let $L(\mathbf{w}, \mathbf{z}) = \frac{\|\mathbf{w}\|^2}{2C} + \sum_i \left[\mathbf{w}^\top \mathbf{F}_i \mathbf{z}_i + \mathbf{c}_i^\top \mathbf{z}_i - \mathbf{w}^\top \mathbf{f}_i(\mathbf{y}_i) \right]$, with gradients given by: $\nabla_{\mathbf{w}} L(\mathbf{w}, \mathbf{z}) = \frac{\mathbf{w}}{C} + \sum_i \mathbf{F}_i \mathbf{z}_i - \mathbf{f}_i(\mathbf{y}_i)$ and $\nabla_{\mathbf{z}_i} L(\mathbf{w}, \mathbf{z}) = \mathbf{F}_i^\top \mathbf{w} + \mathbf{c}_i$. We denote the projection of a vector $\mathbf{z}_i$ onto $\mathcal{Z}_i$ as $\pi_{\mathcal{Z}_i}(\mathbf{z}_i) = \arg\min_{\mathbf{z}'_i \in \mathcal{Z}_i} \|\mathbf{z}'_i - \mathbf{z}_i\|$ and similarly, the projection onto $\mathcal{W}$ as $\pi_{\mathcal{W}}(\mathbf{w}') = \arg\min_{\mathbf{w} \in \mathcal{W}} \|\mathbf{w}' - \mathbf{w}\|$.

A well-known solution strategy for saddle-point optimization is provided by the *extragradient method* [11]. An iteration of the extragradient method consists of two very simple steps, prediction $(\mathbf{w}, \mathbf{z}) \to (\mathbf{w}^p, \mathbf{z}^p)$ and correction $(\mathbf{w}^p, \mathbf{z}^p) \to (\mathbf{w}^c, \mathbf{z}^c)$:

$$\mathbf{w}^p = \pi_{\mathcal{W}}(\mathbf{w} - \beta \nabla_{\mathbf{w}} L(\mathbf{w}, \mathbf{z})); \qquad \mathbf{z}_i^p = \pi_{\mathcal{Z}_i}(\mathbf{z}_i + \beta \nabla_{\mathbf{z}_i} L(\mathbf{w}, \mathbf{z})); \tag{5}$$

$$\mathbf{w}^c = \pi_{\mathcal{W}}(\mathbf{w} - \beta \nabla_{\mathbf{w}} L(\mathbf{w}^p, \mathbf{z}^p)); \qquad \mathbf{z}_i^c = \pi_{\mathcal{Z}_i}(\mathbf{z}_i + \beta \nabla_{\mathbf{z}_i} L(\mathbf{w}^p, \mathbf{z}^p)); \tag{6}$$

where β is an appropriately chosen step size. The algorithm starts with a feasible point $\mathbf{w} = 0$, $\mathbf{z}_i$'s that correspond to the assignments $\mathbf{y}_i$'s and step size $\beta = 1$. After each prediction step, it computes $r = \beta \frac{\|\nabla L(\mathbf{w}, \mathbf{z}) - \nabla L(\mathbf{w}^p, \mathbf{z}^p)\|}{(\|\mathbf{w} - \mathbf{w}^p\| + \|\mathbf{z} - \mathbf{z}^p\|)}$. If r is greater than a threshold ν, the step size is decreased using an Armijo type rule: $\beta = (2/3)\beta \min(1, 1/r)$, and a new prediction step is computed until $r \leq \nu$, where $\nu \in (0, 1)$ is a parameter of the algorithm. Once a suitable β is found, the correction step is taken and $(\mathbf{w}^c, \mathbf{z}^c)$ becomes the new $(\mathbf{w}, \mathbf{z})$. The method is guaranteed to converge linearly to a solution $\mathbf{w}^*, \mathbf{z}^*$ [11, 9]. See the longer version of this paper at http://www.cs.berkeley.edu/~taskar/extragradient.pdf for details. By comparison, Exponentiated Gradient [4] has sublinear convergence rate guarantees, while Structured SMO [18] has none.

The key step influencing the efficiency of the algorithm is the Euclidean projection onto the feasible sets $\mathcal{W}$ and $\mathcal{Z}_i$. In case $\mathcal{W} = \mathbb{R}^n$, the projection is the identity operation; projecting onto $\mathbb{R}^n_+$ consists of clipping negative weights to zero. Additional problem-specific constraints on the weight space can be efficiently incorporated in this step (although linear convergence guarantees only hold for polyhedral $\mathcal{W}$). In case of word alignment, $\mathcal{Z}_i$ is the convex hull of bipartite matchings and the problem reduces to the much-studied minimum cost quadratic flow problem. The projection $\mathbf{z}_i = \pi_{\mathcal{Z}_i}(\mathbf{z}'_i)$ is given by

$$\min_{0 \leq \mathbf{z} \leq 1} \quad \sum_{jk} \frac{1}{2}(z'_{i,jk} - z_{i,jk})^2 \quad \text{s.t.} \quad \sum_j z_{i,jk} \leq 1, \quad \sum_k z_{i,jk} \leq 1.$$

We use a standard reduction of bipartite matching to min-cost flow by introducing a source node s linked to all the nodes in $\mathcal{V}^s_i$ (words in the "source" sentence), and a sink node t linked from all the nodes in $\mathcal{V}^t_i$ (words in the "target" sentence), using edges of capacity 1 and cost 0. The original edges jk have a quadratic cost $\frac{1}{2}(z'_{i,jk} - z_{i,jk})^2$ and capacity 1. Minimum (quadratic) cost flow from s to t is the projection of $\mathbf{z}'_i$ onto $\mathcal{Z}_i$.

The reduction of the projection to minimum quadratic cost flow for the min-cut polytope $\mathcal{Z}_i$ is shown in the longer version of the paper. Algorithms for solving this problem are nearly as efficient as those for solving regular min-cost flow problems. In case of word alignment, the running time scales with the cube of the sentence length. We use publicly-available code for solving this problem [8] (see http://www.math.washington.edu/~tseng/netflowg_nl/).

5 Experiments

We investigate two structured models we described above: bipartite matchings for word alignments and restricted potential Markov nets for 3D segmentation. A commercial QP-solver, MOSEK, runs out of memory on the problems we describe below using the QP formulation [19]. We compared the extragradient method with the averaged perceptron algorithm [6]. A question which arises in practice is how to choose the regularization parameter C. The typical approach is to run the algorithm for several values of the regularization parameter and pick the best model using a validation set. For the averaged perceptron, a standard method is to run the algorithm tracking its performance on a validation set, and selecting the model with best performance. We use the same training regime for the extragradient by running it with $C = \infty$.

Object segmentation. We test our algorithm on a 3D scan segmentation problem using the class of Markov networks with potentials that were described above. The dataset is a challenging collection of cluttered scenes containing articulated wooden puppets [2]. It contains eleven different single-view scans of three puppets of varying sizes and positions, with clutter and occluding objects such as rope, sticks and rings. Each scan consists of around $7,000$ points. Our goal was to segment the scenes into two classes—puppet and background. We use five of the scenes for our training data, three for validation and three for testing. Sample scans from the training and test set can be seen at http://www.cs.berkeley.edu/~taskar/3DSegment/. We computed spin images of size 10×5 bins at two different resolutions, then scaled the values and performed PCA to obtain 45 principal components, which comprised our node features. We used the surface links output by the scanner as edges between points and for each edge only used a

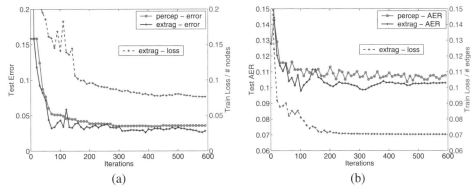

Figure 2: Both plots show test error for the averaged perceptron and the extragradient (left y-axis) and training loss per node or edge for the extragradient (right y-axis) versus number of iterations for (a) object segmentation task and (b) word alignment task.

single feature, set to a constant value of 1 for all edges. This results in all edges having the same potential. The training data contains approximately $37,000$ nodes and $88,000$ edges. Training time took about 4 hours for 600 iterations on a 2.80GHz Pentium 4 machine. Fig. 2(a) shows that the extragradient has a consistently lower error rate (about 3% for extragradient, 4% for averaged perceptron), using only slightly more expensive computations per iteration. Also shown is the corresponding decrease in the hinge-loss upperbound on the training data as the extragradient progresses.

Word alignment. We also tested our learning algorithm on word-level alignment using a data set from the 2003 NAACL set [15], the English-French Hansards task. This corpus consists of 1.1M automatically aligned sentences, and comes with a validation set of 39 sentence pairs and a test set of 447 sentences. The validation and test sentences have been hand-aligned and are marked with both *sure* and *possible* alignments. Using these alignments, *alignment error rate* (AER) is calculated as: $AER(A, S, P) = 1 - \frac{|A \cap S| + |A \cap P|}{|A| + |S|}$. Here, A is a set of proposed index pairs, S is the set of sure gold pairs, and P is the set of possible gold pairs (where $S \subseteq P$).

We used the intersection of the predictions of the English-to-French and French-to-English IBM Model 4 alignments (using GIZA++ [16]) on the first 5000 sentence pairs from the 1.1M sentences. The number of edges for 5000 sentences was about 555,000. We tested on the 347 hand-aligned test examples, and used the validation set to select the stopping point. The features on the word pair (e_j, f_k) include measures of association, orthography, relative position, predictions of generative models (see [22] for details). It took about 3 hours to perform 600 training iterations on the training data using a 2.8GHz Pentium 4 machine. Fig. 2(b) shows the extragradient performing slightly better (by about 0.5%) than average perceptron.

6   Conclusion

We have presented a general solution strategy for large-scale structured prediction problems. We have shown that these problems can be formulated as saddle-point optimization problems, problems that are amenable to solution by the extragradient algorithm. Key to our approach is the recognition that the projection step in the extragradient algorithm can be solved by network flow algorithms. Network flow algorithms are among the most well-developed in the field of combinatorial optimization, and yield stable, efficient algorithmic platforms. We have exhibited the favorable scaling of this overall approach in two concrete, large-scale learning problems. It is also important to note that the general approach extends to a much broader class of problems. In [21], we show how to apply this approach efficiently to other types of models, including general Markov networks and weighted context-free grammars, using Bregman projections.

Acknowledgments

We thank Paul Tseng for kindly answering our questions about his min-cost flow code. This work was funded by the DARPA CALO project (03-000219) and Microsoft Research MICRO award (05-081). SLJ was also supported by an NSERC graduate sholarship.

References

[1] Y. Altun, I. Tsochantaridis, and T. Hofmann. Hidden Markov support vector machines. In *Proc. ICML*, 2003.

[2] D. Anguelov, B. Taskar, V. Chatalbashev, D. Koller, D. Gupta, G. Heitz, and A. Ng. Discriminative learning of Markov random fi elds for segmentation of 3d scan data. In *CVPR*, 2005.

[3] P. Baldi, J. Cheng, and A. Vullo. Large-scale prediction of disulphide bond connectivity. In *Proc. NIPS*, 2004.

[4] P. Bartlett, M. Collins, B. Taskar, and D. McAllester. Exponentiated gradient algorithms for large-margin structured classifi cation. In *NIPS*, 2004.

[5] S. Belongie, J. Malik, and J. Puzicha. Shape matching and object recognition using shape contexts. *IEEE Trans. Pattern Anal. Mach. Intell.*, 24, 2002.

[6] M. Collins. Discriminative training methods for hidden Markov models: Theory and experiments with perceptron algorithms. In *Proc. EMNLP*, 2002.

[7] D. M. Greig, B. T. Porteous, and A. H. Seheult. Exact maximum a posteriori estimation for binary images. *J. R. Statist. Soc. B*, 51, 1989.

[8] F. Guerriero and P. Tseng. Implementation and test of auction methods for solving generalized network fbw problems with separable convex cost. *Journal of Optimization Theory and Applications*, 115(1):113–144, October 2002.

[9] B.S. He and L. Z. Liao. Improvements of some projection methods for monotone nonlinear variational inequalities. *JOTA*, 112:111:128, 2002.

[10] M. Jerrum and A. Sinclair. Polynomial-time approximation algorithms for the Ising model. *SIAM J. Comput.*, 22, 1993.

[11] G. M. Korpelevich. The extragradient method for fi nding saddle points and other problems. *Ekonomika i Matematicheskie Metody*, 12:747:756, 1976.

[12] S. Kumar and M. Hebert. Discriminative fi elds for modeling spatial dependencies in natural images. In *NIPS*, 2003.

[13] J. Lafferty, A. McCallum, and F. Pereira. Conditional random fi elds: Probabilistic models for segmenting and labeling sequence data. In *ICML*, 2001.

[14] E. Matusov, R. Zens, and H. Ney. Symmetric word alignments for statistical machine translation. In *Proc. COLING*, 2004.

[15] R. Mihalcea and T. Pedersen. An evaluation exercise for word alignment. In *Proceedings of the HLT-NAACL 2003 Workshop, Building and Using parallel Texts: Data Driven Machine Translation and Beyond*, pages 1–6, Edmonton, Alberta, Canada, 2003.

[16] F. Och and H. Ney. A systematic comparison of various statistical alignment models. *Computational Linguistics*, 29(1), 2003.

[17] A. Schrijver. *Combinatorial Optimization: Polyhedra and Efficiency*. Springer, 2003.

[18] B. Taskar. *Learning Structured Prediction Models: A Large Margin Approach*. PhD thesis, Stanford University, 2004.

[19] B. Taskar, V. Chatalbashev, D. Koller, and C. Guestrin. Learning structured prediction models: a large margin approach. In *ICML*, 2005.

[20] B. Taskar, C. Guestrin, and D. Koller. Max margin Markov networks. In *NIPS*, 2003.

[21] B. Taskar, S. Lacoste-Julien, and M. Jordan. Structured prediction, dual extragradient and Bregman projections. Technical report, UC Berkeley Statistics Department, 2005.

[22] B. Taskar, S. Lacoste-Julien, and D. Klein. A discriminative matching approach to word alignment. In *EMNLP*, 2005.

[23] L. G. Valiant. The complexity of computing the permanent. *Theoretical Computer Science*, 8:189–201, 1979.

Affine Structure From Sound

Sebastian Thrun

Stanford AI Lab
Stanford University, Stanford, CA 94305
Email: thrun@stanford.edu

Abstract

We consider the problem of localizing a set of microphones together with a set of external acoustic events (e.g., hand claps), emitted at unknown times and unknown locations. We propose a solution that approximates this problem under a far field approximation defined in the calculus of affine geometry, and that relies on singular value decomposition (SVD) to recover the affine structure of the problem. We then define low-dimensional optimization techniques for embedding the solution into Euclidean geometry, and further techniques for recovering the locations and emission times of the acoustic events. The approach is useful for the calibration of ad-hoc microphone arrays and sensor networks.

1 Introduction

Consider a set of acoustic sensors (microphones) for detecting acoustic events in the environment (e.g., a hand clap). The *structure from sound* (SFS) problem addresses the problem of simultaneously localizing a set of N sensors and a set of M external acoustic events, whose locations and emission times are unknown.

The SFS problem is relevant to the spatial calibration problem for microphone arrays. Classically, microphone arrays are mounted on fixed brackets of known dimensions; hence there is no spatial calibration problem. *Ad-hoc microphone arrays*, however, involve a person placing microphones at arbitrary locations with limited knowledge as to where they are. Today's best practice requires a person to measure the distance between the microphones by hand, and to apply algorithms such as multi-dimensional scaling (MDS) [1] for recovering their locations. When sensor networks are deployed from the air [4], manual calibration may not be an option. Some techniques rely on GPS receivers [8]. Others require a capability to emit and sense wireless radio signals [5] or sounds [9, 10], which are then used to estimate relative distances between microphones (directly or indirectly, as in [9]). Unfortunately, wireless signal strength is a poor estimator of range, and active acoustic and GPS localization techniques are uneconomical in that they consume energy and require additional hardware. In contrast, SFS relies on environmental acoustic events such as hand claps, which are *not* generated by the sensor network. The general SFS problem was previously treated in [2] under the name *passive localization*. A related paper [3] describes a technique for *incrementally* localizing a microphone relative to a well-calibrated microphone array through external sound events.

In this paper, the *structure from sound (SFS) problem* is defined as the simultaneous localization problem of N sound sensors and M acoustic events in the environment detected by these sensors. Each event occurs at an unknown time and an unknown location. The sensors are able to measure the detection times of the event. We assume that the clocks of the sensors are synchronized (see [6]); that events are spaced sufficiently far apart in time to make the association between different sensors unambiguous; and we also assume absence of sound reverberation. For the ease of representation, the paper assumes a 2D world; although the technique is easily generalized to 3D.

Under the assumption of independent and identically distributed (iid) Gaussian noise, the SFS problem can be formulated as a least squares problem in a space over three types of variables: the locations of the microphones, the locations of the acoustic events, and their emission times. However, this least squares problem is plagued by local minima, and the number of constraints is quite large.

The gist of this paper transforms this optimization problem into a sequence of simpler problems, some of which can be solved optimally, without the danger of getting stuck in local minima. The key transformation involves a far field approximation, which presupposes that the sound sources are relatively far away from the sensors. This approximation reformulates the problem as one of recovering the incident angle of the acoustic signal, which is the same for all sensors for any fixed acoustic event. The resulting optimization problem is still non-linear; however, by relaxing the laws of Euclidean geometry into the more general calculus of affine geometry, the optimization problem can be solved by singular value decomposition (SVD). The resulting solution is mapped back into Euclidean space by optimizing a matrix of size 2×2, which is easily carried out using gradient descent. A subsequent non-linear optimization step overcomes the far field approximation and enables the algorithm to recover locations and emission times of the defining acoustic events. Experimental results illustrate that our approach reliably solves hard SFS problems where gradient-based techniques consistently fail.

Our approach is similar in spirit to the affine solution to the structure from motion (SFM) problem proposed by a seminal paper by Tomasi&Kanade [11], which was later extended to the non-orthographic case [7]. Like us, these authors expressed the structure finding problem using affine geometry, and applied SVD for solving it. SFM is of course defined for cameras, not for microphone arrays. Camera measure angles, whereas microphones measure range. This paper establishes an affine solution to the structure from sound problem that tends to work well in practice.

2 Problem Definition

2.1 Setup

We are given N sensors (microphones) located in a 2D plane. We shall denote the location of the i-th sensor by $(x_i \ y_i)$, which defined the following sensor location matrix of size $N \times 2$:

$$X = \begin{pmatrix} x_1 & y_1 \\ x_2 & y_2 \\ \vdots & \vdots \\ x_N & y_N \end{pmatrix} \tag{1}$$

We assume that the sensor array detects M acoustic events. Each event has as unknown coordinate and an unknown emission time. The coordinate of the j-th event shall be denoted $(a_j \ b_j)$, providing us with the event location matrix A of size $M \times 2$. The emission time of the j-th acoustic event is denoted t_j, resulting in the vector T of length M:

$$A = \begin{pmatrix} a_1 & b_1 \\ a_2 & b_2 \\ \vdots & \vdots \\ a_M & b_M \end{pmatrix} \qquad T = \begin{pmatrix} t_1 \\ t_2 \\ \vdots \\ t_M \end{pmatrix} \tag{2}$$

X, A, and T, comprise the set of unknown variables. In problems such as sensor calibration, only X is of interest. In general SFS applications, A and T might also be of interest.

2.2 Measurement Data

In SFS, the variables X, A, and T are recovered from data. The *data* establishes the detection times of the acoustic events by the individual sensors. Specifically, the *data matrix* is of the form:

$$D = \begin{pmatrix} d_{1,1} & d_{1,2} & \cdots & d_{1,M} \\ d_{2,1} & d_{2,2} & \cdots & d_{2,M} \\ \vdots & \vdots & \ddots & \vdots \\ d_{N,1} & d_{N,2} & \cdots & d_{N,M} \end{pmatrix} \tag{3}$$

Here each $d_{i,j}$ denotes the detection time of acoustical event j by sensor i. Notice that we assume that there is no *data association problem*. Even if all acoustic events sound alike, the correspondence between different detections is easily established as long as there exists sufficiently long time gaps between any two sound events.

The matrix D is a random field induced by the laws of sound propagation (without reverberation). In the absence of measurement noise, each $d_{i,j}$ is the sum of the corresponding emission time t_j, plus the time it takes for sound to travel from $(a_j\ b_j)$ to $(x_i\ y_i)$:

$$d_{i,j} = t_j + c^{-1} \left| \begin{pmatrix} x_i \\ y_i \end{pmatrix} - \begin{pmatrix} a_j \\ b_j \end{pmatrix} \right| \tag{4}$$

Here $|\cdot|$ denotes the L2 norm (Euclidean distance), and c denoted the speed of sound.

2.3 Relative Formulation

Obviously, we cannot recover the global coordinates of the sensors. Hence, without loss of generality, we define the first sensor's location as $x_1 = y_1 = 0$. This gives us the *relative location matrix* for the sensors:

$$\bar{X} = \begin{pmatrix} x_2 - x_1 & y_2 - y_1 \\ x_3 - x_1 & y_3 - y_1 \\ \vdots & \vdots \\ x_N - x_1 & y_N - y_1 \end{pmatrix} \tag{5}$$

This relative sensor location matrix is of dimension $(N-1) \times 2$.

It shall prove convenient to subtract from the arrival time $d_{i,j}$ the arrival time $d_{1,j}$ measured by the first sensor $i = 1$. This *relative arrival time* is defined as $\Delta_{i,j} := d_{i,j} - d_{1,j}$. In the relative arrival time, the absolute emission times t_j cancel out:

$$\begin{aligned} \Delta_{i,j} &= t_j + c^{-1} \left| \begin{pmatrix} x_i \\ y_i \end{pmatrix} - \begin{pmatrix} a_j \\ b_j \end{pmatrix} \right| - t_j - c^{-1} \left| \begin{pmatrix} a_j \\ b_j \end{pmatrix} \right| \\ &= c^{-1} \left\{ \left| \begin{pmatrix} x_i \\ y_i \end{pmatrix} - \begin{pmatrix} a_j \\ b_j \end{pmatrix} \right| - \left| \begin{pmatrix} a_j \\ b_j \end{pmatrix} \right| \right\} \end{aligned} \tag{6}$$

We now define the matrix of relative arrival times:

$$\Delta = \begin{pmatrix} d_{2,1} - d_{1,1} & d_{2,2} - d_{1,2} & \cdots & d_{2,M} - d_{1,M} \\ d_{3,1} - d_{1,1} & d_{3,2} - d_{1,2} & \cdots & d_{3,M} - d_{1,M} \\ \vdots & \vdots & \ddots & \vdots \\ d_{N,1} - d_{1,1} & d_{N,2} - d_{1,2} & \cdots & d_{N,M} - d_{1,M} \end{pmatrix} \tag{7}$$

This matrix Δ is of dimension $(N-1) \times M$.

2.4 Least Squares Formulation

The relative sensor locations X and the corresponding locations of the acoustic events A can now be recovered through the following least squares problem. This optimization seeks to identify X and A so as to minimize the quadratic difference between the predicted relative measurements and the actual measurements.

$$\langle A^*, X^* \rangle = \operatorname*{argmin}_{X,A} \sum_{i=2}^{N} \sum_{j=1}^{M} \left\{ \left| \begin{pmatrix} x_i \\ y_i \end{pmatrix} - \begin{pmatrix} a_j \\ b_j \end{pmatrix} \right| - \left| \begin{pmatrix} a_j \\ b_j \end{pmatrix} \right| - \Delta_{i,j} \right\}^2 \tag{8}$$

1355

The minimum of this expression is a maximum likelihood solution for the SFS problem under the assumption of iid Gaussian measurement noise.

If emission times are of interest, they are now easily recovered by the following weighted mean:

$$T^* = \frac{1}{N} \sum_{i=1}^{N} d_{i,j} - c \left| \begin{pmatrix} x_i \\ y_i \end{pmatrix} - \begin{pmatrix} a_j \\ b_j \end{pmatrix} \right| \tag{9}$$

The minimum of Eq. 8 is not unique. This is because any solution can be rotated around the origin of the coordinate system, and mirrored through any axis intersecting the origin. This shall not concern us, as we shall be content with *any* solution of Eq. 8; others are then easily generated.

What is of concern, however, is the fact that minimizing Eq. 8 is difficult. A straw man algorithm—which tends to work poorly in practice—involves starting with random guesses for X and A and then adjusting them in the direction of the negative gradient until convergence. As we shall show experimentally, such gradient algorithms work poorly in practice because of the large number of local minima.

3 The Far Field Approximation

The essence of our approximation pertains to the fact that for far range acoustic events— i.e., events that are (infinitely) far away from the sensor array—the incoming sound wave hits each sensor at the same incident angle. Put differently, the rays connecting the location of an acoustic event $(a_j \ b_j)$ with each of the perceiving sensors $(x_i \ y_i)$ are approximately parallel for all i (but *not* for all j!). Under the far field approximation, these incident angles are entirely parallel. Thus, all that matters are the incident angle of the acoustic events.

To derive an equation for this case, it shall prove convenient to write the Euclidean distance between a sensor and an acoustic event as a function of the incident angle α. This angle is given by the four-quadrant extension of the arctan function:

$$\alpha_{i,j} = \text{arctan2} \frac{b_j - y_i}{a_j - x_i} \tag{10}$$

The Euclidean distance between $(a_j \ b_j)$ and $(x_i \ y_i)$ can now be written as

$$\left| \begin{pmatrix} x_i \\ y_i \end{pmatrix} - \begin{pmatrix} a_j \\ b_j \end{pmatrix} \right| = (\cos \alpha_{i,j} \ \sin \alpha_{i,j}) \begin{pmatrix} a_j - x_i \\ b_j - y_i \end{pmatrix} \tag{11}$$

For far-away points $(a_j \ b_j)$, we can safely assume that all incident angles for the j-th acoustic event are identical:

$$\alpha_j := \alpha_{1,j} = \alpha_{2,j} = \ldots = \alpha_{N,j} \tag{12}$$

Hence we substitute α_j for $\alpha_{i,j}$ in Eq. 11. Plugging this back into Eq. 6, this gives us the following expression for $\Delta_{i,j}$:

$$\begin{aligned}
\Delta_{i,j} &= c^{-1} \left\{ \left| \begin{pmatrix} x_i \\ y_i \end{pmatrix} - \begin{pmatrix} a_j \\ b_j \end{pmatrix} \right| - \left| \begin{pmatrix} a_j \\ b_j \end{pmatrix} \right| \right\} \\
&\approx c^{-1} \left\{ (\cos \alpha_j \ \sin \alpha_j) \left[\begin{pmatrix} a_j - x_i \\ b_j - y_i \end{pmatrix} - \begin{pmatrix} a_j \\ b_j \end{pmatrix} \right] \right\} \\
&= c^{-1} (\cos \alpha_j \ \sin \alpha_j) \begin{pmatrix} x_i \\ y_i \end{pmatrix}
\end{aligned} \tag{13}$$

This leads to the following non-linear least squares problem for the desired sensor locations:

$$\langle X^*, \alpha_1^*, \ldots, \alpha_M^* \rangle = \underset{X, \alpha_1, \ldots, \alpha_M}{\text{argmin}} \left| X \begin{pmatrix} \cos \alpha_1 & \cos \alpha_2 & \cdots & \cos \alpha_M \\ \sin \alpha_1 & \sin \alpha_2 & \cdots & \sin \alpha_M \end{pmatrix} - \Delta \right|^2 \tag{14}$$

The reader many notice that in this formulation of the SFS problem, the locations of the sound events (a_j, b_j) have been replaced by α_j, the incident angles of the sound waves.

One might think of this as the "ortho-acoustic" model of sound propagation (in analogy to the orthographic camera model in computer vision). The ortho-acoustic projection reduces the number of variables in the optimization. However, the argument in the quadratic expression is still non-linear, due to the non-linear trigonometric functions involved.

4 Affine Solution for the Sensor Locations

Eq. 14 is trivially solvable in the space of *affine geometry*. Following [11], in affine geometry projections can be arbitrary linear functions, not just rotations and translations. Specifically, let us replace the specialized matrix

$$
\begin{pmatrix}
\cos \alpha_1 & \cos \alpha_2 & \cdots & \cos \alpha_M \\
\sin \alpha_1 & \sin \alpha_2 & \cdots & \sin \alpha_M
\end{pmatrix}
\tag{15}
$$

by a general $2 \times M$ matrix of the form

$$
\Gamma = \begin{pmatrix}
\gamma_{1,1} & \gamma_{1,2} & \cdots & \gamma_{1,M} \\
\gamma_{2,1} & \gamma_{2,2} & \cdots & \gamma_{2,M}
\end{pmatrix}
\tag{16}
$$

This leads to the least squares problem

$$
\langle X^*, \Gamma^* \rangle = \operatorname*{argmin}_{X, \Gamma} |X\Gamma - \Delta|^2
\tag{17}
$$

In the noise free-case case, we know that there must exist a X and a Γ for which $X\Gamma = \Delta$. This suggests that the rank of Δ should be 2, since it is the product of a matrix of size $(N-1) \times 2$ and a matrix of size $2 \times M$.

Further, we can recover both X and Γ via singular value decomposition (SVD). Specifically, we know that the matrix Δ can be decomposed as into three other matrices, U, V, and W:

$$
UVW^T = \operatorname{svd}(\Delta)
\tag{18}
$$

where U is a matrix of size $(N-1) \times 2$, V a diagonal matrix of eigenvalues of size 2×2, and W a matrix of size $M \times 2$. In practice, Δ might be of higher rank because of noise or because of violations of the far field assumption, but it suffices to restrict the consideration to the first two eigenvalues.

The decomposition in Eq. 18 leads to the optimal affine solution of the SFS problem:

$$
X = UV \qquad \text{and} \qquad \Gamma = W^T
\tag{19}
$$

However, this solution is not yet Euclidean, since Γ might not be of the form of Eq. 15. Specifically, Eq. 15 is a function of angles, and each row in Eq. 15 must be of the form $\cos^2 \gamma_j + \sin^2 \gamma_j = 1$. Clearly, this constraint is not enforced in the SVD.

However, there is an easy "trick" for recovering a X and Γ for which this constraint is at least approximately met. The key insight is that for any invertible 2×2 matrix C,

$$
X' = UVC^{-1} \qquad \text{and} \qquad \Gamma' = CW^T
\tag{20}
$$

is equally a solution to the factorization problem in Eq.18. This is because

$$
X'\Gamma' = UVC^{-1}CW^T = UVW^T = X\Gamma
\tag{21}
$$

The remaining search problem, thus, is the problem of finding an appropriate matrix C for which Γ' is of the form of Eq. 15. This is a *non-linear* optimization problem, but it is much lower-dimensional than the original SFS problem (it only involves 4 parameters!).

Specifically, we seek a C for which $\Gamma' = CW^T$ minimizes

$$
C^* = \operatorname*{argmin}_{C} \left| \underbrace{(1 \; 1) \, (\Gamma' \cdot \Gamma')}_{(*)} - (1 \; 1 \; \cdots \; 1) \right|^2
\tag{22}
$$

Here "·" denotes the dot product. The expression labeled $(*)$ evaluates to a vector of expressions of the form

$$
(\gamma_{1,1}^2 + \gamma_{2,1}^2 \quad \gamma_{1,2}^2 + \gamma_{2,2}^2 \quad \cdots \quad \gamma_{1,M}^2 + \gamma_{2,M}^2)
\tag{23}
$$

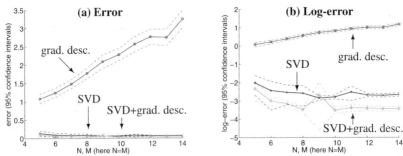

Figure 1: (a) Error and (b) log error for three different algorithms: gradient descent (red), SVD (blue), and SVD followed by gradient descent (green). Performance is shown for different values of N and M, with $N = M$. The plot also shows 95% confidence bars.

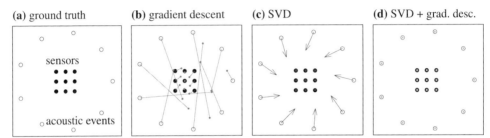

Figure 2: Typical SFS results for a simulated array of nine microphones spaced in a regular grid, surrounded by 9 sounds arranged on a circle. (a) Ground truth; (b) Result of plain gradient descent after convergence; the dashed lines visualize the residual error; (c) Result of the SVD with sound directions as indicated; and (d) Result of gradient descent initialized with our SVD result.

The minimization in Eq. 22 is carried out through standard gradient descent. It involves only 4 variables (C is of the size 2×2), and each single iteration is linear in $O(N + M)$ (instead of the $O(NM)$ constraints that define Eq. 8). In (tens of thousands of) experiments with synthetic noise-free data, we find empirically that gradient descent reliably converges to the globally optimal solution.

5   Recovering the Acoustic Event Locations and Emission Times

With regards to the acoustic events, the optimization for the far field case only yields the incident angles. In the near field setting, in which the incident angles tend to differ for different sensors, it may be desirable to recover the locations A of the acoustic event and the corresponding emission times T.

To determine these variables, we use the vector X^* from the far field case as mere starting points in a subsequent gradient search. The event location matrix A is initialized by selecting points sufficiently far away along the estimated incident angle for the far field approximation to be sound:

$$A \;=\; k\,\Gamma'^* \tag{24}$$

Here $\Gamma'^* = C^* W^T$ with C^* defined in Eq. 22, and k is a multiple of the diameter of the locations in X. With this initial guess for A, we apply gradient descent to optimize Eq. 8, and finally use Eq. 9 to recover T.

6   Experimental Results

We ran a series of simulation experiments to characterize the quality of our algorithm, especially in comparison with the obvious nonlinear least squares problem (Eq. 8) from which it is derived. Fig. 1 graphs the residual error as a function of the number of sensors

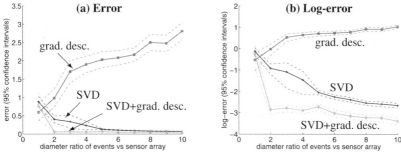

Figure 3: (a) Error and (b) log-error for three different algorithms (gradient descent in red, SVD in blue, and SVD followed by gradient descent in green), graphed here for varying distances of the sound events to the sensor array. An error above 2 means the reconstruction has entirely failed. All diagrams also show the 95% confidence intervals, and we set $N = M = 10$.

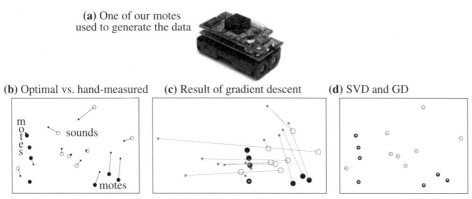

Figure 4: Results using our seven sensor motes as the sensor array, and a seventh mote to generate sound events. (a) A mote; (b) the globally optimal solution (big circles) compared to the hand-measures locations (small circles); (c) a typical result of vanilla gradient descent; and (d) the result of our approach, all compared to the optimal solution given the (noisy) data.

N and acoustic events M (here $N = M$). Panel (a) plots the regular error along with 95% confidence intervals, and panel (b) the corresponding log-error. Clearly, as N and M increase, plain gradient descent tends to diverge, whereas our approach converges. Each data point in these graphs was obtained by averaging 1,000 random configurations, in which sensors were sampled uniformly within an interval of 1×1m; sounds were placed at varying ranges, from 2m to 10m. An example outcome (for a non-random configuration!) is shown in Fig. 2. This figure plots (a) a simulated sensor array consisting of 9 sensors with 9 sound sources arranged in a circle; and (b)-(d) the resulting reconstructions of our three methods. For the SVD result shown in (c), only the directions of the incoming sounds are shown.

An interesting question pertains to the effect of the far field approximation in cases where it is clearly violated. To examine the robustness of our approach, we ran a series of experiments in which we varied the diameter of the acoustic events relative to the diameter of the sensors. If this parameter is 1, the acoustic events are emitted in the same region as the microphones; for values such as 10, the events are far away.

Fig. 3 graphs the residual errors and log-errors. The further away the acoustic events, the better our results. However, even for nearby events, for which the far field assumption is clearly invalid, our approach generates results that are no worse than those of the plain gradient descent technique.

We also implemented our approach using a physical sensor array. Fig. 4 plots empirical results using a microphone array comprised of seven Crossbow sensor motes, one of which is shown in Panel (a). Panels (b-d) compare the recovered structure with the one that globally minimizes the LMS error, which we obtain by running gradient descent using the hand-measured locations as starting point. Panel (a) in Fig. 4 shows the manually measured locations; the relatively high deviation to the LMS optimum is the result of measurement error, which is amplified by the fact that our motes are only spaced a few tens of centimeters apart from each other (the standard deviation in the timing error corresponds to a distance of 6.99cm, and the motes are placed between 14cm and 125cm apart). Panel (b) in Fig. 4 shows the solution of plain gradient descent applied to applied to Eq.8 and compares it to the optimal reconstruction; and Panel (c) illustrates our solution. In all plots the lines indicate residual error. This result shows that our method may work well on real-world data that is noisy and that does not adhere to the far field assumption.

7 Discussion

This paper considered the *structure from sound* problem and presented an algorithm for solving it. Our approach makes is possible to simultaneously recover the location of a collection of microphones, the locations of external acoustic events detected by these microphones, and the emission times for these events. By resorting to affine geometry, our approach overcomes the problem of local minima in the structure from sound problem.

There remain a number of open research issues. We believe the extension to 3-D is mathematically straightforward but requires empirical validation. The current approach also fails to address reverberation problems that are common in confined space. It shall further be interesting to investigate data association problems in the SFS framework, and to develop parallel algorithms that can be implemented on sensor networks with limited communication resources. Finally, of great interest should be the incomplete data case in which individual sensors may fail to detect acoustic events—a problem studied in [2].

Acknowledgement

The motes data was made available by Rahul Biswas, which is gratefully acknowledged. We also acknowledge invaluable suggestions by three anonymous reviewers.

References

[1] S.T. Birchfield and A. Subramanya. Microphone array position calibration by basis-point classical multidimensional scaling. *IEEE Trans. Speech and Audio Processing*, forthcoming.

[2] R. Biswas and S. Thrun. A passive approach to sensor network localization. IROS-04.

[3] J.C. Chen, R.E. Hudson, and K. Yao. Maximum likelihod source localization and unknown sensor location estimation for wideband signals in the near-field. *IEEE Trans. Signal Processing*, 50, 2002.

[4] P. Corke, S. Hrabar, R. Peterson, D. Rus, S. Saripalli, and G. Sukhatme. Deployment and connectivity repair of a sensor net with a flying robot. ISER-04.

[5] E. Elnahrawy, X. Li, and R. Martin. The limits of localization using signal strength: A comparative study. SECON-04.

[6] J. Elson and K. Romer. Wireless sensor networks: A new regime for time synchronization. HotNets-02.

[7] S. Mahamud and M. Hebert. Iterative projective reconstruction from multiple views. CVPR-00.

[8] D. Niculescu and B. Nath. Ad hoc positioning system (APS). GLOBECOM-01.

[9] V.C. Raykar, I.V. Kozintsev, and R. Lienhart. Position calibration of microphones and loudspeakers in distributed computing platforms. *IEEE transaction on Speech and Audio Processing*, 13(1), 2005.

[10] J. Sallai, G. Balogh, M. Maroti, and A. Ledeczi. Acoustic ranging in resource-constrained sensor networks. eCOTS-04.

[11] C. Tomasi and T. Kanade. Shape and motion from image streams under orthography: A factorization method. *IJCV*, 9(2), 1992.

[12] T.L. Tung, K. Yao, D. Chen, R.E. Hudson, and C.W. Reed. Source localization and spatial filtering using wideband music and maxiumum power beam forming for multimedia applications. In SIPS-99.

Predicting EMG Data from M1 Neurons with Variational Bayesian Least Squares

Jo-Anne Ting[1], Aaron D'Souza[1]
Kenji Yamamoto[3], Toshinori Yoshioka[2], Donna Hoffman[3]
Shinji Kakei[4], Lauren Sergio[6], John Kalaska[5]
Mitsuo Kawato[2], Peter Strick[3], Stefan Schaal[1,2]

[1]Comp. Science & Neuroscience, U.of S. California, Los Angeles, CA 90089, USA
[2]ATR Computational Neuroscience Laboratories, Kyoto 619-0288, Japan
[3]University of Pittsburgh, Pittsburgh, PA 15261, USA
[4]Tokyo Metropolitan Institute for Neuroscience, Tokyo 183-8526, Japan
[5]University of Montreal, Montreal, Canada H3C-3J7
[6]York University, Toronto, Ontario, Canada M3J1P3

Abstract

An increasing number of projects in neuroscience requires the statistical analysis of high dimensional data sets, as, for instance, in predicting behavior from neural firing or in operating artificial devices from brain recordings in brain-machine interfaces. Linear analysis techniques remain prevalent in such cases, but classical linear regression approaches are often numerically too fragile in high dimensions. In this paper, we address the question of whether EMG data collected from arm movements of monkeys can be faithfully reconstructed with linear approaches from neural activity in primary motor cortex (M1). To achieve robust data analysis, we develop a full Bayesian approach to linear regression that automatically detects and excludes irrelevant features in the data, regularizing against overfitting. In comparison with ordinary least squares, stepwise regression, partial least squares, LASSO regression and a brute force combinatorial search for the most predictive input features in the data, we demonstrate that the new Bayesian method offers a superior mixture of characteristics in terms of regularization against overfitting, computational efficiency and ease of use, demonstrating its potential as a drop-in replacement for other linear regression techniques. As neuroscientific results, our analyses demonstrate that EMG data can be well predicted from M1 neurons, further opening the path for possible real-time interfaces between brains and machines.

1 Introduction

In recent years, there has been growing interest in large scale analyses of brain activity with respect to associated behavioral variables. For instance, projects can be found in the area of brain-machine interfaces, where neural firing is directly used to control an artificial system like a robot [1, 2], to control a cursor on a computer screen via non-invasive brain signals [3] or to classify visual stimuli presented to a subject [4, 5]. In these projects, the brain signals to be processed are typically high dimensional, on the order of hundreds or thousands of inputs, with large numbers of redundant and irrelevant signals. Linear modeling techniques like linear regression are among the primary analysis tools [6, 7] for such data. However, the computational problem of data analysis involves not only data fitting, but requires that the model extracted from the data has good generalization properties. This is crucial for predicting behavior from future neural recordings, e.g., for continual on-line interpretation of brain activity to control prosthetic devices or for longitudinal scientific studies of information processing in the brain. Surprisingly, robust linear modeling of high dimensional data is non-trivial as the danger of fitting noise and encountering numerical problems is high. Classical techniques like ridge regression, stepwise regression or partial least squares regression are known to be prone to overfitting and require careful human supervision to ensure useful results.

In this paper, we will focus on how to improve linear data analysis for the high dimensional scenarios described above, with a view towards developing a statistically robust "black box" approach that automatically detects the most relevant input dimensions for generalization and excludes other dimensions in a statistically sound way. For this purpose, we investigate a full Bayesian treatment of linear regression with automatic relevance detection [8]. Such an algorithm, called Variational Bayesian Least Squares (VBLS), can be formulated in closed form with the help of a variational Bayesian approximation and turns out to be computationally highly efficient. We apply VBLS to the reconstruction of EMG data from motor cortical firing, using data sets collected by [9] and [10, 11]. This data analysis addresses important neuroscientific questions in terms of whether M1 neurons can directly predict EMG traces [12], whether M1 has a muscle-based topological organization and whether information in M1 should be used to predict behavior in future brain-machine interfaces. Our main focus in this paper, however, will be on the robust statistical analysis of these kinds of data. Comparisons with classical linear analysis techniques and a brute force combinatorial model search on a cluster computer demonstrate that our VBLS algorithm achieves the "black box" quality of a robust statistical analysis technique without any tunable parameters.

In the following sections, we will first sketch the derivation of Variational Bayesian Least Squares and subsequently perform extensive comparative data analysis of this technique in the context of prediction EMG data from M1 neural firing.

2 High Dimensional Regression

Before developing our VBLS algorithm, let us briefly revisit classical linear regression techniques. The standard model for linear regression is:

$$y = \sum_{m=1}^{d} b_m x_m + \epsilon \tag{1}$$

where $\mathbf{b}$ is the regression vector composed of b_m components, d is the number of input dimensions, ϵ is additive mean-zero noise, $\mathbf{x}$ are the inputs and y are the outputs. The Ordinary Least Squares (OLS) estimate of the regression vector is $\mathbf{b} = \left(\mathbf{X}^T\mathbf{X}\right)^{-1}\mathbf{X}^T\mathbf{y}$. The main problem with OLS regression in high dimensional input spaces is that the full rank assumption of $\left(\mathbf{X}^T\mathbf{X}\right)^{-1}$ is often violated due to underconstrained data sets. Ridge regression can "fix" such problems numerically, but introduces uncontrolled bias. Additionally, if the input dimensionality exceeds around 1000 dimensions, the matrix inversion can become prohibitively computationally expensive.

Several ideas exist how to improve over OLS. First, stepwise regression [13] can be employed. However, it has been strongly criticized for its potential for overfitting and its inconsistency in the presence of collinearity in the input data [14]. To

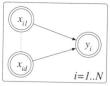
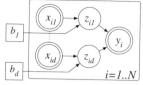
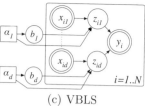

(a) Linear regression (b) Probabilistic backfitting (c) VBLS

Figure 1: Graphical Models for Linear Regression. Random variables are in circular nodes, observed random variables are in double circles and point estimated parameters are in square nodes.

deal with such collinearity directly, dimensionality reduction techniques like Principal Components Regression (PCR) and Factor Regression (FR) [15] are useful. These methods retain components in input space with large variance, regardless of whether these components influence the prediction [16], and can even eliminate low variance inputs that may have high predictive power for the outputs [17]. Another class of linear regression methods are projection regression techniques, most notably Partial Least Squares Regression (PLS) [18]. PLS performs computationally inexpensive $O(d)$ univariate regressions along projection directions, chosen according to the correlation between inputs and outputs. While slightly heuristic in nature, PLS is a surprisingly successful algorithm for ill-conditioned and high-dimensional regression problems, although it also has a tendency towards overfitting [16]. LASSO (Least Absolute Shrinkage and Selection Operator) regression [19] shrinks certain regression coefficients to 0, giving interpretable models that are sparse. However, a tuning parameter needs to be set, which can be done using n-fold cross-validation or manual hand-tuning. Finally, there are also more efficient methods for matrix inversion [20, 21], which, however, assume a well-condition regression problem a priori and degrade in the presence of collinearities in inputs.

In the following section, we develop a linear regression algorithm in a Bayesian framework that automatically regularizes against problems of overfitting. Moreover, the iterative nature of the algorithm, due to its formulation as an Expectation-Maximization problem [22], avoids the computational cost and numerical problems of matrix inversions. Thus, it addresses the two major problems of high-dimensional OLS simultaneously. Conceptually, the algorithm can be interpreted as a Bayesian version of either backfitting or partial least squares regression.

3 Variational Bayesian Least Squares

Figure 1 illustrates the progression of graphical models that we need in order to develop a robust Bayesian version of linear regression. Figure 1a depicts the standard linear regression model. In the spirit of PLS, if we knew an optimal projection direction of the input data, then the entire regression problem could be solved by a univariate regression between the projected data and the outputs. This optimal projection direction is simply the true gradient between inputs and outputs. In the tradition of EM algorithms [22], we encode this projection direction as a hidden variable, as shown in Figure 1b. The unobservable variables z_{im} (where $i = 1..N$ denotes the index into the data set of N data points) are the results of each input being multiplied with its corresponding component of the projection vector (i.e. b_m). Then, the z_{im} are summed up to form a predicted output y_i.

More formally, the linear regression model in Eq. (1) is modified to become:

$$z_{im} = b_m x_{im} \qquad\qquad y_i = \sum_{m=1}^{d} z_{im} + \epsilon$$

For a probabilistic treatment with EM, we make a standard normal assumption of all distributions in form of:

$$y_i|\mathbf{z}_i \sim \text{Normal}\left(y_i; \mathbf{1}^T\mathbf{z}_i, \psi_y\right) \qquad z_{im}|\mathbf{x}_i \sim \text{Normal}\left(z_{im}; b_m x_{im}, \psi_{zm}\right)$$

where $\mathbf{1} = [1, 1, .., 1]^T$. While this model is still identical to OLS, notice that in the graphical model, the regression coefficients b_m are behind the fan-in to the outputs y_i. Given the data $D = \{\mathbf{x}_i, y_i\}_{i=1}^N$, we can view this new regression model as an EM problem and maximize the incomplete log likelihood $\log p(\mathbf{y}|\mathbf{X})$ by maximizing the expected complete log likelihood $\langle \log p(\mathbf{y}, \mathbf{Z}|\mathbf{X}) \rangle$:

$$\log p(\mathbf{y}, \mathbf{Z}|\mathbf{X}) = -\frac{N}{2}\log \psi_y - \frac{1}{2\psi_y}\sum_{i=1}^N \left(y_i - \mathbf{1}^T\mathbf{z}_i\right)^2 - \frac{N}{2}\sum_{m=1}^d \log \psi_{zm}$$
$$- \sum_{m=1}^d \frac{1}{2\psi_{zm}}\left(z_{im} - b_m x_{im}\right)^2 + \text{const} \qquad (2)$$

where $\mathbf{Z}$ denotes the N by d matrix of all z_{im}. The resulting EM updates require standard manipulations of normal distributions and result in:

M-step :

$$b_m = \frac{\sum_{i=1}^N \langle z_{im}\rangle x_{im}}{\sum_{i=1}^N x_{im}^2}$$

$$\psi_y = \frac{1}{N}\sum_{i=1}^N \left(y_i - \mathbf{1}^T\langle\mathbf{z}_i\rangle\right)2 + \mathbf{1}^T\mathbf{\Sigma}_z\mathbf{1}$$

$$\psi_{zm} = \frac{1}{N}\sum_{i=1}^N \left(\langle z_{im}\rangle - b_m x_{im}\right)^2 + \sigma_{zm}^2$$

E-step :

$$\mathbf{1}^T\mathbf{\Sigma}_z\mathbf{1} = \left(\sum_{m=1}^d \psi_{zm}\right)\left[1 - \frac{1}{s}\left(\sum_{m=1}^d \psi_{zm}\right)\right]$$

$$\sigma_{zm}^2 = \psi_{zm}\left(1 - \frac{1}{s}\psi_{zm}\right)$$

$$\langle z_{im}\rangle = b_m\mathbf{x}_i + \frac{1}{s}\psi_{zm}\left(y_i - \mathbf{b}^T\mathbf{x}_i\right)$$

where we define $s = \psi_y + \sum_{m=1}^d \psi_{xm}$ and $\mathbf{\Sigma}_z = \text{Cov}(\mathbf{z}|\mathbf{y}, \mathbf{X})$. It is very important to note that one EM update has a computationally complexity of $O(d)$, where d is the number of input dimensions, instead of the $O(d^3)$ associated with OLS regression. This efficiency comes at the cost of an iterative solution, instead of a one-shot solution for $\mathbf{b}$ as in OLS. It can be proved that this EM version of least squares regression is guaranteed to converge to the same solution as OLS [23].

This new EM algorithm appears to only replace the matrix inversion in OLS by an iterative method, as others have done with alternative algorithms [20, 21], although the convergence guarantees of EM are an improvement over previous approaches. The true power of this probabilistic formulation, though, becomes apparent when we add a Bayesian layer that achieves the desired robustness in face of ill-conditioned data.

3.1 Automatic Relevance Determination

From a Bayesian point of view, the parameters b_m should be treated probabilistically so that we can integrate them out to safeguard against overfitting. For this purpose, as shown in Figure 1c, we introduce precision variables α_m over each regression parameter b_m:

$$p(\mathbf{b}|\boldsymbol{\alpha}) = \prod_{m=1}^d \left(\frac{\alpha_m}{2\pi}\right)^{\frac{1}{2}}\exp\left\{-\frac{\alpha_m}{2}b_m^2\right\}$$
$$p(\boldsymbol{\alpha}) = \prod_{m=1}^d \frac{b_\alpha^{a_\alpha}}{\text{Gamma}(a_\alpha)}\alpha_m^{(a_\alpha-1)}\exp\left\{-b_\alpha\alpha_m\right\} \qquad (3)$$

where $\boldsymbol{\alpha}$ is the vector of all α_m. In order to obtain a tractable posterior distribution over all hidden variables $\mathbf{b}$, z_{im} and $\boldsymbol{\alpha}$, we use a factorial variational approximation of the true posterior $Q(\boldsymbol{\alpha}, \mathbf{b}, \mathbf{Z}) = Q(\boldsymbol{\alpha}, \mathbf{b})Q(\mathbf{Z})$. Note that the connection from the α_m to the corresponding z_{im} in Figure 1c is an intentional design. Under this graphical model, the marginal distribution of b_m becomes a Student t-distribution that allows traditional hypothesis testing [24]. The minimal factorization of the posterior into $Q(\boldsymbol{\alpha}, \mathbf{b})Q(\mathbf{Z})$ would not be possible without this special design.

The resulting augmented model has the following distributions:

$$y_i|\mathbf{z}_i \sim N(y_i; \mathbf{1}^T\mathbf{z}_i, \psi_y) \qquad\qquad b_m|\alpha_m \sim N(w_{bm}; 0, 1/\alpha_m)$$
$$z_{im}|b_m, \alpha_m x_{im} \sim N(z_{im}; b_m x_{im}, \psi_{zm}/\alpha_m) \qquad\qquad \alpha_m \sim \text{Gamma}(\alpha_m; a_\alpha, b_\alpha)$$

We now have a mechanism that infers the significance of each dimension's contribution to the observed output y. Since b_m is zero mean, a very large α_m (equivalent to a very small variance of b_m) suggests that b_m is very close to 0 and has no contribution to the output. An EM-like algorithm [25] can be used to find the posterior updates of all distributions. We omit the EM update equations due to space constraints as they are similar to the EM update above and only focus on the posterior update for b_m and α:

$$\sigma^2_{b_m|\alpha_m} = \frac{\psi_{zm}}{\alpha_m} \left(\sum_{i=1}^{N} x^2_{im} + \psi_{zm} \right)^{-1}$$

$$\langle b_m|\alpha_m \rangle = \left(\sum_{i=1}^{N} x^2_{im} + \psi_{zm} \right)^{-1} \left(\sum_{i=1}^{N} \langle z_{im} \rangle x_{im} \right)$$

$$\hat{a}_\alpha = a_\alpha + \frac{N}{2} \qquad (4)$$

$$\hat{b}_\alpha^{(m)} = b_\alpha + \frac{1}{2\psi_{zm}} \left\{ \sum_{i=1}^{N} \langle z^2_{im} \rangle - \left(\sum_{i=1}^{N} x^2_{im} + \psi_{zm} \right)^{-1} \left(\sum_{i=1}^{N} \langle z_{im} \rangle x_{im} \right)^2 \right\}$$

Note that the update equation for $\langle b_m|\alpha_m \rangle$ can be rewritten as:

$$\langle b_m|\alpha_m \rangle^{(n+1)} = \left(\frac{\sum_{i=1}^{N} x^2_{im}}{\sum_{i=1}^{N} x^2_{im} + \psi_{zm}} \right) \langle b_m|\alpha_m \rangle^{(n)} + \frac{\psi_{zm}}{s\alpha_m} \frac{\sum_{i=1}^{N} \left(y_i - \langle \mathbf{b}|\alpha \rangle^{(n)T} \mathbf{x}_i \right) x_{im}}{\sum_{i=1}^{N} x^2_{im} + \psi_{zm}} \qquad (5)$$

Eq. (5) demonstrates that in the absence of a correlation between the current input dimension and the residual error, the first term causes the current regression coefficient to decay. The resulting regression solution regularizes over the number of retained inputs in the final regression vector, performing a functionality similar to Automatic Relevance Determination (ARD) [8]. The update equations' algorithmic complexity remains $O(d)$. One can further show that the marginal distribution of all b_m is a t-distribution with $t = \langle b_m|\alpha_m \rangle / \sigma_{b_m|\alpha_m}$ and $2\hat{a}_\alpha$ degrees of freedom, which allows a principled way of determining whether a regression coefficient was excluded by means of standard hypothesis testing. Thus, Variational Bayesian Least Squares (VBLS) regression is a full Bayesian treatment of the linear regression problem.

4 Evaluation

We now turn to the application and evaluation of VBLS in the context of predicting EMG data from neural data recorded in M1 of monkeys. The key questions addressed in this application were i) whether EMG data can be reconstructed accurately with good generalization, ii) how many neurons contribute to the reconstruction of each muscle and iii) how well the VBLS algorithm compares to other analysis techniques. The underlying assumption of this analysis is that the relationship between neural firing and muscle activity is approximately linear.

4.1 Data sets

We investigated data from two different experiments. In the first experiment by Sergio & Kalaska [9], the monkey moved a manipulandum in a center-out task in eight different directions, equally spaced in a horizontal planar circle of 8cm radius. A variation of this experiment held the manipulandum rigidly in place, while the monkey applied isometric forces in the same eight directions. In both conditions, movement or force, feedback was given through visual display on a monitor. Neural activity for 71 M1 neurons was recorded in all conditions (2400 data points for each neuron), along with the EMG outputs of 11 muscles.

The second experiment by Kakei et al. [10] involved a monkey trained to perform eight different combinations of wrist flexion-extension and radial-ulnar movements while in three different arm postures (pronated, supinated and midway between the two). The data set consisted of neural data of 92 M1 neurons that were recorded

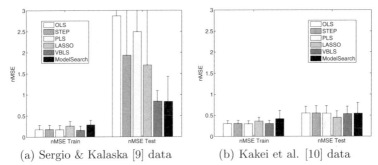

(a) Sergio & Kalaska [9] data　　　　　(b) Kakei et al. [10] data

Figure 2: Normalized mean squared error for Cross-validation Sets (6-fold for [10] and 8-fold for [9])

	VBLS	PLS	STEP	LASSO
Sergio & Kalaska data set	93.6%	7.44%	8.71%	8.42%
Kakei et al. data set	87.1%	40.1%	72.3%	76.3%

Table 1: Percentage neuron matches between baseline and all other algorithms, averaged over all muscles in the data set

at all three wrist postures (producing 2664 data points for each neuron) and the EMG outputs of 7 contributing muscles. In all experiments, the neural data was represented as average firing rates and was time aligned with EMG data based on analyses that are outside of the scope of this paper.

4.2 Methods

For the Sergio & Kalaska data set, a baseline comparison of good EMG reconstruction was obtained through a limited combinatorial search over possible regression models. A particular model is characterized by a subset of neurons that is used to predict the EMG data. Given 71 neurons, theoretically 2^{71} possible models exist. This value is too large for an exhaustive search. Therefore, we considered only possible combinations of up to 20 neurons, which required several weeks of computation on a 30-node cluster computer. The optimal predictive subset of neurons was determined from an 8-fold cross validation. This baseline study served as a comparison for PLS, stepwise regression, LASSO regression, OLS and VBLS. The five other algorithms used the same validation sets employed in the baseline study. The number of PLS projections for each data fit was found by leave-one-out cross-validation. Stepwise regression used Matlab's "stepwisefit" function. LASSO regression was implemented, manually choosing the optimal tuning parameter over all cross-validation sets. OLS was implemented using a small ridge regression parameter of 10^{-10} in order to avoid ill-conditioned matrix inversions.

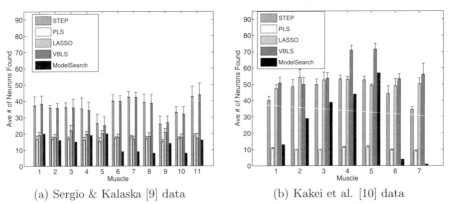

(a) Sergio & Kalaska [9] data　　　　　(b) Kakei et al. [10] data

Figure 3: Average Number of Relevant Neurons found over Cross-validation Sets (6-fold for [10] and 8-fold for [9])

1366

The average number of relevant neurons was calculated over all 8 cross-validation sets and a final set of relevant neurons was reached for each algorithm by taking the common neurons found to be relevant over the 8 cross-validation sets. Inference of relevant neurons in PLS was based on the subspace spanned by the PLS projections, while relevant neurons in VBLS were inferred from t-tests on the regression parameters, using a significance of $p < 0.05$. Stepwise regression and LASSO regression determined the number of relevant neurons from the inputs that were included in the final model. Note that since OLS retained all input dimensions, this algorithm was omitted in relevant neuron comparisons.

Analogous to the first data set, a combinatorial analysis was performed on the Kakei et al. data set in order to determine the optimal set of neurons contributing to each muscle (i.e. producing the lowest possible prediction error) in a 6-fold cross-validation. PLS, stepwise regression, LASSO regression, OLS and VBLS were applied using the same cross-validation sets, employing the same procedure described for the first data set.

4.3 Results

Figure 2 shows that, in general, EMG traces seem to be well predictable from M1 neural firing. VBLS resulted in a generalization error comparable to that produced by the baseline study. In the Kakei et al. dataset, all algorithms performed similarly, with LASSO regression performing a little better than the rest. However, OLS, stepwise regression, LASSO regression and PLS performed far worse on the Sergio & Kalaska dataset, with OLS regression attaining the worst error. Such performance is typical for traditional linear regression methods on ill-conditioned high dimensional data, motivating the development of VBLS. The average number of relevant neurons found by VBLS was slightly higher than the baseline study, as seen in Figure 3. This result is not surprising as the baseline study did not consider all possible combination of neurons. Given the good generalization results of VBLS, it seems that the Bayesian approach regularized the participating neurons sufficiently so that no overfitting occurred. Note that the results for muscle 6 and 7 in Figure 3b seem to be due to some irregularities in the data and should be considered outliers. Table 1 demonstrates that the relevant neurons identified by VBLS coincided at a very high percentage with those of the baseline results, while PLS, stepwise regression and LASSO regression had inferior outcomes.

Thus, in general, VBLS achieved comparable performance with the baseline study when reconstructing EMG data from M1 neurons. While VBLS is an iterative statistical method, which performs slower than classical "one-shot" linear least squares methods (i.e., on the order of several minutes for the data sets in our analyses), it achieved comparable results with our combinatorial model search, which took weeks on a cluster computer.

5 Discussion

This paper addressed the problem of analyzing high dimensional data with linear regression techniques, as encountered in neuroscience and the new field of brain-machine interfaces. To achieve robust statistical results, we introduced a novel Bayesian technique for linear regression analysis with automatic feature detection, called Variational Bayesian Least Squares. Comparisons with classical linear regression methods and a "gold standard" obtained from a brute force search over all possible linear models demonstrate that VBLS performs very well without any manual parameter tuning, such that it has the quality of a "black box" statistical analysis technique.

A point of concern against the VBLS algorithm is how the variational approximation in this algorithm affects the quality of function approximation. It is known that factorial approximations to a joint distribution create more peaked distributions, such that one could potentially assume that VBLS might tend to overfit. However, in the case of VBLS, a more peaked distribution over b_m pushes the regression parameter closer to zero. Thus, VBLS will be on the slightly pessimistic side of function fitting and is unlikely to overfit. Future evaluations and comparisons with Markov Chain Monte Carlo methods will reveal more details of the nature of the variational approximation. Regardless, it appears that VBLS could become a useful drop-in replacement for various classical regression methods. It lends itself to incremental implementation as would be needed in real-time analyses of brain information.

Acknowledgments

This research was supported in part by National Science Foundation grants ECS-0325383, IIS-0312802, IIS-0082995, ECS-0326095, ANI-0224419, a NASA grant AC#98 − 516, an AFOSR grant on Intelligent Control, the ERATO Kawato Dynamic Brain Project funded by the Japanese Science and Technology Agency, the ATR Computational Neuroscience Laboratories and by funds from the Veterans Administration Medical Research Service.

References

[1] M.A. Nicolelis. Actions from thoughts. *Nature*, 409:403–407, 2001.

[2] D.M. Taylor, S.I. Tillery, and A.B. Schwartz. Direct cortical control of 3d neuroprosthetic devices. *Science*, 296:1829–1932, 2002.

[3] J.R. Wolpaw and D.J. McFarland. Control of a two-dimensional movement signal by a noninvasive brain-computer interface in humans. *Proceedings of the National Academy of Sciences*, 101:17849–17854, 2004.

[4] Y. Kamitani and F. Tong. Decoding the visual and subjective contents of the human brain. *Nature Neuroscience*, 8:679, 2004.

[5] J.D. Haynes and G. Rees. Predicting the orientation of invisible stimuli from activity in human primary visual cortex. *Nature Neuroscience*, 8:686, 2005.

[6] J. Wessberg and M.A. Nicolelis. Optimizing a linear algorithm for real-time robotic control using chronic cortical ensemble recordings in monkeys. *Journal of Cognitive Neuroscience*, 16:1022–1035, 2004.

[7] S. Musallam, B.D. Corneil, B. Greger, H. Scherberger, and R.A. Andersen. Cognitive control signals for neural prosthetics. *Science*, 305:258–262, 2004.

[8] R.M. Neal. *Bayesian learning for neural networks*. PhD thesis, Dept. of Computer Science, University of Toronto, 1994.

[9] L.E. Sergio and J.F. Kalaska. Changes in the temporal pattern of primary motor cortex activity in a directional isometric force versus limb movement task. *Journal of Neurophysiology*, 80:1577–1583, 1998.

[10] S. Kakei, D.S. Hoffman, and P.L. Strick. Muscle and movement representations in the primary motor cortex. *Science*, 285:2136–2139, 1999.

[11] S. Kakei, D.S. Hoffman, and P.L. Strick. Direction of action is represented in the ventral premotor cortex. *Nature Neuroscience*, 4:1020–1025, 2001.

[12] E. Todorov. Direct cortical control of muscle activation in voluntary arm movements: a model. *Nature Neuroscience*, 3:391–398, 2000.

[13] N. R. Draper and H. Smith. *Applied Regression Analysis*. Wiley, 1981.

[14] S. Derksen and H.J. Keselman. Backward, forward and stepwise automated subset selection algorithms: Frequency of obtaining authentic and noise variables. *British Journal of Mathematical and Statistical Psychology*, 45:265–282, 1992.

[15] W.F. Massey. Principal component regression in exploratory statistical research. *Journal of the American Statistical Association*, 60:234–246, 1965.

[16] S. Schaal, S. Vijayakumar, and C.G. Atkeson. Local dimensionality reduction. In M.I. Jordan, M.J. Kearns, and S.A. Solla, editors, *Advances in Neural Information Processing Systems*. MIT Press, 1998.

[17] I.E. Frank and J.H. Friedman. A statistical view of some chemometric regression tools. *Technometrics*, 35:109–135, 1993.

[18] H. Wold. Soft modeling by latent variables: The nonlinear iterative partial least squares approach. In J. Gani, editor, *Perspectives in probability and statistics, papers in honor of M. S. Bartlett*. Academic Press, 1975.

[19] R. Tibshirani. Regression shrinkage and selection via the lasso. *Journal of Royal Statistical Society, Series B*, 58(1):267–288, 1996.

[20] V. Strassen. Gaussian elimination is not optimal. *Num Mathematik*, 13:354–356, 1969.

[21] T. J. Hastie and R. J. Tibshirani. *Generalized additive models*. Number 43 in Monographs on Statistics and Applied Probability. Chapman and Hall, 1990.

[22] A. Dempster, N. Laird, and D. Rubin. Maximum likelihood from incomplete data via the em algorithm. *Journal of Royal Statistical Society. Series B*, 39(1):1–38, 1977.

[23] A. D'Souza, S. Vijayakumar, and S. Schaal. The bayesian backfitting relevance vector machine. In *Proceedings of the 21st International Conference on Machine Learning*. ACM Press, 2004.

[24] A. Gelman, J. Carlin, H.S. Stern, and D.B. Rubin. *Bayesian Data Analaysis*. Chapman and Hall, 2000.

[25] Z. Ghahramani and M.J. Beal. Graphical models and variational methods. In D. Saad and M. Opper, editors, *Advanced Mean Field Methods - Theory and Practice*. MIT Press, 2000.

Generalization error bounds for classifiers trained with interdependent data

Nicolas Usunier, Massih-Reza Amini, Patrick Gallinari
Department of Computer Science, University of Paris VI
8, rue du Capitaine Scott, 75015 Paris France
{usunier, amini, gallinari}@poleia.lip6.fr

Abstract

In this paper we propose a general framework to study the generalization properties of binary classifiers trained with data which may be dependent, but are deterministically generated upon a sample of independent examples. It provides generalization bounds for binary classification and some cases of ranking problems, and clarifies the relationship between these learning tasks.

1 Introduction

Many machine learning (ML) applications deal with the problem of *bipartite ranking* where the goal is to find a function which orders relevant elements over irrelevant ones. Such problems appear for example in Information Retrieval, where the system returns a list of documents, ordered by relevancy to the user's demand. The criterion widely used to measure the ranking quality is the Area Under the ROC Curve (AUC) [6]. Given a training set $S = ((x_p, y_p))_{p=1}^{n}$ with $y_p \in \{\pm 1\}$, its optimization over a class of real valued functions $\mathcal{G}$ can be carried out by finding a classifier of the form $c_g(x, x') = sign(g(x) - g(x')), g \in \mathcal{G}$ which minimizes the error rate over pairs of examples $(x, 1)$ and $(x', -1)$ in S [6]. More generally, it is well-known that the learning of scoring functions can be expressed as a classification task over pairs of examples [7, 5].

The study of the generalization properties of ranking problems is a challenging task, since the pairs of examples violate the central i.i.d. assumption of binary classification. Using task-specific studies, this issue has recently been the focus of a large amount of work. [2] showed that SVM-like algorithms optimizing the AUC have good generalization guarantees, and [11] showed that maximizing the margin of the pairs, defined by the quantity $g(x) - g(x')$, leads to the minimization of the generalization error. While these results suggest some similarity between the classification of the pairs of examples and the classification of independent data, no common framework has been established. As a major drawback, it is not possible to directly deduce results for ranking from those obtained in classification.

In this paper, we present a new framework to study the generalization properties of classifiers over data which can exhibit a suitable dependency structure. Among others, the problems of binary classification, bipartite ranking, and the *ranking risk* defined in [5] are special cases of our study. It shows that it is possible to infer generalization bounds for classifiers trained over interdependent examples using generalization results known for binary classification. We illustrate this property by proving a new margin-based, data-dependent bound for SVM-like algorithms optimizing the AUC. This bound derives straightforwardly from the same kind of bounds for SVMs for classification given in [12]. Since learning algorithms aim at minimizing the generalization error of their chosen hypothesis, our results suggest that the design of bipartite ranking algorithms can follow the design of standard classification learning systems.

The remainder of this paper is as follows. In section 2, we give the formal definition of our framework and detail the progression of our analysis over the paper. In section 3, we present a new concentration inequality which allows to extend the notion of Rademacher complexity (section 4), and, in section 5, we prove generalization bounds for binary classification and bipartite ranking tasks under our framework. Finally, the missing proofs are given in a longer version of the paper [13].

2   Formal framework

We distinguish between the *input* and the *training* data. The input data $S = (s_p)_{p=1}^n$ is a set of n independent examples, while the training data $Z = (z_i)_{i=1}^N$ is composed of N binary classified elements where each z_i is in $\mathcal{X}_{tr} \times \{-1, +1\}$, with $\mathcal{X}_{tr}$ the space of characteristics. For example, in the general case of bipartite ranking, the *input data* is the set of elements to be ordered, while the *training data* is constituted by the pairs of examples to be classified. The purpose of this work is the study of generalization properties of classifiers trained using a possibly dependent *training data*, but in the special case where the latter is deterministically generated from the *input data*. The aim here is to select a hypothesis $h \in \mathcal{H} = \{h_\theta : \mathcal{X}_{tr} \to \{-1, 1\} | \theta \in \Theta\}$ which optimizes the empirical risk $L(h, Z) = \frac{1}{N} \sum_{i=1}^N \ell(h, z_i)$, ℓ being the instantaneous loss of h, over the training set Z.

Definition 1 (Classifiers trained with interdependent data). *A classification algorithm over interdependent training data takes as input data a set $S = (s_p)_{p=1}^n$ supposed to be drawn according to an unknown product distribution $\otimes_{p=1}^n \mathcal{D}_p$ over a product sample space $\mathcal{S}^n$[1], outputs a binary classifier chosen in a hypothesis space $\mathcal{H} : \{h : \mathcal{X}_{tr} \to \{+1, -1\}\}$, and has a two-step learning process. In a first step, the learner applies to its input data S a fixed function $\varphi : \mathcal{S}^n \to (\mathcal{X}_{tr} \times \{-1, 1\})^N$ to generate a vector $Z = (z_i)_{i=1}^N = \varphi(S)$ of N training examples $z_i \in \mathcal{X}_{tr} \times \{-1, 1\}, i = 1, ..., N$. In the second step, the learner runs a classification algorithm in order to obtain h which minimizes the empirical classification loss $L(h, Z)$, over its training data $Z = \varphi(S)$.*

Examples   Using the notations above, when $\mathcal{S} = \mathcal{X}_{tr} \times \{\pm 1\}$, $n = N$, φ is the identity function and S is drawn i.i.d. according to an unknown distribution $\mathcal{D}$, we recover the classical definition of a binary classification algorithm. Another example is the ranking task described in [5] where $\mathcal{S} = \mathcal{X} \times \mathbb{R}$, $\mathcal{X}_{tr} = \mathcal{X}^2$, $N = n(n-1)$ and, given $S = ((x_p, y_p))_{p=1}^n$ drawn i.i.d. according to a fixed $\mathcal{D}$, φ generates all the pairs $((x_k, x_l), sign(\frac{y_k - y_l}{2})), k \neq l$.

In the remaining of the paper, we will prove generalization error bounds of the selected hypothesis by upper bounding

$$\sup_{h \in \mathcal{H}} L(h) - L(h, \varphi(S)) \tag{1}$$

with high confidence over S, where $L(h) = \mathbb{E}_S L(h, \varphi(S))$. To this end we decompose $Z = \varphi(S)$ using the dependency graph of the random variables composing Z with a technique similar to the one proposed by [8]. We go towards this result by first bounding

---

[1]It is equivalent to say that the *input data* is a vector of independent, but not necessarily identically distributed random variables.

$\sup_{q \in \mathcal{Q}} \left[\mathbb{E}_{\tilde{S}} \frac{1}{N} \sum_{i=1}^{N} q(\varphi(\tilde{S})_i) - \frac{1}{N} \sum_{i=1}^{N} q(\varphi(S)_i) \right]$ with high confidence over samples S, where $\tilde{S}$ is also drawn according to $\otimes_{p=1}^{n} \mathcal{D}_p$, $\mathcal{Q}$ is a class of functions taking values in $[0, 1]$, and $\varphi(S)_i$ denotes the i-th training example (Theorem 4). This bound uses an extension of the Rademacher complexity [3], the fractional Rademacher complexity (FRC) (definition 3), which is a weighted sum of Rademacher complexities over independent subsets of the training data. We show that the FRC of an arbitrary class of real-valued functions can be trivially computed given the Rademacher complexity of this class of functions and φ (theorem 6). This theorem shows that generalization error bounds for classes of classifiers over interdependent data (in the sense of definition 1) trivially follows from the same kind of bounds for the same class of classifiers trained over i.i.d. data. Finally, we show an example of the derivation of a margin-based, data-dependent generalization error bound (i.e. a bound on equation (1) which can be computed on the training data) for the bipartite ranking case when $\mathcal{H} = \{(x, x') \mapsto sign(K(\theta, x) - K(\theta, x')) | K(\theta, \theta) \le B^2\}$, assuming that the input examples are drawn i.i.d. according to a distribution $\mathcal{D}$ over $\mathcal{X} \times \{\pm 1\}$, $\mathcal{X} \subset \mathbb{R}^d$ and K is a kernel over $\mathcal{X}^2$.

Notations Throughout the paper, we will use the notations of the preceding subsection, except for $Z = (z_i)_{i=1}^{N}$, which will denote an arbitrary element of $(\mathcal{X}_{tr} \times \{-1, 1\})^N$. In order to obtain the dependency graph of the random variables $\varphi(S)_i$, we will consider, for each $1 \le i \le N$, a set $[i] \subset \{1, ..., n\}$ such that $\varphi(S)_i$ depends only on the variables $s_p \in S$ for which $p \in [i]$. Using these notations, if we consider two indices k, l in $\{1, ..., N\}$, we can notice that the two random variables $\varphi(S)_k$ and $\varphi(S)_l$ are independent if and only if $[k] \cap [l] = \emptyset$. The dependency graph of the $\varphi(S)_i$s follows, by constructing the graph $\Gamma(\varphi)$, with the set of vertices $V = \{1, ..., N\}$, and with an edge between k and l if and only if $[k] \cap [l] \ne \emptyset$. The following definitions, taken from [8], will enable us to separate the set of partly dependent variables into sets of independent variables:

- A subset A of V is independent if all the elements in A are independent.
- A sequence $\mathcal{C} = (C_j)_{j=1}^{m}$ of subsets of V is a proper cover of V if, for all j, C_j is independent, and $\bigcup_j C_j = V$
- A sequence $\mathcal{C} = (C_j, w_j)_{j=1}^{m}$ is a proper, exact fractional cover of Γ if $w_j > 0$ for all j, and, for each $i \in V$, $\sum_{j=1}^{m} w_j \mathbf{I}_{C_j}(i) = 1$, where $\mathbf{I}_{C_j}$ is the indicator function of C_j.
- The fractional chromatic number of Γ, noted $\chi(\Gamma)$, is equal to the minimum of $\sum_j w_j$ over all proper, exact fractional cover.

It is to be noted that from lemma 3.2 of [8], the existence of proper, exact fractional covers is ensured. Since Γ is fully determined by the function φ, we will note $\chi(\Gamma) = \chi(\varphi)$. Moreover, we will denote by $\mathcal{C}(\varphi) = (C_j, w_j)_{j=1}^{m}$ a proper, exact fractional cover of Γ such that $\sum_j w_j = \chi(\varphi)$. Finally, for a given $\mathcal{C}(\varphi)$, we denote by κ_j the number of elements in C_j, and we fix the notations: $C_j = \{C_{j1}, ..., C_{j\kappa_j}\}$. It is to be noted that if $(t_i)_{i=1}^{N} \in \mathbb{R}^N$, and $\mathcal{C}(\varphi) = (C_j, w_j)_{j=1}^{\kappa}$, lemma 3.1 of [8] states that:

$$\sum_{i=1}^{N} t_i = \sum_{j=1}^{\kappa} w_j T_j, \text{ where } T_j = \sum_{k=1}^{\kappa_j} t_{C_j k} \tag{2}$$

3   A new concentration inequality

Concentration inequalities bound the probability that a random variable deviates *too much* from its expectation (see [4] for a survey). They play a major role in learning theory as they can be used for example to bound the probability of deviation of the expected loss of a function from its empirical value estimated over a sample set. A well-known inequality is McDiarmid's theorem [9] for independent random variables, which bounds the probability of deviation from its expectation of an arbitrary function with bounded variations over each one of its parameters. While this theorem is very general, [8] proved a large deviation bound for sums of partly random variables where the dependency structure of the variables is known, which can be tighter in some cases. Since we also consider variables with known dependency structure, using such results may lead to tighter bounds. However, we will bound functions like in equation (1), which do not write as a sum of partly dependent variables. Thus, we need a result on more general functions than sums of random variables, but which also takes into account the known dependency structure of the variables.

Theorem 2. *Let* $\varphi : \mathcal{X}^n \rightarrow \mathcal{X}'^N$. *Using the notations defined above, let* $\mathcal{C}(\varphi) = (C_j, w_j)_{j=1}^{\kappa}$. *Let* $f : \mathcal{X}'^N \rightarrow \mathbb{R}$ *such that:*

1. *There exist* κ *functions* $f_j : \mathcal{X}'^{\kappa_j} \rightarrow \mathbb{R}$ *which satisfy* $\forall Z = (z_1, ..., z_N) \in \mathcal{X}'^N$, $f(Z) = \sum_j w_j f_j(z_{C_{j1}}, ..., z_{C_{j\kappa_j}})$.

2. *There exist* $\beta_1, ..., \beta_N \in \mathbb{R}_+$ *such that* $\forall j, \forall Z_j, Z_j^k \in \mathcal{X}'^{\kappa_j}$ *such that* Z_j *and* Z_j^k *differ only in the* k-*th dimension,* $|f_j(Z_j) - f_j(Z_j^k)| \leq \beta_{C_{jk}}$.

Let finally $\mathcal{D}_1, ..., \mathcal{D}_n$ *be* n *probability distributions over* $\mathcal{X}$. *Then, we have:*

$$\mathbb{P}_{X \sim \otimes_{i=1}^n \mathcal{D}_i}(f \circ \varphi(X) - \mathbb{E}f \circ \varphi > \epsilon) \leq \exp(-\frac{2\epsilon^2}{\chi(\varphi)\sum_{i=1}^N \beta_i^2}) \quad (3)$$

and the same holds for $\mathbb{P}(\mathbb{E}f \circ \varphi - f \circ \varphi > \epsilon)$.

The proof of this theorem (given in [13]) is a variation of the demonstrations in [8] and McDiarmid's theorem. The main idea of this theorem is to allow the decomposition of f, which will take as input partly dependent random variables when applied to $\varphi(S)$, into a sum of functions which, when considering $f \circ \varphi(S)$, will be functions of independent variables. As we will see, this theorem will be the major tool in our analysis. It is to be noted that when $\mathcal{X} = \mathcal{X}'$, $N = n$ and φ is the identity function of $\mathcal{X}^n$, the theorem 2 is exactly McDiarmid's theorem. On the other hand, when f takes the form $\sum_{i=1}^N q_i(z_i)$ with for all $z \in \mathcal{X}'$, $a \leq q_i(z) \leq a + \beta_i$ with $a \in \mathbb{R}$, then theorem 2 reduces to a particular case of the large deviation bound of [8].

4 The fractional Rademacher complexity

Let $Z = (z_i)_{i=1}^N \in \mathcal{Z}^N$. If Z is supposed to be drawn i.i.d. according to a distribution $\mathcal{D}_{\mathcal{Z}}$ over $\mathcal{Z}$, for a class $\mathcal{F}$ of functions from $\mathcal{Z}$ to $\mathbb{R}$, the Rademacher complexity of $\mathcal{F}$ is defined by [10] $R_N(\mathcal{F}) = \mathbb{E}_{Z \sim \mathcal{D}_{\mathcal{Z}}} R_N(\mathcal{F}, Z)$, where $R_N(\mathcal{F}, Z) = \mathbb{E}_{\sigma} \sup_{f \in \mathcal{F}} \sum_{i=1}^N \sigma_i f(z_i)$ is the empirical Rademacher complexity of $\mathcal{F}$ on Z, and $\sigma = (\sigma_i)_{i=1}^n$ is a sequence of independent Rademacher variables, i.e. $\forall i, \mathbb{P}(\sigma_i = 1) = \mathbb{P}(\sigma_i = -1) = \frac{1}{2}$. This quantity has been extensively used to measure the complexity of function classes in previous bounds for binary classification [3, 10]. In particular, if we consider a class of functions $\mathcal{Q} = \{q : \mathcal{Z} \mapsto [0, 1]\}$, it can be shown (theorem 4.9 in [12]) that with probability at least $1 - \delta$ over Z, all $q \in \mathcal{Q}$ verify the following inequality, which serves as a preliminary result to show data-dependent bounds for SVMs in [12]:

$$\mathbb{E}_{Z \sim \mathcal{D}_{\mathcal{Z}}} q(z) \leq \frac{1}{N} \sum_{i=1}^N q(z_i) + R_N(\mathcal{Q}) + \sqrt{\frac{\ln(1/\delta)}{2N}} \quad (4)$$

In this section, we generalize equation (4) to our case with theorem 4, using the following definition[2] (we denote $\lambda(q, \varphi(S)) = \frac{1}{N} \sum_{i=1}^{N} q(\varphi(S)_i)$ and $\lambda(q) = \mathbb{E}_S \lambda(q, \varphi(S))$):

Definition 3. *Let $\mathcal{Q}$, be class of functions from a set $\mathcal{Z}$ to $\mathbb{R}$, Let $\varphi : \mathcal{X}^n \to \mathcal{Z}^N$ and S a sample of size n drawn according to a product distribution $\otimes_{p=1}^{n} \mathcal{D}_p$ over $\mathcal{X}^n$. Then, we define the empirical fractional Rademacher complexity [3] of $\mathcal{Q}$ given φ as:*

$$R_n^*(\mathcal{Q}, S, \varphi) = \frac{2}{N} \mathbb{E}_\sigma \sum_j w_j \sup_{q \in \mathcal{Q}} \sum_{i \in C_j} \sigma_i q(\varphi(S)_i)$$

As well as the fractional Rademacher complexity of $\mathcal{Q}$ as $R_n^*(\mathcal{Q}, \varphi) = \mathbb{E}_S R_n^*(\mathcal{Q}, S, \varphi)$

Theorem 4. *Let $\mathcal{Q}$ be a class of functions from $\mathcal{Z}$ to $[0,1]$. Then, with probability at least $1 - \delta$ over the samples S drawn according to $\otimes_{p=1}^{n} \mathcal{D}_p$, for all $q \in \mathcal{Q}$:*

$$\lambda(q) - \frac{1}{N} \sum_{i=1}^{N} q(\varphi_i(S)) \leq R_n^*(\mathcal{Q}, \varphi) + \sqrt{\frac{\chi(\varphi) \ln(1/\delta)}{2N}}$$

And: $\lambda(q) - \frac{1}{N} \sum_{i=1}^{N} q(\varphi_i(S)) \leq R_n^*(\mathcal{Q}, S, \varphi) + 3\sqrt{\frac{\chi(\varphi) \ln(2/\delta)}{2N}}$

In the definition of the fractional Rademacher complexity (FRC), if φ is the identity function, we recover the standard Rademacher complexity, and theorem 4 reduces to equation (4). These results are therefore extensions of equation (4), and show that the generalization error bounds for the tasks falling in our framework will follow from a unique approach.

Proof. In order to find a bound for all q in $\mathcal{Q}$ of $\lambda(q) - \lambda(q, \varphi(S))$, we write:

$$\lambda(q) - \lambda(q, \varphi(S)) \leq \sup_{q \in \mathcal{Q}} \left[\mathbb{E}_{\tilde{S}} \frac{1}{N} \sum_{i=1}^{N} q(\varphi(\tilde{S})_i) - \frac{1}{N} \sum_{i=1}^{N} q(\varphi(S)_i) \right]$$

$$\leq \frac{1}{N} \sum_j w_j \sup_{q \in \mathcal{Q}} \left[\mathbb{E}_{\tilde{S}} \sum_{i \in C_j} q(\varphi(\tilde{S})_i) - \sum_{i \in C_j} q(\varphi(S)_i) \right] \tag{5}$$

Where we have used equation (2). Now, consider, for each j, $f_j : \mathcal{Z}^{\kappa_j} \to \mathbb{R}$ such that, for all $z^{(j)} \in \mathcal{Z}^{\kappa_j}$, $f_j(z^{(j)}) = \frac{1}{N} \sup_{q \in \mathcal{Q}} \mathbb{E}_{\tilde{S}} \sum_{k=1}^{\kappa_j} q(\varphi(\tilde{S})_{C_j k}) - \sum_{k=1}^{\kappa_j} q(z_k^{(j)})$. It is clear that if $f : \mathcal{Z}^N \to \mathbb{R}$ is defined by: for all $Z \in \mathcal{Z}^N$, $f(Z) = \sum_{j=1}^{N} w_j f_j(z_{Cj1}, ..., z_{Cj\kappa_j})$, then the right side of equation (5) is equal to $f \circ \varphi(S)$, and that f satisfies all the conditions of theorem 2 with, for all $i \in \{1, ..., N\}$, $\beta_i = \frac{1}{N}$. Therefore, with a direct application of theorem 2, we can claim that, with probability at least $1 - \delta$ over samples S drawn according to $\otimes_{p=1}^{n} \mathcal{D}_p$ (we denote $\lambda_j(q, \varphi(S)) = \frac{1}{N} \sum_{i \in C_j} q(\varphi(S)_i)$):

$$\lambda(q) - \lambda(q, \varphi(S)) \leq \mathbb{E}_S \sum_j w_j \sup_{q \in \mathcal{Q}} \left[\mathbb{E}_{\tilde{S}} \lambda_j(q, \varphi(\tilde{S})) - \lambda_j(q, \varphi(S)) \right] + \sqrt{\frac{\chi(\varphi) \ln(1/\delta)}{2N}}$$

$$\leq \mathbb{E}_{S,\tilde{S}} \sum_j \frac{w_j}{N} \sup_{q \in \mathcal{Q}} \sum_{i \in C_j} [q(\varphi(\tilde{S})_i) - q(\varphi(S)_i)] + \sqrt{\frac{\chi(\varphi) \ln(1/\delta)}{2N}}$$

$$\tag{6}$$

---

[2] The fractional Rademacher complexity depends on the cover $\mathcal{C}(\varphi)$ chosen, since it is not unique. However in practice, our bounds only depend on $\chi(\varphi)$ (see section 4.1).

[3] this denomination stands as it is a sum of Rademacher averages over independent parts of $\varphi(S)$.

Now fix j, and consider $\sigma = (\sigma_i)_{i=1}^N$, a sequence of N independent Rademacher variables. For a given realization of σ, we have that

$$\mathbb{E}_{S,\tilde{S}}\sup_{q\in\mathcal{Q}}\sum_{i\in C_j}[q(\varphi(\tilde{S})_i) - q(\varphi(S)_i)] = \mathbb{E}_{S,\tilde{S}}\sup_{q\in\mathcal{Q}}\sum_{i\in C_j}\sigma_i[q(\varphi(\tilde{S})_i) - q(\varphi(S)_i)] \quad (7)$$

because, for each σ_i considered, $\sigma_i = -1$ simply corresponds to permutating, in $S, \tilde{S}$, the two sequences $S_{[i]}$ and $\tilde{S}_{[i]}$ (where $S_{[i]}$ denotes the subset of S $\varphi(S)_i$ really depends on) which have the same distribution (even though the s_p's are not identically distributed), and are independent from the other $S_{[k]}$ and $\tilde{S}_{[k]}$ since we are considering $i, k \in C_j$. Therefore, taking the expection over $S, \tilde{S}$ is the same with the elements permuted this way as if they were not permuted. Then, from equation (6), the first inequality of the theorem follow. The second inequality is due to an application of theorem 2 to $R_n^*(\mathcal{Q}, S, \varphi)$. □

Remark 5. The symmetrization performed in equation (7) requires the variables $\varphi(S)_i$ appearing in the same sum to be independent. Thus, the generalization of Rademacher complexities could only be performed using a decomposition in independent sets, and the cover $\mathcal{C}$ assures some optimality of the decomposition. Moreover, even though McDiarmid's theorem could be applied each time we used theorem 2, the derivation of the real numbers bounding the differences is not straightforward, and may not lead to the same result. The creation of the dependency graph of φ and theorem 2 are therefore necessary tools for obtaining theorem 4.

Properties of the fractional Rademacher complexity

Theorem 6. *Let $\mathcal{Q}$ be a class of functions from a set $\mathcal{Z}$ to $\mathbb{R}$, and $\varphi : \mathcal{X}^n \to \mathcal{Z}^N$. For $S \in \mathcal{X}^n$, the following results are true.*

1. *Let $\phi : \mathbb{R} \to \mathbb{R}$, an L-Lipschitz function. Then $R_n^*(\phi \circ \mathcal{Q}, S, \varphi) \leq L R_n^*(\mathcal{Q}, S, \varphi)$*

2. *If there exist $M > 0$ such that for every k, and samples S_k of size k $R_k(\mathcal{Q}, S_k) \leq \frac{M}{\sqrt{k}}$, then $R_n^*(\mathcal{Q}, S, \varphi) \leq M\sqrt{\frac{\chi(\varphi)}{N}}$*

3. *Let K be a kernel over $\mathcal{Z}$, $B > 0$, denote $||x||_K = \sqrt{K(x,x)}$ and define $\mathcal{H}_{K,B} = \{h_\theta : \mathcal{Z} \to \mathbb{R}, h_\theta(x) = K(\theta, x) | ||\theta||_K \leq B\}$. Then:*

$$R_n^*(\mathcal{H}_{K,B}, S, \varphi) \leq \frac{2B\sqrt{\chi(\varphi)}}{N}\sqrt{\sum_{i=1}^N ||\varphi(S)_i||_K^2}$$

The first point of this theorem is a direct consequence of a Rademacher process comparison theorem, namely theorem 7 of [10], and will enable the obtention of margin-based bounds. The second and third points show that the results regarding the Rademacher complexity can be used to immediately deduce bounds on the FRC. This result, as well as theorem 4 show that binary classifiers of i.i.d. data and classifiers of interdependent data will have generalization bounds of the same form, but with different convergence rate depending on the dependency structure imposed by φ.

elements of proof. The second point results from Jensen's inequality, using the facts that $\sum_j w_j = \chi(\varphi)$ and, from equation (2), $\sum_j w_j|C_j| = N$. The third point is based on the same calculations by noting that (see e.g. [3]), if $S_k = ((x_p, y_p))_{p=1}^k$, then

$R_k(\mathcal{H}_{K,B}, S_k) \leq \frac{2B}{k}\sqrt{\sum_{p=1}^k ||x_p||_K^2}$. □

5 Data-dependent bounds

The fact that classifiers trained on interdependent data will "inherit" the generalization bound of the same classifier trained on i.i.d. data suggests simple ways of obtaining bipartite ranking algorithms. Indeed, suppose we want to learn a linear ranking function, for example a function $h \in \mathcal{H}_{K,B}$ as defined in theorem 6, where K is a linear kernel, and consider a sample $S \in (\mathcal{X} \times \{-1, 1\})^n$ with $\mathcal{X} \subset \mathbb{R}^d$, drawn i.i.d. according to some $\mathcal{D}$. Then we have, for input examples $(x, 1)$ and $(x', -1)$ in S, $h(x) - h(x') = h(x - x')$. Therefore, we can learn a bipartite ranking function by applying an SVM algorithm to the pairs $((x, 1), (x', -1))$ in S, each pair being represented by $x - x'$, and our framework allows to immediately obtain generalization bounds for this learning process based on the generalization bounds for SVMs. We show these bounds in theorem 7.

To derive the bounds, we consider ϕ, the 1-Lipschitz function defined by $\phi(x) = \min(1, \max(1 - x, 0)) \geq [[x \leq 0]]$[4]. Given a training example z, we denote by z^l its label and z^f its feature representation. With an abuse of notation, we denote $\phi(h, Z) = \frac{1}{N} \sum_{i=1}^{N} \phi(z_i^l h(z_i^f))$. For a sample S drawn according to $\bigotimes_{p=1}^{n} \mathcal{D}_p$, we have, for all h in some function class $\mathcal{H}$:

$$\mathbb{E}_S \frac{1}{N} \sum_i \ell(h, z_i) \leq \mathbb{E}_S \frac{1}{N} \sum_i \phi(z_i^l h(z_i^f))$$

$$\leq \phi(h, Z) + \mathbb{E}_\sigma \sum_j \frac{2w_j}{N} \sup_{h \in \mathcal{H}} \sum_{i \in C_j} \sigma_i \phi(z_i^l h(z_i^f)) + 3 \sqrt{\frac{\chi(\varphi) \ln(2/\delta)}{2N}}$$

where $\ell(h, z_i) = [[z_i^l h(z_i^f) \leq 0]]$, and the last inequality holds with probability at least $1 - \delta$ over samples S from theorem 4. Notice that when $\sigma_{C_{jk}}$ is a Rademacher variable, it has the same distribution as $z_{C_{jk}}^l \sigma_{C_{jk}}$ since $z_{C_{jk}}^l \in \{-1, 1\}$. Thus, using the first result of theorem 6 we have that with probability $1 - \delta$ over the samples S, all h in $\mathcal{H}$ satisfy:

$$\mathbb{E}_S \frac{1}{N} \sum_i \ell(h, z_i) \leq \frac{1}{N} \sum_i \phi(z^l h(z^f)) + R_n^*(\mathcal{H}, S, \varphi) + 3\sqrt{\frac{\chi(\varphi) \ln(2/\delta)}{2N}} \quad (8)$$

Now putting in equation (8) the third point of theorem 6, with $\mathcal{H} = \mathcal{H}_{K,B}$ as defined in theorem 6 with $\mathcal{Z} = \mathcal{X}$, we obtain the following theorem:

Theorem 7. Let $S \in (\mathcal{X} \times \{-1, 1\})^n$ be a sample of size n drawn i.i.d. according to an unknown distribution $\mathcal{D}$. Then, with probability at least $1 - \delta$, all $h \in \mathcal{H}_{K,B}$ verify:

$$\mathbb{E}_S[[y_i h(x_i) \leq 0]] \leq \frac{1}{n} \sum_{i=1}^{n} \phi(y_i h(x_i)) + \frac{2B}{n} \sqrt{\sum_{i=1}^{n} ||x_i||_K^2} + 3\sqrt{\frac{\ln(2/\delta)}{2n}}$$

$$And \; \mathbb{E}\{[[h(x) \leq h(x')]] | y = 1, y' = -1\} \leq \frac{1}{n_+^S n_-^S} \sum_{i=1}^{n_+^S} \sum_{j=1}^{n_-^S} \phi(h(x_{\sigma(i)}) - h(x_{\nu(j)}))$$

$$+ \frac{2B \sqrt{\max(n_+^S, n_-^S)}}{n_+^S n_-^S} \sqrt{\sum_{i=1}^{n_+^S} \sum_{j=1}^{n_-^S} ||x_{\sigma(i)} - x_{\nu(j)}||_K^2} + 3\sqrt{\frac{\ln(2/\delta)}{2 \min(n_+^S, n_-^S)}}$$

Where n_+^S, n_-^S are the number of positive and negative instances in S, and σ and ν also depend on S, and are such that $x_{\sigma(i)}$ is the i-th positive instance in S and $\nu(j)$ the j-th negative instance.

---

[4] remark that ϕ is upper bounded by the slack variables of the SVM optimization problem (see e.g. [12]).

It is to be noted that when $h \in \mathcal{H}_{K,B}$ with a non linear kernel, the same bounds apply, with, for the case of bipartite ranking, $||x_{\sigma(i)} - x_{\nu(j)}||_K^2$ replaced by $||x_{\sigma(i)}||_K^2 + ||x_{\nu(j)}||_K^2 - 2K(x_{\sigma(i)}, x_{\nu(j)})$.

For binary classification, we recover the bounds of [12], since our framework is a generalization of their approach. As expected, the bounds suggest that kernel machines will generalize well for bipartite ranking. Thus, we recover the results of [2] obtained in a specific framework of algorithmic stability. However, our bound suggests that the convergence rate is controlled by $1/\min(n_+^S, n_-^S)$, while their results suggested $1/n_+^S + 1/n_-^S$. The full proof, in which we follow the approach of [1], is given in [13].

6 Conclusion

We have shown a general framework for classifiers trained with interdependent data, and provided the necessary tools to study their generalization properties. It gives a new insight on the close relationship between the binary classification task and the bipartite ranking, and allows to prove the first data-dependent bounds for this latter case. Moreover, the framework could also yield comparable bounds on other learning tasks.

Acknowledgments

This work was supported in part by the IST Programme of the European Community, under the PASCAL Network of Excellence, IST-2002-506778. This publication only reflects the authors views.

References

[1] Agarwal S., Graepel T., Herbrich R., Har-Peled S., Roth D. (2005) Generalization Error Bounds for the Area Under the ROC curve, *Journal of Machine Learning Research.*

[2] Agarwal S., Niyogi P. (2005) Stability and generalization of bipartite ranking algorithms, *Conference on Learning Theory 18.*

[3] Bartlett P., Mendelson S. (2002) Rademacher and Gaussian Complexities: Risk Bounds and Structural Results, *Journal of Machine Learning Research 3*, pp. 463-482.

[4] Boucheron S., Bousquet O., Lugosi G. (2004) Concentration inequalities, in O. Bousquet, U.v. Luxburg, and G. Rtsch (editors), *Advanced Lectures in Machine Learning*, Springer, pp. 208-240.

[5] Clemençon S., Lugosi G., Vayatis N. (2005) Ranking and scoring using empirical risk minimization, *Conference on Learning Theory 18.*

[6] Cortes C., Mohri M. (2004) AUC optimization vs error rate miniminzation *NIPS 2003,*

[7] Freund Y., Iyer R.D., Schapire R.E., Singer Y. (2003) An Efficient Boosting Algorithm for Combining Preferences, *Journal of Machine Learning Research 4*, pp. 933-969.

[8] Janson S. (2004) Large deviations for sums of partly dependent random variables, *Random Structures and Algorithms 24*, pp. 234-248.

[9] McDiarmid C. (1989) On the method of bounded differences, *Surveys in Combinatorics.*

[10] Meir R., Zhang T. (2003) Generalization Error Bounds for Bayesian Mixture Algorithms, *Journal of Machine Learning Research 4*, pp. 839-860.

[11] Rudin C., Cortes C., Mohri M., Schapire R.E. (2005) Margin-Based Ranking meets Boosting in the middle, *Conference on Learning Theory 18.*

[12] Shawe-Taylor J., Cristianini N. (2004) Kernel Methods for Pattern Analysis, Cambridge U. Prs.

[13] *Long version of this paper*, Available at http://www-connex.lip6.fr/˜usunier/nips05-lv.pdf

TD(0) Leads to Better Policies than Approximate Value Iteration

Benjamin Van Roy
Management Science and Engineering and Electrical Engineering
Stanford University
Stanford, CA 94305
bvr@stanford.edu

Abstract

We consider approximate value iteration with a parameterized approximator in which the state space is partitioned and the optimal cost-to-go function over each partition is approximated by a constant. We establish performance loss bounds for policies derived from approximations associated with fixed points. These bounds identify benefits to having projection weights equal to the invariant distribution of the resulting policy. Such projection weighting leads to the same fixed points as TD(0). Our analysis also leads to the first performance loss bound for approximate value iteration with an average cost objective.

1 Preliminaries

Consider a discrete-time communicating Markov decision process (MDP) with a finite state space $\mathcal{S} = \{1, \ldots, |\mathcal{S}|\}$. At each state $x \in \mathcal{S}$, there is a finite set $\mathcal{U}_x$ of admissible actions. If the current state is x and an action $u \in \mathcal{U}_x$ is selected, a cost of $g_u(x)$ is incurred, and the system transitions to a state $y \in \mathcal{S}$ with probability $p_{xy}(u)$. For any $x \in \mathcal{S}$ and $u \in \mathcal{U}_x$, $\sum_{y \in \mathcal{S}} p_{xy}(u) = 1$. Costs are discounted at a rate of $\alpha \in (0, 1)$ per period. Each instance of such an MDP is defined by a quintuple $(\mathcal{S}, \mathcal{U}, g, p, \alpha)$.

A (stationary deterministic) policy is a mapping μ that assigns an action $u \in \mathcal{U}_x$ to each state $x \in \mathcal{S}$. If actions are selected based on a policy μ, the state follows a Markov process with transition matrix P_μ, where each (x, y)th entry is equal to $p_{xy}(\mu(x))$. The restriction to communicating MDPs ensures that it is possible to reach any state from any other state.

Each policy μ is associated with a cost-to-go function $J_\mu \in \Re^{|\mathcal{S}|}$, defined by $J_\mu = \sum_{t=0}^\infty \alpha^t P_\mu^t g_\mu = (I - \alpha P_\mu)^{-1} g_\mu$, where, with some abuse of notation, $g_\mu(x) = g_{\mu(x)}(x)$ for each $x \in \mathcal{S}$. A policy μ is said to be *greedy* with respect to a function J if $\mu(x) \in \operatorname*{argmin}_{u \in \mathcal{U}_x}(g_u(x) + \alpha \sum_{y \in \mathcal{S}} p_{xy}(u) J(y))$ for all $x \in \mathcal{S}$.

The optimal cost-to-go function $J^* \in \Re^{|\mathcal{S}|}$ is defined by $J^*(x) = \min_\mu J_\mu(x)$, for all $x \in \mathcal{S}$. A policy μ^* is said to be optimal if $J_{\mu^*} = J^*$. It is well-known that an optimal policy exists. Further, a policy μ^* is optimal if and only if it is greedy with respect to J^*. Hence, given the optimal cost-to-go function, optimal actions can computed be minimizing the right-hand side of the above inclusion.

Value iteration generates a sequence J_ℓ converging to J^* according to $J_{\ell+1} = TJ_\ell$, where T is the dynamic programming operator, defined by $(TJ)(x) = \min_{u \in \mathcal{U}_x}(g_u(x) + \alpha \sum_{y \in \mathcal{S}} p_{xy}(u)J(y))$, for all $x \in \mathcal{S}$ and $J \in \Re^{|\mathcal{S}|}$. This sequence converges to J^* for any initialization of J_0.

2 Approximate Value Iteration

The state spaces of relevant MDPs are typically so large that computation and storage of a cost-to-go function is infeasible. One approach to dealing with this obstacle involves partitioning the state space $\mathcal{S}$ into a manageable number K of disjoint subsets $\mathcal{S}_1, \ldots, \mathcal{S}_K$ and approximating the optimal cost-to-go function with a function that is constant over each partition. This can be thought of as a form of state aggregation – all states within a given partition are assumed to share a common optimal cost-to-go.

To represent an approximation, we define a matrix $\Phi \in \Re^{|\mathcal{S}| \times K}$ such that each kth column is an indicator function for the kth partition $\mathcal{S}_k$. Hence, for any $r \in \Re^K$, k, and $x \in \mathcal{S}_k$, $(\Phi r)(x) = r_k$. In this paper, we study variations of value iteration, each of which computes a vector r so that Φr approximates J^*. The use of such a policy μ_r which is greedy with respect to Φr is justified by the following result (see [10] for a proof):

Theorem 1 *If μ is a greedy policy with respect to a function $\tilde{J} \in \Re^{|\mathcal{S}|}$ then*

$$\|J_\mu - J^*\|_\infty \le \frac{2\alpha}{1-\alpha}\|J^* - \tilde{J}\|_\infty.$$

One common way of approximating a function $J \in \Re^{|\mathcal{S}|}$ with a function of the form Φr involves projection with respect to a weighted Euclidean norm $\|\cdot\|_\pi$. The weighted Euclidean norm: $\|J\|_{2,\pi} = \left(\sum_{x \in \mathcal{S}} \pi(x)J^2(x)\right)^{1/2}$. Here, $\pi \in \Re_+^{|\mathcal{S}|}$ is a vector of weights that assign relative emphasis among states. The projection $\Pi_\pi J$ is the function Φr that attains the minimum of $\|J - \Phi r\|_{2,\pi}$; if there are multiple functions Φr that attain the minimum, they must form an affine space, and the projection is taken to be the one with minimal norm $\|\Phi r\|_{2,\pi}$. Note that in our context, where each kth column of Φ represents an indicator function for the kth partition, for any π, J, and $x \in \mathcal{S}_k$, $(\Pi_\pi J)(x) = \sum_{y \in \mathcal{S}_k} \pi(y)J(y)/\sum_{y \in \mathcal{S}_k} \pi(y)$.

Approximate value iteration begins with a function $\Phi r^{(0)}$ and generates a sequence according to $\Phi r^{(\ell+1)} = \Pi_\pi T \Phi r^{(\ell)}$. It is well-known that the dynamic programming operator T is a contraction mapping with respect to the maximum norm. Further, Π_π is maximum-norm nonexpansive [16, 7, 8]. (This is not true for general Φ, but is true in our context in which columns of Φ are indicator functions for partitions.) It follows that the composition $\Pi_\pi T$ is a contraction mapping. By the contraction mapping theorem, $\Pi_\pi T$ has a unique fixed point $\Phi \tilde{r}$, which is the limit of the sequence $\Phi r^{(\ell)}$. Further, the following result holds:

Theorem 2 *For any MDP, partition, and weights π with support intersecting every partition, if $\Phi \tilde{r} = \Pi_\pi T \Phi \tilde{r}$ then*

$$\|\Phi \tilde{r} - J^*\|_\infty \le \frac{2}{1-\alpha} \min_{r \in \Re^K} \|J^* - \Phi r\|_\infty,$$

and

$$(1-\alpha)\|J_{\mu_{\tilde{r}}} - J^*\|_\infty \le \frac{4\alpha}{1-\alpha} \min_{r \in \Re^K} \|J^* - \Phi r\|_\infty.$$

The first inequality of the theorem is an *approximation error bound*, established in [16, 7, 8] for broader classes of approximators that include state aggregation as a special case. The second is a *performance loss bound*, derived by simply combining the approximation error bound and Theorem 1.

Note that $J_{\mu_{\tilde{r}}}(x) \geq J^*(x)$ for all x, so the left-hand side of the performance loss bound is the maximal increase in cost-to-go, normalized by $1 - \alpha$. This normalization is natural, since a cost-to-go function is a linear combination of expected future costs, with coefficients $1, \alpha, \alpha^2, \ldots$, which sum to $1/(1 - \alpha)$.

Our motivation of the normalizing constant begs the question of whether, for fixed MDP parameters $(\mathcal{S}, \mathcal{U}, g, p)$ and fixed Φ, $\min_r \|J^* - \Phi r\|_\infty$ also grows with $1/(1 - \alpha)$. It turns out that $\min_r \|J^* - \Phi r\|_\infty = O(1)$. To see why, note that for any μ,

$$J_\mu = (I - \alpha P_\mu)^{-1} g_\mu = \frac{1}{1 - \alpha} \lambda_\mu + h_\mu,$$

where $\lambda_\mu(x)$ is the *expected average cost* if the process starts in state x and is controlled by policy μ,

$$\lambda_\mu = \lim_{\tau \to \infty} \frac{1}{\tau} \sum_{t=0}^{\tau-1} P_\mu^t g_\mu,$$

and h_μ is the *discounted differential cost function*

$$h_\mu = (I - \alpha P_\mu)^{-1}(g_\mu - \lambda_\mu).$$

Both λ_μ and h_μ converge to finite vectors as α approaches 1 [3]. For an optimal policy μ^*, $\lim_{\alpha \uparrow 1} \lambda_{\mu^*}(x)$ does not depend on x (in our context of a communicating MDP). Since constant functions lie in the range of Φ,

$$\lim_{\alpha \uparrow 1} \min_{r \in \Re^K} \|J^* - \Phi r\|_\infty \leq \lim_{\alpha \uparrow 1} \|h_{\mu^*}\|_\infty < \infty.$$

The performance loss bound still exhibits an undesirable dependence on α through the coefficient $4\alpha/(1 - \alpha)$. In most relevant contexts, α is close to 1; a representative value might be 0.99. Consequently, $4\alpha/(1 - \alpha)$ can be very large. Unfortunately, the bound is sharp, as expressed by the following theorem. We will denote by $\mathbf{1}$ the vector with every component equal to 1.

Theorem 3 *For any $\delta > 0$, $\alpha \in (0, 1)$, and $\Delta \geq 0$, there exists MDP parameters $(\mathcal{S}, \mathcal{U}, g, p)$ and a partition such that $\min_{r \in \Re^K} \|J^* - \Phi r\|_\infty = \Delta$ and, if $\Phi \tilde{r} = \Pi_\pi T \Phi \tilde{r}$ with $\pi = \mathbf{1}$,*

$$(1 - \alpha)\|J_{\mu_{\tilde{r}}} - J^*\|_\infty \geq \frac{4\alpha}{1 - \alpha} \min_{r \in \Re^K} \|J^* - \Phi r\|_\infty - \delta.$$

This theorem is established through an example in [22]. The choice of uniform weights ($\pi = \mathbf{1}$) is meant to point out that even for such a simple, perhaps natural, choice of weights, the performance loss bound is sharp.

Based on Theorems 2 and 3, one might expect that there exists MDP parameters $(\mathcal{S}, \mathcal{U}, g, p)$ and a partition such that, with $\pi = \mathbf{1}$,

$$(1 - \alpha)\|J_{\mu_{\tilde{r}}} - J^*\|_\infty = \Theta\left(\frac{1}{1 - \alpha} \min_{r \in \Re^K} \|J^* - \Phi r\|_\infty\right).$$

In other words, that the performance loss is both lower and upper bounded by $1/(1 - \alpha)$ times the smallest possible approximation error. It turns out that this is not true, at least if we restrict to a finite state space. However, as the following theorem establishes, the coefficient multiplying $\min_{r \in \Re^K} \|J^* - \Phi r\|_\infty$ can grow arbitrarily large as α increases, keeping all else fixed.

Theorem 4 *For any L and $\Delta \geq 0$, there exists MDP parameters $(\mathcal{S}, \mathcal{U}, g, p)$ and a partition such that $\lim_{\alpha \uparrow 1} \min_{r \in \Re^K} \|J^* - \Phi r\|_\infty = \Delta$ and, if $\Phi \tilde{r} = \Pi_\pi T \Phi \tilde{r}$ with $\pi = \mathbf{1}$,*

$$\liminf_{\alpha \uparrow 1} (1 - \alpha) \left(J_{\mu_{\tilde{r}}}(x) - J^*(x)\right) \geq L \lim_{\alpha \uparrow 1} \min_{r \in \Re^K} \|J^* - \Phi r\|_\infty,$$

for all $x \in \mathcal{S}$.

This Theorem is also established through an example [22].

For any μ and x,

$$\lim_{\alpha \uparrow 1} \left((1 - \alpha) J_\mu(x) - \lambda_\mu(x)\right) = \lim_{\alpha \uparrow 1} (1 - \alpha) h_\mu(x) = 0.$$

Combined with Theorem 4, this yields the following corollary.

Corollary 1 *For any L and $\Delta \geq 0$, there exists MDP parameters $(\mathcal{S}, \mathcal{U}, g, p)$ and a partition such that $\lim_{\alpha \uparrow 1} \min_{r \in \Re^K} \|J^* - \Phi r\|_\infty = \Delta$ and, if $\Phi \tilde{r} = \Pi_\pi T \Phi \tilde{r}$ with $\pi = \mathbf{1}$,*

$$\liminf_{\alpha \uparrow 1} \left(\lambda_{\mu_{\tilde{r}}}(x) - \lambda_{\mu^*}(x)\right) \geq L \lim_{\alpha \uparrow 1} \min_{r \in \Re^K} \|J^* - \Phi r\|_\infty,$$

for all $x \in \mathcal{S}$.

3 Using the Invariant Distribution

In the previous section, we considered an approximation $\Phi \tilde{r}$ that solves $\Pi_\pi T \Phi \tilde{r} = \Phi \tilde{r}$ for some arbitrary pre-selected weights π. We now turn to consider use of an invariant state distribution $\pi_{\tilde{r}}$ of $P_{\mu_{\tilde{r}}}$ as the weight vector.[1] This leads to a circular definition: the weights are used in defining $\tilde{r}$ and now we are defining the weights in terms of $\tilde{r}$. What we are really after here is a vector $\tilde{r}$ that satisfies $\Pi_{\pi_{\tilde{r}}} T \Phi \tilde{r} = \Phi \tilde{r}$. The following theorem captures the associated benefits. (Due to space limitations, we omit the proof, which is provided in the full length version of this paper [22].)

Theorem 5 *For any MDP and partition, if $\Phi \tilde{r} = \Pi_{\pi_{\tilde{r}}} T \Phi \tilde{r}$ and $\pi_{\tilde{r}}$ has support intersecting every partition, $(1 - \alpha) \pi_{\tilde{r}}^T (J_{\mu_{\tilde{r}}} - J^*) \leq 2\alpha \min_{r \in \Re^K} \|J^* - \Phi r\|_\infty$.*

When α is close to 1, which is typical, the right-hand side of our new performance loss bound is far less than that of Theorem 2. The primary improvement is in the omission of a factor of $1 - \alpha$ from the denominator. But for the bounds to be compared in a meaningful way, we must also relate the left-hand-side expressions. A relation can be based on the fact that for all μ, $\lim_{\alpha \uparrow 1} \|(1 - \alpha) J_\mu - \lambda_\mu\|_\infty = 0$, as explained in Section 2. In particular, based on this, we have

$$\lim_{\alpha \uparrow 1} (1 - \alpha) \|J_\mu - J^*\|_\infty = |\lambda_\mu - \lambda^*| = \lambda_\mu - \lambda^* = \lim_{\alpha \uparrow 1} \pi^T (J_\mu - J^*),$$

for all policies μ and probability distributions π. Hence, the left-hand-side expressions from the two performance bounds become directly comparable as α approaches 1.

Another interesting comparison can be made by contrasting Corollary 1 against the following immediate consequence of Theorem 5.

Corollary 2 *For all MDP parameters $(\mathcal{S}, \mathcal{U}, g, p)$ and partitions, if $\Phi \tilde{r} = \Pi_{\pi_{\tilde{r}}} T \Phi \tilde{r}$ and $\liminf_{\alpha \uparrow 1} \sum_{x \in \mathcal{S}_k} \pi_{\tilde{r}}(x) > 0$ for all k,*

$$\limsup_{\alpha \uparrow 1} \|\lambda_{\mu_{\tilde{r}}} - \lambda_{\mu^*}\|_\infty \leq 2 \lim_{\alpha \uparrow 1} \min_{r \in \Re^K} \|J^* - \Phi r\|_\infty.$$

The comparison suggests that solving $\Phi \tilde{r} = \Pi_{\pi_{\tilde{r}}} T \Phi \tilde{r}$ is strongly preferable to solving $\Phi \tilde{r} = \Pi_\pi T \Phi \tilde{r}$ with $\pi = \mathbf{1}$.

---

[1] By an *invariant state distribution* of a transition matrix P, we mean any probability distribution π such that $\pi^T P = \pi^T$. In the event that $P_{\mu_{\tilde{r}}}$ has multiple invariant distributions, $\pi_{\tilde{r}}$ denotes an arbitrary choice.

4 Exploration

If a vector $\tilde{r}$ solves $\Phi\tilde{r} = \Pi_{\pi_{\tilde{r}}} T\Phi\tilde{r}$ and the support of $\pi_{\tilde{r}}$ intersects every partition, Theorem 5 promises a desirable bound. However, there are two significant shortcomings to this solution concept, which we will address in this section. First, in some cases, the equation $\Pi_{\pi_{\tilde{r}}} T\Phi\tilde{r} = \Phi\tilde{r}$ does not have a solution. It is easy to produce examples of this; though no example has been documented for the particular class of approximators we are using here, [2] offers an example involving a different linearly parameterized approximator that captures the spirit of what can happen. Second, it would be nice to relax the requirement that the support of $\pi_{\tilde{r}}$ intersect every partition.

To address these shortcomings, we introduce stochastic policies. A stochastic policy μ maps state-action pairs to probabilities. For each $x \in \mathcal{S}$ and $u \in \mathcal{U}_x$, $\mu(x, u)$ is the probability of taking action u when in state x. Hence, $\mu(x, u) \geq 0$ for all $x \in \mathcal{S}$ and $u \in \mathcal{U}_x$, and $\sum_{u \in \mathcal{U}_x} \mu(x, u) = 1$ for all $x \in \mathcal{S}$.

Given a scalar $\epsilon > 0$ and a function J, the ϵ-greedy Boltzmann exploration policy with respect to J is defined by

$$\mu(x, u) = \frac{e^{-(T_u J)(x)(|\mathcal{U}_x|-1)/\epsilon e}}{\sum_{u \in \mathcal{U}_x} e^{-(T_u J)(x)(|\mathcal{U}_x|-1)/\epsilon e}}.$$

For any $\epsilon > 0$ and r, let μ_r^ϵ denote the ϵ-greedy Boltzmann exploration policy with respect to Φr. Further, we define a modified dynamic programming operator that incorporates Boltzmann exploration:

$$(T^\epsilon J)(x) = \frac{\sum_{u \in \mathcal{U}_x} e^{-(T_u J)(x)(|\mathcal{U}_x|-1)/\epsilon e}(T_u J)(x)}{\sum_{u \in \mathcal{U}_x} e^{-(T_u J)(x)(|\mathcal{U}_x|-1)/\epsilon e}}.$$

As ϵ approaches 0, ϵ-greedy Boltzmann exploration policies become greedy and the modified dynamic programming operators become the dynamic programming operator. More precisely, for all r, x, and J, $\lim_{\epsilon \downarrow 0} \mu_r^\epsilon(x, \mu_r(x)) = 1$ and $\lim_{\epsilon \downarrow 1} T^\epsilon J = TJ$. These are immediate consequences of the following result (see [4] for a proof).

Lemma 1 *For any* n, $v \in \Re^n$, $\min_i v_i + \epsilon \geq \sum_i e^{-v_i(n-1)/\epsilon e} v_i / \sum_i e^{-v_i(n-1)/\epsilon e} \geq \min_i v_i$.

Because we are only concerned with communicating MDPs, there is a unique invariant state distribution associated with each ϵ-greedy Boltzmann exploration policy μ_r^ϵ and the support of this distribution is $\mathcal{S}$. Let π_r^ϵ denote this distribution. We consider a vector $\tilde{r}$ that solves $\Phi\tilde{r} = \Pi_{\pi_{\tilde{r}}^\epsilon} T^\epsilon \Phi\tilde{r}$. For any $\epsilon > 0$, there exists a solution to this equation (this is an immediate extension of Theorem 5.1 from [4]).

We have the following performance loss bound, which parallels Theorem 5 but with an equation for which a solution is guaranteed to exist and without any requirement on the resulting invariant distribution. (Again, we omit the proof, which is available in [22].)

Theorem 6 *For any MDP, partition, and* $\epsilon > 0$, *if* $\Phi\tilde{r} = \Pi_{\pi_{\tilde{r}}^\epsilon} T^\epsilon \Phi\tilde{r}$ *then* $(1 - \alpha)(\pi_{\tilde{r}}^\epsilon)^T (J_{\mu_{\tilde{r}}^\epsilon} - J^*) \leq 2\alpha \min_{r \in \Re^K} \|J^* - \Phi r\|_\infty + \epsilon$.

5 Computation: TD(0)

Though computation is not a focus of this paper, we offer a brief discussion here. First, we describe a simple algorithm from [16], which draws on ideas from temporal-difference learning [11, 12] and Q-learning [23, 24] to solve $\Phi\tilde{r} = \Pi_\pi T\Phi\tilde{r}$. It requires an ability to sample a sequence of states $x^{(0)}, x^{(1)}, x^{(2)}, \ldots$, each independent and identically distributed according to π. Also required is a way to efficiently compute $(T\Phi r)(x) = \min_{u \in \mathcal{U}_x}(g_u(x) + \alpha \sum_{y \in \mathcal{S}} p_{xy}(u)(\Phi r)(y))$, for any given x and r. This is typically possible when the action set $\mathcal{U}_x$ and the support of $p_{x.}(u)$ (i.e., the set of states that can follow x if action u is selected) are not too large. The algorithm generates a sequence of vectors $r^{(\ell)}$ according to

$$r^{(\ell+1)} = r^{(\ell)} + \gamma_\ell \phi(x^{(\ell)}) \left((T\Phi r^{(\ell)})(x^{(\ell)}) - (\Phi r^{(\ell)})(x^{(\ell)}) \right),$$

where γ_ℓ is a step size and $\phi(x)$ denotes the column vector made up of components from the xth row of Φ. In [16], using results from [15, 9], it is shown that under appropriate assumptions on the step size sequence, $r^{(\ell)}$ converges to a vector $\tilde{r}$ that solves $\Phi\tilde{r} = \Pi_\pi T\Phi\tilde{r}$.

The equation $\Phi\tilde{r} = \Pi_\pi T\Phi\tilde{r}$ may have no solution. Further, the requirement that states are sampled independently from the invariant distribution may be impractical. However, a natural extension of the above algorithm leads to an easily implementable version of TD(0) that aims at solving $\Phi\tilde{r} = \Pi_{\pi_{\tilde{r}}^\epsilon} T^\epsilon \Phi\tilde{r}$. The algorithm requires simulation of a trajectory $x_0, x_1, x_2, \dots$ of the MDP, with each action $u_t \in \mathcal{U}_{x_t}$ generated by the ϵ-greedy Boltzmann exploration policy with respect to $\Phi r^{(t)}$. The sequence of vectors $r^{(t)}$ is generated according to

$$r^{(t+1)} = r^{(t)} + \gamma_t \phi(x_t) \left((T^\epsilon \Phi r^{(t)})(x_t) - (\Phi r^{(t)})(x_t) \right).$$

Under suitable conditions on the step size sequence, if this algorithm converges, the limit satisfies $\Phi\tilde{r} = \Pi_{\pi_{\tilde{r}}^\epsilon} T^\epsilon \Phi\tilde{r}$. Whether such an algorithm converges and whether there are other algorithms that can effectively solve $\Phi\tilde{r} = \Pi_{\pi_{\tilde{r}}^\epsilon} T^\epsilon \Phi\tilde{r}$ for broad classes of relevant problems remain open issues.

6 Extensions and Open Issues

Our results demonstrate that weighting a Euclidean norm projection by the invariant distribution of a greedy (or approximately greedy) policy can lead to a dramatic performance gain. It is intriguing that temporal-difference learning implicitly carries out such a projection, and consequently, any limit of convergence obeys the stronger performance loss bound.

This is not the first time that the invariant distribution has been shown to play a critical role in approximate value iteration and temporal-difference learning. In prior work involving approximation of a cost-to-go function for a fixed policy (no control) and a general linearly parameterized approximator (arbitrary matrix Φ), it was shown that weighting by the invariant distribution is key to ensuring convergence and an approximation error bound [17, 18]. Earlier empirical work anticipated this [13, 14].

The temporal-difference learning algorithm presented in Section 5 is a version of TD(0), This is a special case of TD(λ), which is parameterized by $\lambda \in [0, 1]$. It is not known whether the results of this paper can be extended to the general case of $\lambda \in [0, 1]$. Prior research has suggested that larger values of λ lead to superior results. In particular, an example of [1] and the approximation error bounds of [17, 18], both of which are restricted to the case of a fixed policy, suggest that approximation error is amplified by a factor of $1/(1 - \alpha)$ as λ is changed from 1 to 0. The results of Sections 3 and 4 suggest that this factor vanishes if one considers a controlled process and performance loss rather than approximation error.

Whether the results of this paper can be extended to accommodate approximate value iteration with general linearly parameterized approximators remains an open issue. In this broader context, error and performance loss bounds of the kind offered by Theorem 2 are unavailable, even when the invariant distribution is used to weight the projection. Such error and performance bounds *are* available, on the other hand, for the solution to a certain linear program [5, 6]. Whether a factor of $1/(1-\alpha)$ can similarly be eliminated from *these* bounds is an open issue.

Our results can be extended to accommodate an average cost objective, assuming that the MDP is communicating. With Boltzmann exploration, the equation of interest becomes

$$\Phi\tilde{r} = \Pi_{\pi_{\tilde{r}}^{\epsilon}}(T^{\epsilon}\Phi\tilde{r} - \tilde{\lambda}\mathbf{1}).$$

The variables include an estimate $\tilde{\lambda} \in \Re$ of the minimal average cost $\lambda^* \in \Re$ and an approximation $\Phi\tilde{r}$ of the optimal differential cost function h^*. The discount factor α is set to 1 in computing an ϵ-greedy Boltzmann exploration policy as well as T^{ϵ}. There is an average-cost version of temporal-difference learning for which any limit of convergence $(\tilde{\lambda}, \tilde{r})$ satisfies this equation [19, 20, 21]. Generalization of Theorem 2 does not lead to a useful result because the right-hand side of the bound becomes infinite as α approaches 1. On the other hand, generalization of Theorem 6 yields the first performance loss bound for approximate value iteration with an average-cost objective:

Theorem 7 *For any communicating MDP with an average-cost objective, partition, and* $\epsilon > 0$, *if* $\Phi\tilde{r} = \Pi_{\pi_{\tilde{r}}^{\epsilon}}(T^{\epsilon}\Phi\tilde{r} - \tilde{\lambda}\mathbf{1})$ *then*

$$\lambda_{\mu_{\tilde{r}}^{\epsilon}} - \lambda^* \leq 2\min_{r \in \Re^K} \|h^* - \Phi r\|_{\infty} + \epsilon.$$

Here, $\lambda_{\mu_{\tilde{r}}^{\epsilon}} \in \Re$ denotes the average cost under policy $\mu_{\tilde{r}}^{\epsilon}$, which is well-defined because the process is irreducible under an ϵ-greedy Boltzmann exploration policy. This theorem can be proved by taking limits on the left and right-hand sides of the bound of Theorem 6. It is easy to see that the limit of the left-hand side is $\lambda_{\mu_{\tilde{r}}^{\epsilon}} - \lambda^*$. The limit of $\min_{r \in \Re^K} \|J^* - \Phi r\|_{\infty}$ on the right-hand side is $\min_{r \in \Re^K} \|h^* - \Phi r\|_{\infty}$. (This follows from the analysis of [3].)

Acknowledgments

This material is based upon work supported by the National Science Foundation under Grant ECS-9985229 and by the Office of Naval Research under Grant MURI N00014-00-1-0637. The author's understanding of the topic benefited from collaborations with Dimitri Bertsekas, Daniela de Farias, and John Tsitsiklis. A full length version of this paper has been submitted to *Mathematics of Operations Research* and has benefited from a number of useful comments and suggestions made by reviewers.

References

[1] D. P. Bertsekas. A counterexample to temporal-difference learning. *Neural Computation*, 7:270–279, 1994.

[2] D. P. Bertsekas and J. N. Tsitsiklis. *Neuro-Dynamic Programming*. Athena Scientific, Belmont, MA, 1996.

[3] D. Blackwell. Discrete dynamic programming. *Annals of Mathematical Statistics*, 33:719–726, 1962.

[4] D. P. de Farias and B. Van Roy. On the existence of fixed points for approximate value iteration and temporal-difference learning. *Journal of Optimization Theory and Applications*, 105(3), 2000.

[5] D. P. de Farias and B. Van Roy. Approximate dynamic programming via linear programming. In *Advances in Neural Information Processing Systems 14*. MIT Press, 2002.

[6] D. P. de Farias and B. Van Roy. The linear programming approach to approximate dynamic programming. *Operations Research*, 51(6):850–865, 2003.

[7] G. J. Gordon. Stable function approximation in dynamic programming. Technical Report CMU-CS-95-103, Carnegie Mellon University, 1995.

[8] G. J. Gordon. Stable function approximation in dynamic programming. In *Machine Learning: Proceedings of the Twelfth International Conference (ICML)*, San Francisco, CA, 1995.

[9] T. Jaakkola, M. I. Jordan, and S. P. Singh. On the Convergence of Stochastic Iterative Dynamic Programming Algorithms. *Neural Computation*, 6:1185–1201, 1994.

[10] S. P. Singh and R. C. Yee. An upper-bound on the loss from approximate optimal-value functions. *Machine Learning*, 1994.

[11] R. S. Sutton. *Temporal Credit Assignment in Reinforcement Learning*. PhD thesis, University of Massachusetts, Amherst, Amherst, MA, 1984.

[12] R. S. Sutton. Learning to predict by the methods of temporal differences. *Machine Learning*, 3:9–44, 1988.

[13] R. S. Sutton. On the virtues of linear learning and trajectory distributions. In *Proceedings of the Workshop on Value Function Approximation, Machine Learning Conference*, 1995.

[14] R. S. Sutton. Generalization in reinforcement learning: Successful examples using sparse coarse coding. In *Advances in Neural Information Processing Systems 8*, Cambridge, MA, 1996. MIT Press.

[15] J. N. Tsitsiklis. Asynchronous stochastic approximation and Q-learning. *Machine Learning*, 16:185–202, 1994.

[16] J. N. Tsitsiklis and B. Van Roy. Feature–based methods for large scale dynamic programming. *Machine Learning*, 22:59–94, 1996.

[17] J. N. Tsitsiklis and B. Van Roy. An analysis of temporal–difference learning with function approximation. *IEEE Transactions on Automatic Control*, 42(5):674–690, 1997.

[18] J. N. Tsitsiklis and B. Van Roy. Analysis of temporal-difference learning with function approximation. In *Advances in Neural Information Processing Systems 9*, Cambridge, MA, 1997. MIT Press.

[19] J. N. Tsitsiklis and B. Van Roy. Average cost temporal-difference learning. In *Proceedings of the IEEE Conference on Decision and Control*, 1997.

[20] J. N. Tsitsiklis and B. Van Roy. Average cost temporal-difference learning. *Automatica*, 35(11):1799–1808, 1999.

[21] J. N. Tsitsiklis and B. Van Roy. On average versus discounted reward temporal-difference learning. *Machine Learning*, 49(2-3):179–191, 2002.

[22] B. Van Roy. Performance loss bounds for approximate value iteration with state aggregation. Under review with *Mathematics of Operations Research*, available at www.stanford.edu/ bvr/psfiles/aggregation.pdf, 2005.

[23] C. J. C. H. Watkins. *Learning From Delayed Rewards*. PhD thesis, Cambridge University, Cambridge, UK, 1989.

[24] C. J. C. H. Watkins and P. Dayan. Q-learning. *Machine Learning*, 8:279–292, 1992.

An aVLSI cricket ear model

André van Schaik[*]
The University of Sydney
NSW 2006, AUSTRALIA
andre@ee.usyd.edu.au

Richard Reeve[+]
University of Edinburgh
Edinburgh, UK
richardr@inf.ed.ac.uk

Craig Jin[*]
craig@ee.usyd.edu.au

Tara Hamilton[*]
tara@ee.usyd.edu.au

Abstract

Female crickets can locate males by phonotaxis to the mating song they produce. The behaviour and underlying physiology has been studied in some depth showing that the cricket auditory system solves this complex problem in a unique manner. We present an analogue very large scale integrated (aVLSI) circuit model of this process and show that results from testing the circuit agree with simulation and what is known from the behaviour and physiology of the cricket auditory system. The aVLSI circuitry is now being extended to use on a robot along with previously modelled neural circuitry to better understand the complete sensorimotor pathway.

1 Introduction

Understanding how insects carry out complex sensorimotor tasks can help in the design of simple sensory and robotic systems. Often insect sensors have evolved into intricate filters matched to extract highly specific data from the environment which solves a particular problem directly with little or no need for further processing [1]. Examples include head stabilisation in the fly, which uses vision amongst other senses to estimate self-rotation and thus to stabilise its head in flight, and phonotaxis in the cricket.

Because of the narrowness of the cricket body (only a few millimetres), the Interaural Time Difference (ITD) for sounds arriving at the two sides of the head is very small (10–20µs). Even with the tympanal membranes (eardrums) located, as they are, on the forelegs of the cricket, the ITD only reaches about 40µs, which is too low to detect directly from timings of neural spikes. Because the wavelength of the cricket calling song is significantly greater than the width of the cricket body the Interaural Intensity Difference (IID) is also very low. In the absence of ITD or IID information, the cricket uses phase to determine direction. This is possible because the male cricket produces an almost pure tone for its calling song.

---

[*]School of Electrical and Information Engineering,
[+]Institute of Perception, Action and Behaviour.

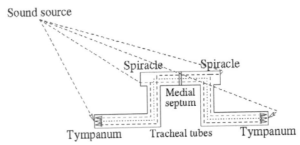

Figure 1: The cricket auditory system. Four acoustic inputs channel sounds directly or through tracheal tubes onto two tympanal membranes. Sound from contralateral inputs has to pass a (double) central membrane (the medial septum), inducing a phase delay and reduction in gain. The sound transmission from the contralateral tympanum is very weak, making each eardrum effectively a 3 input system.

The physics of the cricket auditory system is well understood [2]; the system (see Figure 1) uses a pair of sound receivers with four acoustic inputs, two on the forelegs, which are the external surfaces of the tympana, and two on the body, the prothoracic or acoustic spiracles [3]. The connecting tracheal tubes are such that interference occurs as sounds travel inside the cricket, producing a directional response at the tympana to frequencies near to that of the calling song. The amplitude of vibration of the tympana, and hence the firing rate of the auditory afferent neurons attached to them, vary as a sound source is moved around the cricket and the sounds from the different inputs move in and out of phase. The outputs of the two tympana match when the sound is straight ahead, and the inputs are bilaterally symmetric with respect to the sound source. However, when sound at the calling song frequency is off-centre the phase of signals on the closer side comes better into alignment, and the signal increases on that side, and conversely decreases on the other. It is that crossover of tympanal vibration amplitudes which allows the cricket to track a sound source (see Figure 6 for example).

A simplified version of the auditory system using only two acoustic inputs was implemented in hardware [4], and a simple 8-neuron network was all that was required to then direct a robot to carry out phonotaxis towards a species-specific calling song [5].

A simple simulator was also created to model the behaviour of the auditory system of Figure 1 at different frequencies [6]. Data from Michelsen et al. [2] (Figures 5 and 6) were digitised, and used together with average and "typical" values from the paper to choose gains and delays for the simulation. Figure 2 shows the model of the internal auditory system of the cricket from sound arriving at the acoustic inputs through to transmission down auditory receptor fibres. The simulator implements this model up to the summing of the delayed inputs, as well as modelling the external sound transmission.

Results from the simulator were used to check the directionality of the system at different frequencies, and to gain a better understanding of its response. It was impractical to check the effect of leg movements or of complex sounds in the simulator due to the necessity of simulating the sound production and transmission. An aVLSI chip was designed to implement the same model, both allowing more complex experiments, such as leg movements to be run, and experiments to be run in the real world.

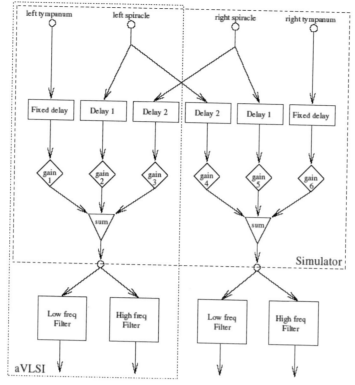

Figure 2: A model of the auditory system of the cricket, used to build the simulator and the aVLSI implementation (shown in boxes).

These experiments with the simulator and the circuits are being published in [6] and the reader is referred to those papers for more details. In the present paper we present the details of the circuits used for the aVLSI implementation.

2 Circuits

The chip, implementing the aVLSI box in Figure 2, comprises two all-pass delay filters, three gain circuits, a second-order narrow-band band-pass filter, a first-order wide-band band-pass filter, a first-order high-pass filter, as well as supporting circuitry (including reference voltages, currents, *etc.*). A single aVLSI chip (MOSIS tiny-chip) thus includes half the necessary circuitry to model the complete auditory system of a cricket. The complete model of the auditory system can be obtained by using two appropriately connected chips.

Only two all-pass delay filters need to be implemented instead of three as suggested by Figure 2, because it is only the relative delay between the three pathways arriving at the one summing node that counts. The delay circuits were implemented with fully-differential gm-C filters. In order to extend the frequency range of the delay, a first-order all-pass delay circuit was cascaded with a second-order all-pass delay circuit. The resulting addition of the first-order delay and the second-order delay allowed for an approximately flat delay response for a wider bandwidth as the decreased delay around the corner frequency of the first-order filter cancelled with the increased delay of the second-order filter around its resonant frequency. Figure 3 shows the first- and second-order sections of the all-pass delay circuit. Two of these circuits were used and, based on data presented in [2], were designed with delays of 28μs and 62μs, by way of bias current manipulation. The operational transconductance amplifier (OTA) in figure 3 is a standard OTA which includes the common-mode feedback necessary for fully differential designs. The buffers (Figure 3) are simple, cascoded differential pairs.

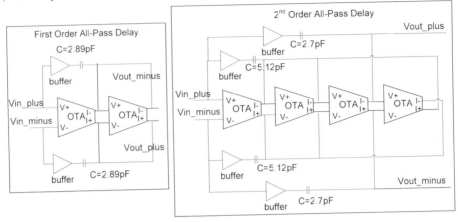

Figure 3: The first-order all-pass delay circuit (left) and the second-order all-pass delay (right).

The differential output of the delay circuits is converted into a current which is multiplied by a variable gain implemented as shown in Figure 4. The gain cell includes a differential pair with source degeneration via transistors N4 and N5. The source degeneration improves the linearity of the current. The three gain cells implemented on the aVLSI have default gains of 2, 3 and 0.91 which are set by holding the *default* input high and appropriately ratioing the bias currents through the value of *vbiasp*. To correct any on-chip mismatches and/or explore other gain configurations a current splitter cell [7] (*p-splitter*, figure 4) allows the gain to be programmed by digital means post fabrication. The current splitter takes an input current (*Ibias*, figure 4) and divides it into branches which recursively halve the current, i.e., the first branch gives ½ *Ibias*, the second branch ¼ *Ibias*, the third branch 1/8 *Ibias* and so on. These currents can be used together with digitally controlled switches as a Digital-to-Analogue converter. By holding *default* low and setting *C5:C0* appropriately, any gain – from 4 to 0.125 – can be set. To save on output pins the program bits (*C5:C0*) for each of the three gain cells are set via a single 18-bit shift register in bit-serial fashion.

Summing the output of the three gain circuits in the current domain simply involves connecting three wires together. Therefore, a natural option for the filters that follow is to use current domain filters. In our case we have chosen to implement log-domain filters using MOS transistors operating in weak inversion. Figure 5 shows the basic building blocks for the filters – the Tau Cell [8] and the multiplier cell – and block diagrams showing how these blocks were connected to create the necessary filtering blocks. The Tau Cell is a log-domain filter which has the first-order response:

$$\frac{I_{out}}{I_{in}} = \frac{1}{s\tau + 1}, \quad \text{where } \tau = \frac{nC_aV_T}{I_a}$$

and n = the slope factor, V_T = thermal voltage, C_a = capacitance, and I_a = bias current. In figure 5, the input currents to the Tau Cell, I_{mult} and $A*I_a$, are only used when building a second-order filter. The multiplier cell is simply a translinear loop where: $I_{out1} * I_{mult} = I_{out2} * AI_a$ or $I_{mult} = AI_a I_{out2}/I_{out1}$. The configurations of the Tau Cell to get particular responses are covered in [8] along with the corresponding equations. The high frequency filter of Figure 2 is implemented by the high-pass filter in Figure 5 with a corner frequency of 17kHz. The low frequency filter, however, is divided into two parts since the biological filter's response (see for example Figure 3A in [9]) separates well into a narrow second-order band-pass filter with a 10kHz resonant frequency and a wide band-pass filter made from a first-order high-pass filter with a 3kHz corner frequency followed by a first-order low-pass filter with a 12kHz corner frequency. These filters are then added together to reproduce the biological filter. The filters' responses can be adjusted post fabrication via their bias currents. This allows for compensation due to processing and matching errors.

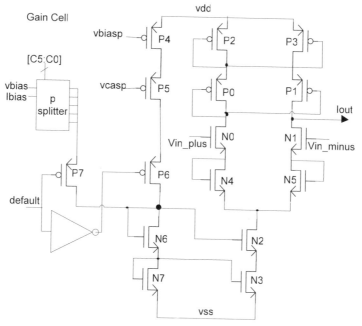

Figure 4: The Gain Cell above is used to convert the differential voltage input from the delay cells into a single-ended current output. The gain of each cell is controllable via a programmable current cell (p_splitter).

An on-chip bias generator [7] was used to create all the necessary current biases on the chip. All the main blocks (delays, gain cells and filters), however, can have their on-chip bias currents overridden through external pins on the chip.

The chip was fabricated using the MOSIS AMI 1.6μm technology and designed using the Cadence Custom IC Design Tools (5.0.33).

3   Methods

The chip was tested using sound generated on a computer and played through a soundcard to the chip. Responses from the chip were recorded by an oscilloscope, and uploaded back to the computer on completion. Given that the output from the chip and the gain circuits is a current, an external current-sense circuit built with discrete components was used to enable the output to be probed by the oscilloscope.

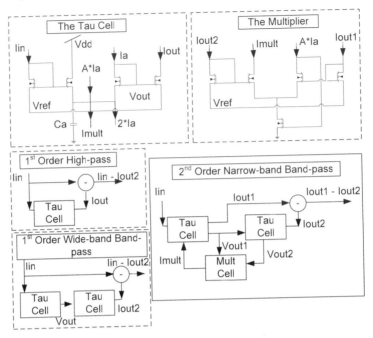

Figure 5: The circuit diagrams for the log-domain filter building blocks – The Tau Cell and The Multiplier – along with the block diagrams for the three filters used in the aVLSI model.

Initial experiments were performed to tune the delays and gains. After that, recordings were taken of the directional frequency responses. Sounds were generated by computer for each chip input to simulate moving the forelegs by delaying the sound by the appropriate amount of time; this was a much simpler solution than using microphones and moving them using motors.

4   Results

The aVLSI chip was tested to measure its gains and delays, which were successfully tuned to the appropriate values. The chip was then compared with the simulation to check that it was faithfully modelling the system. A result of this test at 4kHz (approximately the cricket calling-song frequency) is shown in Figure 6. Apart from a drop in amplitude of the signal, the response of the circuit was very similar to that of the simulator. The differences were expected because the aVLSI circuit has to deal with real-world noise, whereas the simulated version has perfect signals. Examples of the gain versus frequency response of the two log-domain band-pass filters are shown in Figure 7. Note that the narrow-band filter peaks at 6kHz, which is significantly above the mating song frequency of the cricket which is around 4.5kHz. This is not a mistake, but is observed in real crickets as well. As stated in the introduction, a range of further testing results with both the circuit and the simulator are being published in [6].

5 Discussion

The aVLSI auditory sensor in this research models the hearing of the field cricket *Gryllus bimaculatus*. It is a more faithful model of the cricket auditory system than was previously built in [4], reproducing all the acoustic inputs, as well as the responses to frequencies of both the co specific calling song and bat echolocation chirps. It also generates outputs corresponding to the two sets of behaviourally relevant auditory receptor fibres. Results showed that it matched the biological data well, though there were some inconsistencies due to an error in the specification that will be addressed in a future iteration of the design. A more complete implementation across all frequencies was impractical because of complexity and size issues as well as serving no clear behavioural purpose.

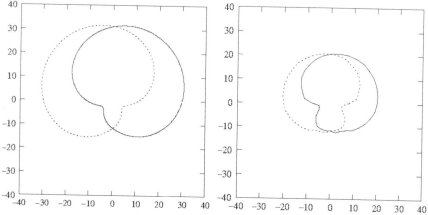

Figure 6: Vibration amplitude of the left (dotted) and right (solid) virtual tympana measured in decibels in response to a 4kHz tone in simulation (left) and on the aVLSI chip (right). The plot shows the amplitude of the tympanal responses as the sound source is rotated around the cricket.

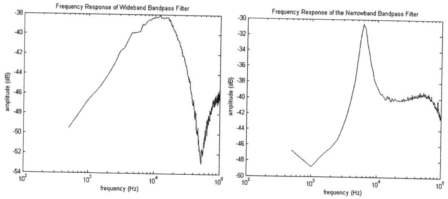

Figure 7: Frequency-Gain curves for the narrow-band and wide-band band-pass filters.

The long-term aim of this work is to better understand simple sensorimotor control loops in crickets and other insects. The next step is to mount this circuitry on a robot to carry out behavioural experiments, which we will compare with existing and new behavioural data (such as that in [10]). This will allow us to refine our models of the neural circuitry involved. Modelling the sensory afferent neurons in hardware is necessary in order to reduce processor load on our robot, so the next revision will include these either onboard, or on a companion chip as we have done before [11]. We will also move both sides of the auditory system onto a single chip to conserve space on the robot.

It is our belief and experience that, as a result of this intelligent pre-processing carried out at the sensor level, the neural circuits necessary to accurately model the behaviour will remain simple.

Acknowledgments

The authors thank the Institute of Neuromorphic Engineering and the UK Biotechnology and Biological Sciences Research Council for funding the research in this paper.

References

[1] R. Wehner. Matched filters – neural models of the external world. J Comp Physiol A, 161: 511–531, 1987.

[2] A. Michelsen, A. V. Popov, and B. Lewis.Physics of directional hearing in the cricket Gryllus bimaculatus. Journal of Comparative Physiology A, 175:153–164, 1994.

[3] A. Michelsen. The tuned cricket. News Physiol. Sci., 13:32–38, 1998.

[4] H. H. Lund, B. Webb, and J. Hallam. A robot attracted to the cricket species Gryllus bimaculatus. In P. Husbands and I. Harvey, editors, Proceedings of 4th European Conference on Artificial Life, pages 246–255. MIT Press/Bradford Books, MA., 1997.

[5] R Reeve and B. Webb. New neural circuits for robot phonotaxis. Phil. Trans. R. Soc. Lond. A, 361:2245–2266, August 2003.

[6] R. Reeve, A. van Schaik, C. Jin, T. Hamilton, B. Torben-Nielsen and B. Webb Directional hearing in a silicon cricket. *Biosystems*, (in revision), 2005b

[7] T. Delbrück and A. van Schaik, Bias Current Generators with Wide Dynamic Range, Analog Integrated Circuits and Signal Processing 42(2), 2005

[8] A. van Schaik and C. Jin, The Tau Cell: A New Method for the Implementation of Arbitrary Differential Equations, IEEE International Symposium on Circuits and Systems (ISCAS) 2003

[9] Kazuo Imaizumi and Gerald S. Pollack. Neural coding of sound frequency by cricket auditory receptors. The Journal of Neuroscience, 19(4):1508–1516, 1999.

[10]Berthold Hedwig and James F.A. Poulet. Complex auditory behaviour emerges from simple reactive steering. Nature, 430:781–785, 2004.

[11]R. Reeve, B. Webb, A. Horchler, G. Indiveri, and R. Quinn. New technologies for testing a model of cricket phonotaxis on an outdoor robot platform. *Robotics and Autonomous Systems*, 51(1):41-54, 2005.

Goal-Based Imitation as Probabilistic Inference over Graphical Models

Deepak Verma
Deptt of CSE, Univ. of Washington,
Seattle WA- 98195-2350
deepak@cs.washington.edu

Rajesh P. N. Rao
Deptt of CSE, Univ. of Washington,
Seattle WA- 98195-2350
rao@cs.washington.edu

Abstract

Humans are extremely adept at learning new skills by imitating the actions of others. A progression of imitative abilities has been observed in children, ranging from imitation of simple body movements to goal-based imitation based on inferring intent. In this paper, we show that the problem of goal-based imitation can be formulated as one of inferring goals and selecting actions using a learned probabilistic graphical model of the environment. We first describe algorithms for planning actions to achieve a goal state using probabilistic inference. We then describe how planning can be used to bootstrap the learning of goal-dependent policies by utilizing feedback from the environment. The resulting graphical model is then shown to be powerful enough to allow goal-based imitation. Using a simple maze navigation task, we illustrate how an agent can infer the goals of an observed teacher and imitate the teacher even when the goals are uncertain and the demonstration is incomplete.

1 Introduction

One of the most powerful mechanisms of learning in humans is learning by watching. Imitation provides a fast, efficient way of acquiring new skills without the need for extensive and potentially dangerous experimentation. Research over the past decade has shown that even newborns can imitate simple body movements (such as facial actions) [1]. While the neural mechanisms underlying imitation remain unclear, recent research has revealed the existence of "mirror neurons" in the primate brain which fire both when a monkey watches an action or when it performs the same action [2].

The most sophisticated forms of imitation are those that require an ability to infer the underlying goals and intentions of a teacher. In this case, the imitating agent attributes not only visible behaviors to others, but also utilizes the idea that others have internal mental states that underlie, predict, and generate these visible behaviors. For example, infants that are about 18 months old can readily imitate actions on objects, e.g., pulling apart a dumbbell shaped object (Fig. 1a). More interestingly, they can imitate this action even when the adult actor accidentally under- or overshot his target, or the hands slipped several times, leaving the goal-state unachieved (Fig. 1b)[3]. They were thus presumably able to infer the actor's goal, which remained unfulfilled, and imitate not the observed action but the intended one.

In this paper, we propose a model for intent inference and goal-based imitation that utilizes probabilistic inference over graphical models. We first describe how the basic problems of planning an action sequence and learning policies (state to action mappings) can be solved through probabilistic inference. We then illustrate the applicability of the learned graphical model to the problems of goal inference and imitation. Goal inference is achieved by utilizing one's own learned model as a substitute for the teacher's. Imitation is achieved by using one's learned policies to reach an inferred goal state. Examples based on the classic maze navigation domain are provided throughout to help illustrate the behavior of the model. Our results suggest that graphical models provide a powerful platform for modeling and implementing goal-based imitation.

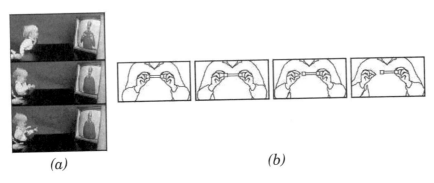

(a)   (b)

Figure 1: **Example of Goal-Based Imitation by Infants:** (a) Infants as young as 14 months old can imitate actions on objects as seen on TV (from [4]). (b) Human actor demonstrating an unsuccessful act. Infants were subsequently able to correctly infer the intent of the actor and successfully complete the act (from [3]).

2 Graphical Models

We first describe how graphical models can be used to plan action sequences and learn goal-based policies, which can subsequently be used for goal inference and imitation. Let Ω_S be the set of states in the environment, Ω_A the set of all possible actions available to the agent, and Ω_G the set of possible goals. We assume all three sets are finite. Each goal g represents a target state $Goal_g \in \Omega_S$. At time t the agent is in state s_t and executes action a_t. g_t represents the current goal that the agent is trying to reach at time t. Executing the action a_t changes the agent's state in a stochastic manner given by the transition probability $P(s_{t+1} \mid s_t, a_t)$, which is assumed to be independent of t i.e., $P(s_{t+1} = s' \mid s_t = s, a_t = a) = \tau_{s'sa}$.

Starting from an initial state $s_1 = s$ and a desired goal state g, planning involves computing a series of actions $a_{1:T}$ to reach the goal state, where T represents the maximum number of time steps allowed (the "episode length"). Note that we do not require T to be *exactly* equal to the shortest path to the goal, just as an upper bound on the shortest path length. We use a, s, g to represent a specific value for action, state, and goal respectively. Also, when obvious from the context, we use s for $s_t = s$, a for $a_t = a$ and g for $g_t = g$.

In the case where the state s_t is fully observed, we obtain the graphical model in Fig. 2a, which is also used in *Markov Decision Process* (MDP) [5] (but with a reward function). The agent needs to compute a stochastic *policy* $\hat{\pi}_t(a \mid s, g)$ that maximizes the probability $P(s_{T+1} = Goal_g \mid s_t = s, g_t = g)$. For a large time horizon ($T \gg 1$), the policy is independent of t i.e. $\hat{\pi}_t(a \mid s, g) = \hat{\pi}(a \mid s, g)$ (a *stationary* policy). A more realistic scenario is where the state s_t is hidden but some aspects of it are visible. Given the current state $s_t = s$, an observation o is produced with the probability $P(o_t = o \mid s_t = s) =$

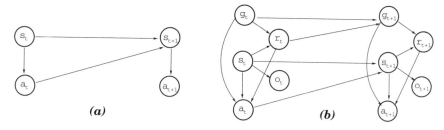

(a) (b)

Figure 2: **Graphical Models:** (a) The standard MDP graphical model: The dependencies between the nodes from time step t to $t+1$ are represented by the transition probabilities and the dependency between actions and states is encoded by the policy. (b) The graphical model used in this paper (note the addition of goal, observation and "reached" nodes). See text for more details.

ζ_{so}. In this paper, we assume the observations are discrete and drawn from the set Ω_O, although the approach can be easily generalized to the case of continuous observations (as in HMMs, for example). We additionally include a goal variable g_t and a "reached" variable r_t, resulting in the graphical model in Fig. 2b (this model is similar to the one used in partially observable MDPs (POMDPs) but without the goal/reached variables). The goal variable g_t represents the current goal the agent is trying to reach while the variable r_t is a boolean variable that assumes the value 1 whenever the current state equals the current goal state and 0 otherwise. We use r_t to help infer the shortest path to the goal state (given an upper bound T on path length); this is done by constraining the actions that can be selected once the goal state is reached (see next section). Note that r_t can also be used to model the switching of goal states (once a goal is reached) and to implement hierarchical extensions of the present model. The current action a_t now depends not only on the current state but also on the current goal g_t, and whether we have reached the goal (as indicated by r_t).

The Maze Domain: To illustrate the proposed approach, we use the standard stochastic maze domain that has been traditionally used in the MDP and reinforcement learning literature [6, 7]. Figure 3 shows the 7×7 maze used in the experiments. Solid squares denote a wall. There are five possible actions: up, down, left, right and stayput. Each action takes the agent into the intended cell with a high probability. This probability is governed by the noise parameter η, which is the probability that the agent will end up in one of the adjoining (non-wall) squares or remain in the same square. For example, for the maze in Fig. 3, $P([3,5] \mid [4,5], \texttt{left}) = \eta$ while $P([4,4] \mid [4,5], \texttt{left}) = 1 - 3\eta$ (we use [i,j] to denote the cell in ith row and jth column from the top left corner).

3 Planning and Learning Policies

3.1 Planning using Probabilistic Inference

To simplify the exposition, we first assume full observability ($\zeta_{so} = \delta(s, o)$). We also assume that the environment model τ is known (the problem of learning τ is addressed later). The problem of planning can then be stated as follows: Given a goal state g, an initial state s, and number of time steps T, what is the sequence of actions $\hat{a}_{1:T}$ that maximizes the probability of reaching the goal state? We compute these actions using the most probable explanation (MPE) method, a standard routine in graphical model packages (see [7] for an alternate approach). When MPE is applied to the graphical model in Fig. 2b, we obtain:

$$\bar{a}_{1:T}, \bar{s}_{2:T+1}, \bar{g}_{1:T}, \bar{r}_{1:T} = \text{argmax } P(a_{1:T}, s_{2:T}, g_{1:T}, r_{1:T} \mid s_1 = s, s_{T+1} = Goal_g) \quad (1)$$

When using the MPE method, the "reached" variable r_t can be used to compute the shortest path to the goal. For $P(a \mid g, s, r)$, we set the prior for the stayput ac-

1395

tion to be very high when $r_t = 1$ and uniform otherwise. This breaks the isomorphism of the MPE action sequences with respect to the `stayput` action, i.e., for $s_1 = [4,6]$, goal=$[4,7]$, and $T = 2$, the probability of `right,stayput` becomes much higher than that of `stayput,right` (otherwise, they have the same posterior probability). Thus, the `stayput` action is discouraged unless the agent has reached the goal. This technique is quite general, in the sense that we can always augment Ω_A with a *no-op* action and use this technique based on r_t to push the *no-op* actions to the end of a T-length action sequence for a pre-chosen upper bound T.

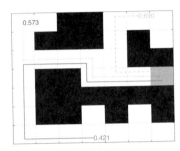

Figure 3: **Planning and Policy Learning:** (a) shows three example plans (action sequences) computed using the MPE method. The plans are shown as colored lines capturing the direction of actions. The numbers denote probability of success of each plan. The longer plans have lower probability of success as expected.

3.2 Policy Learning using Planning

Executing a plan in a noisy environment may not always result in the goal state being reached. However, in the instances where a goal state is indeed reached, the executed action sequence can be used to bootstrap the learning of an optimal policy $\hat{\pi}(a \mid s, g)$, which represents the probability for action a in state s when the goal state to be reached is g. We define optimality in terms of reaching the goal using the shortest path. Note that the optimal policy may differ from the prior $P(a|s, g)$ which counts all actions executed in state s for goal g, regardless of whether the plan was successful.

MDP Policy Learning: Algorithm 1 shows a planning-based method for learning policies for an MDP (both τ and π are assumed unknown and initialized to a prior distribution, e.g., uniform). The agent selects a random start state and a goal state (according to $P(g_1)$), infers the MPE plan $\bar{a}_{1:T}$ using the current τ, executes it, and updates the frequency counts for $\tau_{s'sa}$ based on the observed s_t and s_{t+1} for each a_t. The policy $\hat{\pi}(a \mid s, g)$ is only updated (by updating the action frequencies) if the goal g was reached. To learn an accurate τ, the algorithm is biased towards exploration of the state space initially based on the parameter α (the "exploration probability"). α decreases by a decay factor γ ($0 < \gamma < 1$) with each iteration so that the algorithm transitions to an "exploitation" phase when transition model is well learned and favors the execution of the MPE plan.

POMDP Policy Learning: In the case of partial observability, Algorithm 1 is modified to compute the plan $\bar{a}_{1:T}$ based on observation $o_1 = o$ as evidence instead of $s_1 = s$ in Eq.1. The plan is executed to record observations $o_{2:T+1}$, which are then used to compute the MPE estimate for the hidden states: $\bar{s}^o_{1:T+1}, \bar{g}_{1:T}, \bar{r}_{1:T+1} = $ argmax $P(s_{1:T+1}, g_{1:T}, r_{1:T+1} \mid o_{1:T+1}, \bar{a}_{1:T}, g_{T+1} = g)$. The MPE estimate $\bar{s}^o_{1:T+1}$ is then used instead of $s^o_{1:T+1}$ to update $\hat{\pi}$ and τ.

Results: Figure 4a shows the error in the learned transition model and policy as a function of the number of iterations of the algorithm. Error in $\tau_{s'sa}$ was defined as the squared sum of differences between the learned and true transition parameters. Error in the learned policy was defined as the number of disagreements between the optimal deterministic pol-

Algorithm 1 Policy learning in an unknown environment

1: Initialize transition model $\tau_{s'sa}$, policy $\hat{\pi}(a \mid s, g)$, α, and $numTrials$.
2: **for** $iter = 1$ to $numTrials$ **do**
3:     Choose random start location s_1 based on prior $P(s_1)$.
4:     Pick a goal g according to prior $P(g_1)$.
5:     With probability α:
6:       $a_{1:T}$= Random action sequence.
7:     Otherwise:
8:       Compute MPE plan as in Eq.1 using current $\tau_{s'sa}$.
         Set $a_{1:T} = \bar{a}_{1:T}$
9:     Execute $a_{1:T}$ and record observed states $s^o_{2:T+1}$.
10:    Update $\tau_{s'sa}$ based on $a_{1:T}$ and $s^o_{1:T+1}$.
11:    If the plan was successful, update policy $\hat{\pi}(a \mid s, g)$ using $a_{1:T}$ and $s^o_{1:T+1}$.
12:    $\alpha = \alpha \times \gamma$
13: **end for**

icy for each goal computed via policy iteration and $\operatorname*{argmax}_a \hat{\pi}(a \mid s, g)$, summed over all goals. Both errors decrease to zero with increasing number of iterations. The policy error decreases only after the transition model error becomes significantly small because without an accurate estimate of τ, the MPE plan is typically incorrect and the agent rarely reaches the goal state, resulting in little or no learning of the policy. Figs. 4b shows the maximum probability action $\operatorname*{argmax}_a \hat{\pi}(a \mid s, g)$ learned for each state (maze location) for one of the goals. It is clear that the optimal action has been learned by the algorithm for all locations to reach the given goal state. The results for the POMDP case are shown in Fig. 4c and d. The policy error decreases but does not reach zero because of perceptual ambiguity at certain locations such as corners, where two (or more) actions may have roughly equal probability (see Fig. 4d). The optimal strategy in these ambiguous states is to sample from these actions.

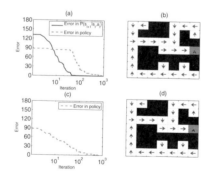

Figure 4: **Learning Policies for an MDP and a POMDP:** (a) shows the error in the transition model and policy w.r.t the true transition model and optimal policy for the maze MDP. (b) The optimal policy learned for one of the 3 goals. (c) and (d) show corresponding results for the POMDP case (the transition model was assumed to be known). The long arrows represent the maximum probability action while the short arrows show all the high probability actions when there is no clear winner.

4 Inferring Intent and Goal-Based Imitation

Consider a task where the agent gets observations $o_{1:t}$ from observing a teacher and seeks to imitate the teacher. We use $P(o_t = o \mid s_t = s) = \zeta_{so}$ in Fig. 2b (for the examples here, ζ_{so} was the same as in the previous section). Also, for $P(a|s, g, r_t = 0)$, we use the policy $\hat{\pi}(a \mid s, g)$ learned as in the previous section. The goal of the agent is to infer the intention of the teacher given a (possibly incomplete) demonstration and to reach the intended goal using its policy (which could be different from the teacher's optimal policy). Using the graphical model formulation the problem of goal inference reduces to finding the marginal $P(g_T \mid o_{1:t'})$, which can be efficiently computed using standard techniques such as belief propagation. Imitation is accomplished by choosing the goal with the highest probability and executing actions to reach that goal.

Fig. 5a shows the results of goal inference for the set of noisy teacher observations in Fig. 5b. The three goal locations are indicated by red, blue, and green squares respectively. Note that the inferred goal probabilities correctly reflect the putative goal(s) of the teacher at each point in the teacher trajectory. In addition, even though the teacher demonstration is incomplete, the imitator can perform goal-based imitation by inferring the teacher's most likely goal as shown in Fig. 5c. This mimics the results reported by [3] on the intent inference by infants.

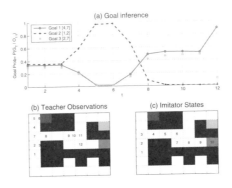

Figure 5: **Goal Inference and Goal-Based Imitation:** (a) shows the goal probabilities inferred at each time step from teacher observations. (b) shows the teacher observations, which are noisy and include a detour while en route to the red goal. The teacher demonstration is incomplete and stops short of the red goal. (c) The imitator infers the most likely goal using (a) and performs goal-based imitation while avoiding the detour (The numbers t in a cell in (b) and (c) represent o_t and s_t respectively).

5   Online Imitation with Uncertain Goals

Now consider a task where the goal is to imitate a teacher online (i.e., simultaneously with the teacher). The teacher observations are assumed to be corrupted by noise and may include significant periods of occlusion where no data is available. The graphical model framework provides an elegant solution to the problem of planning and selecting actions when observations are missing and only a probability distribution over goals is available. The best current action can be picked using the marginal $P(a_t \mid o_{1:t})$, which can be computed efficiently for the graphical model in Fig. 2c. This marginal is equal to $\sum_i P(a_t \mid g_i, o_{1:t}) P(g_i \mid o_{1:t})$, i.e., the policy for each goal *weighted* by the likelihood of that goal given past teacher observations, which corresponds to our intuition of how actions should be picked when goals are uncertain.

Fig. 6a shows the inferred distribution over goal states as the teacher follows a trajectory given by the noisy observations in Fig. 6b. Initially, all goals are nearly equally likely (with a slight bias for the nearest goal). Although the goal is uncertain and certain portions of the teacher trajectory are occluded[1], the agent is still able to make progress towards regions

---

[1]We simulated occlusion using a special observation symbol which carried no information about current state, i.e., $P(\text{occluded} \mid s) = \epsilon$ for all s ($\epsilon \ll 1$)

most likely to contain any probable goal states and is able to "catch-up" with the teacher when observations become available again (Fig.. 6c).

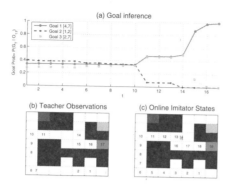

Figure 6: **Online Imitation with Uncertain Goals:** (a) shows the goal probabilities inferred by the agent at each time step for the noisy teacher trajectory in (b). (b) Observations of the teacher. Missing numbers indicate times at which the teacher was occluded. (c) The agent is able to follow the teacher trajectory even when the teacher is occluded based on the evolving goal distribution in (a).

6 Conclusions

We have proposed a new model for intent inference and goal-based imitation based on probabilistic inference in graphical models. The model assumes an initial learning phase where the agent explores the environment (cf. body babbling in infants [8]) and learned a graphical model capturing the sensory consequences of motor actions. The learned model is then used for planning action sequences to goal states and for learning policies. The resulting graphical model then serves as a platform for intent inference and goal-based imitation.

Our model builds on the proposals of several previous researchers. It extends the approach of [7] from planning in a traditional state-action Markov model to a full-fledged graphical model involving states, actions, and goals with edges for capturing conditional distributions denoting policies. The indicator variable r_t used in our approach is similar to the ones used in some hierarchical graphical models [9, 10, 11]. However, these papers do not address the issue of action selection or imitation. Several models of imitation have previously been proposed [12, 13, 14, 15, 16, 17]; these models are typically not probabilistic and have focused on trajectory following rather than intent inference and goal-based imitation.

An important issue yet to be resolved is the scalability of the proposed approach. The Bayesian model requires both a learned environment model as well as a learned policy. In the case of the maze example, these were learned using a relatively small number of trials due to small size of the state space. A more realistic scenario involving, for example, a human or a humanoid robot would presumably require an extremely large number of trials during learning due to the large number of degrees-of-freedom available; fortunately, the problem may be alleviated in two ways: first, only a small portion of the state space may be physically realizable due to constraints imposed by the body or environment; second, the agent could selectively refine its models during imitative sessions. Hierarchical state space models may also help in this regard.

The probabilistic model we have proposed also opens up the possibility of applying Bayesian methodologies such as manipulation of prior probabilities of task alternatives to obtain a deeper understanding of goal inference and imitation in humans. For example, one could explore the effects of biasing a human subject towards particular classes of actions (e.g., through repetition) under particular sets of conditions. One could also manipulate the learned environment model used by subjects with the help of virtual reality environments. Such manipulations have yielded valuable information regarding the type of priors and internal models that the adult human brain uses in perception (see, e.g., [18]) and in motor learning [19]. We believe that the application of Bayesian techniques to imitation could shed new light on the problem of how infants acquire internal models of the people and objects they encounter in the world.

References

[1] A. N. Meltzoff and M. K. Moore. Newborn infants imitate adult facial gestures. *Child Development*, 54:702–709, 1983.

[2] L. Fogassi G. Rizzolatti, L. Fadiga and V. Gallese. From mirror neurons to imitation, facts, and speculations. *In A. N. Meltzoff and W. Prinz (Eds.), The imitative mind: Development, evolution, and brain bases*, pages 247–266, 2002.

[3] A. N. Meltzoff. Understanding the intentions of others: Re-enactment of intended acts by 18-month-old children. *Developmental Psychology*, 31:838–850, 1995.

[4] A. N. Meltzoff. Imitation of televised models by infants. *Child Development*, 59:1221–1229, 1988a.

[5] C. Boutilier, T. Dean, and S. Hanks. Decision-theoretic planning: Structural assumptions and computational leverage. *Journal of AI Research*, 11:1–94, 1999.

[6] R. S. Sutton and A. Barto. *Reinforcement Learning: An Introduction*. MIT Press, Cambridge, MA, 1998.

[7] H. Attias. Planning by probabilistic inference. In *Proceedings of the 9th Int. Workshop on AI and Statistics*, 2003.

[8] R. P. N. Rao, A. P. Shon, and A. N. Meltzoff. A Bayesian model of imitation in infants and robots. In *Imitation and Social Learning in Robots, Humans, and Animals*. Cambridge University Press, 2004.

[9] G. Theocharous, K. Murphy, and L. P. Kaelbling. Representing hierarchical POMDPs as DBNs for multi-scale robot localization. *ICRA*, 2004.

[10] S. Fine, Y. Singer, and N. Tishby. The hierarchical hidden Markov model: Analysis and applications. *Mach. Learn.*, 32(1):41–62, 1998.

[11] H. Bui, D. Phung, and S. Venkatesh. Hierarchical hidden Markov models with general state hierarchy. In *AAAI 2004*, 2004.

[12] G. Hayes and J. Demiris. A robot controller using learning by imitation. *Proceedings of the 2nd International Symposium on Intelligent Robotic Systems, Grenoble, France,*, pages 198–204, 1994.

[13] M. J. Mataric and M. Pomplun. Fixation behavior in observation and imitation of human movement. *Cognitive Brain Research*, 7:191–202, 1998.

[14] S. Schaal. Is imitation learning the route to humanoid robots? *Trends in Cognitive Sciences*, 3:233–242, 1999.

[15] A. Billard and K. Dautenhahn. Experiments in social robotics- grounding and use of communication in robotic agents. *Adaptive Behavior*, 7:3–4, 2000.

[16] C. Breazeal and B. Scassellati. Challenges in building robots that imitate people. *In K. Dautenhahn and C. L. Nehaniv (Eds.), Imitation in animals and artifacts*, pages 363–390, 2002.

[17] K. Dautenhahn and C. Nehaniv. *Imitation in Animals and Artifacts*. Cambridge, MA: MIT Press, 2002.

[18] B. A. Olshausen R. P. N. Rao and M. S. Lewicki (Eds.). *Probabilistic Models of the Brain: Perception and Neural Function*. Cambridge, MA: MIT Press, 2002.

[19] KP. Krding and D. Wolpert. Bayesian integration in sensorimotor learning. *Nature*, 427:244–247, 2004.

Kernels for gene regulatory regions

Jean-Philippe Vert
Geostatistics Center
Ecole des Mines de Paris - ParisTech
Jean-Philippe.Vert@ensmp.fr

Robert Thurman
Division of Medical Genetics
University of Washington
rthurman@u.washington.edu

William Stafford Noble
Department of Genome Sciences
University of Washington
noble@gs.washington.edu

Abstract

We describe a hierarchy of motif-based kernels for multiple alignments of biological sequences, particularly suitable to process regulatory regions of genes. The kernels incorporate progressively more information, with the most complex kernel accounting for a multiple alignment of orthologous regions, the phylogenetic tree relating the species, and the prior knowledge that relevant sequence patterns occur in conserved motif blocks. These kernels can be used in the presence of a library of known transcription factor binding sites, or *de novo* by iterating over all k-mers of a given length. In the latter mode, a discriminative classifier built from such a kernel not only recognizes a given class of promoter regions, but as a side effect simultaneously identifies a collection of relevant, discriminative sequence motifs. We demonstrate the utility of the motif-based multiple alignment kernels by using a collection of aligned promoter regions from five yeast species to recognize classes of cell-cycle regulated genes. Supplementary data is available at http://noble.gs.washington.edu/proj/pkernel.

1 Introduction

In a eukaryotic cell, a variety of DNA switches—promoters, enhancers, silencers, etc.—regulate the production of proteins from DNA. These switches typically contain multiple binding site motifs, each of length 5–15 nucleotides, for a class of DNA-binding proteins known as transcription factors. As a result, the detection of such regulatory motifs proximal to a gene provides important clues about its regulation and, therefore, its function. These motifs, if known, are consequently interesting features to extract from genomic sequences in order to compare genes, or cluster them into functional families.

These regulatory motifs, however, usually represent a tiny fraction of the intergenic sequence, and their automatic detection remains extremely challenging. For well-studied transcription factors, libraries of known binding site motifs can be used to scan the intergenic sequence. A common approach for the *de novo* detection of regulatory motifs is to start from a set of genes known to be similarly regulated, for example by clustering gene expression data, and search for over-represented short sequences in their proximal intergenic regions. Alternatively, some authors have proposed to represent each intergenic sequence by its content in short sequences, and to correlate this representation with gene expression data [1]. Finally, additional information to characterize regulatory motifs can be gained by comparing the intergenic sequences of orthologous genes, i.e., genes from different species that have evolved from a common ancestor, because regulatory motifs are more conserved than non-functional intergenic DNA [2].

We propose in this paper a hierarchy of increasingly complex representations for intergenic sequences. Each representation yields a positive definite kernel between intergenic sequences. While various motif-based sequence kernels have been described in the literature (e.g., [3, 4, 5]), these kernels typically operate on sequences from a single species, ignoring relevant information from orthologous sequences. In contrast, our hierarchy of motif-based kernels accounts for a multiple alignment of orthologous regions, the phylogenetic tree relating the species, and the prior knowledge that relevant sequence patterns occur in conserved motif blocks. These kernels can be used in the presence of a library of known transcription factor binding sites, or *de novo* by iterating over all k-mers of a given length. In the latter mode, a discriminative classifier built from such a kernel not only recognizes a given class of regulatory sequences, but as a side effect simultaneously identifies a collection of discriminative sequence motifs. We demonstrate the utility of the motif-based multiple alignment kernels by using a collection of aligned intergenic regions from five yeast species to recognize classes of co-regulated genes.

From a methodological point of view, this paper can be seen as an attempt to incorporate an increasing amount of prior knowledge into a kernel. In particular, this prior information takes the form of a probabilistic model describing with increasing accuracy the object we want to represent. All kernels were designed before any experiment was conducted, and we then performed an objective empirical evaluation of each kernel without further parameter optimization. In general, classification performance improved as the amount of prior knowledge increased. This observation supports the notion that tuning a kernel with prior knowledge is beneficial. However, we observed no improvement in performance following the last modification of the kernel, highlighting the fact that a richer model of the data does not always lead to better performance accuracy.

2 Kernels for intergenic sequences

In a complex eukaryotic genome, regulatory switches may occur anywhere within a relatively large genomic region near a given gene. In this work we focus on a well-studied model organism, the budding yeast *Saccharomyces cerevisiae*, in which the typical intergenic region is less than 1000 bases long. We refer to the intergenic region upstream of a yeast gene as its *promoter region*. Denoting the four-letter set of nucleotides as $\mathcal{A} = \{A, C, G, T\}$, the promoter region of a gene is a finite-length sequence of nucleotides $x \in \mathcal{A}^* = \bigcup_{i=0}^{\infty} \mathcal{A}^i$. Given several sequenced organisms, *in silico* comparison of genes between organisms often allows the detection of orthologous genes, that is, genes that evolved from a common ancestor. If the species are evolutionarily close, as are different yeast strains, then the promoter regions are usually quite similar and can be represented as a *multiple alignment*. Each position in this alignment represents one letter in the shared ancestor's promoter region. Mathematically speaking, a multiple alignment of length n of p sequences is a sequence $\mathbf{c} = c_1, c_2, \ldots, c_n$, where each $c_i \in \bar{\mathcal{A}}^p$, for $i = 1, \ldots, n$, is a column of p letters in the alphabet $\bar{\mathcal{A}} = \mathcal{A} \cup \{-\}$. The additional letter "$-$" is used to represent gaps in sequences, which represent insertion or deletion of letters during the evolution of the sequences.

We are now in the position to describe a family of representations and kernels for promoter regions, incorporating an increasing amount of prior knowledge about the properties of regulatory motifs. All kernels below are simple inner products between vector representations of promoter regions. These vector representations are always indexed by a set $\mathcal{M}$ of short sequences of fixed length d, which can either be all d-mers, i.e., $\mathcal{M} = \mathcal{A}^d$, or a predefined library of indexing sequences. A promoter region P (either single sequence or multiple alignment) is therefore always represented by a vector $\Phi_{\mathcal{M}}(P) = (\Phi_a(P))_{a \in \mathcal{M}}$.

Motif kernel on a single sequence   The simplest approach to index a *single* promoter region $\mathbf{x} \in \mathcal{A}^*$ with an alphabet $\mathcal{M}$ is to define

$$\Phi_a^{\text{Spectrum}}(\mathbf{x}) = n_a(\mathbf{x}) \,, \quad \forall a \in \mathcal{M} \,,$$

where $n_a(\mathbf{x})$ counts the number of occurrences of a in $\mathbf{x}$. When $\mathcal{M} = \mathcal{A}^d$, the resulting kernel is the spectrum kernel [3] between single promoter regions.

Motif kernel on multiple sequences   When a gene has p orthologs in other species, then a set of p promoter regions $\{\mathbf{x}_1, \mathbf{x}_2, \ldots, \mathbf{x}_p\} \in (\mathcal{A}^*)^p$, which are expected to contain similar regulatory motifs, is available. We propose the following representation for such a set:

$$\Phi_a^{\text{Summation}}(\{\mathbf{x}_1, \mathbf{x}_2, \ldots, \mathbf{x}_p\}) = \sum_{i=1}^{p} \Phi_a^{\text{Spectrum}}(\mathbf{x}_i) \,, \quad \forall a \in \mathcal{M} \,.$$

We call the resulting kernel the *summation* kernel. It is essentially the spectrum kernel on the concatenation of the available promoter regions—ignoring, however, k-mers that overlap different sequences in the concatenation. The rationale behind this kernel, compared to the spectrum kernel, is two-fold. First, if all promoters contain common functional motifs and randomly varying nonfunctional motifs, then the signal-to-noise ratio of the relevant regulatory features compared to other irrelevant non-functional features increases by taking the sum (or mean) of individual feature vectors. Second, even functional motifs representing transcription factor binding sites are known to have some variability in some positions, and merging the occurrences of a similar motif in different sequences is a way to model this flexibility in the framework of a vector representation.

Marginalized motif kernel on a multiple alignment   The summation kernel might suffer from at least two limitations. First, it does not include any information about the relationships between orthologs, in particular their relative similarities. Suppose for example that three species are compared, two of them being very similar. Then the promoter regions of two out of three orthologs would be virtually identical, giving an unjustified double weight to this duplicated species compared to the third one in the summation kernel. Second, although mutations in functional motifs between different species would correspond to different short motifs in the summation kernel feature vector, these varying short motifs might not cover all allowed variations in the functional motifs, especially if the motifs are extracted from a small number of orthologs. In such cases, probabilistic models such as weight matrices, which estimate possible variations for each position independently, are known to make more efficient use of the data.

In order to overcome these limitations, we propose to transform the set of promoter regions into a multiple alignment. We therefore assume that a fixed number of q species has been selected, and that a probabilistic model $p(h, c)$, with $h \in \bar{\mathcal{A}}$ and $c \in \bar{\mathcal{A}}^q$ has been tuned on these species. By "tuned," we mean that $p(h, c)$ is a distribution that accurately describes the probability of a given letter h in the common ancestor of the species, together with the set of letters c at the corresponding position in the set of species. Such distributions are commonly used in computational genomics, often resulting from the estimation of a phylogenetic tree model [6]. We also assume that all sets of q promoter regions of groups of orthologous genes in the q species have been turned into multiple alignments.

Given an alignment $\mathbf{c} = c_1, c_2, \ldots, c_n$, suppose for the moment that we know the corresponding true sequence of nucleotides of the common ancestor $\mathbf{h} = h_1, h_2, \ldots, h_n$. Then the spectrum of the sequence $\mathbf{h}$, that is, $\Phi_{\mathcal{M}}^{\text{Spectrum}}(\mathbf{h})$, would be a good summary for the multiple alignment, and the inner product between two such spectra would be a candidate kernel between multiple alignments. The sequence $\mathbf{h}$ being of course unknown, we propose to estimate its conditional probability given the multiple alignment $\mathbf{c}$, under the model where all columns are independent and identically distributed according to the evolutionary model, that is, $p(\mathbf{h}|\mathbf{c}) = \prod_{i=1}^{n} p(h_i|c_i)$. Under this probabilistic model, it is now possible to define the representation of the multiple alignment as the expectation of the spectrum representation of $\mathbf{h}$ with respect to this conditional probability, that is:

$$\Phi_a^{\text{Marginalized}}(\mathbf{c}) = \sum_{\mathbf{h}} \Phi_a^{\text{Spectrum}}(\mathbf{h}) p(\mathbf{h}|\mathbf{c}), \quad \forall a \in \mathcal{M}. \tag{1}$$

In order to compute this representation, we observe that if $\mathbf{h}$ has length n and $a = a_1 \ldots a_d$ has length d, then

$$\Phi_a^{\text{Spectrum}}(\mathbf{h}) = \sum_{i=1}^{n-d+1} \delta(a, h_i \ldots h_{i+d-1}),$$

where δ is the Kronecker function. Therefore,

$$\Phi_a^{\text{Marginalized}}(\mathbf{c}) = \sum_{\mathbf{h} \in \mathcal{A}^n} \left\{ \left(\sum_{i=1}^{n-d+1} \delta(a, h_i \ldots h_{i+d-1}) \right) \prod_{i=1}^{n} p(h_i|c_i) \right\}$$

$$= \sum_{i=1}^{n-d+1} \left(\prod_{j=0}^{d-1} p(a_{j+1}|c_{i+j}) \right).$$

This computation can be performed explicitly by computing $p(a_{j+1}|c_{i+j})$ at each position $i = 1, \ldots, n$, and performing the sum of the products of these probabilities over a moving window. We call the resulting kernel the *marginalized* kernel because it corresponds to the marginalization of the spectrum kernel under the phylogenetic probabilistic model [7].

Marginalized motif kernel with phylogenetic shadowing   The marginalized kernel is expected to be useful when relevant information is distributed along the entire length of the sequences analyzed. In the case of promoter regions, however, the relevant information is more likely to be located within a few short motifs. Because only a small fraction of the total set of promoter regions lies within such motifs, this information is likely to be lost when the whole sequence is represented by its spectrum. In order to overcome this limitation, we exploit the observation that relevant motifs are more evolutionarily conserved on average than the surrounding sequence. This hypothesis has been confirmed by many studies that show that functional parts, being under more evolutionary pressure, are more conserved than non-functional ones.

Given a multiple alignment c, let us assume (temporarily) that we know which parts are relevant. We can encode this information into a sequence of binary variables $\mathbf{s} = s_1 \ldots s_n \in \{0, 1\}^n$, where $s_i = 1$ means that the ith position is relevant, and irrelevant if $s_i = 0$. A typical sequence for a promoter region consist primarily of 0's, except for a few positions indicating the position of the transcription factor binding motifs. Let us also assume that we know the nucleotide sequence $\mathbf{h}$ of the common ancestor. Then it would make sense to use a spectrum kernel based on the spectrum of $\mathbf{h}$ restricted to the relevant positions only. In other words, all positions where $s_i = 0$ could be thrown away, in order to focus only on the relevant positions. This corresponds to defining the features:

$$\Phi_a^{\text{Relevant}}(\mathbf{h}, \mathbf{s}) = \sum_{i=1}^{n-d+1} \delta(a, h_i \ldots h_{i+d-1}) \delta(s_i, 1) \ldots \delta(s_{i+d-1}, 1), \quad \forall a \in \mathcal{M}.$$

Given only a multiple alignment $\mathbf{c}$, the sequences $\mathbf{h}$ and $\mathbf{s}$ are not known but can be estimated. This is where the hypothesis that relevant nucleotides are more conserved than irrelevant nucleotides can be encoded, by using two models of evolution with different rates of mutations, as in phylogenetic shadowing [2]. Let us therefore assume that we have a model $p(c|h, s = 0)$ that describes "fast" evolution from an ancestral nucleotide h to a column c in a multiple alignment, and a second model $p_1(c|h, s = 1)$ that describes "slow" evolution. In practice, we take these models to be two classical evolutionary models with different mutation rates, but any reasonable pair of random models could be used here, if one had a better model for functional sites, for example. Given these two models of evolution, let us also define a prior probability $p(s)$ that a position is relevant or not (related to the proportion of relevant parts we expect in a promoter region), and prior probabilities for the ancestor nucleotide $p(h|s = 0)$ and $p(h|s = 1)$.

The joint probability of being in state s, having an ancestor nucleotide h and a resulting alignment c is then $p(c, h, s) = p(s)p(h|s)p(c|h, s)$. Under the probabilistic model where all columns are independent from each other, that is, $p(\mathbf{h}, \mathbf{s}|\mathbf{c}) = \prod_{i=1}^{n} p(h_i, s_i|c_i)$, we can now replace (1) by the following features:

$$\Phi_a^{\text{Shadow}}(\mathbf{c}) = \sum_{\mathbf{h},\mathbf{s}} \Phi_a^{\text{Relevant}}(\mathbf{h}, \mathbf{s})p(\mathbf{h}, \mathbf{s}|\mathbf{c}) , \quad \forall a \in \mathcal{M} . \tag{2}$$

Like the marginalized spectrum kernel, this kernel can be computed by computing the explicit representation of each multiple sequence alignment $\mathbf{c}$ as a vector $(\Phi_a(\mathbf{c}))_{a \in \mathcal{M}}$ as follows:

$$\Phi_a^{\text{Shadow}}(\mathbf{c}) = \sum_{\mathbf{h} \in \mathcal{A}^n} \sum_{\mathbf{s} \in \{0,1\}^n} \left\{ \sum_{i=1}^{n-d+1} \delta(a, h_i \ldots h_{i+d-1})\delta(s_i, 1) \ldots \delta(s_{i+d-1}, 1) \prod_{i=1}^{n} p(h_i, s_i|c_i) \right\}$$

$$= \sum_{i=1}^{n-d+1} \left(\prod_{j=0}^{d-1} p(h = a_{j+1}, s = 1|c_{i+j}) \right) .$$

The computation can then be carried out by exploiting the observation that each term can be computed by:

$$p(h, s = 1|c) = \frac{p(s = 1)p(h|s = 1)p(c|h, s = 1)}{p(s = 0)p(c|s = 0) + p(s = 1)p(c|s = 1)} .$$

Moreover, it can easily be seen that, like the marginalized kernel, the shadow kernel is the marginalization of the kernel corresponding to Φ^{Relevant} with respect to $p(\mathbf{h}, \mathbf{s}|\mathbf{c})$.

Incorporating Markov dependencies between positions The probabilistic model used in the shadow kernel models each position independently from the others. As a result, a conserved position has the same contribution to the shadow kernel if it is surrounded by other conserved positions, or by varying positions. In order to encode our prior knowledge that the pattern of functional / nonfunctional positions along the sequence is likely to be a succession of short functional regions and longer nonfunctional regions, we propose to replace this probabilistic model by a probabilistic model with a Markov dependency between successive positions for the variable $\mathbf{s}$, that is, to consider the probability:

$$p^{\text{Markov}}(\mathbf{c}, \mathbf{h}, \mathbf{s}) = p(s_1)p(h_1, c_1|s_1) \prod_{i=2}^{n} p(s_i|s_{i-1}) p(h_i, c_i|s_i).$$

This suggests replacing (2) by

$$\Phi_a^{\text{Markov}}(\mathbf{c}) = \sum_{\mathbf{h},\mathbf{s}} \Phi_a(\mathbf{h}, \mathbf{s})p^{\text{Markov}}(\mathbf{h}, \mathbf{s}|\mathbf{c}) , \quad \forall a \in \mathcal{M} .$$

Once again, this feature vector can be computed as a sum of window weights over sequences by

$$\Phi_a^{\text{Markov}}(\mathbf{c}) = \sum_{i=1}^{n-d+1} \left(p\left(s_i = 1 | \mathbf{c}\right) p\left(h_i = a_{j+1} | c_i, s_i = 1\right) \right.$$
$$\left. \times \prod_{j=1}^{d-1} p(h_{i+j} = a_{j+1}, s_{i+j} = 1 | c_{i+j}, s_{i+j-1} = 1) \right).$$

The main difference with the computation of the shadow kernel is the need to compute the term $P\left(s_i = 1 | \mathbf{c}\right)$, which can be done using the general sum-product algorithm.

3   Experiments

We measure the utility of our hierarchy of kernels in a cross-validated, supervised learning framework. As a starting point for the analysis, we use various groups of genes that show co-expression in a microarray study. Eight gene groups were derived from a study that applied hierarchical clustering to a collection of 79 experimental conditions, including time series from the diauxic shift, the cell cycle series, and sporulation, as well as various temperature and reducing shocks [8]. We hypothesize that co-expression implies co-regulation of a given group of genes by a common set of transcription factors. Hence, the corresponding promoter regions should be enriched for a corresponding set of transcription factor binding motifs. We test the ability of a support vector machine (SVM) classifier to learn to recapitulate the co-expression classes, based only upon the promoter regions. Our results show that the SVM performance improves as we incorporate more prior knowledge into the promoter kernel.

We collected the promoter regions from five closely related yeast species [9, 10]. Promoter regions from orthologous genes were aligned using ClustalW, discarding promoter regions that aligned with less than 30% sequence identity relative to the other sequences in the alignment. This procedure produced 3591 promoter region alignments. For the phylogenetic kernels, we inferred a phylogenetic tree among the five yeast species from alignments of four highly conserved proteins—MCM2, MCM3, CDC47 and MCM6. The concatenated alignment was analyzed with fastDNAml [11] using the default parameters. The resulting tree was used in all of our analyses.

SVMs were trained using Gist (microarray.cpmc.columbia.edu/gist) with the default parameters. These include a normalized kernel, and a two-norm soft margin with asymmetric penalty based upon the ratio of positive and negative class sizes. All kernels were computed by summing over all 4^5 k-mers of width 5. Each class was recognized in a one-vs-all fashion. SVM testing was performed using balanced three-fold cross-validation, repeated five times.

The results of this experiment are summarized in Table 1. For every gene class, the worst-performing kernel is one of the three simplest kernels: "simple," "summation" or "marginalization." The mean ROC scores across all eight classes for these three kernels are 0.733, 0.765 and 0.748. Classification performance improves dramatically using the shadow kernel with either a small (2) or large (5) ratio of fast-to-slow evolutionary rates. The mean ROC scores for these two kernels are 0.854 and 0.844. Furthermore, across five of the eight gene classes, one of the two shadow kernels is the best-performing kernel. The Markov kernel performs approximately as well as the shadow kernel. We tried six different parameterizations, as shown in the table, and these achieved mean ROC scores ranging from 0.822 to 0.850. The differences between the best parameterization of this kernel ("Markov 5 90/90") and "shadow 2" are not significant. Although further tuning

Table 1: **Mean ROC scores for SVMs trained using various kernels to recognize classes of co-expressed yeast genes.** The second row in the table gives the number of genes in each class. All other rows contain mean ROC scores across balanced three-fold cross-validation, repeated five times. Standard errors (not shown) are almost uniformly 0.02, with a few values of 0.03. Values in bold-face are the best mean ROC for the given class of genes. The classes of genes (columns) are, respectively, ATP synthesis, DNA replication, glycolysis, mitochondrial ribosome, proteasome, spindle-pole body, splicing and TCA cycle. The kernels are as described in the text. For the shadow and Markov kernels, the values "2" and "5" refer to the ratio of fast to slow evolutionary rates. For the Markov kernel, the values "90" and "99" refer to the self-transition probabilities (times 100) in the conserved and varying states of the model.

Kernel	ATP 15	DNA 5	Glyc 17	Ribo 22	Prot 27	Spin 11	Splic 14	TCA 16	Mean
single	0.711	0.777	0.814	0.743	0.735	0.716	0.683	0.684	0.733
summation	0.773	0.768	0.824	0.750	0.763	0.756	0.739	0.740	0.764
marginalized	0.799	0.805	0.833	0.729	0.748	0.721	0.676	0.673	0.748
shadow 2	0.881	0.929	**0.928**	0.840	0.867	**0.827**	0.787	**0.770**	**0.854**
shadow 5	**0.889**	**0.935**	0.927	0.819	0.849	0.821	0.766	0.752	0.845
Markov 2 90/90	0.848	0.891	0.908	0.830	0.853	0.801	0.773	0.758	0.833
Markov 2 90/99	0.868	0.911	0.915	0.826	0.850	0.782	0.773	0.758	0.830
Markov 2 99/99	0.869	0.910	0.912	0.816	0.840	0.773	0.752	0.735	0.823
Markov 5 90/90	0.875	0.922	0.924	**0.844**	**0.868**	0.814	**0.788**	0.769	0.851
Markov 5 90/99	0.872	0.916	0.920	0.834	0.858	0.794	0.774	0.755	0.840
Markov 5 99/99	0.868	0.917	0.921	0.830	0.853	0.774	0.751	0.733	0.831

of kernel parameters might yield significant improvement, our results thus far suggest that incorporating dependencies between adjacent positions does not help very much.

Finally, we test the ability of the SVM to identify sequence regions that correspond to biologically significant motifs. As a gold standard, we use the JASPAR database (jaspar.cgb.ki.se), searching each class of promoter regions using MONKEY (rana.lbl.gov/~alan/Monkey.htm) with a p-value threshold of 10^{-4}. For each gene class, we identify the three JASPAR motifs that occur most frequently within that class, and we create a list of all 5-mers that appear within those motif occurrences. Next, we create a corresponding list of 5-mers identified by the SVM. We do this by calculating the hyperplane weight associated with each 5-mer and retaining the top 20 5-mers for each of the 15 cross-validation runs. We then take the union over all runs to come up with a list of between 40 and 55 top 5-mers for each class. Table 2 indicates that the discriminative 5-mers identified by the SVM are significantly enriched in 5-mers that appear within biologically significant motif regions, with significant p-values for all eight gene classes (see caption for details).

4 Conclusion

We have described and demonstrated the utility of a class of kernels for characterizing gene regulatory regions. These kernels allow us to incorporate prior knowledge about the evolution of a set of orthologous sequences and the conservation of transcription factor binding site motifs. We have also demonstrated that the motifs identified by an SVM trained using these kernels correspond to biologically significant motif regions. Our future work will focus on automating the process of agglomerating the identified k-mers into a smaller set of motif models, and on applying these kernels in combination with gene expression, protein-protein interaction and other genome-wide data sets.

This work was funded by NIH awards R33 HG003070 and U01 HG003161.

Table 2: **SVM features correlate with discriminative motifs.** The first row lists the number of non-redundant 5-mers constructed from high-scoring SVM features. Row two gives the number of 5-mers constructed from JASPAR motif occurrences in the 5-species alignments. Row three is a tally of all 5-mers appearing in the sequences making up the class. The fourth row gives the size of the intersection between the SVM and motif-based 5-mer lists. The final two rows give the expected value and p-value for the intersection size. The p-value is computed using the hypergeometric distribution by enumerating all possibilites for the intersection of two sets selected from a larger set given the sizes in the first three rows.

	ATP	DNA	Glyc	Ribo	Prot	Spin	Splic	TCA
SVM	46	40	55	50	49	43	48	50
Motif	180	68	227	38	148	152	52	104
Class	1006	839	967	973	1001	891	881	995
Inter	24	8	23	18	23	19	14	21
Expect	8.23	3.24	12.91	1.95	7.25	7.34	2.83	5.23
p-value	6.19e-8	1.15e-2	1.44e-3	3.88e-15	3.24e-8	1.74e-5	1.15e-7	2.00e-9

References

[1] D. Y. Chiang, P. O. Brown, and M. B. Eisen. Visualizing associations between genome sequences and gene expression data using genome-mean expression profiles. *Bioinformatics*, 17(Supp. 1):S49–S55, 2001.

[2] D. Boffelli, J. McAuliffe, D. Ovcharenko, K. D. Lewis, I. Ovcharenko, L. Pachter, and E. M. Rubin. Phylogenetic shadowing of primate sequences to find functional regions of the human genome. *Science*, 299:1391–1394, 2003.

[3] C. Leslie, E. Eskin, and W. S. Noble. The spectrum kernel: A string kernel for SVM protein classification. In R. B. Altman, A. K. Dunker, L. Hunter, K. Lauderdale, and T. E. Klein, editors, *Proceedings of the Pacific Symposium on Biocomputing*, pages 564–575, New Jersey, 2002. World Scientific.

[4] X. H-F. Zhang, K. A. Heller, I. Hefter, C. S. Leslie, and L. A. Chasin. Sequence information for the splicing of human pre-mRNA identified by support vector machine classification. *Genome Research*, 13:2637–2650, 2003.

[5] A. Zien, G. Rätch, S. Mika, B. Schölkopf, T. Lengauer, and K.-R. Müller. Engineering support vector machine kernels that recognize translation initiation sites. *Bioinformatics*, 16(9):799–807, 2000.

[6] R. Durbin, S. Eddy, A. Krogh, and G. Mitchison. *Biological Sequence Analysis*. Cambridge UP, 1998.

[7] K. Tsuda, T. Kin, and K. Asai. Marginalized kernels for biological sequences. *Bioinformatics*, 18:S268–S275, 2002.

[8] M. Eisen, P. Spellman, P. O. Brown, and D. Botstein. Cluster analysis and display of genome-wide expression patterns. *Proceedings of the National Academy of Sciences of the United States of America*, 95:14863–14868, 1998.

[9] Paul Cliften, Priya Sudarsanam, Ashwin Desikan, Lucinda Fulton, Bob Fulton, John Majors, Robert Waterston, Barak A. Cohen, and Mark Johnston. Finding functional features in Saccharomyces genomes by phylogenetic footprinting. *Science*, 301(5629):71–76, 2003.

[10] Manolis Kellis, Nick Patterson, Matthew Endrizzi, Bruce Birren, and Eric S Lander. Sequencing and comparison of yeast species to identify genes and regulatory elements. *Nature*, 423(6937):241–254, 2003.

[11] GJ Olsen, H Matsuda, R Hagstrom, and R Overbeek. fastDNAmL: a tool for construction of phylogenetic trees of DNA sequences using maximum likelihood. *Comput. Appl. Biosci.*, 10(1):41–48, 1994.

Consistency of one-class SVM and related algorithms

Régis Vert
Laboratoire de Recherche en Informatique
Université Paris-Sud
91405, Orsay Cedex, France
Masagroup
24 Bd de l'Hôpital
75005, Paris, France
Regis.Vert@lri.fr

Jean-Philippe Vert
Geostatistics Center
Ecole des Mines de Paris - ParisTech
77300 Fontainebleau, France
Jean-Philippe.Vert@ensmp.fr

Abstract

We determine the asymptotic limit of the function computed by support vector machines (SVM) and related algorithms that minimize a regularized empirical convex loss function in the reproducing kernel Hilbert space of the Gaussian RBF kernel, in the situation where the number of examples tends to infinity, the bandwidth of the Gaussian kernel tends to 0, and the regularization parameter is held fixed. Non-asymptotic convergence bounds to this limit in the L_2 sense are provided, together with upper bounds on the classification error that is shown to converge to the Bayes risk, therefore proving the Bayes-consistency of a variety of methods although the regularization term does not vanish. These results are particularly relevant to the one-class SVM, for which the regularization can not vanish by construction, and which is shown for the first time to be a consistent density level set estimator.

1 Introduction

Given n i.i.d. copies $(X_1, Y_1), \ldots, (X_n, Y_n)$ of a random variable $(X, Y) \in \mathbb{R}^d \times \{-1, 1\}$, we study in this paper the limit and consistency of learning algorithms that solve the following problem:

$$\arg\min_{f \in \mathcal{H}_\sigma} \left\{ \frac{1}{n} \sum_{i=1}^{n} \phi\left(Y_i f(X_i)\right) + \lambda \| f \|_{\mathcal{H}_\sigma}^2 \right\}, \tag{1}$$

where $\phi : \mathbb{R} \to \mathbb{R}$ is a convex loss function and $\mathcal{H}_\sigma$ is the reproducing kernel Hilbert space (RKHS) of the normalized Gaussian radial basis function kernel (denoted simply Gaussian kernel below):

$$k_\sigma(x, x') = \frac{1}{\left(\sqrt{2\pi}\sigma\right)^d} \exp\left(\frac{-\| x - x' \|^2}{2\sigma^2}\right), \quad \sigma > 0. \tag{2}$$

This framework encompasses in particular the classical support vector machine (SVM) [1] when $\phi(u) = \max(1 - u, 0)$. Recent years have witnessed important theoretical advances aimed at understanding the behavior of such regularized algorithms when n tends to infinity and λ decreases to 0. In particular the consistency and convergence rates of the two-class SVM (see, e.g., [2, 3, 4] and references therein) have been studied in detail, as well as the shape of the asymptotic decision function [5, 6]. All results published so far study the case where λ decreases as the number of points tends to infinity (or, equivalently, where $\lambda\sigma^{-d}$ converges to 0 if one uses the classical non-normalized version of the Gaussian kernel instead of (2)). Although it seems natural to reduce regularization as more and more training data are available –even more than natural, it is the spirit of regularization [7, 8]–, there is at least one important situation where λ is typically held fixed: the one-class SVM [9]. In that case, the goal is to estimate an α-quantile, that is, a subset of the input space $\mathcal{X}$ of given probability α with minimum volume. The estimation is performed by thresholding the function output by the one-class SVM, that is, the SVM (1) with only positive examples; in that case λ is supposed to determine the quantile level[1]. Although it is known that the fraction of examples in the selected region converges to the desired quantile level α [9], it is still an open question whether the region converges towards a quantile, that is, a region of minimum volume. Besides, most theoretical results about the consistency and convergence rates of two-class SVM with vanishing regularization constant do not translate to the one-class case, as we are precisely in the seldom situation where the SVM is used with a regularization term that does not vanish as the sample size increases.

The main contribution of this paper is to show that Bayes consistency can be obtained for algorithms that solve (1) without decreasing λ, if instead the bandwidth σ of the Gaussian kernel decreases at a suitable rate. We prove upper bounds on the convergence rate of the classification error towards the Bayes risk for a variety of functions ϕ and of distributions P, in particular for SVM (Theorem 6). Moreover, we provide an explicit description of the function asymptotically output by the algorithms, and establish converge rates towards this limit for the L_2 norm (Theorem 7). In particular, we show that the decision function output by the one-class SVM converges towards the density to be estimated, truncated at the level 2λ (Theorem 8); we finally show that this implies the consistency of one-class SVM as a density level estimator for the excess-mass functional [10] (Theorem 9).

Due to lack of space we limit ourselves in this extended abstract to the statement of the main results (Section 2) and sketch the proof of the main theorem (Theorem 3) that underlies all other results in Section 3. All detailed proofs are available in the companion paper [11].

2 Notations and main results

Let (X, Y) be a pair of random variables taking values in $\mathbb{R}^d \times \{-1, 1\}$, with distribution P. We assume throughout this paper that the marginal distribution of X is absolutely continuous with respect to Lebesgue measure with density $\rho : \mathbb{R}^d \to \mathbb{R}$, and that is has a support included in a compact set $\mathcal{X} \subset \mathbb{R}^d$. We denote $\eta : \mathbb{R}^d \to [0, 1]$ a measurable version of the conditional distribution of $Y = 1$ given X.

The normalized Gaussian radial basis function (RBF) kernel k_σ with bandwidth parameter $\sigma > 0$ is defined for any $(x, x') \in \mathbb{R}^d \times \mathbb{R}^d$ by:

$$k_\sigma(x, x') = \frac{1}{\left(\sqrt{2\pi}\sigma\right)^d} \exp\left(\frac{-\|x - x'\|^2}{2\sigma^2}\right) ,$$

and the corresponding reproducing kernel Hilbert space (RKHS) is denoted by $\mathcal{H}_\sigma$. We note $\kappa_\sigma = \left(\sqrt{2\pi}\sigma\right)^{-d}$ the normalizing constant that ensures that the kernel integrates to 1.

---

[1]While the original formulation of the one-class SVM involves a parameter ν, there is asymptotically a one-to-one correspondance between λ and ν

Denoting by $\mathcal{M}$ the set of measurable real-valued functions on $\mathbb{R}^d$, we define several risks for functions $f \in \mathcal{M}$:

- The classification error rate, usually refered to as *(true) risk* of f, when Y is predicted by the sign of $f(X)$, is denoted by

$$R(f) = P\left(\mathrm{sign}\left(f(X)\right) \neq Y\right) .$$

- For a scalar $\lambda > 0$ fixed throughout this paper and a convex function $\phi : \mathbb{R} \to \mathbb{R}$, the ϕ-risk regularized by the RKHS norm is defined, for any $\sigma > 0$ and $f \in \mathcal{H}_\sigma$, by

$$R_{\phi,\sigma}(f) = \mathbb{E}_P\left[\phi\left(Yf(X)\right)\right] + \lambda\| f \|_{\mathcal{H}_\sigma}^2$$

Furthermore, for any real $r \geq 0$, we denote by $L(r)$ the Lipschitz constant of the restriction of ϕ to the interval $[-r, r]$. For example, for the hinge loss $\phi(u) = \max(0, 1 - u)$ one can take $L(r) = 1$, and for the squared hinge loss $\phi(u) = \max(0, 1 - u)^2$ one can take $L(r) = 2(r + 1)$.

- Finally, the L_2-norm regularized ϕ-risk is, for any $f \in \mathcal{M}$:

$$R_{\phi,0}(f) = \mathbb{E}_P\left[\phi\left(Yf(X)\right)\right] + \lambda\| f \|_{L_2}^2$$

where,

$$\| f \|_{L_2}^2 = \int_{\mathbb{R}^d} f(x)^2 dx \in [0, +\infty].$$

The minima of the three risk functionals defined above over their respective domains are denoted by R^*, $R_{\phi,\sigma}^*$ and $R_{\phi,0}^*$ respectively. Each of these risks has an empirical counterpart where the expectation with respect to P is replaced by an average over an i.i.d. sample $T = \{(X_1, Y_1), \ldots, (X_n, Y_n)\}$. In particular, the following empirical version of $R_{\phi,\sigma}$ will be used

$$\forall \sigma > 0, f \in \mathcal{H}_\sigma, \quad \widehat{R}_{\phi,\sigma}(f) = \frac{1}{n}\sum_{i=1}^{n}\phi\left(Y_i f(X_i)\right) + \lambda\| f \|_{\mathcal{H}_\sigma}^2 .$$

The main focus of this paper is the analysis of learning algorithms that minimize the empirical ϕ-risk regularized by the RKHS norm $\widehat{R}_{\phi,\sigma}$, and their limit as the number of points tends to infinity and the kernel width σ decreases to 0 at a suitable rate when n tends to ∞, λ being kept fixed. Roughly speaking, our main result shows that in this situation, if ϕ is a convex loss function, the minimization of $\widehat{R}_{\phi,\sigma}$ asymptotically amounts to minimizing $R_{\phi,0}$. This stems from the fact that the empirical average term in the definition of $\widehat{R}_{\phi,\sigma}$ converges to its corresponding expectation, while the norm in $\mathcal{H}_\sigma$ of a function f decreases to its L_2 norm when σ decreases to zero. To turn this intuition into a rigorous statement, we need a few more assumptions about the minimizer of $R_{\phi,0}$ and about P. First, we observe that the minimizer of $R_{\phi,0}$ is indeed well-defined and can often be explicitly computed:

Lemma 1 *For any $x \in \mathbb{R}^d$, let*

$$f_{\phi,0}(x) = \arg\min_{\alpha \in \mathbb{R}} \left\{\rho(x)\left[\eta(x)\phi(\alpha) + (1 - \eta)\phi(-\alpha)\right] + \lambda\alpha^2\right\} .$$

Then $f_{\phi,0}$ is measurable and satisfies:

$$R_{\phi,0}(f_{\phi,0}) = \inf_{f \in \mathcal{M}} R_{\phi,0}(f)$$

Second, we provide below a general result that shows how to control the excess $R_{\phi,0}$-risk of the empirical minimizer of the $R_{\phi,\sigma}$-risk, for which we need to recall the notion of modulus of continuity [12].

Definition 2 (Modulus of continuity) *Let f be a Lebesgue measurable function from $\mathbb{R}^d$ to $\mathbb{R}$. Then its modulus of continuity in the L_1-norm is defined for any $\delta \geq 0$ as follows*

$$\omega(f, \delta) = \sup_{0 \leq \|t\| \leq \delta} \| f(. + t) - f(.) \|_{L_1},\tag{3}$$

where $\|t\|$ is the Euclidian norm of $t \in \mathbb{R}^d$.

Our main result can now be stated as follows:

Theorem 3 (Main Result) *Let $\sigma_1 > \sigma > 0$, $0 < p < 2$, $\delta > 0$, and let $\hat{f}_{\phi,\sigma}$ denote a minimizer of the $\widehat{R}_{\phi,\sigma}$ risk over $\mathcal{H}_\sigma$. Assume that the marginal density ρ is bounded, and let $M = \sup_{x \in \mathbb{R}^d} \rho(x)$. Then there exist constants $(K_i)_{i=1\ldots4}$ (depending only on p, δ, λ, d, and M) such that, for any $x > 0$, the following holds with probability greater than $1 - e^{-x}$ over the draw of the training data:*

$$\begin{aligned}
R_{\phi,0}(\hat{f}_{\phi,\sigma}) - R_{\phi,0}^* \leq\ & K_1 L \left(\sqrt{\frac{\kappa_\sigma \phi(0)}{\lambda}} \right)^{\frac{4}{2+p}} \left(\frac{1}{\sigma} \right)^{\frac{[2+(2-p)(1+\delta)]d}{2+p}} \left(\frac{1}{n} \right)^{\frac{2}{2+p}} \\
& + K_2 L \left(\sqrt{\frac{\kappa_\sigma \phi(0)}{\lambda}} \right)^2 \left(\frac{1}{\sigma} \right)^d \frac{x}{n} \\
& + K_3 \frac{\sigma^2}{\sigma_1^2} \\
& + K_4 \omega(f_{\phi,0}, \sigma_1).
\end{aligned}\tag{4}$$

The first two terms in the r.h.s. of (4) bound the estimation error associated with the gaussian RKHS, which naturally tends to be small when the number of training data increases and when the RKHS is 'small', i.e., when σ is large. As is usually the case in such variance/bias splitings, the variance term here depends on the dimension d of the input space. Note that it is also parametrized by both p and δ. The third term measures the error due to penalizing the L_2-norm of a fixed function in $\mathcal{H}_{\sigma_1}$ by its $\|.\|_{\mathcal{H}_\sigma}$-norm, with $0 < \sigma < \sigma_1$. This is a price to pay to get a small estimation error. As for the fourth term, it is a bound on the approximation error of the Gaussian RKHS. Note that, once λ and σ have been fixed, σ_1 remains a free variable parameterizing the bound itself.

In order to highlight the type of convergence rates one can obtain from Theorem 3, let us assume that the ϕ loss function is Lipschitz on $\mathbb{R}$ (e.g., take the hinge loss), and suppose that for some $0 \leq \beta \leq 1$, $c_1 > 0$, and for any $h \geq 0$, the function $f_{\phi,0}$ satisfies the following inequality

$$\omega(f_{\phi,0}, h) \leq c_1 h^\beta.\tag{5}$$

Then we can optimize the right hand side of (4) w.r.t. σ_1, σ, p and δ by balancing the four terms. This eventually leads to:

$$R_{\phi,0}\left(\hat{f}_{\phi,\sigma} \right) - R_{\phi,0}^* = O_P \left(\left(\frac{1}{n} \right)^{\frac{2\beta}{4\beta + (2+\beta)d} - \epsilon} \right),\tag{6}$$

for any $\epsilon > 0$. This rate is achieved by choosing

$$\sigma_1 = \left(\frac{1}{n} \right)^{\frac{2}{4\beta + (2+\beta)d} - \frac{\epsilon}{\beta}},\tag{7}$$

$$\sigma = \sigma_1^{\frac{2+\beta}{2}} = \left(\frac{1}{n} \right)^{\frac{2+\beta}{4\beta + (2+\beta)d} - \frac{\epsilon(2+\beta)}{2\beta}},\tag{8}$$

$p = 2$ and δ as small as possible (that is why an arbitray small quantity ϵ appears in the rate).

Theorem 3 shows that minimizing the $\widehat{R}_{\phi,\sigma}$ risk for well-chosen width σ is a an algorithm consistant for the $R_{\phi,0}$-risk. In order to relate this consistency with more traditional measures of performance of learning algorithms, the next theorem shows that under a simple additionnal condition on ϕ, $R_{\phi,0}$-risk-consistency implies Bayes consistency:

Theorem 4 *If ϕ is convex, differentiable at 0, with $\phi'(0) < 0$, then for every sequence of functions $(f_i)_{i \geq 1} \in \mathcal{M}$,*

$$\lim_{i \to +\infty} R_{\phi,0}(f_i) = R_{\phi,0}^* \implies \lim_{i \to +\infty} R(f_i) = R^*$$

This theorem results from a more general quantitative analysis of the relationship between the excess $R_{\phi,0}$-risk and the excess R-risk, in the spirit of [13]. In order to state a refined version in the particular case of the support vector machine algorithm, we first need the following definition:

Definition 5 *We say that a distribution P with ρ as marginal density of X w.r.t. Lebesgue measure has a low density exponent $\gamma \geq 0$ if there exists $(c_2, \epsilon_0) \in (0, +\infty)^2$ such that*

$$\forall \epsilon \in [0, \epsilon_0], \quad P\left(\{x \in \mathbb{R}^d : \rho(x) \leq \epsilon\}\right) \leq c_2 \epsilon^{\gamma}.$$

We are now in position to state a quantitative relationship between the excess $R_{\phi,0}$-risk and the excess R-risk in the case of support vector machines:

Theorem 6 *Let $\phi_1(\alpha) = \max(1 - \alpha, 0)$ be the hinge loss function, and $\phi_2(\alpha) = \max(1 - \alpha, 0)^2$, be the squared hinge loss function. Then for any distribution P with low density exponent γ, there exist constant $(K_1, K_2, r_1, r_2) \in (0, +\infty)^4$ such that for any $f \in \mathcal{M}$ with an excess $R_{\phi_1,0}$-risk upper bounded by r_1 the following holds:*

$$R(f) - R^* \leq K_1 \left(R_{\phi_1,0}(f) - R_{\phi_1,0}^*\right)^{\frac{\gamma}{2\gamma+1}},$$

and if the excess regularized $R_{\phi_2,0}$-risk upper bounded by r_2 the following holds:

$$R(f) - R^* \leq K_2 \left(R_{\phi_2,0}(f) - R_{\phi_2,0}^*\right)^{\frac{\gamma}{2\gamma+1}},$$

This result can be extended to any loss function through the introduction of variational arguments, in the spirit of [13]; we do not further explore this direction, but the reader is invited to consult [11] for more details. Hence we have proved the consistency of SVM, together with upper bounds on the convergence rates, in a situation where the effect of regularization does not vanish asymptotically.

Another consequence of the $R_{\phi,0}$-consistency of an algorithm is the L_2-convergence of the function output by the algorithm to the minimizer of the $R_{\phi,0}$-risk:

Lemma 7 *For any $f \in \mathcal{M}$, the following holds:*

$$\| f - f_{\phi,0} \|_{L_2}^2 \leq \frac{1}{\lambda} \left(R_{\phi,0}(f) - R_{\phi,0}^*\right).$$

This result is particularly relevant to study algorithms whose objective are not binary classification. Consider for example the one-class SVM algorithm, which served as the initial motivation for this paper. Then we claim the following:

Theorem 8 *Let ρ_λ denote the density truncated as follows:*

$$\rho_\lambda(x) = \begin{cases} \frac{\rho(x)}{2\lambda} & \text{if } \rho(x) \le 2\lambda, \\ 1 & \text{otherwise.} \end{cases} \tag{9}$$

Let $\hat{f}_\sigma$ denote the function output by the one-class SVM, that is the function that solves (1) in the case ϕ is the hinge-loss function and $Y_i = 1$ for all $i \in \{1, \ldots, n\}$. Then, under the general conditions of Theorem 3, for σ chosen as in Equation (8),

$$\lim_{n \to +\infty} \| \hat{f}_\sigma - \rho_\lambda \|_{L_2} = 0 \, .$$

An interesting by-product of this theorem is the consistency of the one-class SVM algorithm for density level set estimation:

Theorem 9 *Let $0 < \mu < 2\lambda < M$, let C_μ be the level set of the density function ρ at level μ, and $\widehat{C}_\mu$ be the level set of $2\lambda \hat{f}_\sigma$ at level μ, where $\hat{f}_\sigma$ is still the function outptut by the one-class SVM. For any distribution Q, for any subset C of $\mathbb{R}^d$, define the excess-mass of C with respect to Q as follows:*

$$H_Q(C) = Q(C) - \mu Leb(C) \, , \tag{10}$$

where Leb is the Lebesgue measure. Then, under the general assumptions of Theorem 3, we have

$$\lim_{n \to +\infty} H_P(C_\mu) - H_P\left(\widehat{C}_\mu\right) = 0 \, , \tag{11}$$

for σ chosen as in Equation (8).

The excess-mass functional was first introduced in [10] to assess the quality of density level set estimators. It is maximized by the true density level set C_μ and acts as a risk functional in the one-class framework. The proof ef Theorem 9 is based on the following result: if $\hat{\rho}$ is a density estimator converging to the true density ρ in the L_2 sense, then for any fixed $0 < \mu < \sup\{\rho\}$, the excess mass of the level set of $\hat{\rho}$ at level μ converges to the excess mass of C_μ. In other words, as is the case in the classification framework, plug-in estimators built on L_2-consistent density estimators are consistent with respect to the excess mass.

3 Proof of Theorem 3 (sketch)

In this section we sketch the proof of the main learning theorem of this contribution, which underlies most other results stated in Section 2 The proof of Theorem 3 is based on the following decomposition of the excess $R_{\phi,0}$-risk for the minimizer $\hat{f}_{\phi,\sigma}$ of $\widehat{R}_{\phi,\sigma}$, valid for any $0 < \sigma < \sqrt{2}\sigma_1$ and any sample $(x_i, y_i)_{i=1,\ldots,n}$:

$$\begin{aligned}
R_{\phi,0}(\hat{f}_{\phi,\sigma}) - R^*_{\phi,0} &= \left[R_{\phi,0}\left(\hat{f}_{\phi,\sigma}\right) - R_{\phi,\sigma}\left(\hat{f}_{\phi,\sigma}\right) \right] \\
&+ \left[R_{\phi,\sigma}(\hat{f}_{\phi,\sigma}) - R^*_{\phi,\sigma} \right] \\
&+ \left[R^*_{\phi,\sigma} - R_{\phi,\sigma}(k_{\sigma_1} * f_{\phi,0}) \right] \\
&+ \left[R_{\phi,\sigma}(k_{\sigma_1} * f_{\phi,0}) - R_{\phi,0}(k_{\sigma_1} * f_{\phi,0}) \right] \\
&+ \left[R_{\phi,0}(k_{\sigma_1} * f_{\phi,0}) - R^*_{\phi,0} \right] \, .
\end{aligned} \tag{12}$$

It can be shown that $k_{\sigma_1} * f_{\phi,0} \in \mathcal{H}_{\sqrt{2}\sigma_1} \subset \mathcal{H}_\sigma \subset L_{2(\mathbb{R}^d)}$ which justifies the introduction of $R_{\phi,\sigma}(k_{\sigma_1} * f_{\phi,0})$ and $R_{\phi,0}(k_{\sigma_1} * f_{\phi,0})$. By studying the relationship between the Gaussian RKHS norm and the L_2 norm, it can be shown that

$$R_{\phi,0}\left(\hat{f}_{\phi,\sigma}\right) - R_{\phi,\sigma}\left(\hat{f}_{\phi,\sigma}\right) = \lambda \left(\| \hat{f}_{\phi,\sigma} \|^2_{L_2} - \| \hat{f}_{\phi,\sigma} \|^2_{\mathcal{H}_\sigma} \right) \le 0,$$

while the following stems from the definition of $R^*_{\phi,\sigma}$:

$$R^*_{\phi,\sigma} - R_{\phi,\sigma}(k_{\sigma_1} * f_{\phi,0}) \leq 0.$$

Hence, controlling $R_{\phi,0}(\hat{f}_{\phi,\sigma}) - R^*_{\phi,0}$ boils down to controlling each of the remaining three terms in (12).

- The second term in (12) is usually referred to as the sample error or estimation error. The control of such quantities has been the topic of much research recently, including for example [14, 15, 16, 17, 18, 4]. Using estimates of local Rademacher complexities through covering numbers for the Gaussian RKHS due to [4], the following result can be shown:

Lemma 10 *For any $\sigma > 0$ small enough, let $\hat{f}_{\phi,\sigma}$ be the minimizer of the $\widehat{R}_{\phi,\sigma}$-risk on a sample of size n, where ϕ is a convex loss function. For any $0 < p < 2$, $\delta > 0$, and $x \geq 1$, the following holds with probability at least $1 - e^x$ over the draw of the sample:*

$$R_{\phi,\sigma}(\hat{f}_{\phi,\sigma}) - R_{\phi,\sigma}(f_{\phi,\sigma}) \leq K_1 L \left(\sqrt{\frac{\kappa_\sigma \phi(0)}{\lambda}} \right)^{\frac{4}{2+p}} \left(\frac{1}{\sigma} \right)^{\frac{[2+(2-p)(1+\delta)]d}{2+p}} \left(\frac{1}{n} \right)^{\frac{2}{2+p}}$$

$$+ K_2 L \left(\sqrt{\frac{\kappa_\sigma \phi(0)}{\lambda}} \right)^2 \left(\frac{1}{\sigma} \right)^d \frac{x}{n} ,$$

where K_1 and K_2 are positive constants depending neither on σ, nor on n.

- In order to upper bound the fourth term in (12), the analysis of the convergence of the Gaussian RKHS norm towards the L_2 norm when the bandwidth of the kernel tends to 0 leads to:

$$R_{\phi,\sigma}(k_{\sigma_1} * f_{\phi,0}) - R_{\phi,0}(k_{\sigma_1} * f_{\phi,0}) = \| k_{\sigma_1} * f_{\phi,0} \|^2_{\mathcal{H}_\sigma} - \| k_{\sigma_1} * f_{\phi,0} \|^2_{L_2}$$

$$\leq \frac{\sigma^2}{2\sigma_1^2} \| f_{\phi,0} \|^2_{L_2}$$

$$\leq \frac{\phi(0)\sigma^2}{2\lambda\sigma_1^2} .$$

- The fifth term in (12) corresponds to the approximation error. It can be shown that for any bounded function in $L_1(\mathbb{R}^d)$ and all $\sigma > 0$, the following holds:

$$\| k_\sigma * f - f \|_{L_1} \leq (1 + \sqrt{d})\omega(f,\sigma) , \tag{13}$$

where $\omega(f,.)$ denotes the modulus of continuity of f in the L_1 norm. From this the following inequality can be derived:

$$R_{\phi,0}(k_{\sigma_1} * f_{\phi,0}) - R_{\phi,0}(f_{\phi,0})$$

$$\leq \left(2\lambda \| f_{\phi,0} \|_{L_\infty} + L(\| f_{\phi,0} \|_{L_\infty}) M \right) \left(1 + \sqrt{d} \right) \omega(f_{\phi,0}, \sigma_1) .$$

4 Conclusion

We have shown that consistency of learning algorithms that minimize a regularized empirical risk can be obtained even when the so-called regularization term does not asymptotically vanish, and derived the consistency of one-class SVM as a density level set estimator. Our method of proof is based on an unusual decomposition of the excess risk due to the presence of the regularization term, which plays an important role in the determination of the asymptotic limit of the function that minimizes the empirical risk. Although the upper bounds on the convergence rates we obtain are not optimal, they provide a first step toward the analysis of learning algorithms in this context.

Acknowledgments

The authors are grateful to Stéphane Boucheron, Pascal Massart and Ingo Steinwart for fruitful discussions. This work was supported by the ACI "Nouvelles interfaces des Mathématiques" of the French Ministry for Research, and by the IST Program of the European Community, under the Pascal Network of Excellence, IST-2002-506778.

References

[1] B. E. Boser, I. M. Guyon, and V. N. Vapnik. A training algorithm for optimal margin classifiers. In *Proceedings of the 5th annual ACM workshop on Computational Learning Theory*, pages 144–152. ACM Press, 1992.

[2] I. Steinwart. Support vector machines are universally consistent. *J. Complexity*, 18:768–791, 2002.

[3] T. Zhang. Statistical behavior and consistency of classification methods based on convex risk minimization. *Ann. Stat.*, 32:56–134, 2004.

[4] I. Steinwart and C. Scovel. Fast rates for support vector machines using gaussian kernels. Technical report, Los Alamos National Laboratory, 2004. submitted to Annals of Statistics.

[5] I. Steinwart. Sparseness of support vector machines. *J. Mach. Learn. Res.*, 4:1071–1105, 2003.

[6] P. L. Bartlett and A. Tewari. Sparseness vs estimating conditional probabilities: Some asymptotic results. In *Lecture Notes in Computer Science*, volume 3120, pages 564–578. Springer, 2004.

[7] A.N. Tikhonov and V.Y. Arsenin. *Solutions of ill-posed problems*. W.H. Winston, Washington, D.C., 1977.

[8] B. W. Silverman. On the estimation of a probability density function by the maximum penalized likelihood method. *Ann. Stat.*, 10:795–810, 1982.

[9] B. Schölkopf, J. C. Platt, J. Shawe-Taylor, A. J. Smola, and R. C. Williamson. Estimating the support of a high-dimensional distribution. *Neural Comput.*, 13:1443–1471, 2001.

[10] J. A. Hartigan. Estimation of a convex density contour in two dimensions. *J. Amer. Statist. Assoc.*, 82(397):267–270, 1987.

[11] R. Vert and J.-P. Vert. Consistency and convergence rates of one-class svm and related algorithms. *J. Mach. Learn. Res.*, 2006. To appear.

[12] R. A. DeVore and G. G. Lorentz. *Constructive Approximation*. Springer Grundlehren der Mathematischen Wissenschaften. Springer Verlag, 1993.

[13] P.I. Bartlett, M.I. Jordan, and J.D. McAuliffe. Convexity, classification and risk bounds. Technical Report 638, UC Berkeley Statistics, 2003.

[14] A. B. Tsybakov. On nonparametric estimation of density level sets. *Ann. Stat.*, 25:948–969, June 1997.

[15] E. Mammen and A. Tsybakov. Smooth discrimination analysis. *Ann. Stat.*, 27(6):1808–1829, 1999.

[16] P. Massart. Some applications of concentration inequalities to statistics. *Ann. Fac. Sc. Toulouse*, IX(2):245–303, 2000.

[17] P. L. Bartlett, O. Bousquet, and S. Mendelson. Local rademacher complexities. *Annals of Statistics*, 2005. To appear.

[18] V. Koltchinskii. Localized rademacher complexities. Manuscript, september 2003.

Multiple Instance Boosting for Object Detection

Paul Viola, John C. Platt, and Cha Zhang
Microsoft Research
1 Microsoft Way
Redmond, WA 98052
`{viola,jplatt}@microsoft.com`

Abstract

A good image object detection algorithm is accurate, fast, and does not require exact locations of objects in a training set. We can create such an object detector by taking the architecture of the Viola-Jones detector cascade and training it with a new variant of boosting that we call MIL-Boost. MILBoost uses cost functions from the Multiple Instance Learning literature combined with the AnyBoost framework. We adapt the feature selection criterion of MILBoost to optimize the performance of the Viola-Jones cascade. Experiments show that the detection rate is up to 1.6 times better using MILBoost. This increased detection rate shows the advantage of simultaneously learning the locations and scales of the objects in the training set along with the parameters of the classifier.

1 Introduction

When researchers use machine learning for object detection, they need to know the location and size of the objects, in order to generate positive examples for the classification algorithm. It is often extremely tedious to generate large training sets of objects, because it is not easy to specify exactly where the objects are. For example, given a ZIP code of handwritten digits, which pixel is the location of a "5" ? This sort of ambiguity leads to training sets which themselves have high error rates, this limits the accuracy of any trained classifier.

In this paper, we explicitly acknowledge that object recognition is innately a Multiple Instance Learning problem: we know that objects are located in regions of the image, but we don't know exactly where. In MIL, training examples are not singletons. Instead, they come in "bags", where all of the examples in a bag share a label [4]. A positive bag means that at least one example in the bag is positive, while a negative bag means that all examples in the bag are negative. In MIL, learning must simultaneously learn which examples in the positive bags are positive, along with the parameters of the classifier.

We have combined MIL with the Viola-Jones method of object detection, which uses Adaboost [11] to create a cascade of detectors. To do this, we created MILBoost, a new method for folding MIL into the AnyBoost [9] framework. In addition, we show how early stage in the detection cascade can be re-trained using information extracted from the final MIL classifier.

We test this new form of MILBoost for detecting people in a teleconferencing application.

This is a much harder problem then face detection, since the participants do not look at the camera (and sometimes away). The MIL framework is shown to produce classifiers with much higher detection rates and fast computation times.

1.1 Structure of paper

We first review the previous work in two fields: previous related work in object detection (Section 2.1) and in multiple instance learning (Section 2.2). We derive a new MIL variant of boosting in Section 3, called MILBoost. MILBoost is used to train a detector in the Viola-Jones framework in Section 4. We then adapt MILBoost to train an effective cascade using a new criterion for selecting features in the early rounds of training (Section 5). The paper concludes in Section 6 with experimental results on the problem of person detection in a teleconferencing application. The MIL framework is shown to produce classifiers with much higher detection rates and fast computation times.

2 Relationship to previous work

This paper lies at the intersection between the subfields of object detection and multiple instance learning. Therefore, we discuss the relationship with previous work in each subfield separately.

2.1 Previous work in image object detection

The task of object detection in images is quite daunting. Amongst the challenges are 1) creating a system with high accuracy and low false detection rate, 2) restricting the system to consume a reasonable amount of CPU time, and 3) creating a large training set that has low labeling error.

Perona et. al [3, 5] and Schmid [12] have proposed constellation models: spatial models of local image features. These models can be trained using unsegmented images in which the object can appear at any location. Learning uses EM-like algorithms to iteratively localize and refine discriminative image features. However, hitherto, the detection accuracy has not be as good as the best methods.

Viola and Jones [13] created a system that exhaustively scans pose space for generic objects. This system is accurate, because it is trained using AdaBoost [11]. It is also very efficient, because it uses a cascade of detectors and very simple image features. However, the AdaBoost algorithm requires exact positions of objects to learn.

The closest work to this paper is Nowlan and Platt [10], which built on the work of Keeler, et. al [7] (see below). In the Nowlan paper, a convolutional neural network was trained to detect hands. The exact location and size of the hands is approximately truthed: the neural network used MIL training to co-learn the object location and the parameters of the classifier. The system is effective, but is not as fast as Viola and Jones, because the detector is more complex and it does not use a cascade.

This paper builds on the accuracy and speed of Viola and Jones, by using the same architecture. We attempt to gain the flexibility of the constellation models. Instead of an EM-like algorithm, we use MIL to create our system, which does not require iteration. Unlike Nowlan and Platt, we maintain a cascade of detectors for maximum speed.

2.2 Previous work in Multiple Instance Learning

The idea for multiple instance learning was originally proposed 1990 for handwritten digit recognition by Keeler, et. al [7]. Keeler's approach was called Integrated Segmentation and Recognition (ISR). In that paper, the position of a digit in a ZIP code was considered completely unknown. ISR simultaneously learned the positions of the digits and the parameters of a convolutional neural network recognizer. More details on ISR are given below (Section 3.2).

Another relevant example of MIL is the Diverse Density approach of Maron [8]. Diverse Density uses the Noisy OR generative model [6] to explain the bag labels. A gradient-descent algorithm is used to find the best point in input space that explains the positive bags. We also utilize the Noisy OR generative model in a version of our algorithm, below (Section 3.1).

Finally, a number of researchers have modified the boosting algorithm to perform MIL. For example, Andrews and Hofmann [1] have proposed modifying the inner loop of boosting to use linear programming. This is not practically applicable to the object detection task, which can have millions of examples (pixels) and thousands of bags.

Another approach is due to Auer and Ortner [2], which enforces a constraint that weak classifiers must be either hyper-balls or hyper-rectangles in $\Re^N$. This would exclude the fast features used by Viola and Jones.

A third approach is that of Xu and Frank [14], which uses a generative model that the probability of a bag being positive is the mean of the probabilities that the examples are positive. We believe that this rule is unsuited for object detection, because only a small subset of the examples in the bag are ever positive.

3 MIL and Boosting

We will present two new variants of AdaBoost which attempt to solve the MIL problem. The derivation uses the AnyBoost framework of of Mason et al. which views boosting as a gradient descent process [9]. The derivation builds on previous appropriate MIL cost functions, namely ISR and Noisy OR. The Noisy OR derivation is simpler and a bit more intuitive.

3.1 Noisy-OR Boost

Recall in boosting each example is classified by a linear combination of weak classifiers. In MILBoost, examples are not individually labeled. Instead, they reside in bags. Thus, an example is indexed with two indices: i, which indexes the bag, and j, which indexes the example within the bag. The score of the example is $y_{ij} = C(x_{ij})$ and $C(x_{ij}) = \sum_t \lambda_t c^t(x_{ij})$ a weighted sum of weak classifiers. The probability of an example is positive is given by

$$p_{ij} = \frac{1}{1 + \exp(-y_{ij})},$$

the standard logistic function. The probability that the bag is positive is a "noisy OR" $p_i = 1 - \prod_{j \in i}(1 - p_{ij})$ [6] [8]. Under this model the likelihood assigned to a set of training bags is:

$$L(C) = \prod_i p_i^{t_i}(1 - p_i)^{(1-t_i)}$$

where $t_i \in \{0, 1\}$ is the label of bag i.

Following the AnyBoost approach, the weight on each example is given as the derivative of the cost function with respect to a change in the score of the example. The derivative of the log likelihood is:

$$\frac{\partial \log L(C)}{\partial y_{ij}} = w_{ij} = \frac{t_i - p_i}{p_i} p_{ij}. \tag{1}$$

Note, that the weights here are signed. The interpretation is straightforward; the sign determines the example label. Each round of boosting is a search for a classifier which maximizes $\sum_{ij} c(x_{ij}) w_{ij}$ where $c(x_{ij})$ is the score assigned to the example by the weak classifier (for a binary classifier $c(x_{ij}) \in \{-1, +1\}$). The parameter λ_t is determined using a line search to maximize $\log L(C + \lambda_t c_t)$.

Examining the criteria (1) the weight on each example is the product of two quantities: the bag weight $W_{\text{bag}} = \frac{t_i - p_i}{p_i}$ and the instance weight $W_{\text{instance}} = p_{ij}$. Observe that W_{bag} for a negative bag is always -1. Thus, the weight for a negative instance, p_{ij}, is the same that would result in a non-MIL AdaBoost framework (i.e. the negative examples are all equally negative). The weight on the positive instances is more complex. As learning proceeds and the probability of the bag approaches the target, the weight on the entire bag is reduced. Within the bag, the examples are assigned a weight which is higher for examples with higher scores. Intuitively the algorithm selects a subset of examples to assign a higher positive weight, and these example dominate subsequent learning.

3.2 ISR Boost

The authors of the ISR paper may well have been aware of the Noisy OR criteria described above. They chose instead to derive a different perhaps less probabilistic criteria. They do this in part because the derivatives (and hence example weights) lead to a form of instance competition.

Define $\chi_{ij} = \exp(y_{ij})$, $S_i = \sum_{j \in i} \chi_{ij}$ and $p_i = \frac{S_i}{1 + S_i}$. Keeler et al. argue that χ_{ij} can be interpreted as the likelihood that the object occurs at ij. The quantity S_i can be interpreted as a likelihood ratio that *some* (at least one) instance is positive, and finally p_i is the probability that some instance is positive. The example weights for the ISR framework are:

$$\frac{\partial \log L(C)}{\partial y_{ij}} = w_{ij} = (t_i - p_i) \frac{\chi_{ij}}{\sum_{j \in i} \chi_{ij}} \tag{2}$$

Examining the ISR criteria reveals two key properties. The first is the form of the example weight which is explicitly competitive. The examples in the bag compete for weight, since the weight is normalized by sum of the χ_{ij}'s. Though the experimental evidence is weak, this rule perhaps leads to a very localized representation, where a single example is labeled positive and the other examples are labeled negative. The second property is that the negative examples also compete for weight. This turns out to be troublesome in the detection framework since there are many, many more negative examples than positive. How many negative bags should there be? In contrast, the Noisy OR criteria treats all negative examples as independent negative examples.

4 Application of MIL Boost to Object Detection in Images

Each image is divided into a set of overlapping square windows that uniformly sample the space of position and scale (typically there are between 10,000 and 100,000 windows in a training image). Each window is used as an example for the purposes of training and detection. Each training image is labeled to determine the position and scale of the object of interest. For certain types of objects, such as frontal faces, it may be possible to accurately determine the position and scale of the face. One possibility is to localize the eyes and then to determine the single positive image window in which the eyes appear at a given relative location and scale. Even for this type of object the effort in carefully labeling the images is significant.

For many other types of objects (objects which may be visible from multiple poses, or

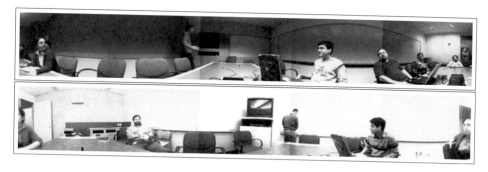

Figure 1: Two example images with people in a wide variety of poses. The algorithm will attempt to detect *all* people in the images, including those that are looking away from the camera.

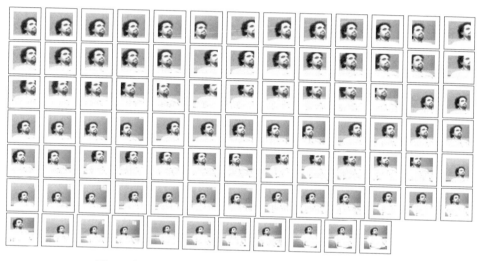

Figure 2: Some of the subwindows in one positive bag.

are highly varied, or are flexible) the "correct" geometric normalization is unclear. It is not clear how to normalize images of people in a conference room, who may be standing, sitting upright, reclining, looking toward, or looking away from the camera. Similar questions arise for most other image classes such as cars, trees, or fruit.

Experiments in this paper are performed on a set of images from a teleconferencing application. The images are acquired from a set of cameras near the center of the conference room (see Figure 1). The practical challenge is to steer a synthetic virtual camera toward the location of the speaker. The focus here is on person detection; determination of the person who is speaking is beyond the scope of this paper.

In every training image each person is labeled by hand. The labeler is instructed to draw a box around the head of the person. While this may seem like a reasonable geometric normalization, it ignores one critical issue, *context*. At the available resolution (approximately 1000x150 pixels) the head is often less than 10 pixels wide. At this resolution, even for clear frontal faces, the best face detection algorithms frequently fail. There are simply too few pixels on the face. The only way to detect the head is to include the surrounding image context. It is difficult to determine the correct quantity of image context (Figure 2 shows many possible normalizations).

If the body context is used to assist in detection, it is difficult to foresee the effect of body pose. Some of the participants are facing right, others left, and still others are leaning far forward/backward (while taking notes or reclining). The same context image is not be appropriate for all situations.

Both of these issues can be addressed with the use of MIL. Each positive head is represented, during training, by a large number of related image windows (see Figure 2). The MIL boosting algorithm is then used to *simultaneously* learn a detector *and* determine the location and scale of the appropriate image context.

5 MIL Boosting a Detection Cascade

In their work on face detection Viola and Jones train a cascade of classifiers, each designed to achieve high detection rates and modest false positive rates. During detection almost all of the computation is performed by the early stages in the cascade, perhaps 90% in the first 10 features. Training the initial stages of the cascade is the key to a fast and effective classifier.

Training and evaluating a detector in a MIL framework has a direct impact on cascade construction, both on the features selected and the appropriate thresholds.

The result of the MIL boost learning process is not only an example classifier, but also a set of weights on the examples. Those examples in positive bags which are assigned high weight have also high score. The final classifier labels these examples positive. The remaining examples in the positive bags are assigned a low weight and have a low score. The final classifier often classifies these examples as negative (as they should be).

Since boosting is a greedy process, the initial weak classifiers do not have any knowledge of the subsequent classifiers. As a result, the first classifiers selected have no knowledge of the final weights assigned to the examples. The key to efficient processing, is that the initial classifiers have a low false negative rate *on the examples determined to be positive by the final MIL classifier*.

This suggests a simple scheme for retraining the initial classifiers. Train a complete MIL boosted classifier and set the detection threshold to achieve the desired false positive and false negative rates. Retrain the initial weak classifier so that it has a zero false negative rate on the examples *labeled positive by the full classifier*. This results in a significant increase in the number of examples which can be pruned by this classifier. The process can be repeated, so that the second classifier is trained to yield a zero false negative rate on the *remaining* examples.

6 Experimental Results

Experiments were performed using a set of 8 videos recorded in different conference rooms. A collection of 1856 images were sampled from these videos. In all cases the detector was trained on 7 video conferences and tested on the remaining video conference. There were a total of 12364 visible people in these images. Each was labeled by drawing a rectangle around the head of each person.

Learning is performed on a total of about 30 million subwindows in the 1856 images. In addition to the monochrome images, two additional feature images are used. One measures the difference from the running mean image (this is something like background subtraction) and the other measures temporal variance over longer time scales. A set of 2654 rectangle filters are used for training. In each round the optimal filter and threshold is selected. In each experiment a total of 60 filters are learned.

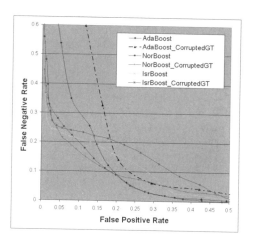

Figure 3: ROC comparison between various boosting rules.

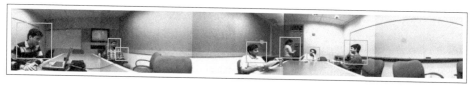

Figure 4: One example from the testing dataset and overlaid results.

We compared classical AdaBoost with two variants of MIL boost: ISR and Noisy-OR. For the MIL algorithms there is one bag for each labeled head, containing those positive windows which overlap that head. Additionally there is one negative bag for each image. After training, performance is evaluated on held out conference video (see Figure 3).

During training a set of positive windows are generated for each labeled example. All windows whose width is between 0.67 times and 1.5 times the head width *and* whose center is within 0.5 times the head width of the center of the head are labeled positive. An exception is made for AdaBoost, which has a tighter definition on positive examples (width between 0.83 and 1.2 times the head width and center within 0.2 times the head width) and produces better performance than the looser criterion. All windows which do not overlap with any head are considered negative. For each algorithm one experiment uses the ground truth obtained by hand (which has small yet unavoidable errors). A second experiment corrupts this ground truth further, moving each head by a uniform random shift such that there is non-zero overlap with the true position. Note that conventional AdaBoost is much worse when trained using corrupted ground truth. Interestingly, Adaboost is worse than NorBoost using the "correct" ground truth, even with a tight definition of positive examples. We conjecture that this is due to unavoidable ambiguity in the training and testing data.

Overall the MIL detection results are practically useful. A typical example of detection results are shown in Figure 4. Results shown are for the noisy OR algorithm. In order to simplify the display, significantly overlapping detection windows are averaged into a single window.

The scheme for retraining the initial classifier was evaluated on the noisy OR strong classifier trained above. Training a conventional cascade requires finding a small set of weak classifiers that can achieve zero false negative rate (or almost zero) and a low false positive rate. Using the first weak classifier yields a false positive rate of 39.7%. Including the first four weak classifiers yields a false positive rate of 21.4%. After retraining the first weak classifier alone yields a false positive rate of 11.7%. This improved rejection rate has the effect of reducing computation time of the cascade by roughly a factor of three.

7 Conclusions

This paper combines the truthing flexibility of multiple instance learning with the high accuracy of the boosted object detector of Viola and Jones. This was done by introducing a new variant of boosting, called MILBoost. MILBoost combines examples into bags, using combination functions such as ISR or Noisy OR. Maximum likelihood on the output of these bag combination functions fit within the AnyBoost framework, which generates boosting weights for each example.

We apply MILBoost to Viola-Jones face detection, where the standard AdaBoost works very well. NorBoost improves the detection rate over standard AdaBoost (tight positive) by nearly 15% (at a 10% false positive rate). Using MILBoost for object detection allows the detector to flexibly assign labels to the training set, which reduces label noise and improves performance.

References

[1] S. Andrews and T. Hofmann. Multiple-instance learning via disjunctive programming boosting. In S. Thrun, L. K. Saul, and B. Schölkopf, editors, *Proc. NIPS*, volume 16. MIT Press, 2004.

[2] P. Auer and R. Ortner. A boosting approach to multiple instance learning. In *Lecture Notes in Computer Science*, volume 3201, pages 63–74, October 2004.

[3] M. C. Burl, T. K. Leung, and P. Perona. Face localization via shape statistics. In *Proc. Int'l Workshop on Automatic Face and Gesture Recognition*, pages 154–159, 1995.

[4] T. G. Dietterich, R. H. Lathrop, and T. Lozano-Pérez. Solving the multiple instance problem with axis-parallel rectangles. *Artif. Intell.*, 89(1-2):31–71, 1997.

[5] R. Fergus, P. Perona, and A. Zisserman. Object class recognition by unsupervised scale-invariant learning. In *Proc. CVPR*, volume 2, pages 264–271, 2003.

[6] D. Heckerman. A tractable inference algorithm for diagnosing multiple diseases. In *Proc. UAI*, pages 163–171, 1989.

[7] J. D. Keeler, D. E. Rumelhart, and W.-K. Leow. Integrated segmentation and recognition of hand-printed numerals. In *NIPS-3: Proceedings of the 1990 conference on Advances in neural information processing systems 3*, pages 557–563, San Francisco, CA, USA, 1990. Morgan Kaufmann Publishers Inc.

[8] O. Maron and T. Lozano-Perez. A framework for multiple-instance learning. In *Proc. NIPS*, volume 10, pages 570–576, 1998.

[9] L. Mason, J. Baxter, P. Bartlett, and M. Frean. Boosting algorithms as gradient descent in function space, 1999.

[10] S. J. Nowlan and J. C. Platt. A convolutional neural network hand tracker. In G. Tesauro, D. Touretzky, and T. Leen, editors, *Advances in Neural Information Processing Systems*, volume 7, pages 901–908. The MIT Press, 1995.

[11] R. E. Schapire and Y. Singer. Improved boosting algorithms using confidence-rated predictions. In *Proc. COLT*, volume 11, pages 80–91, 1998.

[12] C. Schmid and R. Mohr. Local grayvalue invariants for image retrieval. *IEEE Trans. PAMI*, 19(5):530–535, 1997.

[13] P. Viola and M. Jones. Robust real-time object detection. *Int'l. J. Computer Vision*, 57(2):137–154, 2002.

[14] X. Xu and E. Frank. Logistic regression and boosting for labeled bags of instances. In *Lecture Notes in Computer Science*, volume 3056, pages 272–281, April 2004.

Estimating the "wrong" Markov random field: Benefits in the computation-limited setting

Martin J. Wainwright
Department of Statistics, and
Department of Electrical Engineering and Computer Science
UC Berkeley, Berkeley CA 94720
wainwrig@{stat,eecs}.berkeley.edu

Abstract

Consider the problem of joint parameter estimation and prediction in a Markov random field: i.e., the model parameters are estimated on the basis of an initial set of data, and then the fitted model is used to perform prediction (e.g., smoothing, denoising, interpolation) on a new noisy observation. Working in the computation-limited setting, we analyze a joint method in which the *same convex variational relaxation* is used to construct an M-estimator for fitting parameters, and to perform approximate marginalization for the prediction step. The key result of this paper is that in the computation-limited setting, using an inconsistent parameter estimator (i.e., an estimator that returns the "wrong" model even in the infinite data limit) is provably beneficial, since the resulting errors can partially compensate for errors made by using an approximate prediction technique. En route to this result, we analyze the asymptotic properties of M-estimators based on convex variational relaxations, and establish a Lipschitz stability property that holds for a broad class of variational methods. We show that joint estimation/prediction based on the reweighted sum-product algorithm substantially outperforms a commonly used heuristic based on ordinary sum-product. [1]

Keywords: Markov random fields; variational method; message-passing algorithms; sum-product; belief propagation; parameter estimation; learning.

1 Introduction

Consider the problem of joint learning (parameter estimation) and prediction in a Markov random field (MRF): in the learning phase, an initial collection of data is used to estimate parameters, and the fitted model is then used to perform prediction (e.g., smoothing, interpolation, denoising) on a new noisy observation. Disregarding computational cost, there exist optimal methods for solving this problem (Route A in Figure 1). For general MRFs, however, optimal methods are computationally intractable; consequently, many researchers have examined various types of message-passing methods for learning and prediction problems, including belief propagation [3, 6, 7, 14], expectation propagation [5], linear response [4], as well as reweighted message-passing algorithms [10, 13]. Accordingly, it is of considerable interest to understand and quantify the performance loss incurred

[1] Work partially supported by Intel Corporation Equipment Grant 22978, an Alfred P. Sloan Foundation Fellowship, and NSF Grant DMS-0528488.

by using computationally tractable methods versus exact methods (i.e., Route B versus A in Figure 1).

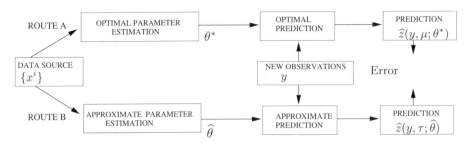

Figure 1. Route A: computationally intractable combination of parameter estimation and prediction. Route B: computationally efficient combination of approximate parameter estimation and prediction.

It is now well known that many message-passing algorithms—including mean field, (generalized) belief propagation, expectation propagation and various convex relaxations—can be understood from a variational perspective; in particular, all of these message-passing algorithms are iterative methods solving relaxed forms of an exact variational principle [12]. This paper focuses on the analysis of variational methods based *convex relaxations*, which includes a broad range of extant algorithms—among them the tree-reweighted sum-product algorithm [11], reweighted forms of generalized belief propagation [13], and semidefinite relaxations [12]. Moreover, it is straightforward to modify other message-passing methods (e.g., expectation propagation [5]) so as to "convexify" them. At a high level, the key idea of this paper is the following: given that approximate methods can lead to errors at both the estimation and prediction phases, it is natural to speculate that these sources of error might be arranged to partially cancel one another. Our theoretical analysis confirms this intuition: we show that with respect to end-to-end performance, it is in fact beneficial, even in the infinite data limit, to learn the "wrong" the model by using an *inconsistent* parameter estimator.

More specifically, we show how any convex variational method can be used to define a surrogate likelihood function. We then investigate the asymptotic properties of parameter estimators based maximizing such surrogate likelihoods, and establish that they are asymptotically normal but inconsistent in general. We then prove that any variational method that is based on a strongly concave entropy approximation is globally Lipschitz stable. Finally, focusing on prediction for a coupled mixture of Gaussians, we prove upper bounds on the increase in MSE of our computationally efficient method, relative to the unachievable Bayes optimum. We provide experimental results using the tree-reweighted (TRW) sum-product algorithm that confirm the stability of our methods, and demonstrate its superior performance to a heuristic method based on standard sum-product.

2   Background

We begin with necessary notation and background on multinomial Markov random fields, as well as variational representations and methods.

Markov random fields: Given an undirected graph $G = (V, E)$ with $N = |V|$ vertices, we associate to each vertex $s \in V$ a discrete random variable X_s, taking values in $\mathcal{X}_s = \{0, 1 \dots, m - 1\}$. We assume that the vector $X = \{X_s \mid s \in V\}$ has a distribution that is

Markov with respect to the graph G, so that its distribution can be represented in the form

$$p(x; \theta) = \exp\{\sum_{s \in V} \theta_s(x_s) + \sum_{(s,t) \in E} \theta_{st}(x_s, x_t) - A(\theta)\} \tag{1}$$

Here $A(\theta) := \log \sum_{x \in \mathcal{X}^N} \exp\{\sum_{s \in V} \theta_s(x_s) + \sum_{(s,t) \in E} \theta_{st}(x_s, x_t)\}$ is the *cumulant generating function* that normalizes the distribution, and $\theta_s(\cdot)$ and $\theta_{st}(\cdot, \cdot)$ are potential functions. In particular, we make use of the parameterization $\theta_s(x_s) := \sum_{j \in \mathcal{X}_s} \theta_{s;j} \mathbb{I}_j[x_s]$, where $\mathbb{I}_j[x_s]$ is an indicator function for the event $\{x_s = j\}$; the quantity θ_{st} is defined analogously. Overall, the family of MRFs (1) is an exponential family with canonical parameter $\theta \in \mathbb{R}^d$. Note that the elements of the canonical parameters are associated with vertices $\{\theta_{s;j}, \; s \in V, j \in \mathcal{X}_s\}$ and edges $\{\theta_{st;jk}, \; (s,t) \in E, (j,k) \in \mathcal{X}_s \times \mathcal{X}_t\}$ of the underlying graph.

Variational representation: We now describe how the cumulant generating function can be represented as the solution of an optimization problem. The constraint set is given by $\text{MARG}(G; \phi) := \{\mu \in \mathbb{R}^d \mid \mu = \sum_{x \in \mathcal{X}^N} p(x) \phi(x) \text{ for some } p(\cdot)\}$, consisting of all globally realizable singleton $\mu_s(\cdot)$ and pairwise $\mu_{st}(\cdot, \cdot)$ marginal distributions on the graph G. For any $\mu \in \text{MARG}(G; \phi)$, we define $A^*(\mu) = -\max_p H(p)$, where the maximum is taken over all distributions that have mean parameters μ. With these definitions, it can be shown [12] that A has the variational representation

$$A(\theta) = \max_{\mu \in \text{MARG}(G;\phi)} \{\theta^T \mu - A^*(\mu)\}. \tag{2}$$

3 From convex surrogates to joint estimation/prediction

In general, solving the variational problem (2) is intractable for two reasons: (i) the constraint set $\text{MARG}(G; \phi)$ is extremely difficult to characterize; and (ii) the dual function A^* lacks a closed-form representation. These challenges motivate approximations to A^* and $\text{MARG}(G; \phi)$; the resulting relaxed optimization problem defines a convex surrogate to the cumulant generating function.

Convex surrogates: Let $\text{REL}(G; \phi)$ be a compact and convex outer bound to the marginal polytope $\text{MARG}(G; \phi)$, and let B^* be a strictly convex and twice continuously differentiable approximation to the dual function A^*. We use these approximations to define a convex surrogate B via the relaxed optimization problem

$$B(\theta) := \max_{\tau \in \text{REL}(G;\phi)} \{\theta^T \tau - B^*(\tau)\}. \tag{3}$$

The function B so defined has several desirable properties. First, since B is defined by the maximum of a collection of functions linear in θ, it is convex [1]. Moreover, by the strict convexity of B^* and compactness of $\text{REL}(G; \phi)$, the optimum is uniquely attained at some $\tau(\theta)$. Finally, an application of Danskin's theorem [1] yields that B is differentiable, and that $\nabla B(\theta) = \tau(\theta)$. Since $\tau(\theta)$ has a natural interpretation as a *pseudomarginal*, this last property of B is analogous to the well-known cumulant generating property of A—namely, $\nabla A(\theta) = \mu(\theta)$.

One example of such a convex surrogate is the tree-reweighted Bethe free energy considered in our previous work [11]. For this surrogate, the relaxed constraint set $\text{REL}(G; \phi)$ takes the form $\text{LOCAL}(G; \phi) := \{\tau \in \mathbb{R}_+^d \mid \sum_{x_s} \tau_s(x_s) = 1, \sum_{x_t} \tau_{st}(x_s, x_t) = \tau_s(x_s)\}$, whereas the entropy approximation B^* is of the "convexified" Bethe form

$$-B^*(\tau) = \sum_{s \in V} H_s(\tau_s) - \sum_{(s,t) \in E} \rho_{st} I_{st}(\tau_{st}). \tag{4}$$

Here H_s and I_{st} are the singleton entropy and edge-based mutual information, respectively, and the weights ρ_{st} are derived from the graph structure so as to ensure convexity (see [11] for more details). Analogous convex variational formulations underlie the reweighted generalized BP algorithm [13], as well as a log-determinant relaxation [12].

Approximate parameter estimation using surrogate likelihoods: Consider the problem of estimating the parameter θ using i.i.d. samples $\{x^1, \ldots, x^n\}$. For an MRF of the form (1), the maximum likelihood estimate (MLE) is specified using the vector $\widehat{\mu}$ of empirical marginal distributions (singleton $\widehat{\mu}_s$ and pairwise $\widehat{\mu}_{st}$). Since the likelihood is intractable to optimize (due to the cumulant generating function A), it is natural to use the convex surrogate B to define an alternative estimator obtained by maximizing the regularized *surrogate likelihood*:

$$\widehat{\theta}^n := \arg\max_{\theta \in \mathbb{R}^d} \left\{ L_B(\theta; \widehat{\mu}) - \lambda^n R(\theta) \right\} = \arg\max_{\theta \in \mathbb{R}^d} \left\{ \theta^T \widehat{\mu} - B(\theta) - \lambda^n R(\theta) \right\}. \ (5)$$

Here $R : \mathbb{R}^d \to \mathbb{R}_+$ is a regularization function (e.g., $R(\theta) = \|\theta\|^2$), whereas $\lambda^n > 0$ is a regularization coefficient. For the tree-reweighted Bethe surrogate, we have shown in previous work [10] that in the absence of regularization, the optimal parameter estimates $\widehat{\theta}^n$ have a very simple closed-form solution, specified in terms of the weights ρ_{st} and the empirical marginals $\widehat{\mu}$. If a regularizing term is added, these estimates no longer have a closed-form solution, but the optimization problem (5) can still be solved efficiently by message-passing methods.

Joint estimation/prediction: Using such an estimator, we now consider the joint approach to estimation and prediction illustrated in Figure 2. Using an initial set of i.i.d. samples, we first use the surrogate likelihood (5) to construct a parameter estimate $\widehat{\theta}^n$. Given a new noisy or incomplete observation y, we wish to perform near-optimal prediction or data fusion using the fitted model (e.g., for smoothing or interpolation of a noisy image). In order to do so, we first incorporate the new observation into the model, and then use the message-passing algorithm associated with the convex surrogate B in order to compute approximate pseudomarginals τ. These pseudomarginals can then be used to construct a prediction $\widehat{z}(y; \tau)$, where the specifics of the prediction depend on the observation model. We provide a concrete illustration in Section 5 using a mixture-of-Gaussians observation model.

4 Analysis

Asymptotics of estimator: We begin by considering the asymptotic behavior of the parameter estmiator $\widehat{\theta}^n$ defined by the surrogate likelihood (5). Since this parameter estimator is a particular type of M-estimator, the following result follows from standard techniques [8]:

Proposition 1. *For a general graph with cycles, $\widehat{\theta}^n$ converges in probability to some fixed $\widehat{\theta} \neq \theta^*$; moreover, $\sqrt{n}[\widehat{\theta}^n - \widehat{\theta}]$ is asymptotically normal.*

A key property of the estimator is its *inconsistency*—i.e., the estimated model $\widehat{\theta}$ differs from the true model θ^* even in the limit of large data. Despite this inconsistency, we will see that $\widehat{\theta}^n$ is useful for performing prediction.

Algorithmic stability: A desirable property of any algorithm—particularly one applied to statistical data—is that it exhibit an appropriate form of stability with respect to its inputs. Not all message-passing algorithms have such stability properties. For instance, the standard BP algorithm, although stable for relatively weakly coupled MRFs [3, 6], can be highly unstable due to phase transitions. Previous experimental work has shown that methods based on convex relaxations, including reweighted belief propagation [10],

Generic algorithm for joint parameter estimation and prediction:

1. Estimate parameters $\widehat{\theta}^n$ from initial data $x^1, \dots, x^n$ by maximizing surrogate likelihood L_B.

2. Given a new set of observations y, incorporate them into the model:

$$\widetilde{\theta}_s(\,\cdot\,; y_s) = \widehat{\theta}_s^n(\,\cdot\,) + \log p(y_s \,|\, \cdot\,). \tag{6}$$

3. Compute approximate marginals τ by using the message-passing algorithm associated with the convex surrogate B. Use approximate marginals to construct prediction $\widehat{z}(y; \tau)$ of z based on the observation y and pseudomarginals τ.

Figure 2. Algorithm for joint parameter estimation and prediction. Both the learning and prediction steps are approximate, but the key is that they are both based on the same underlying convex surrogate B. Such a construction yields a provably beneficial cancellation of the two sources of error (learning and prediction).

reweighted generalized BP [13], and log-determinant relaxations [12] appear to be very stable. Here we provide theoretical support for these empirical observations: in particular, we prove that, in sharp contrast to non-convex methods, any variational method based on a strongly convex entropy approximation is globally stable.

A function $f : \mathbb{R}^n \to \mathbb{R}$ is *strongly convex* if there exists a constant $c > 0$ such that $f(y) \geq f(x) + \nabla f(x)^T (y - x) + \frac{c}{2}\|y - x\|^2$ for all $x, y \in \mathbb{R}^n$. For a twice continuously differentiable function, this condition is equivalent to the eigenspectrum of the Hessian $\nabla^2 f(x)$ being uniformly bounded away from zero by c. With this definition, we have:

Proposition 2. *Consider any variational method based on a strongly concave entropy approximation* $-B^*$; *moreover, for any parameter* $\theta \in \mathbb{R}^d$, *let* $\tau(\theta)$ *denote the associated set of pseudomarginals. If the optimum is attained interior of the constraint set, then there exists a constant* $R < +\infty$ *such that*

$$\|\tau(\theta + \delta) - \tau(\theta)\| \leq R\|\delta\| \qquad \text{for all } \theta, \delta \in \mathbb{R}^d.$$

Proof. By our construction of the convex surrogate B, we have $\tau(\theta) = \nabla B(\theta)$, so that the statement is equivalent to the assertion that the gradient ∇B is a Lipschitz function. Applying the mean value theorem to ∇B, we can write $\nabla B(\theta + \delta) - \nabla B(\theta) = \nabla^2 B(\theta + t\delta)\delta$ where $t \in [0, 1]$. Consequently, in order to establish the Lipschitz condition, it suffices to show that the spectral norm of $\nabla^2 B(\gamma)$ is uniformly bounded above over all $\gamma \in \mathbb{R}^d$. Differentiating the relation $\nabla B(\theta) = \tau(\theta)$ yields $\nabla^2 B(\theta) = \nabla \tau(\theta)$. Now standard sensitivity analysis results [1] yield that $\nabla \tau(\theta) = [\nabla^2 B^*(\tau(\theta)]^{-1}$. Finally, our assumption of strong convexity of B^* yields that the spectral norm of $\nabla^2 B^*(\tau)$ is uniformly bounded away from zero, which yields the claim. $\qquad \square$

Many existing entropy approximations, including the convexifed Bethe entropy (4), can be shown to be strongly concave [9].

5 Bounds on performance loss

We now turn to theoretical analysis of the joint method for parameter estimation and prediction illustrated in Figure 2. Note that given our setting of limited computation, the Bayes optimum is unattainable for two reasons: (a) it has knowledge of the exact parameter value θ^*; and (b) the prediction step (7) involves computing exact marginal probabilities μ. Therefore, our ultimate goal is to bound the performance loss of our method relative to the unachievable Bayes optimum. So as to obtain a concrete result, we focus on the special case of joint learning/prediction for a mixture-of-Gaussians; however, the ideas and techniques described here are more generally applicable.

Prediction for mixture of Gaussians: Suppose that the discrete random vector is a label vector for the components in a finite mixture of Gaussians: i.e., for each $s \in V$, the random variable Z_s is specified by $p(Z_s = z_s \mid X_s = j; \theta^*) \sim N(\nu_j, \sigma_j^2)$, for $j \in \{0, 1, \ldots, m - 1\}$. Such models are widely used in statistical signal and image processing [2]. Suppose that we observe a noise-corrupted version of Z_s—namely $Y_s = \alpha Z_s + \sqrt{1 - \alpha^2} W_s$, where $W_s \sim N(0, 1)$ is additive Gaussian noise, and the parameter $\alpha \in [0, 1]$ specifies the signal-to-noise ratio (SNR) of the observation model. (Here $\alpha = 0$ corresponds to pure noise, whereas $\alpha = 1$ corresponds to completely uncorrupted observations.)

With this set-up, it is straightforward to show that the optimal Bayes least squares estimator (BLSE) of Z takes the form

$$\widehat{z}_s(y; \mu) \quad := \quad \sum_{j=0}^{m-1} \mu_s(j; \theta^*) \Big[\omega_j(\alpha) \big(y_s - \nu_j \big) + \nu_j \Big], \tag{7}$$

where $\mu_s(j; \theta^*)$ is the exact marginal of the distribution $p(y \mid x) p(x; \theta^*)$; and $\omega_j(\alpha) := \frac{\alpha \sigma_j^2}{\alpha^2 \sigma_j^2 + (1 - \alpha^2)}$ is the usual BLSE weighting for a Gaussian with variance σ_j. For this set-up, the approximate predictor $\widehat{z}_s(y; \tau)$ defined by our joint procedure in Figure 2 corresponds to replacing the exact marginals μ with the pseudomarginals $\tau_s(j; \widetilde{\theta})$ obtained by solving the variational problem with $\widetilde{\theta}$.

Bounds on performance loss: We now turn to a comparison of the mean-squared error (MSE) of the Bayes optimal predictor $\widehat{z}(Y; \mu)$ to the MSE of the surrogate-based predictor $\widehat{z}(Y; \tau)$. More specifically, we provide an upper bound on the increase in MSE, where the bound is specified in terms of the coupling strength and the SNR parameter α. Although results of this nature can be derived more generally, for simplicity we focus on the case of two mixture components ($m = 2$), and consider the asymptotic setting, in which the number of data samples $n \to +\infty$, so that the law of large numbers [8] ensures that the empirical marginals $\widehat{\mu}^n$ converge to the exact marginal distributions μ^*. Consequently, the MLE converges to the true parameter value θ^*, whereas Proposition 1 guarantees that our approximate parameter estimate $\widehat{\theta}^n$ converges to the fixed quantity $\widehat{\theta}$. By construction, we have the relations $\nabla B(\widehat{\theta}) = \mu^* = \nabla A(\theta^*)$.

An important factor in our bound is the quantity

$$L(\theta^*; \widehat{\theta}) \quad := \quad \sup_{\delta \in \mathbb{R}^d} \sigma_{\max}\big(\nabla^2 A(\theta^* + \delta) - \nabla^2 B(\widehat{\theta} + \delta)\big), \tag{8}$$

where $\sigma_{\max}$ denotes the maximal singular value. Following the argument in the proof of Proposition 2, it can be seen that $L(\theta^*; \widehat{\theta})$ is finite. Two additional quantities that play a role in our bound are the differences

$$\Delta_\omega(\alpha) := \omega_1(\alpha) - \omega_0(\alpha), \quad \text{and} \quad \Delta_\nu(\alpha) := [1 - \omega_1(\alpha)]\nu_1 - [1 - \omega_0(\alpha)]\nu_0,$$

where ν_0, ν_1 are the means of the two Gaussian components. Finally, we define $\gamma(Y; \alpha) \in \mathbb{R}^d$ with components $\log \frac{p(Y_s \mid X_s = 1)}{p(Y_s \mid X_s = 0)}$ for $s \in V$, and zeroes otherwise. With this notation, we state the following result (see the technical report [9] for the proof):

Theorem 1. *Let* $\mathrm{MSE}(\tau)$ *and* $\mathrm{MSE}(\mu)$ *denote the mean-squared prediction errors of the surrogate-based predictor* $\widehat{z}(y; \tau)$*, and the Bayes optimal estimate* $\widehat{z}(y; \mu)$ *respectively. The MSE increase* $\mathcal{I}(\alpha) := \frac{1}{N}\big[\mathrm{MSE}(\tau) - \mathrm{MSE}(\mu)\big]$ *is upper bounded by*

$$\mathcal{I}(\alpha) \quad \leq \quad \mathbb{E}\left\{\Omega^2(\alpha)\Delta_\nu^2(\alpha) + \Omega(\alpha)\Big[\Delta_\omega^2(\alpha)\sqrt{\frac{\sum_s Y_s^4}{N}} + 2|\Delta_\nu(\alpha)|\,|\Delta_\omega(\alpha)|\sqrt{\frac{\sum_s Y_s^2}{N}}\Big]\right\}$$

where $\Omega(\alpha) := \min\{1, L(\theta^*; \widehat{\theta}) \|\frac{\gamma(Y; \alpha)}{N}\|\}$.

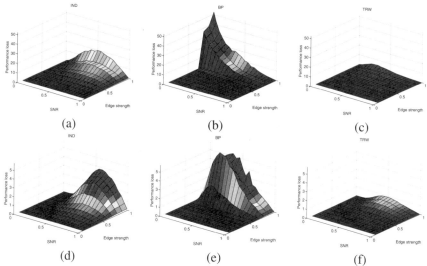

Figure 3. Surface plots of the percentage increase in MSE relative to Bayes optimum for different methods as a function of observation SNR and coupling strength. Top row: Gaussian mixture with components $(\nu_0, \sigma_0^2) = (-1, 0.5)$ and $(\nu_1, \sigma_1^2) = (1, 0.5)$. Bottom row: Gaussian mixture with components $(\nu_0, \sigma_0^2) = (0, 1)$ and $(\nu_0, \sigma_1^2) = (0, 9)$. Left column: independence model (IND). Center column: ordinary belief propagation (BP). Right column: tree-reweighted algorithm (TRW).

It can be seen that $\mathcal{I}(\alpha) \rightarrow 0$ as $\alpha \rightarrow 0^+$ and as $\alpha \rightarrow 1^-$, so that the surrogate-based method is asymptotically optimal for both low and high SNR. The behavior of the bound in the intermediate regime is controlled by the balance between these two terms.

Experimental results: In order to test our joint estimation/prediction procedure, we have applied it to coupled Gaussian mixture models on different graphs, coupling strengths, observation SNRs, and mixture distributions. Although our methods are more generally applicable, here we show representative results for $m = 2$ components, and two different mixture types. The first ensemble, constructed with mean and variance components $(\nu_0, \sigma_0^2) = (0, 1)$ and $(\nu_1, \sigma_1^2) = (0, 9)$, mimics heavy-tailed behavior. The second ensemble is bimodal, with components $(\nu_0, \sigma_0^2) = (-1, 0.5)$ and $(\nu_1, \sigma_1^2) = (1, 0.5)$. In both cases, each mixture component is equally weighted. Here we show results for a 2-D grid with $N = 64$ nodes. Since the mixture variables have $m = 2$ states, the coupling distribution can be written as $p(x; \theta) \propto \exp \left\{ \sum_{s \in V} \theta_s x_s + \sum_{(s,t) \in E} \theta_{st} x_s x_t \right\}$. where $x \in \{-1, +1\}^N$ are spin variables indexing the mixture components. In all trials, we chose $\theta_s = 0$ for all nodes $s \in V$, which ensures uniform marginal distributions $p(x_s; \theta)$ at each node. For each coupling strength $\gamma \in [0, 1]$, we chose edge parameters as $\theta_{st} \sim \mathcal{U}[0, \gamma]$, and we varied the SNR parameter α controlling the observation model in $[0, 1]$. We evaluated the following three methods based on their increase in mean-squared error (MSE) over the Bayes optimal predictor (7): (a) As a baseline, we used the *independence model* for the mixture components: parameters are estimated $\theta_s(x_s) = \log \widehat{\mu}_s(x_s)$, and setting coupling terms $\theta_{st}(x_s, x_t)$ equal to zero. The prediction step reduces to performing BLSE at each node independently. (b) The *standard belief propagation* (BP) approach is based on estimating parameters (see step (1) of Figure 2) using $\rho_{st} = 1$ for all edges (s, t), and using BP to compute the pseudomarginals. (c) The *tree-reweighted method* (TRW) is based on estimating parameters using the tree-reweighted surrogate [10] with weights $\rho_{st} = \frac{1}{2}$ for all edges (s, t), and using the TRW sum-product algorithm to compute the pseudomarginals.

Shown in Figure 3 are 2-D surface plots of the average percentage increase in MSE, taken over 100 trials, as a function of the coupling strength $\gamma \in [0, 1]$ and the observation SNR parameter $\alpha \in [0, 1]$ for the independence model (left column), BP approach (middle column) and TRW method (right column). For weak coupling ($\gamma \approx 0$), all three methods— including the independence model—perform quite well, as should be expected given the weak dependency. Although not clear in these plots, BP outperforms TRW for weak coupling; however, both methods lose than than 1% in this regime. As the coupling is increased, the BP method eventually deteriorates quite seriously; indeed, for large enough coupling and low/intermediate SNR, its performance can be worse than the independence model. Looking at alternative models (in which phase transitions are known), we have found that this rapid degradation co-incides with the appearance of multiple fixed points. In contrast, the behavior of the TRW method is extremely stable, consistent with our theory.

6 Conclusion

We have described and analyzed joint methods for parameter estimation and prediction/smoothing using variational methods that are based on convex surrogates to the cumulant generating function. Our results—both theoretical and experimental—confirm the intuition that in the computation-limited setting, in which errors arise from approximations made both during parameter estimation and subsequent prediction, it is *provably beneficial* to use an inconsistent parameter estimator. Our experimental results on the coupled mixture of Gaussian model confirm the theory: the tree-reweighted sum-product algorithm yields prediction results close to the Bayes optimum, and substantially outperforms an analogous but heuristic method based on standard belief propagation.

References

[1] D. Bertsekas. *Nonlinear programming*. Athena Scientific, Belmont, MA, 1995.

[2] M. Crouse, R. Nowak, and R. Baraniuk. Wavelet-based statistical signal processing using hidden Markov models. *IEEE Trans. Signal Processing*, 46:886–902, April 1998.

[3] A. Ihler, J. Fisher, and A. S. Willsky. Loopy belief propagation: Convergence and effects of message errors. *Journal of Machine Learning Research*, 6:905–936, May 2005.

[4] M. A. R. Leisink and H. J. Kappen. Learning in higher order Boltzmann machines using linear response. *Neural Networks*, 13:329–335, 2000.

[5] T. P. Minka. *A family of algorithms for approximate Bayesian inference*. PhD thesis, MIT, January 2001.

[6] S. Tatikonda and M. I. Jordan. Loopy belief propagation and Gibbs measures. In *Proc. Uncertainty in Artificial Intelligence*, volume 18, pages 493–500, August 2002.

[7] Y. W. Teh and M. Welling. On improving the efficiency of the iterative proportional fitting procedure. In *Workshop on Artificial Intelligence and Statistics*, 2003.

[8] A. W. van der Vaart. *Asymptotic statistics*. Cambridge University Press, Cambridge, UK, 1998.

[9] M. J. Wainwright. Joint estimation and prediction in Markov random fields: Benefits of inconsistency in the computation-limited regime. Technical Report 690, Department of Statistics, UC Berkeley, 2005.

[10] M. J. Wainwright, T. S. Jaakkola, and A. S. Willsky. Tree-reweighted belief propagation algorithms and approximate ML estimation by pseudomoment matching. In *Workshop on Artificial Intelligence and Statistics*, January 2003.

[11] M. J. Wainwright, T. S. Jaakkola, and A. S. Willsky. A new class of upper bounds on the log partition function. *IEEE Trans. Info. Theory*, 51(7):2313–2335, July 2005.

[12] M. J. Wainwright and M. I. Jordan. A variational principle for graphical models. In *New Directions in Statistical Signal Processing*. MIT Press, Cambridge, MA, 2005.

[13] W. Wiegerinck. Approximations with reweighted generalized belief propagation. In *Workshop on Artificial Intelligence and Statistics*, January 2005.

[14] J. Yedidia, W. T. Freeman, and Y. Weiss. Constructing free energy approximations and generalized belief propagation algorithms. *IEEE Trans. Info. Theory*, 51(7):2282–2312, July 2005.

Recovery of Jointly Sparse Signals
from Few Random Projections

Michael B. Wakin
ECE Department
Rice University
wakin@rice.edu

Marco F. Duarte
ECE Department
Rice University
duarte@rice.edu

Shriram Sarvotham
ECE Department
Rice University
shri@rice.edu

Dror Baron
ECE Department
Rice University
drorb@rice.edu

Richard G. Baraniuk
ECE Department
Rice University
richb@rice.edu

Abstract

Compressed sensing is an emerging field based on the revelation that a small group of linear projections of a sparse signal contains enough information for reconstruction. In this paper we introduce a new theory for *distributed compressed sensing* (DCS) that enables new distributed coding algorithms for multi-signal ensembles that exploit both intra- and inter-signal correlation structures. The DCS theory rests on a new concept that we term the *joint sparsity* of a signal ensemble. We study three simple models for jointly sparse signals, propose algorithms for joint recovery of multiple signals from incoherent projections, and characterize theoretically and empirically the number of measurements per sensor required for accurate reconstruction. In some sense DCS is a framework for distributed compression of sources with memory, which has remained a challenging problem in information theory for some time. DCS is immediately applicable to a range of problems in sensor networks and arrays.

1 Introduction

Distributed communication, sensing, and computing [13, 17] are emerging fields with numerous promising applications. In a typical setup, large groups of cheap and individually unreliable nodes may collaborate to perform a variety of data processing tasks such as sensing, data collection, classification, modeling, tracking, and so on. As individual nodes in such a network are often battery-operated, power consumption is a limiting factor, and the reduction of communication costs is crucial. In such a setting, *distributed source coding* [8, 13, 14, 17] may allow the sensors to save on communication costs. In the Slepian-Wolf framework for lossless distributed coding [8, 14], the availability of *correlated side information* at the decoder enables the source encoder to communicate losslessly at the conditional entropy rate, rather than the individual entropy. Because sensor networks and arrays rely on data that often exhibit strong spatial correlations [13, 17], distributed compression can reduce the communication costs substantially, thus enhancing battery life. Unfortunately, distributed compression schemes for sources with memory are not yet mature [8, 13, 14, 17].

We propose a new approach for distributed coding of correlated sources whose signal correlations take the form of a sparse structure. Our approach is based on another emerging field known as *compressed sensing* (CS) [4, 9]. CS builds upon the groundbreaking work of Candès et al. [4] and Donoho [9], who showed that signals that are *sparse* relative to a known basis can be recovered from a small number of nonadaptive linear projections onto a second basis that is incoherent with the first. (A random basis provides such incoherence with high probability. Hence CS with random projections is *universal* — the signals can be reconstructed if they are sparse relative to *any* known basis.) The implications of CS for signal acquisition and compression are very promising. With no a priori knowledge of a signal's structure, a sensor node could simultaneously acquire and compress that signal, preserving the critical information that is extracted only later at a fusion center.

In our framework for *distributed compressed sensing* (DCS), this advantage is particularly compelling. In a typical DCS scenario, a number of sensors measure signals that are each individually sparse in some basis and also correlated from sensor to sensor. Each sensor *independently* encodes its signal by projecting it onto another, incoherent basis (such as a random one) and then transmits just a few of the resulting coefficients to a single collection point. Under the right conditions, a decoder at the collection point can reconstruct each of the signals precisely. The DCS theory rests on a concept that we term the *joint sparsity* of a signal ensemble. We study in detail three simple models for jointly sparse signals, propose tractable algorithms for joint recovery of signal ensembles from incoherent projections, and characterize theoretically and empirically the number of measurements per sensor required for reconstruction. While the sensors operate entirely without collaboration, joint decoding can recover signals using far fewer measurements per sensor than would be required for separable CS recovery. This paper presents our specific results for one of the three models; the other two are highlighted in our papers [1, 2, 11].

2   Sparse Signal Recovery from Incoherent Projections

In the traditional CS setting, we consider a single signal $x \in \mathbb{R}^N$, which we assume to be sparse in a known orthonormal basis or frame $\Psi = [\psi_1, \psi_2, \ldots, \psi_N]$. That is, $x = \Psi\theta$ for some θ, where $\|\theta\|_0 = K$ holds.[1] The signal x is observed indirectly via an $M \times N$ measurement matrix Φ, where $M < N$. We let $y = \Phi x$ be the observation vector, consisting of the M inner products of the measurement vectors against the signal. The M rows of Φ are the measurement vectors, against which the signal is projected. These rows are chosen to be *incoherent* with Ψ — that is, they each have non-sparse expansions in the basis Ψ [4, 9]. In general, Φ meets the necessary criteria when its entries are drawn *randomly*, for example independent and identically distributed (i.i.d.) Gaussian.

Although the equation $y = \Phi x$ is underdetermined, it is possible to recover x from y under certain conditions. In general, due to the incoherence between Φ and Ψ, θ can be recovered by solving the ℓ_0 optimization problem

$$\widehat{\theta} = \arg \min \|\theta\|_0 \quad \text{s.t.} \quad y = \Phi\Psi\theta.$$

In principle, remarkably few random measurements are required to recover a K-sparse signal via ℓ_0 minimization. Clearly, more than K measurements must be taken to avoid ambiguity; in theory, $K + 1$ random measurements will suffice [2]. Unfortunately, solving this ℓ_0 optimization problem appears to be NP-hard [6], requiring a combinatorial enumeration of the $\binom{N}{K}$ possible sparse subspaces for θ.

The amazing revelation that supports the CS theory is that a much simpler problem yields an equivalent solution (thanks again to the incoherence of the bases): we need only solve

---

[1]The ℓ_0 "norm" $\|\theta\|_0$ merely counts the number of nonzero entries in the vector θ. CS theory also applies to signals for which $\|\theta\|_p \leq K$, where $0 < p \leq 1$; such extensions for DCS are a topic of ongoing research.

for the ℓ_1-sparsest vector θ that agrees with the observed coefficients y [4, 9]

$$\widehat{\theta} = \arg\min \|\theta\|_1 \quad \text{s.t.} \quad y = \Phi\Psi\theta.$$

This optimization problem, known also as Basis Pursuit (BP) [7], is significantly more tractable and can be solved with traditional linear programming techniques. There is no free lunch, however; more than $K + 1$ measurements will be required in order to recover sparse signals. In general, there exists a constant oversampling factor $c = c(K, N)$ such that cK measurements suffice to recover x with very high probability [4, 9]. Commonly quoted as $c = O(\log(N))$, we have found that $c \approx \log_2(1 + N/K)$ provides a useful rule-of-thumb [2]. At the expense of slightly more measurements, greedy algorithms have also been developed to recover x from y. One example, known as Orthogonal Matching Pursuit (OMP) [15], requires $c \approx 2\ln(N)$. We exploit both BP and greedy algorithms for recovering jointly sparse signals.

3 Joint Sparsity Models

In this section, we generalize the notion of a signal being sparse in some basis to the notion of an ensemble of signals being *jointly sparse*. We consider three different *joint sparsity models* (JSMs) that apply in different situations. In most cases, each signal is itself sparse, and so we could use the CS framework from above to encode and decode each one separately. However, there also exists a framework wherein a *joint representation* for the ensemble uses fewer total vectors.

We use the following notation for our signal ensembles and measurement model. Denote the *signals* in the ensemble by x_j, $j \in \{1, 2, \ldots, J\}$, and assume that each signal $x_j \in \mathbb{R}^N$. We assume that there exists a known *sparse basis* Ψ for $\mathbb{R}^N$ in which the x_j can be sparsely represented. Denote by Φ_j the *measurement matrix* for signal j; Φ_j is $M_j \times N$ and, in general, the entries of Φ_j are different for each j. Thus, $y_j = \Phi_j x_j$ consists of $M_j < N$ *incoherent measurements* of x_j.

JSM-1: Sparse common component + innovations. In this model, all signals share a *common* sparse component while each individual signal contains a sparse *innovation* component; that is,

$$x_j = z_C + z_j, \quad j \in \{1, 2, \ldots, J\}$$

with

$$z_C = \Psi\theta_C, \quad \|\theta_C\|_0 = K \quad \text{and} \quad z_j = \Psi\theta_j, \quad \|\theta_j\|_0 = K_j.$$

Thus, the signal z_C is common to all of the x_j and has sparsity K in basis Ψ. The signals z_j are the unique portions of the x_j and have sparsity K_j in the same basis. A practical situation well-modeled by JSM-1 is a group of sensors measuring temperatures at a number of outdoor locations throughout the day. The temperature readings x_j have both temporal (intra-signal) and spatial (inter-signal) correlations. Global factors, such as the sun and prevailing winds, could have an effect z_C that is both common to all sensors and structured enough to permit sparse representation. More local factors, such as shade, water, or animals, could contribute localized innovations z_j that are also structured (and hence sparse). Similar scenarios could be imagined for a network of sensors recording other phenomena that change smoothly in time and in space and thus are highly correlated.

JSM-2: Common sparse supports. In this model, all signals are constructed from the same sparse set of basis vectors, but with different coefficients; that is,

$$x_j = \Psi\theta_j, \quad j \in \{1, 2, \ldots, J\},$$

where each θ_j is supported only on the same $\Omega \subset \{1, 2, \ldots, N\}$ with $|\Omega| = K$. Hence, all signals have ℓ_0 sparsity of K, and all are constructed from the same K basis elements, but with arbitrarily different coefficients. A practical situation well-modeled by JSM-2 is where multiple sensors acquire the same signal but with phase shifts and attenuations

1435

caused by signal propagation. In many cases it is critical to recover each one of the sensed signals, such as in many acoustic localization and array processing algorithms. Another useful application for JSM-2 is MIMO communication [16].

JSM-3: Nonsparse common + sparse innovations. This model extends JSM-1 so that the common component need no longer be sparse in any basis; that is,

$$x_j = z_C + z_j, \quad j \in \{1, 2, \ldots, J\}$$

with

$$z_C = \Psi \theta_C \quad \text{and} \quad z_j = \Psi \theta_j, \ \|\theta_j\|_0 = K_j,$$

but z_C is not necessarily sparse in the basis Ψ. We also consider the case where the supports of the innovations are shared for all signals, which extends JSM-2. A practical situation well-modeled by JSM-3 is where several sources are recorded by different sensors together with a background signal that is not sparse in any basis. Consider, for example, a computer vision-based verification system in a device production plant. Cameras acquire snapshots of components in the production line; a computer system then checks for failures in the devices for quality control purposes. While each image could be extremely complicated, the ensemble of images will be highly correlated, since each camera is observing the same device with minor (sparse) variations. JSM-3 could also be useful in some non-distributed scenarios. For example, it motivates the compression of data such as video, where the innovations or differences between video frames may be sparse, even though a single frame may not be very sparse. In general, JSM-3 may be invoked for ensembles with significant inter-signal correlations but insignificant intra-signal correlations.

4 Recovery of Jointly Sparse Signals

In a setting where a network or array of sensors may encounter a collection of jointly sparse signals, and where a centralized reconstruction algorithm is feasible, the number of incoherent measurements required by each sensor can be reduced. For each JSM, we propose algorithms for joint signal recovery from incoherent projections and characterize theoretically and empirically the number of measurements per sensor required for accurate reconstruction. We focus in particular on JSM-3 in this paper but also overview our results for JSMs 1 and 2, which are discussed in further detail in our papers [1, 2, 11].

4.1 JSM-1: Sparse common component + innovations

For this model (see also [1, 2]), we have proposed an analytical framework inspired by the principles of information theory. This allows us to characterize the measurement rates M_j required to *jointly* reconstruct the signals x_j. The measurement rates relate directly to the signals' *conditional sparsities*, in parallel with the Slepian-Wolf theory. More specifically, we have formalized the following intuition. Consider the simple case of $J = 2$ signals. By employing the CS machinery, we might expect that (*i*) $(K + K_1)c$ coefficients suffice to reconstruct x_1, (*ii*) $(K + K_2)c$ coefficients suffice to reconstruct x_2, yet only (*iii*) $(K + K_1 + K_2)c$ coefficients should suffice to reconstruct both x_1 and x_2, since we have $K + K_1 + K_2$ nonzero elements in x_1 and x_2. In addition, given the $(K + K_1)c$ measurements for x_1 as side information, and assuming that the partitioning of x_1 into z_C and z_1 is known, cK_2 measurements that describe z_2 should allow reconstruction of x_2. Formalizing these arguments allows us to establish theoretical lower bounds on the required measurement rates at each sensor; Fig.1(a) shows such a bound for the case of $J = 2$ signals.

We have also established upper bounds on the required measurement rates M_j by proposing a specific algorithm for reconstruction [1]. The algorithm uses carefully designed measurement matrices Φ_j (in which some rows are identical and some differ) so that the resulting measurements can be combined to allow step-by-step recovery of the sparse components. The theoretical rates M_j are below those required for separable CS recovery of each signal x_j (see Fig. 1(a)). We also proposed a reconstruction technique based on a single execution of a linear program, which seeks the sparsest components $[z_C; \ z_1; \ \ldots \ z_J]$ that

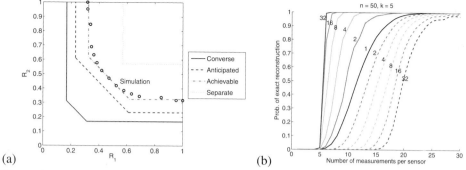

(a)　　　　　　　　　　　　　　　　　　　　　　(b)

Figure 1: *(a) Converse bounds and achievable measurement rates for $J = 2$ signals with common sparse component and sparse innovations (JSM-1). We fix signal lengths $N = 1000$ and sparsities $K = 200$, $K_1 = K_2 = 50$. The measurement rates $R_j := M_j/N$ reflect the number of measurements normalized by the signal length. Blue curves indicate our theoretical and anticipated converse bounds; red indicates a provably achievable region, and pink denotes the rates required for separable CS signal reconstruction. (b) Reconstructing a signal ensemble with common sparse supports (JSM-2). We plot the probability of perfect reconstruction via DCS-SOMP (solid lines) and independent CS reconstruction (dashed lines) as a function of the number of measurements per signal M and the number of signals J. We fix the signal length to $N = 50$ and the sparsity to $K = 5$. An oracle encoder that knows the positions of the large coefficients would use 5 measurements per signal.*

account for the observed measurements. Numerical simulations support such an approach (see Fig.1(a)). Future work will extend JSM-1 to ℓ_p-compressible signals, $0 < p \leq 1$.

4.2　JSM-2: Common sparse supports

Under the JSM-2 signal ensemble model (see also [2, 11]), independent recovery of each signal via ℓ_1 minimization would require cK measurements per signal. However, algorithms inspired by conventional greedy pursuit algorithms (such as OMP [15]) can substantially reduce this number. In the single-signal case, OMP iteratively constructs the sparse support set Ω; decisions are based on inner products between the columns of $\Phi\Psi$ and a residual. In the multi-signal case, there are more clues available for determining the elements of Ω.

To establish a theoretical justification for our approach, we first proposed a simple One-Step Greedy Algorithm (OSGA) [11] that combines all of the measurements and seeks the largest correlations with the columns of the $\Phi_j\Psi$. We established that, assuming that Φ_j has i.i.d. Gaussian entries and that the nonzero coefficients in the θ_j are i.i.d. Gaussian, then with $M \geq 1$ measurements per signal, OSGA recovers Ω with probability approaching 1 as $J \to \infty$. Moreover, with $M \geq K$ measurements per signal, OSGA recovers all x_j with probability approaching 1 as $J \to \infty$. This meets the theoretical lower bound for M_j.

In practice, OSGA can be improved using an iterative greedy algorithm. We proposed a simple variant of Simultaneous Orthogonal Matching Pursuit (SOMP) [16] that we term DCS-SOMP [11]. For this algorithm, Fig. 1(b) plots the performance as the number of sensors varies from $J = 1$ to 32. We fix the signal lengths at $N = 50$ and the sparsity of each signal to $K = 5$. With DCS-SOMP, for perfect reconstruction of all signals the average number of measurements per signal decreases as a function of J. The trend suggests that, for very large J, close to K measurements per signal should suffice. On the contrary, with independent CS reconstruction, for perfect reconstruction of all signals the number of measurements per sensor *increases* as a function of J. This surprise is due to the fact that each signal will experience an independent probability $p \leq 1$ of successful reconstruction; therefore the overall probability of complete success is p^J. Consequently, each sensor must compensate by making additional measurements.

4.3 JSM-3: Nonsparse common + sparse innovations

The JSM-3 signal ensemble model provides a particularly compelling motivation for joint recovery. Under this model, no individual signal x_j is sparse, and so separate signal recovery would require fully N measurements per signal. As in the other JSMs, however, the commonality among the signals makes it possible to substantially reduce this number.

Our recovery algorithms are based on the observation that if the common component z_C were known, then each innovation z_j could be estimated using the standard single-signal CS machinery on the adjusted measurements $y_j - \Phi_j z_C = \Phi_j z_j$. While z_C is not known in advance, it can be *estimated* from the measurements. In fact, across all J sensors, a total of $\sum_j M_j$ random projections of z_C are observed (each corrupted by a contribution from one of the z_j). Since z_C is not sparse, it cannot be recovered via CS techniques, but when the number of measurements is sufficiently large ($\sum_j M_j \gg N$), z_C can be estimated using standard tools from linear algebra. A key requirement for such a method to succeed in recovering z_C is that each Φ_j be different, so that their rows combine to span all of $\mathbb{R}^N$. In the limit, z_C can be recovered while still allowing each sensor to operate at the minimum measurement rate dictated by the $\{z_j\}$. A prototype algorithm, which we name Transpose Estimation of Common Component (TECC), is listed below, where we assume that each measurement matrix Φ_j has i.i.d. $\mathcal{N}(0, \sigma_j^2)$ entries.

TECC Algorithm for JSM-3

1. **Estimate common component:** Define the matrix $\widehat{\Phi}$ as the concatenation of the regularized individual measurement matrices $\widehat{\Phi}_j = \frac{1}{M_j \sigma_j^2}\Phi_j$, that is, $\widehat{\Phi} = [\widehat{\Phi}_1, \widehat{\Phi}_2, \ldots, \widehat{\Phi}_J]$.
   Calculate the estimate of the common component as $\widehat{z_C} = \frac{1}{J}\widehat{\Phi}^T y$.

2. **Estimate measurements generated by innovations:** Using the previous estimate, subtract the contribution of the common part on the measurements and generate estimates for the measurements caused by the innovations for each signal: $\widehat{y}_j = y_j - \Phi_j \widehat{z_C}$.

3. **Reconstruct innovations:** Using a standard single-signal CS reconstruction algorithm, obtain estimates of the innovations $\widehat{z}_j$ from the estimated innovation measurements $\widehat{y}_j$.

4. **Obtain signal estimates:** Sum the above estimates, letting $\widehat{x}_j = \widehat{z_C} + \widehat{z}_j$.

The following theorem shows that asymptotically, by using the TECC algorithm, each sensor need only measure at the rate dictated by the sparsity K_j.

Theorem 1 [2] *Assume that the nonzero expansion coefficients of the sparse innovations z_j are i.i.d. Gaussian random variables and that their locations are uniformly distributed on $\{1, 2, ..., N\}$. Then the following statements hold:*

1. *Let the measurement matrices Φ_j contain i.i.d. $\mathcal{N}(0, \sigma_j^2)$ entries with $M_j \geq K_j + 1$. Then each signal x_j can be recovered using the TECC algorithm with probability approaching 1 as $J \to \infty$.*

2. *Let Φ_j be a measurement matrix with $M_j \leq K_j$ for some $j \in \{1, 2, ..., J\}$. Then with probability 1, the signal x_j cannot be uniquely recovered by any algorithm for any J.*

For large J, the measurement rates permitted by Statement 1 are the lowest possible for *any* reconstruction strategy on JSM-3 signals, even neglecting the presence of the nonsparse component. Thus, Theorem 1 provides a tight achievable and converse for JSM-3 signals. The CS technique employed in Theorem 1 involves combinatorial searches for estimating the innovation components. More efficient techniques could also be employed (including several proposed for CS in the presence of noise [3, 5, 7, 10, 12]).

While Theorem 1 suggests the theoretical gains from joint recovery as $J \to \infty$, practical gains can also be realized with a moderate number of sensors. For example, suppose in the TECC algorithm that the initial estimate $\widehat{z_C}$ is not accurate enough to enable correct identification of the sparse innovation supports $\{\Omega_j\}$. In such a case, it may still be possible for a rough approximation of the innovations $\{z_j\}$ to help refine the estimate $\widehat{z_C}$. This in turn could help to refine the estimates of the innovations. Since each component helps to estimate the others, we propose an iterative algorithm for JSM-3 recovery. The Alternating Common and Innovation Estimation (ACIE) algorithm exploits the observation that once the basis vectors comprising the innovation z_j have been identified in the index set Ω_j, their effect on the measurements y_j can be removed to aid in estimating z_C.

ACIE Algorithm for JSM-3

1. **Initialize:** Set $\widehat{\Omega}_j = \emptyset$ for each j. Set the iteration counter $\ell = 1$.

2. **Estimate common component:** Let $\Phi_{j,\widehat{\Omega}_j}$ be the $M_j \times |\widehat{\Omega}_j|$ submatrix obtained by sampling the columns $\widehat{\Omega}_j$ from Φ_j and construct an $M_j \times (M_j - |\widehat{\Omega}_j|)$ matrix $Q_j = [q_{j,1} \cdots q_{j,M_j-|\widehat{\Omega}_j|}]$ having orthonormal columns that span the orthogonal complement of $\mathrm{colspan}(\Phi_{j,\widehat{\Omega}_j})$. Remove the projection of the measurements into the aforementioned span to obtain measurements caused exclusively by vectors not in $\widehat{\Omega}_j$, letting $\widetilde{y}_j = Q_j^T y_j$ and $\widetilde{\Phi}_j = Q_j^T \Phi_j$. Use the modified measurements $\widetilde{Y} = \begin{bmatrix} \widetilde{y}_1^T & \widetilde{y}_2^T & \cdots & \widetilde{y}_J^T \end{bmatrix}^T$ and modified holographic basis $\widetilde{\Phi} = \begin{bmatrix} \widetilde{\Phi}_1^T & \widetilde{\Phi}_2^T & \cdots & \widetilde{\Phi}_J^T \end{bmatrix}^T$ to refine the estimate of the measurements caused by the common part of the signal, setting $\widetilde{z_C} = \widetilde{\Phi}^\dagger \widetilde{Y}$, where $A^\dagger = (A^T A)^{-1} A^T$ denotes the pseudoinverse of matrix A.

3. **Estimate innovation supports:** For each signal j, subtract $\widetilde{z_C}$ from the measurements, $\widehat{y}_j = y_j - \Phi_j \widetilde{z_C}$, and estimate the sparse support of each innovation $\widehat{\Omega}_j$.

4. **Iterate:** If $\ell < L$, a preset number of iterations, then increment ℓ and return to Step 2. Otherwise proceed to Step 5.

5. **Estimate innovation coefficients:** For each signal j, estimate the coefficients for the indices in $\widehat{\Omega}_j$, setting $\widehat{\theta}_{j,\widehat{\Omega}_j} = \Phi_{j,\widehat{\Omega}_j}^\dagger (y_j - \Phi_j \widetilde{z_C})$, where $\widehat{\theta}_{j,\widehat{\Omega}_j}$ is a sampled version of the innovation's sparse coefficient vector estimate $\widehat{\theta}_j$.

6. **Reconstruct signals:** Estimate each signal as $\widehat{x}_j = \widetilde{z_C} + \widetilde{z}_j = \widetilde{z_C} + \Phi_j \widehat{\theta}_j$.

In the case where the innovation support estimate is correct ($\widehat{\Omega}_j = \Omega_j$), the measurements $\widetilde{y}_j$ will describe only the common component z_C. If this is true for every signal j and the number of remaining measurements $\sum_j M_j - KJ \geq N$, then z_C can be perfectly recovered in Step 2. Because it may be difficult to correctly obtain all Ω_j in the first iteration, we find it preferable to run the algorithm for several iterations.

Fig. 2(a) shows that, for sufficiently large J, we can recover all of the signals with significantly fewer than N measurements per signal. We note the following behavior in the graph. First, as J grows, it becomes more difficult to perfectly reconstruct all J signals. We believe this is inevitable, because even if z_C were known without error, then perfect ensemble recovery would require the successful execution of J *independent* runs of OMP. Second, for small J, the probability of success can decrease at high values of M. We believe this is due to the fact that initial errors in estimating z_C may tend to be somewhat sparse (since $\widehat{z_C}$ roughly becomes an average of the signals $\{x_j\}$), and these sparse errors can mislead the subsequent OMP processes. For more moderate M, it seems that the errors in estimating z_C (though greater) tend to be less sparse. We expect that a more sophisticated algorithm could alleviate such a problem, and we note that the problem is also mitigated at higher J.

Fig. 2(b) shows that when the sparse innovations share common supports we see an even greater savings. As a point of reference, a traditional approach to signal encoding would require 1600 total measurements to reconstruct these $J = 32$ nonsparse signals of length $N = 50$. Our approach requires only about 10 per sensor for a total of 320 measurements.

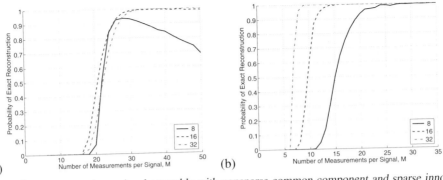

(a)   (b)

Figure 2: *Reconstructing a signal ensemble with nonsparse common component and sparse innovations (JSM-3) using ACIE. (a) Reconstruction using OMP independently on each signal in Step 3 of the ACIE algorithm (innovations have arbitrary supports). (b) Reconstruction using DCS-SOMP jointly on all signals in Step 3 of the ACIE algorithm (innovations have identical supports). Signal length $N = 50$, sparsity $K = 5$. The common structure exploited by DCS-SOMP enables dramatic savings in the number of measurements. We average over 1000 simulation runs.*

Acknowledgments: Thanks to Emmanuel Candès, Hyeokho Choi, and Joel Tropp for informative and inspiring conversations.

References

[1] D. Baron, M. F. Duarte, S. Sarvotham, M. B. Wakin, and R. G. Baraniuk. An information-theoretic approach to distributed compressed sensing. In *Allerton Conf. Comm., Control, Comput.*, Sept. 2005.

[2] D. Baron, M. B. Wakin, M. F. Duarte, S. Sarvotham, and R. G. Baraniuk. Distributed compressed sensing. 2005. Preprint. Available at www.dsp.rice.edu/cs.

[3] E. Candès, J. Romberg, and T. Tao. Stable signal recovery from incomplete and inaccurate measurements. *Comm. Pure Applied Mathematics*, 2005. To appear.

[4] E. Candès and T. Tao. Near optimal signal recovery from random projections and universal encoding strategies. 2004. Preprint.

[5] E. Candès and T. Tao. The Dantzig selector: Statistical estimation when p is much larger than n. 2005. Preprint.

[6] E. Candès and T. Tao. Error correction via linear programming. 2005. Preprint.

[7] S. Chen, D. Donoho, and M. Saunders. Atomic decomposition by basis pursuit. *SIAM Journal on Scientific Computing*, 20(1):33–61, 1998.

[8] T. M. Cover and J. A. Thomas. *Elements of Information Theory*. Wiley, New York, 1991.

[9] D. Donoho. Compressed sensing. 2004. Preprint.

[10] D. Donoho and Y. Tsaig. Extensions of compressed sensing. 2004. Preprint.

[11] M. F. Duarte, S. Sarvotham, D. Baron, M. B. Wakin, and R. G. Baraniuk. Distributed compressed sensing of jointly sparse signals. In *Asilomar Conf. Signals, Sys., Comput.*, Nov. 2005.

[12] J. Haupt and R. Nowak. Signal reconstruction from noisy random projections. 2005. Preprint.

[13] S. Pradhan and K. Ramchandran. Distributed source coding using syndromes (DISCUS): Design and construction. *IEEE Trans. Inform. Theory*, 49:626–643, March 2003.

[14] D. Slepian and J. K. Wolf. Noiseless coding of correlated information sources. *IEEE Trans. Inform. Theory*, 19:471–480, July 1973.

[15] J. Tropp and A. C. Gilbert. Signal recovery from partial information via orthogonal matching pursuit. 2005. Preprint.

[16] J. Tropp, A. C. Gilbert, and M. J. Strauss. Simulataneous sparse approximation via greedy pursuit. In *IEEE 2005 Int. Conf. Acoustics, Speech, Signal Processing*, March 2005.

[17] Z. Xiong, A. Liveris, and S. Cheng. Distributed source coding for sensor networks. *IEEE Signal Proc. Mag.*, 21:80–94, September 2004.

Gaussian Process Dynamical Models

Jack M. Wang, David J. Fleet, Aaron Hertzmann
Department of Computer Science
University of Toronto, Toronto, ON M5S 3G4
{jmwang,hertzman}@dgp.toronto.edu, fleet@cs.toronto.edu

Abstract

This paper introduces Gaussian Process Dynamical Models (GPDM) for nonlinear time series analysis. A GPDM comprises a low-dimensional latent space with associated dynamics, and a map from the latent space to an observation space. We marginalize out the model parameters in closed-form, using Gaussian Process (GP) priors for both the dynamics and the observation mappings. This results in a nonparametric model for dynamical systems that accounts for uncertainty in the model. We demonstrate the approach on human motion capture data in which each pose is 62-dimensional. Despite the use of small data sets, the GPDM learns an effective representation of the nonlinear dynamics in these spaces. **Webpage:** http://www.dgp.toronto.edu/~jmwang/gpdm/

1 Introduction

A central difficulty in modeling time-series data is in determining a model that can capture the nonlinearities of the data without overfitting. Linear autoregressive models require relatively few parameters and allow closed-form analysis, but can only model a limited range of systems. In contrast, existing nonlinear models can model complex dynamics, but may require large training sets to learn accurate MAP models.

In this paper we investigate learning nonlinear dynamical models for high-dimensional datasets. We take a Bayesian approach to modeling dynamics, averaging over dynamics parameters rather than estimating them. Inspired by the fact that averaging over nonlinear regression models leads to a Gaussian Process (GP) model, we show that integrating over parameters in nonlinear dynamical systems can also be performed in closed-form. The resulting Gaussian Process Dynamical Model (GPDM) is fully defined by a set of low-dimensional representations of the training data, with both dynamics and observation mappings learned from GP regression. As a natural consequence of GP regression, the GPDM removes the need to select many parameters associated with function approximators while retaining the expressiveness of nonlinear dynamics and observation.

Our work is motivated by modeling human motion for video-based people tracking and data-driven animation. Bayesian people tracking requires dynamical models in the form of transition densities in order to specify prediction distributions over new poses at each time instant (e.g., [11, 14]); similarly, data-driven computer animation requires prior distributions over poses and motion (e.g., [1, 4, 6]). An individual human pose is typically parameterized with more than 60 parameters. Despite the large state space, the space of activity-specific human poses and motions has a much smaller intrinsic dimensionality; in our experiments with walking and golf swings, 3 dimensions often suffice.

Our work builds on the extensive literature in nonlinear time-series analysis, of which we

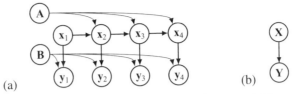

(a)   (b)

Figure 1: Time-series graphical models. (a) Nonlinear latent-variable model for time series. (Hyperparameters $\bar{\alpha}$ and $\bar{\beta}$ are not shown.) (b) GPDM model. Because the mapping parameters $\mathbf{A}$ and $\mathbf{B}$ have been marginalized over, all latent coordinates $\mathbf{X} = [\mathbf{x}_1, ..., \mathbf{x}_N]^T$ are jointly correlated, as are all poses $\mathbf{Y} = [\mathbf{y}_1, ..., \mathbf{y}_N]^T$.

mention a few examples. Two main themes are the use of switching linear models (e.g., [11]), and nonlinear transition functions, such as represented by Radial Basis Functions [2]. Both approaches require sufficient amounts of training data that one can learn the parameters of the switching or basis functions. Determining the appropriate number of basis functions is also difficult. In Kernel Dynamical Modeling [12], linear dynamics are kernelized to model nonlinear systems, but a density function over data is not produced.

Supervised learning with GP regression has been used to model dynamics for a variety of applications [3, 7, 13]. These methods model dynamics directly in observation space, which is impractical for the high-dimensionality of motion capture data. Our approach is most directly inspired by the unsupervised Gaussian Process Latent Variable Model (GPLVM) [5], which models the joint distribution of the observed data and their corresponding representation in a low dimensional latent space. This distribution can then be used as a prior for inference from new measurements. However, the GPLVM is not a dynamical model; it assumes that data are generated independently. Accordingly it does not respect temporal continuity of the data, nor does it model the dynamics in the latent space. Here we augment the GPLVM with a latent dynamical model. The result is a Bayesian generalization of subspace dynamical models to nonlinear latent mappings and dynamics.

2 Gaussian Process Dynamics

The Gaussian Process Dynamical Model (GPDM) comprises a mapping from a latent space to the data space, and a dynamical model in the latent space (Figure 1). These mappings are typically nonlinear. The GPDM is obtained by marginalizing out the parameters of the two mappings, and optimizing the latent coordinates of training data.

More precisely, our goal is to model the probability density of a sequence of vector-valued states $\mathbf{y}_1 ..., \mathbf{y}_t, ..., \mathbf{y}_N$, with discrete-time index t and $\mathbf{y}_t \in \mathbb{R}^D$. As a basic model, consider a latent-variable mapping with first-order Markov dynamics:

$$\mathbf{x}_t = f(\mathbf{x}_{t-1}; \mathbf{A}) + \mathbf{n}_{x,t} \tag{1}$$
$$\mathbf{y}_t = g(\mathbf{x}_t; \mathbf{B}) + \mathbf{n}_{y,t} \tag{2}$$

Here, $\mathbf{x}_t \in \mathbb{R}^d$ denotes the d-dimensional latent coordinates at time t, $\mathbf{n}_{x,t}$ and $\mathbf{n}_{y,t}$ are zero-mean, white Gaussian noise processes, f and g are (nonlinear) mappings parameterized by $\mathbf{A}$ and $\mathbf{B}$, respectively. Figure 1(a) depicts the graphical model.

While linear mappings have been used extensively in auto-regressive models, here we consider the nonlinear case for which f and g are linear combinations of basis functions:

$$f(\mathbf{x}; \mathbf{A}) = \sum_i \mathbf{a}_i \, \phi_i(\mathbf{x}) \tag{3}$$

$$g(\mathbf{x}; \mathbf{B}) = \sum_j \mathbf{b}_j \, \psi_j(\mathbf{x}) \tag{4}$$

for weights $\mathbf{A} = [\mathbf{a}_1, \mathbf{a}_2, ...]$ and $\mathbf{B} = [\mathbf{b}_1, \mathbf{b}_2, ...]$, and basis functions ϕ_i and ψ_j. In order to fit the parameters of this model to training data, one must select an appropriate number of basis functions, and one must ensure that there is enough data to constrain the shape of each basis function. Ensuring both of these conditions can be very difficult in practice.

However, from a Bayesian perspective, the specific forms of f and g — including the numbers of basis functions — are incidental, and should therefore be marginalized out. With an isotropic Gaussian prior on the columns of $\mathbf{B}$, marginalizing over g can be done in closed form [8, 10] to yield

$$p(\mathbf{Y} \mid \mathbf{X}, \bar{\beta}) = \frac{|\mathbf{W}|^N}{\sqrt{(2\pi)^{ND}|\mathbf{K}_Y|^D}} \exp\left(-\frac{1}{2}\mathrm{tr}\left(\mathbf{K}_Y^{-1}\mathbf{Y}\mathbf{W}^2\mathbf{Y}^T\right)\right),\qquad(5)$$

where $\mathbf{Y} = [\mathbf{y}_1, ..., \mathbf{y}_N]^T$, $\mathbf{K}_Y$ is a kernel matrix, and $\bar{\beta} = \{\beta_1, \beta_2, ..., \mathbf{W}\}$ comprises the kernel hyperparameters. The elements of kernel matrix are defined by a kernel function, $(\mathbf{K}_Y)_{i,j} = k_Y(\mathbf{x}_i, \mathbf{x}_j)$. For the latent mapping, $\mathbf{X} \to \mathbf{Y}$, we currently use the RBF kernel

$$k_Y(\mathbf{x}, \mathbf{x}') = \beta_1 \exp\left(-\frac{\beta_2}{2}||\mathbf{x} - \mathbf{x}'||^2\right) + \beta_3^{-1}\delta_{\mathbf{x},\mathbf{x}'}.\qquad(6)$$

As in the SGPLVM [4], we use a scaling matrix $\mathbf{W} \equiv \mathrm{diag}(w_1, ..., w_D)$ to account for different variances in the different data dimensions. This is equivalent to a GP with kernel function $k(\mathbf{x}, \mathbf{x}')/w_m^2$ for dimension m. Hyperparameter β_1 represents the overall scale of the output function, while β_2 corresponds to the inverse width of the RBFs. The variance of the noise term $\mathbf{n}_{y,t}$ is given by β_3^{-1}.

The dynamic mapping on the latent coordinates $\mathbf{X}$ is conceptually similar, but more subtle.[1] As above, we form the joint probability density over the latent coordinates and the dynamics weights $\mathbf{A}$ in (3). We then marginalize over the weights $\mathbf{A}$, i.e.,

$$p(\mathbf{X} \mid \bar{\alpha}) = \int p(\mathbf{X}, \mathbf{A} \mid \bar{\alpha})\,d\mathbf{A} = \int p(\mathbf{X} \mid \mathbf{A}, \bar{\alpha})\,p(\mathbf{A} \mid \bar{\alpha})\,d\mathbf{A}.\qquad(7)$$

Incorporating the Markov property (Eqn. (1)) gives:

$$p(\mathbf{X} \mid \bar{\alpha}) = p(\mathbf{x}_1)\int \prod_{t=2}^N p(\mathbf{x}_t \mid \mathbf{x}_{t-1}, \mathbf{A}, \bar{\alpha})\,p(\mathbf{A} \mid \bar{\alpha})\,d\mathbf{A},\qquad(8)$$

where $\bar{\alpha}$ is a vector of kernel hyperparameters. Assuming an isotropic Gaussian prior on the columns of $\mathbf{A}$, it can be shown that this expression simplifies to:

$$p(\mathbf{X} \mid \bar{\alpha}) = p(\mathbf{x}_1)\frac{1}{\sqrt{(2\pi)^{(N-1)d}|\mathbf{K}_X|^d}} \exp\left(-\frac{1}{2}\mathrm{tr}\left(\mathbf{K}_X^{-1}\mathbf{X}_{out}\mathbf{X}_{out}^T\right)\right),\qquad(9)$$

where $\mathbf{X}_{out} = [\mathbf{x}_2, ..., \mathbf{x}_N]^T$, $\mathbf{K}_X$ is the $(N-1) \times (N-1)$ kernel matrix constructed from $\{\mathbf{x}_1, ..., \mathbf{x}_{N-1}\}$, and $\mathbf{x}_1$ is assumed to be have an isotropic Gaussian prior.

We model dynamics using both the RBF kernel of the form of Eqn. (6), as well as the following "linear + RBF" kernel:

$$k_X(\mathbf{x}, \mathbf{x}') = \alpha_1 \exp\left(-\frac{\alpha_2}{2}||\mathbf{x} - \mathbf{x}'||^2\right) + \alpha_3\mathbf{x}^T\mathbf{x}' + \alpha_4^{-1}\delta_{\mathbf{x},\mathbf{x}'}.\qquad(10)$$

The kernel corresponds to representing g as the sum of a linear term and RBF terms. The inclusion of the linear term is motivated by the fact that linear dynamical models, such as

---

[1]Conceptually, we would like to model each pair $(\mathbf{x}_t, \mathbf{x}_{t+1})$ as a training pair for regression with g. However, we cannot simply substitute them directly into the GP model of Eqn. (5) as this leads to the nonsensical expression $p(\mathbf{x}_2, ..., \mathbf{x}_N \mid \mathbf{x}_1, ..., \mathbf{x}_{N-1})$.

first or second-order autoregressive models, are useful for many systems. Hyperparameters α_1, α_2 represent the output scale and the inverse width of the RBF terms, and α_3 represents the output scale of the linear term. Together, they control the relative weighting between the terms, while α_4^{-1} represents the variance of the noise term $\mathbf{n}_{x,t}$.

It should be noted that, due to the nonlinear dynamical mapping in (3), the joint distribution of the latent coordinates is *not* Gaussian. Moreover, while the density over the initial state may be Gaussian, it will not remain Gaussian once propagated through the dynamics. One can also see this in (9) since $\mathbf{x}_t$ variables occur inside the kernel matrix, as well as outside of it. So the log likelihood is not quadratic in $\mathbf{x}_t$.

Finally, we also place priors on the hyperparameters ($p(\bar{\alpha}) \propto \prod_i \alpha_i^{-1}$, and $p(\bar{\beta}) \propto \prod_i \beta_i^{-1}$) to discourage overfitting. Together, the priors, the latent mapping, and the dynamics define a generative model for time-series observations (Figure 1(b)):

$$p(\mathbf{X}, \mathbf{Y}, \bar{\alpha}, \bar{\beta}) = p(\mathbf{Y} | \mathbf{X}, \bar{\beta}) \, p(\mathbf{X} | \bar{\alpha}) \, p(\bar{\alpha}) \, p(\bar{\beta}) . \tag{11}$$

Multiple sequences. This model extends naturally to multiple sequences $\mathbf{Y}_1, ..., \mathbf{Y}_M$. Each sequence has associated latent coordinates $\mathbf{X}_1, ..., \mathbf{X}_M$ within a shared latent space. For the latent mapping g we can conceptually concatenate all sequences within the GP likelihood (Eqn. (5)). A similar concatenation applies for the dynamics, but omitting the first frame of each sequence from $\mathbf{X}_{out}$, and omitting the final frame of each sequence from the kernel matrix $\mathbf{K}_X$. The same structure applies whether we are learning from multiple sequences, or learning from one sequence and inferring another. That is, if we learn from a sequence $\mathbf{Y}_1$, and then infer the latent coordinates for a new sequence $\mathbf{Y}_2$, then the joint likelihood entails full kernel matrices $\mathbf{K}_X$ and $\mathbf{K}_Y$ formed from both sequences.

Higher-order features. The GPDM can be extended to model higher-order Markov chains, and to model velocity and acceleration in inputs and outputs. For example, a second-order dynamical model,

$$\mathbf{x}_t = f(\mathbf{x}_{t-1}, \mathbf{x}_{t-2}; \mathbf{A}) + \mathbf{n}_{x,t} \tag{12}$$

may be used to explicitly model the dependence of the prediction on two past frames (or on velocity). In the GPDM framework, the equivalent model entails defining the kernel function as a function of the current and previous time-step:

$$\begin{aligned} k_X([\mathbf{x}_t, \mathbf{x}_{t-1}], [\mathbf{x}_\tau, \mathbf{x}_{\tau-1}]) &= \alpha_1 \exp\left(-\frac{\alpha_2}{2}||\mathbf{x}_t - \mathbf{x}_\tau||^2 - \frac{\alpha_3}{2}||\mathbf{x}_{t-1} - \mathbf{x}_{\tau-1}||^2\right) \\ &+ \alpha_4 \mathbf{x}_t^T \mathbf{x}_\tau + \alpha_5 \mathbf{x}_{t-1}^T \mathbf{x}_{\tau-1} + \alpha_6^{-1}\delta_{t,\tau} \end{aligned} \tag{13}$$

Similarly, the dynamics can be formulated to predict velocity:

$$\mathbf{v}_{t-1} = f(\mathbf{x}_{t-1}; \mathbf{A}) + \mathbf{n}_{x,t} \tag{14}$$

Velocity prediction may be more appropriate for modeling smoothly motion trajectories. Using Euler integration with time-step Δt, we have $\mathbf{x}_t = \mathbf{x}_{t-1} + \mathbf{v}_{t-1}\Delta t$. The dynamics likelihood $p(\mathbf{X} | \bar{\alpha})$ can then be written by redefining $\mathbf{X}_{out} = [\mathbf{x}_2 - \mathbf{x}_1, ..., \mathbf{x}_N - \mathbf{x}_{N-1}]^T/\Delta t$ in Eqn. (9). In this paper, we use a fixed time-step of $\Delta t = 1$. This is analogous to using $\mathbf{x}_{t-1}$ as a "mean function." Higher-order features can also be fused together with position information to reduce the Gaussian process prediction variance [15, 9].

3 Properties of the GPDM and Algorithms

Learning the GPDM from measurements $\mathbf{Y}$ entails minimizing the negative log-posterior:

$$\mathcal{L} = -\ln p(\mathbf{X}, \bar{\alpha}, \bar{\beta} \,|\, \mathbf{Y}) \tag{15}$$

$$= \frac{d}{2} \ln |\mathbf{K}_X| + \frac{1}{2} \text{tr} \left(\mathbf{K}_X^{-1} \mathbf{X}_{out} \mathbf{X}_{out}^T \right) + \sum_j \ln \alpha_j \qquad (16)$$

$$- N \ln |\mathbf{W}| + \frac{D}{2} \ln |\mathbf{K}_Y| + \frac{1}{2} \text{tr} \left(\mathbf{K}_Y^{-1} \mathbf{Y} \mathbf{W}^2 \mathbf{Y}^T \right) + \sum_j \ln \beta_j$$

up to an additive constant. We minimize $\mathcal{L}$ with respect to $\mathbf{X}, \bar{\alpha}$, and $\bar{\beta}$ numerically.

Figure 2 shows a GPDM 3D latent space learned from a human motion capture data comprising three walk cycles. Each pose was defined by 56 Euler angles for joints, 3 global (torso) pose angles, and 3 global (torso) translational velocities. For learning, the data was mean-subtracted, and the latent coordinates were initialized with PCA. Finally, a GPDM is learned by minimizing $\mathcal{L}$ in (16). We used 3D latent spaces for all experiments shown here. Using 2D latent spaces leads to intersecting latent trajectories. This causes large "jumps" to appear in the model, leading to unreliable dynamics.

For comparison, Fig. 2(a) shows a 3D SGPLVM learned from walking data. Note that the latent trajectories are not smooth; there are numerous cases where consecutive poses in the walking sequence are relatively far apart in the latent space. By contrast, Fig. 2(b) shows that the GPDM produces a much smoother configuration of latent positions. Here the GPDM arranges the latent positions roughly in the shape of a saddle.

Figure 2(c) shows a volume visualization of the inverse reconstruction variance, i.e., $-2 \ln \sigma_{\mathbf{y}|\mathbf{x}, \mathbf{X}, \mathbf{Y}, \bar{\beta}}$. This shows the confidence with which the model reconstructs a pose from latent positions $\mathbf{x}$. In effect, the GPDM models a high probability "tube" around the data. To illustrate the dynamical process, Fig. 2(d) shows 25 fair samples from the latent dynamics of the GPDM. All samples are conditioned on the same initial state, $\mathbf{x}_0$, and each has a length of 60 time steps. As noted above, because we marginalize over the weights of the dynamic mapping, $\mathbf{A}$, the distribution over a pose sequence cannot be factored into a sequence of low-order Markov transitions (Fig. 1(a)). Hence, we draw fair samples $\tilde{\mathbf{X}}_{1:60}^{(j)} \sim p(\tilde{\mathbf{X}}_{1:60} \,|\, \mathbf{x}_0, \mathbf{X}, \mathbf{Y}, \bar{\alpha})$, using hybrid Monte Carlo [8]. The resulting trajectories (Fig. 2(c)) are smooth and similar to the training motions.

3.1 Mean Prediction Sequences

For both 3D people tracking and computer animation, it is desirable to generate new motions efficiently. Here we consider a simple online method for generating a new motion, called *mean-prediction*, which avoids the relatively expensive Monte Carlo sampling used above. In mean-prediction, we consider the next timestep $\tilde{\mathbf{x}}_t$ conditioned on $\tilde{\mathbf{x}}_{t-1}$ from the Gaussian prediction [8]:

$$\tilde{\mathbf{x}}_t \sim \mathcal{N}(\mu_X(\tilde{\mathbf{x}}_{t-1}); \sigma_X^2(\tilde{\mathbf{x}}_{t-1})\mathbf{I}) \qquad (17)$$

$$\mu_X(\mathbf{x}) = \mathbf{X}_{out}^T \mathbf{K}_X^{-1} \mathbf{k}_X(\mathbf{x}), \qquad \sigma_X^2(\mathbf{x}) = k_X(\mathbf{x}, \mathbf{x}) - \mathbf{k}_X(\mathbf{x})^T \mathbf{K}_X^{-1} \mathbf{k}_X(\mathbf{x}) \qquad (18)$$

where $\mathbf{k}_X(\mathbf{x})$ is a vector containing $k_X(\mathbf{x}, \mathbf{x}_i)$ in the i-th entry and $\mathbf{x}_i$ is the ith training vector. In particular, we set the latent position at each time-step to be the most-likely (mean) point given the previous step: $\tilde{\mathbf{x}}_t = \mu_X(\tilde{\mathbf{x}}_{t-1})$. In this way we ignore the process noise that one might normally add. We find that this mean-prediction often generates motions that are more like the fair samples shown in Fig. 2(d), than if random process noise had been added at each time step (as in (1)). Similarly, new poses are given by $\tilde{\mathbf{y}}_t = \mu_Y(\tilde{\mathbf{x}}_t)$.

Depending on the dataset and the choice of kernels, long sequences generated by sampling or mean-prediction can diverge from the data. On our data sets, mean-prediction trajectories from the GPDM with an RBF or linear+RBF kernel for dynamics usually produce sequences that roughly follow the training data (e.g., see the red curves in Figure 3). This usually means producing closed limit cycles with walking data. We also found that mean-prediction motions are often very close to the mean obtained from the HMC sampler; by

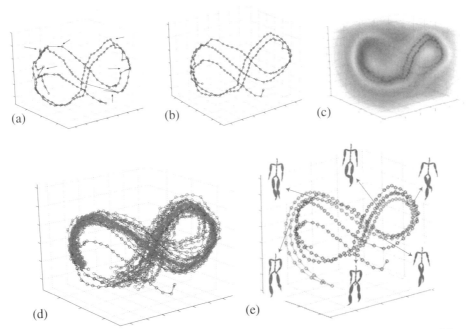

Figure 2: Models learned from a walking sequence of 2.5 gait cycles. The latent positions learned with a GPLVM (a) and a GPDM (b) are shown in blue. Vectors depict the temporal sequence. (c) - log variance for reconstruction shows regions of latent space that are reconstructed with high confidence. (d) Random trajectories drawn from the model using HMC (green), and their mean (red). (e) A GPDM of walk data learned with RBF+linear kernel dynamics. The simulation (red) was started far from the training data, and then optimized (green). The poses were reconstructed from points on the optimized trajectory.

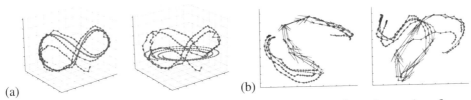

Figure 3: (a) Two GPDMs and mean predictions. The first is that from the previous figure. The second was learned with a linear kernel. (b) The GPDM model was learned from 3 swings of a golf club, using a 2nd order RBF kernel for dynamics. The two plots show 2D orthogonal projections of the 3D latent space.

initializing HMC with mean-prediction, we find that the sampler reaches equilibrium in a small number of interations. Compared to the RBF kernels, mean-prediction motions generated from GPDMs with the linear kernel often deviate from the original data (e.g., see Figure 3a), and lead to over-smoothed animation.

Figure 3(b) shows a 3D GPDM learned from three swings of a golf club. The learning aligns the sequences and nicely accounts for variations in speed during the club trajectory.

3.2 Optimization

While mean-prediction is efficient, there is nothing in the algorithm that prevents trajectories from drifting away from the training data. Thus, it is sometimes desirable to optimize a particular motion under the GPDM, which often reduces drift of the mean-prediction mo-

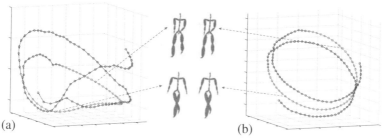

Figure 4: GPDM from walk sequence with missing data learned with (a) a RBF+linear kernel for dynamics, and (b) a linear kernel for dynamics. Blue curves depict original data. Green curves are the reconstructed, missing data.

tions. To optimize a new sequence, we first select a starting point $\tilde{\mathbf{x}}_1$ and a number of time-steps. The likelihood $p(\tilde{\mathbf{X}} \mid \mathbf{X}, \bar{\alpha})$ of the new sequence $\tilde{\mathbf{X}}$ is then optimized directly (holding the latent positions of the previously learned latent positions, $\mathbf{X}$, and hyperparameters, $\bar{\alpha}$, fixed). To see why optimization generates motion close to the traing data, note that the variance of pose $\tilde{\mathbf{x}}_{t+1}$ is determined by $\sigma_X^2(\tilde{\mathbf{x}}_t)$, which will be lower when $\tilde{\mathbf{x}}_t$ is nearer the training data. Consequently, the likelihood of $\tilde{\mathbf{x}}_{t+1}$ can be increased by moving $\tilde{\mathbf{x}}_t$ closer to the training data. This generalizes the preference of the SGPLVM for poses similar to the examples [4], and is a natural consequence of the Bayesian approach. As an example, Fig. 2(e) shows an optimized walk sequence initialized from the mean-prediction.

3.3 Forecasting

We performed a simple experiment to compare the predictive power of the GPDM to a linear dynamical system, implemented as a GPDM with linear kernel in the latent space and RBF latent mapping. We trained each model on the first 130 frames of the 60Hz walking sequence (corresponding to 2 cycles), and tested on the remaining 23 frames. From each test frame mean-prediction was used to predict the pose 8 frames ahead, and then the RMS pose error was computed against ground truth. The test was repeated using mean-prediction and optimization for three kernels, all based on first-order predictions as in (1):

	Linear	RBF	Linear+RBF
mean-prediction	59.69	48.72	36.74
optimization	58.32	45.89	31.97

Due to the nonlinear nature of the walking dynamics in latent space, the RBF and Linear+RBF kernels outperform the linear kernel. Moreover, optimization (initialized by mean-prediction) improves the result in all cases, for reasons explained above.

3.4 Missing Data

The GPDM model can also handle incomplete data (a common problem with human motion capture sequences). The GPDM is learned by minimizing $\mathcal{L}$ (Eqn. (16)), but with the terms corresponding to missing poses $\mathbf{y}_t$ removed. The latent coordinates for missing data are initialized by cubic spline interpolation from the 3D PCA initialization of observations.

While this produces good results for short missing segments (e.g., 10–15 frames of the 157-frame walk sequence used in Fig. 2), it fails on long missing segments. The problem lies with the difficulty in initializing the missing latent positions sufficiently close to the training data. To solve the problem, we first learn a model with a subsampled data sequence. Reducing sampling density effectively increases uncertainty in the reconstruction process so that the probability density over the latent space falls off more smoothly from the data. We then restart the learning with the entire data set, but with the kernel hyperparameters fixed. In doing so, the dynamics terms in the objective function exert more influence over the latent coordinates of the training data, and a smooth model is learned.

With 50 missing frames of the 157-frame walk sequence, this optimization produces models (Fig. 4) that are much smoother than those in Fig. 2. The linear kernel is able to pull the latent coordinates onto a cylinder (Fig. 4b), and thereby provides an accurate dynamical model. Both models shown in Fig. 4 produce estimates of the missing poses that are visually indistinguishable from the ground truth.

4 Discussion and Extensions

One of the main strengths of the GPDM model is the ability to generalize well from small datasets. Conversely, performance is a major issue in applying GP methods to larger datasets. Previous approaches prune uninformative vectors from the training data [5]. This is not straightforward when learning a GPDM, however, because each timestep is highly correlated with the steps before and after it. For example, if we hold x_t fixed during optimization, then it is unlikely that the optimizer will make much adjustment to x_{t+1} or x_{t-1}. The use of higher-order features provides a possible solution to this problem. Specifically, consider a dynamical model of the form $v_t = f(x_{t-1}, v_{t-1})$. Since adjacent time-steps are related only by the velocity $v_t \approx (x_t - x_{t-1})/\Delta t$, we can handle irregularly-sampled datapoints by adjusting the timestep Δt, possibly using a different Δt at each step.

A number of further extensions to the GPDM model are possible. It would be straightforward to include a control signal u_t in the dynamics $f(x_t, u_t)$. It would also be interesting to explore uncertainty in latent variable estimation (e.g., see [3]). Our use of maximum likelihood latent coordinates is motivated by Lawrence's observation that model uncertainty and latent coordinate uncertainty are interchangeable when learning PCA [5]. However, in some applications, uncertainty about latent coordinates may be highly structured (e.g., due to depth ambiguities in motion tracking).

Acknowledgements This work made use of Neil Lawrence's publicly-available GPLVM code, the CMU mocap database (mocap.cs.cmu.edu), and Joe Conti's volume visualization code from mathworks.com. This research was supported by NSERC and CIAR.

References

[1] M. Brand and A. Hertzmann. Style machines. *Proc. SIGGRAPH*, pp. 183-192, July 2000.

[2] Z. Ghahramani and S. T. Roweis. Learning nonlinear dynamical systems using an EM algorithm. *Proc. NIPS 11*, pp. 431-437, 1999.

[3] A. Girard, C. E. Rasmussen, J. G. Candela, and R. Murray-Smith. Gaussian process priors with uncertain inputs - application to multiple-step ahead time series forecasting. *Proc. NIPS 15*, pp. 529-536, 2003.

[4] K. Grochow, S. L. Martin, A. Hertzmann, and Z. Popović. Style-based inverse kinematics. *ACM Trans. Graphics*, 23(3):522-531, Aug. 2004.

[5] N. D. Lawrence. Gaussian process latent variable models for visualisation of high dimensional data. *Proc. NIPS 16*, 2004.

[6] J. Lee, J. Chai, P. S. A. Reitsma, J. K. Hodgins, and N. S. Pollard. Interactive control of avatars animated with human motion data. *ACM Trans. Graphics*, 21(3):491-500, July 2002.

[7] W. E. Leithead, E. Solak, and D. J. Leith. Direct identification of nonlinear structure using Gaussian process prior models. *Proc. European Control Conference*, 2003.

[8] D. MacKay. *Information Theory, Inference, and Learning Algorithms*. 2003.

[9] R. Murray-Smith and B. A. Pearlmutter. Transformations of Gaussian process priors. Technical Report, Department of Computer Science, Glasgow University, 2003

[10] R. M. Neal. *Bayesian Learning for Neural Networks*. Springer-Verlag, 1996.

[11] V. Pavlović, J. M. Rehg, and J. MacCormick. Learning switching linear models of human motion. *Proc. NIPS 13*, pp. 981-987, 2001.

[12] L. Ralaivola and F. d'Alché-Buc. Dynamical modeling with kernels for nonlinear time series prediction. *Proc. NIPS 16*, 2004.

[13] C. E. Rasmussen and M. Kuss. Gaussian processes in reinforcement learning. *Proc. NIPS 16*, 2004.

[14] H. Sidenbladh, M. J. Black, and D. J. Fleet. Stochastic tracking of 3D human figures using 2D motion. *Proc. ECCV*, volume 2, pp. 702-718, 2000.

[15] E. Solak, R. Murray-Smith, W. Leithead, D. Leith, and C. E. Rasmussen. Derivative observations in Gaussian process models of dynamic systems. *Proc. NIPS 15*, pp. 1033-1040, 2003.

Group and Topic Discovery
from Relations and Their Attributes

Xuerui Wang, Natasha Mohanty, Andrew McCallum
Department of Computer Science
University of Massachusetts
Amherst, MA 01003
{xuerui,nmohanty,mccallum}@cs.umass.edu

Abstract

We present a probabilistic generative model of entity relationships and their attributes that simultaneously discovers groups among the entities and topics among the corresponding textual attributes. Block-models of relationship data have been studied in social network analysis for some time. Here we simultaneously cluster in several modalities at once, incorporating the attributes (here, words) associated with certain relationships. Significantly, joint inference allows the discovery of topics to be guided by the emerging groups, and vice-versa. We present experimental results on two large data sets: sixteen years of bills put before the U.S. Senate, comprising their corresponding text and voting records, and thirteen years of similar data from the United Nations. We show that in comparison with traditional, separate latent-variable models for words, or Block-structures for votes, the Group-Topic model's joint inference discovers more cohesive groups and improved topics.

1   Introduction

The field of social network analysis (SNA) has developed mathematical models that discover patterns in interactions among entities. One of the objectives of SNA is to detect salient groups of entities. Group discovery has many applications, such as understanding the social structure of organizations or native tribes, uncovering criminal organizations, and modeling large-scale social networks in Internet services such as Friendster.com or LinkedIn.com. Social scientists have conducted extensive research on group detection, especially in fields such as anthropology and political science. Recently, statisticians and computer scientists have begun to develop models that specifically discover group memberships [5, 2, 7]. One such model is the stochastic Blockstructures model [7], which discovers the latent groups or classes based on pair-wise relation data. A particular relation holds between a pair of entities (people, countries, organizations, etc.) with some probability that depends only on the class (group) assignments of the entities. This model is extended in [4] to support an arbitrary number of groups by using a Chinese Restaurant Process prior.

The aforementioned models discover latent groups by examining only whether one or more relations exist between a pair of entities. The Group-Topic (GT) model presented in this paper, on the other hand, considers both the relations between entities and also the attributes of the relations (e.g., the text associated with the relations) when assigning group memberships. The GT model can be viewed as an extension of the stochastic Blockstructures model [7] with the key addition that group membership is conditioned on a latent variable, which in turn is also associated with the attributes of the relation. In our experiments, the attributes of relations are words, and the latent variable represents the topic responsible for generating those words. Our model captures the *(language) attributes* associated with interactions, and uses distinctions based on these attributes to better assign group memberships.

Consider a legislative body and imagine its members forming coalitions (groups), and voting accordingly. However, different coalitions arise depending on the topic of the resolution up for a vote. In the GT model, the discovery of groups is guided by the emerging topics, and the forming of topics is shaped by emerging groups.Resolutions that would have been assigned the same topic in a model using words alone may be assigned to different topics if they exhibit distinct voting patterns. Topics may be merged if the entities vote very similarly on them. Likewise, multiple different divisions of entities into groups are made possible by conditioning them on the topics.

The importance of modeling the *language* associated with interactions between people has recently been demonstrated in the Author-Recipient-Topic (ART) model [6]. It can measure role similarity by comparing the topic distributions for two entities. However, the ART model does not explicitly discover groups formed by entities. When forming latent groups, the GT model simultaneously discovers salient topics relevant to relationships between entities—topics which the models that only examine words are unable to detect.

We demonstrate the capabilities of the GT model by applying it to two large sets of voting data: one from US Senate and the other from the General Assembly of the UN. The model clusters voting entities into coalitions and simultaneously discovers topics for word attributes describing the relations (bills or resolutions) between entities. We find that the groups obtained from the GT model are significantly more cohesive (p-value < 0.01) than those obtained from the Blockstructures model. The GT model also discovers new and more salient topics that help better predict entities' behaviors.

2   Group-Topic Model

The Group-Topic model is a directed graphical model that clusters entities with relations between them, as well as attributes of those relations. The relations may be either symmetric or asymmetric and have multiple attributes. In this paper, we focus on symmetric relations and have words as the attributes on relations. The graphical model representation of the model and our notation are shown in Figure 1.

Without considering the topics of events, or by treating all events in a corpus as reflecting a single topic, the simplified model becomes equivalent to the stochastic Blockstructures model [7]. Here, each event defines a relationship, *e.g.*, whether in the event two entities' group(s) behave the same way or not. On the other hand, in our model a relation may also have multiple attributes. When we consider the complete model, the dataset is dynamically divided into T sub-blocks each of which corresponds to a topic. The generative process of the GT model is as right.

$$
\begin{aligned}
t_b &\sim \text{Uniform}(1/T) \\
w_{it}|\phi_t &\sim \text{Multinomial}(\phi_t) \\
\phi_t|\eta &\sim \text{Dirichlet}(\eta) \\
g_{it}|\theta_t &\sim \text{Multinomial}(\theta_t) \\
\theta_t|\alpha &\sim \text{Dirichlet}(\alpha) \\
v_{ij}^{(b)}|\gamma_{g_i g_j}^{(b)} &\sim \text{Binomial}(\gamma_{g_i g_j}^{(b)}) \\
\gamma_{gh}^{(b)}|\beta &\sim \text{Beta}(\beta).
\end{aligned}
$$

We want to perform joint inference on (text) attributes and relations to obtain topic-wise group memberships. We employ Gibbs sampling to conduct inference. Note that we adopt conjugate priors in our setting, and thus we can easily integrate out θ, ϕ and γ to decrease

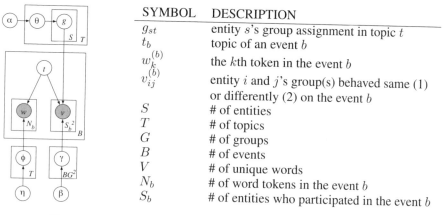

SYMBOL	DESCRIPTION
g_{st}	entity s's group assignment in topic t
t_b	topic of an event b
$w_k^{(b)}$	the kth token in the event b
$v_{ij}^{(b)}$	entity i and j's group(s) behaved same (1) or differently (2) on the event b
S	# of entities
T	# of topics
G	# of groups
B	# of events
V	# of unique words
N_b	# of word tokens in the event b
S_b	# of entities who participated in the event b

Figure 1: The Group-Topic model and notations used in this paper

the uncertainty associated with them.. In our case we need to compute the conditional distribution $P(g_{st}|\mathbf{w}, \mathbf{v}, \mathbf{g}_{-st}, \mathbf{t}, \alpha, \beta, \eta)$ and $P(t_b|\mathbf{w}, \mathbf{v}, \mathbf{g}, \mathbf{t}_{-b}, \alpha, \beta, \eta)$, where $\mathbf{g}_{-st}$ denotes the group assignments for all entities except entity s in topic t, and $\mathbf{t}_{-b}$ represents the topic assignments for all events except event b. Beginning with the joint probability of a dataset, and using the chain rule, we can obtain the conditional probabilities conveniently. In our setting, the relationship we are investigating is always symmetric, so we do not distinguish R_{ij} and R_{ji} in our derivations (only $R_{ij}(i \leq j)$ remain). Thus

$$P(g_{st}|\mathbf{v}, \mathbf{g}_{-st}, \mathbf{w}, \mathbf{t}, \alpha, \beta, \eta)$$

$$\propto \frac{\alpha_{g_{st}} + n_{tg_{st}} - 1}{\sum_{g=1}^{G}(\alpha_g + n_{tg}) - 1} \prod_{b=1}^{B} \left(I(t_b = t) \prod_{h=1}^{G} \frac{\prod_{k=1}^{2} \prod_{x=1}^{d_{g_{st}hk}^{(b)}} (\beta_k + m_{g_{st}hk}^{(b)} - x)}{\prod_{x=1}^{\sum_{k=1}^{2} d_{g_{st}hk}^{(b)}} ((\sum_{k=1}^{2}(\beta_k + m_{g_{st}hk}^{(b)}) - x)} \right),$$

where n_{tg} represents how many entities are assigned into group g in topic t, c_{tv} represents how many tokens of word v are assigned to topic t, $m_{ghk}^{(b)}$ represents how many times group g and h vote same ($k = 1$) and differently ($k = 2$) on event b, $I(t_b = t)$ is an indicator function, and $d_{g_{st}hk}^{(b)}$ is the increase in $m_{g_{st}hk}^{(b)}$ if entity s were assigned to group g_{st} than without considering s at all (if $I(t_b = t) = 0$, we ignore the increase in event b).

$$P(t_b|\mathbf{v}, \mathbf{g}, \mathbf{w}, \mathbf{t}_{-b}, \alpha, \beta, \eta)$$

$$\propto \frac{\prod_{v=1}^{V} \prod_{x=1}^{e_v^{(b)}} (\eta_v + c_{t_b v} - x)}{\prod_{x=1}^{\sum_{v=1}^{V} e_v^{(b)}} (\sum_{v=1}^{V}(\eta_v + c_{t_b v}) - x)} \prod_{g=1}^{G} \prod_{h=g}^{G} \frac{\prod_{k=1}^{2} \Gamma(\beta_k + m_{ghk}^{(b)})}{\Gamma(\sum_{k=1}^{2}(\beta_k + m_{ghk}^{(b)}))},$$

where $e_v^{(b)}$ is the number of tokens of word v in event b.

The GT model uses information from two different modalities whose likelihoods are generally not directly comparable, since the number of occurrences of each type may vary greatly. Thus we raise the first term in the above formula to a power, as is common in speech recognition when the acoustic and language models are combined.

3 Related Work

There has been a surge of interest in models that describe relational data, or relations between entities viewed as links in a network, including recent work in group discovery [2, 5]. The GT model is an enhancement of the stochastic Blockstructures model [7] and

Datasets	Avg. AI for GT	Avg. AI for Baseline	p-value
Senate	0.8294	0.8198	$< .01$
UN	0.8664	0.8548	$< .01$

Table 1: Average AI for GT and Baseline for both Senate and UN datasets. The group cohesion in GT is significantly better than in baseline.

the extended model of Kemp et al. [4] as it takes advantage of information from different modalities by conditioning group membership on topics. In this sense, the GT model draws inspiration from the Role-Author-Recipient-Topic (RART) model [6]. As an extension of ART model, RART clusters together entities with similar roles. In contrast, the GT model presented here clusters entities into groups based on their relations to other entities.

There has been a considerable amount of previous work in understanding voting patterns. Exploring the notion that the behavior of an entity can be explained by its (hidden) group membership, Jakulin and Buntine [3] develop a discrete PCA model for discovering groups, where each entity can belong to each of the k groups with a certain probability, and each group has its own specific pattern of behaviors. They apply this model to voting data in the 108th US Senate where the behavior of an entity is its vote on a resolution. We apply our GT model also to voting data. However, unlike [3], since our goal is to cluster entities based on the similarity of their voting patterns, we are only interested in whether a pair of entities voted the same or differently, not their actual yes/no votes. This "content-ignorant" feature is similarly found in work on web log clustering [1].

4 Experimental Results

We present experiments applying the GT model to the voting records of members of two legislative bodies: the US Senate and the UN General Assembly. For comparison, we present the results of a baseline method that first uses a mixture of unigrams to discover topics and associate a topic with each resolution, and then runs the Blockstructures model [7] separately on the resolutions assigned to each topic. This baseline approach is similar to the GT model in that it discovers both groups and topics, and has different group assignments on different topics. However, whereas the baseline model performs inference serially, GT performs joint inference simultaneously.

We are interested in the quality of both the groups and the topics. In the political science literature, group cohesion is quantified by the *Agreement Index (AI)* [3], which, based on the number of group members that vote Yes, No or Abstain, measures the similarity of votes cast by members of a group during a particular roll call. Higher AI means better cohesion. The group cohesion using the GT model is found to be significantly greater than the baseline group cohesion under pairwise t-test, as shown in Table 1 for both datasets, which indicates that the GT model is better able to capture cohesive groups.

4.1 The US Senate Dataset

Our Senate dataset consists of the voting records of Senators in the 101st-109th US Senate (1989-2005) obtained from the Library of Congress THOMAS database. During a roll call for a particular bill, a Senator may respond *Yea* or *Nay* to the question that has been put to vote, else the vote will be recorded as *Not Voting*. We do not consider *Not Voting* as a unique vote since most of the time it is a result of a Senator being absent from the session of the US Senate. The text associated with each resolution is composed of its index terms provided in the database. There are 3423 resolutions in our experiments (we excluded roll calls that were not associated with resolutions). Since there are far fewer words than

Economic	Education	Military Misc.	Energy
federal	education	government	energy
labor	school	military	power
insurance	aid	foreign	water
aid	children	tax	nuclear
tax	drug	congress	gas
business	students	aid	petrol
employee	elementary	law	research
care	prevention	policy	pollution

Table 2: Top words for topics generated with the mixture of unigrams model on the Senate dataset. The headers are our own summary of the topics.

Economic	Education + Domestic	Foreign	Social Security + Medicare
labor	education	foreign	social
insurance	school	trade	security
tax	federal	chemicals	insurance
congress	aid	tariff	medical
income	government	congress	care
minimum	tax	drugs	medicare
wage	energy	communicable	disability
business	research	diseases	assistance

Table 3: Top words for topics generated with the GT model on the Senate dataset. The topics are influenced by both the words and votes on the bills.

pairs of votes, we raise the text likelihood to the 5th power (mentioned in Section 2) in the experiments with this dataset so as to balance its influence during inference.

We cluster the data into 4 topics and 4 groups (cluster sizes are chosen somewhat arbitrarily) and compare the results of GT with the baseline. The most likely words for each topic from the traditional mixture of unigrams model is shown in Table 2, whereas the topics obtained using GT are shown in Table 3. The GT model collapses the topics **Education** and **Energy** together into **Education and Domestic**, since the voting patterns on those topics are quite similar. The new topic **Social Security + Medicare** did not have strong enough word coherence to appear in the baseline model, but it has a very distinct voting pattern, and thus is clearly found by the GT model. Thus, importantly, GT discovers topics that help predict people's behavior and relations, not simply word co-occurrences.

Examining the group distribution across topics in the GT model, we find that on the topic **Economic** the Republicans form a single group whereas the Democrats split into 3 groups indicating that Democrats have been somewhat divided on this topic. On the other hand, in **Education + Domestic** and **Social Security + Medicare**, Democrats are more unified whereas the Republicans split into 3 groups. The group membership of Senators on **Education + Domestic** issues is shown in Table 4. We see that the first group of Republicans include a Democratic Senator from Texas, a state that usually votes Republican. Group 2 (majority Democrats) includes Sen. Chafee who has been involved in initiatives to improve education, as well as Sen. Jeffords who left the Republican Party to become an Independent and has championed legislation to strengthen education and environmental protection.

Nearly all the Republican Senators in Group 4 (in Table 4) are advocates for education and many of them have been awarded for their efforts. For instance, Sen. Voinovich and Sen. Symms are strong supporters of early education and vocational education, respectively; and

Group 1	Group 3	Group 4	
73 Republicans Krueger (D-TX)	Cohen (R-ME)	Armstrong (R-CO)	Brown (R-CO)
Group 2	Danforth (R-MO)	Garn (R-UT)	DeWine (R-OH)
90 Democrats	Durenberger (R-MN)	Humphrey (R-NH)	Thompson (R-TN)
Chafee (R-RI)	Hatfield (R-OR)	McCain (R-AZ)	Fitzgerald (R-IL)
Jeffords (I-VT)	Heinz (R-PA)	McClure (R-ID)	Voinovich (R-OH)
	Kassebaum (R-KS)	Roth (R-DE)	Miller (D-GA)
	Packwood (R-OR)	Symms (R-ID)	Coleman (R-MN)
	Specter (R-PA)	Wallop(R-WY)	
	Snowe (R-ME)		
	Collins (R-ME)		

Table 4: Senators in the four groups corresponding to **Education + Domestic** in Table 3.

Everything Nuclear	Human Rights	Security in Middle East
nuclear	rights	occupied
weapons	human	israel
use	palestine	syria
implementation	situation	security
countries	israel	calls

Table 5: Top words for topics generated from mixture of unigrams model with the UN dataset. Only text information is utilized to form the topics, as opposed to Table 6 where our GT model takes advantage of both text and voting information.

Sen. Roth has voted for tax deductions for education. It is also interesting to see that Sen. Miller (D-GA) appears in a Republican group; although he is in favor of educational reforms, he is a conservative Democrat and frequently criticizes his own party—even backing Republican George W. Bush over Democrat John Kerry in the 2004 Presidential Election.

Many of the Senators in Group 3 have also focused on education and other domestic issues such as energy, however, they often have a more liberal stance than those in Group 4, and come from states that are historically less conservative. For example, Sen. Danforth has presented bills for a more fair distribution of energy resources. Sen. Kassebaum is known to be uncomfortable with many Republican views on domestic issues such as education, and has voted against voluntary prayer in school. Thus, both Groups 3 and 4 differ from the Republican core (Group 2) on domestic issues, and also differ from each other.

We also inspect the Senators that switch groups the most across topics in the GT model. The top 5 Senators are Shelby (D-AL), Heflin (D-AL), Voinovich (R-OH), Johnston (D-LA), and Armstrong (R-CO). Sen. Shelby (D-AL) votes with the Republicans on **Economic**, with the Democrats on **Education + Domestic** and with a small group of maverick Republicans on **Foreign** and **Social Security + Medicare**. Sen. Shelby, together with Sen. Heflin, is a Democrat from a fairly conservative state (Alabama) and are found to side with the Republicans on many issues.

4.2 The United Nations Dataset

The second dataset involves the voting record of the UN General Assembly[1]. We focus on the resolutions discussed from 1990-2003, which contain votes of 192 countries on 931 resolutions. If a country is present during the roll call, it may choose to vote *Yes*, *No* or

---

[1]http://home.gwu.edu/~voeten/UNVoting.htm

GROUP ↓	Nuclear Nonproliferation	Nuclear Arms Race	Human Rights
	nuclear states united weapons nations	nuclear arms prevention race space	rights human palestine occupied israel
1	Brazil Columbia Chile Peru Venezuela...	UK France Spain Monaco East-Timor	Brazil Mexico Columbia Chile Peru...
2	USA Japan Germany UK... Russia...	India Russia Micronesia	Nicaragua Papua Rwanda Swaziland Fiji...
3	China India Mexico Iran Pakistan...	Japan Germany Italy... Poland Hungary...	USA Japan Germany UK... Russia...
4	Kazakhstan Belarus Yugoslavia Azerbaijan Cyprus...	China Brazil Mexico Indonesia Iran...	China India Indonesia Thailand Philippines...
5	Thailand Philippines Malaysia Nigeria Tunisia...	USA Israel Palau	Belarus Turkmenistan Azerbaijan Uruguay Kyrgyzstan...

Table 6: Top words for topics generated from the GT model with the UN dataset as well as the corresponding groups for each topic (column). The countries listed for each group are ordered by their 2005 GDP (PPP).

Abstain. Unlike the Senate dataset, a country's vote can have one of three possible values instead of two. Because we parameterize *agreement* and not the votes themselves, this 3-value setting does not require any change to our model. In experiments with this dataset, we use a weighting factor 500 for text (adjusting the likelihood of text by a power of 500 so as to make it comparable with the likelihood of pairs of votes for each resolution). We cluster this dataset into 3 topics and 5 groups (chosen somewhat arbitrarily).

The most probable words in each topic from the mixture of unigrams model is shown in Table 5. For example, **Everything Nuclear** constitutes all resolutions that have anything to do with the use of nuclear technology, including nuclear weapons. Comparing these with topics generated from the GT model shown in Table 6, we see that the GT model splits the discussion about nuclear technology into two separate topics, **Nuclear Nonproliferation** (generally about countries obtaining nuclear weapons and management of nuclear waste), and **Nuclear Arms Race** (focused on the historic arms race between Russia and the US, and preventing a nuclear arms race in outer space). These two issues had drastically different voting patterns in the UN, as can be seen in the contrasting group structure for those topics in Table 6. Thus, again, the GT model is able to discover more salient topics—topics that reflect the voting patterns and coalitions, not simply word co-occurrence alone. The countries in Table 6 are ranked by their GDP in 2005.[2]

As seen in Table 6, groups formed in **Nuclear Arms Race** are unlike the groups formed in other topics. These groups map well to the global political situation of that time when, despite the end of the Cold War, there was mutual distrust between Russia and the US with regard to the continued manufacture of nuclear weapons. For missions to outer space and nuclear arms, India was a staunch ally of Russia, while Israel was an ally of the US.

5 Conclusions

We introduce the Group-Topic model that jointly discovers latent groups in a network as well as clusters of attributes (or topics) of events that influence the interaction between entities. The model extends prior work on latent group discovery by capturing not only pair-wise relations between entities but also multiple attributes of the relations (in particular, words describing the relations). In this way the GT model obtains more cohesive groups as well as salient topics that influence the interaction between groups. This paper demonstrates that the Group-Topic model is able to discover topics capturing the group based interactions between members of a legislative body. The model can be applied not just to voting data, but any data having relations with attributes. We are now using the model to analyze the citations in academic papers capturing the topics of research papers and discovering research groups. The model can be altered suitably to consider other categorical, multi-dimensional, and continuous attributes characterizing relations.

Acknowledgments

This work was supported in part by the CIIR, the Central Intelligence Agency, the National Security Agency, the National Science Foundation under NSF grant #IIS-0326249, and by the Defense Advanced Research Projects Agency, through the Department of the Interior, NBC, Acquisition Services Division, under contract #NBCHD030010. We would also like to thank Prof. Vincent Moscardelli, Chris Pal and Aron Culotta for helpful discussions.

References

[1] Doug Beeferman and Adam Berger. Agglomerative clustering of a search engine query log. In *The 6th ACM SIGKDD Int. Conf. on Knowledge Discovery and Data Mining*, 2000.

[2] Indrajit Bhattacharya and Lise Getoor. Deduplication and group detection using links. In *The 10th SIGKDD Conference Workshop on Link Analysis and Group Detection (LinkKDD)*, 2004.

[3] Aleks Jakulin and Wray Buntine. Analyzing the US Senate in 2003: Similarities, networks, clusters and blocs, 2004. http://kt.ijs.si/aleks/Politics/us_senate.pdf.

[4] Charles Kemp, Thomas L. Griffiths, and Joshua Tenenbaum. Discovering latent classes in relational data. Technical report, AI Memo 2004-019, MIT CSAIL, 2004.

[5] Jeremy Kubica, Andrew Moore, Jeff Schneider, and Yiming Yang. Stochastic link and group detection. In *The 17th National Conference on Artificial Intelligence (AAAI)*, 2002.

[6] Andrew McCallum, Andres Corrada-Emanuel, and Xuerui Wang. Topic and role discovery in social networks. In *The 19th International Joint Conference on Artificial Intelligence*, 2005.

[7] Krzysztof Nowicki and Tom A.B. Snijders. Estimation and prediction for stochastic blockstructures. *Journal of the American Statistical Association*, 96(455):1077–1087, 2001.

---

[2]http://en.wikipedia.org/wiki/List_of_countries_by_GDP_%28PPP%29. In Table 6, we omit some countries (represented by ...) in order to show other interesting but relatively low-ranked countries (for example, Russia) in the GDP list.

A Bayes Rule for Density Matrices

Manfred K. Warmuth[*]
Computer Science Department
University of California at Santa Cruz
manfred@cse.ucsc.edu

Abstract

The classical Bayes rule computes the posterior model probability from the prior probability and the data likelihood. We generalize this rule to the case when the prior is a density matrix (symmetric positive definite and trace one) and the data likelihood a covariance matrix. The classical Bayes rule is retained as the special case when the matrices are diagonal.

In the classical setting, the calculation of the probability of the data is an *expected likelihood*, where the expectation is over the prior distribution. In the generalized setting, this is replaced by an *expected variance* calculation where the variance is computed along the eigenvectors of the prior density matrix and the expectation is over the eigenvalues of the density matrix (which form a probability vector). The variances along any direction is determined by the covariance matrix. Curiously enough this expected variance calculation is a quantum measurement where the co-variance matrix specifies the instrument and the prior density matrix the mixture state of the particle. We motivate both the classical and the generalized Bayes rule with a minimum relative entropy principle, where the Kullbach-Leibler version gives the classical Bayes rule and Umegaki's quantum relative entropy the new Bayes rule for density matrices.

1 Introduction

In [TRW05] various on-line updates were generalized from vector parameters to matrix parameters. Following [KW97], the updates were derived by minimizing the loss plus a divergence to the last parameter. In this paper we use the same method for deriving a Bayes rule for density matrices (symmetric positive definite matrices of trace one). When the parameters are probability vectors over the set of models, then the "classical" Bayes rule can be derived using the relative entropy as the divergence (e.g.[KW99, SWRL03]). Analogously we now use the quantum relative entropy, introduced by Umegaki, to derive the generalized Bayes rule.

---
[*]Supported by NSF grant CCR 9821087. Some of this work was done while visiting National ICT Australia in Canberra

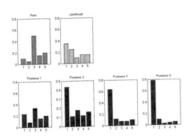

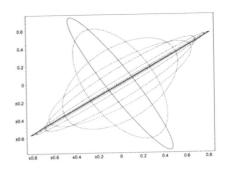

Figure 1: We update the prior four times based on the same data likelihood vector $P(y|M_i)$. The initial posteriors are close to the prior but eventually the posteriors focus their weight on $\operatorname{argmax}_i P(y|M_i)$. The classical Bayes rule may be seen as a soft maximum calculation.

Figure 2: We depict seven iterations of the generalized Bayes rule with the bold NW-SE ellipse as the prior density and the bold-dashed SE-NW ellipse as data covariance matrix. The posterior density matrices (dashed) gradually move from the prior to the longest axis of the covariance matrix.

The new rule uses matrix logarithms and exponentials to avoid the fact that symmetric positive definite matrices are not closed under the matrix product. The rule is strikingly similar to the classical Bayes rule and retains the latter as a special case when the matrices are diagonal. Various cancellations occur when the classical Bayes rule is applied iteratively and similar cancellations happen with the new rule. We shall see that the classical Bayes rule may be seen a soft maximum calculation and the new rule as a soft calculation of the eigenvector with the largest eigenvalue (See figures 1 and 2).

The mathematics applied in this paper is most commonly used in quantum physics. For example, the data likelihood becomes a quantum measurement. It is tempting to call the new rule the "quantum Bayes rule". However, we have no physical interpretation of the this rule. The measurement does not collapse our state and we don't use the unitary evolution of a state to model the rule. Also, the term "quantum Bayes rule" has been claimed before in [SBC01] where the classical Bayes rule is used to update probabilities that happen to arise in the context of quantum physics. In contrast, in this paper our parameters are density matrices.

Our work is most closely related to a paper by Cerf and Adam [CA99] who also give a formula for conditional densities that relies on the matrix exponential and logarithm. However they are interested in the multivariate case (which requires the use of tensors) and their motivation is to obtain a generalization of a conditional quantum entropy. We hope to build on the great body of work done with the classical Bayes rule in the statistics community and therefore believe that this line of research holds great promise.

2   The Classical Bayes Rule

To establish a common notation we begin by introducing the familiar Bayes rule. Assume we have n models $M_1, \ldots, M_n$. In the classical setup, model M_i is chosen with prior probability $P(M_i)$ and then M_i generates a datum y with probability $P(y|M_i)$. After observing y, the *posterior* probabilities of model M_i are calculated via *Bayes Rule*:

$$P(M_i|y) \;=\; \frac{P(M_i)P(y|M_i)}{\sum_j P(M_j)P(y|M_j)}. \tag{1}$$

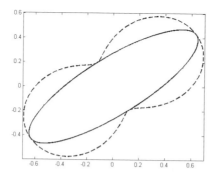

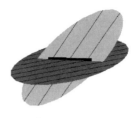

Figure 3: An ellipse $\boldsymbol{S}$ in $\mathbb{R}^2$: The eigenvectors are the directions of the axes and the eigenvalues their lengths. Ellipses are weighted combinations of the one-dimensional degenerate ellipses (dyads) corresponding to the axes. (For unit $\boldsymbol{u}$, the dyad $\boldsymbol{u}\boldsymbol{u}^\top$ is a degenerate one-dimensional ellipse with its single axis in direction $\boldsymbol{u}$.) The solid curve of the ellipse is a plot of $\boldsymbol{S}\boldsymbol{u}$ and the outer dashed figure eight is direction $\boldsymbol{u}$ times the variance $\boldsymbol{u}^\top\boldsymbol{S}\boldsymbol{u}$. At the eigenvectors, this variance equals the eigenvalues and touches the ellipse.

Figure 4: When the ellipse $\boldsymbol{S}$ and $\boldsymbol{T}$ don't have the same span, then $\boldsymbol{S} \odot \boldsymbol{T}$ lies in the intersection of both spans and is a degenerate ellipse of dimension one (bold line). This generalizes the following intersection property of the matrix product when $\boldsymbol{S}$ and $\boldsymbol{T}$ are both diagonal (here of dimension four):

$diag(\boldsymbol{S})$	$diag(\boldsymbol{T})$	$diag(\boldsymbol{ST})$
0	0	0
a	0	0
0	b	0
a	b	ab

See Figure 1 for a bar plot of the effect of the update on the posterior. By the Theorem of Total Probability, the expected likelihood in the denominator equals $P(y)$. In a moment we will replace this expected likelihood by an expected variance.

3   Density Matrices as Priors

We now let our prior $\boldsymbol{D}$ be an arbitrary symmetric positive[1] definite matrix of trace one. Such matrices are called *density matrices* in quantum physics. An outer product $\boldsymbol{u}\boldsymbol{u}^T$, where $\boldsymbol{u}$ has unit length is called a *dyad*. Any *mixture* $\sum_i \alpha_i \boldsymbol{a}_i \boldsymbol{a}_i^\top$ of dyads $\boldsymbol{a}_i \boldsymbol{a}_i^\top$ is a density matrix as long as the coefficients α_i are non-negative and sum to one. This is true even if the number of dyads is larger or smaller than the dimension of $\boldsymbol{D}$. The trace of such a mixture is one because dyads have trace one and $\sum_i \alpha_i = 1$. Of course any density matrix $\boldsymbol{D}$ can be decomposed based on an eigensystem. That is, $\boldsymbol{D} = \boldsymbol{D}\boldsymbol{\delta}\boldsymbol{D}^\top$ where $\boldsymbol{D}\boldsymbol{D}^\top = \boldsymbol{I}$. Now the vector of eigenvalues (δ_i) forms a probability vector equal to the dimension of the density.

In quantum physics, the dyads are called *pure states* and density matrices are mixtures over such states. Note that in this paper we want to address the statistics community and use linear algebra notation instead of Dirac notation. The probability vector $(P(M_i))$ can be represented as a diagonal matrix $diag((P(M_i))) = \sum_i P(M_i) \boldsymbol{e}_i \boldsymbol{e}_i^\top$, where $\boldsymbol{e}_i$ denotes the ith standard basis vector. This means that

---

[1]We use the convention that positive definite matrices have non-negative eigenvalues and *strictly* positive definite matrices have positive eigenvalues.

probability vectors are special density matrices where the eigenvectors are fixed to the standard basis vectors.

4 Co-variance Matrices and Basic Notation

In this paper we replace the (conditional) data likelihoods $P(y|M_i)$ by a data co-variance matrix $\mathcal{D}(y|.)$ (symmetric positive definite matrix). We now discuss such matrices in more detail.

A covariance matrix $\mathcal{S}$ can be depicted as an ellipse $\{\mathcal{S}u : ||u||_2 \leq 1\}$ centered at the origin, where the eigenvectors form the principal axes and the eigenvalues are the lengths of the axes (See Figure 3). Assume $\mathcal{S}$ is the covariance matrix of some random cost vector $c \in \mathbb{R}^n$, i.e. $\mathcal{S} = \mathbb{E}\left((c - \mathbb{E}(c)(c - \mathbb{E}(c))^\top\right)$. Note that a covariance matrix $\mathcal{S}$ is diagonal if the components of the cost vector are independent. The variance of the cost vector c along a unit vector u has the form

$$\mathbb{V}(c^\top u) = \mathbb{E}\left(\left(c^\top u - \mathbb{E}(c^\top u)\right)^2\right) = \mathbb{E}\left(\left((c^\top - \mathbb{E}(c^\top))u\right)^2\right) = u^\top \mathcal{S} u$$

and the variance along an eigenvector is the corresponding eigenvalue (See Figure 3). Using this interpretation, the matrix $\mathcal{S}$ may be seen as a mapping $\mathcal{S}(.)$ from the unit ball to $\mathbb{R}_{\geq 0}$, i.e. $\mathcal{S}(u) = u^\top \mathcal{S} u$.

A second interpretation of the scalar $u^\top \mathcal{S} u$ is the square length of u w.r.t. the basis $\sqrt{\mathcal{S}}$, that is $u^\top \mathcal{S} u = u^\top \sqrt{\mathcal{S}}\sqrt{\mathcal{S}}u = ||\sqrt{\mathcal{S}}u||_2^2$. Thirdly, $u^T \mathcal{S} u$ is a *quantum measurement* of the pure state u with an instrument represented by $\mathcal{S}$. Since the square length of u w.r.t. any orthogonal basis S is one, any such basis turns the unit vector into an n-dimensional probability vector $((u^\top s_i)^2)$. Now $u^\top \mathcal{S} u$ is the expected eigenvalue w.r.t. this probability vector: $u^\top \mathcal{S} u = \sum_i \sigma_i (u^\top s_i)^2$.

The trace $\text{tr}(A)$ of a square matrix A is the sum of its diagonal elements A_{ii}. Recall that $\text{tr}(AB) = \text{tr}(BA)$ for any matrices $A \in \mathbb{R}^{n \times m}$, $B \in \mathbb{R}^{m \times n}$. The trace is *unitarily invariant*, i.e. for any orthogonal matrix U, $\text{tr}(UAU^\top) = \text{tr}(U^\top UA) = \text{tr}(A)$. Also, $\text{tr}(uu^\top A) = \text{tr}(u^\top Au) = u^\top Au$. Therefore the trace of a square matrix may be seen as the total variance along any set of orthogonal directions:

$$\text{tr}(A) = \text{tr}(IA) = \text{tr}(\sum_i u_i u_i^\top A) = \sum_i u_i^\top A u_i.$$

In particular, the trace of a square matrix is the sum of its eigenvalues.

The matrix exponential $\exp(\mathcal{S})$ of the symmetric matrix $\mathcal{S} = S\sigma S^\top$ is defined as $S\exp(\sigma)S^\top$, where $\exp(\sigma)$ is obtained by exponentiating the diagonal entries (eigenvalues). The matrix logarithm $\log(\mathcal{S})$ is defined similarly but now $\mathcal{S}$ must be strictly positive definite. Clearly, the two functions are inverses of each other. It is important to remember that $\exp(\mathcal{S} + \mathcal{T}) = \exp(\mathcal{S})\exp(\mathcal{T})$ only holds iff the two symmetric matrices commute[2], i.e. $\mathcal{S}\mathcal{T} = \mathcal{T}\mathcal{S}$. However, the following trace inequality, known as the Golden-Thompson inequality [Bha97], always holds:

$$\text{tr}(\exp\mathcal{S}\exp\mathcal{T}) \geq \text{tr}(\exp(\mathcal{S} + \mathcal{T})). \tag{2}$$

5 The Generalized Bayes Rule

The following experiment underlies the more general setup: If the prior is $\mathcal{D}(.) = \sum_i \delta_i d_i d_i^\top$, then the dyad (or pure state) $d_i d_i^\top$ is chosen with probability δ_i and a random variable $c^\top d_i$ is observed where c has covariance matrix $\mathcal{D}(y|.)$.

---

[2]This occurs iff the two symmetric matrices have the same eigensystem.

In our generalization we replace the expected data likelihood $P(y) = \sum_i P(M_i)P(y|M_i)$ by the following trace:

$$\mathrm{tr}(\boldsymbol{D}(.)\boldsymbol{D}(y|.)) = \mathrm{tr}(\sum_i \delta_i\, \boldsymbol{d}_i\boldsymbol{d}_i^\top \boldsymbol{D}(y|.)) = \sum_i \delta_i\, \boldsymbol{d}_i^\top \boldsymbol{D}(y|.)\boldsymbol{d}_i.$$

Recall that $\boldsymbol{d}_i^\top \boldsymbol{D}(y|.)\boldsymbol{d}_i$ is the variance of $\boldsymbol{c}$ in direction $\boldsymbol{d}_i$: i.e. $\mathbb{V}(\boldsymbol{c}^\top \boldsymbol{d}_i)$. Therefore the above trace is the expected variance along the eigenvectors of the density matrix weighted by the eigenvalues. Curiously enough, this trace computation is a *quantum measurement*, where $\boldsymbol{D}(y|.)$ represents the instrument and $\boldsymbol{D}(.)$ the mixture state of the particle.

In the generalized Bayes rule we cannot simply multiply the prior density matrix with the covariance matrix that corresponds to the data likelihood. This is because a product of two symmetric positive definite matrices may be neither symmetric nor positive definite. Instead we define the operation $\odot$ on the cone of symmetric positive definite matrices. We begin by defining this operation for the case when the matrices $\boldsymbol{S}$ and $\boldsymbol{T}$ are strictly positive definite (and symmetric):

$$\boldsymbol{S} \odot \boldsymbol{T} := \exp(\log \boldsymbol{S} + \log \boldsymbol{T}). \tag{3}$$

The matrix log of both matrices produces symmetric matrices that sum to a symmetric matrix. Finally the matrix exponential of the sum produces again a symmetric positive matrix. Note that the matrix log is not defined when the matrix has a zero eigenvalue. However for arbitrary symmetric positive definite matrices one can define the operation $\odot$ as the following limit:

$$\boldsymbol{S} \odot \boldsymbol{T} := \lim_{n\to\infty} (\boldsymbol{S}^{1/n}\boldsymbol{T}^{1/n})^n.$$

This limit is the *Lie Product Formula* [Bha97] when $\boldsymbol{S}$ and $\boldsymbol{T}$ are both strictly positive, but it exists even if the matrices don't have full rank and by Theorem 1.2 of [Sim79],

$$range(\boldsymbol{S} \odot \boldsymbol{T}) = range(\boldsymbol{S}) \cap range(\boldsymbol{T}).$$

Assume that k is the dimension of $range(\boldsymbol{S}) \cap range(\boldsymbol{T})$, that $\boldsymbol{B}$ is an orthonormal basis of $range(\boldsymbol{S}) \cap range(\boldsymbol{T})$ (i.e. $\boldsymbol{B} \in \mathbb{R}^{n\times k}$, $\boldsymbol{B}^T\boldsymbol{B} = \boldsymbol{I}_k$, and $range(\boldsymbol{B}) = range(\boldsymbol{S}) \cap range(\boldsymbol{T})$) and that $\log^+$ denotes the modified matrix logarithm that takes logs of the non-zero eigenvalues but leaves zero eigenvalues unchanged. Then by the same theorem[3],

$$\boldsymbol{S} \odot \boldsymbol{T} = \boldsymbol{B} \exp(\boldsymbol{B}^T(\log^+ \boldsymbol{S} + \log^+ \boldsymbol{T})\boldsymbol{B}) \boldsymbol{B}^T. \tag{4}$$

When both matrices have the same eigensystem, then $\odot$ becomes the matrix product. One can show that $\odot$ is associative, commutative, has the identity matrix $\boldsymbol{I}$ as its neutral element and for any strictly positive definite and symmetric matrix $\boldsymbol{S}$, $\boldsymbol{S} \odot \boldsymbol{S}^{-1} = \boldsymbol{I}$. Finally, $(c\boldsymbol{S}) \odot \boldsymbol{T} = c(\boldsymbol{S} \odot \boldsymbol{T})$, for any non-negative scalar.

Using this new product operation, the generalized Bayes rule becomes:

$$\boldsymbol{D}(.|y) = \frac{\boldsymbol{D}(.) \odot \boldsymbol{D}(y|.)}{\mathrm{tr}(\boldsymbol{D}(.) \odot \boldsymbol{D}(y|.))}. \tag{5}$$

Normalizing by the trace assures that the trace of the posterior density matrix is one. As we see in Figure 2, this posterior moves toward the largest axis of the data covariance matrix and the new rule can be interpreted as a soft calculation of the

---

[3]The $\log^+ \boldsymbol{S}$ term in the formula can be replaced by $\tilde{\boldsymbol{B}} \log(\tilde{\boldsymbol{B}}^T\boldsymbol{S}\tilde{\boldsymbol{B}})\tilde{\boldsymbol{B}}^T$, where $\tilde{\boldsymbol{B}}$ is an orthonormal basis of $range(\boldsymbol{S})$, and similarly for $\log^+ \boldsymbol{T}$.

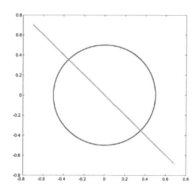

Figure 5: Assume the prior density matrix is the circle $\boldsymbol{D}(.) = \begin{pmatrix} \frac{1}{2} & 0 \\ 0 & \frac{1}{2} \end{pmatrix}$ and the data covariance matrix the degenerate NE-SW ellipse $\boldsymbol{D}(y|.) = \frac{1}{2} \begin{pmatrix} 1 & -1 \\ -1 & 1 \end{pmatrix} = \boldsymbol{U} \begin{pmatrix} 0 & 0 \\ 0 & 1 \end{pmatrix} \boldsymbol{U}^\top$,

where $\boldsymbol{U} = \begin{pmatrix} \frac{1}{\sqrt{2}} & \frac{1}{\sqrt{2}} \\ \frac{1}{\sqrt{2}} & -\frac{1}{\sqrt{2}} \end{pmatrix}$. Now for all diagonal matrices $\boldsymbol{S}(.)$, $\mathrm{tr}(\boldsymbol{S}(.) \ \boldsymbol{D}(y|.)) = \frac{1}{2}$, i.e.

largest eigenvalue is not "visible" in basis $\boldsymbol{I}$. But $\mathrm{tr}\left(\underbrace{\boldsymbol{U} \begin{pmatrix} 0 & 0 \\ 0 & 1 \end{pmatrix} \boldsymbol{U}^\top}_{\boldsymbol{D}(.|y) \text{ of new rule}} \ \boldsymbol{D}(y|.) \right) = 1.$

eigenvector with maximum eigenvalue. When the matrices $\boldsymbol{D}(.)$ and $\boldsymbol{D}(y|.)$ have the same eigensystem, then $\odot$ becomes the matrix multiplication. In particular, when the prior is $diag((P(M_i)))$ and the covariance matrix $diag((P(y|M_i))$, then the new rule realizes the classical rule and computes $diag((P(M_i|y))$. Figure 5 gives an example that shows how the off-diagonal elements can be exploited by the new rule.

In the classical Bayes rule, the normalization factor is the expected data likelihood. In the case of the generalized Bayes rule, the expected variance only upper bounds the normalization factor via the Golden-Thompsen inequality (2):

$$\mathrm{tr}(\boldsymbol{D}(.)\boldsymbol{D}(y|.)) \geq \mathrm{tr}(\boldsymbol{D}(.) \odot \boldsymbol{D}(y|.)). \tag{6}$$

The classical Bayes rule can be applied iteratively to a sequence of data and various cancellations occur. For the sake of simplicity we only consider two data points y_1, y_2:

$$P(M_i|y_2 y_1) = \frac{P(M_i|y_1)P(y_2|M_i, y_1)}{P(y_2|y_1)} = \frac{P(M_i)P(y_1|M_i)P(y_2|M_i, y_1)}{P(y_2 y_1)}.$$

$$P(y_2|y_1)P(y_1) = (\sum_i \underbrace{P(M_i|y_1)}_{use(1)} P(y_2|M_i, y_1))(\sum_i P(M_i)P(y_1|M_i))$$

$$= \sum_i P(M_i)P(y_1|M_i)P(y_2|M_i, y_1) = P(y_2 y_1). \tag{7}$$

Analogously,

$$\boldsymbol{D}(.|y_2 y_1) = \frac{\boldsymbol{D}(.|y_1) \odot \boldsymbol{D}(y_2|., y_1)}{\mathrm{tr}(\boldsymbol{D}(.|y_1) \odot \boldsymbol{D}(y_2|., y_1))} = \frac{\boldsymbol{D}(.) \odot \boldsymbol{D}(y_1|.) \odot \boldsymbol{D}(y_2|., y_1)}{\mathrm{tr}(\boldsymbol{D}(.) \odot \boldsymbol{D}(y_1|.) \odot \boldsymbol{D}(y_2|., y_1))}.$$

Finally, the product of the expected variance for both trials combine in a similar way, except that in the generalized case the equality becomes an inequality:

$$\operatorname{tr}(\boldsymbol{\mathcal{D}}(.|y_1)\boldsymbol{\mathcal{D}}(y_2|.,y_1))\,\operatorname{tr}(\boldsymbol{\mathcal{D}}(.)\boldsymbol{\mathcal{D}}(y_1|.))$$

$$\geq \quad \operatorname{tr}(\underbrace{\boldsymbol{\mathcal{D}}(.|y_1)}_{use(5)} \odot \boldsymbol{\mathcal{D}}(y_2|.,y_1))\,\operatorname{tr}(\boldsymbol{\mathcal{D}}(.) \odot \boldsymbol{\mathcal{D}}(y_1|.))$$

$$= \quad -\log \operatorname{tr}(\boldsymbol{\mathcal{D}}(.) \odot \boldsymbol{\mathcal{D}}(y_1|.) \odot \boldsymbol{\mathcal{D}}(y_2|.,y_1)).$$

The above inequality is an instantiation of the Golden-Thompsen inequality (2) and the above equality generalizes the middle equality in (7).

6 The Derivation of the Generalized Bayes Rule

The classical Bayes rule can be derived[4] by minimizing a relative entropy to the prior plus a convex combination of the log losses of the models (See e.g. [KW99, SWRL03]):

$$\inf_{\gamma_i \geq 0,\, \sum_i \gamma_i = 1} \sum_i \gamma_i \ln \frac{\gamma_i}{P(M_i)} \;-\; \sum_i \gamma_i \log P(y|M_i).$$

Without the relative entropy, the argument of the infimum is linear in the weights γ_i and is minimized when all weight is placed on the maximum likelihood models, i.e. the set of indices $\operatorname{argmax}_i P(y|M_i)$. The negative entropy ameliorates the maximum calculation and pulls the optimal solution towards the prior. Observe that the non-negativity constraints can be dropped since the entropy acts as a barrier. By introducing a Lagrange multiplier for the remaining constraint and differentiating, we obtain the solution $\gamma_i^* = \frac{P(M_i)P(y|M_i)}{\sum_j P(M_j)P(y|M_j)}$, which is the classical Bayes rule (1). By plugging γ_i^* into the argument of the infimum we obtain the optimum value $-\ln P(y)$. Notice that this is minus the logarithm of the normalization of the Bayes rule (1) and is also the log loss associated the standard Bayesian setup.

To derive the new generalized Bayes rule in an analogous way, we use the quantum physics generalizations of the relative entropy between two densities $\boldsymbol{\mathcal{G}}$ and $\boldsymbol{\mathcal{D}}$ (due to Umegaki): $\operatorname{tr}(\boldsymbol{\mathcal{G}}(\log \boldsymbol{\mathcal{G}} - \log \boldsymbol{\mathcal{D}}))$. We also need to replace the mixture of negative log likelihoods by the trace $-\operatorname{tr}(\boldsymbol{\mathcal{G}} \log \boldsymbol{\mathcal{D}}(y|.))$. Now the matrix parameter $\boldsymbol{\mathcal{G}}$ is constrained to be a density matrix and the minimization problem becomes[5] :

$$\inf_{\boldsymbol{\mathcal{G}}\ \text{dens.matr.}} \operatorname{tr}(\boldsymbol{\mathcal{G}}(\log \boldsymbol{\mathcal{G}} - \log \boldsymbol{\mathcal{D}}(.))) \quad - \quad \operatorname{tr}(\boldsymbol{\mathcal{G}} \log \boldsymbol{\mathcal{D}}(y|.))$$

Except for the quantum relative entropy term, the argument of the infimum is again linear in the variable $\boldsymbol{\mathcal{G}}$ and is minimized when $\boldsymbol{\mathcal{G}}$ is a single dyad $\boldsymbol{uu}^\top$, where $\boldsymbol{u}$ is the eigenvector belonging to maximum eigenvalue of the matrix $\log \boldsymbol{\mathcal{D}}(y|.)$. The linear term pulls $\boldsymbol{\mathcal{G}}$ toward a direction of high variance of this matrix, whereas the quantum relative entropy pulls $\boldsymbol{\mathcal{G}}$ toward the prior density matrix. The density matrix constraint requires the eigenvalues of $\boldsymbol{\mathcal{G}}$ to be non-negative and the trace to $\boldsymbol{\mathcal{G}}$ to be one. The entropy works as a barrier for the non-negativity constraints and thus these constraints can be dropped. Again by introducing a Lagrange multiplier for the remaining trace constraint and differentiating (following [TRW05]), we arrive at a formula for the optimum $\boldsymbol{\mathcal{G}}^*$ which coincides with the formula for the $\boldsymbol{\mathcal{D}}(.|y)$ given in the generalized Bayes rule (5), where $\odot$ is defined[6] as in (3). Since the quantum relative entropy is strictly convex [NC00] in $\boldsymbol{\mathcal{G}}$, the optimum $\boldsymbol{\mathcal{G}}^*$ is unique.

---

[4]For the sake of simplicity assume that for all i, $P(M_i)$ and $P(y|M_i)$ are non-negative.
[5]Assume here that $\boldsymbol{\mathcal{D}}(.)$ and $\boldsymbol{\mathcal{D}}(y|.)$ are both strictly positive definite.
[6]With some work, one can also derive the Bayes rule with the fancier $\odot$ operation (4).

7 Conclusion

Our generalized Bayes rule suggests a definition of conditional density matrices and we are currently developing a calculus for such matrices. In particular, a common formalism is needed that includes the multivariate conditional density matrices defined in [CA99] based on tensors.

In this paper we only considered real symmetric matrices. However, our methods immediately generalize to complex Hermitian matrices, i.e square matrices in $\mathbb{C}^{n \times n}$ for which $\boldsymbol{S} = \overline{\boldsymbol{S}}^T = \boldsymbol{S}^*$. Now both the prior density matrix and the data covariance matrix must be Hermitian instead of symmetric.

The generalized Bayes rule for symmetric positive definite matrices relies on computing eigendecompositions ($\Omega(n^3)$ time). Hopefully, there exist $O(n^2)$ versions of the update that approximate the generalized Bayes rule sufficiently well.

Extensive research has been done in the so-called "expert framework" (see e.g.[KW99] for a list of references) where a mixture over experts is maintained by the on-line algorithm for the purpose of performing as well as the best expert chosen in hindsight. In preliminary research we showed that one can maintain a density matrix over the base experts instead and derive updates similar to the generalized Bayes rule given in this paper. Most importantly, the bounds generalize to the case when mixtures over experts are replaced by density matrices.

Acknowledgment: We would like to thank Dima Kuzmin for his extensive help with all aspects of this paper. Thanks also to Torsten Ehrhardt who first proved to us the range intersection and projection properties of the $\odot$ operation.

References

[Bha97] R. Bhatia. *Matrix Analysis*. Springer, Berlin, 1997.

[CA99] N. J. Cerf and C. Adam. Quantum extension of conditional probability. *Physical Review A*, 60(2):893–897, August 1999.

[KW97] J. Kivinen and M. K. Warmuth. Additive versus exponentiated gradient updates for linear prediction. *Information and Computation*, 132(1):1–64, January 1997.

[KW99] J. Kivinen and M. K. Warmuth. Averaging expert predictions. In *Computational Learning Theory: 4th European Conference (EuroCOLT '99)*, pages 153–167, Berlin, March 1999. Springer.

[NC00] M.A. Nielsen and I.L. Chuang. *Quantum Computation and Quantum Information*. Cambridge University Press, 2000.

[SBC01] R. Schack, T. A. Brun, and C. M. Caves. Quantum Bayes rule. *Physical Review A*, 64(014305), 2001.

[Sim79] Barry Simon. *Functional Integration and Quantum Physics*. Academic Press, New York, 1979.

[SWRL03] R. Singh, M. K. Warmuth, B. Raj, and P. Lamere. Classificaton with free energy at raised temperatures. In *Proc. of EUROSPEECH 2003*, pages 1773–1776, September 2003.

[TRW05] K. Tsuda, G. Rätsch, and M. K. Warmuth. Matrix exponentiated gradient updates for on-line learning and Bregman projections. *Journal of Machine Learning Research*, 6:995–1018, June 2005.

Variational Bayesian Stochastic Complexity of Mixture Models

Kazuho Watanabe*
Department of Computational Intelligence
and Systems Science
Tokyo Institute of Technology
Mail Box:R2-5, 4259 Nagatsuta,
Midori-ku, Yokohama, 226-8503, Japan
kazuho23@pi.titech.ac.jp

Sumio Watanabe
P& I Lab.
Tokyo Institute of Technology
swatanab@pi.titech.ac.jp

Abstract

The Variational Bayesian framework has been widely used to approximate the Bayesian learning. In various applications, it has provided computational tractability and good generalization performance. In this paper, we discuss the Variational Bayesian learning of the mixture of exponential families and provide some additional theoretical support by deriving the asymptotic form of the stochastic complexity. The stochastic complexity, which corresponds to the minimum free energy and a lower bound of the marginal likelihood, is a key quantity for model selection. It also enables us to discuss the effect of hyperparameters and the accuracy of the Variational Bayesian approach as an approximation of the true Bayesian learning.

1 Introduction

The Variational Bayesian (VB) framework has been widely used as an approximation of the Bayesian learning for models involving hidden (latent) variables such as mixture models[2][4]. This framework provides computationally tractable posterior distributions with only modest computational costs in contrast to Markov chain Monte Carlo (MCMC) methods. In many applications, it has performed better generalization compared to the maximum likelihood estimation.

In spite of its tractability and its wide range of applications, little has been done to investigate the theoretical properties of the Variational Bayesian learning itself. For example, questions like how accurately it approximates the true one remained unanswered until quite recently. To address these issues, the stochastic complexity in the Variational Bayesian learning of gaussian mixture models was clarified and the accuracy of the Variational Bayesian learning was discussed[10].

---

*This work was supported by the Ministry of Education, Science, Sports and Culture, Grant-in-Aid for JSPS Fellows 4637 and for Scientific Research 15500130, 2005.

In this paper, we focus on the Variational Bayesian learning of more general mixture models, namely the mixtures of exponential families which include mixtures of distributions such as gaussian, binomial and gamma. Mixture models are known to be non-regular statistical models due to the non-identifiability of parameters caused by their hidden variables[7]. In some recent studies, the Bayesian stochastic complexities of non-regular models have been clarified and it has been proven that they become smaller than those of regular models[12][13]. This indicates an advantage of the Bayesian learning when it is applied to non-regular models.

As our main results, the asymptotic upper and lower bounds are obtained for the stochastic complexity or the free energy in the Variational Bayesian learning of the mixture of exponential families. The stochastic complexity is important quantity for model selection and giving the asymptotic form of it also contributes to the following two issues. One is the accuracy of the Variational Bayesian learning as an approximation method since the stochastic complexity shows the distance from the variational posterior distribution to the true Bayesian posterior distribution in the sense of Kullback information. Indeed, we give the asymptotic form of the stochastic complexity as $\overline{F}(n) \simeq \overline{\lambda} \log n$ where n is the sample size, by comparing the coefficient $\overline{\lambda}$ with that of the true Bayesian learning, we discuss the accuracy of the VB approach. Another is the influence of the hyperparameter on the learning process. Since the Variational Bayesian algorithm is a procedure of minimizing the functional that finally gives the stochastic complexity, the derived bounds indicate how the hyperparameters influence the process of the learning. Our results have an implication for how to determine the hyperparameter values before the learning process.

We consider the case in which the true distribution is contained in the learner model. Analyzing the stochastic complexity in this case is most valuable for comparing the Variational Bayesian learning with the true Bayesian learning. This is because the advantage of the Bayesian learning is typical in this case[12]. Furthermore, this analysis is necessary and essential for addressing the model selection problem and hypothesis testing.

The paper is organized as follows. In Section 2, we introduce the mixture of exponential family model. In Section 3, we describe the Bayesian learning. In Section 4, the Variational Bayesian framework is described and the variational posterior distribution for the mixture of exponential family model is derived. In Section 5, we present our main result. Discussion and conclusion follow in Section 6.

2 Mixture of Exponential Family

Denote by $c(x|b)$ a density function of the input $x \in R^N$ given an M-dimensional parameter vector $b = (b^{(1)}, b^{(2)}, \cdots, b^{(M)})^T \in B$ where B is a subset of R^M. The general mixture model $p(x|\theta)$ with a parameter vector θ is defined by

$$p(x|\theta) = \sum_{k=1}^{K} a_k c(x|b_k),$$

where integer K is the number of components and $\{a_k | a_k \geq 0, \sum_{k=1}^{K} a_k = 1\}$ is the set of mixing proportions. The model parameter θ is $\{a_k, b_k\}_{k=1}^{K}$.

A mixture model is called a mixture of exponential family (MEF) model or exponential family mixture model if the probability distribution $c(x|b)$ for each component is given by the following form,

$$c(x|b) = \exp\{b \cdot f(x) + f_0(x) - g(b)\}, \tag{1}$$

where $b \in B$ is called the natural parameter, $b \cdot f(x)$ is its inner product with the vector $f(x) = (f_1(x), \cdots, f_M(x))^T$, $f_0(x)$ and $g(b)$ are real-valued functions of the input x and the parameter b, respectively[3]. Suppose functions $f_1, \cdots, f_M$ and a constant function are linearly independent, which means the effective number of parameters in a single component distribution $c(x|b)$ is M.

The conjugate prior distribution $\varphi(\theta)$ for the MEF model is given by the product of the following two distributions on $\mathbf{a} = \{a_k\}_{k=1}^K$ and $\mathbf{b} = \{b_k\}_{k=1}^K$,

$$\varphi(\mathbf{a}) = \frac{\Gamma(K\phi_0)}{\Gamma(\phi_0)^K} \prod_{k=1}^K a_k^{\phi_0 - 1}, \tag{2}$$

$$\varphi(\mathbf{b}) = \prod_{k=1}^K \varphi(b_k) = \prod_{k=1}^K \frac{\exp\{\xi_0(b_k \cdot \nu_0 - g(b_k))\}}{C(\xi_0, \nu_0)}, \tag{3}$$

where $\xi_0 > 0$, $\nu_0 \in R^M$ and $\phi_0 > 0$ are constants called hyperparameters and

$$C(\xi, \mu) = \int \exp\{\xi(\mu \cdot b - g(b))\}db \tag{4}$$

is a function of $\xi \in R$ and $\mu \in R^M$.

The mixture model can be rewritten as follows by using a hidden variable $y = (y^1, \cdots, y^K) \in \{(1, 0, \cdots, 0), (0, 1, \cdots, 0), \cdots, (0, 0, \cdots, 1)\}$,

$$p(x, y|\theta) = \prod_{k=1}^K \left[a_k c(x|b_k) \right]^{y^k}.$$

If and only if the datum x is generated from the kth component, $y^k = 1$.

3   The Bayesian Learning

Suppose n training samples $X^n = \{x_1, \cdots, x_n\}$ are independently and identically taken from the true distribution $p_0(x)$. In the Bayesian learning of a model $p(x|\theta)$ whose parameter is θ, first, the prior distribution $\varphi(\theta)$ on the parameter θ is set. Then the posterior distribution $p(\theta|X^n)$ is computed from the given dataset and the prior by

$$p(\theta|X^n) = \frac{1}{Z(X^n)} \exp(-nH_n(\theta))\varphi(\theta), \tag{5}$$

where $H_n(\theta)$ is the empirical Kullback information,

$$H_n(\theta) = \frac{1}{n} \sum_{i=1}^n \log \frac{p_0(x_i)}{p(x_i|\theta)}, \tag{6}$$

and $Z(X^n)$ is the normalization constant that is also known as the marginal likelihood or the evidence of the dataset X^n[6]. The Bayesian predictive distribution $p(x|X^n)$ is given by averaging the model over the posterior distribution as follows,

$$p(x|X^n) = \int p(x|\theta)p(\theta|X^n)d\theta. \tag{7}$$

The stochastic complexity $F(X^n)$ is defined by

$$F(X^n) = -\log Z(X^n), \tag{8}$$

which is also called the free energy and is important in most data modelling problems. Practically, it is used as a criterion by which the model is selected and the hyperparameters in the prior are optimized[1][9].

Define the average stochastic complexity $F(n)$ by

$$F(n) = E_{X^n}[F(X^n)], \qquad (9)$$

where $E_{X^n}[\cdot]$ denotes the expectation value over all sets of training samples. Recently, it was proved that $F(n)$ has the following asymptotic form[12],

$$F(n) \simeq \lambda \log n - (m-1) \log \log n + O(1), \qquad (10)$$

where λ and m are the rational number and the natural number respectively which are determined by the singularities of the set of true parameters. In regular statistical models, 2λ is equal to the number of parameters and $m = 1$, whereas in non-regular models such as mixture models, 2λ is not larger than the number of parameters and $m \geq 1$. This means an advantage of the Bayesian learning.

However, in the Bayesian learning, one computes the stochastic complexity or the predictive distribution by integrating over the posterior distribution, which typically cannot be performed analytically. As an approximation, the VB framework was proposed[2][4].

4 The Variational Bayesian Learning

4.1 The Variational Bayesian Framework

In the VB framework, the Bayesian posterior $p(Y^n, \theta|X^n)$ of the hidden variables and the parameters is approximated by the variational posterior $q(Y^n, \theta|X^n)$, which factorizes as

$$q(Y^n, \theta|X^n) = Q(Y^n|X^n)r(\theta|X^n), \qquad (11)$$

where $Q(Y^n|X^n)$ and $r(\theta|X^n)$ are posteriors on the hidden variables and the parameters respectively. The variational posterior $q(Y^n, \theta|X^n)$ is chosen to minimize the functional $\overline{F}[q]$ defined by

$$\overline{F}[q] = \sum_{Y^n} \int q(Y^n, \theta|X^n) \log \frac{q(Y^n, \theta|X^n)p_0(X^n)}{p(X^n, Y^n, \theta)} d\theta, \qquad (12)$$

$$= F(X^n) + K(q(Y^n, \theta|X^n)||p(Y^n, \theta|X^n)), \qquad (13)$$

where $K(q(Y^n, \theta|X^n)||p(Y^n, \theta|X^n))$ is the Kullback information between the true Bayesian posterior $p(Y^n, \theta|X^n)$ and the variational posterior $q(Y^n, \theta|X^n)$ [1]. This leads to the following theorem. The proof is well known[8].

Theorem 1 *If the functional $\overline{F}[q]$ is minimized under the constraint (11) then the variational posteriors, $r(\theta|X^n)$ and $Q(Y^n|X^n)$, satisfy*

$$r(\theta|X^n) = \frac{1}{C_r} \varphi(\theta) \exp \left\langle \log p(X^n, Y^n|\theta) \right\rangle_{Q(Y^n|X^n)}, \qquad (14)$$

$$Q(Y^n|X^n) = \frac{1}{C_Q} \exp \left\langle \log p(X^n, Y^n|\theta) \right\rangle_{r(\theta|X^n)}, \qquad (15)$$

---

[1] $K(q(x)||p(x))$ denotes the Kullback information from a distribution $q(x)$ to a distribution $p(x)$, that is,

$$K(q(x)||p(x)) = \int q(x) \log \frac{q(x)}{p(x)} dx.$$

where C_r and C_Q are the normalization constants[2].

We define the stochastic complexity in the VB learning $\overline{F}(X^n)$ by the minimum value of the functional $\overline{F}[q]$, that is ,

$$\overline{F}(X^n) = \min_{r,Q} \overline{F}[q],$$

which shows the accuracy of the VB approach as an approximation of the Bayesian learning. $\overline{F}(X^n)$ is also used for model selection since it gives an upper bound of the true Bayesian stochastic complexity $F(X^n)$.

4.2 Variational Posterior for MEF Model

In this subsection, we derive the variational posterior $r(\theta|X^n)$ for the MEF model based on (14) and then define the variational parameter for this model.

Using the complete data $\{X^n, Y^n\} = \{(x_1, y_1), \cdots, (x_n, y_n)\}$, we put

$$\overline{y}_i^k = \langle y_i^k \rangle_{Q(Y^n)}, \quad n_k = \sum_{i=1}^n \overline{y}_i^k, \text{and} \quad \nu_k = \frac{1}{n_k} \sum_{i=1}^n \overline{y}_i^k f(x_i),$$

where $y_i^k = 1$ if and only if the ith datum x_i is from the kth component. The variable n_k is the expected number of the data that are estimated to be from the kth component. From (14) and the respective prior (2) and (3), the variational posterior $r(\theta)$ is obtained as the product of the following two distributions[3],

$$r(\mathbf{a}) = \frac{\Gamma(n + K\phi_0)}{\prod_{k=1}^K \Gamma(n_k + \phi_0)} \prod_{k=1}^K a_k^{n_k + \phi_0 - 1}, \tag{16}$$

$$r(\mathbf{b}) = \prod_{k=1}^K r(b_k) = \prod_{k=1}^K \frac{1}{C(\gamma_k, \overline{\mu}_k)} \exp\{\gamma_k(\overline{\mu}_k \cdot b_k - g(b_k))\}, \tag{17}$$

where $\overline{\mu}_k = \frac{n_k \nu_k + \xi_0 \nu_0}{n_k + \xi_0}$ and $\gamma_k = n_k + \xi_0$. Let

$$\overline{a}_k = \langle a_k \rangle_{r(\mathbf{a})} = \frac{n_k + \phi_0}{n + K\phi_0}, \tag{18}$$

$$\overline{b}_k = \langle b_k \rangle_{r(b_k)} = \frac{1}{\gamma_k} \frac{\partial \log C(\gamma_k, \overline{\mu}_k)}{\partial \overline{\mu}_k}, \tag{19}$$

and define the variational parameter $\overline{\theta}$ by $\overline{\theta} = \langle \theta \rangle_{r(\theta)} = \{\overline{a}_k, \overline{b}_k\}_{k=1}^K$. Then it is noted that the variational posterior $r(\theta)$ and C_Q in (15) are parameterized by the variational parameter $\overline{\theta}$. Therefore, we denote them as $r(\theta|\overline{\theta})$ and $C_Q(\overline{\theta})$ henceforth. We define the variational estimator $\overline{\theta}_{vb}$ by the variational parameter $\overline{\theta}$ that attains the minimum value of the stochastic complexity $\overline{F}(X^n)$. Then, putting (15) into (12), we obtain

$$\overline{F}(X^n) = \min_{\overline{\theta}}\{K(r(\theta|\overline{\theta})||\varphi(\theta)) - (\log C_Q(\overline{\theta}) + S(X^n))\}, \tag{20}$$

$$= K(r(\theta|\overline{\theta}_{vb})||\varphi(\theta)) - (\log C_Q(\overline{\theta}_{vb}) + S(X^n)), \tag{21}$$

where $S(X^n) = -\sum_{i=1}^n \log p_0(x)$.

Therefore, our aim is to evaluate the minimum value of (20) as a function of the variational parameter $\overline{\theta}$.

---

[2]$\langle\cdot\rangle_{p(x)}$ denotes the expectation over $p(x)$.

[3]Hereafter, we omit the condition X^n of the variational posteriors, and abbreviate them to $q(Y^n, \theta)$, $Q(Y^n)$ and $r(\theta)$.

5   Main Result

The average stochastic complexity $\overline{F}(n)$ in the VB learning is defined by

$$\overline{F}(n) = E_{X^n}[\overline{F}(X^n)]. \tag{22}$$

We assume the following conditions.

(i) The true distribution $p_0(x)$ is an MEF model $p(x|\theta_0)$ which has K_0 components and the parameter $\theta_0 = \{a_k^*, b_k^*\}_{k=1}^{K_0}$,

$$p(x|\theta_0) = \sum_{k=1}^{K_0} a_k^* \exp\{b_k^* \cdot f(x) + f_0(x) - g(b_k^*)\},$$

where $b_k^* \in R^M$ and $b_k^* \neq b_j^* (k \neq j)$. And suppose that the model $p(x|\theta)$ has K components,

$$p(x|\theta) = \sum_{k=1}^{K} a_k \exp\{b_k \cdot f(x) + f_0(x) - g(b_k)\},$$

and $K \geq K_0$ holds.

(ii) The prior distribution of the parameters is $\varphi(\theta) = \varphi(\mathbf{a})\varphi(\mathbf{b})$ given by (2) and (3) with $\varphi(\mathbf{b})$ bounded.

(iii) Regarding the distribution $c(x|b)$ of each component, the Fisher information matrix $I(b) = \frac{\partial^2 g(b)}{\partial b \partial b}$ satisfies $0 < |I(b)| < +\infty$, for arbitrary $b \in B$ [4]. The function $\mu \cdot b - g(b)$ has a stationary point at $\hat{b}$ in the interior of B for each $\mu \in \{\frac{\partial g(b)}{\partial b}|b \in B\}$.

Under these conditions, we prove the following.

Theorem 2 (Main Result) *Assume the conditions (i),(ii) and (iii). Then the average stochastic complexity $\overline{F}(n)$ defined by (22) satisfies*

$$\underline{\lambda} \log n + E_{X^n}\left[nH_n(\overline{\theta}_{vb})\right] + C_1 \leq \overline{F}(n) \leq \overline{\lambda} \log n + C_2, \tag{23}$$

for an arbitrary natural number n, where C_1, C_2 are constants independent of n and

$$\underline{\lambda} = \begin{cases} (K-1)\phi_0 + \frac{M}{2}, \\ \frac{MK+K-1}{2}, \end{cases} \quad \overline{\lambda} = \begin{cases} (K-K_0)\phi_0 + \frac{MK_0+K_0-1}{2} & (\phi_0 \leq \frac{M+1}{2}), \\ \frac{MK+K-1}{2} & (\phi_0 > \frac{M+1}{2}). \end{cases} \tag{24}$$

This theorem shows the asymptotic form of the average stochastic complexity in the Variational Bayesian learning. The coefficients $\underline{\lambda}, \overline{\lambda}$ of the leading terms are identified by K, K_0, that are the numbers of components of the learner and the true distribution, the number of parameters M of each component and the hyperparameter ϕ_0 of the conjugate prior given by (2).

In this theorem, $nH_n(\overline{\theta}_{vb}) = -\sum_{i=1}^{n} \log p(x_i|\overline{\theta}_{vb}) - S(X^n)$, and $-\sum_{i=1}^{n} \log p(x_i|\overline{\theta}_{vb})$ is a training error which is computable during the learning. If the term $E_{X^n}[nH_n(\overline{\theta}_{vb})]$ is a bounded function of n, then it immediately follows from this theorem that

$$\underline{\lambda} \log n + O(1) \leq \overline{F}_0(n) \leq \overline{\lambda} \log n + O(1),$$

---

[4] $\frac{\partial^2 g(b)}{\partial b \partial b}$ denotes the matrix whose ijth entry is $\frac{\partial^2 g(b)}{\partial b^{(i)} \partial b^{(j)}}$ and $|\cdot|$ denotes the determinant of a matrix.

where $O(1)$ is a bounded function of n. In certain cases, such as binomial mixtures and mixtures of von-Mises distributions, it is actually a bounded function of n. In the case of gaussian mixtures, if $B = R^N$, it is conjectured that the minus likelihood ratio $\min_\theta nH_n(\theta)$, a lower bound of $nH_n(\bar{\theta}_{vb})$, is at most of the order of $\log\log n$[5].

Since the dimension of the parameter θ is $MK + K - 1$, the average stochastic complexity of regular statistical models, which coincides with the Bayesian information criterion (BIC)[9] is given by $\lambda_{\mathrm{BIC}} \log n$ where $\lambda_{\mathrm{BIC}} = \frac{MK+K-1}{2}$. Theorem 2 claims that the coefficient $\bar{\lambda}$ of $\log n$ is smaller than λ_{BIC} when $\phi_0 \leq (M+1)/2$. This implies that the advantage of non-regular models in the Bayesian learning still remains in the VB learning.

(Outline of the proof of Theorem 2)

From the condition (iii), calculating $C(\gamma_k, \bar{\mu}_k)$ in (17) by the saddle point approximation, $K(r(\theta|\bar{\theta})||\varphi(\theta))$ in (20) is evaluated as follows [5],

$$K(r(\theta|\bar{\theta})||\varphi(\theta)) = G(\bar{\mathbf{a}}) - \sum_{k=1}^{K} \log \varphi(\bar{b}_k) + O_p(1), \qquad (25)$$

where the function $G(\bar{\mathbf{a}})$ of $\bar{\mathbf{a}} = \{\bar{a}_k\}_{k=1}^K$ is given by

$$G(\bar{\mathbf{a}}) = \frac{MK + K - 1}{2} \log n + \{\frac{M}{2} - (\phi_0 - \frac{1}{2})\} \sum_{k=1}^{K} \log \bar{a}_k. \qquad (26)$$

Then $\log C_Q(\bar{\theta})$ in (20) is evaluated as follows.

$$nH_n(\bar{\theta}) + O_p(1) \leq -(\log C_Q(\bar{\theta}) + S(X^n)) \leq n\overline{H}_n(\bar{\theta}) + O_p(1) \qquad (27)$$

where

$$\overline{H}_n(\bar{\theta}) = \frac{1}{n} \sum_{i=1}^{n} \log \frac{p(x_i|\theta_0)}{\sum_{k=1}^{K} \bar{a}_k c(x_i|\bar{b}_k) \exp\{-\frac{C'}{n_k + \min\{\phi_0, \xi_0\}}\}},$$

and C' is a constant. Thus, from (20), evaluating the right-hand sides of (25) and (27) at specific points near the true parameter θ_0, we obtain the upper bound in (23). The lower bound in (23) is obtained from (25) and (27) by Jensen's inequality and the constraint $\sum_{k=1}^{K} \bar{a}_k = 1$. **(Q.E.D)**

6 Discussion and Conclusion

In this paper, we showed the upper and lower bounds of the stochastic complexity for the mixture of exponential family models in the VB learning.

Firstly, we compare the stochastic complexity shown in Theorem 2 with the one in the true Bayesian learning. On the mixture models with M parameters in each component, the following upper bound for the coefficient of $F(n)$ in (10) is known [13],

$$\lambda \leq \begin{cases} (K + K_0 - 1)/2 & (M = 1), \\ (K - K_0) + (MK_0 + K_0 - 1)/2 & (M \geq 2). \end{cases} \qquad (28)$$

By the certain conditions about the prior distribution under which the above bound was derived, we can compare the stochastic complexity when $\phi_0 = 1$. Putting $\phi_0 = 1$ in (24), we have

$$\bar{\lambda} = K - K_0 + (MK_0 + K_0 - 1)/2. \qquad (29)$$

---

[5] $O_p(1)$ denotes a random variable bounded in probability.

Since we obtain $\overline{F}(n) \simeq \overline{\lambda} \log n + O(1)$ under certain assumptions[11], let us compare $\overline{\lambda}$ of the VB learning to λ in (28) of the true Bayesian learning. When $M = 1$, that is, each component has one parameter, $\overline{\lambda} \geq \lambda$ holds since $K_0 \leq K$. This means that the more redundant components the model has, the more the VB learning differs from the true Bayesian learning. In this case, $2\overline{\lambda}$ is equal to the number of the parameters of the model. Hence the BIC[9] corresponds to $\overline{\lambda} \log n$ when $M = 1$. If $M \geq 2$, the upper bound of λ is equal to $\overline{\lambda}$. This implies that the variational posterior is close to the true Bayesian posterior when $M \geq 2$. More precise discussion about the accuracy of the approximation can be done for models on which tighter bounds or exact values of the coefficient λ in (10) are given[10].

Secondly, we point out that Theorem 2 shows how the hyperparameter ϕ_0 influence the process of the VB learning. The coefficient $\overline{\lambda}$ in (24) indicates that only when $\phi_0 \leq (M + 1)/2$, the prior distribution (2) works to eliminate the redundant components that the model has and otherwise it works to use all the components.

And lastly, let us give examples of how to use the theoretical bounds in (23). One can examine experimentally whether the actual iterative algorithm converges to the optimal variational posterior instead of local minima by comparing the stochastic complexity with our theoretical result. The theoretical bounds would also enable us to compare the accuracy of the VB learning with that of the Laplace approximation or the MCMC method. As mentioned in Section 4, our result will be important for developing effective model selection methods using $\overline{F}(X^n)$ in the future work.

References

[1] H.Akaike, "Likelihood and Bayes procedure," *Bayesian Statistics*, (Bernald J.M. eds.) University Press, Valencia, Spain, pp.143-166, 1980.

[2] H.Attias, "Inferring parameters and structure of latent variable models by variational bayes," *Proc. of UAI*, 1999.

[3] L.D.Brown, "Fundamentals of statistical exponential families," IMS Lecture Notes-Monograph Series, 1986.

[4] Z.Ghahramani, M.J.Beal, "Graphical models and variational methods," *Advanced Mean Field Methods*, MIT Press, 2000.

[5] J.A.Hartigan, "A Failure of likelihood asymptotics for normal mixtures," *Proc. of the Berkeley Conference in Honor of J.Neyman and J.Kiefer*, Vol.2, 807-810, 1985.

[6] D.J. Mackay, "Bayesian interpolation," *Neural Computation*, 4(2), pp.415-447, 1992.

[7] G.McLachlan, D.Peel,"Finite mixture models," Wiley, 2000.

[8] M.Sato, "Online model selection based on the variational bayes," *Neural Computation*, 13(7), pp.1649-1681, 2001.

[9] G.Schwarz, "Estimating the dimension of a model," *Annals of Statistics*, 6(2), pp.461-464, 1978.

[10] K.Watanabe, S.Watanabe, "Lower bounds of stochastic complexities in variational bayes learning of gaussian mixture models," *Proc. of IEEE CIS04*, pp.99-104, 2004.

[11] K.Watanabe, S.Watanabe, "Stochastic complexity for mixture of exponential families in variational bayes," *Proc. of ALT05*, pp.107-121, 2005.

[12] S.Watanabe,"Algebraic analysis for non-identifiable learning machines," *Neural Computation*, 13(4), pp.899-933, 2001.

[13] K.Yamazaki, S.Watanabe, "Singularities in mixture models and upper bounds of stochastic complexity," *Neural Networks*, 16, pp.1029-1038, 2003.

Distance Metric Learning for Large Margin Nearest Neighbor Classification

Kilian Q. Weinberger, John Blitzer and Lawrence K. Saul
Department of Computer and Information Science, University of Pennsylvania
Levine Hall, 3330 Walnut Street, Philadelphia, PA 19104
{kilianw, blitzer, lsaul}@cis.upenn.edu

Abstract

We show how to learn a Mahanalobis distance metric for k-nearest neighbor (kNN) classification by semidefinite programming. The metric is trained with the goal that the k-nearest neighbors always belong to the same class while examples from different classes are separated by a large margin. On seven data sets of varying size and difficulty, we find that metrics trained in this way lead to significant improvements in kNN classification—for example, achieving a test error rate of 1.3% on the MNIST handwritten digits. As in support vector machines (SVMs), the learning problem reduces to a convex optimization based on the hinge loss. Unlike learning in SVMs, however, our framework requires no modification or extension for problems in multiway (as opposed to binary) classification.

1 Introduction

The k-nearest neighbors (kNN) rule [3] is one of the oldest and simplest methods for pattern classification. Nevertheless, it often yields competitive results, and in certain domains, when cleverly combined with prior knowledge, it has significantly advanced the state-of-the-art [1, 14]. The kNN rule classifies each unlabeled example by the majority label among its k-nearest neighbors in the training set. Its performance thus depends crucially on the *distance metric* used to identify nearest neighbors.

In the absence of prior knowledge, most kNN classifiers use simple Euclidean distances to measure the dissimilarities between examples represented as vector inputs. Euclidean distance metrics, however, do not capitalize on any statistical regularities in the data that might be estimated from a large training set of labeled examples.

Ideally, the distance metric for kNN classification should be adapted to the particular problem being solved. It can hardly be optimal, for example, to use the same distance metric for face recognition as for gender identification, even if in both tasks, distances are computed between the same fixed-size images. In fact, as shown by many researchers [2, 6, 7, 8, 12, 13], kNN classification can be significantly improved by learning a distance metric from labeled examples. Even a simple (global) linear transformation of input features has been shown to yield much better kNN classifiers [7, 12]. Our work builds in a novel direction on the success of these previous approaches.

In this paper, we show how to learn a Mahanalobis distance metric for kNN classification. The metric is optimized with the goal that *k-nearest neighbors always belong to the same class while examples from different classes are separated by a large margin.* Our goal for metric learning differs in a crucial way from those of previous approaches that minimize the pairwise distances between *all* similarly labeled examples [12, 13, 17]. This latter objective is far more difficult to achieve and does not leverage the full power of kNN classification, whose accuracy does *not* require that all similarly labeled inputs be tightly clustered.

Our approach is largely inspired by recent work on neighborhood component analysis [7] and metric learning by energy-based models [2]. Though based on the same goals, however, our methods are quite different. In particular, we are able to cast our optimization as an instance of semidefinite programming. Thus the optimization we propose is convex, and its global minimum can be efficiently computed.

Our approach has several parallels to learning in support vector machines (SVMs)—most notably, the goal of margin maximization and a convex objective function based on the hinge loss. In light of these parallels, we describe our approach as *large margin nearest neighbor* (LMNN) classification. Our framework can be viewed as the logical counterpart to SVMs in which kNN classification replaces linear classification.

Our framework contrasts with classification by SVMs, however, in one intriguing respect: it requires no modification for problems in multiway (as opposed to binary) classification. Extensions of SVMs to multiclass problems typically involve combining the results of many binary classifiers, or they require additional machinery that is elegant but non-trivial [4]. In both cases the training time scales at least linearly in the number of classes. By contrast, our learning problem has no explicit dependence on the number of classes.

2 Model

Let $\{(\vec{x}_i, y_i)\}_{i=1}^n$ denote a training set of n labeled examples with inputs $\vec{x}_i \in \mathcal{R}^d$ and discrete (but not necessarily binary) class labels y_i. We use the binary matrix $y_{ij} \in \{0, 1\}$ to indicate whether or not the labels y_i and y_j match. Our goal is to learn a linear transformation $\mathbf{L}: \mathcal{R}^d \to \mathcal{R}^d$, which we will use to compute squared distances as:

$$\mathcal{D}(\vec{x}_i, \vec{x}_j) = \|\mathbf{L}(\vec{x}_i - \vec{x}_j)\|^2. \tag{1}$$

Specifically, we want to learn the linear transformation that optimizes kNN classification when distances are measured in this way. We begin by developing some useful terminology.

Target neighbors
In addition to the class label y_i, for each input $\vec{x}_i$ we also specify k "target" neighbors—that is, k other inputs with the same label y_i that we wish to have minimal distance to $\vec{x}_i$, as computed by eq. (1). In the absence of prior knowledge, the target neighbors can simply be identified as the k nearest neighbors, determined by Euclidean distance, that share the same label y_i. (This was done for all the experiments in this paper.) We use $\eta_{ij} \in \{0, 1\}$ to indicate whether input $\vec{x}_j$ is a target neighbor of input $\vec{x}_i$. Like the binary matrix y_{ij}, the matrix η_{ij} is fixed and does not change during learning.

Cost function
Our cost function over the distance metrics parameterized by eq. (1) has two competing terms. The first term penalizes large distances between each input and its target neighbors, while the second term penalizes small distances between each input and all other inputs that do not share the same label. Specifically, the cost function is given by:

$$\varepsilon(\mathbf{L}) = \sum_{ij} \eta_{ij} \|\mathbf{L}(\vec{x}_i - \vec{x}_j)\|^2 + c \sum_{ijl} \eta_{ij}(1 - y_{il}) \left[1 + \|\mathbf{L}(\vec{x}_i - \vec{x}_j)\|^2 - \|\mathbf{L}(\vec{x}_i - \vec{x}_l)\|^2\right]_+,$$

$$\tag{2}$$

where in the second term $[z]_+ = \max(z, 0)$ denotes the standard hinge loss and $c > 0$ is some positive constant (typically set by cross validation). Note that the first term only penalizes large distances between inputs and target neighbors, *not between all similarly labeled examples*.

Large margin

The second term in the cost function incorporates the idea of a margin. In particular, for each input $\vec{x}_i$, the hinge loss is incurred by differently labeled inputs whose distances do not exceed, by one absolute unit of distance, the distance from input $\vec{x}_i$ to any of its target neighbors. The cost function thereby favors distance metrics in which differently labeled inputs maintain a large margin of distance and do not threaten to "invade" each other's neighborhoods. The learning dynamics induced by this cost function are illustrated in Fig. 1 for an input with $k = 3$ target neighbors.

Parallels with SVMs

The competing terms in eq. (2) are analogous to those in the cost function for SVMs [11]. In both cost functions, one term penalizes the norm of the "parameter" vector (i.e., the weight vector of the maximum margin hyperplane, or the linear transformation in the distance metric), while the other incurs the hinge loss for examples that violate the condition of unit margin. Finally, just as the hinge loss in SVMs is only triggered by examples near the decision boundary, the hinge loss in eq. (2) is only triggered by differently labeled examples that invade each other's neighborhoods.

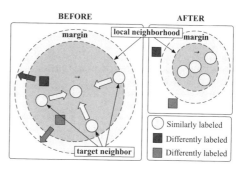

Figure 1: Schematic illustration of one input's neighborhood $\vec{x}_i$ before training (*left*) versus after training (*right*). The distance metric is optimized so that: (i) its $k = 3$ target neighbors lie within a smaller radius after training; (ii) differently labeled inputs lie outside this smaller radius, with a margin of at least one unit distance. Arrows indicate the gradients on distances arising from the optimization of the cost function.

Convex optimization

We can reformulate the optimization of eq. (2) as an instance of semidefinite programming [16]. A semidefinite program (SDP) is a linear program with the additional constraint that a matrix whose elements are linear in the unknown variables is required to be positive semidefinite. SDPs are convex; thus, with this reformulation, the global minimum of eq. (2) can be efficiently computed. To obtain the equivalent SDP, we rewrite eq. (1) as:

$$\mathcal{D}(\vec{x}_i, \vec{x}_j) = (\vec{x}_i - \vec{x}_j)^\top \mathbf{M} (\vec{x}_i - \vec{x}_j), \tag{3}$$

where the matrix $\mathbf{M} = \mathbf{L}^\top \mathbf{L}$, parameterizes the Mahalanobis distance metric induced by the linear transformation $\mathbf{L}$. Rewriting eq. (2) as an SDP in terms of $\mathbf{M}$ is straightforward, since the first term is already linear in $\mathbf{M} = \mathbf{L}^\top \mathbf{L}$ and the hinge loss can be "mimicked" by introducing slack variables ξ_{ij} for all pairs of differently labeled inputs (i.e., for all $\langle i, j \rangle$ such that $y_{ij} = 0$). The resulting SDP is given by:

Minimize $\sum_{ij} \eta_{ij} (\vec{x}_i - \vec{x}_j)^\top \mathbf{M} (\vec{x}_i - \vec{x}_j) + c \sum_{ij} \eta_{ij}(1 - y_{il})\xi_{ijl}$ **subject to:**

(1) $(\vec{x}_i - \vec{x}_l)^\top \mathbf{M}(\vec{x}_i - \vec{x}_l) - (\vec{x}_i - \vec{x}_j)^\top \mathbf{M}(\vec{x}_i - \vec{x}_j) \geq 1 - \xi_{ijl}$

(2) $\xi_{ijl} \geq 0$

(3) $\mathbf{M} \succeq 0.$

The last constraint $\mathbf{M} \succeq 0$ indicates that the matrix $\mathbf{M}$ is required to be positive semidefinite. While this SDP can be solved by standard online packages, general-purpose solvers tend to scale poorly in the number of constraints. Thus, for our work, we implemented our own special-purpose solver, exploiting the fact that most of the slack variables $\{\xi_{ij}\}$ never attain positive values[1]. The slack variables $\{\xi_{ij}\}$ are sparse because most labeled inputs are well separated; thus, their resulting pairwise distances do not incur the hinge loss, and we obtain very few *active* constraints. Our solver was based on a combination of sub-gradient descent in both the matrices **L** and **M**, the latter used mainly to verify that we had reached the global minimum. We projected updates in **M** back onto the positive semidefinite cone after each step. Alternating projection algorithms provably converge [16], and in this case our implementation worked much faster than generic solvers[2].

3   Results

We evaluated the algorithm in the previous section on seven data sets of varying size and difficulty. Table 1 compares the different data sets. Principal components analysis (PCA) was used to reduce the dimensionality of image, speech, and text data, both to speed up training and avoid overfitting. Except for Isolet and MNIST, all of the experimental results are averaged over several runs of randomly generated 70/30 splits of the data. Isolet and MNIST have pre-defined training/test splits. For the other data sets, we randomly generated 70/30 splits for each run. Both the number of target neighbors (k) and the weighting parameter (c) in eq. (2) were set by cross validation. (For the purpose of cross-validation, the training sets were further partitioned into training and validation sets.) We begin by reporting overall trends, then discussing the individual data sets in more detail.

We first compare kNN classification error rates using Mahalanobis versus Euclidean distances. To break ties among different classes, we repeatedly reduced the neighborhood size, ultimately classifying (if necessary) by just the $k = 1$ nearest neighbor. Fig. 2 summarizes the main results. Except on the smallest data set (where over-training appears to be an issue), the Mahalanobis distance metrics learned by semidefinite programming led to significant improvements in kNN classification, both in training and testing. The training error rates reported in Fig. 2 are leave-one-out estimates.

We also computed test error rates using a variant of kNN classification, inspired by previous work on energy-based models [2]. Energy-based classification of a test example $\vec{x}_t$ was done by finding the label that minimizes the cost function in eq. (2). In particular, for a hypothetical label y_t, we accumulated the squared distances to the k nearest neighbors of $\vec{x}_t$ that share the same label in the training set (corresponding to the first term in the cost function); we also accumulated the hinge loss over all pairs of differently labeled examples that result from labeling $\vec{x}_t$ by y_t (corresponding to the second term in the cost function). Finally, the test example was classified by the hypothetical label that minimized the combination of these two terms:

$$y_t = \operatorname{argmin}_{y_t} \sum_j \eta_{tj} \|\mathbf{L}(\vec{x}_t - \vec{x}_j)\|^2 + c \sum_{j,i=t \vee l=t} \eta_{ij} (1 - y_{il}) \left[1 + \|\mathbf{L}(\vec{x}_i - \vec{x}_j)\|^2 - \|\mathbf{L}(\vec{x}_i - \vec{x}_l)\|^2 \right]_+$$

As shown in Fig. 2, energy-based classification with this assignment rule generally led to even further reductions in test error rates.

Finally, we compared our results to those of multiclass SVMs [4]. On each data set (except MNIST), we trained multiclass SVMs using linear and RBF kernels; Fig. 2 reports the results of the better classifier. On MNIST, we used a non-homogeneous polynomial kernel of degree four, which gave us our best results. (See also [9].)

---

[1] A great speedup can be achieved by solving an SDP that only monitors a fraction of the margin conditions, then using the resulting solution as a starting point for the actual SDP of interest.

[2] A matlab implementation is currently available at http://www.seas.upenn.edu/~kilianw/lmnn.

	Iris	Wine	Faces	Bal	Isolet	News	MNIST
examples (train)	106	126	280	445	6238	16000	60000
examples (test)	44	52	120	90	1559	2828	10000
classes	3	3	40	3	26	20	10
input dimensions	4	13	1178	4	617	30000	784
features after PCA	4	13	30	4	172	200	164
constraints	5278	7266	78828	76440	37 Mil	164 Mil	3.3 Bil
active constraints	113	1396	7665	3099	45747	732359	243596
CPU time (per run)	2s	8s	7s	13s	11m	1.5h	4h
runs	100	100	100	100	1	10	1

Table 1: Properties of data sets and experimental parameters for LMNN classification.

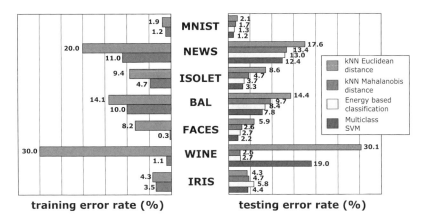

Figure 2: Training and test error rates for kNN classification using Euclidean versus Mahalanobis distances. The latter yields lower test error rates on all but the smallest data set (presumably due to over-training). Energy-based classification (see text) generally leads to further improvement. The results approach those of state-of-the-art multiclass SVMs.

Small data sets with few classes

The wine, iris, and balance data sets are small data sets, with less than 500 training examples and just three classes, taken from the UCI Machine Learning Repository[3]. On data sets of this size, a distance metric can be learned in a matter of seconds. The results in Fig. 2 were averaged over 100 experiments with different random 70/30 splits of each data set. Our results on these data sets are roughly comparable (i.e., better in some cases, worse in others) to those of neighborhood component analysis (NCA) and relevant component analysis (RCA), as reported in previous work [7].

Face recognition

The AT&T face recognition data set[4] contains 400 grayscale images of 40 individuals in 10 different poses. We downsampled the images from to 38×31 pixels and used PCA to obtain 30-dimensional eigenfaces [15]. Training and test sets were created by randomly sampling 7 images of each person for training and 3 images for testing. The task involved 40-way classification—essentially, recognizing a face from an unseen pose. Fig. 2 shows the improvements due to LMNN classification. Fig. 3 illustrates the improvements more graphically by showing how the $k = 3$ nearest neighbors change as a result of learning a Mahalanobis metric. (Though the algorithm operated on low dimensional eigenfaces, for clarity the figure shows the rescaled images.)

---

[3] Available at http://www.ics.uci.edu/~mlearn/MLRepository.html.

[4] Available at http://www.uk.research.att.com/facedatabase.html

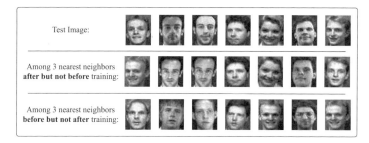

Figure 3: Images from the AT&T face recognition data base. *Top row*: an image correctly recognized by kNN classification ($k = 3$) with Mahalanobis distances, but not with Euclidean distances. *Middle row*: correct match among the $k = 3$ nearest neighbors according to Mahalanobis distance, but not Euclidean distance. *Bottom row*: incorrect match among the $k = 3$ nearest neighbors according to Euclidean distance, but not Mahalanobis distance.

Spoken letter recognition

The Isolet data set from UCI Machine Learning Repository has 6238 examples and 26 classes corresponding to letters of the alphabet. We reduced the input dimensionality (originally at 617) by projecting the data onto its leading 172 principal components—enough to account for 95% of its total variance. On this data set, Dietterich and Bakiri report test error rates of 4.2% using nonlinear backpropagation networks with 26 output units (one per class) and 3.3% using nonlinear backpropagation networks with a 30-bit error correcting code [5]. LMNN with energy-based classification obtains a test error rate of 3.7%.

Text categorization

The 20-newsgroups data set consists of posted articles from 20 newsgroups, with roughly 1000 articles per newsgroup. We used the 18828-version of the data set[5] which has cross-postings removed and some headers stripped out. We tokenized the newsgroups using the rainbow package [10]. Each article was initially represented by the weighted word-counts of the 20,000 most common words. We then reduced the dimensionality by projecting the data onto its leading 200 principal components. The results in Fig. 2 were obtained by averaging over 10 runs with 70/30 splits for training and test data. Our best result for LMNN on this data set at 13.0% test error rate improved significantly on kNN classification using Euclidean distances. LMNN also performed comparably to our best multiclass SVM [4], which obtained a 12.4% test error rate using a linear kernel and 20000 dimensional inputs.

Handwritten digit recognition

The MNIST data set of handwritten digits[6] has been extensively benchmarked [9]. We deskewed the original 28×28 grayscale images, then reduced their dimensionality by retaining only the first 164 principal components (enough to capture 95% of the data's overall variance). Energy-based LMNN classification yielded a test error rate at 1.3%, cutting the baseline kNN error rate by over one-third. Other comparable benchmarks [9] (not exploiting additional prior knowledge) include multilayer neural nets at 1.6% and SVMs at 1.2%. Fig. 4 shows some digits whose nearest neighbor changed as a result of learning, from a mismatch using Euclidean distance to a match using Mahanalobis distance.

4   Related Work

Many researchers have attempted to learn distance metrics from labeled examples. We briefly review some recent methods, pointing out similarities and differences with our work.

---

[5]Available at http://people.csail.mit.edu/jrennie/20Newsgroups/
[6]Available at http://yann.lecun.com/exdb/mnist/

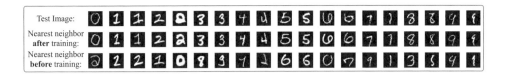

Figure 4: *Top row:* Examples of MNIST images whose nearest neighbor changes during training. *Middle row:* nearest neighbor after training, using the Mahalanobis distance metric. *Bottom row:* nearest neighbor before training, using the Euclidean distance metric.

Xing et al [17] used semidefinite programming to learn a Mahalanobis distance metric for clustering. Their algorithm aims to minimize the sum of squared distances between similarly labeled inputs, while maintaining a lower bound on the sum of distances between differently labeled inputs. Our work has a similar basis in semidefinite programming, but differs in its focus on local neighborhoods for kNN classification.

Shalev-Shwartz et al [12] proposed an online learning algorithm for learning a Mahalanobis distance metric. The metric is trained with the goal that all similarly labeled inputs have small pairwise distances (bounded from above), while all differently labeled inputs have large pairwise distances (bounded from below). A margin is defined by the difference of these thresholds and induced by a hinge loss function. Our work has a similar basis in its appeal to margins and hinge loss functions, but again differs in its focus on local neighborhoods for kNN classification. In particular, we do not seek to minimize the distance between all similarly labeled inputs, only those that are specified as neighbors.

Goldberger et al [7] proposed neighborhood component analysis (NCA), a distance metric learning algorithm especially designed to improve kNN classification. The algorithm minimizes the probability of error under stochastic neighborhood assignments using gradient descent. Our work shares essentially the same goals as NCA, but differs in its construction of a convex objective function.

Chopra et al [2] recently proposed a framework for similarity metric learning in which the metrics are parameterized by pairs of identical convolutional neural nets. Their cost function penalizes large distances between similarly labeled inputs and small distances between differently labeled inputs, with penalties that incorporate the idea of a margin. Our work is based on a similar cost function, but our metric is parameterized by a linear transformation instead of a convolutional neural net. In this way, we obtain an instance of semidefinite programming.

Relevant component analysis (RCA) constructs a Mahalanobis distance metric from a weighted sum of in-class covariance matrices [13]. It is similar to PCA and linear discriminant analysis (but different from our approach) in its reliance on second-order statistics.

Hastie and Tibshirani [?] and Domeniconi et al [6] consider schemes for locally adaptive distance metrics that vary throughout the input space. The latter work appeals to the goal of margin maximization but otherwise differs substantially from our approach. In particular, Domeniconi et al [6] suggest to use the decision boundaries of SVMs to induce a locally adaptive distance metric for kNN classification. By contrast, our approach (though similarly named) does not involve the training of SVMs.

5   Discussion

In this paper, we have shown how to learn Mahalanobis distance metrics for kNN classification by semidefinite programming. Our framework makes no assumptions about the structure or distribution of the data and scales naturally to large number of classes. Ongoing work is focused in three directions. First, we are working to apply LMNN classification to problems with hundreds or thousands of classes, where its advantages are most apparent. Second, we are investigating the kernel trick to perform LMNN classification in nonlinear feature spaces. As LMMN already yields highly nonlinear decision boundaries in the original input space, however, it is not obvious that "kernelizing" the algorithm will lead to significant further improvement. Finally, we are extending our framework to learn locally adaptive distance metrics [6, 8] that vary across the input space. Such metrics should lead to even more flexible and powerful large margin classifiers.

References

[1] S. Belongie, J. Malik, and J. Puzicha. Shape matching and object recognition using shape contexts. *IEEE Transactions on Pattern Analysis and Machine Intelligence (PAMI)*, 24(4):509–522, 2002.

[2] S. Chopra, R. Hadsell, and Y. LeCun. Learning a similiarty metric discriminatively, with application to face verification. In *Proceedings of the IEEE Conference on Computer Vision and Pattern Recognition (CVPR-05)*, San Diego, CA, 2005.

[3] T. Cover and P. Hart. Nearest neighbor pattern classification. In *IEEE Transactions in Information Theory, IT-13*, pages 21–27, 1967.

[4] K. Crammer and Y. Singer. On the algorithmic implementation of multiclass kernel-based vector machines. *Journal of Machine Learning Research*, 2:265–292, 2001.

[5] T. G. Dietterich and G. Bakiri. Solving multiclass learning problems via error-correcting output codes. In *Journal of Artificial Intelligence Research*, number 2 in 263-286, 1995.

[6] C. Domeniconi, D. Gunopulos, and J. Peng. Large margin nearest neighbor classifiers. *IEEE Transactions on Neural Networks*, 16(4):899–909, 2005.

[7] J. Goldberger, S. Roweis, G. Hinton, and R. Salakhutdinov. Neighbourhood components analysis. In L. K. Saul, Y. Weiss, and L. Bottou, editors, *Advances in Neural Information Processing Systems 17*, pages 513–520, Cambridge, MA, 2005. MIT Press.

[8] T. Hastie and R. Tibshirani. Discriminant adaptive nearest neighbor classification. *IEEE Transactions on Pattern Analysis and Machine Intelligence (PAMI)*, 18:607–616, 1996.

[9] Y. LeCun, L. Jackel, L. Bottou, A. Brunot, C. Cortes, J. Denker, H. Drucker, I. Guyon, U. Muller, E. Sackinger, P. Simard, and V. Vapnik. A comparison of learning algorithms for handwritten digit recognition. In F.Fogelman and P.Gallinari, editors, *Proceedings of the 1995 International Conference on Artificial Neural Networks (ICANN-95)*, pages 53–60, Paris, 1995.

[10] A. K. McCallum. Bow: A toolkit for statistical language modeling, text retrieval, classification and clustering. http://www.cs.cmu.edu/ mccallum/bow, 1996.

[11] B. Schölkopf and A. J. Smola. *Learning with Kernels: Support Vector Machines, Regularization, Optimization, and Beyond*. MIT Press, Cambridge, MA, 2002.

[12] S. Shalev-Shwartz, Y. Singer, and A. Y. Ng. Online and batch learning of pseudo-metrics. In *Proceedings of the 21st International Conference on Machine Learning*, Banff, Canada, 2004.

[13] N. Shental, T. Hertz, D. Weinshall, and M. Pavel. Adjustment learning and relevant component analysis. In *Proceedings of the Seventh European Conference on Computer Vision (ECCV-02)*, volume 4, pages 776–792, London, UK, 2002. Springer-Verlag.

[14] P. Y. Simard, Y. LeCun, and J. Decker. Efficient pattern recognition using a new transformation distance. In *Advances in Neural Information Processing Systems*, volume 6, pages 50–58, San Mateo, CA, 1993. Morgan Kaufman.

[15] M. Turk and A. Pentland. Eigenfaces for recognition. *Journal of Cognitive Neuroscience*, 3(1):71–86, 1991.

[16] L. Vandenberghe and S. P. Boyd. Semidefinite programming. *SIAM Review*, 38(1):49–95, March 1996.

[17] E. P. Xing, A. Y. Ng, M. I. Jordan, and S. Russell. Distance metric learning, with application to clustering with side-information. In T. G. Dietterich, S. Becker, and Z. Ghahramani, editors, *Advances in Neural Information Processing Systems 14*, Cambridge, MA, 2002. MIT Press.

Analyzing Auditory Neurons by Learning Distance Functions

Inna Weiner[1]   Tomer Hertz[1,2]   Israel Nelken[2,3]   Daphna Weinshall[1,2]

[1]School of Computer Science and Engineering,
[2]The Center for Neural Computation, [3]Department of Neurobiology,
The Hebrew University of Jerusalem, Jerusalem, Israel, 91904
`weinerin,tomboy,daphna@cs.huji.ac.il,israel@md.huji.ac.il`

Abstract

We present a novel approach to the characterization of complex sensory neurons. One of the main goals of characterizing sensory neurons is to characterize dimensions in stimulus space to which the neurons are highly sensitive (causing large gradients in the neural responses) or alternatively dimensions in stimulus space to which the neuronal response are invariant (defining iso-response manifolds). We formulate this problem as that of learning a geometry on stimulus space that is compatible with the neural responses: the distance between stimuli should be large when the responses they evoke are very different, and small when the responses they evoke are similar. Here we show how to successfully train such distance functions using rather limited amount of information. The data consisted of the responses of neurons in primary auditory cortex (A1) of anesthetized cats to 32 stimuli derived from natural sounds. For each neuron, a subset of all pairs of stimuli was selected such that the responses of the two stimuli in a pair were either very similar or very dissimilar. The distance function was trained to fit these constraints. The resulting distance functions generalized to predict the distances between the responses of a test stimulus and the trained stimuli.

1 Introduction

A major challenge in auditory neuroscience is to understand how cortical neurons represent the acoustic environment. Neural responses to complex sounds are idiosyncratic, and small perturbations in the stimuli may give rise to large changes in the responses. Furthermore, different neurons, even with similar frequency response areas, may respond very differently to the same set of stimuli. The dominant approach to the functional characterization of sensory neurons attempts to predict the response of the cortical neuron to a novel stimulus. Prediction is usually estimated from a set of known responses of a given neuron to a set of stimuli (sounds). The most popular approach computes the spectrotemporal receptive field (STRF) of each neuron, and uses this linear model to predict neuronal responses. However, STRFs have been recently shown to have low predictive power [10, 14].

In this paper we take a different approach to the characterization of auditory cortical neurons. Our approach attempts to learn the non-linear warping of stimulus space that is induced by the neuronal responses. This approach is motivated by our previous observations [3] that different neurons impose different partitions of the stimulus space, which are not necessarily simply related to the spectro-temporal structure of the stimuli. More specifically, we characterize a neuron by learning a pairwise distance function over the stimulus domain that will be consistent with the similarities between the responses to different stimuli, see Section 2. Intuitively a good distance function would assign small values to pairs of stimuli that elicit a similar neuronal response, and large values to pairs of stimuli that elicit different neuronal responses.

This approach has a number of potential advantages: First, it allows us to aggregate information from a number of neurons, in order to learn a good distance function even when the number of known stimuli responses per neuron is small, which is a typical concern in the domain of neuronal characterization. Second, unlike most functional characterizations that are limited to linear or weakly non-linear models, distance learning can approximate functions that are highly non-linear. Finally, we explicitly learn a distance function on stimulus space; by examining the properties of such a function, it may be possible to determine the stimulus features that most strongly influence the responses of a cortical neuron. While this information is also implicitly incorporated into functional characterizations such as the STRF, it is much more explicit in our new formulation.

In this paper we therefore focus on two questions: (1) Can we learn distance functions over the stimulus domain for single cells using information extracted from their neuronal responses?? and (2) What is the predictive power of these cell specific distance functions when presented with novel stimuli? In order to address these questions we used extracellular recordings from 22 cells in the auditory cortex of cats in response to natural bird chirps and some modified versions of these chirps [1]. To estimate the distance between responses, we used a normalized distance measure between the peri-stimulus time histograms of the responses to the different stimuli.

Our results, described in Section 4, show that we can learn compatible distance functions on the stimulus domain with relatively low training errors. This result is interesting by itself as a possible characterization of cortical auditory neurons, a goal which eluded many previous studies [3]. Using cross validation, we measure the test error (or predictive power) of our method, and report generalization power which is significantly higher than previously reported for natural stimuli [10]. We then show that performance can be further improved by learning a distance function using information from pairs of related neurons. Finally, we show better generalization performance for wide-band stimuli as compared to narrow-band stimuli. These latter two contributions may have some interesting biological implications regarding the nature of the computations done by auditory cortical neurons.

Related work   Recently, considerable attention has been focused on spectrotemporal receptive fields (STRFs) as characterizations of the function of auditory cortical neurons [8, 4, 2, 11, 16].   The STRF model is appealing in several respects: it is a conceptually simple model that provides a linear description of the neuron's behavior. It can be interpreted both as providing the neuron's most efficient stimulus (in the time-frequency domain), and also as the spectro-temporal impulse response of the neuron [10, 12]. Finally, STRFs can be efficiently estimated using simple algebraic techniques.

However, while there were initial hopes that STRFs would uncover relatively complex response properties of cortical neurons, several recent reports of large sets of STRFs of cortical neurons concluded that most STRFs are somewhat too simple [5], and that STRFs are typically rather sluggish in time, therefore missing the highly precise synchronization of some cortical neurons [11]. Furthermore, when STRFs are used to predict neuronal responses to natural stimuli they often fail to predict the correct responses [10, 6]. For example, in Machens et al. only 11% of the response power could be predicted by STRFs on average [10]. Similar results were also reported in [14], who found that STRF models account for only $18-40\%$ (on average) of the stimulus related power in auditory cortical neural responses to dynamic random chord stimuli. Various other studies have shown that there are significant and relevant non-linearities in auditory cortical responses to natural stimuli [13, 1, 9, 10]. Using natural sounds, Bar-Yosef et. al [1] have shown that auditory neurons are extremely sensitive to small perturbations in the (natural) acoustic context. Clearly, these non-linearities cannot be sufficiently explained using linear models such as the STRF.

2 Formalizing the problem as a distance learning problem

Our approach is based on the idea of learning a cell-specific distance function over the space of all possible stimuli, relying on partial information extracted from the neuronal responses of the cell. The initial data consists of stimuli and the resulting neural responses. We use the neuronal responses to identify pairs of stimuli to which the neuron responded similarly and pairs to which the neuron responded very differently. These pairs can be formally described by equivalence constraints. Equivalence constraints are relations between pairs of datapoints, which indicate whether the points in the pair belong to the same category or not. We term a constraint *positive* when they points are known to originate from the same class, and *negative* belong to different classes. In this setting the goal of the algorithm is to learn a distance function that attempts to comply with the equivalence constraints.

This formalism allows us to combine information from a number of cells to improve the resulting characterization. Specifically, we combine equivalence constraints gathered from pairs of cells which have similar responses, and train a single distance function for both cells. Our results demonstrate that this approach improves prediction results of the "weaker" cell, and almost always improves the result of the "stronger" cell in each pair. Another interesting result of this formalism is the ability to classify stimuli based on the responses of the total recorded cortical cell ensemble. For some stimuli, the predictive performance based on the learned inter-stimuli distance was very good, whereas for other stimuli it was rather poor. These differences were correlated with the acoustic structure of the stimuli, partitioning them into narrowband and wideband stimuli.

3 Methods

Experimental setup Extracellular recordings were made in primary auditory cortex of nine halothane-anesthetized cats. Anesthesia was induced by ketamine and xylazine and maintained with halothane (0.25-1.5%) in 70% N_2O using standard protocols authorized by the committee for animal care and ethics of the Hebrew University - Haddasah Medical School. Single neurons were recorded using metal microelectrodes and an online spike sorter (MSD, alpha-omega). All neurons were well separated. Penetrations were performed over the whole dorso-ventral extent of the appropriate frequency slab (between about 2 and 8 kHz). Stimuli were presented 20 times using sealed, calibrated earphones at 60-80 dB SPL, at the preferred aurality of the neurons as determined using broad-band noise bursts. Sounds were taken from the Cornell Laboratory of Ornithology and have been selected as in [1]. Four stimuli, each of length 60-100 ms, consisted of a main tonal component with frequency and amplitude modulation and of a background noise consisting of echoes and unrelated components. Each of these stimuli was further modified by separating the main tonal component from the noise, and by further separating the noise into echoes and background. All possible combinations of these components were used here, in addition to a stylized artificial version that lacked the amplitude modulation of the natural sound. In total, 8 versions of each stimulus were used, and therefore each neuron had a dataset consisting of 32 datapoints. For more detailed methods, see Bar-Yosef et al. [1].

Data representation   We used the first 60 ms of each stimulus. Each stimulus was represented using the first d real Cepstral coefficients. The real Cepstrum of a signal x was calculated by taking the natural logarithm of magnitude of the Fourier transform of x and then computing the inverse Fourier transform of the resulting sequence. In our experiments we used the first 21-30 coefficients. Neuronal responses were represented by creating Peri-Stimulus Time Histograms (PSTHs) using 20 repetitions recorded for each stimuli. Response duration was 100 ms.

Obtaining equivalence constraints over stimuli pairs   The distances between responses were measured using a normalized χ^2 distance measure. All responses to both stimuli (40 responses in total) were superimposed to generate a single high-resolution PSTH. Then, this PSTH was non-uniformly binned so that each bin contained at least 10 spikes. The same bins were then used to generate the PSTHs of the responses to the two stimuli separately. For similar responses, we would expect that on average each bin in these histograms would contain 5 spikes. Formally, let N denote the number of bins in each histogram, and let r_1^i, r_2^i denote the number of spikes in the i'th bin in each of the two histograms respectively. The distance between pairs of histograms is given by: $\chi^2(r_1^i, r_2^i) = \sum_{i=1}^{N} \frac{(r_1^i - r_2^i)^2}{(r_1^i + r_2^i)/2}/(N-1)$.

In order to identify pairs (or small groups) of similar responses, we computed the normalized χ^2 distance matrix over all pairs of responses, and used the complete-linkage algorithm to cluster the responses into $8 - 12$ clusters. All of the points in each cluster were marked as similar to one another, thus providing positive equivalence constraints. In order to obtain negative equivalence constraints, for each cluster c_i we used the $2 - 3$ furthest clusters from it to define negative constraints. All pairs, composed of a point from cluster c_i and another point from these distant clusters, were used as negative constraints.

Distance learning method   In this paper, we use the *DistBoost* algorithm [7], which is a semi-supervised boosting learning algorithm that learns a distance function using unlabeled datapoints and equivalence constraints. The algorithm boosts weak learners which are soft partitions of the input space, that are computed using the constrained Expectation-Maximization (cEM) algorithm [15]. The *DistBoost* algorithm, which is briefly summarized in 1, has been previously used in several different applications and has been shown to perform well [7, 17].

Evaluation methods   In order to evaluate the quality of the learned distance function, we measured the correlation between the distances computed by our distance learning algorithm to those induced by the χ^2 distance over the responses. For each stimulus we measured the distances to all other stimuli using the learnt distance function. We then computed the rank-order (Spearman) correlation coefficient between these learnt distances in the stimulus domain and the χ^2 distances between the appropriate responses. This procedure produced a single correlation coefficient for each of the 32 stimuli, and the average correlation coefficient across all stimuli was used as the overall performance measure.

Parameter selection   The following parameters of the *DistBoost* algorithm can be fine-tuned: (1) the input dimensionality $d = 21$-30, (2) the number of Gaussian models in each weak learner $M = 2$-4, (3) the number of clusters used to extract equivalence constraints $C = 8$-12, and (4) the number of distant clusters used to define negative constraints $numAnti = 2$-3. Optimal parameters were determined separately for each of the 22 cells, based *solely* on the training data. Specifically, in the cross-validation testing we used a validation paradigm: Using the 31 training stimuli, we removed an additional datapoint and trained our algorithm on the remaining 30 points. We then validated its performance using the left out datapoint. The optimal cell specific parameters were determined using this approach.

Algorithm 1 The *DistBoost* Algorithm

Input:

Data points: $(x_1, ..., x_n)$, $x_k \in \mathcal{X}$

A set of equivalence constraints: (x_{i_1}, x_{i_2}, y_i), where $y_i \in \{-1, 1\}$

Unlabeled pairs of points: $(x_{i_1}, x_{i_2}, y_i = *)$, implicitly defined by all unconstrained pairs of points

- Initialize $W^1_{i_1 i_2} = 1/(n^2)$ $i_1, i_2 = 1, \ldots, n$ (weights over pairs of points)
  $w_k = 1/n$ $k = 1, \ldots, n$ (weights over data points)

- For $t = 1, .., T$

  1. Fit a constrained GMM (weak learner) on weighted data points in $\mathcal{X}$ using the equivalence constraints.

  2. Generate a weak hypothesis $\tilde{h}_t : \mathcal{X} \times \mathcal{X} \rightarrow [-1, 1]$ and define a weak distance function as $h_t(x_i, x_j) = \frac{1}{2} \left(1 - \tilde{h}_t(x_i, x_j) \right) \in [0, 1]$

  3. Compute $r_t = \sum_{(x_{i_1}, x_{i_2}, y_i = \pm 1)} W^t_{i_1 i_2} y_i h_t(x_{i_1}, x_{i_2})$, only over **labeled** pairs. Accept the current hypothesis only if $r_t > 0$.

  4. Choose the hypothesis weight $\alpha_t = \frac{1}{2} \ln(\frac{1 + r_t}{1 - r_t})$

  5. Update the weights of **all** points in $\mathcal{X} \times \mathcal{X}$ as follows:

$$W^{t+1}_{i_1 i_2} = \begin{cases} W^t_{i_1 i_2} \exp(-\alpha_t y_i \tilde{h}_t(x_{i_1}, x_{i_2})) & y_i \in \{-1, 1\} \\ W^t_{i_1 i_2} \exp(-\alpha_t) & y_i = * \end{cases}$$

  6. Normalize: $W^{t+1}_{i_1 i_2} = \dfrac{W^{t+1}_{i_1 i_2}}{\sum\limits_{i_1, i_2 = 1}^{n} W^{t+1}_{i_1 i_2}}$

  7. Translate the weights from $\mathcal{X} \times \mathcal{X}$ to $\mathcal{X}$: $w^{t+1}_k = \sum_j W^{t+1}_{kj}$

Output: A final distance function $\mathcal{D}(x_i, x_j) = \sum_{t=1}^{T} \alpha_t h_t(x_i, x_j)$

4 Results

Cell-specific distance functions We begin our analysis with an evaluation of the fitting power of the method, by training with the entire set of 32 stimuli (see Fig. 1). In general almost all of the correlation values are positive and they are quite high. The average correlation over all cells is 0.58 with $ste = 0.023$.

In order to evaluate the generalization potential of our approach, we used a Leave-One-Out (LOU) cross-validation paradigm. In each run, we removed a single stimulus from the dataset, trained our algorithm on the remaining 31 stimuli, and then tested its performance on the datapoint that was left out (see Fig. 3). In each histogram we plot the test correlations of a single cell, obtained when using the LOU paradigm over all of the 32 stimuli. As can be seen, on some cells our algorithm obtains correlations that are as high as 0.41, while for other cells the average test correlation is less then 0.1. The average correlation over all cells is 0.26 with $ste = 0.019$.

Not surprisingly, the train results (Fig. 1) are better than the test results (Fig. 3). Interestingly, however, we found that there was a significant correlation between the training performance and the test performance $C = 0.57, p < 0.05$ (see Fig. 2, left).

Boosting the performance of weak cells In order to boost the performance of cells with low average correlations, we constructed the following experiment: We clustered the responses of each cell, using the complete-linkage algorithm over the χ^2 distances with 4 clusters. We then used the $F_{\frac{1}{2}}$ score that evaluates how well two clustering partitions are in agreement with one another ($F_{\frac{1}{2}} = \frac{2 * P * R}{P + R}$, where P denotes precision and R denotes recall.). This measure was used to identify pairs of cells whose partition of the stimuli was most similar to each other. In our experiment we took the four cells with the lowest

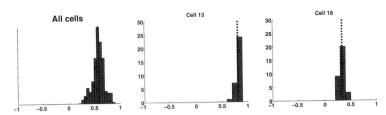

Figure 1: Left: Histogram of train rank-order correlations on the entire ensemble of cells. The rank-order correlations were computed between the learnt distances and the distances between the recorded responses for each single stimulus ($N = 22 * 32$). Center: train correlations for a "strong" cell. Right: train correlations for a "weak" cell. Dotted lines represent average values.

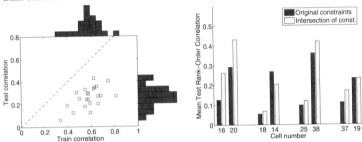

Figure 2: Left: Train vs. test cell specific correlations. Each point marks the average correlation of a single cell. The correlation between train and test is 0.57 with $p = 0.05$. The distribution of train and test correlations is displayed as histograms on the top and on the right respectively. Right: Test rank-order correlations when training using constraints extracted from each cell separately, and when using the intersection of the constraints extracted from a pair of cells. This procedure always improves the performance of the weaker cell, and usually also improves the performance of the stronger cell

performance (right column of Fig 3), and for each of them used the $F_{\frac{1}{2}}$ score to retrieve the most similar cell. For each of these pairs, we trained our algorithm once more, using the constraints obtained by intersecting the constraints derived from the two cells in the pair, in the LOU paradigm. The results can be seen on the right plot in Fig 2. On all four cells, this procedure improved LOUT test results. Interestingly and counter-intuitively, when training the better performing cell in each pair using the intersection of its constraints with those from the poorly performing cell, results deteriorated only for one of the four better performing cells.

Stimulus classification   The cross-validation results induced a partition of the stimulus space into narrowband and wideband stimuli. We measured the predictability of each stimulus by averaging the LOU test results obtained for the stimulus across all cells (see Fig. 4). Our analysis shows that wideband stimuli are more predictable than narrowband stimuli, despite the fact that the neuronal responses to these two groups are not different as a whole. Whereas the non-linearity in the interactions between narrowband and wideband stimuli has already been noted before [9], here we further refine this observation by demonstrating a significant difference between the behavior of narrow and wideband stimuli with respect to the predictability of the similarity between their responses.

5   Discussion

In the standard approach to auditory modeling, a linear or weakly non-linear model is fitted to the data, and neuronal properties are read from the resulting model. The usefulness of this approach is limited however by the weak predictability of A1 responses when using such models. In order to overcome this limitation, we reformulated the problem of char-

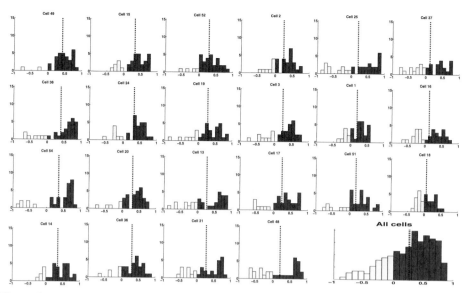

Figure 3: Histograms of cell specific test rank-order correlations for the 22 cells in the dataset. The rank-order correlations compare the predicted distances to the distances between the recorded responses, measured on a single stimulus which was left out during the training stage. For visualization purposes, cells are ordered (columns) by their average test correlation per stimulus in descending order. Negative correlations are in yellow, positive in blue.

acterizing neuronal responses of highly non-linear neurons. We use the neural data as a guide for training a highly non-linear distance function on stimulus space, which is compatible with the neural responses. The main result of this paper is the demonstration of the feasibility of this approach.

Two further results underscore the usefulness of the new formulation. First, we demonstrated that we can improve the test performance of a distance function by using constraints on the similarity or dissimilarity between stimuli derived from the responses of multiple neurons. Whereas we expected this manipulation to improve the test performance of the algorithm on the responses of neurons that were initially poorly predicted, we found that it actually improved the performance of the algorithm also on neurons that were rather well predicted, although we paired them with neurons that were poorly predicted. Thus, it is possible that intersecting constraints derived from multiple neurons uncover regularities that are hard to extract from individual neurons.

Second, it turned out that some stimuli consistently behaved better than others across the neuronal population. This difference was correlated with the acoustic structure of the stimuli: those stimuli that contained the weak background component (wideband stimuli) were generally predicted better. This result is surprising both because background component is substantially weaker than the other acoustic components in the stimuli (by as much as 35-40 dB). It may mean that the relationships between physical structure (as characterized by the Cepstral parameters) and the neuronal responses becomes simpler in the presence of the background component, but is much more idiosyncratic when this component is absent. This result underscores the importance of interactions between narrow and wideband stimuli for understanding the complexity of cortical processing.

The algorithm is fast enough to be used in near real-time. It can therefore be used to guide real experiments. One major problem during an experiment is that of stimulus selection: choosing the best set of stimuli for characterizing the responses of a neuron. The distance functions trained here can be used to direct this process. For example, they can be used to

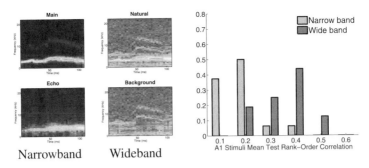

Narrowband   Wideband

Figure 4: Left: spectrograms of input stimuli, which are four different versions of a single natural bird chirp. Right: Stimuli specific correlation values averaged over the entire ensemble of cells. The predictability of wideband stimuli is clearly better than that of the narrowband stimuli.

find surprising stimuli: either stimuli that are very different in terms of physical structure but that would result in responses that are similar to those already measured, or stimuli that are very similar to already tested stimuli but that are predicted to give rise to very different responses.

References

[1] O. Bar-Yosef, Y. Rotman, and I. Nelken. Responses of Neurons in Cat Primary Auditory Cortex to Bird Chirps: Effects of Temporal and Spectral Context. *J. Neurosci.*, 22(19):8619–8632, 2002.

[2] D. T. Blake and M. M. Merzenich. Changes of AI Receptive Fields With Sound Density. *J Neurophysiol*, 88(6):3409–3420, 2002.

[3] G. Chechik, A. Globerson, M.J. Anderson, E.D. Young, I. Nelken, and N. Tishby. Group redundancy measures reveal redundancy reduction in the auditory pathway. In *NIPS*, 2002.

[4] R. C. deCharms, D. T. Blake, and M. M. Merzenich. Optimizing Sound Features for Cortical Neurons. *Science*, 280(5368):1439–1444, 1998.

[5] D. A. Depireux, J. Z. Simon, D. J. Klein, and S. A. Shamma. Spectro-Temporal Response Field Characterization With Dynamic Ripples in Ferret Primary Auditory Cortex. *J Neurophysiol*, 85(3):1220–1234, 2001.

[6] J. J. Eggermont, P. M. Johannesma, and A. M. Aertsen. Reverse-correlation methods in auditory research. *Q Rev Biophys.*, 16(3):341–414, 1983.

[7] T. Hertz, A. Bar-Hillel, and D. Weinshall. Boosting margin based distance functions for clustering. In *ICML*, 2004.

[8] N. Kowalski, D. A. Depireux, and S. A. Shamma. Analysis of dynamic spectra in ferret primary auditory cortex. I. Characteristics of single-unit responses to moving ripple spectra. *J Neurophysiol*, 76(5):3503–3523, 1996.

[9] L. Las, E. A. Stern, and I. Nelken. Representation of Tone in Fluctuating Maskers in the Ascending Auditory System. *J. Neurosci.*, 25(6):1503–1513, 2005.

[10] C. K. Machens, M. S. Wehr, and A. M. Zador. Linearity of Cortical Receptive Fields Measured with Natural Sounds. *J. Neurosci.*, 24(5):1089–1100, 2004.

[11] L. M. Miller, M. A. Escabi, H. L. Read, and C. E. Schreiner. Spectrotemporal Receptive Fields in the Lemniscal Auditory Thalamus and Cortex. *J Neurophysiol*, 87(1):516–527, 2002.

[12] I. Nelken. Processing of complex stimuli and natural scenes in the auditory cortex. *Current Opinion in Neurobiology*, 14(4):474–480, 2004.

[13] Y. Rotman, O. Bar-Yosef, and I. Nelken. Relating cluster and population responses to natural sounds and tonal stimuli in cat primary auditory cortex. *Hearing Research*, 152(1-2):110–127, 2001.

[14] M. Sahani and J. F. Linden. How linear are auditory cortical responses? In *NIPS*, 2003.

[15] N. Shental, A. Bar-Hilel, T. Hertz, and D. Weinshall. Computing Gaussian mixture models with EM using equivalence constraints. In *NIPS*, 2003.

[16] F. E. Theunissen, K. Sen, and A. J. Doupe. Spectral-Temporal Receptive Fields of Nonlinear Auditory Neurons Obtained Using Natural Sounds. *J. Neurosci.*, 20(6):2315–2331, 2000.

[17] C. Yanover and T. Hertz. Predicting protein-peptide binding affinity by learning peptide-peptide distance functions. In *RECOMB*, 2005.

Oblivious Equilibrium: A Mean Field Approximation for Large-Scale Dynamic Games

Gabriel Y. Weintraub, Lanier Benkard, and Benjamin Van Roy
Stanford University
{gweintra,lanierb,bvr}@stanford.edu

Abstract

We propose a mean-field approximation that dramatically reduces the computational complexity of solving stochastic dynamic games. We provide conditions that guarantee our method approximates an equilibrium as the number of agents grow. We then derive a performance bound to assess how well the approximation performs for any given number of agents. We apply our method to an important class of problems in applied microeconomics. We show with numerical experiments that we are able to greatly expand the set of economic problems that can be analyzed computationally.

1 Introduction

In this paper we consider a class of infinite horizon non-zero sum stochastic dynamic games. At each period of time, each agent has a given state and can make a decision. These decisions together with random shocks determine the evolution of the agents' states. Additionally, agents receive profits depending on the current states and decisions. There is a literature on such models which focusses on computation of Markov perfect equilibria (MPE) using dynamic programming algorithms. A major shortcoming of, however, is the computational complexity associated with solving for the MPE. When there are more than a few agents participating in the game and/or more than a few states per agent, the curse of dimensionality renders dynamic programming algorithms intractable.

In this paper we consider a class of stochastic dynamic games where the state of an agent captures its competitive advantage. Our main motivation is to consider an important class of models in applied economics, namely, dynamic industry models of imperfect competition. However, we believe our methods can be useful in other contexts as well. To clarify the type of models we consider, let us describe a specific example of a dynamic industry model. Consider an industry where a group of firms can invest to improve the quality of their products over time. The state of a given firm represents its quality level. The evolution of quality is determined by investment and random shocks. Finally, at every period, given their qualities, firms compete in the product market and receive profits. Many real world industries where, for example, firms invest in R&D or advertising are well described by this model.

In this context, we propose a mean-field approximation approach that dramatically simplifies the computational complexity of stochastic dynamic games. We propose a simple algorithm for computing an "oblivious" equilibrium in which each agent is assumed to make decisions based only on its own state and knowledge of the long run equilibrium distribution of states, but where agents ignore current information about rivals' states. We prove that, if the distribution of agents obeys a certain "light-tail" condition, when the number of agents becomes large the oblivious equilibrium approximates a MPE. We then derive an error bound that is simple to compute to assess how well the approximation performs for any given number of agents.

We apply our method to analyze dynamic industry models of imperfect competition. We conduct numerical experiments that show that our method works well when there are several hundred firms, and sometimes even tens of firms. Our method, which uses simple code that runs in a couple of minutes on a laptop computer, greatly expands the set of economic problems that can be analyzed computationally.

2 A Stochastic Dynamic Game

In this section, we formulate a non-zero sum stochastic dynamic game. The system evolves over discrete time periods and an infinite horizon. We index time periods with nonnegative integers $t \in \mathbb{N}$ ($\mathbb{N} = \{0, 1, 2, \ldots\}$). All random variables are defined on a probability space $(\Omega, \mathcal{F}, \mathcal{P})$ equipped with a filtration $\{\mathcal{F}_t : t \geq 0\}$. We adopt a convention of indexing by t variables that are $\mathcal{F}_t$-measurable.

There are n agents indexed by $S = \{1, \ldots, n\}$. The state of each agent captures its ability to compete in the environment. At time t, the state of agent $i \in S$ is denoted by $x_{it} \in \mathbb{N}$. We define the *system state* s_t to be a vector over individual states that specifies, for each state $x \in \mathbb{N}$, the number of agents at state x in period t. We define the state space $\overline{S} = \left\{ s \in \mathbb{N}^\infty \middle| \sum_{x=0}^\infty s(x) = n \right\}$. For each $i \in S$, we define $s_{-i,t} \in \overline{S}$ to be the state of the *competitors* of agent i; that is, $s_{-i,t}(x) = s_t(x) - 1$ if $x_{it} = x$, and $s_{-i,t}(x) = s_t(x)$, otherwise.

In each period, each agent earns profits. An agent's single period expected profit $\pi_m(x_{it}, s_{-i,t})$ depends on its state x_{it}, its competitors' state $s_{-i,t}$ and a parameter $m \in \Re_+$. For example, in the context of an industry model, m could represent the total number of consumers, that is, the size of the pie to be divided among all agents. We assume that for all $x \in \mathbb{N}$, $s \in S$, $m \in \Re_+$, $\pi_m(x, s) > 0$ and is increasing in x. Hence, agents in larger states earn more profits.

In each period, each agent makes a decision. We interpret this decision as an investment to improve the state at the next period. If an agent invests $\mu_{it} \in \Re_+$, then the agent's state at time $t + 1$ is given by, $x_{i,t+1} = x_{it} + w(\mu_{it}, \zeta_{i,t+1})$, where the function w captures the impact of investment on the state and $\zeta_{i,t+1}$ reflects uncertainty in the outcome of investment. For example, in the context of an industry model, uncertainty may arise due to the risk associated with a research endeavor or a marketing campaign. We assume that for all ζ, $w(\mu, \zeta)$ is nondecreasing in μ. Hence, if the amount invested is larger it is more likely the agent will transit next period to a better state. The random variables $\{\zeta_{it} | t \geq 0, i \geq 1\}$ are i.i.d.. We denote the unit cost of investment by d.

Each agent aims to maximize expected net present value. The interest rate is assumed to be positive and constant over time, resulting in a constant discount factor of $\beta \in (0, 1)$ per time period. The equilibrium concept we will use builds on the notion of a Markov perfect equilibrium (MPE), in the sense of [3]. We further assume that equilibrium is symmetric, such that all agents use a common stationary strategy. In particular, there is a function μ such that at each time t, each agent $i \in S$ makes a decision $\mu_{it} = \mu(x_{it}, s_{-i,t})$. Let $\mathcal{M}$ denote the set of strategies such that an element $\mu \in \mathcal{M}$ is a function $\mu : \mathbb{N} \times S \to \Re_+$.

We define the value function $V(x, s|\mu', \mu)$ to be the expected net present value for an agent at state x when its competitors' state is s, given that its competitors each follows a common strategy $\mu \in \mathcal{M}$, and the agent itself follows strategy $\mu' \in \mathcal{M}$. In particular,

$$V(x, s|\mu', \mu) = E_{\mu', \mu} \left[\sum_{k=t}^{\infty} \beta^{k-t} \left(\pi(x_{ik}, s_{-i,k}) - d\iota_{ik} \right) \bigg| x_{it} = x, s_{-i,t} = s \right],$$

where i is taken to be the index of an agent at state x at time t, and the subscripts of the expectation indicate the strategy followed by agent i and the strategy followed by its competitors. In an abuse of notation, we will use the shorthand, $V(x, s|\mu) \equiv V(x, s|\mu, \mu)$, to refer to the expected discounted value of profits when agent i follows the same strategy μ as its competitors.

An equilibrium to our model comprises a strategy $\mu \in \mathcal{M}$ that satisfy the following condition:

$$(2.1) \qquad \sup_{\mu' \in \mathcal{M}} V(x, s|\mu', \mu) = V(x, s|\mu) \qquad \forall x \in \mathbb{N}, \forall s \in \overline{\mathcal{S}}.$$

Under some technical conditions, one can establish existence of an equilibrium in pure strategies [4]. With respect to uniqueness, in general we presume that our model may have multiple equilibria. Dynamic programming algorithms can be used to optimize agent strategies, and equilibria to our model can be computed via their iterative application. However, these algorithms require compute time and memory that grow proportionately with the number of relevant system states, which is often intractable in contexts of practical interest. This difficulty motivates our alternative approach.

3 Oblivious Equilibrium

We will propose a method for approximating MPE based on the idea that when there are a large number of agents, simultaneous changes in individual agent states can average out because of a law of large numbers such that the normalized system state remains roughly constant over time. In this setting, each agent can potentially make near-optimal decisions based only on its own state and the long run average system state. With this motivation, we consider restricting agent strategies so that each agent's decisions depend only on the agent's state. We call such restricted strategies *oblivious* since they involve decisions made without full knowledge of the circumstances — in particular, the state of the system. Let $\tilde{\mathcal{M}} \subset \mathcal{M}$ denote the set of oblivious strategies. Since each strategy $\mu \in \tilde{\mathcal{M}}$ generates decisions $\mu(x, s)$ that do not depend on s, with some abuse of notation, we will often drop the second argument and write $\mu(x)$.

Let $\tilde{s}_\mu$ be the long-run expected system state when all agents use an oblivious strategy $\mu \in \tilde{\mathcal{M}}$. For an oblivious strategy $\mu \in \tilde{\mathcal{M}}$ we define an *oblivious value function*

$$\tilde{V}(x|\mu', \mu) = E_{\mu'} \left[\sum_{k=t}^{\infty} \beta^{k-t} \left(\pi(x_{ik}, \tilde{s}_\mu) - d\iota_{ik} \right) \bigg| x_{it} = x \right].$$

This value function should be interpreted as the expected net present value of an agent that is at state x and follows oblivious strategy μ', under the assumption that its competitors' state will be $\tilde{s}_\mu$ for all time. Again, we abuse notation by using $\tilde{V}(x|\mu) \equiv \tilde{V}(x|\mu, \mu)$ to refer to the oblivious value function when agent i follows the same strategy μ as its competitors.

We now define a new solution concept: an *oblivious equilibrium* consists of a strategy $\mu \in \tilde{\mathcal{M}}$ that satisfy the following condition:

$$(3.1) \qquad \sup_{\mu' \in \tilde{\mathcal{M}}} \tilde{V}(x|\mu', \mu) = \tilde{V}(x|\mu), \qquad \forall x \in \mathbb{N}.$$

In an oblivious equilibrium firms optimize an oblivious value function assuming that its competitors' state will be $\tilde{s}_\mu$ for all time. The optimal strategy obtained must be μ. It is straightforward to show that an oblivious equilibrium exists under mild technical conditions. With respect to uniqueness, we have been unable to find multiple oblivious equilibria in any of the applied problems we have considered, but similarly with the case of MPE, we have no reason to believe that in general there is a unique oblivious equilibrium.

4   Asymptotic Results

In this section, we establish asymptotic results that provide conditions under which oblivious equilibria offer close approximations to MPE as the number of agents, n, grow. We consider a sequence of systems indexed by the one period profit parameter m and we assume that the number of agents in system m is given by $n^{(m)} = am$, for some $a > 0$. Recall that m represents, for example, the total pie to be divided by the agents so it is reasonable to increase $n^{(m)}$ and m at the same rate.

We index functions and random variables associated with system m with a superscript (m). From this point onward we let $\tilde{\mu}^{(m)}$ denote an oblivious equilibrium for system m. Let $V^{(m)}$ and $\tilde{V}^{(m)}$ represent the value function and oblivious value function, respectively, when the system is m. To further abbreviate notation we denote the expected system state associated with $\tilde{\mu}^{(m)}$ by $\tilde{s}^{(m)} \equiv \tilde{s}_{\tilde{\mu}^{(m)}}$. The random variable $s_t^{(m)}$ denotes the system state at time t when every agent uses strategy $\tilde{\mu}^{(m)}$. We denote the invariant distribution of $\{s_t^{(m)} : t \geq 0\}$ by $q^{(m)}$. In order to simplify our analysis, we assume that the initial system state $s_0^{(m)}$ is sampled from $q^{(m)}$. Hence, $s_t^{(m)}$ is a stationary process; $s_t^{(m)}$ is distributed according to $q^{(m)}$ for all $t \geq 0$. It will be helpful to decompose $s_t^{(m)}$ according to $s_t^{(m)} = f_t^{(m)} n^{(m)}$, where $f_t^{(m)}$ is the random vector that represents the fraction of agents in each state. Similarly, let $\tilde{f}^{(m)} \equiv E[f_t^{(m)}]$ denote the expected fraction of agents in each state. With some abuse of notation, we define $\pi_m(x_{it}, f_{-i,t}, n) \equiv \pi_m(x_{it}, n \cdot f_{-i,t})$. We assume that for all $x \in \mathbb{N}$, $f \in \mathcal{S}_1$, $\pi_m(x, f, n^{(m)}) = \Theta(1)$, where $\mathcal{S}_1 = \{f \in \Re_+^\infty | \sum_{x \in \mathbb{N}} f(x) = 1\}$. If m and $n^{(m)}$ grow at the same rate, one period profits remain positive and bounded.

Our aim is to establish that, under certain conditions, oblivious equilibria well-approximate MPE as m grows. We define the following concept to formalize the sense in which this approximation becomes exact.

Definition 4.1. *A sequence* $\tilde{\mu}^{(m)} \in \mathcal{M}$ *possesses the asymptotic Markov equilibrium (AME) property if for all* $x \in \mathbb{N}$,

$$\lim_{m \to \infty} E_{\tilde{\mu}^{(m)}} \left[\sup_{\mu' \in \mathcal{M}} V^{(m)}(x, s_t^{(m)} | \mu', \tilde{\mu}^{(m)}) - V^{(m)}(x, s_t^{(m)} | \tilde{\mu}^{(m)}) \right] = 0 \,.$$

The definition of AME assesses approximation error at each agent state x in terms of the amount by which an agent at state x can increase its expected net present value by deviating from the oblivious equilibrium strategy $\tilde{\mu}^{(m)}$, and instead following an optimal (non-oblivious) best response that keeps track of the true system state. The system states are averaged according to the invariant distribution.

It may seem that the AME property is always obtained because $n^{(m)}$ is growing to infinity. However, recall that each agent state reflects its competitive advantage and if there are agents that are too "dominant" this is not necessarily the case. To make this idea more concrete, let us go back to our industry example where firms invest in quality. Even when there are a large number of firms, if the market tends to be concentrated — for example, if the market is usually dominated by a single firm with a an extremely high quality —

the AME property is unlikely to hold. To ensure the AME property, we need to impose a "light-tail" condition that rules out this kind of domination.

Note that $\frac{d \ln \pi_m(y, f, n)}{df(x)}$ is the semi-elasticity of one period profits with respect to the fraction of agents in state x. We define the *maximal absolute semi-elasticity function*:

$$g(x) = \max_{m \in \Re_+, y \in \mathbb{N}, f \in \mathcal{S}_1, n \in \mathbb{N}} \left| \frac{d \ln \pi_m(y, f, n)}{df(x)} \right|.$$

For each x, $g(x)$ is the maximum rate of relative change of any agent's single-period profit that could result from a small change in the fraction of agents at state x. Since larger competitors tend to have greater influence on agent profits, $g(x)$ typically increases with x, and can be unbounded.

Finally, we introduce our light-tail condition. For each m, let $\tilde{x}^{(m)} \sim \tilde{f}^{(m)}$, that is, $\tilde{x}^{(m)}$ is a random variable with probability mass function $\tilde{f}^{(m)}$. $\tilde{x}^{(m)}$ can be interpreted as the state of an agent that is randomly sampled from among all agents while the system state is distributed according to its invariant distribution.

Assumption 4.1. *For all states x, $g(x) < \infty$. For all $\epsilon > 0$, there exists a state z such that*

$$E \left[g(\tilde{x}^{(m)}) \mathbf{1}_{\{\tilde{x}^{(m)} > z\}} \right] \le \epsilon,$$

for all m.

Put simply, the light tail condition requires that states where a small change in the fraction of agents has a large impact on the profits of other agents, must have a small probability under the invariant distribution. In the previous example of an industry where firms invest in quality this typically means that very large firms (and hence high concentration) rarely occur under the invariant distribution.

Theorem 4.1. *Under Assumption 4.1 and some other regularity conditions[1], the sequence $\tilde{\mu}^{(m)}$ of oblivious equilibria possesses the AME property.*

5 Error Bounds

While the asymptotic results from Section 4 provide conditions under which the approximation will work well as the number of agents grows, in practice one would also like to know how the approximation performs for a particular system. For that purpose we derive performance bounds on the approximation error that are simple to compute via simulation and can be used to asses the accuracy of the approximation for a particular problem instance.

We consider a system m and to simplify notation we suppress the index m. Consider an oblivious strategy $\tilde{\mu}$. We will quantify approximation error at each agent state $x \in \mathbb{N}$ by $E \left[\sup_{\mu' \in \mathcal{M}} V(x, s_t | \mu', \tilde{\mu}) - V(x, s_t | \tilde{\mu}) \right]$. The expectation is over the invariant distribution of s_t. The next theorem provides a bound on the approximation error. Recall that $\tilde{s}$ is the long run expected state in oblivious equilibrium ($E[s_t]$). Let $a_x(y)$ be the expected discounted sum of an indicator of visits to state y for an agent starting at state x that uses strategy $\tilde{\mu}$.

Theorem 5.1. *For any oblivious equilibrium $\tilde{\mu}$ and state $x \in \mathbb{N}$,*

$$(5.1) \qquad E\left[\Delta V\right] \le \frac{1}{1 - \beta} E[\Delta \pi(s_t)] + \sum_{y \in \mathbb{N}} a_x(y) \left(\pi(y, \tilde{s}) - E\left[\pi(y, s_t)\right] \right),$$

---

[1]In particular, we require that the single period profit function is "smooth" as a function of its arguments. See [5] for details.

where $\Delta V = \sup_{\mu' \in \mathcal{M}} V(x, s_t | \mu', \tilde{\mu}) - V(x, s_t | \tilde{\mu})$ *and* $\Delta \pi(s) = \max_{y \in \mathbb{N}} (\pi(y, s) - \pi(y, \tilde{s}))$.

The error bound can be easily estimated via simulation algorithms. In particular, note that the bound is not a function of the true MPE or even of the optimal non-oblivious best response strategy.

6 Application: Industry Dynamics

Many problems in applied economics are dynamic in nature. For example, models involving the entry and exit of firms, collusion among firms, mergers, advertising, investment in R&D or capacity, network effects, durable goods, consumer learning, learning by doing, and transaction or adjustment costs are inherently dynamic. [1] (hereafter EP) introduced an approach to modeling industry dynamics. See [6] for an overview. Computational complexity has been a limiting factor in the use of this modeling approach. In this section we use our method to expand the set of dynamic industries that can be analyzed computationally.

Even though our results apply to more general models where for example firms make exit and entry decisions, here we consider a particular case of an EP model which itself is a particular case of the model introduced in Section 2. We consider a model of a single-good industry with quality differentiation. The agents are firms that can invest to improve the quality of their product over time. In particular x_{it} is the quality level of firm i at time t. μ_{it} represents represents the amount of money invested by firm i at time t to improve its quality. We assume the one period profit function is derived from a logit demand system and where firms compete setting prices. In this case, m represents the market size. See [5] for more details about the model.

6.1 Computational Experiments

In this section, we discuss computational results that demonstrate how our approximation method significantly expands the range of relevant EP-type models like the one previously introduced that can be studied computationally.

First, we propose an algorithm to compute oblivious equilibrium [5]. Whether this algorithm is guaranteed to terminate in a finite number of iterations remains an open issue. However, in over 90% of the numerical experiments we present in this section, it converged in less than five minutes (and often much less than this). In the rest, it converged in less than fifteen minutes.

Our first set of results investigate the behavior of the approximation error bound under several different model specifications. A wide range of parameters for our model could reasonably represent different real world industries of interest. In practice the parameters would either be estimated using data from a particular industry or chosen to reflect an industry under study. We begin by investigating a particular set of representative parameter values. See [5] for the specifications.

For each set of parameters, we use the approximation error bound to compute an upper bound on the percentage error in the value function, $\frac{E[\sup_{\mu' \in \mathcal{M}} V(x, s | \mu', \tilde{\mu}) - V(x, s | \tilde{\mu})]}{E[V(x, s | \tilde{\mu})]}$, where $\tilde{\mu}$ is the OE strategy and the expectations are taken with respect to s. We estimate the expectations using simulation. We compute the previously mentioned percentage approximation error bound for different market sizes m and number of firms $n^{(m)}$. As the market size increases, the number of firms increases and the approximation error bound decreases.

In our computational experiments we found that the most important parameter affecting the approximation error bounds was the degree of vertical product differentiation, which indicates the importance consumers assign to product quality. In Figure 1 we present our results. When the parameter that measures the level of vertical differentiation is low the approximation error bound is less than 0.5% with just 5 firms, while when the parameter is high it is 5% for 5 firms, less than 3% with 40 firms, and less than 1% with 400 firms.

Figure 1: Percentage approximation error bound for fixed number of firms.

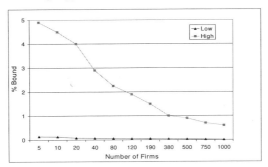

Most economic applications would involve from less than ten to several hundred firms. These results show that the approximation error bound may sometimes be small (<2%) in these cases, though this would depend on the model and parameter values for the industry under study.

Having gained some insight into what features of the model lead to low values of the approximation error bound, the question arises as to what value of the error bounds is required to obtain a good approximation. To shed light on this issue we compare long-run statistics for the same industry primitives under oblivious equilibrium and MPE strategies. A major constraint on this exercise is that it requires the ability to actually compute the MPE, so to keep computation manageable we use four firms here. We compare the average values of several economic statistics of interest under the oblivious equilibrium and the MPE invariant distributions. The quantities compared are: average investment, average producer surplus, average consumer surplus, average share of the largest firm, and average share of the largest two firms. We also computed the actual benefit from deviating and keeping track of the industry state (the actual difference $\frac{E[\sup_{\mu' \in \mathcal{M}} V(x,s|\mu',\tilde{\mu}) - V(x,s|\tilde{\mu})]}{E[V(x,s|\tilde{\mu})]}$). Note that the the latter quantity should always be smaller than the approximation error bound.

From the computational experiments we conclude the following (see [5] for a table with the results):

1. When the bound is less than 1% the long-run quantities estimated under oblivious equilibrium and MPE strategies are very close.

2. Performance of the approximation depends on the richness of the equilibrium investment process. Industries with a relatively low cost of investment tend to have a symmetric average distribution over quality levels reflecting a rich investment process. In this cases, when the bound is between 1-20%, the long-run quantities estimated under oblivious equilibrium and MPE strategies are still quite close. In industries with high investment cost the industry (system) state tends to be skewed, reflecting low levels of investment. When the bound is above 1% and there is little investment, the long-run quantities can be quite different on a percentage basis (5% to 20%), but still remain fairly close in absolute terms.

3. The performance bound is not tight. For a wide range of parameters the performance bound is as much as 10 to 20 times larger than the actual benefit from deviating.

The previous results suggest that MPE dynamics are well-approximated by oblivious equilibrium strategies when the approximation error bound is small (less than 1-2% and in some cases even up to 20 %). Our results demonstrate that the oblivious equilibrium approximation significantly expands the range of applied problems that can be analyzed computationally.

7 Conclusions and Future Research

The goal of this paper has been to increase the set of applied problems that can be addressed using stochastic dynamic games. Due to the curse of dimensionality, the applicability of these models has been severely limited. As an alternative, we proposed a method for approximating MPE behavior using an oblivious equilibrium, where agents make decisions only based on their own state and the long run average system state. We began by showing that the approximation works well asymptotically, where asymptotics were taken in the number of agents. We also introduced a simple algorithm to compute an oblivious equilibrium.

To facilitate using oblivious equilibrium in practice, we derived approximation error bounds that indicate how good the approximation is in any particular problem under study. These approximation error bounds are quite general and thus can be used in a wide class of models. We use our methods to analyze dynamic industry models of imperfect competition and showed that oblivious equilibrium often yields a good approximation of MPE behavior for industries with a couple hundred firms, and sometimes even with just tens of firms.

We have considered very simple strategies that are functions only of an agent's own state and the long run average system state. While our results show that these simple strategies work well in many cases, there remains a set of problems where exact computation is not possible and yet our approximation will not work well either. For such cases, our hope is that our methods will serve as a basis for developing better approximations that use additional information, such as the states of the dominant agents. Solving for equilibria of this type would be more difficult than solving for oblivious equilibria, but is still likely to be computationally feasible. Since showing that such an approach would provide a good approximation is not a simple extension of our results, this will be a subject of future research.

References

[1] R. Ericson and A. Pakes. Markov-perfect industry dynamics: A framework for empirical work. *Review of Economic Studies*, 62(1):53 – 82, 1995.

[2] R. L. Goettler, C. A. Parlour, and U. Rajan. Equilibrium in a dynamic limit order market. Forthcoming, Journal of Finance, 2004.

[3] E. Maskin and J. Tirole. A theory of dynamic oligopoly, I and II. *Econometrica*, 56(3):549 – 570, 1988.

[4] U. Doraszelski and M. Satterthwaite. Foundations of Markov-perfect industry dynamics: Existence, purification, and multiplicity. Working Paper, Hoover Institution, 2003.

[5] G. Y. Weintraub, C. L. Benkard, and B. Van Roy. Markov perfect industry dynamics with many firms. Submitted ofr publication, 2005.

[6] A. Pakes. A framework for applied dynamic analysis in i.o. NBER Working Paper 8024, 2000.

Active Bidirectional Coupling in a Cochlear Chip

Bo Wen and Kwabena Boahen
Department of Bioengineering
University of Pennsylvania
Philadelphia, PA 19104
{wenbo,boahen}@seas.upenn.edu

Abstract

We present a novel cochlear model implemented in analog very large scale integration (VLSI) technology that emulates nonlinear active cochlear behavior. This silicon cochlea includes outer hair cell (OHC) electromotility through active bidirectional coupling (ABC), a mechanism we proposed in which OHC motile forces, through the microanatomical organization of the organ of Corti, realize the cochlear amplifier. Our chip measurements demonstrate that frequency responses become larger and more sharply tuned when ABC is turned on; the degree of the enhancement decreases with input intensity as ABC includes saturation of OHC forces.

1 Silicon Cochleae

Cochlear models, mathematical and physical, with the shared goal of emulating nonlinear active cochlear behavior, shed light on how the cochlea works if based on cochlear micromechanics. Among the modeling efforts, silicon cochleae have promise in meeting the need for real-time performance and low power consumption. Lyon and Mead developed the first analog electronic cochlea [1], which employed a cascade of second-order filters with exponentially decreasing resonant frequencies. However, the cascade structure suffers from delay and noise accumulation and lacks fault-tolerance. Modeling the cochlea more faithfully, Watts built a two-dimensional (2D) passive cochlea that addressed these shortcomings by incorporating the cochlear fluid using a resistive network [2]. This parallel structure, however, has its own problem: response gain is diminished by interference among the second-order sections' outputs due to the large phase change at resonance [3].

Listening more to biology, our silicon cochlea aims to overcome the shortcomings of existing architectures by mimicking the cochlear micromechanics while including outer hair cell (OHC) electromotility. Although how exactly OHC motile forces boost the basilar membrane's (BM) vibration remains a mystery, cochlear microanatomy provides clues. Based on these clues, we previously proposed a novel mechanism, active bidirectional coupling (ABC), for the cochlear amplifier [4]. Here, we report an analog VLSI chip that implements this mechanism. In essence, our implementation is the first silicon cochlea that employs stimulus enhancement (i.e., active behavior) instead of undamping (i.e., high filter Q [5]).

The paper is organized as follows. In Section 2, we present the hypothesized mechanism (ABC), first described in [4]. In Section 3, we provide a mathematical formulation of the

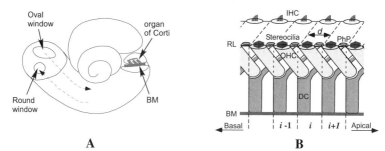

A   **B**

Figure 1: The inner ear. **A** Cutaway showing cochlear ducts (adapted from [6]). **B** Longitudinal view of cochlear partition (CP) (modified from [7]-[8]). Each outer hair cell (OHC) tilts toward the base while the Deiter's cell (DC) on which it sits extends a phalangeal process (PhP) toward the apex. The OHCs' stereocilia and the PhPs' apical ends form the reticular lamina (RL). d is the tilt distance, and the segment size. IHC: inner hair cell.

model as the basis of cochlear circuit design. Then we proceed in Section 4 to synthesize the circuit for the cochlear chip. Last, we present chip measurements in Section 5 that demonstrate nonlinear active cochlear behavior.

2   Active Bidirectional Coupling

The cochlea actively amplifies acoustic signals as it performs spectral analysis. The movement of the stapes sets the cochlear fluid into motion, which passes the stimulus energy onto a certain region of the BM, the main vibrating organ in the cochlea (Figure 1A). From the base to the apex, BM fibers increase in width and decrease in thickness, resulting in an exponential decrease in stiffness which, in turn, gives rise to the passive frequency tuning of the cochlea. The OHCs' electromotility is widely thought to account for the cochlea's exquisite sensitivity and discriminability. The exact way that OHC motile forces enhance the BM's motion, however, remains unresolved.

We propose that the triangular mechanical unit formed by an OHC, a phalangeal process (PhP) extended from the Deiter's cell (DC) on which the OHC sits, and a portion of the reticular lamina (RL), between the OHC's stereocilia end and the PhP's apical tip, plays an active role in enhancing the BM's responses (Figure 1B). The cochlear partition (CP) is divided into a number of segments longitudinally. Each segment includes one DC, one PhP's apical tip and one OHC's stereocilia end, both attached to the RL. Approximating the anatomy, we assume that when an OHC's stereocilia end lies in segment $i - 1$, its basolateral end lies in the immediately apical segment i. Furthermore, the DC in segment i extends a PhP that angles toward the apex of the cochlea, with its apical end inserted just behind the stereocilia end of the OHC in segment $i + 1$.

Our hypothesis (ABC) includes both feedforward and feedbackward interactions. On one hand, the feedforward mechanism, proposed in [9], hypothesized that the force resulting from OHC contraction or elongation is exerted onto an adjacent downstream BM segment due to the OHC's basal tilt. On the other hand, the novel insight of the feedbackward mechanism is that the OHC force is delivered onto an adjacent upstream BM segment due to the apical tilt of the PhP extending from the DC's main trunk.

In a nutshell, the OHC motile forces, through the microanatomy of the CP, feed forward and backward, in harmony with each other, resulting in bidirectional coupling between BM segments in the longitudinal direction. Specifically, due to the opposite action of OHC

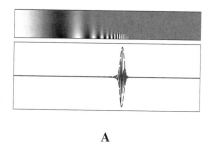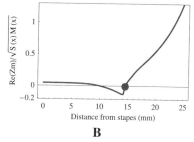

A	**B**

Figure 2: Wave propagation (WP) and basilar membrane (BM) impedance in the active cochlear model with a 2kHz pure tone ($\alpha = 0.15$, $\gamma = 0.3$). **A** WP in fluid and BM. **B** BM impedance Z_m (i.e., pressure divided by velocity), normalized by $\sqrt{S(x)M(x)}$. Only the resistive component is shown; dot marks peak location.

forces on the BM and the RL, the motion of BM segment $i-1$ reinforces that of segment i while the motion of segment $i+1$ opposes that of segment i, as described in detail in [4].

3 The 2D Nonlinear Active Model

To provide a blueprint for the cochlear circuit design, we formulate a 2D model of the cochlea that includes ABC. Both the cochlea's length (BM) and height (cochlear ducts) are discretized into a number of segments, with the original aspect ratio of the cochlea maintained. In the following expressions, x represents the distance from the stapes along the CP, with $x = 0$ at the base (or the stapes) and $x = L$ (uncoiled cochlear duct length) at the apex; y represents the vertical distance from the BM, with $y = 0$ at the BM and $y = \pm h$ (cochlear duct radius) at the bottom/top wall.

Providing that the assumption of fluid incompressibility holds, the velocity potential ϕ of the fluids is required to satisfy $\nabla^2 \phi(x, y, t) = 0$, where ∇^2 denotes the Laplacian operator. By definition, this potential is related to fluid velocities in the x and y directions: $V_x = -\partial\phi/\partial x$ and $V_y = -\partial\phi/\partial y$.

The BM is driven by the fluid pressure difference across it. Hence, the BM's vertical motion (with downward displacement being positive) can be described as follows.

$$P_d(x) + F_{OHC}(x) = S(x)\delta(x) + \beta(x)\dot{\delta}(x) + M(x)\ddot{\delta}(x), \tag{1}$$

where $S(x)$ is the stiffness, $\beta(x)$ is the damping, and $M(x)$ is the mass, per unit area, of the BM; δ is the BM's downward displacement. $P_d = \rho\, \partial(\phi_{SV}(x, y, t) - \phi_{ST}(x, y, t))/\partial t$ is the pressure difference between the two fluid ducts (the scala vestibuli (SV) and the scala tympani (ST)), evaluated at the BM ($y = 0$); ρ is the fluid density.

The $F_{OHC}(x)$ term combines feedforward and feedbackward OHC forces, described by

$$F_{OHC}(x) = s_0\big(\tanh(\alpha\gamma S(x)\delta(x-d)/s_0) - \tanh(\alpha S(x)\delta(x+d)/s_0)\big), \tag{2}$$

where α denotes the OHC motility, expressed as a fraction of the BM stiffness, and γ is the ratio of feedforward to feedbackward coupling, representing relative strengths of the OHC forces exerted on the BM segment through the DC, directly and via the tilted PhP. d denotes the tilt distance, which is the horizontal displacement between the source and the recipient of the OHC force, assumed to be equal for the forward and backward cases. We use the hyperbolic tangent function to model saturation of the OHC forces, the nonlinearity that is evident in physiological measurements [8]; s_0 determines the saturation level.

We observed wave propagation in the model and computed the BM's impedance (i.e., the ratio of driving pressure to velocity). Following the semi-analytical approach in [2], we simulated a linear version of the model (without saturation). The traveling wave transitions from long-wave to short-wave before the BM vibration peaks; the wavelength around the characteristic place is comparable to the tilt distance (Figure 2A). The BM impedance's real part (i.e., the resistive component) becomes negative before the peak (Figure 2B). On the whole, inclusion of OHC motility through ABC boosts the traveling wave by pumping energy onto the BM when the wavelength matches the tilt of the OHC and PhP.

4 Analog VLSI Design and Implementation

Based on our mathematical model, which produces realistic responses, we implemented a 2D nonlinear active cochlear circuit in analog VLSI, taking advantage of the 2D nature of silicon chips. We first synthesize a circuit analog of the mathematical model, and then we implement the circuit in the log-domain. We start by synthesizing a passive model, and then extend it to a nonlinear active one by including ABC with saturation.

4.1 Synthesizing the BM Circuit

The model consists of two fundamental parts: the cochlear fluid and the BM. First, we design the fluid element and thus the fluid network. In discrete form, the fluids can be viewed as a grid of elements with a specific resistance that corresponds to the fluid density or mass. Since charge is conserved for a small sheet of resistance and so are particles for a small volume of fluid, we use current to simulate fluid velocity. At the transistor level, the current flowing through the channel of a MOS transistor, operating subthreshold as a diffusive element, can be used for this purpose. Therefore, following the approach in [10], we implement the cochlear fluid network using a diffusor network formed by a 2D grid of nMOS transistors.

Second, we design the BM element and thus the BM. As current represents velocity, we rewrite the BM boundary condition (Equation 1, without the F_{OHC} term):

$$\dot{I}_{\text{in}} = S(x) \int I_{\text{mem}} dt + \beta(x) I_{\text{mem}} + M(x) \dot{I}_{\text{mem}}, \tag{3}$$

where I_{in}, obtained by applying the voltage from the diffusor network to the gate of a pMOS transistor, represents the velocity potential scaled by the fluid density. In turn, I_{mem} drives the diffusor network to match the fluid velocity with the BM velocity, $\dot{\delta}$. The F_{OHC} term is dealt with in Section 4.2.

Implementing this second-order system requires two state-space variables, which we name I_{s} and I_{o}. And with $s = j\omega$, our synthesized BM design (passive) is

$$\tau_1 I_{\text{s}} s + I_{\text{s}} = -I_{\text{in}} + I_{\text{o}}, \tag{4}$$

$$\tau_2 I_{\text{o}} s + I_{\text{o}} = I_{\text{in}} - b I_{\text{s}}, \tag{5}$$

$$I_{\text{mem}} = I_{\text{in}} + I_{\text{s}} - I_{\text{o}}, \tag{6}$$

where the two first-order systems are both low-pass filters (LPFs), with time constants τ_1 and τ_2, respectively; b is a gain factor. Thus, I_{in} can be expressed in terms of I_{mem} as:

$$I_{\text{in}} s^2 = \left((b+1)/\tau_1 \tau_2 + ((\tau_1 + \tau_2)/\tau_1 \tau_2) s + s^2 \right) I_{\text{mem}}.$$

Comparing this expression with the design target (Equation 3) yields the circuit analogs:

$$S(x) = (b+1)/\tau_1 \tau_2, \quad \beta(x) = (\tau_1 + \tau_2)/\tau_1 \tau_2, \quad \text{and} \quad M(x) = 1.$$

Note that the mass $M(x)$ is a constant (i.e., 1), which was also the case in our mathematical model simulation. These analogies require that τ_1 and τ_2 increase exponentially to

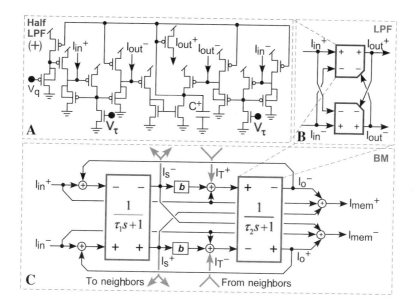

Figure 3: Low-pass filter (LPF) and second-order section circuit design. **A** Half-LPF circuit. **B** Complete LPF circuit formed by two half-LPF circuits. **C** Basilar membrane (BM) circuit. It consists of two LPFs and connects to its neighbors through I_s and I_T.

simulate the exponentially decreasing BM stiffness (and damping); b allows us to achieve a reasonable stiffness for a practical choice of τ_1 and τ_2 (capacitor size is limited by silicon area).

4.2 Adding Active Bidirectional Coupling

To include ABC in the BM boundary condition, we replace δ in Equation 2 with $\int I_{\mathrm{mem}} dt$ to obtain

$$F_{\mathrm{OHC}} = r_{\mathrm{ff}} S(x) \mathcal{T}\big(\int I_{\mathrm{mem}}(x-d)dt\big) - r_{\mathrm{fb}} S(x) \mathcal{T}\big(\int I_{\mathrm{mem}}(x+d)dt\big),$$

where $r_{\mathrm{ff}} = \alpha\gamma$ and $r_{\mathrm{fb}} = \alpha$ denote the feedforward and feedbackward OHC motility factors, and $\mathcal{T}$ denotes saturation. The saturation is applied to the displacement, instead of the force, as this simplifies the implementation. We obtain the integrals by observing that, in the passive design, the state variable $I_s = -I_{\mathrm{mem}}/s\tau_1$. Thus, $\int I_{\mathrm{mem}}(x-d)dt = -\tau_{1\mathrm{f}} I_{\mathrm{sf}}$ and $\int I_{\mathrm{mem}}(x+d)dt = -\tau_{1\mathrm{b}} I_{\mathrm{sb}}$. Here, I_{sf} and I_{sb} represent the outputs of the first LPF in the upstream and downstream BM segments, respectively; $\tau_{1\mathrm{f}}$ and $\tau_{1\mathrm{b}}$ represent their respective time constants. To reduce complexity in implementation, we use τ_1 to approximate both $\tau_{1\mathrm{f}}$ and $\tau_{1\mathrm{b}}$ as the longitudinal span is small.

We obtain the active BM design by replacing Equation 5 with the synthesis result:

$$\tau_2 I_{\mathrm{o}} s + I_{\mathrm{o}} = I_{\mathrm{in}} - b I_s + r_{\mathrm{fb}}(b+1)\mathcal{T}(-I_{\mathrm{sb}}) - r_{\mathrm{ff}}(b+1)\mathcal{T}(-I_{\mathrm{sf}}).$$

Note that, to implement ABC, we only need to add two currents to the second LPF in the passive system. These currents, I_{sf} and I_{sb}, come from the upstream and downstream neighbors of each segment.

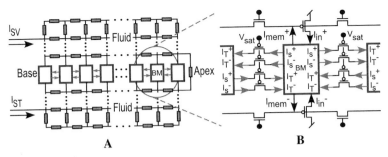

Figure 4: Cochlear chip. **A** Architecture: Two diffusive grids with embedded BM circuits model the cochlea. **B** Detail. BM circuits exchange currents with their neighbors.

4.3 Class AB Log-domain Implementation

We employ the log-domain filtering technique [11] to realize current-mode operation. In addition, following the approach proposed in [12], we implement the circuit in Class AB to increase dynamic range, reduce the effect of mismatch and lower power consumption. This differential signaling is inspired by the way the biological cochlea works—the vibration of BM is driven by the pressure difference across it.

Taking a bottom-up strategy, we start by designing a Class AB LPF, a building block for the BM circuit. It is described by

$$\tau(I_{\text{out}}^+ - I_{\text{out}}^-)s + (I_{\text{out}}^+ - I_{\text{out}}^-) = I_{\text{in}}^+ - I_{\text{in}}^- \ \text{ and } \ \tau I_{\text{out}}^+ I_{\text{out}}^- s + I_{\text{out}}^+ I_{\text{out}}^- = I_q^2,$$

where I_q sets the geometric mean of the positive and negative components of the output current, and τ sets the time constant.

Combining the common-mode constraint with the differential design equation yields the nodal equation for the positive path (the negative path has superscripts $+$ and $-$ swapped):

$$C\dot{V}_{\text{out}}^+ = I_\tau \left((I_{\text{in}}^+ - I_{\text{in}}^-) + (I_q^2 / I_{\text{out}}^+ - I_{\text{out}}^-) \right) / (I_{\text{out}}^+ + I_{\text{out}}^-).$$

This nodal equation suggests the half-LPF circuit shown in Figure 3A. V_{out}^+, the voltage on the positive capacitor (C^+), gates a pMOS transistor to produce the corresponding current signal, I_{out}^+ (V_{out}^- and I_{out}^- are similarly related). The bias V_q sets the quiescent current I_q while V_τ determines the current I_τ, which is related to the time constant by $\tau = C u_T / \kappa I_\tau$ (κ is the subthreshold slope coefficient and u_T is the thermal voltage). Two of these sub-circuits, connected in push–pull, form a complete LPF (Figure 3B).

The BM circuit is implemented using two LPFs interacting in accordance with the synthe-sized design equations (Figure 3C). I_{mem} is the combination of three currents, I_{in}, I_s, and I_o. Each BM sends out I_s and receives I_T, a saturated version of its neighbor's I_s. The saturation is accomplished by a current-limiting transistor (see Figure 4B), which yields $I_T = \mathcal{T}(I_s) = I_s I_{\text{sat}} / (I_s + I_{\text{sat}})$, where I_{sat} is set by a bias voltage V_{sat}.

4.4 Chip Architecture

We fabricated a version of our cochlear chip architecture (Figure 4) with 360 BM circuits and two 4680-element fluid grids (360×13). This chip occupies 10.9mm^2 of silicon area in $0.25 \mu\text{m}$ CMOS technology. Differential input signals are applied at the base while the two fluid grids are connected at the apex through a fluid element that represents the helicotrema.

5   Chip Measurements

We carried out two measurements that demonstrate the desired amplification by ABC, and the compressive growth of BM responses due to saturation. To obtain sinusoidal current as the input to the BM subcircuits, we set the voltages applied at the base to be the logarithm of a half-wave rectified sinusoid.

We first investigated BM-velocity frequency responses at six linearly spaced cochlear positions (Figure 5). The frequency that maximally excites the first position (Stage 30), defined as its characteristic frequency (CF), is 12.1kHz. The remaining five CFs, from early to later stages, are 8.2k, 1.7k, 905, 366, and 218Hz, respectively. Phase accumulation at the CFs ranges from 0.56 to 2.67π radians, comparable to 1.67π radians in the mammalian cochlea [13]. Q_{10} factor (the ratio of the CF to the bandwidth 10dB below the peak) ranges from 1.25 to 2.73, comparable to 2.55 at mid-sound intensity in biology (computed from [13]). The cutoff slope ranges from -20 to -54dB/octave, as compared to -85dB/octave in biology (computed from [13]).

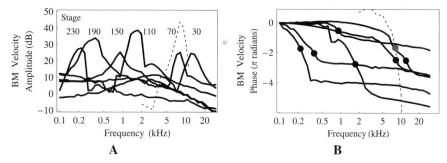

Figure 5: Measured BM-velocity frequency responses at six locations. **A** Amplitude. **B** Phase. Dashed lines: Biological data (adapted from [13]). Dots mark peaks.

We then explored the longitudinal pattern of BM-velocity responses and the effect of ABC. Stimulating the chip using four different pure tones, we obtained responses in which a 4kHz input elicits a peak around Stage 85 while 500Hz sound travels all the way to Stage 178 and peaks there (Figure 6A). We varied the input voltage level and obtained frequency responses at Stage 100 (Figure 6B). Input voltage level increases linearly such that the current increases exponentially; the input current level (in dB) was estimated based on the measured κ for this chip. As expected, we observed linearly increasing responses at low frequencies in the logarithmic plot. In contrast, the responses around the CF increase less and become broader with increasing input level as saturation takes effect in that region (resembling a passive cochlea). We observed 24dB compression as compared to 27 to 47dB in biology [13]. At the highest intensities, compression also occurs at low frequencies.

These chip measurements demonstrate that inclusion of ABC, simply through coupling neighboring BM elements, transforms a passive cochlea into an active one. This active cochlear model's nonlinear responses are qualitatively comparable to physiological data.

6   Conclusions

We presented an analog VLSI implementation of a 2D nonlinear cochlear model that utilizes a novel active mechanism, ABC, which we proposed to account for the cochlear amplifier. ABC was shown to pump energy into the traveling wave. Rather than detecting the wave's amplitude and implementing an automatic-gain-control loop, our biomorphic model accomplishes this simply by nonlinear interactions between adjacent neighbors. Im-

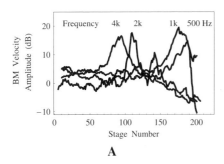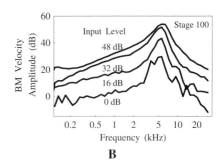

A	B

Figure 6: Measured BM-velocity responses (cont'd). **A** Longitudinal responses (20-stage moving average). Peak shifts to earlier (basal) stages as input frequency increases from 500 to 4kHz. **B** Effects of increasing input intensity. Responses become broader and show compressive growth.

plemented in the log-domain, with Class AB operation, our silicon cochlea shows enhanced frequency responses, with compressive behavior around the CF, when ABC is turned on. These features are desirable in prosthetic applications and automatic speech recognition systems as they capture the properties of the biological cochlea.

References

[1] Lyon, R.F. & Mead, C.A. (1988) An analog electronic cochlea. *IEEE Trans. Acoust. Speech and Signal Proc.*, **36**: 1119-1134.

[2] Watts, L. (1993) *Cochlear Mechanics: Analysis and Analog VLSI*. Ph.D. thesis, Pasadena, CA: California Institute of Technology.

[3] Fragnière, E. (2005) A 100-Channel analog CMOS auditory filter bank for speech recognition. *IEEE International Solid-State Circuits Conference (ISSCC 2005)*, pp. 140-141.

[4] Wen, B. & Boahen, K. (2003) A linear cochlear model with active bi-directional coupling. *The 25th Annual International Conference of the IEEE Engineering in Medicine and Biology Society (EMBC 2003)*, pp. 2013-2016.

[5] Sarpeshkar, R., Lyon, R.F., & Mead, C.A. (1996) An analog VLSI cochlear model with new transconductance amplifier and nonlinear gain control. *Proceedings of the IEEE Symposium on Circuits and Systems (ISCAS 1996)*, **3**: 292-295.

[6] Mead, C.A. (1989) *Analog VLSI and Neural Systems*. Reading, MA: Addison-Wesley.

[7] Russell, I.J. & Nilsen, K.E. (1997) The location of the cochlear amplifier: Spatial representation of a single tone on the guinea pig basilar membrane. *Proc. Natl. Acad. Sci. USA*, **94**: 2660-2664.

[8] Geisler, C.D. (1998) *From sound to synapse: physiology of the mammalian ear*. Oxford University Press.

[9] Geisler, C.D. & Sang, C. (1995) A cochlear model using feed-forward outer-hair-cell forces. *Hearing Research*, **86**: 132-146.

[10] Boahen, K.A. & Andreou, A.G. (1992) A contrast sensitive silicon retina with reciprocal synapses. In Moody, J.E. and Lippmann, R.P. (eds.), *Advances in Neural Information Processing Systems 4 (NIPS 1992)*, pp. 764-772, Morgan Kaufmann, San Mateo, CA.

[11] Frey, D.R. (1993) Log-domain filtering: an approach to current-mode filtering. *IEE Proc. G, Circuits Devices Syst.*, **140** (6): 406-416.

[12] Zaghloul, K. & Boahen, K.A. (2005) An On-Off log-domain circuit that recreates adaptive filtering in the retina. *IEEE Transactions on Circuits and Systems I: Regular Papers*, **52** (1): 99-107.

[13] Ruggero, M.A., Rich, N.C., Narayan, S.S., & Robles, L. (1997) Basilar membrane responses to tones at the base of the chinchilla cochlea. *J. Acoust. Soc. Am.*, **101** (4): 2151-2163.

Neural mechanisms of contrast dependent receptive field size in V1

Jim Wielaard and Paul Sajda
Department of Biomedical Engineering
Columbia University
New York, NY 10027
(djw21, ps629)@columbia.edu

Abstract

Based on a large scale spiking neuron model of the input layers $4C\alpha$ and β of macaque, we identify neural mechanisms for the observed contrast dependent receptive field size of V1 cells. We observe a rich variety of mechanisms for the phenomenon and analyze them based on the relative gain of excitatory and inhibitory synaptic inputs. We observe an average growth in the spatial extent of excitation and inhibition for low contrast, as predicted from phenomenological models. However, contrary to phenomenological models, our simulation results suggest this is neither sufficient nor necessary to explain the phenomenon.

1 Introduction

Neurons in the primary visual cortex (V1) display what is often referred to as "size tuning", i.e. the response of a cell is maximal around a cell-specific stimulus size and generally decreases substantially (30-40% on average) or vanishes altogether for larger stimulus sizes[1−9]. The cell-specific stimulus size eliciting a maximum response, also known as the "receptive field size" of the cell[4], has a remarkable property in that it is not contrast invariant, unlike for instance orientation tuning in V1. Quite the contrary, the contrast-dependent change in receptive field size of V1 cells is profound. Typical is a doubling in receptive field size for stimulus contrasts decreasing by a factor of 2-3 on the linear part of the contrast response function[4]. This behavior is seen throughout V1, including all cell types in all layers and at all eccentricities. A functional interpretation of the phenomenon is that neurons in V1 sacrifice spatial resolution in return for a gain in contrast sensitivity at low contrasts [4]. However, its neural mechanisms are at present very poorly understood. Understanding these mechanisms is potentially important for developing a theoretical model of early signal integration and neural encoding of visual features in V1.

We have recently developed a large-scale spiking neuron model that accounts for the phenomenon and suggests neural mechanisms from which it may originate. This paper provides a technical description of these mechanisms.

2 The model

Our model consists of 8 ocular dominance columns and 64 orientation hypercolumns (i.e. pinwheels), representing a 16 mm^2 area of a macaque V1 input layer $4C\alpha$ or $4C\beta$. The model consists of approximately 65,000 cortical cells in each of the four configurations (see below), and the corresponding appropriate number of LGN cells. Our cortical cells are modeled as conductance based integrate-and-fire point neurons, 75% are excitatory cells and 25% are inhibitory cells. Our LGN cells are rectified spatio-temporal linear filters. The model is constructed with isotropic short-range cortical connections ($< 500\mu m$), realistic LGN receptive field sizes and densities, realistic sizes of LGN axons in V1, and cortical magnification factors and receptive field scatter that are in agreement with experimental observations.

Dynamic variables of a cortical model-cell i are its membrane potential $v_i(t)$ and its spike train $\mathcal{S}_i(t) = \sum_k \delta(t - t_{i,k})$, where t is time and $t_{i,k}$ is its kth spike time. Membrane potential and spike train of each cell obey a set of N equations of the form

$$C_i \frac{dv_i}{dt} = -g_{L,i}(v_i - v_L) - g_{E,i}(t, [\mathcal{S}]_E, \eta_E)(v_i - v_E)$$

$$-g_{I,i}(t, [\mathcal{S}]_I, \eta_I)(v_i - v_I) , \ i = 1, \ldots, N . \tag{1}$$

These equations are integrated numerically using a second order Runge-Kutta method with time step 0.1 ms. Whenever the membrane potential reaches a fixed threshold level v_T it is reset to a fixed reset level v_R and a spike is registered. The equation can be rescaled so that $v_i(t)$ is dimensionless and $C_i = 1$, $v_L = 0$, $v_E = 14/3$, $v_I = -2/3$, $v_T = 1$, $v_R = 0$, and conductances (and currents) have dimension of inverse time.

The quantities $g_{E,i}(t, [\mathcal{S}], \eta_E)$ and $g_{I,i}(t, [\mathcal{S}], \eta_I)$ are the excitatory and inhibitory conductances of neuron i. They are defined by interactions with the other cells in the network, external noise $\eta_{E(I)}$, and, in the case of $g_{E,i}$ possibly by LGN input. The notation $[\mathcal{S}]_{E(I)}$ stands for the spike trains of all excitatory (inhibitory) cells connected to cell i. Both, the excitatory and inhibitory populations consist of two subpopulations $\mathcal{P}_k(E)$ and $\mathcal{P}_k(I)$, $k = 0, 1$, a population that receives LGN input ($k = 1$) and one that does not ($k = 0$). In the model presented here 30% of both the excitatory and inhibitory cell populations receive LGN input. We assume noise, cortical interactions and LGN input act additively in contributing to the total conductance of a cell,

$$g_{E,i}(t, [\mathcal{S}]_E, \eta_E) = \eta_{E,i}(t) + g_{E,i}^{cor}(t, [\mathcal{S}]_E) + \delta_i g_i^{LGN}(t)$$

$$g_{I,i}(t, [\mathcal{S}]_I, \eta_I) = \eta_{I,i}(t) + g_{I,i}^{cor}(t, [\mathcal{S}]_I) , \tag{2}$$

where $\delta_i = \ell$ for $i \in \{\mathcal{P}_\ell(E), \mathcal{P}_\ell(I)\}$, $\ell = 0, 1$. The terms $g_{\mu,i}^{cor}(t, [\mathcal{S}]_\mu)$ are the contributions from the cortical excitatory ($\mu = E$) and inhibitory ($\mu = I$) neurons and include only isotropic connections,

$$g_{\mu,i}^{cor}(t, [\mathcal{S}]_\mu) =$$

$$\int_{-\infty}^{+\infty} ds \sum_{k=0}^{1} \sum_{j \in \mathcal{P}_k(\mu)} \mathcal{C}_{\mu',\mu}^{k',k}(||\vec{x}_i - \vec{x}_j||) G_{\mu,j}(t - s) \mathcal{S}_j(s) , \tag{3}$$

where $i \in \mathcal{P}_{k'}(\mu')$ Here $\vec{x}_i$ is the spatial position (in cortex) of neuron i, the functions $G_{\mu,j}(\tau)$ describe the synaptic dynamics of cortical synapses and the functions $\mathcal{C}_{\mu',\mu}^{k',k}(r)$ describe the cortical spatial couplings (cortical connections). The length scale of excitatory and inhibitory connections is about 200μm and 100μm respectively.

In agreement with experimental findings (see references in [10]), the LGN neurons are modeled as rectified center-surround linear spatiotemporal filters. The LGN temporal kernels are modeled in agreement with [11], and the LGN spatial kernels are of center-surround type.

An important class of parameters are those that define and relate the model's geometry in visual space and cortical space. Geometric properties are different for the two input layers $4C\alpha, \beta$ and depend also on the eccentricity. As said, contrast dependent receptive field size is observed to be insensitive to those differences[4–6,8]. In order to verify that our explanations are consistent with this observation, we have performed numerical simulations for four different sets of parameters, corresponding to the $4C\alpha, \beta$ layers at para-foveal eccentricities ($< 5°$) and at eccentricities around $10°$. These different model configurations are referred to as M0, M10, and P0, P10. Reported results are qualitatively similar for all four configurations unless otherwise noted. The above is only a very brief description of the model, the details can be found in [12].

3 Visual stimuli and data collection

The stimulus used to analyze the phenomenon is a drifting grating confined to a circular aperture, surrounded by a blank (mean luminance) background. The luminance of the stimulus is given by $I(\vec{y}, t) = I_0(1 + \epsilon \cos(\omega t - \vec{k} \cdot \vec{y} + \phi))$ for $||\vec{y}|| \leq r_A$ and $I(\vec{y}, t) = I_0$ for $||\vec{y}|| > r_A$, with average luminance I_0, contrast ϵ, temporal frequency ω, spatial wave vector $\vec{k}$, phase ϕ, and aperture radius r_A. The aperture is centered on the receptive field of the cell and varied in size, while the other parameters are kept fixed and set to preferred values. All stimuli are presented monocularly. Samples consisting of approximately 200 cells were collected for each configuration, containing about an equal number of simple and complex cells. The experiments were performed at "high" contrast, $\epsilon = 1$, and "low" contrast, $\epsilon = 0.3$.

4 Approximate model equations

We find that, to good approximation, the membrane potential and instantaneous firing rate of our model cells are respectively[12,13]

$$\langle v_k(t, r_A) \rangle \approx V_k(r_A, t) \equiv \frac{\langle I_{D,k}(t, r_A) \rangle}{\langle g_{T,k}(t, r_A) \rangle} , \tag{4}$$

$$\langle S_k(t, r_A) \rangle \approx f_k(t, r_A) \equiv \delta_k [\langle I_{D,k}(t, r_A) \rangle - \langle g_{T,k}(t, r_A) \rangle - \Delta_k]_+ , \tag{5}$$

where $[x]_+ = x$ if $x \geq 0$ and $[x]_+ = 0$ if $x \leq 0$, and where, the gain δ_k and threshold Δ_k do not depend on the aperture radius r_A for most cells. The total conductance $g_{T,k}(t, r_A)$ and difference current $I_{D,k}(t, r_A)$ are given by

$$g_{T,k}(t, r_A) = g_L + g_{E,k}(t, [S]_E, r_A) + g_{I,k}(t, [S]_I, r_A) \tag{6}$$

$$I_{D,k}(r_A, t) = g_{E,k}(t, [S]_E, r_A) V_E - g_{I,k}(t, [S]_I, r_A) |V_I| . \tag{7}$$

5 Mechanisms of contrast dependent receptive field size

From Eq. (4) and (5) it follows that a change in receptive field size in general results from a change in behavior of the relative gain,

$$G(r_A) = \frac{\partial g_E/\partial r_A}{\partial g_I/\partial r_A} . \tag{8}$$

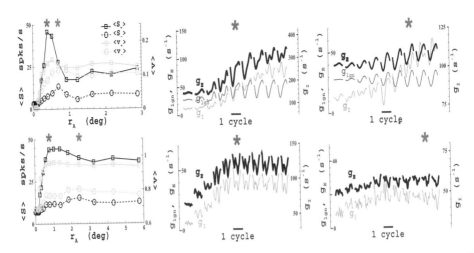

Figure 1: Two example cells, an M0 simple cell which receives LGN input (top) and an M10 complex cell which does not (bottom). (column 1) Responses as function of aperture size. Mean responses are plotted for the complex cell, first harmonic for the simple cell. Apertures of maximum of responses (i.e. receptive field sizes) are indicated with asterisks (dark=high contrast, light=low contrast). (column 2) Conductances for high contrast at apertures near the maximum responses. Conductances are displayed as nine (top) and eleven (bottom) sub-panels giving the cycle-trial averaged conductances as a function of time (relative to cycle) and aperture size. (column 3) Conductances for low contrast at apertures near the maximum responses. Asterisks in the conductance figures (columns 2 and 3) indicate corresponding apertures of maximum response (column 1)

Note that this is a rather different parameter than the "surround gain" parameter (k_s) used in the ratio-of-Gaussians (ROG) model[8]–e.g. unlike for k_s, there is no one-to-one relationship between $G(r_A)$ and the degree of surround suppression. Qualitatively, the conductances show a similar dependence on aperture size as the membrane potential responses and spike responses, i.e. they display surround suppression as well [12]. Receptive field sizes based on these conductances are a measure of the spatial summation extent of excitation and inhibition.

An obvious way to change the behavior of G, and consequently the receptive field size, is to change the spatial summation extent of g_E and/or g_I. However this is not strictly necessary. For example, other possibilities are illustrated by the two cells in Fig. 1. These cells show, both in spike and membrane potential responses, a receptive field growth of a factor of 2 (top) and 3 (bottom) at low contrast. However, for both cells the spatial summation extent of excitation at low contrast is one aperture less than at high contrast.

In a similar way as for spike train responses, we also obtained receptive field sizes for the conductances. As do spike responses (Fig. 2A), both excitation and inhibition (Fig. 2B&C) also show, on the average, an increase in their spatial summation extent as contrast is decreased, but the increase is in general smaller than what is seen for spike responses, particularly for cells that show significant receptive field growth. For instance, we see from Figure 2B and C that for cells in the sample with receptive field growths ~ 2 or greater, the growth for the conductances is always considerably less than the growth based on spike responses. Expressed more rigorously, a Wilcoxon test on ratio of growth ratios larger than unity gives $p < 0.05$ (all cells, excitation, Fig. 2B), $p < 0.15$ (all cells, inhibition, Fig. 2C), $p < 0.001$ (cells with receptive field growth rate $r_+/r_- > 1.5$, both excitation and inhibition.) Although some increase in the spatial summation extent of excitation and inhibition is in general the rule, this increase is rather arbitrary and bears not much relation with the receptive field growth based on spike responses. The same conclusions follow from membrane potential responses (not shown).

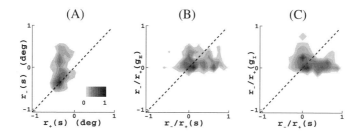

Figure 2: (A) Joint distribution of high and low contrast receptive field sizes, r_+ and r_-, based on spike responses. All scales are logarithmic, base 10. All distributions are normalized to a peak value of one. Receptive field growth at low contrast is clear. Average growth ratio is 1.9 and is significantly greater than unity (Wilcoxon test, $p < 0.001$). (B & C) Joint distributions of receptive field growth and growth of spatial summation extent of excitation (B) and inhibition (C) (computed as ratios). There is no simple relation between receptive field growth and the growth of the spatial summation extent of excitatory or inhibitory inputs. For cells in the sample with larger receptive field growths (factor of ~ 2 or greater) this growth is always considerably larger than the growths of their excitatory and inhibitory inputs.

Fig. 2 thus demonstrates that, contrary to what is predicted by the difference-of-Gaussians (DOG) [4] and ROG models [8] (see Discussion), a growth of spatial summation extent of excitation (and/or inhibition) at low contrast is neither sufficient nor necessary to explain the receptive field growth seen in spike responses. Membrane potential responses give the same conclusion. The fact that a change in receptive field size can take place without a change in the spatial summation extent of g_E or g_I can be illustrated by a simple example.

Consider a situation where both g_E and g_I have their maximum at the same aperture size $r_E = r_I = r_\star$ and are monotonically increasing for $r_A < r_\star$ and monotonically decreasing for $r_A > r_\star$, as depicted in Fig. 3. We can distinguish three classes with respect to the relative location of the maxima in spike responses r_S and the conductances $r_\star$, namely $\{X: r_S < r_\star\}$, $\{Y: r_S = r_\star\}$ and $\{Z: r_S > r_\star\}$. It follows from (5) that if we define the

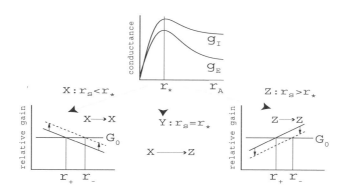

Figure 3: Schematic illustration of mechanisms for receptive field growth under equal and constant spatial summation extent of the conductances ($r_E = r_I = r_\star$).

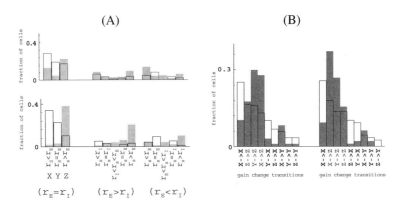

Figure 4: (A) Distributions of the relative positions of the maxima (receptive field sizes) of spike responses r_S and conductances r_E and r_I, for the M0 configuration. A division is made with respect to the maxima in the conductances, this corresponds to the left ($r_E = r_I$), central ($r_E > r_I$), and right ($r_E < r_I$) part of the figure. Each panel is further subdivided with respect to the maximum in the spike response r_S. Upper histograms are for all cells in the sample, lower histograms are for cells that have receptive field growth $r_-/r_+ > 1.5$. Unfilled histograms are for high contrast, shaded histograms are for low contrast. (B) Prevalence of transitions between positions of maxima in spike responses and excitatory conductances (left) and in spike responses and inhibitory conductances (right) for a high $\rightarrow$ low contrast change. See text for definitions of X, Y, Z classes. Data are evaluated for all cells (unfilled histograms) and for cells with a receptive field growth $r_-/r_+ > 1.5$ (shaded histograms).

parameter $G_0(v) = (|v_I| + v)/(v_E - v)$ then we can characterize the difference between classes X and Z by the way that G crosses $G_0(1)$ around r_S as depicted in Fig. 3. For class Y the parameter G is not of any particular interest as it can assume arbitrary behavior around r_S. It follows from (4) that similar observations hold for the maximum in the membrane potential r_v and we need simply to replace $G_0(1)$ with $G_0(v(r_v))$. A growth of receptive field size can occur without any change in the spatial summation extent ($r_\star$) of the conductances. Suppose we wish to remain within the same class X or Z, then receptive field growth, can be induced, for instance, by an overall increase (X) or an overall decrease (Z) in relative gain $G(r_A)$ as shown in Fig. 3 (dashed line). Receptive field growth also can be caused by more drastic changes in G so that the transitions X $\rightarrow$ Y, X $\rightarrow$ Z or Y $\rightarrow$ Z occur for a high $\rightarrow$ low contrast change The situation is somewhat more involved when we allow for non-suppressed responses and conductances, and for different positions of the maxima of g_E and g_I, however, the essence of our conclusions remains the same.

Analysis of our data in the light of the above example is given in Fig. 4. Cells were classified (Fig. 4A) according to the relative positions of their maxima in spike response (r_S) and excitatory (r_E) and inhibitory (r_I) conductances, using F0+F1 (i.e. mean response + first Fourier component of the response). Membrane potential responses yield similar results. Comparing this classification at high and low contrast we observe a striking difference for cells with significant receptive field growths, i.e. with growth ratios >1.5 (Fig. 4A, bottom), indicative of X $\rightarrow$ Y, X $\rightarrow$ Z and Y $\rightarrow$ Z transitions (as discussed in the simplified example above). In this realistic situation there are of course many more transitions (i.e. 13^2), however, that we indeed observe a prevalence for these transitions can be demonstrated in two ways using slightly modified definitions of the X,Y,Z classes. First (Fig. 4B, left), if we redefine the X,Y,Z classes with respect to r_S and r_E while ignoring r_I, i.e. {X: $r_S < r_E$}, {Y: $r_S = r_E$} and {Z: $r_S > r_E$}, then the transition distribution for cells with significant receptive field growth shows that in about 60% of these cells a X $\rightarrow$ Z or

$Y \rightarrow Z$ transition occurs. Taken together with the fact that roughly 10% of the cells with significant receptive field growth (Figure 4A, bottom) have $r_I \leq r_S < r_E$ at high contrast and $r_E < r_S \leq r_I$ at low contrast, we can conclude that for more than 50% of the cells with significant receptive field growth, a transition takes place from a high contrast RF size less or equal to the spatial summation extent of excitation and inhibition, to a low contrast receptive field size which exceeds both (by at least one aperture). Note that these transitions occur in addition to any growth of r_E or r_I. Secondly (Fig. 4B, right), the same conclusion is reached when we redefine the X,Y,Z classes with respect to r_S and r_I while ignoring r_E ($\{X: r_S < r_I\}$, $\{Y: r_S = r_I\}$ and $\{Z: r_S > r_I\}$), Now a $X \rightarrow Z$ or $Y \rightarrow Z$ transition occurs in about 70% of the cells with significant receptive field growth, while about 20% of the cells with significant receptive field growth (Fig. 4A, bottom) have $r_E \leq r_S < r_I$ at high contrast and $r_I < r_S \leq r_E$ at low contrast. Finally, Fig. 4B also demonstrates the presence of a rich diversity in relative gain changes in our model, since all transitions (for all cells, unfilled histograms) occur with some reasonable probability.

6   Discussion

The DOG model suggests that growth in receptive field size at low contrast is due to an increase of the spatial summation extent of excitation[4] (i.e. increase in the spatial extent parameter σ_E). This was partially confirmed experimentally in cat primary visual cortex[7]. Although it has been claimed[8] that the ROG model could explain receptive field growth solely from a change in the relative gain parameter k_s, we believe this is incorrect. Since there is a one-to-one relationship between k_s and surround suppression, this would imply that contrast dependent receptive field size simply results from contrast dependent surround suppression, which contradicts experimental data[4,8]. As does the DOG model, the ROG model, based on analysis of our data, also predicts that contrast dependent receptive field size is due to contrast dependence of the spatial summation extent of excitation. As we have shown, our simulations confirm an average growth of spatial summation extent of excitation (and inhibition) at low contrast. However, this growth is neither sufficient nor necessary to explain receptive field growth. For cells with significant receptive field growth, ($r_+/r_- > 1.5$) we were able to identify an additional property of the neural mechanisms. For more than 50% of such cells, a transition takes place from a high contrast RF size less or equal to the spatial summation extent of excitation and inhibition, to a low contrast receptive field size which exceeds both.

An important characteristic of our model is that it is not specifically designed to produce the phenomenon. Rather, the model parameters are set such that it produces realistic orientation tuning and a realistic distribution of response modulations in response to drifting gratings (simple & complex cells). Constructed in this way, our model then naturally produces a wide variety of realistic response properties, classical as well as extraclassical, including the phenomenon discussed here. A prominent feature of the mechanisms we suggest is that, contrary to common belief, they require neither the long-range lateral connections in V1 [14–18] nor extrastriate feedback [6,8,19,20]. The average receptive field growth we see in our model is about a factor of two $(\overline{r_-/r_+} \sim 2)$. This is a little less than what is observed in experiments [5,8]. This leaves room for contributions from the LGN input. It seems reasonable to assume that contrast dependent receptive field size is not limited to V1 and is also a property of LGN cells. Somewhat surprisingly, this has to our knowledge not been verified yet for macaque. Contrast dependent receptive field size of LGN cells has been observed in marmoset and an average growth ratio at low contrast of 1.3 was reported[21]. Receptive field growth of LGN cells in some sense introduces an overall geometric scaling factor on the entire visual input to V1. This observation ignores a great many details of course. For instance, the fact that the density of LGN cells (LGN receptive fields) is not known to change with contrast. On the other hand, it seems unlikely that a reasonable receptive field expansion of LGN cells would not be at least partially transferred to V1. Thus it seems reasonable to conclude from our work that the phenomenon in V1, in particular that seen in layer 4, may be attributed largely to isotropic short-range (< 0.5 mm) cortical connections and LGN input.

Acknowledgments

This work was supported by grants from ONR (MURI program, N00014-01-1-0625) and NGA (HM1582-05-C-0008).

References

[1] Dow, B, Snyder, A, Vautin, R, & Bauer, R. (1981) *Exp Brain Res* **44**, 213–228.

[2] Schiller, P, Finlay, B, & Volman, S. (1976) *J Neurophysiol* **39**, 1288–1319.

[3] Silito, A, Grieve, K, Jones, H, Cudeiro, J, & Davis, J. (1995) *Nature* **378**, 492–496.

[4] Sceniak, M, Ringach, D, Hawken, M, & Shapley, R. (1999) *Nat Neurosci* **2**, 733–739.

[5] Kapadia, M, Westheimer, G, & Gilbert, C. (1999) *Proc Nat Acad Sci USA* **96**, 12073–12078.

[6] Sceniak, M, Hawken, M, & Shapley, R. (2001) *J Neurophysiol* **85**, 1873–1887.

[7] Anderson, J, Lampl, I, Gillespie, D, & Ferster, D. (2001) *J Neurosci* **21**, 2104–2112.

[8] Cavanaugh, J, Bair, W, & Movshon, J. (2002) *J Neurophysiol* **88**, 2530–2546.

[9] Ozeki, H, Sadakane, O, Akasaki, T, Naito, T, Shimegi, S, & Sato, H. (2004) *J Neurosci* **24**, 1428–1438.

[10] McLaughlin, D, Shapley, R, Shelley, M, & Wielaard, J. (2000) *Proc Nat Acad Sci USA* **97**, 8087–8092.

[11] Benardete, E & Kaplan, E. (1999) *Vis Neurosci* **16**, 355–368.

[12] Wielaard, J & Sajda, P. (2005) *Cerebral Cortex* in press.

[13] Wielaard, J, Shelley, M, McLaughlin, D, & Shapley, R. (2001) *J Neurosci* **21(14)**, 5203–5211.

[14] DeAngelis, G, Freeman, R, & Ohzawa, I. (1994) *J Neurophysiol* **71**, 347–374.

[15] Somers, D, Todorov, E, Siapas, A, Toth, L, Kim, D, & Sur, M. (1998) *Cereb Cortex* **8**, 204–217.

[16] Dragoi, V & Sur, M. (2000) *J Neurophysiol* **83**, 1019–1030.

[17] Hupé, J, James, A, Girard, P, & Bullier, J. (2001) *J Neurophysiol* **85**, 146–163.

[18] Stettler, D, Das, A, Bennett, J, & Gilbert, C. (2002) *Neuron* **36**, 739–750.

[19] Angelucci, A, Levitt, J, Walton, E, Hupé, J, Bullier, J, & Lund, J. (2002) *J Neurosci* **22**, 8633–8646.

[20] Bair, W, Cavanaugh, J, & Movshon, J. (2003) *J Neurosci* **23(20)**, 7690–7701.

[21] Solomon, S, White, A, & Martin, P. (2002) *J Neurosci* **22(1)**, 338–349.

Factorial Switching Kalman Filters for Condition Monitoring in Neonatal Intensive Care

Christopher K. I. Williams and John Quinn
School of Informatics, University of Edinburgh
Edinburgh EH1 2QL, UK
`c.k.i.williams@ed.ac.uk`
`john.quinn@ed.ac.uk`

Neil McIntosh
Simpson Centre for Reproductive
Health, Edinburgh EH16 4SB, UK
`neil.mcintosh@ed.ac.uk`

Abstract

The observed physiological dynamics of an infant receiving intensive care are affected by many possible factors, including interventions to the baby, the operation of the monitoring equipment and the state of health. The Factorial Switching Kalman Filter can be used to infer the presence of such factors from a sequence of observations, and to estimate the true values where these observations have been corrupted. We apply this model to clinical time series data and show it to be effective in identifying a number of artifactual and physiological patterns.

1 Introduction

In a neonatal intensive care unit (NICU), an infant's vital signs, including heart rate, blood pressures, blood gas properties and temperatures, are continuously monitored and displayed at the cotside. The levels of these measurements and the way they vary give an indication of the baby's health, but they can be affected by many different things. The potential factors include handling of the baby, different cardiovascular and respiratory conditions, the effects of drugs which have been administered, and the setup of the monitoring equipment. Each factor has an effect on the dynamics of the observations, some by affecting the physiology of the baby (such as an oxygen desaturation), and some by overwriting the measurements with artifactual values (such as a probe dropout).

We use a Factorial Switching Kalman Filter (FSKF) to model such data. This consists of three sets of variables which we call *factors*, *state* and *observations*, as indicated in Figure 1(a). There are a number of hidden factors; these are discrete variables, modelling for example if the baby is in a normal respiratory state or not, or if a probe is disconnected or not. The state of baby denotes continuous-valued quantities; this models the true values of infant's physiological variables, but also has dimensions to model certain artifact processes (see below). The observations are those readings obtained from the monitoring equipment, and are subject to corruption by artifact etc.

By describing the dynamical regime associated with each combination of factors as a linear Gaussian model we obtain a FSKF, which extends the Switching Kalman Filter (see e.g. [10, 3]) to incorporate multiple independent factors. With this method we can infer the value of each factor and estimate the true values of vital signs during the times that the measurements are obscured by artifact. By using an interpretable hidden state structure for this application, domain knowledge can be used to set some of the parameters.

This paper demonstrates an application of the FSKF to NICU monitoring data. In Section 2 we introduce the model, and discuss the links to previous work in the field. In Section 3 we describe an approach for setting the parameters of the model and in Section 4 we show results from the model when applied to NICU data. Finally we close with a discussion in Section 5.

2 Model description

The Factorial Switching Kalman Filter is shown in Figure 1(a). In this model, M factors $f_t^{(1)} \dots f_t^{(M)}$ affect the hidden continuous state $\mathbf{x}_t$ and the observations $\mathbf{y}_t$. The factor $f^{(m)}$ can take on $K^{(m)}$ different values. For example, a simple factor is 'ECG probe dropout', taking on two possible values, 'dropped out' or 'normal'. As factors in this application can affect the observations either by altering the baby's physiology or overwriting them with artifactual values, the hidden state vector $\mathbf{x}_t$ contains information on both the 'true' physiological condition of the baby and on the levels of any artifactual processes.

The dynamical regime at time t is controlled by the 'switch' variable s_t, which is the cross product of the individual factors,

$$s_t = f_t^{(1)} \otimes \dots \otimes f_t^{(M)} . \tag{1}$$

For a given setting of s_t, the hidden continuous state and the observations are related by:

$$\mathbf{x}_t \sim \mathcal{N}(A(s_t)\mathbf{x}_{t-1} + \mathbf{d}(s_t), Q(s_t)), \qquad \mathbf{y}_t \sim \mathcal{N}(H(s_t)\mathbf{x}_t, R(s_t)), \tag{2}$$

where as in the SKF the system dynamics and observation process are dependent on the switch variable. Here $A(s_t)$ is a square system matrix, $\mathbf{d}(s_t)$ is a drift vector, $H(s_t)$ is the state-observations matrix, and $Q(s_t)$ and $R(s_t)$ are noise covariance matrices. The factors are taken to be a priori independent and first-order Markovian, so that

$$p(s_t|s_{t-1}) = \prod_{m=1}^{M} p(f_t^{(m)}|f_{t-1}^{(m)}) . \tag{3}$$

2.1 Application-specific setup

The continuous hidden state vector $\mathbf{x}$ contains two types of values, the true physiological values, $\mathbf{x}_p$, and those of artifactual processes, $\mathbf{x}_a$. The true values are modelled as independent autoregressive processes, described in more detail in section 3. To represent this as a state space, the vector $\mathbf{x}_t$ has to contain the value of the current state and store the value of the states at previous times.

Note that artifact state values can be affected by physiological state, but not the other way round. For example, one factor we model is the arterial blood sample, seen in Figure 1(b), lower panel. This occurs when a three-way valve is closed in the baby's arterial line, in order for a clinician to draw blood for a sample. While the valve is closed a pump works against the pressure sensor, causing the systolic and diastolic blood pressure measurements to rise artificially. The artifactual values in this case always start at around the value of the baby's diastolic blood pressure.

The factors modelled in these experiments are listed in Table 1. The dropout factors represent the case where probes are disconnected and measurements fall to zero on the channels supplied by that probe. In this case, the true physiological values are completely hidden.

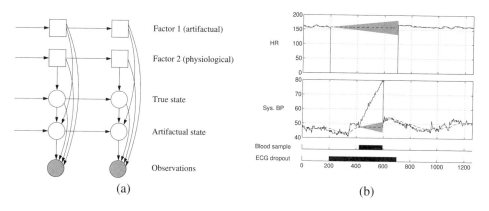

(a)   (b)

Figure 1: (a) shows a graphical representation of a Factorial Switching Kalman Filter, with $M = 2$ factors. Squares are discrete values, circles are continuous and shaded nodes are observed. Panel (b) shows ECG dropout and arterial blood sample events occurring simultaneously. HR denotes heart rate, Sys. BP denotes the systolic blood pressure, and times are in seconds. The dashed line indicates the estimate of true values and the greyscale denotes two standard deviation error bars. We see uncertainty increasing while observations are artifactual. The traces at the bottom show the inferred duration of the arterial blood sample and ECG dropout events.

The transcutaneous probe (TCP) provides measurements of the partial pressure of oxygen ($TcPO_2$) and carbon dioxide ($TcPCO_2$) in the baby's blood, and is recalibrated every few hours. This process has three stages: firstly calibration, where $TcPO_2$ and $TcPCO_2$ are set to known values by applying a gas to the probe, secondly a stage where the probe is in air and $TcPCO_2$ drops to zero, and finally an equilibration phase where both values slowly return to the physiological baseline when the probe is replaced.

As explained above, when an arterial blood sample is being taken one sees a characteristic ramp in the blood pressure measurements. Temperature probe disconnection frequently occurs in conjunction with handling. The core temperature probe is under the baby and can come off when the baby is turned over for an examination, causing the readings to drop to the ambient temperature level of the incubator over the course of a few minutes. When the probe is reapplied, the measurements gradually return to the true level of the baby's core temperature.

Bradycardia is a genuine physiological occurrence where the heart rate temporarily drops, often with a characteristic curve, then a systemic reaction brings the measurements back to the baseline. The final factor models opening of the portals on the baby's incubator. Because the environment within the incubator is closely regulated, an intervention can be inferred from a fall in the incubator humidity measurements. While the portals are open and a clinician is handling the baby, we expect increased variability in the measurements from the probes that are still attached.

2.2 Inference

For the application of real time clinical monitoring, we are interested in filtering, inferring $\mathbf{x}_t$ and s_t from the observations $\mathbf{y}_{1:t}$. However, the time taken for exact inference of the posterior $p(\mathbf{x}_t, s_t | \mathbf{y}_{1:t})$ scales exponentially with t, making it intractable. This is because the probabilities of having moved between every possible combination of switch settings in times $t - 1$ and t are needed to calculate the posterior at time t. Hence the number of

FACTOR	POSSIBLE SETTINGS
5 Probe dropout factors: pulse oximeter, ECG, arterial line, temperature probe, transcutaneous probe	**1**. Dropped out **2**. Normal
TCP recalibration	**1**. O_2 high, CO_2 low **2**. $CO_2 \rightarrow 0$ **3**. Equilibration **4**. Normal
Arterial blood sample	**1**. Blood sample **2**. Normal
Temperature probe disconnection	**1**. Temperature probe disconnection **2**. Reconnection **3**. Normal
Bradycardia	**1**. Bradycardia onset **2**. HR restabilisation **3**. Normal
Incubator open	**1**. Incubator portals opened **2**. Normal

Table 1: Description of factors.

Gaussians needed to represent the posterior exactly at each time step increases by a factor of K, the number of cross-product switch settings, where $K = \prod_{m=1}^{M} K^{(m)}$.

In this experiment we use the Gaussian Sum approximation [1]. At each time step we maintain an approximation of $p(\mathbf{x}_t | s_t, \mathbf{y}_{1:t})$ as a mixture of K Gaussians. Calculating the Kalman updates and likelihoods for every possible setting of s_{t+1} will result in the posterior $p(\mathbf{x}_{t+1} | s_{t+1}, \mathbf{y}_{1:t+1})$ having K^2 mixture components, which can be collapsed back into K components by matching means and variances of the distribution, as described in [6].

For comparison we also use Rao-Blackwellised particle filtering (RBPF) [7] for approximate inference. In this technique a number of particles are propagated through each time step, each with a switch state s_t and an estimate of the mean and variance of $\mathbf{x}_t$. A value for the switch state s_{t+1} is obtained for each particle by sampling from the transition probabilities, after which Kalman updates are performed and a likelihood value can be calculated. Based on this likelihood, particles can be either discarded or multiplied. Because Kalman updates are not calculated for every possible setting of s_{t+1}, this method can give a significant increase in speed when there are many factors, with some tradeoff in accuracy.

Both inference methods can be speeded up by considering the dropout factors. Because a probe dropout always results in an observation of zero on the corresponding measurement channels, the value of y_t can be examined at each step. If it is not equal to zero then we know that the likelihood of a dropout factor being active will be very low, so there is no need to calculate it explicitly. Similarly, if any of the observations are zero then we only perform Kalman updates and calculate likelihoods for those switch states with the appropriate dropout setting.

2.3 Relation to previous work

The SKF and various approximations for inference have been described by many authors, see e.g. [10, 3]. In [5], the authors used a 2-factor FSKF in a speech recognition application; the two factors corresponded to (i) phones and (ii) the phone-to-spectrum transformation. There has also been much prior work on condition monitoring in intensive care; here we give a brief review of some of these studies and the relationship to our own work.

The specific problem of artifact detection in physiological time series data has been approached in a number of ways. For example Tsien [9] used machine learning techniques, notably decision trees and logistic regression, to classify each observation $\mathbf{y}_t$ as genuine or artifactual. Hoare and Beatty [4] describe the use of time series analysis techniques

(ARIMA models, moving average and Kalman filters) to predict the next point in a patient's monitoring trace. If the difference between the observed value and the predicted value was outside a predetermined range, the data point was classified as artifactual. Our application of a model with factorial state extends this work by explaining the specific cause of an artifact, rather than just the fact that a certain data point is artifactual or not. We are not aware of other work in condition monitoring using a FSKF.

3 Parameter estimation

We use hand-annotated training data from a number of babies to estimate the parameters of the model.

Factor dynamics: Using equation 3 we can calculate the state transition probabilities from the transition probabilities for individual state variables, $P(f_t^{(m)} = a | f_{t-1}^{(m)} = b)$. The estimates for these are given by $P(f_t^{(m)} = a | f_{t-1}^{(m)} = b) = (n_{ba} + c) / \left(\sum_{c=1}^{K^{(m)}} (n_{bc} + c) \right)$, where n_{ba} is the number of transitions from state b to state a in the training data. The smoothing constant c (in our experiments we set $c = 1$) is added to stop any of the transition probabilities being zero or very small. While a zero probability could be useful for a sequence of states that we know are impossible, in general we want to avoid it. This solution can be justified theoretically as a maximum a posteriori estimate where the prior is given by a Dirichlet distribution. The factor dynamics can be used to create left-to-right models, e.g. for passing through the sequence O_2 high, CO_2 low; $CO_2 \rightarrow 0$; equilibration in the TCP recalibration case.

System dynamics: When no factor is active (i.e. non-normal), the baby is said to be in a stable condition and has some capacity for self-regulation. In this condition we consider each observation channel separately, and use standard methods to fit AR or ARIMA models to each channel. Most channels vary around reference ranges when the baby is stable and are well fitted by AR(2) models. Heart rate and blood pressure observation channels are more volatile and stationarity is improved after differencing. Heart rate dynamics, for example, are well fitted with an ARIMA(2,1,0) process. Representing trained AR or ARIMA processes in state space form is then straightforward.

The observational data tends to have some high frequency noise on it (see e.g. Fig. 1(b), lower panel) due to probe error and quantization effects. Thus we smooth sections of stable data with a 21-point moving average in order to obtain training data for the system dynamics.

The Yule-Walker equations are then used to set parameters for this moving-averaged data. The fit can be verified for each observation channel by comparing the spectrum of new data with the theoretical spectrum of the AR process (or the spectrum of the differenced data for ARIMA processes), see e.g. [2]. The measurement noise matrix R is estimated by calculating the variance of the differences between the original and averaged training data for each measurement channel.

Above we have modelled the dynamics for a baby in the stable condition; we now describe some of the system models used when the factors are active (i.e. non-normal). The drop and rise in temperature measurements caused by a temperature probe disconnection closely resemble exponential decay and can be therefore be fitted with an AR(1) process. This also applies to the equilibration stage of a TCP recalibration.

The dynamics corresponding to the bradycardia factor are set by finding the mean slope of the fall and rise in heart rate, which is used for the drift term $\mathbf{d}$, then fitting an AR(1) process to the residuals. The arterial blood sample dynamics are modelled with linear drift; note that the variable in $\mathbf{x}_a$ corresponding to the value of the arterial blood sample is tied

	Blood sample		TCP recal.		Bradycardia		TC disconnect		Incu. open	
	AUC	EER	AUC	EER	AUC	EER	AUC	EER	AUC	EER
FHMM	0.97	0.02	0.78	0.25	0.67	0.42	0.75	0.35	0.97	0.07
GS	0.99	0.01	0.91	0.12	0.72	0.39	0.88	0.19	0.97	0.06
RBPF	0.62	0.46	0.90	0.14	0.76	0.37	0.85	0.32	0.95	0.08

Table 2: Inference results on evaluation data. FHMM denotes the Factorial Hidden Markov Model, GS denotes the Gaussian Sum approximation, and RBPF denotes Rao-Blackwellised particle filtering with 560 particles. AUC denotes area under ROC curve and EER denotes the equal error rate.

to the diastolic blood pressure value while the factor is inactive. We also use linear drift to model the drop in incubator humidity measurements corresponding to a clinician opening the incubator portals.

We assume that the measurement noise from each probe is the same for physiological and artifactual readings, for example if the core temperature probe is attached to the baby's skin or is reading ambient incubator temperature.

Combining factors: The parameters $\{A, H, Q, R, \mathbf{d}\}$ have to be supplied for every combination of factors. It might be thought that training data would be needed for each of these possible combinations, but in practice parameters can be trained for factors individually and then combined, as we know that some of the phenomena we want to model only affect a subset of the channels, or override other phenomena [8]. This process of setting parameters for each combination of factor settings can be automated. The factors are arranged in a partially ordered set, where later factors overwrite the dynamics $A, Q, \mathbf{d}$ or observations H, R on at least one channel of their predecessor. For example, the 'bradycardia' factor overwrites the heart rate dynamics of the normal state, while the 'ECG dropout' factor overwrites the heart rate observations; if both these things are happening simultaneously then we expect the same observations as if there was only an ECG dropout, but the dynamics of the true state $\mathbf{x}_p$ are propagated as though there was only a bradycardia. Having found this ordering it is straightforward to merge the trained parameters for every combination of factors.

4 Results

Monitoring data was obtained from eight infants of 28 weeks gestation during their first week of life, from the NICU at Edinburgh Royal Infirmary. The data for each infant was collected every second for 24 hours, on nine channels: heart rate, systolic and diastolic blood pressures, $TcPO_2$, $TcPCO_2$, O_2 saturation, core temperature and incubator temperature and humidity. These infants were the first 8 in the NICU database who satisfied the age criteria and were monitored on all 8 channels for some 24 hour period within their first week. Four infants were used for training the model and four for evaluation. The test data was annotated with the times of occurrences of the factors in Table 1 by a clinical expert and one of the authors.

Some examples of inference under the model are shown in Figures 1(b) and 2. In Figure 1(b) two factors, arterial blood sample and ECG dropout are simultaneously active, and the inference works nicely in this case, with growing uncertainty about the true value of the heart-rate and blood pressure channels when artifactual readings are observed. The upper panel in figure 2(a) shows two examples of bradycardia being detected. In the lower panel, the model correctly infers the times that a clinician enters the incubator and replaces a disconnected core temperature probe. Figure 2(b) illustrates the simultaneous detection of a TCP artifact (the TCP recal state plotted is obtained by summing the probabilities of

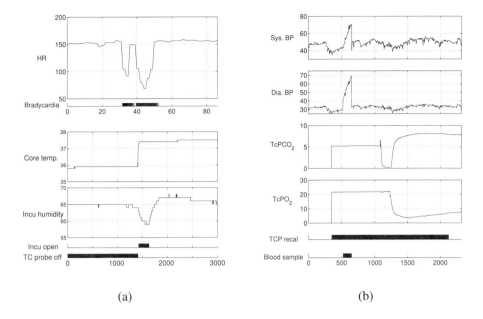

(a)　　　　　　　　　　　　　　　　　　　(b)

Figure 2: Inferred durations of physiological and artifactual states: (a) shows two episodes of bradycardia *(top)*, and a clinician entering the incubator and replacing the core temperature probe *(bottom)*. Plot (b) shows the inference of two simultaneous artifact processes, arterial blood sampling and TCP recalibration. Times are in seconds.

the three non-normal TCP states) and a blood sample spike.

In Table 2 we show the performance of the model on the test data. The inferred probabilities for each factor were compared with the gold standard which has a binary value for each factor setting at each time point. Inference was done using the Gaussian sum approximation and RBPF, where the number of particles was set so that the two inference methods had the same execution time. As a baseline we also used a Factorial Hidden Markov Model (FHMM) to infer when each factor was active. This model has the same factor structure as the FSKF, without any hidden continuous state. The FHMM parameters were set using the same training data as the FSKF.

It can be seen that the FSKF generalised well to the data from the test set. Inferences using the Gaussian Sum approximation had consistently higher area under the ROC curve and lower equal error rates than the FHMM. In particular, the inferred times of blood samples and incubator opening were reliably detected. The lower performance of the FHMM, which has no knowledge of the dynamics, illustrates the difficulty caused by baseline physiological levels changing over time and between babies.

Inference results using Rao-Blackwellised particle filtering were less consistent. For blood sampling and opening of the incubator the performance was worse than the baseline model, though in detecting bradycardia the performance was marginally higher than for inferences made using either the FHMM or the Gaussian Sum approximation.

Execution times for inference on 24 hours of monitoring data with the set of factors listed in Table 1 on a 3.2GHz processor were approximately 7 hours 10 minutes for the FSKF inference, and 100 seconds for the FHMM.

5 Discussion

In this paper we have shown that the FSKF model can be applied successfully to complex monitoring data from a neonatal intensive care unit.

There are a number of directions in which this work can be extended. Firstly, for simplicity we have used univariate autoregressive models for each component of the observations; it would be interesting to fit a multivariate model to this data instead, as we expect that there will be correlations between the channels. Also, there are additional factors that can be incorporated into the model, for example to model a pneumothorax event, where air becomes trapped inside the chest between the chest wall and the lung, causing the lung to collapse. Fortunately this event is relatively rare so it was not seen in the data we have analyzed in this experiment.

Acknowledgements

We thank Birgit Wefers for providing expert annotation of the evaluation data set, and the anonymous referees for their comments which helped improve the paper. This work was funded in part by a grant from the premature baby charity BLISS. The work was also supported in part by the IST Programme of the European Community, under the PAS-CAL Network of Excellence, IST-2002-506778. This publication only reflects the authors' views.

References

[1] D. L. Alspach and H. W. Sorenson. Nonlinear Bayesian Estimation Using Gaussian Sum Approximations. *IEEE Transactions on Automatic Control*, 17(4):439–448, 1972.

[2] C. Chatfield. *The Analysis of Time Series: An Introduction*. Chapman and Hall, London, 4th edition, 1989.

[3] Z. Ghahramani and G. E. Hinton. Variational Learning for Switching State-Space Models. *Neural Computation*, 12(4):963–996, 1998.

[4] S.W. Hoare and P.C.W. Beatty. Automatic artifact identification in anaesthesia patient record keeping: a comparison of techniques. *Medical Engineering and Physics*, 22:547–553, 2000.

[5] J. Ma and L. Deng. A mixed level switching dynamic system for continuous speech recognition. *Computer Speech and Language*, 18:49–65, 2004.

[6] K. Murphy. Switching Kalman filters. Technical report, U.C. Berkeley, 1998.

[7] K. Murphy and S. Russell. Rao-Blackwellised particle filtering for dynamic Bayesian networks. In A. Doucet, N. de Freitas, and N. Gordon, editors, *Sequential Monte Carlo in Practice*. Springer-Verlag, 2001.

[8] A. Spengler. Neonatal baby monitoring. Master's thesis, School of Informatics, University of Edinburgh, 2003.

[9] C. Tsien. *TrendFinder: Automated Detection of Alarmable Trends*. PhD thesis, MIT, 2000.

[10] M. West and P. J. Harrison. *Bayesian Forecasting and Dynamic Models*. Springer-Verlag, 1997. Second edition.

Comparing the Effects of Different Weight Distributions on Finding Sparse Representations

David Wipf and **Bhaskar Rao** *

Department of Electrical and Computer Engineering
University of California, San Diego, CA 92093
dwipf@ucsd.edu, brao@ece.ucsd.edu

Abstract

Given a redundant dictionary of basis vectors (or atoms), our goal is to find maximally sparse representations of signals. Previously, we have argued that a sparse Bayesian learning (SBL) framework is particularly well-suited for this task, showing that it has far fewer local minima than other Bayesian-inspired strategies. In this paper, we provide further evidence for this claim by proving a restricted equivalence condition, based on the distribution of the nonzero generating model weights, whereby the SBL solution will equal the maximally sparse representation. We also prove that if these nonzero weights are drawn from an approximate Jeffreys prior, then with probability approaching one, our equivalence condition is satisfied. Finally, we motivate the worst-case scenario for SBL and demonstrate that it is still better than the most widely used sparse representation algorithms. These include Basis Pursuit (BP), which is based on a convex relaxation of the ℓ_0 (quasi)-norm, and Orthogonal Matching Pursuit (OMP), a simple greedy strategy that iteratively selects basis vectors most aligned with the current residual.

1 Introduction

In recent years, there has been considerable interest in finding sparse signal representations from redundant dictionaries [1, 2, 3, 4, 5]. The canonical form of this problem is given by,

$$\min_{\boldsymbol{w}} \|\boldsymbol{w}\|_0, \qquad \text{s.t. } \boldsymbol{t} = \Phi\boldsymbol{w}, \tag{1}$$

where $\Phi \in \mathbb{R}^{N \times M}$ is a matrix whose columns represent an overcomplete or redundant basis (i.e., rank$(\Phi) = N$ and $M > N$), $\boldsymbol{w} \in \mathbb{R}^M$ is the vector of weights to be learned, and $\boldsymbol{t}$ is the signal vector. The cost function being minimized represents the ℓ_0 (quasi)-norm of $\boldsymbol{w}$ (i.e., a count of the nonzero elements in $\boldsymbol{w}$).

Unfortunately, an exhaustive search for the optimal representation requires the solution of up to $\binom{M}{N}$ linear systems of size $N \times N$, a prohibitively expensive procedure for even modest values of M and N. Consequently, in practical situations there is a need for approximate procedures that efficiently solve (1) with high probability. To date, the two most widely used choices are Basis Pursuit (BP) [1] and Orthogonal Matching Pursuit (OMP) [5]. BP is based on a convex relaxation of the ℓ_0 norm, i.e., replacing $\|\boldsymbol{w}\|_0$ with $\|\boldsymbol{w}\|_1$, which leads to an attractive, unimodal optimization problem that can be readily solved via linear programming. In contrast, OMP is a greedy strategy that iteratively selects the basis

*This work was supported by DiMI grant 22-8376, Nissan, and NSF grant DGE-0333451.

vector most aligned with the current signal residual. At each step, a new approximant is formed by projecting t onto the range of all the selected dictionary atoms.

Previously [9], we have demonstrated an alternative algorithm for solving (1) using a sparse Bayesian learning (SBL) framework [6] that maintains several significant advantages over other, Bayesian-inspired strategies for finding sparse solutions [7, 8]. The most basic formulation begins with an assumed likelihood model of the signal t given weights w,

$$p(t|w) = (2\pi\sigma^2)^{-N/2} \exp\left(-\frac{1}{2\sigma^2}\|t - \Phi w\|_2^2\right). \tag{2}$$

To provide a regularizing mechanism, SBL uses the parameterized weight prior

$$p(w;\gamma) = \prod_{i=1}^{M} (2\pi\gamma_i)^{-1/2} \exp\left(-\frac{w_i^2}{2\gamma_i}\right), \tag{3}$$

where $\gamma = [\gamma_1, \ldots, \gamma_M]^T$ is a vector of M hyperparameters controlling the prior variance of each weight. These hyperparameters can be estimated from the data by marginalizing over the weights and then performing ML optimization. The cost function for this task is

$$\mathcal{L}(\gamma) = -\log \int p(t|w)p(w;\gamma)dw \propto \log|\Sigma_t| + t^T \Sigma_t^{-1} t, \tag{4}$$

where $\Sigma_t \triangleq \sigma^2 I + \Phi \Gamma \Phi^T$ and we have introduced the notation $\Gamma \triangleq \mathrm{diag}(\gamma)$. This procedure, which can be implemented via the EM algorithm (or some other technique), is referred to as evidence maximization or type-II maximum likelihood [6]. Once γ has been estimated, a closed-form expression for the posterior weight distribution is available.

Although SBL was initially developed in a regression context, it can be easily adapted to handle (1) in the limit as $\sigma^2 \to 0$. To accomplish this we must reexpress the SBL iterations to handle the low noise limit. Applying various matrix identities to the EM algorithm-based update rules for each iteration, we arrive at the modified update [9]

$$\begin{aligned}
\gamma_{(\text{new})} &= \mathrm{diag}\left(\hat{w}_{(\text{old})}\hat{w}_{(\text{old})}^T + \left[I - \Gamma_{(\text{old})}^{1/2}\left(\Phi\Gamma_{(\text{old})}^{1/2}\right)^\dagger \Phi\right]\Gamma_{(\text{old})}\right) \\
\hat{w}_{(\text{new})} &= \Gamma_{(\text{new})}^{1/2}\left(\Phi\Gamma_{(\text{new})}^{1/2}\right)^\dagger t,
\end{aligned} \tag{5}$$

where $(\cdot)^\dagger$ denotes the Moore-Penrose pseudo-inverse. Given that $t \in \mathrm{range}(\Phi)$ and assuming γ is initialized with all nonzero elements, then feasibility is enforced at every iteration, i.e., $t = \Phi\hat{w}$. We will henceforth refer to w^{SBL} as the solution of this algorithm when initialized at $\Gamma = I_M$ and $\hat{w} = \Phi^\dagger t$.[1] In [9] (which extends work in [10]), we have argued why w^{SBL} should be considered a viable candidate for solving (1).

In comparing BP, OMP, and SBL, we would ultimately like to know in what situations a particular algorithm is likely to find the maximally sparse solution. A variety of results stipulate rigorous conditions whereby BP and OMP are guaranteed to solve (1) [1, 4, 5]. All of these conditions depend explicitly on the number of nonzero elements contained in the optimal solution. Essentially, if this number is less than some Φ-dependent constant κ, the BP/OMP solution is proven to be equivalent to the minimum ℓ_0-norm solution. Unfortunately however, κ turns out to be restrictively small and, for a fixed redundancy ratio M/N, grows very slowly as N becomes large [3]. But in practice, both approaches still perform well even when these equivalence conditions have been grossly violated. To address this issue, a much looser bound has recently been produced for BP, dependent only on M/N. This bound holds for "most" dictionaries in the limit as N becomes large [3], where "most"

---

[1] Based on EM convergence properties, the algorithm will converge monotonically to a fixed point.

is with respect to dictionaries composed of columns drawn uniformly from the surface of an N-dimensional unit hypersphere. For example, with $M/N = 2$, it is argued that BP is capable of resolving sparse solutions with roughly $0.3N$ nonzero elements with probability approaching one as $N \to \infty$.

Turning to SBL, we have neither a convenient convex cost function (as with BP) nor a simple, transparent update rule (as with OMP); however, we can nonetheless come up with an alternative type of equivalence result that is neither unequivocally stronger nor weaker than those existing results for BP and OMP. This condition is dependent on the relative magnitudes of the nonzero elements embedded in optimal solutions to (1). Additionally, we can leverage these ideas to motivate which sparse solutions are the most difficult to find. Later, we provide empirical evidence that SBL, even in this worst-case scenario, can still outperform both BP and OMP.

2   Equivalence Conditions for SBL

In this section, we establish conditions whereby $\boldsymbol{w}^{\text{SBL}}$ will minimize (1). To state these results, we require some notation. First, we formally define a dictionary $\Phi = [\boldsymbol{\phi}_1, \ldots, \boldsymbol{\phi}_M]$ as a set of M unit ℓ_2-norm vectors (atoms) in $\mathbb{R}^N$, with $M > N$ and rank$(\Phi) = N$. We say that a dictionary satisfies the unique representation property (URP) if every subset of N atoms forms a basis in $\mathbb{R}^N$. We define $w_{(i)}$ as the i-th largest weight magnitude and $\bar{w}$ as the $\|\boldsymbol{w}\|_0$-dimensional vector containing all the nonzero weight magnitudes of $\boldsymbol{w}$. The set of optimal solutions to (1) is $\mathcal{W}^*$ with cardinality $|\mathcal{W}^*|$. The *diversity* (or anti-sparsity) of each $\boldsymbol{w}^* \in \mathcal{W}^*$ is defined as $D^* \triangleq \|\boldsymbol{w}^*\|_0$.

Result 1. For a fixed dictionary Φ that satisfies the URP, there exists a set of $M - 1$ scaling constants $\nu_i \in (0, 1]$ (i.e., strictly greater than zero) such that, for any $\boldsymbol{t} = \Phi \boldsymbol{w}'$ generated with

$$w'_{(i+1)} \leq \nu_i w'_{(i)} \qquad i = 1, \ldots, M - 1, \tag{6}$$

SBL will produce a solution that satisfies $\|\boldsymbol{w}^{\text{SBL}}\|_0 = \min(N, \|\boldsymbol{w}'\|_0)$ and $\boldsymbol{w}^{\text{SBL}} \in \mathcal{W}^*$.

Do to space limitations, the proof has been deferred to [11]. The basic idea is that, as the magnitude differences between weights increase, at any given scale, the covariance Σ_t embedded in the SBL cost function is dominated by a single dictionary atom such that problematic local minimum are removed. The unique, global minimum in turn achieves the stated result.[2] The most interesting case occurs when $\|\boldsymbol{w}'\|_0 < N$, leading to the following:

Corollary 1. Given the additional restriction $\|\boldsymbol{w}'\|_0 < N$, then $\boldsymbol{w}^{\text{SBL}} = \boldsymbol{w}' \in \mathcal{W}^*$ and $|\mathcal{W}^*| = 1$, i.e., SBL will find the unique, maximally sparse representation of the signal $\boldsymbol{t}$.

See [11] for the proof. These results are restrictive in the sense that the dictionary dependent constants ν_i significantly confine the class of signals $\boldsymbol{t}$ that we may represent. Moreover, we have not provided any convenient means of computing what the different scaling constants might be. But we have nonetheless solidified the notion that SBL is most capable of recovering weights of different scales (and it must still find all D^* nonzero weights no matter how small some of them may be). Additionally, we have specified conditions whereby we will find the unique $\boldsymbol{w}^*$ even when the diversity is as large as $D^* = N - 1$. The tighter BP/OMP bound from [1, 4, 5] scales as $O\left(N^{-1/2}\right)$, although this latter bound is much more general in that it is independent of the magnitudes of the nonzero weights.

In contrast, neither BP or OMP satisfy a comparable result; in both cases, simple 3D counter examples suffice to illustrate this point.[3] We begin with OMP. Assume the fol-

---

[2]Because we have effectively shown that the SBL cost function must be unimodal, etc., any proven descent method could likely be applied in place of (5) to achieve the same result.

[3]While these examples might seem slightly nuanced, the situations being illustrated can occur frequently in practice and the requisite column normalization introduces some complexity.

lowing:

$$\boldsymbol{w}^* = \begin{bmatrix} 1 \\ \epsilon \\ 0 \\ 0 \end{bmatrix} \quad \Phi = \begin{bmatrix} 0 & \frac{1}{\sqrt{2}} & 0 & \frac{1}{\sqrt{1.01}} \\ 0 & 0 & 1 & \frac{0.1}{\sqrt{1.01}} \\ 1 & \frac{1}{\sqrt{2}} & 0 & 0 \end{bmatrix} \quad \boldsymbol{t} = \Phi\boldsymbol{w}^* = \begin{bmatrix} \frac{\epsilon}{\sqrt{2}} \\ 0 \\ 1 + \frac{\epsilon}{\sqrt{2}} \end{bmatrix}, \quad (7)$$

where Φ satisfies the URP and has columns ϕ_i of unit ℓ_2 norm. Given any $\epsilon \in (0, 1)$, we will now show that OMP will necessarily fail to find $\boldsymbol{w}^*$. Provided $\epsilon < 1$, at the first iteration OMP will select ϕ_1, which solves $\max_i |\boldsymbol{t}^T \phi_i|$, leaving the residual vector

$$\boldsymbol{r}_1 = \left(I - \phi_1 \phi_1^T\right) \boldsymbol{t} = [\ \epsilon/\sqrt{2} \quad 0 \quad 0\ ]^T. \quad (8)$$

Next, ϕ_4 will be chosen since it has the largest value in the top position, thus solving $\max_i |\boldsymbol{r}_1^T \phi_i|$. The residual is then updated to become

$$\boldsymbol{r}_2 = \left(I - [\ \phi_1 \quad \phi_4\ ][\ \phi_1 \quad \phi_4\ ]^T\right) \boldsymbol{t} = \frac{\epsilon}{101\sqrt{2}}[\ 1 \quad -10 \quad 0\ ]^T. \quad (9)$$

From the remaining two columns, $\boldsymbol{r}_2$ is most highly correlated with ϕ_3. Once ϕ_3 is selected, we obtain zero residual error, yet we did not find $\boldsymbol{w}^*$, which involves only ϕ_1 and ϕ_2. So for all $\epsilon \in (0, 1)$, the algorithm fails. As such, there can be no fixed constant $\nu > 0$ such that if $w_{(2)}^* \equiv \epsilon \leq \nu w_{(1)}^* \equiv \nu$, we are guaranteed to obtain $\boldsymbol{w}^*$ (unlike with SBL).

We now give an analogous example for BP, where we present a feasible solution with smaller ℓ_1 norm than the maximally sparse solution. Given

$$\boldsymbol{w}^* = \begin{bmatrix} 1 \\ \epsilon \\ 0 \\ 0 \end{bmatrix} \quad \Phi = \begin{bmatrix} 0 & 1 & \frac{0.1}{\sqrt{1.02}} & \frac{0.1}{\sqrt{1.02}} \\ 0 & 0 & \frac{-0.1}{\sqrt{1.02}} & \frac{0.1}{\sqrt{1.02}} \\ 1 & 0 & \frac{1}{\sqrt{1.02}} & \frac{1}{\sqrt{1.02}} \end{bmatrix} \quad \boldsymbol{t} = \Phi\boldsymbol{w}^* = \begin{bmatrix} \epsilon \\ 0 \\ 1 \end{bmatrix}, \quad (10)$$

it is clear that $\|\boldsymbol{w}^*\|_1 = 1 + \epsilon$. However, for all $\epsilon \in (0, 0.1)$, if we form a feasible solution using only ϕ_1, ϕ_3, and ϕ_4, we obtain the alternate solution $\boldsymbol{w} = [\ (1 - 10\epsilon) \quad 0 \quad 5\sqrt{1.02}\epsilon \quad 5\sqrt{1.02}\epsilon\ ]^T$ with $\|\boldsymbol{w}\|_1 \approx 1 + 0.1\epsilon$. Since this has a smaller ℓ_1 norm for all ϵ in the specified range, BP will necessarily fail and so again, we cannot reproduce the result for a similar reason as before.

At this point, it remains unclear what probability distributions are likely to produce weights that satisfy the conditions of Result 1. It turns out that the Jeffreys prior, given by $p(x) \propto 1/x$, is appropriate for this task. This distribution has the unique property that the probability mass assigned to any given scaling is equal. More explicitly, for any $s \geq 1$,

$$P\left(x \in [s^i, s^{i+1}]\right) \propto \log(s) \quad \forall i \in \mathbb{Z}. \quad (11)$$

For example, the probability that x is between 1 and 10 equals the probability that it lies between 10 and 100 or between 0.01 and 0.1. Because this is an improper density, we define an approximate Jeffreys prior with range parameter $a \in (0, 1]$. Specifically, we say that $x \sim J(a)$ if

$$p(x) = \frac{-1}{2\log(a)x} \quad \text{for } x \in [a, 1/a]. \quad (12)$$

With this definition in mind, we present the following result.

Result 2. For a fixed Φ that satisfies the URP, let $\boldsymbol{t}$ be generated by $\boldsymbol{t} = \Phi\boldsymbol{w}'$, where $\boldsymbol{w}'$ has magnitudes drawn iid from $J(a)$. Then as a approaches zero, the probability that we obtain a $\boldsymbol{w}'$ such that the conditions of Result 1 are satisfied approaches unity.

Again, for space considerations, we refer the reader to [11]. However, on a conceptual level this result can be understood by considering the distribution of order statistics. For example, given M samples from a uniform distribution between zero and some θ, with probability approaching one, the distance between the k-th and $(k+1)$-th order statistic can be made arbitrarily large as θ moves towards infinity. Likewise, with the $J(a)$ distribution, the relative scaling between order statistics can be increased without bound as a decreases towards zero, leading to the stated result.

Corollary 2. Assume that $D' < N$ randomly selected elements of $\boldsymbol{w}'$ are set to zero. Then as a approaches zero, the probability that we satisfy the conditions of Corollary 1 approaches unity.

In conclusion, we have shown that a simple, (approximate) noninformative Jeffreys prior leads to sparse inverse problems that are optimally solved via SBL with high probability. Interestingly, it is this same Jeffreys prior that forms the implicit weight prior of SBL (see [6], Section 5.1). However, it is worth mentioning that other Jeffreys prior-based techniques, e.g., direct minimization of $p(\boldsymbol{w}) = \prod_i \frac{1}{|w_i|}$ subject to $\boldsymbol{t} = \Phi \boldsymbol{w}$, do *not* provide any SBL-like guarantees. Although several algorithms do exist that can perform such a minimization task (e.g., [7, 8]), they perform poorly with respect to (1) because of convergence to local minimum as shown in [9, 10]. This is especially true if the weights are highly scaled, and no nontrivial equivalence results are known to exist for these procedures.

3 Worst-Case Scenario

If the best-case scenario occurs when the nonzero weights are all of very different scales, it seems reasonable that the most difficult sparse inverse problem may involve weights of the same or even identical scale, e.g., $\bar{w}_1^* = \bar{w}_2^* = \ldots \bar{w}_{D^*}^*$. This notion can be formalized somewhat by considering the $\bar{\boldsymbol{w}}^*$ distribution that is furthest from the Jeffreys prior. First, we note that both the SBL cost function and update rules are independent of the overall scaling of the generating weights, meaning $\alpha \bar{\boldsymbol{w}}^*$ is functionally equivalent to $\bar{\boldsymbol{w}}^*$ provided α is nonzero. This invariance must be taken into account in our analysis. Therefore, we assume the weights are rescaled such that $\sum_i \bar{w}_i^* = 1$. Given this restriction, we will find the distribution of weight magnitudes that is most different from the Jeffreys prior.

Using the standard procedure for changing the parameterization of a probability density, the joint density of the constrained variables can be computed simply as

$$p(\bar{w}_1^*, \ldots, \bar{w}_{D^*}^*) \propto \frac{1}{\prod_{i=1}^{D^*} \bar{w}_i^*} \quad \text{for} \quad \sum_{i=1}^{D^*} \bar{w}_i^* = 1, \quad \bar{w}_i^* \geq 0, \forall i. \tag{13}$$

From this expression, it is easily shown that $\bar{w}_1^* = \bar{w}_2^* = \ldots = \bar{w}_{D^*}^*$ achieves the global minimum. Consequently, equal weights are the absolute *least* likely to occur from the Jeffreys prior. Hence, we may argue that the distribution that assigns $\bar{w}_i^* = 1/D^*$ with probability one is furthest from the constrained Jeffreys prior.

Nevertheless, because of the complexity of the SBL framework, it is difficult to prove axiomatically that $\bar{\boldsymbol{w}}^* \sim \boldsymbol{1}$ is overall the most problematic distribution with respect to sparse recovery. We can however provide additional motivation for why we should expect it to be unwieldy. As proven in [9], the global minimum of the SBL cost function is guaranteed to produce some $\boldsymbol{w}^* \in \mathcal{W}^*$. This minimum is achieved with the hyperparameters $\gamma_i^* = (w_i^*)^2$, $\forall i$. We can think of this solution as forming a collapsed, or degenerate covariance $\Sigma_t^* = \Phi \Gamma^* \Phi^T$ that occupies a proper D^*-dimensional subspace of N-dimensional signal space. Moreover, this subspace must necessarily contain the signal vector $\boldsymbol{t}$. Essentially, Σ_t^* proscribes infinite density to $\boldsymbol{t}$, leading to the globally minimizing solution.

Now consider an alternative covariance $\Sigma_t^\diamond$ that, although still full rank, is nonetheless ill-conditioned (flattened), containing $\boldsymbol{t}$ within its high density region. Furthermore, assume that $\Sigma_t^\diamond$ is not well aligned with the subspace formed by Σ_t^*. The mixture of two flattened, yet misaligned covariances naturally leads to a more voluminous (less dense) form as measured by the determinant $|\alpha \Sigma_t^* + \beta \Sigma_t^\diamond|$. Thus, as we transition from $\Sigma_t^\diamond$ to Σ_t^*, we necessarily reduce the density at t, thereby increasing the cost function $\mathcal{L}(\gamma)$. So if SBL converges to $\Sigma_t^\diamond$ it has fallen into a local minimum.

So the question remains, what values of w^* are likely to create the most situations where this type of local minima occurs? The issue is resolved when we again consider the D^*-dimensional subspace determined by Σ_t^*. The volume of the covariance *within* this subspace is given by $\left| \bar{\Phi}^* \bar{\Gamma}^* \bar{\Phi}^{*T} \right|$, where $\bar{\Phi}^*$ and $\bar{\Gamma}^*$ are the basis vectors and hyperparameters associated with w^*. The larger this volume, the higher the probability that other basis vectors will be suitably positioned so as to both (i), contain t within the high density portion and (ii), maintain a sufficient component that is misaligned with the optimal covariance.

The maximum volume of $\left| \bar{\Phi}^* \bar{\Gamma}^* \bar{\Phi}^{*T} \right|$ under the constraints $\sum_i \bar{w}_i^* = 1$ and $\bar{\gamma}_i^* = (\bar{w}^*)_i^2$ occurs with $\bar{\gamma}_i^* = 1/(D^*)^2$, i.e., all the $\bar{w}_i^*$ are equal. Consequently, geometric considerations support the notion that deviance from the Jeffreys prior leads to difficulty recovering w^*. Moreover, empirical analysis (not shown) of the relationship between volume and local minimum avoidance provide further corroboration of this hypothesis.

4 Empirical Comparisons

The central purpose of this section is to present empirical evidence that supports our theoretical analysis and illustrates the improved performance afforded by SBL. As previously mentioned, others have established deterministic equivalence conditions, dependent on D^*, whereby BP and OMP are guaranteed to find the unique w^*. Unfortunately, the relevant theorems are of little value in assessing practical differences between algorithms. This is because, in the cases we have tested where BP/OMP equivalence is provably known to hold (e.g., via results in [1, 4, 5]), SBL always converges to w^* as well.

As such, we will focuss our attention on the insights provided by Sections 2 and 3 as well as probabilistic comparisons with [3]. Given a fixed distribution for the nonzero elements of w^*, we will assess which algorithm is best (at least empirically) for most dictionaries relative to a uniform measure on the unit sphere as discussed.

To this effect, a number of monte-carlo simulations were conducted, each consisting of the following: First, a random, overcomplete $N \times M$ dictionary Φ is created whose entries are each drawn uniformly from the surface of an N-dimensional hypersphere. Next, sparse weight vectors w^* are randomly generated with D^* nonzero entries. Nonzero amplitudes $\bar{w}^*$ are drawn iid from an experiment-dependent distribution. Response values are then computed as $t = \Phi w^*$. Each algorithm is presented with t and Φ and attempts to estimate w^*. In all cases, we ran 1000 independent trials and compared the number of times each algorithm failed to recover w^*. Under the specified conditions for the generation of Φ and t, all other feasible solutions w almost surely have a diversity greater than D^*, so our synthetically generated w^* must be maximally sparse. Moreover, Φ will almost surely satisfy the URP.

With regard to particulars, there are essentially four variables with which to experiment: (i) the distribution of $\bar{w}^*$, (ii) the diversity D^*, (iii) N, and (iv) M. In Figure 1, we display results from an array of testing conditions. In each *row* of the figure, $\bar{w}_i^*$ is drawn iid from a fixed distribution for all i; the first row uses $\bar{w}_i^* = 1$, the second has $\bar{w}_i^* \sim J(a = 0.001)$, and the third uses $\bar{w}_i^* \sim N(0, 1)$, i.e., a unit Gaussian. In all cases, the signs of the nonzero weights are irrelevant due to the randomness inherent in the basis vectors.

The *columns* of Figure 1 are organized as follows: The first column is based on the values $N = 50$, $D^* = 16$, while M is varied from N to $5N$, testing the effects of an increasing level of dictionary redundancy, M/N. The second fixes $N = 50$ and $M = 100$ while D^* is varied from 10 to 30, exploring the ability of each algorithm to resolve an increasing number of nonzero weights. Finally, the third column fixes $M/N = 2$ and $D^*/N \approx 0.3$

while N, M, and D^* are increased proportionally. This demonstrates how performance scales with larger problem sizes.

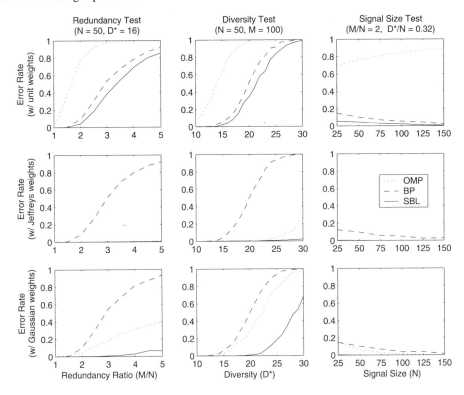

Figure 1: Empirical results comparing the probability that OMP, BP, and SBL fail to find w^* under various testing conditions. Each data point is based on 1000 independent trials. The distribution of the nonzero weight amplitudes is labeled on the far left for each row, while the values for N, M, and D^* are included on the top of each column. Independent variables are labeled along the bottom of the figure.

The first row of plots essentially represents the worst-case scenario for SBL per our previous analysis, and yet performance is still consistently better than both BP and OMP. In contrast, the second row of plots approximates the best-case performance for SBL, where we see that SBL is almost infallible. The handful of failure events that do occur are because a is not sufficiently small and therefore, $J(a)$ was not sufficiently close to a true Jeffreys prior to achieve perfect equivalence (see center plot). Although OMP also does well here, the parameter a can generally never be adjusted such that OMP always succeeds. Finally, the last row of plots, based on Gaussian distributed weight amplitudes, reflects a balance between these two extremes. Nonetheless, SBL still holds a substantial advantage.

In general, we observe that SBL is capable of handling more redundant dictionaries (column one) and resolving a larger number of nonzero weights (column two). Also, column three illustrates that both BP and SBL are able to resolve a number of weights that grows linearly in the signal dimension ($\approx 0.3N$), consistent with the analysis in [3] (which applies only to BP). In contrast, OMP performance begins to degrade in some cases (see the upper right plot), a potential limitation of this approach. Of course additional study is necessary to fully compare the relative performance of these methods on large-scale problems.

Finally, by comparing row one, two and three, we observe that the performance of BP is roughly independent of the weight distribution, with performance slightly below the worst-case SBL performance. Like SBL, OMP results are highly dependent on the distribution; however, as the weight distribution approaches unity, performance is unsatisfactory. In summary, while the relative proficiency between OMP and BP is contingent on experimental particulars, SBL is uniformly superior in the cases we have tested (including examples not shown, e.g., results with other dictionary types).

5 Conclusions

In this paper, we have related the ability to find maximally sparse solutions to the particular distribution of amplitudes that compose the nonzero elements. At first glance, it may seem reasonable that the most difficult sparse inverse problems occur when some of the nonzero weights are extremely small, making them difficult to estimate. Perhaps surprisingly then, we have shown that the exact opposite is true with SBL: The more diverse the weight magnitudes, the better the chances we have of learning the optimal solution. In contrast, unit weights offer the most challenging task for SBL. Nonetheless, even in this worst-case scenario, we have shown that SBL outperforms the current state-of-the-art; the overall assumption here being that, if worst-case performance is superior, then it is likely to perform better in a variety of situations.

For a *fixed* dictionary and diversity D^*, successful recovery of unit weights does not absolutely guarantee that any alternative weighting scheme will necessarily be recovered as well. However, a weaker result does appear to be feasible: For fixed values of N, M, and D^*, if the success rate recovering unity weights approaches one for most dictionaries, where most is defined as in Section 1, then the success rate recovering weights of any other distribution (assuming they are distributed independently of the dictionary) will also approach one. While a formal proof of this conjecture is beyond the scope of this paper, it seems to be a very reasonable result that is certainly born out by experimental evidence, geometric considerations, and the arguments presented in Section 3. Nonetheless, this remains a fruitful area for further inquiry.

References

[1] D. Donoho and M. Elad, "Optimally sparse representation in general (nonorthogonal) dictionaries via ℓ_1 minimization," *Proc. Nat. Acad. Sci.*, vol. 100, no. 5, pp. 2197–2202, March 2003.

[2] R. Gribonval and M. Nielsen, "Sparse representations in unions of bases," *IEEE Transactions on Information Theory*, vol. 49, pp. 3320–3325, Dec. 2003.

[3] D. Donoho, "For most large underdetermined systems of linear equations the minimal ℓ_1-norm solution is also the sparsest solution," *Stanford University Technical Report*, September 2004.

[4] J.J. Fuchs, "On sparse representations in arbitrary redundant bases," *IEEE Transactions on Information Theory*, vol. 50, no. 6, pp. 1341–1344, June 2004.

[5] J.A. Tropp, "Greed is good: Algorithmic results for sparse approximation," *IEEE Transactions on Information Theory*, vol. 50, no. 10, pp. 2231–2242, October 2004.

[6] M.E. Tipping, "Sparse Bayesian learning and the relevance vector machine," *Journal of Machine Learning Research*, vol. 1, pp. 211–244, 2001.

[7] I.F. Gorodnitsky and B.D. Rao, "Sparse signal reconstruction from limited data using FOCUSS: A re-weighted minimum norm algorithm," *IEEE Transactions on Signal Processing*, vol. 45, no. 3, pp. 600–616, March 1997.

[8] M.A.T. Figueiredo, "Adaptive sparseness using Jeffreys prior," *Advances in Neural Information Processing Systems 14*, pp. 697–704, 2002.

[9] D.P. Wipf and B.D. Rao, "ℓ_0-norm minimization for basis selection," *Advances in Neural Information Processing Systems 17*, pp. 1513–1520, 2005.

[10] D.P. Wipf and B.D. Rao, "Sparse Bayesian learning for basis selection," *IEEE Transactions on Signal Processing*, vol. 52, no. 8, pp. 2153–2164, 2004.

[11] D.P. Wipf, To appear in *Bayesian Methods for Sparse Signal Representation*, PhD Dissertation, UC San Diego, 2006 (estimated). http://dsp.ucsd.edu/~dwipf/

Message passing for task redistribution on sparse graphs

K. Y. Michael Wong
Hong Kong U. of Science & Technology
Clear Water Bay, Hong Kong, China
phkywong@ust.hk

David Saad
NCRG, Aston University
Birmingham B4 7ET, UK
D.Saad@aston.ac.uk

Zhuo Gao
Hong Kong U. of Science & Technology, Clear Water Bay, Hong Kong, China
Permanent address: Dept. of Physics, Beijing Normal Univ., Beijing 100875, China
zhuogao@bnu.edu.cn

Abstract

The problem of resource allocation in sparse graphs with *real* variables is studied using methods of statistical physics. An efficient distributed algorithm is devised on the basis of insight gained from the analysis and is examined using numerical simulations, showing excellent performance and full agreement with the theoretical results.

1 Introduction

Optimal resource allocation is a well known problem in the area of distributed computing [1, 2] to which significant effort has been dedicated within the computer science community. The problem itself is quite general and is applicable to other areas as well where a large number of nodes are required to balance loads/resources and redistribute tasks, such as reducing internet traffic congestion [3]. The problem has many flavors and usually refers, in the computer science literature, to finding practical heuristic solutions to the distribution of computational load between computers connected in a predetermined manner.

The problem we are addressing here is more generic and is represented by nodes of some computational power that should carry out tasks. Both computational powers and tasks will be chosen at random from some arbitrary distribution. The nodes are located on a randomly chosen sparse graph of some given connectivity. The goal is to migrate tasks on the graph such that demands will be satisfied while minimizing the migration of (sub-)tasks. An important aspect of the desired algorithmic solution is that decisions on messages to be passed are carried out locally; this enables an efficient implementation of the algorithm in large non-centralized distributed networks. We focus here on the satisfiable case where the total computing power is greater than the demand, and where the number of nodes involved is very large. The unsatisfiable case can be addressed using similar techniques.

We analyze the problem using the Bethe approximation of statistical mechanics in Section 2, and alternatively a new variant of the replica method [4, 5] in Section 3. We then present numerical results in Section 4, and derive a new message passing distributed algorithm on the basis of the analysis (in Section 5). We conclude the paper with a summary and a brief discussion on future work.

2   The statistical physics framework: Bethe approximation

We consider a typical resource allocation task on a sparse graph of N nodes, labelled $i = 1, .., N$. Each node i is randomly connected to c other nodes[1], and has a capacity Λ_i randomly drawn from a distribution $\rho(\Lambda_i)$. The objective is to migrate tasks between nodes such that each node will be capable of carrying out its tasks. The *current* $y_{ij} \equiv -y_{ji}$ drawn from node j to i is aimed at satisfying the constraint

$$\sum_j \mathcal{A}_{ij} y_{ij} + \Lambda_i \geq 0 , \tag{1}$$

representing the 'revised' assignment for node i, where $\mathcal{A}_{ij} = 1/0$ for connected/unconnected node pairs i and j, respectively. To illustrate the statistical mechanics approach to resource allocation, we consider the load balancing task of minimizing the energy function (cost) $E = \sum_{(ij)} \mathcal{A}_{ij} \phi(y_{ij})$, where the summation (ij) runs over all pairs of nodes, subject to the constraints (1); $\phi(y)$ is a general function of the current y. For load balancing tasks, $\phi(y)$ is typically a convex function, which will be assumed in our study. The analysis of the graph is done by introducing the free energy $F = -T \ln \mathcal{Z}_y$ for a temperature $T \equiv \beta^{-1}$, where $\mathcal{Z}_y$ is the partition function

$$\mathcal{Z}_y = \prod_{(ij)} \int dy_{ij} \prod_i \Theta \left(\sum_j \mathcal{A}_{ij} y_{ij} + \Lambda_i \right) \exp\left[-\beta \sum_{(ij)} \mathcal{A}_{ij} \phi(y_{ij}) \right] . \tag{2}$$

The Θ function returns 1 for a non-negative argument and 0 otherwise.

When the connectivity c is low, the probability of finding a loop of finite length on the graph is low, and the Bethe approximation well describes the local environment of a node. In the approximation, a node is connected to c branches in a tree structure, and the correlations among the branches of the tree are neglected. In each branch, nodes are arranged in generations. A node is connected to an ancestor node of the previous generation, and another $c - 1$ descendent nodes of the next generation.

Consider a vertex $V(\mathbf{T})$ of capacity $\Lambda_{V(\mathbf{T})}$, and a current y is drawn from the vertex. One can write an expression for the free energy $F(y|\mathbf{T})$ as a function of the free energies $F(y_k|\mathbf{T}_k)$ of its descendants, that branch out from this vertex

$$F(y|\mathbf{T}) = -T \ln \left\{ \prod_{k=1}^{c-1} \left(\int dy_k \right) \Theta \left(\sum_{k=1}^{c-1} y_k - y + \Lambda_V \right) \right.$$
$$\left. \times \exp\left[-\beta \sum_{k=1}^{c-1} (F(y_k|\mathbf{T}_k) + \phi(y_k)) \right] \right\}, \tag{3}$$

where $\mathbf{T}_k$ represents the tree terminated at the kth descendent of the vertex. The free energy can be considered as the sum of two parts, $F(y|\mathbf{T}) = N_\mathbf{T} F_{\text{av}} + F_V(y|\mathbf{T})$, where $N_\mathbf{T}$ is the number of nodes in the tree $\mathbf{T}$, F_{av} is the average free energy per node, and $F_V(y|\mathbf{T})$ is referred to as the *vertex free energy*[2]. Note that when a vertex is added to a tree, there is a

---

[1]Although we focus here on graphs of fixed connectivity, one can easily accommodate any connectivity profile within the same framework; the algorithms presented later are completely general.

[2]This term is marginalized over all inputs to the current vertex, leaving the difference in chemical potential y as its sole argument, hence the terminology used.

change in the free energy due to the added vertex. Since the number of nodes increases by 1, the vertex free energy is obtained by subtracting the free energy change by the average free energy. This allows us to obtain the recursion relation

$$F_V(y|\mathbf{T}) = -T \ln \left\{ \prod_{k=1}^{c-1} \left(\int dy_k \right) \Theta \left(\sum_{k=1}^{c-1} y_k - y + \Lambda_{V(\mathbf{T})} \right) \right.$$
$$\left. \times \exp \left[-\beta \sum_{k=1}^{c-1} (F_V(y_k|\mathbf{T}_k) + \phi(y_k)) \right] \right\} - F_{\mathrm{av}}, \qquad (4)$$

and the average free energy per node is given by

$$F_{\mathrm{av}} = -T \left\langle \ln \left\{ \prod_{k=1}^{c} \left(\int dy_k \right) \Theta \left(\sum_{k=1}^{c} y_k + \Lambda_V \right) \right. \right.$$
$$\left. \left. \times \exp \left[-\beta \sum_{k=1}^{c} (F_V(y_k|\mathbf{T}_k) + \phi(y_k)) \right] \right\} \right\rangle_\Lambda, \qquad (5)$$

where Λ_V is the capacity of the vertex V fed by c trees $\mathbf{T}_1, \ldots, \mathbf{T}_c$, and $\langle \ldots \rangle_\Lambda$ represents the average over the distribution $\rho(\Lambda)$. In the zero temperature limit, Eq. (4) reduces to

$$F_V(y|\mathbf{T}) = \min_{\{y_k | \sum_{k=1}^{c-1} y_k - y + \Lambda_{V(\mathbf{T})} \geq 0\}} \left[\sum_{k=1}^{c-1} (F_V(y_k|\mathbf{T}_k) + \phi(y_k)) \right] - F_{\mathrm{av}}. \qquad (6)$$

The current distribution and the average free energy per link can be derived by integrating the current y' in a link from one vertex to another, fed by the trees $\mathbf{T}_1$ and $\mathbf{T}_2$, respectively; the obtained expressions are $P(y) = \langle \delta(y - y') \rangle_\star$ and $\langle E \rangle = \langle \phi(y') \rangle_\star$ where

$$\langle \bullet \rangle_\star = \left\langle \frac{\int dy' \exp\left[-\beta \left(F_V(y'|\mathbf{T}_1) + F_V(-y'|\mathbf{T}_2) + \phi(y') \right) \right] (\bullet)}{\int dy' \exp\left[-\beta \left(F_V(y'|\mathbf{T}_1) + F_V(-y'|\mathbf{T}_2) + \phi(y') \right) \right]} \right\rangle_\Lambda. \qquad (7)$$

3   The statistical physics framework: replica method

In this section, we sketch the analysis of the problem using the replica method, as an alternative to the Bethe approximation. The derivation is rathe involved, details will be provided elsewhere. To facilitate derivations, we focus on the quadratic cost function $\phi(y) = y^2/2$. The results confirm the validity of the Bethe approximation on sparse graphs.

An alternative formulation of the original optimization problem is to consider its dual. Introducing Lagrange multipliers, the function to be minimized becomes $L = \sum_{(ij)} \mathcal{A}_{ij} y_{ij}^2 / 2 + \sum_i \mu_i (\sum_j \mathcal{A}_{ij} y_{ij} + \Lambda_i)$. Optimizing L with respect to y_{ij}, one obtains $y_{ij} = \mu_j - \mu_i$, where μ_i is referred to as the *chemical potential* of node i, and the current is driven by the potential difference.

Although the analysis has also been carried out in the space of currents, we focus here on the optimization problem in the space of the chemical potentials. Since the energy function is invariant under the addition of an arbitrary global constant to the chemical potentials of all nodes, we introduce an extra regularization term $\epsilon \sum_i \mu_i^2 / 2$ to break the translational symmetry, where $\epsilon \to 0$. To study the characteristics of the problem one calculates the averaged free energy per node $F_{\mathrm{av}} = -T \langle \ln \mathcal{Z}_\mu \rangle_{A,\Lambda} / N$, where $\mathcal{Z}_\mu$ is the partition function

$$\prod_i \left[\int d\mu_i \, \Theta \left(\sum_j \mathcal{A}_{ij}(\mu_j - \mu_i) + \Lambda_i \right) \right] \exp \left[-\frac{\beta}{2} \left(\sum_{(ij)} \mathcal{A}_{ij}(\mu_j - \mu_i)^2 + \epsilon \sum_i \mu_i^2 \right) \right].$$

The calculation follows the main steps of a replica based calculation in diluted systems [6], using the identity $\ln \mathcal{Z} = \lim_{n \to 0}[\mathcal{Z}^n - 1]/n$. The replicated partition function [5] is averaged over all network configurations with connectivity and capacity distributions $\rho(\Lambda_i)$. We consider the case of intensive connectivity $c \sim O(1) \ll N$. Extending the analysis of [6] and averaging over all connectivity matrices, one finds

$$
\langle \mathcal{Z}_\mu^n \rangle = \quad \exp N \left\{ \frac{c}{2} - c \sum_{\mathbf{r},\mathbf{s}} \hat{Q}_{\mathbf{r},\mathbf{s}} Q_{\mathbf{r},\mathbf{s}} + \ln \int d\Lambda \rho(\Lambda) \prod_\alpha \left(\int d\mu_\alpha \int_\Lambda^\infty d\lambda_\alpha \int \frac{d\hat{\lambda}_\alpha}{2\pi} \right) \right.
$$
$$
\left. \times \exp\left[\sum_\alpha \left(i\hat{\lambda}_\alpha (\lambda_\alpha + c\mu_\alpha) - \frac{\beta}{2}(c + \epsilon)\mu_\alpha^2 \right) \right] X^c \right\}, \tag{8}
$$

where $X = \sum_{\mathbf{r},\mathbf{s}} \hat{Q}_{\mathbf{r},\mathbf{s}} \prod_\alpha (-i\hat{\lambda}_\alpha)^{r_\alpha} \mu_\alpha^{s_\alpha} + \sum_{\mathbf{r},\mathbf{s}} \frac{Q_{\mathbf{r},\mathbf{s}}}{2 \prod_\alpha r_\alpha! s_\alpha!} \prod_\alpha \mu_\alpha^{r_\alpha} (\beta\mu_\alpha - i\hat{\lambda}_\alpha)^{s_\alpha}$. The order parameters $Q_{\mathbf{r},\mathbf{s}}$ and $\hat{Q}_{\mathbf{r},\mathbf{s}}$, are labelled by the somewhat unusual indices $\mathbf{r}$ and $\mathbf{s}$, representing the n-component integer vectors $(r_1, .., r_n)$ and $(s_1, .., s_n)$ respectively. This is a result of the specific interaction considered which entangles nodes of different indices. The order parameters $Q_{\mathbf{r},\mathbf{s}}$ and $\hat{Q}_{\mathbf{r},\mathbf{s}}$ are given by the extremum condition of Eq. (8), i.e., via a set of saddle point equations w.r.t the order parameters. Assuming replica symmetry, the saddle point equations yield a recursion relation for a two-component function R, which is related to the order parameters via the generating function

$$
P_{\mathbf{s}}(\mathbf{z}) = \sum_{\mathbf{r}} Q_{\mathbf{r},\mathbf{s}} \prod_\alpha \frac{(z_\alpha)^{r_\alpha}}{r_\alpha!} = \left\langle \prod_\alpha \left(\int d\mu \, R(z_\alpha, \mu | \mathbf{T}) e^{-\beta\mu^2/2} \mu^{s_\alpha} \right) \right\rangle_\Lambda. \tag{9}
$$

In Eq. (9), $\mathbf{T}$ represents the tree terminated at the vertex node with chemical potential μ, providing input to the ancestor node with chemical potential z, and $\langle \ldots \rangle_\Lambda$ represents the average over the distribution $\rho(\Lambda)$. The resultant recursion relation for $R(z, \mu | \mathbf{T})$ is independent of the replica indices, and is given by

$$
R(z, \mu | \mathbf{T}) = \quad \frac{1}{\mathcal{D}} \prod_{k=1}^{c-1} \left(\int d\mu_k R(\mu, \mu_k | \mathbf{T}_k) \right) \Theta\left(\sum_{k=1}^{c-1} \mu_k - c\mu + z + \Lambda_{V(\mathbf{T})} \right)
$$
$$
\times \exp\left[-\frac{\beta}{2} \left(\sum_{k=1}^{c-1} (\mu - \mu_k)^2 + \epsilon\mu^2 \right) \right], \tag{10}
$$

where the vertex node has a capacity $\Lambda_{V(\mathbf{T})}$; $\mathcal{D}$ is a constant. $R(z, \mu | \mathbf{T})$ is expressed in terms of $c - 1$ functions $R(\mu, \mu_k | \mathbf{T}_k)$ $(k = 1, .., c-1)$, integrated over μ_k. This algebraic structure is typical of the Bethe lattice tree-like representation of networks of connectivity c, where a node obtains input from its $c - 1$ descendent nodes of the next generation, and $\mathbf{T}_k$ represents the tree terminated at the kth descendent.

Except for the regularization factor $\exp(-\beta\epsilon\mu^2/2)$, R turns out to be a function of $y \equiv \mu - z$, which is interpreted as the current drawn from a node with chemical potential μ by its ancestor with chemical potential z. One can then express the function R as the product of a *vertex partition function* Z_V and a normalization factor W, that is, $R(z, \mu | \mathbf{T}) = W(\mu) Z_V(y | \mathbf{T})$. In the limit $n \to 0$, the dependence on μ and y are separable, providing a recursion relation for $Z_V(y | \mathbf{T})$. This gives rise to the *vertex free energy* $F_V(y | \mathbf{T}) = -T \ln Z_V(y | \mathbf{T})$ when a current y is drawn from the vertex of a tree $\mathbf{T}$. The recursive equation and the average free energy expression agrees with the results in the Bethe approximation. These iterative equations can be directly linked to those obtained from a principled Bayesian approximation, where the logarithms of the messages passed between nodes are proportional to the vertex free energies.

4   Numerical solution

The solution of Eq. (6) is obtained numerically. Since the vertex free energy of a node depends on its own capacity and the disordered configuration of its descendants, we generate 1000 nodes at each iteration of Eq. (6), with capacities randomly drawn from the distribution $\rho(\Lambda)$, each being fed by $c-1$ nodes randomly drawn from the previous iteration.

We have discretized the vertex free energies $F_V(y|\mathbf{T})$ function into a vector, whose i^{th} component is the value of the function corresponding to the current y_i. To speed up the optimization search at each node, we first find the *vertex saturation current* drawn from a node such that: (a) the capacity of the node is just used up; (b) the current drawn by each of its descendant nodes is just enough to saturate its own capacity constraint. When these conditions are satisfied, we can separately optimize the current drawn by each descendant node, and the vertex saturation current is equal to the node capacity subtracted by the current drawn by its descendants. The optimal solution can be found using an exhaustive search, by varying the component currents in small discrete steps. This approach is particularly convenient for $c = 3$, where the search is confined to a single parameter.

To compute the average energy, we randomly draw 2 nodes, compute the optimal current flowing between them, and repeat the sampling to obtain the average. Figure 1(a) shows the results as a function of iteration step t, for a Gaussian capacity distribution $\rho(\Lambda)$ with variance 1 and average $\langle \Lambda \rangle$. Each iteration corresponds to adding one extra generation to the tree structure, such that the iterative process corresponds to approximating the network by an increasingly extensive tree. We observe that after an initial rise with iteration steps, the average energies converges to steady-state values, at a rate which increases with the average capacity.

To study the convergence rate of the iterations, we fit the average energy at iteration step t using $\langle E(t) - E(\infty) \rangle \sim \exp(-\gamma t)$ in the asymptotic regime. As shown in the inset of Fig. 1(a), the relaxation rate γ increases with the average capacity. It is interesting to note that a cusp exists at the average capacity of about 0.45. Below that value, convergence of the iteration is slow, since the average energy curve starts to develop a plateau before the final convergence. On the other hand, the plateau disappears and the convergence is fast above the cusp. The slowdown of convergence below the cusp is probably due to the appearance of increasingly large clusters of nonzero currents on the network, since clusters of nodes with negative capacities become increasingly extensive, and need to draw currents from increasingly extensive regions of nodes with excess capacities to satisfy the demand. Figure 1(b) illustrates the current distribution for various average capacities. The distribution $P(y)$ consists of a delta function component at $y = 0$ and a continuous component whose breadth decreases with average capacity. The fraction of links with zero currents increases with the average capacity. Hence at a low average capacity, links with nonzero currents form a percolating cluster, whereas at a high average capacity, it breaks into isolated clusters.

5   Distributed algorithms

The local nature of the recursion relation Eq. (6) points to the possibility that the network optimization can be solved by message passing approaches, which have been successful in problems such as error-correcting codes [8] and probabilistic inference [9]. The major advantage of message passing is its potential to solve a global optimization problem via local updates, thereby reducing the computational complexity. For example, the computational complexity of quadratic programming for the load balancing task typically scales as N^3, whereas capitalizing on the network topology underlying the connectivity of the variables, message passing scales as N. An even more important advantage, relevant to

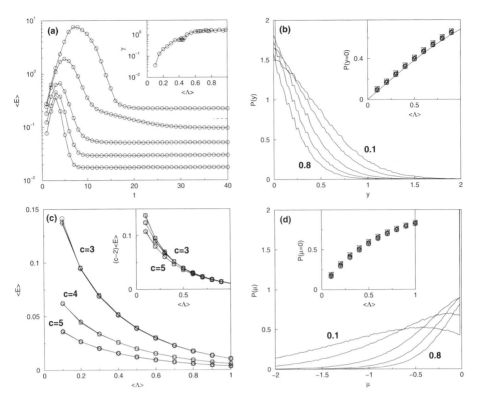

Figure 1: Results for system size $N = 1000$ and $\phi(y) = y^2/2$. (a) $\langle E \rangle$ obtained by iterating Eq. (6) as a function of t for $\langle \Lambda \rangle = 0.1, 0.2, 0.4, 0.6, 0.8$ (top to bottom) and $c = 3$. Dashed line: The asymptotic $\langle E \rangle$ for $\langle \Lambda \rangle = 0.1$. Inset: γ as a function of $\langle \Lambda \rangle$. (b) The distribution $P(y)$ obtained by iterating Eq. (6) to steady states for the same parameters and average capacities as in (a), from right to left. Inset: $P(y=0)$ as a function of $\langle \Lambda \rangle$. Symbols: $c=3$ ($\bigcirc$) and ($\square$), $c=4$ ($\diamond$) and ($\triangle$), $c=5$ ($\triangleleft$) and (∇); each pair obtained from Eqs. (11) and (14) respectively. Line: $\mathrm{erf}(\langle \Lambda \rangle / \sqrt{2})$. (c) $\langle E \rangle$ as a function of $\langle \Lambda \rangle$ for $c=3, 4, 5$. Symbols: results of Eq. (6) ($\bigcirc$), Eq.(11) ($\square$), and Eq. (14) ($\diamond$). Inset: $\langle E \rangle$ multiplied by $(c-2)$ as a function of $\langle \Lambda \rangle$ for the same conditions. (d) The distribution $P(\mu)$ obtained by iterating Eq. (14) to steady states for the same parameters and average capacities as in (b), from left to right. Inset: $P(\mu=0)$ as a function of $\langle \Lambda \rangle$. Symbols: same as (b).

practical implementation, is its distributive nature; it does not require a global optimizer, and is particularly suitable for distributive control in evolving networks.

However, in contrast to other message passing algorithms which pass conditional probability estimates of *discrete variables* to neighboring nodes, the messages in the present context are more complex, since they are *functions* $F_V(y|\mathbf{T})$ of the current y. We simplify the message to 2 parameters, namely, the first and second derivatives of the vertex free energies. For the quadratic load balancing task, it can be shown that a self-consistent solution of the recursion relation, Eq. (6), consists of vertex free energies which are piecewise quadratic with continuous slopes. This makes the 2-parameter message a very precise approximation.

Let $(A_{ij}, B_{ij}) \equiv (\partial F_V(y_{ij}|\mathbf{T}_j)/\partial y_{ij}, \partial^2 F_V(y_{ij}|\mathbf{T}_j)/\partial y_{ij}^2)$ be the message passed from node j to i; using Eq.(6), the recursion relation of the messages become

$$A_{ij} \leftarrow -\mu_{ij}, \quad B_{ij} \leftarrow \Theta(-\mu_{ij}) \left[\sum_{k \neq i} \mathcal{A}_{jk} (\phi''_{jk} + B_{jk})^{-1} \right]^{-1}, \text{ where} \quad (11)$$

$$\mu_{ij} = \min \left[\frac{\sum_{k \neq i} \mathcal{A}_{jk} [y_{jk} - (\phi'_{jk} + A_{jk})(\phi''_{jk} + B_{jk})^{-1}] + \Lambda_j - y_{ij}}{\sum_{k \neq i} \mathcal{A}_{jk} (\phi''_{jk} + B_{jk})^{-1}}, 0 \right], \quad (12)$$

with ϕ'_{jk} and ϕ''_{jk} representing the first and second derivatives of $\phi(y)$ at $y = y_{jk}$ respectively. The forward passing of the message from node j to i is then followed by a backward message from node j to k for updating the currents y_{jk} according to

$$y_{jk} \leftarrow y_{jk} - \frac{\phi'_{jk} + A_{jk} + \mu_{ij}}{\phi''_{jk} + B_{jk}}. \quad (13)$$

We simulate networks with $c = 3$, $\phi(y) = y^2/2$ and compute their average energies. The network configurations are generated randomly, with loops of lengths 3 or less excluded. Updates are performed with random sequential choices of the nodes. As shown in Fig. 1(c), the simulation results of the message passing algorithm have an excellent agreement with those obtained by the recursion relation Eq.(6).

For the quadratic load balancing task considered here, an independent exact optimization is available for comparison. The Kühn-Tucker conditions for the optimal solution yields

$$\mu_i = \min \left[\frac{1}{c} \left(\sum_j \mathcal{A}_{ij} \mu_j + \Lambda_i \right), 0 \right]. \quad (14)$$

It also provides a local iterative method for the optimization problem. As shown in Fig. 1(c), both the recursion relation Eq.(6) and the message passing algorithm Eq.(11) yield excellent agreement with the iteration of chemical potentials Eq.(14).

Both Eqs. (11) and (14) allow us to study the distribution $P(\mu)$ of the chemical potentials μ. As shown in Fig. 1(d), $P(\mu)$ consists of a delta function and a continuous component. Nodes with zero chemical potentials correspond to those with unsaturated capacity constraints. The fraction of unsaturated nodes increases with the average capacity, as shown in the inset of Fig. 1(d). Hence at a low average capacity, saturated nodes form a percolating cluster, whereas at a high average capacity, it breaks into isolated clusters. It is interesting to note that at the average capacity of 0.45, below which a plateau starts to develop in the relaxation rate of the recursion relation Eq. (6), the fraction of unsaturated nodes is about 0.53, close to the percolation threshold of 0.5 for $c = 3$.

Besides the case of $c = 3$, Fig. 1(c) also shows the simulation results of the average energy for $c = 4, 5$, using both Eqs. (11) and (14). We see that the average energy decreases when the connectivity increases. This is because the increase in links connecting a node provides more freedom to allocate resources. When the average capacity is 0.2 or above, an exponential fit $\langle E \rangle \sim \exp(-k\langle \Lambda \rangle)$ is applicable, where k lies in the range 2.5 to 2.7. Remarkably, multiplying by a factor of $(c - 2)$, we find that the 3 curves collapse in this regime of average capacity, showing that the average energy scales as $(c - 2)^{-1}$ in this regime, as shown in the inset of Fig. 1(c).

Further properties of the optimized networks have been studied by simulations, and will be presented elsewhere. Here we merely summarize the main results. (a) When the average capacity drops below 0.1, the energy rises above the exponential fit applicable to the average capacity above 0.2. (b) The fraction of links with zero currents increases with the average capacity, and is rather insensitive to the connectivity. Remarkably, except for very small average capacities, the function $\text{erf}(\langle\Lambda\rangle/\sqrt{2})$ has a very good fit with the data. Indeed, in the limit of large $\langle\Lambda\rangle$, this function approaches the fraction of links with both vertices unsaturated, that is, $[\int_0^\infty d\Lambda\rho(\Lambda)]^2$. (c) The fraction of unsaturated nodes increases with the average capacity, and is rather insensitive to the connectivity. In the limit of large average capacities, it approaches the upper bound of $\int_0^\infty d\Lambda\rho(\Lambda)$, which is the probability that the capacity of a node is non-negative. (d) The convergence time of Eq. (11) can be measured by the time for the r.m.s. of the changes in the chemical potentials to fall below a threshold. Similarly, the convergence time of Eq. (14) can be measured by the time for the r.m.s. of the sums of the currents in both message directions of a link to fall below a threshold. When the average capacity is 0.2 or above, we find the power-law dependence on the average capacity, the exponent ranging from -1 for $c = 3$ to -0.8 for $c = 5$ for Eq. (14), and being about -0.5 for $c = 3, 4, 5$ for Eq. (11). When the average capacity decreases further, the convergence time deviates above the power laws.

6   Summary

We have studied a prototype problem of resource allocation on sparsely connected networks using the replica method, resulting in recursion relations interpretable using the Bethe approximation. The resultant recursion relation leads to a message passing algorithm for optimizing the average energy, which significantly reduces the computational complexity of the global optimization task and is suitable for online distributive control. The suggested 2-parameter approximation produces results with excellent agreement with the original recursion relation. For the simple but illustrative example in this letter, we have considered a quadratic cost function, resulting in an exact algorithm based on local iterations of chemical potentials, and the message passing algorithm shows remarkable agreement with the exact result. The suggested simple message passing algorithm can be generalized to more realistic cases of nonlinear cost functions and additional constraints on the capacities of nodes and links. This constitutes a rich area for further investigations with many potential applications.

Acknowledgments

This work is partially supported by research grants HKUST6062/02P and DAG04/05.SC25 of the Research Grant Council of Hong Kong and by EVERGROW, IP No. 1935 in the FET, EU FP6 and STIPCO EU FP5 contract HPRN-CT-2002-00319.

References

[1] Peterson L. and Davie B.S., *Computer Networks: A Systems Approach*, Academic Press, San Diego CA (2000)

[2] Ho Y.C., Servi L. and Suri R. *Large Scale Systems* **1** (1980) 51

[3] Shenker S., Clark D., Estrin D. and Herzog S. *ACM Computer Comm. Review* **26** (1996) 19

[4] Nishimori H. *Statistical Physics of Spin Glasses and Information Processing*, OUP UK (2001)

[5] Mézard M., Parisi P. and Virasoro M., *Spin Glass Theory and Beyond*, World Scientific, Singapore (1987)

[6] Wong K.Y.M. and Sherrington D. *J. Phys. A***20**(1987) L793

[7] Sherrington D. and Kirkpatrick S. *Phys. Rev. Lett.***35** (1975) 1792

[8] Opper M. and Saad D. *Advanced Mean Field Methods*, MIT press (2001)

[9] MacKay D.J.C., *Information Theory, Inference and Learning Algorithms*, CUP UK(2003)

Modeling Neural Population Spiking Activity with Gibbs Distributions

Frank Wood, Stefan Roth, and Michael J. Black
Department of Computer Science
Brown University
Providence, RI 02912
{fwood,roth,black}@cs.brown.edu

Abstract

Probabilistic modeling of correlated neural population firing activity is central to understanding the neural code and building practical decoding algorithms. No parametric models currently exist for modeling multivariate correlated neural data and the high dimensional nature of the data makes fully non-parametric methods impractical. To address these problems we propose an energy-based model in which the joint probability of neural activity is represented using learned functions of the 1D marginal histograms of the data. The parameters of the model are learned using contrastive divergence and an optimization procedure for finding appropriate marginal directions. We evaluate the method using real data recorded from a population of motor cortical neurons. In particular, we model the joint probability of population spiking times and 2D hand position and show that the likelihood of test data under our model is significantly higher than under other models. These results suggest that our model captures correlations in the firing activity. Our rich probabilistic model of neural population activity is a step towards both measurement of the importance of correlations in neural coding and improved decoding of population activity.

1 Introduction

Modeling population activity is central to many problems in the analysis of neural data. Traditional methods of analysis have used single cells and simple stimuli to make the problems tractable. Current multi-electrode technology, however, allows the activity of tens or hundreds of cells to be recorded simultaneously along with with complex natural stimuli or behavior. Probabilistic modeling of this data is challenging due to its high-dimensional nature and the correlated firing activity of neural populations. One can view the problem as one of learning the joint probability $P(\mathbf{s}, \mathbf{r})$ of a stimulus or behavior $\mathbf{s}$ and the firing activity of a neural population $\mathbf{r}$. The neural activity may be in the form of firing rates or spike times. Here we focus the latter more challenging problem of representing a multivariate probability distribution over spike times.

Modeling $P(\mathbf{s}, \mathbf{r})$ is made challenging by the high dimensional, correlated, and non-Gaussian nature of the data. The dimensionality means that we are unlikely to have sufficient training data for a fully non-parametric model. On the other hand no parametric models currently exist that capture the one-sided, skewed nature of typical correlated neural data. We do, however, have sufficient data to model the marginal statistics of the data. With that observation we draw on the FRAME model developed by Zhu and Mumford for image texture synthesis [1] to represent neural population activity.

The FRAME model represents $P(\mathbf{s}, \mathbf{r})$ in terms of its marginal histograms. In particular we seek the maximum entropy distribution that matches the observed marginals of $P(\mathbf{s}, \mathbf{r})$. The joint is represented by a Gibbs model that combines functions of these marginals and we exploit the method of [2] to automatically choose the optimal marginal directions. To learn the parameters of the model we exploit the technique of contrastive divergence [3, 4] which has been used previously to learn the parameters of Product-of-Experts (PoE) models [5]. We observe that the FRAME model can be viewed as a Product of Experts where the experts are functions of the marginal histograms. The resulting model is more flexible than the standard PoE formulation and allows us to model more complex, skewed distributions observed in neural data.

We train and test the model on real data recorded from a monkey performing a motor control task; details of the task and the neural data are described in the following section. We learn a variety of probabilistic models including full Gaussian, independent Gaussian, product of t-distributions [4], independent non-parametric, and the FRAME model. We evaluate the log likelihood of test data under the different models and show that the complete FRAME model outperforms the other methods (note that "complete" here means the model uses the same number of marginal directions as there are dimensions in the data).

The use of energy-based models such as FRAME for modeling neural data appears novel and promising, and the results reported here are easily extended to other cortical areas. There is a need in the community for such probabilistic models of multi-variate spiking processes. For example Bell and Para [6] formulate a simple model of correlated spiking but acknowledge that what they would really like, and do not have, is what they call a "maximum spikelihood" model. This neural modeling problem represents a new application of energy-based models and consequently suggests extensions of the basic methods. Finally, there is a need for rich probabilistic models of this type in the Bayesian decoding of neural activity [7].

2   Methods

The data used in this study consists of simultaneously recorded spike times from a population of M1 motor neurons recorded in monkeys trained to perform a manual tracking task [8, 9]. The monkey viewed a computer monitor displaying a target and a feedback cursor. The task involved moving a 2D manipulandum so that a cursor controlled by the manipulandum came into contact with a target. The monkey was rewarded when the target was acquired, a new target appeared and the process repeated. Several papers [9, 11, 10] have reported successfully decoding the cursor kinematics from this data using firing rates estimated from binned spike counts.

The activity of a population of cells was recorded at a rate of 30kHz then sorted using an automated spike sorting method; from this we randomly selected five cells with which to demonstrate our method.

As shown in Fig. 1, $\mathbf{r}_{i,k} = [t_{i,k}^{(1)}, t_{i,k}^{(2)}, \ldots, t_{i,k}^{(J)}]$ is a vector of time intervals $t_{i,k}^{(j)}$ that represents the spiking activity of a single cell i at timestep k. These intervals are the elapsed time between the time at timestep k and the time at each of j past spikes. Let $R_k = [\mathbf{r}_{1,k}, \mathbf{r}_{2,k}, \ldots, \mathbf{r}_{N,k}]$ be a vector concatenation of N such spiking activity representations. Let $\mathbf{s}_k = [x_k, y_k]$ be the position of the manipulandum at each timestep. Our

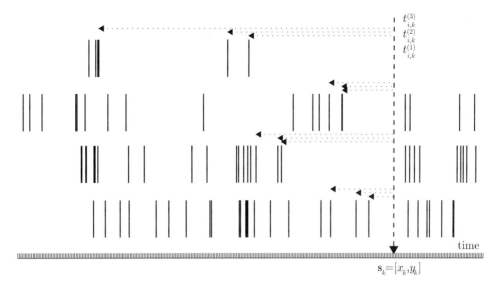

Figure 1: Representation of the data. Hand position at time k, $\mathbf{s}_k = [x_k, y_k]$, is regularly sampled every $50ms$. Spiking activity (shown as vertical bars) is retained at full data acquisition precision (30khz). Sections of spike trains from four cells are shown. The response of a single cell, i, is represented by the time intervals to the three preceding spikes; that is, $\mathbf{r}_{i,k} = [t_{i,k}^{(1)}, t_{i,k}^{(2)}, t_{i,k}^{(3)}]$.

training data consists of 4000 points R_k, s_k sampled at $50ms$ intervals with a history of 3 past spikes ($J = 3$) per neuron. Our test data is 1000 points of the same.

Various empirical marginals of the data (shown in Fig 2) illustrate that the data are not well fit by canonical symmetric parametric distributions because the data is asymmetric and skewed. For such data traditional parametric models may not work well so instead we apply the FRAME model of [1] to this modeling problem. FRAME is a semi-parametric energy based model of the following form:

Let $\mathbf{d}_k = [\mathbf{s}_k, R_k]$, where $\mathbf{s}_k$ and R_k are defined as above. Let $D = [\mathbf{d}_1, \ldots, \mathbf{d}_N]$ be a matrix of N such points. We define

$$P(\mathbf{d}_k) = \frac{1}{Z(\Theta)} e^{-\sum_e \lambda_e^T \phi(\omega_e^T \mathbf{d}_k)} \tag{1}$$

where ω_e is a vector that projects the datum $\mathbf{d}_k$ onto a 1-D subspace, $\phi : \mathbb{R} \to \mathbb{I}^b$ is a "histogramming" function that produces a vector with a single 1 in a single bin per datum according to the projected value of that datum, $\lambda_e \in \mathbb{R}^b$ is a weight vector, Z is a normalization constant sometimes called the partition function (as it is a function of the model parameters), b is the granularity of the histogram, and e is the number of "experts". Taken together, $\lambda_e^T \phi(\cdot)$ can be thought of as a discrete representation of a function. In this view $\lambda_e^T \phi(\omega_e^T \mathbf{d}_k)$ is an energy function computed over a projection of the data. Models of this form are constrained maximum entropy models, and in this case by adjusting λ_e the model marginal projection onto ω_e is constrained to be identical (ideally) to the empirical marginal over the same projection. Fig. 3 illustrates the model.

To relate this to current PoE models, if $\lambda_e^T \phi(\cdot)$ were replaced with a log Student-t function then this FRAME model would take the same form as the Product-of-Student-t formulation of [12]. Distributions of this form are called Gibbs or energy-based distributions as $\sum_e \lambda_e^T \phi(\omega_e^T \mathbf{d}_k)$ is analogous to the energy in a Boltzmann distribution. Minimizing the

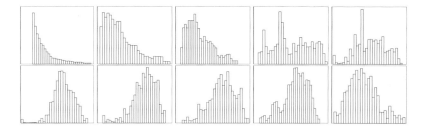

Figure 2: Histograms of various projections of single cell data. The top row are histograms of the values of $t^{(1)}, t^{(2)}, t^{(3)}, x$, and y respectively. The bottom row are random projections from the same data. All these figures illustrate skew or one-sidedness, and motivate our choice of a semi-parametric Gibbs model.

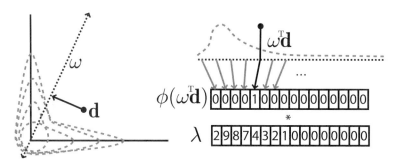

Figure 3: *(left)* Illustration of the projection and weighting of a single point $\mathbf{d}$: Here, the data point $\mathbf{d}$ is projected onto the projection direction ω. The isosurfaces from a hypothetical distribution $p(\mathbf{d})$ are shown in dotted gray. *(right)* Illustration of the projection and binning of $\mathbf{d}$: The upper plot shows the empirical marginal (in dotted gray) as obtained from the projection illustrated in the left figure. The function $\phi(\cdot)$ takes a real valued projection and produces a vector of fixed length with a single 1 in the bin that is mapped to that range of the projection. This discretization of the projection is indicated by the spacing of the downward pointing arrows. The resulting vector is weighted by λ to produce an energy. This process is repeated for each of the projection directions in the model. The constraints induced by multiple projections result in a distribution very close to the empirical distribution.

this energy is equivalent to maximizing the log likelihood.

Our model is parameterized by $\Theta = \{\{\lambda_e, \omega_e\} : 1 < e < E\}$ where E is the total number of projections (or "experts"). We use gradient ascent on the log likelihood to train the λ_e's. As $\phi(\cdot)$ is not differentiable, the ω_e's must be specified or learned in another way.

2.1 Learning the λ's

Standard gradient ascent becomes intractable for large numbers of cells because computing the partition function and its gradient becomes intractable. The gradient of the log probability with respect to $\lambda_{1..E}$ is

$$\nabla_{\Theta_\lambda} \log P(\mathbf{d}_k) = [\frac{\partial \log P(\mathbf{d}_k)}{\partial \lambda_1}, \dots, \frac{\partial \log P(\mathbf{d}_k)}{\partial \lambda_E}]. \tag{2}$$

Besides not being able to normalize the distribution, the right hand term of the partial

$$\frac{\partial \log P(\mathbf{d}_k)}{\partial \lambda_e} = \phi(\omega_e^T \mathbf{d}_k) - \frac{\partial \log Z(\Theta)}{\partial \lambda_e}$$

typically has no closed-form solution and is very hard to compute.

Markov chain Monte Carlo (MCMC) techniques can be used to learn such models. Contrastive divergence [4] is an efficient learning algorithm for energy based models that approximates the gradient as

$$\frac{\partial \log P(\mathbf{d}_k)}{\partial \lambda_e} \approx \left\langle \frac{\partial \log P(\mathbf{d}_k)}{\partial \lambda_e} \right\rangle_{P^0} - \left\langle \frac{\partial \log P(\mathbf{d}_k)}{\partial \lambda_e} \right\rangle_{P_\Theta^m} \tag{3}$$

where P^0 is the training data and P_Θ^m are samples drawn according to the model. The key is that the sampler is started at the training data and does not need to be run until convergence, which typically would take much more time. The superscript indicates that we use m regular Metropolis sampling steps [13] to draw samples from the model for contrastive divergence training ($m = 50$ in our experiments).

The intuition behind this approximation is that samples drawn from the model should have the same statistics as the training data. Maximizing the log probability of training data is equivalent to minimizing the Kullback Leibler (KL) divergence between the model and the true distribution. Contrastive divergence attempts to minimize the difference in KL divergence between the model one step towards equilibrium and the training data. Intuitively this means that the contrastive divergence opposes any tendency for the model to diverge from the true distribution.

2.2 Learning the ω's

Because $\phi(\cdot)$ is not differentiable, we turn to the feature pursuit method of [2] to learn the projection directions $\omega_{1..E}$. This approach involves successively searching for a new projection in a direction where a model with the new projection would differ maximally from the model without. Their approach involves approximating the expected projection using a Parzen window method with Gaussian kernels. Gradient search on a KL-divergence objective function is used to find each subsequent projection. We refer readers to [2] for details.

It was suggested by [2] that there are many local optima in this feature pursuit. Our experience tends to support this claim. In fact, it may be that feature pursuit is not entirely necessary. Additionally, in our experience, the most important aspect of the feature selection algorithm is how many feature pursuit starting points are considered. It may be as effective (and certainly more efficient) to simply guess a large number of projections and estimate the marginal KL-divergence for them all, selecting the largest as the new projection.

2.3 Normalizing the distribution

Generally speaking, the partition function is intractable to compute as it involves integration over the entire domain of the joint; however, in the case where E (the number of experts) is the same as the dimensionality of d then the partition function is tractable. Each expert can be normalized individually. The per-expert normalization is

$$Z_e = \sum_b s_e^{(b)} e^{-\lambda_e^{(b)}}$$

where b indexes the elements of λ_e and $s_e^{(b)}$ is the width of the bth bin of the eth histogramming function. Using the change of variables rule

$$Z = |det(\Omega)| \prod_e Z_e$$

where the square matrix $\Omega = [\omega_1 \omega_2 \ldots \omega_E]$. This is not possible when the number of experts exceeds or is smaller than the dimensionality of the data.

POT	IG	G	RF	I	FP
-31849	-30893	-23573	-23108	-19155	-12509

Table 1: Log likelihoods of test data. The test data consists of the spiking activity of 5 cells and x, y position behavioral variables as illustrated in Fig. 1. Log likelihoods are reported for various models: POT: Product of Student-t, IG: diagonal covariance Gaussian, G: full covariance Gaussian, RF: random filter FRAME, I: 5 independent FRAME models, one per cell, and FP: feature pursuit FRAME

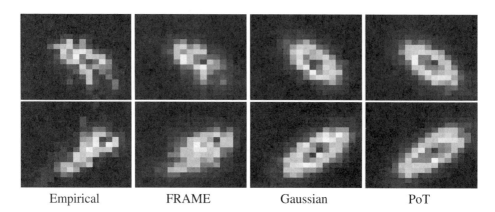

| Empirical | FRAME | Gaussian | PoT |

Figure 4: This figure illustrates the modeling power of the semi-parametric Gibbs distribution over a number of symmetric, fully parametric distributions. Each row shows normalized 2-d histograms of samples projected onto a plane. The first column is the training data, column two is the Gibbs distribution, column three is a Gaussian distribution, and column four is a Product-of-Student-t distribution.

3 Results

We trained several models on several datasets. We show results for complete models of the joint neuronal response of 5 real motor cortex cells plus x, y hand kinematics (3 past spikes for each cell plus 2 behavior variables equals a 17 dimension dataset). A complete model has the same number of experts as dimensions.

Table 1 shows the log likelihood of test data under several models: Product of Student-t, a diagonal covariance multidimensional Gaussian (independent), multivariate Gaussian, a complete FRAME model with random projection directions, a product of 5 complete FRAME single cell models with learned projections, and a complete FRAME model with learned projection directions. Because these all are complete models, we are able to compute the partition function of each. Each model was trained on 4000 points and the log likelihood was computed using 1000 distinct test points.

In Fig. 4 we show histograms of samples drawn from a full covariance Gaussian and energy-based models with two times more projection directions than the data dimensionality. These figures illustrate the modeling power of our approach in that it represents the irregularities common to real neural data better than Gaussian and other symmetric distributions.

Note that the model using random marginal directions does not model the data as well as one using optimized directions; this is not surprising. It may well be the case, however, that with many more random directions such a model would perform significantly better. This overcomplete case however is unnormalized and hence cannot be directly compared here.

4 Discussion

In this work we demonstrated an approach for using Gibbs distributions to model the joint spiking activity of a population of cells and an associated behavior. We developed a novel application of contrastive divergence for learning a FRAME model which can be viewed as a semi-parametric Product-of-Experts model. We showed that our model outperformed other models in representing complex monkey motor cortical spiking data.

Previous methods for probabilistically modeling spiking process have focused on modeling the firing rates of a population in terms of a conditional intensity function (firing rate conditioned on various correlates and previous spiking) [15, 16, 17, 18, 19]. These functions are often formulated in terms of log-linear models and hence resemble our approach. Here we take a more direct approach of modeling the joint probability using energy-based models and exploit contrastive divergence for learning

Information theoretic analysis of spiking populations calls for modeling high dimensional joint and conditional distributions. In the work of [20, 21, 22], these distributions are used to study encoding models, in particular the importance of correlation in the neural code. Our models are directly applicable to this pursuit. Given an experimental design with a relatively low dimension stimulus, where the entropy of that stimulus can be accurately computed, our models are applicable without modification.

Our approach may also be applied to neural decoding. A straightforward extension of our model could include hand positions (or other kinematic variables) at multiple time instants. Decoding algorithms that exploits these joint models by maximizing the likelihood of the observed firing activity over an entire data set remain to be developed. Note that it may be possible to produce more accurate models of the un-normalized joint probability by increasing the number of marginal constraints. To exploit these overcomplete models, algorithms that do not require normalized probabilities are required (particle filtering is a good example).

Not surprisingly the FRAME model performed better on the non-symmetric neural data than the related, but symmetric, Product-of-Student-t model. We have begun exploring more flexible and asymmetric experts which would offer advantages over discrete histogramming inherent to the FRAME model.

Acknowledgments

Thanks to J. Donoghue, W. Truccolo, M. Fellows, and M. Serruya. This work was supported by NIH-NINDS R01 NS 50967-01 as part of the NSF/NIH Collaborative Research in Computational Neuroscience Program.

References

[1] S. C. Zhu, Z. N. Wu, and D. Mumford, "Minimax entropy principle and its application to texture modeling," *Neural Comp.*, vol. 9, no. 8, pp. 1627–1660, 1997.

[2] C. Liu, S. C. Zhu, and H. Shum, "Learning inhomogeneous Gibbs model of faces by minimax entropy," in *ICCV*, pp. 281–287, 2001.

[3] G. Hinton, "Training products of experts by minimizing contrastive divergence," *Neural Comp.*, vol. 14, pp. 1771–1800, 2002.

[4] Y. Teh, M. Welling, S. Osindero, and G. E. Hinton, "Energy-based models for sparse overcomplete representations," *JMLR*, vol. 4, pp. 1235–1260, 2003.

[5] G. Hinton, "Product of experts," in *ICANN*, vol. 1, pp. 1–6, 1999.

[6] A. J. Bell and L. C. Parra, "Maximising sensitivity in a spiking network," in *Advances in NIPS*, vol. 17, pp. 121–128, 2005.

[7] R. S. Zemel, Q. J. M. Huys, R. Natarajan, and P. Dayan, "Probabilistic computation in spiking populations," in *Advances in NIPS*, vol. 17, pp. 1609–1616, 2005.

[8] M. Serruya, N. Hatsopoulos, M. Fellows, L. Paninski, and J. Donoghue, "Robustness of neuroprosthetic decoding algorithms," *Biological Cybernetics*, vol. 88, no. 3, pp. 201–209, 2003.

[9] M. D. Serruya, N. G. Hatsopoulos, L. Paninski, M. R. Fellows, and J. P. Donoghue, "Brain-machine interface: Instant neural control of a movement signal," *Nature*, vol. 416, pp. 141–142, 2002.

[10] W. Wu, M. J. Black, Y. Gao, E. Bienenstock, M. Serruya, A. Shaikhouni, and J. P. Donoghue, "Neural decoding of cursor motion using a Kalman filter," in *Advances in NIPS*, vol. 15, pp. 133–140, 2003.

[11] Y. Gao, M. J. Black, E. Bienenstock, S. Shoham, and J. P. Donoghue, "Probabilistic inference of arm motion from neural activity in motor cortex," *Advances in NIPS*, vol. 14, pp. 221–228, 2002.

[12] M. Welling, G. Hinton, and S. Osindero, "Learning sparse topographic representations with products of Student-t distributions," in *Advances in NIPS*, vol. 15, pp. 1359–1366, 2003.

[13] A. Gelman, J. B. Carlin, H. S. Stern, and D. B. Rubin, *Bayesian Data Analysis*, 2nd ed. Chapman & Hall/CRC, 2004.

[14] S. Roth and M. J. Black, "Fields of experts: A framework for learning image priors," in *CVPR*, vol. 2, pp. 860–867, 2005.

[15] D. R. Brillinger, "The identification of point process systems," *The Annals of Probability*, vol. 3, pp. 909–929, 1975.

[16] E. S. Chornoboy, L. P. Schramm, and A. F. Karr, "Maximum likelihood identification of neuronal point process systems," *Biological Cybernetics*, vol. 59, pp. 265–275, 1988.

[17] Y. Gao, M. J. Black, E. Bienenstock, W. Wu, and J. P. Donoghue, "A quantitative comparison of linear and non-linear models of motor cortical activity for the encoding and decoding of arm motions," in *First International IEEE/EMBS Conference on Neural Engineering*, pp. 189–192, 2003.

[18] M. Okatan, "Maximum likelihood identification of neuronal point process systems," *Biological Cybernetics*, vol. 59, pp. 265–275, 1988.

[19] W. Truccolo, U. T. Eden, M. R. Fellows, J. P. Donoghue, and E. N. Brown, "A point process framework for relating neural spiking activity to spiking history," *J. Neurophysiology*, vol. 93, pp. 1074–1089, 2005.

[20] P. E. Latham and S. Nirenberg, "Synergy, redundancy, and independence in population codes, revisited," *J. Neuroscience*, vol. 25, pp. 5195–5206, 2005.

[21] S. Nirenberg and P. E. Latham, "Decoding neuronal spike trains: How important are correlations?" *PNAS*, vol. 100, pp. 7348–7353, 2003.

[22] S. Panzeri, H. D. R. Golledge, F. Zheng, M. Tovee, and M. P. Young, "Objective assessment of the functional role of spike train correlations using information measures," *Visual Cognition*, vol. 8, pp. 531–547, 2001.

Extracting Dynamical Structure Embedded in Neural Activity

Byron M. Yu[1], Afsheen Afshar[1,2], Gopal Santhanam[1],
Stephen I. Ryu[1,3], Krishna V. Shenoy[1,4]
[1]Department of Electrical Engineering, [2]School of Medicine, [3]Department of
Neurosurgery, [4]Neurosciences Program, Stanford University, Stanford, CA 94305
{byronyu,afsheen,gopals,seoulman,shenoy}@stanford.edu

Maneesh Sahani
Gatsby Computational Neuroscience Unit, UCL
London, WC1N 3AR, UK
maneesh@gatsby.ucl.ac.uk

Abstract

Spiking activity from neurophysiological experiments often exhibits dynamics beyond that driven by external stimulation, presumably reflecting the extensive recurrence of neural circuitry. Characterizing these dynamics may reveal important features of neural computation, particularly during internally-driven cognitive operations. For example, the activity of premotor cortex (PMd) neurons during an instructed delay period separating movement-target specification and a movement-initiation cue is believed to be involved in motor planning. We show that the dynamics underlying this activity can be captured by a low-dimensional non-linear dynamical systems model, with underlying recurrent structure and stochastic point-process output. We present and validate latent variable methods that simultaneously estimate the system parameters and the trial-by-trial dynamical trajectories. These methods are applied to characterize the dynamics in PMd data recorded from a chronically-implanted 96-electrode array while monkeys perform delayed-reach tasks.

1 Introduction

At present, the best view of the activity of a neural circuit is provided by multiple-electrode extracellular recording technologies, which allow us to simultaneously measure spike trains from up to a few hundred neurons in one or more brain areas during each trial. While the resulting data provide an extensive picture of neural spiking, their use in characterizing the fine timescale dynamics of a neural circuit is complicated by at least two factors. First, extracellularly captured action potentials provide only an occasional view of the process from which they are generated, forcing us to interpolate the evolution of the circuit between the spikes. Second, the circuit activity may evolve quite differently on different trials that are otherwise experimentally identical.

The usual approach to handling both problems is to average responses from different trials, and study the evolution of the peri-stimulus time histogram (PSTH). There is little alternative to this approach when recordings are made one neuron at a time, even when the dynamics of the system are the subject of study. Unfortunately, such averaging can obscure important internal features of the response. In many experiments, stimulus events provide the trigger for activity, but the resulting time-course of the response is internally regulated and may not be identical on each trial. This is especially important during cognitive processing such as decision making or motor planning. In this case, the PSTH may not reflect the true trial-by-trial dynamics. For example, a sharp change in firing rate that occurs with varying latency might appear as a slow smooth transition in the average response.

An alternative approach is to adopt latent variable methods and to identify a hidden dynamical system that can summarize and explain the simultaneously-recorded spike trains. The central idea is that the responses of different neurons reflect different views of a common dynamical process in the network, whose effective dimensionality is much smaller than the total number of neurons in the network. While the underlying state trajectory may be slightly different on each trial, the commonalities among these trajectories can be captured by the network's parameters, which are shared across trials. These parameters define how the network evolves over time, as well as how the observed spike trains relate to the network's state at each time point.

Dimensionality reduction in a latent dynamical model is crucial and yields benefits beyond simple noise elimination. Some of these benefits can be illustrated by a simple physical example. Consider a set of noisy video sequences of a bouncing ball. The trajectory of the ball may not be identical in each sequence, and so simply averaging the sequences together would provide little information about the dynamics. Independently smoothing the dynamics of each pixel might identify a dynamical process; however, correctly rejecting noise might be difficult, and in any case this would yield an inefficient and opaque representation of the underlying physical process. By contrast, a hidden dynamical system account could capture the video sequence data using a low-dimensional latent variable that represented only the ball's position and momentum over time, with dynamical rules that captured the physics of ballistics and elastic collision. This representation would exploit shared information from all pixels, vastly simplifying the problem of noise rejection, and would provide a scientifically useful depiction of the process.

The example also serves to illustrate the two broad benefits of this type of model. The first is to obtain a low dimensional summary of the dynamical trajectory in any one trial. Besides the obvious benefits of denoising, such a trajectory can provide an invaluable representation for prediction of associated phenomena. In the video sequence example, predicting the loudness of the sound on impact might be easy given the estimate of the ball's trajectory (and thus its speed), but would be difficult from the raw pixel trajectories, even if denoised. In the neural case, behavioral variables such as reaction time might similarly be most easily predicted from the reconstructed trajectory. The second broad goal is systems identification: learning the rules that govern the dynamics. In the video example this would involve discovery of various laws of physics, as well as parameters describing the ball such as its coefficient of elasticity. In the neural case this would involve identifying the structure of dynamics available to the circuit: the number and relationship of attractors, appearance of oscillatory limit cycles and so on.

The use of latent variable models with hidden dynamics for neural data has, thus far, been limited. In [1], [2], small groups of neurons in the frontal cortex were modeled using hidden Markov models, in which the latent dynamical system is assumed to transition between a set of discrete states. In [3], a state space model with linear hidden dynamics and point-process outputs was applied to simulated data. However, these restricted latent models cannot capture the richness of dynamics that recurrent networks exhibit. In particular, systems that converge toward point or line attractors, exhibit limit cycle oscillations, or even transition into chaotic regimes have long been of interest in neural modeling. If such systems are relevant to real neural data, we must seek to identify hidden models capable of reflecting this range of behaviors.

In this work, we consider a latent variable model having (1) hidden underlying recurrent structure with continuous-valued states, and (2) Poisson-distributed output spike counts (conditioned on the state), as described in Section 2. Inference and learning for this nonlinear model are detailed in Section 3. The methods developed are applied to a delayed-reach task described in Section 4. Evidence of motor preparation in PMd is given in Section 5. In Section 6, we characterize the neural dynamics of motor preparation on a trial-by-trial basis.

2 Hidden non-linear dynamical system

A useful dynamical system model capable of expressing the rich behavior expected of neural systems is the recurrent neural network (RNN) with Gaussian perturbations

$$\mathbf{x}_t \mid \mathbf{x}_{t-1} \sim \mathcal{N}\left(\psi(\mathbf{x}_{t-1}), \mathsf{Q}\right) \tag{1}$$

$$\psi(\mathbf{x}) = (1 - k)\mathbf{x} + kW g(\mathbf{x}), \tag{2}$$

where $\mathbf{x}_t \in \mathbb{R}^{p \times 1}$ is the vector of the node values in the recurrent network at time $t \in \{1, \ldots, T\}$, $W \in \mathbb{R}^{p \times p}$ is the connection weight matrix, g is a non-linear activation function which acts element-by-element on its vector argument, $k \in \mathbb{R}$ is a parameter related to the time constant of the network, and $\mathsf{Q} \in \mathbb{R}^{p \times p}$ is a covariance matrix. The initial state is Gaussian-distributed

$$\mathbf{x}_0 \sim \mathcal{N}\left(\mathbf{p}_0, \mathsf{V}_0\right), \tag{3}$$

where $\mathbf{p}_0 \in \mathbb{R}^{p \times 1}$ and $\mathsf{V}_0 \in \mathbb{R}^{p \times p}$ are the mean vector and covariance matrix, respectively.

Models of this class have long been used, albeit generally without stochastic pertubation, to describe the dynamics of neuronal responses (e.g., [4]). In this classical view, each node of the network represents a neuron or a column of neurons. Our use is more abstract. The RNN is chosen for the range of dynamics it can exhibit, including convergence to point or surface attractors, oscillatory limit cycles, or chaotic evolution; but each node is simply an abstract dimension of latent space which may couple to many or all of the observed neurons.

The output distribution is given by a generalized linear model that describes the relationship between all nodes in the state $\mathbf{x}_t$ and the spike count $y_t^i \in \mathbb{R}$ of neuron $i \in \{1, \ldots, q\}$ in the tth time bin

$$y_t^i \mid \mathbf{x}_t \sim \text{Poisson}\left(h\left(\mathbf{c}^i \cdot \mathbf{x}_t + d^i\right)\Delta\right), \tag{4}$$

where $\mathbf{c}^i \in \mathbb{R}^{p \times 1}$ and $d^i \in \mathbb{R}$ are constants, h is a link function mapping $\mathbb{R} \to \mathbb{R}_+$, and $\Delta \in \mathbb{R}$ is the time bin width. We collect the spike counts from all q simultaneously-recorded physical neurons into a vector $\mathbf{y}_t \in \mathbb{R}^{q \times 1}$, whose ith element is y_t^i. The choice of the link functions g and h is discussed in Section 3.

3 Inference and Learning

The Expectation-Maximization (EM) algorithm [5] was used to iteratively (1) *infer* the underlying hidden state trajectories (i.e., recover a distribution over the hidden sequence $\{\mathbf{x}\}_1^T$ corresponding to the observations $\{\mathbf{y}\}_1^T$), and (2) *learn* the model parameters (i.e., estimate $\theta = \{W, \mathsf{Q}, k, \mathbf{p}_0, \mathsf{V}_0, \{\mathbf{c}^i\}, \{d^i\}\}$), given only a set of observation sequences.

Inference (the E-step) involves computing or approximating $P\left(\{\mathbf{x}\}_1^T \mid \{\mathbf{y}\}_1^T, \theta_k\right)$ for each sequence, where θ_k are the parameter estimates at the kth EM iteration. A variant of the Extended Kalman Smoother (EKS) was used to approximate these joint smoothed state posteriors. As in the EKS, the non-linear time-invariant state system (1)-(2) was transformed into a linear time-variant sytem using local linearization. The difference from EKS arises in the measurement update step of the forward pass

$$P\left(\mathbf{x}_t \mid \{\mathbf{y}\}_1^t\right) \propto P\left(\mathbf{y}_t \mid \mathbf{x}_t\right) P\left(\mathbf{x}_t \mid \{\mathbf{y}\}_1^{t-1}\right). \tag{5}$$

Because $P\left(\mathbf{y}_t \mid \mathbf{x}_t\right)$ is a product of Poissons rather than a Gaussian, the filtered state posterior $P\left(\mathbf{x}_t \mid \{\mathbf{y}\}_1^t\right)$ cannot be easily computed. Instead, as in [3], we approximated this posterior with a Gaussian centered at the mode of $\log P\left(\mathbf{x}_t \mid \{\mathbf{y}\}_1^t\right)$ and whose covariance is given by the negative inverse Hessian of the log posterior at that mode. Certain choices of h, including e^z and $\log\left(1 + e^z\right)$, lead to a log posterior that is strictly concave in $\mathbf{x}_t$. In these cases, the unique mode can easily be found by Newton's method.

Learning (the M-step) requires finding the θ that maximizes $E\left[\log P\left(\{\mathbf{x}\}_1^T, \{\mathbf{y}\}_1^T \mid \theta\right)\right]$, where the expectation is taken over the posterior state distributions found in the E-step. Note that, for multiple sequences that are independent conditioned on θ, we use the *sum* of expectations over all sequences. Because the posterior state distributions are approximated as Gaussians in the E-step, the above expectation is a Gaussian integral that involves non-linear functions g and h and cannot be computed analytically in general. Fortunately, this high-dimensional integral can be reduced to many one-dimensional Gaussian integrals, which can be accurately and reasonably efficiently approximated using Gaussian quadrature [6], [7].

We found that setting g to be the error function

$$g(z) = \frac{2}{\sqrt{\pi}} \int_0^z e^{-t^2} dt \tag{6}$$

made many of the one-dimensional Gaussian integrals involving g analytically tractable. Those that were not analytically tractable were approximated using Gaussian quadrature. The error function is one of a family of sigmoid activation functions that yield similar behavior in a RNN.

If h were chosen to be a simple exponential, all the Gaussian integrals involving h could be computed exactly. Unfortunately, this exponential mapping would distort the relationship between perturbations in the latent state (whose size is set by the covariance matrix $\mathbf{Q}$) and the resulting fluctuations in firing rates. In particular, the size of firing-rate fluctuations would grow *exponentially* with the mean, an effect that would then add to the usual linear increase in spike-count variance that comes from the Poisson output distribution. Since neural firing does not show such a severe scaling in variability, such a model would fit poorly. Therefore, to maintain more even firing-rate fluctuations, we instead take

$$h(z) = \log\left(1 + e^z\right). \tag{7}$$

The corresponding Gaussian integrals must then be approximated by quadrature methods. Regardless of the forms of g and h chosen, numerical Newton methods are needed for maximization with respect to $\{\mathbf{c}^i\}$ and $\{d^i\}$.

The main drawback of these various approximations is that the overall observation likelihood is no longer guaranteed to increase after each EM iteration. However, in our simulations, we found that sensible results were often produced. As long as the variances of the posterior state distribution did not diverge, the output distributions described by the learned model closely approximated those of the actual model that generated the simulated data.

4 Task and recordings

We trained a rhesus macaque monkey to perform delayed center-out reaches to visual targets presented on a fronto-parallel screen. On a given trial, the peripheral target was presented at one of eight radial locations (30, 70, 110, 150, 190, 230, 310, 350°) 10 cm away, as shown in Figure 1. After a pseudo-randomly chosen delay period of 200, 750, or 1000 ms, the target increased in size as the go cue and the monkey reached to the target. A 96-channel silicon electrode array (Cyberkinetics, Inc.) was implanted straddling PMd and motor cortex (M1). Spike sorting was performed offline to isolate 22 single-neuron and 109 multi-neuron units.

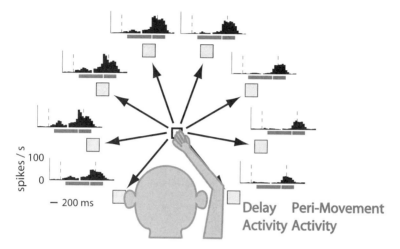

Figure 1: Delayed reach task and average action potential (spike) emission rate from one representative unit. Activity is arranged by target location. Vertical dashed lines indicate peripheral reach target onset (left) and movement onset (right).

5 Motor preparation in PMd

Motor preparation is often studied using the "instructed delay" behavioral paradigm, as described in Section 4, where a variable-length "planning" period temporally separates an instruction stimulus from a go cue [8]–[13]. Longer delay periods typically lead to shorter reaction times (RT, defined as time between go cue and movement onset), and this has been interpreted as evidence for a motor preparation process that takes time [11], [12], [14], [15]. In this view, the delay period allows for motor preparation to complete prior to the go cue, thus shortening the RT.

Evidence for motor preparation at the neural level is taken from PMd (and, to a lesser degree, M1), where neurons show sustained activity during the delay period (Figure 1, delay activity) [8]–[10]. A number of findings support the hypothesis that such activity is related to motor preparation. First, delay period activity typically shows tuning for the instruction (i.e., location of reach target; note that the PMd neuron in Figure 1 has greater delay activity before leftward than before rightward reaches), consistent with the idea that something specific is being prepared [8], [9], [11], [13]. Second, in the absence of a delay period, a brief burst of similarly-tuned activity is observed during the RT interval, consistent with the idea that motor preparation is taking place at that time [12].

Third, we have recently reported that firing rates *across trials* to the same reach target become more consistent as the delay period progresses [16]. The variance of firing rate, measured across trials, divided by mean firing rate (similar to the Fano factor) was computed for each unit and each time point. Averaged across 14 single- and 33 multi-neuron units, we found that this Normalized Variance (NV) declined 24% (t-test, p $<10^{-10}$) from 200 ms before target onset to the median time of the go cue. This decline spanned $\sim$119 ms just after target onset and appears to, at least roughly, track the time-course of motor preparation.

The NV may be interpreted as a signature of the approximate degree of motor preparation yet to be accomplished. Shortly after target onset, firing rates are frequently far from their mean. If the go cue arrives then, it will take time to correct these "errors" and RTs will therefore be longer. By the time the NV has completed its decline, firing rates are consistently near their mean (which we presume is near an "optimal" configuration for the impending reach), and RTs will be shorter if the go cue arrives then. This interpretation assumes that there is a limit on how quickly firing rates can converge to their ideal values (a limit on how quickly the NV can drop) such that a decline during the delay period saves time later. The NV was found to be lower at the time of the go cue for trials with shorter RTs than those with longer RTs [16].

The above data strongly suggest that the network underlying motor preparation exhibits rich dynamics. Activity is initially variable across trials, but appears to settle during the delay period. Because the RNN (1)-(2) is capable of exhibiting such dynamics and may underly motor preparation, we sought to identify such a dynamical system in delay activity.

6 Results and discussion

The NV reveals an average process of settling by measuring the convergence of firing across different trials. However, it provides little insight into the course of motor planning on a single trial. A gradual fall in trial-to-trial variance might reflect a gradual convergence on each trial, or might reflect rapid transitions that occur at different times on different trials. Similarly, all the NV tells us about the dynamic properties of the underlying network is the basic fact of convergence from uncontrolled initial conditions to a consistent pre-movement preparatory state. The structure of any underlying attractors and corresponding basins of attraction is unobserved. Furthermore, the NV is first computed per-unit and averaged across units, thus ignoring any structure that may be present in the correlated firing of units on a given trial. The methods presented here are well-suited to extending the characterization of this settling process.

We fit the dynamical system model (1)–(4) with three latent dimensions ($p = 3$) to training data, consisting of delay activity preceding 70 reaches to the same target (30°). Spike counts were taken in non-overlapping $\Delta = 20$ ms bins at 20 ms time steps from 50 ms after target onset to 50 ms after the go cue. Then, the fitted model parameters were used to infer the latent space trajectories for 146 test trials, which are plotted in Figure 2. Despite the trial-to-trial variability in the delay period neural responses, the state evolves along a characteristic path on each trial. It could have been that the neural variability across trials would cause the state trajectory to evolve in markedly different ways on different trials. Even with the characteristic structure, the state trajectories are not all identical, however. This presumably reflects the fact that the motor planning process is internally-regulated, and its timecourse may differ from trial to trial, even when the presented stimulus (in this case, the reach target) is identical. How these timecourses differ from trial to trial would have been obscured had we combined the neural data across trials, as with the NV in Section 5.

Is this low-dimensional description of the system dynamics adequate to describe the firing of all 131 recorded units? We transformed the inferred latent trajectories into trial-by-trial

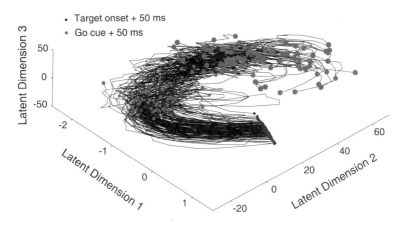

Figure 2: Inferred modal state trajectories in latent (**x**) space for 146 test trials. Dots indicate 50 ms after target onset (blue) and 50 ms after the go cue (green). The radius of the green dots is logarithmically-related to delay period length (200, 750, or 1000ms).

inhomogeneous firing rates using the output relationship from (4)

$$\lambda_t^i = h\left(\mathbf{c}^i \cdot \mathbf{x}_t + d^i\right), \tag{8}$$

where λ_t^i is the imputed firing rate of the ith unit at the tth time bin. Figure 3 shows the imputed firing rates for 15 representative units overlaid with empirical firing rates obtained by directly averaging raw spike counts across the same test trials. If the imputed firing rates truly reflect the rate functions underlying the observed spikes, then the mean behavior of the imputed firing rates should track the empirical firing rates. On the other hand, if the latent system were inadequate to describe the activity, we should expect to see dynamical features in the empirical firing that could not be captured by the imputed firing rates. The strong agreement observed in Figure 3 and across all 131 units suggests that this simple dynamical system is indeed capable of capturing significant components of the dynamics of this neural circuit. We can view the dyamical system approach adopted in this work as a form of *non-linear dynamical embedding* of point-process data. This is in contrast to most current embedding algorithms that rely on continuous data. Figure 2 effectively represents a three-dimensional manifold in the space of firing rates along which the dynamics unfold.

Beyond the agreement of imputed means demonstrated by Figure 3, we would like to directly test the fit of the model to the neural spike data. Unfortunately, current goodness-of-fit methods for spike trains, such as those based on time-rescaling [17], cannot be applied directly to latent variable models. The difficulty arises because the average trajectory obtained from marginalizing over the latent variables in the system (by which we might hope to rescale the inter-spike intervals) is not designed to provide an accurate estimate of the trial-by-trial firing rate functions. Instead, each trial must be described by a distinct trajectory in latent space, which can only be inferred after observing the spike trains themselves. This could lead to overfitting. We are currently exploring extensions to the standard methods which infer latent trajectories using a subset of recorded neurons, and then test the quality of firing-rate predictions for the remaining neurons. In addition, we plan to compare models of different latent dimensionalities; here, the latent space was arbitrarily chosen to be three-dimensional. To validate the learned latent space and inferred trajectories, we would also like to relate these results to trial-by-trial behavior. In particular, given the evidence from Section 5, how "settled" the activity is at the time of the go cue should be predictive of RT.

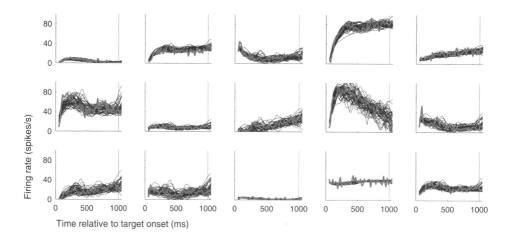

Figure 3: Imputed trial-by-trial firing rates (blue) and empirical firing rates (red). Gray vertical line indicates the time of the go cue. Each panel corresponds to one unit. For clarity, only test trials with delay periods of 1000 ms (44 trials) are plotted for each unit.

Acknowledgments

This work was supported by NIH-NINDS-CRCNS-R01, NSF, NDSEGF, Gatsby, MSTP, CRPF, BWF, ONR, Sloan, and Whitaker. We would like to thank Dr. Mark Churchland for valuable discussions and Missy Howard for expert surgical assistance and veterinary care.

References

[1] M. Abeles, H. Bergman, I. Gat, I. Meilijson, E. Seidemann, N. Tishby, and E. Vaadia. *Proc Natl Acad Sci USA*, 92:8616–8620, 1995.

[2] I. Gat, N. Tishby, and M. Abeles. *Network*, 8(3):297–322, 1997.

[3] A. Smith and E. Brown. *Neural Comput*, 15(5):965–991, 2003.

[4] S. Amari. *Biol Cybern*, 27(2):77–87, 1977.

[5] A. Dempster, N. Laird, and D. Rubin. *J R Stat Soc Ser B*, 39:1–38, 1977.

[6] S. Julier and J. Uhlmann. In *Proc. AeroSense: 11th Int. Symp. Aerospace/Defense Sensing, Simulation and Controls*, pp. 182–193, 1997.

[7] U. Lerner. *Hybrid Bayesian networks for reasoning about complex systems*. PhD thesis, Stanford University, Stanford, CA, 2002.

[8] J. Tanji and E. Evarts. *J Neurophysiol*, 39:1062–1068, 1976.

[9] M. Weinrich, S. Wise, and K. Mauritz. *Brain*, 107:385–414, 1984.

[10] M. Godschalk, R. Lemon, H. Kuypers, and J. van der Steen. *Behav Brain Res*, 18:143–157, 1985.

[11] A. Riehle and J. Requin. *J Neurophysiol*, 61:534–549, 1989.

[12] D. Crammond and J. Kalaska. *J Neurophysiol*, 84:986–1005, 2000.

[13] J. Messier and J. Kalaska. *J Neurophysiol*, 84:152–165, 2000.

[14] D. Rosenbaum. *J Exp Psychol Gen*, 109:444–474, 1980.

[15] A. Riehle and J. Requin. *J Behav Brain Res*, 53:35–49, 1993.

[16] M. Churchland, B. Yu, S. Ryu, G. Santhanam, and K. Shenoy. *Soc. for Neurosci. Abstr.*, 2004.

[17] E. Brown, R. Barbieri, V. Ventura, R. Kass, and L. Frank. *Neural Comput*, 14(2):325–346, 2002.

Soft Clustering on Graphs

Kai Yu[1], Shipeng Yu[2], Volker Tresp[1]
[1]Siemens AG, Corporate Technology
[2]Institute for Computer Science, University of Munich
kai.yu@siemens.com, volker.tresp@siemens.com
spyu@dbs.informatik.uni-muenchen.de

Abstract

We propose a simple clustering framework on graphs encoding pairwise data similarities. Unlike usual similarity-based methods, the approach softly assigns data to clusters in a probabilistic way. More importantly, a *hierarchical clustering* is naturally derived in this framework to gradually merge lower-level clusters into higher-level ones. A random walk analysis indicates that the algorithm exposes clustering structures in various *resolutions*, i.e., a higher level statistically models a longer-term diffusion on graphs and thus discovers a more *global* clustering structure. Finally we provide very encouraging experimental results.

1 Introduction

Clustering has been widely applied in data analysis to group similar objects. Many algorithms are either similarity-based or model-based. In general, the former (e.g., normalized cut [5]) requires no assumption on data densities but simply a similarity function, and usually partitions data exclusively into clusters. In contrast, model-based methods apply mixture models to fit data distributions and assign data to clusters (i.e. mixture components) probabilistically. This *soft* clustering is often desired, as it encodes uncertainties on data-to-cluster assignments. However, their density assumptions can sometimes be restrictive, e.g. clusters have to be Gaussian-like in Gaussian mixture models (GMMs).

In contrast to flat clustering, *hierarchical clustering* makes intuitive senses by forming a tree of clusters. Despite of its wide applications, the technique is usually achieved by heuristics (e.g., single link) and lacks theoretical backup. Only a few principled algorithms exist so far, where a Gaussian or a sphere-shape assumption is often made [3, 1, 2].

This paper suggests a novel graph-factorization clustering (GFC) framework that employs data's affinities and meanwhile partitions data probabilistically. A hierarchical clustering algorithm (HGFC) is further derived by merging lower-level clusters into higher-level ones. Analysis based on graph random walks suggests that our clustering method models data affinities as *empirical transitions* generated by a mixture of latent factors. This view significantly differs from conventional model-based clustering since here the mixture model is not directly for data objects but for their relations. Clusters with arbitrary shapes can be modeled by our method since only pairwise similarities are considered. Interestingly, we prove that the higher-level clusters are associated with longer-term diffusive transitions on the graph, amounting to smoother and more global similarity functions on the data manifold. Therefore, the cluster hierarchy exposes the observed affinity structure gradually in different *resolutions*, which is somehow similar to the *wavelet* method that analyzes signals in different bandwidths. To the best of our knowledge, this property has never been considered by other agglomerative hierarchical clustering algorithms (e.g., see [3]).

The paper is organized as follows. In the following section we describe a clustering algorithm based on similarity graphs. In Sec. 3 we generalize the algorithm to hierarchical clustering, followed by a discussion from the random walk point of view in Sec. 4. Finally we present the experimental results in Sec. 5 and conclude the paper in Sec. 6.

2 Graph-factorization clustering (GFC)

Data similarity relations can be conveniently encoded by a graph, where vertices denote data objects and adjacency weights represent data similarities. This section introduces *graph factorization clustering*, which is a probabilistic partition of graph vertices. Formally, let $G(\mathbf{V}, \mathbf{E})$ be a weighted undirected graph with vertices $\mathbf{V} = \{v_i\}_{i=1}^n$ and edges $\mathbf{E} \subseteq \{(v_i, v_j)\}$. Let $\mathbf{W} = \{w_{ij}\}$ be the adjacency matrix, where $w_{ij} = w_{ji}$, $w_{ij} > 0$ if $(v_i, v_j) \in \mathbf{E}$ and $w_{ij} = 0$ otherwise. For instances, w_{ij} can be computed by the RBF similarity function based on the features of objects i and j, or by a binary indicator (0 or 1) of the k-nearest neighbor affinity.

2.1 Bipartite graphs

Before presenting the main idea, it is necessary to introduce *bipartite graphs*. Let $K(\mathbf{V}, \mathbf{U}, \mathbf{F})$ be the bipartite graph (e.g., Fig. 1–(b)), where $\mathbf{V} = \{v_i\}_{i=1}^n$ and $\mathbf{U} = \{u_p\}_{p=1}^m$ are the two disjoint vertex sets and $\mathbf{F}$ contains all the edges connecting $\mathbf{V}$ and $\mathbf{U}$. Let $\mathbf{B} = \{b_{ip}\}$ denote the $n \times m$ adjacency matrix with $b_{ip} \geq 0$ being the weight for edge $[v_i, u_p]$. The bipartite graph K induces a similarity between v_i and v_j [6]

$$w_{ij} = \sum_{p=1}^m \frac{b_{ip}b_{jp}}{\lambda_p} = \left(\mathbf{B}\boldsymbol{\Lambda}^{-1}\mathbf{B}^\top\right)_{ij}, \quad \boldsymbol{\Lambda} = \mathrm{diag}(\lambda_1, \ldots, \lambda_m) \tag{1}$$

where $\lambda_p = \sum_{i=1}^n b_{ip}$ denotes the degree of vertex $u_p \in \mathbf{U}$. We can interpret Eq. (1) from the perspective of *Markov random walks* on graphs. w_{ij} is essentially a quantity proportional to the stationary probability of direct transitions between v_i and v_j, denoted by $p(v_i, v_j)$. Without loss of generality, we normalize $\mathbf{W}$ to ensure $\sum_{ij} w_{ij} = 1$ and $w_{ij} = p(v_i, v_j)$. For a bipartite graph $K(\mathbf{V}, \mathbf{U}, \mathbf{F})$, there is no direct links between vertices in $\mathbf{V}$, and all the paths from v_i to v_j must go through vertices in $\mathbf{U}$. This indicates

$$p(v_i, v_j) = p(v_i)p(v_j|v_i) = d_i \sum_p p(u_p|v_i)p(v_j|u_p) = \sum_p \frac{p(v_i, u_p)p(u_p, v_j)}{\lambda_p},$$

where $p(v_j|v_i)$ is the conditional transition probability from v_i to v_j, and $d_i = p(v_i)$ the degree of v_i. This directly leads to Eq. (1) with $b_{ip} = p(v_i, u_p)$.

2.2 Graph factorization by bipartite graph construction

For a bipartite graph K, $p(u_p|v_i) = b_{ip}/d_i$ tells the conditional probability of transitions from v_i to u_p. If the size of $\mathbf{U}$ is smaller than that of $\mathbf{V}$, namely $m < n$, then $p(u_p|v_i)$ indicates how likely data point i belongs to vertex p. This property suggests that one can construct a bipartite graph $K(\mathbf{V}, \mathbf{U}, \mathbf{F})$ to approximate a given $G(\mathbf{V}, \mathbf{E})$, and then obtain a soft clustering structure, where $\mathbf{U}$ corresponds to clusters (see Fig. 1–(a) (b)).

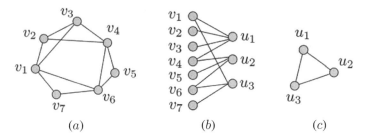

Figure 1: (*a*) The original graph representing data affinities; (*b*) The bipartite graph representing data-to-cluster relations; (*c*) The induced cluster affinities.

Eq. (1) suggests that this approximation can be done by minimizing $\ell(\mathbf{W}, \mathbf{B}\mathbf{\Lambda}^{-1}\mathbf{B}^{\top})$, given a distance $\ell(\cdot, \cdot)$ between two adjacency matrices. To make the problem easy to solve, we remove the coupling between $\mathbf{B}$ and $\mathbf{\Lambda}$ via $\mathbf{H} = \mathbf{B}\mathbf{\Lambda}^{-1}$ and then have

$$\min_{\mathbf{H}, \mathbf{\Lambda}} \ell\left(\mathbf{W}, \mathbf{H}\mathbf{\Lambda}\mathbf{H}^{\top}\right), \qquad \text{s. t. } \sum_{i=1}^{n} h_{ip} = 1, \mathbf{H} \in \mathbb{R}_{+}^{n \times m}, \mathbf{\Lambda} \in \mathbb{D}_{+}^{m \times m}, \qquad (2)$$

where $\mathbb{D}_{+}^{m \times m}$ denotes the set of $m \times m$ diagonal matrices with positive diagonal entries. This problem is a symmetric variant of non-negative matrix factorization [4]. In this paper we focus on the *divergence distance* between matrices. The following theorem suggests an alternating optimization approach to find a local minimum:

Theorem 2.1. *For divergence distance $\ell(\mathbf{X}, \mathbf{Y}) = \sum_{ij}(x_{ij} \log \frac{x_{ij}}{y_{ij}} - x_{ij} + y_{ij})$, the cost function in Eq. (2) is non-increasing under the update rule ($\tilde{}$ denote updated quantities)*

$$\tilde{h}_{ip} \propto h_{ip} \sum_{j} \frac{w_{ij}}{(\mathbf{H}\mathbf{\Lambda}\mathbf{H}^{\top})_{ij}} \lambda_p h_{jp}, \quad normalize \ s.t. \ \sum_{i} \tilde{h}_{ip} = 1; \qquad (3)$$

$$\tilde{\lambda}_p \propto \lambda_p \sum_{ij} \frac{w_{ij}}{(\mathbf{H}\mathbf{\Lambda}\mathbf{H}^{\top})_{ij}} h_{ip} h_{jp}, \quad normalize \ s.t. \ \sum_{p} \tilde{\lambda}_p = \sum_{ij} w_{ij}. \qquad (4)$$

The distance is invariant under the update if and only if $\mathbf{H}$ and $\mathbf{\Lambda}$ are at a stationary point.

See Appendix for all the proofs in this paper. Similar to GMM, $p(u_p|v_i) = b_{ip}/\sum_q b_{iq}$ is the *soft* probabilistic assignment of vertex v_i to cluster u_p. The method can be seen as a counterpart of mixture models on graphs. The time complexity is $\mathcal{O}(m^2 N)$ with N being the number of nonzero entries in $\mathbf{W}$. This can be very efficient if $\mathbf{W}$ is sparse (e.g., for k-nearest neighbor graph the complexity $\mathcal{O}(m^2 nk)$ scales linearly with sample size n).

3 Hierarchical graph-factorization clustering (HGFC)

As a nice property of the proposed graph factorization, a natural affinity between two clusters u_p and u_q can be computed as

$$p(u_p, u_q) = \sum_{i=1}^{n} \frac{b_{ip} b_{iq}}{d_i} = \left(\mathbf{B}^{\top}\mathbf{D}^{-1}\mathbf{B}\right)_{pq}, \qquad \mathbf{D} = \text{diag}(d_1, \dots, d_n) \qquad (5)$$

This is similar to Eq. (1), but derived from another way of two-hop transitions $\mathbf{U} \to \mathbf{V} \to \mathbf{U}$. Note that the similarity between clusters p and q takes into account a weighted average of contributions from *all* the data (see Fig. 1–(*c*)).

Let $G_0(\mathbf{V}_0, \mathbf{E}_0)$ be the initial graph describing the similarities of totally $m_0 = n$ data points, with adjacency matrix $\mathbf{W}_0$. Based on G_0 we can build a bipartite graph $K_1(\mathbf{V}_0, \mathbf{V}_1, \mathbf{F}_1)$, with $m_1 < m_0$ vertices in $\mathbf{V}_1$. A hierarchical clustering method can be motivated from the observation that the cluster similarity in Eq. (5) suggests a new adjacency matrix $\mathbf{W}_1$ for graph $G_1(\mathbf{V}_1, \mathbf{E}_1)$, where $\mathbf{V}_1$ is formed by clusters, and $\mathbf{E}_1$ contains edges connecting these clusters. Then we can group those clusters by constructing another bipartite graph $K_2(\mathbf{V}_1, \mathbf{V}_2, \mathbf{F}_2)$ with $m_2 < m_1$ vertices in $\mathbf{V}_2$, such that $\mathbf{W}_1$ is again factorized as in Eq. (2), and a new graph $G_2(\mathbf{V}_2, \mathbf{E}_2)$ can be built. In principal we can repeat this procedure until we get only one cluster. Algorithm 1 summarizes this algorithm.

Algorithm 1 Hierarchical Graph-Factorization Clustering (HGFC)

Require: given n data objects and a similarity measure
1: build the similarity graph $G_0(\mathbf{V}_0, \mathbf{E}_0)$ with adjacency matrix $\mathbf{W}_0$, and let $m_0 = n$
2: **for** $l = 1, 2, \ldots,$ **do**
3:     choose $m_l < m_{l-1}$
4:     factorize G_{l-1} to obtain $K_l(\mathbf{V}_{l-1}, \mathbf{V}_l, \mathbf{F}_l)$ with the adjacency matrix $\mathbf{B}_l$
5:     build a graph $G_l(\mathbf{V}_l, \mathbf{E}_l)$ with the adjacency matrix $\mathbf{W}_l = \mathbf{B}_l^\top \mathbf{D}_l^{-1} \mathbf{B}_l$, where $\mathbf{D}_l$'s diagonal entries are obtained by summation over $\mathbf{B}_l$'s columns
6: **end for**

The algorithm ends up with a hierarchical clustering structure. For level l, we can assign data to the obtained m_l clusters via a propagation from the bottom level of clusters. Based on the chain rule of Markov random walks, the soft (i.e., probabilistic) assignment of $v_i \in \mathbf{V}_0$ to cluster $v_p^{(l)} \in \mathbf{V}_l$ is given by

$$p\left(v_p^{(l)}|v_i\right) = \sum_{v^{(l-1)}\in\mathbf{V}_{l-1}} \cdots \sum_{v^{(1)}\in\mathbf{V}_1} p\left(v_p^{(l)}|v^{(l-1)}\right) \cdots p\left(v^{(1)}|v_i\right) = \left(\mathbf{D}_1^{-1}\bar{\mathbf{B}}_l\right)_{ip}, \quad (6)$$

where $\bar{\mathbf{B}}_l = \mathbf{B}_1 \mathbf{D}_2^{-1} \mathbf{B}_2 \mathbf{D}_3^{-1} \mathbf{B}_3 \ldots \mathbf{D}_l^{-1} \mathbf{B}_l$. One can interpret this by deriving an *equivalent* bipartite graph $\bar{K}_l(\mathbf{V}_0, \mathbf{V}_l, \bar{\mathbf{F}}_l)$, and treating $\bar{\mathbf{B}}_l$ as the *equivalent* adjacency matrix attached to the *equivalent* edges $\bar{\mathbf{F}}_l$ connecting data $\mathbf{V}_0$ and clusters $\mathbf{V}_l$.

4 Analysis of the proposed algorithms

4.1 Flat clustering: statistical modeling of single-hop transitions

In this section we provide some insights to the suggested clustering algorithm, mainly from the perspective of random walks on graphs. Suppose that from a stationary stage of random walks on $G(\mathbf{V}, \mathbf{E})$, one observes π_{ij} single-hop transitions between v_i and v_j in a unitary time frame. As an intuition of graph-based view to similarities, if two data points are similar or related, the transitions between them are likely to happen. Thus we connect the observed similarities to the *frequency* of transitions via $w_{ij} \propto \pi_{ij}$. If the observed transitions are i.i.d. sampled from a true distribution $p(v_i, v_j) = (\mathbf{H}\mathbf{\Lambda}\mathbf{H}^\top)_{ij}$ where a bipartite graph is behind, then the log likelihood with respect to the observed transitions is

$$\mathcal{L}(\mathbf{H}, \mathbf{\Lambda}) = \log \prod_{ij} p(v_i, v_j)^{\pi_{ij}} \propto \sum_{ij} w_{ij} \log(\mathbf{H}\mathbf{\Lambda}\mathbf{H}^\top)_{ij}. \quad (7)$$

Then we have the following conclusion

Proposition 4.1. *For a weighted undirected graph $G(\mathbf{V}, \mathbf{E})$ and the log likelihood defined in Eq. (7), the following results hold: (i) Minimizing the divergence distance $l(\mathbf{W}, \mathbf{H}\mathbf{\Lambda}\mathbf{H}^\top)$ is equivalent to maximizing the log likelihood $\mathcal{L}(\mathbf{H}, \mathbf{\Lambda})$; (ii) Updates Eq. (3) and Eq. (4) correspond to a standard EM algorithm for maximizing $\mathcal{L}(\mathbf{H}, \mathbf{\Lambda})$.*

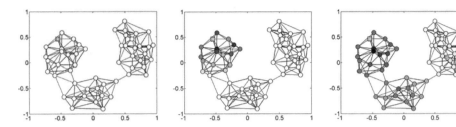

Figure 2: The similarities of vertices to a fixed vertex (marked in the left panel) on a 6-nearest-neighbor graph, respectively induced by clustering level $l = 2$ (the middle panel) and $l = 6$ (the right panel). A darker color means a higher similarity.

4.2 Hierarchical clustering: statistical modeling of multi-hop transitions

The adjacency matrix $\mathbf{W}_0$ of $G_0(\mathbf{V}_0, \mathbf{E}_0)$ only models one-hop transitions that follow direct links from vertices to their neighbors. However, the random walk is a process of diffusion on the graph. Within a relatively longer period, a walker starting from a vertex has the chance to reach vertices faraway through *multi-hop* transitions. Obviously, multi-hop transitions induce a slowly decaying similarity function on the graph. Based on the chain rule of Markov process, the equivalent adjacency matrix for t-hop transitions is

$$\mathbf{A}_t = \mathbf{W}_0(\mathbf{D}_0^{-1}\mathbf{W}_0)^{t-1} = \mathbf{A}_{t-1}\mathbf{D}_0^{-1}\mathbf{W}_0. \tag{8}$$

Generally speaking, a slowly decaying similarity function on the similarity graph captures a global affinity structure of data manifolds, while a rapidly decaying similarity function only tells the local affinity structure. The following proposition states that in the suggested HGFC, a higher-level clustering implicitly employs a more global similarity measure caused by multi-hop Markov random walks:

Proposition 4.2. *For a given hierarchical clustering structure that starts from a bottom graph $G_0(\mathbf{V}_0, \mathbf{E}_0)$ to a higher level $G_k(\mathbf{V}_k, \mathbf{E}_k)$, the vertices $\mathbf{V}_l$ at level $0 < l \leq k$ induces an equivalent adjacency matrix of $\mathbf{V}_0$, which is $\mathbf{A}_t$ with $t = 2^{l-1}$ as defined in Eq. (8).*

Therefore the presented hierarchical clustering algorithm HGFC applies different sizes of time windows to examine random walks, and derives different scales of similarity measures to expose the local and global clustering structures of data manifolds. Fig. 2 illustrates the employed similarities of vertices to a fixed vertex in clustering levels $l = 2$ and 6, which corresponds to time periods $t = 2$ and 32. It can be seen that for a short period $t = 2$, the similarity is very local and helps to uncover low-level clusters, while in a longer period $t = 32$ the similarity function is rather global.

5 Empirical study

We apply HGFC on USPS handwritten digits and Newsgroup text data. For USPS data we use the images of digits 1, 2, 3 and 4, with respectively 1269, 929, 824 and 852 images per class. Each image is represented as a 256-dimension vector. The text data contain totally 3970 documents covering 4 categories, autos, motorcycles, baseball, and hockey. Each document is represented by an 8014-dimension TFIDF feature vector. Our method employs a 10-nearest-neighbor graph, with the similarity measure RBF for USPS and cosine for Newsgroup. We perform 4-level HGFC, and set the cluster number, respectively from bottom to top, to be 100, 20, 10 and 4 for both data sets.

We compare HGFC with two popular agglomerative hierarchical clustering algorithms, single link and complete link (e.g., [3]). Both methods merge two closest clusters at each step.

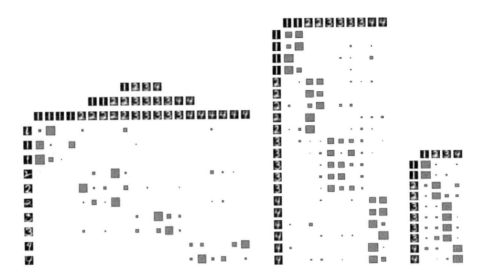

Figure 3: Visualization of HGFC for USPS data set. Left: mean images of the top 3 clustering levels, along with a Hinton graph representing the soft (probabilistic) assignments of randomly chosen 10 digits (shown on the left) to the top 3rd level clusters; Middle: a Hinton graph showing the soft cluster assignments from top 3rd level to top 2nd level; Right: a Hinton graph showing the soft assignments from top 2nd level to top 1st level.

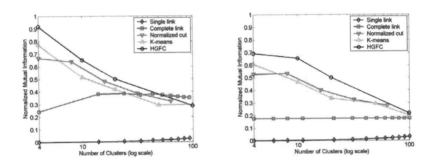

Figure 4: Comparison of clustering methods on USPS (left) and Newsgroup (right), evaluated by normalized mutual information (NMI). Higher values indicate better qualities.

Single link defines the cluster distance to be the smallest point-wise distance between two clusters, while complete link uses the largest one. A third compared method is normalized cut [5], which partitions data into two clusters. We apply the algorithm recursively to produce a top-down hierarchy of 2, 4, 8, 16, 32 and 64 clusters. We also compare with the k-means algorithm, $k = 4, 10, 20$ and 100.

Before showing the comparison, we visualize a part of clustering results for USPS data in Fig. 3. On top of the left figure, we show the top three levels of the hierarchy with respectively 4, 10 and 20 clusters, where each cluster is represented by its mean image via an average over all the images weighted by their posterior probabilities of belonging to this cluster. Then 10 randomly sampled digits with soft cluster assignments to the top 3rd level clusters are illustrated with a Hinton graph. The middle and right figures in Fig. 3 show the assignments between clusters across the hierarchy. The clear diagonal block structure in all the Hinton graphs indicates a very meaningful cluster hierarchy.

	Normalized cut				HGFC				K-means			
"1"	635	630	1	3	**1254**	3	8	4	1265	1	0	3
"2"	2	4	744	179	1	**886**	33	9	17	720	95	97
"3"	2	1	817	4	1	4	**816**	3	10	9	796	9
"4"	10	6	1	835	4	8	2	**838**	58	20	0	774

Table 1: Confusion matrices of clustering results, 4 clusters, USPS data. In each confusion matrix, rows correspond true classes and columns correspond the found clusters.

	Normalized cut				HGFC				K-means			
autos	858	98	30	2	**772**	182	13	21	977	7	4	0
motor.	79	893	16	5	42	**934**	5	12	985	3	5	0
baseball	44	33	875	40	15	33	**843**	101	39	835	114	4
hockey	11	8	893	85	7	21	11	**958**	16	4	900	77

Table 2: Confusion matrices of clustering results, 4 clusters, Newsgroup data. In each confusion matrix, rows correspond true classes and columns correspond the found clusters.

We compare the clustering methods by evaluating the normalized mutual information (NMI) in Fig. 4. It is defined to be the mutual information between clusters and true classes, normalized by the maximum of marginal entropies. Moreover, in order to more directly assess the clustering quality, we also illustrate the confusion matrices in Table 1 and Table 2, in the case of producing 4 clusters. We drop out the confusion matrices of single link and complete link in the tables, for saving spaces and also due to their clearly poor performance compared with others.

The results show that single link performs poorly, as it greedily merges nearby data and tends to form a big cluster with some outliers. Complete link is more balanced but unsatisfactory either. For the Newsgroup data it even gets stuck at the 3601-th merge because all the similarities between clusters are 0. Top-down hierarchical normalized cut obtains reasonable results, but sometimes cannot split one big cluster (see the tables). The confusion matrices indicates that k-means does well for digit images but relatively worse for high-dimension textual data. In contrast, Fig. 4 shows that HGFC gives significantly higher NMI values than competitors on both tasks. It also produces confusion matrices with clear diagonal structures (see tables 1 and 2), which indicates a very good clustering quality.

6 Conclusion and Future Work

In this paper we have proposed a probabilistic graph partition method for clustering data objects based on their pairwise similarities. A novel hierarchical clustering algorithm HGFC has been derived, where a higher level in HGFC corresponds to a statistical model of random walk transitions in a longer period, giving rise to a more global clustering structure. Experiments show very encouraging results.

In this paper we have empirically specified the number of clusters in each level. In the near future we plan to investigate effective methods to automatically determine it. Another direction is hierarchical clustering on directed graphs, as well as its applications in web mining.

Appendix

Proof of Theorem 2.1. We first notice that $\sum_p \lambda_p = \sum_{ij} w_{ij}$ under constraints $\sum_i h_{ip} = 1$. Therefore we can normalize $\mathbf{W}$ by $\sum_{ij} w_{ij}$ and after convergence multiply all λ_p by this quantity to get the solution. Under this assumption we are maximizing $\mathcal{L}(\mathbf{H}, \boldsymbol{\Lambda}) = \sum_{ij} w_{ij} \log(\mathbf{H}\boldsymbol{\Lambda}\mathbf{H}^\top)_{ij}$ with an extra constraint $\sum_p \lambda_p = 1$. We first fix λ_p and show update Eq. (3) will not decrease $\mathcal{L}(\mathbf{H}) \equiv \mathcal{L}(\mathbf{H}, \boldsymbol{\Lambda})$. We prove this by constructing an auxiliary function $f(\mathbf{H}, \mathbf{H}^*)$ such that $f(\mathbf{H}, \mathbf{H}^*) \le \mathcal{L}(\mathbf{H})$ and $f(\mathbf{H}, \mathbf{H}) = \mathcal{L}(\mathbf{H})$. Then we know the update $\mathbf{H}^{t+1} = \arg\max_{\mathbf{H}} f(\mathbf{H}, \mathbf{H}^t)$ will not decrease $\mathcal{L}(\mathbf{H})$ since $\mathcal{L}(\mathbf{H}^{t+1}) \ge f(\mathbf{H}^{t+1}, \mathbf{H}^t) \ge f(\mathbf{H}^t, \mathbf{H}^t) = \mathcal{L}(\mathbf{H}^t)$. Define $f(\mathbf{H}, \mathbf{H}^*) = \sum_{ij} w_{ij} \sum_p \frac{h_{ip}^* \lambda_p h_{jp}^*}{\sum_l h_{il}^* \lambda_l h_{jl}^*} \left(\log h_{ip} \lambda_p h_{jp} - \log \frac{h_{ip}^* \lambda_p h_{jp}^*}{\sum_l h_{il}^* \lambda_l h_{jl}^*} \right)$. $f(\mathbf{H}, \mathbf{H}) = \mathcal{L}(\mathbf{H})$ can be easily verified, and $f(\mathbf{H}, \mathbf{H}^*) \le \mathcal{L}(\mathbf{H})$ also follows if we use concavity of log function. Then it is straightforward to verify Eq. (3) by setting the derivative of f with respect to h_{ip} to be zero. The normalization is due to the constraints and can be formally derived from this procedure with a Lagrange formalism. Similarly we can define an auxiliary function for $\boldsymbol{\Lambda}$ with $\mathbf{H}$ fixed, and verify Eq. (4). $\square$

Proof of Proposition 4.1. (i) follows directly from the proof of Theorem 2.1. To prove (ii) we take u_p as the missing data and follow the standard way to derive the EM algorithm. In the E-step we estimate the *a posteriori* probability of taking u_p for pair (v_i, v_j) using Bayes' rule: $\hat{p}(u_p|v_i, v_j) \propto p(v_i|u_p)p(v_j|u_p)p(u_p)$. And then in the M-step we maximize the "complete" data likelihood $\hat{\mathcal{L}}(G) = \sum_{ij} w_{ij} \sum_p \hat{p}(u_p|v_i, v_j) \log p(v_i|u_p)p(v_j|u_p)p(u_p)$ with respect to model parameters $h_{ip} = p(v_i|u_p)$ and $\lambda_p = p(u_p)$, with constraints $\sum_i h_{ip} = 1$ and $\sum_p \lambda_p = 1$. By setting the corresponding derivatives to zero we obtain $h_{ip} \propto \sum_j w_{ij}\hat{p}(u_p|v_i, v_j)$ and $\lambda_p \propto \sum_{ij} w_{ij}\hat{p}(u_p|v_i, v_j)$. It is easy to check that they are equivalent to updates Eq. (3) and Eq. (4) respectively. $\square$

Proof of Proposition 4.2. We give a brief proof. Suppose that at level l the data-cluster relationship is described by $\bar{K}_l(\mathbf{V}_0, \mathbf{V}_l, \bar{\mathbf{F}}_l)$ (see Eq. (6)) with adjacency matrix $\bar{\mathbf{B}}_l$, degrees $\mathbf{D}_0$ for $\mathbf{V}_0$, and degrees $\boldsymbol{\Lambda}_l$ for $\mathbf{V}_l$. In this case the induced adjacency matrix of $\mathbf{V}_0$ is $\bar{\mathbf{W}}_l = \bar{\mathbf{B}}_l \boldsymbol{\Lambda}_l^{-1} \bar{\mathbf{B}}_l^\top$, and the adjacency matrix of $\mathbf{V}_l$ is $\mathbf{W}_l = \bar{\mathbf{B}}_l^\top \mathbf{D}_0^{-1} \bar{\mathbf{B}}_l$. Let $K_l(\mathbf{V}_l, \mathbf{V}_{l+1}, \mathbf{F}_{l+1})$ be the bipartite graph connecting $\mathbf{V}_l$ and $\mathbf{V}_{l+1}$, with the adjacency $\mathbf{B}_{l+1}$ and degrees $\boldsymbol{\Lambda}_{l+1}$ for $\mathbf{V}_{l+1}$. Then the adjacency matrix of $\mathbf{V}_0$ induced by level $l+1$ is $\bar{\mathbf{W}}_{l+1} = \bar{\mathbf{B}}_l \boldsymbol{\Lambda}_l^{-1} \mathbf{B}_{l+1} \boldsymbol{\Lambda}_{l+1}^{-1} \mathbf{B}_{l+1}^\top \boldsymbol{\Lambda}_l^{-1} \bar{\mathbf{B}}_l^\top = \bar{\mathbf{W}}_l \mathbf{D}_0^{-1} \bar{\mathbf{W}}_l$, where relations $\mathbf{B}_{l+1} \boldsymbol{\Lambda}_{l+1}^{-1} \mathbf{B}_{l+1}^\top = \bar{\mathbf{B}}_l^\top \mathbf{D}_0^{-1} \bar{\mathbf{B}}_l$ and $\bar{\mathbf{W}}_l = \bar{\mathbf{B}}_l \boldsymbol{\Lambda}_l^{-1} \bar{\mathbf{B}}_l^\top$ are applied. Given the initial condition from the bottom level $\bar{\mathbf{W}}_1 = \mathbf{W}_0$, it is not difficult to obtain $\bar{\mathbf{W}}_l = \mathbf{A}_t$ with $t = 2^{l-1}$. $\square$

References

[1] J. Goldberger and S. Roweis. Hierarchical clustering of a mixture model. In L.K. Saul, Y. Weiss, and L. Bottou, editors, *Neural Information Processing Systems 17 (NIPS*04)*, pages 505–512, 2005.

[2] K.A. Heller and Z. Ghahramani. Bayesian hierarchical clustering. In *Proceedings of the 22nd International Conference on Machine Learning*, pages 297–304, 2005.

[3] S. D. Kamvar, D. Klein, and C. D. Manning. Interpreting and extending classical agglomerative clustering algorithms using a model-based approach. In *Proceedings of the 19th International Conference on Machine Learning*, pages 283–290, 2002.

[4] Daniel D. Lee and H. Sebastian Seung. Algorithms for non-negative matrix factorization. In T. K. Leen, T. G. Dietterich, and V. Tresp, editors, *Advances in Neural Information Processing Systems 13 (NIPS*00)*, pages 556–562, 2001.

[5] Jianbo Shi and Jitendra Malik. Normalized cuts and image segmentation. *IEEE Transactions on Pattern Analysis and Machine Intelligence*, 22(8):888–905, 2000.

[6] D. Zhou, B. Schölkopf, and T. Hofmann. Semi-supervised learning on directed graphs. In L.K. Saul, Y. Weiss, and L. Bottou, editors, *Advances in Neural Information Processing Systems 17 (NIPS*04)*, pages 1633–1640, 2005.

Augmented Rescorla-Wagner and Maximum Likelihood estimation.

Alan Yuille
Department of Statistics
University of California at Los Angeles
Los Angeles, CA 90095
yuille@stat.ucla.edu

Abstract

We show that linear generalizations of Rescorla-Wagner can perform Maximum Likelihood estimation of the parameters of all generative models for causal reasoning. Our approach involves augmenting variables to deal with conjunctions of causes, similar to the augmented model of Rescorla. Our results involve genericity assumptions on the distributions of causes. If these assumptions are violated, for example for the Cheng causal power theory, then we show that a linear Rescorla-Wagner can estimate the parameters of the model up to a nonlinear transformtion. Moreover, a nonlinear Rescorla-Wagner is able to estimate the parameters directly to within arbitrary accuracy. Previous results can be used to determine convergence and to estimate convergence rates.

1 Introduction

It is important to understand the relationship between the Rescorla-Wagner (RW) algorithm [1,2] and theories of learning based on maximum likelihood (ML) estimation of the parameters of generative models [3,4,5]. The Rescorla-Wagner algorithm has been shown to account for many experimental findings. But maximum likelihood offers the promise of a sound statistical basis including the ability to learn sophisticated probabilistic models for causal learning [6,7,8].

Previous work, summarized in section (2), showed a direct relationship between the basic Rescorla-Wagner algorithm and maximum likelihood for the ΔP model of causal learning [4,9]. More recently, a generalization of Rescorla-Wagner was shown to perform maximum likelihood estimation for both the ΔP and the noisy-or models [10]. *Throughout the paper, we follow the common practice of studying the convergence of the expected value of the weights and ignoring the fluctuations. The size of these fluctuations can be calculated analytically and precise convergence quantified* [10].

In this paper, we greatly extend the connections between Rescorla-Wagner and ML estimation. We show that two classes of generalized Rescorla-Wagner algorithms can perform ML estimation for all generative models provided genericity assumptions on the causes are satisfied. These generalizations include *augmenting the set of variables to represent conjunctive causes* and are related to the augmented Rescorla-Wagner algorithm [2].

We also analyze the case where the genericity assumption breaks down and pay particular attention to Chengs' causal power model [4,5]. We demonstrate that Rescorla-Wagner can perform ML estimation for this model up to a nonlinear transformation of the model parameters (i.e. Rescorla-Wagner does ML but in a different coordinate system). We sketch how a nonlinear Rescorla-Wagner can estimate the parameters directly.

Convergence analysis from previous work [10] can be directly applied to these new Rescorla-Wagner algorithms. This gives convergence conditions and put bounds on the convergence rate. The analysis assumes that the data consists of i.i.d. samples from the (unknown) causal distribution. But the results can also be applied in the piecewise iid case (such as forward and backward blocking [11]).

2   Summary of Previous Work

We summarize pervious work relating maximum likelihood estimation of generative models with the Rescorla-Wagner algorithm [4,9,10]. This work assumes that there is a binary-valued event E which can be caused by one or more of two binary-valued causes C_1, C_2. The ΔP and Noisy-or theories use generative models of form:

$$P_{\Delta P}(E = 1|C_1, C_2, \omega_1, \omega_2) = \omega_1 C_1 + \omega_2 C_2 \tag{1}$$

$$P_{Noisy-or}(E = 1|C_1, C_2, \omega_1, \omega_2) = \omega_1 C_1 + \omega_2 C_2 - \omega_1 \omega_2 C_1 C_2, \tag{2}$$

where $\{\omega_1, \omega_2\}$ are the model parameters.

The training data consists of examples $\{E^\mu, C_1^\mu, C_2^\mu\}$. The parameters $\{\omega_1, \omega_2\}$ are estimated by Maximum Likelihood

$$\{\omega_1^*, \omega_2^*\} = \arg\max_{\{\omega_1, \omega_2\}} \prod_\mu P(E^\mu|C_1^\mu, C_2^\mu; \omega_1, \omega_2) P(C_1^\mu, C_2^\mu), \tag{3}$$

where $P(C_1, C_2)$ is the distribution on the causes. It is independent of $\{\omega_1, \omega_2\}$ and does not affect the Maximum Likelihood estimation, except for some non-generic cases to be discussed in section (5).

An alternative approach to learning causal models is the Rescorla-Wagner algorithm which updates weights V_1, V_2 as follows:

$$V_1^{t+1} = V_1^t + \Delta V_1^t, \quad V_2^{t+1} = V_2^t + \Delta V_2^t, \tag{4}$$

where the update rule ΔV can take forms like:

$$\Delta V_1 = \alpha_1 C_1(E - C_1 V_1 - C_2 V_2), \quad \Delta V_2 = \alpha_2 C_2(E - C_1 V_1 - C_2 V_2), \text{ basic rule} \tag{5}$$

$$\Delta V_1 = \alpha_1 C_1(1 - C_2)(E - V_1), \quad \Delta V_2 = \alpha_2 C_2(1 - C_1)(E - V_2), \text{ variant rule.} \tag{6}$$

It is known that if the basic update rule (5) is used then the weights converge to the ML estimates of the parameters $\{\omega_1, \omega_2\}$ provided the data is generated by the ΔP model (1) [4,9] (but not for the noisy-or model).

If the variant update rule (6) is used, then the weights converge to the parameters $\{\omega_1, \omega_2\}$ of the ΔP model *or* the noisy-or model (2) depending on which model generates the data [10].

3   Basic Ingredients

This section describes three basic ingredients of this work: (i) the generative models, (ii) maximum likelihood, and (iii) the generalized Rescorla-Wagner algorithms.

Representing the generative models.

We represent the distribution $P(E|\vec{C}; \vec{\alpha})$ by the function:

$$P(E = 1|\vec{C}; \vec{\alpha}) = \sum_i \alpha_i h_i(\vec{C}), \tag{7}$$

where the $\{h_i(\vec{C})\}$ are a set of basis functions and the $\{\alpha_i\}$ are parameters. If the dimension of $\vec{C}$ is n, then the number of basis functions is 2^n. All distributions of binary variables can be represented in this form.

For example, if $n = 2$ we can use the basis:

$$h_1(\vec{C}) = 1, h_2(\vec{C}) = C_1, h_3(\vec{C}) = C_2, h_4(\vec{C}) = C_1 C_2, \tag{8}$$

Then the noisy-or model $P(E = 1|C_1, C_2) = \omega_1 C_1 + \omega_2 C_2 - \omega_1 \omega_2 C_1 C_2$ corresponds to setting $\alpha_1 = 0, \alpha_2 = \omega_1, \alpha_3 = \omega_2, \alpha_4 = -\omega_1 \omega_2$.

Data Generation Assumption and Maximum Likelihood

We assume that the observed data $\{E^\mu, \vec{C}^\mu : \mu \in \Lambda\}$ are i.i.d. samples from $P(E|\vec{C})P(\vec{C})$. It is possible to adapt our results to cases where the data is piecewise i.i.d., such as blocking experiments, but we have no space to describe this here.

Maximum Likelihood (ML) estimates the $\vec{\alpha}$ by solving:

$$\vec{\alpha}^* = \arg\min_{\vec{\alpha}} - \sum_{\mu \in \Lambda} \log\{P(E^\mu|\vec{C}^\mu; \vec{\alpha})P(\vec{C}^\mu)\} = \arg\min_{\vec{\alpha}} - \sum_{\mu \in \Lambda} \log P(E^\mu|\vec{C}^\mu; \vec{\alpha}). \tag{9}$$

Observe that the estimate of $\vec{\alpha}$ is independent of $P(\vec{C})$ provided the distribution is generic. Important non-generic cases are treated in section (5).

Generalized Rescorla-Wagner.

The Rescorla-Wagner (RW) algorithm updates weights $\{V_i : i = 1, ..., n\}$ by a discrete iterative algorithm:

$$V_i^{t+1} = V_i^t + \Delta V_i^t, \quad i = 1, ..., n. \tag{10}$$

We assume a generalized form:

$$\Delta V_i = \sum_j V_j f_{ij}(\vec{C}) + E g_i(\vec{C}), \quad i, j = 1, ..., n \tag{11}$$

for functions $\{f_{ij}(\vec{C})\}, \{g_i(\vec{C})\}$. It is easy to see that equations (5,6) are special cases.

4 Theoretical Results

We now gives sufficient conditions which ensure that the only fixed points of generalized Rescorla-Wagner correspond to ML estimates of the parameters $\vec{\alpha}$ of generative models $P(E|\vec{C}, \vec{\alpha})$. We then obtain two classes of generalized Rescorla-Wagner which satisfy these conditions. For one class, convergence to the fixed points follow directly. For the other class we need to adapt results from [10] to guarantee convergence to the fixed points. Our results assume genericity conditions on the distribution $P(\vec{C})$ of causes. We relax these conditions in section (5).

The number of weights $\{V_i\}$ used by the Rescorla-Wagner algorithm is equal to the number of parameters $\{\alpha_i\}$ that specify the model. But many weights will remain zero unless conjunctions of causes occur, see section (6).

Theorem 1. *A sufficient condition for generalized Rescorla-Wagner (11), to have a unique fixed point at the maximum likelihood estimates of the parameters of a generative model* $P(E|\vec{C};\vec{\alpha})$ *(7), is that* $< f_{ij}(\vec{C}) >_{P(\vec{C})} = - < g_i(\vec{C})h_j(\vec{C}) >_{P(\vec{C})} \forall i,j$ *and the matrix* $< f_{ij}(\vec{C}) >_{P(\vec{C})}$ *is invertible.*

Proof. *We calculate the expectation* $< \Delta V_i >_{P(E|\vec{C})P(\vec{C})}$. *This is zero if, and only if,* $\sum_j V_j < f_{ij}(\vec{C}) >_{P(\vec{C})} + \sum_j \alpha_j < g_i(\vec{C})h_j(\vec{C}) >_{P(\vec{C})} = 0$. *The result follows.*

We use notation that $< . >_{P(\vec{C})}$ is the expectation with respect to the probability distribution $P(\vec{C})$ on the causes. For example, $< f_{ij}(\vec{C}) >_{P(\vec{C})} = \sum_{\vec{C}} P(\vec{C})f_{ij}(\vec{C})$. Hence the requirement that the matrix $< f_{ij}(\vec{C}) >_{P(\vec{C})}$ is invertible usually requires that $P(\vec{C})$ is generic. See examples in sections (4.1,4.2). Convergence may still occur if the matrix $< f_{ij}(\vec{C}) >_{P(\vec{C})}$ is non-invertible. Linear combinations of the weights will remained fixed (in the directions of the zero eigenvectors of the matrix) and the remaining linear co,mbinations will converge.

Additional conditions to ensure convergence to the fixed point, and to determine the convergence rate, can be found using Theorems 3,4,5 in [10].

4.1 Generalized RW class I

We now give prove a corollary of Theorem 1 which will enable us to obtain our first class of generalized RW algorithms.

Corollary 1. *A sufficient condition for generalized RW to have fixed points at ML estimates of the model parameters is* $f_{ij}(\vec{C}) = -h_i(\vec{C})h_j(\vec{C})$, $g_i(\vec{C}) = h_i(\vec{C}) \forall i,j$ *and the matrix* $< h_i(\vec{C})h_j(\vec{C}) >_{P(\vec{C})}$ *is invertible. Moreover, convergence to the fixed point is guaranteed.*

Proof. *Direct verification. Convergence to the fixed point follows from the gradient descent nature of the algorithm, see equation (12).*

These conditions define generalized RW class I (GRW-I) which is a natural extension of basic Rescorla-Wagner (5):

$$\Delta V_i = h_i(\vec{C})\{E - \sum_j h_j(\vec{C})V_j\} = -\frac{\partial}{\partial V_i}(E - \sum_j h_j(\vec{C})V_j)^2, \quad i = 1, ..., n \quad (12)$$

This GRW-I algorithm ia guaranteed to converge to the fixed point because it performs stochastic steepest descent. This is essentially the Widrow-Huff algorithm [12,13].

To illustrate Corollary 1, we show the relationships between GRW-I and ML for three different generative models: (i) the ΔP model, (ii) the noisy-or model, and (iii) the most general form of $P(E|\vec{C})$ for two causes. *It is important to realize that these generative models form a hierarchy and GRW-I algorithms for the later models will also perform ML on the simpler ones.*

1. The ΔP model.

Set $n = 2$, $h_1(\vec{C}) = C_1$ and $h_2(\vec{C}) = C_2$. Then equation (12) reduces to the basic RW algorithm (5) with two weights V_1, V_2. By Corollary 1, we see that it performs ML estimation for the ΔP model (1). This rederives the known relationship between basic RW, ML, and the ΔP model [4,9].

Observe that Corollary 1 requires that the matrix $\begin{pmatrix} < C_1 >_{P(\vec{C})} & < C_1 C_2 >_{P(\vec{C})} \\ < C_1 C_2 >_{P(\vec{C})} & < C_2 >_{P(\vec{C})} \end{pmatrix}$

be invertible. This is equivalent to the genericity condition $< C_1 C_2 >^2_{P(\vec{C})} \neq < C_1 >_{P(\vec{C})} < C_2 >_{P(\vec{C})}$.

2. The Noisy-Or model.

Set $n = 3$ with $h_1(\vec{C}) = C_1, h_2(\vec{C}) = C_2, h_3(\vec{C}) = C_1 C_2$. Then Corollary 1 proves that the following algorithm will converge to estimate $V_1^* = \omega_1$, $V_2^* = \omega_2$ and $V_3^* = -\omega_1 \omega_2$ for the noisy-or model.

$$\Delta V_1 = C_1(E - C_1 V_1 - C_2 V_2 - C_1 C_2 V_3) = C_1(E - V_1 - C_2 V_2 - C_2 V_3)$$
$$\Delta V_2 = C_2(E - C_1 V_1 - C_2 V_2 - C_1 C_2 V_3) = C_2(E - C_1 V_1 - V_2 - C_1 V_3)$$
$$\Delta V_3 = C_1 C_2(E - C_1 V_1 - C_2 V_2 - C_1 C_2 V_3) = C_1 C_2(E - V_1 - V_2 - V_3). \tag{13}$$

This algorithm is a minor variant of basic RW. Observe that this has more weights ($n = 3$) than the total number of causes. The first two weights V_1 and V_2 yield ω_1, ω_2 while the third weight V_3 gives a (redundant) estimate of $\omega_1 \omega_2$. The matrix $< h_i(\vec{C}) h_j(\vec{C}) >_{P(\vec{C})}$ has determinant $(< C_1 C_2 > - < C_1 >)(< C_1 C_2 > - < C_2 >) < C_1 C_2 >$ and is invertible provided $< C_1 > \neq 0, 1$, $< C_2 > \neq 0, 1$ and $< C_1 C_2 > \neq < C_1 >< C_2 >$. This rules out the special case in Cheng's experiments [4,5] where $C_1 = 1$ always, see discussion in section (5).

It is known that basic RW is unable to do ML estimation for the noisy-or model *if there are only two weights* [4,5,9,10]. The differences here is that three weights are used.

3. The general two-cause model.

Thirdly, we consider the most general model $P(E|\vec{C})$ for two causes. This can be written in the form:

$$P(E = 1|C_1, C_2) = \alpha_1 + \alpha_2 C_1 + \alpha_3 C_2 + \alpha_4 C_1 C_2. \tag{14}$$

This corresponds to $h_1(\vec{C}) = 1, h_2(\vec{C}) = C_1, h_3(\vec{C}) = C_2, h_4(\vec{C}) = C_1 C_2$. Corollary 1 gives us *the most general algorithm*:

$$\Delta V_1 = (E - V_1 - C_1 V_2 - C_2 V_3 - C_1 C_2 V_4) = (E - V_1 - C_1 V_2 - C_2 V_3 - C_1 C_2 V_4)$$
$$\Delta V_2 = C_1(E - V_1 - C_1 V_2 - C_2 V_3 - C_1 C_2 V_4) = C_1(E - V_1 - V_2 - C_2 V_3 - C_2 V_4)$$
$$\Delta V_3 = C_2(E - V_1 - C_1 V_2 - C_2 V_3 - C_1 C_2 V_4) = C_2(E - V_1 - C_1 V_2 - V_3 - C_1 V_4)$$
$$\Delta V_4 = C_1 C_2(E - V_1 - C_1 V_2 - C_2 V_3 - C_1 C_2 V_4) = C_1 C_2(E - V_1 - V_2 - V_3 - V_4).$$

By Corollary 1, this algorithm will converge to $V_1^* = \alpha_1, V_2^* = \alpha_2, V_3^* = \alpha_3, V_4^* = \alpha_4$, provided the matrix is invertible. The determinant of the matrix $< h_i(\vec{C}) h_j(\vec{C}) >_{P(\vec{C})}$ is $< C_1 C_2 > (< C_1 C_2 > - < C_1 >)(< C_1 C_2 > - < C_2 >)(1 - < C_1 > - < C_2 > + < C_1 C_2 >)$. This will be zero for special cases, for example if $C_1 = 1$ always.

It is important to realize that the most general GRW-I algorithm will converge if $P(E|\vec{C})$ is the ΔP or the noisy-or model. For ΔP it will converge to $V_1^* = 0, V_2^* = \omega_1, V_3^* = \omega_2, V_4^* = 0$. For noisy-or, it converges to $V_1^* = 0, V_2^* = \omega_1, V_3^* = \omega_2, V_4^* = -\omega_1 \omega_2$.

The learning system which implements the GRW-I algorithm will not know *a priori* whether the data is generated by ΔP, noisy-or, or the general model for $P(E|C_1, C_2)$. It is therefore better to implement the most general algorithm because this works whatever model generated the data.

Note: other functions $\{h_i(\vec{C})\}$ will lead to different ways to parameterize the probability distribution $P(E|\vec{C})$. They will correspond to different RW algorithms. But their basic properties will be similar to those discussed in this section.

4.2 Generalized RW Class II

We can obtain a second class of generalized RW algorithms which perform ML estimation.

Corollary 2. *A sufficient condition for RW to have unique fixed point at the ML estimate of the generative model $P(E|\vec{C})$ is that $f_{ij}(\vec{C}) = -g_i(\vec{C})h_j(\vec{C})$, provided the matrix $< h_i(\vec{C})h_j(\vec{C}) >_{P(\vec{C})}$ is invertible.*

Proof. *Direct verification.*

Corollary 2 defines GRW-II to be of form:

$$\Delta V_i = g_i(\vec{C})\{E - \sum_j h_j(\vec{C})V_j\}. \tag{15}$$

We illustrate GRW-II by applying it to the noisy-or model (2). It gives an algorithm very similar to equation (6).

Set $h_1(\vec{C}) = C_1, h_2(\vec{C}) = C_2, h_3(\vec{C}) = C_1C_2$ and $g_1(\vec{C}) = C_1(1 - C_2), g_2(\vec{C}) = C_2(1 - C_1), g_3(\vec{C}) = C_1C_2$.

Corollary 2 yields the update rule:

$$\Delta V_1 = C_1(1 - C_2)\{E - C_1V_1 - C_2V_2 - C_1C_2V_3\} = C_1(1 - C_2)\{E - V_1\},$$
$$\Delta V_2 = C_2(1 - C_1)\{E - C_1V_1 - C_2V_2 - C_1C_2V_3\} = C_2(1 - C_1)\{E - V_2\},$$
$$\Delta V_3 = C_1C_2\{E - C_1V_1 - C_2V_2 - C_1C_2V_3\} = C_1C_2\{E - V_1 - V_2 - V_3\}. \tag{16}$$

The matrix $< h_i(\vec{C})h_j(\vec{C}) >_{P(\vec{C})}$ has determinant $< C_1C_2 > (< C_1 > - < C_1C_2 >)(< C_2 > - < C_1C_2 >)$ and so is invertible for generic $P(\vec{C})$. The algorithm will converge to weights $V_1^* = \omega_1, V_2^* = \omega_2, V_3^* = -\omega_1\omega_2$. If we change the model to ΔP, then we get convergence to $V_1^* = \omega_1, V_2^* = \omega_2, V_3^* = 0$.

Observe that the equations (16) are largely decoupled. In particular, the updates for V_1 and V_2 do not depend on the third weight V_3. It is possible to remove the update equation for V_3 by setting $g_3(\vec{C}) = 0$. The remaining update equations for $V_1 \& V_2$ will converge to ω_1, ω_2 for both the noisy-or and the ΔP model.

These reduced update equations are identical to those given by equation (6) which were proven to converge to ω_1, ω_2 [10]. We note that the matrix $< h_i(\vec{C})h_j(\vec{C}) >_{P(\vec{C})}$ now has a zero eigenvalue (because $g_3(\vec{C}) = 0$) but this does not matter because it corresponds to the third weight V_3. The matrix remains invertible if we restrict it to $i, j = 1, 2$.

A limitation of GRW-II algorithm of equation (16) is that it only updates the weights if only one cause is active. So it would fail to explain effects such as blocking where both causes are on for part of the stimuli (Dayan personal communication).

5   Non-generic, coordinate transformations, and non-linear RW

Our results have assumed genericity constraints on the distribution $P(\vec{C})$ of causes. They usually correspond to cases where one cause is always present. We now briefly discuss what happens when these constraints are violated. For simplicity, we concentrate on an important special case.

Cheng's PC theory [4,5] uses the noisy-or model for generating the data but cause C_1 is a background cause which is on all the time (i.e. $C_1 = 1$ always). This implies that

$< C_2 >=< C_1 C_2 >$ and so we cannot apply RW algorithms (13), the most general algorithm, or (16) because the matrix determinant will be zero in all three cases. Since $C_1 = 1$ we can drop it as a variable and re-express the noisy-or model as:

$$P(E = 1|\vec{C}) = \omega_1 + \omega_2(1 - \omega_1)C_2. \tag{17}$$

Theorem 1 shows that we can define generalized RW algorithms to find ML estimates of ω_1 and $\omega_2(1 - \omega_1)$ (assuming $\omega_1 \neq 1$). But, conversely, it is impossible to estimate ω_2 directly by any linear generalized RW.

The problem is simply a matter of different coordinate systems. RW estimates the parameters of the generative model in a different coordinate system than the one used to specify the model. There is a non-linear transformation between the coordinates systems relating $\{\omega_1, \omega_2\}$ to $\{\omega_1, \omega_2(1 - \omega_1)\}$. So RW can estimate the ML parameters provided we allow for an additional non-linear transformation. From this perspective, the inability to RW to perfrom ML estimation for Cheng's model is merely an artifact. If we reparameterize the generative model to be $P(E = 1|\vec{C}) = \omega_1 + \hat{\omega}_2 C_2$, where $\hat{\omega}_2 = \omega_2(1 - \omega_1)$, then we can design an RW to estimate $\{\omega_1, \hat{\omega}_2\}$.

The non-linear transformation breaks down if $\omega_1 = 1$. In this case, the generative model $P(E|\vec{C})$ becomes independent of ω_2 and so it is impossible to estimate it.

But suppose we want to really estimate ω_1 and ω_2 directly (for Cheng's model, the value of ω_2 is the causal power and hence is a meaningful quantity [4,5]). To do this we first define a linear RW to estimate ω_1 and $\hat{\omega}_2 = \omega_2(1 - \omega_1)$. The equations are:

$$V_1^{t+1} = V_1^t + \gamma_1 \Delta V_1^t, \quad V_2^{t+1} = V_2^t + \gamma_2 \Delta V_2^t. \tag{18}$$

with $< V_1 > \mapsto \omega_1$ and $< V_2 > \mapsto \omega_2$ for large t. The fluctuations (variances) are scaled by the parameters γ_1, γ_2 and hence can be made arbitrarily small, see [10].

To estimate ω_2, we replace the variable V_2 by a new variable $V_3 = V_2/(1 - V_1)$ which is updated by a nonlinear equation (V_1 is updated as before):

$$V_3^{t+1} = V_3^t + \frac{V_3^t}{1 - V_1^t} \delta V_1^t + \frac{\Delta V_2^t}{1 - V_1^t}, \tag{19}$$

where we use $V_3 = V_2/(1 - V_1)$ to re-express ΔV_1 and ΔV_2 in terms of functions of V_1 and V_3. Provided the fluctuations are small, by controlling the size of the γ's, we can ensure that V_3 converges arbitrarily close to $\hat{\omega}_2/(1 - \omega_1) = \omega_2$.

6 Conclusion

This paper shows that we can obtain linear generalizations of the Rescorla-Wagner algorithm which can learn the parameters of generative models by Maximum Likelihood. For one class of RW generalizations we have only shown that the fixed points are unique and correspond to ML estimates of the parameters of the generative models. But Theorems 3,4 & 5 of Yuille (2004) can be applied to determine convergence conditions. Convergence rates can be determined by these Theorems provided that the data is generated as i.i.d. samples from the generative model. These theorems can also be used to obtain convergence results for piecewise i.i.d. samples as occurs in forward and backward blocking experiments.

These generalizations of Rescorla-Wagner require augmenting the number of weight variables. This was already proposed, on experimental grounds, so that new weights get created if causes occur in conjunction, [2]. Note that this happens naturally in the algorithms presented (13, the most general algorithm,16) – weights remain at zero until we get an event

$C_1 C_2 = 1$. It is straightforward to extend the analysis to models with conjunctions of many causes. We conjecture that these generalizations converge to good approaximation to ML estimates if we truncate the conjunction of causes at a fixed order.

Finally, many of our results have involved a genericity assumption on the distribution of causes $P(\vec{C})$. We have argued that when these assumptions are violated, for example in Cheng's experiments, then generalized RW still performs ML estimation, but with a non-linear transform. Alternatively we have shown how to define a nonlinear RW that estimates the parameters directly.

Acknowledgement

I acknowledge helpful conversations with Peter Dayan, Rich Shiffrin, and Josh Tennenbaum. I thank Aaron Courville for describing augmented Rescorla-Wagner. I thank the W.M. Keck Foundation for support and NSF grant 0413214.

References

[1]. R.A. Rescorla and A.R. Wagner. "A Theory of Pavlovian Conditioning". In A.H. Black andW.F. Prokasy, eds. **Classical Conditioning II: Current Research and Theory.** New York. Appleton-Century-Crofts, pp 64-99. 1972.

[2] R.A. Rescorla. Journal of Comparative and Physiological Psychology. 79, 307. 1972.

[3]. B. A. Spellman. "Conditioning Causality". In D.R. Shanks, K.J. Holyoak, and D.L. Medin, (eds). **Causal Learning: The Psychology of Learning and Motivation, Vol. 34**. San Diego, California. Academic Press. pp 167-206. 1996.

[4]. P. Cheng. "From Covariance to Causation: A Causal Power Theory". *Psychological Review*, **104**, pp 367-405. 1997.

[5]. M. Buehner and P. Cheng. "Causal Induction: The power PC theory versus the Rescorla-Wagner theory". In *Proceedings of the 19th Annual Conference of the Cognitive Science Society"*. 1997.

[6]. J.B. Tenenbaum and T.L. Griffiths. "Structure Learning in Human Causal Induction". Advances in Neural Information Processing Systems 12. MIT Press. 2001.

[7]. D. Danks, T.L. Griffiths, J.B. Tenenbaum. "Dynamical Causal Learning". *Advances in Neural Information Processing Systems 14*. 2003.

[8] A.C. Courville, N.D. Dew, and D.S. Touretsky. "Similarity and discrimination in classical conditioning". NIPS. 2004.

[9]. D. Danks. "Equilibria of the Rescorla-Wagner Model". *Journal of Mathematical Psychology*. Vol. 47, pp 109-121. 2003.

[10] A.L. Yuille. "The Rescorla-Wagner algorithm and Maximum Likelihood estimation of causal parameters". NIPS. 2004.

[11]. P. Dayan and S. Kakade. "Explaining away in weight space". In *Advances in Neural Information Processing Systems 13*. 2001.

[12] B. Widrow and M.E. Hoff. "Adapting Switching Circuits". *1960 IRE WESCON Conv. Record.*, Part 4, pp 96-104. 1960.

[13] A.G. Barto and R.S. Sutton. "Time-derivative Models of Pavlovian Conditioning". In *Learning and Computational Neuroscience: Foundations of Adaptive Networks*. M. Gabriel and J. Moore (eds). pp 497-537. MIT Press. Cambridge, MA. 1990.

The Role of Top-down and Bottom-up Processes in Guiding Eye Movements during Visual Search

Gregory J. Zelinsky[†‡], **Wei Zhang**[‡], **Bing Yu**[‡], **Xin Chen**[†*], **Dimitris Samaras**[‡]

Dept. of Psychology[†], Dept. of Computer Science[‡]
State University of New York at Stony Brook
Stony Brook, NY 11794

Gregory.Zelinsky@stonybrook.edu[†], xichen@ic.sunysb.edu[*]
{wzhang,ybing,samaras}@cs.sunysb.edu[‡]

Abstract

To investigate how top-down (TD) and bottom-up (BU) information is weighted in the guidance of human search behavior, we manipulated the proportions of BU and TD components in a saliency-based model. The model is biologically plausible and implements an artificial retina and a neuronal population code. The BU component is based on feature-contrast. The TD component is defined by a feature-template match to a stored target representation. We compared the model's behavior at different mixtures of TD and BU components to the eye movement behavior of human observers performing the identical search task. We found that a purely TD model provides a much closer match to human behavior than any mixture model using BU information. Only when biological constraints are removed (e.g., eliminating the retina) did a BU/TD mixture model begin to approximate human behavior.

1. Introduction

The human object detection literature, also known as visual search, has long struggled with how best to conceptualize the role of bottom-up (BU) and top-down (TD) processes in guiding search behavior.[1] Early theories of search assumed a pure BU feature decomposition of the objects in an image, followed by the later reconstitution of these features into objects if the object's location was visited by spatially directed visual attention [1]. Importantly, the direction of attention to feature locations was believed to be random in these early models, thereby making them devoid of any BU or TD component contributing to the guidance of attention to objects in scenes.

The belief in a random direction of attention during search was quashed by Wolfe and colleague's [2] demonstration of TD information affecting search guidance. According to their guided-search model [3], preattentively available features from objects not yet bound by attention can be compared to a high-level target description to generate signals indicating evidence for the target in a display. The search process can then use these signals to

---

[1]In this paper we will refer to BU guidance as guidance based on task-independent signals arising from basic neuronal feature analysis. TD guidance will refer to guidance based on information not existing in the input image or proximal search stimulus, such as knowledge of target features or processing constraints imposed by task instruction.

guide attention to display locations indicating the greatest evidence for the target. More recent models of TD target guidance can accept images of real-world scenes as stimuli and generate sequences of eye movements that can be directly compared to human search behavior [4].

Purely BU models of attention guidance have also enjoyed a great deal of recent research interest. Building on the concept of a saliency map introduced in [5], these models attempt to use biologically plausible computational primitives (e.g., center-surround receptive fields, color opponency, winner-take-all spatial competition, etc.) to define points of high salience in an image that might serve as attractors of attention. Much of this work has been discussed in the context of scene perception [6], but recently Itti and Koch [7] extended a purely BU model to the task of visual search. They defined image saliency in terms of intensity, color, and orientation contrast for multiple spatial scales within a pyramid. They found that a saliency model based on feature-contrast was able to account for a key finding in the behavioral search literature, namely very efficient search for feature-defined targets and far less efficient search for targets defined by conjunctions of features [1].

Given the body of evidence suggesting both TD and BU contributions to the guidance of attention in a search task, the logical next question to ask is whether these two sources of information should be combined to describe search behavior and, if so, in what proportion? To answer this question, we adopt a three-pronged approach. First, we implement two models of eye movements during visual search, one a TD model derived from the framework proposed by [4] and the other a BU model based on the framework proposed by [7]. Second, we use an eyetracker to collect behavioral data from human observers so as to quantify guidance in terms of the number of fixations needed to acquire a target. Third, we combine the outputs of the two models in various proportions to determine the TD/BU weighting best able to describe the number of search fixations generated by the human observers.

2. Eye movement model

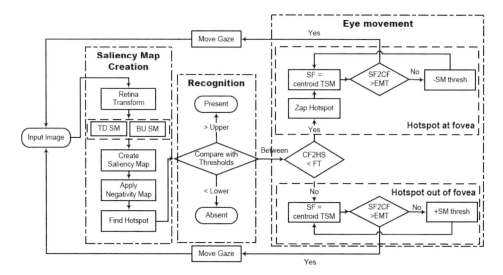

Figure 1: Flow of processing through the model. Abbreviations: TD SM (top-down saliency map); BU SM (bottom-up saliency map); SF(suggested fixation point); TSM (thresholded saliency map); CF2HS (Euclidean distance between current fixation and hotspot); SF2CF(Euclidean distance between suggested fixation and current fixation); EMT (eye movement threshold); FT (foveal threshold).

In this section we introduce a computational model of eye movements during visual search. The basic flow of processing in this model is shown in Figure 1. Generally, we represent search scenes in terms of simple and biologically-plausible visual feature-detector responses (colors, orientations, scales). Visual routines then act on these representations to produce a sequence of simulated eye movements. Our framework builds on work described in [8, 4], but differs from this earlier model in several important respects. First, our model includes a perceptually-accurate simulated retina, which was not included in [8, 4]. Second, the visual routine responsible for moving gaze in our model is fundamentally different from the earlier version. In [8, 4], the number of eye movements was largely determined by the number of spatial scale filters used in the representation. The method used in the current model to generate eye movements (Section 2.3) removes this upper limit. Third, and most important to the topic of this paper, the current model is capable of integrating both BU and TD information in guiding search behavior. The [8, 4] model was purely TD.

2.1. Overview

The model can be conceptually divided into three broad stages: (1) the creation of a saliency map (SM) based on TD and BU analysis of a retinally-transformed image, (2) recognizing the target, and (3) the operations required to generate eye movements. Within each of these stages are several more specific operations, which we will now describe briefly in an order determined by the processing flow.

Input image: The model accepts as input a high-resolution (1280×960 pixel) image of the search scene, as well as a smaller image of the search target. A point is specified on the target image and filter responses are collected from a region surrounding this point. In the current study this point corresponded to the center of the target image.

Retina transform: The search image is immediately transformed to reflect the acuity limitations imposed by the human retina. To implement this neuroanatomical constraint, we adopt a method described in [9], which was shown to provide a good fit to acuity limitations in the human visual system. The approach takes an image and a fixation point as input, and outputs a retina-transformed version of the image based on the fixation point (making it a good front-end to our model). The initial retina transformation assumes fixation at the center of the image, consistent with the behavioral experiment. A new retina transformation of the search image is conducted after each change in gaze.

Saliency maps: Both the TD and the BU saliency maps are based on feature responses from Gaussian filters of different orientations, scales, colors, and orders. These two maps are then combined to create the final SM used to guide search (see Section 2.2 for details).

Negativity map: The negativity map keeps a spatial record of every nontarget location that was fixated and rejected through the application of Gaussian inhibition, a process similar to *inhibition of return* [10] that we refer to as "zapping". The existence of such a map is supported by behavioral evidence indicating a high-capacity spatial memory for rejected nontargets in a search task [11].

Find hotspot: The hotspot (HS) is defined as the point on the saliency map having the largest saliency value. Although no biologically plausible mechanism for isolating the hotspot is currently used, we assume that a standard winner-take-all (WTA) algorithm can be used to find the SM hotspot.

Recognition thresholds: Recognition is accomplished by comparing the hotspot value with two thresholds. The model terminates with a target-present judgment if the hotspot value exceeds a high target-present threshold, set at .995 in the current study. A target-absent response is made if the hotspot value falls below a low target-absent threshold (not used in the current study). If neither of these termination criteria are satisfied, processing passes to the eye movement stage.

Foveal threshold: Processing in the eye movement stage depends on whether the model's simulated fovea is fixated on the SM hotspot. This event is determined by computing the Euclidean distance between the current location of the fovea's center and the hotspot (CF2HS), then comparing this distance to a foveal threshold (FT). The FT, set at 0.5 deg of visual angle, is determined by the retina transform and viewing angle and corresponds to the radius of the foveal window size. The foveal window is the region of the image not blurred by the retina transform function, much like the high-resolution foveola in the human visual system.

Hotspot out of fovea: If the hotspot is not within the FT, meaning that the object giving rise to the hotspot is not currently fixated, then the model will make an eye movement to bring the simulated fovea closer to the hotspot's location. In making this movement, the model will be effectively canceling the effect of the retina transform, thereby enabling a judgment regarding the hotspot pattern. The destination of the eye movement is computed by taking the weighted centroid of activity on the thresholded saliency map (TSM). See Section 2.3 for additional details regarding the centroid calculation of the suggested fixation point (SF), its relationship to the distance threshold for generating an eye movement (EMT), and the dynamically-changing threshold used to remove those SM points offering the least evidence for the target (+SM thresh).

Hotspot at fovea: If the simulated fovea reaches the hotspot (CF2HS < FT) and the target is still not detected (HS < target-present threshold), the model is likely to have fixated a nontarget. When this happens (a common occurrence in the course of a search), it is desirable to inhibit the location of this false target so as not to have it re-attract attention or gaze. To accomplish this, we inhibit or "zap" the hotspot by applying a negative Gaussian filter centered at the hotspot location (set at 63 pixels). Following this injection of negativity into the SM, a new eye movement is made based on the dynamics outlined in Section 2.3.

2.2. Saliency map creation

The first step in creating the TD and BU saliency maps is to separate the retina-transformed image into an intensity channel and two opponent-process color channels (R-G and B-Y). For each channel, we then extract visual features by applying a set of steerable 2D Gaussian-derivative filters, $G(t, \theta, s)$, where t is the order of the Gaussian kernel, θ is the orientation, and s is the spatial scale. The current model uses first and second order Gaussians, 4 orientations (0, 45, 90 and 180 degrees), and 3 scales (7, 15 and 31 pixels), for a total of 24 filters. We therefore obtain 24 feature maps of filter responses per channel, $M(t, \theta, s)$, or alternatively, a 72-dimensional feature vector, F, for each pixel in the retina-transformed image.

The TD saliency map is created by correlating the retina-transformed search image with the target feature vector F_t.[2]

To maintain consistency between the two saliency map representations, the same channels and features used in the TD saliency map were also used to create the BU saliency map. Feature-contrast signals on this map were obtained directly from the responses of the Gaussian derivative filters. For each channel, the 24 feature maps were combined into a single map according to:

$$\sum_{t,\theta,s} \mathcal{N}(|M(t,\theta,s)|) \tag{1}$$

where $\mathcal{N}(\bullet)$ is the normalization function described in [12]. The final BU saliency map is then created by averaging the three combined feature maps. Note that this method of creating a BU saliency map differs from the approach used in [12, 7] in that our filters consisted of 1st and 2nd order derivatives of Gaussians and not center-surround DoG filters. While the two methods of computing feature contrast are not equivalent, in practice they yield very similar patterns of BU salience.

---

[2]Note that because our TD saliency maps are derived from correlations between target and scene images, the visual statistics of these images are in some sense preserved and might be described as a BU component in our model. Nevertheless, the correlation-based guidance signal requires knowledge of a target (unlike a true BU model), and for this reason we will continue to refer to this as a TD process.

Finally, the combined SM was simply a linear combination of the TD and BU saliency maps, where the weighting coefficient was a parameter manipulated in our experiments.

2.3. Eye movement generation

Our model defines gaze position at each moment in time by the weighted spatial average (centroid) of signals on the SM, a form of neuronal population code for the generation of eye movement [13, 14]. Although a centroid computation will tend to bias gaze in the direction of the target (assuming that the target is the maximally salient pattern in the image), gaze will also be pulled away from the target by salient nontarget points. When the number of nontarget points is large, the eye will tend to move toward the geometric center of the scene (a tendency referred to in the behavioral literature as the global effect, [15, 16]); when the number of points is small, the eye will move more directly to the target.

To capture this activity-dependent eye movement behavior, we introduce a moving threshold, ρ, that excludes points from the SM over time based on their signal strength. Initially ρ will be set to zero, allowing every signal on the SM to contribute to the centroid gaze computation. However, with each timestep, ρ is increased by .001, resulting in the exclusion of minimally salient points from the SM (+ SM thresh in Figure 1). The centroid of the SM, what we refer to as the suggested fixation point (SF), is therefore dependent on the current value of ρ and can be expressed as:

$$SF = \sum_{S_p > \rho} \frac{pS_p}{\sum S_p}. \tag{2}$$

Eventually, only the most salient points will remain on the thresholded saliency map (TSM), resulting in the direction of gaze to the hotspot. If this hotspot is not the target, ρ can be decreased (- SM thresh in Figure 1) after zapping in order to reintroduce points to the SM. Such a moving threshold is a plausible mechanism of neural computation easily instantiated by a simple recurrent network [17].

In order to prevent gaze from moving with each change in ρ, which would result in an unrealistically large number of very small eye movements, we impose an eye movement threshold (EMT) that prevents gaze from shifting until a minimum distance between SF and CF is achieved (SF2CF > EMT in Figure 1). The EMT is based on the signal and noise characteristics of each retina-transformed image, and is defined as:

$$EMT = \max{(FT, d(1 + Cd \log \frac{Signal}{Noise}))}, \tag{3}$$

where FT is the fovea threshold, C is a constant, and d is the distance between the current fixation and the hotspot. The $Signal$ term is defined as the sum of all foveal saliency values on the TSM; the $Noise$ term is defined as the sum of all other TSM values. The $Signal/Noise\ log\ ratio$ is clamped to the range of $[-1/C, 0]$. The lower bound of the SF2CF distance is FT, and the upper bound is d. The eye movement dynamics can therefore be summarized as follows: incrementing ρ will tend to increase the SF2CF distance, which will result in an eye movement to SF once this distance exceeds the EMT.

3. Experimental methods

For each trial, the two human observers and the model were first shown an image of a target (a tank). In the case of the human observers, the target was presented for one second and presumably encoded into working memory. In the case of the model, the target was represented by a single 72-dimensional feature vector as described in Section 2. A search image was then presented, which remained visible to the human observers until they made a button press response. Eye movements were recorded during this interval using an ELII eyetracker. Section 2 details the processing stages used by the model. There were 44 images and targets, which were all modified versions of images in the TNO dataset [18]. The images subtended approximately 20° on both the human and simulated retinas.

4. Experimental results

Model and human data are reported from 2 experiments. For each experiment we tested 5 weightings of TD and BU components in the combined SM. Expressed as a proportion of the BU component, these weightings were: BU 0 (TD only), BU .25, BU .5, BU .75, and BU 1.0 (BU only).

4.1. Experiment 1

Table 1: Human and model search behavior at 5 TD/BU mixtures in Experiment 1.

Retina Population	Human subjects		Model				
	H1	H2	TD only	BU: 0.25	BU: 0.5	BU: 0.75	BU only
Misses (%)	0.00	0.00	**0.00**	36.36	72.73	77.27	88.64
Fixations	4.55	4.43	**4.55**	18.89	20.08	21.00	22.40
Std Dev	0.88	2.15	**0.82**	10.44	12.50	10.29	12.58

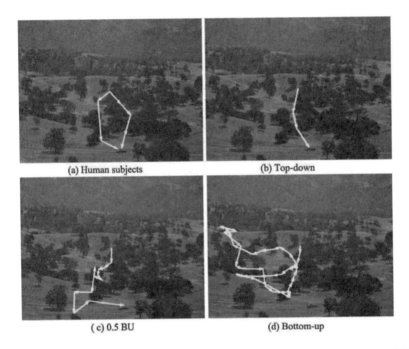

(a) Human subjects

(b) Top-down

(c) 0.5 BU

(d) Bottom-up

Figure 2: Comparison of human and model scanpaths at different TD/BU weightings.

As can be seen from Table 1, the human observers were remarkably consistent in their behavior. Each required an average of 4.5 fixations to find the target (defined as gaze falling within .5 deg of the target's center), and neither generated an error (defined by a failure to find the target within 40 fixations). Human target detection performance was matched almost exactly by a pure TD model, both in terms of errors (0%) and fixations (4.55). This exceptional match between human and model disappeared with the addition of a BU component. Relative to the human and TD model, a BU 0.25 mixture model resulted in a dramatic increase in the miss rate (36%) and in the average number of fixations needed to acquire the target (18.9) on those trials in which the target was ultimately fixated. These high miss and fixation rates continued to increase with larger weightings of the BU contribution, reaching an unrealistic 89% misses and 22 fixations with a pure BU model.

Figure 2 shows representative eye movement scanpaths from our two human observers (a) and the model at three different TD/BU mixtures (b, BU 0; c, BU 0.5; d, BU 1.0) for one image. Note the close agreement between the human scanpaths and the behavior of the

TD model. Note also that, with the addition of a BU component, the model's eye either wanders to high-contrast patterns (bushes, trees) before landing on the target (c), or misses the target entirely (d).

4.2. Experiment 2

Recently, Navalpakkam & Itti [19] reported data from a saliency-based model also integrating BU and TD information to guide search. Among their many results, they compared their model to the purely TD model described in [4] and found that their mixture model offered a more realistic account of human behavior. Specifically, they observed that the [4] model was too accurate, often predicting that the target would be fixated after only a single eye movement. Although our current findings would seem to contradict [19]'s result, this is not the case. Recall from Section 2.0 that our model differs from [4] in two respects: (1) it retinally transforms the input image with each fixation, and (2) it uses a thresholded population-averaging code to generate eye movements. Both of these additions would be expected to increase the number of fixations made by the current model relative to the TD model described in [4]. Adding a simulated retina should increase the number of fixations by reducing the target-scene TD correlations and increasing the probability of false targets emerging in the blurred periphery. Adding population averaging should increase fixations by causing eye movements to locations other than hotspots. It may therefore be the case that [19]'s critique of [4] may be pointing out two specific weaknesses of [4]'s model rather than a general weakness of their TD approach.

To test this hypothesis, we disabled the artificial retina and the population averaging code in our current model. The model now moves directly from hotspot to hotspot, zapping each before moving to the next. Without retinal blurring and population averaging, the behavior of this simpler model is now driven entirely by a WTA computation on the combined SM. Moreover, with a BU weighting of 1.0, this version of our model now more closely approximates other purely BU models in the literature that also lack retinal acuity limitations and population dynamics.

Table 2: Human and model search behavior at 5 TD/BU mixtures in Experiment 2.

NO Retina NO Population	Human subjects		Model				
	H1	H2	TD only	BU: 0.25	BU: 0.5	BU: 0.75	BU only
Misses (%)	0.00	0.00	0.00	9.09	27.27	56.82	68.18
Fixations	4.55	4.43	1.00	8.73	16.60	13.37	14.71
Std Dev	0.88	2.15	0.00	9.15	12.29	9.20	12.84

Table 2 shows the data from this experiment. The first two columns replot the human data from Table 1. Consistent with [19], we now find that the performance of a purely TD model is too good. The target is consistently fixated after only a single eye movement, unlike the 4.5 fixations averaged by human observers. Also consistent with [19] is the observation that a BU contribution may assist this model in better characterizing human behavior. Although a 0.25 BU weighting resulted in a doubling of the human fixation rate and 9% misses, it is conceivable that a smaller BU weighting could nicely describe human performance. As in Experiment 1, at larger BU weightings the model again generated unrealistically high error and fixation rates. These results suggest that, in the absence of retinal and neuronal population-averaging constraints, BU information may play a small role in guiding search.

5. Conclusions

To what extent is TD and BU information used to guide search behavior? The findings from Experiment 1 offer a clear answer to this question: when biologically plausible constraints are considered, any addition of BU information to a purely TD model will worsen, not improve, the match to human search performance (see [20] for a similar conclusion applied to a walking task). The findings from Experiment 2 are more open to interpretation. It may be possible to devise a TD model in which adding a BU component might prove useful, but doing this would require building into this model biologically implausible assumptions.

A corollary to this conclusion is that, when these same biological constraints are added to existing BU saliency-based models, these models may no longer be able to describe human behavior.

A final fortuitous finding from this study is the surprising degree of agreement between our purely TD model and human performance. The fact that this agreement was obtained by direct comparison to human behavior (rather than patterns reported in the behavioral literature), and observed in eye movement variables, lends validity to our method. Future work will explore the generality of our TD model, extending it to other forms of TD guidance (e.g., scene context) and tasks in which a target may be poorly defined (e.g., categorical search).

Acknowledgments

This work was supported by a grant from the ARO (DAAD19-03-1-0039) to G.J.Z.

References

[1] A. Treisman and G. Gelade. A feature-integration theory of attention. *Cognitive Psychology*, 12:97–136, 1980.

[2] J. Wolfe, K. Cave, and S. Franzel. Guided search: An alternative to the feature integration model for visual search. *Journal of Experimental Psychology: Human Perception and Performance*, 15:419–433, 1989.

[3] J. Wolfe. Guided search 2.0: A revised model of visual search. *Psychonomic Bulletin and Review*, 1:202–238, 1994.

[4] R. Rao, G. Zelinsky, M. Hayhoe, and D. Ballard. Eye movements in iconic visual search. *Vision Research*, 42:1447–1463, 2002.

[5] C. Koch and S. Ullman. Shifts of selective visual attention: Toward the underlying neural circuitry. *Human Neurobiology*, 4:219–227, 1985.

[6] L. Itti and C. Koch. Computational modeling of visual attention. *Nature Reviews Neuroscience*, 2(3):194–203, 2001.

[7] L. Itti and C. Koch. A saliency-based search mechanism for overt and covert shift of visual attention. *Vision Research*, 40(10-12):1489–1506, 2000.

[8] R. Rao, G. Zelinsky, M. Hayhoe, and D. Ballard. Modeling saccadic targeting in visual search. In *NIPS*, 1995.

[9] J.S. Perry and W.S. Geisler. Gaze-contingent real-time simulation of arbitrary visual fields. In *SPIE*, 2002.

[10] R. M. Klein and W.J. MacInnes. Inhibition of return is a foraging facilitator in visual search. *Psychological Science*, 10(4):346–352, 1999.

[11] C. A. Dickinson and G. Zelinsky. Marking rejected distractors: A gaze-contingent technique for measuring memory during search. *Psychonomic Bulletin and Review*, In press.

[12] L. Itti, C. Koch, and E. Niebur. A model of saliency-based visual attention for rapid scene analysis. *PAMI*, 20(11):1254–1259, 1998.

[13] T. Sejnowski. Neural populations revealed. *Nature*, 332:308, 1988.

[14] C. Lee, W. Rohrer, and D. Sparks. Population coding of saccadic eye movements by neurons in the superior colliculus. *Nature*, 332:357–360, 1988.

[15] J. Findlay. Global visual processing for saccadic eye movements. *Vision Research*, 22:1033–1045, 1982.

[16] G. Zelinsky, R. Rao, M. Hayhoe, and D. Ballard. Eye movements reveal the spatio-temporal dynamics of visual search. *Psychological Science*, 8:448–453, 1997.

[17] J. L. Elman. Finding structures in time. *Cognitive Science*, 14:179–211, 1990.

[18] A. Toet, P. Bijl, F. L. Kooi, and J. M. Valeton. A high-resolution image dataset for testing search and detection models. Technical Report TNO-NM-98-A020, TNO Human Factors Research Institute,, Soesterberg, The Netherlands, 1998.

[19] V. Navalpakkam and L Itti. Modeling the influence of task on attention. *Vision Research*, 45:205–231, 2005.

[20] K. A. Turano, D. R. Geruschat, and F. H. Baker. Oculomotor strategies for direction of gaze tested with a real-world activity. *Vision Research*, 43(3):333–346, 2003.

Learning Influence among Interacting Markov Chains

Dong Zhang
IDIAP Research Institute
CH-1920 Martigny, Switzerland
zhang@idiap.ch

Daniel Gatica-Perez
IDIAP Research Institute
CH-1920 Martigny, Switzerland
gatica@idiap.ch

Samy Bengio
IDIAP Research Institute
CH-1920 Martigny, Switzerland
bengio@idiap.ch

Deb Roy
Massachusetts Institute of Technology
Cambridge, MA 02142, USA
dkroy@media.mit.edu

Abstract

We present a model that learns the influence of interacting Markov chains within a team. The proposed model is a dynamic Bayesian network (DBN) with a two-level structure: individual-level and group-level. Individual level models actions of each player, and the group-level models actions of the team as a whole. Experiments on synthetic multi-player games and a multi-party meeting corpus show the effectiveness of the proposed model.

1 Introduction

In multi-agent systems, individuals within a group coordinate and interact to achieve a goal. For instance, consider a basketball game where a team of players with different roles, such as attack and defense, collaborate and interact to win the game. Each player performs a set of individual actions, evolving based on their own dynamics. A group of players interact to form a team. Actions of the team and its players are strongly correlated, and different players have different influence on the team. Taking another example, in conversational settings, some people seem particularly capable of driving the conversation and dominating its outcome. These people, skilled at establishing the leadership, have the largest influence on the group decisions, and often shift the focus of the meeting when they speak [8].

In this paper, we quantitatively investigate the influence of individual players on their team using a dynamic Bayesian network, that we call two-level influence model. The proposed model explicitly learns the influence of individual player on the team with a two-level structure. In the first level, we model actions of individual players. In the second one, we model team actions as a whole. The model is then applied to determine (a) the influence of players in multi-player games, and (b) the influence of participants in meetings.

The paper is organized as follows. Section 2 introduces the two-level influence model. Section 3 reviews related models. Section 4 presents results on multi-player games, and Section 5 presents results on a meeting corpus. Section 6 provides concluding remarks.

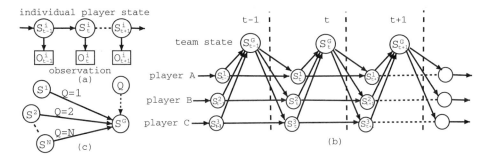

Figure 1: (a) Markov Model for individual player. (b) Two-level influence model (for simplicity, we omit the observation variables of individual Markov chains, and the switching parent variable Q). (c) Switching parents. Q is called a switching parent of S^G, and $\{S^1 \cdots S^N\}$ are conditional parents of S^G. When $Q = i$, S^i is the only parent of S^G.

2   Two-level Influence Model

The proposed model, called two-level influence model, is a dynamic Bayesian network (DBN) with a two-level structure: the *player* level and the *team* level (Fig. 1). The player level represents the actions of individual players, evolving based on their own Markovian dynamics (Fig. 1 (a)). The team level represents group-level actions (the action belongs to the team as a whole, not to a particular player). In Fig. 1 (b), the arrows up (from players to team) represent the influence of the individual actions on the group actions, and the arrows down (from team to players) represent the influence of the group actions on the individual actions. Let O^i and S^i denote the observation and state of the ith player respectively, and S^G denotes the team state. For N players, and observation sequences of identical length T, the joint distribution of our model is given by

$$P(S,O)=\prod_{i=1}^{N} P(S_1^i)\prod_{t=1}^{T}\prod_{i=1}^{N}P(O_t^i|S_t^i)\prod_{t=1}^{T}P(S_t^G|S_t^1 \cdots S_t^N)\prod_{t=2}^{T}\prod_{i=1}^{N}P(S_t^i|S_{t-1}^i,S_{t-1}^G). \quad (1)$$

Regarding the player level, we model the actions of each individual with a first-order Markov model (Fig. 1 (a)) with one observation variable O^i and one state variable S^i. Furthermore, to capture the dynamics of all the players interacting as a team, we add a hidden variable S^G (team state), which is responsible to model the group-level actions. Different from individual player state that has its own Markovian dynamics, team state is not directly influenced by its previous state . S^G could be seen as the aggregate behaviors of the individuals, yet provides a useful level of description beyond individual actions. There are two kinds of relationships between the team and players: (1) The team state at time t influences the players' states at the next time (down arrow in Fig. 1 (b)). In other words, the state of the ith player at time $t + 1$ depends on its previous state as well as on the team state, i.e., $P(S_{t+1}^i|S_t^i, S_t^G)$. (2) The team state at time t is influenced by all the players' states at the current time (up arrow in Fig. 1 (b)), resulting in a conditional state transition distribution $P(S_t^G|S_t^1 \cdots S_t^N)$.

To reduce the model complexity, we add one hidden variable Q in the model, to switch parents for S^G. The idea of switching parent (also called Bayesian multi-nets in [3]) is as follows: a variable -S^G in this case- has a set of parents $\{Q, S^1 \cdots S^N\}$ (Fig. 1(c)). Q is the switching parent that determines which of the other parents to use, conditioned on the current value of the switching parent. $\{S^1 \cdots S^N\}$ are the conditional parents. In Fig. 1(c), Q switches the parents of S^G among $\{S^1 \cdots S^N\}$, corresponding to the distribution

$$P(S_t^G|S_t^1 \cdots S_t^N) \quad = \quad \sum_{i=1}^{N} P(S_t^G, Q=i|S_t^1 \cdots S_t^N) \quad (2)$$

$$= \sum_{i=1}^{N} P(Q=i|S_t^1 \cdots S_t^N) P(S_t^G|S_t^i \cdots S_t^N, Q=i) \quad (3)$$

$$= \sum_{i=1}^{N} P(Q=i) P(S_t^G|S_t^i) = \sum_{i=1}^{N} \alpha_i P(S_t^G|S_t^i). \quad (4)$$

From Eq. 3 to Eq. 4, we made two assumptions: (i) Q is independent of $\{S^1 \cdots S^N\}$; and (ii) when $Q=i$, S_t^G only depends on S_t^i. The distribution over the switching-parent variable $P(Q)$ essentially describes how much influence or contribution the state transitions of the player variables have on the state transitions of the team variable. We refer to $\alpha_i = P(Q=i)$ as the influence value of the ith player. Obviously, $\sum_{i=1}^{N} \alpha_i = 1$. If we further assume that all player variables have the same number of states N_S, and the team variable has N_G possible states, the joint log probability is given by

$$\log P(S,O) = \underbrace{\sum_{i=1}^{N} \sum_{j=1}^{N_S} z_{j,1}^i \cdot \log P(S_1^i = j)}_{initial\ probability} + \underbrace{\sum_{t=1}^{T} \sum_{i=1}^{N} \sum_{j=1}^{N_S} z_{j,t}^i \cdot \log P(O_t^i|S_t^i = j)}_{emission\ probability}$$

$$+ \underbrace{\sum_{t=2}^{T} \sum_{i=1}^{N} \sum_{j=1}^{N_S} \sum_{k=1}^{N_S} \sum_{g=1}^{N_G} z_{j,t}^i \cdot z_{k,t-1}^i \cdot z_{g,t-1}^G \cdot \log P(S_t^i = j|S_{t-1}^i = k, S_{t-1}^G = g)}_{group\ influence\ on\ individual\ transition}$$

$$+ \underbrace{\sum_{t=1}^{T} \sum_{k=1}^{N_S} \sum_{g=1}^{N_G} z_{g,t}^G \cdot z_{k,t}^i \cdot \log\{\sum_{i=1}^{N} \alpha_i P(S_t^G = g|S_t^i = k)\}}_{individual\ influence\ on\ group}, \quad (5)$$

where the indicator variable $z_{j,t} = 1$ if $S_t = j$, otherwise $z_{j,t} = 0$. We can see that the model has complexity $O(T \cdot N \cdot N_G \cdot N_S^2)$. For $T = 2000, N_S = 10, N_G = 5, N = 4$, a total of 10^6 operations is required, which is still tractable.

For the model implementation, we used the Graphical Models Toolkit (GMTK) [4], a DBN system for speech, language, and time series data. Specifically, we used the switching parents feature of GMTK, which greatly facilitates the implementation of the two-level model to learn the influence values using the Expectation Maximization (EM) algorithm. Since EM has the problem of local maxima, good initialization is very important. To initialize the emission probability distribution in Eq. 5, we first train individual action models (Fig. 1 (a)) by pooling all observation sequences together. Then we use the trained emission distribution from the individual action model to initialize the emission distribution of the two-level influence model. This procedure is beneficial because we use data from all individual streams together, and thus have a larger amount of training data for learning.

3 Related Models

The proposed two-level influence model is related to a number of models, namely mixed-memory Markov model (MMM) [14, 11], coupled HMM (CHMM) [13], influence model [1, 2, 6] and dynamical systems trees (DSTs) [10]. MMMs decompose a complex model into mixtures of simpler ones, for example, a K-order Markov model, into mixtures of first-order models: $P(S_t|S_{t-1}S_{t-2} \cdots S_{t-K}) = \sum_{i=1}^{K} \alpha_i P(S_t|S_{t-i})$. The CHMM models interactions of multiple Markov chains by directly linking the current state of one stream with the previous states of all the streams (including itself): $P(S_t^i|S_{t-1}^1 S_{t-1}^2 \cdots S_{t-1}^N)$. However, the model becomes computationally intractable for more than two streams. The influence model [1, 2, 6] simplifies the state transition distribution of the CHMM into a

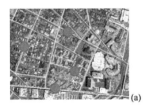 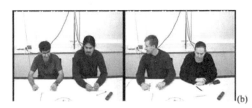

Figure 2: (a) A snapshot of the multi-player games: four players move along the pathes labeled in the map. (b) A snapshot of four-participant meetings.

convex combination of pairwise conditional distributions, i.e., $P(S_t^i|S_{t-1}^1 S_{t-1}^2 \cdots S_{t-1}^N) = \sum_{j=1}^N \alpha_{ji} P(S_t^i|S_{t-1}^j)$. We can see that influence model and MMM take the same strategy to reduce complex models with large state spaces to a combination of simpler ones with smaller state spaces. In [2, 6], the influence model was used to analyze speaking patterns in conversations (i.e., turn-taking) to determine how much influence one participant has on others. In such model, α_{ji} is regarded as the influence of the jth player on the ith player.

All these models, however, limit themselves to modeling the interactions between individual players, *i.e.*, the influence of *one player on another player*. The proposed two-level influence model extends these models by using the group-level variable S^G that allows to model the influence between *all the players and the team*: $P(S_t^G|S_t^1 S_t^2 \cdots S_t^N) = \sum_{i=1}^N \alpha_i P(S_t^G|S_t^i)$, and additionally conditioning the dynamics of each player on the team state: $P(S_{t+1}^i|S_t^i, S_t^G)$.

DSTs [10] have a tree structure that models interacting processes through the parent hidden Markov chains. There are two differences between DSTs and our model: (1) In DSTs, the parent chain has its own Markovian dynamics, while the team state of our model is not directly influenced by the previous team state. Thus, our model captures the emergent phenomena in which the group action is "nothing more" than the aggregate behaviors of individuals, yet it provides a useful level of representation beyond individual actions. (2) The influence between players and team in our model is "bi-direction" (up and down arrows in Fig. 1(b)). In DSTs, the influence between child and parent chains is "uni-direction": parent chains could influence child chains, while child chains could not influence their parent chains.

4 Experiments on Synthetic Data

We first test our model on multi-player synthetic games, in which four players (labeled A-D) move along a number of predetermined paths manually labeled in a map (Fig. 2(a)), based on the following rules:

- Game I: Player A moves randomly. Player B and C are meticulously following player A. Player D moves randomly.
- Game II: Player A moves randomly. Player B is meticulously following player A. Player C moves randomly. Player D is meticulously following player C.
- Game III: All four players, A, B, C and D, move randomly.

A follower moves randomly until it lies on the same path of its target, and after that it tries to reach the target by following the target's direction. The initial positions and speeds of players are randomly generated. The observation of an individual player is its motion trajectory in the form of a sequence of positions, $(x_1, y_1), (x_2, y_2) \cdots (x_t, y_t)$, each of which belongs to one of 20 predetermined paths in the map. Therefore, we set $N_S = 20$. The number of team states is set to $N_G = 5$. In experiments, we found that the final results were not sensitive to the specific number of team states for this dataset in a wide range. The length of each game sequence is $T = 2000$ frames. EM iterations were stopped once

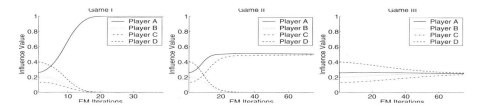

Figure 3: Influence values with respect to the EM iterations in different games.

the relative difference in the global log likelihood was less than 2%.

Fig. 3 shows the learned influence value for each of the four players in the different games with respect to the number of EM iterations. We can see that for `Game I`, player A is the leader player based on the defined rules. The final learned influence value for player A is almost 1, while the influence for the rest three players are almost 0. For `Game II`, player A and player C are both leaders based on the defined rules. The learned influence values for player A and C are indeed close to 0.5, which indicates they have similar influence on the team. For `Game III`, the four players are moving randomly, and the learned influence values are around 0.25, which indicates that all players have similar influence on the team. The results on these toy data suggest that our model is capable of learning sensible values for $\{\alpha_i\}$, in good agreement with the concept of influence we have described before.

5 Experiments on Meeting Data

As an application of the two-level influence model, we investigate the influence of participants in meetings. Status, dominance, and influence are important concepts in social psychology for which our model could be particularly suitable in a (dynamic) conversational setting [8]. We used a public meeting corpus (available at `http://mmm.idiap.ch`), which consists of 30 five-minute four-participant meetings collected in a room equipped with synchronized multi-channel audio and video recorders [12]. A snapshot of the meeting is shown in Fig. 2 (b). These meetings have pre-defined topics and an action agenda, designed to ensure discussions and monologues. Manual speech transcripts are also available. We first describe how we manually collected influence judgements, and the performance measure we used. We then report our results using audio and language features, compared with simple baseline methods.

5.1 Manually Labeling Influence Values and the Performance Measure

The manual annotation of influence of meeting participants is to some degree a subjective task, as a definite ground-truth does not exist. In our case, each meeting was labeled by three independent annotators who had no access to any information about the participants (e.g. job titles and names). This was enforced to avoid any bias based on prior knowledge of the meeting participants (e.g. a student would probably assign a large influence value to his supervisor). After watching an entire meeting, the three annotators were asked to assign a probability-based value (ranging from 0 to 1, all adding up to 1) to meeting participants, which indicated their influence in the meeting (Fig. 5(b-d)). From the three annotations, we computed the pairwise Kappa statistics [7], a commonly used measure for inter-rate agreement. The obtained pairwise Kappa ranges between 0.68 and 0.72, which demonstrates a good agreement among the different annotators. We estimated the ground-truth influence values by averaging the results from the three annotators (Fig. 5(a)).

We use Kullback-Leibler (KL) divergence to evaluate the results. For the jth meeting, given an automatically determined influence distribution $\tilde{P}(Q)$, and the ground truth influence distribution $P(Q)$, the KL divergence is given by: $D^j(\tilde{P}\|P) =$

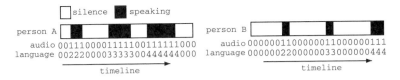

Figure 4: Illustration of state sequences using audio and language features respectively: Using audio, there are two states: speaking and silence. Using language, the number of states equals PLSA topics plus one silence state.

$\sum_{i=1}^{N} \tilde{P}(Q=i) \log_2 \frac{\tilde{P}(Q=i)}{P(Q=i)}$, where N is the number of participants. The smaller D^j, the better the performance (if $\tilde{P} = P \Rightarrow D^j = 0$). Note that KL divergence is not symmetric. We calculate the average KL divergence for all the meetings: $D = \frac{1}{M} \sum_{j=1}^{M} D^j(\tilde{P}\|P)$, where M is the number of meetings.

5.2 Audio and Language Features

We first extract audio features useful to detect speaking turns in conversations. We compute the SRP-PHAT measure using the signals from a 8-microphone array [12], which is a continuous value indicating the speech activity from a particular participant. We use a Gaussian emission probability, and set $N_S = 2$, each state corresponding to speaking and non-speaking (silence), respectively (Fig. 4).

Additionally, language features were extracted from manual transcripts. After removing stop words, the meeting corpus contains 2175 unique terms. We then employed *probabilistic latent semantic analysis* (PLSA) [9], which is a language model that projects documents in the high-dimensional bag-of-words space into a topic-based space of lower dimension. Each dimension in this new space represents a "topic", and each document is represented as a mixture of topics. In our case, a document corresponds to one speech utterance $(t_s, t_e, w_1 w_2 \cdots w_k)$, where t_s is the start time, t_e is the end time, and $w_1 w_2 \cdots w_k$ is a sequence of words. PLSA is thus used as a feature extractor that could potentially capture "topic turns" in meetings.

We embedded PLSA into our model by treating the states of individual players as instances of PLSA topics (similar to [5]). Therefore, the PLSA model determines the emission probability in Eq. 5. We repeat the PLSA topic within the same utterance ($t_s \leq t \leq t_e$). The topic for the silence segments was set to 0 (Fig. 4). We can see that using audio-only features can be seen as a special case of using language features, by using only one topic in the PLSA model (i.e., all utterances belong to the same topic). We set 10 topics in PLSA ($N_S = 10$), and set $N_G = 5$ using simple reasonable a priori knowledge. EM iterations were stopped once the relative difference in the global log likelihood was less than 2%.

5.3 Results and Discussions

We compare our model with a method based on the speaking length (how much time each of the participants speaks). In this case, the influence value of a meeting participant is defined to be proportional to his speaking length: $P(Q = i) = L_i / \sum_{i=1}^{N} L_i$, where L_i is the speaking length of participant i. As a second baseline model, we randomly generated 1000 combinations of influence values (under the constraint that the sum of the four values equals 1), and report the average performance.

The results are shown in Table 1 (left) and Fig. 5(e-h). We can see that the results of the three methods: model + language, model + audio, and speaking-length (Fig. 5 (e-g)) are significantly better than the result of randomization (Fig. 5 (h)). Using language features

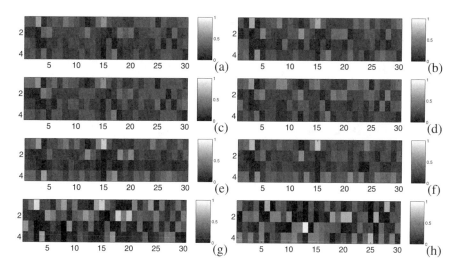

Figure 5: Influence values of the 4 participants (y-axis) in the 30 meetings (x-axis) (a) ground-truth (average of the three human annotations: A_1, A_2, A_3). (b) A_1 : human annotation 1 (c) A_2 : human annotation 2 (d) A_3 : human annotation 3 (e) our model + language (f) our model + audio (g) speaking-length (h) randomization.

Table 1: Results on meetings ("model" denotes the two-level influence model).

Method	KL divergence		Human Annotation	KL divergence
model + Language	0.106		A_i vs. A_j	0.090
model + Audio	0.135		A_i vs. $\overline{A_i}$	0.053
Speaking length	0.226		A_i vs. GT	0.037
Randomization	0.863			

with our model achieves the best performance. Our model (using either audio or language features) outperforms the speaking-length based method, which suggests that the learned influence distributions are in better accordance with the influence distributions from human judgements. As shown in Fig. 4, using audio features can be seen as a special case of using language features. We use language features to capture "topic turns" by factorizing the two states: "speaking, silence" into more states: "topic1, topic2, ..., silence". We can see that the result using language features is better than that using audio features. In other words, compared with "speaking turns", "topic turns" improves the performance of our model to learn the influence of participants in meetings.

It is interesting to look at the KL divergence between any pair of the three human annotations (A_i vs. A_j), any one against the average of the others (A_i vs. $\overline{A_i}$), and any one against the ground-truth (A_i vs. GT). The average results are shown in Table 1 (right). We can see that the result of "A_i vs. GT" is the best, which is reasonable since "GT" is the average of A_1, A_2, and A_3. Fig. 6(a) shows the histogram of KL divergence between any pair of human annotations for the 30 meetings. The histogram has a distribution of $\mu = 0.09, \sigma = 0.11$. We can see that the results of our model (language: 0.106, audio: 0.135) are very close to the mean ($\mu = 0.09$), which indicates that our model is comparable to human performance.

With our model, we can calculate the cumulative influence of each meeting participant over time. Fig. 6(b) shows such an example using the two-level influence model with audio features. We can see that the cumulative influence is related to the meeting agenda: The meeting starts with the monologue of person1 (monologue1). The influence of person1 is almost 1, while the influences of the other persons are nearly 0. When four participants are

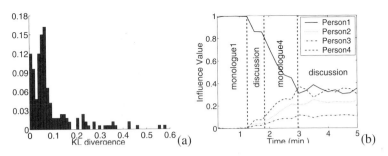

Figure 6: (a) Histogram of KL divergence between any pair of the human annotations (A_i vs. A_j) for the 30 meetings. (b) The evolution of cumulative influence over time (5 minutes). The dotted vertical lines indicate the predefined meeting agenda.

involved in a discussion, the influence of person1 decreases, and the influences of the other three persons increase. The influence of person4 increases quickly during monologue4. The final influence of participants becomes stable in the second discussion.

6 Conclusions

We have presented a two-level influence model that learns the influence of all players within a team. The model has a two-level structure: individual-level and group-level. Individual level models actions of individual players and group-level models the group as a whole. Experiments on synthetic multi-player games and a multi-party meeting corpus showed the effectiveness of the proposed model. More generally, we anticipate that our approach to multi-level influence modeling may provide a means for analyzing a wide range of social dynamics to infer patterns of emergent group behaviors.

Acknowledgements

This work was supported by the Swiss National Center of Competence in Research on Interactive Multimodal Information Management (IM2), and the EC project AMI (Augmented Multi-Party Interaction) (pub. AMI-124). We thank Florent Monay (IDIAP) and Jeff Bilmes (University of Washington) for sharing PLSA code and the GMTK. We also thank the annotators for their efforts.

References

[1] C. Asavathiratham. The influence model: A tractable representation for the dynamics of networked markov chains. *Ph.D. dissertation, Dept. of EECS, MIT, Cambridge*, 2000.

[2] S. Basu, T. Choudhury, B. Clarkson, and A. Pentland. Learning human interactions with the influence model. *MIT Media Laboratory Technical Note No. 539*, 2001.

[3] J. Bilmes. Dynamic bayesian multinets. In *Uncertainty in Artificial Intelligence*, 2000.

[4] J. Bilmes and G. Zweig. The graphical models toolkit: An open source software system for speech and time series processing. *Proc. ICASSP*, vol. 4:3916–3919, 2002.

[5] D. Blei and P. Moreno. Topic segmentation with an aspect hidden markov model. *Proc. of ACM SIGIR conference on Research and development in information retrieval*, pages 343–348, 2001.

[6] T. Choudhury and S. Basu. Modeling conversational dynamics as a mixed memory markov process. *Proc. of Intl. Conference on Neural Information and Processing Systems (NIPS)*, 2004.

[7] J.A. Cohen. A coefficient of agreement for nominal scales. *Educ Psych Meas*, 20:37–46, 1960.

[8] S. L. Ellyson and J. F. Dovidio, editors. *Power, Dominance, and Nonverbal Behavior*. Springer-Verlag., 1985.

[9] T. Hofmann. Unsupervised learning by probabilistic latent semantic analysis. In *Machine Learning, 42:177–196*, 2001.

[10] A. Howard and T. Jebara. Dynamical systems trees. In *Uncertainty in Artificial Intelligence'01*.

[11] K. Kirchhoff, S. Parandekar, and J. Bilmes. Mixed-memory markov models for automatic language identification. *IEEE Int. Conf. on Acoustics, Speech, and Signal Processing*, 2000.

[12] I. McCowan, D. Gatica-Perez, S. Bengio, G. Lathoud, M. Barnard, and D. Zhang. Automatic analysis of multimodal group actions in meetings. In *IEEE Transactions on PAMI*, volume 27(3), 2005.

[13] N. Oliver, B. Rosario, and A. Pentland. Graphical models for recognizing human interactions. *Proc. of Intl. Conference on Neural Information and Processing Systems (NIPS)*, 1998.

[14] L. K. Saul and M. I. Jordan. Mixed memory markov models: Decomposing complex stochastic processes as mixtures of simpler ones. *Machine Learning*, 37(1):75–87, 1999.

Learning Multiple Related Tasks using Latent Independent Component Analysis

Jian Zhang†, Zoubin Ghahramani†‡, Yiming Yang†

† School of Computer Science
Cargenie Mellon University
Pittsburgh, PA 15213

‡ Gatsby Computational Neuroscience Unit
University College London
London WC1N 3AR, UK

{jian.zhang, zoubin, yiming}@cs.cmu.edu

Abstract

We propose a probabilistic model based on Independent Component Analysis for learning multiple related tasks. In our model the task parameters are assumed to be generated from independent sources which account for the relatedness of the tasks. We use Laplace distributions to model hidden sources which makes it possible to identify the hidden, independent components instead of just modeling correlations. Furthermore, our model enjoys a sparsity property which makes it both parsimonious and robust. We also propose efficient algorithms for both empirical Bayes method and point estimation. Our experimental results on two multi-label text classification data sets show that the proposed approach is promising.

1 Introduction

An important problem in machine learning is how to generalize between multiple related tasks. This problem has been called "multi-task learning", "learning to learn", or in some cases "predicting multivariate responses". Multi-task learning has many potential practical applications. For example, given a newswire story, predicting its subject categories as well as the regional categories of reported events based on the same input text is such a problem. Given the mass tandem spectra of a sample protein mixture, identifying the individual proteins as well as the contained peptides is another example.

Much attention in machine learning research has been placed on how to effectively learn multiple tasks, and many approaches have been proposed[1][2][3][4][5][6][10][11]. Existing approaches share the basic assumption that tasks are related to each other. Under this general assumption, it would be beneficial to learn all tasks jointly and borrow information from each other rather than learn each task independently. Previous approaches can be roughly summarized based on how the "relatedness" among tasks is modeled, such as IID tasks[2], a Bayesian prior over tasks[2][6][11], linear mixing factors[5][10], rotation plus shrinkage[3] and structured regularization in kernel methods[4].

Like previous approaches, the basic assumption in this paper is that the multiple tasks are related to each other. Consider the case where there are K tasks and each task is a binary classification problem from the same input space (e.g., multiple simultaneous classifications of text documents). If we were to separately learn a classifier, with parameters θ_k for each task k, we would be ignoring relevant information from the other classifiers. The assumption that the tasks are related suggests that the θ_k for different tasks should be related to each other. It is therefore natural to consider different statistical models for how the θ_k's might be related.

We propose a model for multi-task learning based on Independent Component Analysis (ICA)[9]. In this model, the parameters θ_k for different classifiers are assumed to have been generated from a sparse linear combination of a small set of basic classifiers. Both the coefficients of the sparse combination (the factors or sources) and the basic classifiers are learned from the data. In the multi-task learning context, the relatedness of multiple tasks can be explained by the fact that they share certain number of hidden, independent components. By controlling the model complexity in terms of those independent components we are able to achieve better generalization capability. Furthermore, by using distributions like Laplace we are able to enjoy a sparsity property, which makes the model both parsimonious and robust in terms of identifying the connections with independent sources. Our model can be combined with many popular classifiers, and as an indispensable part we present scalable algorithms for both empirical Bayes method and point estimation, with the later being able to solve high-dimensional tasks. Finally, being a probabilistic model it is always convenient to obtain probabilistic scores and confidence which are very helpful in making statistical decisions. Further discussions on related work are given in Section 5.

2   Latent Independent Component Analysis

The model we propose for solving multiple related tasks, namely the Latent Independent Component Analysis (LICA) model, is a hierarchical Bayesian model based on the traditional Independent Component Analysis. ICA[9] is a promising technique from signal processing and designed to solve the blind source separation problem, whose goal is to extract independent sources given only observed data that are linear combinations of the unknown sources. ICA has been successfully applied to blind source separation problem and shows great potential in that area. With the help of non-Gaussianity and higher-order statistics it can correctly identify the independent sources, as opposed to technique like Factor Analysis which is only able to remove the correlation in the data due to the intrinsic Gaussian assumption in the corresponding model.

In order to learn multiple related tasks more effectively, we transform the joint learning problem into learning a generative probabilistic model for our tasks (or more precisely, task parameters), which precisely explains the relatedness of multiple tasks through the latent, independent components. Unlike the standard Independent Component Analysis where we use observed data to estimate the hidden sources, in LICA the "observed data" for ICA are actually task parameters. Consequently, they are latent and themselves need to be learned from the training data of each individual task. Below we give the precise definition of the probabilistic model for LICA.

Suppose we use $\theta_1, \theta_2, \ldots, \theta_K$ to represent the model parameters of K tasks where $\theta_k \in \mathbb{R}^{F \times 1}$ can be thought as the parameter vector of the k-th individual task. Consider the following generative model for the K tasks:

$$
\begin{aligned}
\theta_k &= \Lambda \mathbf{s}_k + \mathbf{e}_k \\
\mathbf{s}_k &\sim p(\mathbf{s}_k \mid \Phi) \\
\mathbf{e}_k &\sim \mathcal{N}(\mathbf{0}, \Psi)
\end{aligned}
\tag{1}
$$

where $\mathbf{s}_k \in \mathbb{R}^{H \times 1}$ are the hidden source models with Φ denotes its distribution parameters; $\Lambda \in \mathbb{R}^{F \times H}$ is a linear transformation matrix; and the noise vector $\mathbf{e}_k \in \mathbb{R}^{F \times 1}$

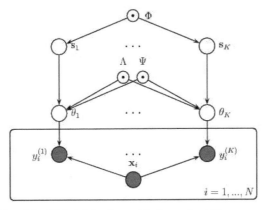

Figure 1: Graphical Model for Latent Independent Component Analysis

is usually assumed to be a multivariate Gaussian with diagonal covariance matrix $\Psi = diag(\psi_{11}, \dots, \psi_{FF})$ or even $\Psi = \sigma^2 \mathbf{I}$. This is essentially assuming that the hidden sources $\mathbf{s}$ are responsible for all the dependencies among θ_k's, and conditioned on them all θ_k's are independent. Generally speaking we can use any member of the exponential families as $p(\mathbf{e}_k)$, but in most situations the noise is taken to be a multivariate Gaussian which is convenient. The graphical model for equation (1) is shown as the upper level in Figure 1, whose lower part will be described in the following.

2.1 Probabilistic Discriminative Classifiers

One building block in the LICA is the probabilistic model for learning each individual task, and in this paper we focus on classification tasks. We will use the following notation to describe a probabilistic discriminative classifier for task k, and for notation simplicity we omit the task index k below. Suppose we have training data $\mathcal{D} = \{(\mathbf{x}_1, y_1), \dots, (\mathbf{x}_N, y_N)\}$ where $\mathbf{x}_i \in \mathbb{R}^{F \times 1}$ is the input data vector and $y_i \in \{0, 1\}$ is the binary class label, our goal is to seek a probabilistic classifier whose prediction is based on the conditional probability $p(y = 1|\mathbf{x}) \overset{\triangle}{=} f(\mathbf{x}) \in [0, 1]$. We further assume that the discriminative function to have a linear form $f(\mathbf{x}) = \mu(\theta^T \mathbf{x})$, which can be easily generalized to non-linear functions by some feature mapping. The output class label y can be thought as randomly generated from a Bernoulli distribution with parameter $\mu(\theta^T \mathbf{x})$, and the overall model can be summarized as follows:

$$y_i \quad \sim \quad \mathcal{B}(\mu(\theta^T \mathbf{x}_i))$$

$$\mu(t) \quad = \quad \int_{-\infty}^{t} p(z)dz \tag{2}$$

where $\mathcal{B}(.)$ denotes the Bernoulli distribution and $p(z)$ is the probability density function of some random variable Z. By changing the definition of random variable Z we are able to specialize the above model into a variety of popular learning methods. For example, when $p(z)$ is standard logistic distribution we will get logistic regression classifier; when $p(z)$ is standard Gaussian we get the probit regression. In principle any member belonging to the above class of classifiers can be plugged in our LICA, or even generative classifiers like Naive Bayes. We take logistic regression as the basic classifier, and this choice should not affect the main point in this paper. Also note that it is straightforward to extend the framework for regression tasks whose likelihood function $y_i \sim \mathcal{N}(\theta^T \mathbf{x}_i, \sigma^2)$ can be solved by simple and efficient algorithms. Finally we would like to point out that although shown in the graphical model that all training instances share the same input vector $\mathbf{x}$, this is mainly for notation simplicity and there is indeed no such restriction in our model. This is convenient since in reality we may not be able to obtain all the task responses for the same training instance.

3   Learning and Inference for LICA

The basic idea of the inference algorithm for the LICA is to iteratively estimate the task parameters θ_k, hidden sources $\mathbf{s}_k$, and the mixing matrix Λ and noise covariance Ψ. Here we present two algorithms, one for the empirical Bayes method, and the other for point estimation which is more suitable for high-dimensional tasks.

3.1   Empirical Bayes Method

The graphical model shown in Figure 1 is an example of a hierarchical Bayesian model, where the upper levels of the hierarchy model the relation between the tasks. We can use an empirical Bayes approach and learn the parameters $\Omega = \{\Phi, \Lambda, \Psi\}$ from the data while treating the variables $\mathcal{Z} = \{\theta_k, \mathbf{s}_k\}_{k=1}^K$ as hidden, random variables. To get around the unidentifiability caused by the interaction between Λ and $\mathbf{s}$ we assume Φ is of standard parametric form (e.g. zero mean and unit variance) and thus remove it from Ω. The goal is to learn point estimators $\hat{\Lambda}$ and $\hat{\Psi}$ as well as obtain posterior distributions over hidden variables given training data.

The log-likelihood of incomplete data $\log p(\mathcal{D} \mid \Omega)$ [1] can be calculated by integrating out hidden variables

$$\log p(\mathcal{D}|\Omega) = \sum_{k=1}^K \log \left\{ \int \prod_{i=1}^N p(y_i^{(k)} \mid \mathbf{x}_i, \theta_k) \left(\int p(\theta_k \mid \mathbf{s}_k, \Lambda, \Psi) p(\mathbf{s}_k|\Phi) d\mathbf{s}_k \right) d\theta_k \right\}$$

for which the maximization over parameters $\Omega = \{\Lambda, \Psi\}$ involves two complicated integrals over θ_k and $\mathbf{s}_k$, respectively. Furthermore, for classification tasks the likelihood function $p(y|\mathbf{x}, \theta)$ is typically non-exponential and thus exact calculation becomes intractable. However, we can approximate the solution by applying the EM algorithm to decouple it into a series of simpler E-steps and M-steps as follows:

1. E-step: Given the parameter $\Omega^{t-1} = \{\Lambda, \Psi\}^{t-1}$ from the $(t-1)$-th step, compute the distribution of hidden variables given Ω^{t-1} and $\mathcal{D}$: $p(\mathcal{Z} \mid \Omega^{t-1}, \mathcal{D})$

2. M-step: Maximizing the expected log-likelihood of complete data $(\mathcal{Z}, \mathcal{D})$, where the expectation is taken over the distribution of hidden variables obtained in the E-step: $\Omega^t = \arg\max_\Omega \mathbb{E}_{p(\mathcal{Z}|\Omega^{t-1}, \mathcal{D})} [\log p(\mathcal{D}, \mathcal{Z} \mid \Omega)]$

The log-likelihood of complete data can be written as

$$\log p(\mathcal{D}, \mathcal{Z} \mid \Omega) = \sum_{k=1}^K \left\{ \sum_{i=1}^N \log p(y_i^{(k)} \mid \mathbf{x}_i, \theta_k) + \log p(\theta_k \mid \mathbf{s}_k, \Lambda, \Psi) + \log p(\mathbf{s}_k \mid \Phi) \right\}$$

where the first and third item do not depend on Ω. After some simplification the M-step can be summarized as $\{\hat{\Lambda}, \hat{\Psi}\} = \arg\max_{\Lambda, \Psi} \sum_{k=1}^K \mathbb{E}[\log p(\theta_k \mid \mathbf{s}_k, \Lambda, \Psi)]$ which leads to the following updating equations:

$$\hat{\Lambda} = \left(\sum_{k=1}^K \mathbb{E}[\theta_k \mathbf{s}_k^T] \right) \left(\sum_{k=1}^K \mathbb{E}[\mathbf{s}_k \mathbf{s}_k^T] \right)^{-1} \quad ; \quad \hat{\Psi} = \frac{1}{K} \left(\sum_{k=1}^K \mathbb{E}[\theta_k \theta_k^T] - (\sum_{k=1}^K \mathbb{E}[\theta_k \mathbf{s}_k^T]) \hat{\Lambda}^T \right)$$

In the E-step we need to calculate the posterior distribution $p(\mathcal{Z} \mid \mathcal{D}, \Omega)$ given the parameter Ω calculated in previous M-step. Essentially only the first and second order

---

[1]Here with a little abuse of notation we ignore the difference of discriminative and generative at the classifier level and use $p(\mathcal{D} \mid \theta_k)$ to denote the likelihood in general.

Algorithm 1 Variational Bayes for the E-step (subscript k is removed for simplicity)

1. Initialize $q(\mathbf{s})$ with some standard distribution (Laplace distribution in our case): $q(\mathbf{s}) = \prod_{h=1}^{H} \mathcal{L}(0, 1)$.

2. Solve the following Bayesian logistic regression (or other Bayesian classifier):

$$q(\theta) \leftarrow \arg\max_{q(\theta)} \left\{ \int q(\theta) \log \frac{\mathcal{N}(\theta; \Lambda \mathbb{E}[\mathbf{s}], \Psi) \prod_{i=1}^{N} p(y_i | \theta, \mathbf{x}_i)}{q(\theta)} d\theta \right\}$$

3. Update $q(\mathbf{s})$:

$$q(\mathbf{s}) \leftarrow \arg\max_{q(\mathbf{s})} \left\{ \int q(\mathbf{s}) \left[\log \frac{p(\mathbf{s})}{q(\mathbf{s})} - \frac{1}{2} \mathbf{Tr} \left(\Psi^{-1} (\mathbb{E}[\theta\theta^T] + \Lambda \mathbf{s}\mathbf{s}^T \Lambda^T - 2\mathbb{E}[\theta](\Lambda \mathbf{s})^T)) \right) \right] d\mathbf{s} \right\}$$

4. Repeat steps 2-5 until convergence conditions are satisfied.

---

moments are needed, namely: $\mathbb{E}[\theta_k]$, $\mathbb{E}[\mathbf{s}_k]$, $\mathbb{E}[\theta_k \theta_k^T]$, $\mathbb{E}[\mathbf{s}_k \mathbf{s}_k^T]$ and $\mathbb{E}[\theta_k \mathbf{s}_k^T]$. Since exact calculation is intractable we will approximate $p(\mathcal{Z} \mid \mathcal{D}, \Omega)$ with $q(\mathcal{Z})$ belonging to the exponential family such that certain distance measure (can be asymmetric) between $p(\mathcal{Z}|\mathcal{D}, \Omega)$ and $q(\mathcal{Z})$) is minimized. In our case we apply the variational Bayes method which applies $\mathcal{KL}(q(\mathcal{Z})||p(\mathcal{D}, \mathcal{Z} \mid \Omega))$ as the distance measure. The central idea is to lower bound the log-likelihood using Jensen's inequality: $\log p(\mathcal{D}) = \log \int p(\mathcal{D}, \mathcal{Z}) d\mathcal{Z} \geq \int q(\mathcal{Z}) \log \frac{p(\mathcal{D}, \mathcal{Z})}{q(\mathcal{Z})} d\mathcal{Z}$. The RHS of the above equation is what we want to maximize, and it is straightforward to show that maximizing this lower bound is equivalent to minimize the KL-divergence $\mathcal{KL}(q(\mathcal{Z})||p(\mathcal{Z}|\mathcal{D}))$. Since given Ω the K tasks are decoupled, we can conduct inference for each task respectively. We further assume $q(\theta_k, \mathbf{s}_k) = q(\theta_k)q(\mathbf{s}_k)$, which in general is a reasonable simplifying assumption and allows us to do the optimization iteratively. The details for the E-step are shown in Algorithm 1.

We would like to comment on several things in Algorithm 1. First, we assume the form of $q(\theta)$ to be multivariate Gaussian, which is a reasonable choice especially considering the fact that only the first and second moments are needed in the M-step. Second, the prior choice of $p(\mathbf{s})$ in step 3 is significant since for each $\mathbf{s}$ we only have one associated "data point" θ. In particular using the Laplace distribution will lead to a more sparse solution of $\mathbb{E}[\mathbf{s}]$, and this will be made more clear in Section 3.2. Finally, we take the parametric form of $q(\mathbf{s})$ to be the product of Laplace distributions with unit variance but known mean, where the fixed variance is intended to remove the unidentifiability issue caused by the interaction between scales of $\mathbf{s}$ and Λ. Although using a full covariance Gaussian for $q(\mathbf{s})$ is another choice, again due to unidentifiability reason caused by rotations of $\mathbf{s}$ and Λ we could make it a diagonal Gaussian. As a result, we argue that the product of Laplaces is better than the product of Gaussians since it has the same parametric form as the prior $p(\mathbf{s})$.

3.1.1 Variational Method for Bayesian Logistic Regression

We present an efficient algorithm based on the variational method proposed in[7] to solve step 2 in Algorithm 1, which is guaranteed to converge and known to be efficient for this problem. Given a Gaussian prior $\mathcal{N}(\mathbf{m}_0, \mathbf{V}_0)$ over the parameter θ and a training set [2] $\mathcal{D} = \{(\mathbf{x}_1, y_1), \ldots, (\mathbf{x}_N, y_N)\}$, we want to obtain an approximation $\mathcal{N}(\mathbf{m}, \mathbf{V})$ to the true posterior distribution $p(\theta|\mathcal{D})$. Taking one data point $(\mathbf{x}, y)$ as an example, the basic idea is to use an exponential function to approximate the non-exponential likelihood function $p(y|\mathbf{x}, \theta) = (1 + \exp(-y\theta^T\mathbf{x}))^{-1}$ which in turn makes the Bayes formula tractable.

---

[2]Again we omit the task index k and use $y \in \{-1, 1\}$ instead of $y \in \{0, 1\}$ to simplify notation.

By using the inequality $p(y|\mathbf{x}, \theta) \geq g(\xi) \exp\left\{(y\mathbf{x}^T\theta - \xi)/2 - \lambda(\xi)((\mathbf{x}^T\theta)^2 - \xi^2)\right\} \overset{\triangle}{=}$ $p(y|\mathbf{x}, \theta, \xi)$ where $g(z) = 1/(1 + \exp(-z))$ is the logistic function and $\lambda(\xi) = tanh(\xi/2)/4\xi$, we can maximize the lower bound of $p(y|\mathbf{x}) = \int p(\theta)p(y|\mathbf{x}, \theta)d\theta \geq \int p(\theta)p(y|\mathbf{x}, \theta, \xi)d\theta$. An EM algorithm can be formulated by treating ξ as the parameter and θ as the hidden variable:

- E-step: $\mathbf{Q}(\xi, \xi^t) = \mathbb{E}\left[\log\left\{p(\theta)p(y|\mathbf{x}, \theta, \xi)\right\} \mid \mathbf{x}, y, \xi^t\right]$
- M-step: $\xi^{t+1} = \arg\max_\xi \mathbf{Q}(\xi, \xi^t)$

Due to the Gaussianity assumption the E-step can be thought as updating the sufficient statistics (mean and covariance) of $q(\theta)$. Finally by using the Woodbury formula the EM iterations can be unraveled and we get the efficient one-shot E-step updating without involving matrix inversion (due to space limitation we skip the derivation):

$$\mathbf{V}_{post} = \mathbf{V} - \frac{2\lambda(\xi)}{1 + 2\lambda(\xi)c}\mathbf{Vx}(\mathbf{Vx})^T$$

$$\mathbf{m}_{post} = \mathbf{m} - \frac{2\lambda(\xi)}{1 + 2\lambda(\xi)c}\mathbf{Vx}\mathbf{x}^T\mathbf{m} + \frac{y}{2}\mathbf{Vx} - \frac{y}{2}\frac{2\lambda(\xi)}{1 + 2\lambda(\xi)c}c\mathbf{Vx}$$

where $c = \mathbf{x}^T\mathbf{Vx}$, and ξ is calculated first from the M-step which is reduced to find the fixed point of the following one-dimensional problem and can be solved efficiently:

$$\xi^2 = c - \frac{2\lambda(\xi)}{1 + 2\lambda(\xi)c}c^2 + \left(\mathbf{x}^T\mathbf{m} - \frac{2\lambda(\xi)}{1 + 2\lambda(\xi)c}c\mathbf{x}^T\mathbf{m} + \frac{y}{2}c - \frac{y}{2}\frac{2\lambda(\xi)}{1 + 2\lambda(\xi)c}c^2\right)^2$$

And this process will be performed for each data point to get the final approximation $q(\theta)$.

3.2 Point Estimation

Although the empirical Bayes method is efficient for medium-sized problem, both its computational cost and memory requirement grow as the number of data instances or features increases. For example, it can easily happen in text or image domain where the number of features can be more than ten thousand, so we need faster methods. We can obtain the point estimation of $\{\theta_k, \mathbf{s}_k\}_{k=1}^K$, by treating it as a limiting case of the previous algorithm. To be more specific, by letting $q(\theta)$ and $q(\mathbf{s})$ converging to the Dirac delta function, step 2 in Algorithm 1 can thought as finding the MAP estimation of θ and step 4 becomes the following lasso-like optimization problem ($\mathbf{m_s}$ denotes the point estimation of $\mathbf{s}$):

$$\hat{\mathbf{m}}_\mathbf{s} = \arg\min_{\mathbf{m_s}}\left\{2||\mathbf{m_s}||_1 + \mathbf{m}_\mathbf{s}^T\Lambda^T\Psi^{-1}\Lambda\mathbf{m_s} - 2\mathbf{m}_\mathbf{s}^T\Lambda^T\Psi^{-1}\mathbb{E}[\theta]\right\}$$

which can be solved numerically. Furthermore, the solution of the above optimization is sparse in $\mathbf{m_s}$. This is a particularly nice property since we would only like to consider hidden sources for which the association with tasks are significantly supported by evidence.

4 Experimental Results

The LICA model will work most effectively if the tasks we want to learn are very related. In our experiments we apply the LICA model to multi-label text classification problems, which are the case for many existing text collections including the most popular ones like Reuters-21578 and the new RCV1 corpus. Here each individual task is to classify a given document to a particular category, and it is assumed that the multi-label property implies that some of the tasks are related through some latent sources (semantic topics).

For Reuters-21578 we choose nine categories out of ninety categories, which is based on fact that those categories are often correlated by previous studies[8]. After some preprocessing[3] we get 3,358 unique features/words, and empirical Bayes method is used to

---

[3]We do stemming, remove stopwords and rare words (words that occur less than three times).

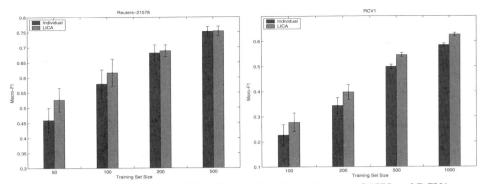

Figure 2: Multi-label Text Classification Results on Reuters-21578 and RCV1

solve this problem. On the other hand, if we include all the 116 TOPIC categories in RCV1 corpus we get a much larger vocabulary size: 47,236 unique features. Bayesian inference is intractable for this high-dimensional case since memory requirement itself is $O(F^2)$ to store the full covariance matrix $\mathbb{V}[\theta]$. As a result we take the point estimation approach which reduces the memory requirement to $O(F)$. For both data sets we use the standard training/test split, but for RCV1 since the test part of corpus is huge (around 800k documents) we only randomly sample 10k as our test set. Since the effectiveness of learning multiple related tasks jointly should be best demonstrated when we have limited resources, we evaluate our LICA by varying the size of training set. Each setting is repeated ten times and the results are summarized in Figure 2.

In Figure 2 the result "individual" is obtained by using regularized logistic regression for each category individually. The number of tasks K is equal to 9 and 116 for the Reuters-21578 and the RCV1 respectively, and we set H (the dimension of hidden source) to be the same as K in our experiments. We use F1 measure which is preferred to error rate in text classification due to the very unbalanced positive/negative document ratio. For the Reuters-21578 collection we report the Macro-F1 results because this corpus is easier and thus Micro-F1 are almost the same for both methods. For the RCV1 collection we only report Micro-F1 due to space limitation, and in fact we observed similar trend in Macro-F1 although values are much lower due to the large number of rare categories. Furthermore, we achieved a sparse solution for the point estimation method. In particular, we obtained less than 5 non-zero sources out of 116 for most of the tasks for the RCV1 collection.

5   Discussions on Related Work

By viewing multitask learning as predicting multivariate responses, Breiman and Friedman[3] proposed a method called "Curds and Whey" for regression problems. The intuition is to apply shrinkage in a rotated basis instead of the original task basis so that information can be borrowed among tasks.

By treating tasks as IID generated from some probability space, empirical process theory[2] has been applied to study the bounds and asymptotics of multiple task learning, similar to the case of standard learning. On the other hand, from the general Bayesian perspective[2][6] we could treat the problem of learning multiple tasks as learning a Bayesian prior over the task space. Despite the generality of above two principles, it is often necessary to assume some specific structure or parametric form of the task space since the functional space is usually of higher or infinite dimension compared to the input space.

Our model is related to the recently proposed Semiparametric Latent Factor Model (SLFM) for regression by Teh et. al.[10]. It uses Gaussian Processes (GP) to model regression through a latent factor analysis. Besides the difference between FA and ICA, its advantage is that GP is non-parametric and works on the instance space; the disadvantage of that model is that training instances need to be shared for all tasks. Furthermore, it is not clear how to explore different task structures in this instance-space viewpoint. As pointed out earlier, the exploration of different source models is important in learning related tasks as the prior often plays a more important role than it does in standard learning.

6   Conclusion and Future Work

In this paper we proposed a probabilistic framework for learning multiple related tasks, which tries to identify the shared latent independent components that are responsible for the relatedness among those tasks. We also presented the corresponding empirical Bayes method as well as point estimation algorithms for learning the model. Using non-Gaussian distributions for hidden sources makes it possible to identify independent components instead of just decorrelation, and in particular we enjoyed the sparsity by modeling hidden sources with Laplace distribution. Having the sparsity property makes the model not only parsimonious but also more robust since the dependence on latent, independent sources will be shrunk toward zero unless significantly supported by evidence from the data. By learning those related tasks jointly, we are able to get a better estimation of the latent independent sources and thus achieve a better generalization capability compared to conventional approaches where the learning of each task is done independently. Our experimental results in multi-label text classification problems show evidence to support our claim.

Our approach assumes that the underlying structure in the task space is a linear subspace, which can usually capture important information about independent sources. However, it is possible to achieve better results if we can incorporate specific domain knowledge about the relatedness of those tasks into the model and obtain a reliable estimation of the structure. For future research, we would like to consider more flexible source models as well as incorporate domain specific knowledge to specify and learn the underlying structure.

References

[1] Ando, R. and Zhang, T. A Framework for Learning Predicative Structures from Multiple Tasks and Unlabeled Data. Technical Rerport RC23462, IBM T.J. Watson Research Center, 2004.

[2] Baxter, J. A Model for Inductive Bias Learning. *J. of Artificial Intelligence Research*, 2000.

[3] Breiman, L. and Friedman J. Predicting Multivariate Responses in Multiple Linear Regression. J. Royal Stat. Society B, 59:3-37, 1997.

[4] Evgeniou, T., Micchelli, C. and Pontil, M. Learning Multiple Tasks with Kernel Methods. *J. of Machine Learning Research*, 6:615-637, 2005.

[5] Ghosn, J. and Bengio, Y. Bias Learning, Knowledge Sharing. *IEEE Transaction on Neural Networks*, 14(4):748-765, 2003.

[6] Heskes, T. Empirical Bayes for Learning to Learn. In *Proc. of the 17th ICML*, 2000.

[7] Jaakkola, T. and Jordan, M. A Variational Approach to Bayesian Logistic Regression Models and Their Extensions. In *Proc. of the Sixth Int. Workshop on AI and Statistics*, 1997.

[8] Koller, D. and Sahami, M. Hierarchically Classifying Documents using Very Few Words. In *Proc. of the 14th ICML*, 1997.

[9] Roberts, S. and Everson, R. (editors). *Independent Component Analysis: Principles and Practice*, Cambridge University Press, 2001.

[10] Teh, Y.-W., Seeger, M. and Jordan, M. Semiparametric Latent Factor Models. In Z. Ghahramani and R. Cowell, editors, *Workshop on Artificial Intelligence and Statistics 10*, 2005.

[11] Yu, K., Tresp, V. and Schwaighofer, A. Learning Gaussian Processes from Multiple Tasks. In *Proc. of the 22nd ICML*, 2005.

Modeling Neuronal Interactivity using Dynamic Bayesian Networks

Lei Zhang†,‡, Dimitris Samaras†, Nelly Alia-Klein‡, Nora Volkow‡, Rita Goldstein‡
† Computer Science Department, SUNY at Stony Brook, Stony Brook, NY
‡ Medical Department, Brookhaven National Laboratory, Upton, NY

Abstract

Functional Magnetic Resonance Imaging (fMRI) has enabled scientists to look into the active brain. However, interactivity between functional brain regions, is still little studied. In this paper, we contribute a novel framework for modeling the interactions between multiple active brain regions, using Dynamic Bayesian Networks (DBNs) as generative models for brain activation patterns. This framework is applied to modeling of neuronal circuits associated with reward. The novelty of our framework from a Machine Learning perspective lies in the use of DBNs to reveal the brain connectivity and interactivity. Such interactivity models which are derived from fMRI data are then validated through a group classification task. We employ and compare four different types of DBNs: Parallel Hidden Markov Models, Coupled Hidden Markov Models, Fully-linked Hidden Markov Models and Dynamically Multi-Linked HMMs (DML-HMM). Moreover, we propose and compare two schemes of learning DML-HMMs. Experimental results show that by using DBNs, group classification can be performed even if the DBNs are constructed from as few as 5 brain regions. We also demonstrate that, by using the proposed learning algorithms, different DBN structures characterize drug addicted subjects vs. control subjects. This finding provides an independent test for the effect of psychopathology on brain function. In general, we demonstrate that incorporation of computer science principles into functional neuroimaging clinical studies provides a novel approach for probing human brain function.

1. Introduction

Functional Magnetic Resonance Imaging (fMRI) has enabled scientists to look into the active human brain [1] by providing sequences of 3D brain images with intensities representing blood oxygenation level dependent (BOLD) regional activations. This has revealed exciting insights into the spatial and temporal changes underlying a broad range of brain functions, such as how we see, feel, move, understand each other and lay down memories. This fMRI technology offers further promise by imaging the dynamic aspects of the functioning human brain. Indeed, fMRI has encouraged a growing interest in revealing brain connectivity and interactivity within the neuroscience community. It is for example understood that a dynamically managed goal directed behavior requires neural control mechanisms orchestrated to select the appropriate and task-relevant responses while inhibiting irrelevant or inappropriate processes [12]. To date, the analyses and interpretation of fMRI data that are most commonly employed by neuroscientists depend on the cognitive-behavioral probes that are developed to tap regional brain function. Thus, brain responses are a-priori labeled based on the putative underlying task condition and are then used to separate a priori defined groups of subjects. In recent computer science research [18][13][3][19], machine learning methods have been applied for fMRI data analysis. However, in these approaches information on the connectivity and interactivity between brain voxels is discarded and brain voxels are assumed to be independent, which is an inaccurate assumption (see use of statistical maps [3][19] or the mean of each fMRI time interval[13]). In this paper, we exploit Dynamic Bayesian Networks for modeling dynamic (i.e., connecting and interacting) neuronal circuits from fMRI sequences. We suggest that through incorporation of graphical models into functional neuroimaging studies we will be able to identify neuronal patterns of connectivity and interactivity that will provide invaluable insights into basic emotional and cognitive neuroscience constructs. We further propose that this interscientific incorporation may provide a valid tool where objective brain imaging data are used for the clinical purpose of diagnosis of psychopathology. Specifically, in our case study we will model neuronal circuits associated with reward processing in drug addiction. We have previously shown loss of sensitivity to the relative value of money in cocaine users [9]. It has also been previously highlighted that the complex mechanism of drug addiction requires the connectivity and interactivity between regions comprising the mesocorticolimbic circuit [12][8]. However, although advancements have been made in studying this circuit's role in inhibitory control and reward processing, inference about the connectivity and interactivity of these regions is at best indirect. Dynamical causal models have been compared in [16]. Compared with dynamic causal models, DBNs admit a class of nonlinear continuous-time interactions among the hidden states and model both causal relationships between brain regions and temporal correlations among multiple processes, useful for both classification and prediction purposes.

Probabilistic graphical models [14][11] are graphs in which nodes represent random variables, and the (lack of) arcs represent conditional independence assumptions. In our case, interconnected brain regions can be considered as nodes of a probabilistic graphical model and interactivity relationships between regions are modeled by probability values on the arcs (or the lack of) between these nodes. However, the major challenge in such a machine learning approach is the choice of a particular structure that models connectivity and interactivity between brain regions in an *accurate* and *efficient* manner. In this work, we contribute a framework of exploiting Dynamic Bayesian Networks to model such a structure for the fMRI data. More specifically, instead of modeling each brain region in isolation, we aim to model the interactive pattern of multiple brain regions. Furthermore, the revealed functional information is validated through a group classification case study: separating drug addicted subjects from healthy non-drug-using controls based on trained Dynamic Bayesian Networks. Both conventional BBNs and HMMs are unsuitable for modeling activities underpinned not only by causal but also by clear temporal correlations among multiple processes [10], and Dynamic Bayesian Networks [5][7] are required. Since the state of each brain region is not known (only observations of activation exist), it can be thought of as a hidden variable[15]. An intuitive way to construct a DBN is to extend a standard HMM to a set of interconnected multiple HMMs. For example, Vogler et al. [17] proposed Parallel Hidden Markov Models (PaHMMs) that factorize state space into multiple independent temporal processes without causal connections in-between. Brand et al. [2] exploited Coupled Hidden Markov Models (CHMMs) for complex action recognitions. Gong et al. [10] developed a Dynamically Multi-Linked Hidden Markov Model (DML-HMM) for the recognition of group activities involving multiple different object events in a noisy outdoor scene. This model is the only one of those models that learns both the structure and parameters of the graphical model, instead of presuming a structure (possibly inaccurate) given the lack of knowledge of human brain connectivity. In order to model the dynamic neuronal circuits underlying reward processing in the human brains, we explore and compare the above DBNs. We propose and compare two learning schemes of

DML-HMMs, one is greedy structure search (Hill-Climbing) and the other is Structural Expectation-Maximization (SEM).

To our knowledge, this is the first time that Dynamic Bayesian Networks are exploited in modeling the connectivity and interactivity among brain regions activated during a fMRI study. Our current experimental classification results show that by using DBNs, group classification can be performed even if the DBNs are constructed from as few as 5 brain regions. We also demonstrate that, by using the proposed learning algorithms, different DBN structures characterize drug addicted subjects vs. control subjects which provides an independent test for the effects of psychopathology on brain function. From the machine learning point of view, this paper provides an innovative application of Dynamic Bayesian Networks in modeling dynamic neuronal circuits. Furthermore, since the structures to be explored are exclusively represented by hidden (cannot be observed directly) states and their interconnecting arcs, the structure learning of DML-HMMs poses a greater challenge than other DBNs [5]. From the neuroscientific point of view, drug addiction is a complex disorder characterized by compromised inhibitory control and reward processing. However, individuals with compromised mechanisms of control and reward are difficult to identify unless they are directly subjected to challenging conditions. Modeling the interactive brain patterns is therefore essential since such patterns may be unique to a certain psychopathology and could hence be used for improving diagnosis and prevention efforts (e.g., diagnosis of drug addiction, prevention of relapse or craving). In addition, the development of this framework can be applied to further our understanding of other human disorders and states such as those impacting insight and awareness, that similarly to drug addiction are currently identified based mostly on subjective criteria and self-report.

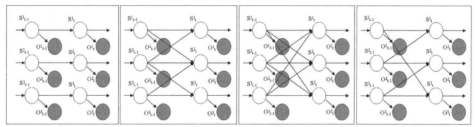

Figure 1: Four types of Dynamic Bayesian Networks: PaHMM, CHMM, FHMM and DML-HMM.

2. Dynamic Bayesian Networks

In this section, we will briefly describe the general framework of Dynamic Bayesian Networks. DBNs are Bayesian Belief Networks that have been extended to model the stochastic evolution of a set of random variables over time [5][7]. As described in [10], a DBN B can be represented by two sets of parameters (m, Θ) where the first set m represents the structure of the DBN including the number of hidden state variables S and observation variables O per time instance, the number of states for each hidden state variable and the topology of the network (set of directed arcs connecting the nodes). More specifically, the ith hidden state variable and the jth observation variable at time instance t are denoted as $S_t^{(i)}$ and $O_t^{(j)}$ with $i \in \{1, ..., N_h\}$ and $j \in \{1, ..., N_o\}$, N_h and N_o are the number of hidden state variables and observation variables respectively. The second set of parameters Θ includes the state transition matrix A, the observation matrix B and a matrix π modeling the initial state distribution $P(S_1^i)$. More specifically, A and B quantify the transition models $P(S_t^{(i)}|Pa(S_t^{(i)}))$ and observation models $P(O_t^{(i)}|Pa(O_t^{(i)}))$ respectively where $Pa(S_t^{(i)})$ are the parents of $S_t^{(i)}$ (similarly $Pa(O_t^{(i)})$ for observations). In this paper, we will examine four types of DBNs: Parallel Hidden Markov Models (PaHMM) [17], Coupled Hidden Markov Models (CHMM)[2], Fully Connected Hidden Markov Models (FHMM) and

Dynamically Multi-Linked Hidden Markov Models (DML-HMM)[10] as shown in Fig 1 where observation nodes are shown as shaded circles, hidden nodes as clear circles and the causal relationships among hidden state variables are represented by the arcs between hidden nodes. Notice that the first three DBNs are essentially three special cases of the DML-HMM.

2.1. Learning of DBNs

Given the form of DBNs in the previous sections, there are two learning problems that must be solved for real-world applications: 1) **Parameter Learning:** assuming fixed structure, given the training sequences of observations O, how we adjust the model parameters $B = (m, \Theta)$ to maximize $P(O|B)$; 2) **Structure Learning:** for DBNs with unknown structure (i.e. DML-HMMs), how we learn the structure from the observation O. Parameter learning has been well studied in [17][2]. Given fixed structure, parameters can be learned iteratively using Expectation-Maximization (EM). The E step, which involves the inference of hidden states given parameters, can be implemented using an exact inference algorithm such as the junction tree algorithm. Then the parameters and maximal likelihood $L(\Theta)$ can be computed iteratively from the M step.

In [10], the DML-HMM was selected from a set of candidate structures, however the selection of candidate structure is non-trivial for most applications including brain region connectivity. For a DML-HMM with N hidden nodes, the total number of different structures is $2^{N^2 - N}$, thus it is impossible to conduct an exhaustive search in most cases. The learning of DBNs involving both parameter learning and structure learning has been discussed in [5], where the scoring rules for standard probabilistic networks were extended to the dynamic case and the Structural EM (SEM) algorithm was developed for structure learning when some of the variables are hidden. The structure learning of DML-HMMs is more challenging since the structures to be explored are exclusively represented by the hidden states and none of them can be directly observed. In the following, we will explain two learning schemes for the DML-HMMs. One standard way is to perform parametric EM within an outer-loop structural search. Thus, our first scheme is to use an outer-loop of the Hill-Climbing algorithm (DML-HMM-HC). For each step of the algorithm, from the current DBN, we first compute a neighbor list by adding, deleting, or reversing one arc. Then we perform parameter learning for each of the neighbors and go to the neighbor with the minimum score until there is no neighbor whose score is higher than the current DBN. Our second learning scheme is similar to the Structural EM algorithm [5] in the sense that the structural and parametric modification are performed within a single EM process. As described in [5][4], a structural search can be performed efficiently given complete observation data. However, as we described above, the structure of DML-HMMs are represented by the hidden states which can not be observed directly. Hence, we develop the DML-HMM-SEM algorithm as follows: given the current structure, we first perform a parameter learning and then, for each training data, we compute the Most Probable Explanation (MPE), which computes the most likely value for each hidden node (similar to Viterbi in standard HMM). The MPE thus provides a complete estimation of the hidden states and a complete-data structural search [4] is then performed to find the best structure. We perform learning iteratively until the structure converges. In this scheme, the structural search is performed in the inner loop thus making the learning more efficient. Pseudo-codes of both learning schemes are described in Table 1. In this paper, we use Schwarz's Bayesian Information Criterion (BIC): $BIC = -2 \log L(\Theta_B) + K_B \log N$ as our score function where for a DBN B, $L(\Theta_B)$ is the maximal likelihood under B, K_B is the dimension of the parameters of B and N is the size of the training data. Theoretically, the DML-HMM-SEM algorithm is not guaranteed to converge since for the same training data, the most probably explanations (S_i, S_j) of two DML-HMMs B_i, B_j might be different. In the worst case, oscillation between two structures is possible. To guarantee halting of the algorithm, a loop detector can be added so that, once any structure is selected in a second time, we stop the learning and select the structure with the minimum score visited during the searching. However, in our experiments, the learning algorithm always converged in a few steps.

Procedure **DML-HMM-HC**	Procedure **DML-HMM-SEM**
$Initial\_Model(B_0);$	$Initial\_Model(B_0);$
Loop $i = 0, 1, ...$ until convergence:	Loop $i = 0, 1, ...$ until convergence:
$\quad [B_i', score_i^0] = Learn\_Parameter(B_i);$	$\quad [B_i', score_i^0] = Learn\_Parameter(B_i);$
$\quad B_i^{1..J} = Generate\_Neighbors(B_i);$	$\quad S = Most\_Prob\_Expl(B_i', O);$
$\quad$ for j=1..J	$\quad B_i^{max} = Find\_Best\_Struct(S);$
$\quad\quad [B_i^{j'}, score_i^j] = Learn\_Parameter(B_i^j);$	$\quad$ if $B_i^{max} == B_i'$
$\quad j = Find\_Minscore(score_i^{1..J});$	$\quad\quad$ return $B_i';$
$\quad$ if $(score_i^j > score_i^0)$	$\quad$ else
$\quad\quad$ return $B_i';$	$\quad\quad B_{i+1} = B_i^{max};$
$\quad$ else	
$\quad\quad B_{i+1} = B_i^j;$	

Table 1: Two schemes of learning DML-HMMs: the left column lists the DML-HMM-HC scheme and the right column lists the DML-HMM-SEM scheme.

3. Modeling Reward Neuronal Circuits: A Case Study

In this section, we will describe our case study of modeling *Reward Neuronal Circuits*: by using DBNs, we aim to model the interactive pattern of multiple brain regions for the neuropsychological problem of sensitivity to the relative value of money. Furthermore, we will examine the revealed functional information encapsulated in the trained DBNs through a group classification study: separating drug addicted subjects from healthy non-drug-using controls based on trained DBNs.

3.1. Data Collection and Preprocess

In our experiments, data were collected to study the neuropsychological problem of loss of sensitivity to the relative value of money in cocaine users[9]. MRI studies were performed on a 4T Varian scanner and all stimuli were presented using LCD-goggles connected to a PC. Human participants pressed a button or refrained from pressing based on a picture shown to them. They received a monetary reward if they performed correctly. Specifically, three runs were repeated twice (T1, T2, T3; and T1R, T2R, T3R) and in each run, there were three monetary conditions (high money, low money, no money) and a baseline condition; the order of monetary conditions was pseudo-randomized and identical for all participants. Participants were informed about the monetary condition by a 3-sec instruction slide, presenting the stimuli: $0.45, $0.01 or $0.00. Feedback for correct responses in each condition consisted of the respective numeral designating the amount of money the subject has earned if correct or the symbol (X) otherwise. To simulate real-life motivational salience, subjects could gain up to $50 depending on their performance on this task. 16 cocaine dependent individuals, 18-55 years of age, in good health, were matched with 12 non-drug-using controls on sex, race, education and general intellectual functioning. Statistical Parametric Mapping (SPM)[6] was used for fMRI data preprocessing (realignment, normalization/registration and smoothing) and statistical analyses.

3.2. Feature Selection and Neuronal Circuit Modeling

The fMRI data are extremely high dimensional (i.e. $53 \times 63 \times 46$ voxels per scan). Prior to training the DBN, we selected 5 brain regions: Left Inferior Frontal Gyrus (Left IFG), Prefrontal Cortex (PFC, including lateral and medial dorsolateral PFC and the anterior cingulate), Midbrain (including substantia nigra), Thalamus and Cerebellum. These regions were selected based on prior SPM analyses random-effects analyses (ANOVA) where the goal was to differentiate effect of money (high, low, no) from the effect of group (cocaine,

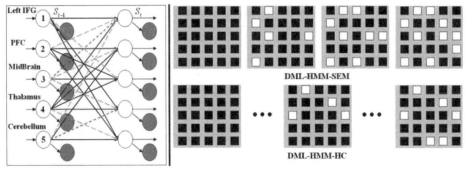

Figure 2: Learning processes and learned structures from two algorithms. The leftmost column demonstrates two (superimposed) learned structures where light gray dashed arcs (long dash) are learned from DML-HMM-HC, dark gray dashed arcs (short dash) from DML-HMM-SEM and black solid arcs from both. The right columns shows the transient structures of the learning processes of two algorithms where black represents existence of arc and white represents no arc.

control) on all regions that were activated to monetary reward in all subjects. In all these five regions, the monetary main effect was significant as evidenced by region of interest follow-up analyses. Of note is the fact that these five regions are part of the mesocorticolimbic reward circuit, previously implicated in addiction. Each of the above brain regions is presented by a k-D feature vector where k is the number of brain voxels selected in this brain region (i.e. $k = 3$ for Left IFG and $k = 8$ for PFC). After feature selection, a DML-HMM with 5 hidden nodes can be learned as described in Sec. 2 from the training data. The leftmost image in Fig. 2 shows two superimposed possible structures of such DML-HMMs. The causal relationships discovered among different brain regions are embodied in the topology of the DML-HMM. Each of the five hidden variables has two states (activated or not) and each continuous observation variable (given by a k-D feature vector) represents the observed activation of each brain region. The Probabilistic Distribution Function (PDF) of each observation variable is a mixture of Gaussians conditioned by the state of its discrete parent node.

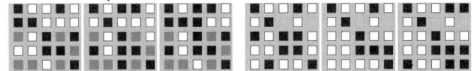

Figure 3: Left three images shows the structures learned from the 3 subsets of Group C and the right three images shows those learned from subsets of Group S. Figure shows that some arcs consistently appeared in Group C but not consistently in Group S (marked in dark gray) and vice versa (marked in light gray), which implies such group differences in the interactive brain patterns may correspond to the loss of sensitivity to the relative value of money in cocaine users.

4. Experiments and Results

We collected fMRI data of 16 drug addicted subjects and 12 control subjects, 6 runs per participant. Due to head motion, some data could not be used. In our experiments, we used a total of 152 fMRI sequences (87 scans per sequence) with 86 sequences for the drug addicted subjects (Group S) and 66 for control subjects (Group C).

First we compare the two learning schemes for DML-HMMs proposed in Sec. 2. Fig. 2 demonstrates the learning process (initialized with the FHMM) for drug addicted subjects. The leftmost column shows two learned structures where red arcs are learned from DML-HMM-HC, green arcs from DML-HMM-SEM and black arcs from both. The right columns show the learning processes of DML-HMM-SEM (top) and DML-HMM-HC (bottom) with black representing existence of arc and white representing no arc. Since in DML-HMM-SEM, structure learning is in the inner loop, the learning process is much faster than that of DML-HMM-HC. We also compared the BIC scores of the learned structures and we found DML-HMM-SEM selected better structures than DML-HMM-HC.

It is also very interesting to examine the structure learning processes by using different training data. For each participant group, we randomly separated the data set into three subsets and trained DBNs are reported in Fig. 3 where the left three images show the structures learned from the 3 subsets of Group C and the right three images show those learned from subsets of Group S. In Fig. 3, we found the learned structures of each group are similar. We also found that some arcs consistently appeared in Group C but not consistently in Group S (marked in red) and vice versa (marked in green), which implies such group differences in the interactive brain patterns may correspond to the loss of sensitivity to the relative value of money in cocaine users. More specifically, in Fig. 3, the average intra-group similarity scores were 80% and 78.3%, while cross-group similarity was 56.7%.

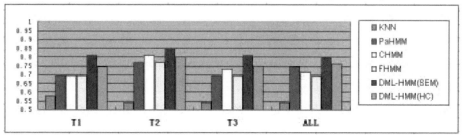

Figure 4: Classification results: All DBN methods significantly improved classification rates compared to K-Nearest Neighbor with DML-HMM performing best.

The second set of experiments was to apply the trained DBNs for group classification. In our data collection, there were 6 runs of fMRI collection: T1, T2, T3, T1R, T2R and T3R with the latter latter repeating the former three, grouped into 4 data sets $\{T1, T2, T3, ALL\}$ with ALL containing all the data. We performed classification experiments on each of the 4 data sets where the data were randomly divided into a training set and a testing set of equal size. During training, the described four DBN type were employed using the training set while during the learning of DML-HMMs, different initial structures (PaHMM, CHMM, FHMM) were used and the structure with the minimum BIC score was selected from the three learned DML-HMMs. For each model, two DBNs $\{B_c, B_s\}$ were trained on the training data of Group C and Group S respectively. During testing, for each testing fMRI sequence O_{test}, we computed two likelihoods $P_c^{test} = P(O_{test}|B_c)$ and $P_s^{test} = P(O_{test}|B_s)$ using the two trained DBNs. Since the two DBNs may have different structures, instead of directly comparing the two likelihoods, we used the difference between these two likelihoods for classification. More specifically, during training, for each training sequence TR_i, we computed the ratio of two likelihoods $R_i^{TR} = P_c^i/P_s^i$ where $P_c^i = P(TR_i|B_c)$ and $P_s^i = P(TR_i|B_s)$. As expected, generally the ratios of Group C training data were significantly greater than those of Group S. During testing, the ratio $R_{test} = P_c^{test}/P_s^{test}$ for each test sequence was also computed and compared to the ratios of the training data for classification. Fig. 4 reports the classification rates of the different DBNs on each data set. For comparison, the k-th Nearest Neighbor (KNN) algorithm was applied on the fMRI sequences directly and Fig. 4 shows that by using DBNs, classification rates are significantly better with DML-HMM outperforming all other models.

5. Conclusions and Future Work

In this work, we contributed a framework of exploiting Dynamic Bayesian Networks to model the functional information of the fMRI data. We explored four types of DBNs: a Parallel Hidden Markov Model (PaHMM), a Coupled Hidden Markov Model (CHMM), a Fully-linked Hidden Markov Model (FHMM) and a Dynamically Multi-linked Hidden Markov Model. Furthermore, we proposed and compared two structural learning schemes of DML-HMMs and applied the DBNs to a group classification problem. To our knowledge, this is the first time that Dynamic Bayesian Networks are exploited in modeling the connectivity and interactivity among brain voxels from fMRI data. This framework of exploring functional information of fMRI data provides a novel approach of revealing brain connectivity and interactivity and provides an independent test for the effect of psychopathology on brain function.

Currently, DBNs use independently pre-selected brain regions, thus some other important interactivity information may have been discarded in the feature selection step. Our future work will focus on developing a dynamic neuronal circuit modeling framework performing feature selection and DBN learning simultaneously. Due to computational limits and for clarity purposes, we explored only 5 brain regions and thus another direction of future work is to develop a hierarchical DBN topology to comprehensively model all implicated brain regions efficiently.

References

[1] S. Anders, M. Lotze, M. Erb, W. Grodd, and N. Birbaumer. Brain activity underlying emotional valence and arousal: A response-related fmri study. In *Human Brain Mapping*.

[2] M. Brand, N. Oliver, and A. Pentland. Coupled hidden markov models for complex action recognition. In *CVPR*, pages 994–999, 1996.

[3] J. Ford, H. Farid, F. Makedon, L.A. Flashman, T.W. McAllister, V. Megalooikonomou, and A.J. Saykin. Patient classification of fmri activation maps. In *MICCAI*, 2003.

[4] N. Friedman. The bayesian structual algorithm. In *UAI*, 1998.

[5] N. Friedman, K. Murphy, and S. Russell. Learning the structure of dynamic probabilistic networks. In *Uncertainty in AI*, pages 139–147, 1998.

[6] K. Friston, A. Holmes, K. Worsley, and et al. Statistical parametric maps in functional imaging: A general linear approach. *Human Brain Mapping*, pages 2:189–210, 1995.

[7] G. Ghahramani. Learning dynamic bayesian networks. In *Adaptive Processing of Sequences and Data Structures, Lecture Notes in AI*, pages 168–197, 1998.

[8] R.Z. Goldstein and N.D. Volkow. Drug addiction and its underlying neurobiological basis: Neuroimaging evidence for the involvement of the frontal cortex. *American Journal of Psychiatry*, (10):1642–1652.

[9] R.Z. Goldstein et al. A modified role for the orbitofrontal cortex in attribution of salience to monetary reward in cocaine addiction: an fmri study at 4t. In *Human Brain Mapping Conference*, 2004.

[10] S. Gong and T. Xiang. Recognition of group activities using dynamic probabilistic networks. In *ICCV*, 2003.

[11] M.I. Jordan and Y. Weiss. *Graphical models: probabilistic inference, Arbib, M. (ed): Handbook of Neural Networks and Brain Theory*. MIT Press, 2002.

[12] A.W. MacDonald et al. Dissociating the role of the dorsolateral prefrontal and anterior cingulate cortex in cognitive control. *Science*, 288(5472):1835–1838, 2000.

[13] T.M. Mitchell, R. Hutchinson, R. Niculescu, F. Pereira, X. Wang, M. Just, and S. Newman. Learning to decode cognitive states from brain images. *Machine Learning*, 57:145–175, 2004.

[14] K.P. Murphy. An introduction to graphical models. 2001.

[15] L.K. Hansen P. Hojen-Sorensen and C.E. Rasmussen. Bayesian modeling of fmri time series. In *NIPS*, 1999.

[16] W.D. Penny, K.E. Stephan, A. Mechelli, and K.J. Friston. Comparing dynamic causal models. *NeuroImage*, 22(3):1157–1172, 2004.

[17] C. Vogler and D. Metaxas. A framework for recognizing the simultaneous aspects of american sign language. In *CVIU*, pages 81:358–384, 2001.

[18] X. Wang, R. Hutchinson, and T.M. Mitchell. Training fmri classifiers to detect cognitive states across multiple human subjects. In *NIPS03*, Dec 2003.

[19] L. Zhang, D. Samaras, D. Tomasi, N. Volkow, and R. Goldstein. Machine learning for clinical diagnosis from functional magnetic resonance imaging. In *CVPR*, 2005.

Analysis of Spectral Kernel Design based Semi-supervised Learning

Tong Zhang
Yahoo! Inc.
New York City, NY 10011

Rie Kubota Ando
IBM T. J. Watson Research Center
Yorktown Heights, NY 10598

Abstract

We consider a framework for semi-supervised learning using spectral decomposition based un-supervised kernel design. This approach subsumes a class of previously proposed semi-supervised learning methods on data graphs. We examine various theoretical properties of such methods. In particular, we derive a generalization performance bound, and obtain the optimal kernel design by minimizing the bound. Based on the theoretical analysis, we are able to demonstrate why spectral kernel design based methods can often improve the predictive performance. Experiments are used to illustrate the main consequences of our analysis.

1 Introduction

Spectral graph methods have been used both in clustering and in semi-supervised learning. This paper focuses on semi-supervised learning, where a classifier is constructed from both labeled and unlabeled training examples. Although previous studies showed that this class of methods work well for certain concrete problems (for example, see [1, 4, 5, 6]), there is no satisfactory theory demonstrating why (and under what circumstances) such methods should work.

The purpose of this paper is to develop a more complete theoretical understanding for graph based semi-supervised learning. In Theorem 2.1, we present a transductive formulation of kernel learning on graphs which is equivalent to supervised kernel learning. This new kernel learning formulation includes some of the previous proposed graph semi-supervised learning methods as special cases. A consequence is that we can view such graph-based semi-supervised learning methods as kernel design methods that utilize unlabeled data; the designed kernel is then used in the standard supervised learning setting. This insight allows us to prove useful results concerning the behavior of graph based semi-supervised learning from the more general view of spectral kernel design. Similar spectral kernel design ideas also appeared in [2]. However, they didn't present a graph-based learning formulation (Theorem 2.1 in this paper); nor did they study the theoretical properties of such methods. We focus on two issues for graph kernel learning formulations based on Theorem 2.1. First, we establish the convergence of graph based semi-supervised learning (when the number of unlabeled data increases). Second, we obtain a learning bound, which can be used to compare the performance of different kernels. This analysis gives insights to what are good kernels, and why graph-based spectral kernel design is often helpful in various applications. Examples are given to justify the theoretical analysis. Due to the space limitations, proofs will not be included in this paper.

2 Transductive Kernel Learning on Graphs

We shall start with notations for supervised learning. Consider the problem of predicting a real-valued output Y based on its corresponding input vector X. In the standard machine learning formulation, we assume that the data (X, Y) are drawn from an unknown underlying distribution D. Our goal is to find a predictor $p(x)$ so that the expected true loss of p given below is as small as possible: $R(p(\cdot)) = E_{(X,Y)\sim D} L(p(X), Y)$, where we use $E_{(X,Y)\sim D}$ to denote the expectation with respect to the true (but unknown) underlying distribution D. Typically, one needs to restrict the hypothesis function family size so that a stable estimate within the function family can be obtained from a finite number of samples. We are interested in learning in Hilbert spaces. For notational simplicity, we assume that there is a feature representation $\psi(x) \in \mathcal{H}$, where $\mathcal{H}$ is a high (possibly infinity) dimensional feature space. We denote $\psi(x)$ by column vectors, so that the inner product in the Hilbert-space $\mathcal{H}$ is the vector product. A linear classifier $p(x)$ on $\mathcal{H}$ can be represented by a vector $w \in \mathcal{H}$ such that $p(x) = w^T \psi(x)$.

Let the training samples be $(X_1, Y_1), \ldots, (X_n, Y_n)$. We consider the following regularized linear prediction method on $\mathcal{H}$:

$$\hat{p}(x) = \hat{w}^T \psi(x), \quad \hat{w} = \arg\min_{w \in \mathcal{H}} \left[\frac{1}{n} \sum_{i=1}^{n} L(w^T \psi(X_i), Y_i) + \lambda w^T w \right]. \qquad (1)$$

If $\mathcal{H}$ is an infinite dimensional space, then it is not be feasible to solve (1) directly. A remedy is to use kernel methods. Given a feature representation $\psi(x)$, we can define kernel $k(x, x') = \psi(x)^T \psi(x')$. It is well-known (the so-called representer theorem) that the solution of (1) can be represented as $\hat{p}(x) = \sum_{i=1}^{n} \hat{\alpha}_i k(X_i, x)$, where $[\hat{\alpha}_i]$ is given by

$$[\hat{\alpha}_i] = \arg\min_{[\alpha_i] \in R^n} \left[\frac{1}{n} \sum_{i=1}^{n} L\left(\sum_{j=1}^{n} \alpha_j k(X_i, X_j), Y_i \right) + \lambda \sum_{i,j=1}^{n} \alpha_i \alpha_j k(X_i, X_j) \right]. \qquad (2)$$

The above formulations of kernel methods are standard. In the following, we present an equivalence of supervised kernel learning to a specific semi-supervised formulation. Although this representation is implicit in some earlier papers, the explicit form of this method is not well-known. As we shall see later, this new kernel learning formulation is critical for analyzing a class of graph-based semi-supervised learning methods.

In this framework, the *data graph* consists of nodes that are the data points X_j. The edge connecting two nodes X_i and X_j is weighted by $k(X_i, X_j)$. The following theorem, which establishes the graph kernel learning formulation we will study in this paper, essentially implies that graph-based semi-supervised learning is equivalent to the supervised learning method which employs the same kernel.

Theorem 2.1 (Graph Kernel Learning) *Consider labeled data $\{(X_i, Y_i)\}_{i=1,\ldots,n}$ and unlabeled data X_j ($j = n+1, \ldots, m$). Consider real-valued vectors $f = [f_1, \ldots, f_m]^T \in R^m$, and the following semi-supervised learning method:*

$$\hat{f} = \arg\inf_{f \in R^m} \left[\frac{1}{n} \sum_{i=1}^{n} L(f_i, Y_i) + \lambda f^T K^{-1} f \right], \qquad (3)$$

where K (often called gram-matrix in kernel learning or affinity matrix in graph learning) is an $m \times m$ matrix with $K_{i,j} = k(X_i, X_j) = \psi(X_i)^T \psi(X_j)$. Let $\hat{p}$ be the solution of (1), then $\hat{f}_j = \hat{p}(X_j)$ for $j = 1, \ldots, m$.

The kernel gram matrix K is always positive semi-definite. However, if K is not full rank (singular), then the correct interpretation of $f^T K^{-1} f$ is $\lim_{\mu \to 0^+} f^T (K + \mu I_{m \times m})^{-1} f$, where $I_{m \times m}$ is the $m \times m$ identity matrix. If we start with a given kernel k and let $K = [k(X_i, X_j)]$, then a semi-supervised learning method of the form (3) is equivalent to the supervised method (1). It follows that with a formulation like (3), the only way to utilize unlabeled data is to replace K by a kernel $\bar{K}$ in (3), or k by $\bar{k}$ in (2), where $\bar{K}$ (or $\bar{k}$) depends on the unlabeled data. In other words, the only benefit of unlabeled data in this setting is to construct a good kernel based on unlabeled data.

Some of previous graph-based semi-supervised learning methods employ the same formulation (3) with K^{-1} replaced by the graph Laplacian operator L (which we will describe in Section 5). However, the equivalence of this formulation and supervised kernel learning (with kernel matrix $K = L^{-1}$) was not obtained in these earlier studies. This equivalence is important for good theoretical understanding, as we will see later in this paper. Moreover, by treating graph-based supervised learning as unsupervised kernel design (see Figure 1), the scope of this paper is more general than graph Laplacian based methods.

Input: labeled data $[(X_i, Y_i)]_{i=1,\ldots,n}$, unlabeled data X_j $(j = n+1, \ldots, m)$
shrinkage factors $s_j \geq 0$ $(j = 1, \ldots, m)$, kernel function $k(\cdot, \cdot)$,
Output: predictive values $\hat{f}'_j$ on X_j $(j = 1, \ldots, m)$
Form the kernel matrix $K = [k(X_i, X_j)]$ $(i, j = 1, \ldots, m)$
Compute the kernel eigen-decomposition:
$\quad K = m \sum_{j=1}^m \mu_j v_j v_j^T$, where (μ_j, v_j) are eigenpairs of K $(v_j^T v_j = 1)$
Modify the kernel matrix as: $\bar{K} = m \sum_{j=1}^m s_j \mu_j v_j v_j^T$ $\quad (*)$
Compute $\hat{f}' = \arg\min_{f \in R^m} \left[\frac{1}{n} \sum_{i=1}^n L(f_i, Y_i) + \lambda f^T \bar{K}^{-1} f \right]$.

Figure 1: Spectral kernel design based semi-supervised learning on graph

In Figure 1, we consider a general formulation of semi-supervised learning method on data graph through spectral kernel design. This is the method we will analyze in the paper. As a special case, we can let $s_j = g(\mu_j)$ in Figure 1, where g is a rational function, then $\bar{K} = g(K/m)K$. In this special case, we do not have to compute eigen-decomposition of K. Therefore we obtain a simpler algorithm with the $(*)$ in Figure 1 replaced by

$$\bar{K} = g(K/m)K. \tag{4}$$

As mentioned earlier, the idea of using spectral kernel design has appeared in [2] although they didn't base their method on the graph formulation (3). However, we believe our analysis also sheds lights to their methods. The semi-supervised learning method described in Figure 1 is useful only when $\hat{f}'$ is a better predictor than $\hat{f}$ in Theorem 2.1 (which uses the original kernel K) – in other words, only when the new kernel $\bar{K}$ is better than K.

In the next few sections, we will investigate the following issues concerning the theoretical behavior of this algorithm: (a) the limiting behavior of $\hat{f}'$ as $m \to \infty$; that is, whether $\hat{f}'_j$ converges for each j; (b) the generalization performance of (3); (c) optimal Kernel design by minimizing the generalization error, and its implications; (d) statistical models under which spectral kernel design based semi-supervised learning is effective.

3 The Limiting Behavior of Graph-based Semi-supervised Learning

We want to show that as $m \to \infty$, the semi-supervised algorithm in Figure 1 is well-behaved. That is, $\hat{f}'_j$ converges as $m \to \infty$. This is one of the most fundamental issues.

Using feature space representation, we have $k(x, x') = \psi(x)^T \psi(x')$. Therefore a change of kernel can be regarded as a change of feature mapping. In particular, we consider a feature transformation of the form $\bar{\psi}(x) = S^{1/2}\psi(x)$, where S is an appropriate positive semi-definite operator on $\mathcal{H}$. The following result establishes an equivalent feature space formulation of the semi-supervised learning method in Figure 1.

Theorem 3.1 *Using notations in Figure 1. Assume $k(x, x') = \psi(x)^T \psi(x')$. Consider $S = \sum_{j=1}^m s_j u_j u_j^T$, where $u_j = \Psi v_j / \sqrt{\mu_j}$, $\Psi = [\psi(X_1), \dots, \psi(X_m)]$, then (μ_j, u_j) is an eigenpair of $\Psi\Psi^T/m$. Let*

$$\hat{p}'(x) = \hat{w}'^T S^{1/2}\psi(x), \qquad \hat{w}' = \arg\min_{w \in \mathcal{H}} \left[\frac{1}{n} \sum_{i=1}^n L(w^T S^{1/2}\psi(X_i), Y_i) + \lambda w^T w \right].$$

Then $\hat{f}'_j = \hat{p}'(X_j)$ $(j = 1, \dots, m)$.

The asymptotic behavior of Figure 1 when $m \to \infty$ can be easily understood from Theorem 3.1. In this case, we just replace $\Psi\Psi^T/m = \frac{1}{m}\sum_{j=1}^m \psi(X_j)\psi(X_j)^T$ by $\mathbf{E}_X \psi(X)\psi(X)^T$. The spectral decomposition of $\mathbf{E}_X \psi(X)\psi(X)^T$ corresponds to the feature space PCA. It is clear that if S converges, then the feature space algorithm in Theorem 3.1 also converges. In general, S converges if the eigenvectors u_j converges and the shrinkage factors s_j are bounded. As a special case, we have the following result.

Theorem 3.2 *Consider a sequence of data $X_1, X_2, \dots$ drawn from a distribution, with only the first n points labeled. Assume when $m \to \infty$, $\sum_{j=1}^m \psi(X_j)\psi(X_j)^T/m$ converges to $\mathbf{E}_X \psi(X)\psi(X)^T$ almost surely, and g is a continuous function in the spectral range of $\mathbf{E}_X \psi(X)\psi(X)^T$. Now in Figure 1 with $(*)$ given by (4) and kernel $k(x, x') = \psi(x)^T \psi(x')$, $\hat{f}'_j$ converges almost surely for each fixed j.*

4 Generalization analysis on graph

We study the generalization behavior of graph based semi-supervised learning algorithm (3), and use it to compare different kernels. We will then use this bound to justify the kernel design method given in Section 2. To measure the sample complexity, we consider m points (X_j, Y_j) for $i = 1, \dots, m$. We randomly pick n distinct integers $i_1, \dots, i_n$ from $\{1, \dots, m\}$ uniformly (sample without replacement), and regard it as the n labeled training data. We obtain predictive values $\hat{f}_j$ on the graph using the semi-supervised learning method (3) with the labeled data, and test it on the remaining $m - n$ data points. We are interested in the average predictive performance over all random draws.

Theorem 4.1 *Consider (X_j, Y_j) for $i = 1, \dots, m$. Assume that we randomly pick n distinct integers $i_1, \dots, i_n$ from $\{1, \dots, m\}$ uniformly (sample without replacement), and denote it by Z_n. Let $\hat{f}(Z_n)$ be the semi-supervised learning method (3) using training data in Z_n: $\hat{f}(Z_n) = \arg\min_{f \in R^m} \left[\frac{1}{n} \sum_{i \in Z_n} L(f_i, Y_i) + \lambda f^T K^{-1} f \right]$. If $|\frac{\partial}{\partial p} L(p, y)| \le \gamma$, and $L(p, y)$ is convex with respect to p, then we have*

$$\mathbf{E}_{Z_n} \frac{1}{m - n} \sum_{j \notin Z_n} L(\hat{f}_j(Z_n), Y_j) \le \inf_{f \in R^m} \left[\frac{1}{m} \sum_{j=1}^m L(f_j, Y_j) + \lambda f^T K^{-1} f + \frac{\gamma^2 \mathrm{tr}(K)}{2\lambda nm} \right].$$

The bound depends on the regularization parameter λ in addition to the kernel K. In order to compare different kernels, it is reasonable to compare the bound with the optimal λ for each K. That is, in addition to minimizing f, we also minimize over λ on the right hand of the bound. Note that in practice, it is usually not difficult to find a nearly-optimal λ through cross validation, implying that it is reasonable to assume that we can choose the optimal λ in the bound. With the optimal λ, we obtain:

$$\mathbf{E}_{Z_n} \frac{1}{m-n} \sum_{j \notin Z_n} L(\hat{f}_j(Z_n), Y_j) \leq \inf_{f \in R^m} \left[\frac{1}{m} \sum_{j=1}^{m} L(f_j, Y_j) + \frac{\gamma}{\sqrt{2n}} \sqrt{R(f, K)} \right],$$

where $R(f, K) = \operatorname{tr}(K/m) f^T K^{-1} f$ is the complexity of f with respect to kernel K.

If we define $\bar{K}$ as in Figure 1, then the complexity of a function f with respect to $\bar{K}$ is given by $R(f, \bar{K}) = (\sum_{j=1}^{m} s_j \mu_j)(\sum_{j=1}^{m} \alpha_j^2/(s_j \mu_j))$. If we believe that a good approximate target function f can be expressed as $f = \sum_j \alpha_j v_j$ with $|\alpha_j| \leq \beta_j$ for some known β_j, then based on this belief, the optimal choice of the shrinkage factor becomes $s_j = \beta_j/\mu_j$. That is, the kernel that optimizes the bound is $\bar{K} = \sum_j \beta_j v_j v_j^T$, where v_j are normalized eigenvectors of K. In this case, we have $R(f, \bar{K}) \leq (\sum_j \beta_j)^2$. The eigenvalues of the optimal kernel is thus independent of K, but depends only on the spectral coefficient's range β_j of the approximate target function.

Since there is no reason to believe that the eigenvalues μ_j of the original kernel K are proportional to the target spectral coefficient range. If we have some guess of the spectral coefficients of the target, then one may use the knowledge to obtain a better kernel. This justifies why spectral kernel design based algorithm can be potentially helpful (when we have some information on the target spectral coefficients). In practice, it is usually difficult to have a precise guess of β_j. However, for many application problems, we observe in practice that the eigenvalues of kernel K decays more slowly than that of the target spectral coefficients. In this case, our analysis implies that we should use an alternative kernel with faster eigenvalue decay: for example, using K^2 instead of K. This has a dimension reduction effect. That is, we effectively project the data into the principal components of data. The intuition is also quite clear: if the dimension of the target function is small (spectral coefficient decays fast), then we should project data to those dimensions by reducing the remaining noisy dimensions (corresponding to fast kernel eigenvalue decay).

5   Spectral analysis: the effect of input noise

We provide a justification on why spectral coefficients of the target function often decay faster than the eigenvalues of a natural kernel K. In essence, this is due to the fact that input vector X is often corrupted with noise. Together with results in the previous section, we know that in order to achieve optimal performance, we need to use a kernel with faster eigenvalue decay. We will demonstrate this phenomenon under a statistical model, and use the feature space notation in Section 3. For simplicity, we assume that $\psi(x) = x$.

We consider a two-class classification problem in R^∞ (with the standard 2-norm inner-product), where the label $Y = \pm 1$. We first start with a noise free model, where the data can be partitioned into p clusters. Each cluster ℓ is composed of a single center point $\bar{x}_\ell$ (having zero variance) with label $\bar{y}_\ell = \pm 1$. In this model, assume that the centers are well separated so that there is a weight vector w_* such that $w_*^T w_* < \infty$ and $w_*^T \bar{x}_\ell = \bar{y}_\ell$. Without loss of generality, we may assume that $\bar{x}_\ell$ and w_* belong to a p-dimensional subspace V_p. Let $V_p^\perp$ be its orthogonal complement. Assume now that the observed input data are corrupted with noise. We first generate a center index ℓ, and then noise δ (which may depend on ℓ). The observed input data is the corrupted data $X = \bar{x}_\ell + \delta$, and the observed output is $Y = w_*^T \bar{x}_\ell$. In this model, let $\ell(X_i)$ be the center corresponding to X_i, the observation can be decomposed as: $X_i = \bar{x}_{\ell(X_i)} + \delta(X_i)$, and $Y_i = w_*^T \bar{x}_{\ell(X_i)}$. Given noise δ, we decompose it as $\delta = \delta_1 + \delta_2$ where δ_1 is the orthogonal projection of δ in V_p, and δ_2 is the orthogonal projection of δ in $V_p^\perp$. We assume that δ_1 is a small noise component; the component δ_2 can be large but has small variance in every direction.

Theorem 5.1 *Consider the data generation model in this section, with observation $X = \bar{x}_\ell + \delta$ and $Y = w_*^T \bar{x}_\ell$. Assume that δ is conditionally zero-mean given ℓ: $\mathbf{E}_{\delta|\ell}\delta = 0$. Let $\mathbf{E}XX^T = \sum_j \mu_j u_j u_j^T$ be the spectral decomposition with decreasing eigenvalues μ_j ($u_j^T u_j = 1$). Then the following claims are valid: let $\sigma_1^2 \geq \sigma_2^2 \geq \cdots$ be the eigenvalues of $\mathbf{E}\delta_2\delta_2^T$, then $\mu_j \geq \sigma_j^2$; if $\|\delta_1\|_2 \leq b/\|w_*\|_2$, then $|w_*^T X_i - Y_i| \leq b$; $\forall t \geq 0$, $\sum_{j\geq 1} (w_*^T u_j)^2 \mu_j^{-t} \leq w_*^T (\mathbf{E} \bar{x}_\ell \bar{x}_\ell^T)^{-t} w_*$.*

Consider m points $X_1, \ldots, X_m$. Let $\Psi = [X_1, \ldots, X_m]$ and $K = \Psi^T \Psi = m \sum_j \mu_j v_j v_j^T$ be the kernel spectral decomposition. Let $u_j = \Psi v_j / \sqrt{m\mu_j}$, $f_i = w_*^T X_i$, and $f = \sum_j \alpha_j v_j$. Then it is not difficult to verify that $\alpha_j = \sqrt{m\mu_j} w_*^T u_j$. If we assume that asymptotically $\frac{1}{m} \sum_{i=1}^m X_i X_i^T \to \mathbf{E}XX^T$, then we have the following consequences:

- $f_i = w_*^T X_i$ is a good approximate target when b is small. In particular, if $b < 1$, then this function always gives the correct class label.
- For all $t > 0$, the spectral coefficient α_j of f decays as $\frac{1}{m} \sum_{j=1}^m \alpha_j^2 / \mu_j^{1+t} \leq w_*^T (\mathbf{E}\bar{x}_\ell \bar{x}_\ell^T)^{-t} w_*$.
- The eigenvalue μ_j decays slowly when the noise spectral decays slowly: $\mu_j \geq \sigma_j^2$.

If the clean data are well behaved in that we can find a weight vector such that $w_*^T (\mathbf{E}_X \bar{x}_{\ell(X)} \bar{x}_{\ell(X)}^T)^{-t} w_*$ is bounded for some $t > 1$, then when the data are corrupted with noise, we can find a good approximate target that has spectral decay faster (on average) than that of the kernel eigenvalues. This analysis implies that if the feature representation associated with the original kernel is corrupted with noise, then it is often helpful to use a kernel with faster spectral decay. For example, instead of using K, we may use $\bar{K} = K^2$. However, it may not be easy to estimate the exact decay rate of the target spectral coefficients. In practice, one may use cross validation to optimize the kernel.

A kernel with fast spectral decay projects the data into the most prominent principal components. Therefore we are interested in designing kernels which can achieve a dimension reduction effect. Although one may use direct eigenvalue computation, an alternative is to use a function $g(K/m)K$ for such an effect, as in (4). For example, we may consider a normalized kernel such that $K/m = \sum_j \mu_j u_j u_j^T$ where $0 \leq u_j \leq 1$. A standard normalization method is to use $D^{-1/2}KD^{-1/2}$, where D is the diagonal matrix with each entry corresponding to the row sums of K. It follows that $g(K/m)K = m \sum_j g(\mu_j)\mu_j u_j u_j^T$. We are interested in a function g such that $g(\mu)\mu \approx 1$ when $\mu \in [\alpha, 1]$ for some α, and $g(\mu)\mu \approx 0$ when $\mu < \alpha$ (where α is close to 1). One such function is to let $g(\mu)\mu = (1-\alpha)/(1-\alpha\mu)$. This is the function used in various graph Laplacian formulations with normalized Gaussian kernel as the initial kernel K. For example, see [5]. Our analysis suggests that it is the dimension reduction effect of this function that is important, rather than the connection to graph Laplacian. As we shall see in the empirical examples, other kernels such as K^2, which achieve similar dimension reduction effect (but has nothing to do with graph Laplacian), also improve performance.

6 Empirical Examples

This section shows empirical examples to demonstrate some consequences of our theoretical analysis. We use the MNIST data set (http://yann.lecun.com/exdb/mnist/), consisting of hand-written digit images (representing 10 classes, from digit "0" to digit "9"). In the following experiments, we randomly draw $m = 2000$ samples. We regard $n = 100$ of them as labeled data, and the remaining $m - n = 1900$ as unlabeled test data.

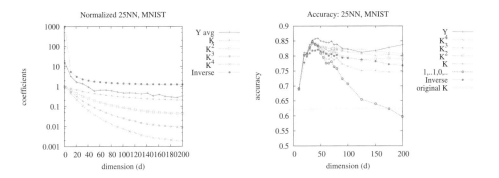

Figure 2: Left: spectral coefficients; right: classification accuracy.

Throughout the experiments, we use the least squares loss: $L(p, y) = (p - y)^2$ for simplicity. We study the performance of various kernel design methods, by changing the spectral coefficients of the initial gram matrix K, as in Figure 1. Below we write $\bar{\mu}_j$ for the new spectral coefficient of the new gram matrix $\bar{K}$: i.e., $\bar{K} = \sum_{i=1}^{m} \bar{\mu}_i v_i v_i^T$. We study the following kernel design methods (also see [2]), with a dimension cut off parameter d, so that $\bar{\mu}_i = 0$ when $i > d$. (a) $[1, \ldots, 1, 0, \ldots, 0]$: $\bar{\mu}_i = 1$ if $i \leq d$, and 0 otherwise. This was used in spectral clustering [3]. (b) K: $\bar{\mu}_i = \mu_i$ if $i \leq d$; 0 otherwise. This method is essentially kernel principal component analysis which keeps the d most significant principal components of K. (c) K^p: $\bar{\mu}_i = \mu_i^p$ if $i \leq d$; 0 otherwise. We set $p = 2, 3, 4$. This accelerates the decay of eigenvalues of K. (d) Inverse: $\bar{\mu}_i = 1/(1 - \rho\mu_i)$ if $i \leq d$; 0 otherwise. ρ is a constant close to 1 (we used 0.999). This is essentially graph-Laplacian based semi-supervised learning for normalized kernel (e.g. see [5]). Note that the standard graph-Laplacian formulation sets $d = m$. (e) Y: $\bar{\mu}_i = |Y^T v_i|$ if $i \leq d$; 0 otherwise. This is the oracle kernel that optimizes our generalization bound. The purpose of testing this oracle method is to validate our analysis by checking whether good kernel in our theory produces good classification performance on real data. Note that in the experiments, we use averaged Y over the ten classes. Therefore the resulting kernel will not be the best possible kernel for each specific class, and thus its performance may not always be optimal.

Figure 2 shows the spectral coefficients of the above mentioned kernel design methods and the corresponding classification performance. The initial kernel is normalized 25-NN, which is defined as $K = D^{-1/2} W D^{-1/2}$ (see previous section), where $W_{ij} = 1$ if either the i-th example is one of the 25 nearest neighbors of the j-th example or vice versa; and 0 otherwise. As expected, the results demonstrate that the target spectral coefficients Y decay faster than that of the original kernel K. Therefore it is useful to use kernel design methods that accelerate the eigenvalue decay. The accuracy plot on the right is consistent with our theory. The near oracle kernel 'Y' performs well especially when the dimension cut-off is large. With appropriate dimension d, all methods perform better than the supervised base-line (original K) which is below 65%. With appropriate dimension cut-off, all methods perform similarly (over 80%). However, K^p with ($p = 2, 3, 4$) is less sensitive to the cut-off dimension d than the kernel principal component dimension reduction method K. Moreover, the hard threshold method in spectral clustering ($[1, \ldots, 1, 0, \ldots, 0]$) is not stable. Similar behavior can also be observed with other initial kernels. Figure 3 shows the classification accuracy with the standard Gaussian kernel as the initial kernel K, both with and without normalization. We also used different bandwidth t to illustrate that the behavior of different methods are similar with different t (in a reasonable range). The result shows that normalization is not critical for achieving high performance, at least for this data. Again, we observe that the near oracle method performs extremely well. The spectral clustering kernel is sensitive to the cut-off dimension, while K^p with $p = 2, 3, 4$ are quite stable. The standard kernel principal component dimension reduction (method K) performs very well with appropriately chosen dimension cut-off. The experiments are consistent with our theoretical analysis.

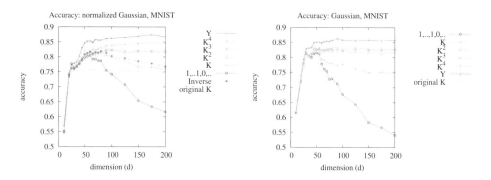

Figure 3: Classification accuracy with Gaussian kernel $k(i, j) = \exp(-\|x_i - x_j\|_2^2/t)$. Left: normalized Gaussian ($t = 0.1$); right: unnormalized Gaussian ($t = 0.3$).

7 Conclusion

We investigated a class of graph-based semi-supervised learning methods. By establishing a graph-based formulation of kernel learning, we showed that this class of semi-supervised learning methods is equivalent to supervised kernel learning with unsupervised kernel design (explored in [2]). We then obtained a generalization bound, which implies that the eigenvalues of the optimal kernel should decay at the same rate of the target spectral coefficients. Moreover, we showed that input noise can cause the target spectral coefficients to decay faster than the kernel spectral coefficients. The analysis explains why it is often helpful to modify the original kernel eigenvalues to achieve a dimension reduction effect.

References

[1] Mikhail Belkin and Partha Niyogi. Semi-supervised learning on Riemannian manifolds. *Machine Learning*, Special Issue on Clustering:209–239, 2004.

[2] Olivier Chapelle, Jason Weston, and Bernhard Sch:olkopf. Cluster kernels for semi-supervised learning. In *NIPS*, 2003.

[3] Andrew Y. Ng, Michael I. Jordan, and Yair Weiss. On spectral clustering: Analysis and an algorithm. In *NIPS*, pages 849–856, 2001.

[4] M. Szummer and T. Jaakkola. Partially labeled classification with Markov random walks. In *NIPS 2001*, 2002.

[5] D. Zhou, O. Bousquet, T.N. Lal, J. Weston, and B. Schlkopf. Learning with local and global consistency. In *NIPS 2003*, pages 321–328, 2004.

[6] Xiaojin Zhu, Zoubin Ghahramani, and John Lafferty. Semi-supervised learning using Gaussian fields and harmonic functions. In *ICML 2003*, 2003.

A Computational Model of Eye Movements during Object Class Detection

Wei Zhang[†]   **Hyejin Yang**[‡*]   **Dimitris Samaras**[†]   **Gregory J. Zelinsky**[†‡]

Dept. of Computer Science[†]   Dept. of Psychology[‡]

State University of New York at Stony Brook

Stony Brook, NY 11794

{wzhang,samaras}@cs.sunysb.edu[†]   hjyang@ic.sunysb.edu[*]

Gregory.Zelinsky@stonybrook.edu[‡]

Abstract

We present a computational model of human eye movements in an object class detection task. The model combines state-of-the-art computer vision object class detection methods (SIFT features trained using AdaBoost) with a biologically plausible model of human eye movement to produce a sequence of simulated fixations, culminating with the acquisition of a target. We validated the model by comparing its behavior to the behavior of human observers performing the identical object class detection task (looking for a teddy bear among visually complex non-target objects). We found considerable agreement between the model and human data in multiple eye movement measures, including number of fixations, cumulative probability of fixating the target, and scanpath distance.

1. Introduction

Object detection is one of our most common visual operations. Whether we are driving [1], making a cup of tea [2], or looking for a tool on a workbench [3], hundreds of times each day our visual system is being asked to detect, localize, or acquire through movements of gaze objects and patterns in the world.

In the human behavioral literature, this topic has been extensively studied in the context of visual search. In a typical search task, observers are asked to indicate, usually by button press, whether a specific target is present or absent in a visual display (see [4] for a review). A primary manipulation in these studies is the number of non-target objects also appearing in the scene. A bedrock finding in this literature is that, for targets that cannot be defined by a single visual feature, target detection times increase linearly with the number of non-targets, a form of clutter or "set size" effect. Moreover, the slope of the function relating detection speed to set size is steeper (by roughly a factor of two) when the target is absent from the scene compared to when it is present. Search theorists have interpreted these findings as evidence for visual attention moving serially from one object to the next, with the human detection operation typically limited to those objects fixated by this "spotlight" of attention [5].

Object class detection has also been extensively studied in the computer vision community, with faces and cars being the two most well researched object classes [6, 7, 8, 9]. The related but simpler task of object class recognition (target recognition without localization) has also been the focus of exciting recent work [10, 11, 12]. Both tasks use supervised learning methods to extract visual features. Scenes are typically realistic and highly cluttered, with object appearance varying greatly due to illumination, view, and scale changes. The task addressed in this paper falls between the class detection and recognition problems. Like object class detection, we will be detecting and localizing class-defined targets; unlike object class detection the test images will be composed of at most 20 objects appearing on a simple background.

Both the behavioral and computer vision literatures have strengths and weaknesses when it comes to understanding human object class detection. The behavioral literature has accumulated a great deal of knowledge regarding the conditions affecting object detection [4], but this psychology-based literature has been dominated by the use of simple visual patterns and models that cannot be easily generalized to fully realistic scenes (see [13, 14] for notable exceptions). Moreover, this literature has focused almost entirely on object-specific detection, cases in which the observer knows precisely how the target will appear in the test display (see [15] for a discussion of target non-specific search using featurally complex objects). Conversely, the computer vision literature is rich with models and methods allowing for the featural representation of object classes and the detection of these classes in visually cluttered real-world scenes, but none of these methods have been validated as models of human object class detection by comparison to actual behavioral data.

The current study draws upon the strengths of both of these literatures to produce the first joint behavioral-computational study of human object class detection. First, we use an eyetracker to quantify human behavior in terms of the number of fixations made during an object class detection task. Then we introduce a computational model that not only performs the detection task at a level comparable to that of the human observers, but also generates a sequence of simulated eye movements similar in pattern to those made by humans performing the identical detection task.

2. Experimental methods

An effort was made to keep the human and model experiments methodologically similar. Both experiments used training, validation (practice trials in the human experiment), and testing phases, and identical images were presented to the model and human subjects in all three of these phases. The target class consisted of 378 teddy bears scanned from [16]. Nontargets consisted of 2,975 objects selected from the Hemera Photo Objects Collection. Samples of the bear and nontarget objects are shown in Figure 1. All objects were normalized to have a bounding box area of 8,000 pixels, but were highly variable in appearance.

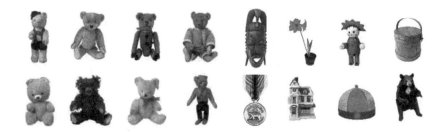

Figure 1: Representative teddy bears (left) and nontarget objects (right).

The training set consisted of 180 bears and 500 nontargets, all randomly selected. In the case of the human experiment, each of these objects was shown centered on a white background and displayed for 1 second. The testing set consisted of 180 new bears and nontargets. No objects were repeated between training and testing, and no objects were repeated within either of the training or testing phases. Test images depicted 6, 13, or 20 color objects randomly positioned on a white background. A single bear was present in half (90) of these displays. Human subjects were instructed to indicate, by pressing a button, whether a teddy bear appeared among the displayed objects. Target presence and set size were randomly interleaved over trials. Each test trial in the human experiment began with the subject fixating gaze at the center of the display, and eye position was monitored throughout each trial using an eyetracker. Eight students from Stony Brook University participated in the experiment.

3. Model of eye movements during object class detection

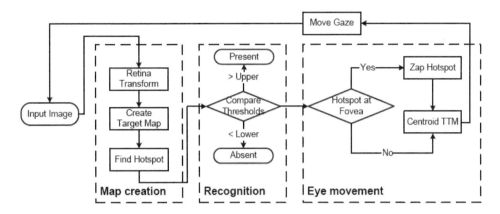

Figure 2: The flow of processing through our model.

Building on a framework described in [17, 14, 18], our model can be broadly divided into three stages (Figure 2): (1) creating a target map based on a retinally-transformed version of the input image, (2) recognizing the target using thresholds placed on the target map, and (3) the operations required in the generation of eye movements. The following sub-sections describe each of the Figure 2 steps in greater detail.

3.1. Retina transform
With each change in gaze position (set initially to the center of the image), our model transforms the input image so as to reflect the acuity limitations imposed by the human retina. We used the method described in [19, 20], which was shown to provide a close approximation to human acuity limitations, to implement this dynamic retina transform.

3.2. Create target map
Each point on the target map ranges in value between 0 and 1 and indicates the likelihood that a target is located at that point. To create the target map, we first compute interest points on the retinally-transformed image (see section 3.2.2), then compare the features surrounding these points to features of the target object class extracted during training. Two types of discriminative features were used in this study: color features and texture features.

3.2.1. Color features
Color has long been used as a feature for instance object recognition [21]. In our study we explore the potential use of color as a discriminative feature for an object class. Specifically, we used a normalized color histogram of pixel hues in HSV space. Because backgrounds in our images were white and therefore uninformative, we set thresholds on the saturation and brightness channels to remove these points. The hue channel was evenly divided into 11 bins and each pixel's hue value was assigned to one of these bins using binary interpolation.

Values within each bin were weighted by $1 - d$, where d is the normalized unit distance to the center of the bin. The final color histogram was normalized to be a unit vector.

Given a test image, I_t, and its color feature, H_t, we compute the distances between H_t and the color features of the training set $\{H_i, i = 1, ..., N\}$. The test image is labeled as: $l(I_t) = l(I_{\arg\min_{1 \leq i \leq N} \chi^2(H_t, H_i)})$, and the distance metric used was: $\chi^2(H_t, H_i) = \sum_{k=1}^{K} \frac{[H_t(k) - H_i(k)]^2}{H_t(k) + H_i(k)}$, where K is the number of bins.

3.2.2. Texture features

Local texture features were extracted on the gray level images during both training and testing. To do this, we first used a Difference-of-Gaussian (DoG) operator to detect interest points in the image, then used a Scale Invariant Feature Transform (SIFT) descriptor to represent features at each of the interest point locations. SIFT features consist of a histogram representation of the gradient orientation and magnitude information within a small image patch surrounding a point [22].

AdaBoost is a feature selection method which produces a very accurate prediction rule by combining relatively inaccurate rules-of-thumb [23]. Following the method described in [11, 12], we used AdaBoost during training to select a small set of SIFT features from among all the SIFT features computed for each sample in the training set. Specifically, each training image was represented by a set of SIFT features $\{F_{i,j}, j = 1, ...n_i\}$, where n_i is the number of SIFT features in sample I_i. To select features from this set, AdaBoost first initialized the weights of the training samples w_i to $\frac{1}{2N_p}$, $\frac{1}{2N_n}$, where N_p and N_n are the number of positive and negative samples, respectively. For each round of AdaBoost, we then selected one feature as a weak classifier and updated the weights of the training samples. Details regarding the algorithm used for each round of boosting can be found in [12]. Eventually, T features were chosen having the best ability to discriminate the target object class from the nontargets. Each of these selected features forms a weak classifier, h_k, consisting of three components: a feature vector, (f_k), a distance threshold, (θ_k), and an output label, (u_k). Only the features from the positive training samples are used as weak classifiers. For each feature vector, F, we compute the distance between it and the training sample, i, defined as $d_i = \min_{1 \leq j \leq n_i} D(F_{i,j}, F_0)$, then apply the classification rule:

$$h(f, \theta) = \left\{ \begin{array}{l} 1, d < \theta \\ 0, d \geq \theta \end{array} \right. \quad . \tag{1}$$

After the desired number of weak classifiers has been found, the final strong classifier can be defined as:

$$H = \sum_{t=1}^{T} \alpha_t h_t \tag{2}$$

where $\alpha_t = log(1/\beta_t)$. Here $\beta_t = \sqrt{\frac{1 - \epsilon_t}{\epsilon_t}}$ and the classification error $\epsilon_t = \sum |u_k - l_k|$.

3.2.3. Validation

A validation set, consisting of the practice trials viewed by the human observers, was used to set parameters in the model. Because our model used two types of features, each having different classifiers with different outputs, some weight for combining these classifiers was needed. The validation set was used to set this weighting.

The output of the color classifier, normalized to unit length, was based on the distance $\chi^2_{min} = \min_{1 \leq i \leq N}$ and defined as:

$$C_{color} = \left\{ \begin{array}{l} 0, l(I_t) = 0 \\ f(\chi^2_{min}), l(I_t) = 1 \end{array} \right. \tag{3}$$

where $f(\chi^2_{min})$ is a function monotonically decreasing with respect to χ^2_{min}. The strong local texture classifier, $C_{texture}$ (Equation 2), also had normalized unit output.

The weights of the two classifiers were determined based on their classification errors on the validation set:

$$W_{color} = \frac{\epsilon_t}{\epsilon_c + \epsilon_t},$$
$$W_{texture} = \frac{\epsilon_c}{\epsilon_c + \epsilon_t} \qquad . \qquad (4)$$

The final combined output was used to generate the values in the target map and, ultimately, to guide the model's simulated eye movements.

3.3. Recognition

We define the highest-valued point on the target map as the *hotspot*. Recognition is accomplished by comparing the hotspot to two thresholds, also set through validation. If the hotspot value exceeds the high target-present threshold, then the object will be recognized as an instance of the target class. If the hotspot value falls below the target-absent threshold, then the object will be classified as not belonging to the target class. Through validation, the target-present threshold was set to yield a low false positive rate and the target-absent threshold was set to yield a high true positive rate. Moreover, target-present judgments were permitted only if the hotspot was fixated by the simulated fovea. This constraint was introduced so as to avoid extremely high false positive rates stemming from the creation of false targets in the blurred periphery of the retina-transformed image.

3.4. Eye movement

If neither the target-present nor the target-absent thresholds are satisfied, processing passes to the eye movement stage of our model. If the simulated fovea is not on the hotspot, the model will make an eye movement to move gaze steadily toward the hotspot location. Fixation in our model is defined as the centroid of activity on the target map, a computation consistent with a neuronal population code. Eye movements are made by thresholding this map over time, pruning off values that offer the least evidence for the target. Eventually, this thresholding operation will cause the centroid of the target map to pass an eye movement threshold, resulting in a gaze shift to the new centroid location. See [18] for details regarding the eye movement generation process. If the simulated fovea does acquire the hotspot and the target-present threshold is still not met, the model will assume that a non-target was fixated and this object will be "zapped". Zapping consists of applying a negative Gaussian filter to the hotspot location, thereby preventing attention and gaze from returning to this object (see [24] for a previous computational implementation of a conceptually related operation).

4. Experimental results

Model and human behavior were compared on a variety of measures, including error rates, number of fixations, cumulative probability of fixating the target, and scanpath ratio (a measure of how directly gaze moved to the target). For each measure, the model and human data were in reasonable agreement.

Table 1: Error rates for model and human subjects.

	Total trials	Misses		False positives	
		Frequency	Rate	Frequency	Rate
Human	1440	46	3.2%	14	1.0%
Model	180	7	3.9%	4	2.2%

Table 1 shows the error rates for the human subjects and the model, grouped by misses and false positives. Note that the data from all eight of the human subjects are shown, resulting in the greater number of total trials. There are two key patterns. First, despite the very high level of accuracy exhibited by the human subjects in this task, our model was able to

Table 2: Average number of fixations by model and human.

Case	Target-present				Target-absent			
	p6	p13	p20	slope	a6	a13	a20	slope
Human	3.38	3.74	4.88	0.11	4.89	7.23	9.39	0.32
Model	2.86	3.69	5.68	0.20	3.97	8.30	10.47	0.46

achieve comparable levels of accuracy. Second, and consistent with the behavioral search literature, miss rates were larger than false positive rates for both the humans and model.

To the extent that our model offers an accurate account of human object detection behavior, it should be able to predict the average number of fixations made by human subjects in the detection task. As indicated in Table 2, this indeed is the case. Data are grouped by target-present (p), target-absent (a), and the number of objects in the scene (6, 13, 20). In all conditions, the model and human subjects made comparable numbers of fixations. Also consistent with the behavioral literature, the average number of fixations made by human subjects in our task increased with the number of objects in the scenes, and the rate of this increase was greater in the target-absent data compared to the target-present data. Both of these patterns are also present in the model data. The fact that our model is able to capture an interaction between set size and target presence in terms of the number of fixations needed for detection lends support for our method.

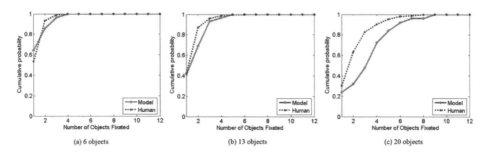

(a) 6 objects   (b) 13 objects   (c) 20 objects

Figure 3: Cumulative probability of target fixation by model and human.

Figure 3 shows the number of fixation data in more detail. Plotted are the cumulative probabilities of fixating the target as a function of the number of objects fixated during the search task. When the scene contained only 6 or 13 objects, the model and the humans fixated roughly the same number of nontargets before finally shifting gaze to the target. When the scene was more cluttered (20 objects), the model fixated an average of 1 additional nontarget relative to the human subjects, a difference likely indicating a liberal bias in our human subjects under these search conditions. Overall, these analyses suggest that our model was not only making the same number of fixations as humans, but it was also fixating the same number of nontargets during search as our human subjects.

Table 3: Comparison of model and human scanpath distance

#Objects	6	13	20
Human	1.62	2.20	2.80
Model	1.93	3.09	6.10
MODEL	1.93	2.80	3.43

Human gaze does not jump randomly from one item to another during search, but instead moves in a more orderly way toward the target. The ultimate test of our model would be to reproduce this orderly movement of gaze. As a first approximation, we quantify this behavior in terms of a scanpath distance. Scanpath distance is defined as the ratio of the total scanpath length (i.e., the summed distance traveled by the eye) and the distance between the target and the center of the image (i.e., the minimum distance that the eye would need to travel to fixate the target). As indicated in Table 3, the model and human data are in close agreement in the 6 and 13-object scenes, but not in the 20-object scenes. Upon closer inspection of the data, we found several cases in which the model made multiple fixations between two nontarget objects, a very unnatural behavior arising from too small of a setting for our Gaussian "zap" window. When these 6 trials were removed, the model data (MODEL) and the human data were in closer agreement.

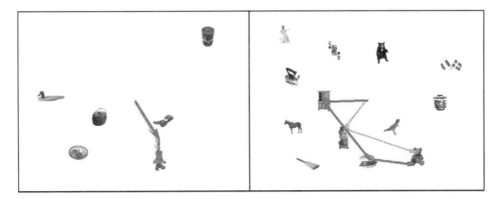

Figure 4: Representative scanpaths. Model data are shown in thick red lines, human data are shown in thin green lines.

Figure 4 shows representative scanpaths from the model and one human subject for two search scenes. Although the scanpaths do not align perfectly, there is a qualitative agreement between the human and model in the path followed by gaze to the target.

5. Conclusion

Search tasks do not always come with specific targets. Very often, we need to search for dogs, or chairs, or pens, without any clear idea of the visual features comprising these objects. Despite the prevalence of these tasks, the problem of object class detection has attracted surprisingly little research within the behavioral community [15], and has been applied to a relatively narrow range of objects within the computer vision literature [6, 7, 8, 9]. The current work adds to our understanding of this important topic in two key respects. First, we provide a detailed eye movement analysis of human behavior in an object class detection task. Second, we incorporate state-of-the-art computer vision object detection methods into a biologically plausible model of eye movement control, then validate this model by comparing its behavior to the behavior of our human observers. Computational models capable of describing human eye movement behavior are extremely rare [25]; the fact that the current model was able to do so for multiple eye movement measures lends strength to our approach. Moreover, our model was able to detect targets nearly as well as the human observers while maintaining a low false positive rate, a difficult standard to achieve in a generic detection model. Such agreement between human and model suggests that simple color and texture features may be used to guide human attention and eye movement in an object class detection task.

Future computational work will explore the generality of our object class detection method to tasks with visually complex backgrounds, and future human work will attempt to use neuroimaging techniques to localize object class representations in the brain.

Acknowledgments

This work was supported by grants from the NIMH (R01-MH63748) and ARO (DAAD19-03-1-0039) to G.J.Z.

References

[1] M. F. Land and D. N. Lee. Where we look when we steer. *Nature*, 369(6483):742–744, 1994.

[2] M. F. Land and M. Hayhoe. In what ways do eye movements contribute to everyday activities. *Vision Research*, 41(25-36):3559–3565, 2001.

[3] G. Zelinsky, R. Rao, M. Hayhoe, and D. Ballard. Eye movements reveal the spatio-temporal dynamics of visual search. *Psychological Science*, 8:448–453, 1997.

[4] J. Wolfe. Visual search. In *H. Pashler (Ed.), Attention*, pages 13–71. London: University College London Press, 1997.

[5] E. Weichselgartner and G. Sperling. Dynamics of automatic and controlled visual attention. *Science*, 238(4828):778–780, 1987.

[6] H. Schneiderman and T. Kanade. A statistical method for 3d object detection applied to faces and cars. In *CVPR*, volume I, pages 746–751, 2000.

[7] P. Viola and M.J. Jones. Rapid object detection using a boosted cascade of simple features. In *CVPR*, volume I, pages 511–518, 2001.

[8] S. Agarwal and D. Roth. Learning a sparse representation for object detection. In *ECCV*, volume IV, page 113, 2002.

[9] Wolf Kienzle, Gökhan H. Bakır, Matthias O. Franz, and Bernhard Schölkopf. Face detection - efficient and rank deficient. In *NIPS*, 2004.

[10] R. Fergus, P. Perona, and A. Zisserman. Object class recognition by unsupervised scale-invariant learning. In *CVPR03*, volume II, pages 264–271, 2003.

[11] A. Opelt, M. Fussenegger, A. Pinz, and P. Auer. Weak hypotheses and boosting for generic object detection and recognition. In *ECCV04*, volume II, pages 71–84, 2004.

[12] W. Zhang, B. Yu, G. Zelinsky, and D. Samaras. Object class recognition using multiple layer boosting with multiple features. In *CVPR*, 2005.

[13] L. Itti and C. Koch. A saliency-based search mechanism for overt and covert shifts of visual attention. *Vision Research*, 40:1489–1506, 2000.

[14] R. Rao, G. Zelinsky, M. Hayhoe, and D. Ballard. Eye movements in iconic visual search. *Vision Research*, 42:1447–1463, 2002.

[15] D. T. Levin, Y. Takarae, A. G. Miner, and F. Keil. Efficient visual search by category: Specifying the features that mark the difference between artifacts and animal in preattentive vision. *Perception and Psychophysics*, 63(4):676–697, 2001.

[16] P. Cockrill. *The teddy bear encyclopedia*. New York: DK Publishing, Inc., 2001.

[17] R. Rao, G. Zelinsky, M. Hayhoe, and D. Ballard. Modeling saccadic targeting in visual search. In *NIPS*, 1995.

[18] G. Zelinsky. *Itti, L., Rees, G. and Tsotos, J.(Eds.), Neurobiology of attention*, chapter Specifying the components of attention in a visual search task, pages 395–400. Elsevier, 2005.

[19] W.S. Geisler and J.S. Perry. A real-time foveated multi-resolution system for low-bandwidth video communications. In *Human Vision and Electronic Imaging, SPIE Proceddings*, volume 3299, pages 294–305, 1998.

[20] J.S. Perry and W.S. Geisler. Gaze-contingent real-time simulation of arbitrary visual fields. In *SPIE*, 2002.

[21] M.J. Swain and D.H. Ballard. Color indexing. *IJCV*, 7(1):11–32, November 1991.

[22] D.G. Lowe. Distinctive image features from scale-invariant keypoints. *IJCV*, 60(2):91–110, November 2004.

[23] Y. Freund and R.E. Schapire. A decision-theoretic generalization of on-line learning and an application to boosting. *Journal of Computer and System Sciences*, 55(1):119–139, 1997.

[24] K. Yamada and G. Cottrell. A model of scan paths applied to face recognition. In *Seventeenth Annual Cognitive Science Conference*, pages 55–60, 1995.

[25] C. M. Privitera and L. W. Stark. Algorithms for defining visual regions-of-interest: comparison with eye fixations. *PAMI*, 22:970–982, 2000.

Separation of Music Signals by Harmonic Structure Modeling

Yun-Gang Zhang
Department of Automation
Tsinghua University
Beijing 100084, China
zyg00@mails.tsinghua.edu.cn

Chang-Shui Zhang
Department of Automation
Tsinghua University
Beijing 100084, China
zcs@mail.tsinghua.edu.cn

Abstract

Separation of music signals is an interesting but difficult problem. It is helpful for many other music researches such as audio content analysis. In this paper, a new music signal separation method is proposed, which is based on harmonic structure modeling. The main idea of harmonic structure modeling is that the harmonic structure of a music signal is stable, so a music signal can be represented by a harmonic structure model. Accordingly, a corresponding separation algorithm is proposed. The main idea is to learn a harmonic structure model for each music signal in the mixture, and then separate signals by using these models to distinguish harmonic structures of different signals. Experimental results show that the algorithm can separate signals and obtain not only a very high Signal-to-Noise Ratio (SNR) but also a rather good subjective audio quality.

1 Introduction

Audio content analysis is an important area in music research. There are many open problems in this area, such as content based music retrieval and classification, Computational Auditory Scene Analysis (CASA), Multi-pitch Estimation, Automatic Transcription, Query by Humming, etc. [1, 2, 3, 4]. In all these problems, content extraction and representation is where the shoe pinches. In a song, the sounds of different instruments are mixed together, and it is difficult to parse the information of each instrument. Separation of sound sources in a mixture is a difficult problem and no reliable methods are available for the general case. However, music signals are so different from general signals. So, we try to find a way to separate music signals by utilizing the special character of music signals. After source separation, many audio content analysis problems will become much easier. In this paper, a music signal means a monophonic music signal performed by one instrument. A song is a mixture of several music signals and one or more singing voice signals.

As we know, music signals are more "ordered" than voice. The entropy of music is much more constant in time than that of speech [5]. More essentially, we found that an important character of a music signal is that its harmonic structure is stable. And the harmonic structures of music signals performed by different instruments are different. So, a harmonic structure model is built to represent a music signal. This model is the fundamental of the separation algorithm. In the separation algorithm, an extended multi-pitch estimation algorithm is used to extract harmonic structures of all sources, and a clustering algorithm is used to calculate harmonic structure models. Then, signals are separated by using these models to distinguish harmonic structures of different signals.

There are many other signal separation methods, such as ICA [6]. General signal separation methods do not sufficiently utilize the special character of music signals. Gil-Jin and Te-Won proposed a probabilistic approach to single channel blind signal separation [7], which is based on exploiting the inherent time structure of sound sources by learning a priori sets of basis filters. In our approach, training sets are not required, and all information are directly learned from the mixture. Feng et al. applied FastICA to extract singing and accompaniment from a mixture [8]. Vanroose used ICA to remove music background from speech by subtracting ICA components with the lowest entropy [9]. Compared to these approaches, our method can separate each individual instrument sound, preserve the harmonic structure in the separated signals and obtain a good subjective audio quality. One of the most important contributions of our method is that it can significantly improve the accuracy of multi-pitch estimation. Compared to previous methods, our method learns models from the primary multi-pitch estimation results, and uses these models to improve the results. More importantly, pitches of different sources can be distinguished by these models. This advantage is significant for automatic transcription.

The rest of this paper is organized as follows: Harmonic structure modeling is detailed in Section two. The algorithm is described in section three. Experimental results are shown in section four. Finally, conclusion and discussions are given in section five.

2 Harmonic structure modeling for music signals

A monophonic music signal $s(t)$ can be represented by a sinusoidal model [10]:

$$s(t) = \sum_{r=1}^{R} A_r(t) \cos[\theta_r(t)] + e(t) \tag{1}$$

where $A_r(t)$ and $\theta_r(t) = \int_0^t 2\pi r f_0(\tau) d\tau$ are the instantaneous amplitude and phase of the rth harmonic, respectively, R is the maximal harmonic number, $f_0(\tau)$ is the fundamental frequency at time τ, $e(t)$ is the noise component.

We divide $s(t)$ into overlapped frames and calculate f_0^l and A_r^l by detecting peaks in the magnitude spectrum. $A_r^l = 0$, if there doesn't exist the rth harmonic. $l = 1, \ldots, L$ is the frame index. f_0^l and $[A_1^l, \ldots, A_R^l]$ describe the position and amplitudes of harmonics. We normalize A_r^l by multiplying a factor $\rho^l = C/A_1^l$ (C is an arbitrary constant) to eliminate the influence of the amplitude. We translate the amplitudes into a log scale, because the human ear has a roughly logarithmic sensitivity to signal intensity. Harmonic Structure Coefficient is then defined as equation (2). The timbre of a sound is mostly controlled by the number of harmonics and the ratio of their amplitudes, so $\mathbf{B}^l = [B_1^l, \ldots, B_R^l]$, which is free from the fundamental frequency and amplitude, exactly represents the timbre of a sound. In this paper, these coefficients are used to represent the harmonic structure of a sound. Average Harmonic Structure and Harmonic Structure Stability are defined as follows to model music signals and measure the stability of harmonic structures.

- Harmonic Structure $\mathbf{B}^l$, B_i^l is Harmonic Structure Coefficient:

$$\mathbf{B}^l = [B_1^l, \ldots, B_R^l], B_i^l = \log(\rho^l A_i^l) / \log(\rho^l A_1^l), i = 1, \ldots, R \tag{2}$$

- Average Harmonic Structure (**AHS**): $\bar{\mathbf{B}} = \frac{1}{L} \sum_{l=1}^{L} \mathbf{B}^l$

- Harmonic Structure Stability (**HSS**):

$$HSS = \frac{1}{R} \cdot \frac{1}{L} \sum_{l=1}^{L} \left\| \mathbf{B}^l - \bar{\mathbf{B}} \right\|^2 = \frac{1}{RL} \sum_{r=1}^{R} \sum_{l=1}^{L} (B_r^l - \bar{B}_r)^2 \qquad (3)$$

AHS and HSS are the mean and variance of $\mathbf{B}^l$. Since timbres of most instruments are stable, $\mathbf{B}^l$ varies little in different frames in a music signal and AHS is a good model to represent music signals. On the contrary, $\mathbf{B}^l$ varies much in a voice signal and the corresponding HSS is much bigger than that of a music signal. See figure 1.

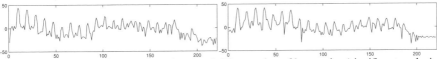

(a) Spectra in different frames of a voice signal. The number of harmonics (significant peaks in the spectrum) and their amplitude ratios are totally different.

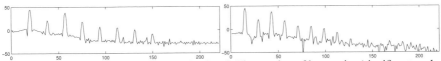

(b) Spectra in different frames of a piccolo signal. The number of harmonics (significant peaks in the spectrum) and their amplitude ratios are almost the same.

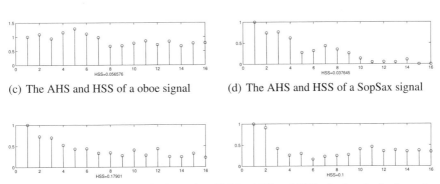

(c) The AHS and HSS of a oboe signal (d) The AHS and HSS of a SopSax signal

(e) The AHS and HSS of a male singing voice (f) The AHS and HSS of a female singing voice

Figure 1: Spectra, AHSs and HSSs of voice and music signals. In (c)-(f), x-axis is harmonic number, y-axis is the corresponding harmonic structure coefficient.

3 Separation algorithm based on harmonic structure modeling

Without loss of generality, suppose we have a signal mixture consisting of one voice and several music signals. The separation algorithm consists of four steps: preprocessing, extraction of harmonic structures, music AHSs analysis, separation of signals.

In preprocessing step, the mean and energy of the input signal are normalized. In the second step, the pitch estimation algorithm of Terhardt [11] is extended and used to extract harmonic structures. This algorithm is suitable for estimating both the fundamental frequency and all its harmonics. In Terhardt's algorithm, in each frame, all spectral peaks exceeding a given threshold are detected. The frequencies of these peaks are $[f_1, \ldots, f_K]$, K is the number of peaks. For a fundamental frequency candidate f, count the number of f_i which satisfies the following condition:

$$floor[(1+d)f_i/f] \geq (1-d)f_i/f \qquad (4)$$

$floor(x)$ denotes the greatest integer less than or equal to x. This condition means whether $r_i f \cdot (1-d) \leq f_i \leq r_i f \cdot (1+d)$. If the condition is fulfilled, f_i is the frequency of the r_i^{th} harmonic component when fundamental frequency is f. For each fundamental frequency candidate f, the coincidence number is calculated and $\hat{f}$ corresponding to the largest coincidence number is selected as the estimated fundamental frequency.

The original algorithm is extended in the following ways: Firstly, not all peaks exceeding the given threshold are detected, only the significant ones are selected by an edge detection procedure. This is very important for eliminating noise and achieving high performances in next steps. Secondly, not only the fundamental frequency but also all its harmonics are extracted, then **B** can be calculated. Thirdly, the original optimality criterion is to select $\hat{f}$ corresponding to the largest coincidence number. This criterion is not stable when the signal is polyphonic, because harmonic components of different sources may influence each other. A new optimality criterion is define as follows (n is the coincidence number):

$$d = \frac{1}{n} \sum_{i=1, f_i \text{ coincident with } f}^{K} \frac{|r_i - f_i/f|}{r_i} \qquad (5)$$

$\hat{f}$ corresponding to the smallest d is the estimated fundamental frequency. The new criterion measures the precision of coincidence. For each fundamental frequency, harmonic components of the same source are more probably to have a high coincidence precision than those of a different source. So, the new criterion is helpful for separation of harmonic structures of different sources. Note that, the coincidence number is required to be larger than a threshold, such as 4-6. This requirement eliminates many errors. Finally, in the original algorithm, only one pitch was detected in each frame. Here, the sound is polyphonic. So, all pitches for which the corresponding d is below a given threshold are extracted.

After harmonic structure extraction, a data set of harmonic structures is obtained. As the analysis in section two, in different frames, music harmonic structures of the same instrument are similar to each other and different from those of other instruments. So, in the data set all music harmonic structures form several high density clusters. Each cluster corresponds to an instrument. Voice harmonic structures scatter around like background noise, because the harmonic structure of the voice signal is not stable.

In the third step, NK algorithm [12] is used to learn music AHSs. NK algorithm is a clustering algorithm, which can cluster data on data sets consisting of clusters with different shapes, densities, sizes and even with some background noise. It can deal with high dimensional data sets. Actually, the harmonic structure data set is such a data set. Clusters of harmonic structures of different instruments have different densities. Voice harmonic structure are background noise. Each data point, a harmonic structure, has a high dimensionality (20 in our experiments). In NK algorithm, first find K neighbors for each point and construct a neighborhood graph. Each point and its neighbors form a neighborhood. Then local PCA is used to calculate eigenvalues of a neighborhood. In a cluster, data points are close to each other and the neighborhood is small, so the corresponding eigenvalues are small. On the contrary, for a noise point, corresponding eigenvalues are much bigger. So noise points can be removed by eigenvalue analysis. After denoising, in the neighborhood graph, all points of a cluster are connected together by edges between neighbors. If two clusters are connected together, there must exist long edges between them. Then the eigenvalues of the corresponding neighborhoods are bigger than others. So all edges between clusters can be found and removed by eigenvalue analysis. Then data points are clustered correctly and AHSs can be obtained by calculate the mean of each cluster.

In the separation step, all harmonic structures of an instrument in all frames are extracted to reconstruct the corresponding music signals and then removed from the mixture. After removing all music signals, the rest of the mixture is the separated voice signal.

The procedure of music harmonic structure detection is detailed as follows. Given a music AHS $[\bar{B}_1, \ldots, \bar{B}_R]$ and a fundamental frequency candidate f, a music harmonic structure is predicted. $[f, 2f, \ldots, Rf]$ and $[\bar{B}_1, \ldots, \bar{B}_R]$ are its frequencies and harmonic structure coefficients. The closest peak in the magnitude spectrum for each predicted harmonic component is detected. Suppose $[f_1, \ldots, f_R]$ and $[B_1, \ldots, B_R]$ are the frequencies and harmonic structure coefficients of these peaks (measured peaks). Formula 6 is defined to calculate the distance between the predicted harmonic structure and the measured peaks.

$$
\begin{aligned}
D(f) = &\sum_{r=1, \bar{B}_r>0, B_r>0}^{R} \left\{ \Delta f_r \cdot (rf)^{-p} + \frac{\bar{B}_r}{\bar{B}_{\max}} \times q \Delta f_r \cdot (rf)^{-p} \right\} \\
&+ a \sum_{r=1, \bar{B}_r>0, B_r>0}^{R} \left(\frac{\bar{B}_r}{\bar{B}_{\max}} \right) (\bar{B}_r - B_r)^2
\end{aligned}
\tag{6}
$$

The first part of D is a modified version of Two-Way Mismatch measure defined by Maher and Beauchamp, which measures the frequency difference between predicted peaks and measured peaks [13], where p and q are parameters, and $\Delta f_r = |f_r - r \cdot f|$. The second part measures the shape difference between the two, a is a normalization coefficient. Note that, only harmonic components with none-zero harmonic structure coefficients are considered. Let $\hat{f}$ indicate the fundamental frequency candidate corresponding to the smallest distance between the predicted peaks and the actual spectral peaks. If $D(\hat{f})$ is smaller than a threshold T_d, a music harmonic structure is detected. Otherwise there is no music harmonic structure in the frame. If a music harmonic structure is detected, the corresponding measured peaks in the spectrum are extracted, and the music signal is reconstructed by IFFT. Smoothing between frames is needed to eliminate errors and click noise between frames.

4 Experimental results

We have tested the performance of the proposed method on mixtures of different voice and music signals. The sample rate of the mixtures is 22.05kHz. Audio files for all the experiments are accessible at the website[1].

Figure 2 shows experimental results. In experiments 1 and 2, the mixed signals consist of one voice signal and one music signal. In experiment 3, the mixture consists of two music signals. In experiment 4, the mixture consists of one voice and two music signals. Table 1 shows SNR results. It can be seen that the mixtures are well separated into voice and music signals and very high SNRs are obtained in the separated signals. Experimental results show that music AHS is a good model for music signal representation and separation. There is another important fact that should be emphasized. In the separation procedure, music harmonic structures are detected by the music AHS model and separated from the mixture, and most of the time voice harmonic structures remain almost untouched. This procedure makes separated signals with a rather good subjective audio quality due to the good harmonic structure in the separated signals. Few existing methods can obtain such a good result because the harmonic structure is distorted in most of the existing methods.

It is difficult to compare our method with other methods, because they are so different. However, we compared our method with a speech enhancement method, because separation

---

[1]http://www.au.tsinghua.edu.cn/szll/bodao/zhangchangshui/bigeye/member/zyghtm/experiments.htm

Table 1: SNR results (DB): snr_v, snr_{m1} and snr_{m2} are the SNRs of voice and music signals in the mixed signal. snr'_e is the SNR of speech enhancement result. snr'_v, snr'_{m1} and snr'_{m2} are the SNRs of the separated voice and music signals.

	snr_v	snr_{m1}	snr_{m2}	snr'_e	snr'_v	snr'_{m1}	snr'_{m2}	Total inc.
Experiment 1	-7.9	7.9	/	-6.0	6.7	10.8	/	17.5
Experiment 2	-5.2	5.2	/	-1.5	6.6	10.0	/	16.6
Experiment 3	/	1.6	-1.6	/	/	9.3	7.1	16.4
Experiment 4	-10.0	0.7	-2.2	/	2.8	8.6	6.3	29.2

of voice and music can be regarded as a speech enhancement problem by regarding music as background noise. Figure 2 (b), (d) give speech enhancement results obtained by a speech enhancement software which tries to estimate the spectrum of noise in the pause of speech and enhance the speech by spectral subtraction [14]. Detecting pauses in speech with music background and enhancing speech with fast music noise are both very difficult problems, so traditional speech enhancement techniques can't work here.

5   Conclusion and discussion

In this paper, a harmonic structure model is proposed to represent music signals and used to separate music signals. Experimental results show a good performance of this method.

The proposed method has many applications, such as multi-pitch estimation, audio content analysis, audio edit, speech enhancement with music background, etc.

Multi-pitch estimation is an important problem in music research. There are many existing methods, such as pitch perception model based methods, and probabilistic approaches [4, 15, 16, 17]. However, multi-pitch estimation is a very difficult problem and remains unsolved. Furthermore, it is difficult to distinguish pitches of different instruments in the mixture. In our algorithm, not only harmonic structures but also corresponding fundamental frequencies are extracted. So, the algorithm is also a new multi-pitch estimation method. It analyzes the primary multi-pitch estimation results and learns models to represent music signals and improve multi-pitch estimation results. More importantly, pitches of different sources can be distinguished by the AHS models. This advantage is significant for automatic transcription. Figure 2 (f) shows multi-pitch estimation results in experiment 3. It can be seen that, the multi-pitch estimation results are fairly good.

The proposed method is useful for melody extraction. As we know, in a mixed signal, multi-pitch estimation is a difficult problem. After separation, pitch estimation on the separated voice signal that contains melody becomes a monophonic pitch estimation problem, which can be done easily. The estimated pitch sequence represents the melody of the song. Then, many content base audio analysis tasks such as audio retrieval and classification become much easier and many midi based algorithms can be used on audio files.

There are still some limitations. Firstly, the proposed algorithm doesn't work for non-harmonic instruments, such as some drums. Some rhythm tracking algorithms can be used instead to separate drum sounds. Fortunately, most instrument sounds are harmonic. Secondly, for some instruments, the timbre in the onset is somewhat different from that in the stable duration. Also, different performing methods (pizz. or arco) produces different timbres. In these cases, the music harmonic structures of this instrument will form several clusters, not one. Then a GMM model instead of an average harmonic structure model (actually a point model) should be used to represent the music.

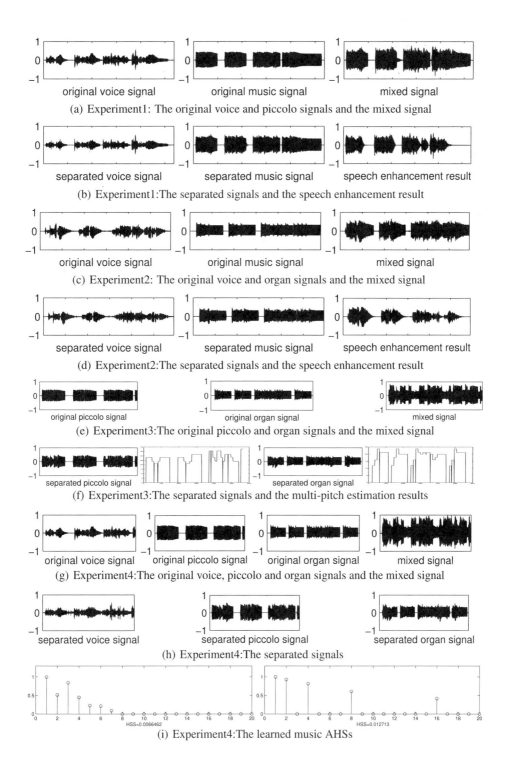

Figure 2: Experimental results.

Acknowledgments

This work is supported by the project (60475001) of the National Natural Science Foundation of China.

References

[1] J. S. Downie, "Music information retrieval," *Annual Review of Information Science and Technology*, vol. 37, pp. 295–340, 2003.

[2] Roger Dannenberg, "Music understanding by computer," in *IAKTA/LIST International Workshop on Knowledge Technology in the Arts Proc.*, 1993, pp. 41–56.

[3] G. J. Brown and M. Cooke, "Computational auditory scene analysis," *Computer Speech and Language*, vol. 8, no. 4, pp. 297–336, 1994.

[4] M.Goto, "A robust predominant-f0 estimation method for real-time detection of melody and bass lines in cd recordings," in *IEEE International Conference on Acoustics, Speech, and Signal Processing (ICASSP2000)*, 2000, pp. 757–760.

[5] J. Pinquier, J. Rouas, and R. Andre-Obrecht, "Robust speech / music classification in audio documents," in *7th International Conference On Spoken Language Processing (ICSLP)*, 2002, pp. 2005–2008.

[6] P. Comon, "Independent component analysis, a new concept?," *Signal Processing*, vol. 36, pp. 287–314, 1994.

[7] Gil-Jin Jang and Te-Won Lee, "A probabilistic approach to single channel blind signal separation," in *Neural Information Processing Systems 15 (NIPS2002)*, 2003.

[8] Yazhong Feng, Yueting Zhuang, and Yunhe Pan, "Popular music retrieval by independent component analysis," in *ISMIR*, 2002, pp. 281–282.

[9] Peter Vanroose, "Blind source separation of speech and background music for improved speech recognition," in *The 24th Symposium on Information Theory*, May 2003, pp. 103–108.

[10] X. Serra, "Musical sound modeling with sinusoids plus noise," in *Musical Signal Processing*, C. Roads, S. Popea, A. Picialli, and G. De Poli, Eds. Swets & Zeitlinger Publishers, 1997.

[11] E. Terhardt, "Calculating virtual pitch," *Hearing Res.*, vol. 1, pp. 155–182, 1979.

[12] Yungang Zhang, Changshui Zhang, and Shijun Wang, "Clustering in knowledge embedded space," in *ECML*, 2003, pp. 480–491.

[13] R. C. Maher and J. W. Beauchamp, "Fundamental frequency estimation of musical signals using a two-way mismatch procedure," *Journal of the Acoustical Society of America*, vol. 95, no. 4, pp. 2254–2263, 1994.

[14] Serguei Koval, Mikhail Stolbov, and Mikhail Khitrov, "Broadband noise cancellation systems: new approach to working performance optimization," in *EUROSPEECH'99*, 1999, pp. 2607–2610.

[15] Anssi Klapuri, "Automatic transcription of music," M.S. thesis, Tampere University of Technology, Finland, 1998.

[16] Keerthi C. Nagaraj., "Toward automatic transcription - pitch tracking in polyphonic environment," Literature survey, Mar. 2003.

[17] Hirokazu Kameoka, Takuya Nishimoto, and Shigeki Sagayama, "Separation of harmonic structures based on tied gaussian mixture model and information criterion for concurrent sounds," in *IEEE International Conference on Acoustics, Speech, and Signal Processing (ICASSP04)*, 2004.

A Domain Decomposition Method for Fast Manifold Learning

Zhenyue Zhang
Department of Mathematics
Zhejiang University, Yuquan Campus,
Hangzhou, 310027, P. R. China
zyzhang@zju.edu.cn

Hongyuan Zha
Department of Computer Science
Pennsylvania State University
University Park, PA 16802
zha@cse.psu.edu

Abstract

We propose a fast manifold learning algorithm based on the methodology of domain decomposition. Starting with the set of sample points partitioned into two subdomains, we develop the solution of the interface problem that can glue the embeddings on the two subdomains into an embedding on the whole domain. We provide a detailed analysis to assess the errors produced by the gluing process using matrix perturbation theory. Numerical examples are given to illustrate the efficiency and effectiveness of the proposed methods.

1 Introduction

The setting of manifold learning we consider is the following. We are given a *parameterized manifold* of dimension d defined by a mapping $f : \Omega \to \mathcal{R}^m$, where $d < m$, and Ω open and connected in $\mathcal{R}^d$. We assume the manifold is well-behaved, it is smooth and contains no self-intersections etc. Suppose we have a set of points $x_1, \cdots, x_N$, sampled possibly with noise from the manifold, i.e.,

$$x_i = f(\tau_i) + \epsilon_i, \quad i = 1, \ldots, N, \tag{1.1}$$

where ϵ_i's represent noise. The goal of manifold learning is to recover the parameters τ_i's and/or the mapping $f(\cdot)$ from the sample points x_i's [2, 6, 9, 12]. The general framework of manifold learning methods involves imposing a connectivity structure such as a k-nearest-neighbor graph on the set of sample points and then turn the embedding problem into the solution of an eigenvalue problem. Usually constructing the graph dominates the computational cost of a manifold learning algorithm, but for large data sets, the computational cost of the eigenvalue problem can be substantial as well.

The focus of this paper is to explore the methodology of domain decomposition for developing fast algorithms for manifold learning. Domain decomposition by now is a well-established field in scientific computing and has been successfully applied in many science and engineering fields in connection with numerical solutions of partial differential equations. One class of domain decomposition methods partitions the solution domain into subdomains, solves the problem on each subdomain and glue the partial solutions on the subdomains by solving an interface problem [7, 10]. This is the general approach we will follow in this paper. In particular, in section 3, we consider the case where the given set of sample points $x_1, \ldots, x_N$ are partitioned into two subdomains. On each of the subdomain, we can use a manifold learning method such as LLE [6], LTSA [12] or any other manifold learning methods to construct an embedding for the subdomain in question. We will then formulate the interface problem the solution of which will allow us to combine the embeddings on the two subdomains together to obtain an embedding over the whole domain. However, it is not always feasible to carry out the procedure described above. In section 2, we give necessary and sufficient conditions under which the embedding on the whole domain can be constructed from the embeddings on the subdomains. In section 4, we analyze the errors produced by the gluing process using matrix perturbation theory. In section 5, we briefly mention how the partitioning of the set of sample points into subdomains can be accomplished by some graph partitioning algorithms. Section 6 is devoted to numerical experiments.

NOTATION. We use e to denote a column vector of all 1's the dimension of which should be clear from the context. $\mathcal{N}(\cdot)$ and $\mathcal{R}(\cdot)$ denote the null space and range space of a matrix, respectively. For an index set $I = [i_1, \ldots, i_k]$, $A(:, I)$ denotes the submatrix of A consisting of columns of A with indices in I with a similar definition for the rows of a matrix. We use $\| \cdot \|$ to denote the spectral norm of a matrix.

2 A Basic Theorem

Let $X = [x_1, \cdots, x_N]$ with $x_i = f(\tau_i) + \epsilon_i, i = 1, \ldots, N$. Assume that the whole sample domain X is divided into two subdomains $X_1 = \{x_i \,|\, i \in I_1\}$ and $X_2 = \{x_i \,|\, i \in I_2\}$. Here I_1 and I_2 denote the index sets such that $I_1 \cup I_2 = \{1, \ldots, N\}$ and $I_1 \cap I_2$ is not empty. Suppose we have obtained the two low-dimensional embeddings T_1 and T_2 of the sub-domains X_1 and X_2, respectively. The domain decomposition method attempts to recover the overall embedding $T = \{\tau_1, \ldots, \tau_N\}$ from the embeddings T_1 and T_2 on the subdomains.

In general, the recovered sub-embedding $T_j, j = 1, 2$, may not be exactly the subset $\{\tau_i \,|\, i \in I_j\}$ of T. For example, it is often the case that the recovered embeddings T_j are approximately affinely equal to $\{\tau_i \,|\, i \in I_j\}$, i.e., up to certain approximation errors, there is an affine transformation such that

$$ T_j = \{F_j \tau_i + c_j \,|\, i \in I_j\}, $$

where F_j is a nonsingular matrix and c_j a column vector. Thus a domain decomposition method for manifold learning should be invariant to affine transformation on the embeddings T_j obtained from subdomains. In that case, we can assume that T_j is just the subset of T, i.e., $T_j = \{\tau_i \,|\, i \in I_j\}$. With an abuse of notation, we also denote by T and T_j the matrices of the column vectors in the set T and T_j, for example, we write $T = [\tau_1, \ldots, \tau_N]$.

Let Φ_j be an orthogonal projection with $\mathcal{N}(\Phi_j) = \text{span}([e, T_j^T])$. Then T_j can be recovered by computing the eigenvectors of Φ_j corresponding to its zero eigenvalues. To recover the whole T we need to construct a matrix Φ with $\mathcal{N}(\Phi) = \text{span}([e, T^T])$ [11].

To this end, for each T_j, let $\Phi_j = Q_j Q_j^T \in \mathcal{R}^{N_j \times N_j}$, where Q_j is an orthonormal basis matrix of $\mathcal{N}([e, T_j^T]^T)$ and N_j is the column-size of T_j. To construct a Φ matrix, Let $S_j \in \mathcal{R}^{N \times N_j}$ be the 0-1 selection matrix defined as $S_j = I_N(:, I_j)$, where I_N is the identity matrix of order N. Let $\hat{\Phi}_j = S_j \Phi_j S_j^T$. We then simply take $\Phi = \hat{\Phi}_1 + \hat{\Phi}_2$, or more flexibly, $\Phi = w_1 \hat{\Phi}_1 + w_2 \hat{\Phi}_2$, where w_1 and w_2 are the weights: $w_i > 0$ and $w_1 + w_2 = 1$. Obviously $\|\Phi\| \le 1$ since $\|\Phi_j\| = 1$. The following theorem gives the necessary and sufficient conditions under which the null space of Φ is just $\text{span}\{[e, T^T]\}$. (In the theorem, we only require the Φ_j to positive semidefinite.)

Theorem 2.1 *Let* Φ_i *be two positive semidefinite matrices such that* $\mathcal{N}(\Phi_i) = \text{span}([e, T_i^T])$, $i = 1, 2$, *and* $T_0 = T_1 \cap T_2$. *Assume that* $[e, T_1^T]$ *and* $[e, T_2^T]$ *are of full column-rank. Then* $\mathcal{N}(\Phi) = \text{span}([e, T^T])$ *if and only if* $[e, T_0^T]$ *is of full column-rank.*

Proof. We first prove the necessity by contradiction. Assume that $\mathcal{N}([e, T_0^T]) \neq \mathcal{N}([e, T_2^T])$, then there is $y \neq 0$ such that $[e, T_0^T]y = 0$ and $[e, T^T(:, I_2)]y \neq 0$. Denote by I_1^c the complement of I_1, i.e., the index set of i's which do not belong to I_1. Then $[e, T^T(:, I_1^c)]y \neq 0$. Now we construct a vector x as

$$x(I_1) = [e, T_1^T]y, \quad x(I_1^c) = 0.$$

Clearly $x(I_2) = 0$ and hence $x \in \mathcal{N}(\Phi)$. By the condition $\mathcal{N}(\Phi) = \text{span}([e, T^T])$, we can write x in the form $x = [e, T^T]z$ for a column vector z. Specially, $x(I_1) = [e, T_1^T]z$. Note that we also have $x(I_1) = [e, T_1^T]y$ by definition. It implies that $z = y$ because $[e, T_1^T]$ is of full rank. Therefor,

$$[e, T^T(:, I_1^c)]y = [e, T^T(:, I_1^c)]z = x(I_1^c) = 0.$$

Using it together with $[e, T_0^T]y = 0$ we have $[e, T^T(:, I_2)]y = 0$, a contradiction.

Now we prove the sufficiency. Let Q be a basis matrix of $\mathcal{N}(\Phi)$. we have

$$w_1 G_1 Q^T \hat{\Phi}_1 Q + w_2 G_2 Q^T \hat{\Phi}_2 Q = Q^T \Phi Q = 0,$$

which implies $\Phi_i Q(I_1, :) = 0$, $i = 1, 2$, because $\hat{\Phi}_i$ is positive semidefinite. So

$$Q(I_i, :) = [e, T_i^T]G_i, \quad i = 1, 2. \tag{2.2}$$

Taking the overlap part $Q(I_0, :)$ of Q with the different representations

$$Q(I_0, :) = [e, T_i(:, I_0)^T]G_i = [e, T_0^T]G_i,$$

we obtain $[e, T_0^T](G_1 - G_2) = 0$. So $G_1 = G_2$ because $[e, T_0^T]$ is of full column rank, giving rise to $Q = [e, T^T]G_1$, i.e., $\mathcal{N}(\Phi) \subset \text{span}([e, T^T])$. It follows together with the obvious result $\text{span}([e, T^T]) \subset \mathcal{N}(\Phi)$ that $\mathcal{N}(\Phi) = \text{span}([e, T^T])$. ∎

The above result states that when the overlapping is large enough such that $[e, T_0^T]$ is of full column-rank (which is generically true when T_0 contains $d + 1$ points or more), the embedding over the whole domain can be recovered from the embeddings over the two subdomains. However, to follow Theorem 2.1, it seems that we will need to compute the null space of Φ. In the next section, we will show this can done much cheaply by considering an interface problem which is of much smaller dimension.

3 Computing the Null Space of Φ

In this section, we formulate the interface problem and show how to solve it to glue the embeddings from the two subdomains to obtain an embedding over the whole domain. To simplify notations, we re-denote by T^* the *actual* embedding over the whole domain and T_j^* the subsets of T^* corresponding to subdomains. We then use T_j to denote affinely transformed versions of T_j^* obtained by LTSA for example, i.e., $T_j^* = c_j e^T + F_j T_j$. Here c_j is a constant column vector in $\mathcal{R}^d$ and F_j is a nonsingular matrix. Denote by T_{0j} the overlapping part of T_j corresponding to $I_0 = I_1 \cap I_2$ as in the proof of Theorem 2.1. We consider the overlapping parts T_{0j}^* of T_j^*,

$$c_1 e^T + F_1 T_{01} = T_{01}^* = T_{02}^* = c_2 e^T + F_2 T_{02}. \tag{3.3}$$

Or equivalently,

$$\left[[e, T_{01}^T], -[e, T_{02}^T] \right] \begin{bmatrix} (c_1, F_1)^T \\ (c_2, F_2)^T \end{bmatrix} = 0.$$

Therefore, if we take an orthonormal basis G of the null space of $\left[[e, T_{01}^T], -[e, T_{02}^T]\right]$ and partition $G = [G_1^T, G_2^T]^T$ conformally, then $[e, T_{01}^T]G_1 = [e, T_{02}^T]G_2$. Let $A_j = G_j^T[e, T_j^T]^T$, $j = 1, 2$. Define the matrix A such that $A(:, I_j) = A_j$. Then since $\Phi_i A_i^T = 0$, the well-defined matrix A^T is a basis of $\mathcal{N}(\Phi)$,

$$\Phi A^T = S_1 \Phi_1 S_1^T A^T + S_2 \Phi_2 S_2^T A^T = S_1 \Phi_1 A_1^T + S_2 \Phi_2 A_2^T = 0.$$

Therefore, we can use A^T to recover the global embedding T.

A simpler alternative way is use a one-sided affine transformation, i.e., fix one of T_i and affinely transform the other; the affine matrix is obtained by fixing one of $\tilde{T}_{0i}$ and transforming the other. For example, we can determine c and F such that

$$T_{01} = ce^T + FT_{02}, \tag{3.4}$$

and transform T_2 to $\hat{T}_2 = ce^T + FT_2$. Clearly, for the overlapping part, $\hat{T}_{02} = T_{01}$. Then we can construct a larger matrix T by $T(:, I_1) = T_1$, $T(:, I_2) = ce^T + FT_2$. One can also readily verify that T^T is a basis matrix of $\mathcal{N}(\Phi)$.

In the noisy case, a least squares formulation will be needed. For example, for the simultaneous affine transformation, we take $G = [G_1^T, G_2^T]^T$ to be an orthonormal matrix in $\mathcal{R}^{2(d+1) \times (d+1)}$ such that

$$\|[e, T_{01}^T]G_1 - [e, T_{02}^T]G_2\| = \min.$$

It is known that the minimum G is given by the right singular vector matrix corresponding to the $d + 1$ smallest singular values of $W = \left[[e, T_{01}^T], -[e, T_{02}^T]\right]$, and the residual $\left\|[e, T_{01}^T]G_1 - [e, T_{02}^T]G_2\right\| = \sigma_{d+2}(W)$. For the one-side approach (3.4), $[c, F]$ can be a solution to the least squares problem

$$\min_{c, F} \left\|T_{01} - (ce^T + FT_{02})\right\| = \min_F \left\|(T_{01} - t_{01}e^T) - F(T_{02} - t_{02}e^T)\right\|,$$

where t_{0j} is the column mean of T_{0j}. The minimum is achieved at $F = (T_{01} - t_{01}e^T)(T_{02} - t_{02}e^T)^+$, $c = t_{01} - Ft_{02}$. Clearly, the residual now reads as

$$\min_{c, F} \left\|T_{01} - (ce^T + FT_{02})\right\| = \left\|(T_{01} - t_{01}e^T)\left(I - (T_{02} - t_{02}e^T)^+(T_{02} - t_{02}e^T)\right)\right\|.$$

Notice that the overlapping parts in the two affinely transformed subsets are not exactly equal to each other in the noisy case. There are several possible choices for setting $A(:, I_0)$ or $\hat{T}(:, I_0)$. For example, one choice is to set $T(:, I_0)$ by a convex combination of T_{0j}'s,

$$T(:, I_0) = \alpha T_{01} + (1 - \alpha)\hat{T}_{02}.$$

with $\alpha = 1/2$ for example.

We summarize discussions above in the following two algorithms for gluing the two subdomains T_1 and T_2.

Algorithm I. [Simultaneously affine transformation]

1. Compute the right singular vector matrix G corresponding to the $d + 1$ smallest singular values of $\left[[e, T_{01}^T], -[e, T_{02}^T]\right]$.

2. Partition $G = [G_1^T, G_2^T]^T$ and set $A_i = G_i^T[e, T_i^T]^T$, $i = 1, 2$, and

$$A(:, I_1 \backslash I_0) = A_{11}, \quad A(:, I_0) = \alpha A_{01} + (1 - \alpha)A_{02}, \quad A(:, I_2 \backslash I_0) = A_{12},$$

where A_{0j} is the overlap part of A_j and A_{1j} is the A_j with A_{0j} deleted.

3 Compute the column mean a of A, and an orthogonal basis U of $\mathcal{N}(a^T)$.

4. Set $T = U^T A$.

Algorithm II. [One-side affine transformation]

1. Compute the least squares problem $\min_W \|T_{01} - W[e, T_{02}^T]^T\|_F$.

2. Affinely transform T_2 to $\hat{T}_2 = W[e, T_2^T]^T$.

3. Set the global coordinate matrix T by

$$T(:, I_1 \backslash I_0) = T_{11}, \quad T(:, I_0) = \alpha T_{01} + (1 - \alpha)\hat{T}_{02}, \quad T(:, I_2 \backslash I_0) = \hat{T}_{12}.$$

4 Error Analysis

As we mentioned before, the computation of $T_j, j = 1, 2$ using a manifold learning algorithm such as LTSA involves errors. In this section, we assess the impact of those errors on the accuracy of the gluing process. Two issues are considered for the error analysis. One is the perturbation analysis of $\mathcal{N}(\Phi^*)$ when the computation of Φ_i^* is subject to error. In this case, $\mathcal{N}(\Phi^*)$ will be approximated by the smallest $(d+1)$-dimensional eigenspace $\mathcal{V}$ of an approximation $\Phi \approx \Phi^*$ (Theorem 4.1). The other issue is the error estimation of $\mathcal{V}$ when a basis matrix of $\mathcal{V}$ is approximately constructed by affinely transformed local embeddings as described in section 3 (Theorem 4.2). Because of space limit, we will not present the details of the proofs of the results.

The distance of two linear subspaces $\mathcal{X}$ and $\mathcal{Y}$ are defined by $\mathrm{dist}(\mathcal{X}, \mathcal{Y}) = \|P_\mathcal{X} - P_\mathcal{Y}\|$, where $P_\mathcal{X}$ and $P_\mathcal{Y}$ are the orthogonal projection onto $\mathcal{X}$ and $\mathcal{Y}$, respectively. Let $\epsilon_i = \|\Phi_i - \Phi_i^*\|$, where Φ_i^* and Φ_i are the orthogonal projectors onto the range spaces $\mathrm{span}([e, (T_i^*)^T])$ and $\mathrm{span}([e, (T_i)^T])$, respectively. Clearly, if $\Phi^* = w_1\Phi_1^* + w_2\Phi_2^*$ and $\Phi = w_1\Phi_1 + w_2\Phi_2$, then

$$\mathrm{dist}\Big(\mathrm{span}([e, (T^*)^T]), \mathrm{span}([e, T^T])\Big) = \|\Phi - \Phi^*\| \le w_1\epsilon_1 + w_2\epsilon_2 \equiv \epsilon.$$

Theorem 4.1 *Let σ be the smallest nonzero eigenvalue of Φ^* and $\mathcal{V}$ the subspace spanned by the eigenvectors of Φ corresponding to the $d + 1$ smallest eigenvalues. If $\epsilon < \sigma/4$, and $4\epsilon^2(\|\Phi^*\| - \sigma + 2\epsilon) < (\sigma - 2\epsilon)^3$, then*

$$\mathrm{dist}(\mathcal{V}, \mathcal{N}(\Phi^*)) \le \frac{\epsilon}{\sqrt{(\sigma/2 - \epsilon)^2 + \epsilon^2}}.$$

Theorem 4.2 *Let σ and ϵ be defined in Theorem 4.1. A is the matrix computed by the simultaneous affine transformation (Algorithm I in section 3) Let $\sigma_i(\cdot)$ be the i-th smallest singular value of a matrix. Denote*

$$\mu = \frac{1}{2}\sigma_{d+2}([[e, T_{01}^T], -[e, T_{02}^T]]), \quad \eta = \frac{\mu}{\sigma_{\min}(A)}.$$

If $\epsilon < \sigma/4$, then

$$\mathrm{dist}(\mathcal{V}, \mathrm{span}(A)) \le \frac{1}{\sigma_{d+2}(\Phi)}\left(\eta + \frac{\epsilon\sigma/2}{(\sigma/2 - \epsilon)^2}\right)$$

From Theorems 4.1 and 4.2 we conclude directly that

$$\mathrm{dist}(\mathrm{span}(A), \mathcal{N}(\Phi^*)) \le \frac{1}{\sigma_{d+2}(\Phi)}\left(\eta + \frac{\epsilon\sigma/2}{(\sigma/2 - \epsilon)^2}\right) + \frac{2\epsilon}{\sqrt{(\sigma - 2\epsilon)^2 + 4\epsilon^2}}.$$

5 Partitioning the Domains

To apply the domain decomposition methods, we need to partition the given set of data points into several domains making use of the k nearest neighbor graph imposed on the data points. This reduces the problem to a graph partition problem and many techniques such as spectral graph partitioning and METIS [3, 5] can be used. In our experiments, we have used a particularly simple approach: we use the reverse Cuthill-McKee method [4] to order the vertices of the k-NN graph and then partition the vertices into domains (for details see Test 2 in the next section).

Once we have partitioned the whole domain into multiple overlapping subdomains we can use the following two approaches to glue them together.

Successive gluing. Here we glue the subdomains one by one as follows. Initially set $T^{(1)} = T_1$ and $I^{(1)} = I_1$, and then glue the patch T_k to $T^{(k-1)}$ and obtain the larger one $T^{(k)}$ for $k = 2, \ldots, K$, and so on. The index set of $T^{(k)}$ is given by $I^{(k)} = I^{(k-1)} \cup I_k$. Clearly the overlapping set of $T^{(k-1)}$ and T_k is $I_0^{(k)} = I^{(k-1)} \cap I_k$.

Recursive gluing. Here at the leaf level, we divide the subdomains into several pairs, say $(T_{2i-1}^{(0)}, T_{2i}^{(0)})$, $1 = 1, 2, \ldots$. Then glue each pair to be a larger subdomain $T_i^{(1)}$ and continue. The recursive gluing method is obviously parallelizable.

6 Numerical Experiments

In this section we report numerical experiments for the proposed domain decomposition methods for manifold learning. This efficiency and effectiveness of the methods clearly depend on the accuracy of the computed embeddings for subdomains, the sizes of the subdomains, and the sizes of the overlaps of the subdomains.

Test 1. Our first test data set is sampled from a Swiss-roll as follows

$$x_i = [t_i \cos(t_i), h_i, t_i \sin(t_i)]^T, \quad i = 1, \ldots, N = 2000, \tag{6.5}$$

where t_i and h_i are uniformly randomly chosen in the intervals $\left[\frac{3\pi}{2}, \frac{9\pi}{2}\right]$ and $[0, 21]$, respectively. Let τ_i be the arc length of the corresponding spiral curve $[t \cos(t), t \sin(t)]^T$ from $t_0 = \frac{3\pi}{2}$ to t_i. $\tau_{\max} = \max_i \tau_i$. To compare the CPU time of the domain decomposition methods, we simply partition the τ-interval $[0, \tau_{\max}]$ into k_τ subintervals $(a_{i-1}, a_i]$ with equal length and also partition the h-interval into k_h subintervals $(b_{j-1}, b_j]$. Let $D_{ij} = (a_{i-1}, a_i] \times (b_{j-1}, b_j]$ and $S_{ij}(r)$ be the balls centered at (a_i, b_j) with radius r. We set the subdomains as

$$X_{ij} = \{x_k \,|\, (\tau_k, h_k) \in D_{ij} \cup S_{ij}(r)\}.$$

Clearly r determines the size of overlapping parts of X_{ij} with $X_{i+1,j}, X_{i,j+1}, X_{i+1,j+1}$. The submatrices X_{ij} are ordered as $X_{1,1}, X_{1,2}, \ldots, X_{1,k_h}, X_{2,1}, \ldots$ and denoted as X_k, $k = 1, \ldots, K = k_\tau k_h$. We first compute the K local 2-D embeddings $T_1, \ldots, T_K$ by applying LTSA on the sample data sets X_k for the subdomains. Then those local coordinate embeddings T_k are aligned by the successive one-sided affine transformation algorithm by adding subdomain T_k one by one.

Table 1 lists the total CPU time for the successive domain decomposition algorithm, including the time for computing the embeddings $\{T_k\}$ for the subdomains, for different parameters k_τ and k_h with the parameter $r = 5$. In Table 2, we list the CPU time for the recursive gluing approach taking into account the parallel procedure. As a comparison, the CPU time of LTSA applying to the whole data points is 6.23 seconds.

Table 1: CPU Time (seconds) of the successive domain decomposition algorithm.

$k_\tau = 3$	$k_h=2$	3	4	5	6
$k_\tau = 3$	1.89	1.70	1.64	1.61	1.64
4	167	1.67	1.61	1.70	1.77
5	1.66	1.59	1.67	1.78	1.86
6	163	1.66	1.75	1.89	2.09
7	1.59	1.70	1.84	2.02	2.23
8	1.58	1.80	1.94	2.22	2.44
9	1.63	1.83	2.06	2.31	2.66
10	1.63	1.86	2.38	2.56	2.94

Table 2: CPU Time (seconds) of the parallel recursive domain decomposition.

$k_\tau = 3$	$k_h=2$	3	4	5	6
$k_\tau = 3$	0.52	0.34	0.27	0.19	017
4	0.53	0.23	0.20	0.17	0.13
5	0.31	0.17	0.19	0.17	0.14
6	0.25	0.19	0.16	0.13	0.14
7	0.20	0.16	0.14	0.14	0.11
8	0.20	0.17	0.16	0.14	0.14
9	0.19	0.16	0.14	0.14	0.14
10	0.19	0.16	0.17	0.19	0.13

Test 2. The symmetric reverse Cuthill-McKee permutation (*symrcm*) is an algorithm for ordering the rows and columns of a symmetric sparse matrix [4]. It tends to move the nonzero elements of the sparse matrix towards the main diagonals of the matrix. We use Matlab's *symrcm* to the adjacency matrix of the k-nearest-neighbor graph of the data points to reorder them. Denote by X the reordered data set. We then partition the whole sample points into $K = 16$ subsets $X_i = X(:, s_i : e_i)$ with $s_i = \max\{1, (i-1)m - 20\}$, $e_i = \min\{im + 20, N\}$, and $m = N/K = 125$.

It is known that the t-h parameters in (6.5) represent an isometric parametrization of the swiss-roll surface. We have shown that within the errors made in computing the local embeddings, LTSA can recover the isometric parametrization up to an affine transformation [11]. We denote by $\tilde{T}^{(k)} = ce^T + FT^{(k)}$ the optimal approximation to $T^*(:, I^{(k)})$ within affine transformations,

$$\|T^*(:, I^{(k)}) - \tilde{T}^{(k)}\|_F = \min_{c,F} \|T^*(:, I^{(k)}) - (ce^T + FT^{(k)})\|_F.$$

We denote by η_k the average of relative errors

$$\eta_k = \frac{1}{|I^{(k)}|} \sum_{i \in I^{(k)}} \frac{\|T^*(:, i) - \tilde{T}^{(k)}(:, i)\|_2}{\|T^*(:, i)\|_2}.$$

In the left panel of Figure 1 we plot the initial embedding errors for the subdomains (blue bar), the error of LTSA applied to the whole data set (red bar), and the errors η_k of the successive gluing (red line). The successive gluing method gives an embedding with an acceptable accuracy comparing with the accuracy obtained by applying LTSA to the whole data set. As shown in the error analysis, the errors in successive gluing will increase when the initial errors for the subdomains increase. To show it more clearly, we also plot the η_k for the recursive gluing method in the right panel of Figure 1.

Acknowledgment. The work of first author was supported in part by by NSFC (project 60372033), the Special Funds for Major State Basic Research Projects (project

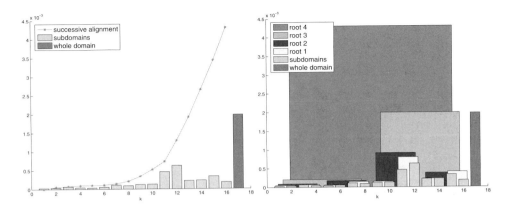

Figure 1: Relative errors for the successive (left) and recursive (right) approaches.

G19990328), and NSF grant CCF-0305879. The work of second author was supported in part by NSF grants DMS-0311800 and CCF-0430349.

References

[1] M. Brand. Charting a manifold. *Advances in Neural Information Processing Systems* 15, MIT Press, 2003.

[2] D. Donoho and C. Grimes. Hessian Eigenmaps: new tools for nonlinear dimensionality reduction. *Proceedings of National Academy of Science*, 5591-5596, 2003.

[3] M. Fiedler. A property of eigenvectors of nonnegative symmetric matrices and its application to graph theory. *Czech. Math. J.* 25:619–637, 1975.

[4] A. George and J. W. Liu. *Computer Solution of Large Sparse Positive Definite Matrices*. Prentice Hall, 1981.

[5] METIS. http://www-users.cs.umn.edu/~karypis/metis/.

[6] S. Roweis and L. Saul. Nonlinear dimensionality reduction by locally linear embedding. *Science*, 290: 2323–2326, 2000.

[7] B. Smith, P. Bjorstad and W. Gropp *Domain Decomposition, Parallel Multilevel Methods for Elliptic Partial Differential Equations*. Cambridge University Press, 1996.

[8] G.W. Stewart and J.G. Sun. *Matrix Perturbation Theory*. Academic Press, New York, 1990.

[9] J. Tenenbaum, V. De Silva and J. Langford. A global geometric framework for nonlinear dimension reduction. *Science*, 290:2319–2323, 2000.

[10] A. Toselli and O. Widlund. *Domain Decomposition Methods - Algorithms and Theory*. Springer, 2004.

[11] H. Zha and Z. Zhang. Spectral analysis of alignment in manifold learning. *Proceedings of IEEE International Conference on Acoustics, Speech, and Signal Processing, (ICASSP)*, 2005.

[12] Z. Zhang and H. Zha. Principal manifolds and nonlinear dimensionality reduction via tangent space alignment. *SIAM J. Scientific Computing*. 26:313-338, 2005.

A Hierarchical Compositional System for Rapid Object Detection

Long Zhu and Alan Yuille
Department of Statistics
University of California at Los Angeles
Los Angeles, CA 90095
{lzhu,yuille}@stat.ucla.edu

Abstract

We describe a hierarchical compositional system for detecting deformable objects in images. Objects are represented by graphical models. The algorithm uses a hierarchical tree where the root of the tree corresponds to the full object and lower-level elements of the tree correspond to simpler features. The algorithm proceeds by passing simple messages up and down the tree. The method works rapidly, in under a second, on 320×240 images. We demonstrate the approach on detecting cats, horses, and hands. The method works in the presence of background clutter and occlusions. Our approach is contrasted with more traditional methods such as dynamic programming and belief propagation.

1 Introduction

Detecting objects rapidly in images is very important. There has recently been great progress in detecting objects with limited appearance variability, such as faces and text [1,2,3]. The use of the SIFT operator also enables rapid detection of rigid objects [4]. The detection of such objects can be performed in under a second even in very large images which makes real time applications practical, see [3].

There has been less progress for the rapid detection of deformable objects, such as hands, horses, and cats. Such objects can be represented compactly by graphical models, see [5,6,7,8], but their variations in shape and appearance makes searching for them considerably harder.

Recent work has included the use of dynamic programming [5,6] and belief propagation [7,8] to perform inference on these graphical models by searching over different spatial configurations. These algorithms are successful at detecting objects but pruning was required to obtain reasonable convergence rates [5,7,8]. Even so, algorithms can take minutes to converge on images of size 320×240.

In this paper, we propose an alternative methods for performing inference on graphical models of deformable objects. Our approach is based on representing objects in a probabilistic compositional hierarchical tree structure. This structure enables rapid detection of objects by passing messages up and down the tree structure. Our approach is fast with a typical speed of 0.6 seconds on a 320×240 image (without optimized code).

Our approach can be applied to detect any object that can be represented by a graphical model. This includes the models mentioned above [5,6,7,8], compositional models [9], constellation models [10], models using chamfer matching [11] and models using deformable blur filters [12].

2 Background

Graphical models give an attractive framework for modeling object detection problems in computer vision. We use the models and notation described in [8].

The positions of feature points on the object are represented by $\{x_i : i \in \Lambda\}$. We augment this representation to include attributes of the points and obtain a representation $\{q_i : i \in \Lambda\}$. These attributes can be used to model the appearance of the features in the image. For example, a feature point can be associated with an oriented intensity edge and q_i can represent the orientation [8]. Alternatively, the attribute could represent the output of a blurred edge filter [12], or the appearance properties of a constellation model part [10].

There is a prior probability distribution on the configuration of the model $P(\{q_i\})$ and a likelihood function for generating the image data $P(D|\{q_i\})$. We use the same likelihood model as [8]. Our priors are similar to [5,8,12], being based on deformations away from a prototype template.

Inference consists of maximizing the posterior $P(\{q_i\}|D) = P(D|\{q_i\})P(\{q_i\})/P(D)$. As described in [8], this corresponds to a maximizing a posterior of form:

$$P(\{q_i\}|D) = \frac{1}{Z} \prod_i \psi_i(q_i) \prod_{i,j} \psi_{ij}(q_i, q_j), \tag{1}$$

where $\{\psi_i(q_i)\}$ and $\{\psi_{ij}(q_i, q_j)\}$ are the unary and pairwise potentials of the graph. The unary potentials model how well the individual features match to positions in the image. The binary potentials impose (probabilistic) constraints about the spatial relationships between feature points.

Algorithms such as dynamic programming [5,6] and belief propagation [7,8] have been used to search for optima of $P(\{q_i\}|D)$. But the algorithms are time consuming because each state variable q_i can take a large number of values (each feature point on the template can, in principle, match any point in the 240×320 image). Pruning and other ingenious techniques are used to speed up the search [5,7,8]. But performance remains at speeds of seconds to minutes.

3 The Hierarchical Compositional System

We define a compositional hierarchy by breaking down the representation $\{q_i : i \in \Lambda\}$ into substructures which have their own probability models.

At the first level, we group elements into K_1 subsets $\{q_i : i \in S_a^1\}$ where $\Lambda = \cup_{a=1}^{K_1} S_a^1$, $S_a^1 \cap S_b^1 = \emptyset$, $a \neq b$. These subsets correspond to meaningful parts of the object, such as ears and other features. See figure (1) for the basic structure. Specific examples for cats and horses will be given later.

For each of these subsets we define a generative model $P_a(D|\{q_i : i \in S_a^1\})$ and a prior $P_a(\{q_i : i \in S_a^1\})$. These generative and prior models are inherited from the full model, see equation (1), by simply cutting the connections between the subset S_a^1 and the Λ/S_a^1 (the remaining features on the object). Hence

$$P_{a^1}(D|\{q_i : i \in S_a^1\}) = \frac{1}{Z_{a^1}} \prod_{i \in S_a^1} \psi_i(q_i)$$

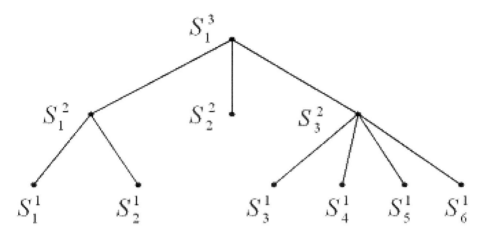

Figure 1: The Hierarchical Compositional structure. The full model contains all the nodes S_1^3. This is decomposed into subsets S_1^2, S_2^2, S_3^2 corresponding to sub-features. These, in turn, can be decomposed into subsets corresponding to more elementary features.

$$P_{a^1}(\{q_i : i \in S_a^1\}) \quad = \quad \frac{1}{\hat{Z}_{a^1}} \prod_{i,j \in S_a^1} \psi_{ij}(q_i, q_j). \tag{2}$$

We repeat the same process at the second and higher levels. The subsets $\{S_a^1 : a = 1, ..., K_1\}$ are composed to form a smaller selection of subsets $\{S_b^2 : b = 1, ..., K_2\}$, so that $\Lambda = \cup_{a=1}^{K_2} S_a^2$, $S_a^2 \cap S_b^2 = \emptyset$, $a \neq b$ and each S_a^1 is contained entirely inside one S_b^2. Again the S_b^2 are selected to correspond to meaningful parts of the object. Their generative models and prior distributions are again obtained from the full model, see equation (1). by cutting them off the links to the remaining nodes Λ/S_b^2.

The algorithm is run using two thresholds T_1, T_2. For each subset, say S_a^1, we define the *evidence* to be $P_{a^1}(D|\{z_i^\mu : i \in S_a^1\})P_{a^1}(\{z_i^\mu : i \in S_a^1\})$. We determine all possible configurations $\{z_i^\mu : i \in S_a^1\}$ such that evidence of each configuration is above T_1. This gives a (possibly large) set of positions for the $\{q_i : i \in S_a^1\}$. We apply non-maximum suppression to reduce many similar configurations in same local area to the one with maximum evidence (measured locally). We observe that a little displacement of position does not change optimality much for upper level matching. Typically, non-maximum suppression keeps around $30 \sim 500$ candidate configurations for each node. These remaining configurations can be considered as *proposals* [13] and are passed up the tree to the subset S_b^2 which contains S_a^1. Node S_b^2 evaluates the proposals to determine which ones are consistent, thus detecting composites of the subfeatures.

There is also top-down message passing which occurs when one part of a node S_b^2 contains high evidence – e.g. $P_{a^1}(D|\{z_i^\mu : i \in S_a^1\})P_{a^1}(\{z_i^\mu : i \in S_a^1\}) > T_2$ – but the other child nodes have no consistent values. In this case, we allow the matching to proceed if the combined matching strength is above threshold T_1. This mechanism enables the high-level models and, in particular, the priors for the relative positions of the sub-nodes to overcome weak local evidence. This performs a similar function to Coughlan and Shen's dynamic quantization scheme [8].

More sophisticated versions of this approach can be considered. For example, we could use the proposals to activate a data driven Monte Carlo Markov Chain (DDMCMC) algorithm [13]. To our knowledge, the use of hierarchical proposals of this type is unknown in the Monte Carlo sampling literature.

4 Experimental Results

We illustrate our hierarchical compositional system on examples of cats, horses, and hands. The images include background clutter and the objects can be partially occluded.

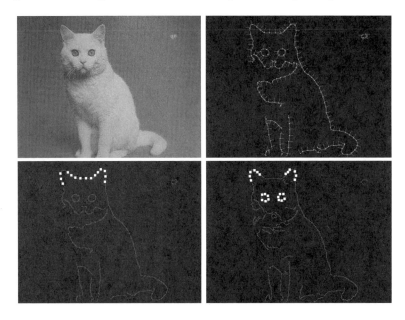

Figure 2: The prototype cat (top left panel), edges after grouping (top right panel), prototype template for ears and top of head (bottom left panel), and prototype for ears and eyes (bottom right panel). 15 points are used for the ears and 24 for the head.

First we preprocess the image using a Canny edge detector followed by simple edge grouping which eliminates isolated edges. Edge detection and edge grouping is illustrated in the top panels of figure (2). This figure is used to construct a prototype template for the ears, eyes, and head – see bottom panels of figure (2).

We construct a graphical model for the cat as described in section (2). Then we define a hierarchical structure, see figure (3).

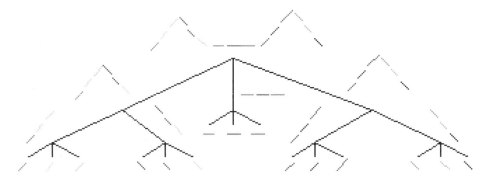

Figure 3: Hierarchy Structure for Cat Template.

Next we illustrate the results on several cat images, see figure (4). Several of these images were used in [8] and we thank Coughlan and Shen for supplying them. In all examples, our algorithm detects the cat correctly despite the deformations of the cat from the prototype, see figure (2). The detection was performed in less than 0.6 seconds (with unoptimized code). The images are 320×240 and the preprocessing time is included.

The algorithm is efficient since the subfeatures give bottom-up proposals which constraint the positions of the full model. For example, figure (5) shows the proposals for ears for the cluttered cat image (center panel of figure (4).

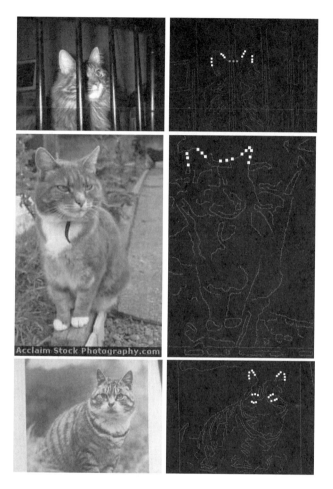

Figure 4: Cat with Occlusion (top panels). Cat with clutter (centre panel). Cat with eyes (bottom panel).

We next illustrate our approach on the tasks of detecting horses. This requires a more complicated hierarchy, see figure (6).

The algorithm succeeds in detecting the horse, see right panels of figure (7), using the prototype template shown in the left panel of figure (7).

Finally, we illustrate this approach for the much studied task of detecting hands, see [5,11]. Our approach detects hand from the Cambridge dataset in under a second, see figure (8). (We are grateful to Thayananthan, Stenger, Torr, and Cipolla for supplying these images).

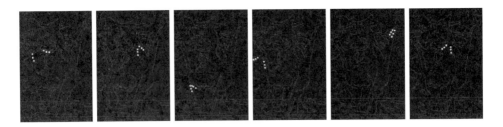

Figure 5: Cat Proposals: Left ears (left three panels). Right ears (right three panels).

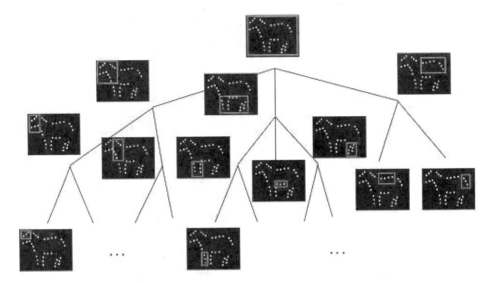

Figure 6: Horse Hierarchy. This is more complicated than the cat.

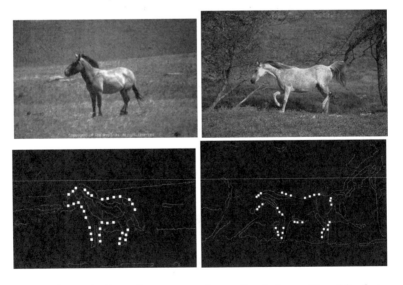

Figure 7: The left panels show the prototype horse (top left panel) and its feature points (bottom left panel). The right panel shows the input image (top right panel) and the position of the horse as detected by the algorithm (bottom right panel).

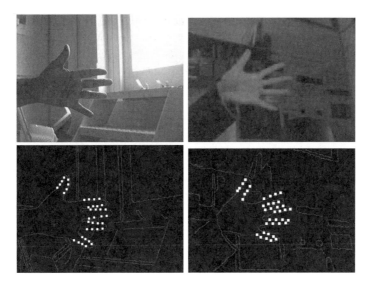

Figure 8: Prototype hand (top left panel), edge map of prototype hand (bottom left panel), Test hand (top right panel), Test hand edges (bottom right panel). 40 points are used.

5   Comparison with alternative methods

We ran the algorithm on image of typical size 320×240. There were usually 4000 segments after edge grouping. The templates had between 15 and 24 points. The average speed was 0.6 seconds on a laptop with 1.6 G Intel Pentium CPU (including all processing: edge detector, edge grouping, and object detection.

Other papers report times of seconds to minutes for detecting deformable objects from similar images [5,6,7,8]. So our approach is up to 100 times faster.

The Soft-Assign method in [15] has the ability to deal with objects with around 200 key points, but requires the initialization of the template to be close to the target object. This requirement is not practical in many applications. In our proposed method, there is no need to initialize the template near to the target.

Our hierarchical compositional tree structure is similar to the standard divide and conquer strategy used in some computer science algorithms. This may roughly be expected to scale as $\log N$ where N is the number of points on the deformable template. But precise complexity convergence results are difficult to obtain because they depend on the topology of the template, the amount of clutter in the background, and other factors.

This approach can be applied to any graphical model such as [10,12]. It is straightforward to design hierarchial compositional structures for objects based on their natural decompositions into parts.

There are alternative, and more sophisticated ways, to perform inference on graphical models by decomposing them into sub-graphs, see for example [14]. But these are typically far more computationally demanding.

6   Conclusion

We have presented a hierarchical compositional system for rapidly detecting deformable objects in images by performing inference on graphical models. Computation is performed by passing messages up and down the tree. The systems detects objects in under a second on images of size 320×240. This makes the approach practical for real world applications.

Our approach is similar in spirit to DDMCMC [13] in that we use proposals to guide the search for objects. In this paper, the proposals are based on a hierarchy of features which enables efficient computation. The low-level features propose more complex features which are validated by the probability models of the complex features. We have not found it necessary to perform stochastic sampling, though it is straightforward to do so in this framework.

Acknowledgments

This research was supported by NSF grant 0413214.

References

[1] Viola, P. and Jones, M. (2001). "Fast and Robust Classification using Asymmetric AdaBoost and a Detector Cascade". In *Proceedings NIPS01*.

[2] Schniederman, H. and Kanade, T. (2000). "A Statistical method for 3D object detection applied to faces and cars". In *Computer Vision and Pattern Recognition*.

[3] Chen, X. and Yuille, A.L. (2004). AdaBoost Learning for Detecting and Reading Text in City Scenes. *Proceedings CVPR*.

[4] Lowe, D.G. (1999). "Object recognition from local scale-invariant features." In *Proc. International Conference on Computer Vision ICCV*. Corfu, pages 1150-1157.

[5] Coughlan, J.M., Snow, D., English, C. and Yuille, A.L. (2000). "Efficient Deformable Template Detection and Localization without User Initialization". Computer Vision and Image Understanding. 78, pp 303-319.

[6] Felzenswalb, P. (2005). "Representation and Detection of Deformable Shapes". *IEEE Transactions on Pattern Analysis and Machine Intelligence*, Vol. 27, No. 2.

[7] Coughlan, J.M., and Ferreira, S. (2002). "Finding Deformable Shapes using Loopy Belief Propoagation". In *Proceedings European Conference of Computer Vision.*. 2002.

[8] Coughlan, J.M., and Shen, H. (2004). "Shape Matching with Belief Propagation: Using Dynamic Quantization to Accomodate Occlusion and Clutter". In GMBV .

[9] Geman, S. Potter, D. and Chi, Z. (2002). " Composition systems". Quarterly of Applied Mathematics, LX, pp 707-736.

[10] Fergus, R., Perona, P. and Zisserman, A. (2003) "Object Class Recognition by Unsupervised Scale-Invariant Learning". *Proceeding CVPR*. (2), pp 264-271.

[11] Thayananthan, A. Stenger, B., Torr, P. and Cipolla, R. (2003). "Shape context and chamfer matching in cluttered scenes," In *Proc. Conf. Comp. Vision Pattern Rec.*, pp. 127–133.

[12] Berg, A.C., Berg, T.L., and Malik, J. (2005). "Shape Matching and Object Recognition using Low Distortion Correspondence". *Proceedings CVPR*.

[13] Tu, Z., Chen, X., Yuille, A.L., and Zhu, S.C. (2003). "Image Parsing: Unifying Segmentation, Detection, and Recognition". In *Proceedings ICCV*.

[14] Wainwright, M.J., Jaakkola, T.S., and Willsky., A.S. "Tree-Based Reparamterization Framework for Analysis of Sum-Product and Related Algorithms". *IEEE Transactions on Information Theory*. Vol. 49, pp 1120-1146. No. 5. 2003.

[15] Chui,H. and Rangarajan, A., A New Algorithm for Non-Rigid Point Matching. In Proceedings CVPR 2000.

Cyclic Equilibria in Markov Games

Martin Zinkevich and Amy Greenwald
Department of Computer Science
Brown University
Providence, RI 02912
{maz,amy}@cs.brown.edu

Michael L. Littman
Department of Computer Science
Rutgers, The State University of NJ
Piscataway, NJ 08854–8019
mlittman@cs.rutgers.edu

Abstract

Although variants of value iteration have been proposed for finding Nash or correlated equilibria in general-sum Markov games, these variants have not been shown to be effective in general. In this paper, we demonstrate by construction that existing variants of value iteration cannot find stationary equilibrium policies in arbitrary general-sum Markov games. Instead, we propose an alternative interpretation of the output of value iteration based on a new (non-stationary) equilibrium concept that we call "cyclic equilibria." We prove that value iteration identifies cyclic equilibria in a class of games in which it fails to find stationary equilibria. We also demonstrate empirically that value iteration finds cyclic equilibria in nearly all examples drawn from a random distribution of Markov games.

1 Introduction

Value iteration (Bellman, 1957) has proven its worth in a variety of sequential-decision-making settings, most significantly single-agent environments (Puterman, 1994), team games, and two-player zero-sum games (Shapley, 1953). In value iteration for Markov decision processes and team Markov games, the value of a state is defined to be the maximum over all actions of the value of the combination of the state and action (or *Q value*). In zero-sum environments, the max operator becomes a minimax over joint actions of the two players. Learning algorithms based on this update have been shown to compute equilibria in both model-based scenarios (Brafman & Tennenholtz, 2002) and Q-learning-like model-free scenarios (Littman & Szepesvári, 1996).

The theoretical and empirical success of such algorithms has led researchers to apply the same approach in general-sum games, in spite of exceedingly weak guarantees of convergence (Hu & Wellman, 1998; Greenwald & Hall, 2003). Here, value-update rules based on select Nash or correlated equilibria have been evaluated empirically and have been shown to perform reasonably in some settings. None has been identified that computes equilibria in general, however, leaving open the question of whether such an update rule is even possible.

Our main negative theoretical result is that an entire class of value-iteration update rules, including all those mentioned above, can be excluded from consideration for computing stationary equilibria in general-sum Markov games. Briefly, existing value-iteration algorithms compute Q values as an intermediate result, then derive policies from these Q values. We demonstrate a class of games in which Q values, even those corresponding to an equilibrium policy, contain insufficient information for reconstructing an equilibrium policy.

Faced with the impossibility of developing algorithms along the lines of traditional value iteration that find stationary equilibria, we suggest an alternative equilibrium concept—cyclic equilibria. A cyclic equilibrium is a kind of non-stationary joint policy that satisfies the standard conditions for equilibria (no incentive to deviate unilaterally). However, unlike conditional non-stationary policies such as tit-for-tat and finite-state strategies based on the "folk theorem" (Osborne & Rubinstein, 1994), cyclic equilibria cycle rigidly through a set of stationary policies.

We present two positive results concerning cyclic equilibria. First, we consider the class of two-player two-state two-action games used to show that Q values cannot reconstruct all stationary equilibrium. Section 4.1 shows that value iteration finds cyclic equilibria for all games in this class. Second, Section 5 describes empirical results on a more general set of games. We find that on a significant fraction of these games, value iteration updates fail to converge. In contrast, value iteration finds cyclic equilibria for nearly all the games.

The success of value iteration in finding cyclic equilibria suggests this generalized solution concept could be useful for constructing robust multiagent learning algorithms.

2 An Impossibility Result for Q Values

In this section, we consider a subclass of Markov games in which transitions are deterministic and are controlled by one player at a time. We show that this class includes games that have no deterministic equilibrium policies. For this class of games, we present (proofs available in an extended technical report) two theorems. The first, a negative result, states that the Q values used in existing value-iteration algorithms are insufficient for deriving equilibrium policies. The second, presented in Section 4.1, is a positive result that states that value iteration does converge to cyclic equilibrium policies in this class of games.

2.1 Preliminary Definitions

Given a finite set X, define $\Delta(X)$ to be the set of all probability distributions over X.

Definition 1 A **_Markov game_** $\Gamma = [S, N, \mathbf{A}, T, R, \gamma]$ _is a set of states_ S, _a set of players_ $N = \{1, \ldots, n\}$, _a set of actions for each player in each state_ $\{A_{i,s}\}_{s \in S, i \in N}$ _(where we represent the set of all state-action pairs as_ $\mathbf{A} \equiv \bigcup_{s \in S} (\{s\} \times \prod_{i \in N} A_{i,s})$), _a transition function_ $T : \mathbf{A} \to \Delta(S)$, _a reward function_ $R : \mathbf{A} \to \mathbf{R}^n$, _and a discount factor_ γ.

Given a Markov game Γ, let $A_s = \prod_{i \in N} A_{i,s}$. A **stationary policy** is a set of distributions $\{\pi(s) : s \in S\}$, where for all $s \in S$, $\pi(s) \in \Delta(A_s)$. Given a stationary policy π, define $V^{\pi,\Gamma} : S \to \mathbf{R}^n$ and $Q^{\pi,\Gamma} : \mathbf{A} \to \mathbf{R}^n$ to be the unique pair of functions satisfying the following system of equations: for all $i \in N$, for all $(s, a) \in \mathbf{A}$,

$$V_i^{\pi,\Gamma}(s) = \sum_{a \in A_s} \pi(s)(a) Q_i^{\pi,\Gamma}(s, a), \tag{1}$$

$$Q_i^{\pi,\Gamma}(s, a) = R_i(s, a) + \gamma \sum_{s' \in S} T(s, a)(s') V_i^{\pi,\Gamma}(s'). \tag{2}$$

A **deterministic** Markov game is a Markov game Γ where the transition function is deterministic: $T : \mathbf{A} \to S$. A **turn-taking game** is a Markov game Γ where in every state, only one player has a choice of action. Formally, for all $s \in S$, there exists a player $i \in N$ such that for all other players $j \in N \setminus \{i\}$, $|A_{j,s}| = 1$.

2.2 A Negative Result for Stationary Equilibria

A **NoSDE** (pronounced "nasty") game is a deterministic turn-taking Markov game Γ with two players, two states, no more than two actions for either player in either state, and no deterministic stationary equilibrium policy. That the set of NoSDE games is non-empty is demonstrated by the game depicted in Figure 1. This game has no deterministic stationary equilibrium policy: If Player 1 sends, Player 2 prefers to send; but, if Player 2 sends, Player 1 prefers to keep; and, if Player 1 keeps, Player 2 prefers to keep; but, if Player 2 keeps, Player 1 prefers to send. No deterministic policy is an equilibrium because one player will always have an incentive to change policies.

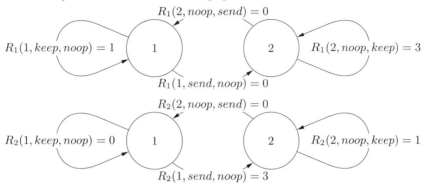

Figure 1: An example of a NoSDE game. Here, $S = \{1, 2\}$, $A_{1,1} = A_{2,2} = \{keep, send\}$, $A_{1,2} = A_{2,1} = \{noop\}$, $T(1, keep, noop) = 1$, $T(1, send, noop) = 2$, $T(2, noop, keep) = 2$, $T(2, noop, send) = 1$, and $\gamma = 3/4$. In the unique stationary equilibrium, Player 1 sends with probability $2/3$ and Player 2 sends with probability $5/12$.

Lemma 1 *Every NoSDE game has a* unique *stationary equilibrium policy.*[1]

It is well known that, in general Markov games, random policies are sometimes needed to achieve an equilibrium. This fact can be demonstrated simply by a game with one state where the utilities correspond to a bimatrix game with no deterministic equilibria (penny matching, say). Random actions in these games are sometimes linked with strategies that use "faking" or "bluffing" to avoid being exploited. That NoSDE games exist is surprising, in that randomness is needed even though actions are always taken with complete information about the other player's choice and the state of the game. However, the next result is even more startling. Current value-iteration algorithms attempt to find the Q values of a game with the goal using these values to find a stationary equilibrium of the game. The main theorem of this paper states that it is not possible to derive a policy from the Q values for NoSDE games, and therefore in general Markov games.

Theorem 1 *For any NoSDE game $\Gamma = [S, N, \mathbf{A}, T, R]$ with a unique equilibrium policy π, there exists another NoSDE game $\Gamma' = [S, N, \mathbf{A}, T, R']$ with its own unique equilibrium policy π' such that $Q^{\pi,\Gamma} = Q^{\pi',\Gamma'}$ but $\pi \neq \pi'$ and $V^{\pi,\Gamma} \neq V^{\pi',\Gamma'}$.*

This result establishes that computing or learning Q values is insufficient to compute a stationary equilibrium of a game.[2] In this paper we suggest an alternative, where we still

---

[1] The policy is both a correlated equilibrium and a Nash equilibrium.

[2] Although maintaining Q values *and* state values and deriving policies from both sets of functions might circumvent this problem, we are not aware of existing value-iteration algorithms or learning algorithms that do so. This observation presents a possible avenue of research not followed in this paper.

do value iteration in the same way, but we extract a *cyclic equilibrium* from the sequence of values instead of a stationary one.

3   A New Goal: Cyclic Equilibria

A **cyclic policy** is a finite sequence of stationary policies $\pi = \{\pi_1, \ldots, \pi_k\}$. Associated with π is a sequence of value functions $\{V^{\pi,\Gamma,j}\}$ and Q-value functions $\{Q^{\pi,\Gamma,j}\}$ such that

$$V_i^{\pi,\Gamma,j}(s) = \sum_{a \in A_s} \pi_j(s)(a)\, Q_i^{\pi,\Gamma,j}(s,a) \quad \text{and} \tag{3}$$

$$Q_i^{\pi,\Gamma,j}(s,a) = R_i(s,a) + \gamma \sum_{s' \in S} T(s,a)(s')\, V_i^{\pi,\Gamma,inc_k(j)}(s') \tag{4}$$

where for all $j \in \{1, \ldots, k\}$, $inc_k(k) = 1$ and $inc_k(j) = j + 1$ if $j < k$.

Definition 2 *Given a Markov game Γ, a **cyclic correlated equilibrium** is a cyclic policy π, where for all $j \in \{1, \ldots, k\}$, for all $i \in N$, for all $s \in S$, for all $a_i, a_i' \in A_{i,s}$:*

$$\sum_{a_{-i} \in A_{-i,s}} \pi_j(s)(a_i, a_{-i})\, Q_i^{\pi,\Gamma,j}(s, a_i, a_{-i}) \geq \sum_{(a_i, a_{-i}) \in A_s} \pi_j(s)(a_i, a_{-i})\, Q_i^{\pi,\Gamma,j}(s, a_i', a_{-i}). \tag{5}$$

Here, a_{-i} denotes a joint action for all players except i. A similar definition can be constructed for Nash equilibria by insisting that all policies $\pi_j(s)$ are product distributions. In Definition 2, we imagine that action choices are moderated by a referee with a clock that indicates the current stage j of the cycle. At each stage, a typical correlated equilibrium is executed, meaning that the referee chooses a joint action a from $\pi_j(s)$, tells each agent its part of that joint action, and no agent can improve its value by eschewing the referee's advice. If no agent can improve its value by more than ϵ at any stage, we say π is an ϵ-**correlated cyclic equilibrium**.

A **stationary correlated equilibrium** is a cyclic correlated equilibrium with $k = 1$. In the next section, we show how value iteration can be used to derive cyclic correlated equilibria.

4   Value Iteration in General-Sum Markov Games

For a game Γ, define $\mathcal{Q}_\Gamma = (\mathbf{R}^n)^{\mathbf{A}}$ to be the set of all state-action (Q) value functions, $\mathcal{V}_\Gamma = (\mathbf{R}^n)^S$ to be the set of all value functions, and Π_Γ to be the set of all stationary policies. Traditionally, value iteration can be broken down into estimating a Q value based upon a value function, selecting a policy π given the Q values, and deriving a value function based upon π and the Q value functions. Whereas the first and the last step are fairly straightforward, the step in the middle is quite tricky. A pair $(\pi, Q) \in \Pi_\Gamma \times \mathcal{Q}_\Gamma$ **agree** (see Equation 5) if, for all $s \in S$, $i \in N$, $a_i, a_i' \in A_{i,s}$:

$$\sum_{a_{-i} \in A_{-i,s}} \pi(s)(a_i, a_{-i})\, Q_i(s, a_i, a_{-i}) \geq \sum_{(a_i, a_{-i}) \in A_s} \pi(s)(a_i, a_{-i})\, Q(s, a_i', a_{-i}). \tag{6}$$

Essentially, Q and π agree if π is a best response for each player given payoffs Q. An **equilibrium-selection rule** is a function $f : \mathcal{Q}_\Gamma \rightarrow \Pi_\Gamma$ such that for all $Q \in \mathcal{Q}_\Gamma$, $(f(Q), Q)$ agree. The set of all such rules is F_Γ. In essence, these rules update values assuming an equilibrium policy for a one-stage game with $Q(s, a)$ providing the terminal rewards. Examples of equilibrium-selection rules are best-Nash, utilitarian-CE, dictatorial-CE, plutocratic-CE, and egalitarian-CE (Greenwald & Hall, 2003). (Utilitarian-CE, which we return to later, selects the correlated equilibrium in which total of the payoffs is maximized.) Foe-VI and Friend-VI (Littman, 2001) do not fit into our formalism, but it can be proven that in NoSDE games they converge to deterministic policies that are neither stationary nor cyclic equilibria. Define $d_\Gamma : \mathcal{V}_\Gamma \times \mathcal{V}_\Gamma \to \mathbf{R}$ to be a distance metric over value functions, such that

$$d_\Gamma(V, V') = \max_{s \in S, i \in N} |V_i(s) - V_i'(s)|. \tag{7}$$

Using our notation, the value-iteration algorithm for general-sum Markov games can be described as follows.

Algorithm 1: ValueIteration(game Γ, $V^0 \in \mathcal{V}_\Gamma$, $f \in \mathbf{F}_\Gamma$, Integer T)

For $t := 1$ to T:

1. $\forall s \in S, a \in A, Q^t(s, a) := R(s, a) + \gamma \sum_{s' \in S} T(s, a)(s') \, V^{t-1}(s')$.

2. $\pi^t = f(Q^t)$.

3. $\forall s \in S, V^t(s) = \sum_{a \in A_s} \pi^t(s)(a) \, Q^t(s, a)$.

Return $\{Q^1, \ldots, Q^T\}, \{\pi^1, \ldots, \pi^T\}, \{V^1, \ldots, V^T\}$.

If a stationary equilibrium is sought, the final policy is returned.

Algorithm 2: GetStrategy(game Γ, $V^0 \in \mathcal{V}_\Gamma$, $f \in \mathbf{F}_\Gamma$, Integer T)

1. Run $(Q^1 \ldots Q^T, \pi^1 \ldots \pi^T, V^1 \ldots V^T) = $ ValueIteration(Γ, V^0, f, T).

2. Return π^T.

For cyclic equilibria, we have a variety of options for how many past stationary policies we want to consider for forming a cycle. Our approach searches for a recent value function that matches the final value function (an exact match would imply a true cycle). Ties are broken in favor of the shortest cycle length. Observe that the order of the policies returned by value iteration is reversed to form a cyclic equilibrium.

Algorithm 3: GetCycle(game Γ, $V^0 \in \mathcal{V}_\Gamma$, $f \in \mathbf{F}_\Gamma$, Integer T, Integer $maxCycle$)

1. If $maxCycle \geq T$, $maxCycle := T - 1$.

2. Run $(Q^1 \ldots Q^T, \pi^1 \ldots \pi^T, V^1 \ldots V^T) = $ ValueIteration(Γ, V^0, f, T).

3. Define $k := \mathrm{argmin}_{t \in \{1, \ldots, maxCycle\}} d(V^T, V^{T-t})$.

4. For each $t \in \{1, \ldots, k\}$ set $\pi_t := \pi^{T+1-t}$.

4.1 Convergence Conditions

Fact 1 *If $d(V^T, V^{T-1}) = \epsilon$ in **GetStrategy**, then **GetStrategy** returns an $\frac{\epsilon\gamma}{1-\gamma}$-correlated equilibrium.*

Fact 2 *If **GetCycle** returns a cyclic policy of length k and $d(V^T, V^{T-k}) = \epsilon$, then **GetCycle** returns an $\frac{\epsilon\gamma}{1-\gamma^k}$-correlated cyclic equilibrium.*

Since, given V^0 and Γ, the space of value functions is bounded, *eventually* there will be two value functions in $\{V^1, \ldots, V^T\}$ that are close according to d_Γ. Therefore, the two practical (and open) questions are (1) how many iterations does it take to find an ϵ-correlated cyclic equilibrium? and (2) How large is the cyclic equilibrium that is found?

In addition to approximate convergence described above, in two-player turn-taking games, one can prove *exact convergence*. In fact, all the members of $\mathbf{F}_\Gamma$ described above can be construed as generalizations of utilitarian-CE in turn-taking games, and utilitarian-CE is proven to converge.

Theorem 2 *Given the utilitarian-CE equilibrium-selection rule f, for every NoSDE game Γ, for every $V^0 \in \mathcal{V}_\Gamma$, there exists some finite T such that **GetCycle**$(\Gamma, V^0, f, T, \lceil T/2 \rceil)$ returns a cyclic correlated equilibrium.*

Theoretically, we can imagine passing infinity as a parameter to value iteration. Doing so shows the limitation of value-iteration in Markov games.

Theorem 3 *Given the utilitarian-CE equilibrium-selection rule f, for any NoSDE game Γ with unique equilibrium π, for every $V^0 \in \mathcal{V}_\Gamma$, the value-function sequence $\{V^1, V^2, \ldots\}$ returned from **ValueIteration**(Γ, V^0, f, ∞) does not converge to V^π.*

Since all of the other rules specified above (except friend-VI and foe-VI) can be implemented with the utilitarian-CE equilibrium-selection rule, none of these rules will be guaranteed to converge, even in such a simple class as turn-taking games!

Theorem 4 *Given the game Γ in Figure 1 and its stationary equilibrium π, given $V_i^0(s) = 0$ for all $i \in N$, $s \in S$, then for any update rule $f \in \mathbf{F}_\Gamma$, the value-function sequence $\{V^1, V^2, \ldots\}$ returned from **ValueIteration**(Γ, V^0, f, ∞) does not converge to V^π.*

5 Empirical Results

To complement the formal results of the previous sections, we ran two batteries of tests on value iteration in randomly generated games. We assessed the convergence behavior of value iteration to stationary and cyclic equilibria.

5.1 Experimental Details

Our game generator took as input the set of players N, the set of states S, and for each player i and state s, the actions $A_{i,s}$. To construct a game, for each state-joint action pair $(s, a) \in \mathbf{A}$, for each agent $i \in N$, the generator sets $R_i(s, a)$ to be an integer between 0 and 99, chosen uniformly at random. Then, it selects $T(s, a)$ to be deterministic, with the resulting state chosen uniformly at random. We used a consistent discount factor of $\gamma = 0.75$ to decrease experimental variance.

The primary dependent variable in our results was the frequency with which value iteration converged to a stationary Nash equilibrium or a cyclic Nash equilibrium (of length less than 100). To determine convergence, we first ran value iteration for 1000 steps. If $d_\Gamma(V^{1000}, V^{999}) \leq 0.0001$, then we considered value iteration to have converged to a stationary policy. If for some $k \leq 100$

$$\max_{t \in \{1, \ldots, k\}} d_\Gamma(V^{1001-t}, V^{1001-(t+k)}) \leq 0.0001, \tag{8}$$

then we considered value iteration to have converged to a cycle.[3]

To determine if a game has a deterministic equilibrium, for every deterministic policy π, we ran policy evaluation (for 1000 iterations) to estimate $V^{\pi, \Gamma}$ and $Q^{\pi, \Gamma}$, and then checked if π was an ϵ-correlated equilibrium for $\epsilon = 0.0001$.

5.2 Turn-taking Games

In the first battery of tests, we considered sets of turn-taking games with x states and y actions: formally, there were x states $\{1, \ldots, x\}$. In odd-numbered states, Player 1 had y

---

[3]In contrast to the **GetCycle** algorithm, we are here concerned with finding a cyclic equilibrium so we check an entire cycle for convergence.

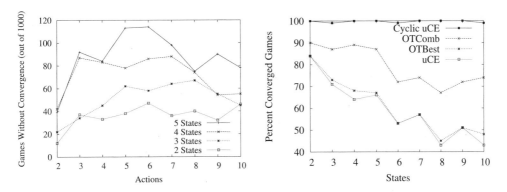

Figure 2: (Left) For each combination of states and actions, 1000 deterministic turn-taking games were generated. The graph plots the number of games where value iteration did not converge to a stationary equilibrium. (Right) Frequency of convergence on 100 randomly generated games with simultaneous actions. **Cyclic uCE** is the number of times utilitarian-CE converged to a cyclic equilibrium. **OTComb** is the number of games where any one of Friend-VI, Foe-VI, utilitarian-NE-VI, and 5 variants of correlated equilibrium-VI: dictatorial-CE-VI (First Player), dictatorial-CE-VI (Second Player), utilitarian-CE-VI, plutocratic-CE-VI, and egalitarian-VI converged to a stationary equilibrium. **OTBest** is the maximum number of games where the best fixed choice of the equilibrium-selection rule converged. **uCE** is the number of games in which utilitarian-CE-VI converged to a stationary equilibrium.

actions and Player 2 had one action: in even-numbered states, Player 1 had one action and Player 2 had y actions. We varied x from 2 to 5 and y from 2 to 10. For each setting of x and y, we generated and tested one thousand games.

Figure 2 (left) shows the number of generated games for which value iteration did *not* converge to a stationary equilibrium. We found that nearly half (48%, as many as 5% of the total set) of these non-converged games had no stationary, deterministic equilibria (they were NoSDE games). The remainder of the stationary, deterministic equilibria were simply not discovered by value iteration. We also found that value iteration converged to cycles of length 100 or less in 99.99% of the games.

5.3 Simultaneous Games

In a second set of experiments, we generated two-player Markov games where both agents have at least two actions in every state. We varied the number of states between 2 and 9, and had either 2 or 3 actions for every agent in every state.

Figure 2 (right) summarizes results for 3-action games (2-actions games were qualitatively similar, but converged more often). Note that the fraction of random games on which the algorithms converged to stationary equilibria decreases as the number of states increases. This result holds because the larger the game, the larger the chance that value iteration will fall into a cycle on some subset of the states. Once again, we see that the cyclic equilibria are found much more reliably than stationary equilibria by value-iteration algorithms. For example, utilitarian-CE converges to a cyclic correlated equilibrium about 99% of the time, whereas with 10 states and 3 actions, on 26% of the games none of the techniques converge.

6 Conclusion

In this paper, we showed that value iteration, the algorithmic core of many multiagent planning reinforcement-learning algorithms, is not well behaved in Markov games. Among other impossibility results, we demonstrated that the Q-value function retains too little information for constructing optimal policies, even in 2-state, 2-action, deterministic turn-taking Markov games. In fact, there are an infinite number of such games with different Nash equilibrium value functions that have identical Q-value functions. This result holds for proposed variants of value iteration from the literature such as updating via a correlated equilibrium or a Nash equilibrium, since, in turn-taking Markov games, both rules reduce to updating via the action with the maximum value for the controlling player.

Our results paint a bleak picture for the use of value-iteration-based algorithms for computing stationary equilibria. However, in a class of games we called NoSDE games, a natural extension of value iteration converges to a limit cycle, which is in fact a cyclic (nonstationary) Nash equilibrium policy. Such cyclic equilibria can also be found reliably for randomly generated games and there is evidence that they appear in some naturally occurring problems (Tesauro & Kephart, 1999). One take-away message of our work is that nonstationary policies may hold the key to improving the robustness of computational approaches to planning and learning in general-sum games.

Acknowledgements

This research was supported by NSF Grant #IIS-0325281, NSF Career Grant #IIS-0133689, and the Alberta Ingenuity Foundation through the Alberta Ingenuity Centre for Machine Learning.

References

Bellman, R. (1957). *Dynamic programming*. Princeton, NJ: Princeton University Press.

Brafman, R. I., & Tennenholtz, M. (2002). R-MAX—a general polynomial time algorithm for near-optimal reinforcement learning. *Journal of Machine Learning Research*, *3*, 213–231.

Greenwald, A., & Hall, K. (2003). Correlated Q-learning. *Proceedings of the Twentieth International Conference on Machine Learning* (pp. 242–249).

Hu, J., & Wellman, M. (1998). Multiagent reinforcement learning:theoretical framework and an algorithm. *Proceedings of the Fifteenth International Conference on Machine Learning* (pp. 242–250). Morgan Kaufman.

Littman, M. (2001). Friend-or-foe Q-learning in general-sum games. *Proceedings of the Eighteenth International Conference on Machine Learning* (pp. 322–328). Morgan Kaufmann.

Littman, M. L., & Szepesvári, C. (1996). A generalized reinforcement-learning model: Convergence and applications. *Proceedings of the Thirteenth International Conference on Machine Learning* (pp. 310–318).

Osborne, M. J., & Rubinstein, A. (1994). *A Course in Game Theory*. The MIT Press.

Puterman, M. (1994). *Markov decision processes: Discrete stochastic dynamic programming*. Wiley-Interscience.

Shapley, L. (1953). Stochastic games. *Proceedings of the National Academy of Sciences of the United States of America*, *39*, 1095–1100.

Tesauro, G., & Kephart, J. (1999). Pricing in agent economies using multi-agent Q-learning. *Proceedings of Fifth European Conference on Symbolic and Quantitative Approaches to Reasoning with Uncertainty* (pp. 71–86).

On the Convergence of Eigenspaces in Kernel Principal Component Analysis

Laurent Zwald
Département de Mathématiques,
Université Paris-Sud,
Bât. 425, F-91405 Orsay, France
`Laurent.Zwald@math.u-psud.fr`

Gilles Blanchard
Fraunhofer First (IDA),
Kékuléstr. 7, D-12489 Berlin, Germany
`blanchar@first.fhg.de`

Abstract

This paper presents a non-asymptotic statistical analysis of Kernel-PCA with a focus different from the one proposed in previous work on this topic. Here instead of considering the reconstruction error of KPCA we are interested in approximation error bounds for the eigenspaces themselves. We prove an upper bound depending on the spacing between eigenvalues but not on the dimensionality of the eigenspace. As a consequence this allows to infer stability results for these estimated spaces.

1 Introduction.

Principal Component Analysis (PCA for short in the sequel) is a widely used tool for data dimensionality reduction. It consists in finding the most relevant lower-dimension projection of some data in the sense that the projection should keep as much of the variance of the original data as possible. If the target dimensionality of the projected data is fixed in advance, say D – an assumption that we will make throughout the present paper – the solution of this problem is obtained by considering the projection on the span S_D of the first D eigenvectors of the covariance matrix. Here by 'first D eigenvectors' we mean eigenvectors associated to the D largest eigenvalues counted with multiplicity; hereafter with some abuse the span of the first D eigenvectors will be called "D-eigenspace" for short when there is no risk of confusion.

The introduction of the 'Kernel trick' has allowed to extend this methodology to data mapped in a kernel feature space, then called KPCA [8]. The interest of this extension is that, while still linear in feature space, it gives rise to *nonlinear* interpretation in original space – vectors in the kernel feature space can be interpreted as nonlinear functions on the original space.

For PCA as well as KPCA, the true covariance matrix (resp. covariance operator) is not known and has to be estimated from the available data, an procedure which in the case of Kernel spaces is linked to the so-called Nyström approximation [13]. The subspace given as an output is then obtained as D-eigenspace $\widehat{S}_D$ of the *empirical* covariance matrix or operator. An interesting question from a statistical or learning theoretical point of view is then, how reliable this estimate is.

This question has already been studied [10, 2] from the point of view of the *reconstruction error* of the estimated subspace. What this means is that (assuming the data is centered in Kernel space for simplicity) the average reconstruction error (square norm of the distance to the projection) of $\widehat{S}_D$ converges to the (optimal) reconstruction error of S_D and that bounds are known about the rate of convergence. However, this does not tell us much about the convergence of S_D to $\widehat{S}_D$ – since two very different subspaces can have a very similar reconstruction error, in particular when some eigenvalues are very close to each other (the gap between the eigenvalues will actually appear as a central point of the analysis to come).

In the present work, we set to study the behavior of these D-eigenspaces themselves: we provide finite sample bounds describing the closeness of the D-eigenspaces of the empirical covariance operator to the true one. There are several broad motivations for this analysis. First, the reconstruction error alone is a valid criterion only if one really plans to perform dimensionality reduction of the data and stop there. However, PCA is often used merely as a *preprocessing* step and the projected data is then submitted to further processing (which could be classification, regression or something else). In particular for KPCA, the projection subspace in the kernel space can be interpreted as a subspace of *functions* on the original space; one then expects these functions to be relevant for the data at hand and for some further task (see e.g. [3]). In these cases, if we want to analyze the full procedure (from a learning theoretical sense), it is desirable to have a more precise information on the selected subspace than just its reconstruction error. In particular, from a learning complexity point of view, it is important to ensure that functions used for learning stay in a set of limited complexity, which is ensured if the selected subspace is stable (which is a consequence of its convergence).

The approach we use here is based on perturbation bounds and we essentially walk in the steps pioneered by Kolchinskii and Giné [7] (see also [4]) using tools of operator perturbation theory [5]. Similar methods have been used to prove consistency of spectral clustering [12, 11]. An important difference here is that we want to study directly the convergence of the whole subspace spanned by the first D eigenvectors instead of the separate convergence of the individual eigenvectors; in particular we are interested in how D acts as a complexity parameter. The important point in our main result is that it does not: only the gap between the D-th and the $(D+1)$-th eigenvalue comes into account. This means that there in no increase in complexity (as far as this bound is concerned: of course we cannot exclude that better bounds can be obtained in the future) between estimating the D-th eigenvector alone or the span of the first D eigenvectors.

Our contribution in the present work is thus

- to adapt the operator perturbation result of [7] to D-eigenspaces.
- to get non-asymptotic bounds on the approximation error of Kernel-PCA eigenspaces thanks to the previous tool.

In section 2 we introduce shortly the notation, explain the main ingredients used and obtain a first bound based on controlling separately the first D eigenvectors, and depending on the dimension D. In section 3 we explain why the first bound is actually suboptimal and derive an improved bound as a consequence of an operator perturbation result that is more adapted to our needs and deals directly with the D-eigenspace as a whole. Section 4 concludes and discusses the obtained results. Mathematical proofs are found in the appendix.

2 First result.

Notation. The interest variable X takes its values in some measurable space $\mathcal{X}$, following the distribution P. We consider KPCA and are therefore primarily interested in the mapping of X into a reproducing kernel Hilbert space $\mathcal{H}$ with kernel function k through the feature mapping $\varphi(x) = k(x, \cdot)$. The objective of the kernel PCA procedure is to recover a D-dimensional subspace S_D of $\mathcal{H}$ such that the projection of $\varphi(X)$ on S_D has maximum averaged squared norm.

All operators considered in what follows are Hilbert-Schmidt and the norm considered for these operators will be the Hilbert-Schmidt norm unless precised otherwise. Furthermore we only consider symmetric nonnegative operators, so that they can be diagonalized and have a discrete spectrum.

Let C denote the covariance operator of variable $\varphi(X)$. To simplify notation we assume that nonzero eigenvalues $\lambda_1 > \lambda_2 > \ldots$ of C are all simple (This is for convenience only. In the conclusion we discuss what changes have to be made if this is not the case). Let $\phi_1, \phi_2, \ldots$ be the associated eigenvectors. It is well-known that the optimal D-dimensional reconstruction space is $S_D = \text{span}\{\phi_1, \ldots, \phi_D\}$. The KPCA procedure approximates this objective by considering the empirical covariance operator, denoted C_n, and the subspace $\widehat{S}_D$ spanned by its first D eigenvectors. We denote $P_{S_D}, P_{\widehat{S}_D}$ the orthogonal projectors on these spaces.

A first bound. Broadly speaking, the main steps required to obtain the type of result we are interested in are

1. A non-asympotic bound on the (Hilbert-Schmidt) norm of the difference between the empirical and the true covariance operators;

2. An operator perturbation result bounding the difference between spectral projectors of two operators by the norm of their difference.

The combination of these two steps leads to our goal. The first step consists in the following Lemma coming from [9]:

Lemma 1 (Corollary 5 of [9]) *Supposing that* $\sup_{x \in \mathcal{X}} k(x, x) \leq M$, *with probability greater than* $1 - e^{-\xi}$,

$$\|C_n - C\| \leq \frac{2M}{\sqrt{n}} \left(1 + \sqrt{\frac{\xi}{2}} \right) .$$

As for the second step, [7] provides the following perturbation bound (see also e.g. [12]):

Theorem 2 (Simplified Version of [7], Theorem 5.2) *Let A be a symmetric positive Hilbert-Schmidt operator of the Hilbert space $\mathcal{H}$ with simple positive eigenvalues $\lambda_1 > \lambda_2 > \ldots$ For an integer r such that $\lambda_r > 0$, let $\widetilde{\delta}_r = \delta_r \wedge \delta_{r-1}$ where $\delta_r = \frac{1}{2}(\lambda_r - \lambda_{r+1})$. Let $B \in HS(\mathcal{H})$ be another symmetric operator such that $\|B\| < \widetilde{\delta}_r/2$ and $(A + B)$ is still a positive operator with simple nonzero eigenvalues.*

Let $P_r(A)$ (resp. $P_r(A + B)$) denote the orthogonal projector onto the subspace spanned by the r-th eigenvector of A (resp. $(A + B)$). Then, these projectors satisfy:

$$\|P_r(A) - P_r(A + B)\| \leq \frac{2\|B\|}{\widetilde{\delta}_r} .$$

Remark about the Approximation Error of the Eigenvectors: let us recall that a control over the Hilbert-Schmidt norm of the projections onto eigenspaces imply a control on the approximation errors of the eigenvectors themselves. Indeed, let ϕ_r, ψ_r denote the (normalized) r-th eigenvectors of the operators above with signs chosen so that $\langle \phi_r, \psi_r \rangle > 0$. Then

$$\|P_{\phi_r} - P_{\psi_r}\|^2 = 2(1 - \langle \phi_r, \psi_r \rangle^2) \geq 2(1 - \langle \phi_r, \psi_r \rangle) = \|\phi_r - \psi_r\|^2 .$$

Now, the orthogonal projector on the direct sum of the first D eigenspaces is the sum $\sum_{r=1}^{D} P_r$. Using the triangle inequality, and combining Lemma 1 and Theorem 2, we conclude that with probability at least $1 - e^{-\xi}$ the following holds:

$$\left\| P_{S_D} - P_{\widehat{S}_D} \right\| \leq \left(\sum_{r=1}^{D} \widetilde{\delta}_r^{-1} \right) \frac{4M}{\sqrt{n}} \left(1 + \sqrt{\frac{\xi}{2}} \right),$$

provided that $n \geq 16M^2 \left(1 + \sqrt{\frac{\xi}{2}} \right)^2 (\sup_{1 \leq r \leq D} \widetilde{\delta}_r^{-2})$. The disadvantage of this bound is that we are penalized on the one hand by the (inverse) gaps between the eigenvalues, and on the other by the dimension D (because we have to sum the inverse gaps from 1 to D). In the next section we improve the operator perturbation bound to get an improved result where only the gap δ_D enters into account.

3 Improved Result.

We first prove the following variant on the operator perturbation property which better corresponds to our needs by taking directly into account the projection on the first D eigenvectors at once. The proof uses the same kind of techniques as in [7].

Theorem 3 *Let A be a symmetric positive Hilbert-Schmidt operator of the Hilbert space $\mathcal{H}$ with simple nonzero eigenvalues $\lambda_1 > \lambda_2 > \ldots$ Let $D > 0$ be an integer such that $\lambda_D > 0$, $\delta_D = \frac{1}{2}(\lambda_D - \lambda_{D+1})$. Let $B \in HS(\mathcal{H})$ be another symmetric operator such that $\|B\| < \delta_D/2$ and $(A + B)$ is still a positive operator. Let $P^D(A)$ (resp. $P^D(A + B)$) denote the orthogonal projector onto the subspace spanned by the first D eigenvectors A (resp. $(A + B)$). Then these satisfy:*

$$\|P^D(A) - P^D(A + B)\| \leq \frac{\|B\|}{\delta_D}. \tag{1}$$

This then gives rise to our main result on KPCA:

Theorem 4 *Assume that $\sup_{x \in \mathcal{X}} k(x, x) \leq M$. Let $S_D, \widehat{S}_D$ be the subspaces spanned by the first D eigenvectors of C, resp. C_n defined earlier. Denoting $\lambda_1 > \lambda_2 > \ldots$ the eigenvalues of C, if $D > 0$ is such that $\lambda_D > 0$, put $\delta_D = \frac{1}{2}(\lambda_D - \lambda_{D+1})$ and*

$$B_D = \frac{2M}{\delta_D} \left(1 + \sqrt{\frac{\xi}{2}} \right).$$

Then provided that $n \geq B_D^2$, the following bound holds with probability at least $1 - e^{-\xi}$:

$$\left\| P_{S_D} - P_{\widehat{S}_D} \right\| \leq \frac{B_D}{\sqrt{n}}. \tag{2}$$

This entails in particular

$$\widehat{S}_D \subset \left\{ g + h, g \in S_D, h \in S_D^{\perp}, \|h\|_{\mathcal{H}_k} \leq 2B_D \, n^{-\frac{1}{2}} \|g\|_{\mathcal{H}_k} \right\}. \tag{3}$$

The important point here is that the approximation error now only depends on D through the (inverse) gap between the D-th and $(D+1)$-th eigenvalues. Note that using the results of section 2, we would have obtained exactly the same bound for estimating the D-th eigenvector only – or even a worse bound since $\widetilde{\delta}_D = \delta_D \wedge \delta_{D-1}$ appears in this case. Thus, at least from the point of view of this technique (which could still yield suboptimal bounds), there is no increase of complexity between estimating the D-th eigenvector alone and estimating the span of the first D eigenvectors.

Note that the inclusion (3) can be interpreted geometrically by saying that for any vector in $\widehat{S}_D$, the tangent of the angle between this vector and its projection on S_D is upper bounded by $B_D/\sqrt{n}$, which we can interpret as a stability property.

Comment about the Centered Case. In the actual (K)PCA procedure, the data is actually first empirically recentered, so that one has to consider the centered covariance operator $\overline{C}$ and its empirical counterpart $\overline{C}_n$. A result similar to Theorem 4 also holds in this case (up to some additional constant factors). Indeed, a result similar to Lemma 1 holds for the recentered operators [2]. Combined again with Theorem 3, this allows to come to similar conclusions for the "true" centered KPCA.

4 Conclusion and Discussion

In this paper, finite sample size confidence bounds of the eigenspaces of Kernel-PCA (the D-eigenspaces of the empirical covariance operator) are provided using tools of operator perturbation theory. This provides a first step towards an in-depth complexity analysis of algorithms using KPCA as pre-processing, and towards taking into account the randomness of the obtained models (e.g. [3]). We proved a bound in which the complexity factor for estimating the eigenspace S_D by its empirical counterpart depends only on the inverse gap between the D-th and $(D+1)$-th eigenvalues. In addition to the previously cited works, we take into account the centering of the data and obtain comparable rates.

In this work we assumed for simplicity of notation the eigenvalues to be simple. In the case the covariance operator C has nonzero eigenvalues with multiplicities $m_1, m_2, \ldots$ possibly larger than one, the analysis remains the same except for one point: we have to assume that the dimension D of the subspaces considered is of the form $m_1 + \cdots + m_r$ for a certain r. This could seem restrictive in comparison with the results obtained for estimating the sum of the first D eigenvalues themselves [2] (which is linked to the reconstruction error in KPCA) where no such restriction appears. However, it should be clear that we need this restriction when considering $D-$eigenspaces themselves since the target space has to be unequivocally defined, otherwise convergence cannot occur. Thus, it can happen in this special case that the reconstruction error converges while the projection space itself does not. Finally, a common point of the two analyses (over the spectrum and over the eigenspaces) lies in the fact that the bounds involve an inverse gap in the eigenvalues of the true covariance operator.

Finally, how tight are these bounds and do they at least carry some correct qualitative information about the behavior of the eigenspaces? Asymptotic results (central limit Theorems) in [6, 4] always provide the correct goal to shoot for since they actually give the limit distributions of these quantities. They imply that there is still important ground to cover before bridging the gap between asymptotic and non-asymptotic. This of course opens directions for future work.

Acknowledgements: This work was supported in part by the PASCAL Network of Excellence (EU # 506778).

A Appendix: proofs.

Proof of Lemma 1. This lemma is proved in [9]. We give a short proof for the sake of completeness. $\|C_n - C\| = \|\frac{1}{n} \sum_{i=1}^{n} C_{X_i} - \mathbb{E}[C_X]\|$ with $\|C_X\| = \|\varphi(X) \otimes \varphi(X)^*\| = k(X, X) \leq M$. We can apply the bounded difference inequality to the variable $\|C_n - C\|$, so that with probability greater than $1 - e^{-\xi}$, $\|C_n - C\| \leq \mathbb{E}\left[\|C_n - C\|\right] + 2M\sqrt{\frac{\xi}{2n}}$.

Moreover, by Jensen's inequality $\mathbb{E}\left[\|C_n - C\|\right] \leq \mathbb{E}\left[\|\frac{1}{n}\sum_{i=1}^{n} C_{X_i} - \mathbb{E}\left[C_X\right]\|^2\right]^{\frac{1}{2}}$, and simple calculations leads to $\mathbb{E}\left[\|\frac{1}{n}\sum_{i=1}^{n} C_{X_i} - \mathbb{E}\left[C_X\right]\|^2\right] = \frac{1}{n}\mathbb{E}\left[\|C_X - \mathbb{E}\left[C_X\right]\|^2\right] \leq \frac{4M^2}{n}$. This concludes the proof of lemma 1. $\qquad\square$

Proof of Theorem 3. The variation of this proof with respect to Theorem 5.2 in [7] is (a) to work directly in a (infinite-dimensional) Hilbert space, requiring extra caution for some details and (b) obtaining an improved bound by considering D-eigenspaces at once.

The key property of Hilbert-Schmidt operators allowing to work directly in a infinite dimensional setting is that $HS(\mathcal{H})$ is a both right and left ideal of $\mathcal{L}_c(\mathcal{H}, \mathcal{H})$, the Banach space of all continuous linear operators of $\mathcal{H}$ endowed with the operator norm $\|.\|_{\mathrm{op}}$. Indeed, $\forall T \in HS(\mathcal{H})$, $\forall S \in \mathcal{L}_c(\mathcal{H}, \mathcal{H})$, TS and ST belong to $HS(\mathcal{H})$ with

$$\|TS\| \leq \|T\|\,\|S\|_{\mathrm{op}} \quad \text{and} \quad \|ST\| \leq \|T\|\,\|S\|_{\mathrm{op}}. \tag{4}$$

The spectrum of an Hilbert-Schmidt operator T is denoted $\Lambda(T)$ and the sequence of eigenvalues in non-increasing order is denoted $\lambda(T) = (\lambda_1(T) \geq \lambda_2(T) \geq \ldots)$. In the following, $P^D(T)$ denotes the orthogonal projector onto the D-eigenspace of T.

The Hoffmann-Wielandt inequality in infinite dimensional setting[1] yields that:

$$\|\lambda(A) - \lambda(A + B)\|_{\ell_2} \leq \|B\| \leq \frac{\delta_D}{2}. \tag{5}$$

implying in particular that

$$\forall i > 0, \qquad |\lambda_i(A) - \lambda_i(A + B)| \leq \frac{\delta_D}{2}. \tag{6}$$

Results found in [5] p.39 yield the formula

$$P^D(A) - P^D(A + B) = -\frac{1}{2i\pi}\int_\gamma (R_A(z) - R_{A+B}(z))dz \in \mathcal{L}_c(\mathcal{H}, \mathcal{H}). \tag{7}$$

where $R_A(z) = (A - z\,Id)^{-1}$ is the resolvent of A, provided that γ is a simple closed curve in $\mathbb{C}$ enclosing exactly the first D eigenvalues of A and $(A + B)$. Moreover, the same reference (p.60) states that for ξ in the complementary of $\Lambda(A)$,

$$\|R_A(\xi)\|_{\mathrm{op}} = dist(\xi, \Lambda(A))^{-1}. \tag{8}$$

The proof of the theorem now relies on the simple choice for the closed curve γ in (7), drawn in the picture below and consisting of three straight lines and a semi-circle of radius L. For all $L > \frac{\delta_D}{2}$, γ intersect neither the eigenspectrum of A (by equation (6)) nor the eigenspectrum of $A + B$. Moreover, the eigenvalues of A (resp. $A + B$) enclosed by γ are exactly $\lambda_1(A), \ldots, \lambda_D(A)$ (resp. $\lambda_1(A + B), \ldots, \lambda_D(A + B)$).

Moreover, for $z \in \gamma$, $T(z) = R_A(z) - R_{A+B}(z) = -R_{A+B}(z)BR_A(z)$ belongs to $HS(\mathcal{H})$ and depends continuously on z by (4). Consequently,

$$\|P^D(A) - P^D(A + B)\| \leq \frac{1}{2\pi}\int_a^b \|(R_A - R_{A+B})(\gamma(t))\|\,|\gamma'(t)|dt.$$

Let $S_N = \sum_{n=0}^{N}(-1)^n (R_A(z)B)^n R_A(z)$. $R_{A+B}(z) = (Id + R_A(z)B)^{-1}R_A(z)$ and, for $z \in \gamma$ and $L > \delta_D$,

$$\|R_A(z)B\|_{\mathrm{op}} \leq \|R_A(z)\|_{\mathrm{op}}\|B\| \leq \frac{\delta_D}{2\,dist(z, \Lambda(A))} \leq \frac{1}{2},$$

1654

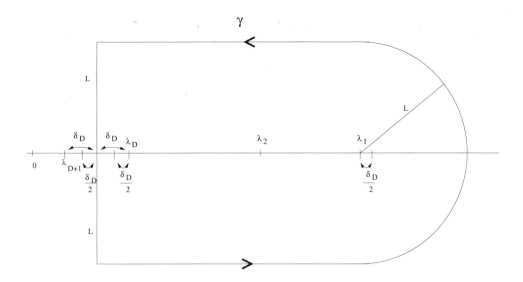

imply that $S_N \overset{\|\cdot\|_{\mathrm{op}}}{\longrightarrow} R_{A+B}(z)$ (uniformly for $z \in \gamma$). Using property (4), since $B \in HS(\mathcal{H})$, $S_N B R_A(z) \overset{\|\cdot\|}{\longrightarrow} R_{A+B}(z) B R_A(z) = R_{A+B}(z) - R_A(z)$. Finally,

$$R_A(z) - R_{A+B}(z) = \sum_{n \geq 1} (-1)^n (R_A(z)B)^n R_A(z)$$

where the series converges in $HS(\mathcal{H})$, uniformly in $z \in \gamma$. Using again property (4) and (8) implies

$$\|(R_A - R_{A+B})(\gamma(t))\| \leq \sum_{n \geq 1} \|R_A(\gamma(t))\|_{\mathrm{op}}^{n+1} \|B\|^n \leq \sum_{n \geq 1} \frac{\|B\|^n}{dist^{n+1}(\gamma(t), \Lambda(A))}$$

Finally, since for $L > \delta_D$, $\|B\| \leq \frac{\delta_D}{2} \leq \frac{dist(\gamma(t), \Lambda(A))}{2}$,

$$\|P^D(A) - P^D(A+B)\| \leq \frac{\|B\|}{\pi} \int_a^b \frac{1}{dist^2(\gamma(t), \Lambda(A))} |\gamma'(t)| dt \,.$$

Splitting the last integral into four parts according to the definition of the contour γ, we obtain

$$\int_a^b \frac{1}{dist^2(\gamma(t), \Lambda(A))} |\gamma'(t)| dt \leq \frac{2\arctan(\frac{L}{\delta_D})}{\delta_D} + \frac{\pi}{L} + 2\frac{\mu_1(A) - (\mu_D(A) - \delta_D)}{L^2} \,,$$

and letting L goes to infinity leads to the result. □

Proof of Theorem 4. Lemma 1 and Theorem 3 yield inequality (2). Together with assumption $n \geq B_D^2$ it implies $\|P_{S_D} - P_{\widehat{S}_D}\| \leq \frac{1}{2}$. Let $f \in \widehat{S}_D$: $f = P_{S_D}(f) + P_{S_D^\perp}(f)$. Lemma 5 below with $F = S_D$ and $G = \widehat{S}_D$, and the fact that the operator norm is bounded by the Hilbert-Schmidt norm imply that

$$\|P_{S_D^\perp}(f)\|_{\mathcal{H}_k}^2 \leq \frac{4}{3} \|P_{S_D} - P_{\widehat{S}_D}\|^2 \|P_{S_D}(f)\|_{\mathcal{H}_k}^2 \,.$$

Gathering the different inequalities, Theorem 4 is proved. □

Lemma 5 *Let F and G be two vector subspaces of $\mathcal{H}$ such that $\|P_F - P_G\|_{\mathrm{op}} \leq \frac{1}{2}$. Then the following bound holds:*

$$\forall f \in G \,, \ \|P_{F^\perp}(f)\|_{\mathcal{H}}^2 \leq \frac{4}{3} \|P_F - P_G\|_{\mathrm{op}}^2 \|P_F(f)\|_{\mathcal{H}}^2 \,.$$

Proof of Lemma 5. For $f \in G$, we have $P_G(f) = f$, hence

$$\|P_{F^\perp}(f)\|^2 = \|f - P_F(f)\|^2 = \|(P_G - P_F)(f)\|^2$$
$$\leq \|P_F - P_G\|_{\text{op}}^2 \|f\|^2$$
$$= \|P_F - P_G\|_{\text{op}}^2 \left(\|P_F(f)\|^2 + \|P_{F^\perp}(f)\|^2\right)$$

gathering the terms containing $\|P_{F^\perp}(f)\|^2$ on the left-hand side and using $\|P_F - P_G\|_{\text{op}}^2 \leq 1/4$ leads to the conclusion. $\square$

References

[1] R. Bhatia and L. Elsner. The Hoffman-Wielandt inequality in infinite dimensions. *Proc.Indian Acad.Sci(Math. Sci.) 104 (3), p. 483-494*, 1994.

[2] G. Blanchard, O. Bousquet, and L. Zwald. Statistical Properties of Kernel Principal Component Analysis. *Proceedings of the 17th. Conference on Learning Theory (COLT 2004)*, p. 594–608. Springer, 2004.

[3] G. Blanchard, P. Massart, R. Vert, and L. Zwald. Kernel projection machine: a new tool for pattern recognition. *Proceedings of the 18th. Neural Information Processing System (NIPS 2004)*, p. 1649–1656. MIT Press, 2004.

[4] J. Dauxois, A. Pousse, and Y. Romain. Asymptotic theory for the Principal Component Analysis of a vector random function: some applications to statistical inference. *Journal of multivariate analysis 12*, 136-154, 1982.

[5] T. Kato. *Perturbation Theory for Linear Operators*. New-York: Springer-Verlag, 1966.

[6] V. Koltchinskii. Asymptotics of spectral projections of some random matrices approximating integral operators. *Progress in Probability*, 43:191–227, 1998.

[7] V. Koltchinskii and E. Giné. Random matrix approximation of spectra of integral operators. *Bernoulli*, 6(1):113–167, 2000.

[8] B. Schölkopf, A. J. Smola, and K.-R. Müller. Nonlinear component analysis as a kernel eigenvalue problem. *Neural Computation*, 10:1299–1319, 1998.

[9] J. Shawe-Taylor and N. Cristianini. Estimating the moments of a random vector with applications. *Proceedings of the GRETSI 2003 Conference*, p. 47-52, 2003.

[10] J. Shawe-Taylor, C. Williams, N. Cristianini, and J. Kandola. On the eigenspectrum of the Gram matrix and the generalisation error of Kernel PCA. *IEEE Transactions on Information Theory 51 (7)*, p. 2510-2522, 2005.

[11] U. von Luxburg, M. Belkin, and O. Bousquet. Consistency of spectral clustering. Technical Report 134, Max Planck Institute for Biological Cybernetics, 2004.

[12] U. von Luxburg, O. Bousquet, and M. Belkin. On the convergence of spectral clustering on random samples: the normalized case. *Proceedings of the 17th Annual Conference on Learning Theory (COLT 2004)*, p. 457–471. Springer, 2004.

[13] C. K. I. Williams and M. Seeger. The effect of the input density distribution on kernel-based classifiers. *Proceedings of the 17th International Conference on Machine Learning (ICML)*, p. 1159–1166. Morgan Kaufmann, 2000.

Subject Index

Author Index